THE
5 MINUTE
VETERINARY
CONSULT

THE
5 MINUTE
VETERINARY
CONSULT

CANINE AND FELINE

Larry Patrick Tilley, D.V.M.

Diplomate, American College of Veterinary Internal Medicine
(Internal Medicine)
Director, Veterinary Specialty Referral Center
President, VET MED FAX Consultation Services
Santa Fe, NM

Francis W.K. Smith, Jr., D.V.M.

Diplomate, American College of Veterinary Internal Medicine
(Internal Medicine)
Chief of Medicine, Cardiopet, Inc.
Little Falls, NJ
Clinical Assistant Professor, Department of Medicine
Tufts University, School of Veterinary Medicine
North Grafton, MA

A. Christine MacMurray, M.A.

Medical Editor
The Animal Medical Center
New York, NY

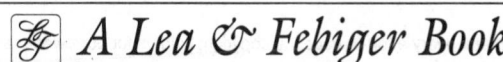 *A Lea & Febiger Book*

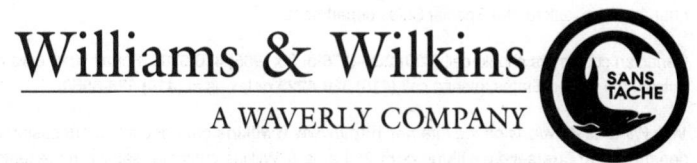 Williams & Wilkins

A WAVERLY COMPANY

BALTIMORE • PHILADELPHIA • LONDON • PARIS • BANGKOK
BUENOS AIRES • HONG KONG • MUNICH • SYDNEY • TOKYO • WROCLAW

Editor: Carroll Cann
Managing Editor: Susan Hunsberger
Production Coordinator: Felecia R. Weber
Book Project Editor: Kathy Gilbert
Designer: Cathy Cotter
Cover *Design:* Darrell L. Russell
Compositor: Donna M. Smith
Printer and Binder: R.R. Donnelley & Sons Company

Copyright © 1997 Williams & Wilkins
351 West Camden Street
Baltimore, Maryland 212012436 USA

Rose Tree Corporate Center
1400 North Providence Road
Building II, Suite 5025
Media, Pennsylvania 19063-2043 USA

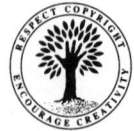

Accurate indications, adverse reactions, and dosage schedules for drugs are provided in this book, but it is possible that they may change. The reader is urged to review the package information data of the manufacturers of the medications mentioned.

Printed in the United States of America

Disclosure:
Medicine is a science that is constantly changing. Changes in treatment and drug therapy are required with new research and clinical experience. The authors and the publisher of this book have made every effort to ensure that the drug dosage schedules are accurate. The drug dosages are based on the standards accepted at the time of publication. The product information sheet included in the package of each drug should be checked before the drug is administered to be certain that changes have not been made in the recommended dosage or in the contraindications for administration. This advice is especially appropriate for new or infrequently used drugs.

Library of Congress Cataloging in Publication Data

Tilley, Lawrence P.
   The 5 minute veterinary consult canine and feline/Larry P. Tilley and Francis W.K. Smith, Jr.
      p. cm.
   Includes index.
   ISBN 0-683-08257-4
   1. Dogs—Diseases—Handbooks, manuals, etc. 2. Cats—Diseases—Handbooks, manuals,
      etc.   I. Smith, Francis W.K.   II. Title.
   [DNLM: 1. Dog Diseases—diagnosis—handbooks. 2. Cat Diseases—diagnosis. 3. Dog
      Diseases—therapy—handbooks. 4. Cat Diseases—therapy—handbooks. 5. Veterinary
      Medicine—handbooks. SF 991 T576z 1997]
   SF991.T55   1997
   636.7'0896—dc20
   DNLM/DLC
   for Library of Congress   96-15334
                                                                             CIP

The Publishers have made every effort to trace the copyright holders for borrowed material. If they have inadvertently overlooked any, they will be pleased to make the necessary arrangements at the first opportunity.

To purchase additional copies of this book, call our customer service department at **(800) 638-0672** or fax orders to **(800) 447-8438.** For other book services, including chapter reprints and large quantity sales, ask for the Special Sales department.

Canadian customers should call **(800) 268-4178** or fax **(905) 470-6780.** For all other calls originating outside the United States, please call **(410) 528-4223** or fax us at **(410) 528-8550.**

Visit Williams & Wilkins on the Internet: **http://www.wwilkins.com** or contact our customer service department at **custser@wwilkins.com**. Williams & Wilkins customer service representatives are available from 8:30 am to 6:00 pm, EST, Monday through Friday, for telephone access.

97 98 99
3 4 5 6 7 8 9 10

To my wife Jeri, my mother Dorothy, and my brother Steve in honor of that secret correspondence and love within our hearts. To my son Kyle, who has opened in me reserves of strength and love I never knew existed.

Larry Patrick Tilley

In loving memory of my mother Jacquelyn and my grandmother Demi. Their love still warms me, their vision guides me, their integrity strengthens me, and their accomplishments inspire me. To my wife May, my son Ben, and my father Frank, who brighten my every day with their zest for life and boundless love.

Francis W.K. Smith, Jr.

PREFACE

Keeping abreast of advances in veterinary internal medicine is extremely difficult, especially for the busy general practitioner. To keep current with all the veterinary journals while practicing medicine is impossible. The veterinarian in practice can be overwhelmed by all of the findings and conclusions of thousands of studies conducted by veterinary specialists. The *5 Minute Veterinary Consult* is designed to provide the busy veterinary practitioner and student of veterinary medicine with concise, practical reviews of almost all the diseases and clinical problems in dogs and cats. Our goal in creating this textbook is also to provide up-to-date information in an easy-to-use format. Emphasis is placed on diagnosis and treatment of problems and diseases likely to be seen by veterinarians.

Several good veterinary internal medicine textbooks are available. The uniqueness and value of the *5 Minute Veterinary Consult* as a quick reference is the consistency of presentation, the breadth of coverage, the contribution of large numbers of experts, and the timely preparation of the manuscript. The format of every clinical problem, laboratory abnormality, and disease is identical, making it easy to find information. An extensive list of topic headings ensures complete coverage of each topic.

The *5 Minute Veterinary Consult* is divided into three basic sections: Presenting Problems and Physical Findings, Diagnostic Tests, and Diseases and Clinical Syndromes. These sections reflect the way one approaches a case. Veterinarians are first confronted with the chief complaints, signs, and abnormal physical findings. The first section deals with the diagnostic approach to problems and physical findings. Emphasis is placed on how to work up the case to determine the cause of the problem and how to provide symptomatic support while working toward a definitive diagnosis. After the veterinarian obtains the history and performs the physical examination, diagnostic tests are performed. The second section of the book is designed to assist the veterinarian in the diagnostic approach to laboratory test abnormalities and electrocardiograms. Diagnostic algorithms are used in these first two sections. The use of algorithms is not designed to encourage cookbook medicine, but rather to provide a logical framework for approaching a specific case. Once the database is complete, a definitive diagnosis is hopefully at hand. The final section covers the diseases likely to be encountered by veterinarians in practice. Common diseases are covered in a two-page, six-column format. Less common diseases are covered in a one-page, three-column format.

As the title implies, one objective of this book is to make information quickly available. To this end, we have organized topics alphabetically within sections. Most topics can be found without using the index. A table of contents is provided at the beginning of each section and a detailed index is provided at the end of the book. Large volumes of useful information are summarized in charts in the appendix. Included in the appendix are a drug formulary, toxicology tables, endocrine testing protocols, normal laboratory values, and conversion tables.

We are delighted and privileged to have had the assistance of numerous experts in veterinary internal medicine. Over 300 veterinary specialists contributed to this text, allowing each chapter to be written by an expert on the subject. In addition to providing outstanding information, this large pool of experts allowed us to publish this major text in a timely manner. Many large textbooks take years to write, making some of the information outdated by the time the book is published. We are indebted to the many contributors and consulting editors, whose hard work allowed us to write, edit, and publish this work in two years. Our goal is to revise the text every two years so that the contents will always be current.

We have also produced a CD-ROM disk to accompany this textbook. This medium combines text, sound, graphics, and video in an interactive format. Now veterinarians can quickly access information about necessary clinical skills and new developments in diagnosis and treatment on their computer. Our *5 Minute Veterinary Consult* CD-ROM offers fast, affordable access to much of the accumulated wisdom in veterinary medicine by use of a simple search and retrieval process. This multimedia computer technology brings to the clinic exam room and doctor's office an-easy-to use, "dynamic textbook" that will markedly improve the quality of continuing education and clinical practice.

This textbook constitutes an important medical reference source for your practice and clinical education. We have strived to make it complete, yet practical and easy to use. Our dreams are realized if this text and CD-ROM help you to quickly locate and use the "momentarily important" information that is essential to the practice of high quality veterinary medicine. We would appreciate your input so that we can make future editions even more useful. If you'd like to see any changes in content or format, additions, or deletions, please let us know. Send comments to:

Drs. Larry Tilley and Frank Smith
c/o Williams & Wilkins
Rose Tree Corporate Center - Building II, Suite 5025
1400 North Providence Road
Media, PA 19063-2043

ACKNOWLEDGMENTS

The completion of this textbook provides a welcome opportunity to recognize in writing the many individuals who have helped along the way. The authors gratefully acknowledge the Consulting Editors and the contributors who, by their expertise, have so unmistakably enhanced the quality of this textbook.

Special gratitude goes to Christine MacMurray of the Animal Medical Center for her editorial supervision of the manuscript and her masterful precision and clarity. The following quotation explains the unique gift she has as an editor and the emotions we share in writing:

> ...Writing is hard work. One has to sit down on that chair and think and transform thought into readable, consecutive, interesting sentences that both make sense and make the reader turn the page. It is laborious, slow, often painful, sometimes agony. It means rearrangement, revision, adding, cutting, rewriting. But it brings a sense of excitement, almost of rapture; a moment on Olympus. In short it is an act of creation.*

We would like to acknowledge and thank our families for their support of this project and the sacrifices they made to allow us the time to complete this book.

We would also like to thank the following people for their secretarial assistance: Mary Ann Romero, Lisa Wilkes, and a special thanks for all those late nights to Willa Porter, office manager at Ved Med Fax. Recognition and thanks should also be given to our colleagues in cardiology and internal medicine at Cardiopet and Vet Med Fax for their support during the preparation of this book.

In addition to thanking veterinarians who have referred patients to us, we would like to express our gratitude to each of the veterinary students, interns, and residents who we have had the privilege of teaching. Their curiosity and intellectual stimulation have enabled us to grow and have prompted us to undertake the task of writing this book.

Finally, a special thank you goes to Carroll Cann, Executive Editor, Williams & Wilkins, whose vision and support were instrumental in the creation of this book. We would also like to thank Susan Hunsberger, Managing Editor, Joanne Husovski, Felecia R. Weber, and their colleagues in the Production Department at Williams & Wilkins. They are all meticulous workers and kind people who have made the final stages of preparing this book both inspiring and fun.

Larry Patrick Tilley
Francis W.K. Smith, Jr.

* Tuchman BW. In search of history. Radcliffe Quarterly 1979;65(1):34.

Consulting Editors

LOWELL ACKERMAN, D.V.M., PH.D.
Diplomate, American College of
Veterinary Dermatology
Scottsdale, AZ
Subject: Dermatology

LARRY G. ADAMS, D.V.M., PH.D.
Diplomate, American College of
Veterinary Internal Medicine (Internal
Medicine)
Department of Veterinary Clinical
Sciences
School of Veterinary Medicine
Purdue University
West Lafayette, IN
Subject: Nephrology and Urology

ALBERT E. JERGENS, D.V.M., M.S.
Diplomate, American College of
Veterinary Internal Medicine (Internal
Medicine)
Department of Veterinary Clinical
Sciences
School of Veterinary Medicine
Iowa State University
Ames, IA
Subject: Hepatology

LYNELLE JOHNSON, D.V.M., M.S.
Diplomate, American College of
Veterinary Internal Medicine (Internal
Medicine)
School of Veterinary Medicine
Missouri State University
Columbia, MO
Subject: Respiratory

BRENT D. JONES, D.V.M.
Veterinary Medicine and Surgery
College of Veterinary Medicine
University of Missouri
Columbia, MO
Subject: Gastroenterology

SARA K. LYLE, D.V.M., M.S.
Diplomate, American College of
Theriogenologists
Referral Practice
Ocala, FL
Subject: Theriogenology

PAUL E. MILLER, D.V.M.
Diplomate, American College of
Veterinary Ophthalmologists
Department of Surgical Sciences

School of Veterinary Medicine
University of Wisconsin
Madison, WI
Subject: Ophthalmology

WALLACE B. MORRISON, D.V.M., M.S.
Diplomate, American College of
Veterinary Internal Medicine (Internal
Medicine)
School of Veterinary Medicine
Veterinary Teaching Hospital
Purdue University
West Lafayette, IN
Subject: Oncology

BRADLEY L. MOSES, D.V.M.
Diplomate, American College of
Veterinary Internal Medicine
(Cardiology)
Roberts Animal Hospital
Hanover, MA
Subject: Respiratory

RHETT NICHOLS, D.V.M.
Diplomate, American College of
Veterinary Internal Medicine (Internal
Medicine)
Director of Internal Medicine
Vet Research
Farmingdale, NY
Subject: Endocrinology

CARL OSBORNE, D.V.M., PH.D.
Diplomate, American College of
Veterinary Internal Medicine (Internal
Medicine)
Small Animal Clinical Sciences
College of Veterinary Medicine
University of Minnesota
St. Paul, MN
Subject: Nephrology and Urology

GARY OSWEILER, D.V.M., PH.D.
Diplomate, American Board of
Veterinary Toxicology
Department of Clinical Sciences
College of Veterinary Medicine
Iowa State University
Ames, IA
Subject: Toxicology

MARK PAPICH, D.V.M., M.S.
Diplomate, American College of
Veterinary Clinical Pharmacology
College of Veterinary Medicine

North Carolina State University
Raleigh, NC
Subject: Drug Formulary

JOANE M. PARENT, D.V.M., M.V.SC.
Diplomate, American College of
Veterinary Internal Medicine
(Neurology)
Ontario Veterinary College
Guelph, ON
Subject: Neurology

ALAN H. REBAR, D.V.M., PH.D.
Diplomate, American College of
Veterinary Pathologists
Dean
School of Veterinary Medicine
Purdue University
West Lafayette, IN
Subject: Hematology

PETER D. SCHWARTZ, D.V.M.
Diplomate, American College of
Veterinary Surgeons
Veterinary Teaching Hospital
College of Veterinary Medicine
University of Colorado
Fort Collins, CO
Subject: Musculoskeletal

FRED W. SCOTT, D.V.M., PH.D.
Diplomate, American College of
Veterinary Microbiologists
Feline Health Center
NYS College of Veterinary Medicine
Cornell University
Ithaca, NY
Subject: Infectious Diseases

FRANCIS W. K. SMITH, JR., D.V.M.
Diplomate, American College of
Veterinary Internal Medicine (Internal
Medicine)
Cardiopet, Inc.
Little Falls, NJ
Subject: Cardiology

LARRY P. TILLEY, D.V.M.
Diplomate, American College of
Veterinary Internal Medicine (Internal
Medicine)
VET MED FAX Consultation Services
Santa Fe, NM
Subject: Cardiology

CONTRIBUTORS

JONATHAN A. ABBOTT, D.V.M.
Diplomate, American College of
Veterinary Internal Medicine
(Cardiology)
Consultant
Cardiopet, Inc.
Little Falls, NJ

LOWELL ACKERMAN, D.V.M., PH.D.
Diplomate, American College of
Veterinary Dermatology
Scottsdale, AZ

LARRY G. ADAMS, D.V.M., PH.D.
Diplomate, American College of
Veterinary Internal Medicine (Internal
Medicine)
Associate Professor of Small Animal
Internal Medicine
Department of Veterinary Clinical
Sciences
Purdue University School of Veterinary
Medicine
West Lafayette, IN

MAX J. G. APPEL, D.V.M., PH.D.
American College of Veterinary
Microbiologists (Virology)
Professor
Baker Institute
College of Veterinary Medicine
Cornell University
Ithaca, NY

LOUIS ARCHBALD, D.V.M., PH.D.
Diplomate, American College of
Theriogenologists
Professor of Reproduction
Department of Large Animal Clinical
Sciences
College of Veterinary Medicine
University of Florida
Gainesville, FL

RODNEY S. BAGLEY, D.V.M.
Diplomate, American College of
Veterinary Internal Medicine (Neurology
and Internal Medicine)
Assistant Professor, Neurology and
Neurosurgery
Department of Clinical Sciences
College of Veterinary Medicine
Washington State University
Pullman, WA

E. MURL BAILEY, D.V.M., PH.D.
Diplomate, American Board of
Veterinary Toxicology
Professor of Toxicology
Department of Veterinary Physiology
and Pharmacology
College of Veterinary Medicine
Texas A & M University
College Station, TX

JEFFREY BARLOUGH, D.V.M., PH.D.
Diplomate, American College of
Veterinary Microbiologists
Postgraduate Researcher
Department of Medicine and
Epidemiology
School of Veterinary Medicine
University of California-Davis
Davis, CA

STEPHEN C. BARR, B.V.SC., M.V.S.,
PH.D.
Diplomate, American College of
Veterinary Internal Medicine (Internal
Medicine)
Associate Professor of Medicine
Department of Clinical Sciences
College of Veterinary Medicine
Cornell University
Ithaca, NY

MARGARET C. BARR, D.V.M., PH.D.
Department of Microbiology and
Immunology
College of Veterinary Medicine
Cornell University
Ithaca, NY

JOSEPH W. BARTGES, D.V.M., PH.D.
Diplomate, American College of
Veterinary Internal Medicine (Internal
Medicine)
Diplomate, American College of
Veterinary Nutrition
Assistant Professor
Clinical Nutritionist
Department of Small Animal Medicine
Department of Physiology and
Pharmacology
Veterinary Teaching Hospital
College of Veterinary Medicine
University of Georgia
Athens, GA

MICHAEL BAUER, D.V.M.
Diplomate, American College of
Veterinary Surgeons
Surgeon
College of Veterinary Medicine
Fort Collins, CO
Colorado State University
Colorado Spring Small Animal Surgery
Referral Service
Colorado Springs, CO

BRIAN BEALE, D.V.M.
Gulf Coast Veterinary Specialists, P.C.
Houston, TX

ANDREW W. BEARDOW, B.V.M. & S.,
M.R.C.V.S.
Diplomate, American College of
Veterinary Internal Medicine
(Cardiology)
Vice-President
Cardiopet, Inc.
Little Falls, NJ

JAMIE R. BELLAH, D.V.M.
Diplomate, American College of
Veterinary Surgeons
Associate Professor
Service Chief, Small Animal Surgery
Department of Small Animal Clinical
Sciences
College of Veterinary Medicine
University of Florida
Gainesville, FL

MARC BERCOVITCH, D.V.M.
Diplomate, American College of
Veterinary Internal Medicine (Internal
Medicine)
Veterinary Referral Associates
Gaithersburg, MD

G. DANIEL BOON, D.V.M., M.S.
Diplomate, American College of
Veterinary Pathologists
Director
Veterinary Pathobiology
College of Veterinary Medicine
University of Missouri
Columbia, MO

SCOTT A. BROWN, V.M.D., PH.D.
Diplomate, American College of Veterinary Internal Medicine (Internal Medicine)
Associate Professor
Department of Physiology and Pharmacology
College of Veterinary Medicine
University of Georgia
Athens, GA

DONALD J. BROWN, D.V.M., PH.D.
Diplomate, American College of Veterinary Internal Medicine (Cardiology)
Assistant Professor
Department of Medicine
School of Veterinary Medicine
Tufts University
North Grafton, MA

JÖRG BUCHELER, D.V.M., PH.D.
Diplomate, American College of Veterinary Internal Medicine (Internal Medicine)
Ross University School of Veterinary Medicine
St. Christopher and Nevis, St. Kitts, West Indies

C.A TONY BUFFINGTON, D.V.M., PH.D.
Diplomate, American College of Veterinary Nutrition
Associate Professor
Department of Clinical Sciences
College of Veterinary Medicine
The Ohio State University
Columbus, OH

COLIN F. BURROWS, D.V.M.
Diplomate, American College of Veterinary Internal Medicine (Internal Medicine)
Professor
Department of Small Animal Clinical Sciences
College of Veterinary Medicine
University of Florida
Gainesville, FL

CATHRYN CALIA, D.V.M.
Diplomate, American College of Veterinary Internal Medicine (Internal Medicine)
Associate Veterinarian
Department of Internal Medicine
Cardiopet Veterinary Associates, P.A.
Little Falls, NJ

CLAY A. CALVERT, D.V.M.
Diplomate, American College of Veterinary Internal Medicine (Internal Medicine)
Diplomate, American College of Veterinary Emergency/Critical Care Medicine
Professor
Department of Small Animal Medicine
College of Veterinary Medicine
University of Georgia
Athens, GA

LELAND CARMICHAEL, D.V.M., PH.D.
Diplomate, American College of Veterinary Microbiologists
John M. Olin Professor of Virology
Baker Institute
College of Veterinary Medicine
Cornell University
Ithaca, NY

LARRY CARPENTER, D.V.M.
Diplomate, American College of Veterinary Surgeons
Chief, Operating Room Services
Mechanical Trauma Research
U.S. Army Institute of Surgical Research
San Antonio, TX

THOMAS L. CARSON, D.V.M., PH.D.
Diplomate, American Board of Veterinary Toxicology
Professor and Toxicologist
Veterinary Diagnostic Laboratory
Iowa State University
Ames, IA

ERIN S. CHAMPAGNE, D.V.M.
Diplomate, American College of Veterinary Ophthalmologists
Assistant Professor
Department of Small Animal Clinical Sciences
Virginia-Maryland Regional College of Veterinary Medicine
Blacksburg, VA

GEORGINA CHILD, B.V.SC.
Diplomate, American College of Veterinary Internal Medicine (Neurology)
Neurology Specialty Practice
Gladesville, New South Wales

MARY M. CHRISTOPHER, D.V.M., PH.D.
Diplomate, American College of Veterinary Pathologists (Clinical Pathology)
Associate Professor
Department of Pathology, Microbiology and Immunology
University of California
School of Veterinary Medicine
Davis, CA

RUTH ANN CHUN, D.V.M.
Department of Veterinary Clinical Sciences
School of Veterinary Medicine
Purdue University
West Lafayette, IN

SUSAN MARY COCHRANE, D.V.M.
Diplomate, American College of Veterinary Internal Medicine (Neurology)
Staff Neurologist
Morningside Animal Clinic
Scarborough, Ontario

ELLEN CODNER, D.V.M.
Diplomate, American College of Veterinary Internal Medicine (Internal Medicine)
Diplomate, American College of Veterinary Dermatology - Board Qualified
Dermatologist, Internist
Animal Dermatology Clinic
Garden Grove, CA

B. KEITH COLLINS, D.V.M., M.S.
Diplomate, American College of Veterinary Ophthalmologists
Associate Professor
A373 Veterinary Teaching Hospital
University of Missouri
Columbia, MO

JAMES L. COOK, D.V.M.
Veterinary Teaching Hospital
University of Missouri College of Veterinary Medicine
Columbia, MO

ROBERT M. CORWIN, D.V.M.
Department of Veterinary Pathobiology
College of Veterinary Medicine
University of Missouri
Columbia, MO

LAINE COWAN, D.V.M., M.S.
Diplomate, American College of Veterinary Internal Medicine (Internal Medicine)
Associate Professor
Department of Veterinary Clinical Sciences
College of Veterinary Medicine
Kansas State University
Manhattan, KS

LARRY COWGILL, D.V.M., PH.D.
Diplomate, American College of Veterinary Internal Medicine (Internal Medicine)
Associate Professor
Department of Medicine & Epidemiology
College of Veterinary Medicine
University of California
Davis, CA

KATHY L. CRENSHAW, D.V.M.
Diplomate, American College of Veterinary Internal Medicine (Internal Medicine)
Staff Veterinarian
Department of Internal Medicine
Rogosin Institute
New York, NY

MITCHELL A. CRYSTAL, D.V.M.
Diplomate, American College of Veterinary Internal Medicine (Internal Medicine)
Assistant Professor
Department of Veterinary Medicine and Surgery
College of Veterinary Medicine
Boren Veterinary Medical Teaching Hospital
Oklahoma State University
Stillwater, OK

PAUL A. CUDDON, B.V.SC
   Diplomate, American College of
   Veterinary Internal Medicine
   (Neurology)
   Associate Professor
   Clinical Sciences
   College of Veterinary Medicine
   Colorado State University
   Fort Collins, CO

ELIZABETH A. CURRY-GALVIN, D.V.M.
   Technical Service Veterinarian
   Sandoz Animal Health
   Sandoz Agro, Inc.
   Des Plains, IL

GEORGE D'ANDREA, B.S., D.V.M., M.S.
   Diplomate, American College of
   Veterinary Pathologists
   Diagnostic Specialist
   Department of Pathology/Toxicology
   Veterinary Diagnostic Laboratory
   Auburn, AL

TOM DAY, D.V.M.
   Diplomate, American College of
   Veterinary Anesthesiologists
   College of Veterinary Medicine
   Mississippi State University
   Mississippi State, MS

HELIO S. AUTRAN DE MORAIS, D.V.M.,
M.S.
   Diplomate, American College of
   Veterinary Internal Medicine
   (Cardiology, Internal Medicine)
   Associate Professor, Departamento de
   Clinicas Veterinarias
   Departmento de Clinicas Veterinarias
   Universidade Estadual de Londrina
   Londrina - Parana

TERRY DE FRANCESCO, D.V.M.
   Diplomate, American College of
   Veterinary Internal Medicine
   (Cardiology)
   Clinical Instructor
   North Carolina State University College
   of Veterinary Medicine
   Raleigh, NC

LINDA J. DEBOWES, D.V.M.
   Diplomate, American College of
   Veterinary Internal Medicine (Internal
   Medicine)
   Associate Professor
   Department of Clinical Sciences
   Veterinary Medical Teaching Hospital
   Kansas State University
   Manhattan, KS

ROBERT C. DENOVO, D.V.M.
   Diplomate, American College of
   Veterinary Internal Medicine (Internal
   Medicine)
   Associate Professor of Medicine
   Department of Small Animal Clinical
   Science
   College of Veterinary Medicine
   University of Tennessee
   Knoxville, TN

NISHI DHUPA, B.V.M., M.R.C.V.S.
   Diplomate, American College of
   Veterinary Internal Medicine (Internal
   Medicine)
   Diplomate, American College of
   Veterinary Emergency and Critical Care
   School of Veterinary Medicine
   Tufts University
   North Grafton, MA

SHARON M. DIAL, D.V.M., PH.D.
   Staff Pathologist and Consultant
   Antech Diagnostics, Inc.
   Phoenix, AZ

STEPHEN P. DIBARTOLA, D.V.M.
   Diplomate, American College of
   Veterinary Internal Medicine (Internal
   Medicine)
   Professor
   Veterinary Clinical Sciences
   College of Veterinary Medicine
   The Ohio State University
   Columbus, OH

KELLY J. DIEHL, D.V.M.
   Diplomate, American College of
   Veterinary Internal Medicine (Internal
   Medicine)
   Post-Doctoral Fellow
   Department of Medicine
   National Jewish Center for Immunology
   and Respiratory Medicine
   Denver, CO

DONNA S. DIMSKI, D.V.M., M.S.
   Diplomate, American College of
   Veterinary Internal Medicine (Internal
   Medicine)
   Staff Internist
   Williamette Veterinarian Referral Center
   Corvallis, OR

BRADFORD C. DIXON, D.V.M.
   Staff Surgeon
   Southwest Veterinary Surgical Service
   Phoenix, AZ

DAVID DORMAN, D.V.M., PH.D.
   Diplomate, American Board of
   Veterinary Toxicology and American
   Board of Toxicology
   Neurotoxicologist
   Chemical Industry Institute of
   Toxicology
   Research Triangle, NC

DAVID DUCLOS, D.V.M.
   Diplomate, American College of
   Veterinary Dermatology
   Animal Skin and Allergy Clinic
   Lynnwood, WA

KAREN R. DYER, D.V.M., PH.D.
   Diplomate, American College of
   Veterinary Internal Medicine
   (Neurology)
   Assistant Professor
   Small Animal Clinical Sciences
   Virginia-Maryland Regional College of
   Veterinary Medicine
   Virginia Polytechnic Institute and State
   University
   Blacksburg, VA

BRUCE E. EILTS, D.V.M., M.S.
   Diplomate, American College of
   Theriogenologists
   Professor
   Department of Veterinary Clinical
   Sciences
   School of Veterinary Medicine
   Louisiana State University
   Baton Rouge, LA

ROBYN ELMSLIE, D.V.M.
   Diplomate, American College of
   Veterinary Internal Medicine (Oncology)
   Clinical Oncologist
   Veterinary Cancer Specialists
   Denver, CO

RICHARD FAYRER-HOSKEN, B.V.SC.,
PH.D., M.R.C.V.S.
   Diplomate, American College of
   Theriogenologists
   Associate Professor
   Department of Large Animal Medicine
   College of Veterinary Medicine
   University of Georgia
   Athens, GA

LINDA S. FINEMAN, D.V.M.
   Department of Veterinary Clinical
   Sciences
   School of Veterinary Medicine
   Purdue University
   West Lafayette, IN

SCOTT D. FITZGERALD, D.V.M.
   Diplomate, American College of
   Veterinary Pathology
   Assistant Professor
   Department of Pathology and Animal
   Health Diagnostic Lab
   Michigan State University
   Lansing, MI

SHARON K. FOOSHEE, M.AG., M.S.,
D.V.M.
   Diplomate, American College of
   Veterinary Internal Medicine (Internal
   Medicine)
   Diplomate, American Board of
   Veterinary Practitioners
   Animal Health Center of Franklin
   Franklin, TN

S. DRU FORRESTER, D.V.M., M.S.
   Diplomate, American College of
   Veterinary Internal Medicine (Internal
   Medicine)
   Associate Professor
   Department of Small Animal Clinical
   Sciences
   Virginia-Maryland Regional College of
   Veterinary Medicine
   Virginia Tech
   Blacksburg, VA

TERESA W. FOSSUM, D.V.M., PH.D.
   Diplomate, American College of
   Veterinary Surgeons
   Department of Small Animal Surgery
   College of Veterinary Medicine
   Texas A & M University
   College Station, TX

JONI L. FRESHMAN, D.V.M., M.S.
Diplomate, American College of
Veterinary Internal Medicine (Internal
Medicine)
East Springs Animal Hospital
Colorado Springs, CO

TAM GARLAND, D.V.M., PH.D.
Research Associate
Diplomate, American Board of
Veterinary Toxicology
Research Associate
Department of Veterinary Physiology
and Pharmacology
College of Veterinary Medicine
Texas A&M University
College Station, TX

BRIAN C. GILGER, D.V.M., M.S.
Diplomate, American College of
Veterinary Ophthalmologists
Associate Professor
Department of Companion Animals
and Special Species Medicine
Veterinary Hospital
The Ohio State University
Columbus, OH

JOHN-KARL GOODWIN, D.V.M.
Diplomate, American College of
Veterinary Internal Medicine
(Cardiology)
Assistant Professor of Cariology
Veterinary Clinical Sciences
Louisiana State University School of
Veterinary Medicine
Baton Rouge, LA

JOANNE C. GRAHAM, D.V.M., M.S.
Diplomate, American College of
Veterinary Internal Medicine (Oncology)
Assistant Professor
Department of Veterinary Clinical
Sciences
College of Veterinary Medicine
Iowa State University
Ames, IA

DUNBAR GRAM, D.V.M.
Diplomate, American College of
Veterinary Dermatology
Animal Allergy and Dermatology
Virginia Beach, VA

GREGORY F. GRAUER, D.V.M., M.S.
Diplomate, American College of
Veterinary Internal Medicine (Internal
Medicine)
Associate Professor and Staff Internist
Department of Clinical Sciences
Veterinary Teaching Hospital
College of Veterinary Medicine and
Biomedical Sciences
Colorado State University
Fort Collins, CO

THOMAS K. GRAVES, D.V.M.
Diplomate, American College of
Veterinary Internal Medicine (Internal
Medicine)
Pharmacology and Physiology
School of Medicine and Dentistry
University of Rochester
Rochester, NY

DEBORAH S. GRECO, D.V.M., PH.D.
Diplomate, American College of
Veterinary Internal Medicine (Internal
Medicine)
Associate Professor
Department of Clinical Sciences
College of Veterinary Medicine
Colorado State University
Fort Collins, CO

AMY M. GROOTERS, D.V.M.
Diplomate, American College of
Veterinary Internal Medicine (Internal
Medicine)
Clinical Instructor
Department of Veterinary Clinical
Sciences
School of Veterinary Medicine
Louisiana State University
Baton Rouge, LA

DEBORAH J. HADLOCK, V.M.D.
Diplomate, American Board of
Veterinary Practitioners
Staff Consultant
Cardiopet, Inc.
Little Falls, NJ

KEVIN A. HAHN, D.V.M., PH.D.
Department of Comparative Medicine
College of Veterinary Medicine
University of Tennessee
Knoxville, TN

JEFFERY O. HALL, D.V.M.
Diplomate, American Board of
Veterinary Toxicology
Department of Veterinary Biosciences
College of Veterinary Medicine
University of Illinois
Urbana, IL

TERRANCE A. HAMILTON, D.V.M.
Diplomate, American College of
Veterinary Internal Medicine (Oncology)
Staff Oncologist
Veterinary Referral Clinic
Cleveland, OH

ROBERT L. HAMLIN, D.V.M., PH.D.
Diplomate, American College of
Veterinary Internal Medicine
(Cardiology, Internal Medicine)
Professor
Department of Physiology and
Pharmacology
The Ohio State University College of
Veterinary Medicine
Columbus, OH

STEVEN R. HANSEN, D.V.M., M.S.
Diplomate, American Board of
Toxicology
Manager, Technical Services
Sandoz Animal Health
Des Plaines, IL

NEIL HARPSTER, D.V.M.
Diplomate, American College of
Veterinary Internal Medicine
(Cardiology)
Director of Cardiology
Department of Cardiology
Angell Memorial Hospital
Boston, MA

DANIEL P. HARRINGTON, D.V.M.
Veterinary Teaching Hospital
University of Missouri College of
Veterinary Medicine
Columbia, MO

JOHN W. HARVEY, D.V.M.
Diplomate, American College of
Veterinary Pathologists (Clinical
Pathology)
Professor and Chair
Physiological Sciences
College of Veterinary Medicine
University of Florida
Gainesville, FL

KAREN HELTON-RHODES, D.V.M.
Diplomate, American College of
Veterinary Dermatology
Staff Dermatologist, Cardiopet
Veterinary Associates, PA
Professional Staff
Cardiopet Inc.
Little Falls, NJ

JOAN C. HENDRICKS, D.V.M.
Diplomate, American College of
Veterinary Internal Medicine (Internal
Medicine)
Department of Veterinary Clinical
Sciences
University of Pennsylvania
Philadelphia, PA

ROSEMARY HENIK, D.V.M., M.S.
Diplomate, American College of
Veterinary Internal Medicine (Internal
Medicine)
Clinical Assistant Professor
Department of Medical Sciences
VMTH/School of Veterinary Medicine
University of Wisconsin - Madison
Madison, WI

MARK E. HITT, D.V.M., M.S.
Diplomate, American College of
Veterinary Internal Medicine (Internal
Medicine)
Atlantic Veterinary Internal Medicine
Annapolis, MD

HARM HOGENESCH, D.V.M., PH.D.
Diplomate, American College of
Veterinary Pathologists
Assistant Professor of
Immunopathology
Department of Veterinary Pathobiology
School of Veterinary Medicine
Purdue University
West Lafayette, IN

MOLLYANN HOLLAND, D.V.M.
Diplomate, American College of
Veterinary Internal Medicine (Internal
Medicine)
Veterinary Teaching Hospital
University of Missouri College of
Veterinary Medicine
Columbia, MO

JOHNNY D. HOSKINS, D.V.M., PH.D.
Diplomate, American College of
Veterinary Internal Medicine (Internal
Medicine)
Professor of Veterinary Internal Medicine
Department of Veterinary Clinical Sciences
School of Veterinary Medicine
Louisiana State University
Baton Rouge, LA

KATHERINE HOUPT, V.M.D., PH.D.
Diplomate, American College of
Veterinary Behaviorists
Professor of Physiology
Department of Physiology
College of Veterinary Medicine
Cornell University
Ithaca, NY

CHRISTINE CAROLYN JENKINS, D.V.M.
Diplomate, American College of
Veterinary Internal Medicine (Internal
Medicine)
Companion Animal Division
Pfizer Animal Health
Exton, PA

ALBERT E. JERGENS, D.V.M., M.S.
Diplomate, American College of
Veterinary Internal Medicine (Internal
Medicine)
Associate Professor
Department of Veterinary Clinical
Sciences
Iowa State University
College of Veterinary Medicine
Ames, IA

LYNELLE JOHNSON, D.V.M., M.S.
Diplomate, American College of
Veterinary Internal Medicine (Internal
Medicine)
Missouri State University
Columbia, MO

SUSAN E. JOHNSON, D.V.M., M.S.
Diplomate, American College of
Veterinary Internal Medicine (Internal
Medicine)
Associate Professor
Department of Veterinary Clinical
Sciences
The Ohio State University
Columbus, OH

KENNETH A. JOHNSON, M.V.SC., PH.D.,
F.A.C.V.SC.
Diplomate, American College of
Veterinary Surgeons
Associate Professor of Surgery
Department of Surgical Sciences
School of Veterinary Medicine
Orthopaedic Surgeon, Veterinary
Teaching Hospital
University of Wisconsin - Madison
Madison, WI

SHIRLEY JOHNSTON, D.V.M., PH.D.
Diplomate, American College of
Theriogenologists
Professor
Department of Small Animal Clinical
Sciences
College of Veterinary Medicine
University of Minnesota
St. Paul, MN

BRENT D. JONES, D.V.M.
Associate Professor of Medicine
Veterinary Teaching Hospital
University of Missouri College of
Veterinary Medicine
Columbia, MO

RICHARD J. JOSEPH, D.V.M.
Diplomate, American College of
Veterinary Internal Medicine (Neurology)
Staff Neurologist/Acupuncturist
Department of Medicine
The Animal Medical Center
New York, NY

BRUCE W. KEENE, D.V.M., M.S.
Diplomate, American College of
Veterinary Internal Medicine
(Cardiology)
Associate Professor of Cardiology
College of Veterinary Medicine
North Carolina State University
Raleigh, NC

MARGARET KERN, D.V.M.
Diplomate, American College of
Veterinary Internal Medicine (Internal
Medicine)
Assistant Professor
Animal Health Center
College of Veterinary Medicine
Mississippi State University
Mississippi State, MS

LESLEY KING, M.V.B., M.R.C.V.S.
Diplomate, American College of
Veterinary Internal Medicine (Internal
Medicine)
Diplomate, American College of
Veterinary Emergency and Critical Care
Assistant Professor, Section of
Medicine
Director, Intensive Care Unit
Department of Clinical Studies
Veterinary Hospital
University of Pennsylvania
Philadelphia, PA

PETER KINTZER, D.V.M.
Diplomate, American College of
Veterinary Internal Medicine (Internal
Medicine)
Clinical Assistant Professor
Department of Lab Animal Medicine
School of Veterinary Medicine
Tufts University
North Grafton, MA

REBECCA KIRBY, D.V.M.
Diplomate, American College of
Veterinary Internal Medicine (Internal
Medicine)
Diplomate, American College of
Veterinary Emergency and Critical Care
Chief of Medicine
Animal Emergency Center
Milwaukee, WI

JEFFREY KLAUSNER, D.V.M.
Diplomate, American College of
Veterinary Internal Medicine (Internal
Medicine, Oncology)
Small Animal Clinical Sciences
College of Veterinary Medicine
University of Minnesota
St. Paul, MN

GARY KOCIBA, D.V.M., PH.D.
Diplomate, American College of
Veterinary Pathologists
Professor
Department of Veterinary Biosciences
Ohio State University
Columbus, OH

JOHN M. KRUGER, D.V.M., PH.D.
Diplomate, American College of
Veterinary Internal Medicine (Internal
Medicine)
Associate Professor
Small Animal Clinical Sciences
Veterinary Clinical Center
Michigan State University
East Lansing, MI

KAREN KUHL, D.V.M.
Diplomate, American College of
Veterinary Dermatology
Animal Allergy and Dermatology
Downers Grove, Illinois

INDIA LANE, D.V.M.
Diplomate, American College of
Veterinary Internal Medicine (Internal
Medicine)
Assistant Professor, Medicine Service
Chief
Department of Companion Animals
Atlantic Veterinary College
University of Prince Edward Island
Charlottetown, Prince Edward Island

ROLF LARSEN, D.V.M.
Diplomate, American College of
Theriogenologists
Associate Professor
Department of Large Animal Clinical
Sciences
College of Veterinary Medicine
University of Florida
Gainesville, FL

KENNETH S. LATIMER, D.V.M., PH.D.
Diplomate, American College of
Veterinary Pathologists (Clinical
Pathology)
Professor of Pathology
Veterinary Pathology
College of Veterinary Medicine
University of Georgia
Athens, GA

DENNIS LAWLER, D.V.M.
Senior Research Veterinarian
Ralston Purina Company, St. Louis
Grocery Products R&D
O'Fallon, IL

GEORGE F. LEES, D.V.M., M.S.
Diplomate, American College of
Veterinary Internal Medicine (Internal
Medicine)
Professor
Small Animal Medicine and Surgery
College of Veterinary Medicine
Texas A&M University
College Station, TX

LINDA B. LEHMKUHL, D.V.M.
Diplomate, American College of
Veterinary Internal Medicine
(Cardiology)
Assistant Professor
Department of Veterinary Clinical
Sciences
The Ohio State University
Columbus, OH

MICHAEL LESSER, D.V.M.
Diplomate, American College of
Veterinary Internal Medicine
(Cardiology)
Animal Medical Center
Los Angeles, CA

STEVEN A. LEVY, V.M.D.
Durham Veterinary Hospital, PC
Durham, CT

DENISE M. LINDLEY, D.V.M.
Diplomate, American College of
Veterinary Ophthalmologists
Department of Veterinary Clinical
Sciences
Animal Eye Consultants
Crestwood, IL

DAVID LIPSITZ, D.V.M.
Diplomate, American College of
Veterinary Internal Medicine (Neurology)
Department of Medical Sciences
School of Veterinary Medicine
University of Wisconsin - Madison
Madison, WI

RANDALL CARL LONGSHORE, D.V.M.
Veterinary Neurological Center
Phoenix, AZ

CARROLL LOYER, D.V.M.
Diplomate, American College of
Veterinary Internal Medicine
(Cardiology)
Animal Medical Specialists of Colorado
Denver, CO

JODY LULICH, D.V.M., PH.D.
Diplomate, American College of
Veterinary Medicine (Internal Medicine)
Department of Small Animal Clinical
Sciences
College of Veterinary Medicine
University of Minnesota
St. Paul, MN

JOHN E. LUND, D.V.M.
Diplomate, American College of
Veterinary Pathologists
Distinguished Research Veterinary
Pathologist
Drug Safety Research
Pharmacia and Upjohn, Inc.
Kalamazoo, MI

PATRICIA J. LUTTGEN, D.V.M., M.S.
Diplomate, American College of
Veterinary Internal Medicine
(Neurology)
Neurological Center for Animals
Lakewood, CO

SARA K. LYLE, D.V.M., M.S.
Diplomate, American College of
Theriogenologists
Referral Practice/Private Practitioner
Ocala, FL

PETER S. MACWILLIAMS, D.V.M., PH.D.
Diplomate, American College of
Veterinary Pathologists
Professor of Clinical Pathology
Chief of Diagnostic Services
Department of Pathobiological

Sciences
School of Veterinary Medicine
University of Wisconsin - Madison
Madison, WI

EDWARD A. MAHAFFEY, D.V.M.
Diplomate, American College of
Veterinary Pathologists
Department of Pathology
College of Veterinary Medicine
University of Georgia
Athens, GA

STEVEN L. MARKS, B.V.SC., M.S.,
M.R.C.V.S.
Diplomate, American College of
Veterinary Internal Medicine (Internal
Medicine)
Assistant Professor
Department of Veterinary Medicine and
Surgery
Louisiana State University
Baton Rouge, LA

STANLEY L. MARKS, B.V.SC., PH.D.
Diplomate, American College of
Veterinary Internal Medicine (Internal
Medicine, Oncology)
Diplomate, American College of
Veterinary Nutrition
Assistant Professor
Medicine and Epidemiology
School of Veterinary Medicine
University of California, Davis
Davis, CA

ROB MASON, D.V.M., D.V.SC.
Diplomate, American Board of
Veterinary Practitioners, (Companion
Animal)
Diplomate, American College of
Veterinary Internal Medicine (Internal
Medicine)
Staff Internist - Director
Oceanview Veterinary Specialists
Vancouver, BC

TERRI L. MCCALLA, D.V.M., M.S.
Diplomate, American College of
Veterinary Ophthalmologists
Associate Veterinary Ophthalmologist
Animal Eye Clinic
Seattle, WA

DUDLEY MCCAW, D.V.M.
Diplomate, American College of
Veterinary Internal Medicine (Internal
Medicine)
Associate Professor
Department of Veterinary Medicine and
Surgery
University of Missouri
Columbia, MO

PATRICK L. MCDONOUGH, D.V.M., M.S.,
PH.D.
Assistant Director
Bacteriology/Mycology
Assistant Professor, Microbiology
Diagnostic Laboratory
College of Veterinary Medicine
Cornell University
Ithaca, NY

CRAIG E. MCINNIS, D.V.M.
Emergency Veterinary Practice
Oxnard, CA

BRENDAN C. MCKIERNAN, D.V.M.
Diplomate, American College of
Veterinary Internal Medicine (Internal
Medicine)
Professor
Department of Veterinary Clinical
Medicine
Veterinary Medicine Teaching Hospital
University of Illinois
Urbana, IL

RONALD MCLAUGHLIN, D.V.M.
Medical Center
University of Missouri
Columbia, MO

LINDA MEDLEAU, D.V.M., M.S.
Diplomate, American College of
Veterinary Dermatology
Professor of Dermatology
Department of Small Animal Medicine
College of Veterinary Medicine
University of Georgia
Athens, GA

MATTHEW MELLEMA, D.V.M.
Consultant
Cardiopet, Inc.
Little Falls, NJ

KATHRYN M. MEURS, D.V.M.
Diplomate, American College of
Veterinary Internal Medicine (Cardiology)
Veterinary Clinical Associate
Small Animal Medicine
College of Veterinary Medicine
Texas A & M University
College Station, TX

DONALD J. MEUTEN, D.V.M., PH.D.
Diplomate, American College of
Veterinary Pathologists
College of Veterinary Medicine
North Carolina State University
Raleigh, NC

VICKI MEYERS-WALLEN, V.M.D., PH.D.
Diplomate, American College of
Theriogenologists
Associate Professor
Department of Anatomy
J.A. Baker Institute
College of Veterinary Medicine
Cornell University
Ithaca, NY

MICHAEL S. MILLER, M.S., V.M.D.
Diplomate, American Board of
Veterinary Practitioners (Canine and
Feline)
Director, Cardiology-Ultrasound Referral
Service
Thornton, PA

PAUL E. MILLER, D.V.M.
Diplomate, American College of
Veterinary Ophthalmologists
Clinical Associate Professor
Department of Surgical Sciences
School of Veterinary Medicine
University of Wisconsin - Madison
Madison, WI

ELLEN MILLER, D.V.M., M.S.
Diplomate, American College of
Veterinary Internal Medicine (Internal
Medicine)
Associate Professor
Department of Clinical Sciences
College of Veterinary Medicine
Colorado State University
Fort Collins, CO

MATTHEW W. MILLER, D.V.M., M.S.
Diplomate, American College of
Veterinary Internal Medicine
(Cardiology)
Associate Professor
College of Veterinary Medicine, Texas
A & M University
College Station, TX
Adjunct Professor of Pediatric
Cardiology
Baylor College of Medicine
Staff Cardiologist
Texas Veterinary Medical Center
College of Veterinary Medicine
Texas A & M University
College Station, TX

LISA E. MOORE, D.V.M.
Diplomate, American College of
Veterinary Internal Medicine (Internal
Medicine)
Associate Staff
Department of Medicine
The Animal Medical Center
New York, NY

WALLACE B. MORRISON, D.V.M., M.S.
Diplomate, American College of
Veterinary Internal Medicine (Internal
Medicine)
Associate Professor
Department of Veterinary Clinical
Sciences
Purdue University
School of Veterinary Medicine
West Lafayette, IN

BRADLEY L. MOSES, D.V.M.
Diplomate, American College of
Veterinary Internal Medicine
(Cardiology)
Staff Clinician and Cardiologist
Roberts Animal Hospital
Hanover, MA
Clinical Assistant Professor
Tufts University School of Veterinary
Medicine
North Grafton, MA

K. MARCIA MURPHY, D.V.M.
Dermatology Resident
College of Veterinary Medicine/
Veterinary Teaching Hospital
North Carolina State University
Raleigh, NC

MICHAEL J. MURPHY, D.V.M., PH.D.
Diplomate, American Board of
Veterinary Practitioners
Veterinary Diagnostic Laboratory
College of Veterinary Medicine
University of Minnesota
St. Paul, MN

MARK NASISSE, D.V.M.
Diplomate, American College of
Veterinary Ophthalmologists
Kraeuch: Professor of Ophthalmology
Medicine and Surgery
University of Missouri
Veterinary Teaching Hospital
Columbia, MO

T. MARK NEER, D.V.M.
Diplomate, American College of
Veterinary Internal Medicine (Internal
Medicine)
Professor of Internal Medicine
Section Chief - Small Animal Medicine
Veterinary Teaching Hospital & Clinic
Department of Clinical Sciences
College of Veterinary Medicine
Louisiana State University
Baton Rouge, LA

REGG D. NEIGER, D.V.M., PH.D.
Associate Professor
Department of Veterinary Science
South Dakota State University
Brookings, SD

RHETT NICHOLS, D.V.M.
Diplomate, American College of
Veterinary Internal Medicine (Internal
Medicine)
Director of Internal Medicine
Antech Diagnostics
Farmingdale, NY

GARY D. NORSWORTHY, D.V.M.
Diplomate, American Board of
Veterinary Practitioners (Feline)
Acres North Animal Hospital
San Antonio, TX

JOYCE OBRADOVICH, D.V.M.
Diplomate, American College of
Veterinary Internal Medicine (Oncology)
Oakland Veterinary Referral Services
Bloomfield Hills, MI

FREDERICK W. OEHME, D.V.M., PH.D.
Diplomate, American Board of
Veterinary Toxicology, American Board
Toxicology, Academy of Toxicological
Sciences
Professor of Toxicology, Medicine and
Physiology; Director, Comparative
Toxicology Laboratories
College of Veterinary Medicine
Kansas State University
Manhattan, KS

CARL A. OSBORNE, D.V.M., PH.D.
Diplomate, American College of
Veterinary Internal Medicine (Internal
Medicine)
Professor
Department of Small Animal Clinical
Sciences
College of Veterinary Medicine
University of Minnesota
St. Paul, MN

GARY OSWEILER, D.V.M., PH.D.
Diplomate, American Board of
Veterinary Toxicology
Director, Veterinary Diagnostic Lab
Veterinary Diagnostic Laboratory

College of Veterinary Medicine
Iowa State University
Ames, IA

KAREN L. OVERALL, M.A., V.M.D., PH.D.
Diplomate, American College of
Veterinary Behaviorists
Department of Clinical Studies
Veterinary Hospital University of
Pennsylvania
Philadelphia, PA

DALE PACCAMONTI, D.V.M., M.S.
Diplomate, American College of
Theriogenologists
Associate Professor of Theriogenology
Department of Clinical Sciences
School of Veterinary Medicine
Louisiana State University
Baton Rouge, LA

PHILIP PADRID, D.V.M.
Assistant Professor
Department of Medicine
University of Chicago
Chicago, IL

MARK G. PAPICH, B.S., D.V.M., M.S.
Diplomate, American College of
Veterinary Clinical Pharmacology
Associate Professor of Clinical
Pharmacology
Advisor of Clinical Pharmacology
Laboratory
North Caroline State University
Clinical Pharmacologist
College of Veterinary Medicine
North Carolina State University
Raleigh, NC

JOANE M. PARENT, D.V.M., M.V.S.C.
Diplomate, American College of
Veterinary Internal Medicine (Neurology)
Professor
Department of Veterinary Clinical
Studies
Ontario Veterinary College
University of Guelph
Guelph, Ontario

ALAN PAUL, D.V.M.
Veterinary Medicine Extension
College of Veterinary Medicine
University of Illinois
Urbana, IL

EDWARD J. PEARCE, D.V.M.
Department of Microbiology
College of Veterinary Medicine
Cornell University
Ithaca, NY

MICHAEL PETERSON, D.V.M.
Animal Medical Clinic
Tucson, AZ

J. PHILLIP PICKETT, D.V.M.
Diplomate, American College of
Veterinary Ophthalmologists
Associate Professor of Ophthalmology
Department of Small Animal Clinical
Sciences
Virginia-Maryland Regional College of
Veterinary Medicine
Blacksburg, VA

JON D. PLANT, D.V.M.
Diplomate, American College of
Veterinary Dermatology
Director
Animal Dermatology Specialty Clinic
Santa Monica, CA

KONSTANZE PLUMLEE, D.V.M.
Diplomate, American College of
Veterinary Internal Medicine (Internal
Medicine)
Diagnostic Toxicologist
Toxicology
California Veterinary Diagnostic
Laboratory System
Davis, CA

DAVID J. POLZIN, D.V.M.
Diplomate, American College of
Veterinary Internal Medicine (Internal
Medicine)
Professor
Department of Small Animal Clinical
Sciences
College of Veterinary Medicine
University of Minnesota
St. Paul, MN

ERIC RUSSELL POPE, D.V.M., M.S.
Diplomate, American College of
Veterinary Surgeons
Associate Professor
Veterinary Medicine and Surgery
Veterinary Teaching Hospital
University of Missouri
Columbia, MO

ROBERT H. POPPENGA, D.V.M., PH.D.
Diplomate, American Board of
Veterinary Toxicology
Assistant Professor of Veterinary
Toxicology
University of Pennsylvania
Kennett Square, PA

KLAAS POST, D.V.M.
Professor
Department of Veterinary Internal
Medicine
Western College of Veterinary
Medicine
University of Saskatchewan
Saskatoon, Saskatchewan

JAMES C. PRUETER, D.V.M.
Diplomate, American College of
Veterinary Internal Medicine (Internal
Medicine)
Director
Veterinary Referral Clinic of Cleveland
Cleveland, OH

BEVERLY J. PURSWELL, D.V.M., PH.D.
Diplomate, American College of
Theriogenologists
Associate Professor
Large Animal Clinical Sciences
College of Veterinary Medicine
Virginia Tech
Blacksburg, VA

ANDREE D. QUESNEL, D.V.M., D.V.SC.
Diplomate, American College of
Veterinary Internal Medicine
(Neurology)

Assistant Professor
Departement des Sciences Clinique
Faculte de Medecine Veterinaire
L'Universite de Montreal
St. Hyacinthe, Quebec

CYNTHIA CRAGER RAMSEY, D.V.M., M.S.
Diplomate, American College of
Veterinary Internal Medicine (Internal
Medicine)
Assistant Professor; Director, Intensive
Care/Emergency Medicine
Small Animal Clinical Sciences
Veterinary Teaching Hospital
Michigan State University
East Lansing, MI

CLARENCE RAWLINGS, D.V.M.
Diplomate, American College of
Veterinary Surgeons
Veterinary Teaching Hospital
University of Georgia College of
Veterinary Medicine
Athens, GA

WILLIAM REAGAN, D.V.M., PH.D.
Diplomate, American College of
Veterinary Pathologists
Associate Professor of Clinical
Pathology
Department of Veterinary Pathobiology
School of Veterinary Medicine
Purdue University
West Lafayette, IN

ALAN H. REBAR, D.V.M., PH.D.
Diplomate, American College of
Veterinary Pathologists
Dean, School of Veterinary Medicine
Department of Veterinary Pathobiology
Purdue University
School of Veterinary Medicine
West Lafayette, IN

JAMES RICHARDS, D.V.M.
Director, Camuti Memorial Feline
Consultation Service
Assistant Director, Cornell Feline
Health Center
Representative-at-Large, American
Association of Feline Practitioners
Cornell Feline Health Center
College of Veterinary Medicine
Cornell University
Ithaca, NY

RALPH C. RICHARDSON, D.V.M.
Diplomate, American College of
Veterinary Internal Medicine (Oncology,
Internal Medicine)
Professor and Department Head
Department of Veterinary Clinical
Sciences
School of Veterinary Medicine
Purdue University
West Lafayette, IN

KEITH P. RICHTER, D.V.M.
Diplomate, American College of
Veterinary Internal Medicine (Internal
Medicine)
Internal Medicine Staff
Veterinary Specialty Hospital of San
Diego
Rancho Santa Fe, CA

MICHAEL J. RINGLE, D.V.M.
Diplomate, American College of
Veterinary Ophthalmologists
The Animal Eye Clinic of New Jersey
Red Bank, NJ

MARK RISHNIW, B.V.SC., M.S.
Diplomate, American College of
Veterinary Internal Medicine (Internal
Medicine)
Resident, Cardiology
Department of Medicine and
Epidemiology
School of Veterinary Medicine
University of California - Davis
Davis, CA

T. ARCH ROBERTSON, D.V.M.
President
Vet Med Consultants
Mesa, Arizona

MARGARET V. ROOT, D.V.M., PH.D.
Diplomate, American College of
Theriogenologists
Department of Small Animal Clinical
Sciences
College of Veterinary Medicine
University of Minnesota
St. Paul, MN

DAVID K. ROSEN, D.V.M.
Glendale, WI

PHILIP ROUDEBUSH, D.V.M.
Diplomate, American College of
Veterinary Internal Medicine (Internal
Medicine)
Veterinary Fellow
Hill's Science and Technology Center
Topeka, KS

JOHN E. RUSH, D.V.M.
Diplomate, American College of
Veterinary Internal Medicine
(Cardiology)
Diplomate, American College of
Veterinary Emergency and Critical Care
Head Cardiologist and Co-Director of
I.C.U./Emergency Services
Department of Medicine
School of Veterinary Medicine
Tufts University
North Grafton, MA

PETER D. SCHWARZ, D.V.M.
Diplomate, American College of
Veterinary Surgeons
Veterinary Teaching Hospital
College of Veterinary Medicine
University of Colorado
Fort Collins, CO

FRED W. SCOTT, D.V.M., PH.D.
Diplomate, American College of
Veterinary Microbiologists; Academy of
Feline Medicine
Professor of Virology
Director, Cornell Feline Health Center
Microbiology and Immunology
College of Veterinary Medicine
Cornell University
Ithaca, NY

DARCY SHAW, D.V.M., M.V.SC.
Diplomate, American College of
Veterinary Internal Medicine (Internal
Medicine)
Associate Professor
Department of Companion Animals
Atlantic Veterinary College
University of Prince Edward Island
Charlottetown, Prince Edward Island

LINDA J. SHELL, D.V.M.
Diplomate, American College of
Veterinary Internal Medicine
(Neurology)
Professor
Small Animal Clinical Sciences
VA-MD Regional College of Veterinary
Medicine
Virginia Tech
Blacksburg, VA

G. DIANE SHELTON, D.V.M., PH.D.
Diplomate, American College of
Veterinary Internal Medicine
(Neurology)
Associate Adjunct Professor
Department of Pathology
School of Medicine
University of California, San Diego
LaJolla, CA

ROBERT M. SHULL, D.V.M.
Diplomate, American College of
Veterinary Pathologists (Clinical
Pathology)
Professor
Department of Pathology
College of Veterinary Medicine
University of Tennessee
Knoxville, TN

BARBARA SIMPSON, D.V.M., PH.D.
Diplomate, American College of
Veterinary Behaviorists
ABS-Certified Applied Animal
Behaviorist
Adjunct Assistant Professor, North
Carolina State College of Veterinary
Medicine
Department of Companion Animal and
Special Species Medicine
Veterinary Behaviorist
The Veterinary Behavior Clinic
Southern Pines, NC

ALLEN FRANKLIN SISSON, D.V.M.
Diplomate, American College of
Veterinary Internal Medicine
(Neurology)
Staff Neurologist
Department of Medicine
Angell Memorial Animal Hospital
Boston, MA

STEPHANIE SMEDES, D.V.M.
Diplomate, American College of
Veterinary Ophthalmologists
Staff Ophthalmologist and Director
Oceanview Veterinary Specialist
Vancouver, British Columbia

FRANCIS W. K. SMITH, JR., D.V.M.
Diplomate, American College of
Veterinary Internal Medicine (Internal

Medicine)
Chief of Medicine, Cardiopet, Inc., Little
Falls, NJ
Clinical Assistant Professor in Medicine,
Tufts University School of Veterinary
Medicine, North Grafton, MA

MARY SMITH, B.V.M.S., PH.D.
Diplomate, American College of
Veterinary Internal Medicine (Neurology)
Assistant Professor
Department of Clinical Sciences
College of Veterinary Medicine
Colorado State University
Fort Collins, CO

PATRICIA J. SMITH, D.V.M., M.S., PH.D.
Diplomate, American College of
Veterinary Ophthalmology
Assistant Professor
Small Animal Clinical Sciences
College of Veterinary Medicine
University of Florida
Gainesville, FL

PATTI S. SNYDER, D.V.M.
Diplomate, American College of
Veterinary Internal Medicine (Internal
Medicine)
Assistant Professor
Small Animal Clinical Sciences
College of Veterinary Medicine
University of Florida
Gainesville, FL

PAUL W. SNYDER, D.V.M., PH.D.
Diplomate, American College of
Veterinary Pathologists
Assistant Professor
Department of Veterinary Pathobiology
School of Veterinary Medicine
Purdue University
West Lafayette, IN

REBECCA L. STEPIEN, D.V.M.
Diplomate, American College of
Veterinary Internal Medicine
(Cardiology)
University of Wisconsin School of
Veterinary Medicine
Madison, WI

J. B. STEVENS, D.V.M., PH.D.
Professor, Clinical Pathology
College of Veterinary Medicine
North Carolina State University
Raleigh, NC

ELIZABETH STONE, D.V.M.
Diplomate, American College of
Veterinary Surgeons
Professor of Surgery
Department of Companion Animal and
Special Species Medicine
North Carolina State University
School of Veterinary Medicine
Raleigh, NC

JUSTIN STRAUS, D.V.M.
Diplomate, American College of
Veterinary Internal Medicine (Internal
Medicine)
Staff Internist
Oradell Animal Hospital
Oradell, NJ

MARGARET SWARTOUT, D.V.M., M.S.
Diplomate, American College of
Veterinary Internal Medicine (Internal
Medicine)
Owner
Veterinary Specialty Consultation
Service
Knoxville, TN

CHERYL L. SWENSON, D.V.M.
Diplomate, American College of
Veterinary Pathologists (Clinical
Pathology)
Assistant Professor
Department of Pathology
Veterinary Medical Center
Michigan State University
East Lansing, MI

JOSEPH TABOADA, D.V.M.
Diplomate, American College of
Veterinary Internal Medicine (Internal
Medicine)
Associate Professor and Chief
Department of Veterinary Clinical
Sciences
School of Veterinary Medicine
Louisiana State University
Baton Rouge, LA

SUSAN M. TAYLOR, D.V.M.
Diplomate, American College of
Veterinary Internal Medicine (Internal
Medicine)
Professor of Small Animal Medicine
and Internist
Department of Veterinary Internal
Medicine
Western College of Veterinary
Medicine
University of Saskatchewan
Saskatoon, Saskatchewan

ROBERT TAYLOR, D.V.M.
Diplomate, American College of
Veterinary Surgeons
Alameda East Veterinary Hospital
Denver, CO

WILLIAM B. THOMAS, D.V.M., M.S.
Diplomate, American College of
Veterinary Internal Medicine
(Neurology)
Assistant Professor
Department of Small Animal Clinical
Sciences
College of Veterinary Medicine
University of Tennessee
Knoxville, TN

LARRY J. THOMPSON, D.V.M., PH.D.
Diplomate, American Board of
Veterinary Toxicology
Clinical Toxicologist
Diagnostic Laboratory
New York State College of Veterinary
Medicine
Ithaca, NY

JAMES P. THOMPSON, D.V.M., PH.D.
Diplomate, American College of
Veterinary Internal Medicine (Internal
Medicine, Oncology)
Diplomate, American College of

Veterinary Microbiologists (Virology, Immunology, Bacteriology, Mycology)
Associate Professor
Small Animal Clinical Sciences
University of Florida College of Veterinary Medicine
Gainesville, FL

LELAND THOMPSON, D.V.M.
College of Veterinary Medicine
Mississippi State University
Mississippi State, MS

JERRY A. THORNHILL, D.V.M.
Diplomate, American College of Veterinary Internal Medicine (Internal Medicine)
Veterinary Medical and Kidney Clinic
Berwyn, IL

MARY ANNA THRALL, D.V.M., M.S.
Diplomate, American College of Veterinary Pathologists
Professor
Department of Pathology
School of Veterinary Medicine and Biomedical Sciences
Colorado State University
Fort Collins, CO

LARRY P. TILLEY, D.V.M.
Diplomate, American College of Veterinary Internal Medicine (Internal Medicine)
Director, Veterinary Specialty Referral Center
President, VET MED FAX Consultation Services
Santa Fe, NM

DAVID C. TWEDT, D.V.M.
Diplomate, American College of Veterinary Internal Medicine (Internal Medicine)
Professor
Clinical Sciences
Veterinary Teaching Hospital
College of Veterinary Medicine
Colorado State University
Fort Collins, CO

RONALD D. TYLER, D.V.M., PH.D.
Diplomate, American College of Veterinary Pathologists (Clinical Pathology and Anatomic Pathology)
Diplomate, American Board of Toxicology
International Head, Strategic Toxicological Sciences Glaxo Wellcome, RTP, NC
Adjunct Professor, College of Veterinary Medicine, Oklahoma State University, Stillwater, OK
Strategic Toxicologic Sciences, Medicines Safety Evaluation
Glaxo Wellcome Inc.
Research Triangle Park, NC

SHELLY L. VADEN, D.V.M.
Diplomate, American College of Veterinary Internal Medicine (Internal Medicine)
Assistant Professor, Internal Medicine
Department of Companion Animal and

Special Species Medicine
North Carolina State University
School of Veterinary Medicine
Raleigh, NC

MARY ANN VONDERHAAR, D.V.M., M.S.
Private Consultant
Guest Instructor
Purdue University College of Veterinary Medicine
West Lafayette, IN

MELISSA WALLACE, D.V.M.
Diplomate, American College of Veterinary Internal Medicine (Internal Medicine)
Staff Internist
Department of Medicine
The Animal Medical Center
New York, NY

MICHELLE JOY WASCHAK, D.V.M.
Veterinary Teaching Hospital
University of Missouri College of Veterinary Medicine
Columbia, MO

ROBERT J. WASHABAU, V.M.D., PH.D.
Diplomate, American College of Veterinary Internal Medicine (Internal Medicine)
Assistant Professor of Medicine
Clinical Studies
School of Veterinary Medicine
University of Pennsylvania
Philadelphia, PA

M. GLADE WEISER, D.V.M.
Diplomate, American College of Veterinary Pathologists (Clinical Pathology)
Professor
Department of Pathology
Colorado State University
Fort Collins, CO

ALEXANDER WERNER, V.M.D.
Diplomate, American College of Veterinary Dermatology
Staff Dermatologist
Valley Veterinary Specialty Services
Studio City, CA

MICHAEL D. WILLARD, D.V.M., M.S.
Diplomate, American College of Veterinary Internal Medicine (Internal Medicine)
Professor of Small Animal Medicine and Surgery
Department of Small Animal Medicine and Surgery
College of Veterinary Medicine
Texas A & M University
College Station, TX

DAVID A. WILLIAMS, M.A., VET. MB, PH.D., M.R.C.V.S.
Diplomate American College of Veterinary Internal Medicine (Internal Medicine)
Chief, Small Animal Medicine
Department of Veterinary Clinical Sciences
School of Veterinary Medicine

Purdue University
West Lafayette, IN

JAMES E. WILLIAMS, JR., D.V.M.
Veterinary Teaching Hospital
University of Missouri College of Veterinary Medicine
Columbia, MO

RONALD B. WILSON, D.V.M.
Diplomate, American College of Veterinary Pathologists
Veterinary Pathologist
C.E. Kord Animal Disease Laboratory
Nashville, TN

J. PAUL WOODS, D.V.M., M.S.
Diplomate, American College of Veterinary Internal Medicine (Internal Medicine)
Canadian Veterinary Medical Association
Certificate of Specialization in Small Animal Internal Medicine
Assistant Professor
College of Veterinary Medicine
Oklahoma State University
Stillwater, OK

KAREN M. YOUNG, V.D.M., PH.D.
Clinical Associate Professor
Department of Pathobiological Sciences
School of Veterinary Medicine
University of Wisconsin - Madison
Madison, WI

DEBRA L. ZORAN, D.V.M., M.S.
Diplomate, American College of Veterinary Internal Medicine (Internal Medicine)
Research Assistant
Department of Animal Science
Texas A&M University
College Station, TX

CONTENTS *by section*

DIAGNOSTICS - LABORATORY TESTS

DIAGNOSTICS - ELECTROCARDIOGRAPHY

DISEASES AND CLINICAL SYNDROMES

TOPIC	

TOPIC	

CONTENTS *by subject*

TOPIC	AUTHOR	

DERMATOLOGY

ENDOCRINOLOGY

GASTROENTEROLOGY

HEMATOLOGY

HEPATOLOGY

MUSCULOSKELETAL

NEPHROLOGY

NEUROLOGY

ONCOLOGY

TOPIC	AUTHOR	

OPHTHALMOLOGY

RESPIRATORY

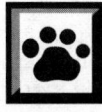

PRESENTING PROBLEMS
AND PHYSICAL FINDINGS

ABORTION, SPONTANEOUS (PREGNANCY LOSS)—CATS

 BASICS

DEFINITION
• Abortion—expulsion of one or more live or dead fetuses that cannot sustain extrauterine life • Pregnancy loss—all pregnancy wastage, including embryonic death, reabsorption of early fetal losses, mummification, abortion, and dystocia

Pathophysiology
• Primary causes kill the embryo or fetus directly. In patients with secondary fetal wastage, death results from defective or compromised placentation, inadequate uterine vascular or nutritional support, or failure of supportive endocrine development and function. Dam-related events such as dystocia, trauma, extreme stress, and metabolic disease usually terminate fetal life indirectly.
• Possible outcomes are reabsorption during early gestation, abortion or mummification during later gestation, and stillbirth at term. Reabsorption, abortion, and mummification occur in descending order of frequency, but reabsorption is more difficult to document. The frequency of early embryonic death in cats is unknown.

Systems Affected
• Reproductive • Other organs if events leading to pregnancy wastage originate in another body system or externally, or if pregnancy wastage leads to complications such as toxemia or shock

SIGNALMENT
Nonspecific, but more common at first parity and in queens > 6 years old, except in animals with infectious cause

SIGNS

General Comments
Animal may be asymptomatic, especially early in gestation

Historical Findings
• Failure to litter on time • Decrease in abdominal size • Expulsion of recognizable fetuses or placental structures • Anorexia • Vomiting and diarrhea

Physical Examination Findings
• Bloody or purulent vulvar discharge (discharge may not be observed in fastidious queens) • Disappearance of vesicles or fetuses previously documented by palpation, ultrasound, or radiography • Abdominal straining and discomfort • Depression • Dehydration • Fever
Note: Not all signs are seen in every animal. Any combination may occur, or none at all.

CAUSES

Infectious Causes
• Viruses—feline panleukopenia virus, feline rhinotracheitis virus, and FeLV • Bacteria—Escherichia coli, Streptococcus spp,

Staphylococcus spp, Salmonella spp, Mycobacterium spp, and Mycoplasma spp • Rickettsia—Coxiella burnetii (Q fever) • Parasite—Toxoplasma gondii

Noninfectious Causes (Reproductive)
• Dystocia (fetal causes)—fetal malposition (relatively uncommon), fetal deformity, excessively large fetal size (i.e., small litter and prolonged gestation), multiple simultaneous fetal presentation, and breed-based fetal-maternal disproportion (i.e., Persian and Himalayan) • Dystocia (maternal causes)—small pelvic diameter because of immaturity, previous injury, or congenital abnormality, insufficient dilation of the soft tissue of the birth canal, fibrosis or malformation of the birth canal, uterine inertia (common), torsion of the uterine horn, prolapse, and metabolic disease predisposing to episodic weakness, pain, and fatigue • Endocrinopathy—endometrial disease (i.e., cystic endometrial hyperplasia) and hypoluteoidism (indirect evidence, but not documented conclusively in cats) • Structural or functional placental inadequacy • Fetal defects—genetic or developmental, including anatomic, metabolic, and chromosomal abnormalities; possibly, gamete aging • Excessive or poorly planned inbreeding and poor choices of breeding stock (usually indirect evidence; difficult diagnosis without thorough family history and test matings) • Abortifacient drugs—luteolytics (e.g., prostaglandin F2-alpha), estrogens, prolactin inhibitors (cabergoline), and glucocorticoids • Additional drugs reported in dogs—prolactin inhibitors (e.g., bromocryptine), antiestrogens (e.g., tamoxifen citrate), progesterone antagonists (e.g., mifepristone), and progesterone synthesis inhibitors (e.g., espostane)

Noninfectious Causes (Nonreproductive)
• Nutrition—taurine < 200 ppm of diet • Severe stress—environmental, physiologic, and psychologic • Trauma • Drugs—various • Consequence of nonreproductive systemic disease

RISK FACTORS
• Previous history of pregnancy loss • Concurrent acute or chronic disease • Possibly, excessive inbreeding

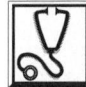 **DIAGNOSIS**

DIFFERENTIAL DIAGNOSIS

Other Causes of Vulvar Discharge
• Impending parturition • Estrus—discharge usually not copious, behavioral signs of estrus present, and vaginal cytologic examination documents estrus (note: sample collection may induce ovulation) • Metritis • Pyometra—neutrophilic leukocytosis, polydipsia and polyuria, and signs of systemic illness characteristic, ultrasonography or radiography reveals large uterus, and vaginal cytologic examination confirms inflammation • Severe

vaginitis • Uterine trauma or hemorrhage—history of recent injury and clinical signs of bloody discharge, weakness, shock, and pallor characteristic, CBC documents acute blood loss, ultrasonography may reveal uterine fluid or suggest blood clots, and vaginal cytologic examination documents bleeding without inflammation • Abnormal vaginal or rectovaginal anatomy—ultrasonography and contrast radiography define abnormal vaginal canal or rectovaginal fistula and discharge of intestinal contents from vulva (fistula) characteristic • Uterine or vaginal neoplasia • Uterine stump infection • Ovarian remnant syndrome—discharge usually not copious, history of ovariohysterectomy and behavioral signs of estrus characteristic, and vaginal cytologic examination documents estrus

Other Causes of Abdominal Signs
• Obstructive uropathy or nonobstructive lower urinary tract disease • Severe renal disease such as pyelonephritis • Pancreatitis • Liver disease • Severe gastrointestinal disease • Peritonitis • Abdominal trauma

CBC/BIOCHEMISTRY/URINALYSIS
• Inflammatory or stress leukocyte response, except in patients with panleukopenia.
• Results of serum biochemistry profile and urinalysis usually are normal, but they may reveal systemic involvement if another disease has led to secondary pregnancy wastage, or if primary pregnancy wastage has resulted in secondary systemic involvement. • Examination of discharge fluid may reveal fetal or placental tissue.

OTHER LABORATORY TESTS

Infectious Causes
• Feline panleukopenia—virus isolated from lungs, kidneys, urine, and feces; rising antibody titer from paired sera, 14 to 21-day interval; histologic changes in gastrointestinal tract. Test affected individuals early in course of disease. • Feline rhinotracheitis—immunofluorescent antibody test of conjunctival scrapings; rising antibody titer from paired sera, 14 to 21-day interval; frozen oropharyngeal, tonsillar, or nasal swabs for virus isolation (probably most practical in catteries because virus is often endemic and serum antibody titers may be positive; contact regional diagnostic laboratory first for instructions or refer to specialized laboratory). Test affected individuals early in course of disease. • FeLV—immunofluorescent antibody and ELISA tests. Test entire cattery or all cats in the household. • Mycoplasma—complement fixation, hemagglutination inhibition, culture (contact laboratory; special media required). Test affected individuals early in course of disease and test unaffected individuals also. Isolation of organismis preferred. • Coxiella—antibody titers from paired sera, 2 to 4-week intervals (contact regional diagnostic laboratory first for instructions or refer to specialized laboratory)

ABORTION, SPONTANEOUS (PREGNANCY LOSS)—CATS

Noninfectious Causes
• Reproductive • Hypoluteoidism—serial serum progesterone determinations starting before time of suspected fetal loss

IMAGING
• Palpation and radiography can establish presence of fetuses if applied at appropriate intervals of gestation. However, ultrasonography is essential for precise evaluation of fetal status. • Radiography and ultrasound are helpful for confirming several differential diagnoses.

OTHER DIAGNOSTIC PROCEDURES
• Bacterial diseases—culture and sensitivity of the cervix, anterior vaginal canal, or uterus; obtain specimen by ultrasound guidance, laparoscopy, or laparotomy (contact laboratory before shipping samples for Salmonella or Mycobacterium culture). Test affected individuals early in course of disease. • Placental inadequacy—histologic and microbiologic evaluation of placenta • Fetal defects—necropsy; karyotype (submit ear tip of necropsied animal shipped in heparinized dam's blood; contact karyotype laboratory, University of Minnesota); screen for inborn metabolic errors (submit urine from necropsy or live subject; contact Medical Genetics Section, University of Pennsylvania); history of involved or related sires and dams. For karyotype subjects, save gonad in Bouin's solution for histopathologic examination.
• Poor reproductive planning—extensive review of breeding records, including inbreeding coefficients, performance records, and records of related individuals. History of high neonatal or pediatric mortality, poor growth of surviving subjects, and increased susceptibility to infectious diseases often suggests excessive inbreeding or poor choice of breeding stock. (Note: Inbreeding coefficient is the probability that two genes that an individual receives from its parents at a randomly chosen autosomal locus are identical by descent; thus, the inbreeding coefficient measures the impact of relatedness on genes found within a single individual.)

TREATMENT
• Patients that are aborting visible fetal and placental material or are likely to do so, and those with clinical illness, usually should be hospitalized for treatment. Abortus or discharge may be infectious. Isolate patient if infectious agent is suspected. Hospitalize patients with potential zoonoses unless safe and effective outpatient management is assured. In all situations, practice strict sanitation for inpatients and outpatients.
• Normally, it is not possible to predict outcome of subsequent pregnancies without a complete diagnosis. Consider ovariohysterectomy for stable patients with no breeding value. Consider prostaglandin or hysterotomy to empty and clean uterus for breeding cats. Potential contraindications for prostaglandin administration include advanced age, live fetuses, mummified fetuses, closed cervix, sepsis, peritonitis, high risk of uterine rupture, and other organ dysfunction. Potential contraindications for surgery include serious risk to the patient and ability to resolve the problem by less invasive means. In catteries, discuss history or possibility of multiple occurrences. Establish monitoring system and encourage careful records of reproductive performance.

MEDICATIONS
DRUGS AND FLUIDS
• Amoxicillin—5-10 mg/lb q12h, pending results of bacterial culture • Normosol or lactated Ringer's solution for management of dehydration, IV or SQ, depending on severity of problem and cooperation of patient
• If ultrasonography demonstrates no live fetuses and significant uterine contents are noted, prostaglandin F2-alpha (Lutalyse, Upjohn; 0.10-0.25 mg/kg SQ q24h for up to 5 days if needed) • Hospitalization for treatment is recommended; obtain informed consent.
• Other treatments are specific according to diagnosis.

CONTRAINDICATIONS
Avoid administration of prostaglandin F2-alpha or other attempts to evacuate the uterus if potentially viable fetuses are present. Use caution if uterine rupture is possible.

PRECAUTIONS
Side effects of prostaglandin include intense grooming, salivation, defecation, vomiting, urination, tachycardia, vocalization, nervousness, panting, mydriasis, lordosis posture, tail flagging and, occasionally, hypotension.

POSSIBLE INTERACTIONS
Between various drugs that might be used in management of specific differential diagnoses

ALTERNATE DRUGS

FOLLOW-UP
PATIENT MONITORING
• Physical examination 7-14 days after treatment • Repeat ultrasound to document complete evacuation of the uterus or to establish continued presence of live fetuses

POSSIBLE COMPLICATIONS
Sepsis, shock, uterine rupture, peritonitis, metritis, pyometra, and subsequent infertility (depending on cause)

MISCELLANEOUS
ASSOCIATED CONDITIONS N/A

AGE RELATED FACTORS
• Fertility declines naturally after age 6 years. • Ovariohysterectomy should be recommended in stable patients > 6 years old.

ZOONOTIC POTENTIAL
Bacterial causes, Coxiella burnetii, and Toxoplasma gondii

PREGNANCY N/A

SYNONYMS N/A

SEE ALSO N/A

ABBREVIATIONS N/A

References
Feldman EC, Nelson RW. Canine and feline endocrinology and reproduction. Philadelphia: WB Saunders, 1987:525-548.
Papich MG. Effects of drugs on pregnancy. In: Kirk RW, Bonagura JD, eds. Current veterinary therapy X. Philadelphia: WB Saunders, 1989:1291-1299.
Troy GC, Herron MA. Infectious causes of infertility, abortion, and stillbirths in cats. In: Morrow DA, ed. Current therapy in theriogenology. Philadelphia: WB Saunders, 1986:834-837.
Author Dennis F. Lawler
Consulting Editor Sara K. Lyle

ABORTION, SPONTANEOUS (PREGNANCY LOSS)—DOGS

BASICS

DEFINITION
Loss of a fetus because of resorption in early stages or expulsion in later stages of pregnancy

Pathophysiology
Direct causes of fetal death include congenital abnormality, infectious disease, and trauma. Indirect causes include infectious placentitis and abnormal ovarian or uterine maternal environment.

Systems Affected
• Reproductive system • Any dysfunction of a major body system can adversely affect pregnancy.

SIGNALMENT Intact bitches

SIGNS N/A

CAUSES

Infectious
• Brucella canis • Canine Herpesvirus • Toxoplasma • Mycoplasma and ureaplasma • Miscellaneous bacteria: E. coli, Streptococci, Campylobacter, Salmonella • Miscellaneous viruses: Distemper virus, Parvovirus

Uterine
• Cystic endometrial hyperplasia and pyometra • Trauma (acute and chronic) • Neoplasia • Embryotoxic drugs • Chemotherapeutic agents • Chloramphenicol (early gestation) • Estrogens • Glucocorticoids (high dosage) • Prostaglandins (lysis of corpora lutea)

Hormonal Dysfunction
• Hypothyroidism • Hypoluteoidism

Fetal Defects
• Lethal chromosomal abnormality • Lethal organ defects

RISK FACTORS
• Exposure of the brood bitch to carrier animals • Old age • Hereditary

DIAGNOSIS

DIFFERENTIAL DIAGNOSIS
• Differentiate infectious causes from noninfectious causes. The immediate concern in dogs is Brucella canis. • Differentiate resorption from infertility. Early diagnosis of pregnancy helps distinguish between pregnancy loss and lack of conception. • History of drug use during pregnancy, particularly during the first trimester or drugs, is known to cause fetal death. • Vulvar discharges during diestrus may only mimic abortion. Evaluation of the discharge and origin helps differentiate uterine from distal reproductive tract disease. • Necropsy of aborted fetus and placenta enhances chances of a definitive diagnosis. Necropsy of apparently stillborn puppies is also indicated. • History of systemic or endocrine disease may indicate problems with the maternal environment.

CBC/BIOCHEMISTRY/URINALYSIS
• Results usually normal • In some patients, results reveal systemic disease such as uterine infection, viral infection, and endocrine abnormality.

OTHER LABORATORY TESTS
• Serologic testing for Brucella canis, canine herpesvirus, and toxoplasma to rule out these infectious causes. Serum for these tests should be collected as soon as possible after an abortion. The slide test for Brucella canis is very sensitive, so negative results are reliable. The prevalence of false positives is as high as 60%. The tube agglutination test gives titers; < 1:200 is considered insignificant. The agar gel immunodiffusion test effectively differentiates between false positives and true positives. • Baseline T_4 serum concentration if no infectious agents are identified. Hypothyroidism is a common endocrine disease in dogs and has been suggested as a cause of fetal wastage. • Progesterone serum concentration if no infectious agents are identified. Hypoluteoidism is a potential cause of abortion because of the dependence of dogs on ovarian progesterone production throughout gestation. The bitch requires a minimum of 2 ng/ml to maintain pregnancy. Progesterone concentration should be determined as soon as possible after abortion. In subsequent pregnancies, after ultrasonographic confirmation of pregnancy, progesterone should be monitored starting at the third week of gestation. • Vaginal culture for Brucella canis if serologic test is positive

IMAGING
• Radiography is useful to identify fetal structures in later stages of pregnancy (> 45 days gestation). Before 45 days, uterine enlargement can be determined but no assessment can be made of uterine contents. • Ultrasonography is useful to identify uterine size and contents. Fluid and its consistency can be assessed. Fetal remains and fetal viability can be assessed by the presence of heartbeats. Fetal heart rates should be > 200 bpm (< 200 bpm indicates fetal stress).

OTHER DIAGNOSTIC PROCEDURES
• Vaginoscopy is useful to identify the source of vulvar discharges as well as any vaginal lesions. A scope should be long enough to examine the entire length of the vagina (16-20 cm in length). • Cytologic examination and bacterial culture of the vagina may reveal the presence of an inflammatory process such as uterine infection. A vaginal culture should be performed with a guarded swab culture instrument to insure an anterior vaginal culture. The distal reproductive tract is normally heavily contaminated with bacteria. • Histopathologic examination of fetal and placental tissue may reveal infectious organisms. Culture of these tissues, particularly stomach contents, is helpful to identify infectious bacterial organisms.

TREATMENT
• Most bitches should be confined and isolated pending diagnosis.
• Brucella canis is highly infective to dogs and is shed in high numbers during an abortion.

MEDICATIONS

DRUG AND FLUIDS
• Uterine evacuation after abortion can be accomplished by administration of prostaglandin F_{2a} (0.1 mg/kg SQ q8h-q24h). This product is not approved for use in dogs, but adequate documentation in the literature legitimizes its use. No analogues should be substituted because of inadequate documentation of safe dosages. Use only if all living fetuses have been expelled.
• Antibiotics are indicated if the bitch has bacterial disease. Broad-spectrum antibiotics should be instituted and changed as needed pending results of vaginal culture and sensitivity testing and necropsy of the fetus.
• In patients that have had a partial abortion, an attempt can be made to salvage the remaining live fetuses. Antibiotics are administered if a bacterial component is identified. Cage rest of the bitch is indicated. Monitoring of the pregnancy by ultrasonography is desirable to document continued fetal viability. Monitoring of the dam (i.e., temperature and CBC) should be ongoing for the remainder of the pregnancy.
• The first recommendation for dogs with confirmed Brucella canis infection is euthanasia. Because of the lack of success of treatment, euthanasia eliminates the possibility of the spread of the organism to other dogs and humans. The second recommendation is ovariohysterectomy and long-term administration of antibiotics. Euthanasia or treatment is strongly encouraged.

CONTRAINDICATIONS
Progesterone (Regu-mate®) 0.088 mg/kg-2 ml/110# PO; progesterone in oil 2mg/kg IM is contraindicated except in those dogs with hypoluteoidism.

PRECAUTIONS
Prostaglandin F_{2a} is metabolized in the lungs. Side effects are related to smooth muscle contraction and are dose related. Panting, salivation, vomition, and defecation are common. Side effects are less severe with each subsequent injection. Dosing is critical. The LD_{50} is 5 mg/kg.

ALTERNATE DRUGS
Oxytocin (1 unit/5 kg SQ q6h-q24h) for uterine evacuation is most effective for the first 24-48 hours after abortion.

ABORTION, SPONTANEOUS (PREGNANCY LOSS)—DOGS

FOLLOW-UP

PATIENT MONITORING

• Vulvar discharges daily for amount, consistency, odor, and inflammatory component. Prostaglandin F_{2a} should be continued for 5 days or until most of the discharge ceases (3-15 days). The amount of discharge should be decreasing with an increasing mucoid component to the discharge. Odors, if present, should diminish over time. Inflammatory component of discharge should diminish over time. • Dogs positive for Brucella canis should be monitored after neutering and antibiotic therapy with yearly serologic testing to identify recrudescence. • Hypothyroidism should be treated appropriately and recommendations made for neutering owing to the hereditary nature of the problem. See Hypothyroidism

POSSIBLE COMPLICATIONS

• Septicemia, toxemia, and death due to untreated pyometra • Discospondylitis, endophthalmitis, and recurrent uveitis may develop over time.

MISCELLANEOUS

ASSOCIATED CONDITIONS N/A

AGE RELATED FACTORS N/A

ZOONOTIC POTENTIAL

Brucella canis can be transmitted to humans, especially when handling the aborting bitch. Massive number of organisms are expelled during the abortion.

PREGNANCY N/A

SYNONYMS N/A

SEE ALSO Infertility-Female

ABBREVIATIONS N/A

References

Carmichael LE, Greene CE. Canine brucellosis. In: Greene CE, ed. Infectious diseases of the dog and cat. Philadelphia: WB Saunders, 1990;573-584.

Evermann JF. Diagnosis of canine herpetic infections. In: Kirk RW, ed. Current veterinary therapy X. Philadelphia: WB Saunders, 1989;1313-1316.

Lein DH. Infertility and reproductive diseases in bitches and queens. In: Roberts SJ, ed. Veterinary obstetrics and genital diseases (theriogenology). Woodstock, VT: SJ Roberts Publisher, 1986;728-734.

Roberts SJ. Diseases and accidents during the gestation period. In: Roberts SJ, ed. Veterinary Obstetrics and Genital Diseases (Theriogenology). Woodstock, VT: S. J. Roberts Publisher, 1986;206-210.

Feldman EC, Nelson RW. Canine and feline endocrinology and reproduction. Philadelphia: WB Saunders, 1987;399-480.

Authors Beverly J. Purswell and Nikola A. Parker
Consulting Editor Sara K. Lyle

ABORTION, TERMINATION OF PREGNANCY

BASICS

DEFINITION
Induced termination of pregnancy can be accomplished by drugs that prevent fertilization, prevent implantation, or terminate an established pregnancy.

Pathophysiology
In dogs, and most likely in cats, maintenance of pregnancy requires a functional corpus luteum throughout pregnancy. It is suggested that pituitary rather than uterine or placental influences are most important for maintenance of the corpus luteum, and that the two principal hormones involved are luteinizing hormone (LH) and prolactin (PRL). Reducing the concentration of LH or PRL may cause regression of the corpus luteum and termination of pregnancy. Compounds that inhibit progesterone secretion or compete with progesterone receptors should work equally as well.

Systems Affected
• Reproductive • Other systems (e.g., gastrointestinal, respiratory, neurologic, and cardiac systems) are affected by drugs used in treatment

SIGNALMENT
Unwanted pregnancies in females

SIGNS
Depending on the stage of gestation, signs vary from no visible signs, to vaginal discharge, to expulsion of a fetus(es).

CAUSES
Termination of pregnancy can be attempted by withdrawing luteotrophic support, inhibiting progesterone synthesis, or using a progesterone receptor antagonist.

RISK FACTORS
• Most of the drugs used have undesirable side effects or require a great deal of time and effort in administration and monitoring of the patient. • Many drugs are not approved for use in therapeutic abortions.

DIAGNOSIS

DIFFERENTIAL DIAGNOSIS
• It is important to establish that a breeding has taken place. • Determine the stage of estrous cycle by examining vaginal smears or measuring the plasma progesterone concentration (see Timing of Breeding). • Look for sperm in vaginal smears, although lack of sperm does not mean that breeding did not take place.
If the dog or cat is presented during estrus with a very high index of suspicion that she is bred, continue examining vaginal smears

daily or every other day, determine day 1 of diestrus, and start treatment on day 6 of diestrus. If the female is presented in very early diestrus, wait 5 days and start treatment.
• The only way to determine that a bitch is pregnant is by ultrasound after day 20-30 of diestrus. Radiographic diagnosis of pregnancy can be made after day 40 of diestrus. • If determined to still be pregnant after earlier treatment, treat again at day 31-35 of diestrus. In most patients, termination of pregnancy is accomplished at this time.

CBC/BIOCHEMISTRY/URINALYSIS
• Only needed as screening tests for some old bitches before treatment • Results normal unless underlying disease is concurrent

OTHER LABORATORY TESTS
• Vaginal cytologic testing to determine stage of estrous cycle and presence of sperm
• Plasma progesterone determination to help differentiate the different stages of the estrous cycle; can also be used to monitor the success of luteoloysis

IMAGING
Ultrasound 4-5 weeks after breeding to determine pregnancy; diagnostic test of choice for documenting pregnancy and documenting uterine evacuation

OTHER DIAGNOSTIC PROCEDURES
N/A

TREATMENT
• Consultation with owner necessary to discuss patient's future; if breeding is not a consideration, ovariohysterectomy might be the best alternative
• Usually as inpatient because of the use of off-label drugs and because of side effects
• If the owner insists on taking patient home, wait at least 1 hour after treatment before discharging the patient.
• Many mismated bitches do not become pregnant and therefore treatment may not be necessary. Since diagnosis of pregnancy by ultrasound is not possible until 4-5 weeks after breeding, knowledge of pregnancy status in early diestrus is unknown. However, in the author's opinion, treatment in midgestation is more unpleasant for veterinarians and technical staff (e.g., more discharge and fetuses may pass) and may have a psychological effect on the dog; therefore, treatment on day 6-10 of diestrus is recommended. Our small study (n = 10) indicated a 100% success rate in suppressing progesterone concentration to < basal concentration by use of a combination of prostaglandin F_{2a} (Lutalyse) and bromocyptine (Parlodel). However, it is best to discuss all options with the owner and to come to a mutually agreeable treatment regimen.

MEDICATIONS

DRUGS AND FLUIDS
• Prostaglandin F_{2a} is luteolytic and causes cervical dilation and intense uterine contractions. Start treatment on day 6 of diestrus (250 mcg/kg SC q12h for 5 days). Perform ultrasound examination at day 28-30 diestrus; if patient is pregnant, repeat regimen on day 31-35.
• Bromocryptine, a prolactin inhibitor, given on day 31-35 of diestrus (30-100 mcg/kg PO for 5-6 days) induces abortion. The lower dosage is given twice daily and the higher dosage once daily.
• A combination of 250 mcg/kg prostaglandin F_{2a} SC q12h and 10 mcg/kg bromocryptine PO q12h produces excellent results when administered on day 6-10 of diestrus. Feed animals 2 hours after morning treatment to reduce side effects (vomiting).
• Miferpreston, a progesterone and glucocorticoid receptor antagonist, and Epistane, an inhibitor of steroid synthesis, have potential but are currently not available to veterinarians in North America.

CONTRAINDICATIONS
• Prostaglandins—because of reports that prostaglandin F_{2a} increases blood pressure and cause bronchoconstriction in some species, it should not be given to animals that suffer from high blood pressure or asthma. Do not attempt treatment with synethetic analogues; safe dosages have not been determined.
• Bromocryptine mesylate (Parlodel)—some animals have sensitivity to ergot alkaloids.
• Estrogens—can cause cystic endometrial hyperplasia, pyometra, and bone marrow suppression leading to pancytopenia.

PRECAUTIONS
• Prostaglandins—side effects are dose-dependent and include hyperpnea, hypersalivation, vomition, and loose stools. High dosage (440 mcg/kg) causes mild locomotor incoordination and slight CNS depression.
• Bromocryptine mesylate (Parlodel)—side effects are minimal except for some vomiting. The actual period of time for evacuation of the uterus is longer than with Prostaglandins F_{2a}.

POSSIBLE INTERACTIONS
Bromocryptine mesylate—concomitant use of erythromycin may increase plasma concentration of bromocryptine

ALTERNATE DRUGS N/A

FOLLOW-UP

PATIENT MONITORING
Ultrasound of the uterus indicates if evacuation of uterine contents has taken place

ABORTION, TERMINATION OF PREGNANCY

POSSIBLE COMPLICATIONS
• May shorten interestrous interval (interval to next estrous cycle) • Treatment with estrogenic compounds is contraindicated.

 MISCELLANEOUS

ASSOCIATED CONDITIONS N/A
AGE RELATED FACTORS N/A
ZOONOTIC POTENTIAL N/A
PREGNANCY N/A
SYNONYMS
• Induced abortion • Mismating—a term that is used when an accidental breeding has taken place

SEE ALSO N/A
ABBREVIATIONS
CNS = central nervous system
LH = luteinizing hormone
PRL = prolactin

References

Braakman A, Okkens AC, van Haaften B. Medical methods to terminate pregnancy in the dog. Comp Cont Educ Pract Vet 1993;15:1505-1512.

Concannon PW. Applied reproductive endocrinology in the dog. In: Proceedings, 12th Annu Forum Am Col Vet Int Med 1994;245-248.

Olson PN, Johnston SD, Root MV et al. Terminating pregnancy in dogs and cats. Ann Reprod Sci 1992;28:399-406.

Post K. Induced pregnancy termination in dogs. In: Proceedings, Annu Meet Soc Theriogenol, 1993;215-221.

Author Klaas Post
Consulting Editor Sara K. Lyle

AGGRESSION—CATS

 BASICS

DEFINITION
Behavioral medicine is concerned with recognizing when behavior becomes maladaptive or abnormal. The categories of aggression are as follows:

Aggression Due to Lack of Socialization
• Cats who have not had contact with humans before 3 months of age have missed sensitive periods important for the development of normal approach responses to people. Cats that are not handled until 14 weeks of age are fearful and aggressive to people. Cats handled for only 5 minutes per day until 7 weeks will interact with people, approach inanimate objects, and play with toys.

Play Aggression
• If weaned early and then hand-raised by humans, cats may never learn to temper their play responses. Social play peaks early and is replaced by predatory activities by weeks 10-12 and social fighting by week 14.

Fearful, Fear or Fear-Induced Aggression
• Fearfully aggressive cats will hiss, spit, arch their backs, and piloerect if flight is not possible. A combination of offensive and defensive postures and overt and covert aggressive behaviors usually is involved. Flight is virtually always a component of fearful aggression in cats. If pursued and cornered, cats will stop, draw their head in, crouch, growl, roll on their back when approached, and paw at the approacher. If pursuit is continued, the cat will try to strike and follow by hold the approacher using the forepaws, while kicking with the back feet and biting around the neck. If threatened, any cat will defend itself, and any cat can learn to become fearfully aggressive.

Pain Aggression
• Cats that are in pain will become aggressive. Aggression can be induced in injured, arthritic, and dysplastic cats. Pain aggression can become fearful aggression with extended painful treatment.

Intercat Aggression
Intercat aggression can involve male-male aggression associated with mating or it may involve hierarchical status within the social group.

Maternal Aggression
Maternal aggression may occur in the periparturient period. Queens may protect nesting areas and kittens by threatening with long approach distances, rather than attack. As the kittens mature, the aggression resolves. It is not known if the kittens learn these aggressive behaviors from the mother.

Predatory Aggression
• Predatory behavior and predatory aggression are different behavioral circumstances. "Normal" predatory behavior is exhibited by free-ranging cats with field moles, house mice, and birds at feeders. Even well-fed cats are predatory, although it is more common in hungry cats. Well-fed cats may kill and only behead their prey. Predatory aggression includes stealth, silence, heightened attentiveness, body postures associated with hunting (slinking, head lowering, tail twitching, and pounce postures), and lunging or springing at prey, exhibiting sudden movement after a quiet period. Solitary predatory behavior develops at 5-7 weeks. Some cats make inappropriate context distinctions about prey. This is a potentially dangerous situation if the prey is the client's foot or hand, or an infant.

Territorial Aggression
Territorial aggression can be exhibited towards other cats, dogs, or people. Turf may be delineated by patrol, chin rubbing, spraying, or nonspraying marking. Due to the transitive nature of social hierarchies, a cat may be aggressive with one housemate and not another. If defending or marking a turf, and an offender crosses into it, threats and a fight may ensue. If the struggle involves social hierarchy, the challenger may be sought out and attacked after the territory is invaded. Territorial aggression can be difficult to treat if there is a social or marking component. Any marking problem is an alert for a possible underlying aggression.

Redirected Aggression
Redirected aggression can be difficult to recognize and may be reported as incidental to another form of aggression. It occurs when a motor pattern appropriate for a specific motivational state is redirected to an accessible target because the primary target is unavailable. Any interruption of an aggressive event between two parties by a third results in redirection of the aggressive behavior to the third party or an uninvolved individual. The interrupted event may only be a threat, so that the person (or animal) interrupting it may not realize what is occurring. This is often precipitated by another inappropriate behavior, so it is important to treat that behavior as well.

Assertion or Status-Related Aggression
This type of aggression has been called the "leave me alone" bite and often occurs during petting and is not provoked. The cat demonstrates a need to control when any attention starts and when it ceases. Cats sometimes bite and leave, while some take the client's hand but don't bite.

Idiopathic Aggression
Idiopathic aggression is poorly understood and poorly defined. It is an unprovoked, unpredictable, toggle-switch aggression and is rare.

Systems Affected
• Cardiovascular—signs may be consistent with sympathetic stimulation (vasodilation and tachycardia) • Endocrine/metabolic • Musculoskeletal—damage to teeth and gums, abscesses, abrasions, and lacerations are common • Nervous—increased motor and repetitive activity, trembling, and increased reactivity may accompany or follow outbursts of aggression • Renal/urologic—urine marking (both spraying and nonspraying) • Skin/exocrine—skin lesions usually are secondary and may result from injury; if consistently stressed, cats may cease to groom

SIGNALMENT
No breed differences, except for those resulting from a lack of socialization/exposure and play. Aggressions appear at the onset of social maturity (2-4 years).

SIGNS

Historical Findings
Abuse can teach any cat to be aggressive as a preemptive strategy.

Physical Examination Findings
Usually nonremarkable except for injuries and a lack of condition associated with increased motor activity and withdrawal. Continuous anxiety will cause decreased grooming.

CAUSES
Excitation of the ventromedial hypothalamus (VMH) causes a defensive response. The arnygdala and the VMH are involved in defensive responses. The medial amygdaloid nucleus is involved in social behavior, including intraspecific aggression, avoidance, and sexual behavior.

RISK FACTORS N/A

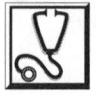 **DIAGNOSIS**

DIFFERENTIAL DIAGNOSIS
Rule-outs include those that cause similar behavioral changes—seizures, brain disease, and metabolic disease. Medical rule-outs include hepatoencephalopathy, feline ischemic encephalopathy, lead poisoning, hyperthyroidism, epilepsy, and rabies.

CBC/BIOCHEMISTRY/URINALYSIS
All should be performed. Urinalysis is important because of the relationship between aggression and elimination disorders.

OTHER LABORATORY TESTS
Clinical signs and serum biochemistry may indicate need to test for thyroid disease. Urine culture and sensitivity and cystoscopy may be indicated when unexplained aggression correlates with urinary tract disease.

IMAGING N/A

OTHER DIAGNOSTIC PROCEDURES
Cardiac disease can produce physical signs of "anxiety." ECG used as a diagnostic rule out or a premedication precaution.

TREATMENT

• Avoid provocation. Teach clients to observe signs (tail flicking, ears flat, pupils dilated, head hunched, claws possibly unsheathed, stillness or tenseness, low growl) and to interrupt the behavior by letting the cat fall from their lap, abandoning it, and refusing to interact until the cat is exhibiting an appropriate behavior. Discourage direct physical correction since this may intensify aggression. Separate cats and keep the active aggressor in a less favored area to passively reinforce more desirable behaviors.
• Desensitization, counterconditioning, flooding, and habituation can be used if the subtleties of cats' social systems and communication are understood

MEDICATIONS

DRUGS AND FLUIDS

• Medications of choice include antianxiety medications that increase central levels of serotonin. These include tricyclic antidepressants (TCA) and the more specific selective serotonin reuptake inhibitors (SSRI). Premedication blood profiles must be obtained before use of any medication.
• Drugs of choice include amitriptyline (Elavil 0.5-1.0 mg/kg [2.5-5.0 mg/cat to start] PO q12h for 30 days); imipramine (Tofranil 0.5-1.0 mg/kg [2.5-5.0 mg/cat to start] PO q12h for 30 days); buspirone (Buspar 0.5-1.0 mg/kg PO q8-24h [2.5-10 mg/day]; clomipramine (Anafranil 0.5 mg/kg PO q24h for 30 days) and fluoxetine (Prozac 0.5 mg/kg PO q24h for 30 days). Nortriptyline can be used to replace amitriptyline or imipramine, at the same dosage, if side effects appear. Buspirone, clomipramine, and fluoxetine can take 3-5 weeks to demonstrate an effect. • These drugs are best for active (not passive) aggressions that are overt. Buspirone

may make some cats more assertive and, thus, works well in cats with anxiety-associated aggression.

CONTRAINDICATIONS

Some drugs are contraindicated in animals with hepatic and renal compromise. Use extreme caution and monitoring when treating cardiac conduction anomalies with TCA. Cats experience more drug-related side effects than dogs. Cats that are fat or have preexisting hepatic disease may develop idiosyncratic, diazepam-induced hepatotoxicity.

PRECAUTIONS

These medications are extralabel, and all HHS recommendations should be followed. All of the benzodiazepines are controlled substances. Use of these drugs may involve premedication ECG evaluation.

POSSIBLE INTERACTIONS

Benzodiazepines are lipophilic and may be potentiated by other lipophilic drugs. These drugs may potentiate each other; if combination treatment is warranted, lower dosages of either medication may be warranted.

ALTERNATE DRUGS None

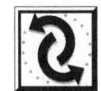
FOLLOW-UP

PATIENT MONITORING

If drug treatment is continuous, semiannual (older patients) or annual (younger patients) CBC and serum biochemistry analyses are desirable. An annual ECG is elective. Dosages should be adjusted accordingly. Monitoring is also indicated by clinical signs (vomiting, GI distress, tachycardia, tachypnea).

POSSIBLE COMPLICATIONS

Use of both behavioral modification and pharmacological intevention is required. If untreated, these disorders always progress.

MISCELLANEOUS

ASSOCIATED CONDITIONS

Many aggressions occur with elimination disorders including substrate and location aversions, substrate and location preferences, and, particularly, spraying and nonspraying marking.

AGE RELATED FACTORS

Social maturity is associated with the development of intercat aggression, fear aggression, territorial aggression, redirected aggression, and status-related aggression.

ZOONOTIC POTENTIAL

Cat scratch disease is a major risk.

PREGNANCY

Most of the drugs used should be avoided in pregnant animals.

SYNONYMS N/A

SEE ALSO N/A

ABBREVIATIONS

VMH = ventromedial hypothalmus
TCA = tricyclic antidepressant
SSRI = selective serotonin reuptake inhibitor

References

Chapman BL. Feline aggression: classification, diagnosis, and treatment. Vet Clin North Am (Small Anim Pract) 1991;21:315-328.
Chapman BL, Voith VL. Cat aggression redirected to people: 14 cases (1981-1987). J Am Vet Med Assoc 1990;196:947-950.
Overall KL. Feline aggression. Part 111. The role of social status in hierarchical systems. Feline Pract 1994;22(6):16-17.

Author Karen L. Overall
Consulting Editor Joane M. Parent

AGGRESSION—DOGS

BASICS

DEFINITION

Aggression in dogs is directed action by one dog against another organism with the result of harming, limiting, or depriving that organism. Aggression is either offensive, defensive, or predatory. Offensive aggression is an unprovoked attempt to gain some resource at the expense of another and includes dominance-related and intermale/interfemale aggression. Defensive aggression is aggression by a victim toward another, perceived as an instigator or threat. These include the functional categories fear-induced, territorial defense, protective, irritable (pain-associated or frustration-related), and parental.

Pathophysiology

Aggressive behavior per se is not a pathologic condition. Recent findings suggest that some type of inappropriate offensive aggression ("rage") may be associated with biochemical differences in the cerebral spinal fluid. Certain pathologic states are associated with an increase in aggression because of their effects on the central nervous system.

Systems Affected

Central nervous system

SIGNALMENT

Any age, sex, or breed. Dominance-related offensive aggression escalates from 1-2 years of age in dogs approaching social maturity. Males (intact or castrate) are more often presented. Most common in the cocker spaniel, springer spaniel, and German shepherd, although regional differences exist. Breeds associated with fatal dog bites include the pit bull, German shepherd, husky, malamute, doberman pinscher, and rottweiler.

SIGNS

General Comments

Aggression is expressed by behavioral signs, including staring, postures, growls, baring the teeth, snapping, or frank attacks.

Historical Findings

Vary according to the situation and the functional type of aggression. The history also forms the basis for risk analysis and for the details of the treatment program. Important historical questions include: When were signs of aggression first noted? How often does the aggression occur? Against whom is the aggression directed? Under what circumstances does the aggression occur?

Common Types of Agression

• Dominance-related—aggression toward household members. Resents reaching toward, patting on head, pushing off favored sleeping sites, approaching food. Head up, tail up, stares, stiff gait. • Intermale/interfemale—aggression toward other dogs. Aggression toward humans only when they interfere with fights. Head up, tail up, stares, stiff gait. • Fear-induced—aggression when approached or reached for. Certain familiar persons may be exempt. Head down, eyes wide, tail tucked. • Territorial—barks, agitated, aggressive toward strangers approaching house, yard, car. May be exacerbated if restrained. Rushes forward, bares teeth. • Protective—aggression more likely if owner is present and owner is approached. Aggression escalates with decreasing distance. • Irritable (pain, frustration)—aggression is restricted to specific context associated with pain such as nail trim, injection. Rule out dominance-related, fear. • Parental (maternal)—aggression occurs when individuals approach whelping area or puppies. Often severity of problem is inversely related to age of puppies.

Physical Examination Findings

• Extreme care should be taken in handling aggressive dogs. Muzzles and other restraints should be used to prevent injury to the examiner. In most dogs, the physical exam will be normal. Dominance-related aggression, fear-related aggression, or irritable aggression may be evident during the exam. • Abnormalities on the neurologic exam may suggest an organic disease process (e.g., rabies).

CAUSES

• Aggression is part of the normal range of behavior, and is strongly influenced by breed, sex, early socialization history, handling, and other variables. • Although rare, aggression can be a manifestation of an organic condition. In all dogs, medical causes of aggression must be ruled out.

RISK FACTORS

Dogs poorly socialized to certain types of stimuli, such as children, may display fear-related aggression to them as adults. Environmental conditions may predispose to aggression of various types, including associating with other dogs in a pack, barrier frustration or tethering, cruel handling and abuse, and dog baiting and fighting.

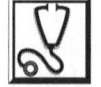

DIAGNOSIS

DIFFERENTIAL DIAGNOSIS

Pathological conditions associated with aggression must be identified before a purely behavioral diagnosis is made.

CBC/BIOCHEMISTRY/URINALYSIS

Usually normal. Abnormalities of these tests may suggest metabolic or endocrine explanations.

OTHER LABORATORY TESTS

Other tests may be indicated, including a thyroid panel or ACTH stimulation test.

IMAGING

May be indicated to identify sources of pain. MRI or CT if cerebral neoplasia is suspected.

OTHER DIAGNOSTIC PROCEDURES

Postmortem fluorescent antibody test should be done on any aggressive dog for which rabies is a differential diagnosis.

RISK ASSESSMENT

The importance of risk analysis in cases of aggression cannot be overemphasized and is therefore considered a separate procedure to be performed before treatment is initiated. Risk analysis consists of historical questions, observation of the animal, and confirmation with supporting data (medical, legal, veterinary records). • Has the dog ever broken the skin or otherwise injured a person? If yes, how many times in the past year? • Has anyone sought medical attention for injuries caused by this dog? If yes, describe the circumstances in detail. • Have the injuries by this dog been reported to authorities, resulting in quarantine or citation? If yes, describe. • Is the weight of this dog over 18.2 kg? • Are there children, elderly persons, or others at high risk in this household? • Is there any doubt that this dog be restrained behind a fence, on a leach, fitted with a muzzle, or in other ways effectively controlled by the owner to protect persons from injury? • Does this dog ever "run free" without being under the owner's strict control? • Does aggression appear to occur unpredictably? • If the owner responds YES to any of these questions, the personal and legal liability risks to the owner and the treating veterinarian should be considered.

TREATMENT

• The first tenet of the management of aggressive dogs is to prevent human injury. Euthanasia is the appropriate solution in cases of vicious dogs and should be offered as the only safe solution. Risk assessment may help the owner objectively evaluate the situation. All parties should understand that aggressive dogs are never "cured," although in some the behavior can be managed. Veterinarians should recommend techniques to reduce human risk from the aggressive dog until the owner seeks treatment.
• Management success combines multiple treatment modalities of environmental control, behavior modification, and pharmacotherapy .

Dominance-Related Aggression

• Environmental control—use of barriers and restraint to prevent human injury
• Devices—train the dog to a muzzle and halter
• Behavior modification (step 1)—withdraw all attention from the dog for two weeks; list situations in which aggression occurs and devise a plan for the owner to avoid each situation; daily list all aggressive incidents and circumstances to avoid in the future
• Behavior modification (step 2)—use non-confrontational means to establish the own-

er's dominance; teach the dog to reliably sit/stay on command in gradually more challenging situations (this means the dog acquiesces to the owner and obtains attention and other benefits); no "free" benefits (dog must sit/stay before eating, being petted, going for walk, etc.; the owner initiates all interactions)
• Behavior modification (step 3)—with greater control, situations that previously elicited aggression are gradually added with the dog controlled in a sit/stay (muzzle if necessary)
• Surgery—neuter

Intermale/Interfemale Aggression
• Environmental control—use barriers to prevent contact between the dogs except when well supervised; note dominance order between dogs, if apparent, and comply with dogs' rules (dominant dog is fed first, travels through doorways first, etc.)
• Devices—halter, muzzle
• Behavior modification (step 1)—the owner must withdraw all attention to both dogs; teach sit/stay program
• Behavior modification (step 2)—desensitize/countercondition by gradually decreasing distance between dogs while under leash control; reinforce acceptable behavior
• Surgery—neuter males; OHE recommended if aggression is associated with the heat cycle; otherwise, OHE will not improve behavior

Fear-Induced Aggression
• Environmental control—use of barriers and restraint to prevent human injury
• Devices—muzzle • Behavior modification (step 1)—list all situations in which the dog appears fearful or exhibits aggression and avoid those situations initially; teach dog basic obedience commands and reinforce under nonfearful conditions (generalize by training in many locations)
• Behavior modification (step 2)—desensitize and countercondition; subject the dog to mildly fearful conditions with the stimulus (e.g., a stranger) far away; keep the dog attentive, performing obedience commands; gradually decrease the distance of the stranger; if the dog exhibits fear, the stranger should withdraw and work should continue at an easier level, then gradually progress
• Surgery—castration or ovariohysterectomy probably will not improve the behavior

Territorial Aggression
• Environmental control—use of barriers and restraint to prevent human injury; initially, prevent the dog from exhibiting the behavior by isolating the dog when visitors come
• Devices—halter, muzzle
• Behavior modification (step 1)—teach the dog sit/stay, first at neutral locations, then near the door and at other sites of territorial aggression; later, the owner should control the dog while a familiar person approaches; the dog should be rewarded for calm, obedient behavior
• Behavior modification (step 2)—gradually introduce strangers (owner can dress in strange garb to represent a stranger); make the exercise more difficult until the dog is under control; move the exercises to the door, add entering the door, ringing the door bell, and other variables
• Surgery—castration or ovariohysterectomy probably will not affect this behavior

MEDICATIONS

DRUGS AND FLUIDS
• There are no drugs approved by the FDA for the treatment of aggression. Inform the client of the experimental nature of these treatments and the risk involved. Document discussion in the medical record.
The following are listed as drug class; drug name; dosage for dogs; frequency; and side effects:
• Azaperone; buspirone hydrochloride; 2.5-10 mg/dog; q8-12h; GI signs
• Tricyclic antidepressant; amitriptyline; 2.2-4.4 mg/kg; q12-24h; sedation, anticholinergic effects • Tricyclic antidepressant; clomipramine; 1-3 mg/kg; q12-24h; sedation, anticholinergic effects, cardiac conduction disturbances if predisposed • Tricyclic antidepressant; imipramine; 2.2-4.4 mg/kg; q12-24h; sedation, anticholinergic effects
• Selective serotonin reuptake inhibitor; fluoxetine; 1mg/kg; q24h; inappetence, irritability

CONTRAINDICATIONS
Tricyclic antidepressants are contraindicated in patients with cardiac conduction disturbances, glaucoma, and fecal or urinary incontinence.

PRECAUTIONS
Use benzodiazepines (e.g., diazepam) with caution in fearfully-aggressive dogs. Drugs in this class can reduce fear but also reduce fear-based inhibition. Dogs can become more aggressive when they lose their fear of the repercussions of biting.

POSSIBLE INTERACTIONS
Drugs listed should not be used with monoamine oxidase inhibitors.

ALTERNATE DRUGS
Megestrol acetate (1 mg/kg PO q24h for 2 weeks then tapered to lowest effective dosage) has been used with success in dominance-related aggression and intermale aggression.

Side effects include obesity, blood dyscrasias, pyometra, polyuria/polydipsia, diabetes mellitus, mammary hyperplasia, and carcinoma.

FOLLOW-UP

PATIENT MONITORING
Weekly to biweekly contact is recommended in the initial phases. Clients frequently need feedback and assistance with behavior modification plans and medication management.

PREVENTION/AVOIDANCE N/A

EXPECTED COURSE AND PROGNOSIS N/A

POSSIBLE COMPLICATIONS
Human injury is a potential complication. Dominance aggression can be directed toward owners. Humans are often seriously injured when interfering with fighting dogs, either by accident or by redirected or irritable aggression. In cases of interdog aggression, owners should not reach for the dogs. Spray the dogs with water or push apart with a broom or a sturdy partition.

MISCELLANEOUS

ASSOCIATED CONDITIONS N/A

AGE RELATED FACTORS
Adult-onset aggression in the absence of any positive historical findings suggests a medical etiology. Sources of pain and sensory acuity should be evaluated carefully.

ZOONOTIC POTENTIAL
Rabies is a potential cause of aggression.

PREGNANCY
Tricyclic antidepressants are contraindicated in pregnant animals.

SYNONYMS N/A

SEE ALSO N/A

ABBREVIATIONS N/A

References
Overall KL. Practical pharmacological approaches to behavior problems. In: Behavioral problems in small animals. St. Louis: Ralston Purina Company, 1992:36-51.
Simpson BS, Simpson DM. Behavioral pharmacotherapy. In: Borchelt P, Voith V, eds. Readings in companion animal behavior. Treton, NJ: Veterinary Learning Systems, 1996:100-115.
Author Barbara S. Simpson
Consulting Editor Joane M. Parent

ALOPECIA

 BASICS

DEFINITION
The loss or lack of hair, ranging from focal to complete hair loss

Pathophysiology
Pathomechanism is related to causative factors and can involve faulty development, and suppression of the hair follicle, destruction and displacement, acute loss of telogen hairs, irritation and self-trauma, leukocytic activity, invasion and weakening of the hair shaft, necrosis and fibrosis of tissue, and immune-mediated responses.

Systems Affected
Skin/Exocrine

SIGNALMENT
Age, breed, and sex predisposition varies with each individual condition causing the alopecia

SIGNS N/A

CAUSES
• Genetics (including hypotrichosis, epitheliogenesis imperfecta, follicular dysplasia, ectodermal defect, color-mutant alopecia • Endocrinopathies (including hypothyroidism, hyperadrenocorticism, growth-hormone responsive dermatosis, sex hormone-related dermatopathies) • Nutrition (e.g., selenium, iodine) • Biologic agents (including parasites and microorganisms) • Physical and chemical factors (e.g., antimitotic agents, thallium, traction alopecia) • Immune-mediated disorders (e.g., lupus erythematosus, alopecia areata) • Stress (e.g. Telogen defluxion) • Therapeutic agents (especially corticosteroids) • Secondary to disorders of other systems

RISK FACTORS
Vary with each of the different causes of alopecia

 DIAGNOSIS

DIFFERENTIAL DIAGNOSIS
Focal
• Demodicosis • Bacterial Pyoderma • Dermatophytosis • Alopecia areata • Cutaneous asthenia • Traction alopecia • Morphea (dogs) • Injection site reaction

Patchy
• Demodicosis • Cheyletiellosis • Lice infestation • Dermatophytosis • Drug Eruption • Lupus erythematosus • Telogen defluxion • Leishmaniasis • Hyperadrenocorticism (cats) • Protein deficiency • Sebaceous adenitis (dogs) • Bronzing syndrome (dogs) • Color-mutant alopecia (dogs) • Spiculosis (dogs)

Regional
• Discoid lupus erythematosus • Hypothyroidism • Feline endocrine alopecia • Hyperadrenocorticism • Growth hormone-responsive alopecia • Adrenal sex-steroid dermatosis • Seasonal alopecia (dogs) • Hyperestrogenism (dogs) • Hypoestrogenism (dogs) • Pattern baldness (dogs) • Testicular neoplasia • Dermatomyositis (dogs) • Follicular dysplasia • Toxicity (e.g., thallium)

Generalized
• Dermatophytosis • Lupus erythematosus • Drug eruption • Demodicosis • Alopecia universalis

CBC/BIOCHEMISTRY/URINALYSIS
For widespread alopecias, the minimum data base should include hemogram and serum biochemistries

OTHER LABORATORY TESTS N/A

IMAGING
• Rarely needed but CT scans may be helpful in diagnosing hyperadrenocorticism.
• Radiographs may also help confirm hyperadrenocorticism in patients with tissue mineralization or enlarged adrenals.

OTHER DIAGNOSTIC PROCEDURES
• For focal alopecias, minimum data base should include examination of skin scrapings, dermatophyte culture and a trichogram
• Additional tests that may be warranted include biopsies for histopathologic assessment and endocrine profiles

 TREATMENT

• Almost always treat as outpatient unless there is some evidence of life-threatening systemic disease
• Treatment must be individualized and based on underlying cause
• Not all patients with alopecia warrant therapy, such as those with alopecia areata, traction alopecia and pattern baldness.

MEDICATIONS

DRUGS AND FLUIDS
Varies with underlying cause of the alopecia.

CONTRAINDICATIONS N/A

PRECAUTIONS
Drugs that have adverse systemic effects (e.g., mitotane, growth hormone, minoxidil)

POSSIBLE INTERACTIONS N/A

ALTERNATE DRUGS N/A

FOLLOW-UP

PATIENT MONITORING
• Patient monitoring varies with each cause of alopecia. • Hair loss aspects of all patients should be re-evaluated 6 weeks after starting therapy, then 12 weeks after starting therapy. • Trichograms or biopsies help monitor response to therapy

POSSIBLE COMPLICATIONS
Some alopecic conditions can be potentially fatal (e.g., systemic lupus erythematosus, drug eruption, hyperadrenocorticism); most are not.

MISCELLANEOUS

ASSOCIATED CONDITIONS N/A

AGE RELATED FACTORS N/A

ZOONOTIC POTENTIAL
• Dermatophytosis is transmissible to people • Mycobacterial infections, sporotrichosis, and other infections are also zoonotic

PREGNANCY N/A

SYNONYMS
Hair loss

SEE ALSO
• Demodicosis • Dermatomyositis • Dermatophytosis • Pyoderma • Dermatoses, Sex and Growth Hormone-Related • Lupus Erythematosus, cutaneous • Feline Symmetrical Alopecia • Follicular Dysplasia • Sebaceous Adenitis • Sporotrichosis

ABBREVIATIONS N/A

References

Ackerman L. Pet skin and haircoat problems: tests and treatments. Trenton, NJ: Veterinary Learning Systems, 1993.
Nesbit GH, Ackerman LJ, Dermatology for the small animal practitioner. Trenton, NJ: Veterinary Learning Systems, 1991.

Author Lowell Ackerman

Consulting Editor Lowell Ackerman

ANISOCORIA

BASICS

DEFINITION Inequality of pupil size

Pathophysiology
Interruption of sympathetic or parasympathetic innervation of the pupil causes altered pupil size. Ocular disease can also cause anisocoria.

Systems Affected
• Nervous • Ophthalmic

SIGNALMENT
Dogs and cats

SIGNS N/A

CAUSES

Neurologic Causes (see Table 1)
Diseases affecting • Optic nerve • Optic tract • Oculomotor nerve • Cerebellum

Ocular Causes (see Table 2)
• Anterior uveitis • Glaucoma • Neoplasia
• Posterior synechia • Iris atrophy or hypoplasia • Pharmacologic blockade
• Spastic pupil syndrome

RISK FACTORS N/A

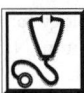

DIAGNOSIS

DIFFERENTIAL DIAGNOSIS
Decide which pupil is abnormal (Algorithm 1). Differentiate neurologic and ocular causes.

CBC/BIOCHEMISTRY/URINALYSIS
N/A

OTHER LABORATORY TESTS N/A

IMAGING
• See Table 1 • Ultrasound useful for identifying ocular and retrobulbar lesions • CT and MRI useful for localizing and identifying CNS lesions

OTHER DIAGNOSTIC PROCEDURES
• See Table 1 • CSF tap to evaluate CNS disease • Electroretinogram (ERG) to evaluate optic nerve function • Pharmacologic testing (Algorithm 1) • Postganglionic lesions cause denervation supersensitivity, and direct acting (para)sympathomimetic drugs cause pupil to constrict or dilate • Preganglionic lesions respond to indirect acting (para)sympathomimetics.

TREATMENT

Depends on underlying disease

MEDICATIONS

DRUGS AND FLUIDS
Depends on underlying disease

CONTRAINDICATIONS N/A

PRECAUTIONS N/A

POSSIBLE INTERACTIONS N/A

ALTERNATE DRUGS N/A

FOLLOW-UP

PATIENT MONITORING N/A

POSSIBLE COMPLICATIONS N/A

MISCELLANEOUS

ASSOCIATED CONDITIONS N/A

AGE RELATED FACTORS N/A

ZOONOTIC POTENTIAL N/A

PREGNANCY N/A

SYNONYMS N/A

SEE ALSO
• Horner's Syndrome • Optic Neuritis
• Anterior Uveitis—Cats • Anterior Uveitis—Dogs • Glaucoma • Iris Atrophy

ABBREVIATIONS
CSF = cerebrospinal fluid
CT = computerized tomography
ERG = electroretinogram
MRI = magnetic resonance imaging
PLR = pupillary light reflex

References
De Lahunta A. Veterinary neuroanatomy and clinical neurology. 2nd ed. Philadelphia: WB Saunders, 1983:115–120.
Neer TM, Carter JD. Anisocoria in dogs and cats. Ocular and neurologic causes. Compend Cont Ed Pract Vet 1987;9: 817–824.
Author David Lipsitz
Consulting Editor Paul E. Miller

Table 1.

Lesion	Neurologic Signs	Differential Diagnosis	Diagnostic Plan
Neurologic Lesions Causing Anisocoria			
optic nerve	ipsilateral mydriasis	optic neuritis	CT/MRI
	ipsilateral monocular anopia	neoplasm	CSF
	(total blindness in 1 eye)		electroretinogram (ERG)
	no direct PLR affected eye		
	consensual PLR affected eye		
optic tract	contralateral blindness in	neoplasm	CT/MRI
	nasal/temporal visual fields	infectious/inflammatory disease	CSF
	ipsilateral pupil smaller in light	trauma	
	other neurologic deficits		
oculomotor nerve parasympathetic nucleus CN III	ipsilateral dilated pupil	neoplasm	CT/MRI
	normal vision/no direct PLR	infectious/ inflammatory disease	CSF
	no consensual PLR from opposite eye	trauma	ultrasound orbit
	ptosis upper eyelid	brain herniation	
	ventrolateral strabismus	retrobulbar mass	
cerebellar disease	contralateral mydriasis	neoplasm	CT/MRI
	normal PLR /normal vision	infectious/inflammatory disease	CSF
	ipsilateral lack of menace response	trauma	
	other cerebellar signs		

Table 2.

Ocular Diseases Causing Anisocoria

Lesion	Associated signs	Causes
anterior uveitis	miosis, aqueous flare, corneal edema conjunctival hyperemia	infectious/inflammatory disease trauma
glaucoma	mydriasis sluggish/absent PLR increased intraocular pressure corneal edema	primary glaucoma secondary glaucoma
neoplasm	miosis/mydriasis change in iridial coloration	lymphoma melanoma
posterior synechia	variable pupil shape sluggish/absent PLR anterior uveitis	secondary to anterior uveitis
iris atrophy iris hypoplasia	variable pupil shape, iridal thinning sluggish/absent PLR irregular pupil margin other ocular abnormalities	old age change congenital
pharmacological blockade	mydriasis absent direct/consensual PLR normal vision	atropine
spastic pupil syndrome	miosis normal vision	FeLV

Algorithm 1.

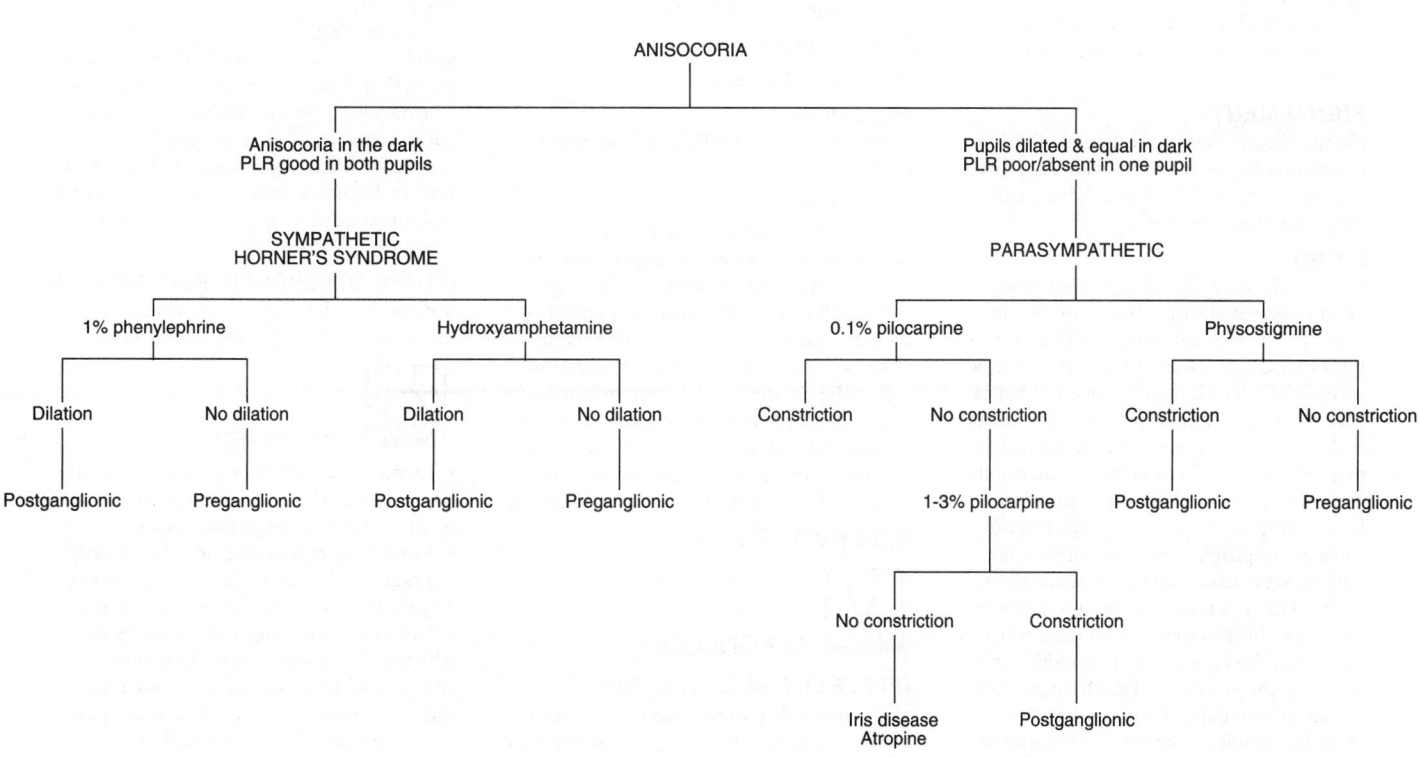

ANOREXIA

 BASICS

DEFINITION

Absence of an appetite for food. The term pseudoanorexia is often used to describe the condition in which an animal does not eat because of an inability to prehend, chew, or swallow food rather than because of a lack of interest in food.

Pathophysiology

Anorexia in dogs and cats is most often associated with systemic disease but can be caused by many different mechanisms. The control of appetite has often been attributed to a satiety center in the medial hypothalamus and a hunger center in the lateral hypothalamus, but recently this idea has been questioned. Many now believe that a combination of neurologic, metabolic, and humoral factors in both the brain and the rest of the body are involved in the control of hunger and satiety. In addition to neurologic regulation, appetite and satiety are influenced by a variety of other factors including gastric and intestinal distension, enteric hormones such as insulin and cholecystokinin, the oxidation of energy rich metabolites in the liver, the amount of adipose tissue in the body, and learned responses related to the taste, texture, and metabolic effects of the food eaten. Any physical or psychologic process that interferes with the mechanisms that stimulate hunger can cause anorexia, and many such processes affect dogs and cats.

Systems Affected

Virtually any body system can be affected by anorexia, especially if it persists more than 2 or 3 days.

SIGNALMENT

No specific age, sex, or breed predisposition to anorexia in general, but signalment predispositions to many of the underlying conditions that cause anorexia

SIGNS

• Often the only clinical sign is not eating, usually associated with a lack of interest in food. This is especially true in animals with a psychologic cause of anorexia. • An anorexic animal may show interest in food but not eat because of pain or other problems associated with eating. Such pseudoanorexic animals may exhibit facial, head or neck pain, inability to prehend food, dropping of prehended food, crying out when eating, reluctance to chew, or dysphagia. They may also display obvious signs associated with trauma involving the face, head, neck, or mouth; periodontal disease; broken teeth; oral foreign body; fracture of the facial bones or mandible; mass involving the oral cavity, face, head, or neck including neoplasm, abscess, or large lymph node; or neurologic deficits involving prehension, mastication, use of the tongue, or swallowing. • Clinical signs in truly anorexic animals are directly related to the underlying cause of the problem. As such, they are numerous and varied. In animals with systemic disease, signs that may accompany anorexia include depression, weight loss, fever, vomiting, diarrhea, coughing, dyspnea, organomegaly, cardiac murmur, muffled heart and lung sounds, and changes in the animal's water consumption.

CAUSES

Psychologic

• Unpalatable diets • Alterations in routine or environment • Stress

Neurologic

• High intracranial pressure—cerebral edema, hydrocephalus, and neoplasia • Intracranial pain • Spinal pain • Peripheral nerve pain • Hypothalamic disorders—neoplasia, infection, and trauma • Loss of sense of smell

Nonneurologic Pain

• Abdominal pain • Thoracic pain • Musculoskeletal pain • Urogenital pain

Disorders Involving Abdominal Organs

• Enlargement or serosal distension • Inflammation • Infectious disease • Neoplasia • Metabolic disease

Endocrine Disease

Neoplasia Involving Any Site

Infectious Disease

Toxicosis

• Exogenous—medications and poisons • Endogenous—toxins from organ failure (e.g., uremia), endotoxins, and pyrogens

Immune-Mediated Disease

Cardiac Failure

Respiratory Disease

Miscellaneous

• Motion sickness • High environmental temperature

Pseudoanorexia

• Oral cavity disorders—abscessed teeth, broken teeth, severe periodontal disease, neoplasia, foreign body, stomatitis, pharyngitis, and tonsillitis • Mandibular dysfunction—fracture, dislocation. and paralysis • Hypoglossal dysfunction • Masticatory myositis • Retrobulbar disease—abscess, inflammation, and neoplasia • Pharyngeal disorders—dysfunction and inflammation • Esophageal disorders—dysfunction, inflammation, neoplasia, and other mass • Tetanus • Blindness

RISK FACTORS N/A

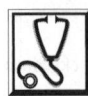 **DIAGNOSIS**

DIFFERENTIAL DIAGNOSIS

• The initial diagnostic decision is to determine whether the anorexia is 1) true anorexia from medical causes such as systemic disease, 2) psychological anorexia with no underlying medical problem, or 3) pseudoanorexia. • A thorough physical examination and history regarding the animal's interest in food and ability to eat helps to identify pseudoanorexia. • A thorough history regarding the animal's environment, diet, other animals and people in the household, and any recent changes involving any of these helps to identify psychologic anorexia. • Clinical signs suggesting medical problems indicate anorexia caused by a disease process. • If oral cavity, head, or neck disease or dysfunction is seen, it should be pursued diagnostically alone or along with pursuit of systemic disease if it seems likely that both may be present. Only if the history strongly suggests psychologic anorexia, the patient has no clinical signs, and the clinician is confident of both of these facts should further diagnostic work-up not be pursued. Otherwise, even if a psychologic cause for the anorexia seems likely, a minimum database should be obtained to better rule out underlying medical disease. Finally, the appropriate diagnostic testing is essential if the patient has any signs of underlying disease.

CBC/BIOCHEMISTRY/URINALYSIS

• Usually normal in patients with psychologic causes of anorexia. • Abnormalites vary with underlying systemic diseases and causes of pseudoanorexia.

OTHER LABORATORY TESTS

Special tests may be necessary to rule out specific diseases suggested by the history, physical examination, or minimum database. (See other topics on specific diseases.)

IMAGING

• If underlying disease is suspected but no abnormalities are revealed by the physical examination or minimum database, it may be worthwhile to perform thoracic and abdominal radiography or ultrasonography in order to identify hidden conditions. • The need for further diagnostic imaging varies with the underlying condition suspected. (See other topics on specific diseases.)

OTHER DIAGNOSTIC PROCEDURES

Vary with underlying condition suspected. (See other topics regarding specific diseases.)

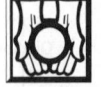 **TREATMENT**

• Identify and correct, if possible, the underlying cause of the problem. Appropriate treatment depends on the underlying cause. • Provide supportive care until the underlying cause is identified. Fluid and electrolyte administration is essential in dehydrated animals and those in danger of becoming so, which includes nearly all patients with anorexia. If the anorexia has persisted more than 2 or 3 days, nutritional support by enteral or parenteral feeding is indicated. Enteral methods include nasogastric tube and percutaneous enterogastric tube, which can be placed by a number of methods. Force feeding is seldom effective in providing adequate caloric intake, can be stressful to patients, and can easily cause aspiration of food by the patient. Total parenteral nutrition is an effective method of parenteral nutritional support if available to the clinician.

MEDICATIONS

DRUGS AND FLUIDS
• The most effective medications for the symptomatic treatment of anorexia have been the benzodiazepines. However, their usefulness is limited by side effects such as sedation and decreasing effectiveness with continued administration. They have been far more effective in cats than dogs.
• Cyproheptadine is effective in anorexic cats without the problems associated with the benzodiazepines.

CONTRAINDICATIONS N/A
PRECAUTIONS N/A
POSSIBLE INTERACTIONS N/A
ALTERNATE DRUGS N/A

FOLLOW-UP

PATIENT MONITORING N/A
POSSIBLE COMPLICATIONS
• Dehydration, malnutrition, and cachexia are most likely and these exacerbate the underlying disease. • Feline hepatic lipidosis is a complication of anorexia in obese cats.

MISCELLANEOUS

ASSOCIATED CONDITIONS N/A
AGE RELATED FACTORS N/A

ZOONOTIC POTENTIAL N/A
PREGNANCY N/A
SYNONYMS Inappetance
SEE ALSO See Causes
ABBREVIATIONS None

References
Lorenz MD. Disturbances of food intake: anorexia and polyphagia. In: Lorenz MD, Cornelius LM, eds. Small animal medical diagnosis. Philadelphia: JP Lippincott, 1987;23-33.
Monroe WE. Anorexia and polyphagia. In: Ettinger SJ, ed. Veterinary internal medicine. 4th ed. Philadelphia: WB Saunders, 1995;18-21.
Author Daniel P. Harrington
Consulting Editor Brent D. Jones

ASCITES

BASICS

DEFINITION
Ascites is the escape of fluid, either transudate or exudate, into the abdominal cavity between the parietal and visceral peritoneum.

Pathophysiology
Ascites can be caused by the following:
• Congestive heart failure (CHF) and associated interference in venous return • Depletion of plasma proteins associated with inappropriate loss of protein from renal or gastrointestinal disease (i.e., protein losing nephropathy or enteropathy, respectively)
• Obstruction of the vena cava or portal vein, or lymphatic drainage due to neoplastic occlusion • Overt neoplastic effusion • Peritonitis (i.e., infective or inflammatory) • Electrolyte imbalance, especially hypernatremia
• Liver cirrhosis

Systems Affected
• Cardiovascular • Gastrointestinal • Renal/Urologic • Hemic/Lymphatic/Immune

SIGNALMENT
Dogs and cats
No species or breed predisposition

SIGNS
• Episodic Weakness • Lethargy • Abdominal fullness • Abdominal discomfort when palpated • Dyspnea from abdominal distention or associated pleural effusion • Anorexia
• Vomiting • Weight gain • Scrotal or penile edema • Groaning when lying down

CAUSES
• Nephrotic syndrome • Cirrhosis of liver
• Right-sided CHF • Heart failure • Hypoproteinemia • Ruptured bladder • Peritonitis
• Abdominal neoplasia • Hemorrhage

RISK FACTORS N/A

DIAGNOSIS

DIFFERENTIAL DIAGNOSIS

Differentiating Similar Signs
Abdominal distention without effusion
• Organomegaly—hepatomegaly, splenomegaly, renomegaly, and hydrouterus • Abdominal neoplasia • Pregnancy • Bladder distention
• Obesity • Gastric dilatation

Differentiating Diseases
• Transudate—nephrotic syndrome, cirrhosis of liver, right-sided congestive heart failure, hypoproteinemia, and ruptured bladder
• Exudate—peritonitis, abdominal neoplasia, and hemorrhage

CBC/BIOCHEMISTRY/URINALYSIS
• Neutrophilic leukocytosis occurs in patients with systemic infection. • Albumin is low in patients with impaired liver synthesis, gastrointestinal loss, or renal loss. • Cholesterol is low in patients with impaired liver synthesis, gastrointestinal loss, or renal loss of albumin

Liver Enzymes
• Low to normal in patients with impaired liver synthesis • High in patients with liver inflammation, hyperadrenocorticism, or gallbladder obstruction

Total and Direct Bilirubin
• Low to normal in patients with impaired liver synthesis • High in patients with biliary obstruction caused by tumor, gallbladder distention, or obstruction

BUN and Creatinine
• High in patients with renal failure • Low in patients with impaired liver synthesis or hyperadrenocorticism

Glucose
• Low in patients with impaired liver synthesis • High in patients with diabetes mellitus

OTHER LABORATORY TESTS
• To detect hypoproteinemia—protein electrophoresis and immune profile • To detect proteinuria—urine protein:creatinine ratio (normal = < 0.5)

IMAGING
• Thoracic and abdominal radiography is sometimes helpful. • Ultrasonography of the liver, spleen, pancreas, kidney, bladder, and abdomen can often determine cause.

OTHER DIAGNOSTIC PROCEDURES
Ascitic fluid evaluation (i.e., exfoliative cytologic examination and bacterial culture and antibiotic sensitivity); remove approximately 3-5 ml abdominal fluid via aseptic technique

Transudate
• Clear and colorless appearance • Protein < 2.5 g/dl • Specific gravity < 1.018 • Cells < 1,000 /mm³ (neutrophils and mesothelial cells)

Modified Transudate
• Red or pink appearance; may be slightly cloudy • Protein 2.5 to 5.0 g/dl • Specific gravity > 1.018 • Cells < 5,000 /mm³ (neutrophils, mesothelial cells, erythrocytes, and lymphocytes)

Exudate (nonseptic)
• Pink or white appearance and cloudy
• Protein 2.5-5.0 g/dl • Specific gravity > 1.018 • Cells 5,000-50,000 /mm³ (neutrophils, mesothelial cells, macrophages, erythrocytes, and lymphocytes)

Exudate (septic)
• Red, white, or yellow appearance and cloudy • Protein > 4.0 g/dl • Specific gravity > 1.018 • Cells 5,000-100,000 /mm³ (neutrophils, mesothelial cells, macrophages, erythrocytes, lymphocytes, and bacteria)

Hemorrhage
• Red appearance; spun supernatant clear and sediment red • Protein > 5.5 g/dl
• Specific gravity 1.007-1.027 • Cells consistent with peripheral blood • Does not clot

Chyle
• Pink, straw, or white appearance • Protein 2.5-7.0 g/dl • Specific gravity 1.007->1.040
• Cells < 10,000 /mm³ (neutrophils, mesothelial cells, and large population of small lymphocytes) • Other—tube of fluid separate into cream-like layer when refrigerated; fat droplets stain with Sudan III

Pseudochyle
• White appearance • Protein > 2.5 g/dl
• Specific gravity 1.007-1.040 • Cells < 10,000 /mm³ (neutrophils, mesothelial cells, and small lymphocytes) • Other—tube of fluid does not separate into cream-like layer when refrigerated; does not stain with Sudan III

Urine
• Clear to pale yellow appearance • Protein > 2.5 g/dl • Specific gravity (1,000 to >1.040
• Cells 5,000-50,000/mm³ (neutrophils, erythrocytes, lymphocytes, and macrophages)
• Other—if the urinary bladder ruptured < 12 hours before, urine glucose and protein could be negative; if bladder ruptured >12 hours before, urine becomes a dialysis medium with ultrafiltrate of plasma, and urine glucose and protein content are positive

Bile
• Slightly cloudy and yellow appearance
• Protein > 2.5 g/dl • Specific gravity > 1.018
• Cells 5,000-750,000/mm³ (neutrophils, erythrocytes, macrophages, and lymphocytes)
• Other —bilirubin confirmed by urine dipstick; nonicteric patient may have gallbladder rupture, biliary tree leakage, or rupture in the proximal bowel

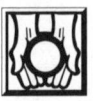

TREATMENT
• Treatment can be designed on an outpatient basis with follow-up or inpatient care depending on physical condition and underlying cause.
• If patients are markedly uncomfortable when lying down or become more dyspnic with stress, consider removing enough ascites to reverse these signs.
• Dietary salt restriction (canine prescription H/D) may help control transudate fluid accumulation due to congestive heart failure, cirrhosis, or hypoproteinemia.
• For exudate ascites control, address the underlying cause. Corrective surgery is often indicated, followed by specific therapeutic management (e.g., patient with splenic tumor: tumor removed, abdominal bleeding controlled, blood transfusion administered).
• Recirculation of nonseptic ascitic fluid in patients with liver insufficiency or nephrotic syndrome that has become refractory to conservative medical and dietary management can be done by use of the LeVeen peritoneovenous shunt concept. A unidirectional shunt conveys ascitic fluid to the jugular vein via a surgically placed one-way catheter from the midabdominal region. This autologous infusion has provided limited success in dogs.

MEDICATIONS

DRUGS AND FLUIDS
• In patients with liver insufficiency or congestive heart failure, sodium restriction (canine prescription H/D or CV) plus diuretic combination of hydrochlorothiazide (2-4 mg/kg ql2h PO) and spironolactone (1-2 mg/kg ql2h PO) should be initiated. If control is inadequate, furosemide (1-2 mg/kg q8h PO) can be substituted for the thiazide with spironalactone continued. Serum potassium concentration must be monitored to prevent hypokalemia-induced metabolic alkalosis.
• Patients with hypoproteinemia attendant with nephrotic syndrome and associated ascitic fluid accumulation can be treated as above with the addition of hetastarch (6% hetastarch in 0.9% NaCl). Administer an IV bolus (dogs, 20 ml/kg; cats, 10-15 ml/kg) slowly over approximately 1 hour. Hetastarch increases plasma oncotic pressure, pulling fluid into the intravascular space for up to 24-48 hours.
• Systemic antibiotic therapy is dictated by bacterial identification and sensitivity testing in patients with septic exudate ascites.

CONTRAINDICATIONS N/A
PRECAUTIONS N/A
POSSIBLE INTERACTIONS N/A
ALTERNATE DRUGS N/A

FOLLOW-UP

PATIENT MONITORING
• Varies with the underlying cause • Monitor sodium, potassium, BUN, creatinine, and weight fluctuations periodically if the patient is maintained on a diuretic

POSSIBLE COMPLICATIONS
Aggressive diuretic administration may cause hypokalemia, which could predispose to metabolic alkalosis and exacerbation of hepatic encephalopathy in patients with underlying liver disease. Alkalosis causes a shift from NH_4 to NH_3.

MISCELLANEOUS

ASSOCIATED CONDITIONS N/A
AGE RELATED FACTORS N/A
ZOONOTIC POTENTIAL N/A

PREGNANCY N/A
SYNONYMS
Abdominal effusion
SEE ALSO
• Nephrotic Syndrome • Cirrhosis and Fibrosis of the Liver • Congestive Heart Failure, Right-sided
ABBREVIATIONS
BUN = blood urea nitrogen
CHF = congestive heart failure

References

Lewis LD, Morris ML Jr, Hand MS: Small animal clinical nutrition. 3rd ed. Topeka, KS:Mark Morris Associates, 1987.
Porayko MK, Wiesner RH: Management of ascites in patients with cirrhosis. Postgrad Med 1992;2:155.
Author Jerry A. Thornhill
Consulting Editors Larry P. Tilley and Francis W.K. Smith, Jr.

ATAXIA

 BASICS

DEFINITION

A sign of sensory dysfunction that produces wobbliness or incoordination of the limbs, head, or trunk. For clinical purposes, ataxia is divided into three types: sensory (proprioceptive), vestibular, and cerebellar. All three produce changes in limb coordination, but vestibular and cerebellar ataxia also produce changes in head and neck movements.

Pathophysiology

• The brain receives information about position (proprioception or position sense) of the limbs, head, and trunk. Proprioceptive pathways in the spinal cord (ie, fasciculus gracilis, fasciculus cuneatus, and spinocerebellar tracts) relay limb and trunk position to the brain. When the spinal cord is slowly compressed, proprioceptive deficits (ataxia) are usually the first signs observed, because these pathways are located more superficially in the white matter and their larger-sized axons are more susceptible to compression than other tracts. Because of the early concomitant upper motor neuron involvement, sensory ataxia is generally accompanied by weakness, although this is not always obvious in the early course of the disease. • Changes in head and neck position are relayed through the vestibulocochlear nerve to the brainstem. Diseases that affect the vestibular receptors or the nerve in the inner ear, or the vestibular nuclei in the brainstem, lead to various degrees of disequilibrium with ensuing vestibular ataxia. The animal leans, tips, falls, or even rolls toward the side of the lesion. This ataxia is accompanied by a head tilt. • The cerebellum regulates, coordinates, smooths motor activity. In patients with cerebellar ataxia, the proprioception is normal, because the ascending proprioceptive pathways to the cortex are intact. Weakness is not characteristic, because the upper motor neurons are also intact. The ataxia is represented by an inadequacy in the performance of motor activity, with strength preservation and an absence of proprioceptive deficits.

Systems Affected

Nervous—specifically the spinal cord (and brainstem), cerebellum, and vestibular system

SIGNALMENT Any age, breed, or sex

SIGNS N/A

CAUSES

Neurologic Causes

• Cerebellar diseases—hypoplasia, canine distemper virus, feline infectious peritonitis virus, neoplasia, granulomatous meningoencephalitis, and storage diseases • Vestibular diseases—otitis interna, geriatric/idiopathic vestibular syndrome, trauma, neoplasia, hypothyroidism, rickettsial diseases, granulomatous meningoencephalitis, canine distemper virus, and FIP • Spinal cord diseases—intervertebral disc herniation, fibrocartilaginous embolism, neoplasia, trauma, discospondylitis, congenital spinal cord and vertebral malformations, and many others

Metabolic Causes

• Anemia • Electrolyte disturbances, especially hypokalemia

Miscellaneous Causes

• Drugs such as acepromazine, antihistamines, and anticonvulsants • Respiratory compromise • Cardiac compromise

RISK FACTORS

• Breeds at risk for intervertebral disc disease—dachshund, poodle, cocker spaniel, and beagle, etc. • Breeds at risk for cervical cord compression—Doberman pinscher and Great Dane • Breeds at risk for fibrocartilaginous embolism—young, large-breed dogs and miniature schnauzer.

 DIAGNOSIS

DIFFERENTIAL DIAGNOSIS

• Must differentiate neurologic ataxia (ie, vestibular, sensory, or cerebellar origin) from other disease processes (ie, musculoskeletal, metabolic, cardiovascular, and respiratory) that can affect gait. Neurologic examination should differentiate between the three types of ataxia. • Musculoskeletal disorders most typically produce lameness and a reluctance to move rather than ataxia. • For unknown reasons, systemic illness endocrine, cardiovascular, and metabolic disorders can cause ataxia, especially of the pelvic limbs. By contrast, this ataxia is often intermittent. Physical examination findings of fever, weight loss, murmurs, arrhythmias, hair loss, or collapse with exercise should make one suspicious of a nonneurologic cause of ataxia and a mimimum data base (ie, hemogram, biochemistry analysis, and urinalysis) should be obtained. • If the patient has head tilt or nystagmus, then the ataxia is likely vestibular in origin. • If ataxia is associated with intention tremors of the head or hypermetria, then cerebellar ataxia should be pursued. • If only limb ataxia is observed, spinal cord dysfunction is likely. If all four limbs are ataxic, the lesion is either in the cervical area or is multifocal to diffuse. If only pelvic limbs are ataxic, the lesion can be located anywhere along the spinal cord, below the second thoracic vertebra.

CBC/BIOCHEMISTRY/URINALYSIS

Results normal unless patient has metabolic causes of ataxia, such as hypoglycemia, electrolyte imbalances, and anemia

OTHER LABORATORY TESTS

• If patient has hypoglycemia, determine serum insulin concentration on the same sample to calculate an amended insulin-glucose ratio (to rule out insulinoma). • If patient has anemia, characterize as nonregenerative or regenerative on the basis of the reticulocyte count • If patient has electrolyte imbalance, correct the problem and see if the ataxia resolves. • If anticonvulsants are being administered, serum concentration should be evaluated to rule -in toxicity.

IMAGING

• Spinal radiographs recommended if spinal cord dysfunction is suspected • Bullae radiographs recommended if peripheral vestibular disease is suspected • CT or MRI recommended if cerebellar disease is suspected • Thoracic radiographs recommended in old patients to establish the possiblity of neoplasia causing or contributing to the ataxia • Abdominal ultrasonography recommended if hepatic, renal, adrenal or pancreatic dysfunction is suspected

OTHER DIAGNOSTIC PROCEDURES

• Cerebrospinal fluid analysis may be helpful in confirming nervous system causes of ataxia. • Myelography may establish evidence of spinal cord compression. • CT or MRI needed to evaluate potential brain diseases

 TREATMENT

• Can usually treat as an outpatient. However, this depends on the severity of the clinical signs and the acuteness of the disease. • Decrease or restrict exercise if spinal cord disease is suspected. • Have owner monitor gait for increasing ataxia or weakness. If paresis worsens or paralysis develops, other testing is warranted. • If possible, avoid drugs that could be contributing to ataxia. This may not be possible in patients on anticonvulsants for seizures.

 MEDICATIONS

DRUGS AND FLUIDS

Ataxia is a sign of many types of diseases. Drugs are not recommended until the source or cause of the ataxia is identified.

CONTRAINDICATIONS N/A

PRECAUTIONS N/A

POSSIBLE INTERACTIONS N/A

ALTERNATE DRUGS N/A

 FOLLOW-UP

PATIENT MONITORING

Periodic neurologic examinations to assess condition.

POSSIBLE COMPLICATIONS

• Progression of ataxia to weakness and possibly paralysis if spinal cord disease exists.

• Seizures if hypoglycemia is a cause of the ataxia. • Head tremors and bobbing if cerebellar disease is causing the ataxia.

☑ **MISCELLANEOUS**

ASSOCIATED CONDITIONS N/A

AGE RELATED FACTORS N/A

ZOONOTIC POTENTIAL N/A

PREGNANCY N/A

SYNONYMS N/A

SEE ALSO
• Cerebellar degeneration • Head tilt
• Weakness (paresis) • Paralysis

ABBREVIATIONS
CT = computerized tomography
MRI = magnetic resonance imaging

References

Oliver JE, Lorenz MD. Handbook of veterinary neurology. 2nd ed. Philadelphia: WB Saunders, 1993:208-228.

Chrisman CL. Vestibular diseases. Vet Clin North Am Small Anim Pract 1980;10:103-129.

Author Linda J. Shell
Consulting Editor Joane M. Parent

BLIND QUIET EYE

BASICS

DEFINITION
Loss of vision in one or both eyes without ocular vascular injection or other externally apparent signs of ocular inflammation

Pathophysiolgy
Vision loss results from abnormalities in focusing images on the retina, retinal image detection, optic nerve transmission, or CNS interpretation of the image.

Systems Affected
• Ophthalmic • Nervous

SIGNALMENT
• Any age, breed, or sex • Many causes (e.g., cataracts and progressive retinal atrophy) have a genetic basis and are often highly breed- and age-specific. • Sudden acquired retinal degeneration syndrome (SARDS) tends to occur in older dogs. • Optic nerve hypoplasia is congenital.

SIGNS

Historical Findings
Bumping into objects

Physical Examination Findings
• Vary with underlying cause • Absent menace response

CAUSES

Lens Associated
Loss of focusing power of the lens—although rarely completely blinding, substantial hyperopia (far-sightedness) occurs after lens extraction in which the optical power of the lens is not replaced, or if the lens luxates posteriorly out of the pupillary plane and into the vitreous.

Retina Associated
• SARDS, progressive retinal atrophy, retinal detachment, taurine deficiency in cats

Optic Nerve Associated
• Optic neuritis, neoplasia of the optic nerve or adjacent tissues, trauma, optic nerve hypoplasia, lead toxicity; excessive traction on the optic nerve during enucleation, resulting in trauma to the contralateral optic nerve or optic chiasm (especially cats and brachycephalic dogs)

CNS Associated (Amaurosis)
• Lesions of the optic chiasm or tract, optic radiation, or visual cortex

RISK FACTORS
• Poorly regulated diabetes mellitus—cataracts • Related animals with genetic cataracts or progressive retinal atrophy • Systemic hypertension—retinal detachment • CNS hypoxia—visual cortical blindness may become apparent after excessively deep anesthesia or revival after cardiac arrest

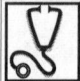

DIAGNOSIS

DIFFERENTIAL DIAGNOSIS

Differential Signs
• Anterior segment inflammation and glaucoma can also cause vision loss, but the conjunctiva typically is injected. • Young animal may lack menace responses but usually successfully navigate a maze or visually track hand movements or cotton balls. • Vision loss in the postictal period is transient. • Abnormal mentation may make it difficult to determine whether an animal is visual, but other neurologic abnormalities help localize the problem.

Differential Causes
• Sudden vision loss (over hours to weeks) suggests optic neuritis, retinal detachment, SARDS, or visual cortex hypoxia. • Polyuria/polydypsia/polyphagia and weight gain often precedes SARDS. • More gradual vision loss, especially in dim light, suggests progressive retinal atrophy; however, vision may appear to be acutely lost if the animal's environment is changed suddenly. • History of either gradual or rapidly increasing opacification and vision loss in a quiet eye suggests cataract. • Optic nerve hypoplasia is congenital and can be unilateral or bilateral. • The presence of other neurologic abnormalities suggests optic neuropathy or CNS disease. • Pupillary light responses are usually normal in animal with cataract or visual cortex lesion but are sluggish to absent in animal with retinal or optic nerve disease. • Results of ophthalmoscopy are normal in animal with SARDS, retrobulbar optic neuritis, and higher visual pathway lesion, and abnormal in animal with retinal detachment and neuropathy of the optic nerve head.

CBC/BIOCHEMISTRY/URINALYSIS
• Usually normal unless vision loss is secondary to a systemic disease. • Hyperglycemia or glucosuria may be present in animal with diabetic cataract. • High alkaline phosphatase and changes consistent with hyperadrenocorticism (Cushing's disease) suggest SARDS. • Mildly High BUN or serum creatinine are common in cats with retinal detachment secondary to systemic hypertension as are changes consistent with hyperthyroidism.

OTHER LABORATORY TESTS
• In animal suspected of having optic neuritis, consider blood lead and serology for deep fungal or viral infection (see optic neuritis). • A low-dose dexamethasone suppression test may help rule out Cushing's syndrome in animal with SARDS.

IMAGING
• Ocular ultrasound may demonstrate a retinal detachment (especially if the ocular media are opaque) or optic nerve mass lesion. • Plain skull radiographs are seldom informative. • CT or MRI are often helpful in animal with orbital or CNS lesion.

OTHER DIAGNOSTIC PROCEDURES
• Ophthalmic examination with a penlight usually permits the diagnosis of cataracts or retinal detachments severe enough to cause blindness. • Ophthalmoscopy may demonstrate progressive retinal atrophy or optic nerve disease. A normal ophthalmoscopic examination suggests SARDS, retrobulbar optic neuritis, or a CNS lesion. • Systemic blood pressure measurement rules in or out systemic hypertension in animal with retinal detachment. • Perform electroretinography to differentiate retinal from optic nerve or CNS disease if the diagnosis is in doubt. • In animal with neurogenic cause of vision loss, a CSF tap may be of value.

TREATMENT
• Try to obtain a definitive diagnosis on outpatient basis before initiating treatment. Consider referral before attempting empirical therapy. • Although most causes of a blind quiet eye are not fatal, a work-up is necessary to rule out potentially fatal diseases. • Assure owner that most causes of a blind quiet eye are not painful, and that a blind animal can lead a relatively normal and functional life. The environment should be examined for potential hazards to a blind animal. • Animal being treated for retinal detachment probably should have severely restricted exercise until the retina is firmly reattached. • Because of reduced activity levels, calorie restriction may be necessary to prevent obesity. • Ensure a diet with adequate concentration of taurine in cats with nutritionally induced retinopathy. • No effective treatment exists for SARDS, progressive retinal atrophy, optic atrophy, or optic nerve hypoplasia. • Cataracts, luxated lenses, and some forms of retinal detachment are best treated surgically. • Animal with progressive retinal atrophy or genetic cataract should not be bred, and related animals should be examined.

MEDICATIONS

DRUGS AND FLUIDS
• Treatment varies with cause. • If a work-up is declined, infectious disease is unlikely, and the diagnosis is narrowed down to SARDS or retrobulbar optic neuritis, prescribe systemic prednisolone (1-2 mg/kg/day for 7-14 days, then taper). Chloramphenicol or other systemic broad-spectrum antibiotics may be administered concurrently.

CONTRAINDICATIONS
Systemic corticosteroids and other immunosuppressive drugs are contraindicated in dogs with infectious optic neuritis and retinal detachments.

PRECAUTIONS
Pretreatment with corticosteroids may mimic or mask liver enzyme changes in dogs with SARDS.

POSSIBLE INTERACTIONS N/A

ALTERNATE DRUGS
• A single dose of flunixin meglumine (0.5 mg/kg, IV) may be used in dogs in place of corticosteroids if infectious causes have not been ruled out. • If systemic corticosteroids are not effective, oral azathioprine (1-2 mg/kg/day for 3-7 days then taper) may be used to treat immune-mediated retinal detachments. If azathioprine is used, a CBC, platelet count, and liver enzyme analysis should be performed q1-2 weeks for the first 8 weeks, then periodically.

FOLLOW-UP

PATIENT MONITORING
Repeated ophthalmic examinations as required to ensure that ocular inflammation is controlled and, if possible, vision maintained. Recurrence of vision loss is common in animal with optic neuritis and may be seen weeks, months, or years after initial examination.

POSSIBLE COMPLICATIONS
• Death • Permanent vision loss • Loss of the eye • Chronic ocular inflammation and pain • Obesity from inactivity or as a sequela of SARDS

MISCELLANEOUS

ASSOCIATED CONDITIONS
• Dogs with SARDS may exhibit signs similar to those of hyperadrenocorticism.
• Animal with neurologic disease may have seizures, behavior or personality changes, and circling or other CNS signs. • Cardiomyopathy has been associated with taurine deficiency in cats.

AGE RELATED FACTORS
Many cataracts and PRA have breed-specific ages of onset. SARDS tends to occur in older dogs. Optic nerve hypoplasia is congenital.

ZOONOTIC POTENTIAL N/A

PREGNANCY
Corticosteroids and immunosuppressive drugs may complicate pregnancy.

SYNONYMS N/A

SEE ALSO See causes

ABBREVIATIONS N/A

References

Rubin LF. Inherited eye disease in purebred dogs. Baltimore: Williams & Wilkins, 1989.

Millichamp NJ. Retinal degeneration in the dog and cat. Vet Clin North Am Small Anim Pract 1990;20:799–835.

Slatter DS. Fundamentals of veterinary ophthalmology. 2nd ed. Philadelphia: WB Saunders, 1990.

Gelatt KN, ed. Veterinary ophthalmology. 2nd ed. Philadelphia: Lea & Febiger, 1991.

Author Paul E. Miller

Consulting Editor Paul E. Miller

Figure 1

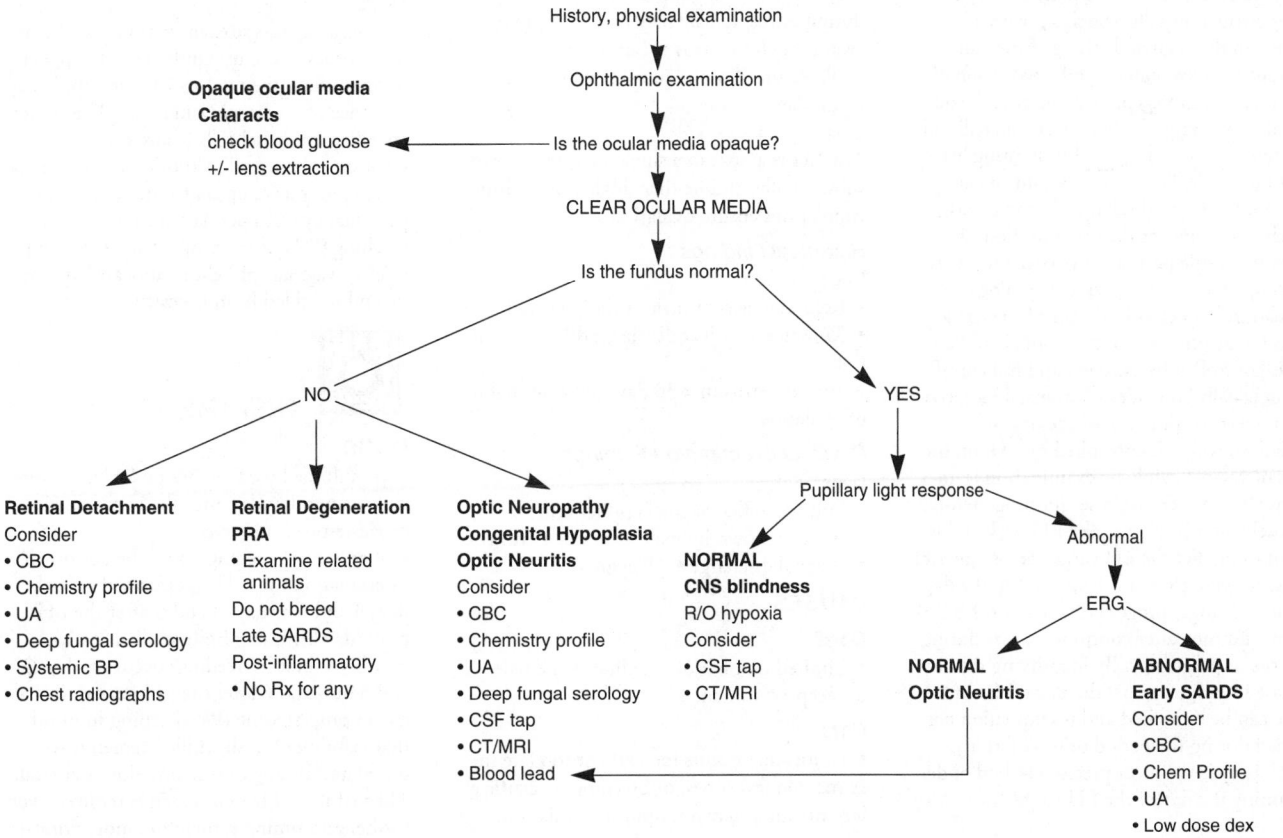

Blind Quiet Eye

BREEDING, TIMING

BASICS

DEFINITION
Timing of inseminations during estrus to maximize fertility

Pathophysiology
Dogs
• If multiple breedings are possible, breeding every other day during the period of estrus maximizes fertility. Use of fresh or frozen, cooled semen usually limits the number of inseminations to one or two and requires insemination to be timed with ovulation for maximum fertility. Variation of the time of ovulation in relation to onset of behavioral or cytologic estrus, in conjunction with reduced longevity of fresh, cooled or frozen semen, requires more precise estimation of the day of ovulation. Timing of artificial insemination is also required in a bitch that refuses to allow natural mating. • Ovulation is controlled by luteinizing hormone (LH). • The LH peak occurs the same day or up to 2 days after full cornification is observed. Ovulation occurs approximately 2 days after the LH surge, and 2-3 more days are required for oocyte maturation. Mature oocytes are viable for another 2-3 days. Therefore, the fertile period is 4-8 days after the LH surge with peak fertility occurring 5-6 days after the LH surge. • Physical signs alone may be unreliable to precisely determine the fertile period. • The onset of estrus is usually associated with a change in the vaginal discharge from sanguinous to straw colored and a reduction of vulvar swelling. Receptivity can often be detected by stroking the bitch near the tailhead. If receptive, she will "flag" by elevating her tail to one side. Some bitches continue to have a sanguinous discharge during estrus which ceases only at the onset of diestrus when the fertile period has passed and she is no longer receptive. • Vaginal cytologic examination is a better indicator of the fertile period. Cornification of the vaginal epithelium is controlled by estrogen and full cornification usually coincides with sexual receptivity. However, estimation of the day of ovulation, which is controlled by LH, on the basis of vaginal cytologic examination is imprecise. • An increase in serum progesterone is closely associated with the LH peak and is useful to predict the LH surge. Before the LH surge, progesterone is < 1 ng/ml. On the day of the LH surge, progesterone rises to 1.5-2.0 ng/ml and thereafter continues to rise during diestrus or pregnancy. By identifying this initial rise in progesterone, the day of the LH surge can be estimated and insemination performed during the period of peak fertility. • LH assay is the most precise method of determining the day of the LH surge.
Cats
Queens are induced ovulators so timing of breeding is not as critical. However, inadequate stimulation, characterized by absence of both a copulatory cry and postcoital reaction, may fail to induce ovulation. Ovulation is dependent on adequate LH release which is triggered by stimulation of the vagina and cervix. Both the peak concentration and the duration of elevation of LH are important in determining whether ovulation occurs. Multiple copulations result in higher concentration of LH in the plasma and are more likely to result in ovulation than single matings. Frequency of coital stimuli is also important in determining the adequacy of coital contact. The LH response to copulation may vary depending on the day of estrus upon which coitus occurs. Because LH release is partially dependent on duration of exposure to estrogen, coitus on day 3 of estrus results in a greater release of LH than coitus on day 1.

Systems Affected
Renal/Urogenital

SIGNALMENT   N/A

SIGNS

General Comments
Dogs
• Normal bitch—sanguinous discharge during proestrus becomes straw colored during estrus; vulvar swelling of proestrus decreases slightly during estrus; bitch is receptive to male during estrus • Problems that may be encountered—sanguinous vulvar discharge during estrus; female may be unreceptive even though in estrus • Limited number of available breedings requires knowing the ovulation day.
Cats
The LH response to a single mating can vary substantially, and neither single nor multiple copulations ensure ovulation.

Historical Findings
Dogs
• Refusal to accept male at the expected time
• Sanguinous vulvar discharge during estrus
Cats
Return to estrus in < 30 days indicates failure of ovulation

Physical Examination Findings
Dogs
• Fully cornified vaginal epithelium
• Interest shown by male • Swollen vulva
• Vaginal discharge • "Flagging"

CAUSES

Dogs
• Limited number of breedings • Female unreceptive to male

Cats
• Coitus that occurs too early or too late in estrus, too few times, or breeding by artificial insemination may not result in ovulation.

RISK FACTORS   N/A

DIAGNOSIS

DIFFERENTIAL DIAGNOSIS
Vaginal discharge—proestrus/estrus, vaginitis, and neoplasia

CBC/BIOCHEMISTRY/URINALYSIS
N/A

OTHER LABORATORY TESTS
Dogs
• In-house semiquantitative progesterone testing can be used as an adjunct to vaginal cytologic examination. Testing should begin when vaginal cytologic examination reveals approximately 60-75% cornification to establish a baseline. If progesterone tests are used without cytologic examination, begin early (3rd or 4th day) in proestrus. Tests should be performed every other day. • In-house LH testing is also available; samples must be run daily to observe the LH peak.

Cats
Submit samples for progesterone testing to verify ovulation.

IMAGING
Although ultrasonographic imaging of the ovaries may help determine ovulation in some circumstances, it is not reliable as the sole method of verifying ovulation.

OTHER DIAGNOSTIC PROCEDURES
Dogs
• Vaginal cytologic examination—at the onset of proestrus, most epithelial cells appear noncornified (the nucleus has the stippled appearance of a normal viable cell). The percent cornified epithelial cells (those cells with angular cytoplasm and pyknotic nuclei or nuclei which fail to take up stain) increases by approximately 10% per day during proestrus reaching 90% or more by estrus. • Vaginoscopy—vaginal epithelium appears hyperplastic and wrinkled from proestrus to estrus

TREATMENT

DOGS
• If multiple breedings are possible, inseminate every other day after the initial rise in progesterone is observed.
• If only two breedings are to be performed, insemination should be performed on either days 3 and 5 or days 4 and 6 after the LH peak (day 0). Using fresh, chilled semen. Fertility is best if breedings occur on days 3 and 5 or 4 and 6 after the LH peak or initial rise in progesterone (P4), keeping in mind that viability of fresh, chilled semen is reduced and timing of insemination is critical. The viability of frozen semen is reduced even further and timing is therefore more critical. Multiple vaginal inseminations with frozen

semen should be performed on days 4, 5 and 6 after the LH rise.

• More commonly, a single surgical insemination is conducted when frozen semen is used. Surgical insemination with frozen semen should be performed on day 5 or 6 after the LH peak or initial rise in P4 (day 0).

• Patients can be treated as outpatients, with every-other-day visits for blood collection and vaginal cytologic examination.

• Normal activity and diet

• Surgical artificial insemination requires routine postoperative care

Cats

• To increase the likelihood of ovulation, maximize the number of matings and breed on successive days of estrus.

• Breed 4 times a day with breedings at least 2-3 hours apart on days 2 and 3 of estrus to maximize LH release. Ovulation can be induced by administration of exogenous hormones. Administration of gonadotropin releasing hormone or human chorionic gonadotropin after mating can be used to increase the likelihood of ovulation.

MEDICATIONS

DRUGS AND FLUIDS

Cats

• hCG (500 IU IM)

• GnRH (25-50 mcg IM or IV)

CONTRAINDICATIONS N/A

PRECAUTIONS N/A

POSSIBLE INTERACTIONS N/A

ALTERNATE DRUGS N/A

FOLLOW-UP

PATIENT MONITORING

Follow-up pregnancy examination at the appropriate time

Dogs

• Vaginal specimens should continue to be obtained through estrus after breeding to determine day 1 (D1) of diestrus. • Another semiquantitative P4 test 3-4 days after the initial rise is recommended to verify a continued rise in P4.

Cats

Progesterone assay to verify ovulation

POSSIBLE COMPLICATIONS

Dogs

• Vaginal cytologic examination to determine Day 1 allows retrospective estimation of the day of ovulation (6 days before Day 1) and comparison to the prospective estimation made on the basis of P4. If the two estimates do not correlate, pregnancy rates are reduced. The semiquantitative P4 kits currently available need to come to room temperature before use. If the test is run with a cold kit, results will be incorrect, often giving a false high progesterone. • Blood should be allowed to clot at a cool temperature and cells should be separated from serum or plasma as soon as possible (within 20 minutes of collection). If serum is allowed to remain with the RBC, progesterone will be bound and test results will be artificially low. • A hemolyzed or lipemic specimen may give a false low progesterone.

MISCELLANEOUS

ASSOCIATED CONDITIONS

Vaginal stricture

AGE RELATED FACTORS

"Split heats" in young dogs

ZOONOTIC POTENTIAL N/A

PREGNANCY N/A

SYNONYMS N/A

SEE ALSO

• Infertility • Vaginal Discharge

ABBREVIATIONS

P4 = progesterone
LH = luteinizing hormone
D1 = day 1 of diestrus
RBC = red blood cells

References

Eilts BE, Paccamonti DL, Causey RC. Reproductive disorders. In: GD Norsworthy, ed. Feline practice. Philadelphia: JB Lippincott, 1993;458-476

Holst PA. Vaginal cytology in the bitch. In: DA Morrow, ed. Current therapy in theriogenology 2. Philadelphia: WB Saunders, 1986;457-462

Olson PN, Nett TM. Reproductive endocrinology and physiology of the bitch. In: DA Morrow, ed. Current therapy in theriogenology 2. Philadelphia: WB Saunders, 1986;453-457.

Author Dale Paccamonti
Consulting Editor Sara K. Lyle

BASICS

DEFINITION
Cessation of effective perfusion and ventilation due to the absence of coordinated cardiac contraction or respiratory muscle function. Cardiac arrest invariably follows respiratory arrest and vice versa if not recognized and treated.

Pathophysiology
• Generalized or localized asphyxia in a particular tissue such as the myocardium is either the cause or the consequence of sudden death. • After 1-4 minutes of airway obstruction (asphyxia), breathing efforts stop while circulation remains intact. • If obstruction continues for 6-9 minutes, severe hypotension and bradycardia lead to dilated pupils, absence of heart sounds, and no pulse. Quick ventilation of the lungs with air is often lifesaving. • After 6-9 minutes, myocardial contractions cease even with a normal ECG (electromechanical dissociation). Drug therapy with artificial ventilation and circulation are required for resuscitation. • Ventricular fibrillation, ventricular asystole, and electromechanical dissociation on the ECG represent cessation of myocardial contractility.

Systems Affected
• All systems are affected, but those requiring the greatest supply of oxygen and nutrients are affected first. • Cardiovascular • Renal/urologic • Nervous

SIGNALMENT
Any age or breed

SIGNS
• Loss of consciousness • Dilated pupils • Agonal gasping or absence of ventilation • Absence of femoral pulse • Absence of auscultable heart sounds • Lack of response to stimulation • Cyanosis

CAUSES
• Hypoxia caused by respiratory failure, anemia, or circulatory failure • Myocardial damage—infectious, inflammatory, infiltrative, traumatic, neoplastic, or embolic • Acid base imbalance • Electrolyte abnormality (e.g., hyperkalemia, hypocalcemia, and hypomagnesemia) • Hypovolemia • Shock • Anesthetics—a common cause • Toxemia • CNS trauma • Electrical shock

RISK FACTORS
• Cardiovascular disease • Polysystemic trauma • Anesthesia • Septicemia • Endotoxemia • Ventricular arrhythmias (e.g., ventricular tachycardia showing R on T phenomenon, ventricular flutter, frequent and multiform ventricular premature complexes) • Parasympathetic activity (e.g., vomiting, abdominal surgery, and manipulation of the eyes, larynx, or trachea) • Prolonged seizing • Invasive cardiovascular manipulation (e.g., pericardiocentesis, surgery, and angiography)

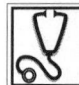

DIAGNOSIS
• Sudden cardiovascular collapse associated with inadequate cardiac output can lead to severe consequences. • A quick diagnosis and approach to treatment is necessary, since more than 4 minutes of cardiac arrest may cause brain damage.

DIFFERENTIAL DIAGNOSIS
• Severe hypovolemia with the absence of palpable pulses • Pericardial effusion; muffling heart sounds and compromising cardiac output • Upper airway obstruction (will rapidly progress to cardiopulmonary arrest [CPA])

CBC/BIOCHEMISTRY/URINALYSIS
N/A

OTHER LABORATORY TESTS N/A

IMAGING
Echocardiography may help identify pericardial effusion but should not interfere with resuscitative attempts once CPA is diagnosed.

OTHER DIAGNOSTIC PROCEDURES
Once CPA has developed, a continuous ECG is used to monitor resuscitative efforts.

TREATMENT
• Artificial ventilation and circulation techniques are instituted until the underlying arrhythmia can be identified and treated. ABCs of resuscitation are as follows: A—airway, B—breathing, C—circulation, D—drugs, defibrillation. The goals are to return spontaneous cardiovascular and respiratory function with minimal damage to vital organs, especially the brain.

A—AIRWAY MANAGEMENT
• The airway can be visualized by extending the patient's head and neck and pulling the tongue forward.
• The airway should be cleared of any secretions, vomit, or foreign material, and a patent airway secured by endotracheal intubation.
• If a complete obstruction exists, an alternative airway can be created with an emergency tracheostomy.

B—BREATHING/VENTILATORY MANAGEMENT
• If spontaneous breathing movements are not seen once the patency of the airway is ensured, artificial ventilation should be initiated.
• Techniques for artificial ventilation include mouth-to-mouth or mouth-to-nose ventilation, which uses exhaled air to provide 16% O_2.
• The preferred technique is endotracheal intubation and ventilation with an ambu bag, the reservoir bag on an anesthesia machine, or a mechanical ventilator. The use of 100% O_2 delivered at a flow rate of 150 ml/kg/min is recommended at this stage.

C—CIRCULATION
• Manual compression of the chest has been shown to provide, at best, only 30% of normal cardiac output; open-chest cardiopulmonary resuscitation (CPR) is consistently two to three times more effective in generating cerebral blood flow.
• The primary goal of cardiac compression is to maintain basal perfusion of the heart and brain.
• Hemodynamic studies in animal models suggest that several different mechanisms exist for the generation of blood flow (artificial systole) during chest compression. The thoracic pump mechanism generates blood flow by changes in intrathoracic pressure. In animals > 15 kg, this mechanism is thought to play the major role in effective CPR.
• Compression of the chest wall during closed-chest CPR causes indirect compression of the cardiac chambers (cardiac pump mechanism) and generates artificial systole. However, in animals > 15 kg, this mechanism is thought to play only a minor role in the forward flow of blood.
• External chest compression is thought to augment circulation largely by the creation of alternating high and low intrathoracic pressure. Sudden, forcible compression of the chest wall generates positive intrathoracic pressure, generating a forward blood flow in the major arteries.

COMPRESSION TECHNIQUES
• Chest compressions should be rapid in order to increase and decrease intrathoracic pressure rapidly. The chest wall should be displaced approximately 30%.
• In small to medium-sized patients (5-15 kg), the cardiac pump effect can be maximized by placing the patient in left lateral recumbency and using the heel of the palm on the lower one-third of the chest at the level of the fifth intercostal space.
• In large patients (> 15 kg), the thoracic pump is maximized when the patient is placed in dorsal recumbency and the heel of the hand is placed over the caudal one-third of the sternum.
• The chest should be compressed at least 60-80 times per minute, with total release between compressions to maximize the diastolic component of the resuscitation cycle. The systolic compressions should take up 40% of the cycle time.
• If mouth-to-mouth or mouth-to-nose ventilation or a face mask is used, ventilation should be interposed with compressions (one ventilation for every five compressions) in order to maximize the efficacy of both.
• For intubated patients, ventilate simultaneously with every second or third compression in order to augment the thoracic pump mechanism.

• Interpose abdominal compression between chest compressions. This has been shown to enhance cerebral and coronary blood flow (by raising aortic diastolic pressure) in dogs.

OPEN-CHEST CPR
• Indicated if closed-chest techniques do not produce a palpable femoral pulse, particularly in patients weighing > 30 kg and those with a flail chest, severe obesity, pericardial effusion, or severe hypovolemia
• Performed through a left thoracotomy at the fifth or sixth intercostal space
• The palmar surface of the fingers and thumb are used to "milk" the ventricular blood toward the great vessels. Digital compression of the descending aorta may help cranial perfusion.

MEDICATIONS

DRUGS AND FLUIDS
• The selection of drugs depends on the underlying arrhythmia.
• Please refer to ventricular fibrillation and ventricular asystole and accompanying flow diagrams for appropriate drug selection and defibrillator use. Refer also to Appendix– Drug Formulary

CONTRAINDICATIONS N/A

PRECAUTIONS N/A

POSSIBLE INTERACTIONS N/A

ALTERNATE DRUGS N/A

FOLLOW-UP

PATIENT MONITORING
• Maintain heart rate and blood pressure with fluids and possible inotropic agents. • Support respiration; assist ventilation and continue O_2 for several hours. • Watch for neurologic deficits from hypoxia (especially blindness). Consider corticosteroids or mannitol.
• Monitor ECG for arrhythmias. • Monitor urine output. • Monitor body temperature, central venous pressure, blood gases, and serum electrolytes. • Radiograph thorax to evaluate for postresuscitative injury.
• Diagnose and correct factors that caused the cardiac arrest.

POSSIBLE COMPLICATIONS
• Vomiting • Aspiration pneumonitis • Fractured ribs or sternebrae • Acute renal failure • Pulmonary contusions and edema • Neurologic deficits • Cardiac arrhythmias following CPR (common) • Pneumothorax

MISCELLANEOUS

ASSOCIATED CONDITIONS N/A

AGE RELATED FACTORS N/A

ZOONOTIC POTENTIAL N/A

PREGNANCY N/A

SYNONYMS
• Cardiac arrest • Heart attack

SEE ALSO
• Ventricular Fibrillation • Ventricular Standstill (Asystole)

ABBREVIATIONS
CPA = cardiopulmonary arrest
CPR = cardiopulmonary resuscitation

References

American Heart Association. Guidelines for cardiopulmonary resuscitation and emergency cardiac care. J Am Med Assoc 1992;268:16.

Henik RA. Basic life support and external cardiac compression in dogs and cats. J Am Vet Med Assoc 1992;200:1925.

Kass PH, Haskins SC. Survival following cardiopulmonary resuscitation in dogs and cats. Vet Emer Crit Care 1992;2:57.

Robello CD, Crowe DT. Cardiopulmonary resuscitation: current recommendations. Vet Clin North Am Small Anim Pract 1989;19:1127.

Beardow AW, Dhupa N. Cardiopulmonary arrest and resuscitation. In: Miller MS, Tilley LP, eds. Manual of canine and feline cardiology. 2nd ed. Philadelphia: WB Saunders, 1995;425.

Author Andrew W. Beardow
Consulting Editors Larry P. Tilley and Francis W. K. Smith, Jr.

CONSTIPATION AND OBSTIPATION

BASICS

DEFINITION
Constipation is infrequent, incomplete, or difficult defecation with passage of hard or dry feces. Obstipation is intractable constipation caused by prolonged retention of hard, dry feces; defecation becomes impossible.

Pathophysiology
Constipation can develop with any disease that impairs passage of feces through the colon. Delayed fecal transit allows removal of additional salt and water producing drier feces. Peristaltic contractions may increase during constipation, but eventually motility diminishes due to smooth muscle degeneration secondary to chronic overdistention.

Systems Affected
Gastrointestinal—vomiting, inappetance, and abdominal discomfort

SIGNALMENT
• Dogs and cats • More common in cats

SIGNS

Historical Findings
Straining to defecate with small fecal volume, hard, dry feces, infrequent defecation, small amount of liquid feces produced after prolonged straining, occasional vomiting, inappetance, and depression

Physical Examination Findings
• Feces filled colon • Other findings depend on the cause • Rectal examination—may palpate a mass, stricture, perianal hernia, anal sac disease, foreign body or material, prostatic enlargement, or narrowed pelvic canal

CAUSES

Dietary
Bones, hair, foreign material, and excessive fiber

Environmental
Lack of exercise, change of environment (e.g., hospitalization and dirty litter box), and inability to ambulate

Drugs
Anticholinergics, antihistamines, opioids, barium sulfate, sucralfate, antacids, kaopectolin, iron supplements, and diuretics

Painful Defecation
• Anorectal disease—anal sacculitis, anal sac abscess, perianal fistula, anal stricture, anal spasm, rectal foreign body, rectal prolapse, and pseudocoprostasis • Trauma—fractured pelvis, fractured limb, dislocated hip, bite wound or laceration, and perineal abscess

Mechanical Obstruction
• Extraluminal—healed pelvic fracture with narrowed pelvic canal, prostatic hypertrophy, prostatitis, prostatic neoplasia, intrapelvic neoplasia, rectal foreign body, pseudocoprostasis, and sublumbar lymphadenopathy
• Intraluminal and intramural—colonic or rectal neoplasia or polyp, rectal stricture, rectal diverticulum, perineal hernia, rectal prolapse, and congenital defect (atresia ani)

Neurologic Disease
• CNS—paraplegia, spinal cord disease, intervertebral disc disease, and cerebral disease (e.g., lead toxicity and rabies) • Peripheral nervous system—dysautonomia and sacral nerve disease • Intrinsic colonic nerve dysfunction—idiopathic megacolon in cats

Metabolic and Endocrinologic Disease
• Impaired colonic smooth muscle function—hyperparathyroidism, hypothyroidism, and hypokalemia (chronic renal failure)
• Debility—general muscle weakness, dehydration, and neoplasia

RISK FACTORS
• Drug therapy • Metabolic disease causing dehydration • Intact male dog with perineal hernia • Low tail carriage causing perianal fistula • Pica (foreign material) • Excessive grooming (hair) • Pelvic fracture

DIAGNOSIS

DIFFERENTIAL DIAGNOSIS
• Must differentiate from dyschezia (painful defecation) and straining caused by colitis. Unlike constipation, these are associated with an increased frequency of attempts to defecate and frequent production of small amounts of liquid feces containing blood or mucus.
• Must differentiate from straining to urinate. Unlike constipation, stranguria can be associated with hematuria and abnormal findings on urinalysis (e.g., pyuria, crystalluria, and bacteriuria).

CBC/BIOCHEMISTRY/URINALYSIS
• Results usually normal • May detect hypokalemia or hypercalcemia (hyperparathyroidism) • High RBC count and total plasma proteins in dehydrated patients • High WBC count in patients with abscess, perianal fistula, and prostatic disease

OTHER LABORATORY TESTS
• If the patient is hypercholesterolemic, consider T_3, T_4, and TSH assay to rule out hypothyroidism. • If the patient is hypercalcemic, consider parathyroid hormone assay.

IMAGING
• Abdominal radiography may reveal colonic or rectal foreign body, colonic or rectal mass, prostatic enlargement, fractured pelvis, or dislocated hip. • After enemas, a barium enema may better define an intraluminal mass or stricture. • Ultrasonography may help define extraluminal mass and prostatic disease.

OTHER DIAGNOSTIC PROCEDURES
Colonoscopy may be needed to identify a mass, stricture, or other colonic or rectal lesion; biopsy specimens can also be obtained.

TREATMENT
• Remove or ameliorate the underlying cause if possible.
• May need to treat as inpatient if the animal has severe impaction of feces or dehydration; adequate hydration and electrolyte balance are important, especially before enemas.
• Diet may need to be altered to include bulking agents such as methylcellulose, canned pumpkin, or bran.
• Manual removal of feces with the animal under general anesthesia may be required if enemas and medication are unsuccessful.
• Subtotal colectomy may be required as a last option in cats with recurring obstipation (aquired megacolon) or idiopathic megacolon.
• Discontinue any medications that may cause constipation.

MEDICATIONS

DRUGS AND FLUIDS
• Dehydrated patients should receive a balanced electrolyte solution with potassium supplementation as needed.
• Dietary supplementation with a bulk forming agent is the mainstay of treatment. Bran, methylcellulose, canned pumpkin,and psyllium can be used.
• Laxatives and cathartics can be given as needed.
• Emollients—docusate sodium and docusate calcium
• Lubricants—mineral oil and white petrolatum not recommended because of danger of lipoid aspiration pneumonia due to lack of taste
• Stimulant laxatives—bisacodyl
• Saline laxatives—isosmotic mixture of polyethylene glycol and poorly absorbable salts; mainly used to prepare the colon for colonoscopy or surgery
• Disaccharide laxatives—lactulose
• Enemas may be needed, either in hospital or periodically by the owners at home. Use warm water with a small amount of mild soap, mineral oil, or docusate sodium. Sodium phosphate retention enemas (e.g., Fleet, C.B. Fleet Co., Inc.) are contraindicated because of their association with severe electrolyte alteration.
• Suppositories can be used as a replacement for enemas. Use glycerol, bisacodyl, or docusate sodium products.
• Motility modifiers can also be tried. Cholinergics such as urecholine may aid in evacuation but are contraindicated in animals with obstruction. Cisapride may also stimulate motility in patients with megacolon.

CONSTIPATION AND OBSTIPATION

CONTRAINDICATIONS
Anticholinergics

PRECAUTIONS
Metoclopramide and cholinergics can be used with caution (contraindicated in patient with an obstructive process).

POSSIBLE INTERACTIONS N/A

ALTERNATE DRUGS N/A

 FOLLOW-UP

PATIENT MONITORING
Frequency of defecation and consistency of feces

POSSIBLE COMPLICATIONS
• Chronic constipation or recurrent obstipation can lead to aquired megacolon.
• Overuse of laxatives and enemas can cause diarrhea. • Colonic mucosa can be damaged by improper enema technique, repeated rough mechanical breakdown of feces, or ischemic necrosis secondary to pressure of hard feces. • Perineal irritation and ulceration can lead to fecal incontinence.

 MISCELLANEOUS

ASSOCIATED CONDITIONS N/A

AGE RELATED FACTORS N/A

ZOONOTIC POTENTIAL N/A

PREGNANCY N/A

SYNONYMS Fecal impaction

SEE ALSO
See Causes

ABBREVIATIONS
CNS = central nervous system
RBC = red blood cells
TSH = thyroid stimulating hormone
WBC = white blood cells

References

Burrows CF, Sherding RG. Constipation and dyschezia. In: Anderson NV, ed. Veterinary gastroenterology. Philadelphia: Lea and Febiger, 1992;484-503.

Bright RM. Management of constipation and megacolon in cats. In: Proceedings. 17th Annu Waltham/OSU Symp, 1993;73-78.

Hoskins JD. Management of fecal impaction. Compend Cont Ed Pract Vet 1990;12:1579-1585.

Burrows CF. Medical diseases of the colon. In: Jones BD, ed. Canine and Feline Gastroenterology. Philadelphia: WB Saunders, 1986;221-256.

Authors Lisa E. Moore and Colin F. Burrows

Consulting Editor Brent D. Jones

COPROPHAGIA

 BASICS

DEFINITION
Ingestion of feces, the animal's own feces or those of another animal including those of another species

Pathophysiology
Coprophagia is common in dogs but rare in cats. The remainder of this section deals with the behavior in dogs . The only circumstance in which coprophagia is considered a normal behavior is when a bitch eats the feces of her pups from the time of their birth until about 3 weeks of age. It is felt that the bitch does this to keep the nest area clean until the pups are able to move away from it to defecate. A clean nest area may be less likely to attract predators in the wild. It may also be considered a natural, although not normal, behavior for dogs to consume the feces of ungulates containing large amounts of nutrients remaining after large intestinal fermentation, which may have helped to sustain dogs in the wild when no other food source was available. Dogs also commonly eat the feces of cats with whom they share a household.

Systems Affected
Gastrointestinal—recurrent infection with intestinal parasites. Gastroenteritis commonly results from consumption of large amounts of ungulate feces.

SIGNALMENT
Nursing bitches frequently exhibit coprophagia, eating the feces of their pups.

SIGNS
• Halitosis • Polyuria, polydipsia, weight loss, vomiting, and small or large bowel diarrhea are signs of the common underlying medical problems associated with coprophagia

CAUSES

Behavioral Causes (Theorized)
• Cleaning of the nest area • Displacement from ungulate feces to those of any species available • Responding to punishment for defecating in inappropriate locations by removing the evidence and imitating the owner's behavior of removing feces • Stressful conditions such as sudden changes in lifestyle or environment

Medical Causes
• Exocrine pancreatic insufficiency • Hyperadrenocorticism • Exogenous glucocorticoid administration • Intestinal malabsorption disorder • Intestinal parasitism • Diabetes mellitus • Hyperthyroidism. • Many have theorized that in some animals, coprophagia may be caused by dietary deficiencies, but there is little information to support this theory.

RISK FACTORS N/A

 DIAGNOSIS

DIFFERENTIAL DIAGNOSIS
• The diagnosis is made on the basis of the owner's historical complaint. • Treatment depends on whether the coprophagia is purely a behavioral problem or is a symptom of an underlying medical problem. This distinction affects prognosis as well as treatment. • A complete history, especially regarding the dog's environment, diet, and handling, is essential. The diet should be examined for nutritional deficiencies. If the physical examination shows evidence of disease, further diagnostic testing is necessary.

CBC/BIOCHEMISTRY/URINALYSIS
• Iron deficiency anemia may be the result of chronic intestinal bleeding caused by parasitism. • Results of biochemical analysis and urinalysis may help diagnose such conditions as diabetes mellitus, hyperadrenocorticism, and intestinal malabsorption disorder.

OTHER LABORATORY TESTS
• Multiple fecal flotations or direct smears may be necessary to rule out intestinal parasitism. • Serum TLI is necessary to diagnose exocrine pancreatic insufficiency. • Specific adrenal function tests are needed to confirm hyperadrenocorticism. • Serum T3 and T4 concentrations can be used to diagnose hyperthyroidism.

IMAGING N/A

OTHER DIAGNOSTIC PROCEDURES
Examination of endoscopically or surgically obtained intestinal biopsy specimen is necessary to diagnose infiltrative bowel disease that may be causing malabsorption.

 TREATMENT

• Treatment varies depending on whether the cause of the coprophagia is behavioral or medical.
• If underlying disease is found and treated, coprophagia may resolve.
• Behavioral coprophagia can be treated in a number of ways. Avoidance of the stools is probably the most reliable solution. One method is to have the owners walk the dog on a leash so that the dog can be taken away from the feces immediately. At the time of defecation, the owner can also give the dog a food reward so that it will become conditioned to expect food at defecation instead of looking for feces. In the case of a dog eating cat feces, litter pans should be cleaned daily and covered or placed in a location unavailable to the dog.
• If the owner is unwilling to leash walk the dog at all times, preferring to let it outside unattended, methods of punishment can be used. Most often a hot or unpleasant tasting substance such as pepper is placed on the feces. However, many dogs learn to eat the untreated feces. Another method is to inject a substance such as hot sauce into the feces to make it more difficult for the dog to avoid treated feces.
• Application of commercial meat tenderizer or pancreatic enzymes to the food also makes the feces taste unpleasant to some dogs, although they may continue to consume the feces of other dogs or animals. Supplementing the diet with pancreatic enzymes is the treatment of choice if exocrine pancreatic insufficiency is diagnosed, although the mechanism by which the enzymes are effective is different.
• A more aggressive method is to inject the feces with apomorphine. Upon ingestion of the feces, the dog will soon become nauseated and vomit. After a few such experiences, many dogs learn to stop eating stools. This is called taste aversion learning by animal behaviorists, and is thought to be most effective if the behavior has recently begun. If the problem is old, the dog may have learned that eating stools is not associated with any adverse effect. Occasionally, making a change in the dog's diet is successful even if dietary deficiency does not play a role. A change in the consistency or flavor of the stools may be the explanation for this method's success.

MEDICATIONS

DRUGS AND FLUIDS

Medications should only be used to treat coprophagia related to an underlying medical condition and should be selected specifically to treat that condition. See sections on specific diseases associated with coprophagia.

CONTRAINDICATIONS N/A

PRECAUTIONS N/A

POSSIBLE INTERACTIONS N/A

ALTERNATE DRUGS N/A

 FOLLOW-UP

PATIENT MONITORING N/A

POSSIBLE COMPLICATIONS

• Reinfection with intestinal parasites
• Gastroenteritis, especially in dogs consuming large amounts of equine feces

 MISCELLANEOUS

ASSOCIATED CONDITIONS
See Causes

AGE RELATED FACTORS N/A

ZOONOTIC POTENTIAL N/A

PREGNANCY N/A

SYNONYMS N/A

SEE ALSO See Causes

ABBREVIATIONS N/A

References

Houpt KA. Feeding and drinking behavior problems. Vet Clin North Am Small Anim Prac 1991;21:288-289.

Lorenz MD. Coprophagy and pica. In: Lorenz MD, Cornelius LM, eds. Small animal medical diagnosis. Philadelphia: JP Lippincott, 1987;63-64.

Author Daniel P. Harrington

Consulting Editor Brent D. Jones

COUGH

BASICS

DEFINITION
A cough is a sudden forceful expiration of air through the glottis, usually accompanied by an audible sound, that is preceded by an exaggerated inspiratory effort.

Pathophysiology
The cough is one of the most powerful reflexes in the body. It is induced by stimulation of either afferent fibers of the pharyngeal distribution of the glossopharyngeal nerves or sensory endings of the vagus nerves located in the larynx, trachea, and larger bronchi. It begins with an inspiratory phase followed in sequence by an inspiratory pause, glottis closure, increased intrathoracic pressure, and glottis opening. The cough serves as an early warning system for the pharynx and respiratory system and as a protective mechanism.

Systems Affected
• Respiratory • Musculoskeletal—because of role played in the reflex by inspiratory and expiratory muscles of respiration • Cardiovascular • Nervous—the result of cough syncope

SIGNALMENT N/A

SIGNS

Historical Findings
Patterns and characteristics of the cough frequently are suggestive of the underlying cause. Nocturnal coughing is commonly associated with early stages of left-sided congestive heart failure (CHF) and tracheal collapse, whereas a cough precipitated by exercise and/or excitement is frequently the result of inflammation or irritation involving the larynx, trachea, and bronchi. Harsh, prolonged coughing is also suggestive of involvement of the major airways, whereas soft, infrequent coughing is more likely the result of pulmonary alveolar disease or CHF. A productive cough suggests the presence of fluid or mucus in the expectorated material, whereas a dry cough indicates an absence of mucus or fluid production.

CAUSES

Upper Respiratory Tract Diseases
• Nasopharyngeal—rhinitis, sinusitis, nasopharyngeal foreign body/tumor, tonsillitis, tonsillar tumor • Laryngeal—inflammation, foreign body, injuries, tumors • Tracheal—inflammation (inhalation of irritating substances, heat), infections (viral, bacterial), foreign body, tracheal collapse, tumor

Lower Respiratory Tract Diseases
• Bronchial—inflammation, infection (viral, bacterial, parasitic), allergy, foreign body, tumor • Pulmonary—inflammation, infection (viral, bacterial, fungal), aspiration pneumonia, pulmonary edema, tumor • Pulmonary vascular—heartworm disease, thrombosis/ embolism, CHF, pulmonary hypertension, tumor

Other Diseases
• Esophageal—inflammation, foreign body, tumor • Pleural—inflammation, infection (bacterial, fungal), hernia, tumor

RISK FACTORS
• Congenital and acquired esophageal, gastroesophageal, and upper gastrointestinal disorders all predispose to aspiration pneumonia. • Hyperadrenocorticism and chronic administration of corticosteroids may increase the incidence of pulmonary thromboembolism. • Genetic predisposition to certain cardiac disorders increases the risk of pulmonary edema secondary to CHF. • Environmental factors include exposure to certain viral, bacterial, fungal, and parasitic diseases and exposure of dogs to mosquitoes without effective heartworm prophylaxis.

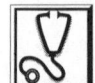

DIAGNOSIS

DIFFERENTIAL DIAGNOSIS
• Both sneezing and coughing are expiratory events that may occur together in certain conditions (i.e., rhinitis, sinusitis, regurgitation) and may confuse both the pet owner and the history. With the forceful expiration of a sneeze the mouth is usually closed, whereas it is normally open with a cough. • A reverse sneeze is another nasopharyngeal event that is commonly misinterpreted as a cough by pet owners. Although nasopharyngeal irritation is the usual cause, some of the same conditions that cause sneezing and coughing may be responsible. A reverse sneeze is associated with both an audible inspiratory and expiratory component without the forceful expiratory event that characterizes both the sneeze and the cough.

CBC/BIOCHEMISTRY/URINALYSIS
• Hemogram may suggest etiologic possibilities—neutrophilia with left shift (e.g., infection, inflammation) or eosinophilia (e.g., allergic response). • High liver enzymes with exaggerated serum alkaline phosphatase (SAP) elevation suggests the presence of hyperadrenocorticism, whereas mild to moderate elevations in SAP may suggest liver congestion secondary to pulmonary disease or right heart failure (R-CHF).

OTHER LABORATORY TESTS
• Filter test for microfilaria and/or filaria serologic test to evaluate for heartworm disease • Low-dose dexamethasone response test to further evaluate elevations in liver enzymes • A coagulation profile should be performed in any patient that presents with a cough associated with either epistaxis or hemoptysis.

IMAGING
• Radiographs are particularly beneficial in evaluating patients with nasal, sinus, tracheal and lower respiratory tract disorders. • Thoracic ultrasound is of use in patients with primary cardiac disease, right heart disease secondary to a pulmonary condition, and pleural effusion.

OTHER DIAGNOSTIC PROCEDURES
• Direct and flotation fecal tests to detect respiratory parasites and ova • Transtracheal aspirate with cytology and culture for evaluation of lower respiratory tract disorders • Laryngoscopy, tracheoscopy, and bronchoscopy for evaluation of suspected foreign body, tumor, or other disorders in these regions (scoping should be combined with biopsy and bronchoalveolar lavage) • Thoracocentesis if pleural effusion is present • Barium swallow when aspiration pneumonia is suspected • CT scan for better evaluation of nasal and sinus disorders

TREATMENT
• Outpatient management is appropriate unless CHF is present or there is marked alteration in pulmonary function or hemoptysis. • Exercise restriction is best enforced until a cause for the cough is established and corrected, especially when activity aggravates the cough. • Inform the owner that a wide variety of conditions can be responsible for the cough, and a fairly extensive workup may be required to define and treat the underlying cause. • Surgical intervention may be indicated for management of certain patients with tracheal collapse and for tumors involving the respiratory system.

MEDICATIONS

DRUGS AND FLUIDS
• Symptomatic treatment of a patient with a cough in which other abnormalities are lacking can include broad-spectrum antibiotics and bronchodilator-expectorant therapy provided appropriate follow-up evaluations are scheduled. • Broad-spectrum antibiotic therapy should be instituted when infection is suspected, pending the results of culture and sensitivity tests. • Bronchodilator (theophylline, terbutaline, etc.) with or without the use of expectorants may be beneficial in a variety of diseases affecting the trachea and lower respiratory airways. • Although cough suppressants (hydrocodone, torbutrol) should be avoided in patients with coughs secondary to bacterial respiratory infections and congestive heart failure, they are frequently beneficial in coughs of other origin. • Therapeutic thoracocentesis should be performed in any patient with a marked pleural effusion.

CONTRAINDICATIONS

Corticosteroids
Should not be used until a definitive allergy is

defined in the absence of infection, parasitic infestation, or cardiac disease. Drugs in this category also potentiate the development of pulmonary thromboembolism and reduce the efficacy of caparsolate therapy in the treatment of heartworm disease.

Cough Suppressants
Should not be used in any patient in which either a respiratory infection or clinically significant heart disease is suspected

PRECAUTIONS

Cough Suppressants
Indiscriminate use may obscure the warning signs of serious cardiac and pulmonary disorders and predispose the patient to serious complications or even death.

Bronchodilator Therapy
Intravenous use of aminophylline may cause in tachyarrhythmias.

POSSIBLE INTERACTIONS N/A

ALTERNATE DRUGS N/A

FOLLOW-UP

PATIENT MONITORING
• Communications with owner concerning

control of the cough • Follow-up thoracic radiographs in 10-14 days when bronchopulmonary disease is present or in 3-4 weeks to monitor tumors of the respiratory tract

POSSIBLE COMPLICATIONS
• Complete control of the cough does not guarantee resolution of the inciting cause.
• Serious respiratory dysfunction and even death can be caused by underlying disease

MISCELLANEOUS

ASSOCIATED CONDITIONS
Heavy breathing, dyspnea

AGE RELATED FACTORS N/A

ZOONOTIC POTENTIAL N/A

PREGNANCY N/A

SYNONYMS N/A

SEE ALSO
• See causes. • Nasal Discharge (Sneezing, Reverse Sneezing, Gagging)

ABBREVIATIONS
SAP = serum alkaline phosphatase
CHF = congestive heart failure

References

Kopos J, Tomori Z. Cough and other respiratory reflexes. Prog Resp Rec 1979;12:15-188.

Langlands J. The dynamics of cough in health and in chronic bronchitis. Thorax 1967;22:88-96.

Yanagihara N, von Ledan H, Werner-Kukuk E. The physical parameters of cough: the larynx in a normal single cough. Acta Otolaryng 1965;61:495-510.

Ettinger SJ. Coughing. In: Ettinger SJ, ed. Textbook of veterinary internal medicine. 3rd ed. Philadelphia: WB Saunders, 1989.

Author Neil K. Harpster

Consulting Editors Lynelle Johnson and Bradley L. Moses

CYANOSIS

BASICS

DEFINITION
Cyanosis is a bluish discoloration of the skin and mucous membranes. This condition usually is associated with an increase in the amount of reduced, or deoxygenated, hemoglobin within the blood. The concentration of deoxygenated hemoglobin must exceed 5 g/dl for cyanosis to be detected.

Pathophysiology
• Central cyanosis is arterial hypoxemia or the presence of abnormal hemoglobin pigments within the circulation.
Arterial hypoxemia is generally associated with one of the following:
• Decreased fraction of inspired oxygen, usually associated with upper airway obstructive disorders, restrictive or obstructive lung disease, pleural space disorders, neuromuscular failure, or high altitude. • Ventilation—perfusion mismatching associated with pulmonary parenchymal diseases • Diffusion impairment associated with a thickening of the alveolar barrier through which oxygen must pass to reach the red blood cell • Addition of venous blood to the arterial circulation as a result of the presence of intrapulmonary or systemic shunting of blood, as with congenital right-to-left shunting cardiac defects (tetralogy of Fallot, transposition of the great vessels, tricuspid valve stenosis, common atrioventricular canal). Reversed shunting cardiac defects caused by high pulmonary vascular resistance (e.g., right-to-left shunting PDA, ASD, VSD) also result in cyanosis. Anatomic shunts are distinguished from the other three causes of hypoxemia by the failure to respond to supplemental oxygen.
• Abnormal heme pigments are most often found in the form of methemoglobin. Methemoglobin results from the oxidation of the iron within hemoglobin from the ferrous to the ferric state. • Methemoglobin is unable to bind oxygen for transport to the tissues.
• Hypoxia occurs when more than 20-40% of hemoglobin has been oxidized to methemoglobin. • Methemoglobin normally is removed from the circulation by a reducing enzyme. • Deficiency of methemoglobin reductase has been reported in the dog.
• Exposure to oxidizing agents such as benzocaine anesthetic spray and acetaminophen are the most common causes of methemoglobinemia in the cat. • Peripheral cyanosis generally is limited to the extremities and is usually the result of increased oxygen extraction from the arterial supply to the area as a result of vasoconstriction, lowered blood flow, obstruction to flow associated with thromboembolism, or stagnation of venous blood within the area.

Systems Affected
All systems are affected by hypoxemia:
• Respiratory • Nervous • Cardiovascular

SIGNALMENT
• Depends upon cause • Young animals more often seen with right-to-left cardiac shunts.
• Older animals more likely present with cyanotic lung disease. • Right-to-left cardiac shunts are recognized in the following breeds: keeshond (tetralogy of Fallot), English bulldog, beagle, keeshond, some cats • Breed associations are recognized for other cardiac conditions; however, no association may be made for those that develop right-to-left shunts in association with Eisenmenger's physiology (high pulmonary vascular resistance and pulmonary hypertension).
• Young or middle-aged animals may present with cyanosis resulting from tracheal collapse. Small-breed dogs (Pomeranians, Yorkshire terriers, poodles) are overrepresented.
• Congenital laryngeal paralysis occurs in young animals and has been reported in the dalmatian, Bouvier des Flandres, and Siberian husky. Acquired laryngeal paralysis is noted in older, large-breed dogs such as the Labrador retriever, Afghan, setter, and greyhound. • English bullterriers—hypoplastic trachea • Bronchial disease in cats is reported to have a higher incidence in the Siamese breed.

SIGNS

Historical Findings
• Stridor • Dyspnea • Cough • Voice change • Episodic weakness • Hindlimb paresis or paralysis • Syncope • Exposure to drugs causing methemoglobinemia

Physical Examination Findings
• Cyanosis may be generalized, causing a bluish tint to all mucous membranes; peripheral (in the extremities), as in aortic thromboembolism; or caudal, as is seen with right-to-left (reversed) PDA.
Auscultation
• Heart murmurs or splitting of the second heart sound, indicating congenital or acquired disease • Pulmonary crackles or wheezes • Muffled heart sounds caused by pleural space disease • Upper airway stridor from laryngeal paralysis • Tracheal palpation may induce the cough typical of tracheal collapse.
Pattern of Respiration
• Stridor—laryngeal disease (paralysis, mass, granulomatous disease, foreign body)
• Dyspnea—lower airway disease or pleural effusion • Abdominal breathing—severe lower airway, thoracic wall, or diaphragmatic disease (neuromuscular)
Examination of Extremities
• Coolness—lack of blood supply (HCM/aortic thrombus) • Paleness • Pain • Edema • Lack of pulses
Neurologic Examination
• Weakness—may be generalized and persistent in severe cardiac diseases; may be episodic, especially with exercise/excitement
• Posterior paresis/paralysis—thrombus

CAUSES

Larynx
• Neoplasia • Granulomatous disease • Paralysis—acquired or congenital • Trauma • Collapse • Spasm

Trachea
• Neoplasia • Foreign body • Collapse • Trauma • Hypoplasia

Lower Airway
• Neoplasia • Foreign body • Pneumonia—viral, bacterial, fungal, allergic, mycobacteria, aspiration • Bronchitis that has evolved to bronchiectasis/emphysema • Parasites—Filarioidea, Paragonimus, protozoa • Pulmonary thromboembolism • Pulmonary contusion or hemorrhage • Noncardiogenic edema—inhalation, snake bite, electric shock • Near drowning

Pleural
• Neoplasia • Trauma—hemothorax, pneumothorax • Infectious—bacterial, fungal • Chylothorax

Thoracic Wall/Diaphragm
• Neuromuscular disease—tick paralysis, coonhound paralysis • Trauma—diaphragmatic hernia, fractured ribs, flail chest • Congenital, pericardial, diaphragmatic hernia

Cardiac
• Congenital defects—PDA, VSD, ASD, tetralogy of Fallot • Acquired disease—mitral valve disease, cardiomyopathy • Pericardial effusion—idiopathic disease and neoplasia

RISK FACTORS N/A

DIAGNOSIS

DIFFERENTIAL DIAGNOSIS

Respiratory
• Chronic obstructive pulmonary disease • Bronchiectasis • Tracheal collapse • Bronchial disease in cats • Laryngeal paralysis/neoplasia • Pulmonary hypertension • Pulmonary thromboembolism

Cardiac
• Tetralogy of Fallot • Tricuspid valve dysplasia • Double outlet right ventricle • Transposition of the great vessels • R-L PDA, VSD, ASD • Chronic valvular fibrosis, HCM in cats, DCM

Neurologic (Lower Motor Neuron Disease)
• Tick paralysis • Botulism • Acute polyradiculoneuritis (coonhound paralysis) • Dysautonomia • Myasthenia gravis

CBC/BIOCHEMISTRY/URINALYSIS
• Cyanotic animals often have noticeably darkened blood. • Methemoglobinemia results in chocolate-brown discoloration of the blood. • Anemia (PCV < 15%) may obscure detection of cyanosis because of lack of sufficient hemoglobin.

OTHER LABORATORY TESTS

• Methemoglobin concentrations may be determined through a human laboratory.
• Arterial blood gas analysis is recommended if available.

IMAGING

• Radiography is essential in defining the cause of cyanosis. • Echocardiography for congenital or acquired cardiac disease and suspected pulmonary hypertension. Doppler ultrasonography may be required in certain conditions.

OTHER DIAGNOSTIC PROCEDURES

• Laryngoscopic exam • Electrocardiography may reveal right heart enlargement changes.
• Bronchoscopy may be used in the diagnosis and treatment of tracheal and pulmonary diseases. Transtracheal wash or fine needle lung aspirate may also be appropriate. • Thoracocentesis is required for the diagnosis and treatment of pleural space disorders.

TREATMENT

• Animals with cyanosis should be hospitalized for immediate diagnostic testing and treatment. Most cases should receive stabilization therapy (e.g., oxygen, thoracocentesis, tracheostomy) before aggressive diagnostics.
• Specific therapy will depend on the ultimate diagnosis. In all likelihood, exercise restriction and dietary modification will be required.
• Owners should be informed on admission that diseases associated with cyanosis can have dire outcomes.
• Surgical treatment will depend upon the primary disease process and the extent of cardiac or respiratory embarrassment as a result of disease.

MEDICATIONS

DRUGS AND FLUIDS

• Oxygen therapy should be provided as soon as possible in animals with cyanosis.
• Specific therapy will depend upon the final diagnosis.

CONTRAINDICATIONS N/A

PRECAUTIONS N/A

POSSIBLE INTERACTIONS N/A

ALTERNATE DRUGS N/A

FOLLOW-UP

PATIENT MONITORING

• While in an oxygen cage, the animal should be disturbed as infrequently as possible for monitoring. Changes in depth and rate of respiration may be used to assess the efficacy of therapy. • Mucous membranes should return to a normal pink color with oxygen therapy if the cause of cyanosis is not an anatomic shunt and patient has adequate reserves.

POSSIBLE COMPLICATIONS

• Follow-up appointments will depend upon the cause of cyanosis. • Owners should be instructed in monitoring of mucous membrane color and respiratory effort. Immediate veterinary care should be sought if cyanosis returns.

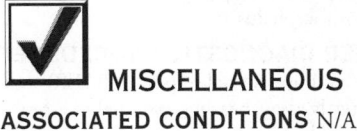

MISCELLANEOUS

ASSOCIATED CONDITIONS N/A

AGE RELATED FACTORS

Congenital cardiac or respiratory abnormalities are usually the cause of cyanosis in the young.

ZOONOTIC POTENTIAL N/A

PREGNANCY

• Advanced pregnancy can exacerbate symptomatology because of pressure on the diaphragm and reduced lung expansion.
• Fetuses are likely to be harmed by the hypoxemia associated with cyanosis.

SYNONYMS N/A

SEE ALSO

Causes

ABBREVIATIONS

DCM = dilated cardiomyopathy
PDA = patent ductus arteriosus
VSD = ventricular septal defect
ASD = atrial septal defect
PCV = packed cell volume
HCM = hypertrophic cardiomyopathy
R-L = right-to-left

Reference

Jacobs G. Cyanosis. In: Ettinger SJ, Feldman EC, eds. Textbook of veterinary internal medicine. 4th ed. Philadelphia: WB Saunders, 1995;192-196.

Author James C. Prueter
Consulting Editors Lynelle Johnson and Bradley L. Moses

DEAFNESS

BASICS

DEFINITION
Lack or loss of sense of hearing, complete or partial.

Pathophysiology
• Caused by either conduction deafness or nerve deafness • Conduction deafness is caused by diseases that obliterate the external ear canal, rupture the tympanum, or interfere with the function of the ear ossicles in the middle ear. • Nerve deafness is caused by acquired or congenital disease. • Congenital deafness is caused by degeneration, hypoplasia, or aplasia of the spiral organ. • Acquired nerve deafness is caused by destruction of the normal inner ear structures. Note: for brainstem disease to cause deafness, extensive damage to auditory pathways is necessary, and such lesions would produce severe neurologic deficits from interference with the other systems adjacent to the auditory pathways.

Systems Affected
Nervous—inner ear

SIGNALMENT
• Congenital deafness—very young age with more than 20 dog breeds now known to be predisposed (Table 1) and white cats with blue iris • Acquired deafness—any age; more common in geriatric dogs

SIGNS
General Comments
Unilateral deafness is difficult for most owners to ascertain; therefore, most animals examined because of this problem have bilateral deafness. Conduction deafness usually causes relatively small hearing losses.

Historical Findings
Owners may notice that their pet no longer responds to everyday sounds, does not respond to its name, cannot be aroused from sleep by a loud noise, and if a puppy, does not respond to the sounds of "squeaky" toys.

CAUSES
Conduction Deafness
• Otitis externa and other external ear canal disease such as stenosis of the canal, neoplasia, or ruptured tympanum • Otitis media

Nerve Deafness
• Degenerative changes in the cochlea of an old dog • Anatomic—hypoplasia or aplasia of the spiral organ; hydrocephalus caused by damage to the auditory cortex • Neoplastic—acoustic neuroma, neurofibroma, and neurofibrosarcoma • Inflammatory and infectious—otitis interna; canine distemper virus can cause alterations in hearing (not complete deafness); in cats, naso-pharyngeal polyps invading inner ear • Trauma

Toxins and Drugs
• Antibiotics—aminoglycosides, polymixin B, erythromycin, vancomycin, chloramphenicol • Antiseptics—ethanol, chlorhexidine, cetrimide • Antineoplastics—cisplatin • Diuretics—furosemide • Heavy metals—arsenic, lead, mercury • Miscellaneous—ceruminolytic agents, propylene glycol, salicylates

RISK FACTORS
• Chronic otitis externa, media, or interna • Merle, piebald gene, or white coat color • Use of certain drugs

DIAGNOSIS

DIFFERENTIAL DIAGNOSIS
• Must attempt to differentiate causes of deafness • History of early age onset usually suggests congenital causes in predisposed breeds • Inquire about the use of ototoxic drug • Inquire about presence of chronic ear disease • Physical examination to assess status of external ear canal and tympanum • Neurologic examination to assess for signs of hydrocephalus or canine distemper

CBC/BIOCHEMISTRY/URINALYSIS
Results usually normal

OTHER LABORATORY TESTS
Bacterial culture and sensitivy testing of ear canal if patient has otitis externa, media, or interna

IMAGING
• Tympanic bullae and skull radiography to detect otitis media or otitis interna • Ultrasonography through open fontanelles to detect hydrocephalus

OTHER DIAGNOSTIC PROCEDURES
Brain auditory evoked response (BAER)—to objectively assess hearing; essential to assess unilateral hearing loss and to select breeding dogs

TREATMENT
• Directed toward acquired causes because congenital deafness is irreversible
• Treat existing otitis externa, media, or interna with medical or surgical approaches on the basis of culture and sensitivity test results and radiographic findings.
• Conduction deafness may improve as otitis externa or media resolves.

MEDICATIONS

DRUGS AND FLUIDS
None specific for deafness; only those used to treat otitis externa, media, and interna

CONTRAINDICATIONS N/A

PRECAUTIONS
• Use aminoglycosides or other ototoxic drugs with caution to prevent additional damage or damage to the normal side if one exists.
• Avoid topical treatment of external ear canal if tympanic membrane is ruptured.

POSSIBLE INTERACTIONS N/A

ALTERNATE DRUGS
Hearing aids have been used. Modifications of apparatus are needed to make their use more practical.

FOLLOW-UP

PATIENT MONITORING
• Weekly to assess treatment of ear disease until resolved. • BAER can be used to assess response to treatment of otitis interna.

POSSIBLE COMPLICATIONS
Patient's environment may have to be controlled for its protection

MISCELLANEOUS

ASSOCIATED CONDITIONS N/A
AGE RELATED FACTORS N/A
ZOONOTIC POTENTIAL N/A
PREGNANCY N/A
SYNONYMS N/A
SEE ALSO Otitis media-interna
ABBREVIATION
BAER = brainstem auditory evoked response

References
Braund KG. Clinical syndromes in veterinary neurology. 2nd ed. St. Louis: Mosby, 1994:100-102.

Hayes HM, et al. Canine congenital deafness: epidemiologic study of 272 cases. J Am Anim Hosp Assoc 1981;17:473-476.

Mansfield PD. Ototoxicity in dogs and cats. Compend Cont Ed Pract Vet 1990;112:331-337.

Marshall AE. Hearing loss in aged dogs. Adv Small Anim Med Surg 1990;2:6.

Oliver JE, Lorenz MD. Handbook of veterinary neurology. 2nd ed. Philadelphia: WB Saunders, 1993:216.

Strain GM. Congenital deafness in dogs and cats. Compend Cont Ed Pract Vet 1991;13:245-254.

Strain GM, et al. Brainstem auditory-evoked potential assessment of congenital deafness in dalmatians: associations with phenotypic markers. J Vet Int Med 1992;5:175-182.

Author Dr. T. Mark Neer
Consulting Editor Joane M. Parent

Table 1

Breeds with Reported Congenital Deafness

Akita	Fox terrier
American Staffordshire terrier	Great Dane
Australian heeler	Great Pyrenees
Australian shepherd	Maltese
Beagle	Miniature poodle
Border collie	Mongrel
Boston terrier	Norwegian dunkerhound
Bullterrier	Old English sheepdog
Catahoula leopard dog	Papillon
Cocker spaniel	Pointer
Collie	Rhodesian Ridgeback
Dalmatian	Scottish terrier
Dappled dachshund	Sealyham terrier
Doberman pinscher	Shetland sheepdog
Dogo Argentino	Shropshire terrier
English bulldog	Walker American foxhound
English setter	West Highland white terrier
Foxhound	

DERMATOSES, EROSIVE-ULCERATIVE

 BASICS

DEFINITION
Skin conditions characterized by the presence of erosions and/or ulcers. Erosions signify cavitation into the epidermis. Ulcers are cavitations that compromise the dermal-epidermal junction.

PATHOPHYSIOLOGY
Pathomechanism is related to causative factors that interfere with the integrity of the epidermis or dermis, and includes faulty development, destruction and displacement, acute loss of dermal/epidermal tissue, irritation and self-trauma, leukocytic activity, invasion and weakening of the epidermis and/or dermis, necrosis and fibrosis of tissue, toxic reactions, and immune-mediated responses.

Systems Affected Skin/Exocrine

SIGNALMENT
Age, breed, and sex predisposition varies with each individual condition causing the erosive-ulcerative dermatosis

CAUSES
• Genetics (e.g., epitheliogenesis imperfecta, cutaneous asthenia, ectodermal defect
• Microbial infections (including pyodermas, cat pox, systemic mycoses, mycetoma)
• Parasites (including fleas, demodicosis, sarcoptic mange, leishmaniasis) • Neoplastic and paraneoplastic syndromes (e.g., squamous-cell carcinoma, Bowen's Disease)
• Physical and chemical factors (e.g., trauma, skin-fold pyoderma, contact eruptions)
• Immune-mediated disorders (e.g., pemphigus, pemphigoid, lupus erythematosus, cutaneous vasculitis) • Toxic syndromes (e.g., drug eruption, toxic epidermal necrolysis)
• Therapeutic agents (especially corticosteroids, contact irritants) • Secondary to disorders of other systems • Miscellaneous (e.g., indolent ulcer, feline hyperadrenocorticism)

RISK FACTORS
Risk factors vary with each of the different causes of erosive-ulcerative dermatosis

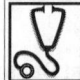 DIAGNOSIS

DIFFERENTIAL DIAGNOSIS

Parasites
• Fleas • Demodicosis • Sarcoptic mange
• Notoedric mange • Leishmaniasis

Microbes
• Bacterial Pyoderma • Skin-fold pyoderma
• Pyotraumatic dermatitis • Perianal pyoderma • Dermatophytosis • Systemic mycoses
• Cat Pox Infection • Bacterial granuloma
• Mycetoma • Atypical mycobacteriosis
• Sporotrichosis • Feline immunodeficiency virus (FIV) infection

Immune-Mediated
• Pemphigus • Pemphigoid • Lupus erythematosus • Lupoid dermatosis • Cutaneous vasculitis

Toxic Syndromes
• Drug eruption • Toxic epidermal necrolysis
• Erythema multiforme majus • Thallium intoxication • Septicemia/toxemia

Neoplastic/Paraneoplastic Syndromes
• Squamous-cell carcinoma • Bowen's disease
• Cutaneous T-cell lymphoma

Genetic Conditions
• Cutaneous asthenia • Dermatomyositis
• Epitheliogenesis imperfecta • Ectodermal defect

Miscellaneous
• Burns • Contact eruptions • Indolent ulcer
• Vesiculopustular dermatoses

CBC/BIOCHEMISTRY/URINALYSIS
For any animal that seems systemically ill, the minimum data base should be extended to include hemogram and serum biochemistries

OTHER LABORATORY TESTS
Special laboratory tests may be indicated based on the results of more conventional assessments.

IMAGING
• Rarely needed but radiographs of the chest may be helpful when systemic mycoses are suspected • Radiographs may also help confirm hyperadrenocorticism in patients with tissue mineralization or enlarged adrenals.

OTHER DIAGNOSTIC PROCEDURES
• Varies with specific cause of the erosive-ulcerative dermatosis • In all cases, minimum data base should include skin scrapings and cytological evaluation (usually impression smear). • Additional tests that may be warranted include biopsies for histopathologic and immunopathologic assessment and microbial cultures (aerobic, anaerobic, fungal).

 TREATMENT

• Treat as outpatient unless there is some evidence of life-threatening systemic disease
• Treatment must be individualized and based on underlying cause
• Not all cases of erosive-ulcerative dermatosis respond to therapy (e.g., ectodermal defect, cutaneous asthenia).

MEDICATIONS

DRUGS AND FLUIDS

• Varies with underlying cause • Fluid therapy is indicated where there has been extensive transdermal fluid loss

CONTRAINDICATIONS N/A

PRECAUTIONS

Drugs that have adverse systemic effects (e.g., immunosuppressive agents, cancer chemotherapy, antimony)

POSSIBLE INTERACTIONS N/A

ALTERNATE DRUGS N/A

 FOLLOW-UP

PATIENT MONITORING

• Patient monitoring varies with each cause of erosive-ulcerative dermatosis. • For outpatients with systemic disease, monitoring should be done on at least a twice-weekly basis until the condition is completely in remission. • Patients with microbial or parasitic disorders should be reevaluated in 14 days to evaluate treatment efficacy. • Animals with systemic disease warranting intravenous fluid therapy are obviously candidates for inpatient care

POSSIBLE COMPLICATIONS

Some conditions can be potentially fatal (e.g., systemic lupus erythematosus, drug eruption, septicemia); most are not.

 MISCELLANEOUS

ASSOCIATED CONDITIONS N/A

AGE RELATED FACTORS N/A

ZOONOTIC POTENTIAL

• Fleas, sarcoptic mange, and notoedric mange are transmissible to people • Mycobacterial infections, sporotrichosis, and other infections are also zoonotic

PREGNANCY N/A

SYNONYMS N/A

SEE ALSO

• Demodicosis • Fleas • Sarcoptic mange • Dermatomyositis • Pyoderma • Systemic lupus erythematosus • Lupus erythematosus, cutaneous (discoid) • Pemphigus • Pemphigoid • Sporotrichosis

ABBREVIATIONS

FIV = feline immunodeficiency virus

References

Ackerman L. Pet skin and haircoat problems: tests and treatments. Trenton, NJ: Veterinary Learning Systems, 1993.

Nesbitt GH, Ackerman LJ. Dermatology for the small animal practitioner. Trenton, NJ: Veterinary Learning Systems, 1991.

Author Lowell Ackerman

Consulting Editor Lowell Ackerman

DERMATOSES, EXFOLIATIVE

BASICS

DEFINITION
Excessive or abnormal shedding of epidermal cells resulting in the clinical presentaton of cutaneous scaling. Clinically significant exfoliation is a clinical sign, not a diagnosis.

Pathophysiology
• An increase in the production, an increase in the desquamation, or a decrease in the cohesion of keratinocytes results in abnormal shedding of epidermal cells individually (fine scale) and in sheets (coarse scale). • Primary exfoliative disorders include keratinization defects, in which the genetic control of epidermal cell proliferation and maturation is abnormal. • Secondary exfoliative disorders result from the affects of disease states on the normal maturation and proliferation of epidermal cells.

SYSTEMS AFFECTED
Skin/Exocrine—Epidermal tissues, including nails.

SIGNALMENT
• Primary keratinization disorders become apparent by two years of age and are characteristic in affected breeds (see causes). • Secondary causes of scaling may be seen in any breed of dog or cat.

SIGNS

Historical Findings
Excessive scaling, malodorous skin, and pruritus are frequently reported.

Physical Examination Findings
• Dry or greasy accumulations of fine scale or coarse rafts of epidermal cells may be located diffusely throughout the hair coat or focally in keratinaceous plaques. A "rancid fat" odor is common. • Comedones, follicular casts (accumulation of adherent debris around the hair shaft), alopecia, pruritus and secondary pyoderma occur frequently. Malassezia overgrowth is an infrequent finding.

CAUSES

Primary Causes
• Primary idiopathic seborrhea (primary keratinization disorder)—a primary cellular defect resulting in accelerated epidermopoiesis and hyperproliferation of the seborrheic epidermis, follicular infundibulum, and sebaceous gland has been identified in some breeds. Breeds at highest risk include the cocker and springer spaniel, West Highland white terrier, basset hound, Doberman pinscher, Irish setter, and Labrador retriever. Both dry (sicca) and greasy (oleosa) forms exist, but determination of type has little prognostic value. • Vitamin A-responsive dermatosis—nutritionally-responsive exfoliative disorder seen primarily in the young cocker spaniel. Clinical signs are similar to those for idiopathic seborrhea, and the syndrome is

distinguished by the response to dietary vitamin A supplementation. • Zinc-responsive dermatosis—nutritionally-responsive exfoliative disorder resulting in alopecia, scaling, crusting, and erythema around the eyes, ears, feet, lips, and other external orifices. Two syndromes are recognized: young adult dogs, especially Siberian huskies and Alaskan malamutes, and rapidly-growing, large-breed puppies. • Ectodermal defects—follicular dysplasias, seen as color mutant or dilution alopecia, represent abnormalities of melanization of the hair shaft and structural hair growth. Blue and fawn colors of Doberman pinschers, Irish setters, dachshunds, chow chows, Yorkshire terriers, poodles, great Danes, whippets, salukis, and Italian greyhounds are commonly affected. Signs include the failure to regrow blue or fawn hair with normal "point" hair growth, excessive scaliness, comedone formation, and secondary pyoderma. • Idiopathic nasodigital hyperkeratosis - Excessive accumulation of scale and crusts on the nasal planum and footpad margins, often of middle-aged spaniels. Lesions are generally asymptomatic unless severe enough to result in cracking and secondary bacterial infection. • Sebaceous adenitis—an inflammatory disease most often seen in middle-aged standard poodles, akitas, and samoyeds. The disease appears distinctly different and granulomatous in the Vizsla. Characteristic diffuse hair loss and excessive scaling with tightly adherent follicular casts occur. With the exception of the akita, most dogs are generally healthy and asymptomatic. The akita frequently develops severe and deep bacterial pyoderma. • Epidermal dysplasia and ichthyosis—rare and severe congenital disorders of keratinization reported in West Highland white terriers and seen as generalized accumulations of scale and crusts at an early age. Secondary infections (bacterial and yeast) are common and the prognosis in severe cases is poor.

Secondary Causes
• Cutaneous hypersensitivity—atopy, flea allergic dermatitis, food allergy, and contact dermatitis produce pruritus and resultant skin trauma and irritation. • Ectoparasitism such as scabies, demodicosis, and cheyletiellosis produce inflammation and exfoliation. • Pyoderma—skin infection produces both bacterial enzymatic mellitus, may also be associated with excessive scaling. • Auto-immune skin diseases, such as pemphigus foliaceus, may appear exfoliative due to rupturing of fragile vesicles and secondary pyoderma. • Dermatophytosis is commonly exfoliative. Increased shedding of affected keratinocytes is a primary skin mechanism in resolving fungal infection. Increased epidermal turnover is also a result of the accompanying inflammation.

Endocrinopathy
• Hypothyroidism and hyperadrenocorticism commonly produce excessive scaling. Thyroid

hormone is critical for normal keratinization, hair growth, and sebum production. Inadequate levels of thyroid hormones result in abnormalities in keratinization, failure to regrow hair, and excessive sebum production. Hypercortisolism interferes with normal keratinization and reduces follicular activity. Secondary pyoderma is common in both syndromes. • Sex hormone abnormalities and diabetes melitus may also be associated with excessive scaling.

RISK FACTORS N/A

DIAGNOSIS

DIFFERENTIAL DIAGNOSIS
• Signalment and history are paramount in distinguishing the possible causes of exfoliation. • The presence or absence of pruritus can assist in determining the possibility of cutaneous hypersensitivity. Primary keratinization defects are often non-pruritic unless secondary pyoderma develops. • Concurrent signs such as lethargy, weight gain, polyuria/polydypsia, reproductive failure, change in body conformation, and lack of hair regrowth, with or without inflammation, can assist in differentiation.

CBC/BIOCHEMISTRY/URINALYSIS
• Routine hemogram, serum chemistry profile, and urinalysis are normal with primary keratinization disorders. • Mild, non-regenerative anemia and hypercholesteremia are consistent with hypothyroidism. • Neutrophilia, monocytosis, eosinopenia, lymphopenia, high serum alkaline phosphatase, hypercholesterolemia, and hyposthenuria are suggestive of hyperadrenocorticism.

OTHER LABORATORY TESTS
• Measurement of basal T_4 is the most common method of evaluation for hypothyroidism. Levels below laboratory normals, in the absence of concurrent illness which might produce a sick euthyroid condition, and in the presence of appropriate clinical signs can be diagnostic. Significance of T_3 and antithyroid antibodies, and calculation of the K-value are controversial. A TSH-stimulation test may be performed to diagnose hypothyroidism. • ACTH-stimulation test or low-dose dexamethasone-suppression test should be performed to diagnose hyperadrenocorticism. A urine cortisol-creatinine ratio can be used to help rule out hyperadrenocorticism, but has a high false-positive rate.

IMAGING N/A

OTHER DIAGNOSTIC PROCEDURES
• Skin scrapings should be performed to diagnose ectoparasitism. • Skin biopsy is often helpful to rule in or rule out a particular differential diagnosis. Histopathologic interpretation by a qualified dermatopathologist is highly recommended. • Intradermal skin

testing or a food elimination trial is performed to diagnose atopy or food allergy, respectively. • Epidermal exudate preparations may be used to determine the type of microflora present on the skin.

TREATMENT

• Frequent and appropriate topical therapy is the cornerstone of proper treatment.
• Underbathing, rather than overbathing, is a common treatment error. • Diagnosis and control of all treatable primary and secondary diseases is required.
• Maintenance of control is often lifelong. Recurrence of secondary pyodermas, etc., may require repeated therapy and further diagnostics.

MEDICATIONS

Shampoos

• Contact time of 10-15 minutes is required for adequate epidermal hydration and shampoo effect.
• Hypoallergenic shampoos (soap-free) are useful only in mild cases of dry scale and to maintain secondary exfoliation after the primary disease has been controlled.
• Sulfur/salicylic acid shampoos are keratolytic, keratoplastic, and bacteriostatic. They are an excellent first choice for the moderately scaley patient and are not overly drying.
• Benzoyl peroxide shampoos are strongly keratolytic, antimicrobial, and follicle-flushing. Irritation and severe dryness can occur. Benzoyl peroxide is best used for animals with recurrent bacterial infection or extreme greasiness.
• Ethyl lactate shampoos are newer and are reported to be as anti-grease and follicle-flushing as benzoyl peroxide without the irritation and extreme dryness associated with benzoyl peroxide. Experience with their use in animals is limited.
• Tar shampoos are keratolytic, keratoplastic and anti-pruritic. They are degreasing, but less so than benzoyl peroxides. Tar shampoos should be used in animals with moderate scale associated with pruritus.

Moisturizers

• The frequent shampooing necessary to remove excessive scale formation can result in excessive dryness and discomfort. Moisturizers

are excellent products to restore skin hydration and also to increase effectiveness of subsequent shampooings.
• Humectants encourage hydration of the stratum corneum by attracting water from the dermis. At high concentrations, humectants can be keratolytic.
• Emollients coat the skin and therefore smooth the roughened surfaces produced by excessive scaling. They are usually combined with occlusives to encourage hydration of the epidermis.

Systemic Therapy

• Specific etiologies for exfoliative disorders each require specific treatments, e.g. thyroxine replacement for hypothyroidism; or zinc supplements for zinc-responsive dermatosis.
• Systemic antibiotics are always indicated when secondary pyoderma is present (see discussion of pyoderma). • Idiopathic or primary seborrhea has been treated with retinoid drugs with limited success. The vitamin A analogs Etretinate and Isotretinoin have been used in limited studies. Results have indicated individual response to retinoids (especially cocker spaniels with a primary keratinization defect). In general, however, all dogs studied improved with the use of topical therapy more than they benefitted from retinoid administration. It is recommended that patients be referred to a dermatologist prior to being treated with these experimental drugs.

DRUGS AND FLUIDS N/A

CONTRAINDICATIONS N/A

PRECAUTIONS

Corticosteroids may be used judiciously to control the inflammation resulting from many exfoliative disorders. However, these drugs will mask signs of pyoderma and prevent accurate diagnosis of primary disease.

POSSIBLE INTERACTIONS N/A

ALTERNATE DRUGS N/A

FOLLOW-UP

PATIENT MONITORING

• Rechecks at three-week intervals are recommended for monitoring response to antibiotics as well as topical therapy. • Seasonal changes, development of additional diseases (especially cutaneous hypersensitivity), and recurrence of pyoderma may cause previously

controlled patients to worsen. Reevaluation is critical to determine if new factors are involved and whether changes in therapy are necessary. • Routine 4-6 hour post-pill thyroid monitoring or ACTH-stimulation test results should be utilized for proper management of endocrinopathies. • Autoimmune disorders require frequent reevaluations during the initial phase of induction, and then less often after remission is achieved.

POSSIBLE COMPLICATIONS N/A

MISCELLANEOUS

ASSOCIATED CONDITIONS N/A

AGE RELATED FACTORS N/A

ZOONOTIC POTENTIAL

Dermatophytosis and several ectoparasites have either zoonotic potential or the ability to produce human lesions. Owners of animals with these diseases should be advised appropriately.

PREGNANCY

• Sulfonamide antibiotics and chloramphenicol, should not be used in the pregnant animal. • Systemic retinoids as well as vitamin A in therapeutic dosages should not be used in the intact female because of their severe and predictable teratogenicity and their extremely long withdrawal period.

SYNONYMS

Keratinization disorders are commonly referred to as seborrhea, idiopathic seborrhea, keratinization defect, and dyskeratinization, as well as by the incorrect human terms "eczema" and "psoriasis."

SEE ALSO

• Pyoderma • Malassezia Dermatitis
• Allergy • Auto-immune Disorders
• Ectoparasitism • Endocrinopathies

ABBREVIATIONS N/A

References
Griffin CE, Kwochka KW, Macdonald JM. Current veterinary dermatology: the science and art of therapy. St. Louis: Mosby Year Book, 1993.
Author Alexander H. Werner
Consulting Editor Lowell Ackerman

DERMATOSES, PAPULONODULAR

 BASICS

DEFINITION
This category includes diseases whose primary lesions may manifest as papules and nodules. Papules and nodules are solid, elevated lesions of the skin.

PATHOPHYSIOLOGY
• Papules are usually formed due to tissue infiltration by inflammatory cells with accompanying intraepidermal edema or epidermal hyperplasia and dermal edema. • Nodules, which are larger than papules, usually are a result of a massive infiltration of inflammatory cells into the dermis or subcutis.

SYSTEMS AFFECTED
Skin/Exocrine

SIGNALMENT
Any age, breed, or sex

CAUSES
Superficial and deep bacterial folliculitis, dermatophytosis, sebaceous adenitis, sterile eosinophilic pustulosis, canine and feline acne, kerions, demodicosis, rhabditic dermatitis, and actinic conditions

RISK FACTORS
• Any disease or medication that causes immune compromise can predispose animals to folliculitis, dermatophytosis, and demodicosis. • Rhabditic dermatitis may be associated with contact with decaying organic debris (straw or hay) containing Pelodera strongyloides. • Actinic conditions are seen more frequently in outdoor, short-haired dogs living in areas with ample sunlight.

 DIAGNOSIS

DIFFERENTIAL DIAGNOSIS
See causes. These diseases can be most easily differentiated based on the following diagnostic tests.

CBC/BIOCHEMISTRY/URINALYSIS
Complete blood count, chemistry screen, and urinalysis should all be within normal range in most patients. A circulating eosinophilia may be present with sterile eosinophilic pustulosis.

OTHER LABORATORY TESTS N/A
IMAGING N/A

OTHER DIAGNOSTIC PROCEDURES
• Skin scrapings should be done to identify possible demodex mites or rhabditiform larvae. • Dermatophyte cultures should be done to identify possible dermatophytosis. • Tzanck preparations should be done to determine if bacteria and degenerative neutrophils are present. This would be compatible with bacterial folliculitis. If eosinophils

are detected, eosinophilic pustulosis or furunculosis is more likely. • Skin biopsy should be done if none of these tests have revealed a definitive diagnosis.

 TREATMENT

• Nearly all causes of this disorder can be treated as outpatients.
• A patient with generalized demodicosis and secondary sepsis would need to be hospitalized.
• Additionally, alteration of activity or diet should not be necessary.

 MEDICATIONS

DRUGS AND FLUIDS

Bacterial Folliculitis
Appropriate antibiotics based on bacterial culture and sensitivity should be given for 3-4 weeks with superficial pyoderma or 6-8 weeks or more with deep pyoderma.

Dermatophytosis
See appropriate section

Sebaceous Adenitis
• First, a 50-75% mixture of propylene glycol and water may be applied once daily as a spray to affected areas. Alternatively, bathing and soaking in baby oil weekly is another option.
• Second, essential fatty acid dietary supplements have been given q12h PO in addition to evening primrose oil (500 mg) q12h PO.
• In refractory cases, isotretinoin may be tried at a dosage of 1 mg/kg q12h-q24h PO. If response is seen, then taper to 1 mg/kg q48h or 0.5 mg/kg q24h.
• Cyclosporine has also been used at a dosage of 5 mg/kg q12h PO.
• Most cases are refractory to corticosteroids.

Sterile Eosinophilic Pustulosis
Prednisolone/prednisone should be used at a dosage of 2.2 to 4.4 mg/kg q24h and then tapered to an alternate day low dosage.

Canine Acne
This may resolve without therapy in mild cases. In more severe cases, benzoyl peroxide shampoos and gels can be used every 24 hours until the lesions are resolved and then as needed. Mupirocin is a topical antibiotic that can be applied every 24 hours or alternated with the benzoyl peroxide therapies. If the acne is recurrent or a very deep infection (furunculosis), then systemic antibiotics and warm water soaks will be necessary. In very refractory cases, topical tretinoin can be applied every 12 hours or isotretinoin PO may be tried at 1-2 mg/kg q24h.

Feline Acne
• An underlying cause should be sought and treated accordingly. If no underlying cause is found, either Stridex pads or benzoyl peroxide gels should be used daily. These can also be alternated daily. Cats can be sensitive to the irritant effects of benzoyl peroxide.
• In refractory patients, systemic antibiotics should be attempted.

Kerion
See section on dermatophytes

Demodicosis
See section on demodicosis

Rhabditic Dermatitis
Bedding should be removed and destroyed. Kennels, beds, or cages should be washed and treated with a premise insecticide or flea spray. Bathe the patient and remove crusts. Then apply a parasiticidal dip at least 2 times at weekly intervals. If a severe infection is present, antibiotics may be necessary.

Actinic Conditions
• Avoid the sun between 10 AM and 4 PM. Sunscreens are also beneficial to filter harmful ultraviolet light. These should have an SPF of 15 or higher and be applied every 12 hours. If inflammation is severe, topical or systemic corticosteroids may provide comfort. Topical corticosteroids of 1-2.5% hydrocortisone are usually sufficient. Prednisone systemically administered may be commenced at 1 mg/kg PO for 3-5 days. If secondary infection is present, antibiotics may be necessary.
• If squamous cell carcinoma has developed, the prognosis is guarded to poor depending on the stage of the disease. Specific therapy for squamous cell carcinoma may include synthetic retinoids, hyperthermia, cryosurgery, photochemotherapy, radiation therapy, and surgical excision.

CONTRAINDICATIONS
Corticosteroids and other immune suppressants should be avoided in cases of folliculitis, dermatophytosis, kerions and demodicosis.

PRECAUTIONS
• Fatty acids should be used with caution in dogs with inflammatory bowel disease or recurrent bouts of pancreatitis.
• Isotretinoin may cause keratoconjunctivitis sicca, hyperactivity, ear pruritus, erythematous mucocutaneous junction, lethargy with vomiting, abdominal distension and erythema, anorexia with lethargy, collapse, and swollen tongue. Complete blood count and chemistry screen abnormalities include high platelet count, hypertriglyceridemia, hypercholesterolemia, and high alanine transaminase.
• Cyclosporine may cause vomiting and diarrhea, gingival hyperplasia, B-lymphocyte hyperplasia, hirsutism, papillomatous skin lesions, and high incidence of infection. Potential toxic reactions include nephrotoxicity and hepatotoxicity.

DERMATOSES, PAPULONODULAR

POSSIBLE INTERACTIONS N/A

ALTERNATE DRUGS N/A

FOLLOW-UP

PATIENT MONITORING

• Monitor complete blood count, chemistry screen and urinalysis monthly for 4-6 months in patients receiving cyclosporine and synthetic retinoid therapy. Tear production should be monitored monthly for 4-6 months, then every 6 months in patients receiving synthetic retinoid therapy. • In patients with demodicosis, skin scrapings are used to monitor therapy. In patients with dermatophytosis, repeat fungal cultures are used to monitor therapy. These are discussed more fully in their respective sections. • Sebaceous adenitis and actinic conditions are monitored via resolution of lesions. All other diseases are monitored by resolution of lesions.

POSSIBLE COMPLICATIONS

Actinic conditions may progress to squamous cell carcinoma.

MISCELLANEOUS

ASSOCIATED CONDITIONS N/A

AGE RELATED FACTORS N/A

ZOONOTIC POTENTIAL

Dermatophytosis is contagious to humans in 30-50% of cases of Microsporum canis.

PREGNANCY

• Synthetic retinoids should not be used in pregnant animals, animals intended for reproduction, or intact animals. Synthetic retinoids should also not be used by women of childbearing age. These medications are very teratogenic. • Corticosteroids should not be used in pregnant animals.

SYNONYMS N/A

SEE ALSO

Pyoderma, Dermatophytosis, Demodicosis

ABBREVIATIONS N/A

References

Griffin CE, Kwochka KW, MacDonald JM, eds. Current veterinary dermatology. St. Louis: Mosby Year Book, 1993.

Gross TL, Ihrke PJ, Walder EJ. Veterinary dermatopatholgy. St. Louis: Mosby Year Book, 1992.

Mueller GH, Kirk RW, Scott DW, eds. Small animal dermatology. 4th ed. Philadelphia: WB Saunders, 1989.

Author Karen A. Kuhl

Consulting Editor Lowell Ackerman

DERMATOSES, VESICULOPUSTULAR

BASICS

DEFINITION
• Pustule—a small, circumscribed elevation of the epidermis filled with pus • Vesicle—a small, circumscribed elevation of the epidermis filled with clear fluid • Pustules and vesicles may be produced by edema, acantholysis (pemphigus), ballooning degeneration (viral infections), proteolytic enzymes from neutrophils (pyoderma), degeneration of basal cells (lupus), or dermoepidermal separation (bullous pemphigoid).

SYSTEMS AFFECTED
• Multiple systems with systemic lupus erythematosus • Skin/Exocrine—integument and muscle with dermatomyositis

SIGNALMENT
• Lupus—collies, shelties and German shepherds may be predisposed • Pemphygus (P.) erythematosus—collies and German shepherds may be predisposed • Pemphigus foliaceus—Akitas, chow chows, dachshunds, bearded collies, Newfoundlands, Ddoberman pinschers, and schipperkes may be predisposed • Bullous pemphigoid—collies and Doberman pinschers may be predisposed • Dermatomyositis—young collies and shelties • Subcorneal pustular dermatosis—schnauzers affected most frequently • Linear IgA dermatosis—dachshunds exclusively • Dermatophytosis—young animals

SIGNS N/A

CAUSES
Pustules
• Superficial pyoderma—impetigo, superficial spreading pyoderma, superficial bacterial folliculitis, acne • Pemphigus complex—P. foliaceus, P. erythematosus, P. vegetans • Subcorneal pustular dermatosis • Dermatophytosis • Sterile eosinophilic pustulosis • Linear IgA dermatosis

Vesicles
• Systemic lupus erythematosus (SLE)
• Discoid lupus erythematosus (DLE)
• Bullous pemphigoid • Pemphigus vulgaris
• Dermatomyositis

RISK FACTORS
• SLE and bullous pemphigoid may be precipitated by drug exposure • Pyodermas are usually secondary to a predisposing factor such as demodicosis, hypothyroidism, allergy, or steroid administration • P. erythematosus, bullous pemphigoid, SLE, DLE and dermatomyositis may be exacerbated by sunlight

DIAGNOSIS

DIFFERENTIAL DIAGNOSIS
PUSTULAR
• Superficial pyodermas are the most common cause of pustular skin disease and readily respond to appropriate antibiotic therapy providing the underlying cause is effectively managed. Direct smear from intact pustule reveals neutrophils engulfing bacteria. Culture of an intact pustule usually yields Staph. intermedius. Biopsy shows intraepidermal neutrophilic pustules or folliculitis. • The pemphigus complex is a group of immune-mediated diseases characterized histologically by acantholysis. Direct smears reveal many acanthocytes, nondegenerate neutrophils, and no bacteria. Culture of an intact pustule is negative. Direct immuno-fluorescence (DIF) shows deposits in the intercellular spaces of the epidermis. Disease tends to wax and wane irrespective of antibiotic therapy, but responds to immunosuppressive therapy. • Subcorneal pustular dermatosis is a rare, idiopathic, pustular dermatosis of dogs that tends to wax and wane. Direct smears from intact pustules reveal numerous neutrophils, no bacteria, and occasional acanthocytes. Cultures from intact pustules are negative. DIF is negative. Poor response to glucocorticoids and antibiotics. • Dermatophytosis is a common disease of both dogs and cats. Dermatophyte culture is positive. Secondary bacterial infection is common. Biopsy reveals folliculitis with fungal elements. • Sterile eosinophilic pustulosis is a rare, idiopathic dermatosis of dogs. Direct smears reveal numerous eosinophils, nondegenerate neutrophils, occasional acanthocytes and no bacteria. Biopsy shows eosinophilic intraepidermal pustules, folliculitis and furunculosis. DIF is negative. Rapid response to glucocorticoids. • Linear IgA dermatosis is a rare, idiopathic dermatosis of dachshunds. Pustules are sterile and subcorneal. DIF is positive for IgA at the basement membrane zone. Tends to wax and wane.

VESICLES/ULCERATION
• Systemic lupus erythematosus is a multisystemic disease with variable clinical signs and cutaneus manifestations including mucocutaneous ulceration. DIF is positive at the basement membrane zone. ANA positive.
• Discoid lupus erythematosus affects only the skin and lesions are usually confined to the face. Depigmentation, erythema and ulceration of the nasal planum is common. Biopsy reveals interface dermatitis. DIF is positive at the basement membrane zone. ANA negative. • Bullous pemphigoid is an ulcerative disorder of the skin and/or mucous membranes. Biopsy shows subepidermal cleft formation and positive DIF at the basement membrane zone. Acantholysis is not seen. • Pemphigus vulgaris is the most severe form of pemphigus and is characterized by ulceration of the oral cavity, mucocutaneous junctions and skin. Biopsy shows suprabasilar acantholysis and cleft formation. DIF is positive at the intercellular spaces of the epidermis. • Dermatomyositis is an idiopathic inflammatory disease of the skin and muscle of young collies and shelties. Lesions affect the face, ear tips, tail tip, and pressure points of the extremities. Alopecia, crusting, pigmentation disturbances, erosions/ulceration, and scarring are characteristic. Biopsy reveals follicular atrophy, perifolliculitis, and hydropic degeneration of the basal cells. DIF negative. Muscle biopsy and EMG show evidence of muscle inflammation.

CBC/BIOCHEMISTRY/URINALYSIS
Hemogram, serum chemistries and urinalysis are usually unremarkable. Anemia, thrombocytopenia or glomerulonephritis may be present in SLE. Most dogs with eosinophilic pustular dermatosis have peripheral eosinophilia.

OTHER LABORATORY TESTS N/A
IMAGING N/A
OTHER DIAGNOSTIC PROCEDURES
• Direct smear from intact pustule • Culture of intact pustule • Biopsy for histopathology • DIF including IgA • ANA • EMG • Muscle biopsy

TREATMENT
• Periodic bathing with an antimicrobial shampoo will help remove surface debris and control secondary bacterial infections.
• Usually treated as an outpatient except for SLE, pemphigus vulgaris, and bullous pemphigoid which may be life threatening and require intensive care.

MEDICATIONS

DRUGS AND FLUIDS
Subcorneal Pustular Dermatosis
• Dapsone—1 mg/kg PO q8h until remission (usually 1-4 weeks) and then tapered to 1 mg/kg q24h or twice weekly.
• Sulfasalazine (Azulfidine)—10-20 mg/kg PO q8h until remission, then as needed.

Sterile Eosinophilic Pustulosis
Prednisolone—2.2-4.4 mg/kg PO q24h until remission (usually 5-10 days) and then as needed to prevent relapses (usually long term, alternate day therapy required).

Linear Iga Dermatosis
• Prednisolone—2.2-4.4 mg/kg PO q24h until remission and then tapered to alternate day therapy.
• Dapsone—1 mg/kg PO q8h until remission, then tapered and given as needed. Individual patients may respond to one drug and not the other.

Other Diseases See specific disease

CONTRAINDICATIONS N/A
PRECAUTIONS

Prednisolone
- Secondary infections
- Iatrogenic Cushings
- Muscle wasting
- Steroid hepatopathy
- Behavioral changes
- Polydipsia, polyuria
- Polyphagia

Dapsone
- In dogs mild anemia, mild leukopenia, and mild elevation of alanine aminotransferase (ALT), which are not associated with clinical signs are frequently seen. These conditions usually return to normal when dosage reduced for maintenance.
- Occasionally, fatal thrombocytopenia or severe leukopenia
- Occasional vomiting, diarrhea, or pruritic skin eruption
- Cats are more susceptible to dapsone toxicity. Hemolytic anemia and neurotoxicity reported.

Sulfasalazine
Keratoconjunctivitis sicca

POSSIBLE INTERACTIONS N/A

ALTERNATE DRUGS N/A

FOLLOW-UP

PATIENT MONITORING
- Monitor hemogram, platelet count, and ALT in patients receiving dapsone every 2 weeks initially and if any clinical side effects develop. • Monitor tear production in patients on long-term sulfasalazine therapy.
- Patients receiving immunosuppressive therapy should be monitored every 1-2 weeks initially and then every 3-4 months during maintenance therapy.

POSSIBLE COMPLICATIONS N/A

MISCELLANEOUS

ASSOCIATED CONDITIONS N/A

AGE RELATED FACTORS N/A

ZOONOTIC POTENTIAL
Dermatophytosis

PREGNANCY N/A

SYNONYMS
Dermatomyositis = Canine familial dermatomyositis

SEE ALSO
- Dermatomyositis • Dermatophytosis • Pyoderma • Acne • Lupus Erythematosus, Cutaneus (Discoid) • Pemphigus • Pemphigoid

ABBREVIATIONS
P = pemphigus
SLE = systemic lupus erythematosus
DLE = discoid lupus erythematosus
DIF = direct immunofluorescence
IgA = immunoglobulin class A
ANA = antinuclear antibody test
EMG = electromyogram
ALT = alanine aminotransferase

References
Muller GH, Kirk RW, Scott DW. Small animal dermatology. 4th ed. Philadelphia: WB Saunders, 1989.

Author Ellen C. Codner

Consulting Editor Lowell Ackerman

DIARRHEA, ACUTE

BASICS

DEFINITION
Abnormal frequency and liquidity of fecal discharges; the most common sign of intestinal disease

Pathophysiology
Diarrhea results when small intestinal absorption decreases or secretion increases or both. One or a combination of the following four mechanisms is responsible.

Osmotic Diarrhea
Poorly absorbed solutes are located in the gut lumen. This can develop with 1) ingestion of poorly absorbed solutes (e.g., fiber), 2) malassimilation of ingested food, or 3) failure to transport a dietary nonelectrolyte that is normally absorbed (e.g., glucose). These solutes retard water absorption and induce a net water movement from plasma to the gut lumen. Osmotic diarrhea is unique in that diarrhea ceases shortly after the patient fasts. Most animals with osmotic diarrheas have chronic disease.

Secretory Diarrhea
Fluids and electrolytes are secreted by mucosal cells at an exaggerated rate. Secretagogues include enterotoxins, gastrointestinal hormones, prostaglandins, parasympathetic stimulation, serotonin, dihydroxy bile acids, hydroxylated fatty acids, and certain laxatives. Pure secretory diarrhea does not resolve when the patient fasts.

Increased Permeability
A change in the surface area or specific abnormalities of the mucosal cell membranes cause an increase in the size of the pores at the epithelial cell junction, thus increasing secretory flux. Increased pore size can be caused by certain chemical mediators and inflammatory processes.

Motility Disorders
Caused by any combination of increased forward peristalsis or decreased reverse peristalsis and rhythmic segmentation

Systems Affected
• Gastrointestinal • Endocrine/Metabolic—fluid, electrolyte, and acid-base imbalances

SIGNALMENT   Dogs and cats

SIGNS

General Comments
• Patients can be placed into one of two categories according to the severity of their illness. The diagnostic work-up and treatment are determined by the category. • Mild illness—patients are alert, active, and have no clinical evidence of dehydration. Most have had less than 3-4 diarrhea episodes in the last 24 hours and there is no blood in the stool. • Moderate illness—patients have more severe clinical signs on examination such as dehydration, depression, listlessness, frequent episodes of diarrhea (> 6 per day), and blood in the stool.

Historical Findings
• Diarrhea, and perhaps vomiting, of acute or peracute onset, with a duration of approximately 24-48 hours or less before examination. • Occasional patients have viral enteritis with clinical signs of depression and anorexia and no diarrhea until after examination.

Physical Examination Findings
• Dehydration is the most common finding. • If the blood volume is low, peripheral vasoconstriction develops and the extremities are cool to the touch. • Depression and listlessness in more severely affected patients

CAUSES

Dietary Indiscretion
Eating spoiled or decomposing food, ingestion of foreign material, overeating, and sudden change of diet

Dietary Intolerance
Lactose, diet high in fat, and certain food additives

Infectious Agents
• Viral—parvovirus, coronavirus, and rotavirus • Bacterial—Salmonella, Clostridium, Campylobactor, Escherichia coli, Yersinia, and Bacillus piliformis • Rickettsial—Neorickettsia • Fungal—may cause acute diarrhea but usually associated with chronic diarrhea

Intestinal Parasites
• Giardia, ascarids, hookworms, strongyloides, coccidia

Drugs and Toxins
• Nonsteroidal anti-inflammatory drugs, digitalis, corticosteroids, anti-cancer drugs, antibiotics, insecticides, heavy metals, and lawn and garden products

Miscellaneous
• Hemorrhagic gastroenteritis, hypoadrenocorticism, and liver, renal, or pancreatic disease

RISK FACTORS
Young patients are more likely to get diarrhea from dietary indiscretion and infectious causes.

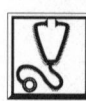

DIAGNOSIS

DIFFERENTIAL DIAGNOSIS
Most patients with mild illness will recover with minimal treatment and therefore only a minimum data base is needed for their assessment. Patients with moderate illness are more likely to have metabolic abnormalities, and thus a more extensive data base is needed.

CBC/BIOCHEMISTRY/URINALYSIS
• Mild illness—examine fecal smears and fecal flotations. Numerous examinations (at least 3) are necessary to rule out parasitic disease. Check for fecal parvovirus antigen in dogs. PCV and total protein are the minimal hematologic values to assess. • Moderate to severe illness—in addtion to fecal examinations, CBC, and electrolyte and biochemical analysis. Azotemia, high WBC count, high liver enzyme activity indicates possibility of more than just gastrointestinal tract disease. Dehydration and electrolyte abnormalities are common. Dogs with parvoviral enteritis are frequently hypoproteinemic after rehydration.

OTHER LABORATORY TESTS   N/A

IMAGING
Seldom contributes to patient management. Imaging has a high cost to benefit ratio. Ileus is seen in many patients. Some patients with parvoviral enteritis have such severe ileus that it is interpreted as obstructive ileus.

OTHER DIAGNOSTIC PROCEDURES
Endoscopy and other special diagnostic procedures seldom needed in patients with acute diarrhea

TREATMENT

• Patients with mild illness are usually treated as outpatients by dietary management and, if needed, oral rehydration. Patients with moderate to severe illness are hospitalized for more intense treatment.
• In most patients with acute diarrhea, pharmacologics are not needed.
• Restrict food intake for at least 24 hours; then gradually increase intake. Frequently offer small portions of a bland diet that consists mainly of carbohydrates and protein. Avoid fats and lactose. Bland diets include commercial prescription diets and boiled rice, tapioca, macaroni, or potatoes, combined with boiled lean meat (e.g., chicken and hamburger), eggs, cottage cheese, or yogurt. Usually the diarrhea resolves in 3-5 days, and the diet can then be gradually changed back to the patient's regular diet. If the diarrhea persists, or if the animal's condition worsens, other diagnostic or therapeutic modalities need to be investigated.

MEDICATIONS

DRUGS AND FLUIDS

Fluid Therapy
Should be part of the treatment protocol in any animal with acute diarrhea. The type of fluid depends on the acid-base and electrolyte status of the patient. Initially, a balanced fluid (e.g., lactated Ringer's solution) is best. The goal is to return the fluid and electrolyte balance to normal status within 18-24 hours. Fluids are administered either intravenously, subcutaneously, or orally depending on the condition of the patient. Animals in shock or severely dehydrated need IV administration. Oral rehydration is effective mostly because of the efficacy of the treatment and the economic benefits it offers. Oral rehydration may not be the treatment of choice if the animal is in severe ionic imbalance, intestinal

obstruction is suspected, or if the dehydration is so severe as to cause shock.

Motility Modulators

• Use only in patients with diarrhea so severe that the fluid and electrolyte status of the animal can not be maintained. When these drugs are used, the goals are to increase rhythmic segmentation contractions (increase resistance) and decrease forward peristalsis (forward driving force). This causes the transit time of the intestinal contents to slow down, allowing time for more water to be reabsorbed. Do not use for longer than a few days because of the side effects associated with these drugs.

• Narcotic analgesics—potent inhibitors of intestinal secretions and stimulators of segmental contractions in the intestine. These drugs increase the resistance to passage of intestinal contents while decreasing fluid influx. This allows fluid absorption from the gastrointestinal tract. The dosages of the various narcotic analgesics are listed in Table I.

• Anticholinergics—decrease intestinal tone. Inhibition of segmental and forward peristaltic contractions produces an open tube that provides no resistance to fecal flow, and thus makes the diarrhea worse in some patients. One beneficial effect is reduction of intestinal secretions.

Antisecretory Agents

• Anticholinergics

• Chlorpromazine is believed to inhibit intracellular calmodulin activity which increases in patients with secretory diarrhea.

• Opiates decrease intestinal secretion and increase absorption. The antisecretory effect may be caused by increased gut capacitance and slowed transit time allowing for increased absorption.

• Salicylates inhibit prostaglandins which may decrease enterotoxin-induced intestinal secretion. Pectin plus salicylates may absorb and inactivate enterotoxins such as those produced by E. coli.

Intestinal Protectants

Except for bismuth subsalicylate (e.g., Pepto-Bismol™), kaolin and pectin type drugs are of doubtful value in patients with severe diarrhea. They have not been shown to alter fluid and electrolyte losses.

Antibiotic Therapy

Indicated in patients with bacterial inflammatory lesions in the gastrointestinal tract evidenced by numerous abnormal bacteria and inflammatory cells seen on a fecal smear. Antibiotics are also indicated in patients with bacterial invasion of the intestinal mucosa evidenced by blood in the feces. If the antibiotics are not effective in killing the pathogenic bacteria, but inhibit the normal bacterial flora, they are detrimental to the recovery of the animal.

CONTRAINDICATIONS

• The use of anticholinergics is contraindicated in patients with intestinal obstruction, gastrointestinal atony, or glaucoma.

• Narcotic analgesics may cause CNS depression, euphoria, confusion, restlessness, and gastrointestinal atony, megacolon, pancreatitis, and anorexia. The use of these drugs is contraindicated in patients with liver disease, enterotoxin-producing bacterial disease, and invasive intestinal bacterial disease.

PRECAUTIONS

A general antibiotic shotgun approach to diarrhea may be ineffective at best and detrimental at worst.

POSSIBLE INTERACTIONS

Do not administer antibiotics orally in conjunction with intestinal protectants. The antibiotics are usually bound to the protectant and are thus ineffective.

ALTERNATE DRUGS N/A

FOLLOW-UP

PATIENT MONITORING

Most animals with uncomplicated acute diarrhea recover spontaneously in 3-5 days. Patients unresponsive to the management outlined require more extensive diagnostic testing and treatment.

POSSIBLE COMPLICATIONS N/A

MISCELLANEOUS

ASSOCIATED CONDITIONS N/A

AGE RELATED FACTORS N/A

ZOONOTIC POTENTIAL

Certain enteritis causing bacteria and parasites have zoonotic potential.

PREGNANCY N/A

SYNONYMS N/A

SEE ALSO See Causes

ABBREVIATIONS

PCV = packed cell volume
WBC = white blood cells

References

Burrows CF, Batt RM, Sherding RG. Diseases of the small intestine. In: Ettinger SJ, Feldman EC, eds. Textbook of veterinary internal medicine. Philadelphia: WB Saunders, 1995;1169-1232.

Jergens AE. Acute diarrhea. In: Bonagura JD, ed. Kirk's current veterinary therapy XII. Philadelphia: WB Saunders, 1995;701-705.

Author Brent D. Jones

Consulting Editor Brent D. Jones

Table 1.

Narcotic Analgesics	
Generic Name	Dosage
Meperidine	10 mg/kg, IV, IM, SQ (C)
Paregoric	0.05-0.06 mg/kg, BID-TID, PO (C&F)
Diphenoxylate	0.05-.01 mg/kg, Q4H-QID, PO (C)
Loperamide	0.08 mg/kg, QID, PO (C)

C=Canine; F=Feline

DIARRHEA, CHRONIC–CATS

BASICS

DEFINITION
A change in the frequency, consistency, and volume of feces for more than 3 weeks or with a pattern of episodic recurrence. Chronic diarrhea can be either small bowel or large bowel in origin.

Pathophysiology
• High solute or fluid secretion • Low solute or fluid absorption • High intestinal permeability • Abnormal gastrointestinal motility

Systems Affected
• Gastrointestinal • Endocrine/metabolic—fluid, electrolyte, and acid-base disturbances

SIGNALMENT
Cats

SIGNS

Historical Findings
Small Bowel
• Larger volume of feces than normal • Frequency of defecation mildly to moderately increased above normal (2-4 per day) • Weight loss and polyphagia with malabsorption and maldigestion • Cat may have melena, but hematochezia and mucus are absent • No tenesmus or dyschezia • Vomiting common
Large Bowel
• Smaller volume of feces per defecation • Frequency of defecation significantly increased over normal (> 4 times per day) • No weight loss • Hematochezia, tenesmus, and mucus in most cats • Dyschezia in cats with rectal or distal colonic disease

Physical Examination Findings
• Poor body condition associated with infiltrative bowel disease, chronic obstruction, and metabolic disorders • Diffuse intestinal thickening suggests infiltrative disease. • Segmental thickening caused by neoplasia (especially lymphoma), foreign body, mesenteric lymphadenopathy, and eosinophilic or granulomatous enteritis (both rare). • Aggregation of bowel loops may be seen in a cat with linear foreign body. • A palpable thyroid nodule suggests hyperthyroidism. • Small kidneys may indicate chronic renal disease. • Hepatomegaly or icterus may indicate hepatic lipidosis, FIP, hepatic neoplasia, or biliary disease. • Rectal palpation may indicate abnormal rectal mucosa, intraluminal or extraluminal rectal mass, or rectal stricture. • Fundic examination may reveal lesions suggestive of toxoplasmosis, FIP, histoplasmosis, or FeLV.

CAUSES
• Inflammatory bowel disease—lymphoplasmacytic enterocolitis, granulomatous enteritis, eosinophilic enteritis/hypereosinophilic syndrome, and idiopathic inflammatory colitis • Neoplasia—lymphoma, adenocarcinoma, mast cell tumor, and polyps • Obstruction—neoplasia, foreign body, inflammatory bowel disease, intussusception, and stricture • Parasitic causes—Giardia, Toxoplasma gondii, Toxocara cati, Dirofilaria immitis, and Cryptosporidium spp. • Metabolic disorders—hyperthyroidism, renal disease, hepatic disease, diabetes mellitus, toxins, and drug administration • Bacterial causes—Campylobacter jejuni, Salmonella spp., Yersinia pseudotuberculosis, and Clostridium perfringes • Viral causes—FeLV, FIV, and FIP • Mycotic causes—histoplasmosis, mycobacteriosis, phycomycosis, and aspergillosis • Noninflammatory malabsorption—lymphangiectasia, small intestinal bacterial overgrowth, short bowel syndrome, villous atrophy, and duodenal ulcer • Maldigestion—hepatobiliary disease and exocrine pancreatic insufficiency (rare in cats) • Dietary—dietary sensitivity, dietary indiscretion, and diet changes • Congenital anomalies—short colon, portosystemic shunt, and persistent pancreaticomesojejunal ligament

RISK FACTORS
Dietary changes and feeding poorly-digestible or high-fat diet

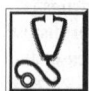

DIAGNOSIS

DIFFERENTIAL DIAGNOSIS
The first step in the evaluation of chronic diarrhea is to localize the origin of the diarrhea to the small or large bowel or both based on historical signs.

CBC/BIOCHEMISTRY/URINALYSIS
• Eosinophilia in some cats with parasitism and eosinophilic enterocolitis/hypereosinophilic syndrome • Macrocytosis in some cats with hyperthyroidism or FeLV infection • Anemia and microcytosis suggest chronic gastrointestinal bleeding and iron deficiency. • Leukopenia in some cats with FeLV or FIV infection • Biochemical abnormalities may suggest renal disease, hepatic disease, or endocrinopathy. • Panhypoproteinemia caused by protein-losing enteropathy is uncommon in cats with intestinal disease.

OTHER LABORATORY TESTS

Fecal Examination
• Direct fecal examination, routine fecal flotation, and zinc sulfate centrifugation (for Giardia) may reveal gastrointestinal parasites. • Cytologic examination of feces may reveal specific organisms such as Histoplasma, Prototheca, or fecal leukocytes, which are associated with inflammatory colitis and with invasive bacteria such as Campylobacter or Salmonella. • Sudan stain for fecal fats may indicate steatorrhea, suggesting malabsorption or maldigestion. • Perform fecal culture if Campylobacter or Salmonella is suspected.

Thyroid Function Tests
• High serum T_4 concentration indicates hyperthyroidism. • If hyperthyroidism is suspected but the T_4 is normal, perform a T_3 suppression test, TRH response test, or thyroid scan.

Serologic Testing
Tests for FeLV and FIV should be performed, especially if the cat has hematologic abnormalities.

Tests of Exocrine Pancreatic Function
• Fecal proteolytic activity should be measured in fecal samples from 3 consecutive days. • Trypsinlike immunoreactivity is not useful in cats because it is species-specific (dogs).

IMAGING
• Survey abdominal radiography may indicate intestinal obstruction, mass, organomegaly, foreign body, or small kidneys. • Contrast radiography (upper gastrointestinal series or barium enema) may indicate bowel wall thickening, mucosal irregularity, mass, radiolucent foreign body, or stricture. • Abdominal ultrasonography may demonstrate bowel wall thickening, gastrointestinal mass, foreign body, ileus, or mesenteric lymphadenopathy.

OTHER DIAGNOSTIC PROCEDURES

Endoscopy
• If maldigestive, metabolic, parasitic, dietary, and infectious causes have been ruled out, endoscopy and mucosal biopsy usually are necessary for definitive diagnosis and treatment of chronic diarrhea. • Upper gastrointestinal endoscopy allows visualization and biopsy of the gastric and duodenal mucosa. Duodenal aspirates should be obtained for quantitative culture if bacterial overgrowth is suspected. Multiple mucosal specimens should always be obtained from both the duodenum and stomach. • Colonoscopy can be performed with either a flexible endoscope, which allows examination of the entire colon and sometimes the distal ileum, or a rigid scope, which is limited to the descending colon and rectum.

TREATMENT
• Treatment of chronic diarrhea often must be specific to the underlying cause to be successful.
• When obtaining a definitive diagnosis is not possible, empirical treatment by dietary management and metronidazole sometimes results in clinical improvement.
• Surgery is necessary for treatment of obstructive disease and gastrointestinal mass.

SURGICAL CONSIDERATIONS
Exploratory laparotomy and surgical biopsy should be pursued if there is evidence of obstruction, an intestinal mass, or distal small bowel disease, or if a diagnosis based on endoscopic biopsy is questioned because of poor response to treatment.

MEDICATIONS

DRUGS AND FLUIDS
• If the cat is dehydrated, replace fluid deficit with balanced electrolyte solution such as normal saline or lactated Ringer's.
• Correct electrolyte (hypokalemia) and acid/base imbalances.
• A bland or hypoallergenic diet may be beneficial.
• A therapeutic trial with metronidazole (10-20 mg/kg PO q8-12h for 10-14 days) often is used to rule out occult Giardia infection. This drug also has nonspecific antiinflammatory gastrointestinal effects and is effective in treating small intestinal bacterial overgrowth.
• Additional treatment as dictated by the the primary disease

CONTRAINDICATIONS
Anticholinergics exacerbate most types of chronic diarrhea and should not be used for empirical treatment.

PRECAUTIONS
Opiate antidiarrheals such as diphenoxylate and loperamide can cause hyperactivity and respiratory depression in cats and should not be used for more than 3 days.

POSSIBLE INTERACTIONS N/A

ALTERNATE DRUGS N/A

FOLLOW-UP

PATIENT MONITORING
• Fecal volume and character, frequency of defecation, and body weight • Resolution of diarrhea usually occurs gradually with treatment. If diarrhea does not resolve, consider reevaluation of the diagnosis.

POSSIBLE COMPLICATIONS N/A

MISCELLANEOUS

ASSOCIATED CONDITIONS N/A

AGE RELATED FACTORS N/A

ZOONOTIC POTENTIAL
Toxoplasma, Giardia, Cryptosporidium

PREGNANCY N/A

SYNONYMS N/A

SEE ALSO
See causes.

ABBREVIATIONS
FeLV = feline leukemia virus
FIV = feline immunodeficiency virus
FIP = feline infectious peritonitis

References

Wolf AM. Diarrhea in the cat. Sem Vet Med Surg (Small Anim) 1989;4:212-218.

Sherding RG. Diseases of the intestines. In: Sherding RG, ed. The cat: diseases and clinical management. New York: Churchill Livingstone, 1989:955-1006.

Jergens AE. Feline idiopathic inflammatory bowel disease. Comp Contin Ed Pract Vet 1992;14:509-518.

Dennis JS, Kruger JM, Mullaney TP. Lymphocytic/plasmacytic colitis in cats: 14 cases (1985-1990). J Am Vet Med Assoc 1993;202:313-318.

Author Amy M. Grooters
Consulting Editor Brent D. Jones

DIARRHEA, CHRONIC–DOGS

BASICS

DEFINITION
A change in the frequency, consistency, and volume of feces for more than 3 weeks or with a pattern of episodic recurrence. Chronic diarrhea can be either small bowel or large bowel in origin.

Pathophysiology
• High solute or fluid secretion • Low solute or fluid absorption • High intestinal permeability • Abnormal gastrointestinal motility

Systems Affected
• Gastrointestinal • Endocrine/metabolic—fluid, electrolyte, and acid-base disturbances

SIGNALMENT
Dogs

SIGNS

Historical Findings
Small Bowel
• Larger volume of feces than normal • Frequency of defecation is mildly to moderately above normal (2-4 per day) • Weight loss • Dog may have melena, but hematochezia and mucus are absent • No tenesmus or dyschezia • Flatulence and borborygmus may be present. • Vomiting in some dogs
Large Bowel
• Smaller volume of feces per defecation • Frequency of defecation significantly increased over normal (> 4 times per day) • No weight loss • Hematochezia and mucus • Tenesmus and urgency • Dyschezia in dogs with rectal or distal colonic disease • Vomiting uncommon

Physical Examination Findings
Small Bowel
• Poor body condition associated with malabsorption, maldigestion, and protein-losing enteropathy • Abdominal palpation may reveal thickened bowel loops associated with infiltrative small bowel disease, abdominal effusion as a result of hypoproteinemia caused by protein-losing enteropathy, or an abdominal mass such as a foreign body, neoplastic mass, intussusception, or large mesenteric lymph node.
Large Bowel
Rectal palpation may reveal irregularity and thickening of the rectal mucosa, intraluminal or extraluminal rectal mass, rectal stricture, or sublumbar lymphadenopathy.

CAUSES

Small Bowel
Primary Small Intestinal Disease
• Inflammatory bowel disease (e.g., lymphoplasmacytic enteritis, eosinophilic enteritis, granulomatous enteritis, immunoproliferative enteropathy in basenjis, and sprue) • Lymphangiectasia • Infiltrative neoplasia (e.g., lymphosarcoma and adenocarcinoma) • Infection (e.g., histoplasmosis, Salmonella spp., Clostridium perfringens, and phycomycosis) • Parasites (e.g., Giardia, ascarids, hookworms, and strongyloides) • Partial obstruction (e.g., foreign body, intussusception, and neoplasia) • Small intestinal bacterial overgrowth • Short bowel syndrome • Duodenal ulcer
Maldigestion
• Exocrine pancreatic insufficiency (e.g., juvenile pancreatic acinar atrophy and chronic pancreatitis) • Hepatobiliary disease
Dietary Causes
• Dietary sensitivity • Gluten-sensitive enteropathy in Irish setters
Metabolic Disorders
• Hepatic disease, hypoadrenocorticism, uremia, toxins, and drug administration (e.g., anticholinergics and antibiotics) • Apudoma (rare)

Large Bowel
Primary Large Intestinal Disease
• Inflammatory causes (e.g., lymphoplasmacytic colitis, eosinophilic colitis, histiocytic ulcerative colitis, and granulomatous colitis) • Parasites (e.g., Trichuris vulpis, Giardi, Ancylostoma caninum, Entamoeba histolytica, and Balantidium coli) • Noninflammatory causes (e.g., ileocolic intussusception and cecal inversion) • Neoplasia (e.g., benign polyp, adenocarcinoma, lymphosarcoma, leiomyoma, and leiomyosarcoma) • Infection (e.g., histoplasmosis, Clostridium perfringes, Salmonella spp., Campylobacter jejuni, and Prototheca)
Dietary and Idiopathic Causes
• Diet—dietary indiscretion, diet changes, and foreign material (e.g., bones and hair) • Fiber-responsive large bowel diarrhea • Irritable bowel syndrome
Metabolic Disorders
Uremia, hypoadrenocorticism, toxins, and drug administration

RISK FACTORS

Small Bowel
• Dietary changes and feeding poorly-digestible or high-fat diet • Large-breed dogs, especially German shepherds, have the highest incidence of exocrine pancreatic insufficiency (EPI).

Large Bowel
• Dietary changes or indiscretion, stress, and psychologic factors may play a role. • Histiocytic ulcerative colitis is seen most often in boxers < 3 years old.

DIAGNOSIS

DIFFERENTIAL DIAGNOSIS
The first step in the evaluation of chronic diarrhea is to localize the origin of the diarrhea to the small or large bowel or both based on historical signs.

CBC/BIOCHEMISTRY/URINALYSIS
• Eosinophilia may be associated with parasitism, eosinophilic enterocolitis, or hypoadrenocorticism. • Lymphopenia and hypocholesterolemia may be associated with lymphangiectasia. • Anemia and microcytosis suggest chronic gastrointestinal bleeding and iron deficiency. • Panhypoproteinemia resulting from protein-losing enteropathy is associated with infiltrative small bowel disorders and lymphangiectasia. • Biochemical abnormalities may suggest renal disease, hepatic disease, or endocrinopathy.

OTHER LABORATORY TESTS

Fecal Examination
• Direct fecal examination, routine fecal flotation, and zinc sulfate centrifugation (for Giardia) may indicate gastrointestinal parasites. • Cytologic examination of feces may reveal specific organisms such as Histoplasma, Prototheca, or fecal leukocytes, which are associated with inflammatory bowel disease or with invasive bacteria such as Campylobacter and Salmonella. • Sudan stain for fecal fats may indicate steatorrhea, suggesting malabsorption or maldigestion. • Perform fecal culture if Campylobacter or Salmonella is suspected.

Tests of Exocrine Pancreatic Function
• Trypsinlike immunoreactivity (TLI)—test of choice for confirming EPI in dogs. Fasted serum TLI < 2.5 mg/L is diagnostic • Oral bentiromide (BT-PABA) test—a negligible rise in plasma PABA is consistent with a diagnosis of EPI

Tests for Malabsorption
• Xylose absorption test—this is an insensitive and nonspecific test of intestinal malabsorption. Peak plasma xylose concentration of < 45 mg/dL indicates malabsorption, but a normal value does not rule it out • Serum folate and cobalamin—low serum cobalamin is associated with EPI and distal small bowel malabsorption; low serum folate is associated with proximal small bowel malabsorption; small intestinal bacterial overgrowth may raise serum folate and lower serum cobalamin

IMAGING
• Survey abdominal radiography may indicate intestinal obstruction, organomegaly, mass, foreign body, or ascites. • Contrast radiography (upper gastrointestinal series or barium enema) may indicate bowel wall thickening, intestinal ulcers, mucosal irregularity, mass, radiolucent foreign body, or stricture. • Abdominal ultrasonography may demonstrate bowel wall thickening, gastrointestinal mass, foreign bodies, ileus, ascites, or mesenteric lymphadenopathy.

OTHER DIAGNOSTIC PROCEDURES

Endoscopy
• If maldigestive, metabolic, parasitic, dietary, and infectious causes have been ruled out, endoscopy and mucosal biopsy usually are necessary for definitive diagnosis and treatment of chronic diarrhea. • Upper gastrointestinal endoscopy allows visualization and biopsy of

the gastric and duodenal mucosa. Duodenal aspirates should be obtained for quantitative culture if bacterial overgrowth is suspected. Multiple mucosal specimens should always be obtained from both the duodenum and stomach. • Colonoscopy can be performed with either a flexible endoscope, which allows examination of the entire colon and often the distal ileum, or a rigid scope, which is limited to the descending colon and rectum.

TREATMENT

SMALL BOWEL
• Treat the underlying cause. Symptomatic or empirical treatment is rarely successful in resolving chronic small bowel diarrhea.
• Inform the owner that complete resolution of signs is not always possible, despite a correct diagnosis and proper treatment. This is especially true for dogs with lymphangiectasia, intestinal neoplasia, and histoplasmosis.

LARGE BOWEL
• Fecal examinations are often negative in whipworm-infested dogs because of intermittent shedding of ova. Because whipworms are a common cause of large bowel diarrhea, therapeutic deworming with fenbendazole should be performed before pursuing additional diagnostic tests.
• Feeding a low-fat, highly-digestible diet for 3-4 weeks may resolve signs of large bowel diarrhea.

SURGICAL CONSIDERATIONS
Exploratory laparotomy and surgical biopsy should be pursued if there is evidence of obstruction, an intestinal mass, or mid-small bowel disease, or if a diagnosis based on endoscopic biopsy is questioned because of poor response to treatment.

MEDICATIONS

DRUGS AND FLUIDS
• If the dog is dehydrated, replace fluid deficit with balanced electrolyte solution such as normal saline or lactated Ringer's solution.
• Correct electrolyte and acid/base imbalances.

CONTRAINDICATIONS
Anticholinergics exacerbate most types of chronic diarrhea. They are, however, sometimes used to relieve cramping associated with irritable bowel syndrome. They should not be used for empiric treatment of diarrhea.

PRECAUTIONS N/A

POSSIBLE INTERACTIONS N/A

ALTERNATE DRUGS N/A

FOLLOW-UP

PATIENT MONITORING
• Fecal volume and character, frequency of defecation, and body weight • In dogs with protein-losing enteropathy, serum proteins and pleural effusion or ascites • Resolution of diarrhea is usually gradual after treatment. If it does not resolve with treatment, consider reevaluation of the diagnosis. • Some dogs with inflammatory bowel disease or EPI have secondary small intestinal bacterial overgrowth, which must be treated along with the primary disorder.

POSSIBLE COMPLICATIONS N/A

MISCELLANEOUS

ASSOCIATED CONDITIONS N/A

AGE RELATED FACTORS N/A

ZOONOTIC POTENTIAL
Giardia

PREGNANCY N/A

SYNONYMS N/A

SEE ALSO
See causes.

ABBREVIATIONS
EPI = exocrine pancreatic insufficiency
TLI = trypsin-like immunoreactivity

References
Leib MS, Monroe WE, Codner EC. A diagnostic approach to chronic large bowel diarrhea in dogs. Vet Med 1991;86:892-899.
Leib MS, Monroe WE, Codner EC. Management of chronic large bowel diarrhea in dogs. Vet Med 1991;86:922-929.
Strombeck DR, Guilford WG. Small animal gastroenterology. Davis, CA: Stonegate Publishing, 1990.
Author Amy M. Grooters
Consulting Editor Brent D. Jones

DYSCHEZIA AND HEMATOCHEZIA

 BASICS

DEFINITION
• Dyschezia is painful or difficult defecation
• Hematochezia is presence of bright red blood in the feces.

Pathophysiology
Associated with diseases of the colon, rectum, and anus

Systems Affected
Gastrointestinal—signs are usually caused by diseases of the rectum or anus, but hematochezia may also be seen in patients with diseases of the colon

SIGNALMENT
• Dogs and cats • No breed or sex predilection

SIGNS

Historical Findings
• Crying and whimpering during defecation in patients with dyschezia • Tenesmus is common. • Lack of defecation with obstipation may occur if pain is severe. • Mucoid, bloody diarrhea in some patients with colonic disease

Physical Examination Findings
• Very hard feces if the patient is constipated
• Polyps or masses may be palpated in the rectum in patients with hematochezia

CAUSES

Rectal and Anal Disease
• Stricture • Anal sacculitis or abscess • Perianal fistula • Rectal or anal foreign body
• Pseudocoprostasis • Perineal hernia
• Rectal prolapse • Trauma—bite wound
• Neoplasia—adenocarcinoma, lymphosarcoma, and anal and anal sac tumor • Rectal polyps • Anal "spasm" • Proctitis

Other
• Fractured pelvis or hind limb • Prostatic disease • Intrapelvic neoplasia

Colonic Disease
• Neoplasia—adenocarcinoma and lymphosarcoma • Idiopathic megacolon (cats)
• Inflammation—inflammatory bowel disease and infectious agents (see Colitis) • Constipation (see Constipation)

RISK FACTORS
• Ingestion of hair, bones, and foreign material contributed to constipation and subsequent dyschezia. • Environmental factor such as a dirty litter pan and infrequent outside walks may contribute to constipation and subsequent dyschezia.

 DIAGNOSIS

DIFFERENTIAL DIAGNOSIS
• Differentiate colonic disease from rectoanal disease; mucoid, bloody diarrhea often seen in patients with colonic disease • Differentiate from dysuria and stranguria

CBC/BIOCHEMISTRY/URINALYSIS
Results usually normal; neutrophilia in patients with infection or inflammation

OTHER LABORATORY TESTS
Fecal examination for parasites and bacteria to rule out infectious causes

IMAGING
Pelvic radiographs may reveal intrapelvic disease, foreign body, or fracture.

OTHER DIAGNOSTIC PROCEDURES
Colonoscopy or proctoscopy to evaluate for inflammatory and neoplastic disease

 TREATMENT

• Usually outpatient
• Consider laxatives to make defecation easier in patients with rectoanal disease.
• Balloon dilation in patient with stricture
• Rectoanal disease (e.g., perianal fistula and perineal hernia) may require surgical correction.

MEDICATIONS

DRUGS AND FLUIDS
- Antibiotics to treat bacterial infection (e.g., anal sac abscess)
- Anti-inflammatory drug (i.e., sulfasalazine or prednisone) to treat colitis
- Laxative—lactulose, docusate, sodium or docusate calcium

CONTRAINDICATIONS
Avoid agents that increase fecal bulk (fiber), unless specifically indicated (e.g., colitis).

PRECAUTIONS N/A

POSSIBLE INTERACTIONS N/A

ALTERNATE DRUGS N/A

FOLLOW-UP

PATIENT MONITORING Clinical signs

POSSIBLE COMPLICATIONS
- Fecal incontinence may develop if aggressive surgery is needed, e.g., for perianal fistula. • Prognosis depends on the disease process involved—e.g., good in patients with anal sac disease, perineal hernia, and wounds; poor in patients with stricture or neoplasia

MISCELLANEOUS

ASSOCIATED CONDITIONS N/A

AGE RELATED FACTORS N/A

ZOONOTIC POTENTIAL N/A

PREGNANCY N/A

SYNONYMS N/A

SEE ALSO
- Constipation and Obstipation • Colitis and Proctitis

ABBREVIATIONS N/A

Reference

Burrows CF, Sherding RG. Constipation and dyschezia. In: Anderson NV, ed. Veterinary gastroenterology. Philadelphia: Lea and Febiger, 1992;484-503.

Authors Lisa E. Moore and Colin F. Burrows

Consulting Editor Brent D. Jones

DYSPHAGIA

BASICS

DEFINITION
Difficulty swallowing, resulting from the inability to prehend, form, and move a bolus of food through the oropharynx into the esophagus. Esophageal dysphagia and regurgitation are discussed under megaesophagus.

Pathophysiology
• Swallowing difficulties can be caused by mechanical obstruction of the oral cavity or pharynx, neuromuscular dysfunction resulting in weak or uncoordinated swallowing movements, or pain associated with prehension, mastication, or swallowing. • Oral dysphagia refers to difficulty with the voluntary components of swallowing, namely prehending and forming a bolus of food at the base of the tongue. • Pharyngeal dysphagia refers to malfunction of the involuntary movement of the food bolus through the oropharynx. • Cricopharyngeal dysphagia refers to abnormal movement of the food bolus from the pharynx through the cricopharyngeus muscle, caused by either failure of the cricopharyngeus to relax (cricopharyngeal achalasia) or asynchrony between pharyngeal contractions and cricopharyngeus opening (cricopharyngeal asynchrony). • Deglutition is coordinated by the swallowing center in the brainstem. Sensory afferents are transmitted to the swallowing center by cranial nerves (CN) V and IX. Motor efferents responsible for swallowing are carried by CN V, VII, XII (prehension and mastication) and IX and X (pharyngeal contraction). Disorders in any of these areas may result in dysphagia.

Systems Affected
• Gastrointestinal • Neuromuscular

SIGNALMENT
Congenital disorders that cause dysphagia, such as cricopharyngeal achalasia and cleft palate, are usually diagnosed in animals < 1 year old. Acquired pharyngeal dysphagias are more common in older patients.

SIGNS

Historical Findings
• Drooling, gagging, weight loss, ravenous appetite, repeated attempts at swallowing, swallowing with the head in an abnormal position, coughing (due to aspiration), regurgitation, painful swallowing, and occasionally anorexia are all possible • Onset and progression of dysphagia should be ascertained. Foreign bodies, for example, cause acute dysphagia while pharyngeal dysphagia may be intermittent.

Physical Examination Findings
• A thorough oral examination, with the patient sedated or anesthetized if necessary, is the most important aspect of the physical examination in dysphagic patients. Observe for asymmetry, anatomic defect, foreign body, inflammation, tumor, edema, abscessed teeth, and loose teeth. • Observing the patient while eating is essential and may identify the abnormal phase of swallowing. • A complete neurologic examination, with emphasis on the cranial nerves, should be performed on all dysphagic patients.

Oral Dysphagia
• Modified eating behavior (e.g., eating with the head tilted to one side and throwing the head back while eating) may be observed as patients learn to compensate for oral dysphagia. • Mandibular paralysis, tongue paralysis, dental disease, masticatory muscle swelling or atrophy, inability to open the mouth and food packed in the buccal folds without retention of saliva suggest oral dysphagia.

Pharyngeal Dysphagia
• Prehension of food is normal. • Repeated attempts at swallowing while repeatedly flexing and extending the head and neck and excessive chewing and gagging suggest pharyngeal dysphagia. • Saliva-coated food retained in the buccal folds, a diminished gag reflex, and nasal discharge from aspiration may be found.

Cricopharyngeal Dysphagia
• Patients with cricopharyngeal dysphagia make repeated efforts to swallow, gag, and cough and then forcibly regurgitate immediately after swallowing. • The gag reflex and prehension are normal. • Emaciation is more common with this form of dysphagia than with others.

CAUSES
• Anatomic or mechanical lesions that cause dysphagia include pharyngeal inflammation (e.g., abscess, inflammatory polyps, and oral eosinophilic granuloma), retropharyngeal lymphadenomegaly, neoplasia, pharyngeal and retropharyngeal foreign body, sialocele, temporomandibular joint disorder (e.g., luxation, fracture, and craniomandibular osteopathy), mandibular fracture, cleft palate, lingual frenulum disorder, and pharyngeal trauma.
• Pain because of dental disease (e.g., tooth fracture and abscess), mandibular trauma, stomatitis and glossitis and pharyngeal inflammation may also disrupt normal prehension, bolus formation, and swallowing.
• Neuromuscular disorders that impair prehension and bolus formation include cranial nerve deficits (e.g., idiopathic trigeminal neuropathy and lingual paralysis-CN XII) and masticatory muscle myositis. Pharyngeal weakness, paresis, or paralysis causing dysphagia can be caused by myasthenia gravis and infectious polymyositis (e.g., toxoplasmosis and neosporosis), immune mediated polymyositis, muscular dystrophy, polyneuropathies, and myoneural junction disorders (e.g., tick paralysis and botulism). Rabies can cause dysphagia by affecting both the brainstem and peripheral nerves. Other CNS disorders, especially those involving the brainstem, can cause dysphagia.

RISK FACTORS
Many of the neuromuscular conditions that cause dysphagia have breed predispositions.

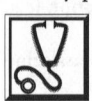

DIAGNOSIS

DIFFERENTIAL DIAGNOSIS
• Dysphagia must be differentiated from vomiting and regurgitation from esophageal disease. • Exaggerated or repeated efforts to swallow, which is characteristic of dysphagic patients, is the most useful means of distinguishing dysphagia from vomiting or regurgitation. Also, vomiting is associated with abdominal contractions whereas dysphagia is not.

CBC/BIOCHEMISTRY/URINALYSIS
• Inflammatory lesions often cause leukocytosis, sometimes with a left shift. • High serum creatine kinase is usually found in patients with muscular disorders that cause dysphagia. • Evidence of renal disease, such as azotemia and low urine concentration, may be found in patients with oral and lingual ulcers.

OTHER LABORATORY TESTS
• Type 2M muscle antibody titers should be obtained if masticatory muscle myositis is suspected. • Acetylcholinesterase receptor antibody titers are high in most patients with acquired myasthenia gravis. • High antinuclear antibody titers may be found in patients with other immune mediated diseases. • Low-dose dexamethasone suppression test or ACTH stimulation test may confirm hyperadrenocorticism in patients with chronic infection or myopathy.

IMAGING
• Survey radiography of the skull and neck, including the hyoid apparatus. Particular attention is given to the mandibles and temporomandibular joint, teeth, pharyngeal and retropharyngeal area, and position of the hyoid apparatus. • Ultrasonography of the pharynx may be useful in patients with mass lesions and for obtaining ultrasound-guided biopsy specimens. • Fluoroscopy, with or without positive contrast, is useful in evaluating pharyngeal movement in patients with suspected pharyngeal or cricopharyngeal dysphagia.

OTHER DIAGNOSTIC PROCEDURES
• Excisional or incisional biopsy of mass lesion • Pharyngoscopy to evaluate the pharynx. Biopsy of a mass lesion and evaluation of the esophagus can also be performed at this time. • Electromyography of the pharyngeal musculature to confirm the presence of a neuromuscular disorder. The patient should also be evaluated for systemic neuromuscular disease. • Repetitive nerve stimulation and

Tensilon® (edrophonium chloride, 0.1-0.2 mg/kg IV) test in patients suspected of having myasthenia gravis • Cerebrospinal fluid analysis in patients with a CNS disorder

TREATMENT

• Determining the underlying cause of dysphagia is important in forming a treatment plan and accurate prognosis.
• Primary treatment should be directed at the underlying cause.
• Nutritional support is an important aspect of managing all dysphagic patients. Patients with oral dysphagia may be able to swallow if a bolus of food is placed in the caudal pharynx. For other patients, a gruel that can be lapped is easier to swallow. Care should be taken to avoid aspiration when feeding orally. Elevating the head and neck may make swallowing easier for patients with pharyngeal or cricopharyngeal dysphagia and help prevent aspiration of food. If nutritional requirements can not be met orally, a parenteral route (e.g., gastrotomy tubes) may be necessary.
• Surgical excision of a mass lesion or foreign body may be curative or temporarily improve signs of dysphagia.
• Cricopharyngeal myotomy may bring about improvement in patients with cricopharyngeal dysphagia. A correct diagnosis is essential before surgery, because cricopharyngeal myotomy performed on patients with oral oropharyngeal dysphagia exacerbates dysphagia.

MEDICATIONS

DRUGS AND FLUIDS

• Dysphagia is not an immediately life-threatening problem and drug therapy should

be directed at the underlying cause after a complete workup.
• Empirical treatment may consist of administration of a broad-spectrum antibiotic and antiinflammatory dosage of corticosteroids if a workup is not possible.

CONTRAINDICATIONS N/A

PRECAUTIONS

Barium sulfate should be used with caution in patients with evidence of aspiration.

POSSIBLE INTERACTIONS N/A

ALTERNATE DRUGS N/A

FOLLOW-UP

PATIENT MONITORING

• Daily for signs of aspiration pneumonia (e.g., depression, fever, coughing, and dyspnea) • Body condition and hydration status daily. If requirements are not being met with enteral nutrition, initiate parental supplementation.

POSSIBLE COMPLICATIONS

Aspiration pneumonia is a common complication in patients with swallowing disorders. Feeding a number of small meals with the patient in an upright position, maintaining this position for 10-15 minutes after feeding, helps prevent aspiration of food.

MISCELLANEOUS

ASSOCIATED CONDITIONS

• Megaesophagus • Pneumonia

AGE RELATED FACTORS

• Young dogs are more likely to ingest foreign objects and suffer facial trauma. • Young cats are more likely to form inflammatory polyps.

ZOONOTIC POTENTIAL

• Rabies should be considered in any patient with dysphagia, especially if the animal's rabies vaccination status is unknown or questionable or it has been exposed to potentially rabid animals. If a dysphagic animal dies of rapidly progressive neurologic disease, the head should be submitted to a qualified laboratory designated by the local or state health department for rabies examination.

PREGNANCY N/A

SYNONYMS N/A

SEE ALSO

• Megaesophagus • Pneumonia, Bacterial

ABBREVIATIONS

ACTH = adrenocorticotrophic hormone
CNS = central nervous system

References

Watrous BJ. Clinical presentation and diagnosis of dysphagia. Vet Clin North Am Small Anim Prac 1983;13:437-459.
Willard MD. Dysphagia and swallowing disorders. In: Kirk's current veterinary therapy XI. Philadelphia: WB Saunders, 1992;572-577.

Author Randall C. Longshore
Consulting Editor Brent D. Jones

DYSPNEA AND TACHYPNEA

 BASICS

DEFINITION

Dyspnea is the distressful feeling associated with difficult or labored breathing, tachypnea is rapid breathing (not necessarily labored), and hyperpnea is deep breathing. In animals, the term dyspnea often is applied to labored breathing that appears to be uncomfortable.

Pathophysiology

• Nonrespiratory causes of dyspnea may include pulmonary vascular tone abnormalities (CNS disease, shock), pulmonary circulation (congestive heart failure, pulmonary thromboebolism), oxygenation (methemoglobinemia, anemia), or ventilation (obesity, ascites, abdominal organomegaly). • Primary respiratory diseases may be divided into upper and lower respiratory tract problems; the latter can be subdivided into obstructive and restrictive causes.

Systems Affected

• Respiratory • Cardiovascular • Nervous (secondary to hypoxia) • Hemic/lymphatic/immune—acid-base disturbances (secondary to hyper- or hypoventilation)

SIGNALMENT

Depends on the underlying cause (i.e., toy breeds with tracheal collapse, older dogs with mitral valvular insufficiency, tomcats with pyothorax)

SIGNS

Historical Findings

• Orthopnea (recumbent dyspnea), restlessness, and poor sleeping may occur in animals with pleural space disease (diaphragmatic hernias, effusions, pneumothorax) or CHF. • Coughing may accompany dyspnea, and the character may relate to the cause (soft and moist in CHF, dry and "honking" in tracheal collapse).

Physical Examination Findings

• Nasal obstruction—impaired nasal airflow • Upper airway obstruction—stridor, stertor, tracheal sensitivity, and honking cough with tracheal collapse • Pulmonary edema—fine inspiratory crackles • Pneumonia—harsh inspiratory and expiratory bronchovesicular sounds • Bronchitis or asthma—harsh wheezes with or without crackles • Pneumothorax—hyperresonant percussion ventrally with absence of lung sounds, lung sounds heard dorsally • Pleural effusion or diaphragmatic hernia—dull percussion and absent lung sounds ventrally, harsh lung sounds dorsally

CAUSES

Nonrespiratory Causes

• Cardiac diseases—CHF (mitral valvular insufficiency), low-output failure (cardiomyopathy, subaortic stenosis), cyanotic heart disease (right-to-left shunts in reverse PDA and tetralogy of Fallot), severe arrhythmias, cardiogenic shock • Neuromuscular disease—severe CNS disease (trauma, neoplasia, inflammation), polyradiculoneuritis (coonhound paralysis), spinal disease (disk extrusion, trauma), myasthenia gravis (aspiration pneumonia, megaesophagus, hypoventilation), polymyopathies • Metabolic disease—acidosis, diabetic ketoacidosis, uremia • Hematologic—methemoglobinemia (acetominophen intoxication), anemia, hyperviscosity syndrome • Other—pain, fever, anxiety, heat stroke, obesity (Pickwickian syndrome - excessive fat in the chest wall, intrathoracic fat, and cranial displacement of the diaphragm due to abdominal obesity), ascites, abdominal organomegaly.

Respiratory Causes

Upper Respiratory Tract (URT)
Brachycephalic syndrome (stenotic nares, elongated soft palate, laryngeal edema, everted laryngeal saccules), nasal obstruction (granuloma, foreign body, neoplasia, cuterebriasis), tonsillar enlargement (hyperplasia or neoplasia), laryngeal paralysis, tracheal stenosis or hypoplasia (bulldogs), cervical tracheal collapse, laryngotracheal foreign body or neoplasia (adenocarcinoma in Siamese cats), traumatic airway rupture, extraluminal compression (mediastinal mass, hilar lymphadenopathy)

Lower Respiratory Tract (LRT)
• Obstructive—intrathoracic tracheal disease (tracheal collapse, foreign body, neoplasia), bronchial disease (bronchial collapse, compression by enlarged left atrium in mitral insufficiency, chronic bronchitis, feline asthma, bronchoconstriction, bronchogenic carcinoma), pulmonary edema (cardiac and noncardiac), pneumonitis (allergic, parasitic), pneumonia (fungal, bacterial, viral), neoplasia (primary, metastatic), pulmonary contusion (trauma), lung lobe torsion • Restrictive—interstitial fibrosis, fibrosing pleuritis, pyothorax, hydrothorax, pleural effusion caused by cardiac or pericardial disease, hemothorax (coagulopathy or trauma), chylothorax, nonseptic exudates (FIP, pancreatitis), pneumothorax (open, closed, tension), hernias (diaphragmatic, pericardioperitoneal), mediastinal masses, rib fractures, and flail chest

RISK FACTORS

Poor ventilation or secondhand smoke (allergic or irritant bronchitis), blunt chest trauma, bite wounds (pyothorax, septic shock), and ingestion of rodenticides (hemothorax)

 DIAGNOSIS

DIFFERENTIAL DIAGNOSIS

• Tachypnea without dyspnea may be a physiologic response to fear, physical exertion, anxiety, fever, heat, pain, or acidosis.
• Primary cardiac disease often presents with a constellation of other signs (e.g., heart murmurs, gallop rhythms, distended jugular veins, pulse deficits, weak femoral pulses, moist cough). • URT dyspnea is often more pronounced on inspiration • LRT obstructions are more often associated with expiratory effort. Fixed obstructions (intraluminal mass or foreign body) may have both inspiratory and expiratory dyspnea. • Pleural space disease often presents as exaggerated chest excursions that generate only minimal airflow at the mouth or nares.

CBC/BIOCHEMISTRY/URINALYSIS

• Hemogram—anemia, polycythemia (cyanotic heart diseases), inflammatory leukocytosis (pneumonia, pyothorax), eosinophilia (allergic or parasitic pneumonitis), and basophilia (heartworm disease) • Biochemistry panel—uremia (azotemia), acidosis (low PCO_2), diabetes (hyperglycemia), hypothyroidism (cholesterol high and T4 low) • Urinalysis—isosthenuria (renal azotemia), proteinuria (predispose to pulmonary thromboembolism [PTE]), pyuria (pyelonephritis, sepsis)

OTHER LABORATORY TESTS

• Heartworm test • Arterial blood gas—assess oxygenation (PaO_2) and ventilation (PCO_2). If unavailable in your clinic, make arrangements with the Stat Lab in local human hospital, and have the owners deliver the sample immediately. • ACTH stimulation (rule out hyperadrenocorticism as a cause of pulmonary thromboembolism)

IMAGING

Radiography

• Skull—nasal obstructions (fungal or neoplastic bony destruction) • Cervical—tracheal collapse; may best be visualized fluoroscopically • Thoracic—tracheal collapse, pleural space disease (effusions, pneumothorax, hernias), pulmonary diseases (peribronchiolar, small airway disease; alveolar, pulmonary edema and pneumonia; pulmonary contusions and interstitial pneumonia) • Cardiac shadow (globose in pericardial effusions, generalized cardiomegaly in cardiomyopthy, valentine-shaped cardiomyopathy in cats, left atrial enlargement in mitral regurgitation). In cardiogenic pulmonary edema, there should be evidence of left atrial enlargement (best seen on the lateral projection), as well as pulmonary venous distension (pulmonary veins > the pulmonary arteries) . This concept does not hold true for noncardiogenic pulmonary edema (i.e., electrocution). • Evaluation of pickwickian syndrome • Severe dyspnea with normal to hyperlucent lungs on radiographs is highly suggestive of pulmonary thromboembolism or asthma.

Ultrasonography

• Echocardiography is a sensitive and noninvasive means of evaluating pericardial effusion, cardiomyopathy, congenital defects, and valvular disease. • Thoracic ultrasound may be beneficial in some animals with mediastinal mass lesions, but the beam is greatly attenuated by any air in surrounding lung lobes.

OTHER DIAGNOSTIC PROCEDURES
• Thoracentesis • Fluid analysis and culture • Lung wash—cytology and culture, specimen retrieved by transtracheal wash or tracheobronchoscopy • Tracheoscopy—assessment and staging of tracheal collapse • Bronchoscopy—allows evaluation of upper and lower airways and collection of specimens for cytology and culture • Others—cerebral spinal fluid (CSF) tap (to rule out CNS disease)

TREATMENT
• Airway—if URT is obstructed, may require intubation (if possible) or tracheostomy • Breathing—supply O$_2$ enrichment (nasal O$_2$, O$_2$ cage, or induction chamber). Ventilate only if animal has bradypnea, pulmonary arrest, or is hypoventilating from exhaustion. If the hypoventilation is from pleural space disease, artificial ventilation and O$_2$ supplementation do little until chest is evacuated.
• Chest tap—this may be both diagnostic and therapeutic in animals with pleural space disease. Should be performed in acutely dyspneic animals, especially trauma patients, before radiography. A negative tap for air or fluid suggests solid pleural space (mass or herniated viscus), primary pulmonary (i.e., contusion in the trauma patient), or cardiac disease. If the tap is positive, remember that small animals may accommodate up to 50 ml/kg free fluid in the chest before becoming dyspneic. Be sure to remove as much fluid as possible; do not stop after you have a diagnostic sample.
• Dyspneic cats are especially fragile. Often, even very stressed cats may be quickly clipped and prepped with minimal restraint and a chest tap performed. If this is not possible, or the tap is "dry," O$_2$, furosemide (IM), nitro-

glycerin topically, and glucocorticoids (IM) are recommended. Status asthmaticus and acute heart failure can appear similar in cats. It is unlikely that this "shotgun" approach will exacerbate either disease. Epinephrine should be reserved for cats with respiratory distress from asthma, once cardiac disease has been ruled out.
• Sedation may be desirable at this time, especially in the frantically air-starved cat. Low dose morphine or butorphanol tartrate have been used safely. This may be prudent before diagnostic procedures (thoracentesis, radiographs, ultrasound, etc.).

MEDICATIONS

FLUIDS AND DRUGS
• Oxygen is the single most underused drug in the treatment of acute severe dyspnea.
• See primary disorder for definitive therapy.

CONTRAINDICATIONS
• In animals with CHF and blunt chest trauma, iatrogenic fluid overload and pulmonary edema is a potential problem. Intravenous administration of crystalloids should be used judiciously.
• Respiratory rate and effort should be monitored carefully and frequently in these patients.

PRECAUTIONS N/A

POSSIBLE INTERACTIONS
Propranolol as an antiarrhythmic may potentiate bronchoconstriction in asthmatic patients.

ALTERNATE DRUGS N/A

FOLLOW-UP

PATIENT MONITORING
• Repeat any abnormal tests • CBC—in inflammatory, infectious, parasitic, anemic, or polycythemic patients • Cardiac ultra-

sound—3-12 weeks, depending on the condition • Radiographs—pulmonary edema should be visibly improved within 12 hours of therapy, if effective therapy is used. Monitoring recurrence of pleural effusion, based upon how quickly the effusion accumulated initially (often unknown).

POSSIBLE COMPLICATIONS
• Relapse, progression of disease and death are common • Depends on the underlying disease

MISCELLANEOUS
ASSOCIATED CONDITIONS N/A

ZOONOTIC POTENTIAL N/A

PREGNANCY N/A

SYNONYMS N/A

SEE ALSO See causes.

ABBREVIATIONS
CHF = congestive heart failure
PDA = patent ductus arteriosus
URT = upper respiratory tract
LRT = lower respiratory tract

References
Keuhn NF, Roudebush P. Dyspnea. In: Allen DG, Kruth SA, Garvey MS, eds. Small animal medicine. Philadelphia: JB Lippincott, 1991:131-145.
Ettinger SJ. Dyspnea and tachypnea. In: Ettinger SJ, ed. Textbook of small animal internal medicine. 3rd ed. Philadelphia: WB Saunders, 1989:88-90.
Ware W. Dyspnea: diagnosis and management. In: August JR, ed. Consultations in feline medicine. 1991:147-169.

Author Robert Mason
Consulting Editors Lynelle Johnson and Bradley L. Moses

DYSTOCIA

BASICS

DEFINITION
Difficult birth

Pathophysiology
Labor has three stages:
Stage 1 begins with onset of uterine contractions and ends when the cervix is fully dilated. It averages from 6-12 hours. Bitches may appear restless, nervous, anorectic, and may shiver, pant, vomit, or pace. Most bitches seek a place to "nest" near the end of this stage. Queens tend to vocalize initially, then purr as delivery approaches.
Stage 2 begins with full dilation of the cervix, entry of the first fetus into the cervical canal, and rupture of the chorioallantois; it ends with delivery of the last puppy. The bitch shows obvious abdominal contractions in her attempt to deliver the puppies. The time between initiation of stage 2 and delivery of the first fetus varies (usually < 4 hours). The time between delivery of subsequent fetuses also varies (usually 20-60 minutes), but can be as long as 2-3 hours in the bitch.
Stage 3 begins after delivery of the fetus(es) and ends with passage of all placentae. If the bitch has multiple puppies, she may alternate between stage 2 and stage 3.
The pathophysiology of dystocia centers around a small or deformed birth canal, fetal oversize, or uterine weakness, i.e., insufficient uterine force to propel fetus through birth canal.

Systems Affected
• Reproductive • Cardiovascular

SIGNALMENT
Common in brachycephalic, miniature, and small dog breeds; occasionally seen in large dog breeds with an extremely large litter; frequently seen in the Persian and Himalayan breeds. • Prevalence increases with age.

SIGNS

Historical Findings
• The bitch or queen has had 30 minutes of persistent, strong, abdominal contractions without expulsion of fetus • More than 4 hours from the onset of stage 2 to delivery of the first fetus • More than 2 hours between delivery of fetuses • Failure to deliver a puppy or kitten 24 hours after rectal temperature falls below 99° F or within 36 hours of serum progesterone < 2 ng/ml • The bitch or queen crys and displays signs of pain and constantly licks the vulvar area when delivering. • Prolonged gestation, i.e., > 70 days from day of first mating, > 59 days from the first day of diestrus (dogs), > 66 days from luteinizing hormone (LH) peak (dogs)

CAUSES

Fetal
Oversize (e.g., one-pup litter, monster, anasarcous fetus, and hydrocephalus) and malposition in birth canal

Maternal
• Abnormal pelvic canal from previous pelvic fracture, congenitally small pelvis (e.g., Welsh corgi and brachycephalic breeds), and pelvic immaturity • Abnormality of the vaginal vault caused by stricture, septae, hyperplasia, intraluminal or extraluminal cyst, or neoplasia. • Insufficient cervical dilation • Lack of adequate lubrication • Uterine torsion • Poor uterine contractions caused by myometrial defect, biochemical imbalance, psychogenic disturbance, or exhaustion (see Uterine inertia). • Ineffective abdominal press due to pain, debility (exhaustion), diaphragmatic hernia, or age

RISK FACTORS
• Age • Brachycephalic and toy breeds • Persian and Himalayan breeds • Obesity • Abrupt change in environment peri-partum • Previous history of dystocia

DIAGNOSIS

DIFFERENTIAL DIAGNOSIS
• Previously diagnosed pelvic or vaginal anomaly and type of breed may help differentiate obstructive dystocia from uterine inertia. • A complete physical examination is essential. Determine concurrent or contributing problem (e.g., hypoglycemia, hypocalcemia, dehydration, and fever). Careful abdominal palpation is used to confirm the presence of fetuses. • A detailed and meticulous, digital vaginal examination can identify the presence of a fetus engaged in the vaginal canal, abnormalities of the maternal pelvic canal or vaginal vault, and the strength of abdominal press in response to stimulation of the roof of the vagina ("feathering"). • Bitches that fail to respond to feathering or to oxytocin with good abdominal contractions are more likely to have uterine inertia than obstructive dystocia unless the obstruction is of several hours' duration.

CBC/BIOCHEMISTRY/URINALYSIS
• Minimum database—PCV, total protein, BUN, and serum glucose and calcium concentrations; results vary from normal to hypoglycemia, dehydration, and hypocalcemia depending on the length of dystocia. • CBC, serum biochemistry, and urinalysis should be done even though results might not be available until after resolution of the dystocia.

OTHER LABORATORY TESTS N/A

Imaging
• Radiography of the abdomen and pelvic area is paramount—determine the presence or absence of pregnancy, pelvic structure, number and malpostion (if present) of fetuses, fetal oversize, and fetal death. • Ultrasonography is recommended to monitor fetal viability and detect the presence of fetal stress (i.e., fetal heart rate <200 bpm).

OTHER DIAGNOSTIC PROCEDURES
N/A

TREATMENT
Treat as inpatient until delivery of all fetuses and stabilization of the dam is accomplished.

MANUAL TREATMENT
Used to deliver a fetus lodged in vaginal vault. Apply lubrication liberally and have the bitch in standing position; use of fingers is the safest and most reliable approach. If the vaginal vault is too small for digital manipulation, instruments can be used provided lubrication is adequate; always place a finger in the vaginal vault to direct the instrument. A spay hook or a nonratcheted forceps is recommended, and traction should be applied in a posterior and ventral direction. One should exercise extreme caution when using instruments to relieve dystocia in the bitch. Undesirable sequelae include mutilation of the fetus and laceration of the dam. Traction on a distal extremity is definitely contraindicated. Use of instruments is not recommended in the queen because of the small size of the vaginal vault. Failure to deliver the fetus with 25-30 minutes is an indication for cesarean section.

SURGICAL TREATMENT
A cesarean section is indicated in the bitch or queen with uterine inertia unresponsive to oxytocin, pelvic or vaginal obstruction, uncorrectable fetal malposition, fetal oversize, fetal stress, or in utero fetal death. Elective cesarean section is indicated in breeds highly prone to dystocia and bitches with a history of dystocia.

MEDICATIONS
• Fluid replacement with balanced electrolyte solutions in clinically dehydrated patients • Initiate medical treatment in a patient with uterine inertia and no evidence of fetal stress.

DRUGS AND FLUIDS

Anesthetic Recommendations
• In a healthy or depressed bitch, premedication should consist of diazepam (0.2-0.4 mg/kg) and butorphanol (0.2-0.4 mg/kg) IM with or without anticholinergics; mask and maintain with isoflurane; administer fluids IV. • In a healthy queen, premedicate with diazepam (0.4 mg/kg) and ketamine (6 mg/kg) IV; administer fluids IV; use 0.5% lidocaine spray for intubation; isoflurane is preferred but halothane can be used. • In a severely depressed queen exhausted from prolonged labor, fluid and electrolyte balance should be restored before anesthetic induction; administer diazepam or midazolam (0.2-0.4 mg/kg) IV, IM with butorphanol (0.4 mg/kg) IV, IM or oxymorphone

(0.2 mg/kg) IM for sedation, low-dose keta-mine (1-2 mg/kg) IV for intubation, and eto-midate or propofol for induction; at the end of surgery, all effects of drugs can be reversed.
• Oxytocin is used to treat uterine inertia; administer balanced electrolyte solution, ad-justed to correct for any electrolyte imbalance identified.

CONTRAINDICATIONS
Oxytocin is contraindicated in patients with obstructive dystocia of fetal or maternal cause, fetal stress, and longstanding in utero fetal death.

PRECAUTIONS N/A

POSSIBLE INTERACTIONS N/A

ALTERNATE DRUGS N/A

FOLLOW-UP

PATIENT MONITORING
Ultrasonography is recommended to monitor fetal heart rate during medical management of uterine inertia.

POSSIBLE COMPLICATIONS
Increased risk of dystocia in future pregnancies

MISCELLANEOUS

ASSOCIATED CONDITIONS N/A

AGE RELATED FACTORS
Old, obese bitches have increased risk of inertia

ZOONOTIC POTENTIAL N/A

PREGNANCY N/A

SYNONYMS N/A

SEE ALSO Uterine Inertia

ABBREVIATIONS
LH = luteinizing hormone

References

Feldman EC, Nelson RW. Dystocia. In: Canine and feline endocrinology and repro-duction. Philadelphia: WB Saunders, 1987; 438-442, 536.

Shille VM. Diagnosis and management of dystocia in the bitch and queen. In: Bojrab MJ, ed. Current techniques in small animal surgery. Philadelphia: Lea & Febiger, 1983.

Paddleford RR. Anesthetic management of the cesarean section. In: Manual of small animal anesthesia. Churchill Livingstone, 1988;290-296.

Tranquilli WJ. Anesthesia for cesarean sec-tion in the cat. Vet Clin North Am Small Anim Pract 1992;22:484-486.

Author Louis F. Archbald
Consulting Editor Sara K. Lyle

DYSURIA AND POLLAKIURIA

BASICS

DEFINITION
Dysuria refers to difficult or painful urination.

Pollakiuria refers to voiding of small quantities of urine more frequently than normal.

Pathophysiology
The urinary bladder and urethra normally serve as a reservoir for storage and periodic release of urine. Inflammatory and noninflammatory disorders of the lower urinary tract may impair bladder compliance and storage capacity by damaging structural components of the bladder wall or by stimulating sensory nerve endings located in the bladder or urethra. Sensations of bladder fullness, urgency, and pain stimulate premature micturition and reduce functional bladder capacity. Dysuria and pollakiuria are caused by lesions of the urinary bladder or urethra and provide unequivocal evidence of lower urinary tract disease. These clinical signs, however, do not exclude concurrent involvement of the upper urinary tract.

Systems Affected
Renal/urologic—bladder, urethra, and prostate gland

SIGNALMENT Dogs and cats

SIGNS N/A

CAUSES

Urinary Bladder
• Urinary tract infection (i.e., bacterial, viral, fungal, parasitic, or mycoplasmal) • Urocystolithiasis • Neoplasia (e.g., transitional cell carcinoma) • Trauma • Anatomic anomaly (e.g., ureterocele, persistent uterus masculinus, perineal hernia containing the urinary bladder, and spay granuloma) • Detrusor atony (e.g., chronic partial obstruction and dysautonomia) • Chemicals/Drugs (e.g., cyclophosphamide) • Iatrogenic (e.g., catheterization, palpation, reverse flushing, overdistension of the bladder during contrast radiography, urohydropropulsion, urethrocystoscopy, and surgery) • Idiopathic (e.g., idiopathic feline lower urinary tract disease)

Urethra
• Urinary tract infection (see previous section) • Urethrolithiasis • Urethral plugs (e.g., matrix and matrix–crystalline) • Neoplasia (see previous section) • Trauma • Anatomic anomaly (e.g., congenital or acquired stricture, urethrorectal fistula, and pseudohermaphrodites) • Urethral sphincter hypertonicity (e.g., upper motor neuron spinal cord lesion, reflex dyssynergia, and urethral spasm) • Iatrogenic (see previous section) • Idiopathic (see previous section)

Prostate Gland
• Prostatitis or prostatic abscess • Neoplasia (e.g., adenocarcinoma and transitional cell carcinoma) • Cystic hyperplasia • Paraprostatic cysts

RISK FACTORS
• Disease , diagnostic procedure, or treatment that (1) alters normal host urinary tract defenses and predisposes animal to infection; (2) predisposes animal to formation of uroliths; (3) damages the urothelium or other tissues composing the lower urinary tract
• Mural or extramural disease that compresses the urethral lumen

DIAGNOSIS

DIFFERENTIAL DIAGNOSIS

Differentiate From Other Abnormal Patterns of Micturition
• Rule out polyuria (increased frequency and volume of urine, greater than 50 ml/kg/day)
• Rule out urethral obstruction (stranguria, anuria, overdistended urinary bladder, signs of post renal uremia) • Rule out urinary incontinence (involuntary urination, urine dribbling, enuresis, incomplete bladder emptying) • Rule out urine spraying or marking (voiding of small amounts of urine on vertical surfaces or other socially significant places)

Differentiate Causes of Dysuria and Pollakiuria
• Rule out urinary tract infection (hematuria, malodorous or cloudy urine, and small, painful, thickened bladder). • Rule out urolithiasis (hematuria and palpable uroliths in urethra or bladder). • Rule out neoplasia (hematuria and palpable masses in urethra or bladder). • Rule out neurogenic disorders (flaccid bladder wall, residual urine in bladder lumen after micturition, and other neurologic deficits of the hind limbs, tail, perineum, and anal sphincter) • Rule out prostatic diseases (urethral discharge, prostatomegaly, pyrexia, depression, tenesmus, caudal abdominal pain, and stiff gait) • Rule out cyclophosphamide cystitis (history) • Rule out iatrogenic disorders (history of catheterization, reverse flushing, contrast radiography, urohydropropulsion, urethrocystoscopy, or surgery)

CBC/BIOCHEMISTRY/URINALYSIS
• Results often normal. However, animals with lower urinary tract disease complicated by urethral obstruction may have azotemia, acidosis, and hyperkalemia. Animals with concurrent pyelonephritis may have impaired urine concentrating capacity, leukocytosis, and azotemia. Animal with acute prostatitis or prostatic abscesses may have leukocytosis.
• Disorders of the urinary bladder are best evaluated by anlaysis of a urine specimen collected by cystocentesis. Urethral disorders are best evaluated by analysis of a voided urine sample or by comparison of results of analysis of voided and cystocentesis samples (caution: cystocentesis can induce hematuria). • Pyuria,

hematuria, and proteinuria indicate urinary tract inflammation; however, they are nonspecific findings and may result from infectious and noninfectious causes of lower urinary tract disease. • Identification of bacteria, fungi, or parasite ova in urine sediment is suggestive but not conclusive evidence that urinary tract infection may be causing or complicating lower urinary tract disease. Contamination of urine during collection and storage must be considered when interpreting urinalysis results. • Identification of neoplastic cells in urine sediment indicates urinary tract neoplasia. Caution should be used in establishing a diagnosis of neoplasia based on urine sediment examination. Urinary tract inflammation or extremes in urine pH or osmolality can cause epithelial cell atypia that is difficult to differentiate from neoplasia. • Crystalluria is observed in normal patients, patients with urolithiasis, and patients with lower urinary tract disease not associated with uroliths. Therefore, caution must be used in interpreting the importantce of crystalluria. • Hematuria, proteinuria, and variable crystalluria are observed in cats with nonobstructive idiopathic lower urinary tract disease. Pyuria is rarely observed in these patients.

OTHER LABORATORY TESTS
• Quantitative urine culture provides the most definitive means of identifying and characterizing bacterial urinary tract infection. Negative urine culture results suggest that dysuria and pollakiuria may be the result of a noninfectious cause (e.g., uroliths and neoplasia) or inflammation associated with urinary tract infection caused by fastidious organisms (e.g., mycoplasmas and viruses).
• Cytologic evaluation of urine sediment, prostatic fluid, urethral or vaginal discharge, or biopsy specimen obtained by catheter or needle aspiration may help to evaluate patients with localized urinary tract disease. Cytologic examination may establish a definitive diagnosis of urinary tract neoplasia; however, negative cytologic findings do not rule out neoplasia.

IMAGING
Survey abdominal radiography, contrast urethrocystography and cystography, urinary tract ultrasonography, and excretory urography are important means of identifying and localizing causes of dysuria and pollakiuria.

OTHER DIAGNOSTIC PROCEDURES
Light microscopic evaluation of tissue specimens is indicated in patients with persistent lesions of the urinary tract for which a definitive diagnosis has not been established by other, less invasive means. Tissue specimens may be obtained by catheter biopsy, by urethrocystoscopy and pinch biopsy, or by surgery.

TREATMENT

- Patients with nonobstructive lower urinary tract disease are typically managed as outpatients. However, diagnostic evaluation may require brief hospitalization.
- Dysuria and pollakiuria associated with systemic signs of illness (e.g., pyrexia, depression, anorexia, vomiting, and dehydration) or laboratory findings of azotemia or leukocytosis warrant aggressive diagnostic evaluation and initiation of supportive and symptomatic treatment.
- Treatment varies depending on the underlying cause and specific sites involved. See specific chapters describing diseases listed in the section on causes.
- Clinical signs of dysuria and pollakiuria resolve quickly after specific treatment of the underlying cause.

MEDICATIONS

DRUGS AND FLUIDS

- Patients with urge incontinence, severe or persistent signs, or untreatable lower urinary tract disease may benefit from symptomatic treatment with propantheline or oxybutynin. Both are anticholinergic agents that reduce the force and frequency of uncontrolled detrusor contractions.
- Patients with transitional cell carcinoma of the urinary bladder or urethra may be symptomatically managed with the nonsteroidal antiinflammatory drug piroxicam, which reduces the severity of clinical signs, improves quality of life, and in some patients, induces tumor remission.

CONTRAINDICATIONS

- Glucocorticoids or other immunosuppressive agents in patients suspected of having urinary or genital tract infection
- Potentially nephrotoxic drugs (e.g., gentamicin) in patients who are febrile, dehydrated, or azotemic or who are suspected of having pyelonephritis, septicemia, or preexisting renal disease

PRECAUTIONS N/A

POSSIBLE INTERACTIONS N/A

ALTERNATE DRUGS N/A

FOLLOW-UP

PATIENT MONITORING

- Response to treatment by clinical signs and by serial physical examinations, laboratory testing, and radiographic and ultrasonographic evaluations appropriate for each specific cause.
- Refer to specific chapters describing diseases listed in the section on causes.

POSSIBLE COMPLICATIONS

- Dysuria and pollakiuria may be associated with formation of macroscopic vesicourachal diverticula.
- Refer to specific chapters describing diseases listed in the section on causes.

MISCELLANEOUS

ASSOCIATED CONDITIONS

- Hematuria, pyuria, and proteinuria
- Disorders predisposing to urinary tract infection
- Disorders predisposing to formation of uroliths

- Macroscopic vesicourachal diverticula

AGE- RELATED FACTORS N/A

ZOONOTIC POTENTIAL N/A

PREGNANCY N/A

SYNONYMS

- Feline urological syndrome (FUS) • Lower urinary tract disease

SEE ALSO

- Lower Urinary Tract Infection • Urolithiasis • Urinary Retention, Functional • Urinary Tract Obstruction • Feline Lower Urinary Tract Disease • Vesicourachal Diverticula

ABBREVIATIONS None

References

Hammer AS, LaRue S. Tumors of the urinary tract. In Textbook of Veterinary Internal Medicine, Ettinger SJ, Feldman EC, editors. 4th ed. Philadelphia, WB Saunders Co. 1995.1788–1796.

Lulich JP, Osborne CA. Bacterial infections of the urinary tract. In Textbook of Veterinary Internal Medicine, Ettinger SJ, Feldman EC, editors. 4th ed. Philadelphia, WB Saunders Co. 1995.1775–1788.

Lulich JP, Osborne CA, Bartges JW, et al. Canine lower urinary tract disorders. In Textbook of Veterinary Internal Medicine. Ettinger SJ, Feldman C, editors. 4th ed. Philadelphia, WB Saunders Co. 1995.1805–1832.

Authors John M. Kruger and Carl A. Osborne
Consulting Editors Larry G. Adams and Carl A. Osborne

EPIPHORA

BASICS

DEFINITION
Abnormal overflow of the aqueous portion of the precorneal tear film

Pathophysiology
Caused by overproduction of the aqueous portion of tears (usually in response to ocular irritation), poor eyelid function secondary to malformation or deformity, or by blockage of the nasolacrimal drainage system

Systems Affected
Ophthalmic—eyelids, nasolacrimal system, periocular skin

SIGNALMENT See causes

SIGNS N/A

CAUSES

Overproduction of Tears Secondary to Ocular Irritants
Congenital malformations
• Distichiasis or trichiasis (common in young sheltie, shih tzu, lhasa apso, cocker spaniel, and miniature poodle) • Entropion (shar pei and chow chow). • Eyelid agenesis (domestic shorthaired cats)
Acquired causes
• Corneal or conjunctival foreign bodies (usually young, large-breed, active dogs). • Eyelid neoplasms (older dogs—all breeds). • Blepharitis (infectious or immune-mediated). • Conjunctivitis (infectious or immune-mediated) • Ulcerative keratitis • Anterior uveitis • Glaucoma

Eyelid Abnormalities/Poor Eyelid Function
Tears never reach the nasolacrimal puncta but instead spill over the eyelid margin.
Congenital malformations
• Macropalpebral fissures (brachiocephalic breeds) • Ectropion (great dane, blood-hound, spaniels) • Entropion (especially of the medial lower lid)
Acquired causes
• Post-traumatic eyelid scarring • Facial nerve paralysis

Obstruction of the Nasolacrimal Drainage System
Congenital malformations
• Imperforate nasolacrimal puncta (cocker spaniel, bulldog, and poodle) • Ectopic nasolacrimal openings (i.e., extra openings along the side of the face ventral to the medial canthus) • Nasolacrimal atresia (i.e., lack of distal openings into the nose)
Acquired nasolacrimal obstructions
• Rhinitis or sinusitis (causes swelling adjacent to the nasolacrimal duct) • Trauma or fractures of the lacrimal or maxillary bones • Foreign bodies (e.g., grass awns, seeds, sand, and parasites) • Neoplasia (of the third eyelid, conjunctiva, medial eyelids, nasal cavi-

ty, maxillary bone, or periocular sinuses) • Dacryocystitis (inflammation of the canaliculi, lacrimal sac, or nasolacrimal ducts)

RISK FACTORS
• Breeds prone to congenital eyelid abnormalities (see previous section). • Active outdoor dogs are at risk for foreign bodies.

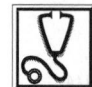

DIAGNOSIS

DIFFERENTIAL DIAGNOSIS
• Differentiate from other ocular discharges (such as mucus or purulent). Epiphora is a watery, serous discharge. • The eye is usually red in animals with epiphora caused by overproduction of tears, and quiet when secondary to impaired outflow. • A thorough ocular examination should help rule out irritative causes of epiphora and some congenital causes of obstruction. • Acute onset, unilateral epiphora with ocular pain (blepharospasm) usually indicates a foreign body or corneal injury. • Chronic, bilateral epiphora usually indicates a congenital problem • Facial pain, swelling, nasal discharge, or sneezing may indicate a nasal or sinus infection or neoplasm which is obstructing the nasolacrimal system. • Mucus or purulent discharge at the medial canthus in addition to epiphora may indicate dacryocystitis.

CBC/BIOCHEMISTRY/URINALYSIS
N/A

OTHER LABORATORY TESTS N/A

IMAGING
• Skull radiographs may show a nasal, sinus, or maxillary bone lesion. • Dacryocystorhinography—radiopaque contrast material helps to localize nasolacrimal obstruction. • Magnetic resonance imaging or computed tomography may help localize the site of nasolacrimal obstruction and characterize associated lesions.

OTHER DIAGNOSTIC PROCEDURES
• If purulent material is seen at the medial canthus (e.g., dacryocystitis), bacterial culture and sensitivity testing and cytologic examination of the material should be performed before instilling any substance into the eye. • Topical fluorescein dye application to the eye—dye will flow though the nasolacrimal system and reach the external nares in approximately 10 seconds in a normal dog. This is the most physiologic test for nasolacrimal function and should be performed first. • Nasolacrimal flush—a nasolacrimal cannula is inserted into the upper nasolacrimal punctum, and eyewash is flushed through the cannula. If fluid does not exit the lower nasolacrimal punctum, the obstruction is in the upper or lower canaliculi, the nasolacrimal sac, or the lower punctum (imperforate). The lower punctum is then manually

obstructed, and further flushing should result in fluid exiting the external nares. If this does not occur, the obstruction is in the nasolacrimal duct or at its distal opening (atresia or blockage from a nasal sinus lesion). • Rhinoscopy (+/- biopsy or bacterial culture) may be indicated if the previous tests suggest a nasal or sinus lesion. • Surgical exploratory may be the only way to obtain a definitive diagnosis. • Temporary tacking out of the lower medial eyelid with suture may help determine whether repair of medial lower entropion or repositioning of the eyelid would reduce epiphora secondary to eyelid conformational abnormalities.

TREATMENT
• Confirmation of the obstruction can be made by performing a nasolacrimal flush, which reveals blockage of fluid or dislodges foreign material.
• Removal of the cause of ocular irritation may involve removing a conjunctival or corneal foreign body or treating the primary ocular disease (e.g., conjunctivitis, ulcerative keratitis, and uveitis).
• Cryosurgery or electroepilation for distichiasis, entropion correction, medial or lateral canthoplasties (for medial trichiasis and macropalpebral fissures), or correction of cicatricial eyelid abnormalities may be needed to relieve ocular irritation.
• Treatment of the primary obstructing lesion (e.g., third eyelid mass, nasal or sinus mass, and infection) should be done initially. Successful management of the primary lesion may allow normal nasolacrimal flow to resume.

IMPERFORATE PUNCTA
Surgical opening of the puncta is indicated. If one of the puncta is patent (usually the upper punctum), flushing eyewash through the upper opening will cause "tenting" of the conjunctiva at the site of the lower punctum. With the animal under topical or general anesthesia, the conjunctiva overlying the lower canaliculi is grasped with forceps and cut with scissors to leave a patent punctum. The same procedure can be done to open puncta closed by conjunctival scarring (symblepharon) caused by severe conjunctivitis (e.g., Herpesvirus conjunctivitis in cats). In animals with recurrent disease, it may be necessary to suture silastic tubing in place to prevent stricture formation.

OBSTRUCTION OF NASOLACRIMAL DUCT
When the more distal nasolacrimal duct is obliterated or obstructed, dacryocystorhinotomy or conjunctivorhinotomy can be used to create an opening to drain the tears into the nasal cavity. See reference for surgical technique.

MEDICATIONS

DRUGS AND FLUIDS
• While awaiting results of diagnostic tests (e.g., bacterial culture and sensitivity testing and diagnostic radiographs), topically applied, broad-spectrum antibiotic ophthalmic solutions can be prescribed (q4-6h); good selections include neomycin, bacitracin, polymyxin triple ophthalmic antibiotic solutions, and ophthalmic chloramphenicol solution.
• Treatment of dacryocystitis should be based on bacterial culture and sensitivity test results, and treatment should be continued for at least 21 days.

CONTRAINDICATIONS
• Topical corticosteriods or antibiotic-corticosteroid combinations should be avoided unless a definitive diagnosis has been made.
• Topical corticosteroids should never be used if the cornea retains fluorescein stain.

PRECAUTIONS N/A

POSSIBLE INTERACTIONS N/A

ALTERNATE DRUGS
• In animals with idiopathic tear staining of the periocular facial hair, tetracycline (5 mg/kg, q24h, PO) may help reduce discoloration. The staining recurs, however, when the drug is discontinued.

FOLLOW-UP

PATIENT MONITORING

Dacryocystitis
• Reevaluation should be done every 7 days until the condition is resolved. • Treatment should be continued for at least 7 days after resolution of clinical signs to help prevent recurrence. • If the problem persists for more than 7-10 days during treatment or if the problem recurs soon after cessation of treatment, a foreign body or nidus of persistent infection is probably present. Further diagnostics, such as a dacryostorhinography, are then indicated. • In many animals with persistent dacryocystitis, a nasolacrimal catheter is needed to maintain patency of the duct and to prevent stricturing. To pass a catheter (silastic or polyethylene [PE90] tubing), 2-0 nylon is passed via the upper punctum and threaded through the nasolacrimal duct to exit the external nares. The silastic tubing is then passed retrograde over the suture. The upper and lower portions of the tubing are then sutured to the face. Most dogs tolerate the tubing well, and it is left in place for 2-4 weeks. Topical antibiotics are continued as before.

Dacryocystorhinotomy/Conjunctivorhinostomy
• Reevaluate every 7 days while silastic tubing is in place to ensure that the tubing remains intact. Resuturing may be needed if the tubing becomes loosened or dislodged.
• After the tubing has been removed, reevaluate in 14 days. At this and future examinations, fluorescein should be placed on the eye and nasolacrimal patency checked by examining the external nares for fluorescein; the nasolacrimal system can be evaluated further by cannulating and flushing with eyewash.
• Three to 4 months after surgery, a dacryocystorhinography contrast study should be repeated to evaluate the size of the nasal opening, and it should be repeated if epiphora returns or if there is no nasolacrimal fluorescein drainage.

POSSIBLE COMPLICATIONS
Recurrence of epiphora is the most common complication. This can happen because of recurrence of ocular irritation (e.g., corneal ulceration, distichiasis, entropion), recurrence of dacryocystitis, or closure of the dacryocystorhinotomy or conjunctivorhinostomy openings into the nasal cavity. Owners should be warned that their animal is predisposed to nasolacrimal obstruction and that recurrence is common. Early detection and intervention provides a better long-term prognosis.

MISCELLANEOUS

ASSOCIATED CONDITIONS
Chronic conjunctivitis, recurrent eye "infections," moist dermatitis ("hot spots") ventral to the medial canthus, nasal discharge

AGE RELATED FACTORS N/A

ZOONOTIC POTENTIAL N/A

PREGNANCY N/A

SYNONYMS N/A

SEE ALSO
• Eyelash Diseases (trichiasis/Distichiasis/Ectopic Cilia) • Third Eyelid, Protruding • Conjunctivitis • Keratitis, Ulcerative

ABBREVIATIONS N/A

Reference
Gelatt KN. Canine lacrimal and nasolacrimal diseases. In: Gelatt KN, ed. Veterinary ophthalmology. 2nd Ed. Philadelphia: Lea & Febiger, 1991;276–289.
Author Brian C. Gilger
Consulting Editor Paul E. Miller

EPISTAXIS

BASICS

DEFINITION
Bleeding from the nose

PATHOPHYSIOLOGY
Nasal hemorrhage results from one of three abnormalities: coagulopathy, space-occupying or destructive lesion, or vascular/systemic disease.

Systems Affected
• Respiratory—hemorrhage, sneezing
• Hemic/lymphatic/immune—anemia
• Gastrointestinal—melena

SIGNALMENT
Variable, depending on underlying cause

SIGNS
Historical Findings
• Nasal hemorrhage • Sneezing • If coagulopathy, owners may report hematochezia, melena, hematuria, and/or hemorrhage from other areas of the body

Physical Examination Findings
• Nasal hemorrhage • If coagulopathy, may see petechia, ecchymosis, hematomas, hematachezia, melena, and/or hematuria • If coagulopathy or hypertension, may see retinal hemorrhages

CAUSES
Coagulopathy
Thrombocytopenia
• Immune-mediated disease (idiopathic, systemic lupus erythematosis [SLE], drug reaction, modified live vaccine reaction)
• Rickettsial disease (Ehrlichia), Rocky Mountain spotted fever (RMSF) • Bone marrow disease (neoplasia, aplastic anemia, infection [fungal, rickettsial, viral]) • Disseminated intravascular coagulation (DIC)
Thrombopathia
Congenital (von Willebrand disease, thrombasthenia, thrombopathia)
Acquired (nonsteriodal antiinfammatory drugs [NSAIDs], hyperglobulinemia [Ehrlichia, multiple myeloma], uremia, DIC)
Coagulation Factor Defects
• Congenital (hemophilia A [factor VIII deficiency], hemophilia B [factor IX deficiency])
• Acquired (anticoagulant rodenticide [warfarin] intoxication, hepatobiliary disease, DIC)
Space-Occupying or Destructive Lesion
• Foreign body, trauma, infection • Bacterial, fungal (aspergillus, cryptococcus, rhinosporidium) • Neoplasia (adenocarcinoma, carcinoma, chondrosarcoma, squamous cell carcinoma, fibrosarcoma, transmissible venereal turmor [TVT])
Vascular/Systemic Disease
• Hypertension (renal disease, hyperthyroidism, hyperadrenocorticism, idiopathic)
• Hyperviscosity (multiple myeloma, Ehrlichia, polycythemia) • Vasculitis (immune-mediated disease, rickettsial disease)

RISK FACTORS
• Coagulopathy—immune-mediated diseases; young to middle-aged, small to mid-sized female dogs • Rickettsial disease—dogs living in or traveling to endemic areas

Congenital Diseases
• Thrombasthenia—otter hounds
• Thrombopathia—basset hounds • Von Willebrand disease—dobermans, shetland sheepdogs, airedales, German shepherds, Scottish terriers, Chesapeake Bay retrievers, many others; cats • Hemophilia A—German shepherds, many others; cats • Hemophilia B—cairn terriers, coonhounds, Saint Bernards, others; cats

Space-Occupying or Destructive Lesions
• Aspergillosis—German shepherds
• Neoplasia—dolicephalic breeds

DIAGNOSIS

DIFFERENTIAL DIAGNOSIS N/A

CBC/BIOCHEMISTRY/URINALYSIS
CBC
All may demonstrate anemia if enough hemorrhage has occurred. Additional findings may include thrombocytopenia (see causes of thrombocytopenia), neutrophilia (infection, neoplasia), or pancytopenia (bone marrow disease).

Biochemistry
All may demonstrate hypoproteinemia if enough hemorrhage has occurred and high BUN with a normal creatinine (as a result of the presence of gastrointestinal blood). Additional findings may include hyperglobulinemia (ehrlichiosis, multiple myeloma), azotemia (renal failure-induced hypertension), or high ALT, AST, and total bilirubin (severe hepatic disease with coagulopathy).

Urinalysis
Usually normal. Additional findings may include hematuria (coagulopathy), isosthenuria (renal failure-induced hypertension), or proteinuria (as a result of SLE or rickettsial disease).

OTHER LABORATORY TESTS
• Coagulation profile—prolonged times in patients with coagulation factor defects (normal in thrombocytopenias and thrombopathias)
• Antinuclear antibody (ANA)—indicated when SLE is suspected • Platelet function testing (bleeding time, von Willebrand factor analysis, others)—indicated when coagulopathy suspected despite normal platelet count and coagulation profile • Ehrlichia and/or RMSF titers—indicated in animals with possible exposure • Thyroid hormone assay—indicated in older cats when coagulopathies and space-occupying lesions have been ruled out

IMAGING
• Thoracic radiographs—to screen for metastasis in animals with suspect neoplasia • Nasal series (under anesthesia and include open mouth view and frontal sinus view)—indicated in animals with suspect space-occupying or destructive lesions. Osteolysis seen with neoplasia and fungal sinusitis. Foreign bodies usually are not visualized.

OTHER DIAGNOSTIC PROCEDURES
• Rhinoscopy • Nasal lavage • Nasal biopsy (blind or via rhinoscopy) • All procedures are indicated to diagnose space-occupying or destructive diseases and are aimed at removing foreign bodies and evaluating and sampling nasal tissue for an etiologic diagnosis (neoplasia, infection) via cytologic and histopathologic examination, and bacterial and fungal culture and sensitivity.
• Bone marrow aspiration biopsy—indicated in cases of pancytopenia (see bone marrow diseases) • Blood pressure evaluation—indicated when coagulopathies and space-occupying lesions have been ruled out and when azotemia is present

TREATMENT
• Coagulopathies are usually treated as inpatients; space-occupying lesions and vascular/systemic diseases may be treated as outpatients or inpatients depending on the disease and its severity.
• Minimize activity or stimuli that precipitate hemorrhage episodes.
• Educate owner about disease process and what constitutes serious hemorrhage (weakness, collapse, pallor, blood loss in excess of 30 ml/kg of body weight).
• Surgery is indicated for foreign bodies not removable by rhinoscopic or blind attempt.
• Fungal rhinitis (aspergillus, rhinosporidium) may be treated via surgical exposure and delayed closure of the nasal cavity with daily application of povidone iodine solution or enilconazole or clotrimazole via surgically placed tubes.
• Radiation therapy provides various response rates depending on tumor type.

MEDICATIONS

DRUGS AND FLUIDS
Whole blood or packed red blood cell transfusion occasionally may be needed if epistaxis leads to severe anemia.

Coagulopathy
• Immune-mediated diseases—prednisone 1.1 mg/kg q12h, taper over 4-6 months. Alternative drugs may be used in addition to prednisone for refractory cases (azothioprine [Immuran] 2.2 mg/kg q24h for 14 days then q48h, danazole [Danocrine] 5 mg/kg q12h).

• Rickettsial diseases—doxycycline 5 mg/kg q12h for 2-3 weeks
• Thrombopathias—no treatment for thrombasthenia and thrombopathia. Plasma or cryoprecipitate for acute bleeding caused by von Willebrand disease; thyroid supplementation for chronic management if hypothyroid. Desmopressin acetate (1 g/kg SC, or IV diluted in 20 ml of 0.9% NaCl given over 10 minutes) may help control hemorrhage in some dogs with von Willebrand disease; the intranasal formulation (less expensive) can be used if first passed through a bacteriostatic filter. Discontinue all NSAIDs. Plasmapharesis if patient is hyperglobulinemic.
• Coagulation factor defects—plasma or cryoprecipitate for acute bleeding resulting from hemophilia A; plasma for acute bleeding resulting from hemophilia B; no long-term treatment for these. Plasma for acute bleeding caused by anticoagulant rodenticide intoxication along with vitamin K (5.0 mg/kg loading dose followed by 1.25 mg/kg q12h for 1 week [warfarin] to 4 weeks [longer-acting formulations]). For patients with liver disease and disseminated intravascular coagulation (DIC), treat/support the underlying cause; plasma may be beneficial.

Space-Occupying Lesions
• Foreign body—N/A
• Trauma—N/A
• Infection—antibiotics for bacterial infections (based on culture and sensitivity). Itraconazole (Sporonox) 5 mg/kg q12h alone for cryptococcus, and with or without surgery for aspergillus, and rhinosporidium for 2-4 weeks past complete clinical remission for fungal infections.
• Neoplasia—chemotherapy for lymphoma and TVT. Cis-platinum improves quality of life but not survival times for adenocarcinomas.

Vascular/Systemic Disease
• Hypertension—treat underlying disease if present (renal disease, hyperthyroidism, hyperadrenocorticism)
• Weight reduction
• Sodium restriction

• Hyperviscosity—treat underlying disease (ehrlichiosis, multiple myeloma); plasmapharesis
• Vasculitis—doxycycline for rickettsial diseases (5 mg/kg q12h for 3-6 weeks), prednisone for immune-mediated disease (1.1 mg/kg q12h, taper over 4-6 months)
Angiotensin-Converting Enzyme Inhibitors
Enalapril (Vasotec)
• Enacard (Merck, Rathway, NJ) 0.25-0.5 mg/kg q12h-q24h
• Benazepril (Lotensin, CIBA, Greensboro, NC) 0.25-0.5 mg/kg q12h-q24h
Beta Blockers
• Propranolol (Inderal) 0.5-1.0 mg/kg q8h
• Atenolol (Tenormin) 2.0 mg/kg q24h
Calcium Channel Blockers
• Diltiazem (Cardizem) 0.5-1.5 mg/kg q8h (dog); 1.75-2.5 mg/kg q8h (cat)
• Amlodipine (Norvasc) 0.625 mg q24h (cat)
Diuretics
• Hydrochlorothiazide (HydroDiuril) 2-4 mg/kg q12h
• Furosemide (Lasix) 0.5-2.0 mg/kg q8h-q12h

CONTRAINDICATIONS
Avoid use of drugs that predispose to hemorrhage (NSAIDs, heparin)

PRECAUTIONS
• When using chemotherapeutic drugs, be sure to monitor weekly neutrophil counts until a pattern has been established that demonstrates that the animal is tolerating the drug.
• Closely monitor patients with renal failure when using enalapril and/or diuretics; avoid severe salt restriction when using enalapril.

POSSIBLE INTERACTIONS N/A

ALTERNATE DRUGS
N/A

FOLLOW-UP
PATIENT MONITORING
• Platelet count—in thrombocytopenic animals • Coagulation profile—in animals with

coagulation factor defects • Blood pressure—in animals with hypertension • All others monitor clinical signs

POSSIBLE COMPLICATIONS
Anemia/collapse is rare.

MISCELLANEOUS
ASSOCIATED CONDITIONS N/A
AGE RELATED FACTORS N/A
ZOONOTIC POTENTIAL N/A
PREGNANCY N/A
SYNONYMS N/A

SEE ALSO
See causes.

ABBREVIATIONS
ANA = antinuclear antibody
DIC = disseminated intravascular coagulation
NSAID = nonsteroidal antiinflammatory drug
RMSF = Rocky Mountain spotted fever
SLE = systemic lupus erythematosis
TVT = transmissible venereal tumor

References
Cowgill LD, Kallet AJ. Systemic hypertension. In: Kirk RW, ed. Current veterinary therapy IX. Philadelphia: WB Saunders, 1986:360-364.
Dodds JW. Hemostasis. In: Kaneko JJ, ed. clinical biochemistry of domestic animals. 4th ed. New York: Academic Press, 1989:274-315.
Feldman BF, ed. Hemostasis, Vet Clin North Am. Philadelphis: WB Saunders, 1988; 18:1-282

Author Mitchell A. Crystal
Consulting Editors Lynelle Johnson and Bradley L. Moses

FEARS AND PHOBIAS—DOGS

BASICS

DEFINITION
Discussions need to include definitions of fears, phobias, and anxieties.
• Fear is a feeling of apprehension associated with the presence or proximity of an object, individual, social situation, or class of the above. Fear is part of normal behavior and can be an adaptive response. Whether the fear or fearful response is abnormal or inappropriate is determined by context. Normal and abnormal fears usually manifest as graded responses, with the intensity of the response proportional to the proximity of the stimulus. Most fear reactions are learned and can be unlearned with gradual exposure. • Phobias are defined as profound and quickly developed fear reactions that do not extinguish with gradual exposure to the object. Phobias involve sudden, all-or-nothing, profound, abnormal responses that result in extremely fearful behaviors (catatonia, panic). An immediate, excessive anxiety response is characteristic of phobias, with little change between bouts. Fears may develop more gradually, and within a bout of fearful behavior, there may be more variation in response than would be seen with a phobic event. It has been postulated that once a phobic event has been experienced, any event associated with it or the memory of it is sufficient to generate the response. Without reinforcement, these phobias can remain at or exceed their former high level for years. Genesis for such events was either extremely scary and traumatic or the dog has profound problems with fear internally, and the fear itself acts as a reinforcer. The most common phobias in dogs are those associated with noises—thunderstorms or firecrackers. • Anxiety is the apprehensive anticipation of future danger or misfortune accompanied by a feeling of dysphoria (in humans) and/or somatic signs of tension (vigilance and scanning, autonomic hyperactivity, increased motor activity, tension).
• Separation anxiety is the most common specific anxiety in companion dogs. When animals are left alone and exhibit anxiety or excessive distress, the condition is called separation anxiety; the most common behaviors (elimination, destruction, excessive vocalization) are the visible signs of anxiety. Question clients with dogs with separation anxiety about their pet's responses to loud noises.

Pathophysiology
• Fears, phobias, and anxieties come to the practitioner's attention because of changes the client perceives in the animal's behavior or because the client feels that the pet has never been normal. • While the underlying pathophysiology is unclear, clinical signs are consistent with alterations in CNS transmitter levels and/or increases in ACTH levels. The latter can be primary or secondary.

Systems Affected
• Cardiovascular—signs can include tachycardia • Endocrine/metabolic • Gastrointestinal—signs can include inappetence, aberrant appetite, and gastrointestinal distress
• Hemic—stress leukograms are not an uncommon sequelae • Musculoskeletal—signs can include poor condition attributable to increased motor activity and self-injury (weight loss, injured pads, damage to teeth and gums, and abrasions and lacerations) • Nervous—increased motor activity, repetitive activity, trembling, and self-injury • Respiratory—high respiratory rate and the attendant metabolic changes • Skin/exocrine—skin lesions usually are secondary and may be a result of self-injury (lick granulomas)

SIGNALMENT
No age, breed, or sex is overrepresented. Most fears, phobias, and anxieties develop at the onset of social maturity (18-36 months of age in dogs). Old-age onset idiopathic separation anxiety that may be a variant of cognitive dysfunction has been reported in elderly dogs.

SIGNS

General Comments
Fears and anxieties are variable, and the diagnosis may be made only on the basis of nonspecific signs for which no discrete, identifiable stimulus is present. Dogs with mild fears tremble, tuck their tails, withdraw, and hide (reduced activity and passive escape behaviors), while those that have progressed to panic show active escape behaviors and increased, out-of-context, and potentially injurious motor activity. Both classes of dogs demonstrate the classic signs of sympathetic autonomic nervous system activity.

Historical Findings
Dogs that exhibit fear may have either had an horrific experience or may just be unfamiliar with the event and subsequently been forced into it. The individual's response is more variable than the historical findings. Dogs with separation anxiety often have histories of abandonment, multiple owners, rehoming, or neglect.

Physical Examination Findings
Physical examination usually is nonremarkable except for self-induced injuries and the lack of condition that may be associated with increased motor activity and withdrawal. The exception to this may be lesions such as lick granulomas, which are more common than has been appreciated in dogs with anxieties, including separation anxiety.

CAUSES
Any illness or painful physical condition can increase an animal's anxieties and contribute to these problems; few of these conditions actually cause fears, phobias, and anxieties.

DIAGNOSIS

DIFFERENTIAL DIAGNOSIS
Common ruleouts include those that would cause similar behavioral changes—seizures, brain disease, and metabolic disease.

CBC/BIOCHEMISTRY/URINALYSIS
All of these should be performed and be within the laboratory's reference range.

OTHER LABORATORY TESTS
Based on clinical signs and serum biochemistry results, thyroid or adrenal tests may be indicated. If there is doubt about whether the signs are "behavioral," nonremarkable results of these tests should confirm this.

IMAGING
SPECT scans, PET scans, and some types of MRI may useful in the future to confirm the behavioral diagnosis and to assay the success of the treatment.

OTHER DIAGNOSTIC PROCEDURES
Biopsies of dermatologic lesions may confirm whether they are primary or secondary, CSF taps can rule out infectious CNS disease, and endoscopy can evaluate primary bowel disease. Cardiac disease can produce physical signs of "anxiety." ECG may be used as a diagnostic ruleout or a premedication precaution.

TREATMENT
• Patients with fears, phobias, and anxieties respond to some extent to a combination of behavior modification and pharmacologic treatment with antianxiety medication. Treat as an outpatient. Exceptions to this include dogs with profound panic and separation anxiety who need to be protected until their antianxiety medications reach effective plasma and CSF levels (days to weeks) and those who must be treated for, or protected from, physical injury (i.e., throwing himself from a window). For these patients, constant day care, dogsitting, or inhospital monitoring, stimulation, and care may be best. Behavior modification should be geared toward teaching the dog to relax in a variety of environmental settings.
• Clients tend to try to reassure the dog when he is experiencing fear or panic, but should understand that the dog could interpret this as a reward for the inappropriate behavior. Attention given to the dog must encourage calmness, not act as a fear reinforcer. Absolutely avoid punishment. Desensitization and counterconditioning are most effective if the fear, anxiety, or phobia is treated early, and the goal is to decrease the reaction to the specific stimulus (i.e., being left alone in the dark, the sound of wind). Clients must understand the subtlety of the signs involved and learn to recognize physical signs associat-

ed with the underlying physiological state characterized by sympathetic stimulation. Any atopic and painful conditions should be diagnosed and controlled because pruritus and pain are both neurochemically related to anxiety and its perception.

MEDICATIONS

DRUGS AND FLUID

• Medications of choice include antianxiety medications that increase central levels of serotonin. These include the tricylcic antidepressants (TCA) and the more specific selective serotonin reuptake inhibitors (SSRI). Do premedication blood profiles before giving medication.

• Drugs of choice include amitriptyline (Elavil 1-2 mg/kg [to start] PO q12h for 30 days); imipramine (Tofranil 1-2 mg/kg PO q12h for 30 days); buspirone (Buspar 1 mg/kg PO q 24h); clomipramine (Anafranil 1 mg/kg PO q12h for 14 days, then 2 mg/kg PO q12h for 14 days, then 3 mg/kg PO q12h for 28 days; if successful this will be the maintenance level), and fluoxetine (Prozac 1 mg/kg PO q24h for 2 months). Clients need to know that buspirone, clomipramine, and fluoxetine can take 3-5 weeks to be effective. Phobias and true panic disorders respond better to benzodiazepines than to the TCA and SSRI. Drugs of choice include diazepam (Valium 0.5 mg/kg PO prn), chlorazepate (Tranxene 0.55-2.2 mg/kg PO q8-12h [prn for phobias]), and alprazolam (Xanax 0.125-1.0 mg/kg prn *not* to exceed 4 mg/day). All benzodiazepines work best if administered before signs of anxiety, fear, or panic and must be given 30-60 minutes before the anticipated stimulus. For separation anxiety that is accompanied by panic (i.e., dogs that break out of crates or throw themselves from windows) and thunderstorm phobia, alprazolam can be used cautiously with other medications on an as-needed basis.

CONTRAINDICATIONS

Some contraindicated in animals with hepatic and renal compromise because these are their main routes of metabolism. Animals with cardiac conduction anomalies should be given TCA with extreme caution and monitoring.

PRECAUTIONS

All of the medications recommended for use are extralabel, and all HHS (Health and Human Services) recommendations should be followed. Clients should know that all benzodiazepines mentioned are controlled substances and are humanly abusable. Overdoses of TCAs can cause profound cardiac conduction disturbances. Premedication ECG evaluation may allow cautious use of these drugs.

POSSIBLE INTERACTIONS

Benzodiazepines are lipophilic and may be potentiated by other lipophilic drugs. These drugs may potentiate each other; if combination treatment is warranted, lower doses of either medication may be warranted.

ALTERNATE DRUGS N/A

FOLLOW-UP

PATIENT MONITORING

If drug treatment is chronic, semiannual or annual CBC and serum biochemistry analyses are desirable. An annual ECG is elective. Dosages should be adjusted accordingly. Monitoring should be warranted by clinical signs (vomiting, GI distress, tachycardia, tachypnea). Advise clients.

POSSIBLE COMPLICATIONS

Early intervention using behavioral modification and pharmacological intervention is key because, if left untreated, these disorders always progress.

MISCELLANEOUS

ASSOCIATED CONDITIONS

Common associated conditions are irritable bowel syndrome and lick granulomas.

AGE RELATED FACTORS

Idiopathic separation anxiety in older dogs is frequently undiagnosed because it is insidious and not associated with social or environmental changes. Changes appear to be in the dog's perception.

ZOONOTIC POTENTIAL N/A

PREGNANCY

Most of the drugs used to treat these conditions are either not evaluated in or contraindicated in pregnant animals. Use should be avoided.

SYNONYMS

Generalized anxiety, neophobia, noise phobia, and thunderstorm phobia

SEE ALSO N/A

ABBREVIATIONS

TCA = tricylcic antidepressants
SSRI = selective serotonin reuptake inhibitors

References

McCrave EA. Diagnostic criteria for separation anxiety in the dog. Vet Clin North Am (Small Anim Pract) 1991;21:247-256.

Tuber DS, Hothersall D, Peters NE. Treatment of fears and phobia in dogs. Vet Clin North Am (Small Anim Pract) 1982;12:607-623.

Young MS. Treatment of fear-induced aggression in dogs. Vet Clin North Am (Small Anim Pract) 1982;12:645-653.

Author Karen L. Overall
Consulting Editor Joane M. Parent

FEVER

BASICS

DEFINITION
A higher than normal body temperature, resulting from a change in the thermoregulatory set point in the hypothalamus. The normal body temperature in dogs and cats is 100.2-102.8° F (37.8-39.3° C). Fever of unknown origin (FUO) is a fever of at least 103.5° F (39.7° C) on at least four occasions over a 14-day period, and illness of 14 days' duration without an obvious cause.

Pathophysiology
During fever, exogenous or endogenous pyrogens cause the release of endogenous substances (e.g., interleukin-1 and prostaglandins) that reset the hypothalamic thermoregulatory center to a higher temperature, thus activating appropriate physiologic responses to raise the body temperature to this new set point. Physiologic consequences include increased metabolic demands, muscle catabolism, bone marrow suppression, heightened fluid and caloric requirements, and, possibly, disseminated intravascular coagulation (DIC) and shock.

Systems Affected Depends on cause

SIGNALMENT N/A

SIGNS

General Comments
• Prolonged fever > 105° F (> 40.5° C) leads to dehydration, anorexia, and depression.
• Fevers > 106° F (> 41.1° C) may lead to cerebral edema, bone marrow depression, and DIC.

Physical Examination Findings
• Hyperthermia • Lethargy • Inappetence • Tachycardia • Hyperpnea • Dehydration • Shock

CAUSES

Infectious Agents (Most Common Cause of Fevers)
• Viruses (e.g., feline leukemia [FeLV], feline immunodeificiency [FIV], parvo, distemper, herpes, and calici) • Bacteria (i.e., gram-positive and gram-negative endotoxins) • Systemic fungi (e.g., Histoplasma, Blastomyces, Coccidioidomyces, and Cryptococcus) • Rickettsia (e.g., Ehrlichia, Rickettsia rickettsii [Rocky Mountain spotted fever], Hemobartonella) • Parasites and protozoa (e.g., Babesia, Toxoplasma, aberrant larva migrans, Dirofilaria thromboemboli, Leishmania)

Immune-Mediated Processes
Systemic lupus erythematosus, immune-mediated hemolytic anemia, immune-mediated thrombocytopenia, pemphigus, polyarthritis, polymyositis, vasculitis, hypersensitivity reactions, transfusion reaction, and infection secondary to inherited or acquired immune defects

Endocrine and Metabolic
Hyperthyroidism, hypoadrenocorticism (rare), pheochromocytoma, hyperlipidemia, and hypernatremia

Neoplasia
Lymphoma, myeloproliferative disease, plasma cell neoplasm, mast cell tumor, metastatic disease, and solid tumor, particularly in liver, kidney, bone, lungs, and lymph nodes

Other Inflammatory Conditions
Cholangiohepatitis, hepatic lipidosis, toxic hepatopathy, cirrhosis, inflammatory bowel disease, pancreatitis, peritonitis, pleuritis, granulomatous diseases, thrombophlebitis, infarctions, pansteatitis, panniculitis, hypertrophic osteodystrophy, blunt trauma, cyclic neutropenia, intracranial lesions (encephalitis, trauma), and pulmonary thromboembolism

Drugs and Toxins
Tetracycline, sulfonamide, penicillins, nitrofurantoin, amphotericin B, barbiturates, iodine, atropine, cimetidine, salicylates (high dosages), antihistamines, procainamide, and heavy metals

Fever of Unknown Origin—Dogs
• Recurrent bacteremia caused by endocarditis or localized abscess of organ or tissue (i.e., liver, pancreas, prostate, retroperitoneal and pleural space [pyothorax], lungs, kidneys and genitourinary system [chronic pyelonephritis and prostatitis], osteomyelitis, arthritis, discospondylitis, and meningitis) • Systemic infection (particularly early, chronic, or latent infection, including brucellosis, systemic mycoses, ehrlichiosis, Rocky Mountain spotted fever, toxoplasmosis) • Neoplasia—as above • Immune disorders—as above • Other causes—chronic hepatic diseases and chronic granulomatous disease

Fever of Unknown Origin—Cats
• Most are virally mediated (e.g., FeLV, FIV, FIP [feline infectious peritonisits], less commonly parvo, herpes, and calici) • Persistent occult bacterial infection with atypical bacteria, sometimes secondary to bite wounds (e.g., Yersinia, Mycobacteria, Nocardia, Actinomyces, and Brucella) • Pyothorax is common. • Additional causes are pyelonephritis, blunt trauma, penetrating intestinal lesion, dental abscess, systemic mycoses (e.g., Histoplasma, Blastomyces, Coccidioides), lymphoma, and solid tumors. • Immune disorders are rare, as are prostatitis, endometritis, discospondylitis, pneumonia, and endocarditis.

RISK FACTORS
• Recent travel • Exposure to biologic agents • Immunosuppression • Very young or old animals

DIAGNOSIS

DIFFERENTIAL DIAGNOSIS
• A good clinical history (e.g., contact with infectious agents, recent vaccination, drug administration, insect bites, allergies, etc.) and thorough physical examination may aid in determining an underlying disease condition. • Elucidation of patterns of fever (e.g., sustained, intermittent, etc.) is rarely helpful in the differential diagnosis. • True fever must be differentiated from hyperthermia. Stress and anxiety in the hospital may cause a mild temperature rise. Temperatures up to 103° F (39.4° C) may be caused by stress or illness. Temperatures > 104° F (> 40° C) are almost always important. Temperatures of > 107° F (> 41.7° C) are usually not fever, but more likely are caused by primary hyperthermia.

CBC/BIOCHEMISTRY/URINALYSIS
• CBC: leukopenia or leukocytosis, left shift, monocytosis, lymphocytosis, and thrombocytopenia or thrombocytosis • Results of biochemistry profile and urinalysis vary with the organ system involved.

OTHER LABORATORY TESTS
• Additional laboratory testing depends on history, physical examination findings, and abnormalities in CBC, serum biochemistry profile, and urinalysis. • If infectious disease is suspected, attempt to culture an organism—urine culture, blood cultures (i.e., three anaerobic and three aerobic cultures, taken during a rise in temperature, or 30 minutes apart), fungal culture, and cultures of CSF, synovial fluid, and biopsy specimens, if clinically indicated. • FeLV and FIV test, serologic tests for Toxoplasma, Lyme disease, systemic mycoses, and rickettsial infection • Fecal examination if gastrointestinal signs are observed • Tracheal wash or bronchoalveolar lavage, if respiratory involvement is observed • Occult heartworm test if pulmonary embolism is suspected • If immune disorders are suspected, cytologic examination of synovial fluid, Coombs', antinuclear antibody, and rheumatoid factor tests, and serum protein electrophoresis • T_4 to rule out hyperthyroidism

IMAGING

Radiography
• Abdominal radiographs to scan for tumors • Thoracic radiographs to rule out pneumonia, neoplasia, and pyothorax • Survey skeletal radiographs to look for bone tumors, multiple myeloma, osteomyelitis, diskospondylitis, panosteiitis, and hypertrophic osteodystrophy • Dental and skull radiographs to look for tooth root abscess, sinus infections, and neoplasia • Contrast radiography (e.g., gastrointestinal and excretory urography) to look for evidence of neoplasia or infection

Ultrasonography
• Abdominal ultrasonography (plus directed biopsy, if indicated) to look for abdominal neoplasia and abscess or other site of infection (e.g., pyelonephritis and pyometra) • Echocardiography if endocarditis is suspected

Nuclear Imaging
Radionuclide scanning procedures to evaluate for bone tumors, osteomyelitis, and pulmonary embolism

OTHER DIAGNOSTIC PROCEDURES
• Endoscopy and biopsy if gastrointestinal signs observed • Bone marrow aspirate and biopsy if malignancy is suspected • Lymph node, skin, or muscle biopsy if clinically indicated • Examination of fine needle aspirate of mass or large organ if present • CSF tap if neurologic signs suggest brain tumor or meningitis • Exploratory laparotomy, as a last resort, if all other diagnostic tests fail to determine the cause, and the patient is not improving

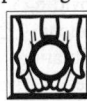

TREATMENT
• Restrict activity.
• Febrile patients are in a hypercatabolic state and require high caloric intake.
• Prepare the owner for the fact that the diagnostic workup of patients with fever of unknown origin is often extensive, expensive, and invasive and does not always provide a definitive diagnosis.
• Surgery may be necessary in some animals with underlying infectious (e.g., pyometra, peritonitis, pyothroax, and liver abscess) or localized neoplasic cause of fever.

MEDICATIONS
DRUGS AND FLUIDS
• The goal of treatment is to reset the thermoregulatory set point to a lower level.
• Drug selection depends on the diagnosis and specific cause.
• Broad spectrum (i.e., "shotgun") treatment should not be used in place of a thorough diagnostic workup, unless the patient's status is critical and deteriorating rapidly.
• Fever may help the body fight the disease condition (e.g., by suppressing bacterial replication and facilitating host defenses). Antipyretic treatment should only be used when fever is prolonged and life threatening (> 106° F, >41.1° C) and if topical cooling is unsuccessful. Impaired patients (e.g., those with heart failure, seizures, or respiratory disease) require antipyretic treatment earlier. Antipyretic treatment may preclude elucidation of the cause, delay correct treatment, and complicate patient monitoring (e.g., reduction of fever is an important indication of response to treatment).

• Fluid administration often lowers the body temperature.
• If the patient is dehydrated, initiate isotonic fluids (i.e., lactated Ringer's or 0.9% saline)

Antibiotics
• Based on results of bacterial culture
• In emergency situations, combination antibiotic therapy can be started after culture specimens have been obtained (e.g., cephalothin, 20 mg/kg IV q6h-q8h; gentamicin 2 mg/kg IV q8h).
• Do not give antibiotics for longer than 1-2 weeks if the response is not favorable.

Antipyretics
• Salicylates—dogs, 10 mg/kg PO q12h; cats, 6 mg/kg PO q48h
• Dipyrone—dogs, 0.2 ml/5kg IM or SC q6h-q12h; cats, 0.1 ml IM or SC q8h-q24h
• Flunixin meglumine—dogs, 0.5-1 mg/kg IV or IM once

Glucocorticoids
• Do not use corticosteroids unless infectious causes have been ruled out.
• May mask clinical signs, lead to immunosuppression, and are not recommended for use as antipyretics. However, the administration of corticosteroids in cats with untractable fever of unknown origin, after ruling out infectious diseases, may promote a favorable response.
• Primarily indicated for treating fever associated with immune-mediated disease and certain steroid responsive tumors (e.g., lymphoma)

CONTRAINDICATIONS N/A
PRECAUTIONS
• Side effects of antipyretics include emesis, diarrhea, gastrointestinal ulceration, renal damage, hemolysis, hepatotoxicity (acetaminophen, particularly dangerous in cats), myelosuppression (dipyrone), and muscle stiffness (flunixin meglumine).
• Dipyrone can reduce the body temperature in cats to a subnormal level for hours to days.

POSSIBLE INTERACTIONS
Combination of nonsteroidal antiinflamatory drugs (NSAIDS) and steroids raises the risk of gastrointestinal hemorrhage

ALTERNATE DRUGS N/A

FOLLOW-UP
PATIENT MONITORING
• The patient's temperature should be monitored at least q12h. • If the cause of the fever continues to elude the clinician, a history and

physical examination along with screening laboratory tests should be repeated. • If a fever develops or worsens during hospitalization, nosocomial infection or superinfection should be considered.

PREVENTION/AVOIDANCE N/A
POSSIBLE COMPLICATIONS
Depend on cause

EXPECTED COURSE AND PROGNOSIS
Vary with cause. In some patients (more commonly in cats), an underlying cause cannot be determined.

MISCELLANEOUS
ASSOCIATED CONDITIONS N/A
AGE RELATED FACTORS
• Young animals—infectious disease more likely than other cause; prognosis better than in old animals • Older animals—common causes are neoplasia and intraabdominal infection; signs tend to be more nonspecific; prognosis often guarded

ZOONOTIC POTENTIAL
Depends on cause

PREGNANCY N/A

SYNONYMS Pyrexia

SEE ALSO
• See Causes • Heatstroke and Hyperthermia

ABBREVIATIONS
CSF = cerebral spinal fluid

References
Hardie EM. Sepsis versus septic shock. In: Murtaugh RJ, Kaplan PM, eds. Veterinary emergency and critical care medicine. Philadelphia: Mosby Year Book, 1992:176-193.
Couto CG. Fever of undetermined origin. In: Nelson RW, Couto CG, eds. Essentials of small animal internal medicine. Philadelphia: Mosby Year Book, 1992:974-977.

Author Jörg Bücheler
Consulting Editors Larry P. Tilley and Francis W. K. Smith, Jr.

FLATULENCE

BASICS

DEFINITION
Flatulence is the distension of the stomach or intestines with gas or air. Flatus is the gas expelled from a body opening. In common usage, these terms usually refer to the release of intestinal gas through the anus.

Pathophysiology
The production and accumulation of gas within the gastrointestinal tract is normal. However, in patients with some gastrointestinal disorders the production of gas increases and the result is excessive flatulence. Nearly all gastrointestinal gas is derived from two sources: swallowed air and bacterial fermentation of ingested nutrients. Any condition that leads to increases in either of these can cause flatulence. Most of the components of intestinal gas are odorless including nitrogen, oxygen, hydrogen, methane, and carbon dioxide. Less than 1% of intestinal gas is composed of odoriferous substances such as hydrogen sulfide, ammonia, indole, skatole, volatile amines, mercaptans, and short-chain fatty acids. The volume and percent composition of flatus are affected by the abundance and type of bacterial flora and by the composition and volume of the diet. Diets high in fiber or legumes often cause flatulence. Disease conditions of the small intestine that cause malabsorption or maldigestion can also cause flatulence because of the increased amounts of carbohydrate available for fermentation.

Systems Affected Gastrointestinal

SIGNALMENT Dogs and cats

SIGNS
• Increased frequency and, possibly, volume of flatulence is reported by the owner.
• Other signs may suggest concurrent digestive system disease including vomiting, diarrhea, weight loss, and evidence of abdominal discomfort (e.g., a hunched posture and adopting a prayer position).

CAUSES

Increased Aerophagia
Seen in animals that are nervous or greedy eaters, especially if there is real, or perceived competition for food.

Diet Related
• Diets that are high in soybeans, fiber (e.g., bran, lactose, and whole wheat products), and fat may cause excessive gas production.
• Diets that are high in protein or fat or that are spoiled are especially likely to cause production of odoriferous intestinal gas. • In lactase deficient animals, diets containing milk products can cause excessive flatus.

Disease Conditions
• Malabsorption caused by small intestinal disease (e.g., viral disease that severely affects the small intestine, severe parasitism, infiltrative bowel disease including inflammatory and neoplastic conditions, and lymphangiectasia) • Maldigestion caused by exocrine pancreatic insufficiency

RISK FACTORS
• Nervous or greedy eating • Diets high in the previously mentioned nutrients that cause excess gas production

DIAGNOSIS

DIFFERENTIAL DIAGNOSIS
• Gastrointestinal disease must be differentiated from dietary or behavioral causes of flatulence. • To determine the cause of the problem, a thorough history of the animal's diet and eating habits is necessary. This information may provide the basis for at least a presumptive diagnosis. • A complete physical examination should be performed with emphasis on searching for signs of gastrointestinal disease, which should be pursued if found. If not, dietary and behavioral etiologic factors should be considered.

CBC/BIOCHEMISTRY/URINALYSIS
Results normal

OTHER LABORATORY TESTS
• Multiple fecal flotation and direct smear examinations to rule out small intestinal parasitism • Examination of feces for undigested fat or protein if malassimilation is suspected
• Serum trypsin-like immunoreactivity (TLI) to rule out maldigestion caused by exocrine pancreatic insufficiency. • See specific topics regarding these problems for further information.

IMAGING N/A

OTHER DIAGNOSTIC PROCEDURES
Small intestinal biopsy with specimen obtained by endoscopy or surgery necessary to diagnose infiltrative bowel disease

TREATMENT
• Treat any underlying gastrointestinal disease that may be causing or related to the flatulence
• If diet is suspected, change the diet to one that is low in fiber and easily digested. A commercial product or homemade diet made up of highly digestible protein and carbohydrate sources, including cottage cheese and rice along with appropriate vitamins and minerals, may be tried. Often this is successful in reducing the frequency of the flatulence.
• Discouraging greedy eating by providing more frequent, smaller meals in a noncompetitive environment and avoiding situations that provoke nervousness may reduce aerophagia.
• Vigorous exercise may also be helpful by causing expulsion of colonic gas and encouraging normal colonic emptying of feces.
• These management practices are often more successful than pharmacologic treatment.

MEDICATIONS

DRUGS AND FLUIDS
• Simethicone is an antifoaming agent that reduces the surface tension of intestinal mucus allowing easier coalescence and release of intestinal gas. It does not reduce gas production, but it helps prevent gas accumulation. It can be used safely in dogs and cats (25-200 mg q6h-q8h). Its effectiveness as an antiflatulent in dogs and cats is unknown.
• Antiflatulent enzyme supplements may reduce the severity of flatulence by aiding in the digestion of poorly digestible fermentable nutrients. Anecdotal evidence suggests that these products may be effective.
• Activated charcoal has commonly been used as an adsorbent to reduce gas production, but its usefulness is questionable.

CONTRAINDICATIONS N/A
PRECAUTIONS N/A
POSSIBLE INTERACTIONS N/A
ALTERNATE DRUGS N/A

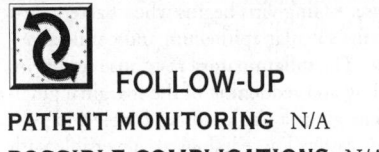 FOLLOW-UP

PATIENT MONITORING N/A
POSSIBLE COMPLICATIONS N/A

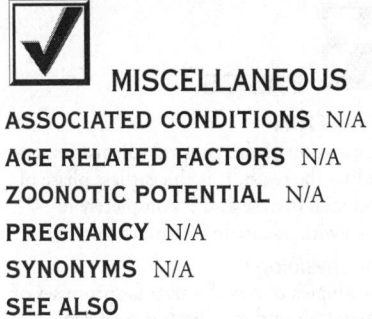 MISCELLANEOUS

ASSOCIATED CONDITIONS N/A
AGE RELATED FACTORS N/A
ZOONOTIC POTENTIAL N/A
PREGNANCY N/A
SYNONYMS N/A
SEE ALSO
• Exocrine Pancreatic Insufficiency • Inflammatory Bowel Disease • Lymphangiectasia

ABBREVIATIONS N/A

References
Guilford GW: Flatulence and borborygmus. In: Ettinger SJ, ed. Veterinary internal medicine. 4th ed. Philadelphia: WB Saunders, 1995;132-133.
Lorenz MD. Flatulence. In: Lorenz MD, Cornelius LM, eds. Small animal medical diagnosis. Philadelphia: JP Lippincott, 1987;243-248.
Author Daniel P. Harrington
Consulting Editor Brent D. Jones

GINGIVITIS

BASICS

DEFINITION
Inflammation of the gingival soft tissues surrounding the teeth. It is the earliest phase of periodontal disease and is completely reversible with adequate treatment.

Pathophysiology
• The gingiva covers the alveolar processes of the mandible and maxilla and conforms closely to the neck of the tooth. The gingiva is divided into attached and free or marginal portions. The attached gingiva is tightly bound to the periosteum overlying the alveolar processes. The marginal gingiva extends above the crest of the alveolar bone and tapers to a knife-like edge which lies in contact with surface of the tooth. The gingival sulcus is the narrow cleft between the inner wall of the marginal gingiva and the tooth. In dogs the gingival sulcus is normally less than 3mm but may be deeper around the canine teeth in large breed dogs. The gingival sulcus in the cat is normally 1 mm or less. The junction between the gingiva and oral mucosa is readily apparent as a distinct line or furrow called the mucogingival line. • The connective tissue of the gingiva (lamina propria) contains an extensive array of blood vessels, lymphatics, nerves and collagen fibers. Plasma cells, lymphocytes, and neutrophils are also abundant and play an important role in the local defense mechanisms. Crevicular fluid is plasma-derived and passes from the gingival connective tissue through the crevicular epithelium to lavage the gingival sulcus. Crevicular fluid flow occurs in response to bacteria (plaque) in the gingival sulcus. It contains immunoglobulins and other nonspecific antibacterial substances. The neutrophil is the predominant cell. The crevicular fluid is an important part of the local defense mechanism to control the bacterial population. • In healthy animals, gram-positive aerobic cocci and rods predominate in supragingival plaque. Anaerobes become more abundant subgingivally and spirochetes are found tightly packed in the apical region of the gingival sulcus. As gingivitis develops, anaerobes and spirochetes become increasingly more abundant in the subgingival sulcus. In dogs the bacteroides orgranisms (Bacteroides sp., Provotella, Porphyromonas sp.) and Fusobacterium sp. appear to be important pathogens. Porphyromonas sp. and Peptostreptococcus sp. are common in samples from cats with gingivitis. Gram-negative organisms, which also increase in numbers as gingivitis develops, invade tissues and elaborate endotoxins that can result in tissue destruction. The fact that these bacteria are present in disease and health and that periodontal disease does not progress in linear fashion (i.e., there are periods of active disease followed by quiescent periods) indicates that the host-bacteria interaction is an important factor in the pathogenesis of periodontal

disease. • Gingivitis begins when bacteria invade the sulcular epithelium and connective tissue. The inflammatory respsonse results in swelling and reddening of the marginal gingiva. The gingiva also becomes friable and bleeds easily. These lesions are reversible with dental prophylaxis and home care. If not controlled at this point, the attached gingiva and attachment apparatus (alveolar bone, periodontal ligament, and tooth root cementum) become involved, signifying the transition to periodontitis. Once periodontitis is established the lesions are generally considered controllable but not reversible. Uncontrolled periodontitis invariably leads to tooth loss.

Systems Affected
Gastrointestinal

Signalment
Dogs and cats

SIGNS

Historical Findings
• Since gingivitis involves only the soft tissues, the owner may not recognize these changes. Gingival swelling or bleeding may be seen if the owner routinely examines the mouth while performing oral hygiene. • In most instances gingivitis is found during routine wellness examinations.

Physical Examination Findings
• Erythema • Gingival swelling (rounding of the marginal gingiva) • Loss of the normal stippling pattern • Bleeding on palpation or probing

CAUSES
Gingivitis is the result of plaque accumulation

RISK FACTORS
• Age • Head shape and occlusive pattern • Size • Diet • Open mouth breathing • Chewing habits • Metabolic disease: uremia, hypothyroidism • Feline leukemia virus (FeLV) • Feline immunodeficiency virus (FIV) • Autoimmune disease: Pemphigus vulgaris, Systemic lupus erythematosus

DIAGNOSIS

DIFFERENTIAL DIAGNOSIS N/A

CBC/BIOCHEMISTRY/URINALYSIS
May be helpful in establishing the etiology

OTHER LABORATORY TESTS
• FeLV and FIV testing • Biopsy and histopathology

IMAGING Radiography

OTHER DIAGNOSTIC PROCEDURES
N/A

TREATMENT
• Modify behavior to avoid chewing hard objects such as rocks and sticks and eliminate repetitive trauma, if possible.

• The importance of good home care or regular dental prophylaxis should be stressed before lesions develop. Daily or at least twice weekly brushing is recommended using an enzymatic toothpaste or zinc-organic acid solution to remove and retard plaque accumulation. If the owner is unwilling to brush the teeth but the patient is manageable, it might be possible to have the owner bring the pet into the clinic for brushing. Rawhide chew strips help to mechanically clean the teeth and exercise the attachment apparatus but should not be relied upon as the sole method of home care.
• Hard food leaves less substrate on the teeth than soft food. Chewing also helps to mechanically clean teeth. Prescription diet t/d® (Hill's Pet Nutrition, Inc., Topeka, KS) is formulated to reduce plaque and tartar accumulation and reduce staining.
• Schedule dental prophylaxis as soon as possible. Dental prophylaxis should include supra- and subgingival scaling followed by polishing and irrigation of the gingival sulcus. Complete examination of the oral cavity including periodontal probing and recording any abnormalities on a dental chart for future reference. Predisposing factors such as retained deciduous teeth and crowded teeth should be eliminated.

MEDICATIONS

DRUGS AND FLUIDS
Medications are unnecessary since the signs will resolve following complete dental prophylaxis.

CONTRAINDICATIONS N/A

PRECAUTIONS N/A

POSSIBLE INTERACTIONS N/A

ALTERNATE DRUGS N/A

FOLLOW-UP

PATIENT MONITORING
Clinical signs generally resolve within several days after dental prophylaxis. The prognosis is excellent if adequate home care is provided. If home care is impossible, regular examinations should be recommended. Examination of the oral cavity should be performed during wellness exams at least once yearly.

POSSIBLE COMPLICATIONS
The temperment of the patient should be considered before recommending home care. Vicious or uncontrollable pets may injure the owner. In all animals appropriate brushing technique should be demonstrated.

MISCELLANEOUS

ASSOCIATED CONDITIONS
Always look for dental resorptive lesions (neck lesions) in cats, especially if gingivitis is focal or has the appearance of granulation tissue.

AGE RELATED FACTORS
Transient gingivitis is a common, self-limiting problem in teething animals. If inflammation persists after adult tooth eruption, the cause should be determined.

ZOONOTIC POTENTIAL N/A

PREGNANCY
For simple gingivitis, dental prophylaxis can be delayed until the puppies or kittens are weaned.

SYNONYMS N/A

SEE ALSO Stomatitis

ABBREVIATIONS
FeLV = feline leukemia virus
FIV = feline immunodeficiency virus

References

Colmery B, Frost P. Periodontal disease: etiology and pathogenesis. Vet Clin N Amer Small Anim Pract 1986;16:817-834.

Emily PP; Penman S. Handbook of small animal dentistry. New York: Pergamon, 1990.

Emily PP, Tholen M. Periodontal therapy. In: Bojrab MJ; Tholen M, eds. Small animal medicine and oral surgery. Philadelphia: Lea & Febiger, 1990.

Harvey CE, Emily PP. Small animal dentistry. St. Louis, MO: Mosby, 1993.

West-Hyde L; Floyd M. Dentistry In: Ettinger SJ; Feldman EC, eds. Textbook of veterinary internal medicine. 4th ed. Philadelphia, WB Saunders, 1995;1097-1121.

Author Eric Russell Pope
Consulting Editor Brent D. Jones

HEAD TILT (VESTIBULAR DISEASE)

BASICS

DEFINITION
Tilting of the head away from its normal orientation with the trunk and limbs; associated with disorders of the vestibular system

Pathophysiology
The vestibular system coordinates the position and movement of the head with that of the eyes, trunk, and limbs by detecting linear acceleration and rotational movements of the head. This system includes the vestibular nuclei in the rostral medulla of the brainstem, the vestibular portion of the vestibulocochlear nerve (CN VIII), and the receptors in the semicircular canals of the inner ear. Diseases affecting the vestibular system and its projections to the cerebellum, spinal cord, cerebral cortex, reticular formation, and extraocular eye muscles via the medial longitudinal fasciculus cause signs associated with vestibular dysfunction. The most consistent of these is a head tilt, usually directed toward the same side as the lesion.

Systems Affected
Nervous—peripheral or CNS

SIGNALMENT N/A

SIGNS N/A

CAUSES

Peripheral Vestibular Disease
• Anatomic—congenital head tilt • Metabolic—hypothyroidism, pituitary chromophobe adenoma, paraneoplastic disease, and cranial nerve polyneuropathy • Neoplastic—nerve sheath tumor of CN VIII and neoplasia of the bone and surrounding tissue (e.g., osteosarcoma, fibrosarcoma, chondrosarcoma, and squamous cell carcinoma) • Inflammatory—otitis media and interna; primarily bacterial but also parasitic (e.g., Otodectes), mycotic, fungal, and foreign body related, and nasopharyngeal polyps • Idiopathic—canine geriatric vestibular disease and feline idiopathic vestibular disease • Immune-mediated—CNS disease; polyneuropathy • Toxic— aminoglycosides, metronidazole, lead, and hexachlorophene • Traumatic—tympanic bulla or petrosal bone fracture and ear flush

Central Vestibular Disease
• Degenerative—storage disease, demyelinating disease, and vascular or embolic event • Anatomic—hydrocephalus • Neoplastic—glioma, choroid plexus papilloma, meningioma lymphosarcoma, nerve sheath tumor, medulloblastoma, skull tumor (e.g., osteosarcoma), metastasis (e.g., hemangiosarcoma and melanoma) • Nutritional—thiamine deficiency • Inflammatory/infectious—viral (e.g., FIP, canine distemper virus), protozoal (e.g., toxoplasmosis), fungal (e.g., cryptococcosis and blastomycosis, histoplasmosis, coc-

cidioidomycosis, and nocardiosis), bacterial (e.g., central erosion caused by otitis media and interna), parasitic (e.g., Cuterebra larvae), rickettsial (e.g., ehrlichiosis), and algae (protothecosis) • Inflammatory noninfectious— granulomatous meningoencephalomyelitis • Trauma—petrosal bone fracture with brainstem injury

RISK FACTORS
• Hypothyroidism • Administration ototoxic drugs • Thiamine deficient diet (e.g., exclusively fish diet) • Otitis externa, media, and interna

DIAGNOSIS

DIFFERENTIAL DIAGNOSIS
• The vestibular head tilt is usually directed toward the side of the lesion and may or may not be accompanied by other vestibular signs. These are abnormal nystagmus (resting, positional) with fast phase in the direction opposite the head tilt, mild ventral deviation of the eye (vestibular strabismus) ipsilateral to the tilt and exacerbated by elevation of the head, and ataxia and disequilibrium with a tendency to fall, lean, or circle toward the side of the head tilt. • If the vestibular disease is bilateral, the head tilt may be absent or mild in the direction of the more severely affected side. The abnormal nystagmus may be present or absent, and the physiologic nystagmus (i.e., normal vestibular nystagmus and conjugate eye movements) may be depressed or absent with wide side-to-side swaying movements of the head (especially evident in cats). Some patients have a wide-based stance, especially in the thoracic limbs or a crouched posture with reluctance to move. • The head tilt must be localized to a peripheral (i.e., vestibular portion of CN VIII or receptors in the inner ear) or central (i.e., vestibular nuclei and their neuronal pathways) nervous system location. • Peripheral vestibular disease deficits include horizontal or rotatory nystagmus with fast phase always in the direction opposite the head tilt; and the patient may have concomitant ipsilateral facial nerve paresis or paralysis or Horner's syndrome, because of the close association of CN VIII and VII in the petrosal bone and the sympathetic nervous system in the tympanic bulla. • Signs of central vestibular disease include vertical, horizontal, or rotatory nystagmus that can change with the position of the head, altered mentation, ipsilateral paresis or proprioceptive deficits, other signs related to the cerebellum, rostral medulla, and caudal pons, and, in some patients, multiple cranial nerve involvement other than CN VII. • Paradoxical vestibular syndrome is caused by lesions in the cerebellar peduncles, cerebellar medulla, or flocculonodular lobes of the cerebellum. With this syndrome, the vestibular signs (e.g., head tilt

and nystagmus) are opposite the side of the lesion, whereas the cerebellar signs and the proprioceptive deficits are ipsilateral to the lesion. • Nonvestibular head tilt and head posture are uncommon but must be differentiated from vestibular head tilt. In rare cases, unilateral lesions of the midbrain cause severe rotation of the head, tilting more than 90° toward the side opposite the lesion. No other vestibular signs are seen, and the tilt corrects when the patient is blindfolded. Circling of adversive syndrome (secondary to rostral thalamic lesions) with a head turn or lean or neck curvature can be misinterpreted as a vestibular tilt. The patient has no vestibular signs, and the contralateral postural, menace, or sensory deficits reflect a thalamic lesion. Circling in adversive syndrome is a compulsive turning, usually in large circles and without the disequilibrium of vestibular circling.

CBC/BIOCHEMISTRY/URINALYSIS
• Results usually normal • May detect mild anemia (hypothyroidism), leucocytosis with neutrophilia (otitis media or interna), thrombocytopenia (ehrlichiosis), hypercholesterolemia (hypothyroidism), and high serum globulin concentration (FIP).

OTHER LABORATORY TESTS
• Thyroid stimulating hormone (TSH) response test if hypothyroidism is suspected on the basis of physical examination findings and unilateral or bilateral involvement of CN VIII and possibly CN VII • Bacterial culture and sensitivity testing of sample from myringotomy or surgical drainage of tympanic bulla if otitis media or interna is suspected • Serologic testing for infectious causes, including canine distemper, FIP, and protozoal, fungal, and rickettsial diseases

IMAGING
• Tympanic bullae and skull radiography. Normal radiographs do not rule out bulla disease. • CT and MRI are valuable in confirming bulla lesions and CNS extension from peripheral disease and to document or localize a tumor, granuloma, or the extent of inflammation.

OTHER DIAGNOSTIC PROCEDURES
• Analysis of CSF collected from the cerebellomedullary cistern. Results valuable in the evaluation of central vestibular disease, especially to rule in or out an inflammatory process. CSF protein electrophoresis and titers to match with serologic testing may be indicated. CSF collection may put the patient at risk for herniation if there is a mass or high intracranial pressure. • Brainstem auditory evoked response (BAER) to assess cochlear portion of CN VIII and brainstem auditory pathways. Particularly valuable in evaluating peripheral vestibular disease, because some diseases may cause ipsilateral deafness (e.g., otitis media and interna), whereas other diseases (e.g., canine geriatric vestibular disease and hypothyroidism) only affect the vestibu-

lar portion of CN VIII • Bone biopsy if a tumor or osteomyelitis is suspected. Brainstem masses (e.g., cerebellomedullary angle) can be biopsied but are difficult to approach, and this is high-risk surgery.

TREATMENT

• Treatment as inpatient or outpatient depends on the severity of the signs (especially vestibular ataxia), size of the patient, and need for supportive care.
• Activity needs to be restricted (e.g., avoid stairs and slippery surfaces) according to the degree of disequilibrium.
• Usually no need for diet modification unless the cause is thiamine deficiency (e.g., exclusively fish diet without vitamin supplementation). Oral intake may need to be restricted if the patient has nausea and vomiting. Beware of aspiration secondary to abnormal body posture in patients with severe head tilt and vestibular disequilibrium or brainstem dysfunction.
• Advise owner that prognosis in patients with central vestibular disorders is usually poorer than for peripheral. Inform owners of risks associated with biopsy, surgery, and radiation of a brainstem mass.
• Surgical treatment may be required to drain bulla in patients with otitis media or interna, to remove nasopharyngeal polyps in cats, and to resect tumor if accessible

MEDICATIONS

DRUGS AND FLUIDS

• Supportive fluids (i.e., replacement or maintenance fluids depending on clinical state) may be required in the acute phase of vestibular syndrome when disorientation, nausea, and vomiting preclude oral intake. Especially important in geriatric patients.
• Otitis media or interna—select broad-spectrum antibiotic (parenteral or oral) that penetrates bone (e.g., trimethoprim sulfa and first generation cephalosporins) while awaiting culture results. Treatment often required for 4-6 weeks.
• Hypothyroidism—T4 replacement may need to be introduced gradually in geriatric patients, especially if cardiac disease is concurrent. Response to treatment varies (e.g., in

some patients, neuropathy is not reversible) depending, in part, on the duration of the signs.
• Drug affecting vestibular function—discontinue offending drug. Signs are usually, but not always, reversible.
• Infectious—specific treatment if indicated: antibiotic that penetrates the blood-brain-barrier for bacterial diseases (e.g., trimethoprim sulfa), sulfa or clindamycin for protozoal diseases, and antifungal for fungal diseases. Prognosis is usually grave for protozoal, fungal, and viral diseases such as canine distemper and FIP.
• Granulomatous meningoencephalomyelitis—usually treated initially with steroids (dexamethasone followed by prednisone) and, pending progress, may require stronger immunosuppression (e.g., azathioprine) or radiation
• Trauma—supportive care (e.g., antiinflammatory drugs, antibiotics, intravenous fluid administration), because specific fracture repair or hematoma removal is difficult considering the location
• Canine geriatric vestibular disease and feline idiopathic vestibular disease—supportive care only
• Cranial polyneuropathy—response to prednisone is usually good if the patient has a primary immune disorder
• Thiamine deficiency—diet modification and thiamine replacement

CONTRAINDICATIONS

Drugs potentially toxic to the vestibular system such as aminoglycoside antibiotics and prolonged high-dose metronidazole

PRECAUTIONS

• Keratoconjunctivitis sicca (dry eye) can result from long-term trimethoprim sulfa administration. • Avoid topical drugs (especially oil-based) if the tympanic membrane is ruptured.

POSSIBLE INTERACTIONS N/A
ALTERNATE DRUGS N/A

FOLLOW-UP

PATIENT MONITORING

• Owner's progress report and repeat of neurologic examination with frequency dictated by the underlying cause. Head tilt may persist. • If hypothyroidism has been diagnosed,

T4 concentration is measured after 4-6 weeks of replacement therapy to evaluate if thyroid dosage needs to be modified. • Repeat CSF and brain imaging indicated in patients with some central vestibular disorders • Monitor tear production (Schirmer tear test) if administering trimethoprim sulfa long-term.

POSSIBLE COMPLICATIONS

• Progression of central vestibular disease with deterioration of mental status • Brain herniation

MISCELLANEOUS

ASSOCIATED CONDITIONS

Facial nerve (CN VII) paresis or paralysis and Horner's syndrome with certain peripheral vestibular diseases

AGE RELATED FACTORS

Canine geriatric vestibular syndrome only affects old dogs.

ZOONOTIC POTENTIAL N/A

PREGNANCY N/A

SYNONYMS N/A

SEE ALSO

• Vestibular disease, geriatric—dogs
• Encephalitis • Vestibular disease, idiopathic—cats • Meningoencephalomyelitis, granulomatous • Nasal and nasopharyngeal polyps
• Otitis media and interna

ABBREVIATIONS

CN = cranial nerve
CNS = central nervous system
CSF = cerebrospinal fluid
CT = computed tomography
FIP = feline infectious peritonitis
MRI = magnetic resonance imaging

References
de Lahunta A. Veterinary neuroanatomy and clinical neurology. 2nd ed. Philadelphia: WB Saunders, 1983:238-254.
Oliver JE, Lorenz MD. Handbook of veterinary neurologic diagnosis. 2nd ed. Philadelphia: WB Saunders, 1993:212-216.
Parent JM, Cochrane SM. Head tilt. In: Allen DG, ed. Small animal medicine. Philadelphia: JB Lippincott, 1991:753-759.
Author Susan M. Cochrane
Consulting Editor Joane M. Parent

HEMATEMESIS

BASICS

DEFINITION
The vomiting of blood

Pathophysiology
A disruption in the esophageal, gastric, or upper small intestinal mucosal barrier leading to inflammation and bleeding. Coagulopathies can also be causative. An animal may vomit blood that originated in the oral cavity or respiratory system (upper or lower) and was swallowed.

Systems Affected
Respiratory—aspiration pneumonia with severe vomiting, especially if patient is debilitated

SIGNALMENT
• Dogs and cats • No age, breed, or sex predilection

SIGNS
• Vomiting • The blood in the vomitus may appear as fresh flecks of blood, blood clots, or digested blood which looks like "coffee grounds." The presence of blood clots or digested blood indicates more serious disease. • Pale mucous membranes if the patient is anemic

CAUSES
Alimentary Tract Causes
• Gastroduodenal erosions and ulcers
• Esophageal erosions and ulcers

Extra-alimentary Tract Causes
• Coagulopathy • Hemoptysis • Upper respiratory disease (e.g., epistaxis) • Oral disease

RISK FACTORS
Gastric, duodenal, and esophageal disease

DIAGNOSIS

DIFFERENTIAL DIAGNOSIS
• Rule out blood coming from the lower gastrointestinal tract, urogenital tract, anal sacs, cutaneous lesion, nasal passages, and oral cavity. • Differentiate from ingestion and vomiting of foreign materials or foods that look like fresh or digested blood.

CBC/BIOCHEMISTRY/URINALYSIS
• Anemia if the patient has severe or chronic blood loss • Thrombocytosis possible in patients with iron deficiency secondary to chronic blood loss • Hypoproteinemia if the patient has severe gastrointestinal blood loss • High BUN in patients with severe gastrointestinal hemorrhage • Acid-base and electrolyte alterations in some patients • Results of urinalysis usually normal

OTHER LABORATORY TESTS
• Fecal occult blood test may be positive (false positive possible) • Coagulation profile if bleeding disorder is suspected

IMAGING
• Abdominal radiography to identify radiodense gastrointestinal foreign object • Abdominal ultrasonography may help identify foreign object and gastric wall abnormality • Thoracic radiography may reveal esophageal abnormality

OTHER DIAGNOSTIC PROCEDURES
• Endoscopy to evaluate esophagus, stomach, and upper small intestinal tract if extra-gastrointestinal causes are ruled out. • Biopsy of abnormal lesions • Positive or double contrast gastrointestinal study usually not indicated. Helpful to identify foreign object, irregularities in the esophageal or gastric mucosa, and gastric ulcer.

TREATMENT
• Vomiting blood clots or digested blood usually indicates serious disease and generally warrants hospitalization, minimum data base collection, and supportive care.
• Supportive care—fluid administraion, correction of acid-base and electrolyte imbalances
• Treat gastric erosions and ulcers
• NPO if the patient is vomiting frequently
• Determine underlying cause and treat specifically.
• Parenteral administrations of antibiotics

MEDICATIONS

DRUGS AND FLUIDS
• Balanced electrolyte fluids used to replace hydration deficits
• If hypoadrenocorticism or renal failure are possibilities, avoid fluids with potassium until serum potassium concentration is determined
• See Gastritis, Acute and Gastric Erosions and Ulcers for specific drug therapy

CONTRAINDICATIONS
Avoid drugs that might damage the gastroduodenal mucosal barrier (e.g., aspirin and corticosteroids)

PRECAUTIONS N/A

POSSIBLE INTERACTIONS N/A

ALTERNATE DRUGS N/A

FOLLOW-UP

PATIENT MONITORING
• PCV and total protein to assess blood loss
• Clinical signs • Laboratory test results associated with primary problem

POSSIBLE COMPLICATIONS
• Severe anemia • Death in patients with severe blood loss

MISCELLANEOUS

ASSOCIATED CONDITIONS
• Anemia • Melena

AGE RELATED FACTORS
• Neoplasia in middle-aged to old animals
• Ingestion of foreign materials in young animals

ZOONOTIC POTENTIAL N/A

PREGNANCY N/A

SYNONYMS N/A

SEE ALSO
• Gastric Erosions and Ulcers • Esophagitis • Regurgitation • Epistaxis • Clotting Factor Deficiency

ABBREVIATIONS N/A

References
DeNovo RC. Medical management of gastritis, ulcers, and erosions. In: Proceedings. 17th Annu Waltham Ohio State Univ Symp. Columbus, Ohio, 1993.
Stanton ME. Gastroduodenal ulceration in dogs. J Vet Int Med, 1989;3:238-244.
Author Linda J. DeBowes
Consulting Editor Brent D. Jones

BASICS

DEFINITION
Hematuria is the presence of blood in the urine.

Pathophysiology
Occurs secondary to loss of endothelial integrity in urinary tract, clotting factor deficiency, or thrombocytopenia.

Systems Affected
Renal/Urologic

SIGNALMENT
• Familial hematuria in young animals, neoplasia in older animals • Females at greater risk for urinary tract infection

SIGNS

Historical Findings
Red-tinged urine with or without pollakiuria

Physical Examination Findings
• Palpable mass in animals with neoplasia • Abdominal pain in some animals • Painful prostate gland in males • Petecchia or ecchymoses in animals with coagulopathy

CAUSES

Systemic Causes
• Coagulopathy • Thrombocytopenia • Vasculitis

Upper Urinary Tract Causes
• Anatomic (e.g., cystic kidney disease and telangiectasia) • Neoplastic (e.g., renal lymphoma and renal adenocarcinoma) • Infectious (e.g., leptospirosis and bacterial disease) • Inflammatory (e.g., glomerulonephritis) • Idiopathic • Trauma (e.g., nephrolithiasis)

Lower Urinary Tract Causes
• Anatomic (e.g., bladder malformations) • Neoplasia (e.g., transitional cell carcinoma) • Infectious (e.g., bacterial, fungal, and viral disease) • Idiopathic (cats) • Trauma (e.g., uroliths) • Cyclophosphamide-induced hemorrhagic cystitis

Genitalia
• Metabolic (e.g., estrous) • Neoplastic (e.g., transmissible venereal tumor and leiomyoma) • Infectious (e.g., bacterial and fungal disease) • Inflammatory (e.g., benign prostatic hyperplasia) • Trauma

RISK FACTORS
• Breed disposed to urolithiasis and coagulopathy • Treatment with cyclophosphamide

DIAGNOSIS

DIFFERENTIAL DIAGNOSIS
Differentiate from other causes of discolored urine (e.g., myoglobinuria and hemoglobinuria)

LABORATORY FINDINGS

Drugs That May Alter Lab Results
None

Disorders That May Alter Lab Results
None

Valid if Run in a Human Lab? Yes

CBC/BIOCHEMISTRY/URINALYSIS
• Thrombocytopenia and severe anemia in some animals • Azotemia in some animals with bilateral renal disease • RBC and possibly infectious agents seen on examination of urine sediment in some animals • Crystalluria in some animals with urolithiasis

OTHER LABORATORY TESTS
• ACT or clotting profile to rule out coagulopathy • Bacterial culture of urine to identify urinary tract infection • Examination of an ejaculation to identify prostatic disease

IMAGING
Ultrasonography, radiography and, possibly, contrast radiography may be useful in obtaining a diagnosis.

OTHER DIAGNOSTIC PROCEDURES
• Biopsy of mass lesion • Vaginoscopy or cystoscopy in females

TREATMENT
• Hematuria may indicate a serious disease process. • Urolithiasis and renal failure require diet modification. • Urinary tract infection may be caused by another disease, local (e.g., neoplasia and urolithiasis) or systemic (e.g., hyperadrenocorticism and diabetes mellitus) that will also require treatment.

MEDICATIONS

DRUGS AND FLUIDS
• Blood transfusion may be necessary if patient is severely anemic. • Crystalloids to treat dehydration • Antibiotics to treat urinary tract infection and septicemia.

CONTRAINDICATIONS
Immunosuppressive drugs except to treat immune-mediated disease

PRECAUTIONS N/A

POSSIBLE INTERACTIONS
Intravenous contrast media can cause acute renal failure.

ALTERNATE DRUGS N/A

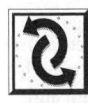

FOLLOW-UP

PATIENT MONITORING
Depends on primary or associated diseases

POSSIBLE COMPLICATIONS
Anemia

MISCELLANEOUS NA

ASSOCIATED CONDITIONS N/A

AGE-RELATED FACTORS N/A

ZOONOTIC POTENTIAL N/A

PREGNANCY N/A

SYNONYMS N/A

SEE ALSO
Dysuria and Pollakiuria, Prostatomegaly, Crystalluria, Cylinduria, Hemoglobinuria and Myoglobinuria, Proteinuria, Urolithiasis, Nephrolithiasis, Feline Lower Urinary Tract Disease, Glomerulonephritis, Prostatitis, Lower Urinary Tract Infection, Pyelonephritis, Thrombocytopenia, Coagulopathies

ABBREVIATIONS
ACT = activated clotting time
RBC = red blood cells

References
Lage AL. Diagnostic approach to canine and feline hematuria. In: Kirk RW, ed. Current veterinary therapy X. Philadelphia: WB Saunders, 1989:1117-1123.
McCall Kaufman G. Hematuria-dysuria. In: Ettinger SJ, ed. Textbook of veterinary internal medicine. 3rd ed. Philadelphia: WB Saunders, 1989:160-164.
Author Joseph W. Bartges
Consulting Editors Larry G. Adams and Carl A. Osborne

HEPATOMEGALY

 BASICS

DEFINITION
A large liver determined by physical examination, radiography, ultrasonography, surgery, or necropsy. A normal liver varies from 1.3 to 6% of body weight.

Pathophysiology
Liver size is determined by several factors, including volume of portal blood flow (which contains growth factors such as insulin and glucagon), amount of hepatic venous pressure and resistance, presence of infiltrative processes (e.g., inflammatory, metabolic, neoplastic, and cystic processes), and patency of bile flow.

Systems Affected
Gastrointestinal—severe hepatomegaly can cause gastric compression and displacement.

SIGNALMENT
• Older animals more commonly affected
• Puppies and kittens normally have a larger liver relative to their body size compared with adults.

SIGNS

Historical Findings
• Abdominal distention or a palpable abdominal mass may be reported by the owner.
• Other historical findings depend on the underlying cause (see below).

Physical Examination Findings
• The liver may be palpable beyond the costal margin (normal or small liver cannot be palpated). • A large liver must be distinguished from gastric, splenic, or other cranial abdominal masses.

CAUSES

Impaired Hepatic Venous Flow
• High central venous pressure caused by right–sided congestive heart failure (e.g., tricuspid valve disease, cardiomyopathy, congenital anomaly, and cardiac neoplasia), pericardial disease, heartworm disease, and severe arrhythmia. • High vena caval or hepatic venous resistance caused by vena caval occlusion (thrombosis, tumor invasion, heartworm disease, stenosis) or hepatic vein occlusion (e.g., thrombosis, tumor invasion, liver lobe torsion, Budd–Chiari syndrome, and veno–occlusive disease).

Neoplasia
Primary hepatic neoplasms including lymphoma, hepatoma, hepatocellular carcinoma, cholangiocarcinoma (i.e., bile duct carcinoma), hemangioma/hemangiosarcoma, fibroma/fibrosarcoma, leiomyoma/leiomyosarcoma, osteosarcoma, and various metastatic tumors.

Cystic Lesions
Hepatic cyst, biliary cyst, cystadenoma, polycystic disease, and hepatic abscess

Inflammatory Diseases
Infectious hepatitis, chronic active hepatitis (early), acute hepatic necrosis (cause by toxin, drug, ischemia, or other), feline cholangiohepatitis complex (cats), and biliary cirrhosis (cats).

Metabolic Abnormalities
Steroid hepatopathy (exogenous or endogenous), lipid accumulation (e.g., diabetes mellitus and feline hepatic lipidosis), glycogen storage disease, and hepatic amyloidosis

Biliary Obstruction
Bile duct obstruction as caused by pancreatitis, pancreatic neoplasia, other neoplasms arising near the common bile duct, bile duct carcinoma, inspissated bile plugs, abscess or granuloma in the area of common bile duct, cholelithiasis, cholecystitis, proximal duodenal foreign body, and parasite migration.

Other Causes
Immune–mediated anemia (i.e., increased hepatic phagocytosis), other regenerative anemia (e.g., extramedullary hematopoiesis), nodular hyperplasia, and certain toxins (e.g., phenobarbital).

RISK FACTORS
• Cardiac disease • Heartworm disease
• Neoplasia with potential for hepatic metastasis • Primary hepatic disease (i.e., inflammatory, neoplastic, or cystic) •
Corticosteroid administration •
Phenobarbital administration •
Hyperadrenocorticism (i.e., Cushing's syndrome) • Poorly controlled diabetes mellitus
• Obesity complicated by anorexia (i.e., hepatic lipidosis in cats) • Disease that causes biliary obstruction • Certain anemias

 DIAGNOSIS

DIFFERENTIAL DIAGNOSIS

Differentiating Similar Signs
• Hepatomegaly must be distinguished from a cranial abdominal mass of nonhepatic origin such as a gastric or splenic mass. Radiographic and ultrasonographic evaluation usually allows definitive identification of the liver.
• Hepatomegaly must be distinguished from peritoneal effusion. Radiographic and ultrasonographic evaluation usually allows definitive identification of the liver and/or effusion. The presence of peritoneal effusion should be verified by abdominocentesis.

Differentiating Causes
• Ultrasonography is useful in documenting the presence of extrahepatic biliary obstruction. • History or physical examination findings indicating cardiac disease (e.g., heart murmur, weak femoral pulses, and jugular venous distention) may suggest this as the cause. • Clinical signs of parenchymal liver disease include depression, lethargy, anorexia,

vomiting, diarrhea, weight loss, jaundice, bleeding tendency, behavior changes, polyuria/polydipsia, and peritoneal effusion.
• Pallor (with or without jaundice) is often seen in animals with immune-mediated anemia. • A history of corticosteroid administration or hyperadrenocorticism is characteristic of animals with steroid hepatopathy. • Long–standing or poorly controlled diabetes mellitus suggests lipid accumulation. • Obese cats that become anorexic are prone to hepatic lipidosis.

CBC/BIOCHEMISTRY/URINALYSIS
• The hemogram helps identify various causes of anemia. • Hepatomegaly caused by impaired hepatic venous flow often associated with mild to moderately high hepatic enzyme activities including those for ALP and ALT
• Primary hepatic neoplasia usually associated with marked increases in serum hepatic enzyme activities and variably high serum total bilirubin concentration. In animals with metastatic hepatic neoplasia, the rise in these values is usually less dramatic and many animals have normal serum hepatic enzymes.
• Animals with cystic hepatic lesions often have normal laboratory findings with the exception of those with hepatic abscess, which is often associated with a marked increase in ALT activity. • Inflammatory hepatic diseases often associated with marked increases in all serum hepatic enzyme activities and serum total bilirubin concentration and a variably inflammatory leukogram • Steroid hepatopathy and lipid accumulation usually associated with a marked increase in ALP activity and lesser increases in other serum hepatic enzyme activities • Extrahepatic biliary obstruction characterized by a marked increase in ALP activity and total bilirubin concentration, with lesser increases in other serum hepatic enzymes.

OTHER LABORATORY TESTS
• Serum bile acid concentration useful to assess hepatobiliary function if total bilirubin concentration is normal • An ACTH response test or low-dose dexamethasone suppression test useful to evaluate the presence of steroid hepatopathy • Heartworm testing may be indicated in endemic areas.

IMAGING

Radiography
• Signs of large hepatic size include extension of the liver margin caudal to the costal arch, rounding of the caudal margins on the lateral view, displacement of the stomach caudally and dorsally on the lateral view, displacement of the stomach caudally and to the left on the ventrodorsal view, and caudal displacement of the cranial duodenal flexure, right kidney, and transverse colon. • Evaluation of the thorax is helpful to determine cardiac causes of hepatomegaly. • Puppies, kittens, and deep inspiration in normal patients may show radiographic signs of large hepatic size.

Ultrasonography
• Useful to estimate liver size and contour
• Allows characterization of the parenchyma as homogeneous, nodular (i.e., focal or multifocal), or infiltrative. The relative echogenicity allows better characterization and narrowing of the differential diagnosis.
• Most reliable noninvasive method of distinguishing intrahepatic from posthepatic (e.g., bile duct obstruction) cholestasis. • Evaluation of the thorax is helpful to determine cardiac causes of hepatomegaly.

OTHER DIAGNOSTIC PROCEDURES
• Hepatic biopsy indicated if laboratory findings suggest primary hepatic disease and imaging rules out extrahepatic biliary obstruction. Coagulation profile recommended before biopsy if functional impairment is suspected. • Hepatic biopsy methods include percutaneous and ultrasound–guided techniques, laparoscopy, and laparotomy.

TREATMENT
• Treatment varies depending on the underlying cause of hepatomegaly. Usually can treat as outpatient unless animal has severe cardiac or hepatic failure.
• Restrict activity and encourage cage rest to facilitate hepatic regeneration.
• Restrict dietary protein if animal has parenchymal hepatic disease and signs of hepatic encephalopathy.
• Restrict sodium intake if animal has parenchymal hepatic disease or cardiac failure.
• Many causes of hepatomegaly are life–threatening, while other less serious causes are amenable to treatment. Thus, an aggressive work-up providing a definitive diagnosis is strongly recommended.
• Hepatotoxic medications should not be administered.
• Surgery is indicated for bile duct obstruction, resection of primary focal hepatic neoplasia, large cystic lesions, hepatic abscess, and certain pericardial diseases.

MEDICATIONS
DRUGS AND FLUIDS OF CHOICE
• If cardiac disease is suspected, a diuretic (e.g., furosemide) is often warranted. Use caution with intravenously administered fluids. Specific pharmacotherapy depends on the cause of cardiac disease.
• General supportive measures for treating hepatic disease include elimination of the inciting cause if possible, providing optimum conditions for hepatic regeneration, preventing complications, and reversing derangements occurring with hepatic failure. Important derangements include dehydration and hypovolemia, hepatic encephalopathy, hypoglycemia, acid–base and electrolyte abnormalities, coagulopathies, gastric ulceration, sepsis, and endotoxemia.
• Infectious (e.g., bacterial) hepatic diseases are treated with appropriate antimicrobial agents.
• Metabolic diseases are managed by treating the underlying cause. Mitotane (Lysodren®) is used to treat hyperadrenocorticism. Insulin and dietary management are used to treat diabetes mellitus. Alternative forms of enteral nutrition are used to treat hepatic lipidosis in cats.

CONTRAINDICATIONS N/A
PRECAUTIONS
Potential hepatotoxic drugs and corticosteroids should be used with caution.

POSSIBLE INTERACTIONS N/A
ALTERNATE DRUGS N/A

FOLLOW-UP
PATIENT MONITORING
• Physical examination and hepatic imaging by abdominal radiography and ultrasonography to reassess hepatic size • Repeat CBC, serum biochemistry analysis, and possibly bile acid concentration to assess progression of hepatic disease. • Repeat thoracic radiography, ECG, and echocardiography to assess progression of cardiac disease. • Repeat endocrine testing in animals with hyperadrenocorticism.

POSSIBLE COMPLICATIONS
Many causes of hepatomegaly are life threatening.

MISCELLANEOUS
ASSOCIATED CONDITIONS N/A
AGE RELATED FACTORS
Puppies and kittens normally have large livers relative to their body size.

ZOONOTIC POTENTIAL N/A
PREGNANCY N/A
SYNONYMS N/A
SEE ALSO See causes.
ABBREVIATIONS
ALP = alkaline phosphatase
ALT = alanine aminotransferase
CBC = complete blood count
ECG = electrocardiogram

References
Strombeck DR, Guilford WG. Small animal gastroenterology. 2nd ed. Davis, Ca: Stonegate Publishing, 1990:529–556.
Center SA. Pathophysiology, laboratory diagnosis, and diseases of the liver. A. pathophysiology and laboratory diagnosis of hepatobiliary disorders. In: Ettinger SJ, Feldman EC, eds. Textbook of veterinary internal medicine. 4th ed. Philadelphia: WB Saunders Company, 1995: 1261–1312.

Author Keith P. Richter
Consulting Editor Albert E. Jergens

HYPOTHERMIA

BASICS

DEFINITION
• A state of body temperature that is below normal in a homoethermic organism • Mild hypothermia—90-99° F (32-35° C) • Moderate hypothermia—82-90° F (28-32° C) • Severe hypothermia—any temperature < 82° F (28° C)

Pathophysiology
• Body temperature is regulated by the hypothalamus in response to changes in blood and skin temperature. Animals conserve heat by behavioral responses as well as physiologic responses, such as peripheral vasoconstriction to reduce heat loss to the environment and piloerection to trap a layer of air next to the skin in order to provide thermal insulation. Active heat production occurs by increases in cardiac output, metabolic rate, and muscle activity (i.e., shivering). • Thermoregulatory responses may be inadequate in neonates and geriatric animals as well as in hypothyroid or anesthetized animals. During prolonged exposure to cold, thermal homeostasis may fail, even in healthy animals. • Hypothermia causes central nervous system depression. Peripheral vasoconstriction and fluid shifts result in increased blood viscosity and reduced cardiac output. Severe hypothermia is associated with hypotension. A reduction in respiratory rate and depth leads to hypercapnia and respiratory acidosis. Alveolar gas exchange is affected by fluid shifts into the alveoli, resulting in hypoxemia. Increased hemoglobin affinity for oxygen causes reduced oxyhemoglodin unloading at the tissue level. Reduction of cellular metabolism may have a protective effect in animals with severe hypothermia.

Systems Affected
• Nervous—imparied consciousness ranging from obtundation to coma • Cardiovascular—arrhythmias, conduction disturbances, changes in vasomotor tone, hypotension, and low cardiac output • Pulmonary—respiratory depression, respiratory acidosis, and hypoxemia • Hemic/lymphatic/immunologic—reversible platelet and coagulation factor dysfunction and DIC

SIGNALMENT
• Any animal exposed to severe cold • Most common in small animals with a predisposition to surface heat loss, neonates, and geriatric, cachectic, and hypothyroid animals with impaired response mechanisms, low body fat and glycogen stores, or reduced metabolic rates.

SIGNS
Historical Findings
• Known prolonged exposure to cold ambient temperatures • Possibly, disappearance from home or a history of trauma • Cold unresponsive animal

Physical Examination Findings
Mild hypothermia (90-99° F)
• Mental depression • Lethargy • Weakness • Shivering
Moderate hypothermia (82-90° F)
• Muscle stiffness • Bradycardia • Hypotension • Reduced respiratory rate and depth • Stupor/obtundation
Severe hypothermia (< 82° F)
• Inaudible heart sounds • Difficulty breathing • Coma • Fixed and dilated pupils

CAUSES
• Cold ambient temperature • Impaired thermoregulation (e.g., neonates, geriatrics, animals with hypothyroidism or hypothalamic disease) • Impaired behavioral responses (as seen in neonates, sick, debilitated, or injured animals) • Predisposition to surface heat loss (as in neonates and small animals) • Inadequate heat generation (as in neonates and cachectic and hypothyroid animals)

RISK FACTORS
• Hypothyroidism • Hypothalamic disease • Very young or old age

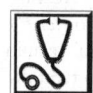

DIAGNOSIS

DIFFERENTIAL DIAGNOSIS
Differentiating Similar Signs
Must differentiate from death in animals with severe hypothermia

Differentiating Causes
• Must differentiate from other causes of CNS depression, including primary CNS disease, metabolic disorders such as hypoglycemia and hepatic encephalopathy, electrolyte disturbances, systemic infection, and neoplasia • Must differentiate from other causes of bradycardia and cardiac arrhythmias such as primary cardiac disease, hyperthyroidism in cats, and anesthetic or sedative agents

CBC/BIOCHEMISTRY/URINALYSIS
• Results usually normal • Mild hemoconcentration and hyperglycemia in some animals

OTHER LABORATORY TESTS
• A platelet count and coagulation panel may reveal thrombocytopenia and prolongation of activated partial thromboplastin and prothrombin times. • Thyroid hormone evaluation may confirm underlying hypothyroidism.

IMAGING N/A

OTHER DIAGNOSTIC PROCEDURES
Rectal or esophageal probes or low recording thermometers may be useful for monitoring body temperatures below 93° F in animals with severe hypothermia.

Electrocardiography
• Sinus bradycardia with lengthening of PR, QRS, and QT intervals • Atrial arrhythmias initially in some animals • Ventricular arrhythmias (e.g., ventricular premature complex and ventricular tachycardia) occur as body temperature decreases further. • Ventricular fibrillation is likely at body temperatures < 82° F.

TREATMENT
• Most animals are treated as inpatients until normothermia is reached.
• Minimize movement in order to prevent lethal cardiac arrhythmias, especially in animals with severe hypothermia.
• Anticipate a further decline in body temperature during initial rewarming because of contact of warmer "core" blood with the colder surface of the body.
• Aim to support vital organ systems, rewarm the patient, and prevent further heat loss.
• Airway management and oxygen supplementation are essential. Ventilatory support may be required in animals with severe hypothermia.
• Passive rewarming techniques, including thermal insulation with blankets, are used to treat mild hypothermia.
• Active external rewarming with heat sources such as heating pads and radiant heat is used to treat moderate hypothermia. Heat should be applied to the trunk to rewarm the body's "core" without causing peripheral vasodilation in the limbs. A protective layer should be provided between the heat source and the patient's skin.
• Core rewarming techniques, including warm water gastric and peritoneal lavage, warm water enemas, warm IV fluid administration, and airway rewarming (using warmed air), are used to treat severe hypothermia.

MEDICATIONS
DRUGS AND FLUIDS
• Oxygen supplementation may be provided via a face mask or endotracheal tube.
• Blood volume support is essential. Most isotonic, balanced electrolyte solutions can be used.
• Fluid solutions should be warm to prevent additional heat loss.
• Supplementation of fluids with dextrose may be helpful.

CONTRAINDICATIONS
• In an animal with severe hypothermia, lactated Ringer's solution should be avoided because the animal has impaired hepatic metabolism of lactate.
• At temperatures < 82° F, the heart is refractory to atropine and antiarrhythmic agents.

PRECAUTIONS N/A

POSSIBLE INTERACTIONS N/A

ALTERNATE DRUGS N/A

FOLLOW-UP

PATIENT MONITORING

• Core body temperature should be monitored closely during rewarming. • ECG and blood pressure should be monitored to assess cardiovascular status during rewarming.

POSSIBLE COMPLICATIONS

• Peripheral vasodilation during rewarming may result in a further drop in body temperature. • Return of cool peripheral blood to the heart may precipitate cardiac arrhythmias. • Severe hypothermia may cause cardiac arrest.

MISCELLANEOUS

ASSOCIATED CONDITIONS N/A

AGE RELATED FACTORS

Sick or hypoglycemic neonates can become markedly hypothermic in normal environments. Treatment may extend to long-term management of ambient temperature of environment.

ZOONOTIC PONTENTIAL N/A

PREGNANCY N/A

SYNONYMS None

SEE ALSO
See causes
Shock

ABBREVIATIONS None

References
Murtaugh RJ, Kaplan PM. Hypothermia. In: Veterinary and emergency critical care medicine. Philadelphia: Mosby Year Book, 1992:199-200.

Dhupa N. Hypothermia in dogs and cats. Compend Contin Educ Pract Vet 1995;17:61-69.

Author Nishi Dhupa

Consulting Editors Larry P. Tilley and Francis W. K. Smith, Jr.

INAPPROPRIATE ELIMINATION—CATS

BASICS

DEFINITION
A behavior problem characterized by failure on the part of a cat to voluntarily urinate or deficate in an available litter box. This chapter addresses problems related to urine. Feline housesoiling includes both inappropriate urination, characterized by simple (squat) urination on horizontal surfaces outside the litter box, and urine spraying on vertical surfaces outside the litter box.

Pathophysiology
With inappropriate urination, the cat's behavior may be entirely normal or a pathophysiological state may underlie the behavior problem. Urine spraying is a normal marking behavior in cats. There are widespread individual differences in the propensity to spray urine, and there may be a heritable component to the behavior.

Systems Affected   Renal/Urologic

SIGNALMENT
• Inappropriate urination can occur in any age, breed, or sex. • Urine spraying is more common but not restricted to intact and neutered males.

SIGNS

Inappropriate urination
• Urination on horizontal surfaces outside the litter box. • The intensity and duration of the problem vary greatly.

Urine spraying
• The owner may have seen the cat display: It orients to a vertical surface, raises and quivers its tail, and directs a stream of urine caudally in the process of urine spraying. • The owner may detect urine around doorways or windows. This urine is sprayed in response to an outdoor cat.

CAUSES
This problem is often strictly behavioral. This is especially true with urine spraying. However, inappropriate urination may be associated with medical conditions, particularly those associated with polyuria and polydipsia, dysuria, and pollakiuria.

Medical Abnormalities Associated with Inappropriate Urination
• Diabetes mellitus • Urolithiasis • Hyperthyroidism • Administraiton of corticosteroids and diuretics • FeLV • FIV • FIP • Lower urinary tract disease • Interstitial cystitis • Intracranial cuterebral migrations • Dysautonomia • Seizures

Environmental Factors Contributing to Inappropriate Urination
Litter Box Characteristics
• Soiled box • Inadequate number of boxes (one box per cat). • Box located in remote or unpleasant surrounding (e.g., a relatively inaccessible basement and noisey laundry room). • Inappropriate type of box. A covered litter box may maintain odors at an offensive level or may be too small for large cats to move around comfortably. A covered litter box allows other cats, pet dogs, and young children to target the cat as it exits. • Wrong litter type. Preference tests indicate that more cats prefer unscented, fine-grained (clumping) type litter over other substrates, but individual differences in litter preference must be considered.

Time Factors
Daily or weekly temporal patterns of inappropriate urination may suggest a patterned, environmental cause. An acute onset in a cat that has previously reliably used the litter box suggests a medical problem. Chronic (months to years) problems have a guarded prognosis for complete resolution.

Substrate
An acute shift from one substrate such as litter to an unusual substrate such as a porcelain sink suggests a lower urinary tract disorder.

Location
Location of the urination may suggest a substrate preference or influential social factor.

Social Dynamics
Consider any concomitant changes in the social world of the cat at the time the problem started.

Environmental Factors Contributing to Urine Spraying
• The more cats in the household, the greater the probability that at least one cat will spray urine. • The presence of outdoor cats, either owned or feral, increases the risk of urine spraying by indoor cats. • Spraying restricted to sites around doorways and windows suggests response to an outdoor cat.

RISK FACTORS
• Multiple-cat households • Households in which the owner travels frequently • Households in which the litter box (or boxes) is infrequently changed

DIAGNOSIS

DIFFERENTIAL DIAGNOSIS
It is extremely important to differentiate inappropriate urination from urine spraying (see signs) because treatment is different. The most common cause of inappropriate urination is dissatisfaction with some quality of the litter box. The most common cause for urine spraying is urine marking in response to the presence of other cats.

CBC/BIOCHEMISTRY/URINALYSIS
Findings vary with the underlying cause. Results are usually normal in cases of urine spraying and inappropriate urination when it is strictly a behavioral problem. Urinalysis is the minimum data base in any cat examined because of inappropriate urination. Serial samples should be collected in cats whose behavioral signs wax and wane.

OTHER LABORATORY TESTS
Cats with refractory inappropriate urination should be tested for thyroid disorders, FeLV, and FIV.

IMAGING   N/A

OTHER DIAGNOSTIC PROCEDURES
In multicat households, it may be difficult to determine which cat is responsible for inappropriate elimination. The offending cat may be identified in one of two ways:
1. Isolate each cat one at a time in a small room to identify the culprit by process of elimination. However, such a protocol may sufficiently alter the social milieu that inappropriate elimination may not occur.
2. Administer the dye fluorescein (6 fluorescein test strips in a gel capsule PO) sequentially to each cat. Urine outside the litter box fluoresces under a Wood's light for approximately 24 hours. If negative after 36 hours, the test can be repeated on another cat.

TREATMENT
• Treat any underlying medical condition. • Intact animals should be neutered, because this curbs spraying behavior in up to 90% of males and 95% of females.

INAPPROPRIATE URINATION
Cats that approach the litter box and eliminate in its vicinity are communicating some dissatisfaction with the litter box.

Recommendations
• Pick out the litter box daily and clean it thoroughly once a week. • Provide at least one litter box per cat, distribute in more than one location, and avoid high traffic or high noise areas. • Move the food bowls away from the litter box. • If the litter box is a covered type, provide an additional large, plain litter box. • Offer unscented, fine-grained clumping type litter in a alternate box. • Do not use a liner in the alternate box. • Place an alternate box over sites of accidents. When in regular use, move the box several inches per day to a site more acceptable to the owner. • Use deterrents at the site of inappropriate elimination. Possibilities include unacceptable substrate such as aluminum foil or plastic sheeting and odor deterrents such as citrus spray. • For problems of long duration, it may be necessary to confine the offending cat in a small room, remote from the sites of elimination. Provide a litter box, food, and other necessities. When regular litter box use has been achieved or when well-supervised, the cat can be let out of the room for increasing periods of time. • Behavior modification techniques include rewarding the cat for the use of the litter box with a favored treat. Punishment with a water pistol or sound alarm is effective only if initiated at the start

of the behavior sequence. Punishment associated with sounds or movements by the owner will condition the cat to avoid the owner. Counterconditioning may be used by feeding or playing with the cat at elimination sites.

MEDICATIONS

DRUGS AND FLUIDS

For inappropriate urination, drugs usually are not indicated. Use environmental management plan.

Cats that are urine spraying may benefit from pharmacotherapy to diminish arousal. Choosing a specific drug depends on a number of variables, including side effects, dosaging, familiarity with the drug, latency to effect, and cost (see Tables 1 and 2)

CONTRAINDICATIONS

• Benzodiazepines are contraindicated in cats with hepatic disease, because a rare but potentially fatal condition, idiopathic hepatic necrosis, can develop spontaneously. • Tricyclic antidepressants have potent antihistamine and anticholinergicside effects and are contraindicated in cats with cardiovascular abnormalities (particularly cardiac conduction disturbances) and glaucoma.

PRECAUTIONS

• Psychotropic drugs have human abuse potential. These medications should be dispensed in small quantities (not more than a 4-week supply) with refills available.
• Explain to the client the experimental nature of these treatments and common side effects (see Table 1). Such a discussion should be documented by a notation in the medical record or use of a dedicated release form.
• Although rare, benzodiazepines can cause idiopathic hepatic necrosis in apparently

healthy cats. • Use tricyclic antidepressants with caution in patients with urinary or fecal retention.

POSSIBLE INTERACTIONS

Benzodiazepine drugs can interact with cimetidine. Monoamine oxidase inhibitors can interact with tricyclic antidepressants and selective serotonin reuptake inhibitors.

ALTERNATE DRUGS

Synthetic progestins. The risk of serious side effects, including blood dyscrasias, pyometra, mammary hyperplasia, mammary carcinoma, diabetes mellitus, and obesity, have diminished their once-common use. Dosage: 5 mg q24h 1-2 weeks, then taper gradually to 2.5 mg 2x/week.

FOLLOW-UP

PATIENT MONITORING

• The owner should keep a detailed log of all elimination patterns to provide more information on the problem and feedback regarding treatment success. Clients on a program of environmental modification need to make adjustments in order to respond to preferences shown by the cat. • Tricyclic antidepressants exacerbate cardiac conduction disturbances in human patients. A screening electrocardiogram is reccommended within 4 weeks of initiation of treatment.

POSSIBLE COMPLICATIONS

Expectations must be realistic. Immediate control of a long-standing problem of inappropriate elimination is unlikely. In many cases, the client has little patience left and treatment failure may result in the cat being euthanatized, given away, or released outside.

MISCELLANEOUS

ASSOCIATED CONDITIONS

Avoidance behavior or aggression toward the owner may be exhibited if the owner punishes the cat.

AGE RELATED FACTORS N/A

ZOONOTIC POTENTIAL

Pregnant women should not clean up cat urine because of the risk of Toxoplasmosis.

PREGNANCY

Tricyclic antidepressants are contraindicated in pregnant animals.

SYNONYMS

Feline housesoiling, squat urination, urination outside the litter box, urine marking, urine spraying.

ABBREVIATIONS

FELV = feline leukemia virus
FIV = feline immunodeficiency virus

References

Borchelt PL, Voith VL. Elimination behavior problems in cats. In: Voith VL, Borchelt PL, eds. Readings in companion animal behavior, Treton, NJ: Veterinary Learning Systems, 1996:179-190.

Marder AR: Psychotropic drugs and behavioral therapy. Vet Clin North Am Small Anim Pract 1991;21:329-342.

Simpson BS, Simpson BS. Behavioral pharmacotherapy. In: Voith VL, Borchelt PL, eds. Readings in companion animal behavior. Trenton, NJ: Veterinary learning systems, 1996:100-115.

Author Barbara S. Simpson
Consulting Editors Larry P. Tilley and Francis W.K.Smith, Jr.

Table 1.

Classes of Drugs Used to Treat Housesoiling in Cats		
Class	*Examples*	*Potential Side Effects*
Benzodiazepines	Diazepam, Alprazolam	Sedation, idiopathic hepatic necrosis
Azaperone	Buspirone	Few
Tricyclic antidepressants	Amitriptyline, Clomipramine	Sedation, anticholinergic effects, cardiac conduction disturbances
Serotonin reuptake inhibitors	Fluoxetine	Sleep disturbances, irritability

Table 2.

Drugs and Doses Used to Manage Feline Housesoiling					
Drug Class	*Drug Name*	*Generic ?*	*Dosage in Cats (PO)*	*Frequency*	*Latency to effect*
Benzodiazepines	Diazepam	Yes	1-2 mg/cat	q12h	Immediate
Benzodiazepines	Alprazolam	Yes	0.125-0.25 mg/cat	q12h	Immediate
Azaperone	Buspirone	No	5-7.5 mg/cat	q12h	3-4 wk
Tricyclic antidepressants	Amitriptyline	Yes	2.5-7.5 mg/cat	q12h-q24h	3-4 wk
Tricyclic antidepressants	Clomipramine	No	1-2.5 mg/cat	q12h-q24h	3-4 wk
Serotonin reuptake inhibitors	Fluoxetine	No	1-5 mg/cat	q24h	3-4 wk

INCONTINENCE, FECAL

BASICS

DEFINITION
Inability to retain feces resulting in involuntary passage of fecal material

Pathophysiology
Reservoir fecal incontinence develops when disease processes reduce the capacity or compliance of the rectum. Sphincter incontinence develops when the external anal sphincter is anatomically disrupted (i.e., nonneurogenic sphincter incontinence) or denervated (i.e., neurogenic sphincter incontinence). Neurogenic sphincter incontinence can be caused by pudendal nerve damage, sacral spinal cord disease, autonomic dysfunction, and generalized peripheral neuropathy or myopathy. Damage to or degeneration of the levator ani and coccygeus muscles can also contribute to fecal incontinence.

Systems Affected
• Nervous • Gastrointestinal

SIGNALMENT
Any age can be affected, but old patients have a higher incidence.

SIGNS

Historical Findings
• Reservoir incontinence promotes an urge to defecate. Signs include frequent, conscious defecation without dribbling of feces. Defecation may be associated with tenesmus, dyschezia, or hematochezia. • Sphincter incontinence is associated with involuntary expulsion or dribbling of fecal material, especially during excitement or barking and coughing. • Owners should be questioned about previous neurologic disease, anorectal surgery, and trauma, house training and deworming, and whether the pet seems to defecate voluntarily or involuntarily. Information regarding the pet's diet, current medication, and concurrent systemic clinical signs, especially neurologic signs, should be obtained. • Concurrent owner complaints of urinary incontinence suggest the presence of neurogenic sphincter incontinence.

Physical Examination Findings
• Reservoir incontinence: Findings may include rectoanal sensitivity or pain on digital palpation. An intrarectal mass or thickening of the rectal mucosa may also be found. External anal sphincter tone and anal reflex is normal. • Non-neurogenic sphincter incontinence: Findings may include evidence of perineal trauma or a perianal fistula. The anal reflex is present, but complete closure of the external anal sphincter may not occur if the sphincter has been anatomically disrupted. • Neurogenic sphincter incontinence: Findings may include loss of tone to the external anal sphincter; however, anal tone is a poor indicator of anal sphincter function.

The anal reflex is absent or diminished. • A complete neurologic examination should be performed in all animals with sphincter incontinence. Additional findings suggesting lumbosacral spinal cord damage include loss of voluntary movement and tone to the tail, lumbosacral pain, flaccid posterior paresis or paralysis, and hyporeflexic myotatic reflexes to the pelvic limbs. Diffuse lower motor neuron signs suggest generalized peripheral neuropathy or myopathy. Upper motor neuron signs to the pelvic limbs suggest CNS disease cranial to the lumbosacral plexus.

CAUSES

Reservoir Incontinence
• Colorectal disease—colitis and neoplasia
• Diarrhea—large volumes of feces from any cause can overwhelm the storage capacity of the colon.

Non-neurogenic Sphincter Incontinence
• Traumatic anal injuries—bite wound, laceration, or gunshot • Iatrogenic—the external anal sphincter and levator ani muscles can be anatomically disrupted during anorectal surgery. • Perianal fistula

Neurogenic Sphincter Incontinence
• CNS—degenerative myelopathy, spinal dysraphism, spina bifida, trauma, intervertebral disc extrusion, brain or spinal cord neoplasia, meningomyelitis (various causes), fibrocartilagenous embolism, and other vascular compromises • Cauda equina syndrome—L6-L7 or L7-S1 intervertebral disc extrusion, spondylosis deformans, congenital spinal canal stenosis, lumbosacral instability, diskospondylitis, and neoplasia •Peripheral neuropathy—infectious, immune-mediated, drug induced (e.g., vincristine sulfate), dysautonomia, and idiopathic • Myopathy, neuromuscular disorder—infectious, immune-mediated, and traumatic • Aging—multiple factors including atrophy of the muscles involved in fecal continence, weakness, degenerative neuropathy, and senility are probably involved.

RISK FACTORS
• Anorectal disease and surgery • CNS disease and peripheral neuropathy

DIAGNOSIS

DIFFERENTIAL DIAGNOSIS
• Gastrointestinal disease from any cause—can induce the urge to defecate without directly altering the reservoir capacity of the colon. Unlike sphincter incontinence, gastrointestinal disease is often associated with weight loss, vomiting, tenesmus, dyschezia, and hematochezia. • Behavior disorders such as separation anxiety—unlike fecal incontinence, behavior disorders that cause inappropriate defecation are often associated with destructive activity or excessive vocalization. • Improper house training—usually occurs in

young dogs or dogs recently introduced to an indoor environment.

CBC/BIOCHEMISTRY/URINALYSIS
• Results usually normal • Urinalysis may show evidence of lower urinary tract infection (e.g., pyuria, hematuria, and high urine pH), especially if the patient has concurrent urinary incontinence.

OTHER LABORATORY TESTS
Fecal flotation should be performed to help rule out parasitism as a cause of diarrhea.

IMAGING
• Lateral and ventrodorsal survey radiography of the lumbosacral spine may show evidence of intervertebral disc extrusion, diskospondylitis, vertebral neoplasia, spina bifida, lumbosacral trauma, and vertebral malformation. • Myelography and epidurography are also useful for demonstrating compressive lesions within the spinal canal. • CT and MRI may be necessary to demonstrate some compressive lesions and intraparenchymal spinal cord lesions.

OTHER DIAGNOSTIC PROCEDURES
• Electromyography to evaluate external anal sphincter, levator ani, and coccygeus muscles for evidence of denervation or myopathy. Evaluation of other muscles is recommended to help localize the neurologic lesion (diffuse denervation versus focal spinal cord lesion). • The pudendal-anal reflex can be evaluated electrophysiologically. • Muscle and nerve biopsies required to diagnose myopathy and peripheral neuropathy • Analysis of cerebrospinal fluid retrieved by lumbar puncture may reveal evidence of a CNS infectious or inflammatory process, neoplasia, or trauma. • Colonoscopy and colorectal mucosal biopsy should be performed if reservoir incontinence is suspected.

TREATMENT
• If possible, the underlying cause of fecal incontinence should be identified. Fecal incontinence may resolve if the underlying cause is successfully treated (e.g., spinal cord decompression).
• Dietary treatment. Fecal volume can be reduced by feeding low-residue diets such as cottage cheese and rice or tofu. Prescription diet i/d may also be used but is less effective than homemade diets in reducing fecal volume.
• Frequent warm water enemas can be applied to diminish the volume of feces in the colon and thus the frequency of inappropriate defecation.
• Environmental changes such as making the pet an outside pet may increase owner satisfaction and thus avoid euthanasia due to fecal incontinence in an otherwise healthy animal.
• Reflex defecation can sometimes be induced in animals with posterior paralysis. For exam-

ple, a mild pinch of the toe on a pelvic limb or tail can stimulate the mass reflex and reflex defecation. Similarly, a warm washcloth applied to the anus or perineum may stimulate defecation.
• Surgical reconstruction of anorectal lesions may markedly improve fecal continence in patients with non-neurogenic sphincter incontinence.
• Fascial slings and silicone elastomer slings have been used with variable success in treatment of neurogenic sphincter incontinence in dogs.
• The prognosis of fecal incontinence is poor if the underlying cause can not be identified and successfully corrected. The prognosis should be discussed with the owner early in the course of evaluation to avoid unrealistic expectations.

MEDICATIONS

DRUGS AND FLUIDS
• Opiate motility modifying drugs such as diphenoxylate hydrochloride (Lomotil) and loperamide hydrochloride (Imodium) increase segmental contraction of the bowel and slow passage of fecal material, thus increasing the amount of water absorbed from the feces.
• Anti-inflammatory agents such as glucocorticoids and sulfasalazine may be beneficial in animals with suspected reservoir incontinence caused by inflammatory bowel disease.

CONTRAINDICATIONS
• Motility modifying drugs should not be used in patients with diarrhea if an infectious or toxic cause is suspected.
• Opiate motility modifiers should not be used in patients with respiratory disease and

with caution in patients with liver disease.
• Use of opiates in cats is generally not recommended.

PRECAUTIONS
Motility modifying drugs can cause constipation and bloat. Opiate motility modifying drugs can cause sedation.

POSSIBLE INTERACTIONS
• Sedation and respiratory depression is possible when opiates are used concurrently with other CNS depressants (e.g., barbiturates, general anesthetics, and tranquilizers).

ALTERNATE DRUGS N/A

FOLLOW-UP

PATIENT MONITORING
• If fecal incontinence is caused by an underlying neurologic cause, serial neurologic examinations are used to monitor patient progress. Radiographic procedures, EMG, CSF analysis, and electrodiagnostic studies can also be used to follow progress. • Fecal consistency and volume should be monitored. Diet and motility modifying drug dosages should be adjusted until the appropriate combination is found for each individual patient.

POSSIBLE COMPLICATIONS
• Neurogenic sphincter incontinence is often not treatable despite appropriate dietary, medical and surgical treatment. Fifty percent of pets with fecal incontinence were euthanized in one recent study.

MISCELLANEOUS

ASSOCIATED CONDITIONS N/A

AGE RELATED FACTORS N/A

ZOONOTIC POTENTIAL
Exposure to animal feces increases the risk of exposure to zoonotic parasites for those living with and caring for a patient with fecal incontinence. Therefore, owners should be advised about zoonotic diseases (e.g., cutaneous and visceral larval migrans and toxoplasmosis).

PREGNANCY N/A

SYNONYMS N/A

SEE ALSO
• Incontinence, Urinary • Intervertebral Disk Disease

ABBREVIATIONS
CT = computed tomography
CNS = central nervous system
MRI = magnetic resonance imaging

References
Guilford WG. Fecal incontinence in dogs and cats. Compend Contin Educ Pract Vet 1990;12:313-326.
Washabau RJ, Brockman DJ. Recto-anal disease. In: Ettinger SJ, Feldman EC, eds. Textbook of veterinary internal medicine. 4th ed. Philadelphia: WB Saunders, 1995;1408-1409.
Richter KP. Diseases of the rectum and anus. In: Kirk RW, Bonagura JD, eds. Kirk's Current veterinary therapy XI. Philadelphia: WB Saunders, 1992:615-616.
Author Randall C. Longshore
Consulting Editor Brent D. Jones

INCONTINENCE, URINARY

BASICS

DEFINITION
Loss of voluntary control of micturition, usually observed as involuntary urine leakage

Pathophysiology
Urinary incontinence is usually a disorder of the storage phase of micturition. Failure of urine storage is caused by failure of urinary bladder accommodation, failure of urethral continence mechanisms, or anatomic bypass of urinary storage structures. Partial outlet obstruction and other causes of urinary bladder overdistension may result in paradoxical, or overflow, urinary incontinence.

Systems Affected
• Renal/Urologic • Nervous • Skin/Exocrine—urine scald and perineal and ventral dermatitis

SIGNALMENT
• Most common in middle-aged to old, neutered female dogs. Also observed in juvenile females and old neutered males
• Medium to large-breed dogs most often affected

SIGNS N/A

CAUSES

Neurologic Causes
• Disruption of local neuroreceptors, peripheral nerves, spinal pathways, or higher centers involved in the control of micturition can disrupt urine storage. • Lesions of the sacral spinal cord, such as a congenital malformation, cauda equina compression, lumbosacral disk disease, or traumatic fracture or dislocation can result in a flaccid, overdistended urinary bladder with weak outlet resistance. Urine retention and overflow incontinence develop. • Lesions of the cerebellum or cerebral micturition center affect inhibition and voluntary control of voiding, usually resulting in frequent, involuntary urination or leakage of small volumes of urine.

Urinary Bladder Storage Dysfunction
• Poor accommodation of urine during storage, or urinary bladder hypercontractility, leads to frequent leakage of small amounts of urine. • Causes include urinary tract infection, chronic inflammatory disorder, infiltrative neoplastic lesion, external compression, and chronic partial outlet obstruction.
• Congenital urinary bladder hypoplasia may accompany ectopic ureters or other developmental disorders of the urogenital tract.
• Idiopathic detrusor instability has been associated with FeLV infection in cats and unknown causes in dogs.

Urethral Disorders
If urethral closure provided by urethral smooth muscle, striated muscle, and connective tissue is inadequate to prevent leakage of urine during storage, intermittent urinary in-

continence will be observed. Examples include congenital urethral hypoplasia or incompetence, acquired urethral incompetence (i.e., reproductive hormone responsive urinary incontinence), urinary tract infection or inflammation, prostatic disease or prostatic surgery (males), and vestibulovaginal anomaly (females).

Anatomic Causes
• Developmental or acquired anatomic abnormality that diverts urine from normal storage mechanisms or interferes with urinary bladder or urethral function and causes incontinence. • Ectopic ureters can terminate in the distal urethra, uterus, or vagina.
• Patent urachal remnants divert urine outflow to the umbilicus. • Vestibulovaginal anomalies, congenital urocystic hypoplasia, and urethral hypoplasia can also interfere with continence.

Urine Retention
Urinary incontinence is observed in animals with a disorder that causes urine retention when intravesicular pressure exceeds outlet resistance.

Mixed Urinary Incontinence
Mixed or multiple causes of urinary incontinence are observed in humans and probably occur in dogs and cats. Combinations of urethral and bladder storage dysfunction and anatomic and functional disorders are most likely.

RISK FACTORS
• Neutering increases the risk of development of urethral incompetence. • Conformational characteristics such as bladder neck position, urethral length, and concurrent vaginal anomalies may increase the risk of urinary incontinence in female dogs.
• Obesity may increase the risk of urinary incontinence in neutered female dogs.

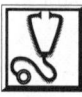

DIAGNOSIS

DIFFERENTIAL DIAGNOSIS

Differentiating Similar Signs
• Must differentiate from voluntary but inappropriate urination • Urethral discharges, often associated with prostatic disease in male dogs and vaginal disorders in female dogs, can be mistaken for urinary incontinence. Evaluation of historical features and physical examination findings is usually sufficient to differentiate. • Urine spraying in cats can be confused with urinary incontinence or inappropriate urination, but spraying is more likely to be done by cats in an upright position, and urine soiling is found on vertical surfaces of furniture, walls, and drapes.

Differentiating Causes
• Polyuria can precipitate or exacerbate urinary incontinence or lead to nocturia and inappropriate urination. Measurement of urine specific gravity in a random urine sample

usually is sufficient to rule in or rule out clinically important polyuria. • Neurogenic causes of urinary incontinence usually cause a large, distended urinary bladder and evidence of other neurologic deficits such as weak anal or tail tone, depressed perineal sensation, and proprioceptive deficits. • Historical signs in dogs with urethral incompetence typically include intermittent occurrences of urinary incontinence, observed most often at night or while the animal is sleeping. A small urinary bladder is found on physical examination and other defects are not observed. • Historical and physical findings in animals with urinary bladder storage dysfunction are similar to those observed in those with urethral incompetence, although increased frequency of urination may be an additional clinical sign.
• Anisocoria is a frequent physical examination finding in cats with urinary incontinence associated with FeLV infection. • Historical signs in male dogs with prostatic disease include tenesmus, hind limb weakness, dysuria, and pollakiuria. Physical findings include prostatomegaly, lumbosacral pain, pain on prostatic palpation, and hind limb trembling or weakness.

CBC/BIOCHEMISTRY/URINALYSIS
• Hematologic and biochemical analyses may be indicated in patients with polyuric disorders (see Polyuria and Polydipsia). • Urinalysis may reveal evidence of urinary tract infection (e.g., WBC, RBC, and bacteria) or polyuria (e.g. low urine specific gravity)

OTHER LABORATORY TESTS
Test for FeLV infection indicated in cats with urinary incontinence

IMAGING

Radiography
• Contrast radiography indicated in juvenile animals and animals exhibiting urinary incontinence shortly after surgical procedures or traumatic incidents • Excretory urography allows visualization of the kidneys, ureteral terminations, and urinary bladder. • Retrograde vaginourethrography allows visualization of the vaginal vault, urethra, and urinary bladder. Ectopic ureters usually fill with contrast media in these retrograde studies as well.
• Double contrast cystography may be required for full visualization of urinary bladder structure and identification of urinary bladder lesions.

Ultrasonography
Ultrasonographic evaluation of the kidneys and urinary bladder can be used to identify uroliths, masses, hydronephrosis or hydroureter, and evidence of pyelonephritis.

OTHER DIAGNOSTIC PROCEDURES

Neurologic Examination
A brief assessment of caudal spinal and peripheral nerve function is provided by examination of anal tone, tail tone, perineal sensation, and bulbospongiosus reflexes.

Urethral Catheterization
May be required to assess patency of the urethra if urine retention is observed

Urodynamic Procedures
Cystometrography, urethral pressure profilometry, and electromyography may be considered to evaluate urinary bladder, urethral, and neurologic function more objectively.

TREATMENT
• Usually as outpatients
• Partial obstructive disorders and primary neurologic disorders should be addressed specifically if possible.
• Urinary tract infection should be identified and treated appropriately.
• Ectopic ureters and congenital urethral hypoplasia can be surgically corrected; however, functional abnormalities of urethral competence or urinary bladder storage function may accompany the anatomic disorder and require ancillary medical treatment.

MEDICATIONS
DRUGS AND FLUIDS
Urethral Incompetence
• Manage with reproductive hormones (e.g., stilbesterol, diethylstilbesterol, and testosterone) or alpha adrenergic agonists (e.g., phenylpropanolamine, phenylephrine, pseudoephedrine).
• Alpha adrenergic agents and reproductive hormones can be administered in combination for a synergistic therapeutic effect.
• Imipramine is a tricyclic antidepressant with anticholinergic and alpha agonist actions that provides an alternative method of treatment.

Detrusor Instability
Manage with anticholinergic or antispasmodic agents (e.g., oxybutynin, propantheline, imipramine, flavoxate, and dicyclomine).

Prostatic Disease
See Prostatomegaly, Prostatitis, and Prostatic Abscesses.

CONTRAINDICATIONS
• Adrenergic agonists are contraindicated in animals with cardiac disease, renal disease, and hypertensive disorders.

• Anticholinergic agents are contraindicated in animals with glaucoma and cardiac disease.

PRECAUTIONS
• Estrogen compounds can (rarely) cause signs of estrus, bone marrow suppression, and exacerbation of immune-mediated disease.
• Testosterone administration can cause signs of aggression or libido, exacerbate prostatic disease, and contribute to the development of perineal hernia or perianal adenoma.
• Adrenergic agonists can cause restlessness, tachycardia, and hypertension.
• Anticholinergic agents can cause nausea, vomiting, and constipation.

POSSIBLE INTERACTIONS N/A

ALTERNATE TREATMENTS
Surgical procedures such as colposuspension, cystourethropexy, teflon or collagen implants, and prosthetic sphincter implantation have been described for the treatment of refractory patients.

FOLLOW-UP
PATIENT MONITORING
• Patients receiving alpha adrenergic agents during initial treatment for adverse effects of the drug including tachycardia, anxiety, and hypertension • Periodic hemogram in patients receiving estrogen • All patients periodically for urinary tract infection • Excellent response to medical treatment can be expected in 60-90% of treated animals. • Once a therapeutic effect has been observed, the dosage and frequency of administration of pharmacologic agents should be slowly reduced to the minimum required.

POSSIBLE COMPLICATIONS
• Recurrent and ascending urinary tract infection • Urine scald and perineal and ventral dermatitis • Refractory and unmanageable incontinence

MISCELLANEOUS
ASSOCIATED CONDITIONS
Urinary tract infection

AGE RELATED FACTORS
See Signalment.

ZOONOTIC POTENTIAL N/A

PREGNANCY
Although urinary incontinence is rarely a disorder of pregnant animals, the use of estrogens or anticholinergic agents is not advised in pregnant animals.

SYNONYMS Enuresis

SEE ALSO
• Polyuria and Polydipsia • Prostatic Disease
• Urinary Tract Obstruction • Urine Retention, Functional

ABBREVIATIONS
FeLV = feline leukemia virus
RBC = red blood cells
WBC = white blood cells

References
Arnold S. Relationship of incontinence to neutering. In: Kirk RW, Bonagura J, eds. Current veterinary therapy XI. Philadelphia: WB Saunders, 1992:875-877.

Barsanti JA. Urinary incontinence. In: Lorenz MD, Cornelius LM. Small animal medical diagnosis. 2nd ed. Philadelphia: JB Lippincott, 1993:345-356.

Holt PE. Pathophysiology and treatment of urethral sphincter mechanism incompetence in the incontinent bitch. Vet International 1992;3:15.

Lane IF, Barsanti JA. Urinary incontinence. In: August J. Consultations in feline internal medicine. 2nd ed. Philadelphia: WB Saunders, 1994:373-382.

Moreau PM, Lappin MR. Pharmacologic manipulation of micturition. In: Kirk RW, ed. Current veterinary therapy X. Philadelphia: WB Saunders, 1989:1214-1222.

Richter K. Use of urodynamics in micturition disorders in dogs and cats. In: Kirk RW, ed. Current veterinary therapy X. Philadelphia, WB Saunders, 1989:1145-1150.

Author India F. Lane
Consulting Editors Larry G. Adams and Carl A. Osborne.

INFERTILITY, FEMALE

BASICS

DEFINITION
Historical complaint that occurs in bitches showing abnormal cycling, copulation failure, conception failure, or pregnancy loss.

Pathophysiology
Normal fertility requires normal estrus cycling with ovulation of normal ova into a patent, healthy reproductive tract, fertilization by normal spermatozoa, implantation of the conceptus into the endometrium, formation of the normal zonary placenta, and maintenance of pregnancy with presence of high progesterone concentration throughout the approximately 2-month gestation. Breakdown in any of these processes causes infertility.

Systems Affected Reproductive

SIGNALMENT
This disorder is seen in animals of all ages but may be more common in old animals. Animals > 6 years old are more likely to have underlying cystic endometrial hyperplasia (CEH) and may be predisposed to uterine infection and failure of conception or implantation. Breeds predisposed to thyroid insufficiency may have a higher prevalence of infertility—golden retriever, doberman pinscher, dachshund, Irish setter, miniature schnauzer, great Dane, poodle, and boxer.

SIGNS

Historical Findings
• Failure to cycle • Failure to copulate • Normal copulation with no subsequent pregnancy or parturition

Physical Examination Findings
Positive pregnancy with no subsequent parturition

CAUSES
• The most common cause in the bitch is insemination at an improper time in the estrous cycle; other causes include subclinical uterine infection, male infertility factors, thyroid insufficiency, hypercortisolism, anatomic abnormality, chromosomal abnormality, and abnormal ovarian function. Brucella canis should always be considered a potential cause of infertility in dogs. • Causes in the queen are similar and include lack of sufficient copulatory stimulus to induce ovulation, subclinical uterine infection, male infertility factors, systemic viral or protozoal infection, anatomic abnormality, chromosomal abnormality, and abnormal ovarian function. • Previous ovariohysterectomy of animals acquired as mature individuals should also be investigated as causative.

RISK FACTORS
• Brucella canis (dogs) • Thyroid insufficiency (dogs) • Hypercortisolism, endogenous or exogenous (dogs and cats) • Systemic viral—canine herpesvirus, FeLV, FIV, and protozoal (e.g., toxoplasmosis) infection (dogs and cats) • Any chronic, debilitating disease condition (dogs and cats) • Congenital vaginal anomaly (dogs and cats)

DIAGNOSIS

DIFFERENTIAL DIAGNOSIS
• Historical information is extremely useful in distinguishing causes of infertility. • Pertinent history questions: Is the bitch or queen cycling? Has the queen or bitch conceived or given birth in the past? If so, how recently has the female given birth, and what was the litter size? Is the bitch or queen free of systemic viral or protozoal infection? Is the bitch or queen capable of normal copulation? Was the bitch or queen bred to a male of proven fertility at the proper time of the estrous cycle? Did the bitch or queen ovulate during the estrous cycle and maintain progesterone concentration consistent with pregnancy during the entire gestation? Is the bitch euthyroid?

CBC/BIOCHEMISTRY/URINALYSIS
Results usually normal

OTHER LABORATORY TESTS

Serologic Test for Brucella Canis (Dogs)
The rapid slide agglutination test is used as a screen. The test is sensitive but not specific; if positive, recheck by an agar gel immunodiffusion test (Cornell University Diagnostic Laboratory, Ithaca, NY, 607 253–3900) or bacterial culture of whole blood or lymph node aspirate is recommended.

Serum Progesterone Measurement
• Dogs—serum progesterone can be measured during proestrus and estrus to predict ovulation time and optimize breeding management. Serum progesterone concentration of 1.0 –1.9 ng/ml indicates ovulation in 3 days, 2.0–2.9 ng/ml in 2 days, 3.0 – 3.9 ng/ml in 1 day, and 4.0 – 8.0 ng/ml that day. The optimal breeding day for maximum litter size is 2 days after ovulation. The day of ovulation is extremely variable in the bitch and is not well correlated with standing behavior (see Breeding, Timing). • Cats—serum progesterone can be measured after breeding to assess induction of ovulation with concentrations of > 2 ng/ml indicating functional luteal tissue. • Dogs and cats—serum progesterone can be measured at the time of examination. If the concentration is > 2 ng/ml, this may indicate "silent heat," estrus with no overt behavioral or physical changes, or pathologic production of progesterone from a luteal ovarian structure, functional ovarian neoplasm, or the adrenal gland. • Dogs and cats—progesterone should remain high throughout gestation. If it falls to < 2 ng/ml in midgestation and pregnancy loss occurs, this indicates insufficient luteal function

OTHER TESTS
• Bacterial culture for uterine organisms (dogs and cats). Collect the vaginal discharge originating in the uterus during proestrus or estrus directly by hysterotomy or indirectly from the anterior vagina by a guarded swab. • Thyroid hormone testing (dogs)—resting concentration of triiodothyronine (T3) or thyroxine (T4) can be measured in serum or serum T4 can be measured after challenge with thyroid stimulating hormone to assess for thyroid insufficiency. • Serologic testing for canine herpesvirus and toxoplasmosis (see Abortion–Dogs). • Serologic testing for FeLV, FIV, and toxoplasmosis (see Abortion—Dogs). • Karyotype (dogs and cats)—this procedure is performed on heparinized blood samples of animals with primary or persistent anestrus to look for chromosomal abnormalities, which can cause abnormal sexual differentiation (University of Minnesota Cytogenetics Laboratory, Minneapolis, MN 612 624–3067; see Sexual Development Disorders). • Serum cortisol assay (dogs and cats)—if the resting serum cortisol concentration is high, the underlying cause should be investigated. • Semen evaluation (dogs and cats)—alternatively, test breeding the male to another queen can be used to prove fertility. Azoospermia in the tom cat can be ruled out after copulation by demonstration of spermatozoa in a vaginal flush or swab specimens from the queen or in urine collected by cystocentesis from the tom.

IMAGING
• Radiography—normal ovaries and a nongravid uterus are not visible radiographically. Large ovaries may indicate cystic ovarian disease or neoplasia. A visible uterus may indicate cystic endometrial hyperplasia. Positive contrast procedures including vaginography in dogs and hysterography in dogs and cats prepuberally or when the animal is in estrus may allow assessment of anatomic abnormality (e.g., abnormal structure and impatency). • Ultrasonography—large ovaries may indicate cystic ovarian disease or neoplasia. A visible uterus may indicate cystic endometrial hyperplasia. Ultrasound can be used for a diagnosis of pregnancy as early as 20–24 days after ovulation and is useful to document pregnancy loss.

OTHER DIAGNOSTIC PROCEDURES
Laparotomy (dogs and cats)— allows assessment of the anatomy of the tubular tract and gonads, hysterotomy for obtaining a direct uterine culture specimen, and biopsy of the uterus or ovaries.

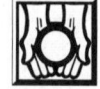

TREATMENT

INPATIENT VERSUS OUTPATIENT
Outpatient unless special procedures performed require anesthesia

CLIENT EDUCATION

Since the most common cause of infertility is improper breeding management, the initial prognosis is good. However, if improper breeding is ruled out, the prognosis for future fertility worsens. Cats are seasonal breeders and are dependent on photoperiod. Queens cycle when exposed to long day length, normally from late January to mid October. Year–round cycling can be induced by exposure to ≥ 12 hours of light daily. If a cat is not cycling during the physiologic breeding season, question the owner as to housing of the queen and exposure to light. In dogs and cats, if the condition causing the infertility is thought to have a heritable basis (e.g., thyroid insufficiency), counseling of the owner regarding the advisability of retaining the animal in a breeding program is recommended.

SURGICAL CONSIDERATIONS

• Surgical resection of vaginal anomalies (dogs)—this procedure may ease natural service and vaginal delivery
• Surgical repair of impatent tubular tract (dogs and cats)—this procedure is difficult, and the prognosis for future fertility is guarded.
• Surgical drainage of ovarian cysts (dogs and cats)—efficacy of this procedure is unknown.
• Unilateral ovariectomy of neoplastic ovary (dogs and cats)—future fertility depends on resumption of normal function of the remaining ovary and lack of metastasis.

MEDICATIONS

DRUGS AND FLUIDS

• Antibiotics for uterine infection (dogs and cats)—choice of drug depends on results of bacterial culture and sensitivity test of the uterus itself or of vaginal discharge during proestrus or estrus. • L–thyroxine for thyroid insufficiency (dogs; 0.01 mg/kg PO q12h). Prognosis for future fertility with return to euthyroid state is guarded. • Gonadotropin therapy for induction of ovulation. The protocol given employs gonadotropin releasing hormone (GnRH), which causes release of endogenous luteinizing hormone from the pituitary, or human chorionic gonadotropin (hCG), which has luteinizing hormone–like activity.

(1) In cats not adequately stimulated to ovulate at the time of copulation—25 mg/cat GnRH IM or 250 IU/cat IM; hCG at the time of breeding
(2) In patients with ovarian cystic disease— cats, 25 mg/cat GnRH IM or 250 IU/cat hCG IM; dogs, 50 mg/dog GnRH IM or 1000 IU/dog hCG, half IV, half IM. This causes ovulation or luteinization of cystic ovarian tissue.

CONTRAINDICATIONS N/A

PRECAUTIONS N/A

POSSIBLE INTERACTIONS N/A

ALTERNATE DRUGS N/A

FOLLOW-UP

PATIENT MONITORING

• L–thyroxine (dogs)—recheck blood concentrations of T3 and T4 after 1 month of supplementation to insure adequate absorption of medication and resumption of a euthyroid state. • Ultrasonography (dogs and cats)— useful to definitively diagnose pregnancy and monitoring gestation. • Progesterone assay (dogs and cats)

POSSIBLE COMPLICATIONS N/A

MISCELLANEOUS

ASSOCIATED CONDITIONS

Infertility caused by endocrinopathy may be associated with a dermatologic abnormality (e.g., alopecia with thyroid insufficiency or hypercortisolism) or systemic signs of disease (e.g., polydipsia and polyuria with hypercortisolism). Bitches with a vaginal anatomic abnormality may have persistent or recurrent urinary tract disease or vaginitis.

AGE RELATED FACTORS N/A

ZOONOTIC POTENTIAL

Brucella canis infection is a zoonotic disease. The organism is less readily shed if affected animals are gonadectomized. Stress good hygiene.

PREGNANCY N/A

SYNONYMS N/A

SEE ALSO See causes.

ABBREVIATIONS

FeLV = feline leukemia virus
FIV = feline immunodeficiency virus
GnRH = gonadotropin releasing hormone
hCG = human chorionic gonadotropin
T3 = triiodothyronine
T4 = thyroxine

References

Johnston SD, Olson PNS, Root MV. Clinical approach to infertility in the bitch. Sem Veter Med Surg Small Anim. 1994;9:2–6.
Freshman JL. Clinical approach to infertility in the cycling bitch. Vet Clin North Am Small Anim Proc Philadelphia: WB Saunders, 1991;21:427–436.
Authors Margaret V. Root and Shirley D. Johnston
Consulting Editor Sara K. Lyle

INFERTILITY, MALE—DOGS

BASICS

DEFINITION
In general terms, infertility in males is diminished or absent fertility; it does not imply sterility. Infertility in male dogs results from a wide range of problems that prevent the delivery of sufficient numbers of spermatozoa to fertilize ovulated, mature oocytes in the bitch.

Pathophysiology
• Spermatogenesis encompasses the formation and development of spermatozoa from primordial germ cells; it is a coordinated, hormonally controlled, cyclic process. Approximately 60 days are required for a complete spermatogenic phase. The testicular phase requires 46 days, the remainder being the epididymal phase. Consequently, testicular problems take at least 60 days to resolve; epididymal problems may take only 2 weeks. • Azoospermia is ejaculate completely devoid of spermatozoa. • Oligozoospermia is low numbers of spermatozoa in an ejaculate. • The primary causes of infertility in male dogs are impaired or arrested spermatogenesis, blockage of the excurrent ducts, genitourinary inflammation, testicular neoplasia, environmental stress, congenital abnormality, and endocrine abnormality.

Systems Affected
• Reproductive • Endocrine • Musculoskeletal • Nervous

SIGNALMENT
• Prevalence increases with age. • Relatively higher prevalence of specific problems seen in certain breeds.

SIGNS

General Comments
The general complaint is usually that no puppies are produced and the owner suspects that the male dog may be infertile. In spite of these observations and initial assumptions, the most common cause of infertility is incorrect timing of breeding.

Historical Findings
Important information includes age of testicular descent, age at first attempted mating, libido and breeding behavior, frequency and number of matings, method used to time breedings, litter size(s), familial history of infertility, degree of inbreeding, fertility status of bitches bred, Brucella canis status of all breeding partners, current and previous drug and dietary therapies, and previous medical or surgical illnesses.

PHYSICAL EXAMINATION FINDINGS
The sheath and penis should be palpated to identify masses or adhesions. The non-erect penis is exteriorized to determine if the superficial mucosa contains any clinically important lesions and if the os penis is undamaged.

The testes and epididymes are palpated and examined, noting the size and symmetry of the epididymis relative to the testes. Location, size, and symmetry of the internal urethra and prostate are determined by digital rectal palpation.

CAUSES

Congenital Infertility
Dogs with chromosomal abnormalities (e.g., XXY syndrome) and those with XX sex reversal ('XX males') are phenotypic males with hypoplastic testes and no spermatogenesis. Biopsy has shown that some male dogs only have Sertoli cells (see Disorders of Sexual Development). Unilateral or bilateral segmental aplasia of the epididymis or vas deferens causes either oligospermia or azoospermia.

Acquired Infertility
• Incomplete ejaculation—unfamiliar surroundings, slippery flooring, absence of an estrous bitch, and presence of a dominant owner or bitch may interfere with the collection of a complete ejaculate. • Obstruction of the efferent system—azoospermia can be caused by obstruction of the efferent ductules, epididymides, or ductus deferens. Causes include sperm granuloma, spermatocele, acute inflammation, chronic inflammatory stenosis, segmental aplasia, neoplasia, previous vasectomy, and attempts to "tack" testes into a scrotal location. Inflammation or infection (particularly by B. canis and Escherichia coli) of the testes or epididymes requires prompt and aggressive treatment if infertility is to be prevented. • Hormonal abnormalities—although the role of hypothyroidism in male infertility of dogs is unclear, thyroid function should be evaluated in males with poor semen quality. Hypothyroidism may be associated with decreased libido. Hyperadrenocorticism causes testicular atrophy; this change is probably reversible. • Drugs and toxins—parasiticides, corticosteroids, anabolic steroids, chemotherapeutic agents, and some antifungal agents can interfere with or interrupt spermatogenesis. It is advisable to assess all topical and systemic therapies. The effect of environmental toxins on canine infertility is unknown. • Miscellaneous causes—trauma, environmental damage, testicular neoplasia, systemic disease, ischemia, and heat stress can cause either transient infertility or sterility. Prostatic disease appears to markedly reduce semen quality. Inbreeding initially reduces fertility until some point at which there is a rebound effect and fertility can start to return to near normal if the breeder selects for fertile individuals. Lymphocytic orchitis is familial in some breeds (e.g., beagles and Borzois); affected animals may be fertile when young, but fertility declines at an accelerated rate with age. • Retrograde ejaculation—during normal ejaculation in dogs, some retrograde flow into the bladder is normal. Complete retrograde ejaculation (aspermia) is rare; diagnosis is aided by urinalysis after ejaculation.

RISK FACTORS
Congenital disorders affecting reproductive function are not uncommon and tend to occur in selected breeds. The risk of problems caused by infectious disease increases when testing of bitches and stud dogs (i.e., serologic test for B. canis and bacterial culture of genital tract) is not performed before breeding.

DIAGNOSIS

DIFFERENTIAL DIAGNOSIS
Before extensive diagnostics are done on the male, it should be determined that the bitches bred to the dog in question are fertile (previous litters) and that breedings were optimally timed (see Infertility - Female, and Breeding, Timing).

CBC/BIOCHEMISTRY/URINALYSIS
• Results usually normal • Dogs with brucellosis or prostatitis have various changes in the leukogram (normal or leukocytosis) and urinalysis (high numbers of leukocytes) depending on the time course of the infection. Systemic illness can impair reproductive function, but infertility is not usually the primary complaint on examination.

OTHER LABORATORY TESTS

Endocrine Profile
The range of resting testosterone in normal, intact dogs is 0.4-10 ng/ml; the most common range of values is 1-4 ng/ml. The presence of androgenic tissue is confirmed if the serum concentration of testosterone increases 100% over the resting value 2-3 hours after injection with either 1-2 mcg/kg gonadotropin releasing hormone (GnRH) or 40 IU/kg human chorionic gonadotropin (hCG). This test is useful to detect bilaterally cryptorchid dogs. Serum follicle stimulating hormone concentration (Cornell Laboratories, Ithaca, NY) rises with marked reduction in spermatogenesis because of loss of inhibin secretion. Serum luteinizing hormone concentration is difficult to interpret because of its episodic secretion. Thyroid function is high according to baseline T_3 and T_4 values and thyroid stimulating hormone stimulation (TSH) test.

IMAGING
Ultrasonography helps identify lesions that alter the testicular and epididymal architecture (e.g., neoplasia and spermatocele) and evaluates the prostate gland for the presence of hyperplasia, chronic prostatitis, cyst, abscess, or neoplasia (see Benign Prostatic hyperplasia, Prostatic Cyst, Prostatitis and Prostatitis Abscess)

OTHER DIAGNOSTIC PROCEDURES

Breeding Soundness Examination
A thorough and comprehensive breeding soundness examination is pivotal to ensure that all appropriate information is collected.

The sperm-rich and prostatic portions of the ejaculate should be collected as separate fractions by use of a sterile artificial vagina and sterile, graduated, nontoxic plastic tubes in the presence of an estrous bitch. Semen volume, concentration and motility of sperm cells, morphologic and cytologic characteristics of sperm cells, and qualitative and quantitative cultures are performed on the sperm-rich fraction. Cytologic examination and qualitative and quantitative cultures are also performed on the prostatic fraction and urine (collected by cystocentesis). Culture results must be correlated with clinical and cytologic evidence of an active infection. Dogs with aprostatic fraction that indicates a clinically important infection should be reevaluated by other sampling techniques that avoid contamination from the penile mucosa and prepuce. Whenever an azoospermic or oligospermic ejaculate is obtained, recollection 1 hour later and then again on several occasions is warranted before the dog is deemed infertile.

Epididymal Markers
The concentration of ALP in seminal fluid (normal, 10,000-40,000 units/ ml), which is of epididymal origin, may indicate obstruction if values are < 5,000 units/ ml and a complete ejaculate was obtained.

Testicular Biopsy
Determines the degree of spermatogenesis and the integrity of the blood-testis barrier and differentiates obstruction of efferent ducts from testicular hypoplasia and degeneration. This information enables one to make an informed prognosis. Incisional biopsy is superior to aspiration or needle biopsy in obtaining a diagnostic sample. Bouin's fixative is required for processing the tissue.

TREATMENT
• The client must be informed that the testis will require time to return to function, at least 60 days.
• Stress patience while the patient is regularly checked to ensure there is no worsening of the condition.
• Supportive regimens include reducing the heat or other stress on the stud dog. Ensure that diet and mineral supplementation are adequate.
• Specific medications must be administered long enough and at a dosage that will ensure tissue penetration.
• Re-anastomosis of blocked excurrent ducts is being attempted; little data is available on success rates.

MEDICATIONS
DRUGS AND FLUIDS
• The antibiotics of choice for penetration and spectrum are chloramphenicol, trimethoprim-sulfa, erythromycin, and enrofloxacin. Usually a minimum of 3-4 weeks of treatment is recommended to allow adequate and sustained levels within the reproductive tract.
• Pseudoephedrine has been used with limited success in men with retrograde ejaculation.

CONTRAINDICATIONS
Trimethoprim-sulfas are contraindicated in dogs predisposed to keratitis sicca. Chloramphenicol and trimethoprim-sulfas reportedly induce blood dyscrasias.

PRECAUTIONS N/A

POSSIBLE INTERACTIONS N/A

ALTERNATE DRUGS N/A

FOLLOW-UP
PATIENT MONITORING
Recheck the stud at intervals that take into account the length of the spermatogenic cycle (60 days) but are frequent enough to allow detection of deterioration in the animal's condition.

POSSIBLE COMPLICATIONS N/A

MISCELLANEOUS
ASSOCIATED CONDITIONS
• Brucellosis infection causes diskospondylitis, polyarthritis, posterior paresis, fever, and uveitis. • Prostatic disease causes obstipation, locomotor difficulties, fever, hematuria, polakiuria, and dysuria. • Lymphocytic orchitis is associated with lymphocytic thyroiditis.

AGE RELATED FACTORS
Although reduction in daily sperm output and morphologically normal sperm cells occurs with age, it is difficult to assess the effect of age alone on fertility. Most old, infertile dogs have concurrent disease (e.g., systemic or prostatic disease and testicular neoplasia) that have documented effects on fertility.

ZOONOTIC POTENTIAL N/A

PREGNANCY N/A

SYNONYMS N/A

SEE ALSO
See Causes

ABBREVIATIONS
GnRH = gonadotropin releasing hormone
hCG = human chorionic gonadotropin

References
Meyers-Wallen, VN. Clinical approach to infertile dogs with sperm in the ejaculate. Vet Clin North Am Small Anim Pract 1991;21:609-633.
Fayrer-Hosken RA, Caudle AB. Canine semen examination, with special reference to proximal cytoplasmic droplets and their relation to fertility. Georgia Vet 1990;42:11-13.
Kennelly JJ. Coyote reproduction. The duration of the spermatogenic cycle and sperm transport. J Reprod Fertil 1972;31:163-170.
Olson PN. Clinical approach for evaluating dogs with azoospermia. In: Proceedings, Annu Meet Soc Theriogenol 1991;202-207.
Wallace MS. Infertility in the male dog. Prob Vet Med 1992;4:531-544.
Authors Richard A. Fayrer-Hosken and Frances O. Smith
Consulting Editor Sara K. Lyle

LAMENESS

BASICS

DEFINITION
A disturbance in gait and locomotion as a response to pain or injury

Pathophysiology
• Severe, sharp pain will cause an animal to carry or non–weight-bear on its affected limb while in motion. • Lesser, dull, or aching pain will result in a limp or off–weight-bearing use of the limb; at rest, the affected limb will bear less weight. • Pain that is produced only during certain phases of movement will cause the animal to adjust its motion and gait during those phases to minimize discomfort.

Systems Affected
• Musculoskeletal • Nervous

SIGNALMENT
• Can affect any age or breed • Certain diseases have specific age, breed, and sex predilections.

SIGNS

General Comments
• Forelimb lameness—animals with unilateral forelimb lameness compensate by moving the head and neck upward as the affected limb is placed on the ground and dropping the head and neck when the sound limb bears the weight. • Hindlimb lameness—movement of the head and neck is less pronounced and more weight is shifted to the forelimbs by dropping the forequarters. With unilateral lameness, animal drops lower on the sound limb when it strikes the ground and elevates its hindquarters when the affected limb is on the ground. • Always assess the neurologic status of the animal, especially if a proximal lesion is suspected.

Historical Findings
• A complete history is mandatory—signalment, identification of affected limb(s), known trauma, changes in weather, exercise, or rest, and responsiveness to previous treatments are important. • Onset of lameness? Acute versus chronic. Progression? Static versus slow versus rapid. • Is the animal demonstrably in pain or just lame?

Physical Examination Findings
• Do a complete routine exam. • Observe gait during a walk, trot, climbing stairs, or figure-of-eights. • Palpate for asymmetry of muscle mass and bony prominences. • Manipulate bones and joints, beginning distally and working proximally. • Assess for instability, incongruency, luxation or subluxation, pain, abnormal range of motion, and abnormal sounds. • Avoid the suspected area of involvement until last. It is better to examine the normal limbs first in order to allow relaxation and to assess normal reactions to maneuvers.
Common Causes of Lameness in Dogs
Forelimb
GROWING DOG (< 12 MONTHS OF AGE)
• Osteochondrosis of the shoulder • Shoulder

luxation/subluxation (congential) • Osteochondrosis of the elbow • Ununited anconeal process • Fragmented medial coronoid process • Elbow incongruity • Avulsion/calcification of the flexor muscles (elbow) • Asymmetric growth of the radius and ulna • Panosteitis • Hypertrophic osteodystrophy • Trauma (soft tissue, bone, joint) • Infection (local or systemic causes) • Nutritional imbalances • Congenital anomalies
MATURE DOG (> 12 MONTHS OF AGE)
• Degenerative joint disease • Bicipital tenosynovitis • Calcification of supra/infraspinatus tendon • Contracture of supra/infraspinatus muscle • Soft tissue or bone neoplasia (primary or metastatic) • Trauma (soft tissue, bone, joint) • Panosteitis • Polyarthropathies • Polymyositis • Polyneuritis
Hindlimb
GROWING DOG (< 12 MONTHS OF AGE)
• Hip dysplasia • Avascular necrosis of femoral head (Legg-Calvé-Perthes) • Osteochondrosis of stifle • Patellar luxation (medial or lateral condyle) • Osteochondrosis of hock • Panosteitis • Hypertrophic osteodystrophy • Trauma (soft tissue, bone, joint) • Infection (local and systemic causes) • Nutritional imbalances • Congenital anomalies
MATURE DOG (> 12 MONTHS OF AGE)
• Degenerative joint disease • Cruciate ligament disease • Avulsion of long digital extensor tendon (stifle) • Soft tissue or bone neoplasia (primary or metastatic) • Trauma (soft tissue, bone, joint) • Panosteitis • Polyarthropathies • Polymyositis • Polyneuritis

RISK FACTORS   N/A

DIAGNOSIS

DIFFERENTIAL DIAGNOSIS
Must differentiate musculoskeletal causes from neurogenic causes of lameness

CBC/BIOCHEMISTRY/URINALYSIS
Hemogram, serum chemistry profile, and urinalysis are usually normal.

OTHER LABORATORY TESTS
Dependent on suspected cause of lameness

IMAGING
• Radiographs are recommended for all suspected causes of musculoskeletal lameness. • CT scans, MRI, and bone scans using radioisotopes are useful in identifying and delineating causative lesions.

OTHER DIAGNOSTIC PROCEDURES
• Cytologic examination of joint fluid is useful in identifying and differentiating intraarticular disease. • EMG is useful for differentiating neuromuscular disease from musculoskeletal disease. • Muscle/nerve biopsies are useful in establishing the presence and identity of neuromuscular disease.

TREATMENT
Dependent on cause of lameness

MEDICATIONS

DRUGS AND FLUIDS

• Analgesic and antiinflammatory drugs (NSAIDs) are often indicated to symptomatically treat the manifestations of lameness.
• Corticosteroids should be used judiciously, unless specifically indicated, due to potential side effects and articular cartilage damage associated with long-term use.

CONTRAINDICATIONS N/A

PRECAUTIONS

Gastrointestinal irritation may occur with the use of NSAIDs and may preclude their use in individual animals.

POSSIBLE INTERACTIONS N/A

ALTERNATE DRUGS

If treating degenerative joint disease, chondroprotective drugs such as polysulfated glycosaminoglycans may be of benefit in limiting cartilage damage and degeneration. They may also help alleviate pain and inflammation.

 FOLLOW-UP

PATIENT MONITORING

Dependent on cause of lameness

POSSIBLE COMPLICATIONS N/A

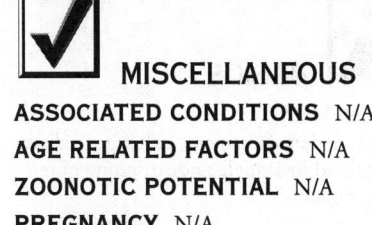 **MISCELLANEOUS**

ASSOCIATED CONDITIONS N/A

AGE RELATED FACTORS N/A

ZOONOTIC POTENTIAL N/A

PREGNANCY N/A

SYNONYMS N/A

SEE ALSO

All chapters in musculoskeletal and neuromuscular section

ABBREVIATION

EMG = electromyographic

Reference

Brinker WO, Piermattei DL, Flo GL. Physical examination for lameness. In: Handbook of small animal orthopedics and fracture treatment. 2nd ed. Philadelphia: WB Saunders, 1990.

Author Peter D. Schwarz

Consulting Author Peter D. Schwarz

LYMPHADENOPATHY

BASICS

DEFINITION
Lymph node enlargement, either generalized or localized to a single node or group of regional nodes.

Pathophysiology
Lymphadenopathy commonly results from hyperplasia of lymphoid elements, inflammatory infiltration, or neoplastic proliferation within the node. Because of their filtration function, lymph nodes often act as sentinels of disease in the tissues that they drain. Inflammation of any tissue is often accompanied by enlargement of the draining nodes. Such enlargement is most likely to result from reactive lymphoid hyperplasia, but may also be due to extension of the inflammatory process into the nodes (lymphadenitis). Reactive hyperplasia involves proliferation of lymphocytes and plasma cells in response to antigenic stimulation. The term "lymphadenitis" implies active migration of neutrophils, activated macrophages, or eosinophils into the node. Neoplastic proliferation may be either primary (malignant lymphoma) or metastatic.

Systems Affected
Hemic/lymphatic/immune

SIGNALMENT
Lymphadenopathy is among the most common of clinical findings in both dogs and cats. Because of the diversity of causes, it has no breed, sex, or age predilection.

SIGNS
Lymphadenopathy typically does not cause clinical signs. Neither is it detected by owners in most cases, although marked node enlargement may be so obvious as to be reported to the veterinarian as a "lump". Severe lympadenopathy may cause mechanical interference with function of adjacent organs. Clinical signs of such interference depend upon the affected node and may include dysphagia, regurgitation, and respiratory distress.

CAUSES
Lymphadenopathy usually is a manifestation of one of three disease processes: lymphoid hyperplasia, lymphadenitis, or neoplasia (either primary or metastatic).

Lymphoid Hyperplasia
• Localized or systemic infections by infectious agents of all categories (bacteria, viruses, fungi, protozoa, algae) commonly cause lymph node hyperplasia when infection does not directly involve the node. Some infectious agents may produce lymphadenitis of certain nodes with concurrent hyperplasia of other nodes that are not directly infected. Other infectious agents such as rickettsia and Brucella canis typically cause marked lymph node hyperplasia without overt lymphadeni-

tis. Feline immunodeficiency virus (FIV) infection stimulates generalized lymph node hyperplasia, although lymphoid depletion may occur late in the course of the disease. • Antigenic stimulation by factors other than infectious agents (e.g., allergens) is a common cause of lymph node hyperplasia. Hyperplastic nodes may also occur in animals with immune-mediated diseases such as systemic lupus erythematosus and rheumatoid arthritis.

Lymphadenitis
• Common infectious causes include bacteria and fungi. Many bacteria are capable of causing purulent lymphadenitis which may progress to abscessation. A few bacteria (e.g. Mycobacterium sp.) induce granulomatous lymphadenitis. • Systemic fungal infections that commonly induce granulomatous lymphadenitis include histoplasmosis, blastomycosis, cryptococcosis, and sporotrichosis. Other infectious agents such as protozoa, algae, and metazoan parasites are uncommon causes. • Lymphadenitis involving several nodes frequently is a manifestation of sytemic infections such as histoplasmosis or blastomycosis. Although primary infections of lymph nodes do occur, lymphadenitis usually is accompanied by (and often results from) infections of other tissues being drained by the affected node. • Eosinophilic lymphadenitis may be associated with allergic inflammation of the organ being drained by the affected node (e.g. skin affected with flea allergy dermatitis). It may also be encountered in multisystemic idiopathic eosinophilic diseases such as feline hypereosinophilic syndrome.

Neoplasia
• Malignant lymphoma in cats results from neoplastic transformation of lymphocytes by feline leukemia virus. • Canine malignant lymphoma and most tumors that metastasize to lymph nodes are of unknown cause.

RISK FACTORS
• Any animal with compromised immune function is predisposed to infection and, therefore, to lymphadenitis. • Animals with allergic diseases are also likely to develop lymph node hyperplasia or eosinophilic lymphadenitis. • The principal risk factor for feline malignant lymphoma is infection with the feline leukemia virus. Risk factors for lymphadenopathy due to metastatic neoplasms vary with the type of primary neoplasm.

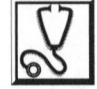

DIAGNOSIS
DIFFERENTIAL DIAGNOSIS
• One must ascertain that a palpable or visible mass is actually a lymph node as opposed to some other inflammatory or neoplastic mass. Lymph nodes that are palpable in normal dogs include the mandibular, prescapular, axillary, superficial inguinal, and popliteal nodes. In addition, the facial, retropharyn-

geal, and iliac nodes are palpable when enlarged. • A mass in a location characteristic of a lymph node usually can be assumed to be one, but cytologic evaluation of a fine needle aspirate will usually resolve any doubts. • Severe lymph node enlargement (>5 times normal size) is most likely to occur with abscessation (lymphadenitis) and with malignant lymphoma. Lesser degrees of enlargement may be attributable to either reactive hyperplasia, lymphadenitis or neoplasia. The extent of enlargement in metastatic disease of nodes varies widely. • Lymphadenopathy affecting nodes throughout the body are likely to be caused by malignant lymphoma or systemic infections that cause either lymphadenitis or lymphoid hyperplasia. Abscessation and metastatic neoplasms more commonly affect a single node.

CBC/BIOCHEMISTRY/URINALYSIS
• Lymphocytosis suggests the possibilities of rickettsial disease (in dogs) and lymphoid neoplasia in dogs and cats. Atypical lymphocytes in the blood, when present, help establish a diagnosis of lymphoid neoplasia. • Eosinophilia may occur in animals with lymphadenopathy due to allergic or parasitic skin disease. • Neutrophilia with or without a left shift may occur with either lymphadenitis, lymphoid hyperplasia, or neoplasia. • Hypercalcemia is relatively common in dogs with lymphoid neoplasia. • Hyperglobulinemia may occur with chronic inflammatory diseases or with lymphoid neoplasia.

OTHER LABORATORY TESTS
• A positive feline leukemia virus test provides supporting evidence for lymphoid neoplasia; however, cats infected with that virus may also develop lymphadenitis because of immunosuppression. • Cats that are positive for FIV may have generalized lymph node hyperplasia as a direct result of the virus or lymphadenitis as a result of immunosuppression. • Serological tests for antibodies against systemic fungal agents such as Blastomyces and Cryptococcus may be helpful in establishing those diagnoses.

IMAGING
• Involvement of deep lymph nodes within the body cavities can be detected. • Lesions may be detected in other organs that can be related to the lymph node enlargement. Examples would include detection of diffuse pneumonia in dogs with blastomycosis and detection of primary tumor masses in animals with lymphadenopathy due to metastatic neoplasia.

OTHER DIAGNOSTIC PROCEDURES
• The single most valuable technique in determining the cause of lymphadenopathy is fine needle aspiration cytology of the affected node(s). Cytologic examination usually allows one to determine which of the three major categories of lymphadenopathy (hyperplasia, inflammation, or neoplasia) exists, and may

provide a specific diagnosis in cases of certain infectious diseases and neoplasms. • Aspirates from hyperplastic nodes contain a mixed cell population in which small lymphocytes predominate. Also present in these specimens are large lymphocytes, plasma cells, occasional neutrophils, and, perhaps, a few eosinophils and mast cells. Hyperplastic nodes and normal nodes are cytologically indistinguishable. • Aspirates from nodes affected with lymphadenitis contain increased proportions of neutrophils, macrophages, and/or eosinophils, depending on the cause of the inflammation. Specific infectious agents such as bacteria and systemic fungi may be evident. Cytologic evaluation frequently is the means of diagnosis in systemic fungal infections such as blastomycosis and cryptococcosis. • Aspirates from nodes affected by malignant lymphoma typically contain increased proportions (usually > 50%) of large lymphocytes. • Aspirates from nodes containing metastatic neoplasms contain populations of cells that do not occur in normal nodes. The appearance of such cells varies widely, depending on the type of neoplasm. • In some individual cases where a diagnosis is not made by cytology, a surgical biopsy may be needed. In such cases, excisional biopsy specimens are preferable to needle biopsy specimens.

TREATMENT

Because of the many disease processes and specific agents that may cause lymphad-enopathy, treatment depends on establishing the reason for node enlargement.

MEDICATIONS

Appropriate medications vary with the cause of the node enlargement.

FOLLOW-UP

PATIENT MONITORING N/A

POSSIBLE COMPLICATIONS N/A

MISCELLANEOUS

ASSOCIATED CONDITIONS

• Both lymph node hyperplasia and lymphadenitis are often components or manifestations of systemic disease. • Malignant lymphoma frequently involves other organs such as the liver, spleen, intestine, kidney, and meninges with a variety of clinical consequences. • Clinical disease in animals with metastatic neoplasms in lymph nodes is usually attributable to the primary tumor rather than the metastasis.

AGE RELATED FACTORS N/A

ZOONOTIC POTENTIAL

Direct transmission of diseases responsible for lymphadenitis to people is unlikely with the exception of sporotrichosis. Caution should be exercised when performing fine needle aspiration in animals that may have systemic fungal disease.

PREGNANCY N/A

SYNONYMS N/A

SEE ALSO

See Causes.

ABBREVIATIONS N/A

References

Day MJ, Whitbread TJ. Pathological diagnoses in dogs with lymph node enlargement. Vet Rec 1988;136:72-73.

Duncan JR. The lymph nodes. In: Cowell RL, Tyler RD, eds. Diagnostic cytology of the dog and cat. Goleta, CA: American Veterinary Publications, 1989; 93-98.

Rogers KS, Barton CL, Landis M: Canine and feline lymph nodes. II. Diagnostic evaluation of lymphadenopathy. Compend Contin Educ Pract Vet 1993;15:1493-1503.

Author Edward A. Mahaffey

Consulting Editor Alan H. Rebar

MELENA

 BASICS

DEFINITION
Presence of digested blood in the feces. Appears as black, tarry stool.

Pathophysiology
Usually the result of upper gastrointestinal bleeding. However, can also be associated with ingested blood from the oral cavity or respiratory tract.

Systems Affected
Gastrointestinal

SIGNALMENT
• More common in dogs than cats • Any age can be affected • No breed or sex predilections

SIGNS
• Melena may be accompanied by vomiting, inappetance, weight loss, and pallor of the mucus membranes. • Physical examination findings depend on the underlying cause.

CAUSES
Gastrointestinal Ulceration And Erosion
• Neoplasia—lymphosarcoma and adenocarcinoma • Infectious—pythiosis, fungal and parasitic infection • Inflammation—foreign body, acute gastitis, hemmorhagic gastroenteritis, and inflammatory bowel disease (i.e., lymphoplasmacytic, eosinophlic, granulomatous, or histiocytic) • Drugs—corticosteroids and nonsteroidal anti-inflammatory drugs (NSAIDs)

Metabolic and Other Diseases That Cause Gastrointestinal Ulceration
• Renal failure • Hepatic disease • Pancreatitis • Hypoadrenocorticism • Neoplasia—gastrinoma and mast cell tumor • Shock

Ingestion of Blood
• Diet • Esophageal lesion—neoplasia or esophagitis • Oral or pharyngeal lesion—neoplasia or abscess • Nasal lesion—neoplasia or fungal rhinitis • Respiratory lesion—lung lobe torsion, neoplasia, hemoptysis, or pneumonia

Coagulopathy
• Thrombocytopenia • Clotting factor abnormality—von Willebrands disease, anticoagulant rodenticide ingestion, or clotting factor deficiency • Disseminated intravascular coagulation (DIC)

RISK FACTORS
Arthritis requiring use of NSAIDs or corticosteroids

 DIAGNOSIS

DIFFERENTIAL DIAGNOSIS
Must differentiate between intestinal and nonintestinal disease

CBC/BIOCHEMISTRY/URINALYSIS
• Hemogram may show microcytic hypochromic anemia if the patient has chronic blood loss; neutrophilia and thrombocytopenia in some patients • Biochemistry analysis may reveal extraintestinal cause of melena (e.g., renal failure and liver disease) • Urinalysis usually normal (isosthenuria in patients with renal failure)

OTHER LABORATORY TESTS
• Coagulation profile may reveal clotting abnormality. • Bleeding time may be prolonged. • Fecal examination may reveal infectious cause (parasites). • ACTH stimulation test if hypoadrenocorticism suspected

IMAGING
• Abdominal radiography may reveal a mass or foreign body. • Ultrasonography may reveal a mass, liver disease, or pancreatitis. • Upper gastrointestinal barium series may delineate gastric, upper small intestinal mass, ulceration, or filling defect.

OTHER DIAGNOSTIC PROCEDURES
Endoscopy allows visualization of gastric, duodenal mass, and ulceration, and retrieval of biopsy specimen.

 TREATMENT

• Inpatient (exception may be animal with intestinal parasites)
• Treat underlying disease (e.g., renal failure and hypoadrenocorticism).
• Temporarily discontinue oral intake (especially if patient is vomiting).
• Surgery may be required for severe gastric or duodenal ulceration and neoplasia.

MEDICATIONS

DRUGS AND FLUIDS

Fluids
• Required if blood loss causes hypovolemia. Use a balanced electrolyte solution with potassium supplementation.
• Whole blood or packed red cell transfusion if anemia is severe
• Whole blood or plasma transfusion if the patient has coagulopathy.
• If the patient has gastric ulceration, treat with mucosal protectants: H_2 receptor antagonists—cimetidine, ranitidine, and famotidine; Sucralfate; Na/K ATPase pump antagonist—omeprazole

CONTRAINDICATIONS

Avoid corticosteroids and NSAIDs in patients with gastric ulceration.

PRECAUTIONS N/A

POSSIBLE INTERACTIONS N/A

ALTERNATE DRUGS N/A

FOLLOW-UP

PATIENT MONITORING

• PCV daily until anemia is stabilized, then weekly • Avoid foreign objects and drugs that cause gastrointestinal ulceration

POSSIBLE COMPLICATIONS

Gastric or duodenal perforation and peritonitis are possible in patients with severe disease.

EXPECTED COURSE AND PROGNOSIS

• Depends on cause • Good prognosis in patients with drug-associated ulceration, parasite infestation, foreign body, inflammatory disease, and hypoadrenocorticism • Guarded prognosis in patients with liver and renal disease and DIC (depends on response to treatment) • Good prognosis with treatment in patients that have ingested anticoagulant rodenticide • Fair prognosis in patients with neoplasia if resectable and no metastasis

MISCELLANEOUS

ASSOCIATED CONDITIONS N/A

AGE RELATED FACTORS N/A

ZOONOTIC POTENTIAL N/A

PREGNANCY N/A

SYNONYMS N/A

SEE ALSO
See Causes

ABBREVIATIONS
DIC = disseminated intravascular coagulation
NSAIDs = nonsteroidal anti-inflammatory drugs

Reference

Willard, MD. Diseases of the stomach. In: Textbook of veterinary internal medicine. SJ Ettinger, EC Feldman, eds. Philadelphia: WB Saunders, 1995;1143-1168.
Author Lisa E. Moore and Colin F. Burrows
Consulting Editor Brent D. Jones

MURMURS, HEART

BASICS

DEFINITION
Vibrations caused by disturbed blood flow

Timing of Murmurs
• Systolic murmurs occur between S1 and S2 (systole). • Diastolic murmurs occur between S2 and S1 (diastole). • Continuous and to-and-fro murmurs occur throughout all or most of the cardiac cycle. • Continuous murmurs are usually accentuated near S2 and to-and-fro murmurs are usually absent near S2.

Grading Scale for Murmurs
• Grade I—barely audible • Grade II—soft, but easily auscultated • Grade III—intermediate loudness. Most hemodynamically important murmurs are at least grade III. • Grade IV—loud with palpable thrill • Grade V—very loud and audible with stethoscope barely touching the chest; palpable thrill • Grade VI—very loud and audible without the stethoscope touching the chest; palpable thrill

Configuration
• Plateau murmurs have uniform loudness and are typical of regurgitant murmurs such as mitral and tricuspid insufficiency and ventricular septal defect. • Crescendo-decrescendo murmurs get louder and then softer and are typical of ejection murmurs such as pulmonic and aortic stenosis and atrial septal defect. • Decrescendo murmurs start loud and then get softer and are typical of diastolic murmurs such as aortic or pulmonic insufficiency.

Location
Dogs
• Mitral area—left fifth intercostal space at costochondral junction • Aortic area—left fourth intercostal space above costochondral junction • Pulmonic area—left second to fourth intercostal space at sternal border • Tricuspid area—right third to fifth intercostal space near costochondral junction
Cats
• Mitral area—left firth to sixth intercostal space 1/4 ventrodorsal distance from sternum • Aortic area—left second to third intercostal space just above the pulmonic area • Pulmonic area—left second to third intercostal space 1/3-1/2 ventrodorsal distance from sternum • Tricuspid area—right fourth to fifth intercostal space 1/4 ventrodorsal distance from sternum

PATHOPHYSIOLOGY
• Disturbed blood flow associated with high flow through normal or abnormal valves or with structures vibrating in the blood flow • Flow disturbances associated with outflow obstruction or forward flow through stenosed valves or into a dilated great vessel • Flow disturbances associated with regurgitant flow through an incompetent valve, septal defect, or patent ductus arteriosus

SYSTEMS AFFECTED Cardiovascular

SIGNALMENT Varies with cause
SIGNS
Relate to cause of the murmur
CAUSES
Systolic Murmurs
• Mitral and tricuspid valve endocardiosis • Cardiomyopathy • Physiologic flow murmurs • Anemia • Congenital cardiac defects • Mitral and tricuspid valve dysplasia • Atrial septal defect • Ventricular septal defect • Pulmonic stenosis • Aortic stenosis • Tetralogy of Fallot • Mitral and tricuspid valve endocarditis • Hyperthyroidism • Heartworm disease

Continuous Murmurs
• Congenital cardiac defects • Patent ductus arteriosus

Diastolic Murmurs
• Congenital cardiac defects • Mitral and tricuspid valve stenosis • Aortic and pulmonic valve endocarditis

RISK FACTORS Cardiac disease

DIAGNOSIS

DIFFERENTIAL DIAGNOSIS
Differential Signs
• Must differentiate murmurs from other abnormal heart sounds (i.e., split sounds, ejection sounds, gallop rhythms, and clicks) • Must differentiate murmurs from abnormal lung sounds and pleural rubs. Listen to see if timing of abnormal sound is correlated with respiration or heart beat.

Differential Causes
• Pale mucous membranes support anemic murmur. • Location and radiation of murmur and timing during cardiac cycle can help determine cause of the murmur. See algorithm.

CBC/BIOCHEMISTRY/URINALYIS
• Anemia in animals with anemic murmurs • Polycythemia in animals with right to left shunting congenital defects • Leukocytosis with left shift in animals with endocarditis

OTHER LABORATORY TESTS N/A
IMAGING
Thoracic Radiography
Useful for evaluating heart size and pulmonary vasculature in hopes of determining cause and significance of the murmur

Echocardiography
• Recommended when a cardiac cause is suspected and the nature of the defect is unknown • Diagnostic test of choice for documenting cardiomyopathy, congenital defects, and valvular disease

Other Diagnostic Procedures
Electrocardiography may be useful in assessing large heart patterns in animals with murmurs.

TREATMENT
• Most animals treated as outpatients unless heart failure is evident • Treatment decisions based on the cause of the murmur and associated clinical signs • No treatment indicated for murmur alone

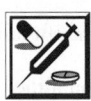

MEDICATIONS

DRUGS AND FLUIDS
Depend on cause of the murmur and associated clinical signs

CONTRAINDICATIONS
Depend on cause of the murmur and associated clinical signs

PRECAUTIONS
Depend on cause of the murmur and associated clinical signs

POSSIBLE INTERACTIONS N/A
ALTERNATE DRUGS N/A

FOLLOW-UP

PATIENT MONITORING
Low-grade systolic ejection murmurs in puppies may be physiologic. Most of these resolve by 6 months of age. If the murmur is still present after 6 months, expand the database to include diagnostic imaging.

POSSIBLE COMPLICATIONS
If the murmur is associated with structural heart disease, signs of congestive heart failure (e.g., coughing, dyspnea, and ascites) or exercise intolerance may develop.

MISCELLANEOUS

ASSOCIATED CONDITIONS N/A
AGE RELATED FACTORS
• Murmurs present since birth generally associated with a congenital defect or physiologic flow murmur • Acquired murmurs in geriatric, small-breed dogs usually associated with degenerative valve disease • Acquired murmurs in large-breed dogs usually associated with dilated cardiomyopathy • Acquired murmurs in geriatric cats usually associated with cardiomyopathy or hyperthyroidism

ZOONOTIC POTENTIAL N/A
PREGNANCY N/A
SYNONYMS N/A
SEE ALSO Causes
ABBREVIATIONS
S1—first heart sound
S2—second heart sound

MURMURS, HEART

Reference

Smith FWK Jr., Tilley LP. Rapid interpretation of heart sounds, murmurs, and arrhythmias. Philadelphia: Lea & Febiger, 1992.

Authors Francis W. K. Smith, Jr and Robert L. Hamlin
Consulting Editors Larry P. Tilley and Francis W. K. Smith, Jr.

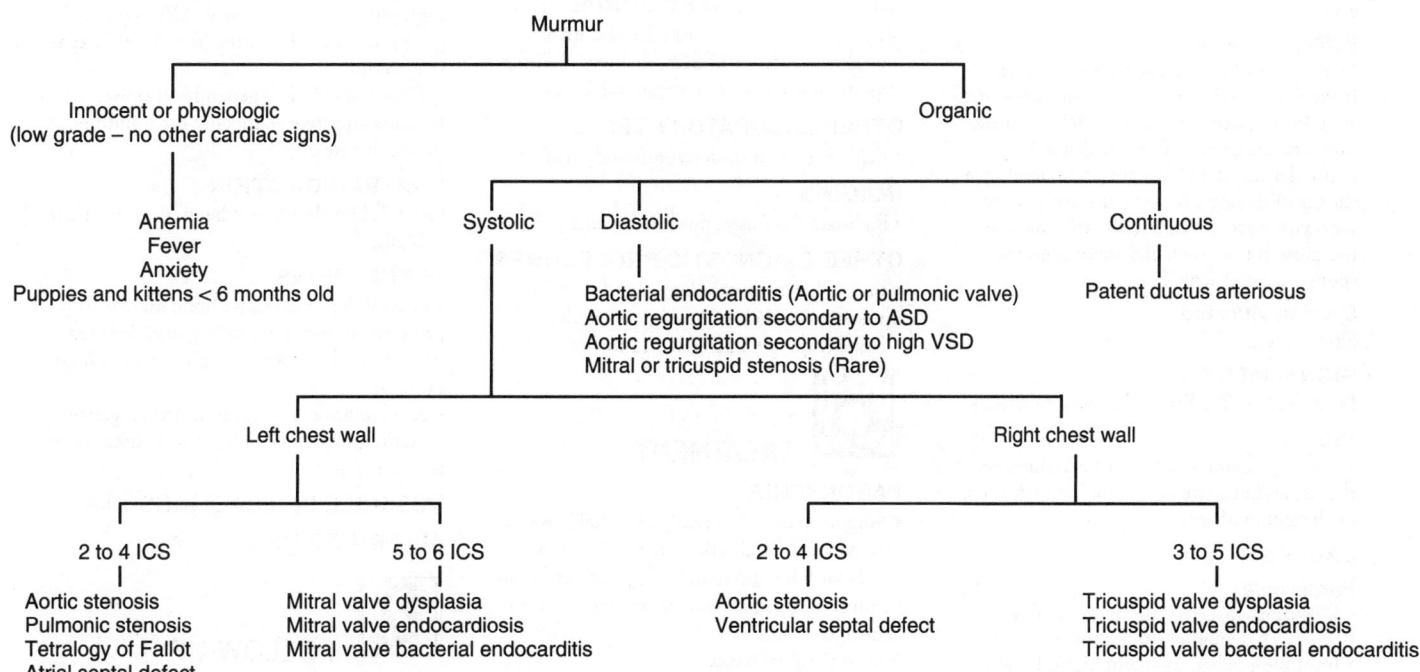

Differential diagnosis of cardiac disease based on the timing and location of murmurs. Adapted from Allen DG. Murmurs and abnormal heart sounds. By permission of Mosby-Year Book, Inc. In: Allen DG, Kruth SA, eds. Small animal cardiopulmonary medicine. Philadelphia: BC Decker, 1988:13.

NAIL AND NAILBED DISORDERS

 BASICS

DEFINITION

• Paronychia—inflammation of soft tissue around the nail • Onychomycosis—fungal infection of the nail • Onychorrhexis—brittle nails that tend to split or break • Onychomadesis—sloughing of the nail • Nail dystrophy—nail deformity caused by abnormal growth

Pathophysiology

Nails and nailfolds are subject to trauma, infection, vascular insufficiency, immune-mediated disease, neoplasia, defects in keratinization, and congenital abnormalities. A particular nail deformity may be caused by a variety of diseases. A single disease can present with various nail lesions. In some cases the cause is unknown and there is no response to treatment.

Systems Affected

Skin/Exocrine

SIGNALMENT

Dachshund—Predisposed to onychorrhexis

SIGNS

• Licking • Lameness • Pain • Swelling, erythema, and exudate of nail fold • Deformity or sloughing of nail

CAUSES

Paronychia

• Infection—bacteria, dermatophyte, yeast (Candida), demodicosis, leishmaniasis • Immune-mediated—pemphigus, bullous pemphigoid, systemic lupus erythematosus (SLE), drug eruption • Neoplasia—squamous cell carcinoma, melanoma, eccrine carcinoma, osteosarcoma, subungual keratoacanthoma, inverted squamous papilloma • Arteriovenous fistula

Onychomycosis

• Dogs—T. mentagrophytes (usually generalized) • Cats—M. canis

Onychorrhexis

• Idiopathic (especially in dachshund)—multiple nails • Trauma • Infection (dermatophytosis, leishmaniasis)

Onychomadesis

• Trauma • Infection • Immune-mediated (pemphigus, bullous pemphigoid, SLE, drug eruption) • Vascular insufficiency (vasculitis, cold agglutinin disease) • Neoplasia (see above) • Idiopathic

Nail Dystrophy

• Acromegaly • Feline hyperthyroidism • Zinc-responsive dermatosis • Congenital malformations

RISK FACTORS

• Paronychia (infectious) - Immunosuppression (endogenous or exogenous), FeLV infection, trauma, and diabetes mellitus • Bacterial onychomadesis—Excessively short nail trimming (into the quick) is postulated to predispose this disorder

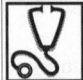 DIAGNOSIS

DIFFERENTIAL DIAGNOSIS

• Trauma or neoplasia often affects a single nail. • Involvement of multiple nails suggests a systemic disease. • Immune-mediated diseases usually have other skin lesions in addition to nail/nailfold lesions.

CBC/BIOCHEMISTRY/URINALYSIS

Hemogram, serum chemistries and urinalysis may show evidence of SLE, diabetes mellitus, hyperthyroidism or other systemic illness.

OTHER LABORATORY TESTS

• FeLV • T_4 • Antinuclear antibody test

IMAGING

• Radiographs—osteomyelitis of third phalanx

OTHER DIAGNOSTIC PROCEDURES

• Biopsy for histopathology and direct immunofluorescence • Cytology of exudate • Skin scraping • Bacterial and fungal culture

 TREATMENT

PARONYCHIA

• Surgical removal of nail plate (shell) to provide adequate drainage. The nail is grasped firmly with hemostat and stripped from its attachments with one swift downward motion. Bandage • Antimicrobial soaks • Identify underlying condition and treat specifically.

ONYCHOMYCOSIS

• Antifungal soaks (captan, chlorhexidine, povidone iodine) • Surgical removal of nail plate may improve response to systemic medication. • Amputation of 3rd phalanx

ONYCHORRHEXIS

• Repair with fingernail glue (type used to attach false nails in humans) • Remove splintered pieces • Amputation of third phalanx • Treat underlying cause

ONYCHOMADESIS

• Antimicrobial soaks • Treat underlying cause

NEOPLASM

• Treatment depends on biologic behavior of specific tumor • Surgical excision • Amputation of digit • Amputation of leg • Chemotherapy • Radiation therapy

NAIL DYSTROPHY

Treat underlying cause

 MEDICATIONS

DRUGS AND FLUIDS

• Bacterial paronychia—systemic antibiotics based on culture and sensitivity; cephalosporins pending culture result. • Candida paronychia—ketoconazole (10 mg/kg PO q12h); topical nystatin or miconazole. • Onychomycosis—Griseofulvin (50-150 mg/kg/day) or ketoconazole (10 mg/kg PO q12h) for several months (6-12) until negative cultures. • Onychomadesis—depends on cause. Immunosuppressive therapy for immune-mediated diseases.

CONTRAINDICATION

Griseofulvin should not be used in pregnant animals.

PRECAUTIONS

• Griseofulvin may cause bone marrow suppression, anorexia, vomiting, and diarrhea. Absorption is enhanced if given with a high fat meal. • Ketoconazole may cause anorexia, gastric irritation, hepatic toxicity, and lightening of the hair coat

POSSIBLE INTERACTIONS N/A

ALTERNATE DRUGS N/A

 FOLLOW-UP

PATIENT MONITORING

Depends on underlying cause

POSSIBLE COMPLICATIONS N/A

EXPECTED COURSE AND PROGNOSIS

• Course of treatment for bacterial or fungal paronychia and onychomycosis may be prolonged and response may be influenced by underlying immunosuppressive factors. • Onychomycosis and onychorrhexis may require amputation of the third phalanx for resolution. • Prognosis for nail dystrophy is good when underlying cause can be effectively treated (hyperthyroidism, zinc-responsive dermatosis). • Prognosis for onychomadesis depends on underlying cause. Immune-mediated diseases and vascular problems carry a more guarded prognosis than trauma or infectious causes. • Some neoplasmas can be totally excised or removed by amputation of the digit. Others are highly malignant and may have already spread at the time of diagnosis.

 MISCELLANEOUS

ASSOCIATED CONDITIONS N/A

AGE RELATED FACTORS N/A

ZOONOTIC POTENTIAL

Dermatophyte infections

PREGNANCY N/A

SYNONYMS

Nailfold = Nailbed

SEE ALSO

- Demodicosis • Dermatophytosis
- Dermatoses, nutritionally responsive
- Pododermatitis • Pyoderma • Cutaneus vasculitis • Pemphigus • Pemphigoid

ABBREVIATIONS

SLE = Systemic lupus erythematosus

References

Muller GH, Kirk RW, Scott DW. Small animal dermatology. 4th ed. Philadelphia: WB Saunders, 1989.

Author Ellen C. Codner

Consulting Editor Lowell Ackerman

NASAL DERMATOSES

BASICS

DEFINITION
Pathologic condition of the nasal skin involving either the haired portion (bridge of the nose) or nonhaired portion (nasal planum).

Pathophysiology N/A

Systems Affected
• Integument • Systemic lupus erythematosus (SLE) - multisystemic.

SIGNALMENT
• Dermatophytosis, zinc responsive dermatosis, dermatomyositis and demodicosis more likely in dogs less than 1 year of age. • Zinc responsive dermatosis - Siberian huskies, Alaskan malamutes. • Dermatomyositis - collies, Shetland sheep dogs. • Uveodermatologic syndrome - Akitas, samoyeds, Siberian huskies. • SLE and Discoid lupus erythematosus (DLE) - Collies, Shetland sheep dogs, German shepherds. • DLE - may occur more often in females

SIGNS
• Depigmentation • Hyperpigmentation • Erythema • Erosion/ulceration • Vesicles/pustules • Crusts • Scarring • Alopecia • Nodules/plaques

CAUSES
• Nasal pyoderma • Demodicosis • Dermatophytosis • Other fungal infections (cryptococcosis, sporotrichosis, aspergillosis) • DLE and SLE • Pemphigus foliaceus (PF) • P. erythematosus (PE) • Nasal solar dermatitis • Dermatomyositis • Zinc-responsive dermatosis • Uveodermatologic syndrome • Vitiligo • Nasal depigmentation • Contact hypersensitivity - plastic dish dermatitis, topical drug hypersensitivity (neomycin) • Tumors - squamous cell carcinoma, basal cell carcinoma, mycosis fungoides, fibrosarcoma • Trauma • Idiopathic sterile granuloma • Idiopathic nasal hyperkeratosis

RISK FACTORS
• Adult cats may be inapparent carriers of dermatophytes • Rooting behavior - pyoderma, dermatophytosis • Sun exposure - nasal solar dermatitis, DLE, SLE, PE • Poorly pigmented nose - nasal solar dermatitis, squamous cell carcinoma • Large, rapidly growing breeds oversupplemented with calcium or fed high cereal diet - zinc responsive dermatosis • Immunosuppression - demodicosis, pyoderma, dermatophytosis

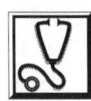

DIAGNOSIS

DIFFERENTIAL DIAGNOSIS
• **Nasal solar dermatitis** - lesions confined to nose and precipitated by heavy sunlight exposure. Begins in poorly pigmented skin at junction of nasal planum and bridge of the nose. Negative for direct immunofluorescence (DIF). • **DLE** - primarily affects nasal area. Exacerbated by sunlight. Positive DIF at basement membrane zone. Biopsy - interface dermatitis. • **SLE** - multisystemic disease. Skin lesions often involve nose, face, mucocutaneous junctions. Multifocal or generalized. ANA positive. Positive DIF at basement membrane zone. • **PF** - lesions usually start on face and ears, commonly involve foot pads and eventually generalize. Biopsy - subcorneal pustules with acantholysis. Positive DIF in intercellular spaces of epidermis. • **PE** - lesions primarily confined to face and ears. Biopsy - intraepidermal pustules with acantholysis. Positive DIF at basement membrane zone and intercellular spaces • **Nasal pyoderma** - acute onset of folliculitis on haired portion of nose • **Dermatophytosis** - haired portion of the nose. Diagnose with culture or biopsy. • **Demodicosis** - often starts on face or forelimbs and may generalize. Diagnose with skin scraping. • **Plastic (or rubber) dish dermatitis** - depigmentation and erythema of anterior nasal planum and anterior lips. No ulceration or crusting. History of exposure. • **Dermatomyositis** - typical breed. Nasal, facial, and extremity lesions characterized by erosion, alopecia, scarring, and hyperpigmentation. Polymyositis or megaesophagus may be present. Biopsy - interface dermatitis with follicular atrophy. DIF Negative. • **Zinc responsive dermatosis** - typical signalment or diet (i.e., high fiber or calcium supplementation). Crusted lesions on face, mucocutaneous junctions, pressure points, foot pads. Biopsy - parakeratotic hyperkeratosis. • **Uveodermatologic syndrome** - typical breed. Uveitis and cutaneous macular depigmentation without inflammation on nose, lips, eyelids. Biopsy of early lesions - interface dermatitis, pigmentary incontinence. • **Vitiligo** - Cutaneus macular depigmentation without inflammation on nose, lips, eyelids, foot pads, and nails. Leukotrichia may be present with leukoderma. • **Nasal depigmentation** - normal black coloration of nasal planum fades to light brown or whitish color. May be seasonal, or wax and wane. • **Idiopathic nasal hyperkeratosis** - dry, horny growths of keratin localized to nasal planum. • **Other diseases** - differentiate with history or biopsy.

CBC/BIOCHEMISTRY/URINALYSIS
• Hemogram, serum chemistry profile and urinalysis are usually normal. • SLE - may see hemolytic anemia, thrombocytopenia or evidence of glomerulonephritis (elevated BUN, proteinuria).

OTHER LABORATORY TESTS N/A

IMAGING N/A

OTHER DIAGNOSTIC PROCEDURES
• Skin scraping for Demodex • Cytology for fungal organisms, bacteria or acantholytic cells (pemphigus) • DTM for dermatophytosis • Culture on Sabouraud's for other fungal infections • Bacterial culture and sensitivity or cytologic evaluation for pyoderma • Joint tap - evidence of polyarthritis in SLE • ANA - positive in most cases of SLE • Ocular examination - uveitis in uveodermatologic syndrome • ECG - Evidence of myocarditis in SLE • EMG - Evidence of polymyositis in SLE and dermatomyositis • DIF - deposition of immunoglobulin at the basement membrane zone in DLE, SLE and PE and intercellular spaces of epidermis in PF and PE. • Skin biopsy

IMAGING N/A

GROSS AND HISTOPATHOLOGIC FINDINGS

Histopathologic Findings
• Folliculitis/furunculosis (± mites, bacteria, or fungal elements) - demodicosis, dermatophytosis, nasal pyoderma. • Follicular atrophy and perifollicular fibrosis - dermatomyositis • Interface dermatitis - DLE, SLE, dermatomyositis, uveodermatologic syndrome • Intraepidermal pustules with acantholysis - PF, PE • Parakeratotic hyperkeratosis - zinc responsive dermatosis • Hypomelanosis - vitiligo, uveodermatologic syndrome • Granulomatous/pyogranulomatous dermatitis - pyoderma, fungal, foreign body, idiopathic sterile granuloma

TREATMENT
• Outpatient except for SLE when severe multi-organ dysfunction is present or for tumors requiring surgical excision or radiation therapy.
• Reduce exposure to sunlight - DLE, SLE, PE, nasal solar dermatitis, squamous cell carcinoma.
• Discourage rooting behavior - pyoderma, dermatophytosis.
• Warm soaks to aid removal of exudate and crusts.
• Replace plastic or rubber dish and avoid contact with topical drug or other agent causing hypersensitivity reaction.

MEDICATIONS

DRUGS AND FLUIDS

Other Fungal Infections
• Systemic antifungals
• Topical enilconazole for aspergillosis
• Surgical excision of early discrete lesions

SLE
Immunosuppressive therapy with prednisolone ± azathioprine (dogs), chlorambucil, or gold salts (cats)

Nasal Solar Dermatitis
• Topical corticosteroids
• Antibiotics for secondary infection
• Sunscreens
• Tattoo hypopigmented skin

NASAL DERMATOSES

Vitiligo/Nasal Depigmentation
No treatment

Tumors
Surgical excision, chemotherapy, or radiation therapy

Idiopathic Sterile Granuloma
• Surgical excision when feasible
• Immunosuppressive therapy with glucocorticoids ± azathioprine

Idiopathic Nasal Hyperkeratosis
Antibiotic-corticosteroid cream for fissures

Other Diseases
See specific disease

CONTRAINDICATIONS
• Avoid crysotherapy in patients with renal disease
• Use azathioprine cautiously in cats - may cause fatal leukopenia or thrombocytopenia.

PRECAUTIONS
• Griseofulvin can cause anorexia, vomiting, diarrhea, and bone marrow suppression. Feed with high fat diet.

• Ketoconazole may cause anorexia, gastric irritation, hepatotoxicity, and lightening of hair coat.

POSSIBLE INTERACTIONS N/A
ALTERNATE DRUGS N/A

FOLLOW-UP

PATIENT MONITORING
Variable with specific disease and treatment prescribed.

POSSIBLE COMPLICATIONS
Scarring with deep infections or overly vigorous cleaning.

MISCELLANEOUS

ASSOCIATED CONDITIONS N/A
AGE RELATED FACTORS N/A

ZOONOTIC POTENTIAL
Dermatophytosis

PREGNANCY
Griseofulvin is teratogenic

SYNONYMS
Uveodermatologic = Vogt-Koyangi-Harada (VKH) syndrome

ABBREVIATIONS
DLE = Discoid lupus erythematosus
SLE = Systemic lupus erythematosus
PF = Pemphigus foliaceus
PE = Pemphigus erythematosus
DIF = Direct immunofluorescence
ANA = Antinuclear antibody
DTM = Dermatophyte test medium

References
Muller GH, Kirk RW, Scott DW. Small animal dermatology. 4th ed. Philadelphia: WB Saunders, 1989.

Author Ellen C. Codner
Consulting Editor Lowell Ackerman

NASAL DISCHARGE (SNEEZING, REVERSE SNEEZING, GAGGING)

BASICS

DEFINITION
• Nasal discharges may be serous, mucoid, mucopurulent, purulent, blood tinged, frank blood (epistaxis), or contain food debris.
• Sneezing is the reflexive expulsion of air through the nasal cavity and is commonly associated with nasal discharge. • Reverse sneezing is the term given to the repetitive, forceful inspiratory efforts elicited after irritation of the caudal-dorsal nasopharynx. • Gagging and retching are involuntary, reflexive attempts to clear secretions from the pharynx or upper respiratory or gastrointestinal tract.

Pathophysiology
• Secretions are produced by mucous cells of the epithelium and glands. Irritation of the nasal mucosa (by mechanical, chemical, or inflammatory stimulation) increases nasal secretion production. • Mucosal irritation and accumulated secretions are a potent stimulus of the sneeze reflex; sneezing may be the first sign of nasal discharge. Sneezing frequency often decreases with chronic disease.
• Reverse sneezing represents irritation of the caudodorsal nasopharynx. • Gagging is a protective reflex elicited by oropharyngeal stimulation, usually functioning to clear material from the oropharynx. Gagging often follows a coughing episode as secretions are brought through the larynx into the oropharynx.
Types of Nasal Discharge and Common Associations
• Serous—mild irritation, viral and parasitic (e.g., nasal mites) disorders • Mucoid—allergic and early neoplastic conditions • Purulent (or mucopurulent)—secondary bacterial and fungal infections • Serosanguinous—destructive processes (primary nasal tumors, aspergillosis in dogs) after violent/paroxysmal sneezing episodes (traumatic capillary rupture) associated with selected systemic diseases (coagulopathy, platelet disorders, hypertension)

Systems Affected
• Respiratory—mucosa of the upper respiratory tract, including the nasal cavities, sinuses, and nasopharynx • Gastrointestinal—these signs also may be observed with extranasal diseases such as swallowing disorders and esophageal or gastrointestinal diseases
• Hemic/lymphatic/immune—systemic diseases may cause in blood tinged nasal discharge or epistaxis due to platelet or primary hemostasis disorders or hypertension

SIGNALMENT
• Young animals—cleft palate, ciliary dyskineasia, immunoglobulin deficiency, nasal polyps • Older animals—nasal tumors, primary dental disease • Hunting dogs—foreign bodies • Dolicocephalic dogs—aspergillosis • Irish wolfhounds—hyperplastic rhinitis
• Nasal aspergillosis and rhinosporidiosis have not been reported in cats. • Male dogs have a higher incidence of nasal fungal infections.

SIGNS

Historical Findings
• Nasal discharge and sneezing are commonly reported as concurrent problems. Information concerning both the initial and present character of the discharge and whether it was originally unilateral or bilateral are important historical findings. • The response to previous antibiotic therapy may be helpful in determining secondary bacterial involvement. Foreign body and dental related disease usually respond initially to antibiotic treatment but commonly relapse days to weeks after treatment; however, nasal tumors and fungal rhinitis typically show little response.

Physical Examination Findings
• Secretions or dried discharge on the hair of the muzzle or front limbs • A reduction in nasal air flow may be noted. • Concurrent dental disease • Bony involvement tumor or fourth premolar abscess may be detected as facial or hard palate swelling or as pain secondary to osteomyelitis with fungal/bacterial infections or tumor invasion.
• Mucosal depigmentation of the nasal cartilages often is observed with chronic nasal discharge, especially with canine nasal aspergillosis. • Physical examination should include regional lymph node palpation, otic examination (for polyps), and a retinal examination (for distemper or cryptococcoccosis-associated chorioretinitis).

CAUSES
Unilateral discharge often is associated with nonsystemic processes:
• Foreign bodies • Dental related disease—abscess, oronasal fistula • Fungal infections (aspergillosis, penicillinosis, cryptococcosis, Sporothrix) • Nasal tumors (adenocarcinoma, squamous cell carcinoma, fibrosarcoma)
Bilateral discharge is most common with:
• Infectious agents—feline viral rhinotracheitis, feline calici virus, canine distemper, and secondary bacterial infection • Airborne irritants • Allergies • Ciliary dyskinesia • IgA deficiency • Lymphoplasmocytictic or hyperplastic rhinitis • Aspergillus and nasal tumors may cause unilateral discharge initially then progress to bilateral discharge as the disease extends through the nasal septum.
Discharge may be unilateral or bilateral with:
• Epistaxis • Foreign body • Nasal parasites • Pneumonyssoides (dogs) • Cuterebra (dogs, cats) • Lingulata (cats) • Capillaria (dogs, cats)

RISK FACTORS
• Dental disease • Exposure to other animals
• Foreign bodies are more common in outdoor animals.
• Infectious causes in poorly vaccinated and kennel situations • Nasal aspergillosis in dogs bedded on straw • Nasal mites in kennel raised dogs • Immunosuppression, chronic corticosteroid use, and FeLV or FIV infection

DIAGNOSIS

DIFFERENTIAL DIAGNOSIS
• Allergic, neoplastic, infectious, inflammatory, and traumatic disorders • Reverse sneezing, occurring on inspiration, must be differentiated from regular sneezing (which occurs on expiration) because it localizes the problem to the caudal dorsal nasopharynx.

CBC/BIOCHEMISTRY/URINALYSIS
Although not specific for any particular cause of nasal discharge, a routine CBC, urinalysis, and chemistry profile are valuable for detecting concurrent problems and as part of a thorough evaluation before general anesthesia for the procedures listed below.

OTHER LABORATORY TESTS
• Serology—aspergillosis and cryptococcosis • Coagulation studies; platelet number and function • Immunoglobulin quantification (IgG, IgM and IgA)—IgA deficiency

IMAGING

Radiography
• Radiography of the nasal cavities can be helpful in cases with nasal discharge. Because of difficulties with overlying structures, the patient should be anesthetized and carefully positioned. • Skull radiography should be performed before rhinoscopy and periodontal probing because these diagnostic tests may lead to nasal bleeding and alter the radiographic density in the nasal cavity • The lateral view is useful in detecting any periosteal reaction over the nasal bone, for gross changes in the maxillary teeth, nasal cavity, and frontal sinus (without identifying which side is involved), and for evaluating the air column of the nasopharynx. • The open mouth ventro dorsal and the intraoral view (using sheet film) are excellent for evaluating the nasal cavities and turbinates; disease may be localized to the affected side. • The lateral oblique views are best for detecting maxillary teeth abnormalities. • The rostrocaudal view is used to evaluate each frontal sinus (e.g., periosteal reaction, filling). • CT scans have proven helpful in detecting the extent of bony changes associated with nasal tumors and fungal rhinitis.

OTHER DIAGNOSTIC PROCEDURES
• Rhinoscopy is indicated in any case of chronic or recurrent nasal discharge and may be indicated in reverse sneezing and acute epistaxis cases. Anterior and posterior rhinoscopy should be performed. Bleeding disorders may be a contraindication. • Nasal cytology—nonspecific inflammation (nondegenerative PMNs) is most commonly found. Large numbers of eosinophils suggest hypersensitivity or allergic rhinitis; hyphae or microconidia are diagnostic for Aspergillus; yeast bodies for Cryptococcus. Neoplastic cells may be seen. • Cultures are difficult to

NASAL DISCHARGE (SNEEZING, REVERSE SNEEZING, GAGGING)

interpret. Up to 40% of normal dogs may have positive fungal cultures. Heavy bacterial growth of a single organism may be significant. Deep cultures obtained by rhinotomy or deep rhinoscopy are more reliable.
• Biopsy of the nasal cavity is indicated in any animal with chronic nasal discharge and cases in which tissue growth (tumor/granuloma) is suspected. Various techniques may be used, including direct endoscopic biopsy, rigid catheter (the "blind" coring technique), or rhinotomy. Multiple samples are required to ensure adequate representation of the process because necrosis of the leading edge of the process is common. Electron microscopy should be performed when ciliary dyskinesia is suspected. • Periodontal probing of all upper teeth should be part of every evaluation of sneezing and nasal discharge; it should follow rhinoscopy. The normal gingival sulcus is < 4.0 mm in dogs and < 1.0 mm in cats.

TREATMENT

• Outpatient treatment is acceptable except for those requiring surgery.
• Surgery may be indicated in selected animals either for an exploratory rhinotomy or to treat Rhinosporidium, nasal foreign body, or placement of tubes to deliver antifungals.
• Symptomatic treatment and nursing care are important in the treatment of dogs and cats with chronic sneezing and nasal discharge. Patient hydration, nutrition, warmth, and hygiene (keeping nares clean) are important

MEDICATIONS

DRUGS AND FLUIDS

• Nasal secretions clear more easily if the animal is well-hydrated; fluid therapy should be considered if hydration is marginal.
• Decongestants may be used in attempt to dry up nasal secretions (oral ephedrine 10-50 mg total q8-12h, maximum of 4 mg/kg [dog] or 2-4 mg/kg q8-12h [cat]; and topical vasoconstrictors, neosynephrine 0.25-0.5% q8-24h or oxymetazoline 0.25% q24h).
• Antibiotics for secondary bacterial infection—to treat culture results, choices include

amoxicillin, Clavamox, clindamycin, and one of the cephalosporins. Tetracyclines are actively secreted into the gingival sulcus and may be used in chronic rhinitis secondary to dental disease.
• There are no drugs that palliatively decrease the frequency of sneezing.
Therapy for specific causes of sneezing and nasal discharge include:
• Dental associated rhinitis—dental work (extractions, gingivectomy, flap closure for fistulas) and antibiotics
• Foreign body—removal and antibiotics
• Nasal parasites—ivermectin 2-300 mg/kg PO weekly for 2-3 weeks to treat Pneumonyssoides; fenbendazole 50 mg/kg q6h for 10 days for Capillaria
• Allergic—prednisolone 1-2 mg/kg PO q6h
• Fungal rhinitis—antifungals (e.g., enilconazole [10 mg/kg q12h in nasal flush; experimental drug in United States] or itraconazole [5-10 mg/kg PO q12-24h]); surgical curretage in selected cases
• Neoplasia—radiation, chemotherapy

CONTRAINDICATIONS

• Ephedrine in cardiac patients • Ivermectin in collies

PRECAUTIONS

• Anorexia, nausea, vomiting, and high liver enzymes (ALT) are commonly noted with ketoconazole, but are reversible when the drug is discontinued. • A rebound phenomenon has been reported with overuse of topical nasal vasoconstrictors.

POSSIBLE INTERACTIONS N/A

ALTERNATE DRUGS

Fungal rhinitis—enilconazole (experimental), ketoconazole, itraconazole, fluconazole, Amphotericin B (caution in cats)

FOLLOW-UP

PATIENT MONITORING

Observe nasal discharge and sneezing; note changes in frequency, volume, and character. Surgically placed nasal tubes require inpatient monitoring; watch for SQ emphysema, local cellulitis.

POSSIBLE COMPLICATIONS

Problems relate to loss of appetite (especially in cats); extension of primary disease (fungal, tumor) into mouth, eye, or brain; dyspnea as a result of nasal obstruction.

MISCELLANEOUS

ASSOCIATED CONDITIONS

Sinusitis • Dental disease • Secondary causes of nasal discharge—coagulopathy, pneumonia, cricopharyngeal disease, megaesophagus
• Cats—immunosuppression from FeLV or FIV; fungal disease (cryptococcosis, Sporothrix); upper respiratory infections

ZOONOTIC POTENTIAL

Sporothrix

PREGNANCY

The safety of most of the drugs recommended for the treatment of sneezing and nasal discharge has not been established in pregnant animals.

SYNONYMS N/A

SEE ALSO

• Epistaxis • Rhinitis • Cilialry Dyskinesia
• Nasal Polyps • Nasopharyngeal Stenosis

ABBREVIATION

References

McKiernan BC. Sneezing and nasal discharge. In: Ettinger SJ, Feldman EC, eds. Textbook of veterinary internal medicine. 4th ed. Philadelphia: WB Saunders, 1994:79-85.

Ogilvie GK, LaRue SM. Canine and feline nasal and paranasal sinus tumors. Vet Clin North Am 1992;22:1133-1144.

Van Pelt DR, Lappin MR. Pathogenesis and treatment of feline rhinitis. Vet Clin North Am 1994;24:807-823.

Van Pelt DR, McKiernan BC. Pathogenesis and treatment of canine rhinitis. Vet Clin North Am 1994;24:789-806.

Author Brendan C. McKiernan
Consulting Editors Lynelle Johnson and Bradley L. Moses

NECK AND BACK PAIN

BASICS

DEFINITION
Discomfort along the spinal column

Pathophysiology
Pain may originate in the epaxial muscle, vertebrae and associated structures, spinal nerves, or meninges.

Systems Affected
• Nervous • Musculoskeletal

SIGNALMENT
• Disk disease usually develops in animals 3-8 years old, but all ages are affected, especially if trauma is involved. • Wobbler syndrome is observed in all large-breed dogs but more often in middle-aged to old Doberman pinschers and young Great Danes. • Atlantoaxial luxation and subluxation occurs in young to middle-aged miniature breeds. • Disk disease is rare in cats.

SIGNS

Historical Findings
Complaints relate to perceived discomfort.

Physical Examination Findings
Head down posture (neck), arched back (neck or back), pain on epaxial palpation, guarded posture, reluctance to walk, epaxial muscle rigidity, palpable heat in the epaxial musculature, and fever (primarily in patients with meningeal involvement)

CAUSES

Epaxial Muscle
Traumatic myositis; exertional rhabdomyolysis; muscle neoplasia (e.g., rhabdomyosarcoma); inflammatory myositis (i.e., parasitic, bacterial, protozoal, or immune-mediated); foreign body myositis (e.g., grass awn migration)

Vertebrae and Associated Structures
Disk disease; osteoarthritis of facets; unstable vertebral anomalies (e.g., hemivertebrae and atlantoaxial luxation or subluxation); vertebral neoplasia (e.g., osteosarcoma, chondrosarcoma, multiple myeloma, and metastatic tumors); diskospondylitis; vertebral osteomyelitis; fracture, luxation, and subluxation; malformation and malarticulation; spondylosis deformans

Spinal Nerves
Entrapment by disk herniation; neoplasia (e.g., neurofibroma and neurofibrosarcoma); traumatic entrapment, tearing, or laceration; neuritis (e.g., viral, bacterial, and parasitic)

Meninges
Meningioma and metastatic neoplasia; meningitis (i.e., bacterial, viral, parasitic, protozoal, rickettsial, immune-mediated, or idiopathic)

RISK FACTORS
• Previous diagnosis of cancer • Highly active animal • Trauma

DIAGNOSIS

DIFFERENTIAL DIAGNOSIS
• Must differentiate from diseases involving thoracic (e.g., pleura, cardiovascular system, and lungs) or abdominal (e.g., kidneys, prostate gland, and intestines) structures in painful patients • Must also rule out limb musculoskeletal pain • Degenerative radiculomyelopathy and fibrocartilaginous myelopathy are nonpainful diseases of the spinal cord. • Neck or back pain in cats is often associated with neoplasia.

CBC/BIOCHEMISTRY/URINALYSIS

Epaxial Muscle
• Creatine kinase can be high in patients with any diseases affecting the muscle. • A high WBC count or myoglobinuria may reflect the etiologic agent and extent of damage.

Vertebrae and Associated Structures
• Results usually are normal in patients with degenerative, anomalous, and neoplastic disease. • Results of hemogram may be abnormal in patients with inflammatory diseases such as acute diskospondylitis and multisystemic involvement.

Spinal Nerves   Results usually normal

Meninges
• Results usually normal, even in patients with severe meningitis • Leucocytosis in some patients with aseptic meningitis

OTHER LABORATORY TESTS

Epaxial Muscle   N/A

Vertebrae and Associated Structures
• Bence Jones protein in the urine of some animals with multiple myeloma • Bone marrow examination may reveal neoplastic cells in patients with multiple myeloma.

Spinal Nerves   N/A

Meninges
• Specific serologic tests, depending on suspected cause (e.g., canine distemper, Rocky Mountain spotted fever, and toxoplasmosis) • Serum IgA is often high in patients with aseptic meningitis.

IMAGING

Epaxial Muscle
• Only applicable in patients with suspected neoplasia or foreign body • Thoracic radiography to detect metastasis

Vertebrae and Associated Structures
• Survey radiography—thoracic to detect metastasis; spinal to detect obvious bony abnormalities such as fracture or luxation, diskospondylitis, neoplasia, osteoarthritis, and extruded calcified disk • Myelography delineates extradural (e.g., disk herniation), intradural-extramedullary (e.g., meningioma) and intramedullary (e.g., spinal neoplasia) lesions. • Discography is best used at the lum-

bosacral junction to identify stenosis and disk herniation. • CT provides cross-sectional and other special views to more clearly define a bony lesion. • MRI provides cross-sectional and other special views to more clearly define a soft tissue lesion.

Spinal Nerves
• Survey radiograph seldom of benefit • Myelography seldom of benefit unless the lesion is pressing or invading the meninges • MRI scanning is the most rewarding imaging technique to identify the location and extent of the lesion.

Meninges
• Myelography can identify neoplastic involvement such as meningioma. • MRI more clearly defines a soft tissue lesion.

OTHER DIAGNOSTIC PROCEDURES

Epaxial Muscle
• Muscle biopsy may reveal neoplastic or inflammatory cells. • Electromyelography (EMG) may identify an irritative or denervative process affecting the muscles.

Vertebrae and Associated Structures
Bone biopsy helps confirm vertebral neoplasia and infection.

Spinal Nerves
Electrodiagnostic testing (e.g., EMG, nerve conduction velocity, and F waves) helps differentiate and confirm muscle versus nerve disease and location of the lesion.

Meninges
CSF analysis is the diagnostic test of choice, including measurement of immunoglobulins, serologic testing, and bacterial culture.

TREATMENT
• Treatment varies widely according to the nature and extent of the tissues involved.
• Symptomatic treatment without first establishing a diagnosis can be dangerous.
• Depending on severity of disease, medical treatment may be provided in or out of the hospital.
• Patients requiring surgical intervention are treated as inpatients.
• Surgical treatment may be indicated in patients with disk herniation, trauma, anomalies, and neoplasia.
• A foreign body may require surgical intervention for removal or drainage to treat an associated abscess.

MEDICATIONS

DRUGS AND FLUIDS

Epaxial Muscle
• Patients with inflammation may require antimicrobial therapy, depending on the causative agent.
• Glucocorticosteroids may be required, depending on the diagnosis.

• Patients with neoplasia may require chemotherapy or radiotherapy, depending on tumor type.

Vertebrae and Associated Structures
• Glucocorticosteroids are indicated in some patients and contraindicated in others. Therefore, a diagnosis should be established if at all possible before initiating steroids.
• Antimicrobials are indicated in patients in which a specific organism can be identified or is suspected, as in patients with diskospondylitis.
• Chemotherapy and radiotherapy may or may not be warranted, depending on the tumor type.

Spinal Nerves
Corticosteroids are useful in patients with trauma, inflammation, and nerve compression and in a few with neoplasia.

Meninges
• Antimicrobials that cross the blood-brain barrier should be chosen when delivery to the CNS is desired.
• Corticosteroids may or may not be indicated; a diagnosis should be established if at all possible before initiating.

CONTRAINDICATIONS
Glucocorticosteroids can be detrimental in patients with many inflammatory conditions and in those with gastroenteritis or cystitis.

PRECAUTIONS
• Look for signs of gastroenteritis or cystitis before initiating and while administering glucocorticosteroids.
• In patients with instability or possible disk disease, cage rest should accompany the use of drugs with analgesic effects to prevent exacerbation of the primary problem and further neurologic damage.

• Do not use steroids and nonsteroidal antiinflammatory drugs (NSAIDs) in combination; life-threatening gastroenteritis may result.

POSSIBLE INTERACTIONS N/A

ALTERNATE DRUGS
• NSAIDs
• Polysulfated glycosaminoglycan
• Methocarbamol for muscle relaxation
• Benzodiazepines such as diazepam for muscle relaxation and antianxiety effects
• Phenylbutazone may alleviate musculoskeletal pain but is ineffective against neurologic pain.

FOLLOW-UP

PATIENT MONITORING
• Response to treatment should be monitored closely and adjustments made as necessary.
• Owners should be instructed to watch for signs of gastroenteritis and cystitis.

POSSIBLE COMPLICATIONS

Epaxial Muscle
Abscess, chronic pain, and fibrous replacement of muscle fibers causing chronic pain and immobility

Vertebrae and Associated Structures
• Frequent recurrence in patients with disk disease that receive medical management only
• Permanent paralysis or dysfunction • Urinary and fecal incontinence • Chronic pain • Spread to adjacent tissues

Spinal Nerves
• Permanent paralysis or dysfunction • Chronic pain

Meninges
• Death • Involvement of surrounding spinal cord and brain tissue

MISCELLANEOUS

ASSOCIATED CONDITIONS
• Cardiac muscle disease (patients with myositis) • Sites of infection in other tissues as a source of CNS or vertebral involvement (e.g., bacterial endocarditis or cystitis as a cause of diskospondylitis) • Metastatic disease from a primary tumor in another organ system • Immunologic incompetence

AGE RELATED FACTORS
• Anomalous conditions usually seen in younger animals • Disk disease most frequently seen in active, middle-aged dogs
• Neoplastic conditions more often seen in middle- to old-aged animals

ZOONOTIC POTENTIAL N/A

PREGNANCY
Use of glucocorticosteroids is contraindicated.

SYNONYMS N/A

SEE ALSO See causes.

ABBREVIATIONS
CNS = central nervous system
CSF = cerebrospinal fluid
EMG = electromyelography
MRI = magnetic resonance imaging
NSAID = nonsteroidal antiinflammatory drug

Reference
Aron DM. Pain. In: Lorenz MD, Cornelius LM, ed. Small animal medical diagnosis. Philadelphia: JB Lippincott, 1987;411-424.
Author Patricia J. Luttgen
Consulting Editor Joane M. Parent

NEONATAL MORTALITY (FADING SYNDROME)

 BASICS

DEFINITION

For the purposes of this topic, the neonatal period will be designated to extend from birth to 2 weeks of age.

Pathophysiology

The neonate's inadequate thermoregulatory mechanisms, immunologic responses, and lack of tight glycemic control allows greater susceptibility to a number of insults that are usually combinations of environmental, infectious, nutritional, and metabolic factors. Hypothermia, hypoglycemia, dehydration, and hypoxia/anoxia are common preludes to neonatal death.

SIGNALMENT

Pedigree animals are more prone to hereditary defects.

SIGNS

General Comments

• Expected preweaning losses range from 10-30%, with about 65% of those losses occurring during the first week (about half of which are stillbirths). Losses in excess of this in a cattery or kennel should be considered abnormal • Because of the limited number of ways neonates can respond to illness, the historical and physical exam findings rarely narrow the differential diagnosis.

Historical Findings

• Low birth weight, loss of weight, and/or failure to gain weight • Decreased activity and appetite • Decreased muscle tone • Constantly vocal or restless early, quiet and inactive later • Tendency to remain separate from the dam and the rest of the litter

Physical Examination Findings

Signs are often nonspecific. Weakness, hypothermia (normal newborn temperature is about 96° F, rising to about 100° F during the first week), hypoglycemia, and dehydration are common and interrelated findings. Respiratory distress, enteric disease, or hemoglobinuria may be present. Gross anatomic defects may be detectable.

CAUSES

Noninfectious causes—more important during the neonatal and early nursing period: • Dam-related causes—dystocia or prolonged labor, cannibalism, lactation disorder, trauma, inattention or overattention, inadequate nutrition, including taurine deficiency in cats • Environmental causes—any factors that discourage nursing and allow hypothermia, including extremes of temperature and humidity, inadequate sanitation, overcrowding, and stress • Nutritional causes—inadequate or ineffective nursing, hypoglycemia, hypothermia-induced digestive malfunction • Birth defects—gross anatomic defects seen more frequently in cats (about 10% of nonsurviv-

ing neonates) than dogs. Examples include gastrointestinal abnormalities such as cleft palate; segmental intestinal agenesis or atresia; craniofacial abnormalities; failure of midline closure, causing herniation; various cardiac defects, including valve disorders, VSD, and AV fistula; and respiratory system defects such as thoracic wall abnormalities and pectus excavatum. Microanatomic defects such as primary ciliary dyskinesia and surfactant deficiency. Inborn errors of metabolism (usually autosomal recessive traits). • Neonatal isoerythrolysis (NI)—blood type-B queen with type-A kitten • **Infectious causes**—more important during late nursing/early weaning period: • Viral infections (cats)—feline calicivirus, feline leukemia virus, feline herpesvirus type 1, feline panleukopenia virus • Viral infections(dogs)—canine adenovirus type 1, canine distemper virus, canine herpesvirus • Bacterial infections—acquired mainly across the placenta, in the birth canal, via the umbilicus, gastrointestinal tract, respiratory tract, urinary tract, or skin wounds • Neonatal sepsis primarily from Escherichia coli, beta-hemolytic streptococcus, coagulase-positive staphylococcus, and gram-negative enteric organisms • Respiratory infections, including Bordetella bronchiseptica and Pasteurella • Enteric infections, including E. coli, Salmonella, and Campylobacter • Brucella canis infections in dogs • Parasitic infections—heavy infection with helminths T. canis, T. cati, Toxascaris leonina, Ancylostoma caninum, or Ancylostoma tubaeforme; coccidian parasites, including Toxoplasma, Isospora, Cryptosporidium, Giardia

RISK FACTORS

• Subnormal birth weight or failure to grow normally. Kittens—minimum daily gain of 7-10 g. Puppies—should double in weight by 10-12 days. Both species—5-10% gain/day is generally acceptable • Dystocia or prolonged labor • Inbreeding causes higher incidence of recessive traits • First to second litter have heavier parasite burden • Kitten with blood type-A sire and type-B queen

 DIAGNOSIS

DIFFERENTIAL DIAGNOSIS

Consideration must be given to the individual sick neonate and the cattery/kennel in which neonatal losses are high. Excessive losses are often a result of a combination of environmental, immunological, nutritional, infectious, and metabolic factors. Detection and correction of problems in each area is necessary to prevent ongoing losses.

CBC/BIOCHEMISTRY/URINALYSIS

Premortem blood samples from affected individuals are usually not obtainable and are rarely pathognomonic.

CBC

• Concurrent dehydration may influence results. • Mild normocytic, normochromic anemia • White cell counts variable. May see thrombocytopenia and mild to moderate neutrophilia (often with left shift) if septic.

Serum Chemistry

• Hypoglycemia or normoglycemia • Other changes dependent on organ system involved

Urinalysis

Hemoglobinuria if NI, bacteria if infection. Urine SG > 1.017 suggests inadequate hydration.

OTHER LABORATORY TESTS

FeLV antigen test

IMAGING N/A

OTHER DIAGNOSTIC PROCEDURES

• Histopathologic examination of multiple tissues harvested at necropsy • Metabolic screening of urine sample to rule out inborn errors of metabolism • Virus isolation • Bacterial culture • Blood typing in pedigree cats

GROSS AND HISTOPATHOLOGICAL FINDINGS

Postmortem examination of a nonsurvivor is extremely important. Examination as soon after death is advisable to minimize autolysis. Special notice given to the following: • A stomach devoid of contents implies lack of nursing. Dam related causes such as inappropriate behavior or lactation must be considered as should neonatal problems such as weakness, trauma, or a physiologic abnormality. A stomach filled with milk suggests sudden death (e.g., trauma, peracute illness) or GI dysfunction (body temperature < 94° F) • A thymus of subnormal size is not pathognomonic and can be a result of multiple causes, including infection, nutrition, and immunology. Petechiation is common. If accompanied by hemorrhage in other organ systems, it suggests coagulopathy or septicemia • Urine in the bladder implies either a degree of renal dysfunction or inadequate care by the dam • Lungs of the normal neonate appear the same as adult lungs. A homogeneous dark red color is typical of a stillborn animal that has not taken a breath. Hemorrhage, edema, congestion, and mottled color are abnormal but nonspecific findings. • Malformations should be noted. • Multiple tissue samples should be submitted to a diagnostic lab for virus isolation, bacterial culture and sensitivity, and histopathologic examination. The lab should be queried on proper submission of specimens.

 TREATMENT

• Correct any underlying deficiencies in husbandry or breeding selection.

• Slowly warm neonate to 97-98° F over several hours if necessary. Provide ambient temperature of 85-95° F with relative humidity of 55-65%. If necessary, supplement with oxygen at 30-40%.
• Do not attempt to feed if body temperature < 94° F. Once warmed, encourage nursing.
• If NI, disallow nursing for first 24 hours after birth.

MEDICATIONS

DRUGS AND FLUIDS

• Consider intravenous administration of warmed isotonic dextrose if hypoglycemic.
• Administer warm LRS or half-strength LRS and D2.5W subcutaneously or intraperitoneally at rate of 1.0 ml/30g body weight. May follow with 5-10% glucose solution via nurser bottle or stomach tube at rate of 0.25 ml/30g body weight.
• Antibiotic choice ideally should be based on culture sensitivity results. Antibiotics commonly used are the penicillins (penicillin G, ampicillin, amoxicillin with or without clavulanic acid) and first generation cephalosporins. Standard adult dose can be used, but lengthened dosage interval may be desirable. The macrolides (erythromycin and tylosin) and the lincosamides (clindamycin and lincomycin) also appear to be safe at adult dosages, but specific dosage guidelines for neonates are lacking.
• Supplement with milk replacer.
• Vitamin K at 0.01-0.1 mg SC or IM

• Prophylactic use of antibiotics is controversial, but low birthweight or colostrum-deprived kittens may benefit from their use.

CONTRAINDICATIONS

Aminoglycosides, tetracyclines, trimethoprim/sulfa, and chloramphenicol should be avoided in the neonate.

PRECAUTIONS

Drug absorption, distribution, metabolism, and excretion in neonates differ significantly from adults. Marginal organ function, dehydration, and other factors further complicate drug therapy and increase the likelihood of adverse reactions.

POSSIBLE INTERACTIONS N/A

ALTERNATE DRUGS N/A

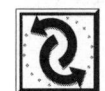

FOLLOW-UP

PATIENT MONITORING

• Body weight should be monitored at least weekly in normal neonates and every 24-48 hours in those that have subnormal weights and/or are failing to thrive. • Make sure nursing and care by dam is adequate. Supplemental feeding of milk replacer if necessary.

POSSIBLE COMPLICATION N/A

MISCELLANEOUS

ASSOCIATED CONDITIONS N/A

AGE RELATED FACTORS N/A

ZOONOTIC POTENTIAL N/A

PREGNANCY N/A

SYNONYMS

Fading or wasting syndrome

SEE ALSO

See causes.

ABBREVIATION

FELV = feline leukemia virus
NI = neonatal isoerythrolysis

References

Jones RL. Special considerations for appropriate antimicrobial therapy in neonates. Vet Clin North Am Small Anim Pract 1987;17:577-602.

Hoskins JD. Clinical evaluation of the kitten: from birth to eight weeks of age. Compend Cont Ed Pract Vet 1990;12:1215-1225.

Lawler DF. Care and diseases of neonatal puppies and kittens. In: Kirk RW, Bonagura JD, eds. Current veterinary therapy X. Philadelphia: WB Saunders, 1989.

Lawler DF. Investigating kitten deaths in catteries. In: August JR, ed. Consultations in feline internal medicine. Philadelphia: WB Saunders, 1991.

Author James R. Richards
Consulting Editor Fred W. Scott

OBESITY

BASICS

DEFINITION
The presence of body fat in sufficient excess to compromise normal physiological function, or predispose to metabolic, surgical and/or mechanical problems. Obesity is a body weight greater than 40% above "optimum" (moderate) body weight

Pathophysiology
• Animal factors: inactivity is an important risk factor in both dogs and cats, as is increasing age and neutering. Breed and sex are also predisposing factors (see Signalment). • Diet factors: no specific diet other than a surfeit of "table scraps" and ``treats'' has been identified to increase risk in dogs. In cats, consumption of high fat diets reportedly increases risk. • Feeding management: many animals are overfed. Reasons for excessive food consumption include: ignorance of proper feeding practices, inappropriately generous feeding recommendations by manufacturers, emphasis on food palatability both by owners and manufacturers, and inadequate explanation of appropriate body condition and how to maintain it by veterinarians. • Owner factors: Many owners of overweight pets are overweight themselves, and engage in feeding as a social activity. Clients also may consider their pet to be "one of the family" and be unwilling to deprive a loved one of food. These factors often are the primary source of failure of simple-minded "eat less and exercise more" approaches to management of obesity. They must be identified and acknowledged by both the client and therapist for long term resolution of obesity to succeed.

Systems Affected
• Cardiovascular (Dogs) • Musculoskeletal (Dogs)—articular and locomotor problems, including developmental orthopedic disease in growing dogs. • Hepatobiliary (Cats)—hepatic lipidosis if food intake ceases is the only documented disease for which obese patients are at increased risk.

SIGNALMENT
Dogs and cats • Breeds predisposed to obesity include the Labrador retriever, cairn terrier, Cocker spaniel, dachshund, Sheltie, basset hound, beagle, King Charles spaniel, collie, and in our practice, Norwegian elkhounds. In cats, mixed breed ancestry increases the risk. • Female dogs and male cats are more likely to be obese.

SIGNS
Excess amounts of body fat for body size, often measured as body condition score of > 4 on a 1–5 scale where 1 = cachectic (>20% underweight), 2 = lean (10–20% underweight), 3 = moderate, 4 = stout (20–40% overweight), 5 = obese (>40% overweight). Sites of adipose tissue to evaluate during physical examination include the rib cage and abdomen. One should be able to feel the ribs easily, and be able to see an abdominal "waist" when viewing the animal either from above or from the side. In cats, excessive inguinal fat often is present.

CAUSES
• Most obesity is caused by excessive access to highly palatable food, usually combined with insufficient activity. • Hypothyroidism • Hyperadrenocorticism (Cushing's disease)

RISK FACTORS
• See Pathophysiology • Owner lifestyle: Two types of owners may be distinguished: "mindless" for whom feeding the animal is an automatic chore, and "timeless," for whom feeding is a significant social and time-filling activity • Diet palatability • Breed (see Signalment) • Activity level

DIAGNOSIS

DIFFERENTIAL DIAGNOSIS
Rule out pregnancy, increased muscle mass, hypothyroidism, and hyperadrenocorticism during history, physical examination and laboratory evaluation. Document body condition score of >4.

CBC/BIOCHEMISTRY/URINALYSIS
Usually normal unless endocrine cause.

OTHER LABORATORY TESTS
Thyroid or adrenal function testing if indicated

IMAGING N/A

DIAGNOSTIC PROCEDURES N/A

TREATMENT
• Successful treatment of obesity is lifelong amelioration of the problem for which treatment was instituted.
• Increase activity level in sedentary animals Prescribe a reduced calorie diet. Changing the diet may assist in psychological re-education of the client with regard to feeding the pet, but diet per se does not cause obesity, and is ancillary to its long term treatment.
• The most important part of obesity therapy is client education, which must be tailored to each particular circumstance.
• Mindless - demonstration of appropriate body condition score, explanation that the pet should be fed whatever amount of food is necessary to achieve this condition in this particular animal, and reduction of food availability to achieve the desired body condition often is sufficient.
• Timeless - much more careful investigation of the circumstances, and consideration of the necessity for maintenance of a lower weight, are necessary for this group. Clients must come to desire that the animal maintain a lower weight for demonstrable reasons, and provided the means and support to permit them to achieve and maintain the reduced weight in their pet, while retaining the desired relationship with it. Therapeutic suggestions include: reasonable, functional weight loss goals, rather than recommendations that a poorly defined "optimal adult weight" be achieved for aesthetic reasons. For example, sufficient weight loss to enhance glycemic control of a non-insulin dependent diabetic, or ability to walk for 20 minutes without exhaustion or lameness. Keeping a food record to identify all food sources may help some clients appreciate the actual number of calories consumed by the animal. Suggesting that "snacks" replace regular food rather than supplement it, and that the snacks consist of a portion of the regularly allotted food.

MEDICATIONS

DRUGS AND FLUIDS
Initiate appropriate therapy for any underlying causes such as hypothyroidism or hyperadrenocorticism

CONTRAINDICATIONS N/A
PRECAUTIONS N/A
POSSIBLE INTERACTIONS N/A
ALTERNATE DRUGS N/A

FOLLOW-UP

PATIENT MONITORING
As with any other chronic metabolic problem, lifelong follow-up is essential for maintenance of the reduced weight. When clients express concern at the small amount of food necessary to maintain moderate body condition, increased activity and/or a reduced calorie diet should be recommended before the animal becomes obese.

POSSIBLE COMPLICATIONS
Cardiovascular and orthopedic complications

MISCELLANEOUS

ASSOCIATED CONDITIONS N/A
AGE RELATED FACTORS N/A
ZOONOTIC POTENTIAL N/A
PREGNANCY N/A
SYNONYMS N/A
SEE ALSO
Hypothyroidism, Hyperadrenocorticism

References
Markwell PJ. Clinical studies in the management of obesity in dogs and cats. Int J Obes Relat Metab Disord 1994;18 Suppl:539-543.
Author C.A. Tony Buffington
Consulting Editor Brent D. Jones

OLIGURIA AND ANURIA

BASICS

DEFINITION
Oliguria is the production of an abnormally small amount of urine (urine production rate of < 0.25 ml/kg/hr). Anuria is the formation of essentially no urine (urine production rate of < 0.08 ml/kg/hr).

Pathophysiology
• Physiologic oliguria occurs when the kidneys limit renal water loss during episodes of low renal perfusion to preserve body fluid and electrolyte balance. High plasma osmolality or low effective circulating fluid volume increase antidiuretic hormone (ADH) synthesis and release. ADH acts on the kidneys to induce formation of small quantities of concentrated urine (the hallmark of physiologic oliguria).
• Pathologic oliguria results from severe renal parenchymal impairment. Factors include (1) high resistance in afferent glomerular vessels, (2) low glomerular permeability, (3) excessive leakage ("back leak") of filtrate from damaged renal tubules, (4) intratubular obstruction, and (5) extensive loss of nephrons resulting in marked reduction in the quantity of glomerular filtrate produced.
• Anuria may be of renal or postrenal origin. Severe renal disease occasionally causes anuria. Mechanisms are the same as for pathologic oliguria. Anuria usually results from postrenal causes (e.g., obstruction of urine flow or rupture of the excretory pathway).

Systems affected
Renal/urologic

SIGNALMENT Dogs and cats

SIGNS N/A

CAUSES
• Physiologic oliguria—renal hypoperfusion (caused by low blood volume or hypotension) or hypertonicity (usually caused by hypernatremia)
• Pathologic oliguria—oliguric acute renal failure or end-stage chronic renal failure
• Anuria—complete urinary tract obstruction, rupture of the urinary excretory pathway, or severe, primary renal failure

RISK FACTORS
• Physiologic oliguria—dehydration, low cardiac output, and hypotension
• Pathologic oliguria and anuria caused by primary renal failure (risk factors for acute renal failure)—preexisting renal disease, exposure to nephrotoxins, dehydration, low cardiac output, hypotension, electrolyte imbalance, acidosis, advanced age, fever, sepsis, liver disease, multiple organ failure, trauma, diabetes mellitus, hypoalbuminemia, and hyperviscosity syndrome
• Anuria—urolithiasis, urinary tract neoplasia, idiopathic feline lower urinary tract disease (obstruction), micturition disorder, and trauma

DIAGNOSIS

DIFFERENTIAL DIAGNOSIS
• Physiologic oliguria is suggested by signs of poor tissue perfusion (e.g., dehydration, slow capillary refill time, pale mucous membranes, weak pulse, rapid or irregular pulse, and cool extremities). Patient may have a history of recent fluid loss (vomiting, diarrhea, polyuria, hemorrhage). Signs of uremia are typically absent and oliguria resolves rapidly when renal hypoperfusion is corrected.
• Pathologic oliguria and renal anuria is suspected in patients with any of the risk factors given. The greater the number of these risk factors, the more likely the patient has or will develop acute renal failure. Patients with pathologic oliguria caused by chronic renal failure typically have a history of progressive renal disease (including long-standing polyuria, polydipsia, poor appetite, and weight loss). Patients with chronic renal failure are at risk of developing acute renal failure. Signs of uremia are commonly observed and fluid therapy and other measures designed to restore adequate renal perfusion often fail to increase urine flow.
• Anuria caused by urinary obstruction or rupture of the excretory pathway is suspected in patients that repeatedly strain to void but are unable to produce urine flow. They may have a previous history of pollakiuria, dysuria, stranguria, hematuria, urolithiasis, trauma, or instrumentation of the urinary tract. In patients with urinary obstruction, physical examination may reveal a large urinary bladder, painful posterior abdomen, and mass or uroliths in the urethra or bladder. Physical examination of patients with rupture of the urinary tract reveals ascites, fluid infiltration in tissues around the urinary tract, painful caudal abdomen, mass or uroliths in the bladder or urethra, or evidence of trauma (e.g., pelvic fracture). Urinary obstruction caused by disorder of micturition may be suspected in patients with a large urinary bladder, high resistance to manual expression of the bladder, and neurologic signs affecting the hind limbs or tail. Signs of uremia may develop. Restoration of urine flow or correcting rents in the excretory pathway rapidly restores adequate urine flow.

CBC/BIOCHEMISTRY/URINALYSIS
• Serum urea nitrogen and creatinine concentrations are typically high unless the onset of oliguria or anuria is very recent.
• Hyperkalemia is common in animals with pathologic oliguria and anuria, less common and less severe in animals with physiologic oliguria (except in those with hypoadrenocorticism).
• Physiologic oliguria is characterized by urine specific gravity values > 1.030 in dogs and > 1.035 in cats. Oliguria associated with

urine specific gravity values below these values suggests primary renal failure. Patients with urine concentrating defects from other diseases or drugs are the exception to this rule.
• Renal anuria and anuria resulting from postrenal causes often is characterized by urine specific gravity values < 1.030 (dogs) or 1.035 (cats). Adequate urine concentrating ability often is lost after urinary obstruction, but may persist with rupture of the excretory pathway.

OTHER LABORATORY TESTS N/A

IMAGING
• Abdominal radiographs and ultrasound are useful to rule out urinary obstruction and rupture of the excretory pathway. Distension of any portion of the excretory pathway or observation of uroliths within the excretory pathway suggests urinary obstruction.
• Detection of fluid within the peritoneal cavity or adjacent to the urinary tract supports a diagnosis of rupture of the excretory pathway.
• Excretory urography, retrograde urethrocystography, and vaginourethrocystography may provide definitive proof of urinary obstruction or rupture of the excretory pathway.

OTHER DIAGNOSTIC PROCEDURES
• Electrocardiography may be used to quickly establish whether patient has clinically important hyperkalemia. Hyperkalemic cardiotoxicity is characterized (in order of progressing hyperkalemia) by: tall, peaked T waves with a narrow base; prolongation of the P-R interval and QRS complex; decreased amplitude and increased width of P waves; bradycardia; atrial standstill; QRS-T fusion causing a wide-complex, idioventricular rhythm; ventricular fibrillation or asystole.
• Urethrocystoscopy may provide evidence of obstruction or rupture of the urinary tract.
• Placing a urinary catheter may provide information concerning the integrity of the lower urinary tract, but this approach is not recommended as a diagnostic procedure because it may be misleading, it may induce additional trauma to the urinary tract, and it may introduce bacteria.

TREATMENT
• Oliguria and anuria are medical emergencies. If untreated, they may lead to death within hours to days. Death typically results from uremia, hyperkalemia, or sepsis (in patients with urinary tract infection).
• Persistent renal hypoperfusion may lead to acute ischemic renal injury and therefore must be rapidly corrected.
• Treatment for primary renal oliguria and anuria is usually limited to symptomatic and supportive care, designed to allow the patient to survive long enough for some recovery of renal function to occur spontaneously.

Elimination of etiologic factors may slow or stop further renal injury (eg, terminating aminoglycoside administration, correcting hypercalcemia, and restoring adequate renal perfusion). However, once oliguria or anuria have developed, few if any renal diseases will be amenable to specific treatment.

• Postrenal causes for anuria may be corrected by nonsurgical or surgical methods. Nonsurgical methods include hydropropulsion of uroliths or urethral plugs or placement of urinary catheters to restore low-pressure urine flow. Surgical methods include removal of uroliths, polyps, or neoplastic tissue and surgical correction of rents, strictures, or malposition of the excretory pathway.

MEDICATIONS

DRUGS AND FLUIDS

• Renal hypoperfusion should be corrected by intravenous administration of normal saline or lactated Ringer's solution. In selected animals, other fluids may be more appropriate (eg, blood to correct hypoperfusion resulting from hemorrhage).

• In patients with renal oliguria, diuretics are usually indicted after correcting renal hypoperfusion. However, diuretics may not improve renal function, and diuretic-induced increase in urine flow rate does not necessarily indicate improved renal function. Nonetheless, diuretics are indicated because converting oliguria to nonoliguria facilitates managing the patient by fluid and electrolyte administration. Increase in urine flow after diuretic administration suggests a more favorable prognosis.

• Furosemide (2 mg/kg IV q8h) is often used initially in patients with oliguric acute renal failure. Urine flow should increase within 1 hour. If diuresis does not ensue within an hour, dosage may be increased to 4 to 6 mg/kg/IV. Infusion of mannitol or infusion of dopamine with furosemide appears to be more effective than furosemide alone.

• Dopamine (1 to 5 µg/kg/minute) is generally administered concurrently with furosemide. Diuresis should ensue within 1 to 2 hours. If urine flow does not increase within 2 hours, discontinue dopamine.

• Mannitol (0.5 to 1.0 gm/kg/IV) can be given as a 10 or 20% solution over 15 to 20 minutes. Urine flow should increase within 1 hour. Administration of mannitol should not be repeated if diuresis does not ensue because it may cause excessive volume expansion.

• A safer but possibly less effective alternative to mannitol is infusion of 10-20% dextrose solution (25 to 50 ml/kg/IV q8h-q12h) over 1-2 hours. Because dextrose is metabolized, the potential for volume expansion is minimized.

CONTRAINDICATIONS

Nephrotoxic Drugs
Precautions

• Administer fluids judiciously to patients that are persistently oliguric or anuric to avoid overhydration. In patients with unresponsive renal oliguria, peritoneal dialysis or hemodialysis may be the only means of correcting severe volume over expansion.

• Correct fluid deficits before initiating diuretic administration. Otherwise, renal hypoperfusion and ischemic renal injury may be exacerbated.

• Drugs requiring renal excretion should be used with caution. If resolution of oliguria or anuria can reasonably be expected within minutes to a few hours (eg, physiologic oliguria and anuria caused by urinary obstruction), standard dosages of drugs requiring renal excretion can be used.

• Avoid electrolyte solutions containing more than 4 mEq/L of potassium in most animals.

• Dopamine can cause cardiac arrhythmias, particularly in animals with hyperkalemia. ECG monitoring is recommended when high dosages are used and in animals with hyperkalemia.

POSSIBLE INTERACTIONS
Furosemide may promote the nephrotoxicity associated with aminoglycoside antibiotics.

ALTERNATE DRUGS
Mannitol can be used in preference to furosemide in patients with aminoglycoside-induced, oliguric acute renal failure.

FOLLOW-UP

PATIENT MONITORING

• Urine flow rate: Urinary catheterization may be necessary for accurate determination of urine volume. However, urinary catheterization can induce bacterial urinary tract infection, an important cause of morbidity and mortality in patients with acute renal failure. Catheters must be placed by aseptic technique. Intermittent catheterization is less likely to cause urinary tract infection than an indwelling catheter. The shorter the interval that a catheter is left indwelling, the lower the risk of urinary tract infection. Indwelling catheters should be attached to a closed, sterile, urinary drainage system.

• Creatinine, serum urea nitrogen and potassium concentrations after 12 to 24 hours. More frequent monitoring of serum potassium concentration may be indicated in animals with severe hyperkalemia.

• ECG monitoring to assess cardiac effects of dopamine, hyperkalemia, and response to treatment.

POSSIBLE COMPLICATIONS

• Hyperkalemia and associated cardiotoxicity
• Uremia leading to death
• Dehydration caused by vomiting, diarrhea, and respiratory losses
• Overhydration caused by excessive fluid intake or administration leading to pulmonary edema
• Bacterial urinary tract infection

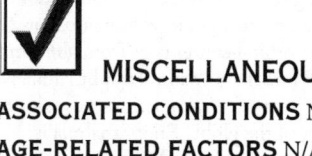

MISCELLANEOUS

ASSOCIATED CONDITIONS N/A

AGE-RELATED FACTORS N/A

ZOONOTIC POTENTIAL N/A

PREGNANCY N/A

SYNONYMS N/A

SEE ALSO

• Creatinine and Blood Urea Nitrogen (BUN)—Azotemia and Uremia
• Hyperkalemia
• Nephrotoxicity, Drug-induced
• Renal failure, Acute and Chronic
• Urinary Tract Obstruction

ABBREVIATIONS
ADH = antidiuretic hormone

References

Grauer GF, Lane IF. Acute renal failure. In: Ettinger SJ, Feldman EC, eds. Textbook of veterinary internal medicine. Philadelphia: WB Saunders, 1995:1720-1733.

DiBartola S. Clinical approach and laboratory evaluation of renal disease. In Textbook of Veterinary Internal Medicine. Ettinger SJ,Feldman EC, editor. Philadelphia, WB Saunders. 1995:1706-1719.

Author David J. Polzin
Consulting Editors Larry Adams and Carl Osborne

ORBITAL DISEASES (EXOPHTHALMUS, ENOPHTHALMUS, STRABISMUS)

BASICS

DEFINITION
Abnormal position of the eye; may take the form of exophthalmos, enophthalmos, or strabismus. Exophthalmos is the anterior displacement of the globe. Enophthalmos is posterior displacement of the globe. Strabismus is a deviation of the globe from the correct position of fixation that the patient cannot correct.

Pathophysiology
The orbit cannot be examined directly, so orbital disease can only be manifested by signs that alter the position, appearance, or function of the globe and adnexa. A malpositioned eye is caused by changes in volume (loss or gain) of the orbital contents or from abnormal extraocular muscle function. Exophthalmia is caused by space-occupying lesions posterior to the equator of the globe. Enophthalmia is caused by loss of orbital volume or space-occupying lesions anterior to the equator of the globe. Strabismus is caused most frequently by imbalance of extraocular muscle tone or lesions that restrict extraocular muscle mobility.

Systems Affected
• Ophthalmic • Respiratory—because of the close proximity, the nasal cavity and frontal and maxillary sinuses are often involved.

SIGNALMENT
• Orbital abscess/cellulitis and myositis are more common in young adult dogs. • German shepherd dog, golden retriever, weimaraner, and English springer spaniel are predisposed to myositis. • Orbital neoplasia is more common in middle-aged to older patients.

SIGNS

Exophthalmia
Secondary signs of space-occupying orbital disease:
• Difficulty in retropulsing the globe
• Serous to mucopurulent ocular discharge
• Chemosis • Eyelid swelling • Lagophthalmos (inability to close the eyelids over the cornea adequately during blinking)
• Exposure keratitis (with or without ulceration) • Pain on opening the mouth • Third eyelid protrusion • Visual impairment caused by optic neuropathy • Fundic abnormalities, including retinal detachment
• Retinal vascular congestion • Focal inward deviation of the posterior globe
• Optic disc swelling • Neurotropic keratitis after damage to the ophthalmic branch of the fifth cranial nerve • Fever and malaise in animals with orbital abscess/cellulitis
• Intraocular pressure rarely high

Enophthalmia
• Ptosis • Third eyelid protrusion
• Extraocular muscle atrophy • Entropion in animals with severe disease

Strabismus
• Deviation of one or both eyes from their normal position • Exophthalmos or enophthalmus in some animals

CAUSES

Exophthalmia
• Neoplasm (primary or secondary)
• Abscess/cellulitis (bacterial or fungal; fungal is more likely in cats). Look for foreign bodies. • Zygomatic mucocele (not described in cats) • Myositis (muscles of mastication or extraocular muscles) • Orbital hemorrhage secondary to trauma • Arteriovenous fistula (rare)

Enophthalmia
• Ocular pain • Microphthalmia • Phthisis bulbi • Collapsed globe • Horner's syndrome • Dehydration • Loss of orbital fat or muscle • Conformational enophthalmos in dolichocephalic breeds

Strabimus
• Abnormality of innervation of extraocular muscle • Restriction of extraocular muscle motility by scar tissue from previous trauma or inflammation • Destruction of extraocular muscle attachments after proptosis
• Convergent strabismus (congenital); results from abnormal crossing of visual fibers in the CNS (Siamese cats)

RISK FACTORS
Proptosis more readily occurs in brachycephalic dogs with shallow orbits.

DIAGNOSTIC

DIFFERENTIAL DIAGNOSIS

Differentiating Similar Signs
• The buphthalmic globe can simulate a space-occupying mass and cause the eye to be displaced anteriorly due to its relative size in relationship to the orbital volume. In affected animals, however, intraocular pressure is usually high and the corneal diameter is greater than normal. • Episcleritis can cause severe diffuse or focal thickening of the fibrous tunic, often imitating a buphthalmic globe. Animals with diffuse episcleritis, however, often have corneal edema, low intraocular pressure, and aqueous flare.

Differentiating Causes
• Acute onset of exophthalmia is often caused by inflammatory orbital disease. Pain, especially on opening the mouth, is more likely the result of an inflammatory orbital disease than orbital neoplasia, which generally is less painful and has a slower onset and progression. • Mucoceles are more variable in speed of onset and degree of patient discomfort. • Myositis can be unilateral but is often bilateral.

CBC/BIOCHEMISTRY/URINALYSIS
• Results are usually normal. • Results of leukogram may show inflammation in animals with abscess/cellulitis or myositis.
• Peripheral eosinophilia is occasionally seen in dogs with masticatory muscle myositis.

OTHER LABORATORY TESTS N/A

IMAGING
• Skull radiographs (especially of the frontal sinuses and nasal cavity), orbital ultrasonography, and computerized tomography are extremely helpful in defining the extent of the lesion. • Thoracic radiographs may help identify metastatic disease.

OTHER DIAGNOSTIC PROCEDURES
• Lack of globe retropulsion confirms a space-occupying mass. • After anesthetizing the patient, oral examination, skull radiographs, and fine needle aspiration of the orbit can be completed. Fine needle aspirate samples (18-20 gauge) should be submitted for aerobic, anaerobic, and fungal cultures, gram stain, and cytologic examination. Results of cytologic examination are often diagnostic for abscess/cellulitis, zygomatic salivary gland mucocele, and neoplasia. If needle aspiration is undiagnostic, biopsy is probably indicated. • Results of biopsy and histopathologic examination of masseter, temporal, or extraocular muscle reveal the presence or absence of myositis. • Forced duction of the globe—by grasping the conjunctiva with a fine pair of forceps with animal under topical anesthesia—allows differentiation of strabismus due to neurologic disease (in which the globe moves freely) from restrictive strabismus (in which the globe cannot be moved manually).

TREATMENT

PROPTOSIS
• An emergency if vision and the globe are to be saved. In the author's experience, when the extraocular muscles are torn, the globe is often blind. If the pupil is miotic or a direct or consensual pupillary light response is present, the prognosis for vision is good. If the pupil is mid-sized, dilated, or unresponsive to light, the prognosis for vision is guarded to poor.
• See chapter on proptosis for treatment details.

ORBITAL ABSCESS/CELLULITIS
• Establish ventral orbital drainage while the patient is anesthetized. The surgically prepared mucosa is incised for approximately 1 cm behind the last molar. A blunt tipped forceps (i.e., Kelly or Carmalt) is pushed into the orbital space and opened. In general, the forceps are advanced to the level of the box lock, or if movement of the eye occurs, with forceps opening. Apparent drainage is seen in less than half of affected animals. Care should be taken to minimize retrobulbar trauma and optic nerve damage. Use only

ORBITAL DISEASES (EXOPHTHALMUS, ENOPHTHALMUS, STRABISMUS)

blunt dissection. Never crush tissue or use scissors to cut.
• Samples for bacterial culture and cytologic examination can also be obtained through this port.
• Hot packing q6h will help lessen swelling and clean discharges.

ORBITAL NEOPLASMS

• Most are primary and malignant. Early exenteration or orbital exploratory surgery and debulking of the mass via a lateral approach to the orbit to save the globe are rational therapeutic choices.
• Chemotherapy or radiotherapy may be employed as adjuncts depending on neoplasm type and extent of the lesion.
• Without adjunct therapy, survival times are weeks to months when malignancy is diagnosed because the patient is usually examined late in the course of disease. Consultation with an oncologist is recommended once the diagnosis is made.

ZYGOMATIC MUCOCELE

May resolve with antibiotic and corticosteroid administration. If not, surgical excision is usually curative.

STRABISMUS

• Neurologic strabismus is best treated by identifying the underlying cause and addressing that, if possible.
• Restrictive or post-traumatic strabismus may be treated surgically by repositioning the attachments of extraocular muscles and by relieving excessive tension on those muscles. This surgical procedure is usually very difficult.

MEDICATIONS

DRUGS AND FLUIDS

• In all animals with exophthalmos, the cornea should be lubricated (i.e., artificial tear ointment q6h) to prevent desiccation and ulceration.
• If ulceration is present, a topically applied antibiotic (e.g., bacitracin-neomycin- polymixin, q8h) and cycloplegic (e.g., 1% atropine

q12h-q24h) should be used to prevent infection and reduce ciliary spasm.

Orbital Abscess/Cellulitis

• In animals suspected of having orbital abscess/cellulitis, administer antibiotics (i.e., sodium ampicillin, 20 mg/kg q6h-q8h IV or chloramphenicol, 25 mg/kg q8h IV) while awaiting results of bacterial culture and cytologic examination or if owners decline diagnostic testing. Bacterial orbital infections can be mixed. Pasteurella multocida and Enterobacteriaceae are common aerobic isolates. After the patient begins to eat, it can be treated according to culture and sensitivity test results with orally administered antibiotics. Most animals recover within approximately 2 weeks of treatment.
• Itraconazole (2.5mg/kg q12h) may be considered in treating orbital aspergillosis.
• Prednisolone acetate (1 mg/kg q24h SQ or IM once or twice) is given to minimize optic neuritis and reduce orbital swelling and globe exposure.
• Animal with orbital abscess/cellulitis should be hospitalized and given fluids intravenously to maintain hydration and replace fluid deficits until it is able to eat.

Acute Myositis

If prehension is difficult, prescribe systemically administered corticosteroids (prednisolone acetate, 2 mg/kg SQ or IM) and then switch to orally administered corticosteroids for the next 4-6 weeks (prednisone, 2 mg/kg q24h until swelling subsides, then taper). Azathioprine (1-2mg/kg q24h PO for 2 weeks, then q48h and taper) should also be prescribed. Azathioprine with or without corticosteroids can be used chronically to manage animals with recurrent disease.

CONTRAINDICATIONS N/A

PRECAUTIONS

• Systemically administered corticosteroids must be used with extreme caution in patients with deep fungal orbital disease.
• Azathioprine may be hepatotoxic and cause myelosuppression.

POSSIBLE INTERACTIONS N/A

ALTERNATE DRUGS N/A

FOLLOW-UP

PATIENT MONITORING

• Patients with inflammatory orbital disease should be examined at least weekly until clinical signs abate. • Owners should be advised to watch for recurrence of signs, especially if an orbital foreign body is likely. • Treat fungal infections with itraconazole for 60 days after signs cease.

POSSIBLE COMPLICATIONS

• Vision loss • Loss of the eye • Permanent malposition of the globe • Death

MISCELLANEOUS

ASSOCIATED CONDITIONS N/A

AGE RELATED FACTORS N\A

ZOONOTIC POTENTIAL N/A

PREGNANCY

Systemically administered corticosteroids, antifungal medications, and azathioprine should be avoided in pregnant animals.

SYNONYMS N\A

SEE ALSO

• Proptosis • Red eye

ABBREVIATIONS N/A

References

Kern TJ. The canine orbit. In: Gelatt KN, ed. Veterinary ophthalmology. Philadelphia: Lea & Febiger, 1991:239–255.
Lindley DM. Disorders of the orbit. In: Kirk RW, Bonagura, JD. CVT XI, 1992:1081–1085.

Author Denise M. Lindley
Consulting Editor Paul E. Miller

PANTING

BASICS

DEFINITION
Rapid, shallow respirations (tachypnea, polypnea) characterized by open-mouthed breathing, often with protrusion of the tongue. May be associated with dyspnea.

Pathophysiology
Hyperthermia stimulates attempts to promote evaporative cooling from the tongue in nonperspiring animals. Evaporative cooling is augmented by circulation of air coming in through the nasopharynx and exiting via the oropharynx. Alterations in respiratory center function resulting from primary neurologic disease can cause panting also. May also be seen in states of excitement, anxiety, or pain. Hypoxemia, hypercapnia, or acidosis leads to attempts to increase alveolar gas exchange.

Systems Affected
• Respiratory • Cardiovascular • Nervous

SIGNALMENT
• Both dogs and cats pant. • Brachycephalic breeds are often quite ineffective with panting.

SIGNS N/A

CAUSES

Respiratory Causes
• Upper respiratory tract obstructions that limit deep inspiratory efforts—nasal obstructions, brachycephalic syndrome, laryngeal dysfunction, nasopharyngeal polyps, collapsed or compressed trachea, and acromegaly • Lower respiratory tract diseases that limit alveolar gas exchange—pulmonary edema or hemorrhage, pneumonitis, pulmonary interstitial fibrosis, bronchiectasis, emphysema, lung lobe torsion, pulmonary neoplasia (primary and metastatic), asthma • Diseases of the pleural cavity—pleural effusions, pneumothorax, mediastinal masses, diaphragmatic hernias

Cardiovascular Causes
• Pulmonary vascular diseases—heartworm disease, pulmonary thromboembolism (PTE), pulmonary vascular dysplasia (with right-left shunting PDA) • Left-sided congestive heart failure—mitral regurgitation, left-to-right congenital shunts, cardiomyopathy, atrial fibrillation • Decreased cardiac output—arrhythmias, subaortic and pulmonic stenosis, severe left heart failure, cardiac tamponade • Right-to-left shunts—PDA, tetralogy of Fallot, dextrapositioned aorta (double-outlet right ventricle), other complicated cardiac anomalies

Hematologic Causes
• Reduced oxygen-carrying capacity—anemia, methemoglobinemia, carbon monoxide poisoning • Hypercapnia—metabolic acidosis as a result of renal disease, diabetes, diarrhea, shock, toxicosis

Neurologic Causes
• Head trauma or brain tumors may affect the respiratory center. • Dysfunction of muscles of respiration—myasthenia gravis, tetanus, polyradiculoneuritis, diabetic neuropathy (diaphragmatic paralysis), hypothyroidism (laryngeal paralysis), various neurotoxicoses that may all lead to inappropriate excursions of the chest and consequent hypoxia/hypercapnia • Seizures cause stimulation of the respiratory center, lactic acidosis, and hyperthermia.

Miscellaneous Causes
• High altitude (decreased inspired O_2 tension) • Abdominal pressure on the diaphragm caused by ascites, abdominal organomegaly, obesity, gestation • Hyperadrenocorticism—resulting from abdominal compression of the diaphragm, PTE • Hyperthermia—fever, exertion, heatstroke, malignant hyperthermia, thyrotoxicosis, excitement, iatrogenic (heating pad), seizures, and poisoning • Anxiety/excitement—often associated with visits to the veterinarian • Hyperactivity—pheochromocytoma, thyrotoxicosis • Pain of all types, especially respiratory pain • Electric shock neurostimulation and pulmonary edema • Drugs—narcotic analgesics and diazepam often cause panting

RISK FACTORS
• Obesity • Diabetes mellitus • Hyperadrenocorticism • Hyperthyroidism • Cardiac disease • Respiratory disease • Neurological disease • Pain

DIAGNOSIS

DIFFERENTIAL DIAGNOSIS
• Determine level of anxiety or stress to rule out physiologic causes. Note: Panting in cats is relatively uncommon; tachypnea in cats often is associated with dyspnea.
• Measure temperature—note that car rides may transiently elevate temperature, so recheck after 15-30 minutes • History of seizures indicates neurologic disease—consider primary cranial and extracranial causes, and toxicosis • History of coughing and exercise intolerance may indicate cardiac or pulmonary disease. • Heart murmurs or arrhythmias may indicate cardiac disease. • Generalized or episodic weakness may indicate a peripheral neuropathy. • Historical polyuria/polydipsia may indicate an endocrinopathy such as hyperadrenocorticism, diabetes mellitus, or hyperthyroidism. • Thoracic auscultation may reveal increased or decreased lung sounds, consistent with primary pulmonary disease or pleural disease. • Laryngeal and tracheal palpation may reveal atrophy of laryngeal muscles or collapsing trachea. Examination of the pharynx may reveal stridorous respiration and obstructive disease. • Mucous membrane color may indicate cyanosis, anemia, or methemoglobinemia. History of exposure to oxidants.

CBC/BIOCHEMISTRY/URINALYSIS
Hemogram may indicate anemia or polycythemia (with right-to-left shunts). Acid-base abnormalities may include low pH or low HCO_3 (TCO_2). Serum chemistry profile may indicate particular endocrinopathy or azotemia.

OTHER LABORATORY TESTS
• Blood gas abnormalities may include low PaO_2 or high $PaCO_2$. • Consider provocative testing (ACTH stimulation, TSH stimulation) if history, clinical signs, and initial laboratory tests are suggestive of endocrinopathy. • Antiacetylcholine receptor antibody titers for myasthenia gravis, especially if weakness is apparent • Heartworm antigen testing if appropriate • Evaluate coagulation profile and fibrin degradation products (FDPs) to diagnose disseminated intravascular coagulopathy (DIC) if heatstroke, malignant hyperthermia, or hemothorax is suspected.

IMAGING
• Thoracic radiography is the technique of choice for evaluation of the pulmonary fields and thoracic cavity. Cardiac silhouette may also be assessed and pleural disease may be diagnosed. Collapsing trachea, redundant dorsal tracheal membrane, or diaphragmatic paralysis may require expiratory film or fluoroscopy. Barium contrast radiography may identify diaphragmatic hernias. • Echocardiography is the technique of choice for cardiac evaluation and should be considered if cardiac disease is suspected. • Pulmonary scintigraphy (ventilatory or perfusatory) may be used to identify pulmonary thromboembolic disease. • Computed tomography or magnetic resonance imaging may be indicated if central nervous system disease is suspected. • Abdominal ultrasound may be indicated if hyperadrenocorticism or abdominal organomegaly/pregnancy is suspected.

OTHER DIAGNOSTIC PROCEDURES
• Examination of the nasooropharynx and larynx under anesthesia may reveal upper respiratory tract obstructive disease. • Bronchoscopy and transtracheal wash/bronchoalveolar lavage may aid in diagnosing lower respiratory disease. Fine needle aspiration of pulmonary and intrathoracic masses may be attempted.
• Thoracocentesis is indicated for pleural effusions. Samples should be submitted for culture and sensitivity if purulent or hemorrhagic.
• An electrocardiogram is necessary to characterize arrhythmias. • If PTE is suspected, oxygen challenge with 100% O_2 may be performed, with analysis of PaO_2 before and after O_2 administration. Patients with severe PTE may have reduced uptake of oxygen at high inspired concentrations. However, any ventilation/perfusion mismatch may affect O_2 uptake.

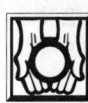

TREATMENT

- May not require treatment if physiologic
- Treat underlying disease—assess severity to determine if hospitalization is necessary
- Correct hypoxemia with O_2 supplementation; blood transfusion if anemia is the cause.
- Correct hypercapnia by treating underlying acid-base imbalance. • Do not attempt to reduce pyrexia unless it is severe (> 106° F).
- Treat hyperthermia with alcohol soaks, cold-water enemas, ice baths.
- Treat any intoxication directly and specifically.
- Consider a reduction in the dosage of corticosteroids or thyroxine if iatrogenic disease has been induced.
- Assist ventilation if respiratory efforts are compromised as a result of neuropathy.

MEDICATIONS

DRUGS AND FLUIDS

- Upper airway disease—treat the specific condition
- Lower airway disease and pleural disease—treat the specific condition. Infectious conditions require appropriate antibiotic therapy. Bronchodilators (aminophylline, theophylline, terbutaline) may be of value.
- Cardiac disease—treat congestive heart failure with diuretics, vasodilators, and inotropes if indicated. Aggressive diuretic therapy will alleviate pulmonary edema in most instances. Arrhythmias should be treated with appropriate antiarrhythmics.
- Neurologic disease—inflammatory and neoplastic disease may respond to a combination of corticosteroid and anticonvulsant

therapy. Idiopathic seizure disorders require anticonvulsant therapy (phenobarbital, potassium bromide, diazepam).
- Pulmonary thromboembolism—treat underlying cause. Heparin administration may prevent further thrombosis.
- Hyperadrenocorticism—mitotane therapy or adrenalectomy if patient is well-stabilized
- Pain—analgesics. Narcotics may reduce generalized pain; however, they also compromise respiration, so care must be taken to avoid further hypoxia. Intrapleural local anesthetics may be used for pain associated with thoracic disease or surgery. Nerve blocks may also be used. Nonsteroidal antiinflammatories also may be considered for more chronic pain. Avoid acetaminophen in small animals.
- Metabolic acidosis—fluid therapy with isoosmolar crystalloid solutions will assist in the correction of most causes of metabolic acidosis. Bicarbonate may be considered if acidosis is severe. Diabetic ketoacidosis requires specific therapy with insulin as well as fluids.

CONTRAINDICATIONS

Acetaminophen should not be used for analgesia in small animals.

PRECAUTIONS

Avoid sedatives/anxiolytics unless panting is a result of anxiety, because these may compromise the respiratory efforts of the patient even further.

POSSIBLE INTERACTIONS N/A

ALTERNATE DRUGS N/A

FOLLOW-UP

PATIENT MONITORING

- Thoracic radiographs to assess resolution of pulmonary or pleural disease or congestive

heart failure • Serial blood-gas analysis to assess ventilation in patients with hypoxemia
- Hematologic evaluation to monitor anemia
- Hydration status and acid-base status in patients with acidosis. • Monitor temperature if hyperthermia exists.

POSSIBLE COMPLICATIONS

Respiratory alkalosis if the panting is associated with nonacidotic or nonhypercapnic causes

MISCELLANEOUS

ASSOCIATED CONDITIONS N/A

AGE RELATED FACTORS N/A

ZOONOTIC POTENTIAL N/A

PREGNANCY N/A

SYNONYMS
Tachypnea, polypnea

SEE ALSO
See causes.

ABBREVIATIONS
PDA = patent ductus arteriosus
PTE = pulmonary thromboembolus
FDP = fibrin degradation product

Reference
Ettinger SJ. Dyspnea and tachypnea. In: Ettinger SJ, ed. Textbook of veterinary internal medicine. 3rd ed. Philadelphia: WB Saunders, 1989.
Author Mark Rishniw
Consulting Editors Lynelle Johnson and Bradley L. Moses

PARALYSIS

BASICS

DEFINITION
Paresis is weakness of voluntary movement, whereas paralysis is lack of voluntary movement. Quadriparesis (tetraparesis) is weakness of voluntary movements in all limbs, whereas quadriplegia (tetraplegia) is an absence of all voluntary limb movement. Paraparesis and paraplegia refer to weakness and paralysis, respectively, of pelvic limbs.

Pathophysiology
• Weakness can be caused by lesions in the upper motor neuron system or the lower motor neuron system. Cell bodies or nuclei for the upper motor neuron system are located within the brain and are responsible for initiating voluntary movement. Axons from these cell bodies form tracts (ie, rubrospinal, corticospinal, vestibulospinal, etc.) that descend from the brain to synapse upon interneurons in the spinal cord. Interneuronal axons then synapse upon the large (alpha) motor neurons in the ventral gray matter of the spinal cord. These large motor neurons are the cell bodies of origin for the lower motor neuron system, which is responsible for spinal reflexes. Collections of lower motor neurons in the cervical and lumbar intumescences give rise to axons that form the ventral nerve roots, the spinal nerves, and, ultimately, the peripheral nerves that innervate limb muscles.
• Evaluation of limb reflexes allows one to determine which system (upper motor neuron or lower motor neuron) is involved. Upper motor neurons and their axons have an inhibitory influence on the large motor neurons of the lower motor neuron system. This inhibitory effect maintains normal muscle tone and normal spinal reflexes. If upper motor neurons or their axons are injured, spinal reflexes are no longer inhibited or controlled. Thus, reflexes become exaggerated or hyperreflexic. If the large alpha motor neurons or their processes (peripheral nerves) are injured, spinal reflexes cannot be elicited (areflexic) or are reduced (hyporeflexic).

Systems Affected Nervous

SIGNALMENT Any animal

SIGNS

General Comments
Limb weakness can have an acute or gradual onset.

Historical Findings
Owners may describe their pets as being unable to move, walk, or get up. Many focal compressive spinal cord diseases begin with ataxia and progress to weakness and finally paralysis.

Physical Examination Findings
• Unless the disease process is systemic, most pets with paresis or paralysis are alert, and physical examination findings are normal. • If the disease process causes pain, many patients resent handling and manipulation during the examination. • Beware that patients with aortic emboli can be paraplegic on examination, but femoral pulses are absent and the limbs should be cold. Nailbeds are often blue in color.

Neurologic Examination Findings
• Should confirm that the problem is weakness or paralysis and should localize it to either lower motor neuron or upper motor neuron system • If the pelvic limbs are paralyzed, it is likely that the bladder is also paralyzed, negating voluntary urination.

CAUSES

Neurologic
Generalized lower motor neuron quadriplegia: Acute onset—coonhound paralysis, botulism, tick paralysis, myasthenia gravis crisis, and protozoal myoneuritis are possibilities; more gradual onset—polyneuropathies and polymyopathies
Generalized upper motor neuron quadriplegia: Cervical spinal cord or multifocal cord diseases are most likely. Causes include disc herniation, trauma, neoplasia, discospondylitis, myelitis of many causes, fibrocartilaginous embolism, and malformations.
Upper motor neuron pelvic limb paralysis: Disc herniation, neoplasia, discospondylitis, trauma, and fibrocartilaginous embolism
Lower motor neuron pelvic limb paralysis Disc herniation, lumbosacral instability, discospondylitis, trauma, neoplasia, and spina bifida
Generalized upper motor neuron quadriplegia with cranial nerve deficits, seizures, or stupor: Consider diseases of the brain such as neoplasia, encephalitis, trauma, vascular accidents, and congenital or inherited disorders.

RISK FACTORS
• Breeds at risk for degenerative disc disease often have disc herniations that cause paralysis. • Breeds of dogs that hunt are at risk for developing coonhound paralysis. • Animals that are allowed to roam are at risk for spinal cord trauma.

DIAGNOSIS

DIFFERENTIAL DIAGNOSIS
• When examining an animal that is weak or paralyzed in the pelvic limbs, make sure that femoral pulses are present and normal. Patients with aortic or femoral artery emboli can have lower motor neuron paraparesis or paraplegia. • Perform spinal reflexes to localize the weakness to the cervical, thoracolumbar, or lower lumbar cord segments. • If the onset was acute, be careful moving the animal because of the possibility of trauma.

CBC/BIOCHEMISTRY/URINALYSIS
Results usually normal unless inflammatory diseases are involved. For example, inflammation may be detected on urinalysis of dogs with discospondylitis.

OTHER LABORATORY TESTS
• If the patient has urinary tract inflammation, perform a bacterial culture of urine. • If discospondylitis is diagnosed by spinal radiography, perform a Brucella titer and consider blood as well as a urine bacterial culture.
• If the weakness is exercise-induced, perform a myasthenia gravis titer and check serum creatine kinase concentration (polymyositis).
• If lower motor neuron weakness or muscle pain, muscle atrophy, or hypertrophy are found, determine creatine kinase concentration to help diagnose polymyositis. • If myelitis is suspected, perform titers for Neospora caninum and Ehrlichia canis.

IMAGING
• If the lesion is localized to the spinal cord, radiographs can diagnose many abnormalities, including disc herniation, discospondylitis, bony tumor, congenital vertebral malformation, and fracture or luxation. • Myelography is required if survey radiography is not diagnostic and if surgery is being considered.

OTHER DIAGNOSTIC PROCEDURES
• CSF analysis should be done before myelography to rule in myelitis and meningitis. • If CSF analysis reveals high protein or numbers of cells, culture is warranted. • If the patient has generalized lower motor neuron signs, needle electromyelography and motor nerve conduction velocity can better characterize the lesion and determine the diagnosis.
• Muscle and nerve biopsy is indicated in patients with generalized lower motor neuron weakness.

TREATMENT
• Patients with severe weakness or paralysis should be treated as inpatients until bladder function can be ascertained.
• In animals with diffuse lower motor neuron signs, swallowing can be affected; thus hand-feeding is recommended until it is certain that the animal can swallow properly. Feeding from an elevated platform is recommended for animals with megaesophagus.
• All activity should be restricted until spinal trauma and disc herniation can be ruled out.
• Physical therapy is important in paralyzed animals to tone muscles and to keep joints flexible.
• Because paralyzed animals are not able to move away from soiled bedding, they must be checked and cleaned frequently to prevent urine scalding and superficial pyoderma.
• Animals that cannot move effectively must be maintained on padded bedding or a waterbed to help prevent decubital ulcer formation.
• Quadriplegic animals must be turned from side to side four to eight times daily to help

prevent hypostatic lung congestion as well as decubital ulcer formation.
• For those with surgical disease (eg, disc herniation, fracture, and some neoplasias and congenital conditions), surgery is often the quickest and most effective method of improving the neurologic status.

MEDICATIONS

DRUGS AND FLUIDS

• If trauma, disc herniation, or fibrocartilaginous embolism is suspected or if the patient has acute upper motor neuron signs, administration of methylprednisolone sodium succinate may be beneficial (30 mg/kg IV followed by 15 mg/kg 2 and 6 hours later).
• Animals with acute generalized lower motor neuron signs should be checked for ticks and dipped with appropriate insecticides if necessary.
• If myasthenia gravis is suspected, pyridostigmine bromide (0.5-3.0 mg/kg PO q8h-q12h) can be administered while waiting for titer results.

CONTRAINDICATIONS

• Corticosteroids should not be used in animals with discospondylitis.
• Corticosteroids should not be used in animals with myasthenia gravis that have aspiration pneumonia.

PRECAUTIONS

Corticosteroid usage is associated with gastrointestinal ulceration and hemorrhage, delayed wound healing, and heightened susceptibility to infection.

POSSIBLE INTERACTIONS N/A

ALTERNATE DRUGS

• Dexamethasone (0.5-1 mg/kg q24h-q48h)
• Prednisolone (1-2 mg/kg q12h-q24h)

FOLLOW-UP

PATIENT MONITORING

• Daily neurologic examinations to monitor patient's neurologic status. Once bladder function has returned, patient can be managed at home. • Bladder evacuation (via manual expression or catheterization) three to four times a day to prevent overdistension and subsequent bladder atony.

POSSIBLE COMPLICATIONS

• Urinary tract infection • Bladder atony
• Urine scalding and pyoderma • Constipation
• Decubital ulcer formation • Aspiration pneumonia in patients with generalized lower motor neuron disease • Myelomalacia in patients with severe cord trauma or disc herniations
• Respiratory compromise or paralysis in patients with myelomalacia or generalized lower motor neuron disease

MISCELLANEOUS

ASSOCIATED CONDITIONS N/A

AGE RELATED FACTORS N/A

ZOONOTIC POTENTIAL N/A

PREGNANCY

Contraindicated in the paralyzed patient

SYNONYMS N/A

SEE ALSO N/A

ABBREVIATION

CSF = cerebrospinal fluid

References

Chrisman CL. Paraplegia, paraparesis, and ataxia of the pelvic limbs. In: Problems in small animal neurology. Philadelphia: Lea & Febiger, 1991:397-431.

Withrow SJ. Localization and diagnosis of spinal cord lesions in small animals. Part 1. Compend Cont Educ Pract Vet 1980;2:464-474.

de Lahunta A. Veterinary neuroanatomy and clinical neurology. 2nd ed. Philadelphia: WB Saunders, 1983:53-93.

Author Linda J. Shell
Consulting Editor Joane M. Parent

PERIPHERAL EDEMA

BASICS

DEFINITION
• Abnormal accumulation of interstitial fluid in subcutaneous tissues • May be localized (one limb), regional (fore- or hind limbs) or generalized (usually midline, dependent surfaces)

PATHOPHYSIOLOGY
• Low plasma oncotic pressure (i.e., hypoproteinemia; albumin <1.5 gm/dl) • High vascular hydrostatic pressure • High capillary permeability • Lymphatic drainage abnormality (e.g., dysgenesis, obstruction, and destruction)

SYSTEMS AFFECTED
• Skin/exocrine—swelling of subcutaneous tissues, especially ventral or dependent aspects; serum exudation or dermal ulceration in affected limbs • Musculoskeletal—gait abnormalities if limb swelling excessive

SIGNALMENT N/A

SIGNS

Historical Findings
• Recent trauma (including surgery) • Exposure to ticks, venomous insects, arachnids, or snakes • History of cardiac or vascular disease

Physical Examination Findings
• Localized or diffuse subcutaneous swelling including limbs and ventral midline • Affected limbs usually not painful but pain may occur if swelling is excessive • Serum exudation from swollen limbs • Dermal ulceration and evidence of self trauma of affected areas (may lead to necrosis) • Subcutaneous edema may be pitting or nonpitting • Local or regional lymph node enlargement • Draining tracts (animal with foreign body or fungal infection)

Causes

Localized Peripheral Edema (Single Limb)
High Hydrostatic Pressure
• Acute arterial or venous thrombosis • Arteriovenous fistula
High Capillary Permeability
• Angioedema (e.g., snake, insect, or arachnid bite or sting and drug reaction at site of injection) • Trauma, burns • Neoplastic infiltration • Cellulitis (e.g., foreign body, infection, and inflammation)
Lymphatic Abnormalities
• Neoplastic infiltration of local lymph node or subcutis (e.g., local or metastatic tumor) • Traumatic lymphatic disruption • Lymphangitis • Congenital malformation of lymphatic system

Regional (Fore- or Hindlimbs) or Generalized Peripheral Edema
Low Oncotic Pressure (Hypoalbuminemia)
• Hepatic disease • Protein-losing renal (i.e., nephrotic syndrome) or gastrointestinal dis-

ease • Severe blood loss with noncolloid fluid replacement • High hydrostatic pressure • Right-sided or biventricular congestive heart failure (CHF) • Pericardial effusion with tamponade • Right atrial mass • Vena cava obstruction • Overhydration, especially if associated with acute oliguric renal failure or hypoproteinemia
High Capillary Permeability
• Sepsis • Vasculitis (e.g., infectious disease and tick-related disease) • Some snake venoms • Trauma, burns
Lymphatic Abnormality (i.e., Lymphedema)
• Infiltration or abcessation of regional or multiple lymph nodes • Traumatic lymphatic disruption • Lymphangitis • Congenital malformation of lymphatic system

Facial
• Jugular catheter thrombosis • Tight cervical bandage or brace • Myxedema (associated with hypothyroidism) • Local lymphadenopathy • Juvenile pyoderma

RISK FACTORS
Vary with underlying cause

DIAGNOSIS

DIFFERENTIAL DIAGNOSIS
• Peripheral edema associated with myxedema and inflammation (i.e., cellulitis) is usually nonpitting. • If animal has peripheral edema with jugular venous distension and ascites, consider cardiac or pericardial disease. • If animal has bilateral forelimb edema, jugular distension, and no ascites, consider cranial vena cava obstruction. • Bilateral hindlimb edema, ascites, no jugular distension: consider hypoproteinemia or caudal vena cava obstruction • Bilateral hindlimb edema, no ascites: consider lymphatic or vascular obstruction • Hyperglobulinemia may be associated with infectious causes • Edematous swelling with palpable fremitus: consider arteriovenous fistula • Sting or snake bite site may be visible • Petechiation or ecchymosis: consider disseminated intravascular coagulation, thrombocytopenia, and vasculitidies • Arteriovenous fistulae and lymphatic obstruction may develop at site of previous trauma

CBC/BIOCHEMISTRY/URINALYSIS
• Inflammatory leukogram—consider infectious disease and inflammation • Thrombocytopenia—consider tick-related disease and DIC • Pancytopenia—consider ehrlichiosis and neoplastic bone marrow infiltration • Hypoalbuminemia (< 1.5 gm/dl)—consider renal or gastrointestinal loss of protein or hepatic failure • Hyperglobulinemia—consider infectious disease • Proteinuria—consider glomerular disease

Other Laboratory Tests
• Measurement resting and post-prandial bile acids to document hepatic disease • Serologic testing for tick-related disease (e.g., ehrlichio-

sis, Rocky Mountain spotted fever) • Bacterial culture and cytologic examination of draining tract exudates (e.g., sporotrichosis, fungal disease, and infected foreign body)

IMAGING
• Thoracic radiography and echocardiography to rule out cardiac disease • Selective angiography to rule out vascular obstruction • Lymphangiography to rule out lymphatic malformation or obstruction

OTHER DIAGNOSTIC PROCEDURES
• Examination of skin or lymph node aspirate to detect infectious or infiltrative disease • Skin or lymph node biopsy to diagnose peripheral lymphatic abnormality, lymphangitis, vasculitis, neoplastic infiltrate, or pyoderma • Central venous pressure measurement to rule out CHF or cranial vena cava obstruction

TREATMENT
• Treat the underlying disease • Secure airway if acute head or cervical edema • Consider hospitalization if patient is nonambulatory • Monitor edematous areas for pressure necrosis if patient is nonambulatory (padded cage or waterbed) • Cage rest not necessary if animal is comfortable • Limb wrapping seldom leads to resolution

MEDICATIONS

DRUGS AND FLUIDS

Acute Severe Angioneurotic Edema (Insect Stings)
Antihistamines (e.g., chlorpheniramine 2-8 mg PO q12h)
Prednisolone (5.5-11 mg/kg IV)
If patient is in anaphylactic shock, epinephrine (1-5 ml of 1:10,000 aqueous epinephrine SC)

Hypoproteinemia
• Minimize use of crystalloid fluids • Use colloids or plasma for vascular reexpansion • Monitor patient carefully for overhydration • Consider initiating treatment for tick-related diseases while serologic tests pending

CONTRAINDICATIONS
Diuretics not helpful unless patient has CHF or oliguria/anuria and may worsen lymphedema

PRECAUTIONS
Beware of overhydration if patient has hypoproteinemia or oliguria

POSSIBLE INTERACTIONS N/A

ALTERNATE DRUGS N/A

PERIPHERAL EDEMA

FOLLOW-UP

PATIENT MONITORING
• Peripheral edema resolves as underlying cause resolves • Monitor edematous areas for trauma or necrosis • Use extreme caution with heating pads in immobilized patients

POSSIBLE COMPLICATIONS
Necrosis may necessitate partial or complete amputation of affected limb

MISCELLANEOUS

ASSOCIATED CONDITIONS
Lymphedema may be associated with chylothorax

AGE RELATED FACTORS
Congenital arteriovenous fistulae and lymphatic malformations usually diagnosed at a young age

ZOONOTIC POTENTIAL
Avoid direct contact with exudates from draining tracts until diagnosis obtained

PREGNANCY N/A

SYNONYMS N/A

SEE ALSO
• See causes • Lymphedema • Congestive Heart Failure, Right Sided • Vasculitis • Snake Venom Toxicity • Anaphylaxis • Albumin, Hypoalbuminemia

ABBREVIATIONS
CHF = congestive heart failure
DIC = disseminated intravascular coagulation

References
Bright JM. Peripheral edema. In: Ettinger SJ, Feldman EC, eds. Textbook of veterinary internal medicine. 4th ed. Philadelphia: WB Saunders, 1995.

Bolton G, Ettinger SJ. Peripheral edema. In: Ettinger SJ, ed. Textbook of veterinary internal medicine. 3rd ed. Philadelphia: WB Saunders, 1989.

Fossum TW, King LA, Miller MW, et al. Lymphedema. Clinical signs, diagnosis and treatment. J Vet Int Med 1992;6:312-319.

Fossum TW, Miller MW. Lymphedema. Etiopathogenesis. J Vet Int Med 1992;6:283-293.

Peterson ME, Meerdink GL. Bites and stings of venomous animals. In: Kirk RW, ed. Current veterinary therapy X, Small animal practice. Philadelphia:WB Saunders, 1989.

Author Rebecca L. Stepien

Consulting Editors Larry P. Tilley and Francis W. K. Smith, Jr.

PETECHIA/ECCHYMOSIS/BRUISING

BASICS

DEFINITION
Disorders of primary hemostasis (platelet- or vessel-wall–mediated) that result in bleeding into the skin or mucous membranes to a degree out of proportion to the trauma

Pathophysiology
• Thrombocytopenia and, less commonly, defective platelet function cause impaired primary hemostasis (ie, failure of platelet plug formation). Thrombocytopenia is caused by shortened platelet life span, decreased thrombopoiesis, or platelet sequestration. Acquired platelet function deficits are most often associated with uremic inhibition of cyclooxygenase, but occasionally are associated with drugs, dysproteinemia, and myeloproliferative disease. Congenital platelet function defects are varied and, other than von Willebrand disease, rare. Sequestration of platelets in a large spleen or liver occurs rarely. • Vascular hemostatic defects generally are caused by one of three mechanisms: increased permeability as in patients with hyperadrenocorticism, decreased vessel strength as in patients with Ehlers-Danlos syndrome or scurvy (seen only in guinea pigs and primates), and lack of contraction.

Systems Affected
• Hemic/lymph/immune • Skin/exocrine—petechia/ecchymosis/bruising • Respiratory—epistaxis • Renal/urologic—hematuria • Gastrointestinal—melena

SIGNALMENT
• Most causes of thrombocytopenia and platelet function defects do not have a breed, age, or sex predisposition. • All are more common in dogs than cats.

SIGNS N/A

CAUSES

Thrombocytopenia
• Increased platelet use or destruction—immune-mediated disease, consumptive coagulopathy, or infectious disease such as ehrlichiosis. Immune-mediated disease can be primary autoimmune, isoimmune in the newborn, secondary to viruses, bacteria, ehrlichia, rickettsia, or protozoa. Some infectious diseases cause thrombocytopenia by immune-mediated mechanisms. • Low platelet production—myelophthisis, aplastic anemia, and drug reactions (e.g., estrogen toxicity) • Sequestration of platelets in a large spleen, liver, or other sizable mass of microvasculature usually does not cause thrombocytopenia to the degree necessary to result in bleeding.

Thrombocytopathy
• Congenital platelet function disorders—von Willebrand disease, Glanzmann's thrombasthenia (rare), and thrombopathia of basset hounds (rare). • Acquired platelet function disorders—uremia, disseminated intravascular coagulation (DIC), liver disease, myeloproliferative and lymphoproliferative disease, paraproteinemia, vitamin C deficiency, congenital heart disease, and treatment with nonsteroidal antiinflammatory drugs

Vascular Disease
Secondary purpura is seen in patients with Cushing's syndrome, uremia, dysproteinemia, drug reaction, and some infectious diseases.

Coagulation Factors
Coagulation factor deficiencies do not result in this type of bleeding disorder. Rather, they are more commonly associated with hematomata and hemarthroses.

RISK FACTORS
The presence of any of the diseases mentioned. Previous administration of aspirin or other nonsteroidal antiinflammatory agent is particularly important to know if bleeding time is to be measured (see below).

DIAGNOSIS

DIFFERENTIAL DIAGNOSIS
• Petechiae, ecchymoses, and bruises usually are not mistaken for anything else. However, injuries causing an expected amount of bleeding or bruising must be ruled out by history and physical examination. • Many breeds are predisposed to von Willebrand disease; those with a high prevalence include Doberman pinscher, standard Manchester terrier, toy Manchester terrier, Pembroke Welsh corgi, miniature schnauzer, Scottish terrier, golden retriever, Shetland sheepdog, and standard poodle.

CBC/BIOCHEMISTRY/URINALYSIS
• Platelets are low either by estimation on a well-made blood smear or by a direct count in patients with thrombocytopenia. If the platelet count is > 100,000/µl, consider other causes of defective primary hemostasis.
• RBC fragmentation suggests DIC or other vascular disease. • Patients with myeloproliferative and lymphoproliferative diseases are leukemic or cytopenic. • Biochemistry analysis is helpful to rule out hepatic, renal, and hormonal (ie, Cushing's syndrome) causes. Hyperproteinemia may be the first indication of paraproteinemia.

OTHER LABORATORY TESTS
• Coagulation studies, including APTT, PT, and FDP, in addition to thrombin time help rule out DIC. • Von Willebrand factor assay is necessary to confirm von Willebrand disease. • Platelet function tests may be necessary to rule out platelet function disorders. • Serum protein electrophoresis and examination of the urine for light chains (i.e., Bence Jones proteins) is indicated if the patient has hyperproteinemia. • Dexamethasone suppression or ACTH stimulation test may be indicated if Cushing's syndrome is suspected.

IMAGING
Abdominal radiography or ultrasonography may be helpful in identifying splenomegaly or hepatomegaly associated with hypersplenism or Cushing's syndrome, respectively.

OTHER DIAGNOSTIC PROCEDURES
• The buccal mucosa simplate bleeding time is long in patients with most of the thrombopathies in addition to thrombocytopenia. • Most invasive procedures are contraindicated in patients with bleeding disorders. • Bone marrow examination is indicated if cytopenia or hyperproteinemia is detected.

TREATMENT
• Usually as an inpatient until a definitive diagnosis is made
• Minimize activity to reduce the risk of even minor trauma.
• Discontinue any medications that may alter platelet function (eg, aspirin and other NSAIDs).

MEDICATIONS

DRUGS AND FLUIDS
• Maintenance of fluid volume by administration of balanced electrolyte solutions is recommended in all conditions. Blood or platelet transfusion may be necessary to survival before a definitive diagnosis is made. Obtain serum, whole blood, and any other samples necessary before initiating such treatment.
• No specific treatment is available for the congenital thrombocytopathies. In patients with an acquired thrombocytopathy, the underlying disease must be treated. See specific diseases for details.

CONTRAINDICATIONS N/A

PRECAUTIONS
Aspirin and other nonsteroidal antiinflammatory drugs should be avoided unless patient has DIC or other cause of platelet activation.

POSSIBLE INTERACTIONS N/A

ALTERNATE DRUGS N/A

FOLLOW-UP

PATIENT MONITORING
In patients with thrombocytopenia, platelet count daily until a response is seen. See specific diseases for details.

POSSIBLE COMPLICATIONS
• Death or morbidity as a result of hemorrhage into the brain or other vital organs
• Shock as a result of hemorrhagic hypovolemia

MISCELLANEOUS

ASSOCIATED CONDITIONS N/A

AGE RELATED FACTORS N/A

ZOONOTIC POTENTIAL N/A

PREGNANCY N/A

SYNONYMS
Hemorrhagic diatheses, bleeding

SEE ALSO
• Disseminated Intravascular Coagulation
• Hyperadrenocorticism (Cushing's Syndrome) • Myeloproliferative Disease

ABBREVIATIONS
ACTH = adrenocortiotrophin hormone
APTT = activated partial thromboplastin time
DIC = disseminated intravascular coagulation
FDP = fibrin degradation products
PT = prothrombin time
RBC = red blood cells

References

Jergens AE, Turrentine MA, Kraus KH, Johnson GS. Buccal mucosa bleeding times of healthy dogs and of dogs in various pathologic states, including thrombocytopenia, uremia, and von Willebrand's disease. Am J Vet Res 1987;48:1337-1342.

Forbes CD, Printice CRM. Vascular and non-thrombocytopenic purpura. In: Bloom AL, Thomas DP, eds. Haemostasis and thrombosis. Edinburgh: Chruchill Livingstone, 1987:321-332.

Boon GD, Rebar AH. The clinical approach to disorders of hemostasis. In: Ettinger SJ, ed. Textbook of veterinary internal medicine. Philadelphia: WB Saunders, 1989:105-107.

Green RA. Hemostatic disorders: coagulopathies and thrombotic disorders. In: Ettinger SJ, ed. Textbook of veterinary internal medicine. Philadelphia: WB Saunders, 1989:2246-2264.

Author G. Daniel Boon

Consulting Editor Alan H. Rebar

PICA

BASICS

DEFINITION
Ingestion of nonfood items

Pathophysiology
Although most cases of pica are not caused by disease, gastrointestinal or hepatic disease may lead to ingestion of nonfood items. The pathophysiology is unknown.

Systems Affected
• CNS system—diseases such as rabies or lead toxicity can cause pica • Gastrointestinal tract—in some animals, diseases of the gastrointestinal tract such as gingivitis and lymphocytic plasmacytic enteritis or enterocolitis, can cause pica. More commonly, however, the gastrointestinal tract is affected when obstruction occurs secondary to pica

SIGNALMENT
Young dog or Siamese cat

SIGNS

Historical Findings
Ingestion of nonfood items. Examples are rocks and feces (dogs), fabrics and plastics (cats).

Physical Examination Findings NA

CAUSES
• Deficiency states or even hunger can lead to pica; the most common are iron deficiency anemia and maldigestion/malabsorption secondary to pancreatic acinar atrophy. • In most animals, there does not appear to be a pathological cause; rather the behavior is a compulsive behavior or a stereotypic behavior.

RISK FACTORS
• Confinement of dogs in barren yards with no environmental stimulation or enrichment predisposes to pica and especially to coprophagia. • Early weaned Oriental breed cats on low roughage diets with no access to prey or grass are most at risk for wool eating.

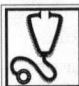

DIAGNOSIS

DIFFERENTIAL DIAGNOSIS
Pica is most often a behavioral abnormality or a secondary effect of disease. Abnormalities found on a physical laboratory evaluation should be worked up. If no abnormalities are found, the problem is probably behavioral.

CBC/BIOCHEMISTRY/URINALYSIS
Used to rule out anemia and to gain a general assessment of organ function. If indicated (e.g., abnormal liver enzyme activity, low BUN, and ammonia biurate crystals on urinalysis), hepatic function tests should be performed.

OTHER LABORATORY TESTS
Hepatic function tests (bile acids and ammonia) can be performed to rule out portocaval or portosystemic shunt. Exocrine pancreatic insufficiency can be diagnosed by measuring serum trypsin-like immunoreactivity (TLI)

IMAGING
Survey abdominal radiography and abdominal ultrasonography may be useful in ruling out some foreign bodies in the gastrointestinal tract.

OTHER DIAGNOSTIC PROCEDURES
Endoscopic examination of the upper gastrointestinal tract rules in or out foreign material in this location.

TREATMENT
• See treatment for the specific disease when a pathologic cause has been identified.
• When there is no pathologic cause, the treatment principles are threefold:
1) limit access to the nonfood items to prevent ingestion
2) find a safe substitute that the animal can ingest with impunity
3) change the animals's motivation to ingest the non-food item.
• Dogs can be kept indoors and walked on leashes to prevent rock chewing and coprophagia. Plastic can be removed from the cat's environment and woolen clothes safely stored away.
• Applying a pungent or bitter taste to objects may discourage consumption. Cats may be given a high roughage diet, tough meat to chew, or a garden of grass or catnip to graze upon. Providing wool fabric which the cat can eat with impunity may reduce the cat's tendency to eat indigestible synthetic materials.
• The animal's motivation can be changed by administration of psychoactive drugs or punishment.

MEDICATIONS

DRUGS AND FLUIDS
• Clomipramine (1 mg/kg q24h)—a tricyclic antidepressant, serotonin reuptake blocker
• Cyproheptadine (4 mg/cat q24h)—an appetite stimulant, serotonin antagonist

CONTRAINDICATIONS N/A

PRECAUTIONS N/A

POSSIBLE INTERACTIONS N/A

ALTERNATE DRUGS N/A

FOLLOW-UP

PATIENT MONITORING
The owner should be contacted in 10 days-2 weeks to determine if the pica has abated and if he or she has complied with the treatments suggested. If the problem has not markedly improved by dietary and management changes, medication should be prescribed.

POSSIBLE COMPLICATIONS
Gastrointestinal complications

MISCELLANEOUS

ASSOCIATED CONDITIONS N/A

AGE-RELATED FACTORS
Chewing and sometimes swallowing objects is normal puppy behavior. The mouth is the best instrument the dog can use to feel and taste its environment during its exploratory period.

ZOONOTIC POTENTIAL N/A

PREGNANCY N/A

SYNONYMS
• Depraved appetite • Wool chewing
• Wool sucking • Coprophagia

SEE ALSO
Gastrointestinal Foreign Bodies

ABBREVIATIONS N/A

References

Bradshaw JWS. The behaviour of the domestic cat. Oxon, U.K.: C.A.B. International, 1992;219.

Houpt KA. Domestic animal behavior for veterinarians and animal scientists. Ames, IA: Iowa State University Press, 1991;408.

Author Katherine A. Houpt
Consulting Editor Brent D. Jones

POISONING (INTOXICATION)

BASICS

- Acutely ill animals are often diagnosed as "poisoned" when no other diagnosis is obvious. The clinician should direct efforts toward stabilizing the patient. The diagnosis should be made and preexisting conditions determined after initial control of clinical signs.
- The goals of treatment include emergency intervention and prevention of further exposure, prevention of further absorption, application of specific antidotes, hastening elimination of the absorbed toxicant, supportive measures, and client education.
- Suspected toxic materials and specimens might be valuable from a medicolegal aspect. A proper chain of physical evidence and good medical records should be kept in cases of suspected intoxication.
- Initial instructions provided to the client may be beneficial to subsequent treatment:
- Transport the affected animal to a veterinarian as soon as possible.
- When transportation is delayed, protect the animal by keeping the animal warm and avoiding any stress.
- Onlookers should be warned about the condition of the animal; it may be desirable to muzzle the animal.
- Transport uncontaminated vomitus and suspected toxic materials and their containers to the hospital. Clean plastic containers or glass jars should be used for the specimens.
- Valuable time can be saved by applying the appropriate treatment for a suspected or known intoxicant.

DIAGNOSIS

DIFFERENTIAL DIAGNOSIS

- Animals come in contact with a vast array of toxicants, often making a definitive diagnosis difficult. Refer to the appendix for a list of toxicants arranged by body system affected.
- The National Poison Control Center, state diagnostic laboratories, and local poison control centers are great resources in toxicologic emergencies. They are of great value to the clinician in cases of suspected intoxication, especially when labels or containers accompany the acutely ill animal.
- When the suspected compound and the signs exhibited by the animal do not concur, the signs should be treated and the label should be disregarded.
- The diagnosis should be confirmed by chemical analysis, even though this may occur after the fact. An accurate diagnosis, as well as detailed records, may help the veterinarian with other animals affected by the same intoxicant. Detailed records also are invaluable in medicolegal proceedings.

TREATMENT

SUPPORTIVE TREATMENT

Important in animals with intoxication:
- Control of body temperature
- Maintenance of respiratory and cardiovascular function
- Control of acid-base imbalances
- Alleviation of pain
- Control of CNS disorders (See specific chapters for information.)

EMERGENCY TREATMENT

- Establishment of a patient airway
- Artificial respiration
- Cardiac massage (external or internal)
- Application of defibrillation techniques
- After patient stabilization, the clinician can proceed with more specific therapeutic measures.

PREVENTING ABSORPTION

- Preventing absorption of additional toxicant(s) is a major factor in treating animals with intoxication.
- Removal of the animal from the affected environment is a necessary first step.
- The judicious use of emetics, gastric lavage techniques, adsorbents, and cathartics aids in preventing further absorption of ingested toxic materials.

Washing Skin
- If an external toxicant is involved, prevention of further absorption may entail washing the animal's skin to remove the noxious agent.
- Caution must be exercised to avoid contamination of persons handling the animal.

Emetics
- Of little value if 4 hours have elapsed since the animal ingested the toxicant, since most material will have passed to the duodenum, rendering emesis ineffective in its removal.
- Emesis should not be induced in unconscious or severely depressed animals or after ingestion of strong acids, alkalis, petroleum distillates, tranquilizers, or other antiemetics.
- Apomorphine is the most effective and most reliable emetic available for use in dogs and cats. However, its availability at any given time is unknown. The effective dosage in small animals is 0.04 mg/kg IV or 0.08 mg/kg IM or SC. Adverse clinical signs caused by apomorphine may be effectively controlled by an appropriate narcotic antagonist injected IV (e.g., naloxone, 0.04 mg/kg).
- Ipecac has little efficacy and it should never be used when activated charcoal is part of the therapeutic regimen.
- Xylazine administered IV has been used with some success as an emetic in dogs and cats.

Activated Charcoal
- Does not detoxify toxicants but prevents absorption of a toxicant if properly used.

- Highly absorptive of many toxicants including organophosphate insecticides, other insecticides, rodenticides, mercuric chloride, strychnine, other alkaloids (e.g., morphine and atropine), barbiturates, and ethylene glycol. Ineffective against cyanide.
- Administration of activated charcoal in combination with emetics increases the efficacy of toxicant elimination by emesis.
- A bathtub or some other easily cleansed area is the best location to use when administering activated charcoal to small animals.
- Dosage—1 to 5 gm/kg body weight in a concentration of 1 g charcoal/5-10 ml water 3 to 4 times a day for 2 to 3 days
- Some charcoal should remain in the stomach and be followed by a cathartic to prevent desorption of the toxicant. A cathartic of sodium sulfate should be administered 30 minutes after administration of the charcoal.

Gastric Lavage
- Gastric lavage is an effective means of emptying the stomach. Use the largest stomach tube possible. A good rule is to use the same size stomach tube as the cuffed endotracheal tube (1 mm = 3 French).
- The volume of water or lavage solution to be used for each washing is 5 to 10 ml/kg body weight. The infusion and aspiration cycle of the lavage solution should be repeated 10 to 15 times. Activated charcoal in the solution enhances the effectiveness of this procedure.
- Some precautions to be taken with this technique:
  1. Use low pressure to prevent forcing the toxicant into the duodenum.
  2. Reduce the infused volume in obviously weakened stomachs (e.g., in an animal that has ingested a caustic or corrosive).
  3. Make sure not to force the stomach tube through either the esophagus or the stomach wall.

Oils
- Mineral oil or vegetable oil is of value if lipid-soluble toxicants are ingested.
- Mineral oil (liquid petrolatum) is inert and is less likely to be absorbed.
- Use oils with a cathartic.
- Sodium sulfate (1 g/kg PO) is a more efficient agent for evacuation of the bowel than is magnesium sulfate, and it is the preferable agent to use with activated charcoal and mineral oil.

Enemas
- A colonic lavage or high enema may be of value to hasten the elimination of toxicants from the gastrointestinal tract.
- Warm water with castile soap makes an excellent enema solution.
- Several commercially available enema preparations are available that act as osmotic agents.
- Care should be taken to avoid the induction of dehydration and electrolyte imbalances with overzealous treatment.
- Hexachlorophene soaps should be avoided in cats.

ENHANCING ELIMINATION
• Absorbed toxicants are generally excreted by the kidneys.
• Some toxicants are excreted by other routes (ie, via bile, feces, lungs, and other body secretions).
• Renal excretion can be manipulated in many animals.
• Urinary excretion of toxicants may be enhanced by the use of diuretics or altering the pH of the urine.

Diuretics
• The use of diuretics to enhance urinary excretion of toxicants requires maintenance of adequate renal function.
• If a minimum urine flow cannot be established, peritoneal dialysis must be performed.
• The diuretics of choice are mannitol (1.0-2.0 gm/kg/ IV q6h)and furosemide (5 mg/kg q6h-q8h)

Manipulation of urine pH
• Alteration of the urinary pH to expedite the excretion of toxicants and foreign chemicals is a classic pharmacologic technique.
• Acidic compounds remain ionized in alkaline urine, while alkaline compounds remain ionized in acidic urine.

• For long-term urinary acidification, ammonium chloride (200 mg/kg/day PO in divided doses) and ethylenediamine dihydrochloride (1 to 2 tablets q8h for the average-sized dog) are available. Physiologic saline is a good, rapid, urinary acidifying agent.
• Sodium bicarbonate (5 mEq/kg/h) may be used as an alkalinizing agent.

Peritoneal dialysis
• Indicated when an intoxicated animal exhibits oliguria or anuria.
• Also indicated for simple removal of absorbed toxicants in animals with normal renal function.
• The pH of the dialyzing solutions can be altered to maintain the ionized state of the offending compound.

MEDICATIONS
Specific antidotes or procedures are available for the more common animal toxicants. These specific antidotal procedures are presented in the sections on specific toxicants.

FOLLOW-UP
Specific monitoring varies according to the toxicant, and the animal's signs and laboratory abnormalities.

MISCELLANEOUS
ABBREVIATIONS N/A

References
Bailey EM, Garland T. Toxicologic Emergencies. In: Murtaugh RJ, Kaplan PM, eds. Veterinary emergency and critical care medicine. St. Louis: Mosby Year Book, 1992;427-452.
Authors E. Murl Bailey and Tom Garland
Consulting Editor Gary D. Osweiler

POLYPHAGIA

 ## BASICS

DEFINITION
The act of eating more times than normal

Pathophysiology
When polyphagia is secondary to diabetes mellitus, the pathophysiology is a lack of insulin causing a paradoxical intracellular glucoprivation despite hyperglycemia. Glucoprivation is one of the stimuli of feeding. The mechanism involved in steroid-induced hyperphagia is unknown. Many diseases characterized by hyperphagia (e.g., hyperthyroidism) increase the energy output of the animal so it must eat more to maintain energy homeostasis.

Systems Affected
Musculoskeletal—overweight patients are susceptible to arthritis and other orthopedic problems.

SIGNALMENT
• Dogs and cats • Young animals are most commonly affected

SIGNS
• Eating more frequently and a greater quantity than normal • Patients may have an excessive amount of body fat, but those with a medical problem causing the polyphagia (e.g., hyperthyroidism, diabetes mellitus, and exocrine pancreatic insufficiency) may be thin.

CAUSES
Physiologic
• Pregnancy • Lactation • Growth
• Response to a cold environment or exercise

Pathologic
• Diabetes mellitus • Insulin shock or insulinoma • Hyperthyroidism • Hyperadrenocorticism • Growth hormone secreting pituitary tumor • Exocrine pancreatic insufficiency
• Lymphocytic cholangitis (cats) • Portocaval shunt • Hepatic or feline spongiform encephalopathy • Neoplasm of the brain
• Megaesophagus • Lymphocytic plasmocytic enteritis • Intestinal neoplasia • Infectious peritonitis

Iatrogenic
Administration of corticosteroid, progestin, or benzodiazepine drugs

RISK FACTORS
See Causes

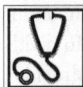 ## DIAGNOSIS

DIFFERENTIAL DIAGNOSIS
A variety of medical problems (see Causes) and behavioral abnormalities can cause polyphagia. A complete behavioral history should be taken to determine the possible cause of compulsive eating (e.g., the addition of a new animal or person to the household).

CBC/BIOCHEMISTRY/URINALYSIS
• Neutrophilia, monocytosis, lymphopenia, and eosinopenia suggest hyperadrenocorticism. • Hyperglycemia in patients with hyperadrenocorticism or diabetes mellitus
• High ALP activity in patients with hyperadrenocorticism, hyperthyroidism (cats), or liver disease and those receiving corticosteroids • High ALT in patients with hyperthyroidism (cats) or liver disease • Low serum proteins may indicate a protein losing enteropathy. • Low BUN may indicate a portocaval shunt or liver disease • Ammonia biurate and urate crystals may indicate portocaval shunts and liver disease • Glucosuria or ketonuria suggests diabetes mellitus

OTHER LABORATORY TESTS
• Serum trypsin-like immunoreactivity (TLI) to rule in or out exocrine pancreatic insufficiency. • Serum T_3 and T_4 and antibodies to T_3 and T_4 to rule in or out hyperthyroidism
• ACTH stimulation or dexamethasone suppression test to rule in or out hyperadrenocorticism

IMAGING
• Abdominal radiology and ultrasonography may identify hepatomegaly, which is associated with hyperadrenocorticism, diabetes mellitus, corticosteroid administration, and hepatopathies. • Microhepatica may indicate portocaval shunt. • An adrenal mass may indicate hyperadrenocorticism. • Thick bowel walls are compatible with infiltrative intestinal disease.

OTHER DIAGNOSTIC PROCEDURES
Endoscopy of the upper gastrointestinal tract indicated to rule out an enteropathy

 ## TREATMENT
The principle is to determine if the cause of polyphagia is medical or iatrogenic. If a new pet or person has been added to the household, polyphagia may be associated with social facilitation. Most animals will eat more in the presence of another animal. This is particularly true for dogs, which may compete for the same food source. Treatment is relatively simple: limit the amount of food available to the dog so that the animal maintains a normal body weight. A low-calorie diet can be given or the animal can be made to work for its food. Chew toys can be used as a substitute for food. If there is polyphagia without weight gain, a medical problem is more likely and the animal should be allowed to eat more to balance its energy input with its energy output.

MEDICATIONS

DRUGS AND FLUIDS
If the feeding appears to be compulsive, drugs such as clomipramine or amitriptyline (1 mg/kg PO q24h) can be used.

CONTRAINDICATIONS N/A

PRECAUTIONS N/A

POSSIBLE INTERACTIONS N/A

ALTERNATE DRUGS N/A

FOLLOW-UP

Care must be taken, especially in cats, that offering only a low-calorie diet does not lead to anorexia and consequent hepatic lipidosis.

MISCELLANEOUS

ASSOCIATED CONDITIONS N/A

AGE-RELATED FACTORS N/A

ZOONOTIC POTENTIAL N/A

PREGNANCY
Polyphagia is a normal physiologic response to pregnancy.

SYNONYMS
• Hyperphagia • Eating disorder

SEE ALSO
See Causes

ABBREVIATIONS N/A

References

Bradshaw JWS. The behaviour of the domestic cat. Oxon, U.K.: C.A.B. International, 1992;219.

Houpt KA. Domestic animal behavior for veterinarians and animal scientists. Ames, IA: Iowa State University Press, 1991;408.

Author Katherine A. Houpt

Consulting Editor Brent D. Jones

POLYURIA AND POLYDIPSIA

BASICS

DEFINITION
• Polyuria is greater than normal urine production (dogs, > 45 ml/kg/day; cats, > 40 ml/kg/day) • Polydipsia is greater than normal water consumption (dogs, > 90 ml/kg/day; cats, > 45 ml/kg/day).

Pathophysiology
• Urine production and water consumption (thirst) are controlled largely by interactions between the kidneys, pituitary gland, and hypothalamus. Volume receptors within the cardiac atria and aortic arch also influence thirst and urine production. Polyuria occurs when the quantity of functional antidiuretic hormone (ADH) synthesized in the hypothalamus or released from the posterior pituitary is limited or the kidneys fail to respond normally to ADH. Polydipsia occurs when the thirst center in the anterior hypothalamus is stimulated. • In most patients, polydipsia occurs as a compensatory response to polyuria to maintain hydration. In such instances, the patient's plasma tends to become relatively hypertonic, activating thirst mechanisms. Occasionally, polydipsia is the primary process with polyuria as the compensatory response. In this situation, the patient's plasma becomes relatively hypotonic due to excessive water intake, and ADH secretion is reduced, resulting in polyuria.

Systems Affected
• Renal/urologic—kidneys • Endocrine/metabolic—pituitary gland and hypothalamus • Cardiovascular—alterations in "effective" circulating fluid volume

SIGNALMENT
• Congenital conditions (e.g., central diabetes insipidus, nephrogenic diabetes insipidus, portal-vascular anomaly, and certain renal diseases), hypoadrenocorticism, and some causes for primary polydipsia predominantly affect young dogs • Renal failure, hyperadrenocorticism, hyperthyroidism, and neoplastic disorders, affecting the pituitary and hypothalamus, predominantly affect middle-aged and older dogs and cats.

SIGNS N/A

CAUSES
• Primary polyuria caused by impaired renal response to ADH—renal failure, hyperadrenocorticism (dogs), hyperthyroidism (cats), pyelonephritis, hypoadrenocorticism (i.e., mineralocorticoid and glucocorticoid deficiency), pyometra, hepatic failure, hypercalcemia, hypokalemia, renal medullary solute washout, dietary protein restriction, drugs, congenital nephrogenic diabetes insipidus
• Primary polyuria caused by osmotic diuresis—diabetes mellitus, primary renal glucosuria, postobstructive diuresis, some diuretics (e.g., mannitol and furosemide), ingestion or administration of large quantities of solute (e.g., sodium chloride or glucose), and hypersomatotropism • Primary polyuria caused by ADH deficiency—idiopathic, traumatic, neoplastic, or congenital origin central diabetes insipidus; some drugs (e.g., alcohol and phenytoin) • Primary polydipsia—behavioral problem, organic disease of the anterior hypothalamic thirst center of neoplastic, traumatic, and inflammatory origin, pyrexia, and pain

RISK FACTORS
• Renal or liver disease • Selected endocrine and electrolyte disorders • Administration of diuretics, corticosteroids, and anticonvulsants • High-sodium, low-protein diet designed for dissolution of struvite uroliths in dogs • Young, hyperactive large-breed dogs appear to be at higher than normal risk for primary polydipsia

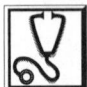

DIAGNOSIS

DIFFERENTIAL DIAGNOSIS

Differentiating Similar Signs
Differentiate polyuria from more than normal frequency of urination (pollakiuria). Pollakiuria is often associated with dysuria, stranguria, or hematuria. Patients with polyuria void large quantities of urine; patients with pollakiuria typically void small quantities of urine. Confirm polyuria/polydipsia by measuring 24-hour water intake or urine output (a 3- to 5-day test is used to enhance reliability). Alternatively, measuring urine specific gravity may provide evidence of adequate urine concentrating ability (dogs, ≥ 1.030; cats, ≥ 1.035), which rules out polyuria/polydipsia.

Differentiating Causes
• Renal failure, hyperadrenocorticism, and diabetes mellitus account for most cases of polyuria/polydipsia in dogs. Renal failure, hyperthyroidism, and diabetes mellitus account for the most cases of polyuria/polydipsia in cats. Rule out these conditions before less common conditions are sought • Progressive weight loss—consider renal failure, diabetes mellitus, hyperthyroidism, hepatic failure, pyometra, pyelonephritis, and malignancy-induced hypercalcemia • Polyphagia—consider diabetes mellitus, hyperthyroidism, and hyperadrenocorticism • Bilateral alopecia and other cutaneous alterations—consider hyperadrenocorticism and other endocrinologic disorders • Uriniferous breath and uremic stomatitis—consider renal failure • Vomiting—consider renal failure, hypoadrenocorticism, pyelonephritis, hepatic failure, hypercalcemia, hypokalemia, and diabetes mellitus. Occasionally, vomiting occurs after rapid consumption of a very large quantity of water. • Recent estrus (within the previous 2 months) in a middle-aged, intact female—consider pyometra • Abdominal distension—consider hepatic failure, hyperadrenocorticism, pyometra, and nephrotic syndrome • Lymphadenopathy or anal sac mass—consider hypercalcemia of malignancy • Palpable thyroid nodule—consider hyperthyroidism • Hypertensive retinopathy—consider renal failure, hyperthyroidism, and hyperadrenocorticism • Behavioral or neurologic disorder—consider hepatic failure and pituitary disorders such as primary polydipsia • Very marked polydipsia wherein patients will almost continuously seek and consume water from any source—consider primary polydipsia, central diabetes insipidus, and congenital nephrogenic diabetes insipidus

CBC/BIOCHEMISTRY/URINALYSIS
• Serum sodium concentration may help differentiate primary polyuria from primary polydipsia. (Measured serum osmolality is the preferred test. Calculated serum osmolality is not an acceptable alternative) • Relative hypernatremia suggests primary polyuria (values typically trend to or exceed the high end of the normal range) • Hyponatremia suggests primary polydipsia (values typically trend to or decline below the low end of the normal range), except in animals with hypoadrenocorticism, which have hyponatremia and primary polyuria. • Azotemia is consistent with renal causes for polyuria/polydipsia, but may also indicate dehydration, resulting from inadequate compensatory polydipsia. Unexpectedly low BUN suggests hepatic failure. • High hepatic enzyme activities are consistent with hyperadrenocorticism (especially when value for ALP is greater than that for ALT), hyperthyroidism, hepatic failure, pyometra, and diabetes mellitus. Some drugs that promote polyuria/polydipsia (e.g., anticonvulsants and corticosteroids) may elevate hepatic enzyme activities. • Persistent hyperglycemia is consistent with diabetes mellitus. • Hyperkalemia, particularly if associated with hyponatremia, suggests hypoadrenocorticism or treatment with potassium-sparing diuretics. • Hypercalcemia and hypokalemia can cause, or occur in association with other diseases that cause, polyuria/polydipsia (e.g., chronic renal failure may be associated with both; hypoadrenocorticism may be associated with hypercalcemia). • Hypercalcemia induces polyuria only when it results from high ionized calcium concentration. • Hypoalbuminemia supports renal or hepatic causes of polyuria/polydipsia. • Neutrophilia is consistent with pyelonephritis, pyometra, hyperadrenocorticism, and corticosteroid administration. • Urine specific gravity values between 1.001 and 1.003 are particularly suggestive of primary polydipsia, central diabetes insipidus, or congenital nephrogenic diabetes insipidus. Glucosuria supports a diagnosis of diabetes mellitus or renal glucosuria. Pyuria, WBC casts, and bacteriuria should prompt consideration of pyelonephritis.

OTHER LABORATORY TESTS

• ACTH stimulation or dexamethasone suppression tests to rule out hyperadrenocorticism in middle-aged to old dogs in which initial findings do not explain polyuria/polydipsia. • Serum thyroxine concentration to rule out hyperthyroidism in middle-aged and old cats. • Urine culture—chronic pyelonephritis cannot be conclusively ruled out by absence of pyuria or bacteriuria.
• Cytologic examination of lymph node aspirate may provide evidence of lymphosarcoma, which induces polyuria by hypercalcemia or direct infiltration of renal tissues.

IMAGING

Abdominal survey radiography and ultrasonography may provide additional evidence of renal (e.g., primary renal disease and urinary obstruction), hepatic (e.g., microhepatica, portal vascular anomaly, and hepatic infiltrate), adrenal (e.g., adrenal mass and bilateral adrenal hypertrophy suggestive of hyperadrenocorticism), or uterine (e.g., pyometra) disorders that can contribute to polyuria/polydipsia.

OTHER DIAGNOSTIC PROCEDURES

Modified Water Deprivation with Antidiureitc Hormone (ADH) Response Testing (see Appendix)

• Differentiates central diabetes insipidus from primary polydipsia and congenital diabetes insipidus. Rule out other causes of polyuria/polydipsia before proceeding.
• Most useful for patients with marked polyuria/polydipsia and hyposthenuric urine
• Water deprivation testing is contraindicated in dehydrated and azotemic patients; however, ADH response testing may be safely performed in these patients. • Patients that concentrate urine adequately in response to water deprivation are presumed to have primary polydipsia. • Patients that fail to concentrate urine adequately in response to water deprivation but further concentrate their urine in response to administration of exogenous ADH have central diabetes insipidus.
• Patients that fail to concentrate urine adequately in response to water deprivation and also fail to further concentrate urine in response to administration of exogenous ADH have nephrogenic diabetes insipidus.

TREATMENT

• Polyuria/polydipsia rarely causes serious medical problems for the patient if free access to water is provided and the patient is willing and able to drink. Until the mechanism of polyuria is understood, it is important to discourage owners from limiting access to water. Treatment is directed at the underlying cause for polyuria/polydipsia.
• Primary polydipsia—primary polydipsia is treated by restricting water intake. Water intake should be limited to a normal daily volume. It may be necessary to gradually reduce water intake over days to weeks in order to avoid undesirable behavior events such as excessive barking, urine consumption, or bizarre behavior. The patient should be closely monitored to avoid inadvertently inducing dehydration. Salt (1 gm/30 kg PO q12h) or sodium bicarbonate (0.6 gm/30 kg PO q12h) may be given to help reestablish the renal medullary solute gradient. Behavior modification may be considered when water restriction alone is unsuccessful.

MEDICATIONS

DRUGS AND FLUIDS

• Free access to water should be provided for all polyuric patients. When conditions limit oral intake or the patient is dehydrated, fluids are to be provided parenterally.
• Fluid selection is based on the underlying cause for fluid loss. In most patients, lactated Ringer's solution is an acceptable replacement fluid.
• When dehydration has resulted from withholding water, or when urine is hyposthenuric, providing 5% dextrose in water orally or parenterally may be preferred to lactated Ringer's solution.

CONTRAINDICATIONS

Antidiuretic hormone (or any of its synthetic analogs such as DDAVP) should not be administered to patients with primary polydipsia because of the risk of inducing water intoxication.

PRECAUTIONS

Until renal and hepatic failure have been excluded as potential causes for polyuria/polydipsia, use caution in administering any drug eliminated via these pathways.

POSSIBLE INTERACTIONS N/A

ALTERNATE DRUGS N/A

FOLLOW-UP

PATIENT MONITORING

• Hydration status by clinical assessment and serial evaluation of body weight. • Monitoring fluid intake and urine output also provides a useful baseline for assessing adequacy of treatment.

POSSIBLE COMPLICATIONS

Dehydration

MISCELLANEOUS

ASSOCIATED CONDITIONS

• Bacterial urinary tract infection. These patients appear to be at particular risk of developing urinary tract infection as a consequence of urinary catheterization. • Urinary incontinence may develop in dogs with concurrent urethral sphincter hypotonus, presumably due to excessive bladder filling associated with polyuria.

AGE RELATED FACTORS N/A

ZOONOTIC POTENTIAL N/A

PREGNANCY N/A

SYNONYMS N/A

SEE ALSO

Renal failure, chronic and acute; congenital/developmental renal disorders, pyelonephritis, urinary tract obstruction, Fanconi's syndrome, hyperadrenocorticism, hypoadrenocorticism, hyperthyroidism, pyometra, hypercalcemia, hypokalemia, diabetes mellitus, and diabetes insipidus.

ABBREVIATIONS

ADH = antidiuretic hormone

References

Lorenz MD: Polydipsia and polyuria. In: Lorenz MD, Cornelius LM, eds. Small animal medical diagnosis. Philadelphia: JB Lippincott, 1993:39-51.
Meric, SM: Polyuria and polydipsia. In: Ettinger SJ, Feldman EC, eds. Textbook of veterinary internal medicine. Philadelphia: WB Saunders, 1995:159-163.
Author David J. Polzin
Consulting Editors Larry G. Adams and Carl A. Osborne

PROSTATOMEGALY

 BASICS

DEFINITION

Abnormally large prostate gland as determined by rectal or abdominal palpation or by abdominal radiography or prostatic ultrasonography; can be symmetrical or asymmetrical, painful or nonpainful. Normal size varies with age, body size, castration status, and breed so that determination of enlargement is subjective.

Pathophysiology

Epithelial cell hyperplasia or hypertrophy (e.g., benign prostatic hyperplasia), neoplasia of prostatic epithelium or stroma, cystic change within the prostatic parenchyma, or inflammatory cell infiltration (e.g., acute and chronic bacterial prostatitis and prostatic abscess)

Systems Affected

- Renal/Urologic
- Reproductive

SIGNALMENT

- Typically, middle-aged to older male dogs
- Benign prostatic hyperplasia not found in neutered dogs
- Bacterial prostatitis uncommon in neutered dogs
- Neutered dogs with prostatomegaly—suspect neoplasia

SIGNS

- Maybe none
- Straining to defecate
- Ribbonlike stools
- Dysuria
- Urethral outflow obstruction

CAUSES

- Benign prostatic hyperplasia
- Squamous metaplasia
- Adenocarcinoma
- Transitional cell carcinoma
- Sarcoma
- Metastatic neoplasia
- Acute bacterial prostatitis
- Prostatic abscess
- Chronic bacterial prostatitis
- Prostatic cyst

RISK FACTORS

- Castration lowers the risk of benign prostatic hyperplasia and bacterial prostatitis.
- Castration lowers the risk of adenocarcinoma.

 DIAGNOSIS

DIFFERENTIAL DIAGNOSIS

- Benign prostatic hyperplasia typically causes nonpainful symmetrical enlargement of the prostate gland.
- Primary or metastatic neoplasia typically causes painful, nonsymmetrical enlargement of the prostate gland; weight loss, impaired appetite, and rear limb weakness observed in some patients.
- Acute bacterial prostatitis typically causes slight to moderate symmetrical or nonsymmetrical enlargement of the prostate gland with prostatic pain; fever, impaired appetite, rear limb weakness, and painful abdomen observed in some patients.
- Chronic bacterial prostatitis causes signs similar to those seen in animals with acute prostatitis or those related to recurrent lower urinary tract infection (e.g., dysuria and hematuria).
- Prostatic abscess may cause signs similar to those in patients with acute or chronic prostatitis; abscess rupture causes fever and caudal abdominal pain.
- Prostatic cysts may cause a palpable caudal abdominal mass, straining to urinate, or straining to defecate; patient may also be asymptomatic.

CBC/BIOCHEMISTRY/URINALYSIS

- CBC normal in patients with benign prostatic hyperplasia
- Leukocytosis in patients with acute and chronic (occasionally) bacterial prostatitis, prostatic abscess, and prostatic neoplasia (occasionally)
- High bilirubin and ALP in some patients with prostatic abscess
- Urinalysis normal or hematuria in patients with benign prostatic hyperplasia
- Pyuria, hematuria, proteinuria, bacteriuria in patients with bacterial prostatitis
- Pyuria, hematuria, proteinuria and, occasionally, neoplastic cells in dogs with prostatic neoplasia

OTHER LABORATORY TESTS

Serum prostatic esterase concentration is high in dogs with benign prostatic hyperplasia.

IMAGING

Radiographic Findings

- Prostatomegaly
- Prostatic mineralization more likely in dogs with prostatic neoplasia

Ultrasonographic Findings

- Abscess or cyst—hypoechoic or anaechoic lesions with distal enhancement
- Acute bacterial prostatitis—uniform prostatic echogenicity
- Benign prostatic hyperplasia—uniform prostatic echogenicity; small fluid-filled cysts in some patients
- Chronic bacterial prostatitis—focal or diffuse hyperechogenicity
- Prostatic neoplasia—focal to multifocal areas of coalescing echogenicity and acoustic shadowing (if mineralization is present)

OTHER DIAGNOSTIC PROCEDURES

- Examination of prostatic fluid obtained by ejaculation or prostatic massage may reveal changes similar to those seen on urinalysis.
- Bacterial culture of prostatic fluid typically reveals >10,000 bacteria/ml in dogs with bacterial prostatitis.
- Transrectal aspiration biopsy (specimen obtained by a Franzen needle guide) or urethral catheter biopsy reveals neoplastic cells in some dogs with prostatic carcinoma.
- Needle biopsy with ultrasound guidance allows visualization of the area to be sampled and increases the likelihood of obtaining a diagnostic sample. Care should be taken to avoid rupturing a prostatic abscess.

 TREATMENT

- Varies with the cause of prostatomegaly
- Surgical castration is indicated in symptomatic dogs with benign prostatic hyperplasia and after resolution of acute infection in dogs with bacterial prostatitis
- Surgical drainage is indicated in dogs with prostatic abscess or large prostatic cysts
- External beam radiotherapy may provide palliative benefit in patients with prostatic carcinoma

 MEDICATIONS

DRUGS AND FLUIDS

Benign prostatic hyperplasia

If castration is not acceptable, the following drugs may produce a temporary response:
- Finasteride (5mg/day)
- Megestrol acetate (0.11 mg/kg PO daily for 3 weeks)
- Medroxyprogesterone (3mg/kg SQ)

Bacterial Prostatitis

Choose antibiotics on the basis of antibacterial sensitivity testing of the isolated organism and ability of the antibiotic to diffuse into prostatic fluid in therapeutic concentrations; good choices for latter include trimethoprim/sulfa, chloramphenicol and enrofloxacin.

Prostatic Carcinoma

Chemotherapy has not been proved beneficial. Combination therapy with cyclophosphamide and doxorubicin can be considered.

CONTRAINDICATIONS N/A

PRECAUTIONS

Chronic administration of megestrol acetate or medroxyprogesterone can cause diabetes mellitus.

POSSIBLE INTERACTIONS N/A

ALTERNATIVE DRUGS N/A

 FOLLOW-UP

PATIENT MONITORING

- Abdominal radiographs or prostatic ultrasonography to assess efficacy of treatment in animals with benign prostatic hyperplasia, prostatic carcinoma, or bacterial prostatitis

• Urine and prostatic fluid culture to access efficacy of treatment in animals with bacterial prostatitis

POSSIBLE COMPLICATIONS
• Urethral obstruction
• Rectal obstruction

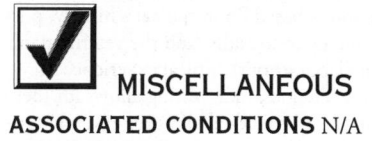

MISCELLANEOUS

ASSOCIATED CONDITIONS N/A

AGE-RELATED FACTORS
Prostatic carcinoma typically diagnosed in 8- to 10-year old dogs

ZOONOTIC POTENTIAL N/A

PREGNANCY N/A

SYNONYMS N/A

SEE ALSO
• Adenocarcinoma, Prostate
• Benign Prostatic Hyperplasia
• Prostatic Cysts
• Prostatitis and Prostatic Abscess

ABBREVIATIONS N/A

References

Barsanti, JA, Finco, DR. Canine prostatic diseases. In: Ettinger SJ, ed. Textbook of veterinary internal medicine. Philadelphia, WB Saunders, 1989:1662-1685.

Kay ND. Diseases of the prostate gland. In: Birchard SJ, Sherding RD, eds. Saunders manual of small animal practice. Philadelphia: WB Saunders, 1994:865-871.

Author Jeffrey S. Klausner
Consulting Editors Larry G. Adams and Carl A. Osborne

PRURITUS

BASICS

DEFINITION
The sensation that provokes the desire to scratch, rub, chew or lick. Pruritus is an indicator of inflamed skin.

Pathophysiology
A specific end-organ for pruritus has not been found. The sensation of itch is conducted by A delta fibers and C fibers of the peripheral nervous system to the dorsal root of the spinal cord. The axons, some of which cross over, ascend via the lateral spinothalamic tract and synapse in the caudal thalmus and then to the sensory cortex. Other factors can modify the perception of pruritus at this level.

Systems Affected
Skin/Exocrine - in severe cases, the mental state of the animal may also be affected.

SIGNALMENT
Highly variable depending on the underlying etiology.

SIGNS
The act of scratching, licking, biting or chewing; in some animals, evidence of self trauma and cutaneous inflammation may be necessary to make the diagnosis if the history is incomplete. In cats, which can be secretive lickers, alopecia without inflammation, may be the only sign.

CAUSES
• Parasitic—fleas, scabies, demodex, otodectes, notoedres, cheyletiella, trombicula, lice, pelodera, endoparasite migration
• Allergic—parasite allergy, atopy, food allergy, contact allergy, drug allergy, "bacterial hypersensitivity" • Bacterial/fungal: pachydermatitis • Miscellaneous—primary and secondary seborrhea, calcinosis cutis, cutaneous neoplasia, immune mediated dermatosis and endocrine dermatosis can be variably pruritic. Psychogenic diseases may also be associated with pruritus.

RISK FACTORS N/A

DIAGNOSIS

DIFFERENTIAL DIAGNOSIS
• Pruritus often causes alopecia. In most cases, a clear history of pruritus is present. Alopecia without pruritus may accompany endocrine diseases. However, some animals may excessively lick themselves without the owner's knowledge. Demodicosis, dermatophytosis, bacterial pyoderma, seborrhea, some cutaneous neoplasms, and unusual diseases such as leismaniasis may cause alopecia with varying degrees of inflamation and pruritus.
• The history is often the most important feature used to determine which tests should

be performed. Severe pruritus that constantly keeps the patient and owner awake is suggestive of scabies, flea allergy/infestation, food allergy, or a cutaneous yeast infection. All but the latter typically have an acute onset. • Uncomplicated atopy is initially a very steroid-responsive disease that manifests itself as an originally seasonal, often progressing to non-seasonal, pruritic disease with a predilection for the face, feet, ears, forelimbs, axilla, and also the rump. Flea allergic and food allergic animals are predisposed to atopy and may show similar signs.

CBC/BIOCHEMISTRY/URINALYSIS
N/A

OTHER LABORATORY TESTS N/A

IMAGING N/A

OTHER DIAGNOSTIC PROCEDURES
• Skin scrapes, epidermal cytology and dermatophyte cultures (with microscopic identification) are very useful in identifying either primary or coexisting diseases caused by parasites or other microrganisms. • Due to large number of false negatives and misinterpretations of florescence, woods lamp examinations should not be used as a sole means of diagnosing or excluding dermatophytosis.

Trial Courses Of Treatment
Scabicidal therapy or a hypoallergenic dietary trial may be appropriate in some animals.
• Canine scabies can be difficult to diagnose and skin scrapes are often negative. A trial course of therapy (lime sulfur, ivermectin) is often necessary to rule out this disease. Ivermectin should be used with caution because it has been associated with idiosyncratic reactions and death • Various tests are available for diagnosing food allergy. Most veterinary dermatologists do not recommend blood or skin tests for the diagnosis of food allergy. A properly performed hypoallergenic dietary trial is the most appropriate test for diagnosing food allergy. Diets containing certain substances such as lamb are not necessarily hypollergenic. Only diets which have undergone clinical trials confirming their hypoallergenic nature should be used during the testing period. The hypoallergenic diet should be continued until the dog improves or for a duration of 8–10 weeks. If a pet improves while eating a hypoallergenic diet, the original diet should be reintroduced and the pet monitored for the return of itching within 7–14 days. Sometimes the itching may return within a matter of hours. Reintroducing the original diet is a critical part of the test and helps prove that the improvement was due to the food and not to coincidence.

Allergy testing
• Two different methods for allergy testing exist. Skin testing, or intradermal skin testing, is similar to the allergy test being used in humans. Blood testing is a relatively new type of test which can also be done and sent to a

laboratory that performs the specialized testing. After the positive reactions identified with the allergy test are correlated with the history, the immunotherapy solution (allergy extract) can be formulated. This solution contains a mixture of specific allergens. The exact mix of allergens is different for each patient and is based upon the pet's history, positive allergy test results, and the veterinarian's (or the laboratory's) clinical experience in treating allergies. Skin testing allows for identification of individual allergens and takes into account the important allergy associated immunoglobulins (IgGd and systemic as well as localized IgE). Commercial blood tests for allergies measure only serum IgE and do not measure IgGd or localized IgE found only in the skin. Some blood tests are at a disadvantage because they test for groups or mixes of allergens. The concentration of the immunotherapy (allergy extract) solution can also vary with the type of test done and can affect the success rate. • Intradermal skin testing is the historical standard and the preferred method for allergy testing. Some veterinary dermatologists, find the combined use of both tests to be useful.

Skin Biopsy
A skin biopsy is useful when the lesions associated with pruritus are unusual and an immune-mediated disease is expected or the history and physical findings do not correlate.

TREATMENT
More than one disease can be contributing to itching. If identification and treatment for one of the causes does not result in adequate improvement, consider other causes. The use of mechanical restraint such as an Elizabethan collar can be a helpful option, but is seldom feasable in the long term.

MEDICATIONS

DRUGS AND FLUIDS

Topical Therapy
Topical therapy is helpful in mildly itchy pets. For localized areas, sprays, lotions and creams are most appropriate. If the itching involves many areas, shampoos are the preferred means of application. Colloidal oatmeal can be found in virtually all forms of topical therapy. In some cases, it is very beneficial, but its duration of effect is usually less than two days. Topical antihistamines may be found alone or in combination with other ingredients. They have not been shown to have a beneficial effect. Topical anesthetics may offer only a very short duration of effect. Antibacterial shampoos help control bacterial infections that cause itching. However, some antibacterial shampoos such as those containing benzoyl peroxide or iodine can cause

increased itching. Lime sulfer (which has a bad odor and can stain) can be antipruritic while also having antiparisitic, antibacterial, and antifungal properties. Topical steroids are probably the most useful topical medication, but there is risk involved. If used excessively, they can cause localized and systemic side effects. Hydrocortisone is the mildest and most common topical steroid. Stronger steroids such as betamethasone are usually more effective, more expensive, and have more side effects. Some topical steroid medications also contain ingredients such as alcohol which can irritate already irritated skin. In some animals, the application of any substance, including water (especially warm water), can result in an increased level of itch. Cool water is often soothing.

Systemic Therapy

• It helps to think of the three separate and individual pathways that lead to inflammation and itching. Steroids block all three pathways, but because of their side effects, drugs that help block the individual pathways should be considered.

• Antihistamines, which include drugs such as hydroxyzine, diphenhydramine, and chlorpheniramine, block only one of the three main pathways that lead to inflammation and itching.

• Fatty acids are available in powder, liquid, and capsules. They help block individual pathways that lead to inflammation, but may require 6-8 weeks of use until maximum effect is observed. Fatty acids work better as a preventative rather than stopping the inflammation once it has become a problem. They also help control dry or flaky skin which can also cause itching. Many different brand names of this type of drug are available.

• Drugs with psychogenic actions can also be helpful in controlling itch. Amitriptyline (Elevil®), a drug used as an antidepressant in humans, has rather potent antihistaminic actions in dogs and can be as beneficial as antihistamines in treating allergy induced itching. Side effects are similar to antihistamines. Flyoxetine (Prozac®) has been used successfully in treating only some dogs with "lick

granuloma" or acral lick dermatitis. Diazepam (Valium®) has also been beneficial in a few cases. However, recent reports of acute hepatotoxicity in cats should be taken into account.

• The use of drugs other than steroids to control itching is less convenient, but reduces the potential for serious side effects. If these other drugs are not totally effective in controlling clinical signs, they often help reduce the amount of steroids that are necessary to decrease itching.

CONTRAINDICATIONS

In some cases, the application of anything topically, including water and products containing alcohol, iodine, and benzoyl peroxide, can exacerbate pruritus. Cool water may be soothing. Steroids should be avoided in cases of pruritus caused by an infectious etiology.

PRECAUTIONS

Steroids are the most well known drug used to control itching but have significant long-term and not always obvious side effects. To help decrease side effects with long term use, daily administration of oral corticosteroids (including prednisone or methylprednisone) should be avoided. Steroids, used wisely, are usually safe. Short term use seldom causes serious problems. They should be avoided in cases with a history of pancreatitis, diabetes mellitus, calcinosis cutis, demodicosis, dermatophytois and other infectious diseases.

ALTERNATIVE DRUGS

In extremely rare cases, immunosupressive drugs such as azathioprine may be utilized. Because of the potential profound side effects, this should be reserved for instances where euthanasia is being considered or because all other treatment has failed.

FOLLOW-UP

PATIENT MONITORING

Patient monitoring as well as client communications are imperative. Many different unrelated diseases may contribute to pruritus

and the erradication or control of one disease does not mean that other causes cannot occur. Multiple etiologies such as flea allergy, inhalant allergy, and pyoderma are commonly present in a single patient. Elimination of the pyoderma and flea-associated disease may not be enough to significantly reduce the pruritus. Food allergy and inhalant-allergic animals may do well during the winter season with a hypoallergenic diet only to become pruritic during the warmer months in association with inhalant allergies. Patients receiving chronic steroids should be evaluated every 3-6 months for signs of iatrogenic Cushing's disease.

POSSIBLE COMPLICATIONS

Due to the chronic nature of pruritus, client frustration is common. For example, demodicosis, dermatophytosis, pyoderma, endocrine disease, or food allergy may occur spontaneously in a patient who has been suffering from a single disease such as inhallant allergies. Skin scrapes and other tests may have been negative or normal during the original workup, but that does not imply that they will remain undiagnostic. Complications are also common with chronic steroid use.

MISCELLANEOUS

AGE RELATED FACTORS N/A

ZOONOTIC POTENTIAL N/A

PREGNANCY N/A

SYNONYMS N/A

SEE ALSO See causes

ABBREVIATIONS N/A

Reference

Bevier DE. Long-term management of atopic disease in the dog. In: DeBoer DJ. ed. The Veterinary Clinics of North America Small Animal Practice: advances in clinical dermatology. Philadelphia: WB Saunders, 1995;25:1487-1505.

Author Dunbar Gram
Consulting Editor Lowell Ackerman

PTYALISM

BASICS

DEFINITION
Excessive production of saliva. Pseudoptyalism is the excessive release of saliva that has accumulated in the oral cavity.

Pathophysiology
Saliva is constantly being produced and secreted into the oral cavity from the salivary glands. Normal saliva production may appear excessive in patients with an anatomic abnormality that allows saliva to dribble out of the mouth or a condition that affects swallowing. Salivation increases as a result of excitation of the salivary nuclei in the brain stem. Stimuli that lead to this are taste and tactile sensations involving the mouth and tongue. Higher centers in the CNS can also excite or inhibit the salivary nuclei. Lesions involving the CNS as well as those of the oral cavity can cause excessive salivation. Diseases that affect the pharynx, esophagus, and gastric mucosa can also stimulate excessive production of saliva.

Systems Affected N/A

SIGNALMENT
• Dogs and cats • Young animals are more likely to have ptyalism caused by a congenital problem such as portosystemic shunt and from ingestion of a toxin, caustic agent, or foreign body. • Yorkshire terrier, Maltese terrier, Australian cattle dog, miniature schnauzer, and Irish wolfhound breeds have a relatively higher incidence of congenital portosystemic shunt. • Giant breeds such as Saint Bernard and mastiff are known for excessive drooling of saliva.

SIGNS

Historical Findings
• Anorexia—seen most often in patients with oral lesions, gastrointestinal disease, and systemic disease • Eating behavior changes—refusing to eat hard food, not chewing with the affected side in animals with unilateral lesions, holding the head in an unusual position while eating, and dropping prehended food. Any of these may be seen, especially in patients with oral disease. • Other behavioral changes—irritability, aggressiveness, and reclusiveness are common, especially in animals with a painful condition • Dysphagia—may be seen if the ptyalism causes inability to swallow • Regurgitation—in patients with esophageal disease • Vomiting— secondary to gastrointestinal or systemic disease • Pawing at the face or muzzle—in patients with oral discomfort or pain • Neurologic signs including seizures—especially in patients that have been exposed to drugs or toxins causing ptyalism; also, patient with hepatic encephalopathy

Physical Examination Findings
• Periodontal disease—may cause ptyalism due to inflammation • Stomatitis—ulceration and inflammation of many different causes is associated with ptyalism • Mass in the oral cavity • Lesions of the tongue—inflammation, ulceration, mass, and foreign body • Lesions of the oropharynx—inflammation, ulceration, and mass, especially involving the soft palate and glossopalatine arch • Blood in the saliva—suggests bleeding from the oral cavity, pharynx, or esophagus • Halitosis—caused most often by oral cavity disease but also by esophageal and gastric disease • Facial pain—caused by oral cavity or pharyngeal disease • Dysphagia—caused by oral cavity, pharyngeal, or neuromuscular disease or abnormally large retropharyngeal lymph nodes • Cranial nerve deficits—lesions of the trigeminal nerve can cause drooling due to inability to close the mouth; facial nerve palsy can cause drooling from the affected side; glossopharyngeal, vagus, and hypoglossal nerve lesions can cause a loss of the gag reflex or inability to swallow • Salivary gland problem—inflamed, enlarged, necrotic, or painful salivary glands can cause ptyalism (rare)

CAUSES

Conformational Disorder of the Lips
(seen particularly in giant-breed dogs)

Oral and Pharyngeal Diseases
• Foreign body • Neoplasm • Gingivitis or stomatitis—secondary to periodontal disease, FeLV infection in cats, viral upper respiratory infection, immune-mediated disease (e.g., pemphigus vulgaris), uremia, ingestion of a caustic agent, and burns such as those resulting from biting on an electrical cord • Neurologic or functional disorder of the pharynx

Esophageal or Gastrointestinal Disorders Metabolic Disorders
Hepatoencephalopathy—caused by congenital or acquired portosystemic shunt or hepatic failure • Hyperthermia • Uremia

Neurologic Disorders
• Rabies • Pseudorabies in dogs • Disorders that cause dysphagia • Disorders that cause facial nerve palsy or a dropped jaw • Disorders that cause seizures—ptyalism may occur during a seizure due to autonomic discharge or reduced swallowing of saliva and may be exacerbated by chomping of the jaws

Drugs and Toxins
• Those that are caustic including many household cleaning products and some common house plants • Those that have a disagreeable taste. • Those that induce hypersalivation including organophosphate compounds, cholinergic drugs, insecticides containing boric acid, pyrethrin and pyrethroid insecticides, ivermectin dogs, fluids containing benzoic acid derivatives in cats, caffeine, and illicit drugs such as amphetamines, cocaine, and opiates. • Animal venom including that from black widow spiders, Gila monsters, and North American scorpions

RISK FACTORS N/A

DIAGNOSIS

DIFFERENTIAL DIAGNOSIS
Differentiating causes of ptyalism and pseudoptyalism requires a thorough history (including vaccination status, current medications, and possible toxin exposure) and complete physical examination with special attention to the oral cavity and neck and neurologic examination.

CBC/BIOCHEMISTRY/URINALYSIS
• Results of CBC often normal. Leukocytosis in patients with immune-mediated or infectious disease. A stress leukogram is common in animals that have ingested a caustic agent or organophosphate. FeLV-infected cats may have leukopenia and nonregenerative anemia. • Results of biochemical analysis usually normal except in patients with uremia and hepatoencephalopathy.

OTHER LABORATORY TESTS
• FeLV testing is essential in cats with oral lesions. • Bile acid testing when hepatoencephalopathy is suspected. • Serum cholinesterase concentration to detect organophosphate toxicosis. • Postmortem fluorescent antibody testing of the brain if rabies is suspected.

IMAGING
• Survey radiography of the oral cavity, neck, and thorax when foreign body or neoplasm is suspected. • Ultrasonographic evaluation, portal venography, or portal scintigraphy may be helpful in diagnosing a portosystemic shunt. • Fluoroscopic evaluation of swallowing may be useful in dysphagic patients.

OTHER DIAGNOSTIC PROCEDURES
• Biopsy of mucocutaneous lesions and immunofluorescence testing when immune-mediated disease such as pemphigus vulgaris is suspected. • Cytologic examination of oral lesions or fine needle aspiration of oral mass • Biopsy of oral lesion or mass

TREATMENT
• Treat the underlying cause. (See topics pertaining to specific conditions.)
• Symptomatic treatment to reduce the flow of saliva is generally unnecessary, may be of little value to the patient, and may mask other signs of the underlying cause, resulting in a delayed diagnosis. It is only recommended when hypersalivation is prolonged and severe and, if possible, only after the underlying condition has been diagnosed.

MEDICATIONS

DRUGS AND FLUIDS
• Atropine (0.05 mg/kg PO or SQ q8h) can be given symptomatically to reduce the flow of saliva. • Petroleum jelly can be applied to areas of the face that are constantly wet from saliva to help prevent moist dermatitis.
• Astringent solutions applied for 10 minutes q8h-q12h can be used to treat any area that develops moist dermatitis.
• The most appropriate crystalloid fluid should be given IV or SQ to treat dehydration caused by prolonged or severe ptyalism.

CONTRAINDICATIONS N/A

PRECAUTIONS N/A

POSSIBLE INTERACTIONS N/A

ALTERNATE DRUGS N/A

FOLLOW-UP

PATIENT MONITORING
• Depends on the underlying cause (see Causes) • For all patients with ptyalism, it is essential to continually monitor hydration and nutritional status, especially in dysphagic or anorexic animals.

POSSIBLE COMPLICATIONS
Dehydration, moist dermatitis

MISCELLANEOUS

ASSOCIATED CONDITIONS N/A

AGE RELATED FACTORS N/A

ZOONOTIC POTENTIAL N/A

PREGNANCY N/A

SYNONYMS
• Hypersalivation • Drooling

SEE ALSO
• Gingivitis • Stomatitis • Hepatic Encephalopathy.

ABBREVIATIONS
CNS = central nervous system
FeLV = feline leukemia virus

References

Cornelius LM. Ptyalism. In: Lorenz MD, Cornelius LM, eds. Small animal medical diagnosis. Philadelphia: JP Lippincott, 1987:243-248.
DeBowes LJ. Ptyalism. In: Ettinger SJ, ed. Veterinary internal medicine. 4th ed. Philadelphia: WB Saunders, 1995;125-128.

Author Daniel P. Harrington
Consulting Editor Brent D. Jones

RED EYE

BASICS

DEFINITION
Hyperemia of the eyelids or ocular vasculature or hemorrhage within the eye

Pathophysiology
Active dilation of ocular vessels occurs in response to extra- or intraocular inflammation, as well as passive congestion. Hemorrhage from existing or newly formed blood vessels also occurs.

Systems Affected
Ophthalmic—the eye or ocular adnexa

SIGNALMENT Any

SIGNS N/A

CAUSES
Virtually every red eye fits into one or more of the following categories:
• Blepharitis • Conjunctivitis • Keratitis
• Episcleritis and scleritis • Anterior uveitis
• Glaucoma • Hyphema • Orbital disease—usually the orbital abnormality is more prominent

RISK FACTORS
• Systemic infectious or inflammatory disease
• Immunocompromise • Coagulopathies
• Systemic hypertension • Topically applied ophthalmic medications (e.g., aminoglycosides, pilocarpine, and epinephrine) • Neoplasia
• Trauma

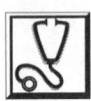

DIAGNOSIS

DIFFERENTIAL DIAGNOSIS
More than one cause of ocular injection may occur simultaneously.

DIFFERENTIATING SIMILAR SIGNS
Rule out normal variations:
• Palpebral conjunctiva is normally redder than bulbar conjunctiva. • One or two large episcleral vessels may be normal if the eye is otherwise quiet. • Transient, mild hyperemia occurs with excitement, exercise, and straining. • Horner's syndrome may cause very mild conjunctival vascular dilation. Other signs of Horner's and pharmacologic testing permit differentiation.

DIFFERENTIATING CAUSES
• Superficial (conjunctival) vessels originate near the fornix, move with the conjunctiva, branch repeatedly, and blanch quickly with topically applied 2.5% phenylephrine or 1:100,000 epinephrine. They suggest an ocular surface disorder such as conjunctivitis, superficial keratitis, or blepharitis. • Deep (episcleral) vessels originate near the limbus, branch infrequently, do not move with the conjunctiva, and blanch slowly or incompletely with topically applied sympath-

omimetics. They suggest episcleritis or intraocular disease such as anterior uveitis or glaucoma. • Mucopurulent to purulent discharge is typical of an ocular surface disorder and blepharitis, whereas a serous discharge, if any, is associated with an intraocular disorder. • Swollen or inflamed eyelids are associated with blepharitis. • Corneal opacification, neovascularization, or fluorescein stain retention suggests keratitis. • Aqueous flare or cell (excessive protein or cells in the anterior chamber) confirms a diagnosis of anterior uveitis. • The pupil is often miotic in animals with anterior uveitis, dilated in those with glaucoma, and normal in those with blepharitis and conjunctivitis. • Abnormally shaped or colored irides suggests anterior uveitis. • Luxated or cataractous lenses suggests glaucoma or anterior uveitis. • High intraocular pressure is diagnostic for glaucoma, whereas lower than normal intraocular pressure suggests anterior uveitis. • Loss of vision suggests glaucoma, anterior uveitis, or severe keratitis. • Glaucoma and anterior uveitis may complicate hyphema.

CBC/BIOCHEMISTRY/URINALYSIS
• Typically normal except in animals with anterior uveitis and hyphema secondary to systemic disease. See anterior uveitis/hyphema.

OTHER LABORATORY TESTS
Vary depending on cause

IMAGING
• Consider thoracic radiographs in animals with anterior uveitis and for which intraocular neoplasia is a possibility. Abdominal radiography and ultrasonography may aid in ruling out infectious or neoplastic causes.
• Ocular ultrasonography (if the ocular media are opaque) may define the extent and nature of intraocular disease or identify an intraocular tumor.

OTHER DIAGNOSTIC PROCEDURES
Tonometry must be performed in every animal with an unexplained red eye. In animals with ocular surface disorders:
• Bacterial culture and sensitivity test in animals with purulent discharge if the problem is chronic or poorly responsive to treatment
• Schirmer tear test • Cytologic examination of affected tissue (i.e., lid, conjunctiva, or cornea). In cats, also consider an immunofluorescent antibody test of conjunctival or corneal scraping for feline herpes virus and chlamydia. Collect sample before fluorescein staining to avoid false/positive results.
• Fluorescein stain • Tonometry • Biopsy of mass lesion or conjunctiva in animals with chronic conjunctivitis • See definitive work-ups for specific diseases, e.g., conjunctivitis and blepharitis
In animals with intraocular disorders:
• Fluorescein stain • Tonometry • See definitive work-ups for specific diseases (e.g., uveitis and hyphema)

TREATMENT

• Most animals with red eyes can be treated as outpatients.
• Consider use of an Elizabethan collar.
• Avoid dirty environments or those that may lead to ocular trauma, especially if administering corticosteroids topically.
• There is a narrow margin for error. Consider referring the patient if it is impossible to attribute the condition to one of the above causes or rule out glaucoma during the initial visit, or if the diagnosis is so uncertain that administering a corticosteroid or topical antibiotic by itself would be questionable.
• Although few causes of a red eye are fatal, a work-up may be indicated (especially in animals with anterior uveitis and hyphema) to rule out potentially fatal systemic diseases that require specific treatment.
• Deep corneal ulcers and glaucoma may be best treated surgically.

MEDICATIONS

DRUGS AND FLUIDS
• Treatment varies with specific cause of the ocular disease. In general, ocular pain, inflammation, infection, and intraocular pressure should be controlled.
• Aspirin (10-15 mg/kg q8h-q12h PO) may control mild ocular inflammation and pain pending test results.
• Flunixin meglumine (0.5 mg/kg IV) one time may be used in dogs with severe ocular inflammation pending test results.

CONTRAINDICATIONS
• Topically applied corticosteroids are contraindicated if the cornea retains fluorescein stain.
• Avoid systemically administered corticosteroids until infectious systemic causes have been ruled out.

PRECAUTIONS
• Topically applied aminoglycosides may be irritating and may impede re-epithelization if used frequently or used at high concentrations.
• Topically applied solutions may be preferable to ointments if corneal perforation is possible.
• Atropine may exacerbate keratoconjunctivitis sicca and glaucoma.
• NSAIDS should be used with caution in animals with hyphema.

POSSIBLE INTERACTIONS N/A

ALTERNATE DRUGS N/A

FOLLOW-UP

PATIENT MONITORING

• Varies greatly depending on cause. Repeat ophthalmic examination as required to ensure that ocular inflammation is well controlled.
• The greater the risk of loss of vision, the more closely the patient needs to be observed. This may mean daily or more frequent examinations in select animals.

POSSIBLE COMPLICATIONS

• Death • Loss of the eye or permanent vision loss • Chronic ocular inflammation and pain

MISCELLANEOUS

ASSOCIATED CONDITIONS

Numerous systemic diseases can be associated with a red eye.

AGE RELATED FACTORS N/A

ZOONOTIC POTENTIAL

See uveitis chapters

PREGNANCY

Systemic corticosteroids may complicate pregnancy.

SYNONYMS N/A

SEE ALSO See causes

ABBREVIATIONS

NSAIDS = nonsteroidal antiinflammatory drugs

References

Glaze MB. Ocular manifestations of systemic disease. In: Kirk RW, Bonagura JD, eds. Current veterinary therapy XI. Philadelphia: WB Saunders, 1992:1061–1070.

Slatter DS. Fundamentals of veterinary ophthalmology. 2nd ed. Philadelphia: WB Saunders, 1990.

Gelatt KN, ed. Veterinary ophthalmology. 2nd ed. Philadelphia: Lea & Febiger, 1991.

Author Paul E. Miller

Consulting Editor Paul E. Miller

Figure 1.

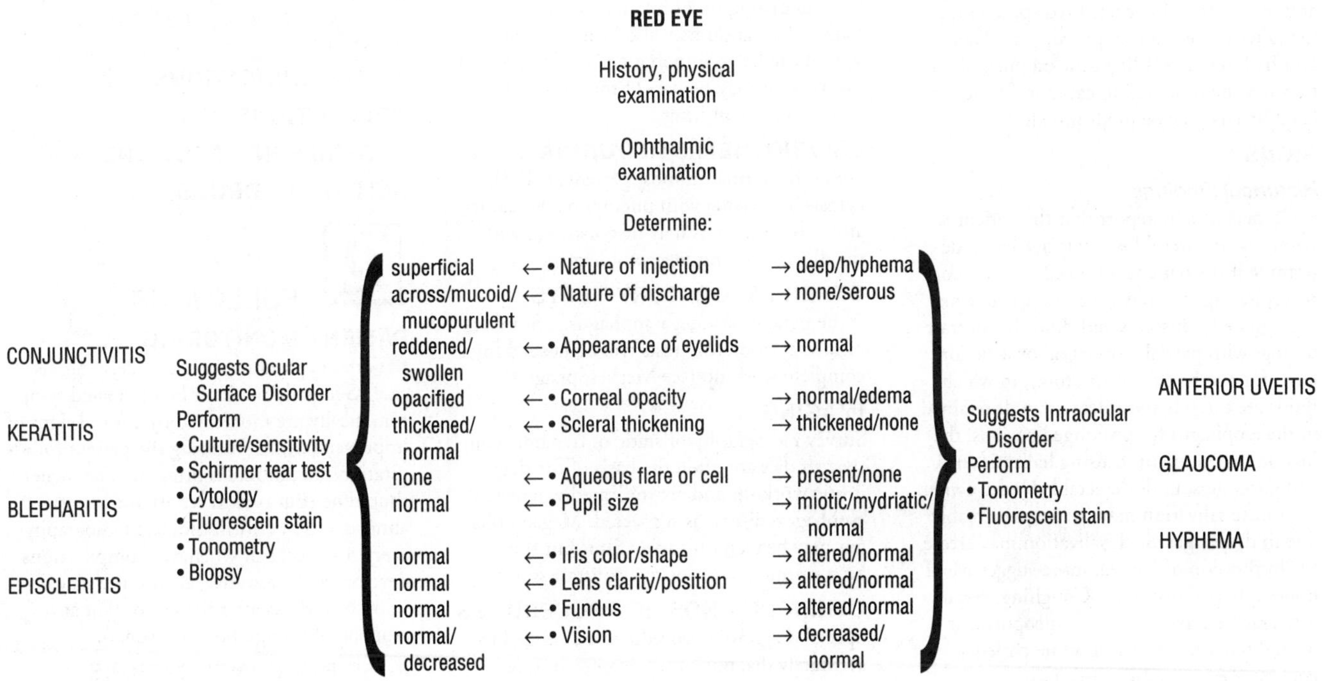

RED EYE

History, physical examination

Ophthalmic examination

Determine:

CONJUNCTIVITIS	Suggests Ocular Surface Disorder Perform • Culture/sensitivity • Schirmer tear test • Cytology • Fluorescein stain • Tonometry • Biopsy	superficial ←	• Nature of injection	→ deep/hyphema		
		across/mucoid/ ← mucopurulent	• Nature of discharge	→ none/serous		
KERATITIS		reddened/ ← swollen	• Appearance of eyelids	→ normal	Suggests Intraocular Disorder Perform • Tonometry • Fluorescein stain	ANTERIOR UVEITIS
		opacified ←	• Corneal opacity	→ normal/edema		
		thickened/ ← normal	• Scleral thickening	→ thickened/none		GLAUCOMA
BLEPHARITIS		none ←	• Aqueous flare or cell	→ present/none		
		normal ←	• Pupil size	→ miotic/mydriatic/ normal		HYPHEMA
		normal ←	• Iris color/shape	→ altered/normal		
EPISCLERITIS		normal ←	• Lens clarity/position	→ altered/normal		
		normal ←	• Fundus	→ altered/normal		
		normal/ ← decreased	• Vision	→ decreased/ normal		

REGURGITATION

BASICS

DEFINITION
• A backward flowing, as in the casting up of undigested food • Usually implies dysphagia • Most commonly associated with the esophageal stage of swallowing

Pathophysiology
Swallowing consists of a series of sequential, well coordinated events that transport food and liquids from the mouth to the stomach. This process is divided into three major phases: oropharyngeal, esophageal, and gastroesophageal. Altered motility of food from the mouth to the stomach allows food to accumulate in the esophagus, and eventually it is regurgitated out the oral cavity.

Systems Affected
Respiratory—aspiration pneumonia

SIGNALMENT
• **After weaning, dogs have a higher prevalence of regurgitation, because idiopathic megaesophagus is frequently diagnosed in younger animals.** • Idiopathic megaesophagus is inherited in the wirehaired fox terrier and miniature schnauzer. Predisposed breeds include the German shepherd, great Dane, and Irish setter. • Idiopathic esophageal dilation may be inherited in cats and Siamese-related breeds may be predisposed.

SIGNS

Historical Findings
• Owners usually report that the patient is vomiting. A careful history is needed to determine if the patient is indeed vomiting or regurgitating. • Dogs with megaesophagus regurgitate both solids and fluids in contrast to dogs with partial esophageal obstruction (e.g., foreign body and stricture), in which fluids are often better tolerated. • If retained in the esophagus for prolonged periods, the ingesta may ferment, causing halitosis and and gurgling sounds detectable by the owner. • Profuse salivation may occur, presumably due to dysphagia. Such salivation may create the impression of nausea, more suggestive of nonesophageal disease. • Coughing, respiratory crackles, dyspnea, and mucopurulent nasal discharge are seen in some patients.

Physical Examination Findings
• The condition of the animal may vary from normal to emaciated, depending on the severity of the disease process. • A cervical mass or esophageal foreign body may be palpable in the neck or thoracic inlet • A dilated cervical esophagus may be visualized or palpated, especially when examined during respiration or if the animal's thorax is forcibly compressed while its nostrils are occluded. • Coarse crackles (moist rales), associated with aspiration pneumonia or fluid movement in a dilated esophagus may be detected.

• Pyrexia if pneumonia is present.

CAUSES
• Congenital—idiopathic megaesophagus, vascular ring anomaly, and esophageal stenosis • Acquired—secondary megaesophagus, adult onset idiopathic megaesophagus, esophagitis, and esophageal stricture • Congenital or acquired—esophageal diverticulum, hiatal hernia, periesophageal hiatal hernia, gastroesophageal intussusception, and diaphragmatic hernia

RISK FACTORS
Many diseases cause megaesophagus (see Megaesophagus)

DIAGNOSIS

DIFFERENTIAL DIAGNOSIS
• Vomiting must be differentiated from regurgitation. A good history helps to differentiate. Vomiting is an active process, whereas regurgitation is more passive. Characteristics of vomiting include retching with involuntary abdominal contractions. Vomiting causes the expulsion of digested and bile-stained food or liquid. Regurgitation involves less forceful casting up of bile-free, undigested food. • Salivation may also be a confusing sign. It can be an important sign of esophageal disease or it may be part of the nausea that accompanies vomiting.

CBC/BIOCHEMISTRY/URINALYSIS
• Results normal in most patients • Leukocytosis in patients with pneumonia • Laboratory abnormalities may be consistent with the disease causing megaesophagus.

OTHER LABORATORY TESTS
If the patient has megaesophagus, a number of special laboratory tests will be needed for a complete work-up (see Megaesophagus).

IMAGING
Survey radiography or static or dynamic contrast studies are often the basis of the diagnostic work-up and are indicated whenever esophageal disease is suspected. Megaesophagus may be seen on survey films but should be confirmed by a positive contrast study.

OTHER DIAGNOSTIC PROCEDURES
Special diagnostic procedures are needed to accurately diagnosis megaesophagus (see Megaesophagus).

TREATMENT
• Whenever possible, treatment is aimed at the primary cause. For example, an esophageal foreign body must be removed; immune-mediated polymyositis and polyneuritis and SLE may respond to immune suppression; regurgitation caused by an esophageal diverticulum usually responds well to surgical removal of the diverticulum; sec-

ondary megaesophagus may respond to treating the primary disease.
• For idiopathic megaesophagus and for most patients with megaesophagus caused by neurologic disease, treatment is entirely symptomatic. The objectives are to reduce the frequency and severity of the common complications of megaesophagus (e.g., aspiration pneumonia) and provide adequate nutrition to maintain the patient in a positive calorie and protein balance. The cornerstone of symptomatic treatment is feeding and watering the affected animal from a raised position. Some patients do better with a liquid diet, whereas others do better with solid food. Antibiotics may be part of symptomatic treatment, especially if the patient frequently gets aspiration pneumonia.

MEDICATIONS

DRUGS AND FLUIDS
If the patient is dehydrated, a balanced electrolyte solution may be used to replace fluid deficits. Although certain drugs have been advocated by some for the treatment of megaesophagus, there is no generally accepted protocol for their use by the veterinary profession.

CONTRAINDICATIONS N/A
PRECAUTIONS N/A
POSSIBLE INTERACTIONS N/A
ALTERNATE DRUGS N/A

FOLLOW-UP

PATIENT MONITORING
• Varies depending on the underlying disease. Generally, patients being treated symptomatically are monitored by clinical signs of improvement. Monitoring the patient for aspiration pneumonia is prudent. The owner should be educated to report any respiratory abnormality. Perform thoracic radiography every 3-4 weeks or whenever complications develop. • An esophageal stricture may develop 6-8 weeks after the removal of an esophageal foreign body (unusual).

POSSIBLE COMPLICATIONS
Aspiration pneumonia

MISCELLANEOUS

ASSOCIATED CONDITIONS
• Aspiration pneumonia • If the regurgitation is caused by acquired secondary megaesophagus, the patient may also exhibit clinical signs of the primary disease.

AGE RELATED FACTORS
Congenital diseases (e.g., vascular ring abnor-

mality and idiopathic megaesophagus) diseases are seen in young patients.

ZOONOTIC POTENTIAL N/A

PREGNANCY N/A

SYNONYMS

Achalasia is a term that has been used as a synonym for megaesophagus; however, achalasia is a specific disease in humans in which esophageal dilation is classically associated with loss of primary peristalsis, a hypertonic lower esophageal sphincter that does not relax in response to swallowing, and evidence of denervation of the esophagus. Achalasia, so defined, has yet to be proven to exist in dogs or cats.

SEE ALSO Megaesophagus

ABBREVIATIONS None

References

Jones BD, Jergens AE, Guilford WG. Diseases of the esophagus. In: Ettinger SJ, ed. Textbook of veterinary internal medicine. 3rd ed. Philadelphia: WB Saunders, 1989.

Author Brent D. Jones

Consulting Editor Brent D. Jones

RENOMEGALY

BASICS

DEFINITION
One or both kidneys are abnormally large as detected by abdominal palpation or radiography.

Pathophysiology
The kidneys may become abnormally large because of abnormal cellular infiltration (e.g., inflammation, infection, and neoplasia), urinary tract obstruction, acute tubular necrosis, or development of renal cysts or pseudocysts.

Systems Affected
• Renal/Urologic
• Nervous, gastrointestinal, and other systems affected secondarily if uremia develops.

SIGNALMENT
Dogs and cats

SIGNS

Historical Findings
• Lethargy
• Loss of appetite
• Weight loss
• Vomiting
• Diarrhea
• Polyuria and polydipsia
• Discolored urine
• Lameness in rare patients because of hypertrophic osteopathy associated with renal neoplasia

Physical Examination Findings
• Abnormally large abdomen
• Abdominal mass
• One or both kidneys palpably large
• Dehydration
• Pale mucous membranes
• Oral ulcers
• Foul-smelling breath

CAUSES

Neoplasia
• Lymphoma—most often occurs in cats and causes bilateral renomegaly.
• Renal carcinoma—most common renal tumor in dogs; often causes unilateral renomegaly. Very malignant and rapidly metastatic to distant sites such as lungs.
• Nephroblastoma—also called Wilm's tumor; a congenital renal tumor that affects young dogs and cats, although it may not be diagnosed until the patient is much older. Biologic behavior varies; usually unilateral.
• Sarcoma—usually causes unilateral renomegaly and behaves malignantly.
• Cystadenocarcinoma—bilateral renal tumor that occurs in German shepherd dogs; often associated with skin lesions (i.e., nodular dermatofibrosis).

Inflammation/Infection
• Leptospirosis—may cause bilateral renomegaly and acute renal failure in dogs.
• Feline infectious peritonitis—causes bilateral renomegaly in cats.
• Renal abscess—localized abscess within renal parenchyma usually causes unilateral renomegaly in dogs and cats.

Developmental/Acquired Disorders
• Hydronephrosis—can cause unilateral or bilateral renomegaly in dogs and cats; develops secondarily to ureteral obstruction (e.g., urolithiasis, ureteral strictures, and neoplasia at trigone of urinary bladder) and ectopic ureters
• Polycystic kidney disease—causes bilateral renomegaly in cats and often leads to chronic renal failure; may be more common in Persians and domestic longhair cats
• Hematoma—occurs secondarily to trauma; infrequent cause of renomegaly in dogs and cats
• Compensatory hypertrophy—causes unilateral renomegaly and occurs secondarily to abnormality of the other kidney (e.g., renal hypoplasia, renal dysplasia, and nephrectomy)
• Ethylene glycol toxicosis—can cause bilateral renomegaly secondary to renal tubular swelling and renal infiltration by calcium oxalate crystals

RISK FACTORS
• Feline leukemia virus infection predisposes cats to development of renal lymphoma.
• Exposure to infectious diseases such as leptospirosis and feline infectious peritonitis increases risk of developing renomegaly associated with these disorders.

DIAGNOSIS

DIFFERENTIAL DIAGNOSIS
• Renomegaly must be distinguished from other abdominal masses.
• Confirming origin of an abdominal mass as renomegaly may require diagnostic imaging procedures or exploratory celiotomy.

CBC/BIOCHEMISTRY/URINALYSIS
• Leukocytosis in patients with infectious, inflammatory, and neoplastic causes of renomegaly
• Nonregenerative anemia secondary to chronic renal failure or inflammatory disorder in some patients
• Polycythemia and extreme leukocytosis accompany some renal neoplasms (rare)
• Azotemia, hyperphosphatemia, and low urine specific gravity (dogs, < 1.030; cats, < 1.035) in patients with renal failure
• Hyperglobulinemia in some patients with infectious or inflammatory disorder (e.g., feline infectious peritonitis)
• Hematuria and proteinuria in some patients with renal neoplasia
• Neoplastic cells rarely observed in urine of patients with renal neoplasia

OTHER LABORATORY TESTS
• Cats with renomegaly should be tested for feline leukemia virus infection.
• Serum protein electrophoresis should be done to distinguish between polyclonal and monoclonal hyperglobulinemia in patients with hyperglobulinemia.
• If leptospirosis is suspected, paired serum titers should be evaluated at 3- to 4-week intervals.

IMAGING

Radiography
• Survey abdominal radiographs indicated to confirm renomegaly.
• Patient has renomegaly if the kidneys on the ventrodorsal view are > 3 or 3.5 times the length of the second lumbar vertebra in dogs and cats, respectively.
• Excretory urography also can be used to confirm renomegaly, hydronephrosis, and space-occupying mass of the kidneys.
• Thoracic radiography is indicated to detect metastases in patients with renal neoplasia.

Ultrasonography
It is helpful to confirm presence of renomegaly and to identify potential causes such as polycystic kidney disease, perirenal pseudocysts, hydronephrosis, neoplastic mass, abscess, and subcapsular hematoma.

OTHER DIAGNOSTIC PROCEDURES
• Examination of fine-needle aspirate may be used to confirm presence of renal cyst, abscess, and neoplasia (especially lymphoma).
• If a definitive diagnosis is not made by cytologic evaluation of renal aspirate, renal biopsy may be indicated.

TREATMENT
• Diagnose and treat underlying cause for renomegaly if possible.
• Usually treat as an outpatient unless patient is dehydrated or has decompensated renal failure.
• If the patient is healthy otherwise, feed normal diet and allow normal exercise.

MEDICATIONS

DRUGS AND FLUIDS
• If the patient can not maintain hydration, administer lactated Ringer's or a maintenance fluid either subcutaneously or intravenously.
• If the patient has dehydration or continuing fluid losses such as vomiting or diarrhea, administer fluids intravenously to correct hydration deficits, maintain daily fluid requirements, and replace ongoing losses.

CONTRAINDICATIONS
Avoid nephrotoxic drugs

PRECAUTIONS N/A

POSSIBLE INTERACTIONS N/A

ALTERNATE DRUGS N/A

FOLLOW-UP

PATIENT MONITORING
Perform physical examination and weigh patient to assess hydration status.

POSSIBLE COMPLICATIONS
• Renal failure depending on underlying cause of renomegaly
• Paraneoplastic syndromes because of production of hormone-like substances by renal neoplasms.

MISCELLANEOUS

ASSOCIATED CONDITIONS N/A

AGE RELATED FACTORS N/A

ZOONOTIC POTENTIAL
Leptospirosis can be spread by contact with infected urine.

PREGNANCY N/A

SYNONYMS None

SEE ALSO
• Ethylene glycol toxicity
• Feline infectious peritonitis
• Hydronephrosis
• Leptospirosis
• Lymphosarcoma—feline
• Polycystic kidneys
• Renal carcinoma

ABBREVIATIONS None

References

Osborne C, Stevens J, Perman V. Kidney biopsy. Vet Clin N Am Small Anim Pract 1974; 4:351-365.

Lulich JP, Osborne CA, Walter PA, et al. Feline idiopathic polycystic kidney disease. Compend Contin Educ Pract Vet 1988; 10:1030-1041.

Klein MK, Cockerell GL, Harris CK, et al. Canine primary renal neoplasms: A retrospective review of 54 cases. J Am Anim Hosp Assoc 1988; 24:443-452.

Mooney SC, Hayes AA, Matus RE, et al. Renal lymphoma in cats: 28 cases (1977-1984). J Am Vet Med Assoc 1987; 191:1473-1477.

Author S. Dru Forrester

Consulting Editor Larry G. Adams and Carl Osborne

SEIZURES (CONVULSIONS, STATUS EPILEPTICUS)—CATS

BASICS

DEFINITION
Clinically detectable manifestation of paroxysmal cerebral dysrhythmia including consciousness alteration, involuntary excessive or reduced motor function, alteration of sensations, autonomic signs, and behavioural disturbances in any combination

PATHOPHYSIOLOGY
Seizures caused by a hypersynchronous discharge of a large population of thalamocortical neurons due to an imbalance between inhibitory and excitatory mechanisms.

SYSTEMS AFFECTED
Central nervous system

SIGNALMENT N/A

SIGNS
• Seizures start suddenly, are transient, end abruptly, and are often followed by postictal disturbances. • Seizures can be generalized with bilateral motor signs or partial (focal) with unilateral motor or stereotypical behavioral signs. • Seizures can be convulsive with generalized and violent motor activity or nonconvulsive with only minor or subtle motor signs (e.g., facial twitching). • Nonconvulsive, bizarre, and atypical seizures are common in cats.

CAUSES
Extracranial Causes
• Metabolic—severe hypoglycemia, polycythemia, and advanced hepatic encephalopathy • Toxicity— many intoxications in advanced stages of disease

Intracranial Causes
• Functional (idiopathic and genetic) epilepsy —poorly documented in cats • Structural brain diseases—by far the most common in cats. • The structural abnormality may be an active or inactive lesion leading to secondary epilepsy: • Active—meningoencephalitis of unknown but suspected viral or perhaps immune-mediated origin, feline ischemic encephalopathy, and brain tumors (e.g., meningioma) are the most common causes. Infectious encephalitides (e.g., FIP, toxoplasmosis, bacterial and fungal infection, and cuterebral myiasis) are much less common. • Inactive—postencephalitic lesion, postinfarction (feline ischemic encephalopathy), and postanoxia or ischemia (e.g., birth related), and post-traumatic epilepsy.

RISK FACTORS
Any brain disease involving the cerebrum

DIAGNOSIS

DIFFERENTIAL DIAGNOSIS
• Syncope—sudden loss of consciousness

and muscle tone resulting in recumbency and flaccidity. May be followed by a secondary stage of seizure-like features (rare). With true seizure activity, recumbency is caused by abnormal motor activity. The history and physical examination usually reveal clues (e.g., cardiovascular abnormalities such as heart murmur or arrythmias) that enable differentiation. Cats with true seizure activity may have abnormal behavior at the onset, autonomic signs such as salivation, piloerection, urination during the seizure, and the seizure is often followed by a period of disorientation. • Sleep-disorders—seizure-like features occurring exclusively during sleep. The cat exhibits a normal waking behavior upon arousal in contrast to the postictal disturbances seen after true seizures. • Extracranial (metabolic and toxic) causes are rare in cats. Characterized by acute onset of multiple or continuous generalized seizures and no focal neurologic deficits. Cats with metabolic disorders have other historical, clinical, and laboratory signs. Cats with seizurogenic toxins have progression from shaking to trembling and finally to sustained convulsive seizures until treatment is provided. • Signs of structural brain disease should be carefully looked for if the cat has (1) an acute onset of multiple or high-frequency seizures in the absence of extracranial causes; (2) partial seizures; (3) subtle neurologic deficits of thalamocortical origin (i.e., menace response, nasal septum sensation, and hopping and proprioceptive positioning).

CBC/BIOCHEMISTRY/URINALYSIS
• Results usually normal unless cat has a multisystemic disease such as fungal, bacterial, and protozoal encephalitides. • In cats with polycythemia, the PCV is usually >60%.

OTHER LABORATORY TESTS
• Serologic testing for FeLV, FIV, FIP and Toxoplasma gondii is usually non-contributory unless cat has concurrent systemic signs. • Bile acid testing is indicated only when cat has classical signs of hepatic encephalopathy (i.e., episodic depression, dementia, and salivation that last hours).

IMAGING
• Skull radiography usually unrewarding; may reveal calcified meningioma or associated calvarial hyperostosis. • Brain imaging (i.e., computed tomography and especially magnetic resonance imaging) most useful for identifying and defining structural brain lesions

OTHER DIAGNOSTIC PROCEDURES
CSF analysis useful for detecting a brain disease but the findings are often nonspecific.

TREATMENT
• Treat the cause if possible.
• Prompt and aggressive anticonvulsant therapy if the cat has (1) more than 1 single

seizure every 6 to 8 weeks, (2) cluster seizures (> 1 seizure/24 hours), or (3) status epilepticus, whether convulsive or nonconvulsive.
• The goal of treatment is < 1 single seizure every 6-8 weeks.
• Cats having severe cluster seizures or status epilepticus should be hospitalized until control is achieved.
• Since seizures in cats are usually the result of a structural disease, the owner should be encouraged to permit a diagnostic work-up so a specific treatment can be applied if needed. In cats with active structural disease, the antiepileptic medication is only a symptomatic treatment.

MEDICATIONS

DRUGS AND FLUIDS
Chronically Recurrent Seizures
Phenobarbital (2-5 mg/kg PO divided q12h). Second choice, diazepam (0.5-1.0 mg/kg divided q12h or q8h)

Severe Cluster Seizures and Status Epilepticus
(1) Diazepam (1-2 mg/kg IV bolus); may be repeated if gross seizure activity has not stopped within 5 minutes; (2) immediately start a diazepam infusion (0.5-1.0 mg/kg/h in maintenance fluids in an in-line burette; cover the line and burette with foil paper; prepare only 1-2 hours of infusion at a time); (3) if seizures persist, increase diazepam dosage and/or add phenobarbital (0.5-1.0 mg/kg/h) to the diazepam infusion; (4) when seizures have been controlled for at least several hours, slowly decrease the infusion rate over many hours; (5) initiate phenobarbital orally as soon as possible; (6) may give dexamethasone (0.25 mg/kg) for extremely severe seizures (i.e., prolonged or frequent, convulsive or nonconvulsive). This may be contraindicated in cats with infectious disease and interferes with CSF analysis.

CONTRAINDICATIONS
• Thiamine, glucose, and calcium should not be administered unless a deficiency is documented.
• Do not administer acepromazine, ketamine, or xylazine to patients with historical, actual, or potential seizure disorders.

PRECAUTIONS
Intensive parenteral anticonvulsant therapy requires constant monitoring and care (e.g., hypothermia common, persistent subtle seizure activity difficult to recognize, and potential cardiovascular and respiratory depression with overdosage).

POSSIBLE INTERACTIONS
• Do not use cimetidine and chloramphenicol with phenobarbital.
• Corticosteroids can reduce the serum concentration of phenobarbital (dose-related).

ALTERNATE DRUGS
Reports of other safe and effective antiepileptic drugs in cats have not been published.

FOLLOW-UP

PATIENT MONITORING
Measure serum antiepileptic drug concentration: (1) at 10-14 days for phenobarbital or 5-7 days for diazepam after treatment start; adjust the dosage if necessary to reach an optimal concentration 100-130 µmol/L (23-30 µg/ml) (phenobarbital) or (200-500 ng/L) (diazepam); (2) verify serum concentration 2 weeks after any dosage modification. • Benzodiazepine assays are not readily available and therapeutic serum concentrations are less well defined compared to phenobarbital making the latter preferable. • Monitor CBC, biochemistry analysis, and serum antiepileptic drug concentration every 6-12 months. • If the cat is seizure-free for > 12 consecutive months, may attempt antiepileptic drug weaning over a few-month period. If seizures recur at a frequency higher than one single seizure every 6-8 weeks, resume treatment.

POSSIBLE COMPLICATIONS
• Hypersensitivity to phenobarbital—thrombocytopenia, neutropenia, dermatitis, and swelling of the feet have been observed in a few cats); repeat CBC may be desirable within a few weeks after treatment starts. May necessitate the discontinuation of the drug (substitute diazepam). • A marked increase in serum phenobarbital concentration without dosage modification, accompanied by sedation and perhaps better seizure control may be the first signs of liver failure. • If high frequency seizures are refractory to single-drug regimen, add diazepam to phenobarbital or vice versa; consult a veterinary neurologist for third-line drugs.

MISCELLANEOUS

ASSOCIATED CONDITIONS N/A

AGE RELATED FACTORS
Brain tumor, especially meningioma more common in cats >10 years old

ZOONOTIC POTENTIAL N/A

PREGNANCY N/A

SYNONYMS
Convulsions (convulsive seizures)

SEE ALSO
• Syncope
• Feline ischemic encephalopathy

ABBREVIATIONS
CSF = cerebrospinal fluid
FeLV = feline leukemia virus
FIP = feline infectious peritonitis
FIV = feline immunodeficiency virus

References
Quesnel AD. A descriptive study on feline seizure disorders (DVSc thesis No. 34669). Guelph, Ontario, Canada: University of Guelph, 1994.
Rand JS, Parent JM, Jacobs R, et al. Reference intervals for feline cerebrospinal fluid: cell counts and cytologic features. Am J Vet Res 1990;51:1044-1048.
Rand JS, Parent JM, Percy D, et al. Clinical, cerebrospinal fluid and histologic data from twenty-seven cats with primary inflammatory disease of the central nervous system. Can Vet J 1994;35:103-110.
Author Andrée D. Quesnel
Consulting Editor Joane M. Parent

SEIZURES (CONVULSIONS, STATUS EPILEPTICUS)—DOGS

 BASICS

DEFINITION
• A seizure is the clinical manifestation of abnormal neuronal hyperactivity involving the cerebral cortical neurons. The clinical appearance of the seizure depends on the extent and location of the neuronal hyperactivity.
• Status epilepticus is a life-threatening medical emergency that results from continuous clinical seizures lasting at least 30 minutes, or seizures repeated at brief intervals for 30 minutes or more, without complete recovery of consciousness between individual attacks.

Pathophysiology
Seizure activity originates from the thalamocortex and results in a paroxysmal disorganization of one or several brain functions. The entire brain, or parts of it, may be involved; the extent of involvement largely determines the type of seizure. The basic disorder most commonly is localized in the brain, but failure of important organ systems and the associated metabolic abnormalities may lead to seizures secondary to encephalopathies. As more seizures occur, the tendency for neuronal damage and the propensity for developing more seizures or status epilepticus increases.

Systems Affected
Nervous

SIGNALMENT Any

SIGNS
General Comments
• Seizures can be generalized or partial.
• Generalized seizures can be convulsive and violent or mild with alteration of consciousness and subtle motor signs. The abnormalities are bilateral and symmetrical. Generalized seizures are more common in the dog.
• Partial seizures have a localized onset and asymmetry in the motor activity. They are called "partial complex" when there is alteration of consciousness or "simple partial" if there is not. Stereotypical behavioral seizures are partial complex seizures.

CAUSES
Extracranial
• Metabolic—hypoglycaemia (insulinoma), hypocalcemia (eclampsia, idiopathic parathyroiditis), renal failure, and hepatic encephalopathy • Toxic—numerous seizurogenic toxins (e.g., metaldehyde in slug bait) and toxicities that result in seizures in the advanced stages of poisoning

Intracranial
• Degenerative—storage diseases, anoxia, vascular accident • Anomalous—hydrocephalus • Neoplasia—primary (gliomas, meningioma) and secondary (metastatic) • Inflammatory infectious—viral (canine distemper, other), fungal, protozoal (Neospora, Toxoplasma), rickettsial (erhlichiosis, Rocky Mountain spotted fever), and bacterial diseases • Idiopathic,

immune-mediated—granulomatous meningoencephalomyelitis, eosinophilic meningoencephalomyelitis, and pug encephalitis
• Primary (idiopathic/genetic) epilepsy and secondary epilepsy (postencephalitic or post-traumatic glial scar) • Head trauma

RISK FACTORS
• Any disease affecting the thalamocortex can cause in seizure activity. • Ketamine and acepromazine may unmask/potentiate seizures in dogs that are otherwise clinically normal.

 DIAGNOSIS

DIFFERENTIAL DIAGNOSIS
• The clinician must ensure that the event is a seizure. Altered mentation, salivation, urination, and defecation during the ictal phase and aimless pacing, blindness, polydipsia, or polyphagia during the postictal phase are clues that seizure activity has occurred.
• Other altered states of consciousness such as syncope must be differentiated. A syncope is a sudden loss of consciousness and muscle tone, resulting in recumbency and flaccidity, whereas with seizure activity, recumbency results from involuntary tonic-clonic muscle activity. In syncope, the recovery is rapid and complete, whereas the seizure often is followed by a period of disorientation, confusion, and apparent blindness. • Obsessive-compulsive behaviors are complex and goal-directed. • With extracranial causes, the seizures are generalized. There are no lateralizing neurologic deficits. • With seizurogenic toxins, there is progression from shaking to trembling to status epilepticus. The seizures usually continue until treated or death of the animal occurs. • Intracranial active structural causes should be carefully sought if there is an acute onset of multiple seizures (more than two seizures within the first week) in the absence of extracranial causes, occurrence of partial seizures, and presence of neurologic deficits interictally. • Idiopathic epilepsy, the most common cause of seizures in dogs, is differentiated by the age and breed of the animal, the pattern of seizures (type and frequency), and results of laboratory testing.

CBC/BIOCHEMISTRY/URINALYSIS
• Combined with the history, signalment of the animal, seizure pattern, and the physical examination, the hemogram, serum chemistry profile, and urinalysis usually identify the extracranial causes of seizures. • Primary diseases of the brain have a normal hemogram, serum chemistry profile, and urinalysis. • Abnormalities related to severe cluster seizures or status epilepticus—metabolic acidosis is a frequent finding; hyperglycemia may occur in the early stages and gives way to hypoglycaemia in the advanced stages, especially in the small breeds; mild to marked creatinine kinase elevations with or without myoglobulinuria may occur as a result of

muscular necrosis. • Infectious intracranial diseases are associated with abnormal standard laboratory tests as a result of multisystemic involvement.

OTHER LABORATORY TESTS
• Bile acid testing is indicated if hepatic encephalopathy is suspected. However, seizures are rare and accompanied interictally by marked abnormal behavior such as dementia and aimless pacing. • Serology for viral, fungal, rickettsial, and protozoal diseases is indicated if there are systemic signs suggestive of these diseases.

IMAGING
• Skull radiographs are usually unrewarding.
• Brain imaging (magnetic resonance and computerized tomography) are the most useful modalities to define the location, extent, and nature of the structural abnormalities.

OTHER DIAGNOSTIC PROCEDURES
• CSF analysis is indicated every time an intracranial structural cause is suspected. • EEG is useful to detect the presence of cerebral disease, but the findings are nonspecific.

 TREATMENT

INPATIENT VERSUS OUTPATIENT
• The patient that has recurrence of isolated seizures can be treated as an outpatient.
• The dog experiencing severe cluster seizures or status epilepticus is treated rapidly and aggressively as an inpatient with constant monitoring. The more seizures occur, the more drugs are required for control and the more time necessitated for the animal to recover.

ACTIVITY
Avoid swimming because drowning may occur.

DIET
Regular diet

CLIENT EDUCATION
The importance of a diagnostic workup must be emphasized to the owner if a metabolic or intracranial structural cerebral disease is suspected, because the antiepileptic treatment in such cases is symptomatic and may not help until the primary cause is specifically treated.

 MEDICATIONS

DRUGS AND FLUID
• Treatment with phenobarbital is initiated if there is more than one seizure per 6-8 weeks, acute cluster seizures, or status epilepticus. PB does not interfere with the diagnostic tests.
• Chronic maintenance therapy—the initial phenobarbital dose is 2-5 mg/kg PO divided twice daily. The dosage is increased until optimal serum levels are reached (15-45 µg/ml).

SEIZURES (CONVULSIONS, STATUS EPILEPTICUS)—DOGS

• Dogs with cluster seizures and status epilepticus—administer diazepam as a bolus IV 0.5-1.0 mg/kg. This can be repeated safely 5 minutes later if gross motor activity has not stopped. Immediately, follow with a constant-rate infusion of diazepam, 0.5-1.0 mg/kg/hour, added to the maintenance fluids in an in-line burette (prepare only 1-2 hours of infusion at a time to avoid adsorption of diazepam to the plastic). If seizures persist, phenobarbital IV bolus 2-5 mg/kg is given, followed by an infusion 2-6 mg/dog/hour added to diazepam. Once seizures have been controlled for several hours (at least 4-6 hours), slowly decrease the infusion rate over many hours. Start oral phenobarbital as soon as possible.
• Dexamethasone 0.25 mg/kg, 1-3 times a day for 1 day. It is contraindicated in infectious diseases. Also alter the CSF.

CONTRAINDICATIONS

Do not administer acepromazine, ketamine, aminophylline, or xylazine to patients with historical, ongoing, or potential seizure disorders because of the lowering effect on the seizure threshold.

PRECAUTIONS

• Phenobarbital should never be abruptly discontinued as it may precipitate seizure activity.
• In the treatment of status epilepticus, phenobarbital must be added cautiously to diazepam because these drugs potentiate each other, and cardiac and respiratory depression may ensue.

POSSIBLE INTERACTIONS

• Cimetidine, ranitidine, and chloramphenicol interfere with the metabolism of phenobarbital, potentially resulting in toxic levels of phenobarbital.
• Each time a drug is added to phenobarbital, refer to pharmacology texts for possible interactions.

ALTERNATE DRUGS

• If the animal is diagnosed with a seizure disorder that requires long-term antiepileptic treatment, potassium bromide (Kbr) is used as a second drug.
• Dogs that do not respond to diazepam and phenobarbital infusion are anaesthetized. Ideally, this should be combined with EEG

monitoring to inform the clinician of the necessity for further depth anaesthesia based on the presence of seizure activity.

FOLLOW-UP

PATIENT MONITORING

Cerebrospinal fluid analysis may need to be repeated if a diagnosis of encephalitis is made to monitor response to treatment.
• If the dog requires long-term antiepileptic treatment, serum phenobarbital levels should be measured 2 weeks after onset of treatment and the dosage adjusted accordingly. The optimal serum levels to reach are 15-45 µg/ml. Once the desired levels have been reached, the levels should be repeated every 6-12 months. Hemogram and chemistry profile should be done before onset of medication and every 6-12 months thereafter to monitor for drug-induced side effects. • If the animal is treated as an inpatient, monitor for presence of seizures. Beware of eyelid or lip twitching on an otherwise heavily sedated dog as this also is a sign of ongoing seizure activity. Inpatients with seizures should be under constant supervision. • It may be 7-10 days before the animal returns to normal after status epilepticus. Vision is last to return. • If the dog is not epileptic, he can be slowly (months) and gradually be weaned off the antiepileptic drug after 6 seizure-free months. If seizures recur at more than one seizure per 6-8 weeks, reinstate the antiepileptic drug.

POSSIBLE COMPLICATIONS

• phenobarbital-induced hepatotoxicity may occur after chronic treatment with serum drug levels in the upper therapeutic range (> 45 µg/ml). • Rarely, acute neutropenia is observed in the first few weeks of phenobarbital introduction. Permanent phenobarbital withdrawal is necessary. • The seizures may continue despite adequate antiepileptic treatment. Refractoriness may develop. • The animal may develop status epilepticus and die.
• Permanent neurologic deficits such as blindness, abnormal behavior, and cerebellar signs may follow status epilepticus regardless of the cause.

MISCELLANEOUS

ASSOCIATED CONDITIONS

Hyperthermia, acid-base and electrolyte imbalances, anoxia, pulmonary edema, arrhythmias, aspiration pneumonia, renal failure, cardiovascular collapse, and death may all occur as a result of status epilepticus.

AGE RELATED FACTORS

• Idiopathic epilepsy is observed in dogs that are 6 months to 5 years of age. The disease is also more severe, often refractory, in dogs that are less than 2 years of age at onset. • Phenobarbital has a shorter half-life in the puppy compared to the adult. An initial dose of 5 mg/kg twice daily is advised. phenobarbital serum levels should be measured every 5 days until optimal levels are reached.

ZOONOTIC POTENTIAL N/A

PREGNANCY N/A

SYNONYMS N/A

SEE ALSO
• Epilepsy • See causes.

ABBREVIATIONS
CSF = cerebrospinal fluid
EEG = electroencephalography
PB = phenobarbital
DZ = diazepam

References
Indrieri RJ. Status epilepticus. Prob Vet Med. Philadelphia: JB Lippincott, 1989;1:606-618.
Oliver JE. Seizure disorders and narcolepsy. In: Oliver JE, Hoerlein BF, Mayhew IG, eds. Veterinary neurology. Philadelphia: WB Saunders, 1987:285-303.
Parent JM. Seizures. In: Allen DG, Kruth SA, Garvey MS, eds. Small animal medicine. Philadelphia: JB Lippincott, 1991:735-741.
Author Joane M. Parent
Consulting Editor Joane M. Parent

SEPSIS AND BACTEREMIA

BASICS

DEFINITION
Transient, intermittant, or continuous shedding of bacteria or other organisms into the blood. When it occurs in the normal individual, bacteremia is usually transient. Invasion of the circulatory system with bacteria as a result of concurrent infection or vascular access devices may lead to prolonged bacteremia and disastrous or overwhelming infection.

Pathophysiology
• In most healthy individuals, bacteria are removed from the circulatory system rapidly and effectively through phagocytosis by fixed-tissue macrophages in the spleen and liver. Persistent bacteremia only ensues when bacteria multiply at a rate that exceeds the ability of the reticuloendothelial system to remove them. Neutrophils are not a major component of the host defense mechanism in the circulation. • Three patterns of bacteremia are possible: 1) transient—occurs frequently as during routine dentistry and is of no consequence in healthy patients; 2) intermittent—characterized by periodic showering of bacteria into the bloodstream, the most common scenario; 3) continuous—characterized by persistent showering of bacteria into the bloodstream

Systems Affected
• Cardiovascular—the circulatory system is affected most adversely, resulting in septic shock. Bacteremia may lead to endocardial or renal manifestations of disease. Development of endocardial disease requires prior damage to heart valves in combination with bacteremia for disease development. • Ultimately, any organ system may be impaired as a result of effects from intermittent or continuous bacteremia.

SIGNALMENT
There is no sex, age, or breed predilection. Critically ill individuals and those with underlying disease are at greater risk.

SIGNS
Signs may be varied and include generalized depression, fever, tachycardia, and tachypnea. With the advent of septic shock, hypothermia, low blood pressure, low urine output, and low toe-web temperature indicate more severe disease, but these signs are not specific for septicemia. Gastrointestinal signs may appear early as anorexia, progressing to vomiting, and severe bloody diarrhea later in the course of disease.

CAUSES
• Dogs—gram-negative bacteria are the most common cause of bacteremia, followed by gram-positive cocci and obligate anaerobes. Mixed infections are also common and may account for as many as 17% of cases. The most common isolates in dogs are Escherichia coli and coagulase-positive staphylococci (S. aureus or S. intermedius). Rare in both dogs and cats are isolates of Pseudomonas. • Cats—either gram-negative bacteria of the Enterobacteriaceae family or obligate anaerobes are most common. Salmonella has been a common finding and may indicate this organism as an important but overlooked cause of infection in cats. Polymicrobial infections in cats are common. • Dow and others did not find evidence that any particular type of bacterial pathogen increased mortality, once the severity of the underlying disease was taken into account.

RISK FACTORS
• Many factors have been cited as predisposing to bacteremia and sepsis. Patients presenting with established infections are at greatest risk. Diseases that can progress to septicemia and shock include pyothorax, peritonitis, pyometra, prostatic abscess, mastitis, biliary tract infection, pyelonephritis, urinary tract infection, and occasionally, hepatic or lung abscess. • Any patient with depression of the immune response is at higher risk for developing bacteremia and sepsis. Noninfectious diseases that may predispose to bacteremia include hematologic malignancy, solid tumors, glucocorticoid therapy, trauma, surgery, diabetes mellitus, Cushing's disease, renal failure, hepatic failure, low body total protein, cytotoxic therapy (for neoplastic or inflammatory diseases), intravenous and urinary tract catheters, and burns. • The most important factor influencing mortality from bacteremia and sepsis is the extent and severity of the underlying disease. Mortality as a result of bacteremia is less likely to occur in previously healthy individuals. • In humans, as many as 25-30% of sources are never identified. • Efforts to prevent the development of bacteremia should be directed toward the most seriously ill patients because these patients are at greatest risk and the most likely to die after becoming bacteremic.

DIAGNOSIS

DIFFERENTIAL DIAGNOSIS
• Must differentiate from other causes of fever, cardiac or renal disease, gastrointestinal disease, and abdominal pain or distension such as that caused by organ enlargement, neoplasia, cystic structures, pancreatitis, and peritonitis. • Must differentiate from other causes such as hypovolemic shock.

CBC/BIOCHEMISTRY/URINALYSIS
• Hemogram—neutrophilia progressing to neutropenia in severe cases. Thrombocytopenia. Severe hemoconcentration. • Biochemistry—hyperkalemia secondary to acidosis, shock, poor renal perfusion, and tissue necrosis. Hypoglycemia may occur early in septic patients because of the presumed "insulinlike" effect of endotoxin. Electrolyte abnormalities vary depending on the etiology and duration of disease. High BUN and liver enzymes. • Urinalysis—presence of bacteria in urine or positive urine cultures • Metabolic alterations, including metabolic acidosis, occur rapidly.

OTHER LABORATORY TESTS N/A

IMAGING N/A

OTHER DIAGNOSTIC PROCEDURES
Blood cultures are indicated in any critically ill animal that develops fever, neutropenia, left shift, shifting leg lameness, recent or changing cardiac murmur, or other signs of sepsis that cannot be explained by a preexisting condition. Blood culture is indicated in patients with suspected bacteremia to confirm that infection exists, to identify the causative organism, and to facilitate optimal antimicrobial therapy.

Guidelines for Blood Culture
• A minimum of two and preferably three cultures should be obtained. This increases the chances of obtaining a positive culture and also facilitates accurate interpretation of cultures. • Three blood samples should be taken over a 24-hour period for patients without severe sepsis. For animals with advanced sepsis, three blood samples should be taken over a 2-hour period. • Whenever possible, 10 ml of blood should be cultured each time because total numbers of organisms in circulation is often low. • Results are usually available after 48 hours for isolates pathogens. • Prior administration of antibiotics or other antimicrobial agents does not reduce the frequency of positive cultures. Prior or concurrent antimicrobial therapy, therefore, should not preclude use of blood cultures. • Documentation of bacteremia requires that bacteria be recovered from properly collected and cultured blood specimens.

Collecting Cultures
• Thorough skin disinfection before venipuncture is the most effective means of avoiding culture contamination. Hair should be clipped. After the vein is located, the site should be thoroughly cleansed, first with 70% alcohol, followed by swabbing with either tincture of iodine or an iodophor. Iodine should contact the skin for at least one minute. If the vein must be palpated after skin disinfection, a sterile glove should be worn. • To minimize the risk of contamination, blood should be drawn through a sterile needle and syringe. An indwelling catheter is not recommended unless venipuncture is impossible. • A blood-to-culture broth ratio of 1:10 must be maintained to counteract the bacteriocidal activity of serum. Commercially available blood culture bottles are available in 25-, 50-, and 100-ml sizes. • Arterial blood samples offer no advantage over venous samples. • Blood is inoculated directly into culture media using either a syringe or blood transfer set. A new needle should be used to

introduce the blood into the culture bottle after the diaphragm has been disinfected with alcohol or iodine. Air must not be allowed to enter the bottles during injection. • Cultures should be maintained at room temperature to avoid killing temperature-sensitive bacteria. • Complementary cultures of urine and any other sources of infection should be done concurrently.

Culture Media

• Commercial multipurpose nutrient broth media are recommended for blood culture. Tryptic soy broth, Columbia broth, and brain-heart infusion broth are suitable for routine culture of aerobic and anaerobic bacteria. • Most liquid media are bottled under vacuum with carbon dioxide added and will support the growth of anaerobic organisms. • Only commercial culture bottles should be used for routine blood cultures.

Interpretation of Cultures

• Recovery of Enterobacteriaceae, Bacteroidaceae, Pseudomonas aeruginosa, Staphylococcus aureus, Staphylococcus intermedius, hemolytic streptococci, or yeasts in the bloodstream is almost always clinically significant. • Contamination is best distinguished from actual bacteremia by culturing multiple blood specimens. • Multiple isolations of the same organism imply significance because of repeatability. • Negative blood culture results (no growth) from two or three successive cultures generally rules out bacteremia caused by common pathogens.

TREATMENT

GENERAL CONSIDERATIONS

• Successful treatment of septicemia and septic shock depends on early diagnosis, identification and elimination of the bacterial nidus and aggressive hemodynamic support.
• Physical examination may reveal superficial abscesses. Blood, sputum, urine, and wound discharges should be obtained for bacterial culture.
• Wounds should be debrided aggressively and abscesses drained.
• Surgical management should be elected when indicated (e.g., pyometra, prostatic

abscess, peritonitis, gastrointestinal tract perforation).
• Appropriate antibiotic treatment is necessary to eliminate the source of bacterial byproducts such as endotoxins and exotoxins.
• Nutritional support should be instituted to combat the catabolic effects of sepsis.
• The owner should be made aware that the fatality rate, even with appropriate therapy, is high and related to the underlying cause of sepsis and physical condition of the patient.

MEDICATIONS

DRUGS AND FLUIDS

• Hypovolemia/shock is treated by intravenous fluids to correct hypovolemia as well as metabolic changes (acidosis, electrolyte abnormalities). Volume replacement at a rate up to 90 ml/kg is started based on extent of disease. Isotonic fluids such as lactated Ringer's or Normosol-R are recommended. If the patient is hypoglycemic, the use of 5% dextrose in a polyionic replacement fluid is indicated. Plasma and dextran solutions are fluids of choice because protein loss to the extravascular space is extensive.
• Infection—antibiotic therapy is warranted and should be started as soon as a diagnosis of septicemia is made. The antibiotic should be broad spectrum and initially should be administered in high doses by the intravenous route. Aminoglycosides, chloramphenicol, and cephalosporins are good first choice antibiotics alone or in combination. Secondary choices include penicillins, erythromycin and metronidazole. Ultimately, antibiotic choice should be based on results of culture and sensitivity testing.
• Controversy exists regarding the use of corticosteroids in sepsis. Most authors agree that the properties of corticosteroids (stabilizing lysosomal membranes, decreasing vascular permeability, protecting against endotoxin, restoring of intestinal wall permeabiltiy) make them a useful adjunct to therapy for peritonitis.
• Nonsteroidal antiinflammatory drugs have been documented to be beneficial in the treatment of septicemia in dogs.

CONTRAINDICATIONS/POSSIBLE INTERACTIONS

The use of corticosteriods and nonsteroidal

inflammatory medications (flunixin meglumine) is controversial.

PRECAUTIONS

Care should be taken to evaluate renal function and ensure adequate renal perfusion in patients treated with aminoglycosides.

POSSIBLE INTERACTIONS N/A

ALTERNATE DRUGS N/A

FOLLOW-UP

PATIENT MONITORING

• Feeding should begin via feeding tube after enterostomy or gastrotomy tube placement.
• Evaluation of serum albumin with replacement of protein losses if albumin falls below 2.0 gm/dl

POSSIBLE COMPLICATIONS

Death from septicemia, hypovolemia, and electrolyte disturbances occurs in a high percentage of patients.

MISCELLANEOUS

ASSOCIATED CONDITIONS

See risk factors.

AGE RELATED FACTORS N/A

ZOONOTIC POTENTIAL N/A

PREGNANCY N/A

SYNONYMS

Septic shock

SEE ALSO

• Shock • Endocarditis • Abcessation
• Peritonitis

ABBREVIATIONS N/A

Reference

Dow SW. Diagnosis of bacteremia in critically ill dogs and cats. In: Bonagura JD, ed. Current veterinary therapy XII. Philadelphia, WB Saunders, 1995:137-139.
Author David K. Rosen
Consulting Editor Fred W. Scott

SHOCK

 BASICS

DEFINITION

Loss of effective circulating blood volume, causing low tissue perfusion and therefore inadequate oxygen delivery to meet the demands of tissue metabolism. Included are a diverse group of life-threatening circulatory conditions such as hypovolemic, cardiogenic, and septic shock.

PATHOPHYSIOLOGY

• Hypovolemic shock may result from fluid losses such as blood loss, vomiting, diarrhea, burns, and third body space fluid accumulation. The reduction in blood volume results in reduced cardiac filling, reduced cardiac output, and low systemic blood pressure. Peripheral blood flow is compromised and oxygen delivery to the tissues is affected. In conditions of hypoxemia, cellular integrity is affected and organ failure ensues. • Cardiogenic shock is caused by cardiac "pump" failure resulting in greatly diminished stroke volume and cardiac output. Severe hypotension causes tissue hypoperfusion. Compensatory neuroendocrine responses cause peripheral vasoconstriction and fluid retention. Rises in left atrial pressure and pulmonary venous pressure may lead to pulmonary edema. • Septic shock is the result of cardiovascular and/or vasomotor failure caused by circulating endotoxin and inflammatory mediator release. A source of systemic infection is the underlying cause. The primary event is hypovolemia caused by pyrexia, dehydration, and vascular fluid leakage, which are the result of increases in microvascular permeability. Differential vasoconstriction and vasodilatation of microvascular beds causes pooling of blood and differential tissue perfusion. Vasculitis and thromboembolic events further compromise tissue perfusion. The ultimate result is tissue hypoxemia and metabolic acidosis.

SYSTEMS AFFECTED

Cardiovascular

• Primary cardiac dysfunction causes cardiogenic shock. • Cardiac dysfunction (i.e., reduced myocardial contractility) may occur secondary to sepsis. • Differential vasoconstriction and vasodilatation in capillary beds is characteristic of sepsis. • Vascular endothelial damage in animals with sepsis results in permeability changes, fluid leakage, and disseminated intravascular coagulation (DIC). • Compensatory responses to all forms of early shock involve increases in heart rate and contractility and peripheral vasoconstriction in an attempt to raise systemic blood pressure.

Gastrointestinal

In dogs, impaired gastric mucosal perfusion may cause mucosal sloughing and bacterial

translocation. Therefore, sepsis may be a complication of hypovolemic shock.

Hepatobiliary

Hepatic ischemia causes high hepatocellular enzyme concentrations, hyperbilirubinemia, and possible coagulation factor deficiency. Reduced bacterial clearance may predispose to sepsis.

Renal /Urologic

Acute renal failure may occur in response to reduced renal blood flow and ischemic tubular damage.

Respiratory

Pulmonary edema may be associated with cardiogenic shock. • Pulmonary edema and pulmonary thromboembolism may be associated with sepsis.

SIGNALMENT N/A

SIGNS

Historical Findings

• Hypovolemic shock may be associated with a history of trauma and blood loss, burn injury, or severe vomiting and diarrhea.
• Cardiac decompensation may be associated with a history of previously compensated cardiac disease and cardiac drug administration.
• Septic shock may be associated with a history of known infection.

Physical Examination Findings

Early or Compensatory Shock
• Tachycardia • Normal or high arterial blood pressure • Bounding peripheral pulses • Hyperemic mucous membranes • Rapid capillary refill time • Tachypnea • Pyrexia in animals with septic shock
Late or Decompensatory Shock
• Tachycardia or bradycardia • Poor peripheral pulses • Pale mucous membranes • Prolonged capillary refill time • Coolness of extremities • Hypothermia • Mental depression or stupor • Oliguria • Dyspnea • Petechiation and peripheral edema in septic shock

CAUSES

Hypovolemic Shock

• Traumatic blood loss into body cavities or lungs, into fracture sites, or from wounds
• Severe gastrointestinal bleeding associated with corticosteroids or nonsteroidal antiinflammatory drug therapy or neoplasia
• Fluid loss from extensive burn injury; severe vomiting or diarrhea

Cardiogenic Shock

• Primary cardiac disease such as dilated cardiomyopathy in large-breed dogs or cats with taurine deficiency; hypertrophic cardiomyopathy in cats; severe mitral insufficiency in dogs • Reduced cardiac contractility secondary to sepsis

Septic Shock

• Infectious focus causing bacteremia and endotoxemia • Gastrointestinal mucosal compromise caused by hypovolemia or ischemia resulting in bacterial translocation and endotoxemia.

RISK FACTORS

• Exposure to possible trauma or burn injury
• Concurrent illness causing immunocompromise or inadequate compensatory response and predisposing to sepsis
• Old or young age

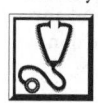 **DIAGNOSIS**

DIFFERENTIAL DIAGNOSIS

• Hypovolemic shock associated with circulatory collapse must be differentiated from compensated hypovolemia or dehydration.
• Cardiogenic shock associated with circulatory collapse must be differentiated from compensated cardiac failure. • Septic shock associated with circulatory collapse must be differentiated from systemic infection with inadequate compensatory cardiovascular response. • Circulatory collapse is associated with tachycardia or bradycardia, reduced cardiac output, hypotension, reduced tissue perfusion and evidence of multiorgan dysfunction such as mental depression, oliguria, and DIC.

CBC/BIOCHEMISTRY/URINALYSIS

Hypovolemic shock

• Anemia and hypoproteinemia in animals with blood loss • Hemoconcentration and electrolyte disturbances in animals with fluid loss caused by gastrointestinal disease or burns

Cardiogenic shock

• Results usually normal • Hyponatremia and high hepatocellular enzyme concentrations in some animals

Septic shock

• Leukocytosis with a left shift and hemoconcentration • High hepatocellular enzyme concentrations • Azotemia

OTHER LABORATORY TESTS

• Coagulation profile may show prolongation of the activated partial thromboplastin and prothrombin times, increased fibrin degradation products, and thrombocytopenia, all consistent with DIC. • Blood gas analysis may reveal hypoxemia and acid-base disturbances.

IMAGING

• Thoracic radiography may reveal evidence of heart failure (cardiogenic shock), pneumonia/pyothorax (septic shock), or microcardia (hypovolemic shock).• Echocardiography may document cardiomyopathy or valvular disease (cardiogenic shock) or depressed myocardial contractility (septic shock).

OTHER DIAGNOSTIC PROCEDURES

• Blood pressure measurement may document hypotension. • Aerobic and anaerobic blood cultures may identify an infectious source of sepsis.

TREATMENT

• Treat as inpatient because of circulatory collapse.
• If a source or sepsis such as an abscess is identified, it should be surgically excised.
• Aggressive treatment and life-support may be required.
• Inform the owner of the danger of imminent cardiac arrest in all patients.

MEDICATIONS

DRUGS AND FLUIDS

• For patient in hypovolemic or septic shock, vigorous fluid therapy is required in order to increase effective circulating volume.
• Use balanced electrolyte solution at initial rate of up to 90 ml/kg/h for dogs and 40 ml/kg/h for cats. Colloidal solutions such as whole blood, Hetastarch®, or dextrans may be used in combination with crystalloid solutions in order to retain fluid within the vascular space. Synthetic colloids may be used (20 ml/kg), allowing the concurrent crystaloid fluid dosage to be reduced to 1/4-1/2 of the usual dosage for shock. A 7.5% solution of hypertonic saline may also be used (5ml/kg IV bolus) for rapid volume resuscitation.
• For patient in cardiogenic shock, minimal fluids are given intravenously. Treatment involves the provision of positive inotropic cardiac support with digoxin (0.005 mg/kg hourly for up to 4 doses) or dobutamine (5-20 mcg/kg/min).
• For patients in refractory hypovolemia or septic shock, vasopressors such as dopamine (5-20 mcg/kg/min) may be used to raise systemic blood pressure.
• Oxygen supplementation is as important as fluid replacement. This can be administered by oxygen cage, mask or nasal cannula.
• Glucocorticosteroids can be used in the early stages of noncardiogenic shock, although their use is controversial. Suggested drugs and dosages are prednisolone sodium succinate (10-30 mg/kg q8h) and dexamethasone sodium phosphate (6-15 mg/kg q12h).

• Broad-spectrum antibiotics administered intravenously are essential in the treatment of septic shock. While awaiting results of blood, urine, or tissue cultures, initiate treatment with one of the following broad-spectrum combinations: ampicillin and gentacin or cephalexin and gentacin. Metronidazole can be used with either of these combinations.
• Sodium bicarbonate may be given intravenously to a patient with severe metabolic acidosis associated with septic shock. Calculate the bicarbonate dose using the following equation: 0.3 mEq X body weight (kg) X (base deficit). Give 1/2 the dose slowly IV over a 20-minute period. Give the rest of the dose in crystaloid fluids over 4 hours. If unable to calculate the plasma bicarbonate, administer 0.5-1 mEq/kg as directed above.
• For patient with congestive heart failure and pulmonary edema, diuretics may be required.

CONTRAINDICATIONS N/A

PRECAUTIONS

Use of diuretics to treat pulmonary edema will further lower cardiac output

POSSIBLE INTERACTIONS

Sodium bicarbonate and dopamine cannot be administered in the same intravenous line.

ALTERNATE DRUGS

Vasopressor agents such as epinephrine of phenylephrine may be used instead of dopamine.

FOLLOW-UP

PATIENT MONITORING

• Heart rate, pulse intensity, mucous membrane color, respiratory rate, lung sounds, urine output, mentation, and rectal temperature should be monitored closely during aggressive treatment with fluids or inotropic drugs. • Cardiovascular monitoring by ECG and measurement of central venous pressure and blood pressure is useful. • Blood gas analysis and pulse oximetry can be used for monitoring tissue oxygenation and acid-base balance. • PCV, serum total protein, serum

electrolytes, hepatocellular enzymes, blood urea nitrogen, and serum creatinine should be monitored.

POSSIBLE COMPLICATIONS

• Electrolyte and acid-base disturbances
• Cardiac arrhythmias • Pulmonary edema or acute respiratory distress syndrome • Pulmonary thromboembolism • DIC • Renal dysfunction • Hepatic dysfunction • Gastrointestinal ischemia and bacterial translocation • Cerebral edema and seizures • Pancreatitis • Vasculitis and peripheral edema
• Cardiac arrest

MISCELLANEOUS

ASSOCIATED CONDITIONS N/A

AGE RELATED FACTORS N/A

ZOONOTIC POTENTIAL N/A

PREGNANCY N/A

SYNONYMS N/A

SEE ALSO
• DIC • Hypoxemia • Dilated Cardiomyopathy—Dogs and Cats • Hypertrophic Cardiomyopathy—Cats • Bacteremia and Septicemia

ABBREVIATIONS
DIC = disseminated intravascular coagulation
PCV = packed cell volume

References

Goodwin J, Schaer M. Septic shock. In: Kirby R, Stamp GL, eds. Veterinary clinics of North America. Small animal practice: critical care. Philadelphia: WB Saunders, 1989:1239-1258.

Shoemaker WC, Kram HB. Shock states: pathophysiology, monitoring, outcome, prediction and therapy. In: WC Shoemaker, et al., eds. Textbook of critical care. Philadelphia: WB Saunders, 1989;425-453.

Author Nishi Dhupa
Consulting Editors Larry P. Tilley and Francis W. K. Smith Jr.

SPLENOMEGALY

BASICS

DEFINITION
Enlargement, diffuse or asymmetric, of the spleen

Pathophysiology
Mechanisms of splenomegaly are often related to its varied functions, which include hematopoiesis, providing a blood reservoir, filtering and removing RBC, phagocytosis of microorganisms, and antibody synthesis.

Diffuse Enlargement
• Inflammation (splenitis) caused by the infiltration of cells, usually in response to an infectious agent. The cells can be neutrophils, eosinophils, lymphocytes, plasma cells, or macrophages. • Hyperplasia caused by increased demand for splenic function. This can be from bacterial infection or destruction of RBC. • Congestion because the spleens of dogs and cats have a large capacity for storing blood. Relaxation of the splenic capsule or high venous pressure causes pooling of blood in the spleen. • Extramedullary hematopoiesis in response to anemia (uncommon in cats) • Infiltration by neoplastic cells

Asymmetric Enlargement
• Neoplasms caused by uncontrolled cell growth. • Hematomas caused by intrasplenic bleeding. This can be caused by trauma, but this is uncommon. • Regenerative hyperplasia caused by injury to the spleen.

Systems Affected N/A

SIGNALMENT
• Varies depending on the cause • Hemangiosarcomas in older, large-breed dogs; male German shepherd dogs and golden retrievers are most common.

SIGNS

General Comments
Most signs are related to the conditions causing the enlargement.

Historical Findings
• Primary splenic disease such as splenic torsion causes anorexia, weight loss, weakness, abdominal distention, vomiting, diarrhea, and polyuria/polydipsia. • Some tumors, particularly hemangiosarcoma, can bleed into the abdominal cavity causing abdominal enlargement, pallor, and weakness.

Physical Examination Findings
• A uniformly enlarged spleen may be felt in some animals with diffuse enlargement.
• A round enlargement with part of the spleen normal may be palpated in some animals with asymmetric splenomegaly.
• Pallor, petechiae, and ecchymoses in some animals depending on the cause • Hepatomegaly in some animals with hypertension or hemolymphatic neoplasm • Large lymph nodes in conjunction with splenomegaly suggest lymphosarcoma.

CAUSES
• Inflammation—bacterial endocarditis, infectious canine hepatitis, salmonellosis, ehrlichiosis, pyometra, brucellosis, hemobartonellosis, systemic mycosis, feline infectious peritonitis, migrating foreign bodies, toxoplasmosis, mycobacteria, eosinophilic gastroenteritis, hypereosinophilic syndrome (cats), histoplasmosis, blastomycosis, leishmaniasis, and sporotrichosis • Hyperplasia—subacute bacterial endocarditis, chronic bacteremia (e.g., discospondylitis and brucellosis), systemic lupus erythematosus, immune hemolytic anemia, and other causes of RBC destruction • Congestion—administration of tranquilizers or anesthetics, portal hypertension, splenic torsion, right-sided heart failure, and heartworms • Infiltration—leukemia, mastocytosis, malignant histocytosis, lymphosarcoma, multiple myeloma, and extramedullary hematopoiesis • Asymmetric enlargement—most commonly, hemangiosarcoma, hemangioma, and hematoma; also, fibrosarcoma, leiomyosarcoma, leiomyoma, myelolipoma, malignant fibrous histiocytoma, and abscess

RISK FACTORS N/A

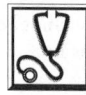

DIAGNOSIS

DIFFERENTIAL DIAGNOSIS
A large spleen must be differentiated from hepatic or other cranial abdominal mass.

CBC/BIOCHEMISTRY/URINALYSIS
The CBC is markedly affected by splenic function; results vary depending on the cause.
• High WBC count in animals with inflammation or abscess • Abnormal cells in the peripheral blood (e.g., neoplastic lymphocytes, mast cells, and eosinophils) in animals with infiltration • Anemia or thrombocytopenia in animals with hyperactivity • Spherocytes suggest immune hemolytic anemia. • Nucleated RBC in the peripheral blood in animals with splenic tumor • Hemoglobinemia resulting in hemoglobinuria in animals with splenic torsion

OTHER LABORATORY TESTS
• Hemangiosarcoma is frequently associated with disseminated intravascular coagulation (DIC). • Abnormalities in animals with DIC include anemia with schistocytes present, thrombocytopenia, high FDP, hypofibrinogenemia, and prolonged clotting times.

IMAGING

Radiography
• Useful to evaluate and sometimes to detect large spleen that can not be palpated • When splenomegaly is asymmetric, masses are usually seen in the caudal or midabdomen on abdominal radiographs. • Can also identify other problems such as gastric dilatation-volvulus, hepatomegaly, large lymph nodes, and ascites. • Thoracic radiographs are recommended to look for pulmonary metastasis or evidence of heart disease in animals suspected of having a splenic tumor or splenomegaly secondary to congestive heart failure.

Ultrasonography
• Useful to determine the size of the spleen and also its contour • Especially helpful to evaluate the parenchyma. Normal or hypoechogenicity without parenchymal abnormalities is seen in animals with congestive and diffuse infiltrative disorders. • Focal abnormalities such as cysts, hematomas, abscesses, and neoplasia can be readily visualized.
• Distension of vessels can also be detected—splenic vessels with torsion and portal vessels with portal hypertension • Useful in animals with peritoneal effusion in which the fluid obscures good radiographic detail of the abdomen.

OTHER DIAGNOSTIC PROCEDURES

Splenic Aspirate
• Cytologic evaluation of splenic aspirate is a safe and reliable procedure for evaluating splenomegaly. • Can usually be obtained blindly, but ultrasound guidance can also be used. • Anesthetics and phenothiazine tranquilizers cause aspirate to be blood contaminated. Diazepam (with or without ketamine) is preferred.

TREATMENT
Splenectomy—the main consideration in most animals is whether the animal will benefit from surgical removal of the spleen.

Diffuse Enlargement
• Of little benefit in most animals
• Indicated in cats with mast cell tumor

Asymmetric Splenomegaly
• Evaluate for spread of a malignant neoplasm before surgery
• Since the spleen is a site of extramedullary hematopoiesis and might be providing cells necessary for the life of the animal, the bone marrow must be evaluated before surgical removal in animals with cytopenias.
• Gross observation of splenic mass can not accurately differentiate between hematoma, hemangioma, and hemangiosarcoma. Previous splenic trauma can cause fragmentation of spleen with splenic nodules growing in omentum. Grossly, these nodules appear like tumor spread. Decisions concerning euthanasia should be made only after histopathologic examination has been performed.

MEDICATIONS

DRUGS AND FLUIDS
Vary with underlying cause

CONTRAINDICATIONS N/A

PRECAUTIONS N/A

POSSIBLE INTERACTIONS N/A

ALTERNATE DRUGS N/A

 FOLLOW-UP

PATIENT MONITORING N/A

POSSIBLE COMPLICATIONS
Overwhelming sepsis after removal of the spleen and its phagocytic functions (uncommon)

 MISCELLANEOUS

ASSOCIATED CONDITIONS
See Causes

AGE RELATED FACTORS N/A

ZOONOTIC POTENTIAL N/A

PREGNANCY N/A

SYNONYMS N/A

SEE ALSO See causes

ABBREVIATIONS
DIC = disseminated intravascular coagulation
FDP = fibrin degradation products
RBC = red blood cells
WBC = white blood cells

References

Couto CG, Hammer AS. Diseases of the lymph nodes and the spleen. In: Ettinger SJ, Feldman EC, eds. Textbook of veterinary internal medicine. 4th edition. Philadelphia: WB Saunders, 1995:1930-1946.

McEntee MC, Page RL. Diseases of the spleen. In: Birchard SJ, Sherding RG, eds. Saunders manual of small animal practice. Philadelphia: WB Saunders, 1994:178-184.
Author Dudley L. McCaw
Consulting Editor Albert E. Jergens

STEREOTYPES—CATS

BASICS

DEFINITION
Stereotypic behaviors are repetitive, relatively invariant behavior patterns without apparent function. Although controversial in their classification and interpretation, stereotypic behaviors such as psychogenic alopecia, compulsive pacing, repetitive vocalizing, and fabric sucking/chewing may be included under this heading when other causes of these behaviors cannot be identified.

Pathophysiology
This is a diagnosis of exclusion. Pathophysiologic etiologies must be ruled out before the diagnosis of stereotypic behavior may be made. Stereotypic behavior may be a behavioral response to undefined environmental conditions such as "stress" or "boredom." Over time, the behavior becomes fixed and independent of the environment. There may be species, breed, and family lines predisposed to stereotypic behaviors. The behaviors may be self-reinforcing, possibly caused by the release of endogenous opioids in the CNS. These behaviors may allow some animals to cope with otherwise intolerable conditions.

Systems Affected
• Nervous/skin—psychogenic alopecia
• Nervous/musculoskeletal—repetitive vocalization, compulsive pacing • Nervous/gastrointestinal—fabric sucking/chewing

SIGNALMENT
Any age, sex, or breed. Siamese and other Oriental breeds and crosses may be overrepresented for the behaviors of repetitive vocalization and fabric sucking/chewing.

SIGNS

General Comments
Stereotypic behaviors, when started, may quickly increase in frequency if they are reinforced in some way by the owner. The owner's response to the cat's behavior is an important part of the history.

Historical Findings
• Psychogenic alopecia—the owner may have observed excessive grooming to the exclusion of other activities or the behavior may occur secretly. Duration of the problem is variable. Frequently the owner reports that the problem started coincident with an environmental change such as a move or a new household member. • Compulsive pacing—the owner may complain that the behavior began intermittently and has increased in frequency. Initiation of the problem may have occurred at a time of confinement, as when restricted from going outdoors. • Repetitive vocalization • Fabric sucking/chewing—often the behavior spontaneously appears in the animal's repertoire, although it has been suggested that

affected cats may have been weaned early. Some cats show preference for a specific fabric type such as wool. Some cats suck the fabric in a manner reminiscent of suckling behavior; other cats chew the fabric and ingest it. With time, the cat may become adept at detecting opportunities for fabric sucking/chewing.

Physical Examination Findings
• Psychogenic alopecia—focal partial to complete alopecia is evident, most commonly in the groin, ventrum, and medial thigh regions. The appearance of the skin at the site of alopecia is variable and may appear normal or abnormal, from erythematous to abraded.
• Compulsive pacing—typically, within normal limits. Rule out neurologic abnormalities. • Repetitive vocalization—typically, within normal limits • Fabric sucking/chewing—typically, within normal limits. Secondary gastrointestinal inflammation or obstruction may occur.

CAUSES
The exact cause or causes in otherwise normal animals have not been identified. Organic causes must be ruled out before a psychogenic etiology is presumed.

RISK FACTORS
• Cats experiencing changes in their surroundings are predisposed. These disorders are more commonly reported in cats living indoors, although this may be an artifact of the higher level of attention such cats receive. • Alternately, these behaviors may be related to the stress of confinement or social isolation, as with pacing and other forms of barrier frustration seen in felids in zoological parks.

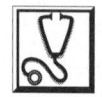

DIAGNOSIS

DIFFERENTIAL DIAGNOSIS
Medical differentials must be ruled out before a behavioral diagnosis can be made.

Psychogenic Alopecia
• Skin conditions, especially those associated with pruritus • External parasites • Fungal dermatitis • Bacterial dermatitis • Allergic dermatitis (including food allergy) • Cutaneous neoplasia • Eosinophilic granuloma complex • Nervous system disorders • Disk rupture and associated neuritis • Feline hyperesthesia syndrome • Pain

Compulsive Pacing
• Normal sexual behavior of the queen or tom • Nervous system disorders • Chronic pain • Focal brain lesions such as tumor and stroke • Postictal, seizure disorder • Metabolic/endocrine disorders • Biotin deficiency • Hepatic encephalopathy • Hyperthyroidism • Lead intoxication • Renal failure • Thiamin deficiency

Repetitive Vocalization
• Normal sexual behavior • Deafness

• Hyperthyroidism • Lead intoxication

Fabric Sucking/Chewing
• Lead intoxication • Hyperthyroidism • Thiamin deficiency

CBC/BIOCHEMISTRY/URINALYSIS
Used to rule out metabolic abnormalities

OTHER LABORATORY TESTS
• Psychogenic alopecia—microscopic exam of hairs typically reveals shafts to be cleanly broken off at variable length as a result of trauma from the cat's tongue. Other tests to rule out dermatologic conditions include skin scraping, fungal culture, bacterial culture, skin biopsy, and intradermal allergy testing.
• Compulsive pacing—cerebral spinal fluid analysis if indicated by abnormal neurologic exam, serum T4, T3. • Repetitive vocalization—cerebral spinal fluid analysis if indicated by abnormal neurologic exam; serum T4, T3. • Fabric sucking/chewing—serum lead titre; T4, T3 if indicated in cats with pica

IMAGING
Abnormalities on the neurologic exam may indicate the need for computerized tomography or magnetic resonance imaging. Questionable serum thyroid levels may indicate thyroid imaging.

OTHER DIAGNOSTIC PROCEDURES
In cats with psychogenic alopecia, examination for fleas and their products or an elimination diet may be indicated.

TREATMENT

ENVIRONMENTAL AND SURGICAL CONTROL
• Reduce environmental "stress" by increasing the predictability of household events, including feeding, play, exercise, and time available for social interactions with the owner. Eliminate unpredictable events as much as possible. Confinement is contraindicated.
• Psychogenic alopecia—topical agents as deterrents are usually ineffective
• Compulsive pacing—allowing the cat to go outside after the start of this behavior may reinforce it. Instead, if permitted, let out the cat before the behavior begins.
• Repetitive vocalizations—breed or spay the cat if an intact female; castrate an intact male
• Fabric chewing/sucking—keep fabrics of interest out of the cat's reach. Increase dietary roughage.

BEHAVIOR MODIFICATION
• The behavior should not be rewarded with attention by the owner. Instead, the owner should be instructed to ignore the behavior as much as possible. Note details of the time, place, and social milieu so that an alternative behavior such as play or feeding may be scheduled then.
• Punishment associated with the owner's voice, movement, and touch will increase the

unpredictability of the environment. Such interactions may increase fear or aggressive behavior toward the owner and disrupt the human/animal bond.

MEDICATIONS

DRUGS AND FLUIDS

• Environmental control is the preferred method of management, but psychoactive drugs may be needed concurrently. The goal is to use the drugs until control is achieved for 2 months, then attempt gradual withdrawal.

Drugs; dosage used to manage stereotypic behaviors; latency; and side effects:

• Benzodiazepine (diazepam); 1-2 mg/cat q12h; immediate; sedation, idiopathic hepatic necrosis

• Phenothiazine (acepromazine); 0.125-0.25 mg/cat PO q12h; immediate; sedation, paradoxical excitation

• Azaperone (buspirone); 5-7.5 mg/cat PO q12h; 3-4 weeks; GI signs

• Tricyclic antidepressant (amitriptyline); 2.5-7.5 mg/cat PO q12-24h; 3-4 weeks; sedation, anticholinergic effects

• Tricyclic antidepressant (clomipramine); 1-2.5 mg/cat PO q12-24h; 3-4 weeks; sedation, anticholinergic effects, cardiac conduction disturbances

• Selective serotonin reuptake inhibitor (fluoxetine); 1-5 mg/cat PO q24h; 3-4 weeks; inappetence, irritability

• Narcotic antagonist (naltrexone); 25-50 mg/cat PO q24h; immediate

CONTRAINDICATIONS

• Benzodiazepines—a rare but potentially fatal condition, idiopathic hepatic necrosis, may develop spontaneously after short term use of the benzodiazepine diazepam

• Tricyclic antidepressants—these drugs have potent antihistamine and anticholinergic (atropine-like) side effects. Cardiovascular abnormalities, particularly cardiac conduction disturbances, glaucoma, and urinary and fecal retention, are contraindications for the use of tricyclic antidepressants.

PRECAUTIONS

• Drug abuse—psychotropic drugs have hu-

man abuse potential. Sensible precautions should be taken to ensure that prescriptions for pets are not abused by humans. When taken in overdose (as in ingesting a bottle of pills) by pets or humans, the tricyclic antidepressants can cause fatal cardiac disturbances. There is no antidote. These medications should be dispensed in small quantities (not more than a 4-week supply) with refills to decrease the risk of fatalities.

• Extralabel drug use—there are no drugs approved by the FDA for the treatment of stereotypic behaviors in cats. Explain to the client the experimental nature of these treatments and the risk involved. Such a discussion should be documented by a notation in the medical record or by the use of a dedicated release form.

• Side effects—instructions and common side effects should be given in writing to the client. For example, the benzodiazepines and tricyclic antidepressants may cause sedation until drug tolerance develops. The use of psychotropic drugs should be initiated when the owner is present to monitor the patient.

• Phenothiazines—these drugs may cause akathisia, expressed as motor restlessness and paradoxical excitation, in some individuals. Extrapyramidal side effects include ataxia and tremors.

• Benzodiazepines—although rare, idiopathic hepatic necrosis may occur in apparently healthy cats given therapeutic doses of the benzodiazepine diazepam, both in the generic and proprietary (Valium) formulations

• Tricyclic antidepressants—although they are generally well-tolerated, tricyclic antidepressants have numerous potential side effects. These include anticholinergic (atropine-like) and antihistaminic effects. These drugs should be used with caution in patients with urinary or fecal retention.

POSSIBLE INTERACTIONS

Benzodiazepine drugs can interact with cimetidine.

ALTERNATE DRUGS N/A

FOLLOW-UP

PATIENT MONITORING

• Treatment of behavioral problems requires a schedule of follow-ups for success. • Clients on a program of environmental modification or psychoactive medications will need to make adjustments according to the responses of the patient. • If one medication is not effective after dosage adjustment, selection of an agent from another drug class is recommended.

POSSIBLE COMPLICATIONS

Realistic expectations must be made. Immediate control of a long-standing problem is unlikely. Before treatment, a baseline of the frequency of stereotypic bouts occurring each week should be established so that progress can be monitored.

MISCELLANEOUS

ASSOCIATED CONDITIONS

Avoidance behavior or aggression toward the owner may be exhibited if the owner punishes the cat when it exhibits a stereotypic behavior.

AGE RELATED FACTORS N/A

ZOONOTIC POTENTIAL N/A

PREGNANCY

Tricyclic antidepressants are contraindicated in pregnant animals.

SYNONYMS

• Compulsive behavior • Obsessive-compulsive behavior • Stereotypies • Psychogenic alopecia • Neurodermatitis • Psychic eczema • Pacing • Repetitive vocalizations • Crying • Vocalizing • Fabric chewing/sucking • Wool chewing/sucking

ABBREVIATIONS N/A

References

Beaver BV. Feline behavior: a guide for veterinarians. Philadelphia: WB Saunders, 1992.
Overall KL. Practical pharmacological approaches to behavior problems. In: Behavioral problems in small animals. St. Louis; Ralston Purina Company, 1992:36-51.
Simpson BS, Simpson DM. Behavioral pharmacotherapy. In: Borchelt P, Voith V, eds. Readings in companion animal behavior. Trenton, NJ: Veterinary Learning Systems, 1996:100-115.

Author Barbara S. Simpson
Consulting Editor Joane M. Parent

STEREOTYPES—DOGS

BASICS

DEFINITION

• Stereotypy is a repetitious, relatively unvaried sequence of movements which have no obvious purpose or function, usually derived from contextually normal maintenance behaviors (e.g., grooming, eating, walking). Inherent in the classification is that the behavior interferes with normal functioning.
• Obsessive-compulsive disorder (OCD) is an American Psychiatric Association classification of abnormal behavior that is characterized by recurrent, frequent thoughts or actions that are out of context to the situations in which they occur. These behaviors can involve cognitive or physical rituals and are deemed excessive (given the context) in duration, frequency, and intensity of the behavior. One of the hallmarks of this condition that distinguishes it from motor tics, etc. is that OCD behaviors follow a set of rules created by the patient. The most common stereotypies/OCD in dogs include spinning, tail chasing, self-mutilation, hallucinating ("fly biting"), circling, fence running, hair/air biting, pica, pacing, staring and vocalizing, self-directed vocalization, and, potentially, some aggressions.

Pathophysiology

Stereotypies/OCD come to the practitioner's attention because the client perceives changes in the animal's behavior or because the client feels that the pet has never been normal. While the underlying pathophysiology is unclear, clinical signs are consistent with alterations in CNS transmitter function. The main neurotransmitters implicated in stereotypic behavior include dopamine, serotonin, and, for conditions involving mutilation, endorphins.

Systems Affected

• Cardiovascular—can include tachycardia
• Endocrine/metabolic—in dogs with anxieties, signs can include those caused by alterations in the hypothalamus axis • Gastrointestinal—inappetence, aberrant appetite (including pica and coprophagia), and gastrointestinal distress • Hemic—stress leukograms are common • Musculoskeletal—poor condition attributable to increased motor activity and self-injury • Nervous—increased motor activity, repetitive activity, trembling, and self-injury are common • Skin/exocrine—skin lesions usually are secondary and may be a result of self-injury, overgrooming, barbering, sucking, or abrasion from repetitive activity. Lick granulomas are not uncommon concomitant signs and may be a dermatologic manifestation.

SIGNALMENT

No age, breed, or sex is overrepresented. These conditions, like other anxiety disorders, begin to develop at the onset of social maturity (18-36 months in dogs). Tail chasing is not uncommon in bull terriers and seems to run in families. German shepherds have been reported to be overrepresented in animals with OCD that spin. Some lines of great Danes and German shorthaired pointers display self-mutilation, stereotypic motor behavior (fence running), or hallucinations. Not all family members show the same manifestation of OCD (i.e., spinning versus grooming versus hallucinating). In fact, the opposite may be true. In humans, the presence of any one manifestation of OCD is associated with an increased risk of another manifestation in first-degree relatives.

SIGNS

General Comments

Signs associated with OCD can be nonspecific. Regardless of the presenting sign, the particular class of behavior may be a manifestation of an OCD if the client cannot interrupt the behavior, if it intensifies over time, increases in frequency or duration, and interferes with normal functioning.

Historical Findings

Clients may report that the dog began to chase his tail as part of play but now the tip is missing and even physical restraint does not stop the dog. While young dogs can exhibit OCD, its onset is more common during social maturity. Play decreases with age and OCD increases (i.e., the conditions worsen with time).

Physical Examination Findings

Usually nonremarkable except for self-induced injuries and the lack of condition that may be associated with increased motor activity and the repetitive behaviors. The exception to this is self-mutilation with a focus on the tail, forelimbs, and distal extremities.

CAUSES

Although any illness or painful physical condition can increase an animal's anxieties and be contributory to these problems, few of these conditions actually cause OCD. The possible exception to this is the extent to which kenneling or incarceration may be associated with dogs that spin. Abnormal behavior is likely to be rooted in either primary or secondary aberrant neurochemical activity.

RISK FACTORS N/A

DIAGNOSIS

DIFFERENTIAL DIAGNOSIS

Common ruleouts include those that would cause similar behavioral changes—seizures, brain disease, and metabolic disease. Behavioral conditions, including play and attention seeking, could look like the early stages of OCD.

CBC/BIOCHEMISTRY/URINALYSIS

All should be performed and be within the laboratory's reference range.

OTHER LABORATORY TESTS

Based on clinical signs and serum biochemistry results. It may be beneficial to test for thyroid disease and liver disease, but these are not mandatory. If there is doubt about whether the signs are "behavioral," nonremarkable results of these tests should confirm a behavioral diagnosis.

IMAGING N/A

OTHER DIAGNOSTIC PROCEDURES

Biopsies of dermatologic lesions may confirm whether they are primary or secondary, CSF taps may rule out infectious CNS disease, and endoscopy can evaluate primary bowel disease. Cardiac disease can produce physical signs of "anxiety." ECG may be useful as a diagnostic ruleout or as a premedication precaution. The extent to which endorphin metabolism may be driving OCD can be evaluated by the administration of naloxone (11-22 mg/kg IV). If the behavior has not decreased dramatically in intensity or frequency within 15-20 minutes, it is unlikely that the main driving mechanism is one of aberrant endorphin metabolism.

TREATMENT

Most patients respond to a combination of behavior modification and pharmacologic treatment with antianxiety medication. Pharmacologic intervention should be implemented early and may be a prerequisite to effecting any behavioral therapy.
• Treat as an outpatient. Exceptions to this include dogs with severe self-mutilation and self-induced injury, or those who need to be protected from the environment until their antianxiety medications reach effective plasma and CSF levels (days to weeks). For these patients, use constant day care, dogsitting, or in-hospital monitoring, stimulation, and care.
• Sedation may be an option in profound cases, but is only a stop-gap measure. Behavior modification should be geared toward teaching the dog to relax in a variety of environmental settings, and to substitute a calm, competitive behavior for the stereotypic one. Do not encourage the client to reassure the dog that he does not have to spin, chew, etc., because this will inadvertently reward the repetitive behaviors.
• Desensitization and counterconditioning are most effective if instituted early and can be coupled to a verbal cue that signals the dog to execute the behavior that is competitive with the ones that interfere with normal functioning. For example, instead of circling, the dog is taught to relax and lie down with his head and neck stretched prone on the floor when the client says "Head down."
• Punishment is contraindicated. It could make the behavior worse and render the dog more secretive.

• Any painful conditions should be diagnosed and controlled because pruritus and pain are both neurochemically related to anxiety and its perception. Amputation should be avoided when possible because it eliminates the outward signs of the condition while doing nothing to alleviate it.

MEDICATIONS

DRUGS AND FLUIDS

• Medications of choice include antianxiety medications that increase central levels of serotonin. These include the tricyclic antidepressants (TCA) and the more specific selective serotonin reuptake inhibitors (SSRI). Before any medication, perform blood profiles.

• Continuous treatment mandates follow-up laboratory evaluations as indicated by clinical signs or annually for younger patients and semiannually for older ones.

• Drugs of choice include amitriptyline (Elavil 1-2 mg/kg [to start] PO q12h for 30 days) and imipramine (Tofranil 1-2 mg/kg PO q12h for 30 days) for animals with mild OCD. OCD that has been ongoing for a long time will require clomipramine (Anafranil 1 mg/kg PO q12h for 14 days, then 2 mg/kg PO q12h for 14 days, then 3 mg/kg PO q12h for 28 days; if successful this will be the maintenance dosage) or fluoxetine (Prozac 1 mg/kg PO q24h for 2 months), or some combination of the above. Clients need to know that both clomipramine and fluoxetine can take 3-5 weeks to demonstrate an effect. If the signs of OCD revolve primarily around self-mutilation, narcotic antagonists (naltrexone; Trexan 2.2 mg/kg PO q8-12-24h) may be useful. The drugs are unlikely to work if the behavior was not blocked by intravenous naloxone administration. Thioridazine (Thorazine) occasionally has been used as an adjuvant treatment, but newer, more specific treatments appear more effective.

CONTRAINDICATIONS

Some medications are contraindicated in animals with hepatic and renal compromise because these are their main routes of metabolism. Animals with cardiac conduction anomalies should only be given TCA with extreme caution and monitoring.

PRECAUTIONS

• All of the medications recommended are extralabel. Follow all recommendations. Human and animal overdoses of TCA can cause profound cardiac conduction disturbances.

• Perform premedication ECG.

POSSIBLE INTERACTIONS

• Any medication that impairs glucuronidation may cause increases of active metabolites in these medications.

• Most TCA and SSRI have active intermediate metabolites, and their pharmacokinetics may differ from that of the parent compound. Combination therapy using two antianxiety agents may potentiate either or both medications, so dosages should be low.

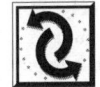

FOLLOW-UP

PATIENT MONITORING

• With continuous treatment, semiannual or annual CBC and serum biochemistry analyses are desirable. Annual ECG is elective. Adjust dosage accordingly. Monitor as warranted by clinical signs and advise clients.

POSSIBLE COMPLICATIONS

Early intervention using behavioral modification and pharmacologic intervention is key. Little is understood about the neurochemistry of these disorders, but left untreated they always progress.

MISCELLANEOUS

ASSOCIATED CONDITIONS

As with other anxiety-related conditions, the most common associated conditions are irritable bowel syndrome and lick granulomas.

AGE RELATED FACTORS

OCD appears most frequently at social maturity. We know little about contributory and developmental factors, but any condition that can contribute to the dog's underlying anxiety or to his perception of it can worsen the condition.

ZOONOTIC POTENTIAL N/A

PREGNANCY

Most of the drugs used to treat these conditions are either not evaluated in or contraindicated in pregnant animals. Their use probably should be avoided.

SYNONYMS

Stereotypies and OCD are now used interchangeably.

SEE ALSO N/A

ABBREVIATIONS

OCD = obsessive-compulsive disorder
TCA = tricyclic antidepressants
SSRI = selective serotonin reuptake inhibitors

References

Brown SA, Crowell-Davis ST, Edwards P. Naloxone-responsive compulsive tail chasing in a dog. J Am Vet Med Assoc 1987;190:884-886.

Dodman NH, Shuster L, White SD, et al. Use of narcotic antagonists to modify stereotypic self-licking, self-chewing, and scratching behavior in dogs. J Am Vet Med Assoc 1988;193:815-819.

Luescher UA, McKeown DB, Halip J. Stereotypic or obsessive-compulsive disorders in dogs and cats. Vet Clin NA (Small Anim Pract) 1991;21:401-414.

Overall KL. Recognition, diagnosis, and management of obsessive-compulsive disorders. Part 1. Canine Pract 1992;17(2): 40-44.

Overall KL. Use of clomipramine to treat ritualistic stereotypic motor behavior in three dogs. J Am Vet Med Assoc 1994;205: 1733-1741.

Author Karen L. Overall
Consulting Editor Joane M. Parent

STERTOR AND STRIDOR

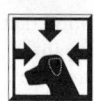

BASICS

DEFINITION
• Stertor and stridor are abnormally loud sounds that result from air passing through the abnormally narrowed pharynx or larynx as a result of increased resistance arising from partial obstruction of these regions. • Stertor refers to the low-pitched snoring sound that usually arises from the vibration of flaccid tissue or fluid; stridor describes the higher-pitched sounds that occur when relatively rigid tissues are vibrated by the passage of air. • In most situations, stertor arises from pharyngeal airway obstructions, while stridor is commonly the result of nasal or laryngeal obstructions.

Pathophysiology
• When airway obstruction is present, turbulence arises as the air passes through the narrowed passage. With increasing obstruction or air velocity, the amplitude of the sound will rise as the tissue, secretion, or foreign body comprising the obstruction is vibrated. • If the obstruction is sufficient to increase the work of breathing, the respiratory muscles will increase their effort and the turbulence will be exacerbated. Inflammation and edema of the tissues in the region of the obstruction may occur, further reducing the airway lumen and further increasing the work of breathing, leading to a vicious cycle.

Systems Affected
Respiratory

SIGNALMENT
• Brachycephalic dogs and cats • Affected dogs are typically less than 1 year of age when owners detect a problem. Cats have been diagnosed less commonly than dogs, so that no obvious pattern of age is apparent. • There is no sex predilection for any of the causes. • Inherited laryngeal paralysis has been identified in Bouvier des Flandres, Siberian husky crosses, and dalmatians. • If the cause of the obstruction is a tumor, the animal usually is older.

SIGNS
• The presence of a partial obstruction will produce an increase in airway sounds before it produces an obvious change in respiratory pattern and long before it produces a change in the respiratory function of gas exchange. Thus, the increased sound can be present without any obvious change in behavior. • Owners may report that the sound has been present for as long as several years. • Whenever breath sounds are audible from a distance without a stethoscope, the veterinarian should suspect a narrowing of the upper airway. • The nature of the sound may range from abnormally loud airway sounds to obvious fluttering to high-pitched squeaking, depending on the degree of airway narrowing. • An increased respiratory effort may be present. "Paradoxical" respiratory movements, with the chest wall collapsing inward during inspiration and springing outward during expiration, can be noted when the effort is extreme. These movements often are accompanied by obvious postural changes (abducted forelimbs, extended head and neck, and open-mouth breathing).

CAUSES
• Brachycephalic syndrome • Laryngeal paralysis (inherited or acquired) • Airway tumors and middle ear polyps • Acromegaly • Neuromuscular dysfunction (myasthenia gravis, brain stem disease, polyneuropathy, polymyopathy, hypothyroidism) • Anesthesia/sedation, but only if predisposing anatomy exists • Edema or inflammation of palate, pharynx, larynx (including everted mucosal lining of the laryngeal ventricles) secondary to: • Coughing, vomiting/regurgitation, turbulent airflow, upper respiratory infections, hemorrhage; Secretions such as pus, mucus, blood in the airway lumen (e.g., acutely after surgery; normal conscious animal would cough these out or swallow them) or foreign bodies

RISK FACTORS
• High ambient temperature • Fever • High metabolic rate such as occurs with hyperthyroidism or sepsis • Exercise • Anxiety • Any respiratory or cardiovascular disease that increases ventilation • The turbulence caused by the increased airflow actually may lead to swelling and worsen the airway obstruction.

DIAGNOSIS

DIFFERENTIAL DIAGNOSIS
• Sounds from pharyngeal and laryngeal narrowing must be differentiated from sounds arising elsewhere in the respiratory system. Nasal and tracheal narrowing can lead to increased respiratory sounds, as can severe or extensive narrowing of the bronchi. If the sound persists when the animal opens its mouth, a nasal cause can virtually be ruled out. If the sound occurs only during expiration, it is likely that an intrathoracic narrowing is the cause. • If the owners describe a change in voice, this directs attention immediately to the larynx as the abnormal site. In the absence of these helpful indicators, auscultation over the nose, pharynx, larynx, and trachea should be carried out systematically to identify the point of maximal intensity of any abnormal sound, as well as to identify the phase of respiration when it is most obvious. • It is important, in addition to identifying the anatomic location from which the abnormal sound arises, to seek exacerbating causes as described above in risk factors. Thus, a chronic airway obstruction may become manifest when an animal is exposed to extremely high ambient temperatures.

CBC/BIOCHEMISTRY/URINALYSIS
N/A

OTHER LABORATORY TESTS N/A

IMAGING
Lateral films of the head and neck can be helpful for identifying abnormal soft tissues of the airway such as an elongated soft palate or a nasal polyp. Their usefulness for indicating laryngeal disease is limited, although experienced radiographers can identify abnormally dilated or swollen laryngeal saccules. External masses compressing the upper airway may be further evaluated. Radiography and fluoroscopy are important to assess the cardiorespiratory system, generally to rule out other or additional causes of respiratory difficulty. Such conditions may add to an underlying upper airway obstruction, causing a subclinical condition to become symptomatic.

OTHER DIAGNOSTIC PROCEDURES
• If the origin of the abnormal sounds is identified as the pharynx or larynx, the definitive diagnostic test is direct visualization (pharyngoscopy/laryngoscopy). Because this assessment requires general anesthesia, the patient's anesthetic risk must be considered. • It is important to realize that the animal's ability to use muscles to open the airway will be compromised by anesthesia. Thus, the veterinarian and the clients must consider whether they are prepared to carry out surgical remedies if these are indicated. If no remediable condition is identified and corrected, the animal's recovery from anesthesia may be complicated by severe airway obstruction. At the very least, preparations must be in place for a tracheostomy in case the airway is found to be obstructed and a definitive surgical remedy cannot be pursued immediately. • The timing and degree of movement of the vocal folds during light anesthesia must be assessed to evaluate whether laryngeal paralysis is present. • The normal palate is thin and just barely overlaps the tip of the epiglottis. It is easily displaced dorsally using the blade of the laryngoscope. In contrast, the overlong soft palate is thick, usually inflamed, and may lie as much as 1 cm or more past the tip of the epiglottis. • While the patient should be as stable as possible before undergoing general anesthesia, this procedure should not be unduly delayed because appropriate surgical treatment is the only means of reducing the airway obstruction in most patients. • Appropriate measures to stabilize the patient may include administration of oxygen if cyanosis or syncope is present, cooling if the body temperature is high, and control of edema (corticosteroids or diuretics).

TREATMENT
• Hypoxia and hypoventilation occur only after prolonged severe obstruction. Provision

of oxygen is therefore not always critical to sustain life in the patient with partial airway collapse. Keeping the patient cool, quiet, and calm is extremely important. Anxiety, exertion, and pain lead to increased ventilation, potentially worsening the obstruction. All sedatives, however, may relax the upper airway muscles and worsen the obstruction. Thus, if a sedative is to be administered, its effect should be monitored closely and the clinician should be prepared with emergency means for securing the airway in the event of complete obstruction.

• In extreme cases of airway obstruction, an emergency intubation should be attempted. If the obstruction prevents intubation, emergency tracheostomy or passage of a tracheal catheter to administer oxygen may be the only available means for sustaining life. A tracheal catheter can only serve briefly to sustain oxygenation while more a permanent solution is sought.

• Serious complications may occur and persist despite efforts to relieve the obstruction. These include airway edema, pulmonary edema, which can progress to life-threatening acute lung injury, and hypoventilation. All of these problems may result in the need to provide a tracheostomy and/or to provide artificial ventilation.

MEDICATIONS

DRUGS AND FLUIDS

• Medical approaches to stertor and stridor will only be appropriate if the underlying cause is infection, edema, inflammation, or hemorrhage. Anatomic or neurologic causes are not amenable to symptomatic medical treatment.

• If edema or inflammation is thought to be an important contributor, steroids may be indicated. Any effect of intravenous steroids should be apparent in approximately 1 hour. Diuretics may be administered, although their efficacy is doubtful.

CONTRAINDICATIONS N/A

PRECAUTIONS

• Atropine, while reducing fluid secretions, will make mucus more tenacious and is thus not advisable other than as an adjunct to emergency resuscitative procedures.

• Sedatives and anesthetics

POSSIBLE INTERACTIONS N/A

ALTERNATE DRUGS N/A

FOLLOW-UP

If the owners have elected to try medical treatment, phone follow-up may be the most prudent course, as the excitement of an office visit can precipitate a crisis. Even after surgical treatment, some degree of obstruction may remain. In that case, owners should be advised to avoid exercise, high ambient temperature, and extreme excitement.

POSSIBLE COMPLICATIONS

Particular care should be taken when inducing general anesthesia or when using sedatives in any patient with upper airway obstruction

CLIENT EDUCATION

An obstructed patient can make the transition from a noisy breather to an obstructed emergency in a few minutes or even seconds.

If an owner chooses to take an apparently stable patient home, or if continual observation is not feasible, the possibility that complete obstruction can occur must be considered and discussed.

MISCELLANEOUS

ASSOCIATED CONDITIONS N/A

AGE RELATED FACTORS N/A

ZOONOTIC POTENTIAL N/A

PREGNANCY N/A

SYNONYM
Snoring

SEE ALSO
See causes.

ABBREVIATIONS N/A

References

Hendricks JC. Brachycephalic airway syndrome. Update on respiratory disease. Vet Clin of N Am (Sm Anim Prac) 1992;22:1145-1153.

Hendricks JC. Respiratory condition in critical patients. Critical care. Vet Clin of N Am (Sm Anim Prac) 1989;19:1167-1188.

Nelson AW. Upper respiratory system. In: Slatter D, ed. Textbook of small animal surgery. 2nd ed. Philadelphia: WB Saunders, 1993:733–776.

Author Joan C. Hendricks
Consulting Editors Lynelle Johnson and Bradley L. Moses

STOMATITIS

BASICS

DEFINITION
Inflammation of the oral mucosa. It may involve any area of the mouth and can be due to local or systemic factors. It is a sign of disease rather than a specific disease entity.

Pathophysiology
The location and severity of lesions is largely influenced by the underlying cause. Secondary bacterial infection may worsen the clinical signs.

Systems Affected
Gastrointestinal

SIGNALMENT
• Dogs and cats • Feline juvenile-onset gingivitis-periodontitis occurs more frequently in Siamese, Maine coon, and domestic short-hair breeds. • Ulcerative stomatitis is a familial problem in some lines of Maltese dogs • Varies with the underlying cause

SIGNS
• Halitosis • Pain • Reluctance to open mouth or prehend food • Anorexia • Bleeding from gums or mouth • Ptyalism • Inflamed or ulcerated lesions in the oral cavity • Plaque and tartar accumulation

CAUSES

Degenerative

Anatomic (Congenital)
• Malocclusion • Retained decidous teeth • Cleft palate - primary or secondary • Gray collie syndrome

Metabolic
• Uremia • Diabetes mellitus • Hypoparathyroidism

Nutritional
• Protein-calorie malnutrition • Hypervitaminosis A (cats)

Neoplastic
• Malignant melanoma • Squamous cell carcinoma • Fibrosarcoma

Immune Mediated
Hypersensitivity Reactions
• Drug induced (toxic epidermal necrolysis—most severe form) • Insect bites
Autoimmune Diseases
• Pemphigus vulgaris • Bullous pemphigoid • Systemic lupus erythematosus • Discoid lupus erythematosus

Infectious
Bacterial
• Periodontal disease • Ulceromembranous stomatitis due to Fusobacterium and Spirochetes (trench mouth, St. Vincent's stomatitis) • Actinomyces • Nocardia • Mycobacterium lepraemurium • Leptospira spp.
Mycotic
• Candida albicans • Aspergillus and Penicillium (extension from nasal cavity)

• Blastomycosis • Histoplasmosis
Viral
• Feline viral rhinotracheitis • Feline calicivirus • Feline leukemia virus • Feline immunodeficiency virus • Feline infectious peritonitis • Feline panleukopenia • Canine distemper

Idiopathic
• Eosinophilic granuloma • Vasculitis

Traumatic
• Lacerations • "Cheek-chewers" lesion • Electrical cord injuries • Foreign bodies such as plant materials, bones, and string • Snakebite

Toxic
• Chemical irritants (e.g., Lye ingestion) • Chemotherapy • Radiation therapy • Chrysotherapy • Poisons (e.g., Thallium, Dieffenbachia)

RISK FACTORS N/A

DIAGNOSIS

DIFFERENTIAL DIAGNOSIS N/A

CBC/BICHEMISTRY/URINALYSIS
Useful to detect systemic diseases

OTHER LABORATORY TESTS
• Immunologic testing • Bacterial and fungal cultures • Serology • Virus isolation • Toxicologic studies • Serum protein electrophoresis

IMAGING
Radiography to identify dental or osseus abnormalities

OTHER DIAGNOSTIC PROCEDURES
Biopsy for histopathology and immunofluorescence testing

GROSS AND HISTOPATHOLOGIC FINDINGS
Focal or diffuse lesions in the oral cavity and/or oropharynx. Severity can range from erythema and swelling to deep necrotizing ulcers with severe tissue loss

TREATMENT
• Anorexic patients should be hospitalized to correct nutritional and hydration deficits. Others can be treated on an outpatient basis. • Soft foods are more readily eaten than hard foods. Anorexic patients should have their nutritional needs met by the placing of a feeding tube • Make clients aware that identifying a specific etiology may be difficult or impossible in some cases and that prolonged or intermittent treatment may be necessary. • Dental prophylaxis, periodontal therapy, or extraction of severely affected teeth are an integral part of the treatment protocol.

MEDICATIONS

DRUGS AND FLUIDS

Antimicrobials
• Treat primary and secondary infections with a broad-spectrum antibiotic with activity against gram-positive cocci and anaerobes • Amoxicllin-clavulanate (12.5–25 mg/kg q12h PO) • Clindamycin (11 mg/kg q12h PO) • Metronidazole (10 mg/kg q8h PO or 30mg/kg q24h PO) (anaerobic activity only)

Anti-inflammatory Drugs
• Improve patient comfort and may improve appetite • Prednisilone (0.5-1.0 mg/kg q12h-q24h PO then taper to q48h)

Topical Therapy
• Chlorhexidine solution or gel (CHX®, VRx Products®, Harbor City, CA) applied 2–3 times daily • Zinc-organic acid solutions or gels (e.g., Maxi-Guard®, Addison Biological Laboratory, Fayette, MO)—plaque retardant action in addition to promoting tissue healing

Immunosuppressive Drugs
Treat immune mediated diseases. See specific disease topic

CONTRAINDICATIONS
All of the antimicrobials listed are contraindicated in animals with known hypersensitivity. Glucocorticoids are contraindicated in patients with systemic fungal infections.

PRECAUTIONS
The most common adverse effects of the antimicrobials are gastrointestinal signs. Prolonged use or high dosages of amoxicillin and metronidazole can cause neurologic signs.

POSSIBLE INTERACTIONS
Cimetidine may slow metabolism of metronidazole

ALTERNATE DRUGS
See specific disease conditions

FOLLOW-UP

PATIENT MONITORING
Clinical response to treatment. Daily or frequent brushing with toothpaste or oral hygiene gels or solution are important in controlling periodontal lesions.

POSSIBLE COMPLICATIONS
Bacteremia has been implicated as a cause of renal, cardiac (myocardial and valvular disease), hepatic, and pulmonary disease

✓ MISCELLANEOUS

ASSOCIATED CONDITIONS N/A

AGE RELATED FACTORS N/A

ZOONOTIC POTENTIAL N/A

PREGNANCY

None of the antimicrobials listed have been proven safe for use in pregnant dogs and cats, but only metronidazole has been shown to have teratogenic effects (in laboratory animals)

SYNONYMS N/A

SEE ALSO

Individual diseases listed under Causes

ABBREVIATIONS N/A

References

Harvey CE, Emily PP. Veterinary dentistry. St. Louis: Mosby, 1993.

McKeever PJ. Stomatitis. In: Kirk RW, ed. Current veterinary therapy IX. Philadelphia: WB Saunders, 1986;846-848.

Sarkiala E, Harvey CE. Systemic antimicrobials in the treatment of periodontitis in dogs. Sem Vet Med Surg (Small Anim) 1993;8:197-203.

Smith MM. Oral and salivary gland disorders. In: Ettinger SJ, Feldman EC, eds. Textbook of veterinary internal medicine. 4th ed. Philadelphia: WB Saunders, 1995;1084-1096.

Wolf AM. Feline gingivitis, stomatitis, and pharyngitis. In: Kirk RW, Bonagura JD, eds. Current veterinary therapy XI. Philadelphia: WB Saunders, 1992;568-572.

Author Eric Russell Pope

Consulting Editor Brent D. Jones

STUPOR AND COMA

BASICS

DEFINITION
• Stupor—unconscious but arousable with noxious stimuli • Coma—unconscious and not arousable with noxious stimuli

Pathophysiology
The ascending reticular activating system (ARAS) processes peripheral sensory input through the brain stem reticular formation with pathways to the thalamus and cerebral cortex. It functions as the arousal system. Any severe pathologic change, either anatomic or metabolic, that causes interruption of neuronal function within the ARAS can lead to stupor or coma.

Systems Affected
• Nervous • Cardiovascular • Respiratory • Ophthalmic

SIGNALMENT
No breed, age, or sex predilection

SIGNS

Historical Findings
• The possibility of trauma or unsupervised roaming • Past medical problems of significance include diabetes mellitus and insulin therapy, hypoglycemia, cardiovascular problems, hypoxic episodes, renal failure, liver failure, and neoplasia. • A description of the animal's environment is recorded to identify possible heatstroke, hypothermia, drowning, or exposure to drugs, narcotics, and toxins (e.g., ethylene glycol, lead, anticoagulants), including owner's medications that could have been ingested by the animal. • Acute onset of stupor and coma is most commonly caused by toxins, drugs, trauma, or vascular or hematologic disorders. • Slow progression of neurologic signs, without systemic abnormalities, suggests primary neurologic disorders of inflammatory, neoplastic, or anatomic causes.

Physical Examination Findings
• Look for external and internal evidence of trauma. • Examine for severe hypothermia or hyperthermia. • Evidence of hypoxia or cyanosis, ecchymosis or petechiation, or cardiac or respiratory insufficiency warrants investigation for metabolic etiologies. • Careful palpation for evidence of neoplasia leads to pursuing neoplasia as a likely etiology. • Retinal hemorrhages or distended vessels suggest hypertension; papilledema suggests cerebral edema; retinal detachment suggests infectious, neoplastic, or hypertensive causes; chorioretinitis suggests infectious etiologies such as distemper, feline leukemia virus related diseases, toxoplasmosis, cryptococcosis, or feline infectious peritonitis. • Bradycardia suggests midbrain, pontine, or medullary lesion.

Neurologic Examination Findings
• Determine level of consciousness and whether animal is arousable. • Evaluate pupillary light reflexes—normal or miotic responsive pupils indicate cerebral or diencephalic lesion; dilated unresponsive pupils (unilateral or bilateral) or midpoint fixed unresponsive pupils reflect midbrain lesion, and miotic or normal pupils indicate pontine and medullary lesion • Perform oculocephalic reflex (cervical manipulation is possible)—loss of normal vestibular nystagmus indicates midbrain, pons, or medullary involvement • Observe respiratory patterns—Cheyne-Stokes respiration is observed with severe, diffuse, cerebral or diencephalic lesion, hyperventilation with the midbrain, and ataxic or apneustic breathing with associated pons or medulla • Evaluate cranial nerves—the exam is normal with lesion of cerebrum-diencephalon; deficits of cranial nerve III with midbrain; deficits of cranial nerves V-XII with the pons and medulla • Examine for postural changes—decerebrate rigidity indicates midbrain pathology

CAUSES
• Drugs—narcotics, depressants, and ivermectin • Anatomic—hydrocephalus • Metabolic—severe hypoglycemia, hyperglycemia; hyperosmolar syndromes; hypernatremia; hyponatremia; hepatic encephalopathy; hypoxemia; hypercarbia; hypothermia; hyperthermia, hypotension, coagulopathies, renal failure, lysosomal storage disease • Nutritional—hypoglycemia; thiamine deficiency • Neoplastic (primary)—meningioma, astrocytoma, gliomas, choroid plexus papilloma, pituitary adenoma, others • Metastatic—lymphosarcoma, mammary carcinoma, others • Inflammatory noninfectious—granulomatous meningoencephalomyelitis (GME) • Infectious—bacterial, viral (distemper, feline infectious peritonitis), parasitic (toxoplasmosis, aberrant larva migrans) fungal (cryptococcosis, blastomycosis, histoplasmosis, coccidioidomycosis, actinomycosis), and rickettsial disease • Idiopathic—epilepsy (poststatus epilepticus) • Immune-mediated— vasculitis and thrombocytopenia leading to hemorrhage • Traumatic • Toxins—ethylene glycol, lead, rodenticide anticoagulants, and others • Vascular—hemorrhage (bleeding disorders, hypertension), and infarction (feline ischemic encephalopathy, microfilaria, or migrating adult heartworm)

RISK FACTORS
• Diabetes mellitus—insulin therapy • Insulinomas • Severe heat or cold exposure without protection • Free roaming animals—trauma • Young and unvaccinated animals

DIAGNOSIS

DIFFERENTIAL DIAGNOSIS
• Differentiate from other altered states of consciousness, including narcolepsy, syncope, collapse, and severe depression. • Unlike stupor and coma, the animal that is collapsed or severely depressed is conscious with depressed mentation and depressed motor activity. • Narcolepsy causes intermittent episodes of deep sleep with spontaneous recovery. • Unlike stupor and coma, syncope is a temporary loss of consciousness with spontaneous recovery.

CBC/BIOCHEMISTRY/URINALYSIS
• Hemogram may show nucleated red blood cells or basophilic stippling if lead toxicity. An inflammatory hemogram may be present with severe infection. Severe anemia suggests hypoxemia. • Serum chemistry profile may show hypoglycemia, hyperglycemia, hypernatremia, renal failure, hepatoencephalopathy, hyperosmolarity, and other metabolic derangements. • Urinalysis can show glycosuria with diabetes mellitus, ammonium biurate crystals with hepatic encephalopathy, or ethylene glycol or hippurate crystals with ethylene glycol toxicity.

OTHER LABORATORY TESTS
• Serum ethylene glycol test or measure osmolar gap with acute onset of stupor or coma • Serum ammonia concentrations and pre- and postprandial bile acids diagnose hepatoencephalopathy as cause. • Serum and CSF titres for infectious diseases (e.g., distemper, feline infectious peritonitis, rickettsial diseases, cryptococcosis, blastomycosis, histoplasmosis, neospora caninum, toxoplasmosis) when inflammatory etiologies are suspected. • Arterial blood gases are measured for evidence of hypoxemia, severe pH changes, or hypercarbia. • When intracranial bleeding or thrombosis is suspected, a coagulogram (i.e., PT, PTT, fibrinogen, FDPs, platelet count, antithrombin III, buccal bleeding time) is performed. • Cite testing for FeLV, FIV, and heartworm disease to aid in detecting these infectious diseases.

IMAGING
• Survey radiographs of the chest and abdomen for evidence of organ compromise, inflammation, infiltration, or neoplasia • Skull radiographs are evaluated for fractures in trauma. • Computed tomography and magnetic resonance imaging scans are the best imaging modalities for detection of acute hemorrhage within the cranial vault or brain.

OTHER DIAGNOSTIC PROCEDURES
• CSF should be obtained (with the analysis including immunoglobulin concentrations and titres if infectious diseases are suspected) if there is no evidence of trauma and high intracranial pressure, coagulopathies, or metabolic disease. • Brain stem auditory evoked potentials are evaluated to determine brain stem function. • Electrocardiographic evaluation aids in determining cardiac dysfunction. The abnormalities may be contributing to the stupor or coma, or may be caused by the brain disease.

TREATMENT

• The head should be leveled with the body or elevated to a 20° angle. The head should never be lower than the body to avoid marked elevation in intracranial pressure (ICP). • The arterial pCO_2 should be maintained between 35-45 mm Hg. If ICP is high, hyperventilating to arterial pCO_2 of 25-30 mm Hg may reduce cerebral blood flow and ICP.
• Arterial pO_2 must be above 50 mm Hg to maintain cerebral blood flow autoregulation. A cough or sneeze reflex must be avoided during intubation or oxygen supplementation by nasal cannula because this can severely elevate ICP.
• Use peripheral veins, leaving the jugular vein blood flow unobstructed. Shifting of blood volume into the jugular veins is an important compensatory mechanism during ICP elevation.
• Thrashing seizures, or any other form of uncontrolled motor activity is to be prevented because this can elevate ICP. Infusion of diazepam (0.5-1mg/kg/hour) may be required to control the seizures.
• Meticulous nursing care prevents secondary complications of recumbency.
• Serious consideration of surgical decompression and exploration must be given when there is worsening of neurologic signs; cerebral dysfunction that is progressing to midbrain signs with a history of trauma or bleeding (tentorial herniation); high ICP not responsive to medical therapy (if monitoring instrumentation available); depressed skull fracture fragments; or penetrating foreign body.
• Nutrition must be maintained during the unconscious period, with nutritional requirements adjusted to compensate for metabolic demands.

MEDICATIONS

DRUGS AND FLUIDS

• Poor perfusion—resuscitation should be done with a minimal amount of crystalloids because these contribute to brain edema. A combination of large molecular weight colloids (i.e., hetastarch) with crystalloids will allow small fluid volume resuscitation. However, colloids should not be used if there is intracranial hemorrhage.

• Hydration is maintained with a balanced electrolyte crystalloid solution.
• Mean arterial blood pressure is maintained around 80 mm Hg using crystalloids and/or colloids. Avoid hypertension.
• Intracranial pressure elevations can be treated by hyperventilation and drug therapy. Furosemide decreases CSF production and lowers ICP. Mannitol improves brain blood flow and lowers ICP, and should be given after furosemide. As an alternative, hypertonic saline (7.5%) can be used in combination with a colloid such as hetastarch.
• Underlying disease—glucocorticosteroids can be given soon after brain trauma to reduce brain inflammation and prevent brain edema. Glucose supplementation is required for hypoglycemia. Hepatic encephalopathy requires lactulose enemas and fluid support. Renal failure requires fluid diuresis. Diabetes mellitus with hyperosmolality warrants rehydration and lowering of glucose slowly with insulin. Hyperthermic animals should have their intravascular volume supported and cooled. Hypothermic animals should have their intravascular volume supported and warmed. Suspected toxic ingestion warrants gastric lavage and instillation of activated charcoal with a cathartic. Specific toxins may require specific therapeutics (e.g., ethylene glycol treated with ethanol and peritoneal dialysis). Suspected bacterial infections are treated with antibiotics that cross the blood-brain barrier (e.g., trimethoprim-sulfa, chloramphenicol, and metronidazole) or broad spectrum antibiotics (e.g., first generation cephalosporins) if the blood-brain barrier is interrupted.

CONTRAINDICATIONS N/A

PRECAUTIONS

• Avoid hypertension.
• Avoid intravascular volume overload.
• Do not allow head to lie below plane of body.
• Do not use colloids when there is intracranial hemorrhage.
• Mannitol and hypertonic saline can worsen neurologic status when there is intracranial hemorrhage.
• When hyperventilating, maintain pCO_2 > 25 mm Hg. Do not hyperventilate for extended time periods (> 48 hours).

POSSIBLE INTERACTIONS N/A

ALTERNATE DRUGS N/A

FOLLOW-UP

PATIENT MONITORING

• Repeat neurologic exams to detect deterioration of function that warrants aggressive therapeutic intervention. • Blood gases to assess need for oxygen supplementation or ventilation and to monitor pCO_2 when hyperventilation is required • Blood glucose to ensure an adequate blood level to maintain brain functions and avoid hyperosmolality from high amounts • Electrocardiograms to detect arrhythmias that may affect perfusion, oxygenation, and cerebral blood flow • ICP monitoring to detect marked elevations and monitor success of therapeutics.

POSSIBLE COMPLICATIONS N/A

MISCELLANEOUS

ASSOCIATED CONDITIONS N/A

AGE RELATED FACTORS N/A

ZOONOTIC POTENTIAL N/A

PREGNANCY N/A

SYNONYMS N/A

SEE ALSO

Brain Injury

ABBREVIATIONS

ARAS = ascending reticular activating system
CSF = cerebrospinal fluid
FDP = fibrin degradation products
ICP = intracranial pressure
PT = prothrombin time
PTT = partial thromboplastin time

Reference
Chrisman CL. Coma and altered states of consciousness. In: Problems in small animal neurology. Philadelphia: Lea & Febiger, 1991:219-233.
Author Rebecca Kirby
Consulting Editor Joane M. Parent

SYNCOPE

 BASICS

DEFINITION
Temporary loss of consciousness and vascular tone associated with loss of postural tone, and spontaneous recovery.

PATHOPHYSIOLOGY
Inadequate cerebral perfusion and delivery of oxygen and metabolic substrates leads to loss of consciousness and motor tone. Impaired cerebral perfusion can result from changes in vasomotor tone, cerebral disease, and low cardiac output caused by structural heart disease or arrhythmias.

SYSTEMS AFFECTED
• Nervous • Cardiovascular

SIGNALMENT
More common in old animals

SIGNS N/A

CAUSES
Cardiac Causes
• Bradyarrhythmias—sinus bradycardia, sinus arrest, second degree atrioventricular (AV) block, complete AV block, atrial standstill
• Tachyarrhythmias—ventricular tachycardia, atrial tachycardia, atrial fibrillation • Reduced cardiac output (nonarrhythmic)—cardiomyopathy, AV valve endocardiosis, subaortic stenosis, pulmonic stenosis, heartworm disease, pulmonary embolism, cardiac tumor, cardiac tamponade

Neurologic and Vasomotor Instability
• Vasovagal syncope—emotional stress and excitement may cause heightened sympathetic stimulation followed by a compensatory rise in vagal tone. This results in excessive vasodilation without a compensatory rise in heart rate and cardiac output. Bradycardia may occur. • Situational syncope refers to syncope associated with coughing, defecation, urination, and swallowing. • Carotid sinus hyperactivity may cause hypotension and bradycardia; this is often the cause of syncope when one pulls on a dog's collar

Miscellaneous Causes
• Drugs that affect blood pressure and regulation of autonomic tone • Hypoglycemia, hypocalcemia, and hyponatremia (rare)
• Hyperviscosity syndromes (e.g., polycythemia and paraproteinemia) cause sludging of blood and impaired cerebral perfusion (rare)

RISK FACTORS
• Heart disease • Sinus node disease (e.g., sick sinus syndrome). Breeds at risk include cocker spaniel, miniature schnauzer, pug, and dachshund. Most common in old females.
• Drug therapy—vasodilators (i.e., calcium channel blockers, ACE inhibitors, hydralazine, and nitrates), phenothiazines (i.e., acepromazine), antiarrhythmics, and diuretics

 DIAGNOSIS

DIFFERENTIAL DIAGNOSIS
Differential Signs
• Must differentiate syncope from other altered states of consciousness, including seizures and narcolepsy • Unlike syncope, seizures are often associated with a prodromal and post-ictal period; syncope occurs without warning, and animal usually has rapid spontaneous recovery. • Unlike syncope, seizure activity is usually associated with tonic clonic muscle activity rather than flaccidity. • Must differentiate syncope from other causes of collapse such as musculoskeletal disease and neuromuscular disease (e.g., myasthenia gravis). These causes of collapse are not associated with a loss of consciousness.

Differential Causes
• Syncope with excitement or stress suggests vasovagal syncope. • Syncope with coughing, urination, or defecation suggests situational syncope. • Syncope with exercise suggests low output states associated with arrhythmias or structural heart disease. • Presence of a murmur supports heart disease but does not confirm cardiac cause for syncope.

CBC/BIOCHEMISTRY/URINALYSIS
• Results usually normal • Hypoglycemia or electrolyte disturbance in some animals

OTHER LABORATORY TESTS
• If animal is hypoglycemic, measure insulin concentration on same sample. Calculate an amended insulin:glucose ratio to rule out insulinoma. • If animal is hyponatremic or hyperkalemic, consider an ACTH stimulation test. • If you suspect low cardiac output, rule out occult heartworm disease.

IMAGING
Echocardiography
Diagnostic test of choice for documenting cardiomyopathy, congenital defects, and valvular disease

OTHER DIAGNOSTIC PROCEDURES
• Have owner monitor heart rate during any syncopal episode • Electroencephologram, computed tomography of the head, CSF tap if CNS origin is suspected

Electrocardiographic Findings
• Postexercise ECG may reveal intermittent arrhythmia • Holter monitoring (24-hour ECG recording) or use of an ECG event (loop) recorder useful for evaluating arrhythmic causes of syncope • Carotid sinus massage with ECG and blood pressure monitoring useful in evaluating carotid sensitivity

 TREATMENT

• Treat as outpatient unless important heart disease evident

• Minimize stimuli that precipitate syncopal episodes:
• Low CO—minimize activity
• Vasovagal—minimize excitement and stress
• Cough—remove collar, avoid inhaled respiratory irritants
• Defecation—use stool softeners to minimize straining
• Assure the owner that most noncardiac causes of syncope are not life-threatening, and most cardiac causes can be treated.
• Avoid or discontinue medications likely to precipitate syncope.

 MEDICATIONS

DRUGS AND FLUIDS
Bradyarrhythmias
• Correct metabolic causes
• Anticholinergics (e.g., atropine, propantheline bromide, and isopropamide iodide)
• Sympathomimetics (e.g., isoproterenol and bronchodilators)
• Pacemaker implantation in refractory animals

Tachyarrhythmias
• Atrial arrhythmias (administer digoxin, propranolol, or diltiazem).
• Ventricular arrhythmias (administer lidocaine, procainamide, quinidine, mexiletine, tocainide, sotalol, or propranolol).

Low Cardiac Output
Institute treatment to improve cardiac output., which varies according to specific cardiac disease.

Vasovagal
• Beta blockers (e.g., atenolol, propranolol, and metoprolol) may indirectly prevent vagal stimulation.
• Anticholinergics (e.g., propantheline bromide and scopolamine) may blunt the vagal response.
• Theophylline or aminophylline are sometimes helpful. Mechanism of action in this setting is unclear.

CONTRAINDICATIONS N/A
PRECAUTIONS
Drugs that lower blood pressure

POSSIBLE INTERACTIONS N/A
ALTERNATE DRUGS N/A

 FOLLOW-UP

PATIENT MONITORING
ECG or Holter monitoring to assess efficacy of antiarrhythmic therapy

POSSIBLE COMPLICATIONS
• Death • Trauma when collapse occurs

SYNCOPE

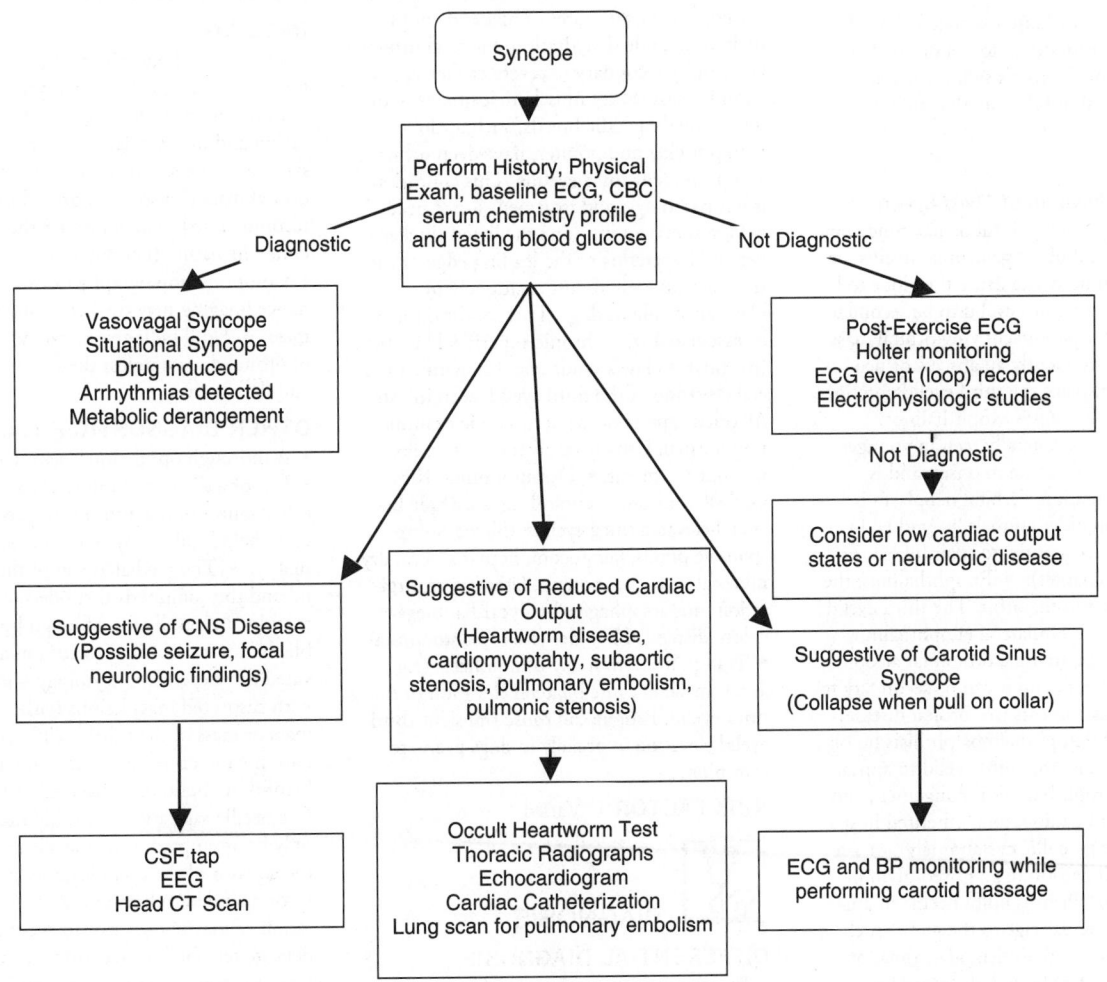

✓

MISCELLANEOUS

ASSOCIATED CONDITIONS N/A

AGE RELATED FACTORS N/A

ZOONOTIC POTENTIAL N/A

PREGNANCY N/A

SYNONYMS Fainting

SEE ALSO

• Seizures • Narcolepsy/cataplexy • Myasthenia Gravis

ABBREVIATIONS

ACE = angiotensin

References

Lusk RH, Ettinger SJ. Cardiovascular syncope. In: Fox PR, ed. Canine and feline cardiology. New York: Churchill Livingstone, 1988;335-339.

Kapoor WN. Hypotension and syncope. In: Braunwald E, ed. Heart disease: a textbook of cardiovascular medicine. 4th ed. Philadelphia:WB Saunders, 1992;875-886.

Author Francis W. K. Smith, Jr.

Consulting Editors Larry P. Tilley and Francis W. K. Smith, Jr

Syncope

Perform History, Physical Exam, baseline ECG, CBC serum chemistry profile and fasting blood glucose

Diagnostic

Not Diagnostic

Vasovagal Syncope
Situational Syncope
Drug Induced
Arrhythmias detected
Metabolic derangement

Post-Exercise ECG
Holter monitoring
ECG event (loop) recorder
Electrophysiologic studies

Not Diagnostic

Consider low cardiac output states or neurologic disease

Suggestive of CNS Disease (Possible seizure, focal neurologic findings)

Suggestive of Reduced Cardiac Output
(Heartworm disease, cardiomyoptahty, subaortic stenosis, pulmonary embolism, pulmonic stenosis)

Suggestive of Carotid Sinus Syncope
(Collapse when pull on collar)

CSF tap
EEG
Head CT Scan

Occult Heartworm Test
Thoracic Radiographs
Echocardiogram
Cardiac Catheterization
Lung scan for pulmonary embolism

ECG and BP monitoring while performing carotid massage

THIRD EYELID, PROTRUDING

 BASICS

DEFINITION

Abnormal protrusion of the third eyelid

Pathophysiology

In dogs, the movement of the third eyelid is passive, but cats have partial sympathetic nervous control of the third eyelid. Elevation (protrusion) of the third eyelid results from a space-occupying mass in the orbit pushing the third eyelid forward, enophthalmia, sympathetic denervation of the eye, or a painful eye.

Systems Affected

- Ophthalmic—third eyelid(s), orbit, eyeball
- Nervous—autonomic nervous system

SIGNALMENT See causes

SIGNS

Occurs with or without associated clinical signs, such as exophthalmos, enophthalmos, blepharospasm, Horner's syndrome (see below). Unilateral or bilateral, depending on the cause.

CAUSES

Unilateral Elevation of Third Eyelid

- Blepharospasm: a painful ocular condition such as a corneal ulcer, glaucoma, uveitis, or ocular foreign body can cause the globe to be retracted and the third eyelid to be secondarily elevated. • Space-occupying orbital mass: orbital mass (frequently an abscess or neoplasm) may displace the third eyelid anteriorly, and it usually causes exophthalmos. Orbital abscess is generally seen in younger animals, is usually acute in onset, and is painful on palpation. Orbital neoplasm is usually seen in older animals, is gradual in onset, and is frequently not painful (see orbital diseases chapter). • Enophthalmos: the globe recedes into the orbit. The third eyelid appears elevated. Unilateral enophthalmos can be caused by trauma, orbital fat atrophy, and inflammation, and it can be secondary to orbital neoplasia in cats (see orbital diseases chapter). • Microphthalmos/phthisis bulbi: small globes allow the third eyelid to appear elevated. Microphthalmos is congenital, and the defect can be idiopathic, inherited in specific breeds (e.g., collie eye anomaly), or a result of toxin ingestion (e.g., griseofulvin in pregnant cats). Phthisis bulbi occurs in animals with severe damage to the globe, such as that caused by severe uveitis, glaucoma, or trauma. The ciliary body fails to produce aqueous humor, intraocular pressure diminishes, and the globe becomes smaller and fibrotic as a sequela of chronic inflammation. • Horner's syndrome: clinical signs develop after sympathetic denervation, including elevated third eyelid, enophthalmos, ptosis (drooping of the upper eyelid), and miosis. (See Horner's syndrome) • Neoplasia of the third eyelid: adenocarcinoma of the gland of the third eyelid and squamous cell carcinoma of eyelid are the most common. • Cherry eye: see chapter on prolapsed gland of the third eyelid. • Everted or "scrolled" cartilage of the third eyelid: seen in wiemaraners, great Danes, German short-haired pointers, and other breeds in which T-shaped cartilage of the third eyelid is rolled away from the surface of the eye instead of conforming to the corneal surface. • Symblepharon: postinflammatory adhesions between the third eyelid and cornea or conjunctiva may cause third eyelid elevation.

Bilateral Elevation of Third Eyelid

- Blepharospasm • Exophthalmos: space-occupying lesions of both orbits can cause bilateral third eyelid elevation. Inflammatory lesions such as eosinophilic myositis and extraocular muscle polymyositis are the most common cause of bilateral exophthalmos. • Enophthalmos: causes of bilateral enophthalmos include dehydration, bilateral orbital fat atrophy secondary to severe cachexia, and chronic masticatory muscle myositis. • Conformational: specific breeds, such as doberman pinscher and pointer, have deep orbits and prominent third eyelids. This condition is not pathologic and treatment is not needed. • Plasmoma: an immune-mediated thickening and hyperemia of the leading edge of the third eyelids seen almost exclusively in German shepherd dogs. This condition may be associated with chronic superficial keratitis (pannus). • Haw's syndrome: Idiopathic bilateral elevation of the third eyelids seen in cats. All other aspects of the ophthalmic examination normal. Usually resolves in 3-4 weeks without treatment. • Dysautonomia (Key-Gaskell syndrome): clinical signs include bilateral elevated third eyelids, dilated nonresponsive pupils, keratoconjunctivitis sicca, dry mucosal surfaces, anorexia, lethargy, regurgitation, megaesophagus, bradycardia, megacolon, distended bladder (see Dysautonomia) • Tranquilization: many tranquilizers (e.g., acepromazine) cause bilateral elevation of the third eyelid. Fatigue can cause transient third eyelid elevation, especially in dogs prone to ectropion.

RISK FACTORS Varied

 DIAGNOSIS

DIFFERENTIAL DIAGNOSIS

- In animals with acute onset of unilateral elevation of the third eyelid, the most common causes are ocular pain (e.g., corneal ulcer and uveitis) and orbital inflammation (e.g., orbital abscess and cellulitis). • If the animal is middle-aged or older and has a unilateral, nonpainful elevation of the third eyelid, a third eyelid or orbital neoplasm is likely. In all cases, a small eye (microphthalmos or phthisis bulbi) and Horner's syndrome need to be ruled out. • Bilateral elevation of the third eyelid is more likely to be caused by systemic illness (e.g., dehydration, cachexia, and dysautonomia) or associated with conformational abnormalities. • A prolapsed gland of the third eyelid can also cause elevation of the third eyelid, but in this case, the medial aspect of the third eyelid is swollen whereas the third eyelid itself is usually normal.

CBC/BIOCHEMISTRY/URINALYSIS

- Leukocytosis and a left shift may be seen in animals with orbital inflammatory processes.
- Blood work is generally unrewarding in differentiating causes.

OTHER LABORATORY TESTS

- Measurement of urine and plasma catecholamine concentrations and pharmacologic testing of the autonomic nervous system can help confirm dysautonomia.

IMAGING

- Thoracic radiography should be considered in all animals with Horner's syndrome to rule out intrathoracic cause of sympathetic denervation and in animals with suspected neoplasia to evaluate for metastatic disease. • If an orbital mass is suspected, orbital ultrasound is recommended to help localize the mass and define its nature (i.e., solid or cystic).
- Computed tomography or magnetic resonance imaging may further define the orbital mass. • Skull radiographs rarely show signs of orbital disease unless the lesion is very large and destructive.

OTHER DIAGNOSTIC PROCEDURES

- A thorough ophthalmic examination.
- Use of a slit-lamp biomicroscope or some other source of magnification is recommended to help localize any potential ocular abnormality. • The medial aspect of the third eyelid and the conjunctival cul-de-sac should be examined carefully for a foreign body or symblepharon in all animals with unilateral elevated third eyelid. • Cytology—in animals with suspected mass lesions (either an orbital mass or mass of the third eyelid itself), examination with a fine needle aspirate may be helpful in obtaining a diagnosis. Unguided fine needle aspiration of orbital masses should only be attempted if the mass is anterior to the equator of the eye. Ultrasonography is recommended to help guide fine needle aspiration of masses posterior to the eye so that delicate retrobulbar structures are avoided. Examination of third eyelid scrapings of German shepherd dogs with suspected plasmoma reveals plasma cells and lymphocytes.
- Pharmacologic testing to localize the lesion(s) in animals with Horner's syndrome (see Horner's syndrome) • In some animals with a suspected orbital or third eyelid mass, the only means to a definitive diagnosis is exploratory surgery and biopsy.

THIRD EYELID, PROTRUDING

TREATMENT

• Treatment of an elevated third eyelid that is caused by pain consists of removing the cause of the irritation (e.g., foreign body) or treating the primary ocular condition.

• Treatment of an orbital mass depends on the cause. Orbital cellulitis and abscess generally respond well to systemically administered antibiotics. Wide surgical excision via an orbital exenteration is usually recommended for orbital neoplasms. Adjunct therapeutic modalities such as radiotherapy or chemotherapy may also be needed if the neoplasm is not removed entirely.

• Microphthalmic eyes do not usually require treatment unless the animal has pain or recurrent conjunctivitis. In these patients, the globes should be removed. Enucleate pathologic globes to prevent formation of intraocular sarcomas.

• If a cause of Horner's syndrome is found, treat that cause. If no cause is found (which is the case in approximately 50% of dogs and cats), signs of Horner's syndrome usually resolve without treatment in 4-12 weeks.

• Surgical removal of the entire third eyelid is indicated in animals with third eyelid neoplasia. If the surgical margins are not free of neoplasm, adjunct therapy such as radiotherapy or cryosurgery is also indicated. Radiotherapy around the eye may result in severe keratitis, dry eye, and cataracts; therefore, enucleation should be discussed with the owners before initiating treatment. Orbital exenteration may also be warranted if the mass extends into the orbit.

• Plasmomas can usually be controlled with topically applied medications, but not cured. Therefore, owners should be informed that some form of treatment is usually needed for the life of the animal. Topically applied corticosteroids (0.1% dexamethasone or 1% prednisolone acetate) are given q6h initially and reduced to q24d when the lesion appears resolved. Topically applied 1% cyclosporine q12h has also been shown to be effective.

• "Haws syndrome" usually resolves in 3-4 weeks without treatment.

• Management of dysautonomia—see dysautonomia.

MEDICATIONS

DRUGS AND FLUIDS See above

CONTRAINDICATIONS

Topically applied corticosteroids should never be used if a corneal ulcer is present.

PRECAUTIONS N/A

POSSIBLE INTERACTIONS N/A

ALTERNATIVE DRUGS N/A

FOLLOW-UP

PATIENT MONITORING

• Animal with malignant neoplasm should have thoracic radiographs taken every 3-6 months to monitor for metastatic disease.

POSSIBLE COMPLICATIONS

• Extension of the neoplasm or infection to adjacent orbital structures (e.g., eye, orbit, orbital sinuses, and cranial cavity) is possible. Metastasis to distant sites (usually the thorax or liver) is also possible with malignant neoplasms (approximately 90% of orbital neoplasms are malignant). • Vision loss can result from the lesion itself, from the third eyelid being elevated, or from treatment (e.g., radiotherapy and exenteration).

MISCELLANEOUS

ASSOCIATED CONDITIONS N/A

AGE RELATED FACTORS

• Middle aged to older animals are at risk for neoplastic diseases of the third eyelid and orbit. • Younger animals with elevated third eyelid are at risk for congenital abnormalities and have inflammatory conditions of the third eyelid more frequently than older animals.

ZOONOTIC POTENTIAL N/A

PREGNANCY N/A

SYNONYMS

• Elevated third eyelid • Haw's syndrome (cats)

SEE ALSO

• Ectropion • Entropion • Horner's Syndrome • Orbital Diseases (Exophthalmus, Enophthalmus, Strabismus) • Prolapsed Gland of the Third Eyelid (Cherry Eye)

ABBREVIATIONS N/A

References

Brooks DE. Canine conjunctiva and nictitating membrane. In: Gelatt KN, ed. Veterinary ophthalmology. 2nd ed. Philadelphia: Lea & Febiger, 1991:290–306.

Sharp NH, Nash AS, Griffiths IR. Feline dysautonomia (the Key-Gaskell syndrome): a clinical and pathological study of forty cases. J Small Anim Pract 1985;25:599–615.

Author Brian C. Gilger
Consulting Editor Paul E. Miller

TREMORS

BASICS

DEFINITION
Rhythmic, oscillatory, involuntary movement of all or part of the body

Pathophysiology
Abnormal movement caused by the alternate or synchronous contraction of reciprocally innervated, antagonistic muscles. If these antagonistic muscles contract synchronously, then the force or duration of contraction is slightly different in the opposing muscles to result in the biphasic, to-and-fro, movement.

Systems Affected
• Nervous • Musculoskeletal—muscle weakness or pain

SIGNALMENT
• Dogs and cats of a variety of ages depending on cause • Dogs with generalized tremor syndrome are usually young to middle-aged and often have white hair coats. • Hypomyelination occurs in dogs 6-8 weeks old. Affected breeds include the chow chow, springer spaniel, samoyed, weimaraner, and dalmatian. • Idiopathic head tremor affects the Doberman pinscher and Labrador retriever.

SIGNS N/A

CAUSES
Localized tremor—most often involves the head or the pelvic limbs

Head Tremor
• Cerebellar abnormalities—degenerative, congenital, inflammatory, immune-mediated, and toxic causes • Idiopathic and genetic causes • Inflammatory—encephalitides • Trauma • Drug administration—doxorubicin, diphenhydramine, and metoclopromide • Abnormalities of the vestibular system, both central and peripheral

Pelvic Limb Tremor
• May be a sign of weakness or pain in the lumbosacral area • Metabolic—renal failure, hypoparathyroidism, and hypoglycemia • Compressive lesions of the spine or nerve roots—lumbosacral stenosis, cauda equina syndrome, spinal cord tumor, and diskospondilitis • Peripheral neuropathy, neuromuscular junction abnormality, and myopathy • Poor perfusion to pelvic muscles—right-to-left shunting patent ductus arteriosus and other cardiopulmonary diseases • Unknown—pelvic limbs in older dogs (senile tremor)

Generalized Tremor
• Hypomyelination • Intoxications including organophosphates, hexachlorophene, and bromethalin • Degenerative neurologic disease such as storage disease and spongiform encephalopathy • Idiopathic generalized tremor syndrome (white shaker dog syndrome)

RISK FACTORS
• Any encephalitis or degenerative neurologic disease such as storage disease and spongiform encephalopathy • Treatment with doxorubicin, diphenhydramine, metoclopramide • White hair coat possibly a risk factor for development of generalized tremor syndrome

DIAGNOSIS

DIFFERENTIAL DIAGNOSIS
Differentiate tremor from shaking, shuddering, myotonia, myoclonus, weakness, tetany, reflex myoclonus, and seizure:
• In comparison to shaking, shuddering, myotonia, and myoclonus, tremor is usually more consistent, rhythmic, to-and-fro movements of similar amplitude that persist throughout the waking state. True tremor stops during sleep. • Tremor associated with weakness usually occurs when the muscles are forced to work (eg, during standing, walking, and running). • Tetany is usually a more consistent extension of the limbs and facial muscles without an extension-flexion cycle of movement. • Seizures are intermittent and associated with autonomic disturbances (eg, urination, defecation, and salivation) and alterations of consciousness. • Reflex myoclonus of the Labrador retriever and dalmatian is characterized by prolonged episodes of extensor rigidity with tactile or auditory stimulus and voluntary exercise.
Next, determine if the tremor is localized or generalized:
• If localized to the pelvic limbs, concentrate on diseases of the lumbosacral spinal cord and associated peripheral nerves. If localized to the head, assess for additional neurologic deficits suggesting cerebellar disease. Tremor of the head is often a clinical sign of cerebellar disease. This type of tremor is an intention tremor that worsens when the animal attempts to move the head in a goal-oriented manner. Cerebellar tremor may also involve the whole body. Other clinical signs of cerebellar disease such as ataxia and dysmetria should be helpful in determining the neuroanatomic diagnosis. • Head tremor occurs as an idiopathic condition in some breeds such as Doberman pinscher. Dogs are usually young at onset of signs. The tremor is sporadic and occurs at a frequency between 2 and 4 Hz. It can be in an up-and-down (yes) or side-to-side (no) direction. • In a 6-8-week-old dog with generalized tremor, consider congenital myelination abnormality and check breed incidences. In a young adult with generalized tremor, assess history for toxin exposure. Consider generalized tremor syndrome in young adults, especially those with white hair coats.

CBC/BIOCHEMISTRY/URINALYSIS
• Results usually normal in animals with tremor associated with a primary brain disease • In animals with localized tremor of the head or the pelvic limbs, assess for occult metabolic disease. Hypoglycemia, hypocalcemia, and abnormal renal function may be found. • Some of the myopathies are characterized by high creatine kinase.

OTHER LABORATORY TESTS N/A

IMAGING
• In patients with localized tremor of the pelvic limbs, radiography, myelography, epidurography, CT, and MRI may reveal lumbosacral, spinal, or vertebral abnormalities. • In patients with generalized tremors and localized tremor of the head, CT and MRI of the brain and radiography of the spine are usually normal. In some Maltese dogs with generalized tremor syndrome, CT reveals hydrocephalus. The importance of this finding is uncertain. MRI may show evidence of lack of myelin in animals with hypomyelination.

OTHER DIAGNOSTIC PROCEDURES
• CSF analysis is usually helpful in establishing a diagnosis in patients with generalized tremor syndrome and other causes of encephalitis. • If a lumbosacral syndrome is suspected, perform survey radiography, CSF analysis, electromyelography of limb muscles, myelography, epidurography, +/- discography, CT, and MRI for evidence of a lumbar spinal compressive lesion. • If a primary brain disease is suspected, CSF analysis gives information about underlying brain inflammation. Consider CT or MRI to assess intracranial structures. Brainstem auditory evoked potentials can be used to assess central auditory pathways and also evaluate overall brainstem function.

TREATMENT
• Treat the underlying primary disease.
• Animals can be treated as outpatients unless surgical treatment is required such as in patients with lumbosacral disease. Decompression and stabilization may be necessary.
• Avoid excitement and exercise—many tremors are worsened by these
• Animals with generalized tremor of primary brain origin may lose weight. Monitor weight and modify oral intake accordingly.
• Most of the causes of tremor in adult dogs are treatable, which is based on results of the diagnostic workup. No treatment is available for degenerative neurologic diseases such as storage disease and spongiform encephalopathy.
• Hypomyelination is generally not treatable but some breeds improve with maturity (eg, chow chow).
• No effective treatment is available for idiopathic head tremor; this is a benign tremor that occurs sporadically and has little health consequences.

• Consider an alternate drug if the tremor is drug-induced.
• If the history suggests intoxication, remove from further exposure. Consult with a poison control center for possible antidotes.

MEDICATIONS

DRUGS AND FLUIDS
• Tremors usually do not respond to muscle relaxants or anticonvulsants such as phenobarbital or valium.
• Immunosuppression with corticosteroids is used to treat generalized tremor syndrome.
• Diskospondilitis—antibiotics are chosen on the basis of culture and sensitivity of the lesion, blood, or urine.
• Cerebellar diseases are treated according to the diagnosis.

CONTRAINDICATIONS
Tremors may be worsened by sympathomimetic drugs.

PRECAUTIONS N/A

POSSIBLE INTERACTIONS N/A

ALTERNATE DRUGS N/A

FOLLOW-UP

PATIENT MONITORING
• Monitor the primary disease. • Animals receiving corticosteroids for generalized tremor syndrome should be monitored weekly initially to assess response to treatment.

POSSIBLE COMPLICATIONS N/A

MISCELLANEOUS

ASSOCIATED CONDITIONS N/A

AGE RELATED FACTORS N/A

ZOONOTIC POTENTIAL N/A

PREGNANCY N/A

SYNONYMS Shaking, shuddering

SEE ALSO
Hypomyelination • Cerebellar degeneration • See causes.

ABBREVIATIONS
CSF = cerebrospinal fluid
CT = computerized tomography
MRI = magnetic resonance imaging

References
Farrow BH. Generalized tremor syndrome. In: Kirk RW, ed. Current veterinary therapy IX. Philadelphia: WB Saunders, 1986:880-881.
de Lahunta A. Veterinary neuroanatomy and clinical neurology. 2nd ed. Philadelphia: WB Saunders, 1983:145-151.
Kornegay JN, Thomson CE. Trembling and shaking. In: Ettinger SJ, ed. Textbook of veterinary internal medicine: diseases of the dog and cat. 3rd ed. Philadelphia: WB Saunders, 1989:54-56.
Cuddon PA. Tremor syndromes. Prog Vet Neurol 1990;1:285-299.
Bagley RS. Tremor syndromes in dogs: diagnosis and treatment. J Small Anim Pract 1992;33:485-490.
Author Rodney S. Bagley
Consulting Editor Joane M. Parent

URINE RETENTION, FUNCTIONAL

BASICS

DEFINITION
Functional urine retention is incomplete voiding not associated with urinary obstruction.

Pathophysiology
Usually a disorder of the voiding phase of micturition. Incomplete voiding results from hypocontractility of the urinary bladder (detrusor atony) or from inappropriately excessive outlet resistance (functional urinary obstruction).

Systems Affected
• Renal/urologic
• Endocrine/metabolic
• Nervous

SIGNALMENT
More common in male than female dogs and cats. See causes.

SIGNS
• Palpably distended resting urinary bladder. After attempts by the animal to void, palpable distension may persist or inappropriate residual urine can be measured (normal < 0.5 ml/kg).
• Affected animals may demonstrate ineffective attempts to void, frequent attempts to void, or no attempts to void.

CAUSES

Hypocontractility of the Urinary Bladder Detrusor Muscle (detrusor atony)
• Most commonly develops as a sequela to acute or chronic urinary bladder overdistension. Many patients have a history of neurologic dysfunction or previous urinary obstruction.
• Neurogenic causes of functional urine retention include lesions of the pelvic nerves, sacral spinal cord, and suprasacral spinal cord.
• Lesions of the sacral spinal cord (e.g., congenital malformations, cauda equina compression, lumbosacral disk disease, and vertebral fractures/dislocations) can result in a flaccid, overdistended urinary bladder with weak outlet resistance. Urine retention and overflow (paradoxical) urinary incontinence are observed.
• Lesions of the suprasacral spinal cord (e.g., intervertebral disk protrusion, spinal fractures, and compressive neoplasms) can result in a distended, firm urinary bladder that is difficult to express.
• Electrolyte disturbances, including hyperkalemia, hypokalemia, hypocalcemia and hypercalcemia and other metabolic disturbances associated with generalized muscle weakness can also affect detrusor muscle contractility.
• Detrusor atony with urine retention may be a feature of dysautonomia, a disturbance of autonomic ganglia primarily encountered in cats in Great Britain. The disorder has also been described in dogs in the United States.

Functional Urinary Obstruction
• Occurs when excessive or inappropriate outlet resistance prevents complete voiding during urinary bladder contraction.
• In patients with suprasacral spinal lesions or midbrain disorders, urethral outlet resistance becomes uninhibited and remains inappropriately excessive or fails to coordinate with voiding contractions (detrusor-urethral dyssynergia). This condition has been associated with sacral lesions, local neuropathy, and idiopathic causes.
• Excessive urethral resistance, usually attributed to smooth or striated muscular components of the urethra, may be seen after urethral obstruction or as a sequela to urethral or pelvic surgery, urethral inflammation, or prostatic disease.

RISK FACTORS
• Feline lower urinary tract disease
• Urethral obstruction
• Pelvic or urethral surgery
• Anticholinergic medications

DIAGNOSIS

DIFFERENTIAL DIAGNOSIS
• Must be differentiated from physical and mechanical obstruction. Clinical signs of urinary obstruction include pollakiuria, stranguria, and hematuria. Animals with mechanical obstruction may void a few drops of urine after long periods of straining.
• Neurologic findings in dogs with supraspinal lesions affecting micturition include paralysis or paresis of pelvic +/- thoracic limbs, hyperreflexia of affected limbs, and cervical, thoracolumbar, and lumbar pain. The urinary bladder is usually distended, firm, and difficult to express. In animals with chronic or partial lesions, reflexive voiding may return, characterized by incomplete, involuntary detrusor contractions with spasticity of the outlet.
• Neurologic findings in dogs with sacral lesions affecting micturition include pelvic limb paresis with hyporeflexia, depressed anal and tail tone, perineal sensory loss, and depressed bulbospongiosus reflexes. The urinary bladder is typically distended, flaccid, and fairly easy to express.
• A urine stream that can be initiated but is abruptly tapered or halted is typical of idiopathic detrusor-urethral dyssynergia. Manual palpation may confirm detrusor contractions, which persist after flow terminates, and may indicate a high residual volume of urine.
• In animals recovering from urinary obstruction, inability to void may result from re-obstruction, functionally high urethral resistance, or detrusor atony caused by overdistension. If the urinary bladder can be expressed with gentle manual compression of the urinary bladder, detrusor atony is likely. If resistance to manual expression is encoun-

tered and urethral obstruction can be ruled out by examination or catheterization, then functional resistance is likely.
• Clinical signs accompanying urine retention in patients with dysautonomia include mydriasis, prolapsed third eyelids, regurgitation or vomiting, and diarrhea or constipation.

CBC/BIOCHEMISTRY/URINALYSIS
• Results of hemogram and serum biochemical profile may rule in or rule out metabolic causes of muscle weakness; also used to assess potential for postrenal azotemia.
• Urinalysis and urine sediment examination may reveal evidence of urinary tract infection or inflammation.

OTHER LABORATORY TESTS N/A

IMAGING
• Contrast cystourethrography or vaginourethrography may be required to rule out obstructive lesions.
• Myelography or epidurography may be indicated to localize neurologic lesions.

OTHER DIAGNOSTIC PROCEDURES
• Neurologic examination— A brief assessment of caudal spinal and peripheral nerve function is provided by examination of anal tone, tail tone, perineal sensation, and bulbospongiosus reflexes.
• Urethral catheterization may be required to rule out urethral obstruction. Urethral catheters should pass easily in animals with no mechanical obstruction and in those with extramural urethral compression, such as that caused by a smooth bladder neck mass, a large prostate gland, or a caudal abdominal mass.
• Testing for dysautonomia includes a number of tests of autonomic responses.
• Urodynamic procedures may be used to confirm detrusor atony or functional urethral obstruction or to document detrusor-urethral dyssynergia. Detrusor areflexia may be documented by cystometrographic studies, whereas inappropriate urethral resistance may be documented by resting urethral profilometry, combined cystometry and urethral pressure measurements, or uroflow studies, which are not readily adaptable for animal subjects.

TREATMENT
• Affected animals are usually managed as inpatients until adequate voiding function returns.
• Primary disorders such as electrolyte disturbances and neurologic lesions should be addressed and corrected if possible.
• The urinary bladder must be kept small by intermittent or indwelling catheterization or frequent manual compression. Intermittent or indwelling urinary catheterization may be required temporarily to ensure urine flow.
• Azotemia, electrolyte imbalances, and acid-base disturbances associated with acute urine retention should be managed appropriately.

URINE RETENTION, FUNCTIONAL

- Urinary tract infection should be identified and treated appropriately.
- Surgical options for salvaging urethral patency may be considered in some animals. Perineal urethrostomy may be required in male cats with unmanageable distal urethral resistance.

MEDICATIONS

DRUGS AND FLUIDS

Detrusor Atony
- Bethanechol is a cholinergic, parasympathomimetic agent that may increase detrusor contractile input in partially denervated or acutely overdistended urinary bladders.
- Metoclopramide is a dopamine antagonist with prokinetic activity in the gastrointestinal tract that may stimulate detrusor contraction as well.

Functional Urethral Obstruction
- Phenoxybenzamine is an alpha adrenergic antagonist that reduces smooth muscle contraction in the urethra. The agent is more effective in dogs than in cats. Prazosin is an alternative alpha antagonist.
- Diazepam is a short-acting, central skeletal muscle relaxant that relaxes striated muscle.
- Acepromazine, a phenothiazine tranquilizer, has general muscle relaxant and alpha blocking effects on urethral tone and may be effective in cats with excessive urethral resistance.
- Dantrolene is another striated muscle relaxant that acts via calcium antagonist properties and appears to be effective in reducing distal urethral resistance in cats.
- Baclofen is a spinal reflex inhibitor that acts as a skeletal muscle relaxant. Clinical use of this agent in small animals has been limited.

CONTRAINDICATIONS
- Baclofen is contraindicated in cats.
- Acepromazine and phenoxybenzamine can have vasodilatory effects and should be avoided in volume depleted or azotemic animals as well as in animals with cardiac disease.

- Acepromazine and diazepam can cause sedation and should be avoided in lethargic patients.

PRECAUTIONS
- An adequate outlet for urine flow must be ensured before administration of bethanechol. Phenoxybenzamine or prazosin is frequently administered concurrently, since bethanechol can increase muscular contraction of the urinary bladder neck and proximal urethra.
- Acute hepatopathy has been described recently as a rare complication of prolonged oral administration of diazepam in cats.

POSSIBLE INTERACTIONS N/A

ALTERNATE DRUGS N/A

FOLLOW-UP

PATIENT MONITORING
- As treatment progresses, assess residual urine volume by urinary bladder palpation or by periodic urinary catheterization.
- In most patients, medications can be slowly withdrawn after primary causes are corrected and adequate voiding function has been sustained for several days.
- Periodic urinalysis should be performed in animals with chronic urine retention to detect urinary tract infection.
- Clients should be advised that complete voiding function may not return, and that pets should be monitored for signs of complete obstruction or uremia.

POSSIBLE COMPLICATIONS
- Lower urinary tract and ascending infection
- Permanent detrusor muscle injury and atony; urinary bladder or urethral rupture
- Postrenal azotemia

MISCELLANEOUS

ASSOCIATED CONDITIONS
- Urinary tract infection
- Azotemia

AGE-RELATED FACTORS N/A

ZOONOTIC POTENTIAL N/A

PREGNANT ANIMAL
Bethanechol is contraindicated in pregnant animals.

SYNONYMS
- Voiding disability
- Neuropathic bladder
- Reflex dyssynergia
- Urethrospasm

SEE ALSO
- Urinary Tract Obstruction
- Intervertebral Disk Disease, Thoracolumbar
- Prostate Disease
- Feline Lower Urinary Tract Disease
- Dysuria and Pollakiuria
- Creatinine and Blood Urea Nitrogen (BUN)—Azotemia and Uremia

ABBREVIATIONS N/A

References

Barsanti JA. Urinary incontinence. In: Lorenz MD, Cornelius LM, eds. Small animal medical diagnosis, 2nd ed. Philadelphia: JB Lippincott, 1993:345-356.

Lees GE. August J, ed. Management of voiding disability following relief of urethral obstruction. In: Consultations in feline internal medicine. 2nd ed. Philadelphia, WB Saunders, 1994:365-372.

Moreau PM, Lees GE. Ettinger SJ, ed. Urinary obstruction and atony. In: Textbook of veterinary internal medicine. 3rd ed. Philadelphia: WB Saunders, 1989:155-159.

Moreau PM, Lappin MR. Pharmacologic manipulation of micturition. In: Kirk RW, ed. Current veterinary therapy X. Small animal practice. Philadelphia: WB Saunders, 1989:1214-1222.

Author India F. Lane
Consulting Editors Larry G. Adams and Carl A. Osborne

URINARY TRACT OBSTRUCTION

BASICS

DEFINITION
Restricted flow of urine from the kidneys through the urinary tract to the external urethral orifice

Pathophysiology
Excess resistance to urine flow through the urinary tract develops because of lesions affecting the excretory pathway. This causes an increase in pressure in the urinary space proximal to the obstruction and may cause abnormal distention of this space with urine. Pathophysiologic consequences ensue depending on the site, degree, and duration of obstruction. Complete urinary obstruction causes pathophysiologic state equivalent to oliguric acute renal failure. Perforation of the excretory pathway with extravasation of urine is functionally equivalent to urinary tract obstruction.

Systems Affected
• Renal/Urologic • Gastrointestinal, cardiovascular, nervous, and respiratory systems as uremia develops

SIGNALMENT
More common in males than females

SIGNS

Urinary Signs
• Bladder neck or urethral obstruction
• Pollakiuria (common) • Stranguria
• Reduced velocity or caliber of the urine stream or no urine flow during voiding
• Gross or microscopic hematuria • Palpable distention of the urinary bladder that is excessive (i.e., overly large or turgid) or inappropriate (i.e., remains after voiding efforts)
• Uroliths often palpated in the urethras of obstructed male dogs • Ureteral obstruction
• Occasionally, palpable renomegaly is discovered in an animal with chronic partial ureteral obstruction, especially when the lesion is unilateral.

Extraurinary Signs
• Signs of uremia develop when urinary tract obstruction is complete (or nearly complete): lethargy, dull attitude, reduced appetite, vomiting, dehydration • Signs of severe uremia: weakness, hypothermia, bradycardia with moderate hyperkalemia, high rate of shallow respirations, stupor or coma, seizures may occur terminally, tachycardia resulting from ventricular dysrhythmias induced by severe hyperkalemia • Signs of perforation of the excretory pathway: leakage of urine into the peritoneal cavity causes abdominal pain and distention; leakage of urine into periurethral spaces causes pain and swelling in intrapelvic or perineal tissues, depending on the site of the urethral injury; fever

CAUSES

Intraluminal Causes
• Solid or semi-solid structures including uroliths, urethral plugs in cats, blood clots, and sloughed tissue fragments • The most common site of urinary tract obstruction is the urethra. • Urolithiasis is the most common cause of urethral obstruction in male dogs. • Urethral plugs are the most common cause of urethral obstruction in male cats.

Intramural Causes
• Neoplasia of the bladder neck or urethra is a common cause of urinary obstruction, particularly in dogs. • Pyogranulomatous inflammatory lesions in the urethra are seen occasionally in dogs. • Fibrosis at a site of a previous injury or inflammation can cause stricture or stenosis, which may impede urine flow or may be a site where intraluminal debris becomes lodged. • Prostatic disorders in male dogs • Edema, hemorrhage, or spasm of muscular components can occur at sites of intraluminal (e.g., urethral) obstruction and contribute to persistent or recurrent obstruction to urine flow after removal of the intraluminal material. Tissue changes might develop because of injury inflicted by the obstructing material, by the manipulations used to remove the obstructing material, or both. • Ruptures, lacerations, and punctures of the excretory pathway are usually caused by traumatic incidents.

Miscellaneous Causes
• Displacement of the urinary bladder into a perineal hernia • Neurogenic (see Urinary Retention, Functional)

RISK FACTORS
• Urolithiasis, particularly in males • Feline lower urinary tract disease, particularly in males. • Prostatic disease in male dogs

DIAGNOSIS

DIFFERENTIAL DIAGNOSIS
• Repeated, unproductive squatting in the litterbox by a cat that has a urethral obstruction can be misinterpreted as constipation.
• Animals whose efforts to urinate are not observed by their owners can be examined because of signs referable to uremia without a history of possible obstruction. • Evaluation of any patient with azotemia should include consideration of possible postrenal causes (e.g., urinary obstruction). See Creatinine and Blood Urea Nitrogen (BUN)—Azotemia and Uremia for differential diagnosis of this problem. • Animals with a ruptured urinary bladder can exhibit clinical signs (e.g., anorexia, vomiting, diarrhea, depression, lethargy, weakness, and collapse) and laboratory test results (azotemia, hyperkalemia, and hyponatremia) similar to that commonly seen in patients with hypoadrenocorticism (Addison's disease). • Once urinary obstruction is recognized, diagnostic efforts focus on detecting the presence and evaluating the magnitude of abnormalities secondary to obstruction, and identifying the location, cause, and completeness of the impediment(s) to urine flow.

CBC/BIOCHEMISTRY/URINALYSIS
• Results of a hemogram are usually normal, but a stress leukogram may be seen. • Biochemistry analysis reveals azotemia, hyperphosphatemia, metabolic acidosis, and hyperkalemia proportional to the degree and duration of the obstruction. • Hematuria and proteinuria are common. Crystalluria supports a diagnosis of urolithiasis and atypical epithelial cells may be seen in patients with neoplasia.

OTHER LABORATORY TESTS
Uroliths that are passed or retrieved should be sent for crystallographic analysis to determine their composition.

IMAGING

Radiography
• Uroliths are often demonstrated by survey radiography; however, some are difficult or impossible to see because of their size, composition, or location. • Positive-contrast urethrography is the most sensitive method of detecting intraluminal and intramural lesions of the urethra, and double-contrast cystography is the most sensitive method of detecting lesions of the bladder lumen and wall.
• Upper urinary tract (i.e., ureter or renal pelvis) obstruction can be detected by excretory urography if renal function is adequately preserved on the affected side(s) so that the radiographic contrast media is excreted and sufficiently concentrated to be seen proximal to the obstruction.

Ultrasonography
Ultrasonography is highly sensitive for detecting lesions of the bladder and proximal urethra (including the prostate gland in male dogs) and upper urinary tract (i.e., ureter or renal pelvis) obstruction.

OTHER DIAGNOSTIC PROCEDURES
• Electrocardiography may detect abnormalities secondary to hyperkalemia including tall T waves, prolonged PR interval, and bradycardia • Urinary catheterization has diagnostic and therapeutic value. As the catheter is inserted, the location and nature of obstructing material may be determined. Some or all of the obstructing material (e.g., small uroliths and feline urethral plugs) may be induced to pass out of the urethra distally for identification and analysis. Retrograde irrigation of the urethral lumen may propel intraluminal debris toward the bladder. Although intramural lesions sometimes are detected during catheterization, catheter insertion can be normal. Animals that cannot urinate despite generating adequate intravesical pressure (i.e., have excessive outlet resistance) and have urethras that can be readily catheterized and irrigated either have intramural lesions or

functional urinary retention. • Cytologic evaluation of specimens obtained from the urinary tract with the assistance of catheters may be diagnostic, particularly for carcinoma of the urethra or bladder and some prostatic diseases. • Prostatic massage or physical manipulation of the catheter tip positioned near the suspected lesion is used to produce cell-rich specimens that are retrieved through the catheter by aspiration or washing with saline in an attached syringe. • Cystoscopy can be helpful, particularly in female dogs with intramural lesions of the bladder neck or urethra.

TREATMENT

• Complete urinary tract obstruction is a medical emergency that can be life-threatening; treatment should be started immediately
• Partial urinary obstruction is not necessarily an emergency; however, animals with partial obstruction may be at risk for developing complete obstruction. Partial obstruction can cause irreversible urinary tract damage if not treated promptly.
• Treat as an inpatient until the animal's ability to urinate has been restored.
• Surgery is sometimes required to relieve obstruction
• Long-term management and prognosis depend on the cause of the obstruction
• Treatment has three major components: combating the metabolic derangements associated with postrenal uremia (e.g., dehydration, hypothermia, acidosis, hyperkalemia, and azotemia); restoring and maintaining a patent pathway for urine outflow; and implementing specific treatment for the underlying cause of urine retention.

MEDICATIONS

DRUGS AND FLUIDS

• Fluid therapy is indicated in patients with dehydration or azotemia. Give fluids intravenously if systemic derangements are moderately severe or worse. Lactated Ringer's solution is the fluid of choice, except for patients with severe hyperkalemia (i.e., > 8.0 mEq/L and/or ECG changes), in which the fluid of choice is 0.45% saline and 2.5% dextrose solution with addition of sodium bicarbonate (1-2 mEq/kg slow bolus). Cardiotoxic effects of hyperkalemia that are immediately life-threatening should be combated by giving

calcium gluconate (2-10 ml 10% solution IV slowly to effect). As soon as hyperkalemia and its effects have abated, lactated Ringer's solution should be used.
• Procedures for relief of obstruction often require or are facilitated by giving sedatives or anesthetics. When substantial systemic derangements exist, fluid administration and other supportive measures should be started first. Careful decompression of the bladder by cystocentesis may be performed before anesthesia and catheterization. The dosage of sedative or anesthetic drug should be calculated by the low end of the recommended range or given only to effect. Isoflurane is the anesthetic of choice; however, satisfactory results can be obtained with a variety of other anesthetic or sedatives.

CONTRAINDICATIONS

Intramuscular ketamine should be avoided in patients with complete obstruction, because it is excreted through the kidneys. If the obstruction can not be eliminated, prolonged sedation will result.

PRECAUTIONS

Drugs that reduce blood pressure or induce cardiac dysrhythmia should be avoided until dehydration or hyperkalemia are resolved.

POSSIBLE INTERACTIONS None

ALTERNATE DRUGS

Normal saline with added dextrose (2.5% IV) is an alternative fluid choice for patients with dehydration and hyperkalemia.

FOLLOW-UP

PATIENT MONITORING

• Check urine production and hydration status frequently; adjust fluid administration rate accordingly. • Verify ability to urinate adequately or use urinary catheterization to combat urine retention. Indwelling catheterization with closed drainage is appropriate if catheter insertion requires chemical restraint or is unduly traumatic, but frequent brief catheterization is a better choice if catheter insertion can readily be done repeatedly (e.g., as in some male dogs). • When the ECG indicates life-threatening changes, continuous monitoring is needed initially to guide treatment and evaluate response.

POSSIBLE COMPLICATIONS

• Death • Injury to the excretory pathway while trying to relieve obstruction • Hypo-

kalemia during postobstruction diuresis
• Recurrence of obstruction

MISCELLANEOUS

ASSOCIATED CONDITIONS

• Bradycardia secondary to hyperkalemia
• Azotemia, hyperphosphatemia, and metabolic acidosis

AGE RELATED FACTORS

In old dogs, the underlying cause of obstruction (e.g., tumor and prostate disease) often is difficult to treat effectively.

ZOONOTIC POTENTIAL N/A

PREGNANCY N/A

SYNONYMS Urethral obstruction

SEE ALSO

• Creatinine and Blood Urea Nitrogen (BUN)—Azotemia and uremia • Hydronephrosis • Hyperkalemia • Feline Lower Urinary Tract Disease

ABBREVIATIONS None

References

Littman MP. Urinary obstruction and atony. In: Ettinger SJ, Feldman EC, eds. Textbook of veterinary internal medicine. 4th ed. Philadelphia: WB Saunders, 1995:169-172.

Labato MA. Urologic emergencies. In: Murtaugh RJ, Kaplan PM, eds. Veterinary emergency and critical care medicine. St Louis: Mosby-Year Book, 1992:295-320.

Barsanti JA, Finco DR, Brown SA. Feline urethral obstruction: medical management. In: Kirk RW, Bonagura JD, eds. Current veterinary therapy XI. Philadelphia: WB Saunders, 1992:883-885.

Osborne CA, Kruger JM, Lulich JP, et al. Feline lower urinary tract diseases. In: Ettinger SJ, Feldman EC, eds. Textbook of veterinary internal medicine. 4th ed. Philadelphia: WB Saunders, 1995:1805-1832.

Stone EA, Barsanti JA. Urologic surgery of the dog and cat. Philadelphia: Lea & Febiger, 1992.

Author George E. Lees
Consulting Editors Larry G. Adams and Carl A. Osborne

VAGINAL DISCHARGE

BASICS

DEFINITION
Any substance emanating from the vulvar labia

Pathophysiology
Discharge observed from the vulva can originate from several distinct sources and depends in part on the age and reproductive status of the animal. Discharges can be from the urinary tract, uterus, vagina, vestibule, clitoris, or perivulvar skin and can be normal or abnormal.

Systems Affected
• Urogenital • Dermatologic

SIGNALMENT
• Anomalies and prepubertal vaginitis more likely to be seen in prepubertal bitches
• Normal discharges commonly seen in estrual and postpartum bitches, whereas some discharges seen in postestrual, pregnant, and postpartum bitches can be more serious.

SIGNS

Historical Findings
• Discharge from the vulva, "spotting," "scooting," attracting males • Parturition in animal with postpartum discharge • Estrus during the preceding two months in animal with pyometra

Physical Examination Findings
• Blood • Lochia • Pus • Urine • Feces

CAUSES

Serosanguinous
• Normal during proestrus and sometimes into estrus • Urinary tract infection • Foreign body • Vaginal neoplasia—transmissable venereal tumor, leiomyoma • Vaginal trauma • Fetal death • Vaginal hematoma • Ovarian neoplasia

Lochia and Postpartum
• Normal postpartum discharge for 6-8 weeks • Subinvolution of placental sites (SIPS) if discharge lasts longer • Retained placentas • Metritis
Purulent Exudate
• Normal in early diestrus (slight) • Prepubertal vaginitis • Primary vaginitis
• Vaginitis secondary to inciting causes such as anomaly, foreign body, urinary tract infection, clitoral hypertrophy, vaginal neoplasia, and fetal death • Pyometra • Embryonic and fetal death • Postpartum metritis • Perivulvar dermatitis • Zinc toxicity has been reported
Other
• Urine or feces in patient with congenital anomaly or acquired perivulvar dermatitis can be mistaken for a vaginal discharge
• Urine from ectopic ureters or incontinence from "hypoestrogenism" • Normal mucus discharge during pregnancy

RISK FACTORS
• Exogenous androgens can cause clitoral hypertrophy. • Prophylactic antibiotics can alter the normal vaginal flora • Exogenous estrogens given during late estrus and diestrus predispose to pyometra

DIAGNOSIS

DIFFERENTIAL DIAGNOSES
• History and signalment establish risk of anomaly and hormonal influences such as estrus, diestrus, pregnancy, and parturition.
• Source and type of the discharge must be identified by appropriate diagnostics.

CBC/BIOCHEMISTRY/URINALYSIS
• Leukocytosis with a left shift if the patient has pyometra or metritis. • High BUN and creatinine if the patient has pyometra • Isosthenuria if the patient has polyuria and polydypsia associated with pyometra. Urinary tract infection revealed by urinalysis in some patients. • Otherwise, results unremarkable

OTHER LABORATORY TESTS
• Serum progesterone concentration determines if the bitch is in diestrus and more likely to have pyometra. • A rapid slide agglutination test helps rule out Brucella canis.

IMAGING
• Radiography to detect a large uterus in patients with metritis or pyometra and later stages of fetal death, but early pregnancy cannot be differentiated from pyometra. Contrast radiography of the vagina can help rule out vaginal neoplasia, urethrovaginal stricture, and rectovaginal stricture. • Ultrasonography can determine pregnancy as early as the 14th day of diestrus and heartbeats can be seen as early as the 20th day of diestrus. Fetal heartbeats and movement rule out fetal death. Fetal distress is considered if the fetal heart rate is < 200 beats per minute.

OTHER DIAGNOSTIC PROCEDURES
• Vaginal bacterial culture by use of a guarded culturette (AccuCulShure, Accu-med Corporation, Pleasantville, NY); should be performed before any other vaginal procedure is done • Vaginal cytologic examination to determine if the discharge is purulent, blood, or feces. The extent of cornification determines the estrogen influence and helps establish whether the bitch is in proestrus or estrus. • Vaginoscopy to reveal anomalies and bands. An endoscope may be needed to see the anterior vagina. The cervix cannot usually be seen by endoscopy, except possibly in large dogs. Fluid emanating from the uterus can be differentiated from vaginal and vestibular discharges. • Digital examination of the vagina to help identify vaginal anomalies such as bands, strictures, and persistent hymen. Tumors may also be palpated. • Cystocentesis and bacterial culture to help rule out urinary tract infection • Biopsy of vaginal mass to rule out neoplasia

TREATMENT
• Unless the bitch is sick with metritis or pyometra, the animal can be treated as an outpatient; otherwise an ovariohysterectomy may be indicated. Medical treatment of a sick bitch with pyometra should be performed in a hospital and with great care.
• Remove or treat any inciting cause (e.g., foreign body, neoplasia, anomaly or urinary tract infection, and exogenous androgens or estrogens).
• Prepubertal vaginitis usually resolves spontaneously after the first estrus or with ovariohysterectomy.
• Subinvolution of placental sites (SIPS)

MEDICATIONS

DRUGS AND FLUIDS
• Pyometra—prostaglandin, systemic antibiotics, and supportive fluids are indicated if the bitch is not extremely ill (see Pyometra and Cystic Endometrial Hyperplasia)
• Prepubertal vaginitis—estrus induction using diethylstilbestrol (DES) may be helpful, although long-term effects have not been documented. Dosage: 5 mg PO q24h for up to 7 days. Count day 1 of bleeding as day 1 of the induced cycle and continue treatment for an additional 2 days.
• Primary vaginitis—systemic antibiotics and vaginal douches
• Metritis—systemic antibiotics and supportive fluids if the bitch is ill
• Transmissable venereal tumor—vincristine

CONTRAINDICATIONS
Many antibiotics are contraindicated during pregnancy.

PRECAUTIONS
• Estrogens given during diestrus increase the risk of pyometra • Prostaglandins cause transient vomiting, diarrhea and, possibly, hypotension.

POSSIBLE INTERACTIONS
Estrogen during diestrus associated with increased risk of pyometra

ALTERNATE DRUGS N/A

FOLLOW-UP

PATIENT MONITORING
Ultrasonography or radiography to determine uterine size and contents if patient has pyometra or metritis

POSSIBLE COMPLICATIONS
Toxic shock in patients with severe pyometra or metritis

MISCELLANEOUS

ASSOCIATED CONDITIONS N/A

AGE RELATED FACTORS

• Puppies—prepubertal vaginitis, anomalies, and ectopic ureters • Aged—pyometra

ZOONOTIC POTENTIAL

Brucella canis—common in patients with postpartum lochia caused by abortion or stillbirth; rare in patients with vaginitis

PREGNANCY

Many antibiotics are contraindicated during pregnancy.

SYNONYMS N/A

SEE ALSO See causes

ABBREVIATIONS

SIPS - Subinvolution of the Placental Sites

References

Bouchard G. Estrus induction in the bitch using DES. In: Proceedings. Annu Meet Soc Theriogenol 1994;176-184.

Johnson CA. Diagnosis and treatment of chronic vaginitis in the bitch. Vet Clin North Am Small Anim Pract 1991;21:523-531.

Memon MA, Mickelson WD. Clinical management of bitches with vaginal discharge during pregnancy. Sem Vet Med Surg Small Anim 1994;9:38-40.

Reberg SR, Peter AT, Blevins WE. Subinvolution of placental sites in dogs. Compend Cont Educ Pract Vet 1992;14:789-793.

Romagnoli SE, Johnston SD. Vulvar discharge. In:Allen DG, ed. Small animal medicine. Philadelphia: JB Lippincott, 1991:763-779.

Wykes PM, Soderberg SF. Disorders of the canine vagina. In: Morgan RV, ed. Handbook of small animal practice. 2nd ed. New York: Churchill Livingstone, 1992:661-666.

Author Bruce E. Eilts

Consulting Editor Sara K. Lyle

VOMITING, CHRONIC

BASICS

DEFINITION
A complex reflex act that results in the expulsion of fluid and or food from the alimentary tract through the oral cavity. Chronic vomiting is defined as persistent vomiting of long duration (> 10 days) with variable frequency.

Pathophysiology
Chronic vomiting can be caused by diseases of the alimentary tract or can occur secondary to toxic, neurologic, metabolic, infectious, and noninfectious causes. Vomiting occurs when the vomiting center, located in the medulla, is stimulated by input from various receptor sites throughout the body. Vomiting can be stimulated by peripheral receptors located in the gastrointestinal tract or in various organs such as the pancreas, urinary bladder, pharynx, and liver. Vomiting can also be initiated directly by stimulation of the receptors in the vomiting center in animals with CNS disease. Stimulation of the chemoreceptor trigger zone by metabolic or bacterial toxins or by various drugs such as digitalis or morphine also stimulates the vomiting center. Motion sickness and vestibulitis stimulate the chemoreceptor trigger zone via cranial nerve VIII, which then activates the vomiting center.

Systems Affected
• Endocrine/Metabolic—electrolyte abnormalities, prerenal azotemia, and dehydration • Gastrointestinal—reflux esophagitis and gastroesophageal reflux • Cardiovascular—hypovolemia can cause tachycardia. Electrolyte abnormalities such as hypokalemia can cause arrhythmias. • Respiratory—aspiration pneumonia • Nervous—altered mental attitude

SIGNALMENT
• Dogs and cats • Basenji breed is prone to immunoproliferative enteritis • Rottweiler breed is prone to gastric eosinophilic granuloma • Chinese shar-pei breed is prone to food intolerances and inflammatory bowel disease

SIGNS

Historical Findings
Vomiting and regurgitation or both of food, clear liquid, or either stained with bile or blood; weight loss, variable appetite, polydipsia, diarrhea, clinical signs related to underlying disease, and melena

Physical Examination Findings
• Include poor hair coat, weight loss, thickened bowel loops on abdominal palpation, masses, and pain. • Dry, pale, mucous membranes if the patients is dehydrated. • Possibly, loud gut sounds. • Diarrhea, blood, or melena may be seen on rectal examination.

CAUSES

Causes in Dogs and Cats
• Infectious—histoplasmosis, disseminated aspergillosis, oömycosis, and bacterial overgrowth • Metabolic diseases—renal disease, hepatic disease, hypoadrenocorticism, chronic recurrent, pancreatitis, ketoacidotic diabetes mellitus, metabolic acidosis, and electrolyte abnormalities (e.g., hypokalemia, hyperkalemia, hyponatremia, and hypercalcemia) • Nervous—cerebral edema, CNS tumor, encephalomeningitis, vestibulitis, and labyrinthitis • Congenital—pyloric antral hypertrophy • Neoplastic—gastric adenocarcinoma, pancreatic adenocarcinoma, lymphosarcoma, fibrosarcoma, polyps, gastrinoma, and mastocytosis • Inflammatory Bowel Disease—lymphocytic, plasmacytic, and eosinophilic gastritis, enteritis, and colitis • Miscellaneous—motility disorders, intussusception, lymphangiectasia, gastrointestinal surgery, drugs (e.g., NSAIDs and glucocorticoids), gastric duodenal ulcer disease, congestive heart failure, food intolerance, and chronic foreign body

Causes Specific In Cats
• Infections—dirofilariasis and giardiasis • Hepatic disease—chlolecystitis and cholangiohepatitis • Hyperthyroidism

RISK FACTORS
Breed-associated disease (see Signalment)

DIAGNOSIS

DIFFERENTIAL DIAGNOSES
• Chronic vomiting is distinguished from acute vomiting by history and physical examination. • Differentiate primary alimentary tract disease from diseases of other organ systems. • It is important to distinguish vomiting from regurgitation, since regurgitation is usually caused by primary esophageal disease. Vomiting is often preceded by restlessness, salivation, and retching and requires abdominal contraction. Vomitus may be digested food, mucus, or liquid with bile staining; fresh or digested blood may be present. Regurgitation is a passive act that results in the expulsion of food into the oronasal cavities. The contents may be tubular in shape and typically composed of undigested food or clear or frothy liquids. Esophageal disorders can occur concurrently with diseases of the stomach and small intestine. Chronic vomiting patients may begin to regurgitate because of concurrent reflux esophagitis.

CBC/BIOCHEMISTRY/URINALYSIS
• Hemogram may be normal or reveal nonregenerative anemia secondary to chronic disease. • High PCV and total protein if the patient is dehydrated • Microcytic hypochromic anemia in some patients with chronic loss of blood from the gastrointestinal tract. Regenerative anemia is typical of an acute loss of blood from the gastrointestinal tract. • Nonregenerative anemia with high BUN and creatinine and low urine specific gravity in some patients with chronic renal disease • **Leukon** may be normal or show signs of inflammation; monocytosis may indicate chronic inflammatory disease. • High liver enzyme activity, hypoglycemia, or hypoalbuminemia in some patients with hepatic insufficiency • High urine and blood glucose with or without ketonemia supports diabetes mellitus. • Hyperglobulinemia may indicate chronic inflammation or infection. • Hypoalbuminemia and or lymphopenia may be secondary to protein-losing enteropathy (usually associated with diarrhea) in dogs with severe infiltrative disease such as lymphocytic plasmacytic gastroenteritis, neoplasia of the gastrointestinal tract, and lymphangiectasia. • Eosinophilia in some patients with eosinophilic gastroenteritis • Metabolic acidosis is common. Hypochloremic metabolic alkalosis may develop if loss of gastric fluid predominates.

OTHER LABORATORY TESTS
ACTH stimulation test is indicated if hypoadrenoadrenocorticism is suspected.

IMAGING
• Survey abdominal radiography; survey thoracic radiography to evaluate for pulmonary metastasis and infectious pulmonary lesions • Contrast radiography of the alimentary tract to evaluate for large mucosal lesion, mass, obstruction, and motility disorder • Ultrasonography of the abdomen to evaluate for parenchymal abnormalities of the liver, kidneys, pancreas, and gastrointestinal tract that might indicate an underlying cause of the chronic vomiting • CT and MRI to evaluate for abnormal parenchymal structures in the abdomen

OTHER DIAGNOSTIC PROCEDURES
• Gastroscopy, duodenoscopy, and laparoscopy • Gross lesions can be identified and biopsied by endoscopy, laparoscopy, or exploratory laparotomy. • Microscopic infiltrative disease my not be indicated by gross lesions, requiring histopathologic evaluation for diagnosis.

TREATMENT
• In patients with clinically important disease of the gastrointestinal tract, parenteral nutrition should be considered while the gastrointestinal tract recovers.
• Dietary trial (6-weeks) of a hypoallergenic diet is recommended in patients with inflammatory cell infiltrate according to biopsy.

MEDICATIONS

DRUGS AND FLUIDS
• If the patient is hypochloremic with metabolic alkalosis, normal saline or lactated Ringer's solution are the fluids of choice.
• It the patient has metabolic acidosis, lactated Ringer's solution or normal saline can be used.
• Potassium should be supplemented in patients with hypokalemia. Hypokalemia is common in vomiting patients unless the patient has acute renal failure, hypoadrenocorticism, or gastrointestinal disease.
• Animals with chronic gastrointestinal bleeding that develop microcytic hypochromic anemia may require iron supplementation
• Patients with lymphocytic, plasmacytic, or esosinophilic gastroenteritis diagnosed by histopathologic examination may require immunosuppressive therapy. Prednisone is the drug of choice; azathioprine and cyclophosphamide can also be used if patients are intolerant of steroids or as maintenance therapy.
• Antiulcer medication is indicated in patients with evidence of upper gastrointestinal bleeding caused by erosive or ulcer disease. Options include H_2-receptor blockers (e.g., cimetidine, ranitidine, and famotidine), proton-pump inhibitors (i.e., omeprazole), and coating agents (i.e., sucralfate).
• Treatment for neoplasia depends on the location of the tumor and the tumor type. Most gastrointestinal tumors should be surgically resected if possible and follow-up

chemotherapy considered. Gastrointestinal lymphosarcoma can be treated by chemotherapy alone without surgical resection. Patients with tumors that increase secretion of hydrochloric acid by the stomach such as mast cell tumor and gastrinoma should be given antacids as listed.
• Antiemetics should be reserved for patients with refractory vomiting that have not responded to treatment of the underlying disease. Options include phenothiazines (e.g., chlorpromazine) and metoclopromide.

CONTRAINDICATIONS
• Alpha-adrenergic blockers such as chlorpromazine should not be used in dehydrated patients, since they can cause hypotension.
• Anticholinergics should be avoided since they can cause gastric atony and retention, which can exacerbate vomiting.
• Metoclopramide is contraindicated in patients with gastrointestinal obstruction and is associated with signs such as restlessness and depression.

PRECAUTIONS
Antiemetics should be used with caution since they can mask an underlying problem.

POSSIBLE INTERACTIONS N/A
ALTERNATE DRUGS N/A

FOLLOW-UP

PATIENT MONITORING N/A
POSSIBLE COMPLICATIONS
Aspiration pneumonia

MISCELLANEOUS

ASSOCIATED CONDITIONS N/A
AGE RELATED FACTORS N/A
ZOONOTIC POTENTIAL N/A
PREGNANCY N/A
SYNONYMS N/A
ABBREVIATIONS N/A
SEE ALSO
See Causes

ABBREVIATIONS
BUN = blood urea nitrogen
CNS = central nervous system
CT = computed tomography
MRI = magnetic resonance imaging
NSAIDs = nonsteroidal anti-inflammatory drugs
PCV = packed cell volume

References
Strombeck DR, Guilford WG. Small animal gastroenterology. 2nd ed. Davis, CA: Stonegate, 1990;186-207.
Willard M. Diseases of the stomach. In: Ettinger SJ, Feldman ED, eds. Textbook of veterinary internal medicine. 4th ed. Philadelphia: WB Saunders, 1995:1143-1167.
Authors Christine C. Jenkins and Robert C. DeNovo
Consulting Editor Brent D. Jones

WEIGHT LOSS AND CACHEXIA

BASICS

DEFINITION
Weight loss is considered clinically important when it exceeds 10% of the normal body weight and is not associated with bodily fluid loss. Cachexia is defined as the state of extreme poor health and is associated with anorexia, weight loss, weakness, and mental depression.

Pathophysiology
Weight loss can result from many different pathophysiologic mechanisms, but they all share the common feature: insufficient caloric intake or availability to meet metabolic needs. This can be caused by high energy demand such as that characteristic of a hypermetabolic state; inadequate energy intake including insufficient quantity or quality of food; inadequate nutrient assimilation as in patients with anorexia, dysphagia, regurgitation, and malassimilation disorders; and excessive loss of nutrients or fluid, which can occur in patients with glucosuria, proteinuria, or dehydration.

Systems Affected
Any body system can be affected by weight loss, especially if severe or the result of systemic disease.

SIGNALMENT Dogs and cats

SIGNS

Historical Findings
• Clinical signs of particular diagnostic value in patients with weight loss are whether the appetite is normal, increased, decreased, or absent and the presence or absence of fever.
• Historical information is very important, especially regarding type of diet, duration of storage of diet, the patient's daily activity or use, environment, pregnancy, appetite, signs of gastrointestinal disease including dysphagia, regurgitation, vomiting, and diarrhea, and signs of any specific disease.

Physical Examination Findings
The clinician should look especially for signs of systemic disease, gastrointestinal disease, cardiac disease, neoplasia, and neuromuscular disease.

CAUSES AND RISK FACTORS

Dietary Causes
• Inadequate quantity • Poor quality
• Inedible food • Spoiled diets • Diets that have lost nutrients due to prolonged storage

Anorexia (See Anorexia)

Pseudoanorexia
• Inability to smell, prehend, or chew food
• Dysphagia (See Dysphagia)

Regurgitation (See Regurgitation)

Vomiting (See Vomiting)

Maldigestive Disorders
Exocrine pancreatic insufficiency

Malabsorptive Disorders
Small intestinal disease including infiltrative and inflammatory bowel disease and severe parasitism

Metabolic Disorders
• Organ failure—cardiac failure, hepatic failure, and renal failure • Hypoadrenocorticism
• Cancer cachexia syndrome

Excessive Nutrient Loss
• Protein-losing enteropathy • Protein-losing nephropathy • Diabetes mellitus

Neuromuscular Disease
• Lower motor neuron disease • CNS disease (usually associated with anorexia or pseudoanorexia)

Excessive Use of Calories
• Increased physical activity • Extremely cold environment • Hyperthyroidism
• Pregnancy or lactation • Increased catabolism—fever, inflammation

DIAGNOSIS

• The first step is to confirm, if possible, the weight loss. This is easily done by comparing the current weight to previous weights. If previous weights are not available, the patient must be subjectively assessed for the presence of cachexia, emaciation, dehydration or other clues that would confirm the owner's complaint of weight loss. • Once weight loss is confirmed, the underlying cause must be sought.

DIFFERENTIAL DIAGNOSIS
• The initial diagnostic step is to categorize the weight loss as occurring with a normal, increased, or decreased appetite. The list of likely differential diagnoses for a patient with weight loss despite a normal or increased appetite is much different and much shorter than it is for patients with a decreased appetite or anorexia. It is important to determine what the patient's appetite was at the onset of weight loss, because any condition can lead to anorexia if it persists long enough for the patient to become debilitated. • The animal's age may provide a clue as to the underlying cause (e.g., portosystemic shunt in a young dogs and hyperthyroidism in an old cats). • Causes of pseudoanorexia should also be sought such as loss of sense of smell, dysphagia, and disorders of the oral cavity, head and neck. • The presence of a fever suggests that the underlying cause is infectious, inflammatory including immune-mediated disease and pancreatitis, neoplastic, or toxic. The absence of fever is more consistent with metabolic causes of weight loss such as cardiac, renal, or hepatic failure.

CBC/BIOCHEMISTRY/URINALYSIS
• Laboratory tests are chosen on the basis of the clinician's list of most likely differential diagnoses after the history is taken and physical examination performed, and thus depend on specific findings. • Usually the initial minimum database includes CBC, serum biochemical analysis, and urinalysis. These tests help to identify infectious, inflammatory, and metabolic diseases including organ failure. They may be especially helpful in patients in which the history and physical examination do not provide much useful information. • Examination of a fecal flotation and direct smear are indicated if intestinal parasitism is suspected. • FeLV and FIV testing should be performed in any cat with weight loss of unknown cause. • Measurement of serum T4 concentration is indicated in any cat > 5 years old with weight loss of unknown cause, especially but not restricted to cats with a normal or increased appetite.

OTHER LABORATORY TESTS
Specific organ function tests are necessary if indicated by historical, physical examination, and initial database findings. Examples include a serum TLI if exocrine pancreatic insufficiency is suspected, an ACTH stimulation test if hypoadrenocorticism is suspected, and ammonia tolerance test or serum bile acids if hepatic disease is suspected.

IMAGING
• Similarly, the most useful diagnostic imaging techniques vary depending on other clinical findings and suspected underlying causes.
• Thoracic radiography, including both left and right lateral views, may be particularly helpful in diagnosing thoracic disease including cardiac failure and metastatic neoplasia. Abdominal radiography may be necessary if abdominal palpation is difficult.

OTHER DIAGNOSTIC PROCEDURES
• Vary depending on initial diagnostic findings and the suspected underlying cause of weight loss. • If gastrointestinal disease is probable but unconfirmed, examination of multiple biopsy specimens taken from the indicated portions of the gastrointestinal tract by endoscopy or exploratory laparotomy is necessary. • Indications for exploratory laparotomy are many and, if performed, it is essential to obtain multiple biopsy specimens of the suspected organ or organs as well as of other routinely biopsied abdominal organs.

TREATMENT

• The most important treatment principle is, as always, to treat the underlying cause of the weight loss.
• The other important principle is to provide sufficient caloric nutrition in the form of adequate amounts of an appropriate, high-quality diet fed in the form or manner that best allows for patient utilization. This requires precise calculation of the patient's caloric needs and may require enteral feeding such as through a nasogastric or pharyngostomy tube or by parenteral feeding.

MEDICATIONS

DRUGS AND FLUIDS
• These depend on the underlying cause of the weight loss. See specific topic for each of these conditions, including anorexia.
• See other sections regarding specific disorders or problems.

CONTRAINDICATIONS N/A

PRECAUTIONS N/A

POSSIBLE INTERACTIONS N/A

ALTERNATE DRUGS N/A

FOLLOW-UP

PATIENT MONITORING
The necessity for frequent patient monitoring and the methods required depends on the underlying cause of the weight loss; however, the patient should be weighed regularly and often.

POSSIBLE COMPLICATIONS
See Causes and Risk Factors

MISCELLANEOUS

ASSOCIATED CONDITIONS
See Causes and Risk Factors

AGE RELATED FACTORS N/A

ZOONOTIC POTENTIAL N/A

PREGNANCY
As mentioned, pregnancy and lactation can be associated with weight loss due to increased calorie expenditure.

SYNONYMS N/A

SEE ALSO See Causes, Anorexia

ABBREVIATIONS N/A

References

Greco DS. Changes in body weight. In: Ettinger SJ, ed. Veterinary internal medicine. 4th ed. Philadelphia: WB Saunders, 1995;2-5.

Lorenz MD. Weight loss. In: Lorenz MD, Cornelius LM, eds. Small animal medical diagnosis. Philadelphia: JP Lippincott, 1987;90-97.

Willard M: Clinical manifestations of gastrointestinal disorders. In: Nelson RW, Couto CG, eds. Essentials of small animal internal medicine. St. Louis: Mosby Year Book, 1992;274-275.

Author Daniel P. Harrington
Consulting Editor Brent D. Jones

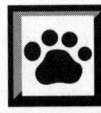

DIAGNOSTICS—
LABORATORY TESTS

ACIDOSIS, METABOLIC

BASICS

DEFINITION

Primary decrease in plasma bicarbonate concentration (HCO_3^-; dogs, < 18 mEq/L; cats, < 16 mEq/L) with high hydrogen ion concentration ($[H^+]$), low pH, and a compensatory decrease in carbon dioxide tension (PCO_2)

Pathophysiology

Loss of HCO_3^--rich fluid, addition of acid, acid production by metabolism, or diminished renal excretion of acid. Loss of HCO_3^--rich fluids (which have low chloride concentration) is associated with retention of chloride, which causes hyperchloremic metabolic acidosis. Addition of acids containing chloride (e.g., NH_4Cl and cationic amino acids) and chloride retention by the kidneys (e.g., renal tubular acidosis and administration of carbonic anhydrase inhibitors) also cause hyperchloremic metabolic acidosis. Addition (e.g., ethylene glycol toxicity), excessive production (e.g., lactate caused by prolonged anaerobic metabolism), or renal retention (e.g., renal failure) of anions other than chloride causes metabolic acidosis without increasing chloride concentration (so-called normochloremic or high anion gap metabolic acidosis).

Systems Affected

• Respiratory—the increase in $[H^+]$ stimulates peripheral and central chemoreceptors to increase alveolar ventilation. Hyperventilation decreases PCO_2, which counters the effect of decreased plasma HCO_3^- concentration on the pH. In dogs, a decrease of approximately 0.7 mm Hg in PCO_2 is expected for each 1 mEq/L decrease in plasma HCO_3^- concentration. Little is known about the degree of compensation in cats, but it is not as effective as in dogs.
• Renal/Urologic—the kidneys increase net acid excretion, primarily by increasing excretion of NH_4^+.
• Cardiovascular—myocardial contractility is diminished and acidosis may predispose the heart to ventricular arrhythmias and ventricular fibrillation when the pH falls below 7.1-7.2.

SIGNALMENT

Any breed, age, or sex

SIGNS

Historical Findings

Chronic disease process that leads to metabolic acidosis (e.g., renal failure, diabetes mellitus, and hypoadrenocorticism), exposure to toxins (e.g., ethylene glycol, salicylate, and paraldehyde), diarrhea, administration of carbonic anhydrase inhibitors (e.g., acetazolamide and dichlorphenamide).

Physical Examination Findings

• Signs generally relate to the underlying disease responsible for the metabolic acidosis

• Depression in animals with severe acidosis
• Tachypnea in some animals resulting from compensatory increase in ventilation
• Kussmaul's respiration, typically seen in humans with metabolic acidosis, is not observed in dogs and cats.

Causes

Associated with hyperchloremia (hyperchloremic metabolic acidosis)
• Diarrhea
• Renal tubular acidosis
• Administration of carbonic anhydrase inhibitors, amiloride, spironolactone, potassium chloride, or NH_4Cl
• Total parenteral nutrition with fluids containing cationic amino acids lysine, arginine, and histidine
• Posthypocapnia (patients in which chronic respiratory alkalosis is corrected too fast).
Associated with normochloremia (high anion-gap metabolic acidosis)
• Uremic acidosis
• Diabetic ketoacidosis
• Lactic acidosis
• Ethylene glycol, salicylate, paraldehyde, and methanol intoxication
• Hyperphosphatemia

RISK FACTORS

• Patients with chronic renal failure, diabetes mellitus, and hypoadrenocorticism are at high risk of developing metabolic acidosis as a complication of the chronic disease process.
• Patients with poor tissue perfusion or hypoxia are at risk of developing lactic acidosis.

DIAGNOSIS

DIFFERENTIAL DIAGNOSIS

• Low plasma HCO_3^- concentration may also be compensatory in animals with chronic respiratory alkalosis. In this setting, PCO_2 is low and pH is high or near normal, despite low HCO_3^- concentration.

LABORATORY FINDINGS

Drugs That May Alter Laboratory Results

• Potassium bromide is measured as chloride in most analyzers. Administration of potassium bromide, therefore, artificially decreases the anion gap.

Disorders That May Alter Laboratory Results

• Too much heparin (> 10% of the sample) reduces HCO_3^- concentration.
• Samples stored at room temperature for more than 20 minutes have low pH because of an increase in PCO_2.
• Some blood gas analyzers only report pH and PCO_2. Bicarbonate has to be calculated separately, which is a potential source of human error.

Valid if Run in Human Lab? Yes

CBC/BIOCHEMISTRY/URINALYSIS

Metabolic acidoses are traditionally divided into hyperchloremic and high anion gap by means of the anion gap. Anion gap is the difference between the measured cations and the measured anions and is calculated as AG = $Na^+ - (HCO_3^- + Cl^-)$ or AG = $(Na^+ + K^+) - (HCO_3^- + Cl^-)$ according to the preference of the clinician or laboratory. Normal values when potassium is included in the calculation are usually from 12 to 24 mEq/L (dogs) and from 13 to 27 mEq/L (cats). The negative charges of albumin are the major contributors to the normal anion gap. Therefore, estimation of anion gap is not reliable in patients with hypoalbuminemia.

Acidosis is suspected in an animal with the following:
• Normal anion gap (i.e., hyperchloremic metabolic acidosis)—the most common cause is diarrhea; also, hypoadrenocorticism
• High anion gap (i.e., normochloremic metabolic acidosis)—the most common causes are renal failure, diabetes mellitus, lactic acidosis (caused by tissue hypoperfusion), and hypoadrenocorticism (caused by lactic acidosis).
• Hyperglycemia—consider diabetes mellitus.
• Azotemia—consider renal failure.
• Hyperphosphatemia—consider renal failure, hypertonic sodium phosphate enema toxicity, and toxicity caused by urinary acidifiers containing phosphate.
• High lactate concentration—consider lactic acidosis caused by poor tissue perfusion or poor metabolism of lactate (e.g., liver disease and lymphoma).
• Hyperkalemia—the only form of metabolic acidosis that can lead clinically to hyperkalemia is acute hyperchloremic acidosis. Otherwise, hyperkalemia results from the disease process causing the metabolic acidosis (e.g., renal failure and diabetes mellitus) and not from the acidosis itself.

OTHER LABORATORY TESTS

Total CO_2 in samples handled aerobically closely approximates the HCO_3^- concentration. Patients with metabolic acidosis have low total CO_2. Unfortunately, patients with chronic respiratory alkalosis also have low total CO_2, and the distinction cannot be made without a blood gas analysis.

IMAGING N/A

OTHER DIAGNOSTIC PROCEDURES
N/A

TREATMENT

• Acid-base disturbances are secondary phenomena. Diagnosis and treatment of the underlying disease process are integral to the successful resolution of acid-base disorders. Treatment varies depending on the underlying cause and severity of the metabolic acidosis.

• Patients with blood pH < 7.1 should be aggressively treated while pursuing the definitive diagnosis.
• Drugs that can cause metabolic acidosis should be discontinued if possible.

MEDICATIONS

DRUG AND FLUIDS

• Lactated Ringer's solution is the fluid of choice for patients with mild metabolic acidosis and normal liver function.
• Patients with metabolic acidosis and pH < 7.2 should receive $NaHCO_3$. Patients with high anion gap metabolic acidosis should receive enough $NaHCO_3$ to bring the pH to 7.2. In these patients, organic anions are metabolized to HCO_3^- and administration of HCO_3^- may predispose the patient to metabolic alkalosis. Patients with hyperchloremic acidosis are less likely to develop overshoot metabolic alkalosis.
• Estimation of HCO_3^- dose: dogs, 0.3 x body weight (kg) x (21 - patient HCO_3^-); cats, 0.3 x body weight (kg) x (19 - patient HCO_3^-). Half of this dose is given slowly intravenously, and blood gases should be reevaluated before a decision is made about the need for additional administration. An empirical dose of 2 mEq/Kg followed by reevaluation of blood gas status is safe in most patients.
• Potential complications of $NaHCO_3$ administration include volume overload resulting from administered sodium, tetany from low ionized calcium concentration, high affinity of hemoglobin for O_2, paradoxical CNS acidosis, overshoot metabolic alkalosis, and hypokalemia.

CONTRAINDICATIONS

• Avoid $NaHCO_3$ in patients with respiratory acidosis because it generates CO_2. Patients with respiratory acidosis cannot adequately excrete CO_2, and the rise in PCO_2 will further decrease the pH.
• Avoid certain diuretics that act in the distal nephron (e.g., spironolactone, triamterene, and amiloride).
• Avoid carbonic anhydrase inhibitors (e.g., acetazolamide and dichlorphenamide).

PRECAUTIONS

$NaHCO_3$ should be used cautiously in patients with congestive heart failure because the sodium load may cause cardiac decompensation.

POSSIBLE INTERACTIONS N/A

ALTERNATE DRUGS

Carbicarb, an equimolar mixture of Na_2CO_3 and $NaHCO_3$, can be used as an alternative to bicarbonate. Carbicarb does not generate CO_2 and is especially useful in patients with concurrent respiratory acidosis.

FOLLOW-UP

PATIENT MONITORING

Recheck acid-base status, with frequency dictated by the underlying disease

POSSIBLE COMPLICATIONS

• Hyperkalemia
• Myocardial depression and ventricular arrhythmia

MISCELLANEOUS

ASSOCIATED CONDITIONS

• Hyperkalemia
• Hyperchloremia.

AGE-RELATED FACTORS N/A

PREGNANCY N/A

SYNONYMS

• Nonrespiratory acidosis

• Hyperchloremic acidosis = normal anion gap acidosis
• Normochloremic acidosis = high anion gap acidosis
• Hyperphosphatemic acidosis—metabolic acidosis resulting from high phosphate concentration
• Organic acidosis—metabolic acidosis resulting from accumulation of organic anions (e.g., ketoacidosis, uremic acidosis, and lactic acidosis)
• Dilutional acidosis—metabolic acidosis resulting from high free water in plasma

SEE ALSO

• Diabetes Mellitus, Ketoacidotic
• Potassium, Hyperkalemia
• Chloride, Hyperchloremia

ABBREVIATIONS

• HCO_3^- = bicarbonate
• $NaHCO_3$ = sodium bicarbonate
• PCO_2 = carbon dioxide tension
• H+ = Hydrogen ion
• O_2 = Oxygen

References

de Morais, HSA, Muir, WW. Strong ions and acid-base disorders. In Kirk's current veterinary therapy XII. Bonagura, JD, Kirk, RW, editors. Philadelphia: WB Saunders, 1995:121–127.

DiBartola, SP. Metabolic acidosis. In Fluid therapy in small animal practice. DiBartola SP, editor. Philadelphia: WB Saunders, 1992:216–243.

DiBartola, SP, Green, RA, de Morais, HSA. Electrolytes and acid base disorders. In Small animal clinical diagnosis by laboratory methods. Willard MD, Tvedten H, Turnwald GH, editors. 2nd ed. Philadelphia, WB Saunders, 1994.97-113.

Author Helio Autran de Morais
Consulting Editors Larry G. Adams and Carl A. Osborne

ALANINE AMINOTRANSFERASE (ALT)/ASPARTATE AMINOTRANSFERASE (AST)

BASICS

DEFINITION
The plasma activities of alanine aminotransferase (ALT) and aspartate aminotransferase (AST) are useful indicators of hepatocellular injury. These markers are not specific for primary liver disease, since their elevation can be induced by disease in other tissues, drugs, or liver injury secondary to another primary disease such as diabetes. The magnitude of their elevation may be proportional to the number of hepatocytes affected, so the absolute concentrations of the aminotransferases and their temporal elevation provide useful clinical clues to the cause of the liver disease.

Pathophysiology
ALT and AST are involved in gluconeogenesis and are present in a variety of tissues in addition to the liver. ALT is present as a cytosolic enzyme; largest quantities are found in the liver, although it can be found in striated muscle and in the brain. In contrast, AST is found in both the mitochondrial and cytosolic fractions of the liver and in large quantities in striated muscle (i.e., skeletal and cardiac), the brain, kidneys, lungs, and RBC. In general, ALT is felt to be liver-specific in both dogs and cats. In cats, AST may actually be more sensitive than ALT to hepatocellular changes, but it is not liver specific. Thus, to evaluate AST more specifically, the clinician should also measure the muscle enzyme creatinine kinase in addition to ALT and other biochemical elements. Both AST and ALT are cleared from plasma by the monocyte-macrophage system; the plasma half-life of ALT is 4-72 hours in dogs and 4-6 hours in cats, and the half-life of AST is 5 hours in dogs and 77 minutes in cats.

Systems Affected N/A

SIGNALMENT
• No breed or sex differences in the expression of ALT and AST reported in dogs or cats • ALT and AST in neonates may be 1-2 times higher than in adults.

SIGNS

Historical Findings N/A

Physical Examination Findings
The cause of high activities of AST and ALT determines historical and physical examination findings. High ALT or AST activity is not directly responsible for clinical signs. In patients with high ALT or AST activity due to hepatocellular disease, clinical signs can range from nonspecific lethargy to those associated with fulminant hepatic failure.

CAUSES
• Degenerative disease—chronic active hepatitis, cirrhosis • Congenital anomaly—portosystemic vascular abnormality, glycogen storage disease • Metabolic disease—hypoxia, shock, severe dehydration, anesthesia, endocrinopathy (e.g., hyperthyroidism, hyperadrenocorticism, hypothyroidism, and diabetes mellitus), severe gastrointestinal disease (acute or chronic) • Nutritional/Neoplastic—hepatic lipidosis, primary or secondary neoplasia • Immunologic/Infectious—bacterial, viral, parasitic, protozoal, fungal, inflammatory-noninfectious (e.g., cholangiohepatitis), amyloidosis, systemic lupus erythematosus • Traumatic/Toxic—drugs (e.g., acetaminophen, phenobarbital, primidone, glucocorticoids, tetracycline [cats], benzimadazole anthelmintics, and halothane anesthesia), chemicals (e.g., arsenicals, ethylene glycol)

RISK FACTORS
See causes; high ALT or AST activity can be associated with any disease, disorder, syndrome, or condition that results in a change in hepatocyte membrane permeability or other tissue cells that contain this enzyme.

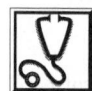

DIAGNOSIS

DIFFERENTIAL DIAGNOSIS
Generally, no specific aspects of the history or physical examination consistently help differentiate causes of high ALT or AST activity. If either is high, the clinician should first attempt to establish the presence of liver disease, whether it is primary or secondary, and the underlying cause.

LABORATORY FINDINGS

Drugs That May Alter Lab Results
Numerous drugs and chemicals (see causes) can cause high ALT and AST activity, but do not interfere with the validity of the laboratory results.

Disorders That May Alter Lab Results
Hemolysis causes falsely high ALT and AST activities.

Valid If Run in a Human Lab? Yes

CBC/BIOCHEMISTRY/URINALYSIS
Results of all these tests should be evaluated together with the finding of high ALT or AST activities to help confirm the presence of liver disease, determine if it is primary or secondary (if possible), and assess the overall clinical status of the patient.

CBC
• Alterations in RBC morphology (e.g., poikilocytes, target cells, microcytosis often associated with portosystemic shunt, and nonregen-erative anemia of chronic disease) • Quantitative or qualitative defects in platelets also occur in association with some liver diseases.

Serum Biochemistry Profile
• Albumin—low • Globulins—high or low • ALP—high in patients with hepatobiliary disease, but finding is nonspecific due to the numerous isoenzymes of ALP • Bilirubin—normal to high due to cholestasis, hemolysis, or hepatocellular dysfunction • BUN—low in patients with severe protein malnutrition, end-stage liver disease, or portosystemic abnormality • Glucose—high in patients with diabetes, stress and other causes of adrenaline release, low with end-stage liver disease or severe fulminant hepatitis, endotoxemia, and septicemia • Creatine kinase—high when ALT and AST activities are high secondary to muscle injury

Urinalysis
• Bilirubinuria (always abnormal in cats; male dogs are able to conjugate bilirubin in the kidneys, thus some bilirubin is normally present) • Uric acid crystals (portosystemic shunt) • Impaired urine concentrating ability

OTHER LABORATORY TESTS
• Bile acid assay (BAA)—To assess function of the enterohepatic circulation, the adequacy of hepatocellular perfusion, and overall functioning of the hepatobiliary tree; uses pre- and 2-hour post-prandial serum samples and is a highly sensitive test of liver function. • Sulfobromophthalein and indocyanine green-cholephilic water-soluble dyes used to evaluate hepatic perfusion and hepatobiliary function; these tests have been largely replaced by the more sensitive BAA. • Ammonia tolerance test and fasting blood ammonia—used to provide evidence of hepatic encephalopathy and to assess liver function. The blood ammonia test has a high specificity, but it is limited by its moderate sensitivity in the diagnosis of liver disease. This assay is also technically demanding (requires the ability to perform assay within minutes), and it is dangerous in animals with hepatoencephalopathy (may induce hepatic coma). As a result of these problems and the equal sensitivity of the BAA, the ammonia tolerance test has been replaced by the BAA for the laboratory diagnosis of portosystemic vascular anomalies. • Endocrine function tests—low-dose dexamethasone suppression test, thyroid stimulation test, and others. Many endocrinopathies can cause high activities of ALT and AST, and must be ruled out. • Serologic tests—in animals with suspected bacterial (e.g., leptospirosis and brucellosis), viral (e.g., feline infectious peritonitis virus and canine infectious hepatitis) or fungal disease (e.g., blastomycosis), serologic tests may be useful in determining the cause of high serum enzyme concentrations. • Coagulation

ALANINE AMINOTRANSFERASE (ALT)/ASPARTATE AMINOTRANSFERASE (AST)

assays—prothrombin time, activated partial thromboplastin time, and activated clotting time should be evaluated in animals with severe or chronic liver disease to assess the liver's ability to produce coagulation factors.

IMAGING

Radiography
Evaluation of liver size, position, and shape, variations in density of abdominal structures, and detection of mineralization or calcification of intrahepatic structures, intrahepatic gas, abdominal masses, and abdominal fluid are all important features of radiographic evaluation.

Ultrasonography
• Allows evaluation of the hepatic parenchyma, biliary system, and vascular structures by assessing density, size, and architecture by noninvasive means. • Can detect focal or multifocal lesions that may not be apparent grossly or radiographically. • The gallbladder and biliary tree are easily examined by this technique because of the anechoic features of this segment of the hepatobiliary system.

OTHER DIAGNOSTIC PROCEDURES
• Ultrasound guided biopsy of the liver allows more specific diagnosis of liver disease than is afforded by blind percutaneous biopsy alone. • Hepatic biopsy—indicated on the basis of history, physical examination findings, clinicopathologic findings, and other tests (e.g., BAA) as a means of obtaining a definitive diagnosis, planning treatment, and establishing an accurate prognosis. • Laparoscopy—an alternative to exploratory laparotomy for evaluation and diagnosis of liver disease; allows visualization of the liver for inspection, biopsy site selection, and post-biopsy observation.

TREATMENT
• The nonpharmacologic treatment of an animal with high ALT and AST activities must be tailored to the individual patient and based on the clinical findings and severity of the laboratory abnormalities. No specific therapeutic approaches are recommended to reduce high enzyme concentrations, because this will only occur over time and with the removal of the inciting cause.
• Nutritional support may be needed in patients unwilling or unable to eat.
• Some hepatopathies such as portosystemic vascular anomalies require specific nutritional intervention to control clinical signs.

MEDICATIONS
DRUGS AND FLUIDS
Fluids
• If fluids are indicated, balanced polyionic solutions such as lactated Ringer's solution are a safe choice for rehydration, correction of acid/base abnormalities associated with vomiting and diarrhea, and supportive care.
• In animals with severe liver failure, fluids containing reduced amounts or no lactate may be indicated, such as 0.9% sodium chloride, 1/2 strength saline, or a combination lactated Ringer's plus dextrose solution.
• The fluid rate is based on the patient's hydration status and clinical condition.

Drugs
• Choice of drugs for supportive treatment should be based on a presumptive or tentative diagnosis, unless the patient is in shock and broad spectrum antibiotics and glucocorticosteroids are indicated.
• Broad-spectrum, bacteriocidal antibiotics effective against gram-negative and anaerobic bacteria (primarily from the gastrointestinal tract) should be used to treat animals in shock.
• Antiemetics or H2 blocking drugs should be used if indicated.

CONTRAINDICATIONS N/A
PRECAUTIONS N/A
POSSIBLE INTERACTIONS N/A
ALTERNATE DRUGS N/A

FOLLOW-UP
PATIENT MONITORING
• The primary concerns are fluid and acid/base status, response to treatment, and progression of clinical signs or disease. The degree of concern about these depends on the individual and the cause of the high liver enzyme activity. • High ALT and AST activities in some patients are associated with mild disease, and the animals are stable. Treatment may not be necessary, or may consist of outpatient supportive care or drug administration and periodic monitoring of liver enzymes. Treatment is then adjusted or initiated as needed to achieve a decline in enzyme concentrations over time. • High ALT and AST activities in other patients are associated with fulminant hepatic necrosis and impending hepatic failure, requiring aggressive, supportive, symptomatic, and specific tratment. Patients require more frequent and extensive monitoring of liver enzymes and other biochemical components.

POSSIBLE COMPLICATIONS
High ALT or AST activity may indicate severe liver disease which can cause severe debilitation and death.

MISCELLANEOUS
ASSOCIATED CONDITIONS N/A
AGE RELATED FACTORS
In neonates, the activities of ALT and AST may be 1-2 times higher than those in normal adults.

ZOONOTIC POTENTIAL
Leptospirosis, brucellosis, salmonellosis

PREGNANCY N/A

SYNONYMS
• ALT was previously known as SGPT (serum glutamic pyruvate transaminase).
• AST was previously known as SGOT (serum glutamic oxaloacetate transaminase).

SEE ALSO
See causes

ABBREVIATIONS
ALP = alkaline phosphatase
ALT = alanine aminotransferase
APT = aspartate transaminase
AST = aspartate aminotransferase
BAA = bile acid assay
BUN = blood urea nitrogen
RBC = red blood cells

References
Murray RL. Liver function. In: Kaplan LA and Pesce AJ, eds. Clinical chemistry: theory, analysis, and correlation. St. Louis: CV Mosby Co., 1989.

Blei AT. Liver and biliary tract. In: Noe DA, Rock RC, eds. Laboratory medicine: the selection and interpretation of clinical laboratory studies. Baltimore: Williams & Wilkins, 1994.

Hall RL. Laboratory evaluation of liver disease. Vet Clin North Am Small Anim Pract 1985;15:3-19.

Strombeck DR, Guilford WG. Laboratory evaluation for hepatic disease. In: Strombeck DR, Guilford WG, eds. Small animal gastroenterology. 2nd ed. Davis: Stonegate Publishing, 1990.

Author Debra L. Zoran
Consulting Editor Albert E. Jergens

ALBUMIN, HYPOALBUMINEMIA

BASICS

DEFINITION
Serum albumin concentration < 2.6 gm/dl

Pathophysiology
• Albumin creates 75-80% of plasma colloid oncotic pressure, which maintains vascular volume by preventing movement of fluid from the intravascular to the extravascular space. • Hypoalbuminemia causes low oncotic pressure, loss of fluid from vascular spaces, edema, and effusions. Effusions are most likely to occur when albumin is < 1.5 gm/dl • Hypoalbuminemia in the range of 1.5 to 2.6 gm/dl does not cause effusions unless accompanied by other factors that promote extravasation of fluid (e.g., high hydrostatic pressure caused by portal hypertension, renal retention of sodium, and volume overload). • Albumin is produced exclusively in the liver. Chronic liver disease can cause hypoalbuminemia. • Loss of albumin can occur in the intestinal tract in animals with severe diffuse infiltrative disorder that causes protein losing enteropathy. Both albumin and globulins are lost. • Renal loss of albumin occurs in animals with glomerular disease.

Systems Affected
• Cardiovascular—transudative body cavity effusions (e.g., pleural effusion and ascites); peripheral edema azotemia pulmonary edema • Renal/ urologic—prerenal secondary to low plasma volume and reduced renal perfusion. • Endocrine/metabolism—altered binding of drugs • Musculoskeletal—delayed wound healing

SIGNALMENT N/A

SIGNS

Historical Findings
• Abdominal distention caused by ascites • Dyspnea caused by pleural effusion or pulmonary edema • Swollen limbs caused by peripheral edema.

Physical Examination Findings
• Ascites • Muffled heart sounds caused by pleural effusion • Pulmonary crackles caused by pulmonary edema • Peripheral edema • Dyspnea

CAUSES

Decreased Production of Albumin
• Chronic liver disease (e.g., chronic hepatitis and cirrhosis) • Inadequate intake (e.g., protein-restricted diet and malnutrition) • Maldigestion • Malabsorption

Increased Loss of Albumin
• Protein losing nephropathy caused by amyloidosis or glomerulonephritis • Small intestinal disorder causing protein-losing enteropathy (e.g., lymphangiectasia, lymphoma, inflammatory bowel disease, and histoplasmosis) • Exudative skin lesion

• Blood loss (e.g., external hemorrhage). • Repeated abdominocentesis of high protein effusions

Sequestration in Body Cavities or Tissues
• Inflammatory effusion (e.g., acute pancreatitis or peritonitis) • Vasculopathy

Miscellaneous
• Hyperglobulinemia • Dilution

RISK FACTORS
Hepatic, renal, and intestinal disorders

DIAGNOSIS

DIFFERENTIAL DIAGNOSIS
• Chronic small bowel diarrhea is a consistent finding in an animal with any intestinal disorder that causes protein-losing enteropathy, except lymphangiectasia. Thickened bowel loops also suggest protein-losing enteropathy. • Icterus, hepatic encephalopathy, and PU/PD suggest chronic liver disease. • PU/PD and palpably small kidneys suggest underlying renal disease. • Skin lesions must be severe and extensive to account for marked exudative protein loss (e.g., severe burns). • Animal with external blood loss may have pale mucous membranes and evidence of hemorrhage (e.g., hemorrhage in the skin and mucous membranes, hematuria, and melena). • Protein-restricted diet may cause mild to moderate hypoalbuminemia. • Aggressive fluid therapy may exacerbate hypoalbuminemia by dilutional effects.

LABORATORY FINDINGS

Drugs That May Alter Lab Results
Ampicillin may cause spurious elevations.

Disorders That May Alter Lab Results
Extreme lipemia or excessive hemolysis causes artificially high values with the bromcresol green (BCG) method.

Valid in Human Lab?
Yes, if the BCG method is used.

CBC/BIOCHEMISTRY/URINALYSIS
• Severe hypoalbuminemia (< 1.0 gm/dl) is most likely associated with protein losing enteropathy, protein-losing nephropathy, or chronic liver disease. • If hypoalbuminemia is associated with hypoglobulinemia, consider protein-losing enteropathy, hemorrhage, dilution, and exudation from severe skin lesions. • If associated with normal serum globulins, consider low albumin production (e.g., liver disease and low intake), protein-losing nephropathy, or sequestration. • If associated with hyperglobulinemia, consider compensatory hypoalbuminemia (i.e., low hepatic albumin production in response to hyperglobulinemia). • If associated with high serum bilirubin and ALT or ALP activity, consider liver disease. • If associated with azotemia, nonregenerative anemia, and hy-

percholesterolemia, consider protein-losing nephropathy. • If associated with proteinuria in the absence of hematuria or pyuria, consider protein-losing nephropathy. • If associated with hypocholesterolemia and lymphopenia, consider lymphangiectasia. • If associated with regenerative anemia, consider external blood loss. • Low total calcium concentration develops secondary to hypoalbuminemia.

OTHER LABORATORY TESTS
• If fasting and 2 hour postprandial serum bile acids are normal, liver disease is unlikely to be the cause of hypoalbuminemia. • If the urine protein: creatinine ratio is less than 1.0 in dogs and cats, protein-losing nephropathy can be excluded. • Body cavity effusions that form as a result of hypoalbuminemia are characterized as a transudate.

IMAGING
• Thoracic radiographs can be useful to document pleural effusion and pulmonary edema. • Abdominal radiographs and ultrasonography can be useful to confirm ascites and to help identify underlying hepatic, renal, or intestinal disorder. • Contrast studies of the gastrointestinal tract may show thickened bowel loops in patients with infiltrative disorder, causing protein-losing enteropathy.

OTHER DIAGNOSTIC PROCEDURES
• Liver biopsy to confirm primary liver disease; evaluate coagulation profile before biopsy • Kidney biopsy to confirm cause of protein-losing nephropathy • Intestinal biopsy by endoscopy or exploratory laparotomy to identify cause of protein losing enteropathy • Careful postoperative management essential after laparotomy because of delayed wound healing in hypoalbuminemic patients.

TREATMENT
• Specific treatment requires identification of the underlying cause. • Perform thoracocentesis or place a chest tube to aid in removal of thoracic effusions causing dyspnea.. • IV infusion of colloid solutions can be used on a short-term basis for symptomatic treatment. • Nutritional support and treatment of the underlying cause is required on a long-term basis.

MEDICATIONS

DRUGS AND FLUIDS
• Plasma can be used to replace albumin and raise plasma oncotic pressure; however, multiple transfusions are required to markedly increase serum albumin concentration, which can be expensive. • Dextran 70, a polysaccharide with a molec-

ular weight of 70,000, is an alternative colloid solution (1ml/kg/hr [6% solution in 0.9% NaCl] IV CRI).

• Hetastarch, a synthetic polymer, also increases oncotic pressure (25-30 ml/kg [6% solution in 0.9% NaCl] IV over 6- 8 hours). At least two doses are given 12-24 hours apart. Hetastarch is more expensive than Dextran 70.

• Consider diuretic therapy (furosemide, 2-4 mg/kg IV, IM, PO q4h-q8h) for treatment of pulmonary edema. Use judiciously so as not to seriously decrease blood volume and further compromise perfusion

• Consider aspirin to prevent thromboembolism in patients with protein-losing nephropathy, which causes low concentration of antithrombin III.

CONTRAINDICATIONS

• Large doses of hetastarch can cause volume overload and affect blood coagulation. Do not use in dogs with anuric renal failure, congestive heart failure, severe coagulopathy, or von Willebrand's disease.

PRECAUTIONS

• In animals with severe hypoalbuminemia, avoid volume overload with crystalloid fluids since they are not retained within the vascular system and may worsen pulmonary edema and effusions.

• Plasma transfusion can be complicated by a tranfusion reaction.

• Administration of Dextran 70 may be associated with hemorrhagic tendencies.

• Diuretics further reduce circulatory blood volume, predisposing the patient to azotemia and hypotension.

POSSIBLE INTERACTIONS N/A
ALTERNATE DRUGS N/A

FOLLOW-UP
PATIENT MONITORING
• Serum albumin concentration to evaluate response to treatment. • Thoracic radiographs to reassess pulmonary edema and pleural effusion.

POSSIBLE COMPLICATIONS
• Severe protein-losing nephropathy can be complicated by emboli formation (pulmonary, aortic, or other vessels). • Low plasma volume may cause reduced renal perfusion and prerenal uremia.

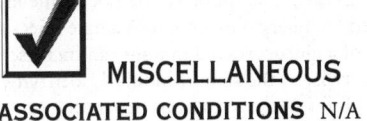

MISCELLANEOUS
ASSOCIATED CONDITIONS N/A

AGE RELATED FACTORS N/A
PREGNANCY N/A
SYNONYMS N/A
SEE ALSO
• Amyloidosis • Cirrhosis/Fibrosis of the Liver • Glomerulonephritis • Protein-losing Enteropathies

ABBREVIATIONS
ALP = alkaline phosphatase
ALT = alanine aminotransferase
PU/PD = polyuria/polydipsia

References
Turnwald GH, Barta O. Immunologic and plasma protein disorders. In: Willard MD, Tvedten H, Turnwald GH. Small animal clinical diagnosis by laboratory mMethods. Philadelphia, PA: WB Saunders Co., 1989.
Smiley LE, Garvey MS. The use of hetastarch as adjunct therapy in 26 dogs with hypoalbuminemia: a phase two clinical trial. J Vet Int Med 1994;8:195–202.
Author Susan E. Johnson
Consulting Editor Albert E. Jergens

ALKALINE PHOSPHATASE (ALP) AND GAMMA GLUTAMYL TRANSFERASE (GGT)

BASICS

DEFINITION
The normal serum alkaline phosphatase (ALP) activity is between 30-150 IU/L for most commercial laboratories. The normal serum gamma glutamyl transferase (GGT) activity is between 1-7 IU/L for most commercial laboratories.

Pathophysiology
Serum ALP activity usually increases in animals with biliary stasis, steroid hepatopathy and, occasionally, bone lesions. ALP is found in many tissues, including the liver, bone, intestine, placenta, and kidneys. In a clinical setting, only isoenzymes found in the liver and in bone are important. The serum activity of ALP increases in animals with hepatic disease primarily when there is intrahepatic or extrahepatic biliary obstruction. Like ALP, serum activity of GGT increases in animals with biliary stasis and steroid hepatopathy. In most patients, the activity of serum GGT parallels that of ALP, and its measurement is only occasionally of value in dogs and cats.

Systems Affected
High serum activities of either ALP or GGT cause no damage to the body but indicate disease.

SIGNALMENT
• The serum activity of ALP is much lower in cats than in dogs. The half-life is much shorter in cats (6 hours in cats versus 3 days in dogs), and cats have less ALP produced secondary to biliary obstruction. • In cats, even mild elevations of serum ALP activity indicate important hepatobiliary disease. • In cats, serum GGT activity has a higher sensitivity but lower specificity than ALP activity for the detection of hepatobiliary disease. In dogs, serum GGT activity is generally more specific but less sensitive than serum ALP activity for the detection of hepatobiliary disease. • In contrast to dogs, cats rarely have high serum activities of ALP or GGT associated with glucocorticoid administration. • Bone ALP increases with osteoblastic activity and is often high in young, growing animals.

SIGNS
• High serum activities of either ALP or GGT cause no damage to the body, but indicate disease. • Clinical signs relate to the underlying disease process.

CAUSES
• ALP activity usually increases in animals with biliary stasis, steroid hepatopathy, and significant bone lesions. • Serum GGT activity increases with biliary stasis and steroid hepatopathy. • The most common drugs that increase ALP activity are glucocorticoids, barbiturates, and anticonvulsant drugs, including phenobarbital, primidone, and phenytoin. In general, serum GGT activity is less

influenced by enzyme-inducing drugs. • The activity of ALP increases in animals with hepatic disease when there is biliary obstruction (intrahepatic or extrahepatic). Cells lining the bile canaliculi produce ALP when biliary obstruction occurs. In animals with primary hepatocellular disease (e.g., inflammation, cloudy swelling, lipid accumulation, and neoplastic infiltration) serum ALP activity may also increase because of swelling of hepatocytes resulting in intrahepatic cholestasis.
• Diseases that are periportal versus centrilobular in location tend to cause greater increases in serum ALP activity, because they tend to affect bile flow through canaliculi more. Diseases often associated with high serum ALP and GGT activity include chronic active hepatitis, steroid hepatopathy (dogs), cholangiohepatitis (cats), hepatic lipidosis (cats; mainly ALP), primary hepatic neoplasia, bile duct obstruction, hepatic necrosis, and hyperthyroidism (cats). Diseases with minimal or inconsistent elevations of serum ALP and GGT activity include metastatic neoplasia, portosystemic shunt, and cirrhosis. • Dogs have a steroid-induced isoenzyme of ALP (rare in cats) in addition to the isoenzyme induced by biliary obstruction. A single injection of a glucocorticoid in dogs can increase the activity of the steroid-induced isoenzyme of ALP for weeks to months depending on the pharmacologic preparation. The magnitude of elevation depends on the dose administered, duration, route, and individual animal sensitivity. Spontaneous hyperadrenocorticism (Cushing's syndrome) causes high serum ALP activity approximately 80% of the time. Serum GGT activity often parallels ALP activity in regard to the effect of glucocorticoids. Other drugs including barbiturates and anticonvulsant drugs (e.g., phenobarbital, primidone, and phenytoin) may also induce increases in serum ALP activity. In general, serum GGT activity is less influenced by nonhepatic disease or enzyme-inducing drugs. • Bone ALP activity increases with osteoblastic activity, and high values are often observed in young, growing animals. Less common causes for high ALP activity of bone origin include bone tumors, severe osteomalacia, and hyperparathyroidism.

RISK FACTORS
• ALP and GGT activities increase with a variety of hepatobiliary diseases. Isoenzyme induction may also occur with the use of certain drugs (see above). • Young animals (primarily dogs) and those having aggressive bone disorders (e.g., neoplasia, osteomalacia, and hyperparathyroidism) are at risk for bone ALP isoenzyme elevations.

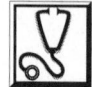

DIAGNOSIS

DIFFERENTIAL DIAGNOSIS
• Mild to moderate increase in ALP activity is

normal in young growing animals. • High ALP activity (and to a lesser extent serum GGT activity) is common in dogs with historical or physical examination findings of hyperadrenocorticism or after glucocorticoid, anticonvulsant drug, or barbiturate administration. • Primary hepatobiliary disease as a cause for high ALP or GGT activity may be suggested by physical examination findings (e.g., icterus, hepatomegaly, and ascites) or other laboratory tests (i.e., high in ALT, AST, serum total bilirubin, and bile acids; low serum albumin, BUN, and glucose concentrations) indicating hepatobiliary disease.

LABORATORY FINDINGS

Drugs that May Alter Lab Results N/A
Numerous drugs affect ALP activity but do not interfere with laboratory procedures.

Disoders that May Alter Lab Results
N/A

Valid if Run in Human Lab? Yes

CBC/BIOCHEMISTRY/URINALYSIS
• Results of a serum biochemical profile are rarely specific, but help to verify the presence of hepatobiliary disease. • High serum concentrations of total bilirubin and activities of ALT and AST are commonly seen in animals with high ALP and GGT. • Changes seen in animals with chronic hepatobiliary disorders include low serum concentrations of urea nitrogen, glucose, and albumin.
• Once hepatobiliary disease is identified, a specific cause is pursued with hepatobiliary imaging or hepatic biopsy.

OTHER LABORATORY TESTS
• Serum bile acid or plasma ammonia concentrations are often high in animals with hepatobiliary disease cause by impaired hepatic function. • Hyperadrenocorticism should be ruled out by an ACTH stimulation test or a low–dose dexamethasone suppression test when ALP and GGT are the only hepatic enzymes that are markedly high (e.g., normal or mild increases in activities of ALT and AST). • Hyperthyroidism should be ruled out by a serum T4 measurement (or possibly T3 suppression test if borderline or clinically suspicious) in cats with high ALP. • Specific determination of the steroid–induced isoenzyme is of little value, since many hepatobiliary diseases cause marked increases in this isoenzyme.

IMAGING

Abdominal Radiographic Findings
• Diseases that cause small hepatic size include cirrhosis, portosystemic shunt, and acute and subacute necrosis; this is normal in deep chested breeds of dog. • Diseases that cause large hepatic size include neoplasia (primary and metastatic), congestion, fatty infiltration, diffuse inflammation, hyperadrenocorticism, storage disease, and hepatic abscess or biliary cyst; this is normal in puppies/kittens and during deep inspiration.

ALKALINE PHOSPHATASE (ALP) AND GAMMA GLUTAMYL TRANSFERASE (GGT)

Ultrasonographic Findings
• Hepatobiliary ultrasonography is currently the most reliable noninvasive method of distinguishing intrahepatic from posthepatic (e.g., common bile duct obstruction) cholestasis.
• Findings may include a large gall bladder, large common bile duct, and large intrahepatic bile ducts (demonstrated by irregular branching patterns and variable diameter compared with blood vessels).

OTHER DIAGNOSTIC PROCEDURES
• Hepatic biopsy is indicated if laboratory findings suggest primary hepatobiliary disease and imaging rules out extrahepatic biliary obstruction. • Hepatic biopsy methods include percutaneous and ultrasound–guided techniques, laparoscopy, and laparotomy.

TREATMENT
• Specific treatment varies depending on the underlying cause of high ALP or GGT.
• An aggressive diagnostic and therapeutic approach is usually warranted, because animals with high activity of ALP or GGT may have a serious underlying disease. Surgery is often required to correct extrahepatic biliary obstruction. Symptomatic and supportive medical treatment is usually warranted to treat intrahepatic disease. Since a variety of hepatic diseases can cause high ALP or GGT activity, hepatic biopsy is often warranted so that specific treatment can be instituted.
• General supportive measures for treating hepatic disease include eliminating the incit-ing cause if possible, providing cage rest for hepatic regeneration, preventing complications (e.g., ascites and thromboembolism), and reversing metabolic derangements that occur with hepatic failure. Important derangements include dehydration and hypovolemia, hepatic encephalopathy, hypoglycemia, acid/base and electrolyte abnormalities, coagulopathies, gastric ulceration, sepsis, and endotoxemia.

MEDICATIONS

DRUGS AND FLUIDS OF CHOICE
Vary depending on the underlying disease process

CONTRAINDICATIONS
Vary depending on the underlying disease process

PRECAUTIONS
Vary depending on the underlying disease process

POSSIBLE INTERACTIONS
Vary depending on the underlying disease process

ALTERNATE DRUGS
Vary depending on the underlying disease process

FOLLOW-UP

PATIENT MONITORING
Recheck serum chemistry profile, bile acids, and hepatic imaging with frequency dictated by the underlying disease.

POSSIBLE COMPLICATIONS
Many causes of increased activities of ALP/GGT are life threatening.

MISCELLANEOUS

ASSOCIATED CONDITIONS N/A

AGE RELATED FACTORS
High ALP activity is normal in growing puppies.

ZOONOTIC POTENTIAL N/A

PREGNANCY N/A

SYNONYMS N/A

SEE ALSO N/A

ABBREVIATIONS
ALT = alanine aminotransferase
AST = aspartate aminotransferase
BUN = blood urea nitrogen

References
Strombeck DR, Guilford WG. Small animal gastroenterology. 2nd ed. Davis, Calif: Stonegate Publishing Company, 1990;529–556.
Center SA. Pathophysiology and laboratory diagnosis of hepatobiliary disorders. In: Ettinger SJ, Feldman EC, eds. Textbook of veterinary internal medicine. 4th ed. Philadelphia: WB Saunders, 1995;1261–1312.

Author Keith P. Richter
Consulting Editor Albert E. Jergens

ALKALOSIS, METABOLIC

 BASICS

DEFINITION

Metabolic alkalosis results in a primary increase in plasma bicarbonate (HCO_3^-) (> 24 mEq/L in dogs and > 22 mEq/L in cats) with low hydrogen ion concentration ($[H^+]$), high pH, and a compensatory increase in carbon dioxide tension (PCO_2).

Pathophysiology

Loss of chloride and hydrogen ion-rich fluid via the alimentary tract or kidneys is usually accompanied by volume depletion. Loss of H^+ is associated with an increase in plasma HCO_3^- concentration. With chloride loss and volume depletion, the kidneys reabsorb sodium and HCO_3^- instead of chloride, perpetuating the metabolic alkalosis. Chronic administration of alkali also may result in transient metabolic alkalosis. Renal excretion of exogenous-administered alkali is effective, and it is difficult to create metabolic alkalosis by increasing HCO_3^- intake, unless the patient has renal dysfunction.

Systems Affected

• Respiratory—Low $[H^+]$ concentration reduces alveolar ventilation. Hypoventilation increases PCO_2 and helps offset the effect of high plasma HCO_3^- concentration on pH. In dogs, an increase of approximately 0.7 mm Hg in PCO_2 can be expected for each 1 mEq/L increase in plasma HCO_3^- concentration.
• Renal/Urologic—the kidneys rapidly and effectively excrete excessive alkali. In a patient with chloride deficiency (and less importantly, volume depletion), the kidneys are unable to excrete the excessive alkali and metabolic alkalosis will be maintained.
• Nervous—muscle twitching and seizures occur rarely in dogs.

SIGNALMENT

Any breed, age, or sex of dog and cat.

SIGNS

Historical Findings

• Administration of loop diuretics (e.g., furosemide) or thiazides
• Vomiting

Physical Findings

• Signs related to the underlying disease or accompanying potassium depletion (e.g., weakness, cardiac arrhythmias, and ileus)
• Muscle twitching caused by a low ionized calcium concentration
• Dehydration in volume-depleted patients
• Muscle twitching and seizures in patients with neurologic involvement (rare)

CAUSES

• Chloride-responsive—diuretic administration, vomiting of stomach contents, and rapid correction of hypercapnia (respiratory acidosis)
• Chloride-resistant—hyperadrenocorticism and primary hyperaldosteronism
• Oral administration of alkali—administration of sodium bicarbonate or other organic anion with sodium (e.g., lactate, acetate, and gluconate). Administration of cation exchange resin with nonabsorbable alkali (e.g., phosphorus binder).
• Miscellaneous—hypoalbuminemia; administration of large doses of sodium penicillin or carbenicillin.

RISK FACTORS

• Administration of loop or thiazide diuretics
• Vomiting

 DIAGNOSIS

DIFFERENTIAL DIAGNOSIS

• High plasma HCO_3^- concentration can also be compensatory in animals with chronic respiratory acidosis, in which PCO_2 is high and pH is low despite high HCO_3^- concentration. Blood gas determination required to differentiate
• In animals with high bicarbonate associated with hypochloremia, consider hypochloremic metabolic alkalosis. This is the most common reason for metabolic alkalosis in dogs and cats and usually results from diuretic administration or vomiting of stomach contents.
• In animals with high bicarbonate associated with hypoalbuminemia, consider hypoalbuminemic metabolic alkalosis. Albumin is a weak acid. In human beings, a decrease in 1 g/dl in albumin is associated with a 3.7 mEq/L increase in HCO_3^- concentration.
• In animals with high bicarbonate associated with normal chloride but high sodium concentration, consider chloride-resistant metabolic alkalosis (e.g., hyperadrenocorticism and primary hyperaldosteronism) or administration of alkali.
• In animals with high bicarbonate associated with hypokalemia, the hypokalemia is probably the result of the metabolic alkalosis or the underlying problem (e.g., vomiting of stomach contents or loop diuretic administration). Hypokalemic-induced metabolic alkalosis does not occur in dogs and cats.

LABORATORY FINDINGS

Drugs That May Alter Lab Results
N/A

Disorders That May Alter Lab Results

• Too much heparin (>10% of the sample) decreases HCO_3^- concentration.
• Samples stored at room temperature for more than 20 minutes have low pH because of an increase PCO_2.
• Some blood gas analyzers only report pH and PCO_2. Bicarbonate has to be calculated and this is a potential source for error.

Valid if Run in Human Lab?
Yes

CBC/BIOCHEMISTRY/URINALYSIS

• High total CO_2 (total CO_2 in samples han-
dled aerobically closely approximates the HCO_3^- concentration)
• Low ionized calcium
• Electrolyte abnormalities vary with underlying cause (see differential diagnosis)

OTHER LABORATORY TESTS

Blood gas analysis reveals a high HCO_3^-, low PCO_2, and low pH

IMAGING N/A

OTHER DIAGNOSTIC PROCEDURES
N/A

 TREATMENT

• Acid-base disturbances are secondary phenomena. Diagnosis and treatment of the underlying disease process is integral to the successful resolution of acid-base disorders.
• Discontinue drugs that may cause metabolic alkalosis

 MEDICATIONS

DRUG AND FLUIDS

• The fluids of choice contain chloride. Patients with volume depletion are given an intravenous infusion of 0.9% NaCl supplemented with KCl. Patients with hypokalemia may require large doses of KCl (see hypokalemia).
• If the underlying cause cannot be corrected (e.g., chronic heart failure patients receiving diuretics), compounds containing chloride without sodium (e.g., KCl and NH4Cl) can be tried. Simultaneous use of distal tubule blocking agents (e.g., spironolactone, triamterene, and amiloride) can also be considered.
• Chloride-resistant metabolic alkalosis can only be corrected by resolution of the underlying disease. Metabolic alkalosis is usually mild in these patients.

CONTRAINDICATIONS

• Avoid chloride-free fluids, because they may correct volume depletion but will not correct metabolic alkalosis.
• Avoid drugs containing sodium without chloride (e.g., sodium penicillin and sodium bicarbonate), because they may worsen metabolic alkalosis.
• Avoid using salts of potassium without chloride (e.g., potassium phosphate), because potassium will be excreted in the urine and will correct neither the alkalosis nor the potassium deficit.

PRECAUTIONS

Distal tubule blocking agents (e.g., spironolactone, triamterene, and amiloride) should not be used in volume-depleted patients.

POSSIBLE INTERACTIONS N/A

ALTERNATE DRUGS N/A

FOLLOW-UP

PATIENT MONITORING
Recheck acid-base status, with frequency dictated by the underlying disease and patient response to treatment.

POSSIBLE COMPLICATIONS
• Hypokalemia
• Neurologic signs

MISCELLANEOUS

ASSOCIATED CONDITIONS
Hypokalemia and hypochloremia

AGE- RELATED FACTORS N/A

PREGNANCY N/A

SYNONYMS
• Nonrespiratory alkalosis
• Chloride-responsive metabolic alkalosis—metabolic alkalosis that responds to chloride administration
• Chloride-resistant metabolic alkalosis—metabolic alkalosis that does not respond to chloride administration.
• Hypoalbuminemic alkalosis—metabolic alkalosis caused by low albumin concentration
• Hypochloremic alkalosis—metabolic alkalosis caused by low chloride concentration
• Concentration alkalosis—metabolic alkalosis caused by high sodium concentration
• Contraction alkalosis—metabolic alkalosis formerly attributed to volume-contraction but now known to be caused by chloride depletion.

SEE ALSO
• Hypokalemia
• Hypochloremia

ABBREVIATIONS
HCO_3^- = bicarbonate
PCO_2 = carbon dioxide tension
H^+ = Hydrogen ion

References
de Morais, HSA. Chloride ion in small animal practice: The forgotten ion. J Vet Emerg Crit Care 1992;2:11-24

DiBartola, SP. Metabolic alkalosis. In Fluid therapy in small animal practice. DiBartola, SP, editor. Philadelphia: WB Saunders, 1992:244-257.

DiBartola, SP, Green, RA, de Morais, HSA. Electrolytes and acid base disorders. In: Willard MD, Tvedten H, Turnwald GH, eds. Small animal clinical diagnosis by laboratory methods. 2nd ed. Philadelphia: WB Saunders, 1994:97-113.

Robinson, EP, Hardy, RM. Clinical signs, diagnosis, and treatment of alkalemia in dogs: 20 cases (1982-1984). J Am Vet Med Assoc 1988;192:943-949.

Authors Helio Autran de Morais and Stephen P. DiBartola
Consulting Editor Larry G. Adams and Carl A. Osborne

AMMONIA

BASICS

DEFINITION
Ammonia (NH_3) is a nonprotein nitrogen compound. Its physiologic state is the ammonium ion (NH_4^+). In order to eliminate waste nitrogen as ammonia, the mammalian body converts it to an excretable form, urea. To a lesser extent, ammonia is eliminated by conversion to glutamine. Normal plasma values for ammonia are 45–120 ug/dl in dogs and 30–100 ug/dl in cats.

Pathophysiology
The liver is the primary site of urea synthesis. Ammonia derives from dietary amino acids, catabolism of glutamine and protein, and skeletal muscle exertion. It is delivered to the liver via the portal vein or hepatic artery. Urea synthesis occurs by means of the urea cycle, or Krebs–Henseleit cycle. If liver function is inadequate, ammonia is not converted to urea, and plasma ammonia concentrations rise. Serum urea concentrations also rise when glomerular filtration is inadequate.

Systems Affected
Nervous—ammonia is cytotoxic. The brain is most affected by high plasma concentrations. Ammonia interferes with the blood brain barrier, cerebral blood flow, cellular excitability, neurotransmitter metabolism, and ratios of neurotransmitter precursor amino acids. Degenerative changes of the neurons and supporting cells have been observed in chronically affected animals.

SIGNALMENT
The presence of hyperammonemia is most often associated with diseases of the liver. These diseases may be associated with specific breed, age, and sex.

SIGNS

General Comments
• Clinical signs of hyperammonemia are primarily those of hepatic encephalopathy.
• Owners often commment on the sporadic nature of the signs and progressive course.
• Owners may have observed signs worsening after feeding.

Historical Findings
• Ptyalism • Behavior changes • Visual deficits (blindness) • Circling • Pacing • Anxiety • Head pressing • Stupor • Coma

Physical Examination Findings
• Stunted growth • Loss of body condition • Mentation changes and aberrant behavior as listed • Similar findings as discussed in topics on liver disease, e.g., icterus, may also be observed. • In animals affected chronically, neuron degeneration occurs and signs become persistent.

CAUSES
• Abnormalities of the urea cycle, abnormal portal blood flow, or any disorder that causes markedly impaired liver function can cause hyperammonemia. • Rare congenital problems of urea cycle enzyme deficiencies have been reported in two dogs. • Cats require dietary arginine (part of the urea cycle). Dietary restriction of this amino acid can cause hyperammonemia and coma in cats. Since most dietary protein contains adequate arginine, this is currently thought not to play a crucial role in clinical cases.

RISK FACTORS
• Use of improperly stored or out-of-date RBC products. • Gastrointestinal hemorrhage. Blood is digested, providing a high protein meal and nitrogen substrate for ammonia production. • Constipation raises ammonia concentrations by increasing time for absorption of ammonia by the colon and production by bacteria.

DIAGNOSIS

DIFFERENTIAL DIAGNOSIS
• Must differentiate from primary neurologic disease and behavior problems. • Evaluation of the history, signalment, and results of serum biochemistry, hemogram, urinalysis, hepatic biopsy, sonography, and possibly contrast portography or technetium–assisted imaging usually results in an appropriate diagnosis.

LABORATORY FINDINGS

Drugs That May Alter Lab Results
The following drugs alter blood ammonia concentration without affecting validity of test results:
• Antibiotics that reduce bacterial intestinal flora may decrease plasma ammonia concentration. • Lactulose and diphenhydramine decrease the ammonia concentration • Enemas decrease the ammonia concentration. • High concentrations of ammonia have been reported after blood transfusion and administration of parenteral amino acids, narcotics, and diuretics.

Disorders That May Alter Lab Results
Prolonged occlusion of a vein during sampling may cause high values, especially if there is muscle exertion during restraint.

Valid if Run in Human Lab?
This test can be performed in human labs. Samples must be kept in an ice bath and analysis performed within 30 minutes. In–house dry chemistry analysis accounts for a resurgence of interest in plasma ammonia. This requires adequate controls, paired samples, and proper sample handling.

CBC/BIOCHEMISTRY/URINALYSIS
• Findings vary with the nature of the liver disease. • CBC—microcytosis in animals with portosystemic shunt, RBC morphologic changes • Biochemistry—results may be normal in animals with portosystemic shunt.

Findings in animals with liver disease may include high liver enzymes and bilirubin, hypoglycemia, hyper- or hypocholesterolemia, hypoalbuminemia, and low BUN. • Urinalysis—ammonia biurate crystals and low urine specific gravity because of underlying liver disease in some animals.

OTHER LABORATORY TESTS
Measurement of serum bile acids is advised if the animal is not icteric.

IMAGING
• Abdominal radiographs can be helpful in assessing hepatic size. • Sonographic evaluation of the liver and portal vessels is advised. • The use of radioisotope technetium perfusion techniques for assessment of portal blood flow is limited to large referral centers.

OTHER DIAGNOSTIC PROCEDURES
• Hepatic biopsy is often necessary. • The ammonia tolerance test can be used when measurement of bile acids is not available, but this test can precipitate hepatic encephalopathy. Ammonium chloride is administered by enema catheter or gelatin capsule and a heparinized blood sample taken before and 30 minutes after. A 3-10-fold elevation from the baseline value indicates insufficient hepatic function.

TREATMENT
• Most animals with clinical signs should be treated as inpatients.
• Restrict activity.
• Feed a very low protein diet, or fast the patient initially, and then institute a protein-restricted diet when the patient is stable.

MEDICATIONS

DRUGS AND FLUIDS
• Fluid administration is needed to correct dehydration.
• Lactulose is used to lower plasma ammonia concentration. Lactulose acts as a cathartic laxative and "traps" ammonia in the lumen by keeping it in its ammonium ion, nonabsorbable form.
• Antibiotics with a broad spectrum against intestinal flora are administered orally. Nonabsorbable aminoglycoside (e.g., neomycin) and metronidazole is a good combination. In less severely affected animals, amoxicillin with clavulanic acid can be administered.
• Cleansing enemas are advocated in patients with clinical signs or constipation.

CONTRAINDICATIONS
Any drugs that affect the CNS must be used with caution because of the common association of hyperammonemia with hepatic encephalopathy and possibly impaired hepat-

ic metabolism. Barbiturates and benzodi-azepam-like drugs are of particular concern.

PRECAUTIONS N/A

POSSIBLE INTERACTIONS

Because of impaired hepatic metabolism, any drugs that inhibit metabolism by the liver must be considered carefully, e.g., cimetidine.

ALTERNATE DRUGS N/A

FOLLOW-UP

PATIENT MONITORING

Repeated assessment of plasma ammonia can be helpful. Monitoring of serum potassium and glucose is advised in critical patients.

POSSIBLE COMPLICATIONS

Inaccuracy is the biggest problem because of the labile nature of ammonia in blood samples. Delay in processing results in falsely high ammonia concentration.

MISCELLANEOUS

ASSOCIATED CONDITIONS N/A

AGE RELATED FACTORS N/A

ZOONOTIC POTENTIAL N/A

PREGNANCY N/A

SYNONYMS N/A

SEE ALSO
• Hepatic encephalopathy
• Refer to specific liver diseases.

ABBREVIATIONS

BUN = blood urea nitrogen
CNS = central nervous system
RBC = red blood cells

References

Willard MD, Tvedten H, Turnwald GH. Small animal clinical diagnosis by laboratory methods. Philadelphia: WB Saunders, 1989;224–225.

Hitt ME, Jones BD. Effects of storage temperature and time on canine plasma ammonia concentrations. Am J Vet Res 1986;47:363–364.

Dimski DS. Ammonia metabolism and the urea cycle: function and clinical implications. J Vet Intern Med 1994;8:73–78.

Author Mark E. Hitt
Consulting Editor Albert E. Jergens

AMYLASE AND LIPASE

BASICS

DEFINITION
Serum amylase and lipase activities higher than laboratory reference ranges.

Pathophysiology
• Only alpha amylase is present in animals. The pancreas, liver, and small intestine serve as sources of serum amylase. In healthy animals, serum amylase is derived primarily from extrapancreatic sources. Considerable serum amylase activity (up to 1000 IU/L) is normal in healthy animals. Hyperamylasemia can develop in animals with pancreatitis, gastrointestinal inflammation, and renal disease. • Serum lipase is derived from the pancreas and gastric mucosa, and its activity is optimal when the pH is alkaline. Hyperlipasemia can develop in animals with pancreatitis, renal disease, hepatic disease, and after the administration of dexamethasone. • Both amylase and lipase are inactivated by the kidneys and eliminated from the body in urine.

Systems Affected
Hyperamylasemia and hyperlipasemia have little to no effect on other organ systems.

SIGNALMENT
Breeds at risk for acute pancreatitis:
• Dogs—middle-aged and older miniature schnauzers, miniature poodles, and cocker spaniels • Cats—middle-aged Siamese cats

SIGNS

General Comments
Clinical signs vary depending on the cause and organ system involved.

Historical Findings
• Pancreatitis—lethargy, depression, anorexia, vomiting, and diarrhea • Hepatic disease—anorexia, altered mentation, icterus, weight loss, vomiting, diarrhea, PU/PD, and abdominal distention • Renal disease—PU/PD, lethargy, anorexia, weight loss, vomiting, and diarrhea • Gastrointestinal disease—vomiting, diarrhea, anorexia, and weight loss • Exogenous glucocorticoids—PU/PD, polyphagia, and weight gain

Physical Examination Findings
• Pancreatitis—lethargy, dehydration, abdominal pain, fever, and icterus (more common in cats) • Hepatic disease—icterus, hepatomegaly, depression, abdominal pain, weight loss, and peritoneal effusion • Renal disease—weight loss, mucus membrane pallor, dehydration, and normal-sized to small, irregular kidneys • Gastrointestinal disease—weight loss, dehydration, palpable mass lesion or foreign body, and variable fecal consistency

CAUSES

Pancreatitis and Hyperamylasemia
• Serum amylase activity increases in most dogs with pancreatitis; activity > 5000 IU/L is highly suggestive of acute pancreatitis. • Although high amylase activity is a sensitive indicator of pancreatic inflammation, it can also be caused by nonpancreatic disease (poor specificity). • Serum amylase activity is best interpreted in light of serum lipase activity. Amylase activity in dogs with pancreatitis does not correlate with lipase activity until serum lipase values exceed 800 IU/L. • Serum amylase activity in cats with acute pancreatitis decreases, and therefore is not recommended.

Pancreatitis and Hyperlipasemia
• Serum lipase activity consistently increases several fold in dogs with pancreatitis. If serum lipase activity of > 500 IU/L is used as a cutoff, the sensitivity of the test for pancreatitis is 98%. • Serum lipase activity is also affected by a variety of nonpancreatic disorders The specificity of the test for pancreatitis is 78% if a value of 500 IU/L is used as a cutoff. • Serum lipase activity in cats with pancreatitis is normal to high. • Normal serum lipase activity does not rule out pancreatic disease. Up to 15-20% of animals with acute pancreatitis have normal lipase and/or amylase activity. • In general, lipase activity is a more reliable marker of pancreatitis in dogs and cats than amylase activity.

Renal Disease
• Renal failure is associated with hyperamylasemia and hyperlipasemia. • High serum activities may result from impaired renal degradation or inadequate clearance due to a reduction in glomerular filtration.

Hepatic Disease
• The source of high lipase activity observed in animals with liver disease is not known.

Gastrointestinal Disease
• High serum amylase activity is observed in some dogs with enteritis, small intestinal obstruction, and gastrointestinal perforation.

Miscellaneous
• A 3-fold or more increase in serum lipase activity may occur after routine laparotomy in dogs without clinical signs or gross evidence of pancreatitis. • Hyperlipasemia and decreases in serum amylase activity have been reported in dogs after the administration of corticosteroids.

RISK FACTORS
• Obesity and the ingestion of high–fat diets in animals with pancreatitis • Presence of underlying renal disease • Presence of underlying hepatic disease • Nonspecific gastrointestinal inflammation • Previous administration of dexamethasone

DIAGNOSIS

DIFFERENTIAL DIAGNOSIS
• If vomiting, depression, fever, and abdominal pain are observed, rule out pancreatitis. • If PU/PD, anorexia, weight loss, vomiting, anemia are observed, rule out chronic renal disease. • If icterus, hepatomegaly, vomiting, PU/PD, and altered mentation are observed, rule out hepatic disease. • If vomiting, diarrhea, anorexia, and palpable abnormalities of intestinal loops are observed, rule out gastrointestinal disease.

LABORATORY FINDINGS

Drugs That May Alter Lab Results
• Corticosteroids increase serum lipase activity and decrease serum amylase activity, but do not alter validity of laboratory results.

Disorders That May Alter Lab Results
• Serum amylase activity should be measured by an amyloclastic method that measures the disappearance of starch from the assay. Maltase activity in the plasma of dogs is high; and use of a saccharogenic method (measuring the appearance of glucose in the assay) indicates falsely high amylase activity, since maltase contributes to glucose formed in the assay. • Measurement of serum lipase activity requires more time and the test is technically more cumbersome to perform. • Hemolysis inhibits lipase activity. • Lipemia falsely decreases serum lipase activity as measured by kinetic assays.

Valid if Run in Human Lab? Yes

CBC/BIOCHEMISTRY/URINALYSIS
• Pancreatitis—leukocytosis with a left shift, anemia in cats, hyperlipidemia, high ALT and ALP activities and total bilirubin, and prerenal azotemia • Renal disease—anemia (nonregenerative), renal azotemia, hyperphosphatemia, hypokalemia (cats), and impaired urinary concentrating ability. • Hepatic disease—high ALT and ALP activities and total bilirubin, hypoproteinemia, hypoalbuminemia, low BUN, and impaired urinary concentrating ability • Gastrointestinal disease—vary depending on cause.

OTHER LABORATORY TESTS
• Measurement of serum trypsin–like immunoreactivity or ELISA for trypsinogen activation peptide in dogs with pancreatitis • Bile acid assay to assess hepatobiliary function in dogs and cats with hepatic disease • Tests to assess gastrointestinal inflammation including serologic testing for infectious agents and fecal culture

IMAGING
• Pancreatitis—abdominal radiographs show peritoneal effusion, focal soft tissue opacity in right cranial abdominal compartment, and gas retention in proximal duodenum; ultrasound shows the presence of a pancreatic mass and loss of normal pancreatic echogenicity. • Renal disease—abdominal radiographs may show normal sized to small kidneys, irregularity of renal cortical margins, and skeletal osteodystrophy; ultrasound may show small, irregular kidneys and increased

renal cortical echogenicity. • Hepatic disease—abdominal radiographs may show peritoneal effusion or hepatomegaly; ultrasound may show hepatomegaly and alterations in hepatic parenchymal echogenicity. • Gastrointestinal disease—abdominal radiographs may show radiopaque foreign body, obstructive lesion, increase in diameter of bowel loops, mucosal irregularity (contrast), and ulcer (contrast); ultrasound findings vary but may show foreign body, obstructive lesion, and intramural infiltrative lesion.

OTHER DIAGNOSTIC PROCEDURES
• Renal biopsy (via laparotomy, laparoscopy, or ultrasound-guidance) to confirm diagnosis of renal disease • Hepatic biopsy (via laparotomy, laparoscopy, or ultrasound–guidance) to confirm diagnosis of liver disease • Laparotomy for full thickness intestinal biopsy • Endoscopy for intestinal mucosal biopsy

TREATMENT
• Treatment varies depending on the underlying cause for high serum amylase and/or lipase activity.
• Patients should be hospitalized for initial medical management.
• Restricted activity is required in most patients.
• Dietary management and fluid therapy are important treatment modalities in these patients.
• Surgical considerations include laparotomy to remove gastrointestinal foreign body, drain pancreatic abscesses, or provide open peritoneal drainage.

MEDICATIONS
DRUGS AND FLUIDS
• Patients with pancreatitis—NPO; lactated Ringer's solution is the fluid of choice and should be given IV; add potassium chloride to fluids in animals with profuse vomiting; use parenteral antibiotics (penicillin or ampicillin) if sepsis is present; use antiemetics (phenothiazine derivatives) if intractable vomiting occurs; use corticosteroids if patient is in shock.
• Renal Disease—lactated Ringer's solution or 0.9% saline are appropriate, first-choice

rehydration fluids; fluids should be given IV in severely azotemic patients; treat signs of uremia with antiemetics (metoclopramide) and antihistamines (ie, H2-blockers such as cimetidine); transfusion may be required in animals with severe anemia.
• Hepatic disease—lactated Ringer's solution is used in animals with acute hepatopathy; use 0.45% saline in animals with chronic liver disorder; potassium supplementation in fluids is important in patients with chronic liver disease; lactulose and metronidazole can be used to reduce signs of hepatic encephalopathy.
• Gastrointestinal disease—NPO if patient is vomiting; lactated Ringer's solution should be used to correct hydration and electrolyte deficits; add potassium to fluids if necessary; avoid antibiotics unless hemorrhagic diarrhea is present; avoid anticholinergic drugs which can cause ileus; avoid antiemetics unless profuse vomiting is present.

CONTRAINDICATIONS
• Avoid the use of azathioprine, chlorothiazide, estrogens, furosemide, tetracycline, and sulfamethazole in patients with pancreatitis.
• Avoid aminoglycosides in patients with renal disease. Adjust the dosage or dosing interval appropriately for all other drugs that are eliminated by the kidneys.
• In animals with liver disease, adjust the dosage of drugs that require hepatic biotransformation or hepatic degradation.
• Avoid metoclopramide in animals with gastrointestinal obstruction.

PRECAUTIONS
• Since pancreatitis is the most common cause of markedly high activity of both serum amylase and lipase, the following drugs should be used cautiously:
(1) Corticosteroids since they may aggravate lesions of pancreatitis
(2) Phenothiazine antiemetics since they have hypotensive properties and may exacerbate pancreatic ischemia
(3) Dextrans since high dosages may promote bleeding in patients with hemorrhagic pancreatitis

POSSIBLE INTERACTIONS N/A
ALTERNATE DRUGS N/A

FOLLOW-UP
PATIENT MONITORING
Pancreatitis
• Evaluate patient's hydration status closely for the first 48 hours. • Repeat biochemistry analysis and measurement of lipase activity as needed. • Gradually reintroduce oral alimentation.

Other Conditions
Patient follow–up is extremely variable depending on the organ system involved and extent of disease.

POSSIBLE COMPLICATIONS
Severe episodes of pancreatitis can cause death.

MISCELLANEOUS
ASSOCIATED CONDITIONS N/A
AGE–RELATED FACTORS N/A
ZOONOTIC POTENTIAL N/A
PREGNANCY N/A
SYNONYMS N/A
SEE ALSO
Pancreatitis
ABBREVIATIONS
ALP = alkaline phosphatase
ALT = alanine aminotransferase
BUN = blood urea nitrogen
NPO = nothing per os
PU/PD = polyuria/polydipsia

References
Strombeck DR, Guilford WG. The pancreas. In: Strombeck DR, Guilford WG eds. Small animal gastroenterology. 1st Ed. Davis, CA: Stonegate Publishing, 1990.
Polzin DJ, Osborne CA, Stevens JB, et al. Serum amylase and lipase activities in dogs with chronic primary renal failure. Am J Vet Res 1983; 44:404–410.
Murtaugh RJ. Acute pancreatitis: diagnostic dilemmmas. Sem Vet Med Surg Small Anim 1987; 2:282–295.
Author Albert E. Jergens
Consulting Editor Albert E. Jergens

ANEMIA, NONREGENERATIVE

 BASICS

DEFINITION
A decrease in the RBC mass without concurrent evidence of a regenerative response (increased polychromasia or reticulocytosis) in the peripheral blood

Pathophysiology
• The key feature is low or inadequate erythroid production or release. Unless RBC survival is concurrently shortened (eg, hemorrhage and hemolysis), the onset of anemia and its related signs is insidious. • The anemia may be caused by a selective alteration in erythropoiesis (suggested by nonregenerative anemia with normal or normally-responding peripheral blood leukocytes or platelets) or generalized bone marrow injury (suggested by nonregenerative anemia with peripheral blood decreases or abnormal responses by leukocytes or platelets). • Mechanisms for selectively altered erythropoiesis in patients with nonregenerative anemia include deficient hormonal stimulation, deficient or defective nutriture, and disturbed metabolism in or destruction of precursors. Generalized bone marrow injury usually is caused by a toxin, infection, or infiltrative process.These distinctions are not absolute. For instance, a cat with FeLV infection can have nonregenerative anemia alone, pancytopenia, or leukemia/erythroleukemia.

Systems Affected
• Cardiovascular—heart murmur associated with low blood viscosity • Hepatobiliary—centrilobular degeneration associated with hypoxic injury

SIGNALMENT
Varies with the primary cause

SIGNS

General Comments
Usually a secondary condition. Signs associated with the primary disease often precede signs directly attributable to the anemia.

Historical Findings
• Lack of energy, exercise intolerance, inappetance, and cold intolerance resulting from anemia • Other findings reflect the primary condition such as polyuria and polydipsia (e.g., chronic renal failure), exposure to paint from remodeling old houses (e.g., lead poisoning), living in multicat households (e.g., FeLV), and treating female dogs for mismating or feminization in male dogs (e.g., hyperestrogenism).

Physical Examination Findings
• Pallor, heart murmur (in patients with relatively severe anemia) and, possibly, tachycardia or polypnea resulting from anemia • Other signs reflect the primary condition such as uremic breath and oral ulcerations (e.g., chronic renal failure), cachexia (e.g.,

cancer), lymphadenopathy (e.g., lymphosarcoma), gastrointestinal or CNS signs (e.g., lead poisoning), symmetrical alopecia (e.g., endocrinopathy).

CAUSES

NRA without Other Cytopenias
• Deficient hormonal stimulation—low erythropoietin associated with chronic renal failure and endocrine deficiencies (e.g., hypothyroidism, hypoadrenocorticoidism, and hypopituitarism) • Defective or deficient nutriture—anemia of chronic inflammation (iron sequestration in macrophages), iron deficiency (late and early stages are regenerative), and copper deficiency • Disturbed metabolism of precursors—lead toxicity and, possibly, aluminum and cadmium toxicity • Destruction of precursors—immune-mediated and infectious (although usually > 1 cell line is involved; e.g., FeLV, FIV, and ehrlichiosis)

NRA with Other Cytopenias
• Toxicities—drugs or chemicals (e.g., cancer chemotherapeutics, chloramphenical, phenylbutazone, trimethoprim-sulfadiazine, and benzene), hormones (e.g., estrogen toxicity secondary to abortifacient therapy and sertoli cell tumor) • Infections—FeLV, FIV, ehrlichiosis, and parvoviral infection (although recovery usually precedes development of anemia) • Infiltrative processes—myelodysplasia, myeloproliferative disease, lymphoproliferative disease, metastatic neoplasia, myelofibrosis, and osteosclerosis

RISK FACTORS
Renal failure, inflammatory disease, chronic disease process, cancer, chronic blood loss, cats from multicat households (FeLV), and lead exposure

 DIAGNOSIS

DIFFERENTIAL DIAGNOSIS
Sudden onset of signs is more consistent with regenerative than nonregenerative anemia. However, the latter can appear to have an acute onset if associated with a sudden exacerbation of a chronic primary condition.

LABORATORY FINDINGS

Drugs That May Alter Lab Results N/A

Disorders That May Alter Lab Results
Factors causing turbidity (lipemia) can falsely elevate hemoglobin and MCHC values.

Valid If Run in Human Lab?
Valid. However, electronic counters used for human RBC may underestimate counts of smaller RBC present in most domestic animals other than the dog. This falsely reduces the PCV (calculated from the RBC count and MCV). A centrifuged, manual PCV is preferred.

CBC/BIOCHEMISTRY/URINALYSIS

CBC and Blood Smear

• An inflammatory leukogram or evidence of a chronic disease process associated with mild to moderate nonregenerative anemia supports anemia associated with inflammatory disease. • A high number of nucleated RBC without polychromasia or disproportionate to the degree of anemia and polychromasia is seen in patients with lead toxicity. (Bone marrow stromal injury by endotoxemia or hypoxia and extramedullary hematopoiesis are other sources of metarubricytosis.) • Presence of RBC or WBC precursors in the peripheral blood, without orderly progression to more mature forms, suggests myelodysplasia or myeloproliferative disease (leukemia). • Macrocytosis (high MCV) without polychromasia suggests a nuclear maturation defect (cells skip a division). It is seen in cats with FeLV. Macrocytosis caused by vitamin B_{12} or folate deficiency is uncommon in domestic animals. • Microcytosis (low MCV) suggests a cytoplasmic maturation defect (cells undergo an extra division). Iron deficiency is the most common cause. In late stages, concurrent hypochromasia (low MCHC) is common in dogs, but not in cats. Microcytosis is also seen (~ 1/3 of patients) with hepatic insufficiency or vascular shunting. • Concurrent cytopenia in other cell lines without evidence of marrow responsiveness (e.g., band neutrophils and macroplatelets) suggests generalized bone marrow injury.

Serum Biochemistry and Urinalysis
• High BUN and creatinine with inadequate urine concentration (dogs, < 1.030; cats, < 1.035) supports anemia associated with renal failure. • High serum cholesterol (> 500 mg/dl) strongly suggests hypothyroidism. • Hyponatremia with concurrent hyperkalemia and a lack of stress responses (e.g., lymphopenia and eosinopenia) in ill dogs is seen in those with hypoadrenocorticoidism.

OTHER LABORATORY TESTS
• Reticulocyte count—value of < 60,000/μl accompanied by a low PCV is confirmatory. Because it takes the bone marrow 3-5 days to increase erythropoiesis in response to an acute demand, patients in the early stage of acute hemorrhage or hemolysis may appear to have nonregenerative anemia. • Direct antiglobulin test (Coomb's)—in some patients, immune-mediated destruction of erythroid precursors can lead to anemia without reticulocytosis. Spherocytes in the peripheral blood or autoagglutination may provide a clue to consider immune-mediated hemolytic anemia. A positive Coomb's test with species-specific reagents provides support for immune-mediated anemia. • Serum iron profile—indicated for evaluation of microcytic anemia. In dogs, evaluation of iron stores in a bone marrow aspirate should precede iron assay. In patients with iron deficiency, serum iron is low, TIBC varies, and serum ferritin is low. In patients with anemia associated with inflammatory disease, serum iron is low but

serum ferritin is high (MCV and MCHC are usually normal). • Serum lead—indicated when metarubricytosis develops, especially when the patient has concurrent gastrointestinal or CNS signs. A value > 0.30 µg/dl (30 ppm) strongly supports lead intoxication. • Serologic testing—for FeLV and FIV test in any cat with nonregenerative anemia. Ehrlichia canis titer is indicated in dogs with unexplained anemia, especially when concurrent with other cytopenias or hyperglobulinemia. E. canis titer ≥ 1:20 is diagnostic. • Endocrine testing—indicated when clinical signs and laboratory tests suggest a possible endocrine disorder; thyroid, T3, T4, TSH stimulation test, and TSH concentration; adrenal, dexamethasone suppression test and ACTH stimulation test

IMAGING N/A

OTHER DIAGNOSTIC PROCEDURES

Cytologic Examination of Bone Marrow and Core Biopsy

• Cytologic examination of an aspirate is indicated in any patient with nonregenerative anemia, unless the primary cause is readily apparent (e.g., anemia of inflammatory disease and chronic renal failure). Erythroid hypoplasia or aplasia confirms nonregenerative anemia. • Myeloid hyperplasia and high iron stores support anemia associated with inflammatory disease. • Absence of bone marrow iron stores, which occurs before microcytosis, supports iron deficiency. Classically, iron deficiency is associated with an expanded erythron and high numbers of metarubricytes. • Increased erythrophagocytosis suggests injury to cells (e.g., immune-mediated and toxic disease), preventing release into the circulation. • An incomplete maturation sequence suggests injury to a specific maturation stage (e.g., immune-mediated and toxic causes) or, possibly, incomplete recovery from a previous injury (recheck in 3-5 days). • High numbers of blast cells, abnormal cell morphology, and a disorderly maturation sequence indicate hematopoietic neoplasia. Morphologic examination of cells and cytochemical stains are used to identify the affected cell line(s).

Circulating neoplastic cells may or may not be seen. The presence of nonmarrow cells (e.g., epithelial cells) indicates metastatic neoplasia. • If specimens are hypocellular, core biopsy should be done to evaluate marrow cellularity and to look for conditions such as myelofibrosis.

TREATMENT

• Nonregenerative anemia usually resolves with successful treatment of the underlying disease. Conditions associated with severe nonregenerative anemia or pancytopenia often carry a guarded to poor prognosis and may involve long-term treatment without complete resolution.
• Metabolic compensation occurs with slowly developing nonregenerative anemia. Thus, mild to moderately severe nonregenerative anemia (PCV ≥ 15%) generally requires no supportive intervention. However, in patients with severe anemia (PCV < 10-15%), the degree of hypoxia will probably require restricted exercise or transfusion therapy, or both.

MEDICATIONS

DRUGS AND FLUIDS

• Blood transfusion with cross-matched, packed RBC (if available) resuspended in normal saline, if signs warrant • If blood volume and tissue perfusion are compromised by concurrent blood loss or shock, lactated Ringer's solution

CONTRAINDICATIONS N/A

PRECAUTIONS N/A

POSSIBLE INTERACTIONS N/A

ALTERNATE DRUGS N/A

FOLLOW-UP

PATIENT MONITORING

• In patients with severe anemia, the PCV and blood smear examination every 1-2 days
• In stabilized animals with chronic or slowly improving disease course, reevaluation every 1-2 weeks

POSSIBLE COMPLICATIONS N/A

MISCELLANEOUS

ASSOCIATED CONDITIONS N/A

AGE RELATED FACTORS N/A

ZOONOTIC POTENTIAL N/A

PREGNANCY

A mildly low PCV caused by dilution of RBC mass by a high blood volume may be seen in some pregnant animals. This is common in humans.

SYNONYMS

Nonresponsive anemia

SEE ALSO

See Causes

ABBREVIATIONS

CNS = central nervous system
FeLV = feline leukemia virus
FIV = feline immunodeficiency virus
IMHA = immune-mediated hemolytic anemia
MCHC = mean cell hemoglobin concentration
MCV = mean cell volume
TIBC = total iron binding capacity

References

Rogers K. Anemia. In: Ettinger SJ, Feldman EC, eds. Textbook of veterinary internal medicine: diseases of the dog and cat, vol. 1. 4th ed. Philadelphia: WB Saunders, 1995:187.
Kristensen AT, Feldman BF. Blood banking and transfusion medicine. In: Ettinger SJ, Feldman EC, eds. Textbook of veterinary internal medicine: diseases of the dog and cat, vol. 1. 4th ed. Philadelphia: WB Saunders, 1995:347.
Author John A. Christian
Consulting Editor Alan H. Rebar

ANEMIA, REGENERATIVE

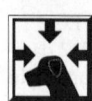

BASICS

DEFINITION

Syndrome characterized by a low circulating RBC mass (as indicated by reductions in PCV, hemoglobin, and total RBC count) accompanied by appropriate, compensatory increase in RBC production by the bone marrow. Evidence of increased RBC production includes polychromasia, reticulocytosis in the peripheral blood, and RBC hyperplasia in the bone marrow. A regenerative response may not be evident until several days after the onset of anemia.

Pathophysiology

Regenerative anemia is caused by two basic mechanisms: blood loss and hemolysis. In patients with blood loss anemia, circulating RBC lifespan is normal and RBC are lost from the body as a result of vascular injury. In contrast, in patients with hemolytic anemia, vessels are intact but there is increased intravascular or extravascular destruction of RBC with shortened circulating RBC lifespan. Hemolytic anemias usually are more regenerative than blood loss anemias. In patients with blood loss anemia, both cells and iron are lost from the body, whereas in those with hemolytic anemia, iron is generally conserved and readily available for reutilization in RBC production. It is this availability of iron that makes hemolytic anemia generally more responsive.

Systems Affected

• Hemic/lymph/immune—marked RBC hyperplasia in the bone marrow. Even in adults, bone marrow of the long bones may be red throughout. Splenomegaly also can be a feature of extravascular hemolytic anemia.
• Cardiovascular—murmurs with significant anemia. Tachycardia with severe, rapid-onset anemia • Hepatic—significant regenerative anemia of rapid onset causes centrilobular degeneration of the liver as a result of anoxia. Hemolytic anemia may cause icterus. Hemolytic icterus is generally prehepatic, but hepatic injury secondary to anoxia may also contribute.

SIGNALMENT

• No breed, age, or sex predilections for the broad category of regenerative anemia • Cats are more likely to develop Heinz body hemolytic anemia than dogs. • Some breeds of dogs have a genetic predisposition to certain heritable coagulopathies such as factor VIII deficiency and von Willebrand syndrome.
• Some authors propose that middle-aged female dogs have a predisposition to immune-mediated syndromes such as immune-mediated hemolytic anemia and lupus erythematosus.
• See specific diseases for details.

DIAGNOSIS

DIFFERENTIAL DIAGNOSIS

Differentiated from nonregenerative anemia by high reticulocyte count

LABORATORY FINDINGS

Drugs That May Alter Lab Results N/A

Disorders That May Alter Lab Results

Lipemia in the sample can cause in vitro hemolysis, resulting in a falsely low PCV and total RBC count and falsely high MCHC.

Valid If Run in Human Lab?

Valid

CBC/BIOCHEMISTRY/URINALYSIS

• PCV, RBC count, and hemoglobin are low.
• Mean corpuscular volume (MCV) is normal to high and mean corpuscular hemoglobin concentration (MCHC) is normal to low in most patients. In patients with intravascular hemolytic anemia with hemoglobinemia, MCHC actually may be high. • Total protein is normal in patients with hemolytic anemia, and may be low in those with blood loss anemia. • Anisocytosis with increased polychromasia • In patients with hemolytic anemia, specific morphologic RBC changes suggest etiologic diagnoses. For example, significant spherocytosis suggests immune-mediated disease, Heinz bodies suggest oxidant injury, and numerous schizocytes suggest microangiopathy.

OTHER LABORATORY TESTS

• Absolute reticulocyte count > 60,000/ul in conjunction with low PCV suggests regenerative anemia. If reticulocyte count is low in a patient with suspected regenerative anemia, it may mean that the anemia is in the early stages of response. Cytologic examination of one marrow may be indicated. • Ctyologic examination of bone marrow reveals RBC hyperplasia. This test is only needed when there is no evidence of RBC responsiveness in the peripheral blood (i.e., no polychromasia and no reticulocytosis) and regenerative anemia is still suspected. Absence of RBC hyperplasia means that the anemia is nonregenerative.
• Direct antiglobulin test (e.g., DAT and Coomb's test) is indicated when immune-mediated hemolytic anemia is suspected. A positive test with species-specific reagents and evidence of spherocytosis and polychromasia in the peripheral blood is confirmatory. Both false-negatives and false-positives are possible, so the test must be used judiciously and interpreted cautiously.

IMAGING N/A

OTHER DIAGNOSTIC PROCEDURES

Bone marrow biopsy

TREATMENT

Emergency situation if anemia is severe and develops rapidly. With massive hemorrhage, the main problems are hypovolemic shock and anoxia. With sudden onset hemolysis, the main problems are anoxia and systemic toxemia. In both instances, cage rest and careful observation may be indicated depending on severity of clinical signs. Fluid therapy may be warranted, particularly in blood loss patients (see below).

MEDICATIONS

DRUGS AND FLUIDS

Blood Loss Anemias

• Fluid therapy to correct hypovolemia may be indicated in the early stages of traumatic blood loss anemia (24-72 hours after onset).
• If signs of hypoxia are severe (i.e., extremely pale mucous membranes, labored breathing, and patient standing with neck extended and elbows turned out), RBC replacement either by cross-matched transfusion or packed RBC may be indicated, but this will slow down the natural regenerative response.
• Administration of iron also may be of benefit—oral administration acceptable in patients with no gastrointestinal problems; injectable administration preferred in patients with gastrointestinal problems.

Hemolytic Anemias

• Blood transfusion or packed RBC may be indicated. Use caution in patients with an immune-mediated process in which the addition of RBC may actually accelerate RBC destruction. Addition of RBC also delays the natural regenerative response.
• Administration of iron is of no value in patients with hemolytic anemia.
• Control the cause of the hemolysis. See the individual hemolytic disease for specific treatment.

FOLLOW-UP

PATIENT MONITORING

• Measurements of RBC mass (i.e., PCV, RBC count, or hemoglobin) and morphologic evaluation of peripheral blood film to monitor effectiveness of treatment and bone marrow responsiveness • Initially, patients should be checked every 24 hours. As regeneration becomes apparent as indicated by rising RBC values and polychromasia, patients should be checked every 3-5 days. Return to normal values should occur about 14 days after the initial insult.

POSSIBLE COMPLICATIONS

None

✓ **MISCELLANEOUS**

ASSOCIATED CONDITIONS None

AGE RELATED FACTORS None

ZOONOTIC POTENTIAL None

PREGNANCY N/A

SYNONYMS

Responsive anemias

SEE ALSO

See individual causes.

ABBREVIATIONS

FeLV = feline leukemia virus

FIP = feline infectious peritonitis

FIV = feline immunodeficiency virus

MCHC = mean corpuscular hemoglobin concentration

MCV = mean corpuscular volume

PCV = packed cell value

RBC = red blood cells

Reference

Weiser MG. Erythrocyte responses and disorders. In: Ettinger SJ, Feldman EC, eds. Textbook of veterinary internal medicine. Philadelphia: WB Saunders, 1995:1876-1886.

Author Alan H. Rebar

Consulting Editor Alan H. Rebar

BILE ACIDS

BASICS

DEFINITION
• Fasting serum bile acid concentration > 5 uM/L • Postprandial serum bile acid concentration >15 uM/L

Pathophysiology
• Bile acids are synthesized in the liver by cholesterol metabolism and secreted into bile. Feeding is a normal stimulus for bile acid secretion. Bile acids enter the intestines and undergo an efficient enterohepatic circulation after active absorption from the ileum. Once absorbed, bile acids are removed from the portal circulation by the liver and reexcreted into bile. Only small amounts of bile acids are lost in the feces. • Abnormal hepatic function or abnormal portal circulation can interrupt the normal enterohepatic circulation and lead to a high serum bile acid concentration. A variety of hepatobiliary disorders may be involved. • Animals with hepatic parenchymal disease have reduced extraction of bile acids from the portal circulation. • In animals with a portosystemic shunt, the enterohepatic circulation is directly interrupted and bile acids fail to be extracted by the bypassed liver. • In animals with intra- or extrahepatic cholestasis, bile acids diffuse from bile into the systemic circulation in a manner similar to that of bilirubin. • Bile acid concentration is a sensitive and specific indicator of hepatic function in dogs and cats. The magnitude of elevation does not distinguish the cause of disease because of the wide overlap among disease processes. The determination of a 2–hour postprandial concentration further increases the sensitivity of this test for some diseases, especially portosystemic shunt.

Systems Affected
• Hepatobiliary—retained bile acids are hepatotoxic and can cause hepatocyte damage and hepatic inflammation. • Gastrointestinal—bile acids can cause secretory diarrhea if abnormal concentrations reach the colon because of poor reabsorption from the ileum. High bile acid concentration can cause abnormally high gastric acidity and contribute to gastrointestinal ulceration.

SIGNALMENT
• Some breeds have a high prevalence of congenital portosystemic shunt (resulting in high serum bile acid concentration), including the Yorkshire terrier, miniature schnauzer, miniature poodle, dachshund, golden retriever, Labrador retriever, and Irish setter. • Breeds predisposed to abnormal hepatic copper storage (Bedlington terrier, West Highland white terrier, Skye terrier, and doberman pinscher) frequently have high bile acid concentration in association with hepatic failure.

SIGNS
• Diarrhea is a potential direct effect of high bile acid concentration. • Bile acid concentration reflects hepatic function. Signs associated with hepatic dysfunction include icterus, PU/PD, lethargy, anorexia, altered mentation, vomiting, and ascites.

CAUSES
• Measurement of serum bile acid concentration should be performed in patients suspected of having hepatobiliary dysfunction. Indications include to detect occult hepatic disease when enzyme determinations are normal (as can occur in animals with portosystemic shunt, cirrhosis, and metastatic hepatic neoplasia), to evaluate the possibility of a portosystemic shunt, to monitor hepatobiliary function and assess progression of hepatic disease, and to identify abnormal hepatic function in animals whose high hepatic enzyme may be due to extrahepatic causes.
• The most common diseases associated with high serum bile acid concentration are congenital or acquired portosystemic shunt, chronic active hepatitis, cholestasis, hepatic necrosis, steroid hepatopathy, infectious hepatitis, primary and metastatic hepatic neoplasia, cirrhosis, toxic hepatopathy, feline cholangiohepatitis, feline hepatic lipidosis, and hepatic infection with FIP virus. • Hepatotoxic drugs can cause high serum bile acid concentration, including acetaminophen, anabolic steroids, anticonvulsant drugs (e.g., phenobarbitol, primadone, and phenytoin), antineoplastic drugs (e.g., methotrexate, L-asparaginase, 6-mercaptopurine, and azathioprine), arsenicals (e.g., thiacetarsamide), diethylcarbamazine, furosemide, glipazide, glucocorticoids, griseofulvin, inhalation anesthetics (e.g., halothane and methoxyflurane), itraconazole, ketoconazole, mebendazole, methimazole, mitotane (i.e., o,p–DDD), sulfonamides, tetracycline, and trimethoprim-sulfadiazine.

RISK FACTORS
• Diseases that affect the liver and cause abnormal hepatic function cause high serum bile acid concentration. • Pancreatitis can cause bile duct obstruction and subsequent high serum bile acid concentration.

DIAGNOSIS

DIFFERENTIAL DIAGNOSIS
• Primary hepatobiliary disease as a cause of high bile acid concentration may be suggested by physical examination findings (e.g., icterus, hepatomegaly, and ascites) or results of laboratory tests (e.g., high ALT, AST, and total bilirubin; low serum albumin, BUN, and glucose concentrations). • Results of hepatic imaging and hepatic biopsy usually reveal the nature of the hepatobiliary disease. • Portosystemic shunt should be strongly considered in young dogs with signs of hepatic disease. • Portosystemic shunt unlikely In

patients with jaundice; consider cholestatic disease • Determine whether hepatotoxic drugs or chemicals have been administered • The presence of ascites with hepatobiliary disease suggests portal hypertension (e.g., cirrhosis, chronic inflammation, and other infiltrative process).

LABORATORY FINDINGS

Drugs That May Alter Lab Results N/A

Disorders That May Alter Lab Results
• Inadequate meal consumption lessens the utility of the 2–hour postprandial sample. • Delayed gastric emptying may cause failure to stimulate gall bladder contraction and lessen the utility of the 2–hour postprandial sample. • Abnormal intestinal transit or malabsorption reduces the amount of reabsorbed bile acids and lessens the utility of the 2–hour postprandial sample. • Ileal disease causes poor bile acid reabsorption and lessens the utility of the test. • Inadequate dietary fat and protein causes inadequate gall bladder contraction and lessens the utility of the 2–hour postprandial sample. • Serum bile acid concentration is normal when high serum total bilirubin concentration is caused solely by hemolytic disease.

Valid If Run in Human Lab? Yes

CBC/BIOCHEMISTRY/URINALYSIS
• Results of a serum biochemical analysis are rarely specific but help to verify the presence of hepatobiliary disease. High serum concentration of bilirubin and high activities of ALT and AST are commonly seen in animals with various hepatobiliary diseases. Additional biochemical changes seen in animals with chronic hepatobiliary disease include low serum concentrations of urea nitrogen, glucose, and albumin. • When hepatic enzyme activities and total bilirubin are normal and bile acid concentration is high, portosystemic shunt, cirrhosis, or metastatic neoplasia should be suspected. • Animals with steroid hepatopathy have markedly high ALP activity, normal total bilirubin concentration, and normal to moderately high serum bile acid concentration. • Animals with cholestatic disease usually have markedly high serum hepatic enzyme activities (especially ALP) and high serum total bilirubin concentration along with markedly high serum bile acid concentration. • Animals with congenital portosystemic shunt may have normal serum biochemical profile, with high bile acid concentration the only indicator of hepatic failure. • When serum bilirubin concentration is high because of hepatobiliary disease, bile acid concentration is always high. In this circumstance, there is no need to measure the serum bile acid concentration. The main value of the measuring serum bile acids is to evaluate hepatic function in animals that may have anicteric hepatic disease.

OTHER LABORATORY TESTS
Plasma ammonia concentration usually paral-

lels serum bile acid concentration.

IMAGING

Abdominal Radiography
• Abdominal radiographs often nonspecific but may help to substantiate hepatobiliary disease • Diseases that cause radiographic signs of small hepatic size include cirrhosis, portosystemic shunt, and acute and subacute necrosis; in deep-chested breeds of dogs, this may be normal. • Diseases that cause radiographic signs of large hepatic size include neoplasia (primary and metastatic), congestion, fatty infiltration, diffuse inflammation, hyperadrenocorticism, storage disease, hepatic abscess, and biliary cyst; this is normal in puppies and kittens and on deep inspiration.

Abdominal Ultrasonography
• Useful for evaluating the hepatic parenchyma • Abnormalities include heterogeneous mottling or nodularity suggesting infiltrative disease and changes in overall echogenicity. • Diffuse hyperechogenicity in animals with fatty change, steroid hepatopathy, fibrosis, and cirrhosis • Hypoechogenicity in animals with passive congestion, lymphoma, and suppurative hepatitis • Most reliable noninvasive modality to distinguish intrahepatic from posthepatic (i.e., bile duct obstruction) cholestasis. Findings with posthepatic cholestasis include large gall bladder with dilated gall bladder neck, large common bile duct, and large intrahepatic bile ducts shown by irregular branching patterns and variable diameter compared with blood vessels.

Nuclear Scintigraphy
• Nuclear scintigraphy after transcolonic ^{99m}technetium administration is very sensitive for detecting a portosystemic shunt.

OTHER DIAGNOSTIC PROCEDURES
• Hepatic biopsy is indicated to obtain a definitive diagnosis when laboratory findings and hepatic imaging suggest hepatic disease without evidence of portosystemic shunt or extrahepatic bile duct obstruction. • Hepatic biopsy methods include blind percutaneous and ultrasound– guided techniques, laparoscopy, and laparotomy. • Laparoscopy is indicated to evaluate biliary patency if ultrasound is nondiagnostic or unavailable and to obtain hepatic biopsy specimens if other methods are unavailable.

TREATMENT
• Treatment varies depending on the underlying cause of the high serum bile acid concentration. Surgery is usually warranted to treat extrahepatic biliary obstruction and congenital portosystemic shunt. Medical treatment is usually warranted to treat intrahepatic disease.
• General supportive measures for treating hepatic disease include elimination of the inciting cause if possible, providing optimum conditions for hepatic regeneration, preventing complications, and reversing derangements occurring with hepatic failure. The important derangements seen in some patients include dehydration and hypovolemia, hepatic encephalopathy, hypoglycemia, acid–base and electrolyte abnormalities, coagulopathy, gastric ulceration, sepsis, and endotoxemia.

MEDICATIONS

DRUGS AND FLUIDS OF CHOICE
Vary depending on the underlying disease process

CONTRAINDICATIONS
Vary depending on the underlying disease process

PRECAUTIONS
Vary depending on the underlying disease process

POSSIBLE INTERACTIONS
Vary depending on the underlying disease process

ALTERNATE DRUGS
Vary depending on the underlying disease process

FOLLOW-UP

PATIENT MONITORING
Recheck serum chemistry profile, bile acid concentration, and hepatic imaging, with frequency dictated by the underlying disease.

POSSIBLE COMPLICATIONS
Many causes of high serum bile acid concentration are life threatening.

MISCELLANEOUS

ASSOCIATED CONDITIONS N/A

AGE RELATED FACTORS
High serum bile acid concentration in puppies and kittens with congenital portosystemic shunts

ZOONOTIC POTENTIAL N/A

PREGNANCY N/A

SYNONYMS N/A

SEE ALSO N/A

ABBREVIATIONS
ALP = serum alkaline phosphatase activity
ALT = alanine aminotransferase
AST = aspartate aminotransferase
BUN = blood urea nitrogen
FIP = feline infectious peritonitis
PU/PD = polyuria/polydipsia

References
Strombeck DR, Guilford WG. Laboratory evaluation for hepatic disease. Small animal gastroenterology. 2nd ed. Davis, Calif: Stonegate Publishing Company, 1990;529–556.
Center SA. Pathophysiology and laboratory diagnosis of hepatobiliary disorders. In: Ettinger SJ, Feldman EC, eds. Textbook of veterinary internal medicine. 4th ed. Philadelphia: WB Saunders, 1995; 1261–1312.
Author Keith P. Richter
Consulting Editor Albert E. Jergens

BILIRUBIN, HIGH

 BASICS

DEFINITION
Serum total bilirubin concentration higher than reference range

Pathophysiology
Bilirubin originates from senescent erythrocytes (about 80%) processed by macrophages in the spleen, liver, and bone marrow and from nonhemoglobin sources (about 20%). Unconjugated bilirubin is transported in plasma bound to albumin. Hepatocellular uptake of bilirubin is followed by conjugation, principally with glucuronic acid. Conjugated bilirubin is transported into the biliary system and expelled into the intestines where most is converted by intestinal microflora to urobilinogen. Hyperbilirubinemia is caused by excessive bilirubin production, impaired processing of bilirubin by hepatocytes, or interference with bilirubin excretion into the intestines.

Systems Affected
• Skin/exocrine—discoloration of the skin (jaundice) occurs when serum bilirubin values exceed 2 mg/dl. • Hepatobiliary—bilirubin toxicity may contribute to hepatocellular injury and cholestasis. • Renal/urologic—hyperbilirubinemia may cause renal tubular injury through the development of bile casts. Bilirubinuria commonly precedes hyperbilirubinemia. • Nervous—kernicterus may cause degenerative lesions in the brain (rare).

SIGNALMENT
• All ages and breeds affected. • Young, unvaccinated dogs at risk for infectious disease including canine hepatitis and leptospirosis. • Middle-aged, female doberman pinschers predisposed to chronic active hepatitis • Bedlington terriers, West Highland white terriers, and cocker spaniels at risk for copper toxicosis • Miniature schnauzers at risk for recurrent pancreatitis and extra–hepatic biliary obstruction • Anorectic, obese cats prone to hepatic lipidosis

SIGNS

Historical Findings
• Lethargy • Anorexia • Icterus • Altered mentation • Weakness • Dyspnea • Vomiting • PU/PD • Recent blood transfusion

Physical Examination Findings
In addition to historical findings, the following may be observed:
• Pale mucous membranes • Ascites • Weight loss • Hepatomegaly • Abdominal pain • Melena • Peripheral lymphadenopathy

CAUSES
Hyperbilirubinemia in dogs and cats can usually be classified as prehepatic, primary hepatic, or posthepatic.

Prehepatic jaundice
Results from excessive production of bilirubin that exceeds the liver's capacity for metabolism and excretion. Hemolytic disorders are the primary causes. Hemolytic causes include:
• Consumptive coagulopathy (i.e., disseminated intravascular coagulation [DIC])
• Immune -mediated disease (e.g., drugs and systemic lupus erythematosus) • Infectious causes (e.g., feline leukemia virus, heartworms, erlichiosis, and leptospirosis)
• Oxidative injury

Hepatic jaundice
Occurs from the abnormal uptake, conjugation, or secretion of bilirubin by hepatocytes. Hepatic causes include:
• Shock • Disseminated intravascular coagulation • Infectious agents (i.e., viral, bacterial, or mycotic) • Neoplasia • Drugs (e.g., anticonvulsants, acetaminophen, androgens, and thiacetarsamide) • Cholangitis • Cirrhosis • Chronic active hepatitis • Feline hepatic lipidosis • Hepatic necrosis • Infiltrative diseases

Posthepatic jaundice
Denotes mechanical interference with the excretion of bilirubin through intra- or extra-hepatic bile ducts. Posthepatic causes include:
• Cholecystitis • Cholangitis • Biliary neoplasia • Intraluminal bile duct occlusion • Pancreatic disease • Ruptured biliary tract.

RISK FACTORS
• Young dogs for infectious disease • Breed predispositions for primary liver disease • Middle-aged, obese dogs for development of pancreatitis • Anorectic, obese cats for development of hepatic lipidosis • Use of hepatotoxic drugs or anticonvulsants • Presence of hemolytic disease

 DIAGNOSIS

DIFFERENTIAL DIAGNOSIS
The following history and physical findings will help differentiate between the different categories of jaundice.

Prehepatic Jaundice
Usually abrupt onset of mucous membrane pallor, mild jaundice, weakness, and respiratory complications such as tachypnea or dyspnea. Murmurs may be heard on thoracic auscultation in some patients.

Hepatic Jaundice
Breeds at risk for hepatic disease, moderate jaundice, nonpale mucous membranes, hepatomegaly, ascites, polyuria and polydipsia, and behavioral abnormalities.

Posthepatic Jaundice
Chronic and/or recurrent bouts of pancreatitis, moderate to severe jaundice, nonpale mucous membranes, and abdominal pain or masses

LABORATORY FINDINGS

Drugs That May Alter Lab Results N/A

Disorders That May Alter Lab Results
• Methods of bilirubin assay are based on the diazo reaction which, following the addition of reagents, assesses the quantity of direct and total bilirubin in the serum. • Most methods yield reasonable total bilirubin results, but values for direct bilirubin may vary.
• Sample management is important, since serum total bilirubin may decrease by 50%/hour in direct exposure to sunlight or artificial fluorescent lighting. • Hemolysis has variable effects on total bilirubin values measured by spectrophotometry. • Lipemia falsely increases total bilirubin values measured by endpoint assays.

Valid If Run in Human Lab? Yes

CBC/BIOCHEMISTRY/URINALYSIS

Prehepatic Jaundice
• Severe anemia (often regenerative), spherocytes, Heinz bodies, and normal total protein.
• Normal to slightly high ALT and ALP, normal albumin, normal to high BUN, and normal glucose and cholesterol. • Bilirubinuria

Hepatic Jaundice
• Mild non-regenerative anemia and low total protein. • Moderate to severely high ALT and ALP, normal to low albumin and BUN, and normal to low glucose and cholesterol • Dilute urine, normal to low urobilinogen normal to low, and high bilirubinuria

Posthepatic Jaundice
• Mild nonregenerative anemia and normal total protein • Mildly high ALT and moderate to severely high ALP; albumin, BUN, glucose, and cholesterol often normal • Normal to low urobilinogen and bilirubinuria

OTHER LABORATORY TESTS
• Perform saline agglutination, direct Coomb's test, osmotic fragility test, examination of blood smears for hemoparasites, and antinuclear antibody test if you suspect a prehepatic cause for jaundice. • Measuring serum bile acids is typically not indicated once prehepatic causes for jaundice are eliminated. • Serology for infectious diseases (e.g., FeLV, leptospirosis, and mycoses) may be indicated in patient with hepatic jaundice.

IMAGING

Radiography
• Abdominal radiographs might reveal hepatomegaly, abdominal effusion, or the presence of mineral densities within the gall bladder or hepatic parenchyma in association with hepatic jaundice. Metallic foreign bodies (e.g., zinc and copper) which can cause hemolysis may be seen. • Thoracic radiography should be performed to screen for metastatic disease in animals suspected of having hepatic neoplasia.

Ultrasonography
• Abdominal ultrasound is indicated in the icteric patient in which differentiation of extrahepatic obstruction from intrahepatic disease is imperative. • Ultrasound is also useful to identify hepatic parenchymal lesions, determine the origin of abdominal effusion, and obtain hepatic biopsy specimens via ultrasound guidance.

OTHER DIAGNOSTIC PROCEDURES
• Liver biopsy and bacterial culture to confirm the cause(s) of hepatic jaundice. Tissue specimens may be obtained by laparotomy or by using blind percutaneous, laparoscopic, or ultrasound–guided biopsy techniques.
• Laparotomy and surgical intervention is required to correct most causes of posthepatic jaundice.

TREATMENT
• Varies depending on underlying cause of hyperbilirubinemia.
• Patients should be hospitalized for initial medical management. Cage rest facilitates liver regeneration.
• Restricted activity is required in most patients.
• Dietary management is a cornerstone of treatment in patients with hepatic and posthepatic jaundice; diets should be nutritionally balanced, carbohydrate–based (dogs), and restricted in protein and sodium.
• Animals with hyperbilirubinemia should be given a guarded prognosis.
• Hepatic biopsy is indicated in patients with hepatic jaundice.

MEDICATIONS

DRUGS AND FLUIDS

Prehepatic Jaundice
• Eliminate inciting cause if possible.
• Treatment of immunohemolytic anemia includes steroid suppression of erythrophagocytosis. Use prednisone or prednisolone (1–2 mg/kg PO q12h).
• Whole blood transfusion if patient has life–threatening anemia.
• Use Normosol–R or Plasma–Lyte if patient has mild dehydration but normal electrolytes. Maintenance flow rates (60 ml/kg/24h) are usually adequate.

Hepatic/Posthepatic Jaundice
• Treat specific causes of hepatic jaundice as determined by results of liver biopsy.
• Manage clinical signs of hepatic en-

cephalopathy with lactulose (cats, 1–5 ml PO q12h; dogs, 2–10 ml PO q12h) and metronidazole (10 mg/kg q12h); lactulose inhibits function of urease-producing bacteria, speeds intestinal transport, and alters gut pH to decrease absorption of ammonia; metronidazole kills urease–producing bacteria in the gut.
• Treat ascites with lasix (2 mg/kg PO q12h–q24h). Spironolactone (1–2 mg/kg PO q12h) can also be used.
• Miscellaneous treatment may include use of antiemetics (e.g., metoclopramide or low-dose phenothiazines) for intractable vomiting and histamine receptor antagonists (e.g., cimetidine 10 mg/kg PO q6h–q8h) to reduce gastrointestinal ulceration.
• Lactated Ringer's solution is the rehydration fluid of choice in patients with acute liver disease.
• Use 0.45% saline in animals with chronic liver disorders. Potassium supplementation is important in these animals and is best guided by measurement of serum potassium concentration.

CONTRAINDICATIONS
• Avoid the use of known hepatotoxic drugs such as anticonvulsants, acetaminophen, androgens, thiacetarsamide in animals with hepatic and/or posthepatic causes for jaundice.
• Avoid tetracyclines which suppress hepatic protein synthesis. Also avoid chloramphenicol, lincomycin, erythromycin, and clindamycin since they are hepatotoxic.
• Avoid analgesics, anesthetics, and barbiturates in patients with hepatic failure.

PRECAUTIONS
• Fortunately, most commonly used drugs are well tolerated in patients with liver disease and hyperbilirubinemia.
• Use antibiotics cautiously for specific hepatic therapy only. Avoid the antibiotics listed under contraindications.
• Sedatives should be avoided since their use may precipitate hepatic coma. Seizures are best controlled with diazepam at reduced dosages.
• Use corticosteroids cautiously since they may increase the chance of intercurrent infections and may aggravate ascites by promoting sodium retention.

POSSIBLE INTERACTIONS
• Use all drugs cautiously since the liver is the most important organ involved with drug metabolism. For many drugs requiring hepatic biotransformation, their duration and intensity of action may be increased with hepatobiliary disease.

ALTERNATE DRUGS N/A

FOLLOW-UP

PATIENT MONITORING

Prehepatic Jaundice
• Recheck PCV as needed. • Repeat transfusions may be required. • Gradually taper patient off immunosuppressive drugs.

Hepatic/Posthepatic Jaundice
• Recheck liver enzymes and bilirubin with frequency dictated by underlying disease.
• Continue symptomatic and specific treatment for hepatic disease.

POSSIBLE COMPLICATIONS
• Diseases causing hyperbilirubinemia may cause death.

MISCELLANEOUS

ASSOCIATED CONDITIONS
• Regenerative anemia in some patients
• High ALT, ALP, and GGT in many patients

AGE RELATED FACTORS N/A

ZOONOTIC POTENTIAL
• Leptospirosis may cause disease in humans.

PREGNANCY N/A

SYNONYMS
• Icterus • Jaundice

SEE ALSO
• See causes for topics on liver diseases.
• Anemia, Immune-Mediated • Pancreatitis

ABBREVIATIONS
ALP = alkaline phosphatase
ALT = alanine aminotransferase
BUN = blood urea nitrogen
DIC = disseminated intravascular coagulation
FeLV = feline leukemia virus
GGT = gamma–glutamyl transferase
PCV = packed cell volume

References

Strombeck DR, Guilford WG. Liver: normal function and pathophysiology. In: Strombeck DR, Guilford WG, eds. Small animal gastroenterology. Davis, CA: Stonegate Publishing, 1990.

Duncan JR, Prasse KW, Mahaffey EA. Liver. In: Duncan RJ, Prasse KW, and Mahaffey EA, eds. Veterinary laboratory medicine. 3rd ed. Ames, IA: Iowa State University Press, 1994.

Author Albert E. Jergens
Consulting Editor Albert E. Jergens

CALCIUM, HYPERCALCEMIA

BASICS

DEFINITION
• Serum total calcium > 11.5 mg/dl (dogs)
• Serum total calcium > 10.5 mg/dl (cats)

Pathophysiology
Control of calcium is complex and is influenced by the actions of PTH and vitamin D, and by the interaction of these hormones with the gut, bone, kidneys, and parathyroid glands. Derangement in the function of these can lead to hypercalcemia. Calcium homeostasis can also be disturbed by secretory products of neoplastic cells.

Systems Affected
• Renal/Urologic—high levels of calcium are toxic to the renal tubules and can cause polyuria and polydipsia (PU/PD) and renal failure. Hypercalcemia can also lead to urolithiasis and associated lower urinary tract disease. • Gastrointestinal—hypercalcemia reduces excitability of smooth muscle and can alter gastrointestinal function. • Neuromuscular—depressed skeletal muscle contractility causes weakness • Cardiovascular—hypertension and altered cardiac contractility

SIGNALMENT
Primary hyperparathyroidism in the keeshond

SIGNS

General Comments
Signs depend on the cause of hypercalcemia. Animals with neoplasia, renal failure, or hypoadrenocorticism as underlying causes generally appear ill. In animals with primary hyperparathyroidism, clinical signs are usually mild and due solely to the effects of hypercalcemia. Signs become apparent when hypercalcemia is severe and chronic.

Historical Findings
• PU/PD (most common in dogs) • Anorexia • Lethargy (most common in cats) • Vomiting • Constipation • Weakness • Stupor and coma (severe cases)

Physical Examination Findings
• Lymphadenopathy or abdominal organomegaly in patients with lymphosarcoma • In dogs with primary hyperparathyroidism, results are usually unremarkable. • Parathyroid gland adenoma not palpable in dogs but sometimes palpable in cats with primary hyperparathyroidism

CAUSES
• Neoplasia—lymphosarcoma (most common), anal sac apocrine gland adenocarcinoma, multiple myeloma, lymphocytic leukemia, and metastatic bone tumor • Primary hyperparathyroidism • Renal failure (acute and chronic) • Blastomycosis • Hypoadrenocorticism • Vitamin D rodenticide intoxication

RISK FACTORS
• Keeshond breed (hyperparathyroidism)
• Renal failure • Neoplasia • Use of calcium supplements or intestinal phosphate binders

DIAGNOSIS

DIFFERENTIAL DIAGNOSIS
• History should include exposure to rat poison and any previous response to steroids. • History of waxing/waning illness suggests hypoadrenocorticism. • Complete lymph node, rectal, and abdominal palpation may raise index of suspicion for lymphosarcoma or other neoplasia. • Assessment of hydration status, renal palpation, and urinary history points toward lower urinary tract disease or renal failure.

LABORATORY FINDINGS

Drugs That May Alter Lab Results
• Oxalate, citrate, and EDTA anticoagulants bind calcium and falsely lower calcium measurement. • Vitamin D preparations and thiazide diuretics can raise serum calcium concentration.

Disorders That May Alter Lab Results
• Hemolysis and lipemia can falsely raise calcium concentration. • Hypoalbuminemia can falsely lower total calcium concentration.

Valid If Run In Human Lab? Yes

CBC/BIOCHEMISTRY/URINALYSIS
• Serum calcium—total calcium concentration depends on binding proteins. Adjusted (corrected) calcium can be estimated by the following formulas:

$$\text{Corrected Ca} = \text{Ca (mg/dl)} - \text{albumin (g/dl)} + 3.5$$
or
$$\text{Corrected Ca} = \text{Ca (mg/dl)} - [0.4 \times \text{total protein (g/dl)}] + 3.3$$

• Azotemia and isosthenuria help define degree of renal impairment. • Serum phosphorus is usually low or low-normal in patients with primary hyperparathyroidism or hypercalcemia associated with malignancy. • Hyperphosphatemia in absence of azotemia suggests a nonparathyroid cause of hypercalcemia. • Combination of hyperphosphatemia and azotemia is difficult to interpret, since renal failure can be the cause or effect of hypercalcemia. • Hyperkalemia and hyponatremia suggest hypoadrenocorticism. • Hyperglobulinemia is associated with multiple myeloma. • Cytopenias are seen in patients with myelophthisic disease.

OTHER LABORATORY TESTS
• Serum ionized calcium is high in patients with primary hyperparathyroidism or hypercalcemia associated with malignancy. It is usually normal or low in patients with hypercalcemia associated with renal failure.

• Serum PTH measurement—intact molecule and two-site assay methods have the greatest specificity. High normal or high concentrations suggests primary hyperparathyroidism; low concentration suggests neoplasia. • Serum PTH-rp measurement is often high in patients with hypercalcemia associated with malignancy. • Vitamin D assays are not readily available.

IMAGING
• Radiography useful to assess renal size and shape, urolithiasis, bone lysis, and occult neoplasia • Ultrasonography valuable to assess renal architecture, abdominal lymphadenopathy, and urolithiasis

OTHER DIAGNOSTIC PROCEDURES
• Cytologic examination of fine needle aspirate of lymph nodes to confirm lymposarcoma • Examination of bone marrow aspirate to confirm occult hematopoietic neoplasia • ACTH stimulation testing to confirm hypoadrenocorticism

TREATMENT
Because of the deleterious effects of hypercalcemia and the need for fluid therapy, inpatient care is necessary. Severe hypercalcemia should be considered a medical emergency.

MEDICATIONS

DRUGS AND FLUIDS
• Normal saline is the fluid of choice.
• Calcium-containing fluids should be avoided.
• Diuretics (furosemide) and corticosteroids can be useful in the treatment of hypercalcemia.

CONTRAINDICATIONS
• Until the diagnosis of lymphoma has been excluded, glucocorticoids should not be used since they can obfuscate the diagnosis. If hypoadrenocorticism is suspected, glucocorticoids should not be given until after ACTH stimulation testing has been performed.
• Thiazide diuretics can cause calcium retention

PRECAUTIONS N/A

POSSIBLE INTERACTIONS
Avoid use of calcium or phosphorus-containing compounds since they can cause soft tissue mineralization in severely hypercalcemic and hyperphosphatemic patients.

ALTERNATIVE DRUGS
• Sodium bicarbonate (1-4 mEq/kg) may be useful in combination with other treatments.
• Mithramycin has been used in severe hypercalcemic crises. Its use should be avoided if possible because of associated nephrotoxicity and hepatotoxicity.
• Calcitonin may be useful in treatment of hypervitaminosis D.

FOLLOW-UP

PATIENT MONITORING
• Serum calcium every 12 hours • Renal function tests (the first sign of tubular damage may be casts in the urine sediment) • Urine output and hydration

POSSIBLE COMPLICATIONS
• Irreversible renal failure • Soft tissue calcification

MISCELLANEOUS

ASSOCIATED CONDITIONS
Calcium-containing urolithiasis

AGE RELATED FACTORS
• Mild elevations in calcium and phosphorus may be normal in a growing dog. • Middle-aged to old patients are at a higher risk for cancer.

ZOONOTIC POTENTIAL None

PREGNANCY
A fetus would be at the same risk as the dam. Treatment should not be altered on the basis of pregnancy.

SYNONYMS None

SEE ALSO See Causes

ABBREVIATIONS
PTH = parathyroid hormone
PTH-rp = parathyroid hormone-related peptide

References
Chew DJ, Nagode LA, Carothers M. Disorders of calcium: hypercalcemia and hypocalcemia. In: DiBartola SP, ed. Fluid therapy in small animal practice. Philadelphia: WB Saunders, 1992;116-176.
Feldman EC. Disorders of the parathyroid glands. In: Ettinger SJ, Feldman EC. eds. Textbook of veterinary internal medicine. Philadelphia: WB Saunders, 1994;1437-1464.
Author Thomas K. Graves
Consulting Editor Rhett Nichols

CALCIUM, HYPOCALCEMIA

BASICS

DEFINITION
Low total serum calcium concentration

Pathophysiology
Of the total circulating serum calcium, 50% is protein bound, 40% is ionized, and 10% is complexed with other substances. Protein-bound calcium cannot diffuse through membranes and, thus, is unusable by the tissues. Complexed calcium is diffusable through membranes but is unavailable for use by tissues. Only the ionized form is available to tissues and, thus, only changes in this fraction of total serum calcium are responsible for clinical problems (hypo- and hypercalcemia). However, measurement of ionized calcium is too difficult for routine performance and, thus, biochemical profiles record only total serum calcium. Mechanisms involved in hypocalcemia include the following:
• Low concentrations of binding proteins (hypoalbuminemia) • Reduced intestinal absorption (deficient vitamin D [renal disease, severe intestinal disease]) • Reduced renal and bone resorption (hypoparathyroidism) • Inadequate dietary intake • Excessive loss (lactation) • Sequestration (soaponification [acute pancreatitis]) • Binding/complexing with administered or ingested chemicals (administration of phosphate-containing enemas, citrate toxicity, ethylene glycol toxicity, low calcium/high phosphorus diet [nutritional secondary hyperparathyroidism]) • Impaired synthesis or refractoriness to PTH (hypomagnesemia)

Systems Affected
• Nervous/neuromuscular—seizures, tetany, ataxia, and weakness • Cardiovascular—ECG changes and bradycardia • Gastrointestinal—anorexia and vomiting (especially cats) • Respiratory—panting

SIGNALMENT
Varies depending on the underlying cause

SIGNS
• Signs of the underlying disease may be seen without clinical signs of hypocalcemia because the latter do not occur until total serum calcium falls below 6.7 mg/dl. • Seizures • Muscle trembling or twitching or fasciculations • Ataxia or stiff gait • Weakness • Panting • Facial rubbing • Vomiting • Anorexia • Fever • Posterior lenticular cataracts in patients with primary hypoparathyroidism

CAUSES

Nonpathologic Hypocalcemia
• Laboratory error—occurs up to 13% of the time. Repeat serum calcium determination is recommended to confirm true hypocalcemia, especially if results indicate clinically important hypocalcemia despite absence of clinical

signs. • Hypoalbuminemia—most common cause of hypocalcemia, accounting for over 50% of patients. Leads to reduction of protein-bound calcium without affecting ionized calcium. Therefore, it is important to correct for hypoalbuminemia by use of one of the following formulas:

$$Corrected\ Ca = Ca\ (mg/dl) - albumin\ (g/dl) + 3.5$$
or
$$Corrected\ Ca = Ca\ (mg/dl) - [0.4 \times total\ protein\ (g/dl)] + 3.3$$

• Note: In cats, hypoalbuminemia causes the calcium concentration to fall, but these formulas were developed in dogs and cannot be applied to cats. • Alkalosis—causes a shift from protein-bound calcium to ionized calcium as well as a reduction in measured calcium. Not associated with clinical signs.

Pathologic Hypocalcemia
• Primary hypoparathyroidism • Hypoparathyroidism secondary to thyroidectomy and parathyroid damage • Renal failure (acute or chronic) • Ethylene glycol toxicity • Acute pancreatitis • Puerperal tetany (eclampsia) • Phosphate-containing enemas • Nutritional secondary hyperparathyroidism • Hypomagnesemia • Intestinal malabsorption • Citrate toxicity (multiple blood transfusions or improper citrate-blood ratio)

RISK FACTORS
Puerperal tetany (eclampsia)—usually seen in small-breed bitches during the first 21 days of nursing a litter

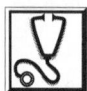

DIAGNOSIS

DIFFERENTIAL DIAGNOSIS
• Clinical signs of hypocalcemia—rule out primary hypoparathyroidism, hypoparathyroidism secondary to thyroidectomy and parathyroid damage, and puerperal tetany (eclampsia) • Polyuria and polydipsia—rule out renal failure • Neurologic signs—rule out ethylene glycol toxicity • Vomiting and diarrhea—rule out acute pancreatitis, intestinal malabsorption, renal failure, and ethylene glycol toxicity • Bone pain or fractures—rule out nutritional secondary hyperparathyroidism

LABORATORY FINDINGS

Drugs That May Alter Lab Results
Sodium bicarbonate may cause alkalosis and lower the serum calcium. Samples collected in EDTA tubes may have a falsely low serum calcium concentration because of calcium chelation.

Disorders That May Alter Lab Results
Lipemia can significantly raise the serum calcium. Any cause of hypoalbumenia can falsely lower the serum calcium (see causes of nonpathogenic hypocalcemia).

Valid If Run in Human Lab?
Valid

CBC/BIOCHEMISTRY/URINALYSIS
• Results usually normal • Mild to moderate anemia possible in patients with chronic renal failure, nutritional secondary hyperparathyroidism, and intestinal malabsorption • Leukocytosis possible in patients with acute pancreatitis • Low calcium • Hypoalbuminemia in patients with hypoproteinemia-induced hypocalcemia and intestinal malabsorption • High total CO_2 in patients with alkalosis-induced hypocalcemia • High BUN and creatinine in patients with acute and chronic renal failure and ethylene glycol toxicity • High phosphorus in patients with acute and chronic renal failure, ethylene glycol toxicity, primary hypoparathyroidism, and those receiving phosphate-containing enemas • High amylase and lipase in many but not all patients with acute pancreatitis • Isosthenuria in patients with chronic renal failure, moderate to advanced acute renal failure, and ethylene glycol toxicity • Glucosuria in patients with acute renal failure and ethylene glycol toxicity

OTHER LABORATORY TESTS
• Ethylene glycol test—indicated in patients suspected of ingesting ethylene glycol within the previous 12-16 hours • PTH assay—indicated when primary hypoparathyroidism is suspected • Serum magnesium concentration—hypomagnesemia is a rare cause of hypocalcemia. Indicated when all other causes of hypocalcemia have been ruled out.

IMAGING
Radiography usually normal. Possibly, small kidneys in patients with acute or chronic renal failure and ethylene glycol toxicity and low bone density in patients with nutritional secondary hyperparathyroidism.

OTHER DIAGNOSTIC PROCEDURES
ECG changes include prolongation of the ST and Q-T segments. Sinus bradycardia and wide T waves or T wave alternans in a few patients.

TREATMENT
• Animals with clinical hypocalcemia and whose underlying disease requires support should be treated as inpatients.
• Emergency treatment is usually only needed for patients with primary hypoparathyroidism, hypoparathyroidism secondary to thyroidectomy and parathyroid damage, puerperal tetany (eclampsia), and citrate toxicity (rare). Short-term and long-term treatment are usually only needed to treat primary hypoparathyroidism and puerperal tetany (ecclampsia).
• Diet change is recommended in patients with nutritional secondary hyperparathyroidism (to a balanced diet) and renal failure (see Renal Failure, Chronic).

MEDICATIONS

DRUGS AND FLUIDS

Emergency Treatment
• Calcium gluconate 10% solution—5-15 mg/kg (0.5-1.5 ml/kg) slowly to effect over a 10-minute period. Heart rate should be monitored and administration stopped temporarily if bradycardia occurs. If ECG monitoring is possible, Q-T interval shortening is an indication to temporarily stop administration.
• Calcium chloride 10% solution—also effective but extremely caustic if administered extravascularly and is three times more potent than calcium gluconate. The mg/kg dosage is the same, but one third the volume is needed (0.15-0.5 ml/kg).
• If the patient has puerperal tetany (eclampsia), remove the puppies from the mother and hand nurse until weaned.

Short-Term Treatment Immediately after Correction of Tetany
Calcium gluconate 10% solution—relapse of clinical signs after emergency treatment can be prevented by use of one of the following:
• Constant rate IV infusion of 60-90 mg/kg/day (6.5-9.75 ml/kg/day) added to the fluids • Subcutaneous administration 3-4 times daily of the dosage determined to be needed to initially control tetany. This dose should be diluted in an equal volume of saline.

Long-Term Treatment
See Hypoparathyroidism.

CONTRAINDICATIONS N/A

PRECAUTIONS
See Hypoparathyroidism.

POSSIBLE INTERACTIONS
See Hypoparathyroidism.

ALTERNATE DRUGS N/A

FOLLOW-UP

PATIENT MONITORING
Serum calcium concentration monthly for the first 6 months then every 2-4 months. Goal is to maintain serum calcium concentration between 8 and 10 mg/dl.

POSSIBLE COMPLICATIONS
Hypocalcemia and hypercalcemia (which can lead to renal failure) are both concerns in patients on long-term hypocalcemic therapy.

MISCELLANEOUS

ASSOCIATED CONDITIONS N/A

AGE RELATED FACTORS N/A

ZOONOTIC POTENTIAL N/A

PREGNANCY
• Hypocalcemia can lead to weakness and dystocia. • Clinical hypocalcemia caused by puerperal tetany (eclampsia) usually is seen in small-breed bitches during the first 21 days of nursing a litter.

SYNONYMS None

SEE ALSO See causes.

ABBREVIATIONS
Ca = calcium
PTH = parathyroid hormone

References
Feldman EC, Nelson RW. Hypocalcemia and primary hypoparathyroidism. In: Feldman EC, Nelson RW, eds. Canine and feline endocrinology and reproduction. Philadelphia: WB Saunders, 1996:497-516.
Waters CB, Scott-Moncrieff JCR. Hypocalcemia in cats. Compend Contin Educ Pract Vet 1992;14:497-507.
Meuten DJ, Armstrong PJ. Parathyroid disease and calcium metabolism. In: Ettinger SJ, ed. Textbook of veterinary internal medicine. Philadelphia: WB Saunders, 1989:1610-1631.

Author Mitchell A. Crystal
Consulting Editor Rhett Nichols

CHLORIDE, HYPERCHLOREMIA

BASICS

DEFINITION
Serum chloride concentration > 122 mEq/L in dogs and >129 mEq/L in cats

Pathophysiology
• Chloride is the most abundant anion in the extracellular fluid. • Hypercholemia is associated with similar conditions that cause hypernatremia (i.e., water loss in excess of sodium and chloride or excessive NaCl intake). • Chloride concentration varies inversely to bicarbonate concentration; high bicarbonate loss (i.e., gastrointestinal or renal wasting) followed by low renal chloride resorption in excess of bicarbonate can cause hyperchloremia.

Systems Affected
Relates to underlying cause

SIGNALMENT
Dogs and Cats

SIGNS

General Comments
• Clinical signs of hyperchloremia are related to concurrent hypernatremia or the underlying disorder or both. • Severity of neurologic signs is related to the degree of hypernatremia and the rate at which hypernatremia develops.

History and Physical Examination Findings
• Polydipsia • Disorientation • Coma • Seizures

CAUSES

High Total Body Chloride
• Oral ingestion (rare) • NaCl administered IV during cardiovascular resuscitation

Normal Total Body Chloride with Water Deficit
• Low intake (e.g., no access to water) • High urinary water loss (e.g., diabetes insipidus) • High insensible water loss (e.g., panting)

Low Total Body Chloride with Hypotonic Fluid Loss
Urinary loss—diabetes mellitus, osmotic diuresis, and diuresis after urinary obstruction

Hyperchloremic Metabolic Acidosis
• Renal tubular acidosis (renal tubular disorders that cause renal wasting of bicarbonate or low hydrogen ion secretion) • Diarrhea associated with gastrointestinal loss of bicarbonate and renal resorption of chloride

RISK FACTORS N/A

DIAGNOSIS

DIFFERENTIAL DIAGNOSIS
• Normal anion gap metabolic acidosis (e.g., renal tubular acidosis and gastrointestinal bicarbonate loss) • Diabetes insipidus • Hypertonic dehydration • Severe forms of diabetes mellitus (e.g., diabetic ketoacidosis and hyperosmolar nonketotic syndrome) • Salt ingestion (rare)

LABORATORY FINDINGS

Drugs That May Alter Lab Results
• A wide variety of drugs can interfere with renal capacity to concentrate urine, leading to water loss in excess of sodium and high sodium and chloride concentrations. These drugs include lithium, demeclocycline, and amphotericin. • Other drugs that may increase chloride concentration include acetazolamide, ammonium chloride, androgens, and cholestyramine. • A falsely high chloride concentration can occur with a high serum concentration of iodide or bromide—most commonly seen in patients with epilepsy treated with potassium bromide.

Disorders That May Alter Lab Results
Hemoglobin and bilirubin cause falsely high chloride readings if colorimetric tests are used.

Valid If Run In A Human Lab? Yes

CBC/BIOCHEMISTRY/URINALYSIS
• High chloride, often coupled with high sodium • Diabetes insipidus—low urine specific gravity, polyuria, and low urine sodium • Diabetic ketoacidosis and hyperosmolar nonketotic syndrome—high blood glucose • Hypertonic dehydration—low urine sodium and high urine specific gravity (usually > 1.030) • Renal tubular acidosis—hyperchloremic acidosis, urine ph > 5.3, serum potassium often low, and other causes of metabolic acidosis have been ruled out

OTHER LABORATORY TESTS
• Renal tubular acidosis—response to $NaHCO_3$ or NH_4CL.

IMAGING
CT scan or MRI in patients with diabetes insipidus to rule out pituitary tumor

OTHER DIAGNOSTIC PROCEDURES
N/A

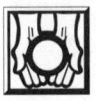

TREATMENT

INPATIENT VS. OUTPATIENT
Depends on underlying disorder.

DIET
No need to alter diet.

CLIENT EDUCATION
Depends on underlying disorder.

SURGICAL CONSIDERATIONS N/A

MEDICATIONS

DRUGS AND FLUIDS
• Hypovolemia—isotonic saline (normal saline or lactated Ringer's solution) or isotonic fluid (5% dextrose with half-normal saline) • Hyperchloremia with hypernatremia—hypotonic fluids (5% dextrose in water); decrease sodium by 0.5 meq/hour or by no more than 20 meq/L/day • Central diabetes insipidus—DDAVP (1-2 drops in the conjunctival sac q12h-q24h) • Nephrogenic diabetes insipidus—chlorothiazide 10-40 mg/kg PO q12h • Hyperchloremic metabolic acidosis—treat underlying cause; consider bicarbonate and potassium replacement if needed

CONTRAINDICATIONS N/A

Precautions
• Rapid correction of hyperchloremia with hypernatremia can cause pulmonary edema. • Hypocalcemia may develop during correction of hyperchloremia.

POSSIBLE INTERACTIONS N/A

ALTERNATE DRUGS N/A

FOLLOW-UP

PATIENT MONITORING
• Electrolytes, body weight, and hydration status

POSSIBLE COMPLICATIONS
Related to associated hypernatremia or the underlying disorder • Neurologic complications include CNS thrombosis or hemorrhage, seizures, and hyperactivity

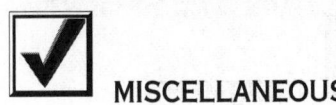

MISCELLANEOUS

ASSOCIATED CONDITIONS N/A

AGE RELATED FACTORS N/A

ZOONOTIC POTENTIAL N/A

PREGNANCY N/A

SYNONYMS N/A

SEE ALSO
Sodium, Hypernatremia

ABBREVIATIONS
CNS = central nervous system
DDAVP = brand name for desmopressin, a synthetic ADH preparation

References
DiBartola SP. Fluid therapy in small animal practice. Philadelphia: WB Saunders, 1992.
Ross DB. Clinical physiology of acid-base and electrolyte disorders. 3rd ed. New York: McGraw-Hill, 1989.

Author Rhett Nichols
Editor Rhett Nichols

CHLORIDE, HYPOCHLOREMIA

 BASICS

DEFINITION

Serum chloride concentration below the lower limit of normal (dogs, < 105 mEq/L; cats, < 117 mEq/L)

Pathophysiology

Chloride is the most abundant anion in the extracellular fluid. Chloride concentration is controlled by electrochemical gradients that correspond to the active transport of sodium. In general, chloride concentration varies directly with sodium concentration and inversely with bicarbonate concentration.

Systems Affected

Depends on the underlying disorder

SIGNALMENT

Dogs and Cats

SIGNS

Depends on the underlying disorder; none result from hypochloremia

CAUSES

• Gastric vomiting • Hypoadrenocorticism • Metabolic alkalosis • Salt-losing nephropathy • Diuretic administration • Severe hypokalemia (rare)

RISK FACTORS N/A

 DIAGNOSIS

DIFFERENTIAL DIAGNOSIS

If the degree of hypochloremia exceeds the degree of hyponatremia, this suggests selective chloride loss as seen in patients with gastric vomiting.

LABORATORY FINDINGS

Drugs That May Alter Lab Results

Furosemide, thiazides, bicarbonate, and laxatives lower the serum chloride concentration.

Disorders That May Alter Lab Results

Lipemia and hyperproteinemia can falsely lower chloride concentration if ion-specific electrodes are not used.

Valid If Run in Human Lab? Valid

CBC/BIOCHEMISTRY/URINALYSIS

• Low chloride • Other abnormalities depend on the underlying disorder; possibly, hyponatremia, hyperkalemia, and high bicarbonate.

OTHER LABORATORY TESTS

• Measurement of urine fractional excretion of chloride may demonstrate high excretion.
• Blood gas measurement may reveal metabolic alkalosis.

IMAGING N/A

OTHER DIAGNOSTIC PROCEDURES
N/A

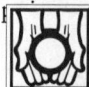 TREATMENT

INPATIENT VERSUS OUTPATIENT

Depends on the underlying disorder

DIET

No need to alter diet

CLIENT EDUCATION

Depends on the underlying disorder

SURGICAL CONSIDERATIONS N/A

MEDICATIONS

DRUGS AND FLUIDS
• 0.9% NaCl if fluid administration indicated
• Other fluid therapy and medication as dictated by the underlying cause

CONTRAINDICATIONS N/A

PRECAUTIONS N/A

POSSIBLE INTERACTIONS N/A

ALTERNATE DRUGS N/A

FOLLOW-UP

PATIENT MONITORING
Serum electrolyte concentrations as needed to assure appropriate response to treatment

PREVENTION/AVOIDANCE
Depends on the underlying disorder

POSSIBLE COMPLICATIONS
Depends on the underlying disorder

EXPECTED COURSE AND PROGNOSIS
Depends on the underlying disorder

MISCELLANEOUS

ASSOCIATED CONDITIONS
Often accompanied by hyponatremia

AGE RELATED FACTORS N/A

ZOONOTIC POTENTIAL N/A

PREGNANCY N/A

SYNONYMS N/A

SEE ALSO N/A

ABBREVIATIONS N/A

References
Rose DB. Clinical physiology of acid-base and electrolyte disorders. 3rd ed. New York: McGraw-Hill, 1989.
DiBartola SP. Fluid therapy in small animal practice. Philadelphia: WB Saunders, 1992.
Author Peter P. Kintzer
Consulting Editor Rhett Nichols

CLOTTING FACTOR DEFICIENCIES

BASICS

DEFINITION
Hemostatic defects characterized by deficient activity of one or more coagulation factors

Pathophysiology
The coagulation mechanism involves a series of sequential enzyme activations leading to the generation of thrombin, which converts fibrinogen to fibrin monomers, and subsequent polymerization of the monomers into fibrin strands, which stabilize the platelet plugs at sites of vessel injury. A defect in any of the coagulation factors can result in defective hemostasis.

Systems Affected
Coagulation defects can cause hemorrhages in any tissue or organ and anemia. The most common types are hemorrhages in and around the joints and major muscle masses, causing large swellings, and into the body cavities. Hemorrhages in the region of the larynx or pleural cavity are of special concern because of the risk of asphyxia. The other hemorrhages of major concern are those in the brain or spinal cord, because the rigid bony case limits expansion, and the risk for permanent damage is high.

SIGNALMENT
• Factor VIII deficiency and factor IX deficiency are severe defects usually recognized as spontaneous hemorrhages before 10 weeks of age. Both are sex-linked recessive defects; males are clinically affected, whereas females are carriers and clinically normal. • Von Willebrand disease is an autosomal defect, and both males and females are affected clinically. It is the most common inherited coagulation defect with high prevalence in many breeds. • Factor X deficiency has been detected mostly in American cocker spaniels. It manifests as stillborn puppies or neonatal deaths related to internal hemorrhage. It is an autosomal defect with a severe defect in homozygotes, whereas heterozygotes may be clinically normal or have only a mild bleeding tendency. • Factor XI deficiency is a rare defect described in English springer spaniels and a few dogs of other breeds. This autosomal defect is mild with bleeding after surgery or injury. • Factor XII deficiency is fairly common in cats but is rarely detected because no bleeding tendency is associated with the defect.

SIGNS
• Inactivity, swollen joints, subcutaneous swellings, or abnormal bleeding from cuts or mucous membranes • Hemorrhages in deeper tissues or body cavities

CAUSES
Coagulation defects can be caused by true deficiency of clotting factors, synthesis of defective factors, or the presence of inhibitors.

RISK FACTORS
• Aspirin or nonsteroidal antiinflammatory drugs can potentiate a bleeding defect. • If rodenticide anticoagulants are suspected, the possibility of environmental exposure should be investigated.

DIAGNOSIS

DIFFERENTIAL DIAGNOSIS
• Spontaneous bleeding noticed in young males but not female littermates should lead to suspicion of factor VIII deficiency or factor IX deficiency. • Von Willebrand disease or factor XI deficiency is usually detected as abnormal bleeding after injury or surgery in males or females. • Factor XII-deficient animals do not have a clinical bleeding defect. • Disseminated intravascular coagulation (DIC) is secondary to severe systemic disease and may be associated with thrombocytopenia or platelet function defects causing petechiae. • Rodenticide anticoagulants often are associated with major bleeding into body cavities.

LABORATORY FINDINGS

Drugs That May Alter Lab Results
Heparin and other anticoagulants used in treatment or from samples collected through heparinized catheters cause abnormal coagulation test results.

Disorders That May Alter Lab Results
• Shortening or prolonging of coagulation test results can be caused by contamination of blood with tissue fluid during problems with venipuncture. The presence of hemolysis should raise concern about possible tissue fluid contamination or prolonged time before testing. • Extreme lipemia may interfere with clot detection by some automated coagulation analyzers. • Because of lability of some coagulation factors, especially factor VIII, plasma should be separated from the rest of the sample and sent on ice or frozen to the laboratory.

Valid If Run in Human Lab?
• Coagulation assays vary in sensitivity but generally should yield valid data. It is important to interpret the results in relation to concurrent data from samples of normal plasma from the same species. • Some of the activators used in the APTT are not as effective on domestic animal samples compared with human samples. • Some tests for FDP are species-specific.

CBC/BIOCHEMISTRY/URINALYSIS
• Regenerative anemia proportional to the blood loss is caused by bleeding episodes. • Platelet count is normal unless the patient has severe bleeding. • Large hematomas may cause high bilirubin.

OTHER LABORATORY TESTS
• Measurement of PT is the test of choice for screening for extrinsic mechanism defects.

• Measurement of APTT is the test of choice for screening for intrinsic mechanism defects. Although not as sensitive or precise, the activated coagulation test is a practical substitute for the APTT test. Specific assays for coagulation factors are required for diagnosis of most of the inherited defects. These assays can be run with human deficient plasma as substrate, but the assays must be performed with dilutions of species-specific normal plasma for the activity curves.

IMAGING N/A

OTHER DIAGNOSTIC PROCEDURES
Bleeding time with a gauze tourniquet on the folded lip over the maxilla is prolonged in patients with von Willebrand disease. The bleeding time is normal in patients with most other coagulation defects with the exception of DIC.

TREATMENT
Most bleeding episodes in animals with inherited coagulation defects can be effectively treated by transfusion of fresh blood, fresh plasma, or fresh frozen plasma. Because repeated transfusions may be required in future, plasma is recommended unless the need for RBC replacement is severe. In patients with factor VIII deficiency, the short half-life of this factor (10-12 hours) may necessitate repeat transfusions at 24-hour intervals.

MEDICATIONS

DRUGS AND FLUIDS
Vitamin K_1 is an effective treatment for patients with anticoagulant rodenticide poisoning or vitamin K deficiency. If the PT is normal, there is no rationale for vitamin K_1 administration.

CONTRAINDICATIONS
Aspirin and nonsteroidal antiinflammatory drugs should be avoided because of possible adverse effects on platelet function.

PRECAUTIONS
• Intramuscular injections should be avoided because of the risk of inducing additional bleeding. • Intravenous administration of vitamin K is not recommended because of the risk of anaphylaxis.

POSSIBLE INTERACTIONS N/A

ALTERNATE DRUGS
Desmopressin acetate (1ug/kg SC) just before surgery may increase the concentration of vWF and shorten the bleeding time in dogs with von Willebrand disease. Results, however, are inconsistent.

CLOTTING FACTOR DEFICIENCIES

FOLLOW-UP

PATIENT MONITORING

• The PT can be used to monitor the effectiveness of vitamin K administration in animals with anticoagulant toxicity. With appropriate treatment, the prolonged PT should be corrected within 24 hours. Prolongations after this time suggest an incorrect diagnosis or undertreatment of poisonings. The activated coagulation test is a less sensitive but reasonable substitute for monitoring response to vitamin K. • Most inherited defects can be monitored by clinical arrest of bleeding and improvement in results of coagulation screening tests.

POSSIBLE COMPLICATIONS

Animals with inherited defects are at continual risk for repeated hemorrhagic episodes.

MISCELLANEOUS

ASSOCIATED CONDITIONS N/A

AGE RELATED FACTORS N/A

ZOONOTIC POTENTIAL N/A

PREGNANCY

Pregnancy may cause fluctuations in clotting factor activity, but these generally do not lead to bleeding episodes.

SYNONYMS

Coagulation defects
Coagulopathies

SEE ALSO

• Von Willebrand Disease • Disseminated Intravascular Coagulation

ABBREVIATIONS

APTT = activated partial thromboplastin time
DIC = disseminated intravascular coagulation
PT = prothrombin time

RBC = red blood cells
vWF = von Willebrand factor

References

Dodds WJ. Hemostasis. In: Kaneko JJ, ed. Clinical biochemistry of domestic animals. New York: Academic Press, 1989:274-315.

Fogh JM, Fogh IT. Inherited coagulation disorders. Vet Clin North Am Small Anim 1988;18:231-243.

Jain NC. Coagulation and its disorders. In: Jain NC, ed. Essentials of veterinary hematology. Philadelphia: Lea & Febiger, 1993:82-104.

Johnstone IB. Clinical and laboratory diagnosis of bleeding disorders. Vet Clin North Am Small Anim 1988;18:231-33.

Parry BW. Laboratory evaluation of hemorrhagic coagulopathies in small animal practice. Vet Clin North Am Small Anim 1989;19:729-742.

Author Gary J. Kociba

Consulting Editor Alan H. Rebar

O.S.P.T.
→ Normal
→ Prolonged

Normal → APTT
→ Normal → Von Willebrand Disease / Normal
→ Prolonged → Factor VIII deficiency / Factor IX deficiency / Factor XI deficiency / Factor XII deficiency

Prolonged → APTT
→ Normal → Factor VII deficiency
→ Prolonged → Anticoagulants / Liver Disease / Factor X deficiency / Vitamin K deficiency

CREATINE KINASE

BASICS

DEFINITION
Serum creatine kinase (CK) above the reference range for the laboratory in use.

Pathophysiology
There are three clinically important isoenzymes of CK; isoenzymes are found in skeletal and cardiac muscle and a third isoenzyme is found in brain tissue. Serum CK does not usually reflect the brain isoenzyme unless the blood-brain barrier is broken, and high serum CK associated with CNS disease is often secondary to muscle trauma and degeneration. CK is a leakage enzyme, and increases in serum CK indicate reversible or irreversible injury to muscle cells. Serum increases occur within a few hours of the muscle injury and peak by 12 hours. Serum activity returns to normal within 24-48 hours unless the damage is ongoing, in which case the CK remains persistently high.

SIGNALMENT
• Any age, breed, or sex of dog or cat, depending on the underlying cause of high CK • Certain breeds may be predisposed to hereditary myopathies (see below).

SIGNS

Historical Findings
Trauma, vigorous exercise, recent IM injections, paralysis/persistent recumbency, exercise intolerance, dysphagia, dysphonia, dyspnea, regurgitation, discolored urine

Physical Examination Findings
• Bruising, muscle pain, paralysis/persistent recumbency, gait abnormality such as stiff gait or hopping, ventroflexion of neck in cats, muscle atrophy or hypertrophy, pain opening mouth, and fever • Conscious proprioception and spinal reflexes are usually normal with primary myopathies. • Neuropathies are more commonly associated with spinal reflex abnormalities, hyperesthesias/paresthesias, and diminished conscious proprioception.

CAUSES
• Degenerative—inherited (muscular dystrophy, Labrador myopathy, Irish terrier myopathy, chow chow myotonia) or acquired (atrophy, myotonia associated with hyperadrenocorticism) • Immune-mediated—idopathic, systemic lupus erythematous, masticatory muscle myositis, dermatomyositis • Metabolic/endocrine—hyperadrenocorticism, hypothyroidism, hyperthermia (malignant or exercise induced) • Metabolic/endocrine—hyperadrenocorticism, hypothyroidism, hyperthermia (malignant or exercise induced) • Neoplastic—paraneoplastic myopathy • Nutritional—hypokalemia (cats), vitamin E and/or selenium deficiency • Infectious—toxoplasmosis, clostridial myositis, neosporosis • Trauma—this is the most common cause of high serum CK and is associated with vigorous exercise or exertional rhabdomyolysis, blunt trauma, IM injections, hypothermia, hyperthermia (exercise induced, malignant, or environmental), persistent recumbency, electric shock, seizures, and lacerations.

RISK FACTORS
• Breeds predisposed to inherited myopathies such as Labradors, Irish terriers, golden retrievers, and chows or immune-mediated myopathies (collies for dermatomyositis) • Hypokalemia in cats • Endocrinopathies such as hyperadrenocorticism and hypothyroidism • Neurologic disease resulting in prolonged recumbency • Muscle trauma, IM injections • Vigorous exercise, seizures • Hyperthermia or hypothermia

DIAGNOSIS

DIFFERENTIAL DIAGNOSIS
• The signalment may suggest one of the inherited myopathies or immune-mediated myositides. • Pain opening the mouth/involvement of muscle of the head suggests masticatory muscle myositis • Systemic signs such as polyuria/polydipsia and alopecia may suggest hyperadrenocorticism; obesity, lethargy, and cold intolerance suggest hypothyroidism • Older cats with polyuria/polydipsia and evidence of primary renal failure may have hypokalemic polymyopathy • History of trauma, injections, electric shock, seizures or vigorous exercise may suggest the cause.

LABORATORY FINDINGS
• Drugs that may alter lab results: clofibrate, succinylcholine, and any drug given by IM injection; penicillin, D-penicillamine, sulfonamides, and phenytoin may cause an immune-mediated polymyositis and increase serum CK • Disorders that may alter lab results: hemolysis falsely increases CK (controversial and only if severe); lipemia does not significantly affect results; ethylenediaminetetraacetic acid (EDTA), citrate, fluoride, exposure to sunlight, and delayed analysis falsely decrease serum CK; icterus falsely increases serum CK; electromyography will cause increased serum CK

CBC/BIOCHEMISTRY/URINALYSIS
• CBC may be inflammatory with infectious or immune-mediated myositis; a stress leukogram is consistent with hyperadrenocorticism • Eosinophilia can be associated with masticatory muscle myositis • Aspartate transaminase (AST)—if increased without evidence of liver disease supports the diagnosis of muscle disease • Hyperadrenocorticism should be considered if alkaline phosphatase (ALP) is increased without significant evidence of liver disease • Hypokalemia and azotemia in cats can result in polymyositis • Hypercholes-terolemia may suggest hyperadrenocorticism or hypothyroidism • Myoglobinuria may accompany exertional rhabdomyolysis

OTHER LABORATORY TESTS
• Antinuclear antibody test, if positive, is supportive of a diagnosis of systemic lupus erythematosus (SLE) if multisystemic disorder is identified • A positive type II muscle fiber antibody test will help confirm masticatory muscle myositis • Thyroid-stimulating hormone (TSH) stimulation test will definitively diagnose hypothyroidism (see hypothyroidism) • Adrenocorticotropic hormone (ACTH) stimulation test or low-dose dexamethasone suppression test will determine if hyperadrenocorticism is present (see hyperadrenocorticism) • Serology for Toxoplasma gondii may support toxoplasmal myositis • Pre- and post- exercise plasma lactate concentrations can identify metabolic myopathy associated with mitochondrial enzyme deficiencies

IMAGING
Radiographs of the chest and abdomen may help identify underlying neoplasia, assess kidney size (hypokalemic nephropathy in cats), confirm traumatic injuries (i.e. fractures), and support endocrinopathies (i.e. hepatomegaly or adrenomegaly with hyperadrenocorticism)

OTHER DIAGNOSTIC PROCEDURES
• Muscle biopsy and electromyography can be pursued when trauma, exercise, hyperthermia, hypothermia, seizures, IM injections, and drugs have been ruled out as a cause for the high CK; these diagnostic tests should be used when increases in serum CK are persistent and unexplained. • Muscle biopsy will help definitively diagnose a primary underlying etiology such as toxoplasmosis, neosporosis, and immune-mediated myositis unless long-standing disease has resulted in fibrosis and atrophy; muscle specimens should be preserved in formalin for routine histopatholic examination, cryopreserved for histochemical staining, and in glutaraldehyde for electron microscopy; in addition, muscle tissue can be cultured if bacterial myositis is suspected. • Electromyography may support the diagnosis of a primary muscle versus primary neurologic disorder in some cases; although overlap is present depending on the duration of the illness, spontaneous discharges are associated with primary myopathies, whereas prolonged insertional activity, positive sharp waves, and fibrillation potentials are more common with primary neuropathies; endocrine disorders often result in pseudomyotonic discharges

TREATMENT
• Specific treatment will depend on the underlying etiology (see specific disease) • Supportive care such as soft bedding, turning the patient, and passive range of motion

exercises is beneficial in the recumbent animal so that pressure sores do not develop and atrophy is minimized
• The traumatized animal may need emergency treatment for shock and/or wound and fracture management

MEDICATIONS

DRUGS AND FLUIDS
There is no specific treatment necessary to lower the CK because it is not dangerous to the animal in high serum concentration.

FOLLOW-UP

PATIENT MONITORING
Serum CK can be monitored to assess response to treatment or recovery from a traumatic incident; however, clinical response to therapy is a better indicator of the efficacy of treatment

POSSIBLE COMPLICATIONS N/A

MISCELLANEOUS

ASSOCIATED CONDITIONS
Hypokalemia in cats with renal disease is associated with polymyositis and high serum CK

AGE-RELATED FACTORS
None known

ZOONOTIC POTENTIAL
High serum CK as a result of toxoplasmosis may have some zoonotic potential depending on the species (dog or cat) and phase of disease

PREGNANCY N/A

SYNONYMS
• Creatine phosphokinase (CPK) • ATP-creatine transphoshorylase

SEE ALSO
See individual causes

ABBREVIATIONS
CK = creatine kinase
CNS = central nervous system
EDTA = ethylenediaminetetraacetic acid
AST = aspartate transaminase
ALP = alkaline phosphatase
SLE = systemic lupus erythematosus
TSH = thyroid-stimulating hormone
ACTH = adrenocorticotropic hormone

References
DiBartola SP, Tasker JB. Elevated serum creatine phosphokinase: A study of 53 cases and a review of its diagnostic significance in clinical veterinary medicine. J Am Anim Hosp Assoc 1977;13:744-753.

Kornegay JN, Gorgacz EJ, Dawe DL, et al. Polymyositis in dogs. J Am Vet Med Assoc 1980;176:431-438.

Scott-Moncrieff JC, Hawkings EC, Cook JR. Canine muscle disorders. Comp Cont Educ Pract Vet 1990;12:31-38.

Wilson JW. Serum creatine phosphokinase in the canine. J Am Anim Hosp Assoc 1976;12:522-524.
Author Ellen Miller
Consulting Editor Peter D. Schwarz

CREATININE AND BLOOD UREA NITROGEN (BUN)—AZOTEMIA AND UREMIA

BASICS

DEFINITION

Azotemia is an excess of urea, creatinine, or other nonprotein, nitrogenous substance in blood, plasma, or serum. Uremia is the polysystemic toxic syndrome that occurs as a result of abnormal renal function in animals with azotemia. Uremia occurs simultaneously in animals with high quantities of urine constituents in blood.

Pathophysiology

• Azotemia can be caused by 1) high production of nonprotein nitrogenous substances, 2) low glomerular filtration rate, or 3) reabsorption of formed urine into the bloodstream. High production of nonprotein nitrogenous waste substances may be caused by high intake of protein (diet or gastrointestinal bleeding) or accelerated catabolism of endogenous proteins. Glomerular filtration rate may decline because of reduced renal perfusion (prerenal azotemia), renal insufficiency or failure due to primary renal disease (renal azotemia), or urinary obstruction (postrenal azotemia). Reabsorption of urine may result from leakage of urine from the excretory pathways (also termed postrenal azotemia). • The pathophysiology of uremia is incompletely understood but may be related to 1) metabolic and toxic systemic effects of waste products retained because of renal excretory failure, 2) deranged renal regulation of fluids, electrolytes, and acid-base balance, and 3) impaired renal production of hormones and other substances (eg, erythropoietin and 1,25-dihydroxycholecalciferol).

Systems Affected

• Generalized or systemic effects—depression, fatigue, weakness, dehydration, and weight loss • Gastrointestinal—anorexia, nausea, vomiting, diarrhea, uremic stomatitis, xerostomia, uriniferous breath, and constipation • Neuromuscular—dullness, drowsiness, lethargy, irritability, tremors, gait imbalance, flaccid muscle weakness, myoclonus, behavioral changes, dementia, isolated cranial nerve deficits, seizures, stupor, and coma • Endocrine/metabolic—renal secondary hyperparathyroidism and inadequate production of 1,25-dihydroxycholecalciferol and erythropoietin • Cardiovascular—arterial hypertension, left ventricular hypertrophy, heart murmur, cardiomegaly, and cardiac rhythm disturbance • Respiratory—dyspnea • Hemic/lymph/immune—hypoproliferative (normocytic, normochromic) anemia and immunodeficiency • Ocular—scleral and conjunctival injection, retinopathy, and acute-onset blindness • Skin/exocrine—pallor, bruising, excessive shedding, unkempt appearance, and loss of normal sheen to coat.

SIGNALMENT Dogs and cats

SIGNS

General Comments

Azotemia may or may not be associated with historical or physical abnormalities. Unless animal has uremia, clinical findings are limited to the disease responsible for azotemia (eg, hypoadrenocorticism and urinary obstruction). Findings described here are those of uremia.

Historical Findings

• Weight loss • Declining appetite or anorexia • Reduced activity • Depression • Fatigue • Weakness • Vomiting • Diarrhea • Halitosis • Constipation • Poor haircoat or unkempt appearance

Physical Examination Findings

• Cachexia • Depression • Dehydration • Weakness • Pallor • Petechia and ecchymosis • Dull and unkempt haircoat • Uriniferous breath • Uremic stomatitis • Scleral and conjunctival injection

CAUSES

Prerenal Azotemia

• Reduced renal perfusion due to low blood volume or low blood pressure • Accelerated production of nitrogenous waste products because of enhanced catabolism of tissues in association with infection, fever, trauma, corticosteroid excess, or burns. • Increased gastrointestinal digestion and absorption of protein sources (diet or gastrointestinal hemorrhage).

Renal Azotemia

Acute or chronic renal failure (ie, primary renal disease affecting glomeruli, renal tubules, renal interstitium, or renal vasculature that impairs renal function by at least 75%)

Postrenal Azotemia

Urinary obstruction; rupture of the excretory pathway.

RISK FACTORS

• Medical conditions—renal disease, hypoadrenocorticism, low cardiac output, hypotension, fever, sepsis, polyuria, liver disease, pyometra, hypoalbuminemia, dehydration, acidosis, exposure to chemicals that are nephrotoxic, gastrointestinal hemorrhage, urolithiasis, urethral plugs in cats, urethral trauma, and neoplasia. • Advanced age may be a risk factor. • Drugs—potentially nephrotoxic drugs, nonsteroidal anti-inflammatory drugs, diuretics, and antihypertensive medications.

DIAGNOSIS

DIFFERENTIAL DIAGNOSIS

• Dehydration, poor peripheral perfusion, low cardiac output, history of recent fluid loss, high protein diet, or black, tarry stools—rule out prerenal azotemia. • Recent onset of altered urine output (high or low), clinical signs consistent with uremia, exposure to possible nephrotoxicants or ischemic renal injury, or kidney size normal or large—rule out acute renal failure • Progressive weight loss, polyuria, polydipsia, small kidneys, pallor, and signs of uremia that have developed over several weeks to months—rule out chronic renal failure • Abrupt decline in urine output and onset of signs of uremia; occasionally dysuria, stranguria and hematuria; large urinary bladder or fluid-filled abdomen—rule out postrenal azotemia

LABORATORY FINDINGS

Drugs That May Alter Lab Results N/A
Disorders That May Alter Lab Results N/A

Valid If Run in Human Lab? Yes

CBC/BIOCHEMISTRY/URINALYSIS

Urinalysis

• A urine specific gravity ≥ 1.030 in dogs and ≥ 1.035 in cats supports a diagnosis of prerenal azotemia. Administration of fluids or diuretics before urine collection may render low urine specific gravity value uninterpretable.
• Azotemic patients that have not received fluids and have a urine specific gravity < 1.030 in dogs and < 1.035 in cats typically have primary renal azotemia. A notable exception to this rule is dogs and cats with glomerular disease. Glomerulopathy is sometimes characterized by glomerulotubular imbalance with urine concentrating ability persisting despite sufficient renal glomerular damage to cause primary renal azotemia. These patients are recognized by moderate to marked proteinuria in the absence of hematuria and pyuria. • Urine specific gravity is not of value in differentiating postrenal azotemia from prerenal or primary renal azotemia.

Biochemistry

• Serial determinations of serum urea nitrogen and creatinine concentrations may be of diagnostic value in differentiating the cause of azotemia. Appropriate treatment to restore renal perfusion typically results in a dramatic reduction in azotemia in patients with prerenal azotemia (typically within 24- to 48 hours). Correcting obstruction to flow or a rent in the excretory pathway typically results in a rapid reduction in the magnitude of azotemia in patients with postrenal azotemia. • Concurrent hyperkalemia may be consistent with postrenal azotemia, primary renal azotemia caused by oliguric renal failure, or prerenal azotemia associated with hypoadrenocorticism.

OTHER LABORATORY TESTS

Endogenous or exogenous creatinine clearances or other specific tests of glomerular filtration rate used to confirm that azotemia is caused by reduced glomerular filtration rate

IMAGING

• Abdominal radiographs are used to determine kidney size (small kidneys are consistent with chronic renal failure; large kidneys may

CREATININE AND BLOOD UREA NITROGEN (BUN)—AZOTEMIA AND UREMIA

be consistent with acute renal failure or urinary obstruction) and to rule out urinary obstruction (dilation of the urinary bladder or mineral densities within the excretory pathway). • Renal ultrasonography may detect changes in echogenicity of renal parenchymal and size and shape of kidneys that support a diagnosis of primary renal azotemia. • Ultrasonography is useful to rule out postrenal azotemia characterized by distension of the excretory pathway and uroliths or mass within or impinging on the excretory pathway and intraabdominal fluid accumulation (with rupture of the excretory pathway). • Excretory urography or cystourethrography may be useful in establishing the diagnosis of postrenal azotemia caused by urinary obstruction or rupture of the excretory pathway.

OTHER DIAGNOSTIC PROCEDURES

Renal biopsy can be used to confirm the diagnosis of primary renal failure, differentiate acute from chronic renal failure, and attempt to establish the underlying disease process responsible for renal failure.

TREATMENT

• Treatment for prerenal azotemia caused by impaired renal perfusion directed at correcting the underlying cause for renal hypoperfusion. The aggressiveness of treatment depends on the severity of the underlying condition and the probability that persistent renal hypoperfusion will lead to primary renal injury or failure.
• Treatment for primary renal azotemia and associated uremia includes 1) specific measures directed at halting or reversing the primary disease process affecting the kidneys, and 2) symptomatic, supportive, and palliative treatment that a) ameliorates clinical signs of uremia, b) minimizes the clinical impact of fluid, electrolyte, and acid-base imbalances, c) minimizes the effects of inadequate renal biosynthesis of hormones and other substances, and d) maintains adequate nutrition.
• Treatment for postrenal azotemia directed at eliminating urinary obstruction or correcting leakage from the urinary system. Supplemental fluid administration is often required to prevent dehydration which may develop during the solute diuresis that follows correction of postrenal azotemia.

MEDICATIONS

DRUGS AND FLUIDS

• Fluid therapy is indicated for most azotemic patients. Preferred fluid selections include 0.9% saline and lactated Ringer's solution. The quantity of fluid administered should be estimated on the basis of severity of dehydration or volume depletion. If clinical dehydration is not evident, it may cautiously be assumed that the patient is < 5% dehydrated and a corresponding volume of fluid administered. The bulk of volume replacement should generally be provided over 2–6 hours, except in patients with overt or suspected cardiac failure.
• Patients in shock should be treated appropriately (see shock).

CONTRAINDICATIONS

Administration of nephrotoxic drugs to patients with azotemia

PRECAUTIONS

• Use caution when administering drugs requiring renal excretion. If they must be administered, be aware of the possible adverse or toxic effects of these drugs. Consult appropriate references concerning dose-reduction schedules.
• Use caution in administering fluids to patients that may be oliguric or anuric. Urine production rates and body weight should be monitored during fluid therapy to minimize the likelihood of inducing overhydration.
• Use caution in administering drugs that may promote hypovolemia or hypotension (eg, diuretics) in patients with azotemia. The response to such drugs should be carefully monitored by assessing hydration status, peripheral perfusion, blood pressure, and result of serial renal function tests.
• Corticosteroid administration will likely worsen azotemia by increasing catabolism of endogenous proteins.

POSSIBLE INTERACTIONS N/A

ALTERNATE DRUGS N/A

FOLLOW-UP

PATIENT MONITORING

Serum urea nitrogen and creatinine concentrations 24 hours after initiating fluid administration; also urine production, body weight, and hydration status.

POSSIBLE COMPLICATIONS

• Failure to rapidly correct prerenal azotemia caused by renal hypoperfusion could result in ischemic primary renal failure. • Primary renal azotemia can progress to uremia. • Failure to restore normal urine flow in patients with postrenal azotemia can result in progressive renal damage or death due to hyperkalemia and uremia.

MISCELLANEOUS

ASSOCIATED CONDITIONS

• An association may exist between hypokalemia and azotemia in cats. Preliminary findings suggest that hypokalemia may be associated with functional or structural renal changes leading to azotemia.

AGE RELATED FACTORS

Primary renal failure may occur in animals of any age, but geriatric dogs and cats appear to be at substantially higher risk for both acute and chronic renal failure. However, azotemia in geriatric dogs and cats should not be assumed to indicate primary renal failure, because these patients are also at higher risk for prerenal and postrenal causes for azotemia.

ZOONOTIC POTENTIAL Leptospirosis

PREGNANCY

• Data on azotemia and pregnancy in dogs and cats is very limited. In humans, minimal renal disease may be well-tolerated during pregnancy. However, ability to sustain a viable pregnancy declines as renal function declines. Women with severe renal dysfunction are usually infertile. • In pregnant azotemic animals, pharmacologic agents excreted by nonrenal pathways are preferred.

SYNONYMS N/A

SEE ALSO

• Renal Failure, Acute • Renal Failure, Chronic • Urinary Tract Obstruction

ABBREVIATIONS N/A

References

Osborne CA, Polzin DJ. Azotemia: a review of what's old and what's new. Part I. Definition of terms and concepts. Compend Cont Ed Pract Vet 1983;5:497-508.

Osborne CA, Polzin DJ. Azotemia: a review of what's old and what's new. Part II. Localization. Compend Cont Ed Pract Vet 1983;5:561-5743.

DiBartola S. Clinical approach and laboratory evaluation of renal disease. In: Ettinger SJ, Feldman EC, eds. Textbook of veterinary internal medicine. Philadelphia: WB Saunders, 1995;1706-1719.

Author David J. Polzin
Consulting Editors Larry G. Adams and Carl A. Osborne

CRYSTALLURIA

 BASICS

DEFINITION
Appearance of crystals in the urine

Pathophysiology
• Crystals only form in urine that is, or recently has been, supersaturated with crystallogenic substances. Therefore, crystalluria represents a risk factor for urolithiasis. However, detection of urine crystals is not synonymous with uroliths, nor are urine crystals irrefutable evidence of a stone-forming tendency.
• Certain types of crystalluria are a manifestation of underlying disease. Proper identification and interpretation of urine crystals is important in formulating medical protocols to dissolve uroliths. Evaluation of urine crystals may aid in 1) detection of disorders predisposing animals to urolith formation, 2) estimation of the mineral composition of uroliths, and 3) evaluation of the effectiveness of medical protocols initiated to dissolve or prevent urolithiasis. • Crystalluria that occurs in individuals with anatomically and functionally normal urinary tracts is usually harmless, because the crystals are eliminated before they grow to sufficient size to interfere with normal urinary function. • Crystals that form after elimination or removal of urine from the patient often are of little clinical importance. Identification of crystals that have formed in vitro does not justify treatment.
• Detection of some types of crystals (e.g.,cystine and ammonium urate) in clinically asymptomatic patients, frequent detection of large aggregates of crystals (e.g.,calcium oxalate and magnesium ammonium phosphate) in apparently normal individuals, or detection of any form of crystals in fresh urine collected from patients with confirmed urolithiasis may be of diagnostic, prognostic, or therapeutic importance.

Systems Affected
Renal/urologic—upper and lower urinary tract

SIGNALMENT
• Calcium oxalate in miniature schnauzer, Yorkshire terrier, Lhasa apso, and miniature poodle • Calcium oxalate in Burmese, Himalayan, and Persian • Cystine in dachshund, English bulldog, and Newfoundland
• Ammonium urate in dalmatian and English bulldog

SIGNS
None or those caused by concomitant urolithiasis

CAUSES

In Vivo Variables
• The concentration of crystallogenic substances in the urine, which in turn is influenced by their rate of excretion and the concentration of water in the urine • Urine pH

(struvite and calcium phosphate crystals are most common in neutral to alkaline urine; ammonium urate, sodium urate, calcium oxalate, cystine, and xanthine crystals are most common in acid to neutral urine) • The solubility of crystallogenic substances in urine • Excretion of diagnostic agents (e.g.,radiopaque contrast agent) and medications (e.g.,sulfonamide) • Dietary influence—influence of hospital diet versus home diet on formation of urine crystals may differ

In Vitro Variables
• Temperature • Evaporation • pH • Technique of specimen preparation (e.g.,centrifugation versus noncentrifugation and volume of urine examined) • Important in vitro changes that occur after urine collection may enhance formation or dissolution of crystals. When knowledge of in vivo urine crystal type and quantity is especially important, fresh specimens should be examined. Ideally they should be body temperature. If this is not possible, they should be room temperature, not refrigeration temperature.

RISK FACTORS
See discussion about in vivo and in vitro crystalluria

 DIAGNOSIS

DIFFERENTIAL DIAGNOSIS

Bilirubin Crystalluria
• Observed in some clinical normal dogs with highly concentrated urine. Large numbers in serial samples of urine should arouse suspicion of an abnormality in bilirubin metabolism. • Usually associated with underlying disease in cats

Calcium Oxalate Dihydrate and Calcium Oxalate Monohydrate Crystalluria
• Observed in some clinically normal dogs and cats and in dogs and cats with uroliths composed primarily of calcium oxalate
• Observed in some dogs intoxicated with ethylene glycol, but calcium oxalate monohydrate crystals (incorrectly termed hippurate crystals) more common. Ethylene glycol toxicity can also occur without crystalluria.

Struvite Crystalluria
Observed in some clinically normal dogs and cats or those with infection-induced struvite uroliths, sterile struvite uroliths, nonstruvite uroliths, uroliths of mixed composition (e.g.,a nucleus composed of calcium oxalate and a shell composed of struvite), or urinary tract disease without uroliths

Ammonium Urate and Amorphous Urate Crystalluria
Uncommon crystal observed in some clinically normal dogs and cats. Frequently observed in dogs with portal vascular anomaly with or without concomitant ammonium urate uroliths. Also observed in some dogs and cats

with ammonium urate uroliths caused by disorders other than portal vascular anomaly.

Uric Acid Crystalluria
• Uncommon in dogs and cats • Same importance as that described for ammonium and amorphous urates

Xanthine Crystalluria
• Suggests administration of excessive dosage of allopurinol in conjunction with a relatively high amount of purine precursors in the diet
• Primary xanthinuria and xanthine uroliths rare in cats

Calcium Phosphate Crystalluria
• Large numbers of crystals presumed to be composed of calcium phosphate have been observed in clinically normal dogs, dogs with persistently alkaline urine, dogs with calcium phosphate uroliths, and dogs with uroliths composed of a mixture of calcium phosphate and calcium oxalate. • Small numbers of calcium phosphate crystals may occur in association with infection-induced struvite crystalluria.

Miscellaneous Crystals
• Cystine uroliths develop in some dogs and cats with cystinuria. • Cholesterol crystals have been reported in humans with excessive tissue destruction, nephrotic syndrome, and chyluria. They have been observed in clinically normal dogs. • True hippuric acid crystals are rare in dogs and cats and are of unknown importance. • Tyrosine crystals occur in association with severe liver disease in humans. They are uncommon in cats and dogs with liver disease. • The importance of leucine crystals in dogs has not been determined.

LABORATORY FINDINGS

Drugs That May Alter Lab Results
Urinary acidifiers (e.g.,d,l-methionine and ammonium chloride) and acidifying diets

Disorders That May Alter Lab Results
N/A

Valid If Run in Human Lab? Yes

CBC/BIOCHEMISTRY/URINALYSIS
• Bilirubin crystals may be associated with bilirubinemia and other laboratory abnormalities in animals with liver disease. • Most dogs and cats with calcium oxalate and calcium phosphate crystalluria are normocalcemic; some are hypercalcemic. • When knowledge of in vivo urine crystal type is especially important, fresh specimens should be serially examined. The number, size, and structure of crystals should be evaluated as well as their tendency to aggregate. • Microscopic evaluation of the appearance of urine crystals represents only a tentative indicator of their composition, because variable conditions associated with their formation, growth, and dissolution may alter their appearance. Definitive identification of crystal composition depends on optical crystallography, infrared spectrophotometry, thermal analysis, x-ray diffraction, electron microprobe analysis, or a combination of these. • To confirm the composition of microscopic crystalluria,

prepare a large pellet of crystals by centrifugation of an appropriate volume of urine in a cone-tipped centrifuge tube. Evaluate the pellet by a quantitative method designed for quantitative urolith analysis. Identification by this method may only reflect the outer portions of uroliths.

OTHER LABORATORY TESTS

• Cystine crystalluria usually associated with a positive urine cyanide-nitroprusside reaction • Sulfonamide crystalluria may be associated with a positive lignin test. • Ammonium urate and amorphous urate crystals are insoluble in acetic acid. However, addition of 10% acetic acid to urine sediment containing these crystals often results in the appearance of uric acid and, sometimes, sodium urate crystals. • Most dogs and a few cats with struvite crystalluria have urinary tract infection caused by urease producing bacteria (e.g.,Staphylococci and Proteus spp.). • Dogs and cats with ammonium urate crystalluria and a portovascular shunt often have high serum bile acid concentration and hyperammonemia. • Dogs and cats with calcium oxalate crystalluria secondary to ethylene glycol intoxication have detectable levels of ethylene glycol in serum and urine up to 48 hours after ingestion.

IMAGING

Crystalluria associated with radiographically or ultrasonographically detectable uroliths in some animals

OTHER DIAGNOSTIC PROCEDURES

Catheter-assisted retrieval of small concomitant uroliths for quantitative analysis

TREATMENT

• Clinically important in vivo crystalluria should be managed by eliminating or controlling the underlying cause(s) or associated risk factors.
• Clinically important crystalluria can be minimized by increasing urine volume, encouraging complete and frequent voiding, dietary modification, and, in some animals, by appropriate drug administration or modifying the pH.
• See chapters on specific urolith types for treatment of concomitant urolithiasis.

MEDICATIONS

DRUGS AND FLUIDS N/A
CONTRAINDICATIONS N/A
PRECAUTIONS N/A
POSSIBLE INTERACTIONS N/A
ALTERNATE DRUGS N/A

FOLLOW-UP

PATIENT MONITORING
• Recheck urinalysis to determine if crystalluria is persistent. • See chapters on specific urolith types for monitoring urolithiasis.

POSSIBLE COMPLICATIONS
• Persistent crystalluria may contribute to for-

mation and growth of uroliths. • Crystalluria may solidify crystalline-matrix plugs, resulting in urethral obstruction.

MISCELLANEOUS

ASSOCIATED CONDITIONS N/A
AGE RELATED FACTORS N/A
ZOONOTIC POTENTIAL N/A
PREGNANCY N/A
SYNONYMS N/A

SEE ALSO
• Nephrolithiasis • Urolithiasis, Calcium Oxalate • Urolithiasis, Calcium Phosphate • Urolithiasis, Cystine • Urolithiasis, Struvite— dogs • Urolithiasis, Struvite—Cats • Urolithiasis, Urate • Urolithiasis, Xanthine

ABBREVIATIONS None

References

Osborne CA, Davis LS, Sanna J, et al. Identification and interpretation of crystalluria in domestic animals. A light and scanning electron microscopic study. Vet Med 1990;85:18-37.

Osborne CA, O' Brien TD, Davenport MP, et al. Crystalluria: causes, detection, and interpretation. In: Kirk RW, ed. Current veterinary therapy X. Philadelphia: WB Saunders, 1989:1127-1133.

Author Carl A. Osborne
Consulting Editors Larry G. Adams and Carl A. Osborne

BASICS

DEFINITION

Abnormally high number of casts (> 2 casts/lpf) detected on examination of urine sediment

Pathophysiology

May develop in animals with primary renal disease or systemic disorder that secondarily affects the kidneys. Presence of high number of casts indicates accelerated renal cellular degeneration, glomerular leakage of protein, hemorrhage, or exudation into renal tubular lumens.

Systems Affected   Renal/urologic

SIGNALMENT   Dogs and cats

SIGNS   None

CAUSES

Nephrotoxicosis

• Toxin (e.g., ethylene glycol) • Nephrotoxic drug (e.g., aminoglycoside, intravenously administered tetracycline, amphotericin-B, cisplatin, thiacetarsamide, nonsteroidal anti-inflammatory drug, and angiotensin-converting enzyme inhibitor) • Diagnostic agent (e.g., intravenously administered radiocontrast agent)

Renal Ischemia

• Dehydration • Hypovolemia • Low cardiac output (e.g., animals with congestive heart failure, cardiac arrhythmia, or pericardial disease) • Renal vessel thrombosis (e.g., animals with emboli from bacterial endocarditis or disseminated intravascular coagulation [DIC]) • Hemoglobinuria (e.g., animals with intravascular hemolysis) • Myoglobulinuria (e.g., animals with rhabdomyolysis) • Renal inflammation • Infectious diseases (e.g., animals with pyelonephritis, leptospirosis, FIP, Rocky Mountain spotted fever, or ehrlichiosis) • Glomerular disease: (ie, animals with glomerulonephritis or amyloidosis) • Renal trauma

RISK FACTORS

• Any disorder that causes impaired renal perfusion • Exposure to nephrotoxins

DIAGNOSIS

DIFFERENTIAL DIAGNOSIS

• History of potential exposure to toxins or nephrotoxic drugs—rule out acute tubular necrosis. • Recent onset of vomiting or diarrhea—rule out renal ischemia caused by dehydration. • Recent inhalation anesthesia—rule out tubular necrosis caused by ischemia. • Potential for exposure to infectious disease—rule out nephritis • Fever—rule out infectious, inflammatory, and neoplastic diseases • Cardiac murmur, especially if diastolic and of recent onset—rule out bacterial endocarditis. • Petechiae and ecchymoses—rule out systemic thrombosis

LABORATORY FINDINGS

Drugs That May Alter Lab Results   N/A

Disorders That May Alter Lab Results

• Waiting longer than 2 hours to perform urinalysis may result in disappearance of casts. • Alkaline urine causes dissolution of casts. • Dilute urine (specific gravity < 1.003) causes dissolution of casts. Therefore, interpret numbers of casts in light of urine specific gravity.

Valid If Run in Human Lab?   Yes

CBC/BIOCHEMISTRY/URINALYSIS

• Anemia, hemoconcentration, leukocytosis, and thrombocytopenia in some animals. • High concentrations of urea nitrogen, creatinine, and phosphorus in patients with dehydration or renal failure • Epithelial, granular, or waxy casts indicate diseases that cause degeneration and necrosis or renal tubular epithelial cells; granular casts can result from disintegration of WBC casts. • RBC casts indicate severe glomerular disease or hemorrhage into renal tubules. • WBC casts indicate renal inflammation, most often caused by pyelonephritis; however, most patients with pyelonephritis do not have WBC casts. • Hyaline casts commonly are associated with disorders that cause proteinuria; they also may be observed during diuresis and after dehydration.

Laboratory Test Patterns

• Cylindruria plus azotemia and adequately concentrated urine (specific gravity > 1.030 in dogs and > 1.040 in cats)—consider prerenal disorders such as dehydration. • Cylindruria plus azotemia and inadequately concentrated urine (specific gravity < 1.030 in dogs and < 1.035 in cats)—consider renal failure. • Cylindruria plus leukocytosis—consider infectious and inflammatory disorders. • Cylinduria plus thrombocytopenia—consider DIC. • Cylindruria plus glucosuria and proteinuria—consider renal tubular necrosis.

OTHER LABORATORY TESTS

• If the patient has thrombocytopenia or RBC casts, perform coagulation studies (e.g., APTT, PT, and FDP) to rule out consumptive coagulopathy such as DIC. • If the patient has proteinuria , perform urine protein:creatinine ratio to determine magnitude of proteinuria. • If the patient has pyuria or WBC casts, perform urine culture to rule out urinary tract infection. • If systemic infectious disease is suspected, submit serum for titers.

IMAGING   N/A

OTHER DIAGNOSTIC PROCEDURES

Consider renal biopsy if renal disease is persistent and progressive and the cause cannot be determined from routine and special laboratory tests.

TREATMENT

• Treat as outpatient unless the patient is dehydrated or has decompensated renal failure.
• If the patient is healthy otherwise, allow normal diet and exercise.

MEDICATIONS

DRUGS AND FLUIDS

• If the patient cannot maintain hydration, administer lactated Ringer's solution or a maintenance fluid either subcutaneously or intravenously. • If the patient has dehydration or continuing fluid losses such as vomiting or diarrhea, administer fluids intravenously to correct hydration deficits, maintain daily fluid requirements, and replace ongoing losses.

CONTRAINDICATIONS

Avoid nephrotoxic drugs.

PRECAUTIONS N/A

POSSIBLE INTERACTIONS N/A

ALTERNATE DRUGS N/A

FOLLOW-UP

PATIENT MONITORING

Physical examination including patient's weight to assess hydration status

POSSIBLE COMPLICATIONS

Renal failure depending on underlying cause of cylindruria

MISCELLANEOUS

ASSOCIATED CONDITIONS N/A

AGE RELATED FACTORS N/A

ZOONOTIC POTENTIAL N/A

PREGNANCY N/A

SYNONYMS N/A

SEE ALSO N/A

ABBREVIATIONS

DIC = disseminated intravascular coagulation
FDP = fibrin degradation products
PTT = partial thromboplastin time
PT = prothrombin time
RBC = red blood cells
WBC = white blood cells

References

Osborne CA, Stevens JB. Handbook of canine and feline urinalysis. St. Louis: Ralston Purina Company, 1981:91-118.

Lees GE, Willard MD, Green RA. Urinary disorders. In: Willard MD, Tvedten H, Turnwald GH, eds. Small animal clinical diagnosis by laboratory methods. Philadelphia: WB Saunders, 1994:115-146.

Chew DJ, DiBartola SP. Diagnosis and pathophysiology of renal disease. In: Ettinger SJ, ed. Textbook of veterinary internal medicine., Philadelphia: WB Saunders, 1994;1893-1961.

Author S. Dru Forrester
Consulting Editors Larry G. Adams and Carl A. Osborne

EOSINOPHILIA AND BASOPHILIA

 BASICS

DEFINITION
• Peripheral blood eosinophil count > 750-1000/µL (reference range may vary regionally) • Peripheral blood basophil count > 200/µL or a minimum of 3-6% of the differential count

Pathophysiology
• Eosinophilia develops in response to a primary disease process. Highest counts are seen in patients with hypereosinophilic syndrome, disseminated mast cell tumor, flea allergy, asthma, and some parasitic diseases. The level of eosinophilia does not predict the degree of eosinophilic infiltration of tissues, which can be significant even in the absence of eosinophilia. Eosinophilia results from heightened bone marrow production in response to specific stimuli (e.g., allergens, parasitic antigens, and products of tumor cells). Repeated exposure to an antigen produces a more rapid and dramatic eosinophilia. Eosinophils can kill parasites and may contribute to host defense against tumors. Eosinophil-derived products can also cause destruction of host tissue. Whether eosinophilic inflammation is beneficial or harmful varies according to the situation. • Basophils play a role in immune-mediated inflammation, especially anaphylaxis and cutaneous hypersensitivity, but specific stimuli are not well characterized. Basophils may participate in host rejection of parasites (especially ticks) and may play a role in tumor cytotoxicity. Basophilia often accompanies eosinophilia, especially in patients with ectoparasites (mites) and dirofilariasis. Basophil numbers may increase when there is sustained lipemia or altered lipid metabolism.

Systems Affected
• Skin, respiratory tract, gastrointestinal tract, and urogenital tract during estrus commonly affected • In patients with hypereosinophilic syndrome or eosinophilic leukemia, common sites of eosinophilic infiltration are the gastrointestinal tract, liver, spleen, and lymph nodes, especially mesenteric lymph nodes.

SIGNALMENT N/A

SIGNS

General Comments
Signs usually relate to underlying disease process, not eosinophilia or basophilia per se.

Historical Findings
• Signs associated with skin (e.g., pruritus, flea infestation, alopecia, and crusty lesions), respiratory tract (e.g., coughing and dyspnea), and gastrointestinal tract (vomiting, diarrhea, anorexia, and weight loss) • Lethargy and depression

Physical Examination Findings
• Physical abnormalities associated with the primary disease • Skin disease—pruritus, alopecia, miliary dermatitis, oral lesions, other cutaneous lesions, regional lymphadenopathy, and plaques, granulomas, or indolent ulcers • Respiratory disease—abnormal lung sounds, coughing, tachypnea, and dyspnea • Gastrointestinal disease—thickened intestines and mesenteric lymphadenopathy • Reproductive conditions—estrus or vaginal discharge with fluid-filled uterus (e.g., pyometra) • Neoplasia—mass lesions and lymphadenopathy

CAUSES

Eosinophilia
Causes listed are associated with tissue infiltrates of eosinophils with or without accompanying basophilic infiltration. Circulating eosinophilia is a variable finding.
Parasitism
Especially parasites that invade tissues; migrating helminthic parasites, particularly Toxocara spp, Strongyloides stercoralis, and Ancylostoma spp; Dirofilaria immitis and Dipetalonema reconditum; respiratory helminths (dogs and cats)—Capillaria aerophila, Paragonimus kellicotti; cats—Aleurostrongylus abstrusus; dogs—Oslerus osleri, Filaroides hirthi, Crenosoma vulpis, and Andersonstrongylus milksi; ectoparasites (e.g., mites and fleas), protozoa (e.g., Giardia, Coccidia, Toxoplasma, and Neosporum), Trichinella spiralis, and Cuterebra
Hypersensitivity Reactions and Other Inflammatory Conditions
• Skin—hypersensitivity to fleas and mites, reaction to insect bites (e.g., hymenoptera), food allergy, inhalant allergic dermatitis (ie, atopy), eosinophilic granuloma complex (indolent ulcer, plaque, granuloma) in cats, eosinophilic granuloma in dogs, sterile eosinophilic folliculitis in cats, sterile eosinophilic pustulosis in dogs, and chronic inflammation of skin • Respiratory tract—chronic upper respiratory infection and rhinitis or sinusitis in cats, allergic bronchopulmonary disease (asthma, bronchitis, pneumonitis) in cats; less commonly seen in dogs as part of chronic obstructive pulmonary disease), parasitic pneumonia, granulomatous disease in dogs (mostly dirofilariasis), pulmonary infiltrates with eosinophilia (PIE—nonspecific term that includes pulmonary eosinophilic granulomatosis, eosinophilic pneumonia, bronchitis, bronchioloitis, and alveolitis caused by parasitism, allergic disease, dirofilariasis, drug reactions, bacterial and fungal infection, neoplasia, and idiopathic disease), focal pneumonia, pneumothorax, foreign body, chronic inflammation of the lung, and lymphomatoid granulomatosis • Gastrointestinal tract—endoparasitism, oral or gastrointestinal eosinophilic granuloma, eosinophilic gastroenterocolitis (caused by dietary, bacterial, toxic, parasitic, and altered mucosal antigens) in dogs may be isolated to one segment of the GI tract, eosinophilic gastroenteritis in cats may be part of the hypereosinophilic syndrome, and bacterial infection (including Helicobacter) • Urogenital tract—estrus (occasionally in dogs), pyometra, chronic inflammation of the reproductive tract, and urologic syndrome in cats • Musculoskeletal system (dogs)—eosinophilic myositis, panosteitis, immune-mediated polyarthritis, idiopathic eosinophilic polyarthritis, diskospondylitis (Airedale) • Other inflammatory conditions—chronic fungal (e.g., gastric phycomycosis, disseminated coccidioidomycosis, and cryptococcosis of CNS) and protozoal (e.g., hepatozoonosis and granulomatous meningoencephalitis) diseases • Tumor-associated eosinophilia (paraneoplastic syndrome)—most commonly observed in patients with mast cell tumor (visceral or disseminated) and lymphoma and occasionally other neoplasms (e.g., carcinoma and sarcoma) • Myeloproliferative disease—dogs and cats • Hypereosinophilic syndrome (including gastroentiritis in cats) • FeLV-associated eosinophilia (Rickard strain) and eosinophilic leukemia (rare) • Miscellaneous—hypoadrenocorticism, eosinophilic meningoencephalitis (e.g., idiopathic steroid-responsive, protozoal, migrating helminths), immune-mediated disease (e.g., systemic lupus erythematosus and AIHA), vaccine reaction (e.g., SQ rabies inoculation with granulomatous response), drug reaction (e.g., cyclophosphamide and phenol), administration of IL-2 or GM-CSF • Miscellaneous (cats)—eosinophilic keratitis and conjunctivitis, hyperthyroidism, panleukopenia, infectious peritonitis, chronic gingivitis, infections with Staphylococcus and Streptococcus spp, and cardiac disease • Most common diseases inciting eosinophilia in cats—flea allergy dermatitis, eosinophilic granuloma complex, allergic bronchitis, chronic upper respiratory infection, chronic rhinitis and sinusitis, and gastrointestinal disease with endoparasitism

Basophilia
• Parasitism—dirofilariasis (especially occult), tick infestation, other ectoparasites, and tracheal parasites • Often accompanies eosinophilia (e.g., caused by chronic inflammation of mucosal and skin surfaces, disseminated mast cell tumor, and PIE) • Lymphomatoid granulomatosis • Basophilic leukemia • Possibly in animals with altered lipid metabolism that have sustained lipemia (e.g., chronic liver disease, nephrotic syndrome, genetic hyperlipoproteinemia, and endocrinopathy such as hyperadrenocorticism, diabetes mellitus, and hypothyroidism)

RISK FACTORS
Parasitism, hypersensitivity disorder, inflammation, and neoplasia

EOSINOPHILIA AND BASOPHILIA

DIAGNOSIS

DIFFERENTIAL DIAGNOSIS

• Pruritus, alopecia, dermatitis, ulcer/plaque/granuloma, flea infestation—rule out atopy, flea or food allergy, eosinophilic granuloma complex, other disorders of hypersensitivity, and other inflammatory disorders of the skin • Coughing, dyspnea, tachypnea—rule out allergic diseases of respiratory tract (e.g., bronchitis and asthma), parasitic diseases (e.g., dirofilariasis and lungworm), PIE, and chronic inflammation • Nodular lung lesions with eosinophilia—rule out mycotic infection, idiopathic eosinophilic granuloma, primary or metastatic neoplasia, and lymphomatoid granulomatosis • Vomiting, diarrhea, weight loss—rule out eosinophilic gastroenterocolitis, parasitism, and hypereosinophilic syndrome • Lymphadenopathy or mass lesion—rule out mast cell tumor, lymphoma, other neoplasms, and hypereosinophilic syndrome

LABORATORY FINDINGS

Drugs That May Alter Lab Results

Corticosteroid-induced eosinopenia can mask eosinophilia.

Disorders That May Alter Lab Results

N/A

Valid If Run in Human Lab?

Valid; laboratory should be informed that basophils in cats have beige-gray or mauve, round granules.

CBC/BIOCHEMISTRY/URINALYSIS

• Eosinophilia and basophilia • Biochemical analysis may detect organ dysfunction.

OTHER LABORATORY TESTS

• Fecal flotation test to identify parasitic ova; repeat examination • Baermann sedimentation test to identify parasite larvae (especially nematode lungworms) • Heartworm identification (e.g., Knott test and ELISA to detect Dirofilaria antigen) • Cytologic examination of tracheobronchial fluid to identify eosinophilic inflammation, ova, and larvae • Examination of skin, mucosal (e.g., oral and rectal) and corneal or conjunctival scrapings for eosinophilic infiltrates and possible cause of eosinophilia? • Examination of buffy coat

for mast cells, presence of which may indicate disseminated mast cell tumor

IMAGING

• Survey radiography of thorax to detect lung disease (e.g., diffuse, peribronchial, interstitial, or alveolar patterns) and of abdomen to detect mass lesions • Contrast studies of gastrointestinal tract to identify mucosal irregularities and wall thickenings • Ultrasonography of thoracic or abdominal mass

OTHER DIAGNOSTIC PROCEDURES

• Intradermal skin testing (atopy) • Transtracheal wash or bronchoalveolar lavage (respiratory disease) • Examination of fine needle aspirate or biopsy of mass lesion, skin, gastrointestinal tract, lung, or lymph nodes to rule out bone marrow neoplasia • Endoscopy (gastrointestinal disease) • Laparotomy • Exclusion diet, flea eradication, or medical trial of corticosteroids or other medications

TREATMENT

• Treatment varies with the primary cause. • Because eosinophils can cause damage to host cells, treatment aimed at decreasing or eliminating eosinophilic infiltrates may be required.

MEDICATIONS

DRUGS AND FLUIDS

• Specific medications for the primary disease (e.g., hyposensitization to treat atopy, anthelminthic and other parasiticidal drugs, hypoallergenic diet, chemotherapy for neoplasia) • Corticosteroids are the most effective antiinflammatory drug for treating eosinophil-related disorders (e.g., prednisolone—1 mg/kg q12h, then taper by giving q24h, then alternate days to lowest dose that is still effective). • For some conditions, cytotoxic drugs such as hydroxyurea may be required.

CONTRAINDICATIONS

In general, corticosteroids are contraindicated in patients with sepsis.

PRECAUTIONS

• Corticosteroids are associated with hepatopathy and pancreatitis and affect the pituitary-adrenal axis.

• Chemotherapeutic agents have toxic effects (e.g., myelosuppression).

POSSIBLE INTERACTIONS N/A

ALTERNATE DRUGS N/A

FOLLOW-UP

PATIENT MONITORING

Monitor primary disease as indicated; recheck CBC for eosinophil and basophil counts.

POSSIBLE COMPLICATIONS

Eosinophilic infiltrates can cause severe tissue damage.

MISCELLANEOUS

ASSOCIATED CONDITIONS

Basophilia is often associated with eosinophilia.

AGE RELATED FACTORS N/A

ZOONOTIC POTENTIAL

Some parasitic diseases

PREGNANCY

Corticosteroids and chemotherapeutic agents may be contraindicated in pregnant animals.

SYNONYMS N/A

SEE ALSO

Hypereosinophilic syndrome

ABBREVIATIONS

CNS = central nervous system
PIE = pulmonary infiltrates with eosinophilia

References

Center SA, Randolph JF. Eosinophilia. In: August JR, ed. Consultations in feline internal medicine. Philadelphia: WB Saunders, 1991.

Taboada J. Pulmonary diseases of potential allergic origin. Sem Vet Med Surg 1991;6:278-285.

Tvedten H. Leukocyte disorders. In: Willard MD, Tvedten H, Turnwald GH, eds. Small animal clinical diagnosis by laboratory methods. Philadelphia: WB Saunders, 1994:63-66.

Author Karen M. Young
Consulting Editor Alan H. Rebar

GLOBULIN

BASICS

DEFINITION
Hyperglobulinemia is a higher than normal concentration of globulins, which are the serum proteins excluding albumin. Hypoglobulinemia is a lower than normal concentration of globulins proteins. Globulin types include alpha-1, alpha-2, beta-1, beta-2, and gamma globulins, and are differentiated by electrophoretic mobility. Gamma globulins include the immunoglobulins.

Pathophysiology
Hyperglobulinemia can be either relative (ie, secondary to hemoconcentration) or absolute. Absolute hyperglobulinemia occurs in animals with marked immunostimulation, which promotes hepatic synthesis of acute phase reactants and plasma cell synthesis of immunoglobulins, and in animals with neoplastic diseases that synthesize a single type of immunoglobulin in very large quantities (i.e., monoclonal gammopathy). In animals with marked hyperglobulinemia, serum viscosity increases resulting in impaired circulation and hypertension.
Hypoglobulinemia occurs when inadequate globulin is synthesized or globulins are lost from the body. Inadequate synthesis of globulin is seen in animals with deficiencies of the humoral immune system. Globulins may be lost via blood loss or through the gastrointestinal tract in patients with protein-losing enteropathy.

Systems Affected
Hyperglobulinemia
• Cardiovascular—marked hyperglobulinemia can cause hyperviscosity which results in high cardiac afterload and hypertension.
• Ophthalmic—hyperviscosity can cause tortuous retinal vessels, retinal hemorrhage, retinal detachment, and blindness. • Nervous—hyperviscosity can cause depression, dementia, seizures, and loss of consciousness.
Hypoglobulinemia
Hemic/Lymphatic/Immune—hypoglobulinemia associated with impaired humoral function is often accompanied by recurrent infection of the respiratory tract, skin, and gastrointestinal tract.

SIGNALMENT
• Hyperglobulinemia associated with neoplasia is more commonly seen in older animals. • Mild hypoglobulinemia is a normal finding in young puppies and kittens. • Puppies show early signs of immunodeficiency associated with hypoglobulinemia. • Breeds with deficiencies in humoral immunity that may lead to hypoglobulinemia include beagle, German shepherd dog, shar pei, doberman pinscher, and samoyed.

SIGNS

Hyperglobulinemia
• Depression, seizures, and other central nervous system signs • Blindness

Hypoglobulinemia
• Diarrhea • Recurrent upper respiratory infections • Pneumonia • Dermatitis

CAUSES

Hyperglobulinemia: Polyclonal Gammopathy
Infection/inflammation
Chronic bacterial diseases
• Pyoderma • Pneumonia • Pyometra
Chronic fungal diseases
• Blastomycosis • Histoplasmosis
• Coccidioidomycosis • Cryptococcosis
Chronic protozoal/ rickettsial diseases
• Ehrlichiosis • Babesiosis • Leishmaniasis
• Typanosomiasis (Chagas' disease) • Hemobartonellosis
Chronic viral diseases
Feline infectious peritonitis • Feline leukemia virus • Feline immunodeficiency virus
Neoplasia
• Lymphoma • Mast cell tumor • Other tumors
Autoimmune disorders
• Systemic lupus erythematosus • Chronic polyarthritis • Others

Hyperglobulinemia: Monoclonal Gammopathy
Neoplasia
• Multiple myeloma • Lymphoma
• Chronic lymphocytic leukemia
Inflammation/infection
• Ehrlichiosis • Leishmaniasis
Idiopathic
• Waldenstrom macroglobulinemia • Benign monoclonal gammopathy

Hypoglobulinemia
• Normal in puppy/kitten • Blood loss
Gastrointestinal loss
Lymphangiectasia • Intestinal neoplasia
• Inflammatory bowel disease • Intestinal histoplasmosis • Other severe protein-losing enteropathy
Humoral immunodeficiency
IgA deficiency • IgM deficiency • Transient hypogammaglobulinemia

RISK FACTORS:
• Hyperglobulinemia is often associated with either chronic inflammation or neoplasia.

DIAGNOSIS

DIFFERENTIAL DIAGNOSIS

Hyperglobulinemia
• Evidence of chronic infection or inflammation (eg, dermatitis, nasal discharge, cough, fever) supports inflammation or infection as the cause. • Splenomegaly, weight loss, neurologic abnormalities, and pale mucous membranes support neoplasia as the cause.

Hypoglobulinemia
• Evidence of blood loss or diarrhea support loss of globulins. • Chronic infection and fever support immunologic impairment.

LABORATORY FINDINGS

Drugs that may alter lab results N/A

Disorders that may alter lab results
• Dehydration and hemoconcentration increase globulins • Lipemia increases globulins • Hemolysis increases globulins

Valid if run in a human lab? Yes

CBC/BIOCHEMISTRY/URINALYSIS
• Evidence of leukemia—may cause hyperglobulinemia • Anemia, neutropenia, and thrombocytopenia may be associated with bone marrow neoplasia or some infections (eg, ehrlichiosis) that cause hyperglobulinemia
• Hypoalbuminemia in some animals with hyperglobulinemia • Hypoalbuminemia and hypoglobulinemia associated with gastrointestinal protein loss or blood loss • Proteinuria in animal with hyperglobulinemia associated with multiple myeloma or accompanying glomerular diseases

OTHER LABORATORY TESTS
• Serum protein electrophoresis differentiates polyclonal from monoclonal gammopathy as a cause of hyperglobulinemia. • Immunoelectrophoresis identifies increases in specific immunoglobulins (important in animals with monoclonal gammopathy) or decreases in a specific immunoglobulin in animals with hypoglobulinemia. • Serum viscosity testing to assess hyperviscosity seen in animals with some monoclonal (and occasional polyclonal) gammopathies resulting in severe hyperglobulinemia. • Appropriate tests for infectious/inflammatory diseases that may cause polyclonal or monoclonal gammopathies

IMAGING
• Thoracic radiographs may identify neoplasia, fungal diseases, or pneumonia. • Radiographs of bones may identify lesions associated with multiple myeloma.

OTHER DIAGNOSTIC PROCEDURES
• Examination of bone marrow aspirate is indicated in patients with monoclonal gammopathy to identify leukemia or multiple myeloma as cause of hyperglobulinemia.
• Intestinal biopsy may be indicated in patients with hypoglobulinemia associated with protein-losing enteropathy.

TREATMENT
• Hyperglobulinemia associated with signs of hyperviscosity is a medical emergency. Phlebotomy with crystalloid fluid replacement is indicated immediately to reduce serum viscosity.
• Hyperglobulinemia not associated with hyperviscosity should be thoroughly evaluated before any treatment is instituted. Supportive care should be given if the patient is clinically ill.
• Animals with hypoglobulinemia associated with humoral immunodeficiency should receive treatment for opportunistic infection while being diagnosed.

MEDICATIONS

DRUGS AND FLUIDS
• Animals undergoing phlebotomy to relieve hyperviscosity should receive a balanced electrolyte solution (eg, lactated Ringer's solution) during and after phlebotomy.
• Additional treatment varies with the underlying cause

CONTRAINDICATIONS N/A
PRECAUTIONS N/A
POSSIBLE INTERACTIONS N/A
ALTERNATE DRUGS N/A

FOLLOW-UP

PATIENT MONITORING
• Animals with hyperglobulinemia and hyperviscosity should have serum globulin concentrations monitored hourly until clinical signs resolve. • Animals with hyperglobulinemia should have serum globulins monitored every 1-2 months if the animal is not symptomatic. • Animals with hypoglobulinemia associated with humoral immunodeficiency should be monitored by the owner for recurrent infection.

POSSIBLE COMPLICATIONS
• Hyperglobulinemia may cause neurologic abnormalities and sudden blindness if hyperviscosity occurs. • Hypoglobulinemia associated with humoral immunodeficiency may allow recurrent infection to occur.

MISCELLANEOUS

ASSOCIATED CONDITIONS
• Hyperglobulinemia is often associated with hypoalbuminemia. • Hypoglobulinemia associated with gastrointestinal protein loss or blood loss is often accompanied by hypoalbuminemia

AGE RELATED FACTORS
• Older animals are more prone to neoplasia as a cause of hyperglobulinemia. • Young animals normally have low globulin concentrations. • Young animals may show signs compatible with humoral immunodeficiency.

ZOONOTIC POTENTIAL N/A
PREGNANCY N/A
SYNONYMS
• Gammopathy • Hypergammaglobulinemia
• Hypogammaglobulinemia

SEE ALSO:
Refer to diseases causing hypo- and hyperglobulinemia

ABBREVIATIONS N/A

References

Dimski DS. Paraproteinemias in small animal medicine. Comp Cont Ed Pract Vet 1992; 14:1259-1262.
Guilford WG. Primary immunodeficiency diseases of dogs and cats. Comp Cont Ed Pract Vet 1987; 9: 641-650.
Author Donna S. Dimski
Consulting Editor Albert E. Jergens

GLUCOSE, HYPERGLYCEMIA

BASICS

DEFINITION
High concentration of glucose in whole blood, plasma, or serum

Pathophysiology
Hyperglycemia may result from absolute or relative insulin deficiency, reduced utilization of glucose in peripheral tissue, increased gluconeogenesis in the liver, and increased glycogenolysis. Insulin antagonists or counterregulatory hormones (e.g., cortisol, adrenocorticotropic hormone [ACTH], growth hormone, epinephrine, and glucagon) also contribute to hyperglycemia.

Systems Affected
• Endocrine/metabolic—primarily because of regulating carbohydrate metabolism • Renal/urologic—osmotic diuresis caused by hyperglycemia causes polyuria with secondary polydipsia • Nervous—severe hyperglycemia may cause CNS dysfunction by increasing serum osmolality • Ophthalmic—persistent hyperglycemia (e.g., diabetes mellitus) can cause cataracts in dogs

SIGNALMENT N/A

SIGNS

General Comments
Clinical signs vary and often reflect underlying disease. Some patients are asymptomatic, especially those with transient stress-induced and postprandial hyperglycemia.

Historical Findings
• Variable • Polydipsia • Polyuria • Depression • Weight loss • Obesity • Polyphagia • CNS depression (severe hyperglycemia)

Physical Examination Findings
Often normal, but can include:
• Nonhealing wounds • Abscesses • Obesity • Cataracts • Hepatomegaly

CAUSES
• Low glucose utilization—diabetes mellitus, acute pancreatitis, acromegaly (excessive growth hormone) in cats, high progesterone during diestrus (dogs), renal insufficiency, and following pancreatectomy to treat insulinoma • High glucose production—hyperadrenocorticism, pheochromocytoma, glucagonoma, and exocrine pancreatic neoplasia • Physiologic—postprandial fluctuation, exertion or excitement, and stress (epinephrine-induced), especially in cats • Drugs—thiazide diuretics, morphine, dextrose-containing fluids, progestens (e.g., megestrol acetate [Ovaban]), growth hormone, glucocorticoids, and ACTH • Insulin administration problems in confirmed diabetics—Somogyi phenomenon, antiinsulin antibodies, and poor insulin absorption • Parenteral administration of nutritional solutions • Laboratory error

RISK FACTORS
• Concurrent disease—hyperadrenocorticism, acromegaly, and acute pancreatitis • Diabetogenic drugs • Dextrose-containing fluids

DIAGNOSIS

DIFFERENTIAL DIAGNOSIS
Mild, transiently high blood glucose can be associated with stress and epinephrine-induced excitement or normal postprandial fluctuation. In patients with mild hyperglycemia and no history of polydipsia/polyuria, repeat blood glucose after 12-hour fast and eliminate or minimize stress (i.e., allow time for acclimation to hospital environment).

LABORATORY FINDINGS

Drugs That May Alter Lab Results
• High blood glucose concentration—glucocorticoids, ACTH, dextrose-containing fluids, epinephrine, asparaginase, beta adrenergic agonists, and diazoxide • Low blood glucose concentration determined by enzymatic methods—aspirin, ascorbic acid, and acetaminophen

Disorders That May Alter Lab Results
• Lipemia, hemolysis, and icterus may interfere with spectrophotometric assays. • Delayed serum separation artificially lowers glucose concentration. Serum must be separated within 1 hour of collection to prevent cellular utilization of glucose. Refrigerate or freeze serum sample if not analyzed within 12 hours. Blood glucose reagent strips require whole blood. Whole blood glucose concentration should be measured within 30 minutes of collection. • Sodium fluoride collection tubes allow more stable readings and can prevent artificially low readings by spectrophotometry. Do not use for enzymatic assays.

Valid If Run in Human Lab?
Valid

CBC/BIOCHEMISTRY/URINALYSIS
• Hyperglycemia may be the only abnormal finding. • CBC may be normal; possible inflammatory leukogram in patients with infection. • Urinalysis may be normal; possible abnormalties include glucosuria, pyuria, bacteruria, and ketonuria. • Fasting hyperglycemia plus glucosuria suggests diabetes mellitus, although mild hyperglycemia and glucosuria can be physiologic in cats. • Lipemia is associated with low lipoprotein lipase, hyperadrenocorticism, acute pancreatitis, and postprandial blood sampling. • High amylase and lipase activity suggest acute pancreatitis, especially in nonazotemic patients. • High liver enzyme activity may accompany fatty infiltration.

OTHER LABORATORY TESTS
• ACTH stimulation or low-dose dexametha-sone suppression test to rule out hyperadrenocorticism • Serum insulin concentration. Normally, hyperglycemia is accompanied by hyperinsulinemia. Hyperglycemia with low serum insulin suggests diabetes mellitus. • Although rarely indicated, IV glucose and a glucagon tolerance test may help demonstrate carbohydrate intolerance. Blood glucose should return to normal within 60 minutes and serum insulin should increase after IV glucose or glucagon administration. • Serum osmolarity should be determined in patients with moderate to severe hyperglycemia.

IMAGING
Abdominal radiography and ultrasonography may provide valuable information regarding underlying causes.

OTHER DIAGNOSTIC PROCEDURES
N/A

TREATMENT
• Minimize or eliminate stress.
• Avoid abrupt decreases in blood glucose.
• Diabetogenic drugs should be discontinued or the dosage adjusted to normalize blood glucose while maintaining therapeutic concentration.
• Avoid semimoist commercial foods because of the higher content of simple sugars.
• Institute a high-protein, low-carbohydrate, low-fat, high-fiber diet.

MEDICATIONS

DRUGS AND FLUIDS
• Insulin—regular (crystalline) insulin has a more rapid onset of effect but a shorter duration of action than other types of insulin • Dextrose-free fluids

CONTRAINDICATIONS
• Diabetogenic drugs (e.g., glucocorticoids) • Dextrose-containing fluids

PRECAUTIONS
Avoid abruptly lowering blood glucose and causing hypoglycemia.

POSSIBLE INTERACTIONS N/A

ALTERNATE DRUGS
Oral administration of hypoglycemic agents—sulfonylureas (e.g., glipizide [Glucotrol]) and biguanides are most useful in cats with type II (noninsulin dependent) diabetes mellitus.

FOLLOW-UP

PATIENT MONITORING
• Blood glucose after initiating treatment and discontinuing diabetogenic drugs • Glucose curves by measuring blood glucose hourly or

every 2 hours for 12-24 hours after insulin administration • Glycosylated hemoglobin and fructosamine on an outpatient basis to monitor long-term glucose control • Insulin concentrations after treatment • For return of clinical signs such as polyuria, polydipsia, and polyphagia

POSSIBLE COMPLICATIONS

• High incidence of sepsis (and infection) • Severe hyperglycemia may be associated with CNS depression and coma as a result of hyperosmolarity.

MISCELLANEOUS

ASSOCIATED CONDITIONS

• Severe hyperglycemia associated with hyperosmolarity • Uremia may be associated with hyperglycemia. • Hyperglycemia associated with acidosis, hyponatremia, hypokalemia, and hypophosphatemia. Although total body concentrations of these electrolytes are low, serum chemistry measurements of these electrolytes may be normal, high, or low.

AGE RELATED FACTORS N/A

ZOONOTIC POTENTIAL N/A

PREGNANCY

Pregnancy-induced diabetes mellitus caused by high progesterone concentration reported in humans

SYNONYM

"High blood sugar"

SEE ALSO

• Diabetes Mellitus • Hyperosmolarity

ABBREVIATION

ACTH = adrenocorticotropic hormone

References

Willard MD, Tvedten H, Turnwald GH. Small animal clinical diagnosis by laboratory methods. 2nd ed. Philadelphia: WB Saunders, 1994:154-160.

Rich LJ, Coles EH. Tables of abnormal blood values as a guide to disease syndromes. In: Ettinger SJ, Feldman EC, eds. Textbook of veterinary internal medicine. 4th ed. Philadelphia: WB Saunders, 1995:11-17.

Kaneko JJ. Carbohydrate metabolism and its diseases. In: Clinical biochemistry of domestic animals. 4th ed. San Diego: Academic Press, 1989:44-85.

Author Margaret R. Kern
Consulting Editor Rhett Nichols

GLUCOSE, HYPOGLYCEMIA

BASICS

Abnormally low blood glucose concentration

Pathophysiology

Mechanisms responsible for hypoglycemia:
• Excess insulin or insulinlike factors (e.g., insulinoma, extrapancreatic paraneoplasia, and iatrogenic insulin overdose) • Reduction of hormones needed for maintenance of normal serum glucose (e.g., hypoadrenocorticism)
• Reduced hepatic gluconeogenesis (e.g., hepatic disease, glycogen storage diseases, and sepsis) • Excessive utilization (e.g., hunting dogs, pregnancy, neoplasia, polycythemia, and sepsis) • Reduced intake or underproduction (e.g., puppies and kittens, toy breeds, and severe malnutrition or starvation)

Systems Affected

• Nervous • Musculoskeletal

SIGNALMENT

Variable depending on the underlying cause

SIGNS

• Seizures • Posterior paresis • Weakness
• Collapse • Muscle fasciculations
• Abnormal behavior • Lethargy and depression • Ataxia • Polyphagia • Weight gain
• Polyuria and polydipsia (PU/PD) • Exercise intolerance • Some animals appear normal aside from findings associated with underlying disease.

CAUSES

Endocrine

• Insulinoma • Extrapancreatic paraneoplasia
• Iatrogenic insulin overdose • Hypoadrenocorticism

Hepatic Disease

• Portosystemic shunt • Cirrhosis • Severe hepatitis (e.g., toxic and inflammatory) • Glycogen storage diseases

Overutilization

• Hunting dog hypoglycemia • Pregnancy
• Polycythemia • Neoplasia • Sepsis

Reduced Intake/Underproduction

• Young puppies and kittens • Toy breed dogs • Severe malnutrition or starvation

RISK FACTORS

• Low energy intake predisposes hypoglycemia in patients with conditions causing overutilization and underproduction.
• Fasting, excitement, exercise, and eating may or may not increase the risk of hypoglycemic episodes in patients with insulinoma.

DIAGNOSIS

DIFFERENTIAL DIAGNOSIS

• Patients with hyperinsulinism have signs of hypoglycemia or a normal physical examination. • Patients with hypoadrenocorticism have waxing and waning and nonspecific

signs (e.g., vomiting, diarrhea, melena, and weakness). Crisis in patients on examination usually is caused by hypovolemia and hyperkalemia rather than hypoglycemia (e.g., shock, bradycardia, and dehydration).
• Patients with portosystemic shunts are usually young to middle-aged and are often thin or appear to have stunted growth. PU/PD is more common in patients with hypoglycemia; rarely, animals have ascites or edema. • Patients with cirrhosis and severe hepatitis usually have other signs of their disease (e.g., gastrointestinal signs, icterus, and ascites or edema). • Patients with sepsis are very sick, usually in shock, have pyrexia or hypothermia on examination, and may have gastrointestinal signs. • Glycogen storage diseases are rare and usually seen in animals < 1 year old. • Hypoglycemia caused by extrapancreatic paraneoplasia and large neoplastic processes is often identifiable by physical examination.

LABORATORY FINDINGS

Drugs That May Alter Lab Results N/A

Disorders That May Alter Lab Results

Delayed separation of serum causes falsely low serum glucose. If blood cannot be centrifuged and the serum separated within 30 minutes of collection, blood should be collected in a sodium fluoride tube.

Valid If Run in Human Lab? Valid

CBC/BIOCHEMISTRY/URINALYSIS

• Patients with hypoadrenocorticism may have lymphocytosis, eosinophilia, hyperkalemia, hyponatremia, azotemia, and hypercalcemia. • Patients with portosystemic shunts may have microcytosis, hypoalbuminemia, low BUN, mildly high activity of liver enzymes, urate crystals, and low urine specific gravity. • Patients with cirrhosis, severe hepatitis, and neoplasia may have anemia associated with chronic disease, high activity of liver enzymes, hyperbilirubinemia, hypoalbuminemia, bilirubinuria, and low urine specific gravity. • Patients with polycythemia have a PCV > 65.

OTHER LABORATORY TESTS

• Simultaneous fasting glucose/insulin determination—indicated when insulinoma is suspected. High plasma insulin in the face of hypoglycemia suggests insulinoma. • Amended insulin-glucose ratio (AIGR)—indicated when insulinoma is suspected. • AIGR = (plasma insulin [mU/ml] x 100)/(plasma glucose [mg/dl] - 30); use 1 as denominator if glucose is < 30 • AIGR > 30 suggests insulinoma • AIGR = 19-30 gray zone, repeat test • AIGR < 19 insulinoma unlikely • Note: False-positive results are possible, especially when the blood glucose concentration is < 40 mg/dl. • ACTH stimulation test—indicated when hypoadrenocorticism is suspected
• Fasting and postprandial serum bile acids— indicated when a portosystemic shunt or functional hepatic disease is suspected • Bacterial

culture of blood—indicated when sepsis is suspected

IMAGING

• Abdominal radiography and ultrasonography—useful in patients with extrapancreatic paraneoplasia and large neoplastic processes (may see organomegaly or masses), as well as portosystemic shunt (microhepatica), cirrhosis (microhepatica, hyperechogenicity), and severe hepatitis (hepatomegaly) • Thoracic radiography—to detect metastasis if neoplasia is suspected • Technetium 99m per rectal quantitative hepatic scintigraphy—useful to detect portosystemic shunt • Mesenteric portography—useful to detect portosystemic shunt (requires surgery)

OTHER DIAGNOSTIC PROCEDURES

• ECG—useful to evaluate bradycardia in patients with hypoadrenocorticism • Ultrasound-guided or surgical biopsy—useful to evaluate patient for cirrhosis, hepatitis, and glycogen storage diseases

TREATMENT

• Animals with clinical hypoglycemia and whose underlying disease needs support should be treated as inpatients.
• If able to eat (i.e., responsive, no vomiting), feeding should be part or all of initial treatment for hypoglycemia.
• Surgery is indicated if a portosystemic shunt or insulinoma is the cause of hypoglycemia.

MEDICATIONS

DRUGS AND FLUIDS

Emergency/Acute Treatment

• In hospital—administer 50% dextrose, 1 ml/kg IV
• At home—do not attempt to have the owner administer medication orally during a seizure; hypoglycemic seizures usually abate within 1-2 minutes. In the case of a prolonged seizure, recommend transportation to hospital. If a short seizure has occurred and ceased or other signs of a hypoglycemic crisis are present, recommend rubbing corn syrup or 50% dextrose on the buccal mucosa followed by 2 ml/kg of the same solution orally once the patient can swallow. Then, seek immediate attention.
• Frequent feeding of a diet low in simple sugars or, if unable to eat, continuous fluid therapy with 2.5% dextrose should be initiated.

Long-Term Treatment

• See Insulinoma for treatment of insulinoma and extrapancreatic paraneoplasia.
• Hunting dog hypoglycemia—feed moderate meal of fat, protein, and complex carbohydrates a few hours before hunting. Snacks (e.g., dog biscuits) can be fed during the hunt every 3-5 hours.

GLUCOSE, HYPOGLYCEMIA

• Toy breed hypoglycemia—increase the frequency of feeding
• Puppy and kitten hypoglycemia—increase the frequency of feeding (i.e., nursing or hand feeding)
• Other causes of hypoglycemia require treatment of the underlying disease and do not usually need long-term treatment.

CONTRAINDICATIONS

• Insulin • Barbiturates and diazepam in patients with hypoglycemic seizures because they do not treat the cause of the seizure and worsen hepatoencephalopathy in patients with portosystemic shunt and cirrhosis

PRECAUTIONS

• 50% dextrose causes tissue necrosis and sloughing if given extravascularly. Never give dextrose in concentrations over 5% without a confirmed vascular access.
• Administration of a dextrose bolus without following with frequent feedings or continuous IV fluids with dextrose can predispose to subsequent hypoglycemic episodes.

POSSIBLE INTERACTIONS N/A

ALTERNATE DRUGS N/A

FOLLOW-UP

PATIENT MONITORING

• At home for return or progression of clinical signs of hypoglycemia. Serum glucose should be assessed if signs recur. • Single, intermittent serum glucose determinations may not truly reflect the glycemic status of the patient because of normal production of counteregulatory hormones. • Other patient monitoring is based on the underlying disease.

POSSIBLE COMPLICATIONS

Recurrent, progressive episodes of hypoglycemia

MISCELLANEOUS

ASSOCIATED CONDITIONS N/A

AGE RELATED FACTORS

Neonatal animals have a poor glycogen storage capacity and a reduced ability to perform gluconeogenesis. As a result, short periods of fasting (6-12 hours) can cause hypoglycemia.

ZOONOTIC POTENTIAL N/A

PREGNANCY

• Hypoglycemia can lead to weakness and dystocia. • Pregnancy coupled with fasting causes hypoglycemia in rare instances.

SYNONYMS N/A

SEE ALSO

See causes

ABBREVIATION

AIGR = amended insulin-glucose ratio
PU/PD = polyuria and polydipsia

References

Leifer CE. Hypoglycemia. In: Kirk RW, ed. Current veterinary therapy IX. Philadelphia: WB Saunders, 1986:982-987.
Nelson RW. Disorders of the endocrine pancreas. In: Ettinger SJ, ed. Textbook of veterinary internal medicine. Philadelphia: WB Saunders, 1989:1676-1720.

Author Mitchell A. Crystal
Consulting Editor Rhett Nichols

HEMOGLOBINURIA AND MYOGLOBINURIA

BASICS

DEFINITION
Loss of hemoglobin or myoglobin through the glomeruli in an amount sufficient to cause a positive reaction to a test for blood in the urine when the patient is tested by the pseudophosphatase-orthotoluidine method.

Pathophysiology
• Intravascular hemolysis causes release of free hemoglobin into the plasma. Hemoglobin forms a complex with haptoglobin. Once haptoglobin is saturated, free hemoglobin appears in the blood, divides into subunits, and is cleared from the blood by the kidneys. Some unbound plasma hemoglobin releases ferriheme, which reversibly binds to either albumin (methemalbumin) or hemopexin, a plasma protein. Free hemoglobin, hemoglobin-haptoglobin complex, hemoglobin subunits, methemalbumin, ferriheme-hemopexin complex, and bilirubin all contribute to the color of plasma. Hemoglobin complexes, when in concentrations > about 50 mg/dl of plasma, are detectable as pink plasma. • Myoglobin released from damaged muscle does not bind to serum proteins, is rapidly cleared by the liver and kidneys, and is not associated with pink plasma. • Both hemoglobin and myoglobin are recovered and metabolized by the proximal renal tubule cells. Only after the renal tubular uptake mechanism is saturated will these proteins appear in the urine.

Systems Affected
• Renal/Urologic—hemoglobin and myoglobin can be nephrotoxic, particularly when renal perfusion is compromised. • Hemic/ Lymph/Immune—intravascular hemolysis, extensive muscle damage, and hypoxia can precipitate disseminated intravascular coagulopathy (DIC). • Low oxygen carrying capacity (acute) can lead to secondary central lobular liver cell damage, lactic acid acidosis, and shock, which in turn exacerbates hypoxia.

SIGNALMENT
• Copper associated liver disease in the Bedlington and West Highland white terrier
• Exertional lactic acidosis in the Old English sheepdog (i.e., hemoglobinuria)
• Exertional myopathy in the racing greyhound. Hematuria should clear within 6-12 hours; If not, myoglobinuria from muscle damage should be suspected. • Neonatal isoerythrolysis (blood type A queen with type B kitten) in the British shorthair, Doven rex, Abyssinian, Birman, Himalayan, Persian, Scottish fold, and Somali breeds. Neonates die within 2 days of birth. • Phosphofructokinase deficiency in the English springer spaniel male • Pyruvate kinase deficiency in the basenji and beagle; affected dogs < 3 years old

SIGNS

General Comments
A wide variety of clinical signs are associated with specific causes. See Causes.

Historical Findings
Breed and drug administration history are particularly important. See Signalment.

Physical Examination Findings
• Signs associated with anemia such as tachycardia, easy fatigue, pale mucous membrane, fever, and icterus are not seen in patients with muscle damage or hematuria. • Fever may be associated with intravascular hemolysis.
• DIC secondary to intravascular hemolysis or muscle trauma may induce hematuria.
• Patients with muscle damage have muscle tenderness or bruising.

CAUSES

Hemoglobinuria
Genetic Associated
• Pyruvate kinase deficiency • Phosphofructokinase deficiency • Exertional lactic acidosis in the Old English sheepdog • Copper-associated liver disease
Toxins And Drugs
• Chlorates • Benzocaine • Copper • Dimethyl sulfoxide (DMSO) • Menadione (Vitamin K3) • Mercury • Methylene blue • Nitrates • Methionine • Phenazopyridine • Paracetamol (acetaminophen) • Phenylhydrazine • Propylene glycol • Propylthiouracil • Snake venom (Elapidae) • Zinc
Plants
Onions
Physical Agents
• Burns (severe) • Crush injury • Electric shock • Extreme exercise • Heatstroke
• Hypoosomotic solution • Microangiopathy (e.g., caval syndrome and DIC)
Infectious Agents
• Babesiasis (i.e., B. canis but usually not B. gibsoni or B. vogeli) • Feline hemobartinellosis (rarely causes intravascular hemolysis)
• Leptospirosis (i.e., L. icterohemorhagica)
Immune-Mediated
• Idiopathic immune-mediated hemolytic anemia • Incompatible blood transfusion • Isoerythrolyis—blood type A queen with type B kittens • Systemic lupus erythematosis
Deficiencies
Hypophosphatemia (induced by hyperalimentation or diabetes mellitus).

Myoglobinuria
• Acute myositis (e.g., toxoplasmosis)
• Compartment syndrome • Crush injury
• Extreme exercise • Tourniquet syndrome
• Seizures (prolonged)

RISK FACTORS
• Genetic predisposition (see Signalment)
• Exposure to selected drugs and toxins (e.g., zinc cage bolts and copper and zinc coins)
• Extreme physical exertion

DIAGNOSIS

DIFFERENTIAL DIAGNOSIS
• Blood in the urine can be caused by hematuria, hemoglobinuria, and myoglobinuria; also, test results can be false. • RBC or ghost cells in the sediment suggests hematuria.
• Clear plasma suggests myoglobinuria or hematuria. • Pink plasma with positive blood test in urine suggests intravascular hemolysis. • Chocolate colored whole blood and a positive test for blood in the urine suggests specific hemolyzing-methemoglobin producing toxins (oxidants). • Hemoglobinuria without icterus suggests acute hemolytic anemia while both findings suggest chronic hemolytic anemia. • Icterus without hemoglobinuria suggests extravascular hemolysis or liver disease. • False positive results (see below)

LABORATORY FINDINGS
Drugs That May Alter Lab Results
• Vitamin C (ascorbic aid) administration
• Resusitation fluids containing polymerized hemoglobin

Disorders That May Alter Lab Results
• Low specific urine gravity (polyuric syndromes) lyses RBC • Bacteriuria (bacterial peroxidase) causes false positive • Formalin preservative causes false negative

VALID IF RUN IN HUMAN LAB? Yes

CBC/BIOCHEMISTRY/URINALYSIS
Intravascular Hemolysis
• Low and falling PCV, often accompanied by leukocytosis • Blood smear evaluation— possibly spherocytes, parasites, and Heinz bodies • Bilirubinemia and high ALT • Bilirubinuria

Rhabdomyolysis
• High creatine kinase
• High AST

OTHER LABORATORY TESTS
• Ammonium sulfate precipitation test— 5 ml of urine is mixed well with 2.8 mg of ammonium sulfate and centrifuged. Hemoglobin precipitates, myoglobin does not. If the supernatant remains dark after centrifugation, suspect myoglobinuria.
• New methylene blue stained blood film to detect Heinz bodies • Methemoglobin in RBC helps identify toxin as an oxidant.
• Haptoglobin concentration is low if the patient has acute or chronic progressive intravascular hemolysis. • Liver biopsy for copper concentration • Serum copper and zinc concentrations

IMAGING
• Abdominal radiography may reveal coins or cage bolts or nuts in the gastrointestinal tract. • Abnormal liver size and conformation in patients with copper-associated liver disease

HEMOGLOBINURIA AND MYOGLOBINURIA

OTHER DIAGNOSTIC PROCEDURES
• Forced exercise (Old English sheepdog)
• Liver biopsy (copper-associated liver disease) • Bone marrow (pyruvate kinase and phosphofructokinase deficiencies)

 TREATMENT

• Copious amounts of fluids to maintain renal function especially in the face of shock
• Exercise induced hematuria has a benign, self-limiting course.
• Avoid stress and excitement if the patient has anemia or copper-associated liver disease.
• Avoid hyperventilation if the patient has phosphofructokinase deficiency. • See suspected causes for specific treatment.

 MEDICATIONS

DRUGS AND FLUIDS
Lactated Ringer's solution if the patient is dehydrated; maintenance fluids if not

CONTRAINDICATIONS
See list of causes for contraindicated drugs

PRECAUTIONS N/A

POSSIBLE INTERACTIONS N/A

ALTERNATE DRUGS
Isotonic saline

 FOLLOW-UP

PATIENT MONITORING
PCV, pO_2, urinalysis, serum creatinine, and ALT (copper associated liver disease)

POSSIBLE COMPLICATIONS
Renal damage (failure) can develop, especially in patients in shock.

 MISCELLANEOUS

ASSOCIATED CONDITIONS N/A

AGE RELATED FACTORS
Neonatal isoerythrolysis

ZOONOTIC POTENTIAL
• Leptospirosis • Toxoplasmosis

PREGNANCY N/A

SYNONYMS
• Hemosiderinuria • Pigmenturia

SEE ALSO See causes

ABBREVIATIONS
ALT = alanine aminotransferase
AST = aspartate aminotransferase
DIC = disseminated intravascular coagulopathy
RBC = red blood cells

References

Ettinger S, ed. Textbook of veterinary internal medicine: Disease of the dog and cat. 4th ed. Philadelphia: WB Saunders, 1995.
Jain NC, ed. Schalm's veterinary hematology. 4th ed. Philadelphia: Lea & Febiger, 1986.
Kaneko JJ. ed. Clinical biochemistry of domestic animals. 4th ed. San Diego: Academic Press, 1989.
Osborne CO, Stevens JB. Handbook of canine & feline urinalysis. Saint Louis: Ralston Purina, 1981.
Sherding RG, ed. The cat: diseases and clinical management. 2nd ed. New York: Churchill Livingstone, 1994.

Author J. B. Stevens
Consulting Editors Carl A. Osborne and Larry G. Adams

HYPERCAPNIA

BASICS

DEFINITION
An increase in the partial pressure of carbon dioxide (CO_2) in arterial blood ($PaCO_2$). Normal $PaCO_2$ values range from 35-45 mm Hg.

Pathophysiology
• CO_2 is an end product of aerobic cellular metabolism. • CO_2 is carried in the blood in three forms: bicarbonate (65%), bound to hemoglobin (30%), and dissolved in plasma (5%). • The portion of CO_2 dissolved in plasma is the source of $PaCO_2$ values. CO_2 is constantly being added to alveolar gas from the pulmonary circulation and removed by alveolar ventilation. • It is uncommon to encounter a $PaCO_2$ above the normal range in nonanesthetized, normal patients. Increases in $PaCO_2$ are the result of hypoventilation.

Systems Affected
• Nervous—the primary organ that is affected by hypercapnia is the brain. Cerebral blood flow is related to the $PaCO_2$ in a linear fashion. An increase in the $PaCO_2$ results in increased cerebral blood flow and an increase in intracranial pressure. • Hemic/lymphatic/immune—increases in $PaCO_2$ can also alter acid base balance. Acute increases in $PaCO_2$ result in production of excess hydrogen ions and a decrease in pH (respiratory acidosis). • Cardiovascular—increases in $PaCO_2$ can also result in endogenous catecholamine release with the possibility of inducing cardiac arrhythmias

SIGNALMENT
Any breed, age, and sex of dogs and cats can develop hypercapnia.

SIGNS

Historical Findings N/A

Physical Examination Findings
• Usually, anesthetized patients show no obvious clinical signs. • Severe hypercapnia in anesthetized patients can lead to tachypnea.

CAUSES
• Hypoventilation—this is defined as an increase in the arterial partial pressure of carbon dioxide ($PaCO_2$) as a result of a decrease in alveolar ventilation. Any cause of decreased alveolar ventilation can result in an increase in $PaCO_2$, including anesthesia, muscular paralysis, upper airway obstruction, air or fluid in the pleural space, restriction of the thoracic cage, diaphragmatic hernia, pulmonary parenchymal disease, and CNS disease. • Animals breathing spontaneously during surgical planes of inhalation anesthesia have elevated $PaCO_2$ values. • Increased inspired CO_2—rebreathing of exhaled gases as a result of exhausted CO_2 absorbent in an anesthesia machine is the most common cause of increased inspired CO_2. Inadequate fresh gas flow using a nonrebreathing anesthesia circuit will also result in increased inspired CO_2 as a result of rebreathing of expired gases.

RISK FACTORS
Deep planes of anesthesia, inadequate fresh gas flow of oxygen with nonrebreathing circuits, bronchial disease (chronic obstructive pulmonary disease [COPD], asthma in cats), upper airway obstruction bronchopneumonia, and pleural disease are risk factors.

DIAGNOSIS

DIFFERENTIAL DIAGNOSIS
• Conscious patients that show signs of tachypnearule out excitement/anxiety, hyperthermia , hypoxia, hyperpyrexia, head trauma, and pain • Anesthetized patients that show tachypnea—rule out light plane of anesthesia and hypoxia

LABORATORY FINDINGS

Drugs That May Alter Lab Results N/A

Disorders That May Alter Lab Results
Air bubbles in the arterial blood sample and/or improper packaging of arterial blood sample will result in falsely low $PaCO_2$ values.

Valid If Run in Human Lab? N/A

CBC/BIOCHEMISTRY/URINALYSIS
N/A

OTHER LABORATORY TESTS
The diagnosis of hypercapnia can be determined by analyzing blood gases from an arterial blood sample that was collected in an anaerobic manner. The syringe should be heparanized with enough heparin to coat the needle and inside of the syringe. A rubber stopper should be placed on the needle or covering the hub of the syringe to prevent room air from entering the blood sample. The sample should be analyzed within 15 minutes if left at room temperature. Placing the sample on ice will extend safe and accurate analysis to 2-4 hours.

IMAGING N/A

OTHER DIAGNOSTIC PROCEDURES
An alternative method of analysis during anesthesia is with a capnometer. End-expired gas is almost entirely alveolar gas. Arterial CO_2 closely approximates the mean value of perfused alveoli and, therefore, end-expired CO_2 is nearly the same value as arterial CO_2.

TREATMENT
• The most important aspect of treating hypercapnia is to provide adequate alveolar ventilation. During anesthesia, this can be accomplished manually or with a mechanical ventilator. Providing mechanical ventilation to the nonanesthetized patient with severe pulmonary disease requires heavy sedation, muscle relaxation, or general anesthesia. Supplemental oxygen may not be indicated based on the patient's primary disease. • Treatment of the underlying disease process that causes hypoventilation and hypercapnia is the definitive therapy. • Discontinuing inhalation anesthesia is definitive treatment of anesthesia-induced hypoventilation.

MEDICATIONS

DRUGS AND FLUIDS
Respiratory stimulants, such as doxapram (5-10 mg/kg, IV), can be administered. Doxapram is a nonspecific stimulant of the respiratory center and does not provide definitive therapy.

CONTRAINDICATIONS
Anesthetic drugs or other respiratory depressants are contraindicated, in patients with CNS disease if adequate ventilatory support cannot be provided. Increases in the $PaCO_2$ in these patients could result in dangerous elevations in intracranial pressure and predispose the patient to herniation of the brain stem.

PRECAUTIONS N/A
POSSIBLE INTERACTIONS N/A
ALTERNATE DRUGS N/A

FOLLOW-UP

PATIENT MONITORING
• The effectiveness of supportive (ventilation) and definitive treatment can be assessed by physical examination findings of decreased respiratory effort. • Reevaluation of the arterial blood gas will indicate improvement of hypercapnia. • Capnometry also assesses adequacy of ventilation.

POSSIBLE COMPLICATIONS
Hypercapnia in patients with CNS disease can cause high intracranial pressure and predispose to herniation of the brain stem.

MISCELLANEOUS

ASSOCIATED CONDITIONS N/A
AGE RELATED FACTORS N/A
ZOONOTIC POTENTIAL N/A
PREGNANCY N/A
SYNONYM
Hypercarbia

SEE ALSO
See causes.

ABBREVIATIONS
COPD = chronic obstructive pulmonary disease

$PaCO_2$ = carbon dioxide in arterial blood

References

Nunn JE. Applied respiratory physiology. 3rd ed. London: Butterworths, 1987:207-226.

Benumof JL. Respiratory physiology and respiratory function during anesthesia. In: Miller RD, ed. Anesthesia. 3rd ed. New York: Churchill Livingstone, 1990:529-532.

Author Thomas Kevin Day

Consulting Editors Lynelle Johnson and Bradley L. Moses

HYPOSTHENURIA

 ## BASICS

DEFINITION
Urine specific gravity between 1.000 and 1.006

Pathophysiology
The ability to concentrate urine normally (dogs, >1.030; cats, >1.035) depends on a complex interaction between antidiuretic hormone (ADH), the protein receptor for ADH on the renal tubule, and a hypertonic renal medullary interstitium. Interference with the synthesis, release, or actions of ADH, damage to the renal tubule, and altered tonicity of the medullary interstitium (medullary washout) can cause hyposthenuria.

Systems Affected
Depends on the underlying disorder

SIGNALMENT
Dogs and Cats

SIGNS
• Polyuria and polydipsia • Urinary incontinence (occasional) • Other signs depend on the underlying disorder

CAUSES
Any disorder or drug that intereferes with the release or action of ADH, damages the renal tubule, causes medullary washout, or causes a primary thirst disorder (see Differential Diagnosis).

RISK FACTORS N/A

 ## DIAGNOSIS

DIFFERENTIAL DIAGNOSIS
• Pyometra • Cushing's disease
• Diabetes insipidus • Pyelonephritis
• Hypercalcemia • Early renal failure
• Primary liver disease • Hypokalemia
• Hypoadrenocorticism • Primary polydipsia (compulsive water drinking)

LABORATORY FINDINGS

Drugs That May Alter Lab Results
Cortisone, lithium, demeclocycline, methoxyfluorane, thiazide diuretics, and intravenous administration of fluids can all lower urine specific gravity into the hyposthenuric range.

Disorders That May Alter Lab Results
N/A

Valid If Run in a Human Lab? Yes

CBC/BIOCHEMISTRY/URINALYSIS
• Low urine specific gravity (1.000 to 1.006). Other abnormalities may point to the underlying cause. • High SAP activity suggests hyperadrenocorticism or primary liver disease. •High cholesterol common in patients with hyperadrenocorticism • Leukocytosis with a left shift in some patients with pyometra or pyelonephritis • Hyperkalemia and hyponatremia suggest hypoadrenocorticism. • Low serum potassium confirms hypokalemia.
• Inflammatory sediment or bacteriuria consistent with pyelonephritis • Proteinuria common in patients with pyelonephritis, pyometra, and hyperadrenocorticism

OTHER LABORATORY TESTS
ACTH levels to determine the cause of hyperadrenocorticism (i.e., pituitary dependent versus adrenal tumor)

IMAGING
• Radiography to assess renal size and shape and to detect calcified adrenal tumor or large uterus • Intravenous pyelogram to help diagnose pyelonephritis • Ultrasonography to assess adrenal size, renal and hepatic size and architecture, and uterine size • MRI or CT scan to assess a pituitary or hypothalamic mass that may be the cause of central diabetes insipidus or hyperadrenocorticism

OTHER DIAGNOSTIC PROCEDURES
• ACTH stimulation test to screen for hyperadrenocorticism and hypoadrenocorticism
• Low-dose dexamethasone suppression test and urine/cortisol creatinine test to screen for hyperadrenocorticism • Serum bile acids to evaluate liver function. Note: dogs with hyperadrenocoticism often have mildly high bile acids. • Modified water deprivation test to differentiate diabetes insipidus from psychogenic polydipsia. See appendix for test protocol.

GROSS AND HISTOPATHOGIC FINDINGS N/A

 ## TREATMENT

INPATIENT VERSUS OUTPATIENT
Depends on the underlying disorder

DIET
No need to alter

CLIENT EDUCATION
Do not restrict patient's water intake unless appropriate to the definitive diagnosis

SURGICAL CONSIDERATIONS
Depends on the underlying disorder

MEDICATIONS

DRUGS AND FLUIDS
Depends on the underlying disorder

CONTRAINDICATIONS N/A

PRECAUTIONS N/A

POSSIBLE INTERACTIONS N/A

ALTERNATE DRUGS N/A

FOLLOW-UP

PATIENT MONITORING
Urine specific gravity, hydration status, renal function, and electrolytes

POSSIBLE COMPLICATIONS
Dehydration

MISCELLANEOUS

ASSOCIATED CONDITIONS
See Differential Diagnosis

AGE RELATED FACTORS N/A

ZOONOTIC POTENTIAL N/A

PREGNANCY N/A

SYNONYMS N/A

SEE ALSO
• Hyperadrenocorticism • Diabetes Insipidus

ABBREVIATIONS
ACTH = adrenocorticotrophic hormone
ALP = alkaline phosphatase
ADH = antidiuretic hormone
CT = computed tomography
MRI = magnetic resonance imaging

References

Rose DB. Clinical physiology of acid-base and electrolyte disorders. 3rd ed. New York: McGraw-Hill, 1989.
DiBartola SP. Fluid therapy in small animal practice. Philadelphia: WB Saunders, 1992.

Author Rhett Nichols
Consulting Editor Rhett Nichols

HYPOXIA

BASICS

DEFINITION
A decrease in the partial pressure of oxygen in arterial blood (PaO_2), resulting in significant desaturation of hemoglobin. Clinically significant desaturation of hemoglobin begins at a $PaO_2 < 60$ mm Hg.

Pathophysiology
The six physiologic causes of hypoxia: 1) low fractional percentage of inspired oxygen (F_IO_2); 2) hypoventilation; 3) mismatching of alveolar ventilation and perfusion, such that areas of the lung that are not ventilated properly are still perfused adequately; 4) alveolar-capillary membrane diffusion defect; 5) right-to-left cardiac or pulmonary shunting; and 6) low cardiac output.

Systems Affected
• All organs can be adversely affected by hypoxia. Oxygen is essential for normal cellular function. Individual tissue oxygen requirements vary from organ to organ. • Nervous—the most important organs to consider during hypoxia are the brain and CNS. Cerebral hypoxia can result in irreversible brain damage.

SIGNALMENT
Any breed, age, and sex of dogs and cats can develop hypoxia.

SIGNS

Historical Findings
The owners may describe breathing problems, trauma, coughing, gagging, exercise intolerance, or collapse.

Physical Examination Findings
Tachypnea, dyspnea, orthopnea, pale mucous membranes, cyanosis, coughing, tachycardia, and shock

CAUSES
• Low F_IO_2—high elevations have low F_IO_2 values; the higher the elevation, the lower the F_IO_2. Suffocation or small enclosed areas with poor ventilation also cause low F_IO_2. • Hypoventilation is defined as an increase in the arterial partial pressure of carbon dioxide ($PaCO_2$) caused by a decrease in alveolar ventilation. Muscular paralysis, upper airway obstruction, air or fluid in the pleural space, restriction of the thoracic cage, diaphragmatic hernia, pulmonary parenchymal disease, and CNS disease can cause decreased alveolar ventilation. • Mismatching of alveolar ventilation and perfusion—this usually occurs during anesthesia or prolonged recumbency in which a large area of the lung is atelectatic. Pulmonary edema of any etiology and pulmonary thromboembolus also have been described in this manner as a cause of hypoxia. • Alveolar-capillary membrane diffusion defect—pulmonary parenchymal disease (infectious or neoplastic), lower airway disease, pulmonary edema, pulmonary throm-

boembolus, and acute respiratory distress syndrome. • Right-to-left cardiac or pulmonary shunting—ventricular septal defect, reversed patent ductus arteriosus, and intrapulmonary arteriovenous shunts • Low cardiac output—cardiac failure of any cause and shock of any cause can cause arterial hypoxia

RISK FACTORS
Sudden change in environment to higher elevations, bronchial disease (COPD, asthma in cats), trauma, bronchopneumonia, pleural disease, anesthesia, cardiac disease, and geriatric pulmonary changes

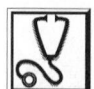

DIAGNOSIS

DIFFERENTIAL DIAGNOSIS
• Signs of tachypnea and/or dyspnea
• Excitement/anxiety, hyperthermia, hyperpyrexia, head trauma, and pain

LABORATORY FINDINGS

Drugs That May Alter Lab Results N/A

Disorders That May Alter Lab Results
Air bubbles in the arterial blood sample and improper packaging of arterial blood sample will result in falsely high PaO_2 values.

Valid If Run in Human Lab N/A

CBC/BIOCHEMISTRY/URINALYSIS
N/A

OTHER LABORATORY TESTS
The diagnosis of hypoxia can only be determined by analyzing blood gases from an arterial blood sample that was collected in an anaerobic manner. The syringe should be heparinized with enough heparin to coat the needle and inside of the syringe. A rubber stopper should be placed on the needle or covering the hub of the syringe to prevent room air from entering the blood sample. The sample should be analyzed within 15 minutes if left at room temperature. Placing the sample on ice will extend safe and accurate analysis to 2-4 hours.

IMAGING N/A

OTHER DIAGNOSTIC PROCEDURES
An alternative method of analysis is with a pulse oximeter. This monitoring device will indirectly determine the saturation of oxygen in arterial blood (SaO_2). The PaO_2 and SaO_2 are related based on the oxyhemoglobin dissociation curve. The SaO_2 remains greater than 90% when PaO_2 values are greater than 60 mm Hg. SaO_2 values below 85-90% are considered abnormal. The probe of the pulse oximeter is most accurate on the tongue of animals; therefore, pulse oximetry may be limited to the anesthetized or severely traumatized patient. Another disadvantage is inaccurate measurements during low flow states (hypotension).

TREATMENT
• The most important aspect of treating hypoxia is to determine the primary cause and direct definitive treatment to the primary cause. The most common supportive treatment of hypoxia is to provide supplemental oxygen therapy. Oxygen therapy usually will be successful in treatment of hypoxia caused by low inspired oxygen, hypoventilation, and alveolar-capillary membrane diffusion defects. Supplemental oxygen therapy will not be successful in the treatment of hypoxia caused by severe mismatching of ventilation and perfusion or right-to-left shunts.
• Oxygen can be delivered to the patient from an anesthetic machine via an oxygen face mask placed securely around the muzzle or head. Other methods of oxygen administration include from an oxygen tank and regulator through a cannula placed in the nares. The increase in F_IO_2 by any of the above methods will be determined by the oxygen flow rate and exposure of oxygen to room air.
• Higher oxygen flow rates delivers 40% F_IO_2 via nasal cannula or up to 80% F_IO_2 with intratracheal administration.
• Effectiveness of oxygen therapy can be assessed accurately by repeating arterial blood gas analysis. Compensatory responses to hypoxia, including tachycardia and tachypnea, may persist in the face of improvements in the PaO_2 values.

MEDICATIONS

DRUGS AND FLUIDS
• Fluid therapy and inotropic support are important treatment modalities for hypoxia caused by low cardiac output.
• Cardiac failure as a cause of hypoxia requires aggressive medical therapy that may include diuretic therapy, afterload reduction, inotropic support, and oxygen supplementation. Aggressive fluid therapy is not a component of treatment for hypoxia caused by cardiac failure.
• Hypoxia resulting from hypovolemic, hemorrhagic, or septic shock require aggressive fluid therapy with 0.9% saline or LRS (90 ml/kg, IV).
• Oxygen supplementation may not be beneficial until circulating blood volume is restored.
• Inotropic support (dobutamine or dopamine) may be required if aggressive fluid therapy is not adequate.

CONTRAINDICATIONS
• Aggressive fluid therapy is contraindicated in patients with hypoxia caused by cardiac failure and pulmonary edema.
• Diuretic therapy is not indicated in patients with hypoxia caused by shock, low F_IO_2,

alveolar-capillary membrane diffusion defects, mismatching of alveolar ventilation and perfusion, and right-to-left shunts.

PRECAUTIONS

• Electrocardiographic monitoring is recommended during administration of inotropic support. A common side effect of dopamine or dobutamine administration is the production of arrhythmias.
• Oxygen toxicity can result from prolonged exposure (> 12 hours) and high F_IO_2 (> 70%). Signs include pulmonary edema, seizures, and death. Reevaluate the arterial blood test for effective F_IO_2.

POSSIBLE INTERACTIONS N/A

ALTERNATE DRUGS N/A

 FOLLOW-UP

PATIENT MONITORING

• The effectiveness of supportive (oxygen therapy) and definitive treatment can be assessed by physical examination findings of reduced respiratory effort and improvement of cyanotic mucous membranes (if present initially). • Reevaluation of the arterial blood gas will indicate status of hypoxia.
• Pulse oximetry is an alternative diagnostic tool.

POSSIBLE COMPLICATIONS

• Partial or complete loss of neuronal function can be a result of prolonged hypoxia. Severity of brain damage depends on severity and duration of hypoxia. Clinical signs may include dementia, seizures, loss of conciousness. • Arrhythmias can be caused by prolonged hypoxia to the heart.

 MISCELLANEOUS

ASSOCIATED CONDITIONS N/A

AGE RELATED FACTORS N/A

ZOONOTIC POTENTIAL N/A

PREGNANCY

Hypoxia can adversely affect the fetus, especially during the first trimester of pregnancy.

SYNONYM

Hypoxemia

SEE ALSO

See causes.

ABBREVIATIONS

F_IO_2 = fractional percentage of inspired oxygen
$PaCO_2$ = arterial partial pressure of carbon dioxide
SaO_2 = saturation of oxygen in arterial blood

References

Nunn JE. Applied respiratory physiology. 3rd ed. London: Butterworths, 1987:471-478.

Taylor AE, Rehder K, Hyatt RE, Parker JC. Clinical respiratory physiology. Philadelphia: WB Saunders, 1989:157-158.

Benumof JL. Respiratory physiology and respiratory function during anesthesia. In: Miller RD, ed. Anesthesia. 3rd ed. New York: Churchill Livingstone, 1990:523-529.

Mann FA, Wagner-Mann C, Allert JA, Smith J. Comparison of intranasal and intratracheal oxygen administration in healthy awake dogs. Am J Vet Res 1992;53:856-860.

Author Thomas Kevin Day
Consulting Editors Lynelle Johnson and Bradley L. Moses

LEUKOPENIA (NEUTROPENIA)

BASICS

DEFINITION
Leukocyte count ≤ 5000 cells/ml in dogs and ≤ 5500 cells/μl in cats. Leukopenia is usually synonymous with neutropenia (≤ 2900 neutrophils/ml in dogs and ≤ 2500 neutrophils/ml in cats) because neutrophils are the most numerous leukocyte in healthy blood. Neutropenia can develop alone or as a component of pancytopenia. Neutropenia is often accompanied by a left shift and toxic change (e.g., cytoplasmic basophilia, cytoplasmic vacuolation, Döhle's bodies, and toxic granulation).

Pathophysiology
Neutropenia results from one of three mechanisms: 1) deficient neutrophil production in the bone marrow; 2) cells shifting from the circulating neutrophil pool to the marginal neutrophil pool in the blood; and 3) reduced neutrophil survival because of excessive tissue demand or immune-mediated destruction of cells. It is most commonly associated with infection because emigration of neutrophils from the blood into the tissues exceeds the rate at which the bone marrow can replace them.

Systems Affected
Neutropenia predisposes the patient to systemic infection by a variety of pathogens. Many body systems can be affected in any combination depending upon the site(s) of infection.

SIGNALMENT
• No specific signalment for generalized infection • Giant schnauzer with inherited B₁₂ malabsorption • Gray collie with cyclic neutropenia

SIGNS
• Signs of localized or systemic infection
• Pyrexia

CAUSES

Deficient Neutrophil Production
Stem Cell Death or Inhibition
• Infectious agents—parvoviruses in dogs and cats, FeLV and FIV in cats, Ehrlichia canis in dogs, and Bacterial-induced myelonecrosis in dogs and cats • Drugs, chemicals, and toxins—chemotherapy agents in dogs and cats, estrogen in dogs, chloramphenicol and benzene-ring compounds in cats, phenylbutazone in dogs, cephalosporins in dogs and cats, trimethoprim-sulfadiazine in dogs, griseofulvin in cats, Noxema ingestion in dogs, thiacetarsamide administration (idiosyncratic) in dogs, and T-2 mycotoxin ingestion in cats
• Lack of trophic factors—inherited malabsorption of vitamin B₁₂ (giant schnauzer) and ionizing radiation
Reduced Hematopoietic Space Secondary to Myelophthisis
• Bone marrow necrosis • Myelofibrosis
• Osteopetrosis • Disseminated neoplasia,

leukemia, and myelodysplastic syndrome
• Disseminated granulomatous disease (histoplasmosis)
Cyclic Stem Cell Proliferation
• Inherited cyclic hematopoiesis (gray collie)
• FeLV infection • Cyclophosphamide treatment • Idiopathic disease
Immune-Mediated Suppression of Granulopoiesis
Poorly documented in dogs and cats

Neutrophil Migration
A shift in neutrophils from the circulating neutrophil pool (where they can be quantitated by the WBC count) to the marginal neutrophil pool (where they cannot be counted) occurs in patients with endotoxemia.

Reduced Survival Neutropenia
• Severe bacterial infection (most common cause)—pneumonia, peritonitis, and pyothorax • Immune-mediated destruction • Drug-induced destruction • Hypersplenism (sequestration) • Paraneoplastic syndrome (precise mechanism unknown)

RISK FACTORS
• Inherited disease—cyclic hematopoiesis in the gray collie and neutropenia in the giant schnauzer • Drug and chemical exposure—estrogen overdose in dogs (pancytopenia) and chloramphenicol and benzene-ring compounds in cats • Exposure to various infectious agents—overwhelming bacterial infection in cats and dogs, acute Ehrlichia canis infection in dogs (pancytopenia), parvovirus infection in dogs, and FeLV infection in cats
• Middle-aged and old animals are less effective at repopulating the bone marrow after a severe toxic insult.

DIAGNOSIS

DIFFERENTIAL DIAGNOSIS
• Breed of dog may promote suspicion of inherited disease (e.g., cyclic hematopoiesis in the gray collie and neutropenia in the giant schnauzer) • History should include information concerning drugs, toxins, and radiation exposure.

LABORATORY FINDINGS

Drugs That May Alter Laboratory Results
None

Disorders That May Alter Laboratory Results
• Failure to properly mix the blood specimen before sampling for the CBC (laboratory error) • Obtaining blood specimen from an IV catheter used for fluid administration (diluted specimen) • Partial clotting of the blood specimen with leukocyte entrapment or aggregation (poor anticoagulation)

Valid If Run in Human Lab?
Automated leukocyte counts are valid; how-

ever, technicians identify too many bands in animal blood (left shift) and cannot reliably recognize some leukocyte types (e.g., basophils in cats).

CBC/BIOCHEMISTRY/URINALYSIS
• Neutropenia is verified by CBC and leukocyte differential counts. • Multiple CBC are necessary to confirm or exclude a diagnosis of cyclic hematopoiesis.

OTHER LABORATORY TESTS
• Serologic test to exclude ehrlichiosis in dogs and FeLV and FIV infections in cats
• Demonstration of antineutrophil antibodies is essential to diagnose immune-mediated neutropenia.

IMAGING
Survey radiography and ultrasonography may help locate occult sites of infection not apparent during physical examination.

OTHER DIAGNOSTIC PROCEDURES
• Examination of a bone marrow aspirate and core biopsy is indicated to evaluate neutrophil production and exclude myelophthisis, myelonecrosis, myelofibrosis, and osteopetrosis. • Provocative exposure to parenteral vitamin B₁₂ should reverse anemia, neutropenia, and neutrophil hypersegmentation in affected giant schnauzers.
• Cytologic examination of preparations can be used to document excess tissue demand for neutrophils, verify sequestration of neutrophils in body cavities or between tissue planes, confirm bacterial infection, and identify sites of insensible or occult loss of neutrophils from mucous membranes or skin lesions.

TREATMENT

INPATIENT VERSUS OUTPATIENT
• Primary concern in a patient with neutropenia is development of secondary infection. In the absence of pyrexia, broad-spectrum antibiotics should be given prophylactically on an outpatient basis.
• Pyrexia, indicating current infection, is treated more aggressively. Inpatient treatment is recommended for administration of parenteral medications until the infection is contained.
• Transfusion may be indicated in patients with severe pancytopenia (PCV < 10%).

MEDICATIONS

DRUGS AND FLUIDS
• Dogs and cats (nonfebrile)—trimethoprim-sulfadiazine (14 mg/kg PO q12h)
• Dogs and cats (febrile)—ampicillin (20 mg/kg IV q6h-q8h) and gentamycin sulfate (1-2 mg/kg IV q6h-q8h)
• Dogs and cats—rC G-CSF 5 mcg/kg/day
• rC G-CSF may be of benefit in minimizing the duration of neutropenia.

• rH G-CSF may be effective short term; however, development of antibodies to the protein takes place in 14-21 days.
• rC G-CSF is effective in dogs for prolonged periods and in cats for 42+ days.
• Neutrophilia subsides within 5 days after drug administration is discontinued.

CONTRAINDICATIONS
• Drugs listed should be used in pregnant animals only if the benefits supercede the inherent risks.
• Sulfa drugs cross the placenta and can cause jaundice, hemolytic anemia, and kernicterus. Trimethoprim also crosses the placenta. No harm accompanies drug administration in early pregnancy; however, this drug should not be used near term because of folic acid inhibition. Gentamycin sulfate crosses the placenta and may be associated with fetal ototoxicity. Adequately controlled safety studies of rC G-CSF and rH G-CSF have not been performed in dogs and cats (including pregnant animals). High-dose administration (80 (mcg/kg/day) of rH G-CSF in pregnant rabbits was associated with fetal resorption, abortion, and increased genitourinary tract hemorrhage.

PRECAUTIONS
• Maintain hydration when administering sulfa drugs to prevent renal crystallization.
• Gentamycin sulfate may be nephrotoxic and ototoxic.
• Risk of nephrotoxicity increases in dehydrated and overdosed animals.

POSSIBLE INTERACTIONS N/A

ALTERNATE DRUGS

Enrofloxacin can be substituted for gentamycin.

ALTERNATE DRUGS N/A

FOLLOW-UP

PATIENT MONITORING
Periodic CBC. Improvement is denoted by a rising leukocyte or neutrophil count, resolution of left shift, and disappearance of toxic change. Rebound neutrophilic leukocytosis is expected during recovery from neutropenia.

POSSIBLE COMPLICATIONS
Secondary infections

MISCELLANEOUS

ASSOCIATED CONDITIONS
Secondary infection

AGE RELATED FACTORS
Repopulation of bone marrow with hematopoietic cells is more difficult in middle-aged and older animals because of age-related reduction in stem cell numbers.

ZOONOTIC POTENTIAL
None

PREGNANCY
N/A

SYNONYM
Neutropenia

SEE ALSO
• Ehrlichiosis • Estrogen Toxicity • Feline Immunodeficiency (FIV) • Feline Leukemia Virus Infection • Parvovirus Infection—Dogs

ABBREVIATIONS
FeLV = feline leukemia virus
FIV = feline immunodeficiency virus
PCV = packed cell volume
rG-CSF = recombinant granulocyte colony-stimulating factor
rC G-CSF = recombinant canine granulocyte colony-stimulating factor
rH G-CSF = recombinant human granulocyte colony-stimulating factor
WBC = white blood cells

References
August JR. Consultations in feline internal medicine. 2nd ed. Philadelphia: WB Saunders, 1994.
Duncan JR, Prasse KW, Mahaffey EA. Veterinary laboratory medicine. 3rd ed. Ames: Iowa State University Press, 1994.
Ettinger SJ, Feldman EC. Textbook of veterinary internal medicine. 4th ed. Philadelphia: WB Saunders, 1994.
Sherding RG. Cat diseases and clinical management. New York: Churchill Livingstone, 1989.

Author Kenneth S. Latimer
Consulting Editor Alan H. Rebar

LIPIDS, HYPERLIPIDEMIA

BASICS

DEFINITIONS
• Concentration of lipid in the blood of a fasted (> 12 hours) patient that exceeds the upper range of normal for that species; includes both hypercholesterolemia and hypertriglyceridemia • Lipemic—serum or plasma separated from blood that contains an excess concentration of triglycerides (> 200 mg/dl) • Lactescence—opaque milklike appearance of serum or plasma that contains even higher concentration of triglycerides (> 1000 mg/dl) than lipemic serum

Pathophysiology
Primary Hyperlipidemia
• Idiopathic hyperchylomicronemia—defect in lipid metabolism causing hypertriglyceridemia and hyperchylomicronemia. Possibly caused by a defect in lipoprotein lipase activity or the absence of the surface apoprotein CII. Familial disorder in the miniature schnauzer. • Hyperchylomicronemia in cats—familial, autosomal recessive defect in lipoprotein lipase activity • Idiopathic hypercholesterolemia—occurs in some families of Doberman pinschers and rottweilers. Low-density lipoprotein (LDL) cholesterol is high.
Secondary Hyperlipidemia
• Postprandial—absorption of chylomicrons from the gastrointestinal tract occurs 30-60 minutes after ingestion of a meal containing fat; may increase serum triglycerides for 3-10 hours • Diabetes mellitus—low lipoprotein lipase (LPL) activity; high synthesis of very-low-density lipoprotein (VLDL) by the liver • Hypothyroidism—low LPL activity and lipolytic activity by other hormones (e.g., catecholamines). Reduced hepatic degradation of cholesterol to bile acids. • Hyperadrenocorticism—increased synthesis of VLDL by the liver and low LPL activity causes both hypercholesterolemia and hypertriglyceridemia • Liver disease—hypercholesterolemia caused by reduced excretion of cholesterol in the bile • Nephrotic syndrome—common synthetic pathway for albumin and cholesterol and possibly low oncotic pressure leads to increased cholesterol synthesis. • Obesity—excessive hepatic synthesis of VLDL

Systems Affected
• Opthalmic • Nervous • Endocrine/metabolism • Gastrointestinal • Hepatobiliary

SIGNALMENT
• Variable, depending on the cause • Heriditary hyperlipidemias—age of onset 8 months in cats and > 4 years in predisposed breeds of dog such as the miniature schnauzer

SIGNS

Historical Findings
• Recent ingestion of a meal • Seizures • Abdominal pain and distress • Neuropathies

Physical Examination Findings
• Lipemia retinalis • Lipemic aqueous • Neuropathy • Cutaneous xanthomata • Lipid granulomas in abdominal organs

CAUSES

Increased Absorption of Triglycerides or Cholesterol
Postprandial

Increased Production of Triglycerides or Cholesterol
• Nephrotic syndrome • Pregnancy • Defects in lipid clearance enzymes or lipid carrier proteins • Idiopathic hyperchylomicronemia • Hyperchylomicronemia in cats • Idiopathic hypercholesterolemia

Decreased Clearance of Triglycerides or Cholesterol
• Hypothyroidism • Hyperadrenocorticism • Diabetes mellitus • Pancreatitis • Cholestasis

RISK FACTORS
• Obesity • High dietary intake of fats • Genetic predisposition in miniature schnauzer and Himalayan cat • Idiopathic hypercholesterolemia observed in families of Doberman pinschers and rottweilers

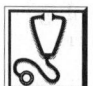

DIAGNOSIS

DIFFERENTIAL DIAGNOSIS

Fasting Hyperlipidemia
Rule out postprandial lipemia with a 12-hour fast.

Primary Hyperlipoproteinemia
• Idiopathic hyperchylomicronemia is observed most commonly in the miniature schnauzer breed. • Hyperchylomicronemia in cats often manifests as polyneuropathies and lipogranulomas. • Idiopathic hypercholesterolemia is observed most frequently in the Doberman pinscher and rottweiler breeds and animals are often asymptomatic.

Secondary Hyperlipidemia
• Diabetes mellitus—signs include polyphagia, weight loss, polydipsia, and polyuria • Glycosuria and fasting hyperglycemia confirm the diagnosis. • Hypothyroidism—signs include lethargy, hypothermia, heat-seeking, and dermatologic changes (e.g., alopecia and hyperpigmentation) • Pancreatitis—signs include abdominal pain, vomiting, diarrhea, and anorexia. Often hyperlipidemia is accompanied by high liver enzyme activites and high lipase and amylase. • Hyperadrenocorticism—signs include polydypsia, polyuria, polyphagia, dermatologic changes (e.g., alopecia and thin skin), and hepatomegaly. Hypercholesterolemia often is attended by high ALP isoenzyme. • Hepatic disease and cholestatic disorders—signs include anorexia, weight loss, and icterus • Nephrotic syndrome—signs include ascites and peripheral edema. Hypercholes-

terolemia is observed in conjunction with hypoproteinemia and proteinuria.

LABORATORY FINDINGS

Sample Handling
Submit serum. Lipemia causes hemolysis if serum remains on RBC for a long time. Inquire about the laboratory method of clearing lipemic samples before submission. Two samples may be submitted; one for biochemical analysis, which may be cleared, and one for triglycerides and cholesterol concentrations.

Drugs That May Alter Lab Results
• Corticosteroids • Phenytoin • Prochlorperazine • Thiazides • Phenothiazines

Disorders That May Alter Lab Results
Falsely High Cholesterol
• Nonfasted samples (< 12 hours) • Icterus (spectrophotometric techniques) • Fluoride and oxalate anticoagulants (enzymatic techniques) • Lipemia

Valid If Run in Human Lab? Valid

CBC/BIOCHEMISTRY/URINALYSIS
• Results of hemogram usually normal • Hyperadrenocorticism—polycythemia and nucleated RBC • Hypothyroidism—mild normocytic, normochromic anemia • High triglycerides—dogs, > 150 mg/dl; cats, > 100 mg/dl • High cholesterol—dogs, > 300 mg/dl; cats, > 200 mg/dl • Nephrotic syndrome—low albumin • Diabetes mellitus—high serum glucose • Hyperadrenocorticism—high ALP activity • Pancreatitis—high serum lipase • Results of urinalysis often normal • Nephrotic syndrome—proteinuria

OTHER LABORATORY TESTS
• HDL and LDL determinations—used in human medicine. Values reported for HDL and LDL in dogs and cats cannot be assumed to be reliable. • Chylomicron test—obtain serum sample after a 12-hour fast and refrigerate for 12-14 hours. *Do not freeze.* Chylomicrons rise to the surface and form a creamy layer. • Lipoprotein electrophoresis—seprates LDL, VLDL, HDL$_1$, and HDL$_2$ • LPL activity—collect serum for triglycerides and cholesterol concentrations and lipoprotein electrophoresis before and 15 minutes after IV administration of heparin (90 IU/kg). If there is no change in values before and after heparin administration, a defective LPL enzyme system should be suspected. • Thyroxine (T$_4$) and triiodothyronine (T$_3$) determinations indicated if hypothyroidism is suspected • Adrenocorticotropic hormone (ACTH) stimulation test indicated if hyperadrenocorticism is suspected

IMAGING N/A

OTHER DIAGNOSTIC TESTS N/A

LIPIDS, HYPERLIPIDEMIA

TREATMENT

Diet should contain 8-12% fat (e.g., Hill's r/d, Hill's Pet Products)

MEDICATIONS

DRUGS AND FLUIDS

Initial management is dietary. See alternate drugs if diet fails to control hyperlipidemia.

CONTRAINDICATIONS N/A

PRECAUTIONS N/A

POSSIBLE INTERACTIONS N/A

ALTERNATE DRUGS

• Gemfibrozil—7.5 mg/kg PO q12h
• Fish oils—linolenic acid (omega-3 polyunsaturated fat)
• Clofibrate and niacin—not currently recommended in cats or dogs

FOLLOW-UP

PATIENT MONITORING

• Triglyceride concentrations should be kept < 500 mg/dl to avoid possibly fatal episodes of acute pancreatitis. • Cholesterol monitoring often is not necessary because hypercholesterolemia is not associated with clinical signs.

POSSIBLE COMPLICATIONS

• Pancreatitis and seizures are common complications of hyperlipidemia in the miniature schnauzer. • In cats with hereditary chylomicronemia, xanthoma formation, lipemia retinalis, and neuropathies have been reported. Peripheral neuropathies usually resolve 2-3 months after institution of a low-fat diet.

MISCELLANEOUS

ASSOCIATED CONDITIONS

• Pancreatitis • Seizures • Neuropathies

AGE RELATED FACTORS N/A

ZOONOTIC POTENTIAL N/A

PREGNANCY

Potential cause of high cholesterol

SYNONYMS

• Lipemia • Hyperlipoproteinemia

SEE ALSO

See causes.

ABBREVIATIONS

ACTH = adrenocorticotropic hormone
HDL = high-density lipoproteins
LDL = low-density lipoproteins
LPL = lipoprotein lipase
VLDL = very-low-density lipoproteins
T_4 = thyroxine
T_3 = triiodithyronine

References

Armstrong PJ, Ford RB. Hyperlipidemia. In: Kirk RW, ed. Current veterinary therapy X. Philadelphia: WB Saunders, 1989:1046-1050.

Jones B. Feline hyperlipidemias. In: Ettinger ST, Feldman EC, eds. Textbook of veterinary internal medicine. 4th ed. Philadelphia: WB Saunders, 1994:1410-1413.

Ford R. Canine hyperlipidemias. In: Ettinger ST, Feldman EC, eds. Textbook of veterinary internal medicine. 4th ed. Philadelphia: WB Saunders 1994:1414-1418.

Author Deborah S. Greco
Consulting Editor Rhett Nichols

LYMPHOCYTOSIS

BASICS

DEFINITION
Absolute number of circulating lymphocytes greater than reference range:
• Dogs, > 5 x 10⁹/l or >5000 ml • Cats, > 7 x 10⁹/l or > 7000 ml • Absolute lymphocyte counts are greater in puppies and kittens than adults.

Pathophysiology
Lymphocytes are imperative for humoral (B lymphocytes) and cell-mediated immunity (T lymphocytes). B lymphocytes are derived from lymphoid stem cells in the bone marrow and are responsible for the production of antibodies. T lymphocytes are derived from lymphoid stem cells in the bone marrow; they develop under the influence of the thymus and/or thymosin and are responsible for cell-mediated immunity and regulation of the immune system. T lymphocytes recirculate from blood to the lymph nodes. Under the proper stimulus, lymphocytes transform into lymphoblasts and then proliferate to make a clonal population of cells. B and T lymphocytes are responsible for approximately 95% of all lymphocytes; the remainder are "null" lymphocytes (i.e., large, granular lymphocytes) that serve as natural killer cells and other diverse functions. Generally, the different types of lymphocytes cannot be identified on a blood film. Infrequently, activated B lymphocytes can be recognized (i.e., immunoblasts) by their large size, deep blue cytoplasm, and perinuclear clear zone. Large, granular lymphocytes can be recognized by the presence of small, red cytoplasmic granules.

Systems Affected
• Hemic/lymph/immune—Spleen, liver, and bone marrow as a result of hyperplasia or neoplasia • Lymphosarcoma can involve all systems and produce specific problems such as ocular, CNS, gastrointestinal, and renal. In dogs, lymphosarcoma frequently causes hypercalcemia, which affects multiple systems.

SIGNALMENT Dogs and cats

SIGNS
• If cause is physiologic, excited, vicious, or scared cat • If cause is lymphosarcoma, lymph node enlargement and, possibly, splenomegaly and hepatomegaly

CAUSES

Physiologic
Epinephrine surge, especially common in excited cats. The change occurs in minutes and lasts about 30 minutes. The effect can be produced by exogenous adrenaline injection, excitement, and fear. Usually seen in young, healthy animals. Can be induced by difficulty collecting a blood sample. The change is much less common in cats that are sick. The absolute lymphocyte count can rise to > 10,000/ml and is much greater than the relatively mild increase in mature neutrophils that accompanies this type of lymphocytosis.

Lymphosarcoma or Lymphocytic Leukemia
Peripheral blood lymphocyte count can range from lymphopenia to counts >100,000 lymphocytes/ml. Significantly high counts (i.e., > 30,000/ml) are uncommon. Lymphocytosis is found in approximately 20% of dogs with lymphosarcoma. In fact, lymphopenia is more common than lymphocytosis in dogs with lymphosarcoma, resulting from the release of endogenous corticosteroids caused by the stress of the disease. Lymphopenia occurs in > 50% of dogs with lymphosarcoma that also have concurrent hypercalcemia. Lymphopenia occurs in > 50% of dogs with LSA and these 50% also have hypercalcemia OR. If a patient does have lymphocytosis it is usually mild to moderate (i.e., 5000-15,000/ml). The critical feature, however, is that the lymphocyte count is high in the face of an obvious or even severe systemic illness, when the "appropriate" or "expected" response would be lymphopenia. Immature and abnormal appearing lymphocytes should be searched for in a blood film. Careful examination of the feathered edge or lateral margins of the blood smear is a good place to search for these cells.

Antigenic Stimulation
• Chronic inflammation—often with a suppurative component such as pyometra and pyoderma • Immune mediated diseases, acquired and autoimmune • Canine ehrlichiosis • Vaccination • The increase in lymphocyte numbers associated with these problems is relatively mild and can range from the higher end of reference range to approximately 10,000/ml. It is important, however, that there are lymphocytes in circulation or that the count is even high, in the face of what may be an obvious clinical disease (when lymphopenia would be a more common response because of the stress of the disease). The presence of immunocytes and immunoblasts, which are plasma cells (B lymphocytes), in the circulation indicates antigenic stimulation.

Hypoadrenocorticism
Lymphocytosis occurs in approximately 25-33% of dogs with hypoadrenocorticism as a result of the absence of glucocorticoids. Classically, lymphocytosis is accompanied by mild eosinophilia and the absence of neutrophilia or monocytosis in a sick and stressed animal. A normal lymphocyte count in a sick and stressed animal suggests low glucocorticoids and, therefore, the possibility of hypoadrenocorticism.

Hyperthyroidism
Approximately 10% of cats with hyperthyroidism have lymphocytosis.
Germ Free Cats
Lymphocyte count, 4000-14,000/ml.

Feline Immunodeficiency Virus
Although listed as a cause of lymphocytosis, FIV causes lymphopenia, an inversion of the CD4⁺:CD8⁺ ratio, and "lymphocytosis" of CD8⁺ T lymphocytes.

Drugs
Methimazole is associated with lymphocytosis in 7% of cats treated for hyperthyroidism.

RISK FACTORS N/A

DIAGNOSIS

DIFFERENTIAL DIAGNOSIS
• Ill, lethargic dog—consider hypoadrenocorticism and lymphosarcoma • Lymphadenosis or lymphadenopathy—consider lymphosarcoma • Thin, hyperactive, polyphagic cat—consider hyperthyroidism • Thin, lethargic animal—consider lymphosarcoma and FIV

LABORATORY FINDINGS

Drugs That May Alter Lab Results
Epinephrine and other beta-adrenergic agonists, corticosteroids, and methimazole

Disorders That May Alter Lab Results
Incorrect identification of nucleated RBC or monocytes as lymphocytes

Valid If Run in Human Lab? Valid

CBC/BIOCHEMISTRY/URINALYSIS
• Severe lymphocytosis (> 15,000/ml)—consider lymphocytic leukemia; > 30,000/ml, diagnose lymphocytic leukemia
• Immature, bizarre, and abnormal lymphocytes in circulation—consider lymphocytic leukemia • Mature neutrophilia—consider physiologic epinephrine response and chronic inflammation • Nonregenerative anemia, leukopenia, and/or thrombocytopenia—consider intramarrow disease such as lymphosarcoma and lymphocytic leukemia • Eosinophilia—consider hypoadrenocorticism • Polycythemia—consider hyperthyroidism • Hypercalcemia—consider lymphosarcoma

OTHER LABORATORY TESTS
• Serum protein electrophoresis—monoclonal gammopathy suggests lymphosarcoma and ehrlichiosis • Thyroid testing—high resting T_3, T_4, diagnose hyperthyroidism

IMAGING
Hepatosplenomegaly—consider lymphosarcoma

OTHER DIAGNOSTIC PROCEDURES
Biopsy helpful to confirm lymphosarcoma

TREATMENT
Treatment must be directed at the primary disease causing lymphocytosis.

MEDICATIONS

DRUGS AND FLUIDS
Lymphosarcoma—chemotherapy (see appropriate topics)

CONTRAINDICATIONS N/A

PRECAUTIONS N/A

POSSIBLE INTERACTIONS
Levamisole is an immunomodulator and restores depressed immune function. Complex interactions between levamisole and B and T lymphocytes affect their function.

ALTERNATE DRUGS N/A

 FOLLOW-UP

PATIENT MONITORING N/A

POSSIBLE COMPLICATIONS N/A

 MISCELLANEOUS

ASSOCIATED CONDITIONS N/A

AGE RELATED FACTORS
• Young puppies—lymphocyte count increases from birth to a maximum at approximately 6 weeks of age of 6 x 10^9/l; value is within adult reference range for adults by 8 weeks of age • Young kittens—absolute lymphocyte count increases from birth to a maximum at approximately 12-14 weeks of age of 10.5 x 10^9/l; value is within reference range for adults by 16-20 weeks of age

ZOONOTIC POTENTIAL N/A

PREGNANCY N/A

SYNONYMS N/A

SEE ALSO
• Hypoadrenocorticism • Leukemia, Chronic Lymphocytic • Lymphosarcoma—Dogs • Lymphosarcoma—Cats

ABBREVIATIONS
CNS = central nervous system
FIV = feline immunodeficiency virus

References

Breitschwerdt EB, et al. Monoclonal gammopathy associated with naturally occurring canine ehrlichiosis. J Vet Intern Med 1987;1:2-9.

Jain NC. Schalm's veterinary hematology. 4th ed. Philadelphia: Lea & Febiger, 1986:109-111,132-134.

Tompkins M, et al. Early events in the immunopathogenesis of feline retrovirus infections. J Am Vet Med Assoc 1991;199:1311-1316.

Author Donald J. Meuten
Consulting Editor Alan H. Rebar

MAGNESIUM, HYPERMAGNESEMIA

BASICS

DEFINITION
• Dogs—serum magnesium > 2.1 mg/dl
• Cats—serum magnesium > 2.3 mg/dl

Pathophysiology
• Magnesium is the second most abundant intracellular cation. Its presence is critical to many cellular enzymatic reactions. • Magnesium homeostasis is largely controlled by renal elimination; any condition that causes severely low glomerular filtration rate can result in hypermagnesemia. • High magnesium concentration impairs transmission of nerve impulses and decreases the postsynaptic response at the neuromuscular junction.

Systems Affected
• Cardiovascular—bradycardia and prolonged QRS duration • Musculoskeletal—impaired reflexes, weakness, and paralysis • Nervous—depression and somnolence

SIGNALMENT N/A

SIGNS

General Comments
Hypermagnesemia usually develops with disorders that cause azotemia. Most signs are referable to causes of azotemia rather than to hypermagnesemia per se.

Historical and Physical Examination Findings
• Bradycardia • Weakness • Hyporeflexia • Depression

CAUSES
• Renal failure • Excessive magnesium administration

RISK FACTORS
• Renal disease • Magnesium hydroxide administration

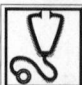

DIAGNOSIS

DIFFERENTIAL DIAGNOSIS
• The signs of hypermagnesemia are most similar to those of hypocalcemia, which often occurs simultaneously in hypermagnesemic patients. • Bradycardia can be caused by neurologic disease, hyperkalemia, hypertension, hypothyroidism, sick sinus syndrome, and various drugs.

LABORATORY FINDINGS

Drugs That May Alter Lab Results N/A

Disorders That May Alter Lab Results
Hemolysis can cause a spurious high value

Valid if Run in Human Lab? Yes

CBC/BIOCHEMISTRY/URINALYSIS
• Serum magnesium > 2.1 mg/gl (dogs) or > 2.3 mg/dl (cats) • Hypocalcemia a common finding • Azotemia in some patients

OTHER LABORATORY TESTS N/A

IMAGING N/A

OTHER DIAGNOSTIC PROCEDURES
Electrodiagnostics (e.g., electromyelography and ECG) reveal effects of hypermagnesemia but do not help differentiate the cause.

TREATMENT
• Depends on the the underlying cause of the abnormality
• Discontinue all magnesium-containing compounds.
• Experience treating veterinary patients with hypermagnesemia is extremely limited, so recommendations are difficult.

MEDICATIONS

DRUGS AND FLUIDS

• Fluid therapy to treat azotemia
• Enteral calcium administration to reverse clinical manifestations of hypermagnesemia and to correct concurrent hypocalcemia. Any calcium preparation can be used (25-50 mg/kg/day PO). Severe hypermagnesemia can be treated by 10% calcium gluconate (1-2 ml/kg [diluted 1:1 with saline] IV or SC administered very slowly q8h).

CONTRAINDICATIONS

Magnesium-containing compounds

PRECAUTIONS

Monitor ECG during calcium infusions.

POSSIBLE INTERACTIONS N/A

ALTERNATE DRUGS N/A

 FOLLOW-UP

PATIENT MONITORING

• Serum magnesium and calcium concentrations 2-3 times daily • ECG continuously if possible, at least every 2-4 hours • Vitals (TPR) frequently

POSSIBLE COMPLICATIONS

Severe hypermagnesemia and hypocalcemia can be fatal.

 MISCELLANEOUS

ASSOCIATED CONDITIONS

• Hypocalcemia • Hyperphosphatemia
• Azotemia

AGE RELATED FACTORS N/A

ZOONOTIC POTENTIAL N/A

PREGNANCY

Effects on the fetus identical to the effects on the dam

SYNONYMS None

SEE ALSO

Calcium, Hypocalcemia

ABBREVIATIONS

ECG = electrocardiogram

References

Brautbar N, Massry SG. Hypomagnesemia and hypermagnesemia. In: Maxwell MH, Kleeman CR, Narins RG, eds. Clinical disorders of fluid and electrolyte metabolism. 4th ed. New York: McGraw-Hill, 1987.

Quamme GA, Dirks JH. Magnesium metabolism. In: Maxwell MH, Kleeman CR, Narins RG, eds. Clinical disorders of fluid and electrolyte metabolism. 4th ed. New York: McGraw-Hill, 1987.

Martin LG, Matteson VL, Wingfield WE, et al. Abnormalities of serum magnesium in critically ill dogs: incidence and implications. J Vet Emerg Crit Care 1994;4:15-20.
Author Thomas K. Graves
Editor Rhett Nichols

MAGNESIUM, HYPOMAGNESEMIA

 BASICS

DEFINITION
•Serum magnesium < 1.3 mg/dl

Pathophysiology
• Magnesium is the second most abundant intracellular cation. Its presence is critical in many cellular enzymatic reactions. Serum magnesium concentration does not always reflect the magnesium status of the whole body. • Many causes of hypomagnesemia are documented, and although it is usually ignored in veterinary practice, it is one of the most common electrolyte abnormalities in critical care patients. • Cardiac arrhythmias are assocated with magnesium depletion; these arrythmias can be life threatening. ECG changes including ventricular arrythmias, QT prolongation, ST segment shortening, and widening of T waves. Hypomagnesemia enhances the danger of digoxin toxicity, and can also cause hypertension. • Hypomagnesemia alters the function of the skeletal muscles and the CNS. • Hypomagnesemia blunts the calcemic effect of PTH by altering its effect on bone and by inhibiting its secretion.

SIGNALMENT N/A

SIGNS
Hypomagnesemia occurs with a variety of diseases with diverse signs:
• Weakness • Muscle fibrillation • Ataxia and depression • Hyperreflexia • Tetany • Behavior changes • Arrhyhthmias

CAUSES
• Since small intestinal absorption is essential to the maintenance of magnesium balance, severe malnutrition or clinically important intestinal disease causing malabsorption can lead to hypomagnesemia. • Magnesium homeostasis is also controlled by renal elimination, and any condition that causes excessive renal magnesium loss can result in hypomagnesemia. These include hypercalcemia, renal tubular acidosis, diabetes mellitus, hyperthyroidism, gentamicin toxicity, cisplatin nephrotoxicity, and the use of loop diuretics. Hypomagnesemia in heart failure patients treated with diuretics does not appear to be as common a problem in dogs as in humans.
• Hypomagnesemia can be caused by redistribution of magnesium such as can occur with refeeding after starvation, parathyroidectomy, the use of total parenteral nutrition formulations with inadequate magnesium content, and in patients with acute pancreatitis.
• Hypomagnesemia can occur after excessive loss of body fluids as in patients with severe, prolonged diarrhea. This has not been well-documented in veterinary patients.

RISK FACTORS
• Total parenteral nutrition • Diuretic administration • Intestinal lymphangiectasia

 DIAGNOSIS

DIFFERENTIAL DIAGNOSIS
The signs of hypomagnesemia are vague and multisystemic, and other causes of neuromuscular abnormalities, especially other electrolyte abnormalities, must be investigated. Cardiac abnormalities, intoxications, and renal diseases are important considerations.

LABORATORY FINDINGS
Drugs That May Alter Lab Results N/A

Disorders That May Alter Lab Results
Hemolysis can cause a spurious high concentration

Valid If Run In Human Lab? Yes

CBC/BIOCHEMISTRY/URINALYSIS
• If patient is azotemic, consider renal causes.
• Tubular casts in urinary sediment may indicate nephrotoxicity. • Hypokalemia, hyponatremia, and hypocalcemia are common findings regardless of the cause of hypomagnesemia.

OTHER LABORATORY TESTS
Urine magnesium determination may help differentiate conditions associated with high urinary magnesium loss versus conditions of low intake or absorption.

IMAGING N/A

OTHER DIAGNOSTIC PROCEDURES
Electrodiagnostics (e.g., electromyelography and ECG) may reveal effects of hypomagnesemia but will not help differentiate the cause.

 TREATMENT

Treatment depends on the underlying cause of the abnormality and on the severity of hypomagnesemia. Since experience in treating veterinary patients with hypomagnesemia is extremely limited, recommendations are difficult. Mild hypomagnesemia may resolve with treatment of the underlying disorder. However, if hypomagnesemia is severe, intensive care is needed.

MEDICATIONS

DRUGS AND FLUIDS

Magnesium sulfate can be diluted in 5% dextrose in water and administered at a dosage of 1 mEq/kg/day as a constant rate intravenous infusion. The solution of magnesium sulfate should be less than 20%. The magnesium infusion should be done via an intravenous line separate from other fluids to minimize interactions with other minerals.

CONTRAINDICATIONS

• Aminoglycosides should not be used since hypomagnesemia potentiates their nephrotoxicity. • Cisplatin chemotherapy should not be used.

PRECAUTIONS

• Digoxin should be discontinued if possible.
• Diuretics should be used with caution.
• Hypermagnesemia is possible with overzealous treatment.

POSSIBLE INTERACTIONS

• Magnesium sulfate is incompatible with sodium bicarbonate, hydrocortisone, and dobutamine HCl. In general, mixing of other drugs with magnesium sulfate solution should be avoided.
• Calcium-containing compounds lower the serum magnesium concentration and should be avoided.
• The effects of CNS depressants, sedatives, neuromuscular blocking agents, and anesthetics are enhanced by hypomagnesemia.

ALTERNATE DRUGS N/A

FOLLOW-UP

PATIENT MONITORING

• Serum magnesium and calcium concentrations 2-3 times daily • ECG continuously if possible; at least every 2-4 hours. • Vitals (TPR) frequently

POSSIBLE COMPLICATIONS

Severe hypomagnesemia can be fatal.

MISCELLANEOUS

ASSOCIATED CONDITIONS

• Hypokalemia • Hyponatremia • Hypocalcemia
• Hypophosphatemia

AGE RELATED FACTORS N/A

ZOONOTIC POTENTIAL N/A

PREGNANCY

Effects on the fetus are identical to the effects on the dam.

SYNONYMS None

SEE ALSO See Causes

ABBREVIATIONS

CNS = central nervous system
ECG = electrocardiography
PTH = parathyroid hormone

References

Brautbar N, Massry SG. Hypomagnesemia and hypermagnesemia. In: Maxwell MH, Kleeman CR, Narins RG, eds. Clinical disorders of fluid and electrolyte metabolism. 4th ed. New York: McGraw-Hill, 1987.

Quamme GA, Dirks JH. Magnesium metabolism. In: Maxwell MH, Kleeman CR, Narins RG, eds. Clinical disorders of fluid and electrolyte metabolism. 4th ed. New York: McGraw-Hill, 1987.

Martin LG, Matteson VL, Wingfield WE, et al. Abnormalities of serum magnesium in critically ill dogs: incidence and implications. J Vet Emerg Crit Care 1994;4:15-20.

Author Thomas K. Graves
Consulting Editor Rhett Nichols

METHEMOGLOBINEMIA

BASICS

DEFINITION
Methemoglobin differs from hemoglobin in that the iron moiety of heme groups has been oxidized from the ferrous (+2) to the ferric (+3) state. Methemoglobinemia refers to methemoglobin content of the blood > 1.5% of total hemoglobin.

Pathophysiology
About 3% of hemoglobin is oxidized to methemoglobin each day in clinically normal animals as a result of autoxidation of hemoglobin or secondarily to oxidants produced in normal metabolic reactions. Methemoglobin usually accounts for less than 1% of total hemoglobin because it is constantly reduced back to hemoglobin by a NADH-dependent methemoglobin reductase (cytochrome-b$_5$-reductase) enzyme reaction present within RBC. Methemoglobinemia is caused by either increased production of methemoglobin by oxidants or decreased reduction of methemoglobin associated with a deficiency in the RBC methemoglobin reductase enzyme.

Systems Affected
Methemoglobinemia causes reduced oxygen carrying capacity of the blood because methemoglobin cannot bind oxygen. If methemoglobin content reaches high values (e.g., > 50% of total hemoglobin), various organs may suffer hypoxic injury.

SIGNALMENT
• Dogs and cats
• Deficiency in RBC methemoglobin reductase has been recognized in the Chihuahua, borzoi, English setter, terrier mix, cockapoo, poodle, corgi, Pomeranian, toy Eskimo dog, and, recently, in a domestic shorthair cat.

SIGNS

Signs Caused by Methemoglobinemia
• Possibly none in animals with mild to moderate methemoglobinemia • Cyanotic mucous membranes • Lethargy, tachycardia, tachypnea, ataxia, and stupor as a result of hypoxia when methemoglobin content reaches 50%
• Coma-like state and death when methemoglobin content reaches 80%

Signs Caused by Diseases Associated with Methemoglobinemia
• Vomiting, anorexia, and diarrhea possible in patients with drug toxicity • Hemoglobinuria secondary to severe intravascular hemolysis in some patients with concomitant Heinz body hemolytic anemia • Subcutaneous edema, especially involving the face, and salivation in patients with acetaminophen toxicity

CAUSES
• Benzocaine, acetaminophen, and phenazopyridine toxicities in dogs and cats. These drugs also can cause Heinz body

hemolytic anemia. • Deficiency in RBC methemoglobin reductase

RISK FACTORS
• Application of benzocaine to traumatized skin or mucous membranes enhances the likelihood of systemic absorption and methemoglobinemia. • Cats are much more likely to develop clinically important methemoglobinemia than are dogs after acetaminophen administration. This drug is not recommended for use in cats. • Methemoglobinemia secondary to methemoglobin reductase deficiency is presumed to be an inherited disorder, but family studies have not been reported.

DIAGNOSIS

DIFFERENTIAL DIAGNOSIS
Both low blood oxygen tension and methemoglobinemia can cause cyanotic-appearing mucous membranes and dark-colored blood samples. Hypoxemia is documented by measuring low pO$_2$ in an arterial blood sample. Methemoglobinemia is suspected when arterial blood with normal or high pO$_2$ is dark-colored.

LABORATORY FINDINGS

Drugs That Alter Lab Results N/A

Disorders That May Alter Lab Results
Hemolysis in the sample may raise the methemoglobin value, especially if the methemoglobin assay is not conducted quickly after sample collection.

Valid If Run in Human Lab?
Valid, as long as the method to lyse RBC does not cause methemoglobin formation in the animal being tested. Saponin should not be used to lyse RBC because it raises the methemoglobin value in some species.

CBC/BIOCHEMISTRY/URINALYSIS
• Chronic methemoglobinemia secondary to methemoglobin reductase deficiency can result in a slightly high PCV. In contrast, anemia may accompany methemoglobinemia that is caused by oxidant drugs. • If methemoglobinemia is severe or induced by oxidant drugs, evidence of injury to various organs (e.g., high BUN or ALT) may be seen.

OTHER LABORATORY TESTS
• A spot test can be used to determine if the patient's methemoglobin concentration is clinically important. One drop of blood from the patient is placed on a piece of absorbent white paper and a drop of normal control blood is placed next to it. If the methemoglobin content is 10% or greater, the patient's blood should have a noticeably brown coloration compared with a bright red color of the control blood. • Accurate determination of methemoglobin content requires that blood be quickly submitted to an appropriate laboratory. Methemoglobin content in dogs with methemoglobin reductase deficiency varies from 13-41%. The methemoglobin

content in the deficient cat was 50%. • A definitive diagnosis of methemoglobin reductase deficiency is made by measuring enzyme activity in RBC. This assay is done in a few research laboratories and requires that arrangements be made before blood samples are submitted.

IMAGING N/A

OTHER DIAGNOSTIC PROCEDURES
Blood should be stained for Heinz bodies if evidence of toxicity is seen. The presence of Heinz bodies indicates exposure to an oxidant drug that may also cause hemolytic anemia.

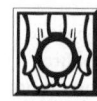

TREATMENT
• Mild to moderate methemoglobinemia does not require specific treatment to reduce the methemoglobin content.
• If methemoglobinemia is drug-induced, the use of the drug should be discontinued. RBC can convert much of the methemoglobin back to hemoglobin within 24 hours after elimination of drug exposure.
• Animals with inherited methemoglobin reductase deficiency do not require treatment and have normal life expectancy.

MEDICATIONS

DRUGS AND FLUIDS
• Methylene blue, given slowly over several minutes as a 1% solution (1 mg/kg IV), may be administered in patients with severe methemoglobinemia. A dramatic response should occur during the first 30 minutes after treatment. While this dose can be repeated if necessary, use methylene blue cautiously in dogs and cats because it can cause Heinz body hemolytic anemia.
• In patients with drug-induced methemoglobinemia, additional supportive treatment may be required. Whole blood transfusions should be given to patients with severe anemia and to those with a rapidly decreasing PCV and clinical signs suggesting that their condition is deteriorating. If severe intravascular hemolysis devlops, IV fluid therapy is recommended to minimize the chance of hemoglobin nephrosis. Treatment of electrolyte or acid-base imbalances may also be indicated in patients with severe vomiting or diarrhea, concomitant renal injury, or impending shock.
• N-acetylcysteine is efficacious in the treatment of acetaminophen toxicity in cats if given within a few hours after exposure. The recommended dosage is 140 mg/kg PO followed by 70 mg/kg q6h for 7 treatments.
• Administration of oxygen is of limited value because methemoglobin cannot bind oxygen, and an increase in dissolved oxygen results in only a small increase in blood oxygen content.

CONTRAINDICATIONS N/A

METHEMOGLOBINEMIA

PRECAUTIONS

In patients that have been given drugs that cause substantial Heinz body formation and methemoglobinemia, methylene blue treatment can potentiate the formation of Heinz bodies and anemia. Consequently, it is prudent to measure the PCV for 3 days after methylene blue treatment to assure that clinically important anemia does not develop.

POSSIBLE INTERACTIONS N/A

ALTERNATE DRUGS N/A

 ## FOLLOW-UP

PATIENT MONITORING

• The cyanotic-appearance of skin and mucous membranes should disappear after reduction of methemoglobin to a concentration that does not cause clinical signs. • Blood on the spot test should appear bright red after reduction of methemoglobin to values below 10% of total hemoglobin. • If methylene blue treatment is given or Heinz bodies are seen within RBC, the PCV should be monitored closely because it usually does not reach its lowest point until approximately 3 days after initial exposure to oxidant.

POSSIBLE COMPLICATIONS

Coma and death if methemoglobin content reaches 80% of total hemoglobin

 ## MISCELLANEOUS

ASSOCIATED CONDITIONS

Heinz body anemia

AGE RELATED FACTORS N/A

ZOONOTIC POTENTIAL N/A

PREGNANCY N/A

SYNONYMS N/A

SEE ALSO

• Anemia, Heinz Body • Acetaminophen Toxicity

ABBREVIATIONS

PCV = packed cell volume
RBC = red blood cells

References

Harvey JW. Methemoglobinemia and Heinz body hemolytic anemia. In Kirk RW, Bonagura J, eds. Current veterinary therapy XII. Philadelphia: WB Saunders, 1994.

Cullison RF. Acetaminophen toxicosis in small animals: clinical signs, mode of action, and treatment. Comp Cont Ed Pract Vet 1984;6:315-321.

Harvey JW, King RR, Berry CR, Blue JT. Methaemoglobin reductase deficiency in dogs. Comp Haematol Int 1991;1:55-59.

Harvey JW, Dahl M, High ME. Methemoglobin reductase deficiency in a cat. J Am Vet Med Assoc 1994;205:1290-1291.

Author John W. Harvey
Consulting Editor Alan H. Rebar

MONOCYTOSIS

BASICS

DEFINITION
Absolute number of circulating monocytes greater than the reference range—dogs, > 1.3 x 10^9/l or >l300/µl or mm³; cats, > 0.9 x 10^9/l or 900/µl or mm³

Pathophysiology
• Monocytes are derived from hematopoietic stem cells named the colony-forming unit – granulocyte, monocyte (CFU-GM). The CFU-GM is responsible for neutrophil and monocyte production. With the appropriate stimulus, cells from this unit differentiate into monoblasts (or myeloblasts) and then into monocytes. • The production, differentiation, and release of monocytes is regulated by a variety of substances, including colony stimulating factor, antichalones, PGE_2, and various interleukins. Production to release of monocytes takes approximately 6 hours, and thus cells in circulation are relatively young.
• Monocytes exit the circulation to reside in various tissues, begin another phase of differentiation, and then become part of the mononuclear phagocyte system. Along with their differentiation, they undergo various "name changes" and are referred to as macrophages and histiocytes. They reside in lymph nodes, bone marrow, spleen, liver (Kupffer cells), lungs (alveolar macrophages), bone (osteoclasts), pleural and peritoneal cavities, and CNS (microglial cells). • Several macrophages may fuse to form multinucleated giant cells. This is a common response to fungi, mycobacterium, syncytial virus, and foreign material. • In tissues, the ratio of macrophages to circulating monocytes is approximately 400:1. The accumulation of monocytes in an area of acute or chronic inflammation is caused by chemotactic factors that attract monocytes to these specific foci. Most macrophages in a region are migrating circulating monocytes but under specific microenvironmental stimuli, they can be derived from local production. • Some of the many functions of the mononuclear phagocyte system are phagocytosis, microbicidal activity, tumor cytolysis, regulation of the immune system, coagulation, fibrinolysis, and bone repair. The mononuclear phagocyte system is vital in controlling certain pathogens, including intracellular bacteria (e.g., Mycobacteria, Listeria, and Brucella), mycotic agents, protozoa, and viruses.

Systems Affected
• Respiratory—alveolar macrophages
• Hemic/lymph/immune—lymph nodes (histiocyte proliferation), spleen (proliferation of red pulp and mononuclear phagocyte system proliferation), and bone marrow • Hepatobiliary—Kupffer cells • Musculoskeletal—osteoclasts
• Nervous—microglial cells • Thoracic and abdominal cavities—macrophage and mesothelial proliferation

SIGNALMENT
• Irish setter—chronic granulocytopathy syndrome • Young animals have higher monocyte counts than adults. • Geriatric dogs have monocytosis.

SIGNS
Referable to primary cause of the monocytosis or proliferation of mononuclear phagocyte system

CAUSES
• General—any process that stimulates neutrophilia because monocytes and neutrophils share the same stem cell precursor CFU-GM
• Glucocorticoids—corticosteroids stimulate absolute monocytosis in dogs and less frequently in cats. Monocytosis develops within hours of steroid exposure and resolves within 24 hours after removing the corticosteroid stimulus. Causes include glucocorticoid treatment, stress of a disease, and hyperadrenocorticism. • Inflammation (infectious)—mycotic (e.g., Aspergillus and Blastomycosis), protozoal (e.g., Toxoplasma), viral (e.g., FIP), bacterial (e.g., Mycobacteria, Brucella) • Inflammation (noninfectious)—foreign material, necrotic tissue, malignant tumor, hemolytic anemia, trauma, neutropenia with compensatory monocytosis, and immune mediated disease
• Monocytic or myelomonocytic leukemia—neoplastic proliferation of the monocyte cell line or a combined myeloid and monocyte cell line produces monocytosis. Immature, bizarre cells are present in the circulation. Careful examination of the feathered edge of the blood smear should permit identification of these cells. • Granulocytopathy syndrome (dogs)—cellular defect in monocytes of Irish setters and familial disease • Cylichematopoiesis (silver-gray collies)—the cyclic neutropenia at 11-14 day intervals is usually followed by high numbers of other cell lines, including monocytes, thrombocytes, and neutrophils • Older dogs—absolute monocytosis, lymphopenia, and eosinopenia can be seen

RISK FACTORS N/A

DIAGNOSIS

DIFFERENTIAL DIAGNOSIS
• Severely stressed or ill dogs—consider endogenous glucocorticoids • Concurrent alopecia, "potbelly," thin skin, and muscle atrophy—consider hyperadrenocorticism
• Fever of undetermined origin—consider endocarditis and immune-mediated disease
• Draining cutaneous wound—consider mycotic infection and foreign body • Splenomegaly, hepatomegaly, or lymphadenopathy—consider leukemia

LABORATORY FINDINGS

Drugs That May Alter Lab Results N/A
Disorders That May Alter Lab Results N/A

Valid If Run in Human Lab?
Vaild, but certain techniques for counting monocytes can yield errors. Mechanical blood-spreading devices shift larger cells (monocytes) into the "counting area," with absolute, artifactual monocytosis reported. Incorrect identification of metamyelocytes and other immature neutrophils in a left shift also can result in erroneous monocytosis.

CBC/BIOCHEMISTRY/URINALYSIS
• Severe monocytosis (i.e., > 20,000 monocytes/ml)—consider leukemia or rebound phase of cyclic hematopoiesis • Immature, bizarre, and abnormal cells in circulation—consider monocytic leukemia and myelomonocytic leukemia • Mature neutrophilia, lymphopenia, and eosinopenia—consider stress and hyperadrenocorticism
• Neutrophilia—consider pyogranulomatous diseases • Anemia—consider immune hemolytic anemia

OTHER LABORATORY TESTS N/A

IMAGING N/A

OTHER DIAGNOSTIC PROCEDURES N/A

TREATMENT
Treatment is directed at the underlying cause of the monocytosis.

MEDICATIONS

DRUGS AND FLUIDS N/A
CONTRAINDICATIONS N/A
PRECAUTIONS N/A
POSSIBLE INTERACTIONS
Levamisole—increases rate of migration of monocytes, enhances chemotaxis, and increases phagocytosis

ALTERNATE DRUGS N/A

FOLLOW-UP

PATIENT MONITORING N/A
POSSIBLE COMPLICATIONS N/A

MISCELLANEOUS

ASSOCIATED CONDITIONS
Other diseases that effect the mononuclear phagocyte system but do not cause consistent monocytosis:
• Malignant and systemic histiocytosis of Bernese mountain dogs • Lysosomal storage diseases • Recovery from leukopenia and neutropenia can cause monocytosis of > 20,000/µl.

The rapid induction of monocytes with their uniquely short marrow transit time causes monocytosis that precedes the rebound neutrophilia.

AGE RELATED FACTORS

Old dogs—monocytosis often seen in patients with lymphopenia and eosinopenia; possibly related to stress

PREGNANCY N/A

SYNONYMS N/A

SEE ALSO N/A

ABBREVIATIONS

CFU-GM = colony-forming unit – granulocyte, monocyte
CNS = central nervous system
FeLV = feline leukemia virus

References
Renshaw HW, Davis WC. Canine granulocytopathy syndrome. Am J Pathol 1979;95:731-744.
Giger U, et al. Deficiency of leukocyte surface glycoproteins Mo1, LFA-1 and Leu M5 in a dog. Blood 1987:1622-1630.
Author Donald J. Meuten
Consulting Editor Alan H. Rebar

NEUTROPHILIA

 BASICS

DEFINITION
An increase in absolute numbers of circulating neutrophils. In adult dogs and cats, neutrophil counts exceed 12,000-13,000/μl.

Pathophysiology
Neutrophils are produced in the bone marrow, released into the blood, circulate briefly, and migrate into tissue spaces and onto epithelial surfaces. Injury or bacterial invasion of tissue causes production and release of colony-stimulating factors, which increase proliferation and maturation of neutrophilic progenitor cells in the bone marrow. Other mediators of inflammation stimulate bone marrow release and promote margination and adhesion of neutrophils to vascular endothelium at the site of inflammation. Transit time for bone marrow granulopoiesis is approximately 4-6 days. Neutrophils circulate for about 10 hours and are compartmentalized into a circulating neutrophil pool (CNP) and a marginal neutrophil pool (MNP). Neutrophils in the CNP circulate with other blood cells and are measured in the CBC. The MNP consists of neutrophils that are intermittently adherent to endothelium, especially in small veins and capillaries. Migration of neutrophils into tissues occurs randomly and is unidirectional. Neutrophils are destroyed in the spleen, liver, and bone marrow. Numbers of circulating neutrophils are affected by the rate of bone marrow production and release, the rate of exchange between CNP and MNP, and the rate of migration into tissue. Neutrophilia results when one or more of the following occurs: 1) the rate of marrow production and release increases, 2) neutrophils demarginate from the MNP into the CNP, 3) tissue demand for neutrophils increases, 4) neoplasia of granulopoiesis develops.

Systems Affected Hemic/lymph/immune

SIGNALMENT N/A

SIGNS Vary with cause

CAUSES

Physiologic Neutrophilia
Fear, excitement, and vigorous exercise cause epinephrine release. Neutrophils demarginate from MNP into CNP, resulting in a transient (1 hour), mature neutrophilia. In cats, severe lymphocytosis (6,000-15,000/ml) occurs concurrently.

Corticosteroid- or Stress-Induced Neutrophilia
Corticosteriods cause increased bone marrow release of mature neutrophils, demargination into the CNP, and decreased tissue migration. Leukocytosis (15,000-35,000/ml) and neutrophilia occur 4-8 hours after administration and return to normal 1-3 days after

treatment. Lymphopenia, eosinopenia, and monocytosis (dogs) occur concurrently. Pain, traumatic injury, boarding, transport, and other stressful conditions are common causes.

Neutrophilia of Acute Inflammation
Inflammation, sepsis, necrosis, and immune-mediated disease cause increased tissue demand and increased bone marrow release of segmented and band neutrophils. Leukocytosis (15,000-30,000/ml), neutrophilia with a left shift, toxic neutrophils, lymphopenia, eosinopenia, and variable monocytosis are usual responses. Surgical removal or drainage of a septic focus may increase neutrophilia.

Neutrophilia of Chronic Inflammation
Chronic suppuration (e.g., pyometra, abscesses, pyothorax, and pyoderma) and some neoplasms cause granulocytic hyperplasia that results in severe leukocytosis (50,000-120,000/ml), neutrophilia with a left shift, variable numbers of toxic neutrophils, monocytosis, and hyperglobulinemia. Anemia associated with chronic disease may be present. Leukemoid response is a term used to describe inflammatory neutrophilia with WBC count >100,000/μl because of its similarity to chronic granulocytic leukemia.

Hemolytic or Hemorrhagic Anemia
Neutrophilia with a left shift is common in dogs with immune-mediated hemolytic anemia. Mature neutrophilia develops 3 hours after acute hemorrhage.

Chronic Granulocytic Leukemia
Hematologic response in dogs is similar to neutrophilia associated with chronic inflammation. Severe neutrophilic leukocytosis (> 80,000/μl), disordered left shift, and variable degrees of thrombocytopenia and anemia are observed. Splenomegaly and hepatomegaly may be pronounced.

Other Causes
Metabolic disease, granulocytopathy, and cyclic hematopoiesis

RISK FACTORS N/A

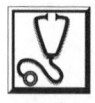 **DIAGNOSIS**

DIFFERENTIAL DIAGNOSIS
• Animals with inflammatory neutrophilia usually have historical or clinical evidence of septic or nonseptic inflammatory disease such as pyrexia, weight loss, loss of appetite, and specific organ system involvement. • Stress neutrophilia commonly develops in dogs and cats examined because of noninflammatory disorders. • Physiologic neutrophilia affects young healthy animals, especially cats.

LABORATORY FINDINGS

Drugs That May Alter Lab Results
Corticosteroid administration causes stress leukogram. Neutrophilia subsides with long-term therapy but lymphopenia persists.

Disorders That May Alter Lab Results
Electronic WBC counts can be falsely high because of large platelets, platelet clumps, and Heinz bodies. Leukocyte clumping causes a false decrease in the count.

Valid If Run in Human Lab?
Valid, but some human laboratories overestimate the number of band cells at the expense of mature neutrophils. Clinically normal animals will appear to have left shifts.

CBC/BIOCHEMISTRY/URINALYSIS
• Assessment of sequential leukograms is important because numbers of segmented and band neutrophils can change dramatically in a few hours. Trends that are persistent, increasing, or decreasing are important in diagnosis and prognosis. • Toxic neutrophils are observed in animals with inflammation, especially when associated with toxemia. Toxic neutrophils are observed in blood and bone marrow and are characterized by diffuse cytoplasmic basophilia, foamy vacuolated cytoplasm, Döhle's bodies, and giant forms with bizarre nuclear shapes.

OTHER LABORATORY TESTS
• Blood culture • Bacterial or fungal culture of urine, tissue samples, and body fluids • Serologic tests for fungi, protozoa, and rickettsia. Genera of special interest include Blastomyces, Histoplasma, Coccidioides, Actinomyces, Nocardia, Toxoplasma, Hepatozoon, and Rickettsia. • Coombs' test, antinuclear antibody test, or rheumatoid factor test indicated if immune-mediated disease is suspected

IMAGING
Radiography and ultrasonography of abdomen, thorax, soft tissue, or skeleton to detect inflammatory or neoplastic lesions (e.g., abscesses, granulomatous lesions, effusions, foreign bodies, and organomegaly)

OTHER DIAGNOSTIC PROCEDURES
N/A

 TREATMENT

• Treatment varies with the identity and severity of underlying cause.
• Animals with acute sepsis or hemolytic anemia require aggressive intervention.
• Those with chronic granulocytic leukemia require chemotherapy.
• Those with inflammatory neutrophilia may require surgical intervention to remove or drain sites of sepsis.

 MEDICATIONS

DRUGS AND FLUIDS
• Appropriate antimicrobial therapy for septic inflammation after identification of causative agent and sensitivity testing

CONTRAINDICATIONS

Corticosteroids should be avoided if fungal or protozoal infection is suspected.

PRECAUTIONS N/A

POSSIBLE INTERACTIONS N/A

ALTERNATE DRUGS N/A

 FOLLOW-UP

PATIENT MONITORING

Animals with inflammatory neutrophilia, especially of acute onset, may require daily or twice-daily hematologic assessment.

POSSIBLE COMPLICATIONS

Animals with acute inflammatory neutrophilia may become neutropenic if migration into the inflammed tissue exceeds the bone marrow production rate. If neutropenia develops, prognosis is grave.

 MISCELLANEOUS

ASSOCIATED CONDITIONS N/A

AGE RELATED FACTORS N/A

ZOONOTIC POTENTIAL N/A

PREGNANCY N/A

SYNONYMS N/A

SEE ALSO

• Infectious Diseases Topics • Myeloproliferative Disorders • Hyperadrenocorticism

ABBREVIATIONS

CNP = circulating neutrophil pool
MNP = marginal neutrophil pool

Reference

Latimer KS. Leukocytes in health and disease. In: Ettinger SJ, Feldman EC, eds. Textbook of veterinary internal medicine. Philadelphia: WB Saunders, 1995:1892-1929.

Author Peter S. MacWilliams
Consulting Editor Alan H. Rebar

OSMOLARITY, HYPEROSMOLARITY

BASICS

DEFINITION
• Osmolarity is expressed in mOsm/L and represents the number of solute particles per liter of solution. Osmolality is expressed in mOsm/kg and represents the number of solute particles per kilogram of solution.
• Hyperosmolarity is defined as a high concentration of solute particles per liter of solution. Serum concentrations > 310 mOsm/L in dogs and > 330 mOsm/L in cats are usually considered hyperosmolar.

Pathophysiology
• Serum sodium is responsible for most of the osmotically active particles that contribute to serum osmolarity. Serum glucose and urea also contribute to serum osmolarity. Anything that causes water loss increases concentrations of solutes in plasma or serum, thereby increasing serum osomolarity. Blood volume, hydration status, and antidiuretic hormone (ADH) are intimately involved in controlling extracellular fluid volume. • Low circulating blood volume stimulates carotid and aortic baroreceptors to respond to changes in blood pressure, causing ADH secretion. • Hyperosmolarity affects the osmoreceptors in the hypothalamus and stimulates ADH secretion from the neurohypophysis. The hypothalamic thirst center is also stimulated and causes an increase in water consumption to counteract serum hyperosmolarity by solute dilution. • Rapid increases in serum osmolarity cause water movement along its concentration gradient from intracellular to extracellular spaces resulting in neuronal dehydration, cell shrinkage, and cell death. Cerebral vessels may weaken and hemorrhage.

Systems Affected
• Nervous—excessive thirst may be the first sign of hyperosmolarity. • Cardiovascular—hypotension and depressed ventricular contractility • Renal/Urinologic—low urine output

SIGNALMENT
• Dogs and cats • Hypodipsia and hyperosmolarity have been reported in young female miniature schnauzers.

SIGNS

General Comments
• Signs are primarily neurologic and behavioral. • The severity of signs is related more to how quickly hyperosmolarity occurs rather than to the absolute magnitude of change. • Signs most likely to develop if serum osmolarity is > 350 mOsm/L and are usually severe if value is > 375 mOsm/L

Historical Findings
Anorexia, lethargy, vomiting, weakness, disorientation, ataxia, seizures, and coma; polydipsia followed by hypodipsia.

Physical Examination Findings
• Findings normal or abnormalities reflect underlying disease • In addition to historical findings, dehydration, tachycardia, hypotension, weak pulses, and fever may be detected.

CAUSES

Increased Solutes
Hypernatremia, hyperglycemia, severe azotemia, ethylene glycol toxicosis, salt poisoning, sodium phosphate enemas in cats and small dogs, aspirin toxicosis, shock, and administration of ethanol, mannitol, radiographic contrast solution, liquid enteral nutrition and parenteral nutrition solutions, lactate in patients with lactic acidosis, and acetoacetate and beta-hydroxybutyrate in patients with ketoacidosis

Decreased Extracellular Fluid Volume
Dehydration—gastrointestinal loss, cutaneous loss, third space loss, low water consumption, and polyuria without adequate compensatory polydipsia

RISK FACTORS
• Medical conditions that predispose—renal failure, diabetes insipidus, diabetes mellitus, hyperadrenocorticism, hyperaldosteronism, and heat stroke • Therapeutic hyperosmolar solutions—hypertonic saline, sodium bicarbonate, sodium phosphate enemas in cats and small dogs, and mannitol • High environmental temperatures • Fever

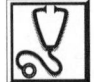

DIAGNOSIS

DIFFERENTIAL DIAGNOSIS
• Primary CNS disease and neoplasia may be characterized by altered mentation, but serum osmolarity is usually normal • Physical evidence or history of injury usually help to rule out CNS depression caused by cranial trauma. • Perform a thorough physical examination to assess hydration status and obtain information regarding previous treatment that may have included sodium-containing fluids or hyperosmolar solutions.

LABORATORY FINDINGS

Drugs That May Alter Lab Results
Excessive administration of sodium-containing fluids or hyperosmolar solutions increases serum osmolarity.

Disorders That May Alter Lab Result N/A

Valid If Run In Human Lab? Yes

CBC/BIOCHEMISTRY/URINALYSIS
• High PCV, hemoglobin, and plasma proteins in dehydrated patients. Serum electrolytes may also be high. • Hyperosmolarity is an indication to evaluate serum sodium and glucose concentrations. • Estimated serum osmolarity can be calculated from serum biochemistries as follows:

$$2(Na) + \frac{BUN}{3} + \frac{glucose}{20}$$

• Normally, the calculated osmolarity should not be greater than measured osmolarity. If it is, the osmolar gap should be determined. Osmolar gap = measured osmolarity - calculated osmolarity. • High measured osmolarity with a high osmolar gap and normal calculated osmolarity indicates the presence of unmeasured solutes (not Na, K, glucose, or BUN). • High measured osmolarity and high calculated osmolarity with a normal osmolar gap usually indicates that the hyperosmolarity is caused by hyperglycemia or hypernatremia. • Serum sodium may be artificially low in patients with severe hyperglycemia and hyperosmalarity. • Fasting hyperglycemia and glucosuria support a diagnosis of diabetes mellitus. • Numerous calcium oxalate crystals in the urine suggests ethylene gylcol toxicosis. • High urine specific gravity rules out diabetes insipidus. • Low urine specific gravity, especially hyposthenuria, suggests diabetes insipidus.

OTHER LABORATORY TESTS
Urine osmolarity lower than serum osmolarity suggests diabetes insipidus, whereas concentrated urine rules out diabetes insipidus.

IMAGING
Renal ultrasonography may reveal bright, hyperechoic kidneys in patients with ethylene glycol toxicosis.

OTHER DIAGNOSTIC PROCEDURES
N/A

TREATMENT
• Mild hyperosmolarity without clinical signs may not warrant specific treatment. However, underlying diseases should be diagnosed and treated.
• Patients with moderate to high osmolarity (> 350 mOsm/L) or patients exhibiting clinical signs should be hospitalized and serum osmolarity gradually lowered with intravenous administration of fluids while a definitive diagnosis is persued.

MEDICATIONS

DRUGS AND FLUIDS
• D$_5$W or 0.45% saline should be administered slowly IV.
• 0.9% saline may be used initially to restore normal hemodynamics and replace dehydration deficits. Replace one half of dehydration deficits over 12 hours and the remainder over 24 hours. Then switch to D$_5$W or 0.45% saline.
• Seizures can be controlled with diazepam, phenobarbital, or pentobarbital.

CONTRAINDICATIONS
Hypertonic saline and hyperosmolar solutions are contraindicated.

PRECAUTIONS
• Normal saline may be used initally, but rapid administration may result in worsening of neurologic signs. • Rapid administration of hypotonic fluids (e.g., D_5W and 0.45% saline) may also cause cerebral edema and worsening of neurologic signs.

POSSIBLE INTERACTIONS N/A

ALTERNATE DRUGS N/A

FOLLOW-UP

PATIENT MONITORING
• Hydration status; avoid overhydration
• Bladder size, urine output, and breathing patterns during IV administration of fluids

• Anuria and irregular breathing patterns may be signs of deterioration.

POSSIBLE COMPLICATIONS
Altered consciousness and abnormal behavior.

MISCELLANEOUS

ASSOCIATED CONDITIONS
Hypernatremia and hyperglycemia

AGE RELATED FACTORS N/A

ZOONOTIC POTENTIAL N/A

PREGNANCY N/A

SYNONYMS
Hyperosmolality

SEE ALSO
• Sodium, Hypernatremia • Glucose, Hyperglycemia • Diabetes Mellitus, Nonketotic Hyperosmolar Syndrome

ABBREVIATIONS
ADH = antidiurectic hormone
CNS = central nervous system
BUN = blood urea nitrogen

References
Riley JH, Cornelius LM. Osmolality, In: Loeb WF, Quimby FW, eds. The clinical chemistry of laboratory animals. New York: Pergamon Press, 1989:395–397.
DiBartola SP, Green RA, Autran de Morais HS. Osmolarity and osmolal gap. In: Willard MD, Tvedten H, Turnwald GH, eds. Small animal clinical diagnosis by laboratory methods. 2nd ed. Philadelphia: WB Saunders, 1994:106–107.
DiBartola SP, ed. Fluid therapy in small animal practice. Philadelphia: WB Saunders, 1992.

Author Margaret R. Kern
Consulting Editor Rhett Nichols

PANCYTOPENIA

BASICS

DEFINITION
Concurrently low peripheral blood concentrations of WBC, RBC, and platelets

Pathophysiology
• Pathophysiologic mechanisms are destruction, utilization, loss, sequestration, and reduced production of WBC, RBC, and platelets. Depending on the situation, these mechanisms may act alone or together.
• Reduced production occurs when pluripotent, multipotent, or committed stem cells are destroyed, their proliferation or differentiation is suppressed, or the maturation of differentiated cells is delayed or arrested. If pluripotent stems cells are affected, pancytopenia develops. If committed stem cells are affected, cytopenia of the cell type of affected stem cells develops. • Destruction, utilization, or loss of mature WBC, RBC, and platelets in excess of their production causes pancytopenia. WBC, RBC, and platelet production can significantly increase in response to demand. About 2 days are required before increased production begins to have an effect on the peripheral blood counts, and peak output usually takes about a week. As a result, the rate of destruction necessary to cause cytopenia is not as great during the first few days of disease as later. • Sequestration of WBC, RBC, or platelets in the microcirculation, especially that of the spleen, intestine, and lungs, can cause cytopenia of the sequestered cell type.

Systems Affected
Hemic/lymph/immune—bone marrow, spleen, lymph nodes, and lymphoid tissues. Depending on the cause of pancytopenia, these organs can be affected by cellular depletion, degeneration, necrosis, hyperplasia, dysplasia, or dyscrasia. These changes may occur alone or in combination.

SIGNALMENT Dogs and cats

SIGNS

Historical Findings
• History reflects the underlying cause of pancytopenia • Lethargy or pallor (anemia) • Petechial hemorrhage or mucosal bleeding (thrombocytopenia) • Repeated febrile episodes or frequent or persistent infection (leukopenia) • Extremely rapid onset with severe clinical signs is more consistent with conditions that cause necrosis, destruction, or sequestration than with conditions that cause reduced cell production resulting from bone marrow suppression. Slow, insidious onset is more consistent with bone marrow suppression.

Physical Examination Findings
Lethargy, pale mucous membranes, petechial hemorrhage, hematuria, hemoptysis, melena, and fever or other evidence of infection

CAUSES
• Infectious diseases (most common)—FeLV infection, FIV infection, FIP, feline and canine parvovirus, infectious canine hepatitis virus, ehrlichiosis, histoplasmosis, and endotoxemia and septicemia (especially that caused by the gram-negative organisms or tularemia) • Toxic agents—griseofulvin, chloramphenicol, trimethoprim-sulfadiazine, estrogen, Fusarium T-2 toxin, radiation and radiomimetic chemotherapeutics, and thallium • Proliferative and infiltrative diseases—myeloproliferative disease, myelofibrosis, and severe diffuse infiltration of the bone marrow by metastatic tumor cells • Immune-mediated disease—immune-mediated mechanisms that may cause or contribute to pancytopenia involve antibodies against mature or stem cells. Causes of pancytopenia that may have an immune-mediated component include lymphoproliferative disease, ehrlichiosis, FeLV infection, FIV infection, and the various immune-mediated disorders. Immune-mediated disease is suspected in many patients with aplastic anemia. • Idiopathic pancytopenia with hypocellular bone marrow that contains abundant fat is called aplastic pancytopenia or aplastic anemia. • Disseminated intravascular coagulation contributes to pancytopenia in some patients.

RISK FACTORS
Risk factors for pancytopenia are those for the different causes of pancytopenia.

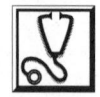

DIAGNOSIS

DIFFERENTIAL DIAGNOSIS
See causes.

LABORATORY FINDINGS

Drugs That May Alter Lab Results
Glucocorticoids often increase the neutrophil count by two times or more and can, therefore, obscure an otherwise decrease neutrophil count.

Disorders That May Alter Lab Results
In vitro hemolysis, platelet aggregation, and leukocyte aggregation artificially decrease RBC, leukocyte, and platelet counts, respectively.

Valid If Run in Human Lab?
Valid, but human laboratories inexperienced in performing differential WBC counts on animal samples may report excessive numbers of band neutrophils and atypical lymphocytes.

CBC/BIOCHEMISTRY/URINALYSIS
• WBC, RBC, and platelet counts are low.
• Rapid, sudden onset and toxic changes in leukocytes suggest bone marrow injury (eg, parvovirus and chemical agents), septicemia, or endotoxemia. • Atypical or blastic leukocytes, rubricytes, and megakaryoblasts suggest myeloproliferative disease. • High ALT, AST, ALP, and GGT activities suggest myeloproliferative or lymphoproliferative disease with bone marrow and hepatic involvement.

OTHER LABORATORY TESTS
• Reticulocyte count to determine if bone marrow is regenerative. A regenerative response to the anemia suggests that the pancytopenia is caused by destruction, utilization, or sequestration. A nonregenerative response suggests bone marrow suppression and merits examination of a bone marrow aspirate or punch biopsy. • Serologic tesing to detect suspected infectious agents (eg, FIV, FeLV, and Erhrlichia spp) • Blood smear examination to detect infectious organisms (eg, Ehrlichia spp and Histoplasma capsulatum)

IMAGING N/A

OTHER DIAGNOSTIC PROCEDURES

Bone Marrow Examination
• Examination of bone marrow aspirate or punch biopsy is indicated when the diagnosis is not otherwise apparent, especially in patients with a reticulocyte count indicating that the bone marrow is not appropriately responding to the anemia. • Pancytopenia associated with hypercellular bone marrow can be caused by ineffective hematopoiesis, peripheral destruction (reticulocyte count is high), myelodysplasia, and myelophthisis.
• Pancytopenia associated with hypocellular bone marrow can be caused by bone marrow necrosis (e.g., toxins and parvovirus), fibrosis, or suppression (e.g., drugs, hormones, and idiopathic disease). • If the bone marrow is unaspirable, fibrosis or necrosis of the bone marrow should be considered. Bone marrow necrosis is usually associated with rapid onset of severe clinical signs, often including emesis and diarrhea.

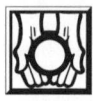

TREATMENT
• Supportive treatment depends on the clinical situation and includes aggressive antibiotic therapy, blood transfusion, and transfusion of platelet rich plasma.
• Treat the underlying condition.

MEDICATIONS

DRUGS AND FLUIDS
Treatment should be appropriate for the clinical situation (e.g., the degree to which each cell population is low, whether the patient has fever or infection, and established or suspected specific diagnoses). The topics on these diseases and on the specific cytopenias should be reviewed to develop an appropriate therapeutic plan.

CONTRAINDICATIONS N/A

PRECAUTIONS
Because of the patient's compromised immune status, glucocorticoids and other immunosuppressive drugs should be used only

when absolutely necessary and with extreme care.

POSSIBLE INTERACTIONS N/A

ALTERNATE DRUGS N/A

FOLLOW-UP

PATIENT MONITORING

Monitoring procedures include daily physical examination with special attention to lymph node palpation, body temperature, and periodic CBC. The frequency of hematologic testing depends upon factors such as the degree to which the different cell types and platelets are low, age and general physical condition of the patient, and underlying cause of pancytopenia. Generally, CBC is performed daily, biweekly, or weekly.

POSSIBLE COMPLICATIONS

Patients should be monitored for development of lethargy, fever, and hemorrhage; these may represent recurrence of anemia, leukopenia, and thrombocytopenia, respectively.

MISCELLANEOUS

ASSOCIATED CONDITIONS

Infection in patients with leukopenia

AGE RELATED FACTORS N/A

ZOONOTIC POTENTIAL

Tularemia has zoonotic potential. The owner can contract histoplasmosis from the same source as the patient.

PREGNANCY

Stress associated with pancytopenia can cause abortion. See the respective topic for the effects of different causes of pancytopenia on pregnancy.

SYNONYMS N/A

SEE ALSO

• Anemia, Nonregenerative • Anemia, Regenerative • Leukopenia • Lymphopenia • Thrombocytopenia • Specific causes of pancytopenia

ABBREVIATIONS

ALP = alkaline phosphatase
ALT = alanine aminotransferase
AST = aspartate aminotransferase
FeLV = feline leukemia virus
FIV = feline immunodeficiency virus
GGT = gamma gultamyltransferase
RBC = red blood cells
WBC = white blood cells

References

Baldwin CJ, Ledet, AE. Pancytopenia. In: August JR, ed. Consultations in feline internal medicine. 2nd ed. Philadelphia: WB Saunders, 1993:495-502.

Shelly SM. Causes of canine pancytopenia. Compend Contin Educ Pract Vet 1988;10:9-16.

Tvedten H. Erythrocyte disorders. In: Willard MD, Tvedten H, Turnwald GH, eds. Small animal clinical diagnosis by laboratory methods. 2nd ed. Philadelphia: WB Saunders, 1994:31-51

Author Ronald D. Tyler

Consulting Editor Alan H. Rebar

PARAPROTEINEMIA

 BASICS

DEFINITION
• An immunoglobulin produced by a clone of neoplastic immune cells, either plasma cells in patients with multiple myeloma or macroglobulinemia or lymphosarcoma • In any single patient, the paraprotein is a single class and subclass of immunoglobulin with a single light chain class.

Pathophysiology
Primary signs of disease are referable to the primary effects of the tumor in the bone and bone marrow. The abnormal immunoglobulin also can produce a variety of effects.

Systems Affected
• Musculoskeletal—bone lysis by the neoplastic cells can cause lameness • Nervous—bone lysis of the axial skeleton by the neoplastic cells can cause neurologic signs. If the paraprotein reaches a sufficient concentration, hyperviscosity syndrome will develop, usually resulting in neurologic signs. • Hemic/lymph/immune—myelophthisis can cause anemia, leukopenia, and thrombocytopenia. Hemostasis compromised by paraprotein interference with platelet and coagulation factor function

SIGNALMENT
• Dogs and cats • Middle-aged to old dogs more frequently affected • No sex predilection

SIGNS
• Lameness • Paresis • Weakness • Weight loss • Epistaxis • Gingival bleeding • Petechia • Ecchymoses • Melena

CAUSES
• No carcinogenic agent has been associated with multiple myeloma, macroglobulinemia, or lymphoproliferative disorders in dogs. • FeLV causes lymphosarcoma in cats.

RISK FACTORS N/A

 DIAGNOSIS

DIFFERENTIAL DIAGNOSIS
• Other causes of a narrow-based gammopathy that resemble paraprotein or monoclonal gammopathy are ehrlichiosis, acute phase reactants in the alpha-2 region, leishmania, amyloidosis, plasmacytic gastroenterocolitis, and benign monclonal gammopathy. • Bleeding disorders concurrent with paraproteinemia can be assumed to be caused by the paraproteinemia. Primary bleeding disorders probably do not need to be considered initially.

LABORATORY FINDINGS

Drugs That May Alter Lab Results N/A
Disorders That May Alter Lab Results N/A

Valid If Run in Human Lab? Valid

CBC/BIOCHEMISTRY/URINALYSIS
• Total protein and globulin usually high in patients with disease severe enough to cause clinical signs • Proteinuria caused by light chains (i.e., Bence Jones protein) is not detected by routine tests. Immunoassay or electrophoresis of a urine sample that has been concentrated in the laboratory increases the likelihood of detection. Urinary light chains are not seen in the "pseudoparaproteinemias." • Hypercalcemia in some patients is generally correlated with bone lysis.

OTHER LABORATORY TESTS
• Examination of bone marrow aspirate reveals > 5% plasma cells, often with criteria of malignancy. The distribution of multiple myeloma is patchy. Aspiration of a lytic lesion might be necessary to detect maligant plasma cells. • Viscosimetry may help define hyperviscosity syndrome but is usually not necessary. • Serologic tests to help rule out Ehrlichia canis

IMAGING
Radiography of affected bones is indispensible to identify lytic bone lesions and sometimes a site for aspiration.

OTHER DIAGNOSTIC PROCEDURES
Cytologic or histopathologic examination of affected organs may identify lymphoproliferative diseases that cause true paraproteinemia and other diseases that cause narrow-based gammopathy, which is not a true paraproteinemia.

 TREATMENT

• Supportive treatment varies depending on the manifestations of disease and the organ systems affected.
• Patients are probably immunocompromised and may need aggressive antibiotic therapy.
• Hyperviscosity syndrome may present as a neurologic emergency. Plasmapheresis can be lifesaving even if done by removal of whole blood, manual centrifugation, and replacement with fluid and the retrieved cells.

 MEDICATIONS

DRUGS AND FLUIDS
See Multiple Myeloma.

CONTRAINDICATIONS N/A

PRECAUTIONS N/A

POSSIBLE INTERACTIONS N/A

ALTERNATE DRUGS N/A

 FOLLOW-UP

PATIENT MONITORING
• Observe clinical signs and repeat abnormal laboratory tests and radiographs at 2 to 4-week intervals. • Patients that respond improve clinically before results of radiography and laboratory testing improve.

POSSIBLE COMPLICATIONS
Vertebral involvement can result in fracture and severe neurologic compromise.

 MISCELLANEOUS

ASSOCIATED CONDITIONS
Immunologic incompetence

AGE RELATED FACTORS N/A

ZOONOTIC POTENTIAL N/A

PREGNANCY N/A

SYNONYMS
Monoclonal gammopathy, M-protein

SEE ALSO
• Multiple Myeloma • Lymphosarcoma—Dogs • Lymphosarcoma—Cats

ABBREVIATIONS
FELV = Feline leukemia virus

References

Matus RE, Leifer CE. Immunoglobulin-producing tumors. Vet Clin North Am Small Anim Pract 1985;15:741-752.

Matus RE, Leifer CE, MacEwen EG, Hurvitz AI. Prognostic factors for multiple myeloma in the dog. J Amer Vet Med Assoc 1986;188:1288-1292.

Breitschwerdt EB, Woody BJ, Zerbe CA, De Buysscher EV, Barta O. Monoclonal gammopathy associated with naturally occurring canine ehrlichiosis. J Vet Int Med 1987;1:2-9.

Author G. Daniel Boon
Consulting Editor Alan H. Rebar

PHOSPHORUS, HYPERPHOSPHATEMIA

BASICS

DEFINITION

High serum phosphorus—dogs, >5.5 mg/dl; cats, >6.0 mg/dl

Pathophysiology

High serum phosphorus is caused by excessive gastrointestinal absorption of phosphorus, excessive bone resorption of phosphorus, and reduced renal excretion of phosphorus.

Systems Affected

• Endocrine/metabolic • Renal

SIGNALMENT

Any age, but commonly in young, growing animals or old animals with renal insufficiency

SIGNS

• Depend on the underlying cause • No specific signs directly attributable to hyperphosphatemia • Acute hyperphosphatemia causes hypocalcemic tetany or vascular collapse. • Chronic hyperphosphatemia causes calcification of soft tissues resulting in chronic renal failure and tumoral calcinosis.

CAUSES

• Hyperphosphatemia secondary to reduced glomerular filtration rate • Prerenal azotemia • Renal azotemia • Post-renal azotemia • Hyperphosphatemia secondary to excessive bone resorption or muscle breakdown • Young growing dogs • Hypoparathyroidism • Osteolysis • Disuse osteoperosis • Osseous neoplasia • Hyperthyroidism • Hypersomatotropism • Hyperphosphatemia caused by excessive gastrointestinal absorption of phosphorus • Phosphorus-containing enemas • Vitamin D toxicosis • Nutritional secondary hyperparathyroidism • Phosphorus dietary • supplementation • Hyperthyroidism • Hypersomatotropism

RISK FACTORS

Administration of phosphate-containing enemas to small animals such as cats

DIAGNOSIS

DIFFERENTIAL DIAGNOSIS

• Hypoparathyroidism—also characterized by clinical signs of hypocalcemia such as seizures and tetany • Pre-renal azotemia as a cause of hyperphosphatemia—associated with disease states that result in low cardiac output such as congestive heart failure, dehydration, hypoadrenocorticism, and shock • Renal insufficiency, either acute or chronic renal failure—attended by azotemia and abnormal findings on urinalysis • Young, growing animals—can have serum phosphorus concentration twice that of adults. • Vitamin D intoxication—history of vitamin D supplementation or ingestion of rodenticides (Rampage) • Nutritional secondary hyperparathyroidism—history of dietary calcium/phosphorus imbalance • Hyperthyroidism in cats—patients exhibit classic clinical signs such as weight loss, polyphagia, and polydypsia and polyuria • Hypersomatotropism—attended by a history of progesterone administration in dogs and insulin-resistant diabetes mellitus in cats • Nonazotemic tumoral calcinosis—observed in human beings as an autosomal dominant disorder. Large periarticular masses of soft tissue calcification are identified. • Osteolysis and osseous neoplasia—rare causes of hyperphosphatemia associated with large bone lesions • Jasmine toxicity—history of plant ingestion • Facticious

LABORATORY FINDINGS

Drugs That May Alter Lab Results

• Phosphate-containing enemas in cats or obstipated small dogs • Intravenous KPO_4 supplementation • Anabolic steroids • Furosemide • Hydrochlorthiazide • Minocycline

Disorders That May Alter Lab Results

• Hemolysis • Lipemia • Collection in citrate, oxalate, or EDTA

VALID IF RUN A HUMAN LAB? Yes

CBC/BIOCHEMISTRY/URINALYSIS

• Serum phosphorus > 5.5-6.0 mg/dl • Low serum calcium in some patients

OTHER LABORATORY TESTS

• Parathyroid hormone assay—indicated in patients with hyperphosphatemia and hypocalcemia. Concentration low in animals with hypoparathyroidism • Thyroxine (T_4) determination—indicated in cats with hyperphosphatemia and clinical signs consistent with hyperthyroidism. Concentration high in cats with hyperthyroidism • IGF-1 determination—indicated in a dog or cat with unexplained hyperphosphatemia and clinical signs consistent with acromegaly. Concentration high in animal with acromegaly

IMAGING

• Abdominal radiography to assess renal size and symmetry or renal ultrasonography to detect soft-tissue mineralization. • Radiography of long bones to detect osteoporosis or neoplasia

OTHER DIAGNOSTIC PROCEDURES

• Parathyroid gland biopsy if PTH concentration cannot be determined. • Renal biopsy to assess source and extent of renal disease. • Thyroid scan to rule out hyperthyroidism if serum T_4 is normal.

TREATMENT

• Patients generally treated as outpatients • Restrict dietary phosphorus. • Restrict protein if hyperphosphatemia is secondary to renal failure

PHOSPHORUS, HYPERPHOSPHATEMIA

MEDICATIONS

DRUGS AND FLUIDS

Acute Hyperphosphatemia
Life support: 0.9% NaCl diuresis; dextrose (1G/kg IV) and insulin (0.5 units/kg IV)

Chronic Hyperphosphatemia
Oral administration of phosphorus binders

CONTRAINDICATIONS N/A

PRECAUTIONS N/A

POSSIBLE INTERACTIONS None

ALTERNATE DRUGS N/A

FOLLOW-UP

PATIENT MONITORING
- Resolution of azotemia by fluid therapy
- Calcium concentration in patients with acute hyperphosphatemia

POSSIBLE COMPLICATIONS
Hypophosphatemia resulting in hemolysis

MISCELLANEOUS

ASSOCIATED CONDITIONS
Hypocalcemia

AGE RELATED FACTORS
Hyperphosphatemia can be twice the normal concentration in young animals, especially young, large-breed dogs, but should resolve by 12 months of age.

ZOONOTIC POTENTIAL N/A

PREGNANCY N/A

SYNONYMS N/A

SEE ALSO
Hypoparathyroidism

ABBREVIATIONS
IGF = Insulin-like growth factor 1
PTH = parathyroid hormone

References
Willard MD, Tvedten H, Turnwald GH. Clinical diagnosis by laboratory methods. Philadelphia: WB Saunders, 1989.
Aurbach GD, Marx SJ, Spiegel AM. Parathyroid hormone, calcitonin, and the calciferols. In: Wilson JD, Foster DW, eds. Williams textbook of endocrinology. 7th ed. Philadelphia: WB Saunders, 1985;1208-1209.

Author Deborah S. Greco
Consulting Editor Rhett Nichols

PHOSPHORUS, HYPOPHOSPHATEMIA

BASICS

DEFINITION
Serum phosphorus concentration < 2.5 mg/dl

Pathophysiology
A low phosphorus concentration can be caused by shifts of phosphorus from the extracellular fluid into body cells, reduced intestinal absorption of phosphorus, or reduced renal phosphorus reabsorption. Because phosphorus is an important component of adenosine triphosphate (ATP), low serum phosphorus concentration can cause ATP depletion and affect cells that are high energy users, including RBC, skeletal muscle cells, and brain cells.

Systems Affected
• Hemic/lymphatic/immune—hemolysis
• Musculoskeletal—weakness and respiratory paralysis • Nervous—seizures

SIGNALMENT N/A

SIGNS

Historical Findings
Consistent with the primary disease that is responsible for the hypophosphatemia rather than relating to the phosphate concentration itself

Physical Examination Findings
• Pallor from hemolytic anemia (severe hypophosphatemia) • Red or dark colored urine as a result of hemoglobinuria (severe hypophosphatemia) • Tachypnea, dyspnea, and anxiety secondary to hypoxia • Muscle weakness • Mental depression • Rapid, shallow respirations as a result of poor respiratory muscle function

CAUSES
• Laboratory error • Mannitol administration

Transcellular Shift (Maldistribution)
• Enteral nutrition and total parenteral nutrition • Ketoacidotic diabetes mellitus • Carbohydrate loading with insulin administration
• Respiratory alkalosis

Reduced Intestinal Absorption of Phosphorus
• Phosphorus poor diet • Vitamin D deficiency • Phosphate binding agent
• Malabsorption syndrome

Reduced Renal Phosphate Reabsorption
• Primary hyperparathyroidism • Renal tubular defects (e.g., Fanconi's syndrome) • Hyperadrenocorticism • Proximal tubular diuretics (e.g., carbonic anhydrase inhibitors) • Hypocalcemic tetany (eclampsia) • Sodium bicarbonate administration

RISK FACTORS
• Undiagnosed or poorly regulated diabetes mellitus • Prolonged anorexia, starvation, or malnutrition

DIAGNOSIS

DIFFERENTIAL DIAGNOSIS
• Severe hypophosphatemia (< 1.0 mg/dl) is seen most often as a complication of diabetic ketoacidosis. Monitor severely ill diabetics closely during the first few days of treatment for the development of hypophosphatemia.
• Patients with prolonged anorexia, starvation, or severe intestinal malabsorption may develop hypophosphatemia if given hyperalimentation, especially if the formulas used are marginal in phosphorus content.

LABORATORY FINDINGS

Drugs That May Alter Results
Mannitol interferes with analysis, falsely lowering serum phosphorus concentration.

Disorders That May Alter Lab Results
Hemolysis, hyperlipidemia, and hyperproteinemia may falsely elevate serum phosphorus.

Valid If Run in Human Lab?
Valid

CBC/BIOCHEMISTRY/URINALYSIS
• Concurrent findings of hyperglycemia, glucosuria, ketonuria, and a high anion gap metabolic acidosis confirm that the hypophosphatemia is a complication of diabetic ketoacidosis. • Hypercalcemia in association with hypophosphatemia suggests primary hyperparathyroidism. • Hypocalcemia with hypophosphatemia is reported in patients with eclampsia. • Moderate hypophosphatemia with high serum SAP activity suggests hyperadrenocorticism. • Panhypoproteinemia suggests an intestinal malabsorption disorder.
• Hypophosphatemia in association with glucosuria, normoglycemia, isosthenuria, or azotemia suggests a renal tubular defect such as Fanconi's syndrome.

OTHER LABORATORY TESTS
• PTH assay—useful to diagnosis primary hyperparathyroidism • Measurement of vitamin D metabolites, particularly cholecalciferol—useful to diagnose vitamin D deficiency

IMAGING
Radiology may reveal poor bone quality or pathologic fractures in patients with disorders of calcium, phosphorus, and vitamin D.

OTHER DIAGNOSTIC PROCEDURES
Exploratory surgery of the cervical region confirms hyperparathyroidism.

TREATMENT

Patients with severe hypophosphatemia (phosphorus concentration < 1.5 mg/dl) require hospitalization to observe for hemolysis and to provide treatment as needed. If the condition is caused by initiation of insulin therapy or hyperalimentation, these treatments should be suspended until phosphate has been administered for a few hours. Obtain fresh whole blood in case a transfusion is required. Patients with moderate hypophosphatemia (1.5-2.5) can be evaluated as outpatients if other conditions are stable.

MEDICATIONS

DRUGS AND FLUIDS
• If the serum phosphorus is < 1.5 mg/dl, a balanced electrolyte solution (e.g., 0.9 % saline, lactated Ringer's solution, Normasol-R, or Plasma-Lyte) should be administered intravenously, supplemented with either sodium or potassium phosphate. Potassium phosphate for injection has 3 mmol/ml of phosphate and 4.4 mEq/ml of potassium. The dose of phosphate is 0.01-0.03 mmol/kg/hr for 6 hours. However, many cats with diabetic ketoacidosis who develop hypophosphatemia often require higher dosages and a longer duration of therapy. A rate of 0.06-0.12 mmol/kg/hr for 6-24 hours is typical.
• Oral supplementation of phosphate may be useful in animals with moderate hypophosphatemia. Sodium and potassium phosphate powders and tablets are commercially available, but current dosaging in veterinary medicine is empirical.

CONTRAINDICATIONS
• Avoid diuretics, especially carbonic anhydrase inhibitors.
• Avoid phosphate poor enteral feeding formulas and total parenteral nutrition solutions in patients with hypophosphatemia and patients with predisposing disorders.
• Intravenous supplementation of phosphate is contraindicated in hypercalcemic patients because precipitation of calcium and phosphate causes soft tissue mineralization and renal damage.

PRECAUTIONS
Oversupplementation, especially in patients with renal impairment or inadequate hydration, can cause hyperphosphatemia. Acute hyperphosphatemia can result in hypocalcemia.

ALTERNATE DRUGS
If an oral or parenteral phosphate supplement is unavailable, skim or low-fat milk may be administered. This will be insufficient in severely affected patients.

FOLLOW-UP

PATIENT MONITORING
• Measure serum phosphorus every 12-24 hours until the concentration is stable within the normal range. • If hyperphosphatemia develops, stop all supplementation and provide

PHOSPHORUS, HYPOPHOSPHATEMIA

intravenous fluid diuresis until the phosphorus returns to normal. Administer calcium gluconate intravenously *only* if tetany from hypocalcemia develops. Hyperphosphatemic animals should be monitored for acute renal failure. The serum potassium should be monitored daily until stable.

POSSIBLE COMPLICATIONS

• Hemolysis from hypophosphatemia may be acute and severe, requiring transfusion. Fresh blood is preferred over stored blood products because stored RBC may use serum phosphate and exacerbate the condition. • Cardiac arrest and respiratory failure are life-threatening complications of severe hypophosphatemia. Respiratory support with positive pressure ventilation is an option. See patient monitoring for other complications.

 MISCELLANEOUS

ASSOCIATED CONDITIONS

Hypokalemia is often concurrent, especially in animals with diabetic ketoacidosis

AGE RELATED FACTORS N/A

ZOONOTIC POTENTIAL N/A

PREGNANCY

• Hypophosphatemia in the periparturient animal may be associated with hypocalcemia caused by secretion of PTH to mobilize calcium for neonatal bone growth and lactation. • PTH promotes phosphaturia and hypophosphatemia.

SYNONYMS N/A

SEE ALSO

• Diabetes Mellitus, Ketoacidotic • Hyperparathyroidism

ABBREVIATIONS

ALP = alkaline phosphatase
PTH = parathyroid hormone
RBC = red blood cells

References

DiBartola SP. Disorders of phosphorus: hypophosphatemia and hyperphosphatemia. In: DiBartola SP, ed. Fluid therapy in small animal practice. Philadelphia: WB Saunders, 1992.

Forrester SD, Moreland RJ. Hypophosphatemia: causes and clinical consequences. J Vet Intern Med 1989;3:149-159.

Willard MD, Zerbe CA, Schall WD, et al. Severe hypophosphatemia associated with diabetes mellitus in six dogs and one cat. J Am Vet Med Assoc 1987;190:1007-1010.

Author Melissa S. Wallace
Consulting Editor Rhett Nichols

POLYCYTHEMIA

BASICS

DEFINITION
Values for PCV, hemoglobin concentration, and RBC count are higher than reference ranges because of a relative or absolute increase in the number of circulating RBC.

Pathophysiology
Numbers of circulating RBC are affected by changes in plasma volume, rate of RBC destruction or loss, splenic contraction, erythropoietin (EPO) secretion, and the rate of bone marrow production. Erythropoiesis also is affected by hormones from the adrenal cortex, thyroid gland, ovary, testis, and anterior pituitary gland. A normal PCV is maintained by an endocrine loop.

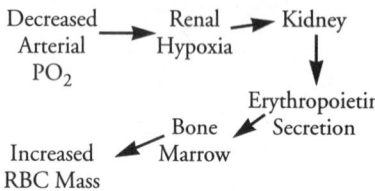

Polycythemias can be classified as relative, transient, or absolute. Relative polycythemia develops when a decrease in plasma volume, usually caused by dehydration, produces a relative increase in circulating RBC. Transient polycythemia is caused by splenic contraction, which injects concentrated RBC into the circulation. Absolute polycythemia is characterized by an absolute increase in the circulating RBC mass as a result of increased marrow production, and is either primary or secondary to increased production of EPO. Primary absolute polycythemia (polycythemia rubra vera) is a myeloproliferative disorder characterized by the uncontrolled but orderly production of excessive numbers of mature RBC. Secondary absolute polycythemia is caused by a physiologically appropriate release of EPO resulting from chronic hypoxemia, or by an inappropriate and excessive production of EPO or an EPO-like substance in an animal with normal arterial oxygen saturation.

Systems Affected
Cardiovascular, pulmonary, nervous, renal—hyperviscosity and poor perfusion and oxygenation of tissues are features of polycythemic animals that are related directly to the high PCV, especially values > 60%

SIGNALMENT
• Reference values for PCV, hemoglobin, and RBC count vary with geographic location and breed. • Animals at altitudes > 6000 ft have higher values than those at sea level. • Brachycephalic breeds have higher PCV values than normocephalic breeds. • Large, excitable breeds are prone to splenic contraction.

SIGNS

General Comments
Vary with the degree of polycythemia

Historical Findings
• Transient polycythemia—excitement or vigorous exercise • Absolute polycythemia—lethargy, anorexia, epistaxis, or stunted growth

Physical Examination Findings
• Relative polycythemia—dehydration as a result of vomiting, diarrhea, or lack of water intake and oliguria • Absolute polycythemia—lethargy, low exercise tolerance, behavioral change, brick red or cyanotic mucous membranes, sneezing, bilateral epistaxis, large size and tortuosity of retinal and sublingual vessels, and cardiopulmonary impairment • Primary absolute polycythemia (polycythemia vera)—characterized by variable degrees of splenomegaly, hepatomegaly, thrombosis, and hemorrhage • Secondary absolute polycythemia caused by tissue hypoxia—clinical signs of hypoxemia as a result of chronic pulmonary disease, cardiac disease or anomaly with right to left shunting, or hemoglobinopathy. • Secondary absolute polycythemias caused by inappropriate EPO secretion—signs associated with neoplasia, space-occupying renal lesion, or endocrine disorder

CAUSES
• Relative polycythemia (common)—vomiting, diarrhea, diminished water intake, diuresis, hyperventilation, renal disease, and shift of plasma H_2O to interstitium or gastrointestinal lumen • Transient polycythemia—excitement, anxiety, seizures, and restraint • Primary absolute polycythemia (polycythemia vera)—rare myeloproliferative disorder • Secondary absolute polycythemia caused by tissue hypoxia—chronic pulmonary disease, cardiac disease or anomaly with right to left shunting, high altitude, brachycephalic breeds, methemoglobinemia, and impairment of renal blood supply • Secondary absolute polycythemia caused by inappropriate EPO secretion (rare)— renal cyst or tumor, hydronephrosis, hyperadrenocorticism, hyperthyroidism, pheochromocytoma, nasal fibrosarcoma, hepatic neoplasia, and hyperandrogenism

RISK FACTORS N/A

DIAGNOSIS

DIFFERENTIAL DIAGNOSIS
• A moderately high PCV and total plasma protein with concurrent dehydration suggest relative polycythemia. • Secondary absolute polycythemia is caused by diseases that produce chronic hypoxemia or by space-occupying lesions of the kidney, endocrine disorders, and neoplasms that produce EPO or an EPO-like substance independent of hypoxia.

• Polycythemia vera is diagnosed by elimination of other causes.

LABORATORY FINDINGS

Drugs That May Alter Lab Results
Dilutional effect of fluid therapy on PCV and total plasma protein

Disorders That May Alter Lab Results
Concurrent anemia, hypoproteinemia, or dehydration can affect interpretation of PCV and total plasma protein values.

Valid If Run in Human Lab? Valid

CBC/BIOCHEMISTRY/URINALYSIS
Assessment of polycythemia begins with CBC and total plasma protein measurement. Additional tests are selected as indicated.

	Relative	Absolute		
Mechanism	Dehydration	Primary Myeloproliferative	Secondary Hypoxemia	Secondary Excess EPO
PCV	Inc	Marked Inc > 60%	Marked Inc > 60%	Marked Inc > 60%
TPP	Inc	N	N	N
Arterial O_2 Sat		N > 90%	Dec << 90%	N > 90%
EPO		N/Dec	Inc	Inc
Bone Marrow		------- Erythroid Hyperplasia -------		
Other	Prerenal Azotemia	Inc WBC Inc Plat		

OTHER LABORATORY TESTS
• Arterial PO_2 and EPO determinations to diagnosis absolute polycythemia. • Hormone assays are available for assessment of endocrine dysfunction.

IMAGING
Radiology and ultrasonography to detect cardiopulmonary disease and space-occupying lesions of the kidneys

OTHER DIAGNOSTIC PROCEDURES
N/A

TREATMENT
• Rehydration and treatment of underlying disease in patients with relative polycythemia • Removal of excess RBC by repeated phlebotomy is the usual treatment for absolute polycythemia.

MEDICATIONS

DRUGS AND FLUIDS
• Relative polycythemia—rehydration with IV administration of fluids appropriate for the primary cause. Assessment of renal function, gastrointestinal system, acid/base status, and electrolyte balance are important to the selection of the fluid.

• Absolute polycythemia—phlebotomy recommended (20 ml/kg over several days) to reduce the RBC mass to a PCV of 55%. Blood volume should be replaced concurrently with isotonic fluids to prevent hypotension, cardiovascular collapse, and thrombosis.
• Polycythemia caused by inappropriate EPO production is treated by phlebotomy and removal of the EPO source.
• In patients with polycythemia caused by hypoxemia, the high PCV is an appropriate compensatory response, and phlebotomy may be dangerous. If indicated, blood is removed at a slower rate (5ml/kg); a higher PCV (60-65%) may be necessary to sustain life until the cause of hypoxemia can be corrected.
• Polycythemia vera is treated by phlebotomy (20 ml/kg) and hydroxyurea (30 mg/kg PO q24h). Frequency of bleeding and dosage are adjusted to maintain a PCV of 55%.

CONTRAINDICATIONS
Phlebotomy may be contraindicated in patients with hypoxemia.

PRECAUTIONS
Removal of blood at a rapid rate can cause hypotension and cardiovascular collapse.

POSSIBLE INTERACTIONS N/A

ALTERNATE DRUGS
Polycythemia vera—chlorambucil (0.2 mg/kg PO q24h) or busulfan (4.0 mg/m^2 PO q24h)

FOLLOW-UP
PATIENT MONITORING
• PCV, TPP, urine output, and body weight 2-3 times daily in severely dehydrated animals until normal hydration is maintained
• Patients being treated for polycythemia vera by chemotherapy monitored weekly for changes in PCV, WBC, and platelets during the initial treatment, and then monthly for adjustment of chemotherapy and periodic phlebotomy

POSSIBLE COMPLICATIONS
• Hyperviscosity of absolute polycythemias, especially polycythemia vera, may cause thrombosis, infarction, or hemorrhage.
• Chemotherapy may cause bone marrow suppression.

MISCELLANEOUS
ASSOCIATED CONDITIONS N/A

AGE RELATED FACTORS N/A

ZOONOTIC POTENTIAL N/A

PREGNANCY N/A

SYNONYM Erythrocytosis

SEE ALSO
Hyperviscosity Syndrome

ABBREVIATIONS
EPO = erythropoietin
PCV = packed cell volume
RBC = red blood cells
TPP = total plasma protein

Reference

Morrison WB. Polycythemia. In: Ettinger SJ, Feldman EC, eds. Textbook of veterinary internal medicine. Philadelphia: WB Saunders, 1995:197-199.
Author Peter S. MacWilliams
Consulting Editor Alan H. Rebar

POTASSIUM, HYPERKALEMIA

BASICS

DEFINITION
Serum potassium concentration higher than the testing laboratory's upper limit of normal, generally > 5.7 mEq/L (mmol/L)

Pathophysiology
Potassium is primarily intracellular, so serum concentrations do not accurately reflect tissue concentrations. Hyperkalemia is often associated with cellular injury (e.g., trauma and ischemia) and other causes of translocation of potassium out of the intracellular space (e.g., acidosis). Potassium is eliminated in the kidneys and elimination is enhanced by aldosterone.

Systems Affected
• Cardiovascular—cardiac conduction is affected by potassium, and changes are reflected on the ECG. With rising potassium, the T waves become tall and spiked with a narrow base. The QRS complexes widen and the P-R intervals lengthen. The P waves become smaller and wider and, in animals with severe hyperkalemia, disappear (atrial standstill). Higher concentrations of potassium cause fusion of the QRS-T, which causes a wide complex idioventricular rhythm followed by ventricular fibrillation or asystole. ECG changes in animals with hyperkalemia vary and are diminished by hypernatremia, hypercalcemia, and alkalosis. • Nervous—neuromuscular function affected

SIGNALMENT
• Dogs and cats • Pseudohyperkalemia in akita

SIGNS

Historical Findings
• Weakness • Collapse • Flaccid paralysis • Death

Physical Examination Findings
In addition to historical findings, arrhythmias, especially bradyarrhythmias, in some animals

CAUSES
• Pseudohyperkalemia—some blood cells (i.e., platelets, WBC, and RBC in akita), contain high concentrations of potassium. If the blood sample is not analyzed or separated promptly, this intracellular potassium is released into the serum, causing the potassium concentration to be artificially high (pseudohyperkalemia). • Low potassium elimination—anuric or oliguric renal failure, ruptured bladder, administration of potassium sparing diuretics, ACE inhibitors, or nonsteroidal antiinflammatory drugs (causing hypoaldosteronism), and urinary tract rupture or urethral obstruction • Translocation of potassium—acidosis, muscle trauma, severe digitalis overdose, infusion of mannitol, and hyperglycemia causing hyperosmolality • High potassium intake—oral or parenteral potassium supplements • Miscellaneous—pleural effusion and ascites

RISK FACTORS
• Akita breed (pseudohyperkalemia) • Fluid therapy with potassium supplementation • Administration of potassium sparing diuretics • Conditions associated with acidosis • Trauma • Renal disease • Lower urinary tract disease in male cats • Cystic calculi in male dogs

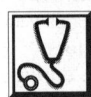

DIAGNOSIS

DIFFERENTIAL DIAGNOSIS
• Waxing and waning history of gastrointestinal complaints, weakness, collapse; consider hypoadrenocorticism • Straining to urinate or low urine output; consider urinary obstruction or oliguric/anuric renal failure

LABORATORY FINDINGS

Drugs That May Alter Lab Results None

Disorders That May Alter Lab Results
• Thrombocytosis (> 1,000,000 cells/mm³), leukocytosis (> 200,000 cells /mm³), and abnormal (leukemic) leukocytes can cause release of a large amount of potassium into the serum if not separated quickly.

Valid If Run in Human Lab? Yes

CBC/BIOCHEMISTRY/URINALYSIS
• In animals with Na:K ratio of < 27, consider hypoadrenocorticism. Realize that some animals with nonspecific diarrhea may also have a low Na:K ratio. • In animals with azotemia, consider hypoadrenocorticism, anuric or oliguric renal failure, and ruptured or obstructed urinary tract. • In animals with high creatine kinase, aspartate aminotransferase, and lactic dehydrogenase, consider muscle injury. • In animals with severe thrombocytosis or leukocytosis or if the animal is an akita, consider pseudohyperkalemia.

OTHER BLOOD TESTS
ACTH response test to rule out hypoadrenocorticism

IMAGING None

OTHER DIAGNOSTIC PROCEDURES
None

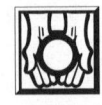

TREATMENT
• Varies depending on the underlying cause of hyperkalemia
• Aggressiveness dictated by patient's appearance and severity of ECG abnormalities
• Initiate supportive measures to lower potassium while pursuing definitive diagnosis.

MEDICATIONS

DRUGS AND FLUIDS
• Saline (0.9%) is the fluid of choice for lowering potassium concentrations and blunting the effects of hyperkalemia on cardiac conduction. If the animal is dehydrated or hypotensive, fluids can be administered rapidly (dogs, up to 90 ml/kg/hr; cats, 60 ml/kg/hr).
• Sodium bicarbonate can be administered in animals with severe hyperkalemia to induce translocation of potassium into cells. If blood pH and base deficit can not be determined, administer 1-2 mEq/kg slowly IV.
• Dextrose and regular insulin can be administered in animals with severe hyperkalemia to induce translocation of potassium into cells (regular insulin, 0.5 units/kg IV with 50% dextrose, 1 G/kg IV). Dextrose can also be used without insulin.
• In animals with life-threatening hyperkalemia, administer calcium gluconate (0.5-1 ml/kg very slowly IV) while monitoring the ECG. Calcium has no effect on potassium concentration but antagonizes the effect of potassium on the conduction system.

CONTRAINDICATIONS
• Avoid potassium-containing fluids and fluids that cause hyponatremia, acidosis, or hypocalcemia.
• Avoid drugs containing potassium or that interfere with potassium elimination (e.g., ACE inhibitors and potassium sparing diuretics).

PRECAUTIONS
Kayexalate and sodium bicarbonate cause a sodium load that may lead to fluid retention in patients with cardiac or renal failure.

POSSIBLE INTERACTIONS N/A

ALTERNATE DRUGS
Sodium polystyrene sulfonate (Kayexalate) per os or rectum binds potassium within the intestinal tract, limiting absorption and reabsorption; rarely used in veterinary practice.

FOLLOW-UP

PATIENT MONITORING
• Recheck potassium, with frequency dictated by the underlying disease. • Monitor ECG frequently until rhythm disturbances resolve.

POSSIBLE COMPLICATIONS
Death in animals with severe hyperkalemia

MISCELLANEOUS

ASSOCIATED CONDITIONS N/A

AGE RELATED FACTORS N/A

ZOONOTIC POTENTIAL N/A

PREGNANCY N/A

SYNONYMS N/A

SEE ALSO
• Atrial standstill • Causes of hyperkalemia

ABBREVIATIONS
ACE = angiotensin converting enzyme

POTASSIUM, HYPERKALEMIA

References

DiBartola SP, Autran de Morais HS.
Disorders of potassium: hypokalemia and
hyperkalemia. In: DiBartola SP, ed. Fluid
therapy in small animal practice.

Philadelphia: WB Saunders, 1992.
Willard MD. Electrolyte and acid-base abnormalities. In: Willard MD, Tvedten H,
Turnwald GH, eds. Small animal clinical
diagnosis by laboratory methods.

Philadelphia: WB Saunders, 1989.
Author Francis W.K. Smith, Jr.
Consulting Editors Larry P. Tilley and
Francis W. K. Smith, Jr.

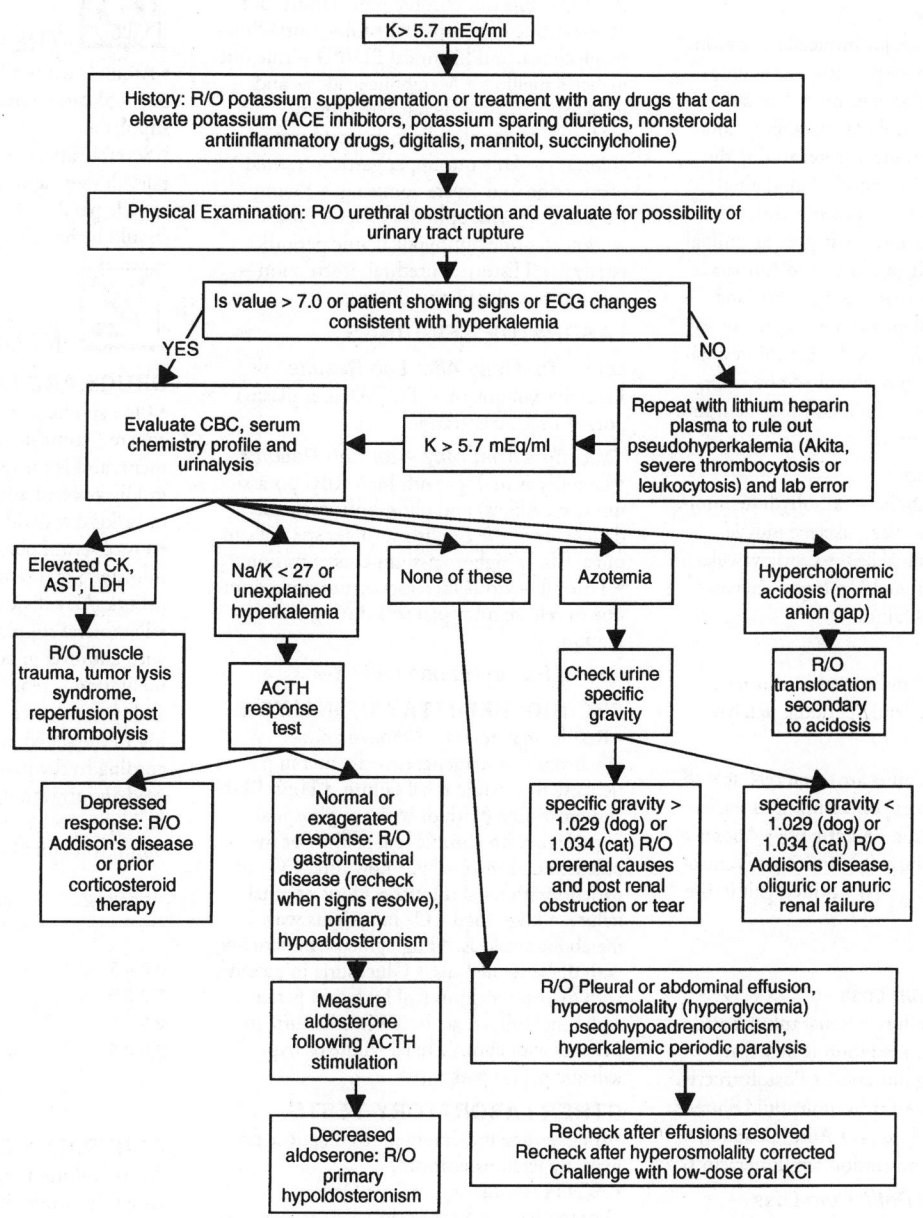

K> 5.7 mEq/ml

History: R/O potassium supplementation or treatment with any drugs that can elevate potassium (ACE inhibitors, potassium sparing diuretics, nonsteroidal antiinflammatory drugs, digitalis, mannitol, succinylcholine)

Physical Examination: R/O urethral obstruction and evaluate for possibility of urinary tract rupture

Is value > 7.0 or patient showing signs or ECG changes consistent with hyperkalemia

YES — Evaluate CBC, serum chemistry profile and urinalysis

NO — Repeat with lithium heparin plasma to rule out pseudohyperkalemia (Akita, severe thrombocytosis or leukocytosis) and lab error

K > 5.7 mEq/ml

- Elevated CK, AST, LDH → R/O muscle trauma, tumor lysis syndrome, reperfusion post thrombolysis

- Na/K < 27 or unexplained hyperkalemia → ACTH response test
  - Depressed response: R/O Addison's disease or prior corticosteroid therapy
  - Normal or exagerated response: R/O gastrointestinal disease (recheck when signs resolve), primary hypoaldosteronism → Measure aldosterone following ACTH stimulation → Decreased aldoserone: R/O primary hypoldosteronism

- None of these → R/O Pleural or abdominal effusion, hyperosmolality (hyperglycemia) psedohypoadrenocorticism, hyperkalemic periodic paralysis → Recheck after effusions resolved, Recheck after hyperosmolality corrected, Challenge with low-dose oral KCl

- Azotemia → Check urine specific gravity
  - specific gravity > 1.029 (dog) or 1.034 (cat) R/O prerenal causes and post renal obstruction or tear
  - specific gravity < 1.029 (dog) or 1.034 (cat) R/O Addisons disease, oliguric or anuric renal failure

- Hypercholoremic acidosis (normal anion gap) → R/O translocation secondary to acidosis

POTASSIUM, HYPOKALEMIA

BASICS

DEFINITION
Serum potassium concentration < 3.5 mEq/L

Pathophysiology
• Potassium is the major intracellular cation and thereby largely responsible for maintenance of intracellular volume. • The ratio of intracellular to extracellular potassium concentration is important in determining the cellular membrane potential. Rapid alterations in extracellular potassium concentration alter this ratio and predispose an animal to arrhythmias and conduction disturbances in excitable tissues (e.g., heart, nerve, and muscle) • Hypokalemia can be caused by excessive potassium loss via the gastrointestinal tract or kidneys or movement of potassium from the extracellular fluid compartment into cells (i.e., translocation).

Systems Affected
• Endocrine/Metabolic—carbohydrate intolerance • Neuromuscular—skeletal muscle weakness and intestinal ileus • Cardiovascular—arrhythmias • Renal/Urologic—hyposthenuria and renal failure

SIGNALMENT
Burmese cats 4-12 months old; recurrent episodes of hypokalemic periodic paralysis

SIGNS
• Historical complaints are often referable to the disease or factors contributing to the hypokalemia • Weakness • Lethargy • Anorexia • Polyuria • Polydipsia • Vomiting • Ventroflexion of the neck (cats) • Stilted gait in the forelimbs (cats)

CAUSES

Urinary Potassium Loss
• Chronic renal railure • Renal tubular acidosis • Diuretic administration (other than potassium sparing diuretics) • Postobstructive diuresis • Dialysis • Intravenous fluid diuresis • Mineralcorticoid excess • Administration penicillins • Administration amphoteracin B

Gastrointestinal Potassium Loss
• Vomiting • Diarrhea

Insufficient Potassium Intake
• Anorexia • Potassium deficient diet • Potassium free fluids

Translocation (Extracellular Fluid to Intracellular Fluid)
• Insulin and glucose administration • Sodium bicarbonate administration • Catecholamine administration • Alkalemia • Hypokalemic periodic paralysis

RISK FACTORS
Feeding cats acidifying diet that is marginal in potassium.

DIAGNOSIS

DIFFERENTIAL DIAGNOSIS
• Azotemia, isosthenuria, and historical PU/PD—rule out chronic renal failure and hypokalemic nephropathy. • Glucosuria, hyperglycemia, and historical PU/PD—rule out diabetes mellitus • Metabolic acidosis and urine pH > 6.5—rule out renal tubular acidosis • Metabolic alkalosis, and hypochloremia—rule out upper gastrointestinal obstruction and severe vomiting. • Young Burmese cat with episodes of severe musele weakness—rule out hypokalemic periodic paralysis • Historical urethral obstruction—rule out postobstructive diuresis

LABORATORY FINDINGS

Drugs That May Alter Lab Results
Excessive volume of K_3EDTA raises plasma potassium concentration.

Disorders That May Alter Lab Results
• Hemolysis in dogs with high RBC potassium (e.g., Akitas) and phosphofructokinase deficiency in the English springer spaniel can cause falsely high potassium concentration. • Thrombocytosis increases serum potassium due to release from platelets during clot formation.

Valid If Run in Human Lab? Yes

CBC/BIOCHEMISTRY/URINALYSIS
• Results may reveal normocytic normochromic nonregenerative anemia in patients with chronic renal failure. • High BUN and creatinine (with or without phosphate) in patients with chronic renal failure or hypokalemic nephropathy. • Low total CO_2 in patients with renal tubular acidosis or renal failure. • High total CO_2 in patients with metabolic alkalosis. • High glucose in patients with diabetes mellitus. • Glucosuria in patients with diabetes mellitus • pH > 6.5 in patients with renal tubular acidosis • Isosthenuria in patients with chronic renal failure or hypokalemic nephropathy

OTHER LABORATORY TESTS
• Aldosterone measurement to diagnose primary hyperaldosteronism. • ACTH stimulation or Low Dose Dexamethasone Suppression Test to diagnose hyperadrenocoritcism (cause of mineralcorticoid excess). • Urinary fractional excretion of K+ is elevated in chronic renal failure and hypokealmic nephropathy.

IMAGING
• Ultrasonography may reveal an adrenal tumor - R/O hyperaldosteronism or hyperadrenocorticism. • Radiographs and ultrasonography - useful in chronic renal failure work-up. • Upper G.I. barium studies - to diagnose upper G.I. disorders (anatomic or functional) causing metabolic alkalosis

OTHER DIAGNOSTIC PROCEDURES
Gastroscopy is useful in diagnosis of upper G.I. disorders resulting in metabolic alkalosis, such as pyloric hypertrophy or gastric neoplasia.

TREATMENT
• Animals with mild hypokalemia (potassium 3.0-3.5) can be treated as outpatients by oral supplementation
• Severely affected patients should be hospitalized; these animals are at risk of respiratory muscle paralysis and cardiac arrhythmias and should be handled with minimal stress.

MEDICATIONS

DRUGS AND FLUIDS
• Oral supplementation—potassium gluconate (Tumil-K, Kaon) is an effective treatment, and is the only treatment required in mildly affected animals (initial dosage, 1-3 mEq/kg/day divided q8h).
• Once serum potassium has normalized, administer a maintenance dosage (1.0 mEq/kg/day divided q12h).
• Parenteral supplementation—in patients with anorexia or vomiting, parenteral supplementation is required. Potassium chloride is added to maintenance fluid therapy according to the schedule below and is adjusted according to the patient's response. Do not exceed an intravenous rate of 0.5 mEq/kq/hr. At high rates of supplementation, an infusion pump is required to avoid overdosage.

SERUM K+	SUPPLEMENT (mEq/L)
3.5-4.5	20
3.0-3.5	30
2.5-3.0	40
2.0-2.5	60
< 2.0	80

CONTRAINDICATIONS
Avoid sodium bicarbonate, insulin, and glucose (if possible) in patients with severe hypokalemia.

PRECAUTIONS
See above

POSSIBLE INTERACTIONS
Potassium supplementation in conjunction with ACE inhibitor, potassium-sparing diuretic, prostaglandin inhibitor, or beta blocker may cause hyperkalemia.

ALTERNATE DRUGS
Potassium phosphate is used in patients with concurrent hypophosphatemia. Dosage is based on phosphate content (see Phosphorus, Hypophosphatemia).

FOLLOW-UP

PATIENT MONITORING
Serum potassium with the frequency dictated by the degree of hypokalemia and the severity of clinical signs

POSSIBLE COMPLICATIONS
Arrhythmias

MISCELLANEOUS

ASSOCIATED CONDITIONS
• Hypomagnesemia • Hypophosphatemia

AGE RELATED FACTORS N/A

ZOONOTIC POTENTIAL N/A

PREGNANCY N/A

SYNONYMS N/A

SEE ALSO
See Causes

ABBREVIATIONS
ECF = extracellular fluid
ICF = intracellular fluid
PU/PD = polyuria/polydipsia
ACE = angiotensin converting enzyme

References
DiBartola SP, Autran de Morais HS. Disorders of potassium: hypokalemia and hyperkalemia. In: DiBartola SP, ed. Fluid therapy in small animal practice. Philadelphia: WB Saunders Co., 1992:89-115.

DiBartola SP, Green RA, Autran de Morais HS. Electrolytes and acid-base. In: Willard MD, Tvedten H, Turnwald GH, eds. Small animal clinical diagnosis by laboratory methods. 2nd ed. Philadelphia: WB Saunders Co., 1994:97-113.

Willard MD. Disorders of potassium homeostasis. Vet Clin North Am Small Anim Pract 1989;19:241-263.

Author Melissa S. Wallace
Consulting Editor Rhett Nichols

PROTEINURIA

BASICS

DEFINITION
Proteinuria is a subjective increase in urine protein detected by dipstick analysis. The urine protein to creatinine ratio is > 1; 24-hour urine protein > 20 mg/kg.

Pathophysiology
• Greater than normal delivery of low molecular weight plasma proteins to the glomerulus
• Excessive leakage of proteins across the glomerular basement membrane secondary to altered permselectivity of the glomerulus
• Reduced tubular reabsorptive capacity for proteins or exudation of blood or serum into the lower urinary tract

Systems affected
Cardiovascular—circulating plasma volume can be reduced if proteinuria is of large enough magnitude to rapidly reduce serum albumin. This can lead to sodium retention, which causes formation of edema and hypertension. Severe proteinuria with loss of antithrombin III can lead to a hypercoagulable state.

SIGNALMENT
• Dogs and cats
• Familial renal diseases associated with proteinuria occur in the following breeds: soft-coated wheaten terrier, lhasa apso, shih tzu, bull terrier, English cocker spaniel, samoyed, doberman pinscher, standard poodle, basenji, Norwegian elkhound, and Chinese shar pei.

SIGNS
• Vary with severity of the proteinuria and the underlying cause
• None directly attributed to proteinuria

CAUSES

Preglomerular Proteinuria
• Functional proteinuria—strenuous exercise, fever, hypothermia, seizures, or venous congestion.
• Overload proteinuria—tubular resorptive capacity exceeded by large amounts of low molecular weight plasma proteins in the glomerular filtrate (e.g., neoplastic production of paraproteins and excessive hemolysis or rhabdomyolysis).

Glomerular Proteinuria
• Glomerulonephritis
• Amyloidosis
• Glomerulosclerosis
• In general, amyloidosis results in the heaviest proteinuria, although dogs with glomerulonephritis can also have massive proteinuria.

Postglomerular Proteinuria
• Hemorrhage or inflammation of the urogenital tract
• Tubular dysfunction resulting in failure of tubular protein reabsorption can cause mild or moderate proteinuria

RISK FACTORS
• Many chronic inflammatory (e.g., infectious and immune-mediated) and neoplastic diseases can lead to development of glomerulonephritis and perhaps amyloidosis, including dirofilariasis, ehrlichiosis, borelliosis, chronic bacterial infections (including endocarditis), pyometra, FeLV, FIV, pancreatitis, and systemic lupus erythematosus.
• Hematuria and pyuria
• Multiple myeloma can produce paraproteins resulting in Bence Jones proteinuria.

DIAGNOSIS

DIFFERENTIAL DIAGNOSIS
• Need to differentiate preglomerular, glomerular, and postglomerular causes of proteinuria:
• Animals with glomerular proteinuria frequently asymptomatic or have signs attributable to the underlying disease process; many have vague signs of weight loss and lethargy; some have signs of uremia, hypertension, edema, ascites, and thromboembolism.
• Animals with lower urinary tract disorders and postglomerular proteinuria may have dysuria, pollakiuria, inappropriate urination, and hematuria.

LABORATORY FINDINGS

Drugs That May Alter Lab Results
• Contamination with quartenary ammonium compounds causes false-positive urine dipstick colorimetric (tetrabromphenol blue) test results.
• Results of the sulfosalicylic acid (SSA) turbidimetric test (Bumintest Tabs®) are falsely increased by radiographic contrast media, penicillins, cephalosporins, sulfa drugs or the urine preservative thymol.

Disorders That May Alter Lab Results
• False-positive urine dipstick test results occur when urine is highly alkaline (pH > 8-9).
• The SSA test results are falsely decreased by very alkaline or dilute urine and increased by uncentrifuged urine.

Valid if Run in Human Labs? Yes

CBC/BIOCHEMISTRY/URINALYSIS
• The urine dipstick and the SSA tests allow for qualitative and semiquantitative assessment of urine protein content, respectively. These screening tests are quick and inexpensive. However, results of both the urine dipstick and SSA are affected by urine concentration and must be interpreted in light of urine specific gravity. Low urine protein (trace or 1+) may be normal in a concentrated urine sample. High protein in dilute urine may not be detected by these methods. If proteinuria is detected by these methods, the urine sediment should be evaluated for hematuria, pyuria, or bacteriuria
• The urine protein screening test should be repeated in dogs that initially have a normal

urine sediment examination or have been treated for urinary tract inflammation or hemorrhage. If proteinuria is transient and the urine sediment is normal, functional proteinuria or false-positive test results should be considered.

OTHER LABORATORY TESTS
• Urine protein should be quantified by urine protein:creatinine ratio or 24-hour urine protein determination in dogs and cats that are hypoalbuminemic or have repeatedly positive urine dipstick or SSA tests in the absence of lower urinary tract hemorrhage or inflammation.
• Glomerular disease should be suspected if the urine protein:creatinine ratio or 24-hour urine protein content is abnormal, concurrent hypoalbuminemia is detected, little evidence supports primary tubular disease, or a large amount of albuminuria is detected by electrophoresis. In these dogs, aggressive attempts should be made to identify an underlying disease (e.g., neoplasia, ehrlichiosis, dirofilariasis, systemic lupus erythematosus, and chronic bacterial infection).

IMAGING
Ultrasound and radiographs may identify an underlying infectious, inflammatory, or neoplastic disease process. Ultrasound may provide information about structural changes suggesting primary renal disease (e.g., loss of corticomedullary distinction, hyperechogenicity, and irregular surface margin).

OTHER DIAGNOSTIC PROCEDURES
Renal biopsy is needed to differentiate glomerulosclerosis, glomerulonephritis, and amyloidosis when an underlying disease can not be identified or proteinuria has persisted for several months after treatment of the underlying disease.

TREATMENT
• Animals do not need to be hospitalized or have their activity altered if proteinuria is the only laboratory abnormality.
• If glomerular disease is suspected, a diet that is moderately reduced in protein should be fed.

MEDICATIONS

DRUGS AND FLUIDS
See chapters describing azotemia and uremia, nephrotic syndrome, glomerulonephritis, and amyloidosis.

CONTRAINDICATIONS N/A

PRECAUTIONS
Drugs that are highly bound to albumin may have an altered effect if proteinuria is of sufficient magnitude to cause hypoalbuminemia. Lower dosages of coumadin may be required

for effective anticoagulation. Higher doses of furosemide may be required to effectively mobilize edema. See hypoalbuminemia.

POSSIBLE INTERACTIONS N/A

ALTERNATE DRUGS

See chapters describing azotemia and uremia, nephrotic syndrome, glomerulonephritis, amyloidosis.

FOLLOW-UP

PATIENT MONITORING

• The urine protein:creatinine ratio or 24-hour urine protein content should be followed for months after resolution of any treatable underlying disease. Protein quantitation can be used to monitor progression of glomerular disease and response to treatment.
• Serum creatinine should be monitored concurrently. In some animals, reduction in proteinuria may reflect deteriorating renal function. Assessment of disease progression and subsequent therapeutic changes should be made on the basis of trends noticed in repeat urine protein:creatinine ratio or 24-hour urine protein content rather than on the basis of one or two data points.

POSSIBLE COMPLICATIONS

Those associated with severe proteinuria:
• Edema
• Thromboembolism
• Systemic hypertension
• Poor wound healing

MISCELLANEOUS

ASSOCIATED CONDITIONS

Heavy proteinuria can be associated with hypoalbuminuria, hypoglobulinemia (rare), hypercholesterolemia, low antithrombin III, thrombocytosis, and hyperfibriginonemia.

AGE-RELATED FACTORS N/A

ZOONOTIC POTENTIAL N/A

PREGNANCY

Some drugs used in the treatment of diseases associated with proteinuria may be contraindicated in pregnancy. See specific sections.

SYNONYMS N/A

SEE ALSO

• Albumin, Hypo-albuminemia
• Amyloidosis
• Creatinine and Blood Urea Nitrogen (BUN)—Azotemia and Uremia
• Glomerulonephritis
• Hematuria
• Nephrotic Syndrome
• Pyuria

ABBREVIATIONS

SSA = sulfosalicylic acid

References

Lulich JP, Osborne CA. Interpretation of urine protein-creatinine ratios in dogs with glomerular and nonglomerular disorders. Comp Cont Ed Pract Vet 1990; 12:59-72.

Grauer GF. Clinical manifestations of urinary disorders. In Essentials of small animal internal medicine. Nelson RW, Couto CG, editors. Baltimore, Mosby Year Book, 1992;449-465.

Authors Shelly L. Vaden

Consulting Editors Larry G. Adams and Carl A. Osborne

PYURIA

BASICS

DEFINITION

• The presence of WBC (i.e., neutrophils, eosinophils, monocytes, lymphocytes, or plasma cells) in the urine • More than five WBC per high power field is generally considered abnormal. However, the total number of WBC found in urine sediment depends on the method of collection, sample volume and concentration, degree of cellular destruction after collection, and laboratory technique.

Pathophysiology

• High numbers of WBC in voided urine samples indicates active inflammation anywhere along the urinary or genital tract.
• Can be associated with any pathologic process (infectious or noninfectious) that causes cellular injury or death. Tissue damage evokes exudative inflammation that is characterized by evidence of leukocyte extravasation (pyuria) and increased vascular permeability (hematuria, proteinuria).

Systems Affected

• Renal/Urologic—urethra, urinary bladder, ureters, and kidneys • Genital—prepuce, prostate, vagina, and uterus

SIGNALMENT   Dogs and cats

SIGNS

General Comments

Inflammation can cause clinical signs localized to the site(s) of injury or be accompanied by systemic manifestations. Historical and physical examination findings depend on the underlying cause, organ(s) affected, degree of organ dysfunction, and magnitude of systemic inflammatory response. Nonobstructive lesions confined to the urinary bladder, urethra, vagina, or prepuce rarely cause systemic signs of inflammation. Systemic signs may accompany inflammatory lesions of the kidneys, prostate, or uterus.

Historical And Physical Examination Findings

Local Effects of Inflammation
• Erythema of mucosal surfaces (e.g., redness of vaginal or prepucial mucosa) • Swelling of tissues (e.g., renomegaly, prostatomegaly, and mural thickening of urinary bladder or urethra) • Exudation of leukocytes and protein–rich fluid (e.g., pyuria, purulent urethral or vaginal discharge, pyometra, and prostatic abscess) • Pain (e.g., adverse response to palpation, dysuria, pollakiuria, and stanguria) • Loss of function (e.g., polyuria, dysuria, pollakiuria, and urinary incontinence)
Systemic Effects of Inflammation
• Fever • Depression • Anorexia • Dehydration

CAUSES

Kidney

• Pyelonephritis—e.g., bacterial, fungal, par-

asitic, and mycoplasmal • Nephrolith(s) • Neoplasia • Trauma • Immune–mediated

Ureter

• Ureteritis—e.g., bacterial • Ureterolith(s) • Neoplasia

Urinary Bladder

• Cystitis—e.g., bacterial, mycoplasmal, fungal, and parasitic • Urocystolith(s) • Neoplasia • Trauma • Overdistention—urethral obstruction

Urethra

• Urethritis—e.g., bacterial, fungal, and mycoplasmal • Urethrolith(s) • Neoplasia • Trauma • Foreign body

Prostate Gland

• Prostatitis/abscess—e.g., bacterial and fungal • Neoplasia

Penis and prepuce

Balanoposthitis • Neoplasia • Foreign body

Uterus

• Pyometra/metritis—e.g., bacterial

Vagina

Vaginitis—bacterial, mycoplasmal, viral, or fungal • Neoplasia • Foreign body • Trauma

RISK FACTORS

• Any disease process, diagnostic procedure, or treatment that alters normal host urinary tract defenses and predisposes to infection
• Any disease process, dietary factor, or treatment that predisposes to the formation of uroliths

DIAGNOSIS

DIFFERENTIAL DIAGNOSIS

Voided Specimens

• Rule out vaginitis (signs include vaginal discharge, erythema of vaginal mucosa, licking of vulva, and attracting male dogs).
• Rule out pyometra, metritis (signs include vaginal discharge, a large uterus, pyrexia, depression, anorexia, polyuria, polydipsia, and a recent history of estrus, parturition, or progestin administration). • Rule out balanoposthitis (signs include prepucial discharge, erythema of the prepucial or penile mucosa, and licking the prepuce). • Rule out prostatitis, prostatic abscess, and prostatic neoplasia (signs include urethral discharge, prostatomegaly, pyrexia, depression, dysuria, tenesmus, caudal abdominal pain, and stiff gait) • Rule out urethritis, urethroliths, and urethral neoplasia (signs include dysuria, pollakiuria, stranguria, and palpable uroliths or mass lesion in the urethra) • Rule out inflammatory disorder of the urinary bladder and kidneys

Specimens Collected By Cystocentesis

• Rule out urethral obstruction (signs include stranguria, anuria, and a large, overdistended urinary bladder). • Rule out prostatic and urethral disorders (see previous text).

Purulent prostatic or urethral exudates can reflux into the urinary bladder. • Rule out cystitis, urocystoliths, and neoplasia of the urinary bladder (signs include dysuria, pollakiuria, stranguria, and palpable uroliths or mass lesion in the urinary bladder) • Rule out pyelonephritis (signs include pyrexia, depression, anorexia, polyuria, polydipsia, renal pain, and renomegaly) • Rule out post–trauma pyuria (signs include history of trauma and including iatrogenic)

LABORATORY FINDINGS

Drugs That May Alter Lab Results

• WBC rapidly lyse in hypotonic or alkaline urine. Administration of alkalinizing agents (e.g., sodium bicarbonate, potassium citrate, chlorothiazide, and acetazolamide) or agents that produce hypotonic urine (e.g., diuretics and glucocorticoids) may falsely decrease urine WBC concentration. • Nitrofurantoin, cephalosporins, and gentamicin can cause false positive leukocyte esterase reaction when urine is tested by the reagent strip (dipstick) method. • Urine WBC concentration can be substantially low in patients with inflammatory disorders that have been given steroidal or nonsteroidal anti–inflammatory drugs.

Disorders That May Alter Lab Results

• Disorders associated with diminished WBC function or absolute neutropenia can artificially lower values. • Disorders associated with production of hypotonic urine or alkaline urine can artificially lower values.

Miscellaneous Factors That May Alter Lab Results

• False negative leukocyte esterase reaction in dogs when the urine is tested by the reagent strip (dipstick) method. • False positive and false negative leukocyte esterase reaction in cats when the urine is tested by the reagent strip (dipstick) method.

Valid If Run In Human Lab?

• Valid if microscopic examination of urine sediment is performed to detect pyuria.
• Invalid if only leukocyte esterase reagent strip (dipstick) method is used to detect pyuria.

CBC/BIOCHEMISTRY/URINALYSIS

• Pyuria in specimens collected by voiding, manual compression, or catheterization indicates an inflammatory lesion involving the urinary or genital tracts • Pyuria in specimens collected by cystocentesis localizes the site of inflammation to the urinary tract. It does not exclude the urethra and genital tract. Reflux of prostatic exudates into the urinary bladder can cause pyuria in patients with prostatic disease. • Pyuria associated with WBC casts is unequivocal evidence of renal parenchymal inflammation. Generalized renal injury may be associated with concomitant leukocytosis, isosthenuria, and azotemia. • Pyuria associated with bacteria, fungi, or parasite ova in sufficient numbers to be seen by microscopic sediment examination indicate that the inflammatory lesion has been caused or complicated by urinary tract infection. • Pyuria associated with neoplastic cells indicates neoplasia. Diagnosis of urinary tract neoplasia by cytologic examination of urine may be complicated by epithelial cell hyperplasia and atypia caused by urinary tract inflammation or the physiochemical properties of urine (pH and tonicity).

OTHER LABORATORY TESTS
• Quantitative urine culture should be performed in all patients with pyuria, because it provides the most definitive means of identifying and characterizing bacterial urinary tract infection. Negative urine culture results suggest a noninfectious cause of inflammation (e.g., uroliths and neoplasia) or inflammation associated with urinary tract infection caused by fastidious organisms (e.g., mycoplasmas and viruses).
• Cytologic evaluation of urine sediment, prostatic fluid, urethral or vaginal discharges, or biopsy specimens obtained by catheter or needle aspiration may be of value in evaluating patients with localized urinary or genital tract disease. Cytologic examination may establish a definitive diagnosis of urinary tract neoplasia; however, negative cytologic findings do not rule out the possibility of neoplasia.

IMAGING
Survey abdominal radiography, contrast urethrocystography and cystography, urinary tract ultrasonography, and excretory urography are important means of identifying and localizing causes of pyuria.

OTHER DIAGNOSTIC PROCEDURES
Light microscopic evaluation of larger tissue biopsy specimens is indicated in patients with lesions of the urinary or genital tract for which a definitive diagnosis has not been established by less invasive means. Tissue specimens can be obtained by catheter biopsy, cystoscopy and pinch biopsy, or exploratory laparotomy.

TREATMENT
• Treatment varies depending on the underlying cause and specific organs involved.

• Pyuria associated with systemic signs of illness (i.e., pyrexia, depression, anorexia, vomiting, dehydration, leukocytosis, polyuria and polydipsia) or urinary obstruction warrants aggressive diagnostic evaluation and initiation of supportive and symptomatic treatment.

MEDICATIONS
DRUGS AND FLUIDS: N/A
CONTRAINDICATIONS
• Glucocorticoids or other immunosuppressive agents should be avoided in patients suspected of having urinary or genital tract infection.
• Potentially nephrotoxic drugs (e.g., gentamicin) should be avoided in patients that are febrile, dehydrated, or azotemic or are suspected of having pyelonephritis, septicemia, or preexisting renal disease.

PRECAUTIONS N/A
POSSIBLE INTERACTIONS N/A
ALTERNATE DRUGS N/A

FOLLOW-UP
PATIENT MONITORING
Response to treatment by serial urinalysis including examination of urine sediment. In most patients, urine specimens should be collected by cystocentesis to avoid contamination by preputial or vaginal exudates.

POSSIBLE COMPLICATIONS
• Infectious and noninfectious inflammatory disorders of the urinary tract can cause primary renal failure, urinary obstruction, uremia, septicemia, and death. • Pyuria is a potential risk factor for the formation of matrix or matrix–crystalline urethral plugs and subsequent urethral obstruction in male cats.

MISCELLANEOUS
ASSOCIATED CONDITIONS
Hematuria, proteinuria, and bacteriuria

AGE RELATED FACTORS N/A

ZOONOTIC POTENTIAL N/A

PREGNANCY N/A

SYNONYMS Leukocyturia

SEE ALSO
• Dysuria and Pollakiuria • Hematuria
• Lower Urinary Tract Infection
• Proteinuria • Pyelonephritis

ABBREVIATIONS None

References
Lulich JP, Osborne CA. Bacterial infections of the urinary tract. In: Ettinger SJ, Feldman EC, eds. Textbook of veterinary internal medicine, 4th ed. Philadelphia: WB Saunders, 1994:1775–1788.
Lulich JP, Osborne CA, Bartges JW, et al. Canine lower urinary tract disorders. In: Ettinger SJ, Feldman EC, eds. Textbook of veterinary internal medicine, 4th ed. Philadelphia: WB Saunders, 1994:1833–1861.
Osborne CA, Kruger JM, Lulich JP, et al. Feline lower urinary tract diseases. In: Ettinger SJ, Feldman EC, eds. Textbook of veterinary internal medicine, 4th ed. Philadelphia: WB Saunders, 1994:1805–1832.
Osborne CA, Stevens JB. Handbook of Canine and Feline Urinalysis. St. Louis: Ralston Purina Co., 1981:91–118.
Polzin D, Osborne C, O'Brien T. Diseases of the kidneys and ureters. In: Ettinger SJ, ed. Textbook of veterinary internal medicine, 3rd ed. Philadelphia: WB Saunders, 1989:1962–2046.

Authors John M. Kruger, Carl A. Osborne and Cheryl L. Swenson
Consulting Editors Larry G. Adams and Carl A. Osborne

SODIUM, HYPERNATREMIA

 BASICS

DEFINITION

A serum sodium concentration > 158 mEq/L in dogs or >165 mEq/L in cats

Pathophysiology

Sodium is the most abundant cation in the extracellular fluid. Therefore, hypernatremia usually reflects hyperosmolality. Common causes of hypernatremia include renal or gastrointestinal loss of water in excess of sodium loss and low water intake.

Systems Affected

• Endocrine/metabolic • Nervous

SIGNALMENT

Dogs and cats

SIGNS

• Polydypsia • Disorientation • Coma
• Seizures • Other findings depend on underlying cause • Severity of signs usually correlates to the degree of hypernatremia

CAUSES

• Total body sodium high: Oral ingestion (rare); IV administration of NaCl during cardiovascular resuscitation; hyperaldosteronism (rare) •Total body sodium normal plus water deficit: Low water intake (e.g., no access to water and adipsia or hypodypsia); high urinary water loss (e.g., diabetes insipidus); high insensible water loss (e.g., panting and hyperthermia) • Total body sodium low and hypotonic fluid loss (i.e., loss of fluid containing sodium without adequate water replacement): Urinary loss (e.g., diabetes mellitus, osmotic diuresis, and diuresis after acute urinary obstruction); gastrointestinal sodium loss (e.g., administration of osmotic cathartic, vomiting, and diarrhea)

RISK FACTORS N/A

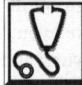 DIAGNOSIS

DIFFERENTIAL DIAGNOSIS

• Diabetes insipidus • Hyperosmolar nonketotic syndrome • Hypertonic dehydration
• Salt ingestion (rare)

LABORATORY FINDINGS

Drugs That May Alter Lab Results

A wide variety of drugs interfere with renal capacity to concentrate urine leading to water loss in excess of sodium and high serum sodium concentration. These drugs include lithium, demeclocycline, and amphotericin.

Disorders That May Alter Lab Results

Lipemia or hyperproteinemia (> 11 g/dl) can artifactually raise sodium concentration when the flame photometry method is used.

Valid If Run In A Human Lab? Yes

CBC/BIOCHEMISTRY/URINALYSIS

• High serum sodium concentration
• Diabetes insipidus—polyuria, low urine specific gravity, and low urine sodium
• Hyperomolar nonketotic syndrome—high blood glucose, low urine output, and high urine specific gravity (usually > 1.025)
• Hypertonic dehydration—low urine sodium and high urine specific gravity (usually > 1.030)

OTHER LABORATORY TESTS

• Modified water deprivation test (see appendix for test protocol) to differentiate diabetes insipidus from other causes of polyuria and polydipsia. Performed after results of CBC, biochemical analysis, urinalysis, and endocrine testing are evaluated to rule out hyperadrenocorticism. • After water restriction, patients with diabetes insipidus have little or no increase in urine specific gravity or urine osmolality. • After ADH or DDAVP administration, patients with nephrogenic diabetes insipidus have < 10% increase in urine specific gravity and those with central diabetes insipidus have a 10-800% increase in urine specific gravity.

IMAGING

CT scan or MRI in patients with diabetes insipidus to rule out pituitary tumor

OTHER DIAGNOSTIC PROCEDURES

N/A

 TREATMENT

• After resolution of the hypernatremia, consider sodium restricted diet (especially in patients with nephrogenic diabetes insipidus).
• Water must be available at all times for patients with diabetes insipidus

MEDICATIONS

DRUGS AND FLUIDS

• If hypovolemia is severe—volume replacement with isotonic saline (i.e., lactated Ringer's or normal saline) or isotonic fluids (i.e., 5% dextrose with half-normal saline)
• Hypernatremia—administer hypotonic fluids (e.g., 5% dextrose in water) to reduce serum sodium by 0.5 mEq/hour or by no more than 20 mEq/L/day. Supplement with potassium and phosphate if needed
• Central diabetes insipidus—DDAVP (1-2 drops in subconjunctival sac q12h-q24h)
• Nephrogenic diabetes insipidus—chlorothiazide (10-40 mg/kg PO q12h)

CONTRAINDICATIONS

Refer to manufacturer's literature

PRECAUTIONS

• Rapid correction of hypernatremia can cause pulmonary edema. • Hypocalcemia may develop during correction of hypernatremia.

POSSIBLE INTERACTIONS N/A

ALTERNATE DRUGS N/A

 FOLLOW-UP

PATIENT MONITORING

• Acute setting—electrolytes, urine output, and body weight • Diabetes insipidus—water intake

POSSIBLE COMPLICATIONS

• CNS thrombosis or hemorrhage • Hyperactivity • Seizures • Serum sodium > 180 meq/L often associated with residual CNS damage • Many patients recover but possibility of neurologic damage is high

 MISCELLANEOUS

ASSOCIATED CONDITIONS N/A

AGE RELATED FACTORS N/A

ZOONOTIC POTENTIAL N/A

PREGNANCY N/A

SYNONYMS None

SEE ALSO

• Diabetes Insipidus • Hyposthenuria

ABBREVIATIONS

ADH = antidiuretic hormone
CNS = central nervous system
DDAVP = brand name of desmopression, a synthetic ADH preparation

REFERENCES

DiBartola SP. Fluid therapy in small animal practice. Philadelphia: WB Saunders, 1992.
Ross DB Clinical physiology of acid-base and electrolyte disorders. 3rd ed. New York: McGraw-Hill, 1989.

Author Rhett Nichols
Consulting Editor Rhett Nichols

SODIUM, HYPONATREMIA

 BASICS

DEFINITION

Serum sodium concentration below the lower limit of normal. Usually associated with low total body sodium.

Pathophysiology

Sodium is the most abundant cation in the extracellular fluid and, therefore, hyponatremia usually reflects hypoosmolality. Either solute loss or water retention can theoretically cause hyponatremia. Most solute loss occurs in isoosmotic solutions (e.g., vomit and diarrhea) and, as a result, water retention in relation to solute is the underlying cause in almost all patients with hyponatremia. In general, hyponatremia occurs only when a defect in renal water excretion is present.

Systems Affected

Nervous—severe neurologic dysfunction is not usually seen until serum sodium concentration falls below 110-115 mEq/L. Overly rapid correction of hyponatremia can also cause neurologic damage.

SIGNALMENT

Dogs and cats.

SIGNS

• Lethargy • Seizures • Obtundation • Coma • Other findings depend on the underlying cause.

CAUSES

Disorders Associated with Normal Renal Water Excretion

• Primary polydipsia • Reset osmostat

Disorders Associated with Reduced Renal Water Excretion

• Low effective circulating volume—gastrointestinal losses, renal losses (including mineralocorticoid deficiency), skin losses, and edematous states (e.g., heart failure, end stage liver disease, and nephrotic syndrome)
• Diuretic administration • Renal failure
• ADH excess with normovolemia—syndrome of inappropriate ADH secretion, hypocortisolemia, and hypothyroidism
• Low solute intake

RISK FACTORS N/A

 DIAGNOSIS

DIFFERENTIAL DIAGNOSIS N/A

LABORATORY FINDINGS

Drugs That May Alter Lab Results

Mannitol can cause pseudohyponatremia.

Disorders That May Alter Lab Results.

Hyperlipidemia, hyperglycemia, and hyperproteinemia can cause pseudohyponatremia.

Valid If Run In A Human Lab? Yes

CBC/BIOCHEMISTRY/URINALYSIS

• Low serum sodium concentration. • Other abnormalities may point to the underlying cause.

OTHER LABORATORY TESTS

• Plasma osmolality is low; if plasma osmolality is normal or high, exclude renal failure or causes of pseudohyponatremia (e.g., hyperlipidemia, hyperglycemia, hyperproteinemia, and mannitol administration). • Urine osmolality < 100-150 mosmol/kg indicates primary polydipsia or reset osmostat. Urine osmolality > 150-200 mosmol/kg indicates impaired renal water excretion. • Urine sodium concentration < 15-20 mEq/L indicates low effective circulating volume, pure cortisol deficiency, primary polydipsia with high urine output. Urine sodium concentration > 20 to 25 mEq/L indicates syndrome of inappropriate ADH secretion, adrenal insufficiency, renal failure, reset osmostat, diuretic administration, or vomiting with marked bicarbonate loss.

IMAGING N/A

DIAGNOSTIC PROCEDURES N/A

GROSS AND HISTOPATHOLOGIC FINDINGS N/A

 TREATMENT

INPATIENT VERSUS OUTPATIENT

Depends on severity of hyponatremia, associated neurologic dysfunction, and the underlying disorder

DIET N/A

CLIENT EDUCATION

Depends on the underlying disorder

SURGICAL CONSIDERATIONS N/A

MEDICATIONS

DRUGS AND FLUIDS

Treatment consists of increasing the serum sodium concentration and treating the underlying cause. Hyponatremia is corrected by administering NaCl if the patient has hypovolemia (e.g., volume depletion, adrenal insufficiency, and diuretic administration) and by restricting water if the patient has normovolemia or edema (e.g., renal failure, SIADH, primary polydipsia, and edematous states). Hypertonic saline administration is usually indicated if the patient has clinical signs or serum sodium concentration < 105-110 mEq/L. The sodium deficit is estimated by 0.5 x lean BW (kg) x (120 - serum sodium concentration). If the patient has no to mild clinical signs, increase sodium concentration at a rate of 0.5 mEq/L per hour until sodium concentration is 120-125 mEq/L, then discontinue hypertonic saline and normalize serum sodium concentration over several days with isotonic saline or water restriction as dictated by the cause of hyponatremia. If the patient has seizures or coma, a rate of 1-1.5 mEq/L per hour for the first 10 mEq/L may be indicated. True volume depletion must also be corrected. In edematous patients with symptomatic hyponatremia, administration of a loop diuretic in addition to hypertonic saline may be necessary. Other medications are dictated by the underlying cause.

CONTRAINDICATIONS N/A

PRECAUTIONS

Overly rapid correction of hyponatremia can result in neurologic damage (demyelination); avoid increasing serum sodium concentration by more than 25 mEq/L in the first 48 hours.

POSSIBLE INTERACTIONS N/A

ALTERNATE DRUGS N/A

 FOLLOW-UP

PATIENT MONITORING

Serum electrolyte concentrations as needed to assure appropriate response to NaCl and other indicated therapies.

PREVENTION/AVOIDANCE

Depends on the underlying disorder

POSSIBLE COMPLICATIONS

Depends on the underlying disorder

EXPECTED COURSE/PROGNOSIS

Depends on the underlying disorder

 MISCELLANEOUS

ASSOCIATED CONDITIONS

Other electrolyte and acid-base abnormalities are often associated with the clinical disorders that cause hyponatremia.

AGE RELATED FACTORS

Depends on the underlying cause

ZOONOTIC POTENTIAL N/A

PREGNANCY N/A

SYNONYMS N/A

SEE ALSO N/A

ABBREVIATIONS

ADH = antidiuretic hormone

References

Rose DB. Clinical physiology of acid-base and electrolyte disorders. 3rd ed. New York: McGraw-Hill, 1989.

DiBartola SP. Fluid therapy in small animal practice. Philadelphia: WB Saunders, 1992.

Author Peter P. Kintzer

Consulting Editor Rhett Nichols

THROMBOCYTOPENIA

BASICS

DEFINITION
Platelet count below the lower limit of the reference range. Purdue University Teaching Hospital reference range for dogs is 200,000-900,000/μl; cats is 300,000-700,000/μl.

Pathophysiology
Platelets are produced by megakaryocytes in the bone marrow, released into the bloodstream, and circulate for a few to several days. In the normal state, the platelet count remains stable because production of platelets is equivalent to the removal of platelets from the circulation. In addition, there is a fairly large reserve of platelets in the spleen. A low number of platelets can be caused by decreased production, sequestration, increased destruction, or increased utilization.

Systems Affected
If the platelet count is low enough (< 40,000/μl), hemorrhage can occur into any organ system. Hemorrhage is commonly recognized in the integumentary, gastrointestinal, urinary, and respiratory systems. Hemorrhage is more difficult to document in the nervous and cardiovascular systems.

SIGNALMENT
• Primary immune-mediated thrombocytopenia is more common in female dogs than male dogs and cats • Primary immune-mediated thrombocytopenia is more common in the poodle, Old English sheepdog, cocker spaniel, and, possibly, German shepherd than other breeds. • Non–immune-mediated thrombocytopenia is more common in the Doberman pinscher than other breeds.

SIGNS

General Comments
Signs typically are not present until the platelet count is < 40,000/μl.

Historical Findings
• Spontaneous and inappropriate mucous membrane, cutaneous, nasal, urinary, and gastrointestinal bleeding • Weakness and collapse • Dyspnea

Physical Examination Findings
• Petechial and ecchymotic hemorrhages in the skin and mucous membranes • Epistaxis • Melena and hematochezia or hematemesis • Hematuria • Pale mucous membranes • Lethargy, weakness, and collapse • Scleral hemorrhages, retinal hemorrhages, and hyphema • Dyspnea • Heart murmur • Neurologic signs

CAUSES
• Decreased production—infectious agents, neoplasia, drugs, and immune-mediated causes • Increased sequestration—splenomegaly or hepatomegaly • Increased utilization—disseminated intravascular coagulation (DIC), vasculitis, and blood loss. Blood loss alone does not cause severe thrombocytopenia. Increased destruction—primary or secondary immune-mediated thrombocytopenia • Miscellaneous—infectious agents

RISK FACTORS
• Potentially any drug, but gold compounds, cephalosporins, and estrogens are featured in well-documented causes of immune-mediated thrombocytopenia in dogs
• Recent vaccination

DIAGNOSIS

DIFFERENTIAL DIAGNOSIS
• Splenomegaly or hepatomegaly and mild thrombocytopenia—consider sequestration of platelets • Blood loss associated with traumatic event—consider increased utilization
• Exposure to vitamin K antagonist—consider increased utilization • Drug history—consider secondary immune-mediated thrombocytopenia • Mass—consider neoplasia associated secondary immune-mediated thrombocytopenia • Primary immune-mediated thrombocytopenia by exclusion of other causes

LABORATORY FINDINGS

Drugs That May Alter Lab Results
N/A

Disorders That May Alter Lab Results
• Poor venipuncture technique can cause clumping of platelets in vitro and provide a falsely low platelet count. • It is difficult to obtain platelet counts from cat blood with some automated blood analyzers. Good commercial laboratories perform manual counts to obtain accurate results.

Valid If Run in Human Lab?
Because of the large size of cat platelets, they will not be measured accurately by most automated hematology analyzers.

CBC/BIOCHEMISTRY/URINALYSIS
• If results reveal anemia and leukopenia, consider decreased production. • If results reveal anemia with spherocytosis with or without agglutination, consider secondary immune-mediated thrombocytopenia. • If morulae are detected in platelets, consider E. platys. • If morulae are detected in neutrophils, consider granulocytic ehrlichiosis. • If morulae are detected in monocytes, consider E. canis.

OTHER LABORATORY TESTS
• Serum titers to rule out ehrlichiosis and Rocky Mountain spotted fever • Coagulation profile (e.g., PT and APTT or ACT). Normal clotting times rule out DIC and exposure to vitamin K antagonists. • Antiplatelet antibody or antimegakaryocyte antibody test to evaluate immune-mediated mechanism • ANA test to screen for systemic lupus erythematosis
• Coombs' test to help document concurrent immune-mediated hemolytic anemia

IMAGING
To identify splenomegaly, hepatomegaly, internal bleeding, and internal neoplasms

OTHER DIAGNOSTIC PROCEDURES
Examination of bone marrow aspirate to rule out primary bone marrow disease

TREATMENT
• If thrombocytopenia is severe, restrict activity to prevent fatal bleeding.
• Minimize bleeding caused by diagnostic procedures (e.g., minimize or eliminate jugular venipunctures and apply extended pressure after venipunctures). Bone marrow aspirate usually is safe.
• Once stabilized, treat as outpatient

MEDICATIONS

DRUGS AND FLUIDS
• If anemia as a result of blood loss is severe, give blood transfusion
• Immune-mediated thrombocytopenia—corticosteroids and other immunosuppressive drugs (see Thrombocytopenia, Immune-Mediated)
• Rickettsial diseases—doxycycline or tetracycline (see Ehrlichiosis, Rocky Mountain Spotted Fever)
• DIC—heparin (see Disseminated Intravascular Coagulation).

CONTRAINDICATIONS
Nonsteroidal antiinflammatory drugs that interfere with platelet function

PRECAUTIONS None

POSSIBLE INTERACTIONS None

ALTERNATE DRUGS None

FOLLOW-UP

PATIENT MONITORING
• Amount of bleeding • Platelet counts daily initially until patient is stable, then weekly until platelet count returns to normal range
• Serial coagulation profile if DIC is suspected

POSSIBLE COMPLICATIONS
Excessive bleeding, which can be fatal

MISCELLANEOUS

ASSOCIATED CONDITIONS
Immune-mediated hemolytic anemia

AGE RELATED FACTORS None

ZOONOTIC POTENTIAL None

PREGNANCY

• Treatment of pregnant animals with immune-mediated thrombocytopenia with corticosteroids should be done with caution.
• Treatment of rickettsial diseases with tetracycline or doxycycline can cause fetal abnormalities.

SYNONYMS None

SEE ALSO See causes.

ABBREVIATIONS

ACT = activated clotting time
APTT = activated partial thromboplastin time
DIC = disseminated intravascular coagulation
PT = prothrombin time

References

Reagan WJ, Rebar AH. Platelet disorders. In: Ettinger SL, Feldman EC, eds. Textbook of veterinary internal medicine. Philadelphia: WB Saunders, 1994.

Thompson JP. Immunologic diseases. In: Ettinger SL, Feldman EC, eds. Textbook of veterinary internal medicine. Philadelphia: WB Saunders, 1994.

Grindem CB, Breischwerdt EB, Corbett WT, Jans HE. Epidemiologic survey of thrombocytopenia in dogs: a report of 987 cases. Vet Clin Pathol 1991;20:38-43.

Williams DA, Maggio-Price L. Canine idiopathic thrombocytopenia: clinical observations and long-term follow-up in 54 cases. J Am Vet Med Assoc 1984;185:660-663.

Author William J. Reagan
Consulting Editor Alan H. Rebar

THROMBOCYTOSIS

 BASICS

DEFINITION
A platelet count above the upper end of the reference range. Purdue University Teaching Hospital reference range for dogs is 200,000-900,000/μl; cats is 300,000-700,000/μl.

Pathophysiology
Thrombocytosis can be caused by increased production of platelets, decreased clearance of platelets, and decreased sequestration of platelets. For most disease states in which thrombocytosis occurs, the exact mechanisms are not well-documented.

Systems Affected
• Usually does not cause systemic abnormalities • Thrombosis is not commonly observed. If the patient has concurrent alterations in blood flow and endothelial cell damage, thrombosis can develop and cause organ dysfunction. • Bleeding is not commonly observed. If the patient has a concurrent platelet functional defect, hemorrhage can occur and cause organ dysfunction.

SIGNALMENT
Excitement-induced thrombocytosis is more common in cats, especially kittens, than in dogs.

SIGNS
Usually no signs directly attributed to the thrombocytosis

CAUSES
Primary Thrombocytosis
Essential thrombocythemia

Secondary Thrombocytosis
• Neoplasia, including both bone marrow and non–bone-marrow origin • Corticosteroids—impede the removal of platelets from the circulation • Vincristine—increases platelet production • Antineoplastic drugs that suppress the bone marrow. A "rebound" thrombocytosis may occur during the recovery phase of the bone marrow. • Antibiotics • Gastrointestinal diseases such as pancreatitis, hepatitis, gingivitis, and colitis • Endocrine disorders such as diabetes mellitus, hyperadrenocorticism, and hypothyroidism • Immune-mediated disorders such as immune-mediated hemolytic anemia, immune-mediated thrombocytopenia, systemic lupus erythematosus, and immune-mediated polyarthritis • Iron deficiency • Fractures or soft tissue trauma • Hemorrhage • Myelofibrosis • Splenectomy • Splenic contraction

RISK FACTORS None

 DIAGNOSIS

DIFFERENTIAL DIAGNOSIS
• Mass—consider thrombocytosis associated with neoplasia • Diarrhea and vomiting—consider thrombocytosis associated with inflammatory conditions of the gastrointestinal tract • Polydipsia and polyuria—consider thrombocytosis associated with hyperadrenocortism and diabetes mellitus • Weight gain, bilateral alopecia, and dry hair coat—consider thrombocytosis associated with hypothyroidism • Gastrointestinal or integumentary chronic blood loss—consider thrombocytosis associated with iron deficiency • Splenectomy—consider reduced sequestration of platelets • Drug therapy (e.g., corticosteroids, vincristine, antibiotics, and antineoplastic drugs)—consider drug-induced thrombocytosis • Bone fracture or soft tissue trauma—consider thrombocytosis associated with trauma • Excited patients during venipuncture—consider excitement-induced splenic contraction

LABORATORY FINDINGS
Drugs That May Alter Lab Results N/A

Disorders That May Alter Lab Results
Excessively large platelets such as in cats or in dogs or cats with a myeloproliferative disorder may disallow an accurate platelet count with some automated hematology analyzers. Most good laboratories recognize this abnormality and perform a manual count.

Valid If Run in Human Lab?
Because of large size of cat platelets, accurate counts by use of most automated hematology analyzers may not be attainable.

CBC/BIOCHEMISTRY/URINALYSIS
• Mild, normocytic normochromic nonregenerative anemia—consider hypothyroidism or neoplasia • Severe nonregenerative anemia with or without dacryocytes and with or without neutropenia—consider myelofibrosis • Regenerative anemia with spherocytosis with or without agglutination—consider immune-mediated hemolytic anemia • Microcytic hypochromic anemia—consider iron deficiency • Concurrent neutrophilia and lymphocytosis—consider excitement-induced thrombocytosis • Inflammatory leukogram—consider secondary thrombocytosis associated with an inflammatory response • Blast cells or bone marrow precursor cells in the circulation—consider myeloproliferative disorders, including megakaryoblastic leukemia and basophilic leukemia • Extremely high platelet count, macroplatelets, and hypo- or hypergranulation with or without basophilia—consider the myeloproliferative disorder essential thrombocythemia. Diagnosis is made by ruling out all other causes of thrombocytosis. • Stress leukogram, fasting hyperglycemia, high liver enzyme activity, including alkaline phosphatase—consider hyperadrenocorticism • High hepatocellular and cholestatic liver enzymes with or without high bilirubin—consider hepatic disease • Fasting hyperglycemia and glucosuria—consider diabetes mellitus • High lipase and amylase—consider pancreatitis

OTHER LABORATORY TESTS
• Serum iron, ferritin, and total iron-binding capacity to detect iron deficiency • Serum T_4 concentration with or without TSH levels to detect hypothyroidism • ACTH levels or low-dose dexamethasone suppression test to detect hyperadrenocorticism • FIV and FeLV testing in cats with myeloproliferative disorders

IMAGING
To detect internal neoplasm, organomegaly, and inflammatory disease

OTHER DIAGNOSTIC PROCEDURES
• Examination of bone marrow aspirate and core biopsy to detect myeloproliferative disorder, iron deficiency, and myelofibrosis • Endoscopy to detect gastrointestinal disease • Biopsy of any internal or external mass

 TREATMENT

• Usually, no specific treatment is necessary. • Excitement-induced thrombocytosis usually is transient. • Treat underlying disease and platelet count will return to normal.

 MEDICATIONS

DRUGS AND FLUIDS
• Immediate treatment is not necessary to correct laboratory abnormality. • Treat underlying disease and platelet count will return to normal.

CONTRAINDICATIONS
If platelet function is abnormal, do not use nonsteroidal antiinflammatory drugs.

PRECAUTIONS N/A
POSSIBLE INTERACTIONS N/A
ALTERNATE DRUGS N/A

 FOLLOW-UP

PATIENT MONITORING
Complete blood counts should be done as needed to monitor the underlying disease process. Thrombocytosis will resolve once the primary disease is eliminated.

POSSIBLE COMPLICATIONS
Bleeding abnormality as a result of concurrent platelet function defect

 MISCELLANEOUS

ASSOCIATED CONDITIONS
Hyperkalemia is sometimes associated with severe thrombocytosis. The hyperkalemia is caused by release of potassium from platelets during clotting in vitro. Plasma potassium concentration should be normal.

AGE RELATED FACTORS

Excitement-induced thrombocytosis is more common in cats, especially kittens, than in dogs.

ZOONOTIC POTENTIAL None

PREGNANCY N/A

SYNONYM Thrombocythemia

SEE ALSO See Causes.

ABBREVIATIONS

ACTH = adrenocorticotropic hormone
FeLV = feline leukemia virus
FIV = feline immunodeficiency virus
T_4 = thyroxine
TSH = thyroid stimulating hormone

References

Reagan WJ, Rebar AH. Platelet disorders. In: Ettinger SL, Feldman EC, eds. Textbook of veterinary internal medicine. Philadelphia: WB Saunders, 1994.

Hammer AS. Thrombocytosis in dogs and cats: a retrospective study. Comparative Haematology International 1991;1:181-186.

Jain NC. The platelets. In: Jain NC, ed. Essentials of veterinary hematology. Philadelphia: Lea & Febiger, 1993.

Author William J. Reagan
Consulting Editor Alan H. Rebar

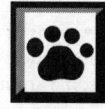

DIAGNOSTICS–
ELECTROCARDIOGRAPHY

ATRIAL FIBRILLATION AND ATRIAL FLUTTER

BASICS

OVERVIEW
• With atrial fibrillation, atrial and ventricular rates are rapid and totally irregular. At very rapid ventricular rates, the ventricular rhythm appears less irregular. There are no P waves. With coarse atrial fibrillation, large oscillations (f waves) of varying amplitude replace normal sinus P waves (Figure). Sometimes these prominent f waves resemble atrial flutter (Figure) ("atrial flutter fibrillation"). • Atrial fibrillation is caused by numerous disorganized atrial impulses frequently bombarding the AV node. • Atrial flutter is caused by a single wave moving in a continuous reentry circuit throughout the atrial myocardium, frequently and regularly stimulating the AV node.

ECG Features
• For atrial flutter, atrial rhythm (f waves) is regular, with a rate usually > 300 bpm. Ventricular rhythm and rate depend on the atrial rate and state of AV conduction (same as the atrial rate 1:1 conduction; half the atrial 2:1; 3:1; 4:1; etc.). Atrial fibrillation has a rapid and totally irregular atrial and ventricular rate. • Normal P waves are replaced by sawtooth flutter (f) waves, a combination of ectopic and pronounced atrial repolarization (Ta) waves, or by oscillations (f waves) with atrial fibrillation. • The QRS configuration is normal or wide and bizarre due to ventricular conduction abnormalities. • For atrial flutter, when conduction through the AV node is constant, the interval between the QRS complex and the F wave is of constant duration. All of the atrial impulses sometimes cannot be conducted to the ventricles. With atrial fibrillation, ventricular rate is totally irregular.

SIGNALMENT
• Commonly seen in dogs and cats with conditions associated with atrial enlargement, or dilated cardiomyopathy. • Irish wolfhound is prone to benign atrial fibrillation

SIGNS

Historical Findings
• Congestive heart failure • Coughing and dyspnea • Exercise intolerance • Syncope

Physical Examination Findings
• Sustained irregular or regular tachycardia • Pulse deficits • Gallop rhythm • Signs of congestive heart failure • Atrial fibrillation in the absence of cardiac disease in some animals (e.g., Irish wolfhounds)

CAUSES AND RISK FACTORS
• Cardiomyopathy • Chronic valvular disease • Congenital heart defects • Atrial myocarditis • Atrial neoplasia • Hyperthyroidism (cats) • Ventricular preexcitation (animals with Wolff-Parkinson-White syndrome)—associated with atrial flutter.

DIAGNOSIS

DIFFERENTIAL DIAGNOSIS
• Frequent atrial premature complexes • AV junctional tachycardia with or without AV block • Sinus tachycardia with or without AV block

CBC/BIOCHEMISTRY/URINALYSIS
N/A

OTHER LABORATORY TESTS N/A

IMAGING
Echocardiography may reveal the type and severity of the underlying heart disease.

OTHER DIAGNOSTIC PROCEDURES
Ocular or carotid sinus pressure slows the ventricular rate by lessening the number of conducted flutter waves into the ventricle.

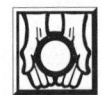

TREATMENT
• Treat the underlying congestive heart failure or other causes.
• Electrical cardioversion with precordial shock (for atrial flutter) is indicated only when a rapid ventricular rate is unresponsive to drugs and the animal has clinical signs.
• A thump on the chest for atrial flutter, in an emergency, may be effective.

MEDICATIONS

DRUGS AND FLUIDS
Correct electrolyte or acid/base imbalance if present.

Dogs
• Digoxin (0.005-0.01 mg/kg q12h mainte- nance or 0.01-0.02 mg/kg q12h for the first day, then maintenance dosage)
• If digoxin is administered alone and the heart rate remains > 160 beats per minute after 5 days, then diltiazem (0.5-1.5 mg/kg q8h titrated), propranolol (0.2-1 mg/kg q8h), or atenolol (0.25-1 mg/kg q12h) can be added.

Cats
• Cats with hypertrophic cardiomyopathy, diltiazem (1-2.5 mg/kg PO q8h) or atenolol (6.25-12.5 mg q24h)
• If the heart rate remains high, add digoxin (0.005 mg/kg q24h-q48h).

CONTRAINDICATIONS/POSSIBLE INTERACTIONS
• Use diltiazem, digoxin, atenolol, or propranolol cautiously with underlying AV block.
• Beware of digoxin-quinidine interaction requiring a reduction in the digoxin dosage.
• Negative inotropic agents (e.g., verapamil, quinidine, and diltiazem) should not be used with congestive heart failure.
• Digoxin and verapamil should not be given for atrial flutter and Wolff-Parkinson-White syndrome.

FOLLOW-UP
• Monitor heart rate and rhythm with serial ECG. • If the condition is associated with cardiac disease, the long-term prognosis is poor.

MISCELLANEOUS

SEE ALSO
• Atrial tachycardia • Atrial premature complexes

ABBREVIATIONS
AV = atrioventricular

References
Tilley LP. Essentials of canine and feline electrocardiography, 3rd ed. Baltimore: Williams & Wilkins, 1992.
Author Michael S. Miller
Consulting Editors Larry P. Tilley and Francis W. K. Smith, Jr.

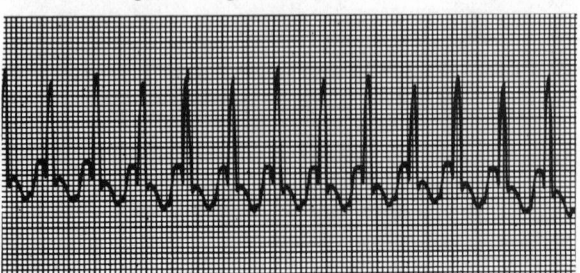

Atrial Flutter

Atrial flutter with 2:1 conduction at a ventricular rate of 330/min in a dog with an atrial septal defect. This supraventricular tachycardia was associated with a Wolff-Parkinson-White pattern. (From Tilley LP. Essentials of canine and feline electrocardiography. 3rd ed. Baltimore: Williams & Wilkins, 1992, with permission).

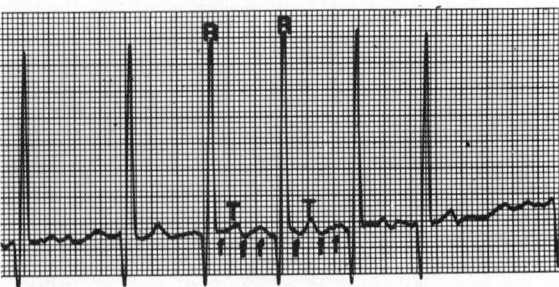

Atrial Fibrillation

"Coarse" atrial fibrillation in a dog with patent ductus arteriosus. The f waves are prominent. (From Tilley LP. Essentials of canine and feline electrocardiography. 3rd ed. Baltimore: Williams & Wilkins, 1992, with permission).

ATRIAL PREMATURE COMPLEXES

BASICS

OVERVIEW
Arrhythmia caused by supraventricular impulses originating from an atrial focus (ectopic focus) other than the sinus node. An increase in automaticity of atrial myocardial fibers or a single reentrant circuit are mechanisms for this arrhythmia.

ECG Features
• The heart rate is usually normal, and the rhythm is irregular due to the premature P wave (called a P' wave) that disrupts the normal P wave rhythm (figure). • The ectopic P' wave is premature, and its configuration is different from that of the sinus P waves. It may be negative, positive, biphasic, or superimposed on the previous T wave.
• The QRS complex is premature, and its configuration is usually normal (same as that of the sinus complexes). It is absent when the P' wave occurs too early (non-conducted atrial premature complexes). The AV node is not completely recovered (refractory), so ventricular conduction does not occur. If there is partial recovery in the AV node or intraventricular conduction systems, the peak P' wave is conducted with a long P'-R interval or is conducted with an abnormal QRS configuration (aberrant conduction). The more premature the complex, the more marked the aberration. • In the P-QRS relationship, the P'-R interval is usually as long as or longer than the sinus P-R interval. • A noncompensatory pause (i.e., when the R to R interval of the two normal sinus complexes enclosing atrial premature complex is less than the R to R intervals of three consecutive sinus complexes) usually follows an APC. The ectopic atrial impulse discharges the sinus node and resets the cycle.

SIGNALMENT
• Commonly seen in dogs with atrial enlargement secondary to chronic mitral valvular insufficiency • May also be observed in dogs or cats with any atrial disease

SIGNS

Historical Findings
• No signs • Congestive heart failure • Coughing and dyspnea • Exercise intolerance • Syncope

Physical Examination Findings
• Irregular heart rhythm • Cardiac murmur • Gallop rhythm • Signs of congestive heart failure

CAUSES AND RISK FACTORS
• Chronic valvular disease • Congenital heart disease • Cardiomyopathy • Atrial myocarditis • Electrolyte disorders • Neoplasia • Hyperthyroidism • Toxemias • Drug toxicity (e.g., digitalis) • Atrial premature complexes can be of normal variation in aged animals.

DIAGNOSIS

DIFFERENTIAL DIAGNOSIS
• Marked sinus arrhythmia • Ventricular premature complexes when aberrant ventricular conduction follows an atrial premature complex

CBC/BIOCHEMISTRY/URINALYSIS
N/A

OTHER LABORATORY TESTS N/A

IMAGING
Echocardiography and Doppler ultrasound may reveal the type and severity of the underlying heart disease.

OTHER DIAGNOSTIC PROCEDURES
N/A

TREATMENT
• Treat animal as inpatient or outpatient.
• Treat the underlying congestive heart failure, cardiac disease, or other causes.

MEDICATIONS

DRUGS AND FLUIDS
Treat congestive heart failure and correct electrolyte or acid/base imbalances if present.

Dogs
• Digoxin (0.005-0.01 mg/kg PO q12h—maintenance dosage), diltiazem (0.5-1.5 mg/kg PO q8h), propranolol (0.2-1 mg/kg PO q8h), atenolol (0.25-1 mg/kg PO q12h)
• Digoxin is treatment of choice and is also indicated to treat the cardiac decompensation that is usually present.
• Congestive heart failure is treated with appropriate dosage of diuretic, angiotensin converting enzyme inhibitor, and vasodilator.

Cats
• Cats with hypertrophic cardiomyopathy—diltiazem at (1-2.5 mg/kg PO q8h) or atenolol (6.25-12.5 mg PO q24h)
• Cats with dilated cardiomyopathy—digoxin (1/4 of a 0.125-mg digoxin tablet q24h or q48h)

CONTRAINDICATIONS/POSSIBLE INTERACTIONS
• Use digoxin, diltiazem, atenolol, or propranolol with caution in animals with underlying atrioventricular block or hypotension.
• In animals with congestive heart failure, negative inotropic agents (e.g., propranolol and quinidine) should be avoided.

FOLLOW-UP
Monitor heart rate and rhythm with serial ECG.

MISCELLANEOUS

SEE ALSO Atrial Tachycardia

ABBREVIATIONS None

Reference
Miller MS, Tilley LP, eds. Manual of canine and feline cardiology. 2nd ed. Philadelphia: WB Saunders, 1995.

Author Michael S. Miller

Consulting Editors Larry P. Tilley and Francis W. K. Smith, Jr.

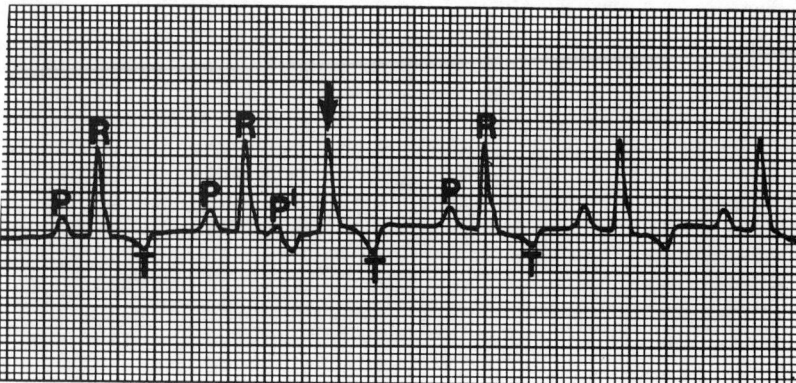

One atrial premature complex (arrow). Heart rate is 160 beats/min. (From: Tilley LP. Essentials of canine and feline electrocardiography. 3rd ed. Baltimore: Williams & Wilkins, 1992, with permission.)

ATRIAL STANDSTILL

 BASICS

OVERVIEW

ECG Features

• P waves are absent (figure). • Heart rate is usually slow (< 60 bpm). • Rhythm is often regular. • QRS complexes are usually normal if the animal has persistent atrial standstill or hyperkalemia and may be wide if the animal has severe hyperkalemia or bundle branch block. • Heart rate does not increase with atropine administration. • Condition can be temporary (e.g., associated with hyperkalemia or drug-induced), terminal (e.g., associated with severe hyperkalemia or dying heart), or persistent • Hyperkalemic patients with atrial standstill have sinus node function, but impulses do not cause atrial myocyte activation. • Persistent atrial standstill (PAS) is caused by inherited atrial myopathy. Skeletal muscle involvement is common.

SIGNALMENT

• PAS is most common in English springer spaniels, but occasionally other breeds are affected. Most affected animals are young.

SIGNS

Historical Findings

• Vary with underlying cause • Letheragy common • Patients with PAS may show signs of congestive heart failure (CHF).

Physical Examination Findings

• Vary with underlying cause • Bradycardia common • Patients with persistent atrial standstill may have skeletal muscle wasting of the antebrachium and scapula.

CAUSES AND RISK FACTORS

• Hyperkalemia • Atrial disease, often associated with atrial distenstion (cats with cardiomyopathy) • Atrial myopathy (English springer spaniels)

 DIAGNOSIS

DIFFERENTIAL DIAGNOSIS

• Slow atrial fibrillation • Sinus bradycardia with small P waves lost in the baseline

CBC/BIOCHEMISTRY/URINALYSIS

N/A

OTHER LABORATORY TESTS

• Rule out hyperkalemia. • ACTH stimulation test if hypoadrenocorticism is suspected • Echocardiogram and electromyography if PAS is suspected—cardiomegaly and depressed contractility may be seen. • Skeletal muscle biopsy in animals with PAS

IMAGING   N/A

OTHER DIAGNOSTIC PROCEDURES

N/A

 TREATMENT

Persistent Atrial Standstill

• PAS is not a life-threatening condition and the animal can be treated as an outpatient. • Implant permanent ventricular pacemaker to regulate rate and rhythm. • Signs of CHF may develop and weakness and lethargy may persist even after heart rate and rhythm are corrected with the pacemaker.

Temporary Atrial Standstill

• Potentially life-threatening condition often requiring aggressive treatment • If underlying cause can be corrected and hyperkalemia reversed, long-term prognosis is excellent.

MEDICATIONS

DRUGS AND FLUIDS

Persistent Atrial Standstill

Treat with diuretics, digoxin (after pacemaker is implanted), and ACE inhibitor if CHF develops.

Temporary Atrial Standstill

• If the animal is hyperkalemic, treat the underlying cause and institute treatment with 0.9% saline and possibly insulin: dextrose or sodium bicarbonate as discussed under the topic hyperkalemia.
• Calcium gluconate counters the effects of hyperkalemia and can be used in life-threatening situations to reestablish a sinus rhythm while instituting treatment to lower potassium concentration.
• If the animal has digoxin toxicity, discontinue medication and provide supportive care.

CONTRAINDICATIONS/POSSIBLE INTERACTIONS

Avoid potassium-containing fluids or medications that increase potassium concentration in hyperkalemic patients.

 ## FOLLOW-UP

Monitor ECG during treatment to correct hyperkalemia and periodically in animals that have a permanent ventricular pacemaker implanted.

Persistent Atrial Standstill

• Warn owners that this condition is generally associated with muscular dystrophy affecting heart and skeletal muscle.
• Monitor patients for signs of CHF.

 ## MISCELLANEOUS

ASSOCIATED CONDITIONS

• Diseases causing hyperkalemia (e.g., hypoadrenocorticism, urethral obstruction or urinary tract tear, acidosis, and drugs)

SEE ALSO

• Hyperkalemia • Digoxin Toxicity • Hypoadrenocorticism • Urethral Obstruction

ABBREVIATIONS

ACE = angiotensin converting enzyme
CHF = congestive heart failure
PAS =- persistent atrial standstill

Reference

Tilley LP. Essentials of canine and feline electrocardiograph. 3rd ed. Philadelphia:. Lea & Febiger, 1992.
Author Francis W. K. Smith, Jr.
Consulting Editors Larry P. Tilley and Francis W. K. Smith, Jr.

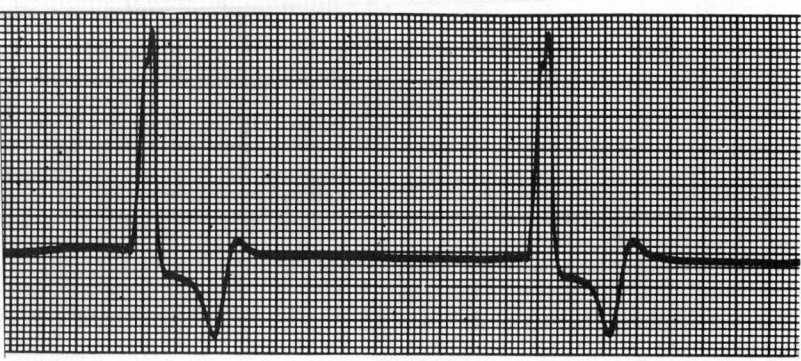

Persistent atrial standstill in an English springer spaniel. No P waves were present in this lead II strip or on any of the other leads. (From Tilley LP. Essentials of canine and feline electrocardiography, 3rd ed. Baltimore: Williams & Wilkins, 1992, with permission.)

ATRIAL TACHYCARDIA

BASICS

OVERVIEW
• Supraventricular impulses originating from an atrial site other than the sinus node • The atrium and atrioventricular (AV) junctional areas are also involved; a reentrant circuit allows the impulse to restimulate the atrium and to pass to the ventricles. • An abnormal automatic focus in the atrium can also be causative.

ECG Features
• The heart rate is rapid (dogs, > 160-180 bpm; cats, > 240 bpm). The rhythm is regular in most animals but may be slightly irregular. The atrial tachycardia can be either intermittent (paroxysmal) (figure) or continuous. • The P′ waves are usually positive in lead II with regular P′-P′ intervals. They may not be easy to see because of the fast ventricular rate or prolonged P′-R interval. • Configuration of the P′ waves is generally somewhat different than that of the sinus P waves. If the atrial rhythm is irregular and the P′ waves are of varying configuration, the term multifocal atrial tachycardia applies. The ectopic rhythm is caused by the rapid firing of two or more ectopic atrial foci. • The QRS configuration is usually normal (same as for the sinus complexes) or wide and bizarre because of bundle branch block, aberrant ventricular conduction, or ventricular preexcitation. • The P′-R interval of the P-QRS is usually constant (1:1 AV conduction). At very high heart rates, various degrees of AV block can occur (2:1; i.e., ventricular rate is half the atrial rate; 3:1, 4:1, etc.).

SIGNALMENT
• Dogs with severe heart disease (common) • Cats with cardiomyopathy and hyperthyroidism • Associated with Wolff-Parkinson-White syndrome, which is congenital in cats and dogs • Same as signalment of animals with atrial premature complexes

SIGNS

Historical Findings
• Congestive heart failure • Syncope • Coughing and dyspnea • Exercise intolerance

Physical Examination Findings
• Regular or intermittently irregular heart rhythm • Heart murmur • Gallop rhythm • Signs of congestive heart failure • Syncope

CAUSES AND RISK FACTORS
• Chronic valvular disease • Congenital heart disease • Cardiomyopathy • Atrial myocarditis • Digoxin toxicity • Systemic disorders • Hyperthyroidism • Electrolyte imbalances • Neoplasia (right atrial hemangiosarcoma) • Ventricular preexcitation (Wolff-Parkinson-White syndrome)

DIAGNOSIS

DIFFERENTIAL DIAGNOSIS
• Sinus tachycardia • AV junctional tachycardia • Atrial flutter

CBC/BIOCHEMISTRY/URINALYSIS
N/A

OTHER LABORATORY TESTS N/A

IMAGING
• Long-term ambulatory (Holter) recording of the ECG can be used to detect paroxysmal atrial tachycardia with unexplained syncope. • Echocardiography and Doppler ultrasonography may reveal the type and severity of underlying heart disease.

OTHER DIAGNOSTIC PROCEDURES
It is important to distinguish atrial tachycardia from sinus tachycardia. Atrial tachycardia is usually terminated immediately with ocular pressure.

TREATMENT
• Vagal maneuver (mild ocular or carotid sinus pressure) may effectively terminate reentrant atrial tachycardia and should be considered if signs of weakness or syncope are evident. • Treat as inpatient initially; treat the underlying congestive heart failure, cardiac disease, or other cause. • Electrical cardioversion or intracardial pacing may be necessary if drugs fail or if the animal is critical. • A thump on the chest often corrects the arrhythmia and is especially useful in an emergency. • Electrophysiologic pacing methods such as overdrive suppression and premature atrial stimulation or electrical cardioversion may be effectively used by clinicians experienced with these methods.

MEDICATIONS

DRUGS AND FLUIDS
Treat congestive heart failure and correct electrolyte and acid/base imbalances if present.

Dogs
• Esmolol (0.1-0.5 mg/kg IV slowly), adenosine (1-12 mg IV rapidly), verapamil (0.05-0.15 mg/kg IV slowly, 5 mg total dose), diltiazem (0.15-0.25 mg/kg IV slowly), or digoxin (0.01 mg/kg IV slowly)
• Digoxin (0.01-0.02 mg/kg PO divided q12h), diltiazem (0.5-1.5 mg/kg PO q8h), propranolol (0.2-1 mg/kg PO q8h), or atenolol (0.25-1 mg/kg PO q12h). Digoxin and diltiazem or digoxin and propranolol or atenolol can be administered orally in combination.
• Quinidine gluconate (IM) has been used in isolated cases.

Cats
Diltiazem (1-2 mg/kg PO q8h), atenolol (6.25-12.5 mg PO q12h), or digoxin (1/4 of 0.125-mg tablet PO q12h or q48h)

CONTRAINDICATIONS/POSSIBLE INTERACTIONS
• Use combination therapy with caution; monitor the heart rate and rhythm with serial ECG.

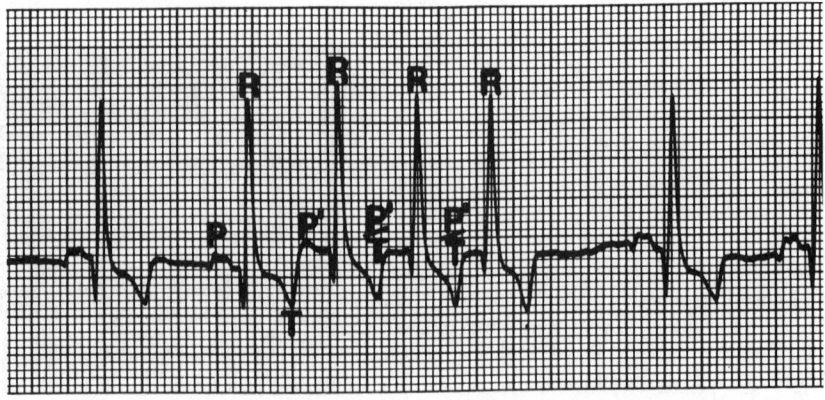

Paroxysms of atrial tachycardia in a dog with severe left atrial enlargement from mitral valvular insufficiency. A hint of a P′ wave can be seen in the previous T wave at the start of each brief period of tachycardia. (From Tilley LP. Essentials of canine and feline electrocardiography, 3rd ed. Baltimore: Williams & Wilkins, 1992, with permission.)

• Verapamil is a potent negative inotropic agent and should be reserved for patients with nonresponsive sustained atrial tachycardia.

FOLLOW-UP

• Monitor with serial ECG. • If associated with primary cardiac disease, prognosis is guarded

MISCELLANEOUS

ABBREVIATIONS

AV = atrioventricular
WPW = Wolff-Parkinson-White

References

Miller MS, Tilley LP, eds. Manual of canine

and feline cardiology. 2nd ed. Philadelphia: WB Saunders, 1995.

Atkins CE, Wright KN. Supraventricular tachycardia associated with accessory pathways in dogs. In: Bonagura JD ed. Current veterinary therapy XII. Phildelphia: WB Saunders, 1995:807.

Author Michael S. Miller

Consulting Editors Larry P. Tilley, Francis W. K. Smith, Jr.

ATRIOVENTRICULAR BLOCK, COMPLETE (THIRD DEGREE)

BASICS

OVERVIEW
• The cardiac impulse is completely blocked in the region of the atrioventricular (AV) junction and/or all bundle branches. • The atrial rate (P to P interval) is normal. • The idioventricular escape rhythm is slow.

ECG Features
• The ventricular rate is slower than the atrial rate (more P waves than QRS complexes). The ventricular escape rhythm (idioventricular) usually has a rate < 40 beats per minute, whereas a junctional escape rhythm (idiojunctional) has a rate of 40-60 in dogs and 60-100 in cats. • The P waves are usually normal in configuration (figure). • The QRS complex is wide and bizarre when the pacemaker is located in the ventricle, or in the lower AV junction in a patient with bundle branch block. The QRS complex is normal when the escape pacemaker is located in the lower AV junction (above the bifurcation of the bundle of His) in a patient without bundle branch block. • There is no conduction between the atria and the ventricles. The P waves have no constant relationship with the QRS complexes. The P to P and R to R intervals are relatively constant (except for a sinus arrhythmia).

SIGNALMENT
• Isolated congenital defect • Idiopathic fibrosis in older dogs, especially cocker spaniels • Geriatric cats with hypertrophic cardiomyopathy • Pugs and Doberman pinschers can have associated sudden death and AV conduction defects and bundle of His lesions

SIGNS
Historical Findings
• Exercise tolerance • Weakness or syncope • Occasionally, congestive heart failure

Physical Examination Findings
• Bradycardia • Variable third and fourth heart sounds • Variation in intensity of the first heart sounds • Signs of congestive heart failure • Intermittent "cannon" waves in jugular venous pulses

CAUSES AND RISK FACTORS
• Isolated congenital defect • Idiopathic fibrosis • Infiltrative cardiomyopathy (amyloidosis or neoplasia) • Hypertrophic cardiomyopathy • Digitalis toxicity • Myocarditis • Endocarditis • Electrolyte disorder • Myocardial infarction • Other congenital heart defects • Lyme disease

DIAGNOSIS

DIFFERENTIAL DIAGNOSIS
• Advanced second degree AV block • Atrial standstill • Slow ventricular tachycardia

CBC/BIOCHEMISTRY/URINALYSIS
• Abnormal serum electrolytes (e.g., hyperkalemia, hypokalemia) • High WBC with a left shift in animals with bacterial endocarditis

OTHER LABORATORY TESTS
• High serum digoxin concentration • Positive Lyme titer and accompanying clinical signs

IMAGING
Echocardiography and Doppler ultrasound to assess cardiac structure and function

OTHER DIAGNOSTIC PROCEDURES
• His bundle electrogram to determine the site of the AV block • Long-term (Holter) ambulatory recording if AV block is intermittent

TREATMENT
• A temporary or permanent cardiac pacemaker is the only effective treatment in symptomatic patients.
• Asymptomatic patients without a pacemaker implanted must be carefully monitored for the development of clinical signs.

MEDICATIONS

DRUGS AND FLUIDS
• Treatment with drugs is usually of no value.
• Traditional drugs used to treat complete AV block include atropine, isoproterenol, theophylline, and corticosteroids.
• An intravenous isoproterenol infusion may help increase the rate of the ventricular escape rhythm to stabilize hemodynamics.

CONTRAINDICATIONS/POSSIBLE INTERACTIONS
Avoid digoxin, xylazine, acepromazine, beta-blockers (e.g., propranolol and atenolol) and calcium channel blockers (e.g., verapamil and diltiazem).

FOLLOW-UP
• Monitor pacemaker function with serial ECG. • A poor long-term prognosis must be given if a cardiac pacemaker is not implanted, especially when the animal has clinical signs.

MISCELLANEOUS

SEE ALSO Atrioventricular Dissociation

Reference
Miller MS, Tilley LP, eds. Manual of canine and feline cardiology. 2nd ed. Philadelphia: WB Saunders, 1995.
Author Michael S. Miller
Consulting Editors Larry P. Tilley and Francis W. K. Smith, Jr.

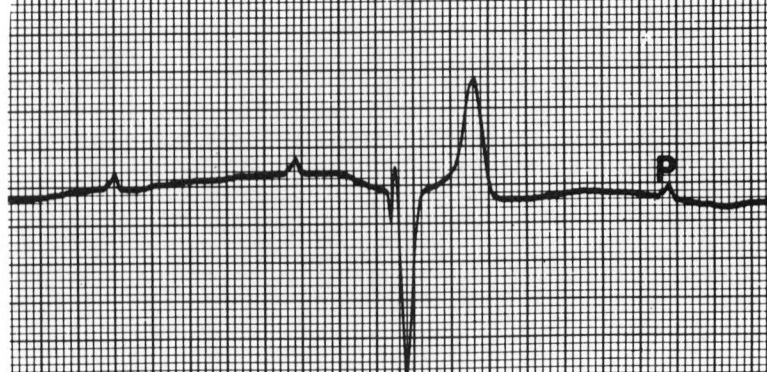

Complete (third-degree) AV block. Atrial heart rate is 125 beats/min. Regular occurring P waves were not associated with the QRS complexes. (From Tilley LP. Essentials of canine and feline electrocardiography, 3rd ed. Baltimore: Williams & Wilkins, 1992, with permission.)

ATRIOVENTRICULAR BLOCK, FIRST DEGREE

BASICS

OVERVIEW
• Caused by delay of conduction of a supraventricular impulse through the atrioventricular (AV) junction and bundle of His • Benign finding often unaccompanied by clinical signs • If caused by primary conduction system disease, may progress to a more serious conduction disturbance

ECG Features
• Rate usually normal • P wave normal (figure) • QRS usually normal • Prolongation of P-R interval > .13 seconds dogs, > .09 seconds cats, in the presence of normal sinus rhythm

SIGNALMENT
• Generally seen in older patients secondary to degenerative changes in the conduction system • Common as an aging change in cocker spaniels and dachshunds

SIGNS

Historical Findings
• Asymptomatic • If secondary to digoxin toxicity, may see signs of lethargy, anorexia, vomiting, and diarrhea

Physical Examination Findings Normal

CAUSES AND RISK FACTORS
• Reflex vagal stimulation (generally results in cyclic increase in P-R interval) • Drug therapy (e.g., digoxin, propranolol, quinidine, procainamide) • Degenerative disease of the conduction system • Potassium imbalance • Hypothyroidism • Protozoal myocarditis • Low dosages of atropine—initially prolong the P-R interval • Lengthening of the P-R interval should not be as an indicator of digoxin serum concentration; approximately 50% of digitalized dogs have a prolonged P-R interval.

DIAGNOSIS

DIFFERENTIAL DIAGNOSIS
• When P waves occur so close to the T wave that they appear as a complex T wave form, differentiate from other supraventricular rhythms such as junctional tachycardia. Generally, when rate slows, P-waves emerge from previous T-waves.
• Long P-R interval with an trial premature complex is not called first degree AV block.

CBC/BIOCHEMISTRY/URINALYSIS
Hyperkalemia and hypokalemia predispose animal to first degree AV block

OTHER LABORATORY TESTS
• Serum digoxin concentration may be high. • Protozoal titer may be positive. • TSH-response test may be abnormal; serum T_4 and free T_4 values may be low.

IMAGING N/A

OTHER DIAGNOSTIC PROCEDURES
N/A

TREATMENT
• Treat any underlying cause.
• Recognize association with certain antiarrhythmic drugs.

MEDICATIONS

DRUGS AND FLUIDS
Correct hypokalemia or hyperkalemia if present.

CONTRAINDICATIONS/POSSIBLE INTERACTIONS
Drugs that intensify vagal stimulation may exaggerate the AV conduction defect.

FOLLOW-UP
Monitor with serial ECG for progression to higher degrees of AV block, especially if first degree AV block is present with bundle branch block.

MISCELLANEOUS

ABBREVIATION
AV = atrioventricular

Reference
Tilley LP. Essentials of canine and feline electrocardiography. 3rd ed. Baltimore: Williams & Wilkins, 1992.

Author Deborah J. Hadlock
Consulting Editors Larry P. Tilley and Francis W. K. Smith, Jr.

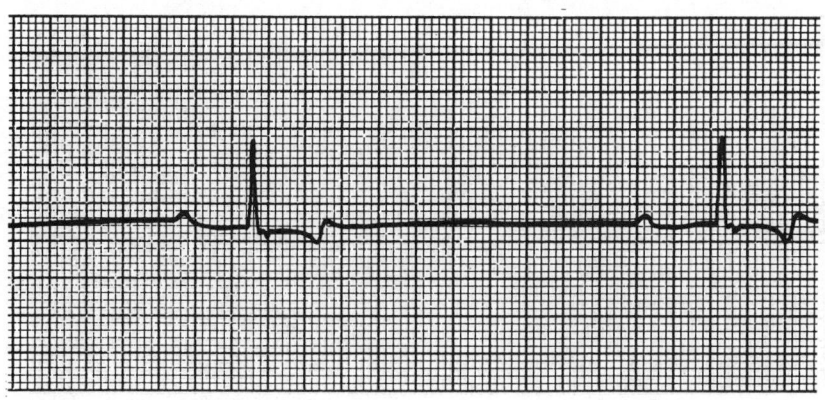

Sinus bradycardia with first-degree AV block. Heart rate is approximately 50 beats/min. Complete (third-degree) AV block. Atrial heart rate is 125 beats/min. From Tilley LP. Essentials of canine and feline electrocardiography, 3rd ed. Baltimore: Williams & Wilkins, 1992, with permission).

ATRIOVENTRICULAR BLOCK, SECOND DEGREE, MOBITZ TYPE I

 BASICS

OVERVIEW
• Usually transient in nature because of causes other than primary heart disease • Does not markedly affect cardiac output in most animals because the ventricular rate remains nearly normal

ECG Features
• Conduction disturbance in which tissues of the atrioventricular (AV) node conduct each successive impulse earlier and earlier in the refractory period. • Eventually, an impulse arrives during the absolute refractory period and is not conducted. The next impulse is conducted normally and the cycle begins again. Typically, the PR interval lengthens with each cycle until a P wave appears without a QRS complex (figure). • Rhythm is regularly irregular. • P waves and QRS are usually normal.

SIGNALMENT
• May be a normal finding in dogs because of increased vagal tone • Seen in older dogs (especailly cocker spaniels and dachshunds) and as a hereditary defect in pugs • Uncommon in cats

SIGNS

Historical Findings
• Most animals are asymptomatic. • Hypotension and syncope can occur if ventricular rate is slow.

Physical Examination Findings
First heart sound may become progressively softer with intermittent pauses.

CAUSES AND RISK FACTORS
• Vagal stimulation • Electrolyte imbalance • Digitalis toxicity • Quinidine or procainamide administration • Xylazine as anesthetic

 DIAGNOSIS

DIFFERENTIAL DIAGNOSIS
• Physiologic AV block, sometimes seen in animals with atrial tachycardia or atrial flutter, should be differentiated from true AV block. This type of AV block is not caused by an abnormality of the conduction system but rather by a physiologic response to impulse overload from atrial excitation. • Type II AV block is not characterized by variation in PR interval of conducted beats.

CBC/BIOCHEMISTRY/URINALYSIS
Electrolyte abnormalities in some animals

OTHER LABORATORY TESTS
Serum digoxin concentration may be high.

IMAGING N/A

OTHER DIAGNOSTIC PROCEDURES
N/A

 TREATMENT

• Usually not necessary
• Correct any underlying electrolyte imbalances.
• If drug induced, discontinue medications
• If wide QRS complexes coexist with second degree AV block, treatment may be necessary. These animals often have tendency to develop third degree AV block and accompanying signs.

 MEDICATIONS

DRUGS AND FLUIDS
• No treatment is necessary for most patients.
• Correct electrolyte imbalance, if present.

• Atropine and a temporary pacemaker may be used if the patient is symptomatic.

CONTRAINDICATIONS/POSSIBLE INTERACTIONS
Avoid drugs that may further enhance the conduction disturbance (e.g., phenothiazines, calcium channel blockers, and beta blockers).

 FOLLOW-UP

Although this type of block is generally transient, it is prudent to monitor the patient with serial ECG for possible progression to a higher degree of block.

 MISCELLANEOUS

SEE ALSO
Atrioventricular Block, Second Degree, Mobitz Type II

ABBREVIATION
AV = atrioventricular

Reference
Tilley LP. Essentials of canine and feline electrocardiography. 3rd ed. Baltimore: Williams & Wilkins, 1992.
Author Deborah J. Hadlock
Consulting Editors Larry P. Tilley and Francis W. K. Smith, Jr.

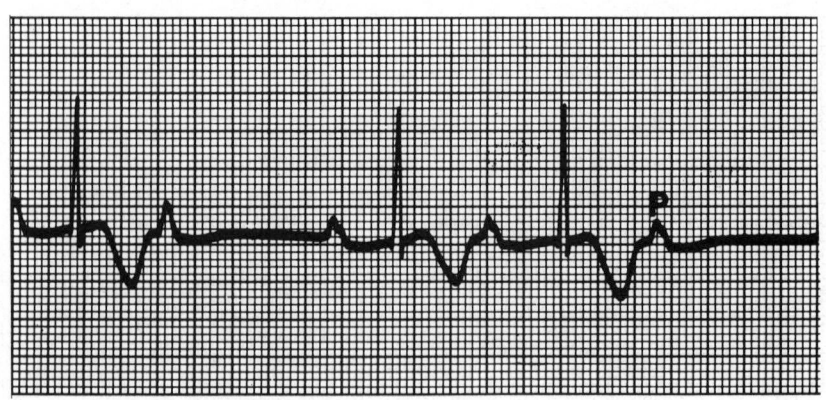

Typical Wenckebach phenomenon (Mobitz Type I). The longest PR interval preceded the nonconducted P waves. (From Tilley LP. Essentials of canine and feline electrocardiography, 3rd ed. Baltimore: Williams & Wilkins, 1992, with permission.)

ATRIOVENTRICULAR BLOCK, SECOND DEGREE, MOBITZ TYPE II

BASICS

OVERVIEW
• Type II, second degree atrioventricular (AV) block almost never occurs in a patient with a healthy heart. • More serious than type I second degree AV block (Wenckebach) because frequency and severity of the block is unpredictable. Frequently, this block progresses to third degree AV block, especially if associated with wide QRS complexes (block below bifurcation of the His bundle).

ECG Features
• Block in conduction at the level of the AV node. A conduction abnormality in the bundle of His or the bundle branches may also occur. • P-R intervals do not vary preceding a blocked beat. • A fixed relationship between the atria and ventricles may occur (i.e., 2:1, 3:1, 4:1 AV block) (Figure). • Advanced second degree AV block occurs when two or more consecutive P waves are blocked. • QRS complexes are often abnormal, an indication that the conduction defect involves the bundle branches. • Second degree AV block may be further categorized into type A and type B block on the basis of the width of QRS complexes. • Type A block involves conduction failure above the bifurcation of the His bundle; QRS duration is normal. • Type B block occurs below the bifurcation with a wide QRS complex; it indicates more serious and extensive cardiac disease.

SIGNALMENT
• Older dogs, especially cocker spaniels and dachshunds, because of fibrosis • In pugs caused by hereditary stenosis of the bundle of His • Cats with hypertrophic cardiomyopathy • Animals with infiltrative cardiomyopathy caused by neoplasia • Cats with hyperthyroid heart disease

SIGNS

Historical Findings
• May be asymptomatic • If overall ventricular rate is slow, signs of low cardiac output may be present (e.g., fainting and weakness). • If digoxin toxicity is the cause; vomiting, diarrhea, and anorexia may be seen.

Physical Examination Findings
• May be normal • Hypotension • Bradycardia • In cats, signs of congestive heart failure (CHF) may be present if block is associated with hypertrophic cardiomyopathy (HCM) or hyperthyroidism.

CAUSES AND RISK FACTORS
• Microscopic idiopathic fibrosis in older dogs • Myocarditis, including Lyme disease • Cardiomyopathy, especially HCM in cats • Drug administration, including digoxin, propranolol, diltiazem, and lidocaine • Hyperthyroidism (cats) • Cardiac neoplasia

DIAGNOSIS

DIFFERENTIAL DIAGNOSIS
• Physiologic AV block, sometimes seen in animals with atrial tachycardia or atrial flutter, should be differentiated from AV block secondary to AV node disease. This type of AV block is not caused by an abnormality of the conduction system but rather a physiologic response to impulse overload from atrial excitation. • Advanced, second degree AV block (consistent blocking of two or more consecutive P waves) should be differentiated from complete AV block, in which no impulses are conducted through the AV node.

CBC/BIOCHEMISTRY/URINALYSIS
Serum electrolyte abnormalities may be present, especially hyperkalemia.

OTHER LABORATORY TESTS
• High T4 (cats) if condition is secondary to hyperthyroidism • High serum digoxin concentration if condition caused by digoxin toxicity

IMAGING
Echocardiography may indicate structural heart disease.

OTHER DIAGNOSTIC PROCEDURES
N/A

TREATMENT
• Intervention dependent on clinical signs; treatment may be required
• If animal is symptomatic, long-term management may require pacemaker insertion.

MEDICATIONS

DRUGS AND FLUIDS
• Correct electrolyte abnormalities if present.
• Discontinue digoxin or other drugs that depress AV conduction.
• Atropine (0.01-0.04 mg/kg IV, IM) or glycopyrrolate (0.005-0.01 mg/kg IV, IM) can be given for short-term treatment of bradycardia.
• Isoproterenol (0.04-0.09 microgram/kg/min IV, titrate to effect) or dopamine (2-5 microgram/kg/min of Intropin) can be given in an emergency attempt to stimulate AV node conduction and enhance the ventricular escape rhythm. Dopamine is preferable because it prevents arterial vasodilation.

CONTRAINDICATIONS/POSSIBLE INTERACTIONS
Avoid drugs (e.g., digitalis, procainamide, lidocaine, propranolol, and phenothiazines) that may further suppress impulse conduction or depress ventricular escape focus.

FOLLOW-UP
• Monitor with serial ECG to detect progression to higher degree of AV block • Some patients with chronic heart disease may develop this type of AV block without signs. No treatment is required as long as they remain stable, particularly in older dogs with idiopathic fibrosis. • Most cats progress to more advanced forms of AV block. Without pacemaker implantation, prognosis is poor; most affect cats are resistant to medical management.

MISCELLANEOUS

SEE ALSO
Atrioventricular Block, Second Degree, Mobitz Type I

ABBREVIATIONS
AV = atrioventricular
CHF = congestive heart failure
HCM = hypertrophic cardiomyopathy

Reference
Tilley LP. Essentials of canine and feline electrocardiography. 3rd ed. Baltmore: Williams & Wilkins, 1992.

Author Deborah J. Hadlock

Consulting Editors Larry P. Tilley and Francis W. K. Smith, Jr.

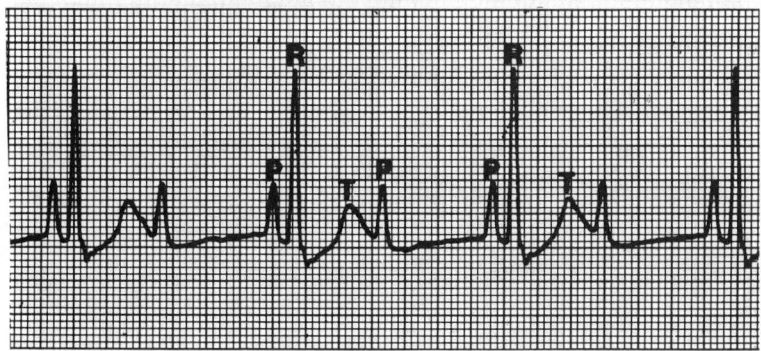

Second-degree 2:1 AV block (Mobitz type II) and possible right atrial enlargement. (From Tilley LP. Essentials of canine and feline electrocardiography, 3rd ed. Baltimore: Williams & Wilkins, 1992, with permission.)

ATRIOVENTRICULAR DISSOCIATION

BASICS

OVERVIEW

• Separate atrial and ventricular pacemakers that are independent of each other. • Possible causes are complete pathologic interruption of conduction between the atria and ventricles (complete atrioventricular [AV] block), temporary physiologic interruption, and variable AV conduction refractoriness. • Mechanisms include depressed sinus node automatically with an AV junctional or ventricular pacemaker controlling the ventricular rhythm; enhanced AV junctional or ventricular automatically (an ectopic focus controls the ventricles while the sinus node controls the atria); disturbed AV conduction with AV junctional or ventricular pacemaker controlling the ventricles and sinus node controlling the atria.

ECG Features

• The sinus P waves have no constant relationship to the QRS complexes (figure).
• The P waves may precede the QRS complex, be in the middle of it, or follow it without changing their usually normal form.
• The P wave rate is usually slower than the QRS complex rate.

SIGNALMENT

The clinician should remember that AV dissociation is never a primary disturbance of rhythm but rather the result of a basic abnormality of impulse formation or conduction.

SIGNS

Historical Findings

• No signs • Congestive heart failure • Exercise intolerance • Syncope

Physical Examination Findings

• Jugular venous pulsations • Regular or irregular rhythm • Gallop rhythm • Signs of congestive heart failure

CAUSES AND RISK FACTORS

• Digoxin toxicity • Myocarditis • Cardiomyopathy • Chronic valvular insufficiency • Congenital heart disease • Halothane anesthesia in cats

DIAGNOSIS

DIFFERENTIAL DIAGNOSIS

• Atrial or ventricular premature complexes • Ventricular tachycardia • Complete AV block

CBC/BIOCHEMISTRY/URINALYSIS
N/A

OTHER LABORATORY TESTS   N/A

IMAGING

Echocardiography may reveal the type and severity of heart disease.

OTHER DIAGNOSTIC PROCEDURES
N/A

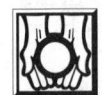

TREATMENT

• Treat as an inpatient or outpatient, based on severity of clinical signs.
• Treat the underlying congestive heart failure or other causes.

MEDICATIONS

DRUGS AND FLUIDS

• Correct electrolyte and acid/base disturbances.
• Treat the underlying cardiac disease with appropriate medication.
• See treatment sections for complete AV block and ventricular tachycardia.

CONTRAINDICATIONS/POSSIBLE INTERACTIONS   N/A

FOLLOW-UP

Monitor the heart rate and rhythm with serial ECG.

MISCELLANEOUS

SEE ALSO

• Idioventricular Rhythm • Atrioventricular Block, Complete • Ventricular Tachycardia

ABBREVIATION

AV = atrioventricular

Reference

Tilley LP. Essentials of canine and feline electrocardiography. 3rd ed. Baltimore: Williams & Wilkins, 1992.

Author Michael S. Miller

Consulting Editors Larry P. Tilley and Francis W. K. Smith, Jr.

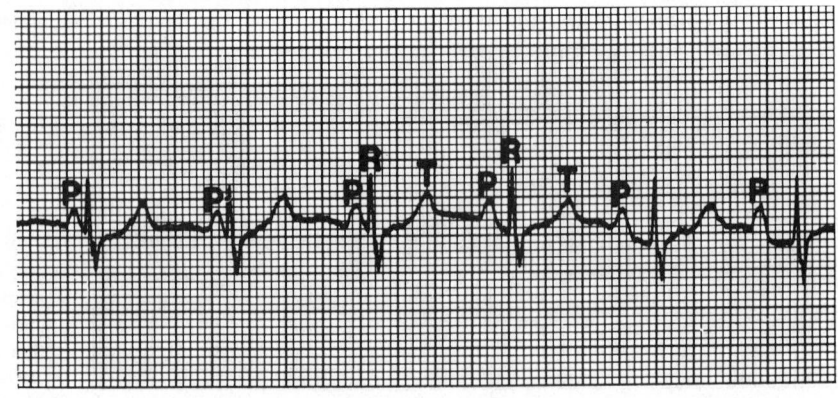

Atrioventricular dissociation bewteen the SA node and the AV junction, probably from an accelerated AV junctional focus. The P waves travel away from and then toward and finally merge with the QRS complexes. This dog had severe digitalis intoxication. (From Tilley LP. Essentials of canine and feline electrocardiography, 3rd ed. Baltimore: Williams & Wilkins, 1992, with permission.)

IDIOVENTRICULAR RHYTHM

BASICS

OVERVIEW
If conduction of sinus node pacemaker impulses to the ventricles are blocked or the impulses decrease in frequency, the lower regions of the heart will automatically take over the role of pacemaker for the ventricles, which results in ventricular escape complexes or an idioventricular rhythm.

ECG Features
• Heart rate < 65 bpm in dogs and less that 100 bpm in cats • P waves may be absent or, if present, may precede, be hidden within, or follow the ectopic QRS complex. P waves are unrelated to the QRS complexes (figure).
• QRS configuration is wide and bizarre, similar to that of a ventricular premature complex.

SIGNALMENT
• Dogs and cats • Atrial standstill in English springer spaniels and Siamese cats • Pugs, miniature schnauzers, and dalmatians prone to conduction abnormalities

SIGNS

Historical Findings
• Some animals asymptomatic • Weakness • Lethargy • Exercise intolerance • Syncope • Heart failure

Physical Examination Findings
• Irregular rhythm associated with pulse deficits • Variation in heart sounds • Possible intermittent "cannon" waves in the jugular venous pulses (with atrioventricular [AV] block)

CAUSES AND RISK FACTORS
An idioventricular rhythm is not a primary disease, but a secondary result of a primary disease. The escape rhythm is a safety mechanism to maintain cardiac output.

Causes of Sinus Bradycardia and Sinus Arrest
• Increased vagal tone (high intracranial pressure, high ocular pressure) • Drugs—digoxin, tranquilizers, propranolol, quinidine, and anesthetics • Addison's disease • Hypoglycemia • Renal failure • Hypothermia • Hyperkalemia • Hypothyroidism

Causes of AV block
• Congenital cause • Neoplasia • Fibrosis • Lyme disease

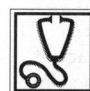

DIAGNOSIS

DIFFERENTIAL DIAGNOSIS
• Ventricular tachycardia—animals with this cardiac rhythm have a cardiac rate > 100 bpm (dogs) and > 150 bpm (cats) • Slow heart rate in animals with right bundle branch block, left bundle branch block, or left anterior fascicular block. In animals with these disturbances, the P waves are associated with the QRS complexes.

CBC/BIOCHEMISTRY/URINALYSIS
• No specific findings • Complete blood testing may suggest a metabolic abnormality

OTHER LABORATORY TESTS
• Test for drug toxicity • Lyme's titer in animals with complete AV block

IMAGING
Echocardiography may show structural heart disease

OTHER DIAGNOSTIC PROCEDURES
N/A

TREATMENT
• An idioventricular rhythm is an escape or safety mechanism for maintaining cardiac output. Treatment is *not* directed toward suppressing this escape rhythm, but toward the primary disease process that allows the escape rhythm to take over pacemaker control of the heart.
• Symptomatic treatment is directed toward increasing the heart rate.

MEDICATIONS

DRUGS AND FLUIDS
• In most animals, atropine or glycopyrrolate is indicated to block vagal tone or increase the heart rate.
• If those drugs are ineffective, isoproterenol, dopamine, dobutamine, or artificial pacing may be needed.

CONTRAINDICATIONS/POSSIBLE INTERACTIONS
Lidocaine, procainamide, quinidine, propranolol, diltiazem, or any other drug that would slow the cardiac rate or reduce contractility

FOLLOW-UP
• Serial ECG may show clearing of the lesion or progression to complete heart block.
• Serial blood profiles may be needed to monitor progress of the primary disease process. • Serial echocardiograms may show improvement or progressive changes in cardiac structure. • Prognosis is guarded if the condition is associated with cardiac or metabolic disorder.

MISCELLANEOUS

SEE ALSO
• Atrioventricular Dissociation • Atrial Standstill • Atrioventricular Block, Complete

ABBREVIATION
AV = atrioventricular

Reference
Tilley LP. Essentials of canine and feline electrocardiography. 3rd ed. Baltimore: Williams & Wilkins, 1992.
Author Craig E. McInnis and Larry P. Tilley
Consulting Editors Larry P. Tilley and Francis W. K. Smith, Jr.

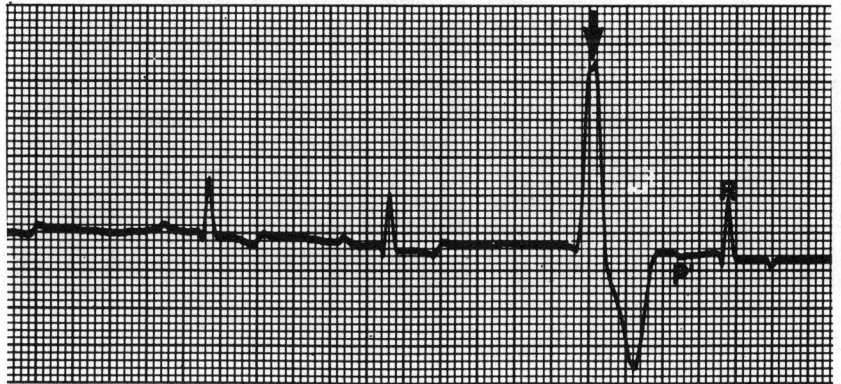

Ventricular escape complexes (arrow) during various phases in the dominant sinus rhythm in a dog during anesthesia. The sinus rate increased (not shown) after the anesthesia was stopped. (From Tilley LP. Essentials of canine and feline electrocardiography, 3rd ed. Baltimore: Williams & Wilkins, 1992, with permission.)

LEFT ANTERIOR FASCICULAR BLOCK

BASICS

OVERVIEW
• Conduction delay or block in the anterior fascicle of the left bundle branch • Activation of the left ventricle is then altered or delayed toward the blocked fascicle and corresponding papillary muscle.

ECG features
• The QRS complex is of normal duration. • A left axis deviation is present (dogs, <+40°; cats, <0°). • Small q waves and tall R waves in leads I and aVL (small q not essential). • Deep S waves (exceeding the R waves) in leads II, III, and aVF.

SIGNALMENT
• Most commonly described form of bundle branch block in cats • Uncommon in dogs

SIGNS

Historical Findings
• Usually an incidental ECG finding • Does not cause hemodynamic abnormalities • Any observed signs are usually associated with the underlying cause.

Physical Examination Findings
No associated signs or hemodynamic compromise

CAUSES AND RISK FACTORS
• Hypertrophic cardiomyopathy (cats) • Causes of left ventricular hypertrophy (e.g., mitral insufficiency, aortic stenosis, aortic body tumor, hypertension, and hyperthyroidism) • Causes of hyperkalemia (e.g., urethral obstruction, acute renal insufficiency, and Addison's disease) • Ischemic cardiomyopathy (e.g., arteriosclerosis of the coronary arteries, myocardial infarction, and myocardial hypertrophy that obstructs coronary arteries) • Surgical repair of a cardiac defect (e.g., repair of ventricular septal defect caused by aortic valvular disease) • Restrictive cardiomyopathy (cats) • Fibrosis

DIAGNOSIS

DIFFERENTIAL DIAGNOSIS
• Left ventricular enlargement. Absence of left ventricular enlargement on thoracic radiograph or cardiac ultrasound lends support to a diagnosis of left anterior fascicular block. • Right bundle branch block—deep and wide S-waves in leads I, II, III and aVF causing a right axis deviation. In animals with left anterior fascicular block, leads I and aVL are positive, whereas leads II, III, and aVF have deep S waves resulting in a left axis deviation. • Altered position of the heart within the thorax; thoracic radiographs will help identify mass or foreign body that may be displacing the heart. • Hyperkalemia should be suspected in an animal with signs of uretheral obstruction, renal insufficiency, or Addison's disease. Serum potassium concentration should be determined. • Ventricular pre-excitation—on ECG, a delta wave is usually present and the PR interval is short.

CBC/BIOCHEMISTRY/URINALYSIS
Hyperkalemia possible

OTHER LABORATORY TESTS N/A

IMAGING
• Echocardiogram may show structural heart disease. • Thoracic and abdominal radiographs may show mass, pulmonary metastatic lesion, foreign body, or abnormal cardiac position.

OTHER DIAGNOSTIC PROCEDURES
Long-term ambulatory monitoring (Holter) may reveal intermittent bundle branch block.

TREATMENT
Insertion of pacemaker may become necessary to correct progressive conduction disturbances and accompanying clinical signs.

MEDICATIONS

DRUGS AND FLUIDS
Treatment directed toward the underlying cause

CONTRAINDICATIONS/POSSIBLE INTERACTIONS N/A

FOLLOW-UP
The causative lesion could progress leading to a more serious arrhythmia or complete heart block. ECG should be done regularly.

MISCELLANEOUS

ABBREVIATIONS None

Reference
Tilley LP. Essentials of canine and feline electrocardiography. 3rd ed. Baltimore: Williams & Wilkins, 1992

Authors Larry P. Tilley and Craig E. McInnis
Consulting Editors Larry P. Tilley and Francis W.K. Smith, Jr.

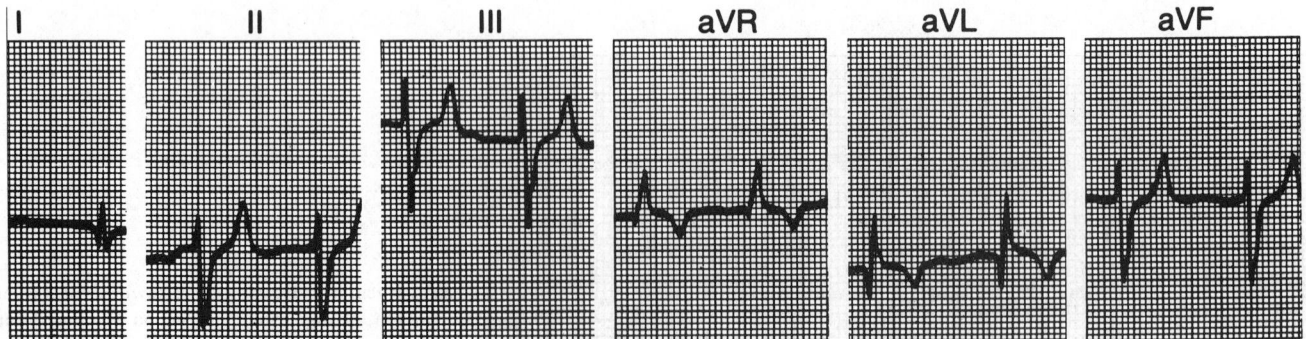

Left anterior fascicular block with right bundle branch block in a cat with hypertrophic cardiomyopathy. Atrial fibrillation is also present, explaining the lack of P waves. (From Tilley LP. Essentials of canine and feline electrocardiography, 3rd ed. Baltimore: Williams & Wilkins, 1992, with permission.)

LEFT BUNDLE BRANCH BLOCK

BASICS

OVERVIEW

Conduction delay or block in both the left posterior and left anterior fascicles of the left bundle. A supraventricular impulse activates the right ventricle first through the right bundle branch. The left ventricle is then activated late, causing the QRS to become wide and bizarre.

ECG Features

• The QRS is prolonged (> 0.08 sec in dogs, > 0.06 sec in cats). • The QRS is wide and positive in leads I, II, III, and aVF. • Because the left bundle branch is thick and extensive, the lesion is required to be large. • The lesion causing the block could progress, leading to more serious arrhythmias or complete heart block. • The block can be intermittent or constant.

SIGNALMENT

Uncommon in cats and dogs

SIGNS

Historical Findings

• Usually an incidental ECG finding—does not cause hemodynamic abnormalities
• Observed signs are usually associated with the underlying condition.

Physical Examination Findings

• Does not cause signs or hemodynamic compromise

CAUSES AND RISK FACTORS

• Direct or indirect cardiac trauma (e.g., hit by car and cardiac needle puncture). • Neo-plasia • Congenital defect • Fibrosis • Cardiomyopathy • Ischemic cardiomyopathy (e.g., arteriosclerosis of the coronary arteries, myocardial infarction, and myocardial hypertrophy which obstructs coronary arteries)

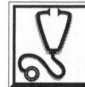

DIAGNOSIS

DIFFERENTIAL DIAGNOSIS

• Left ventricular enlargement • Absence of left ventricular enlargement on thoracic radiograph or cardiac ultrasound studies lends support to diagnosis of isolated left bundle branch block • It can also be confused with ventricular ectopic beats, but the PR interval is usually constant and there are no pulse deficits with left bundle branch block.

CBC/BIOCHEMISTRY/URINALYSIS

N/A

OTHER LABORATORY TESTS N/A

IMAGING

• Echocardiography may reveal structural heart disease. Absence of left heart enlargement lends support to a diagnosis of left bundle branch block. • Thoracic and abdominal radiographs may show masses or pulmonary metastatic lesions. • Traumatic injuries could result in localized or diffuse pulmonary densities.

OTHER DIAGNOSTIC PROCEDURES

Long-term ambulatory (Holter) monitoring may reveal intermittent left bundle branch block.

TREATMENT

Treatment is directed toward the underlying cause.

MEDICATIONS

DRUGS AND FLUIDS N/A

CONTRAINDICATIONS/POSSIBLE INTERACTIONS N/A

FOLLOW-UP

• Serial ECG may show clearing or progression to complete heart block. • Presence of first- or second-degree AV block may indicate involvement of the right bundle branch.

MISCELLANEOUS

ABBREVIATIONS None

Reference

Tilley, L P. Essentials of canine and feline electrocardiography. 3rd ed. Baltimore: Williams & Wilkins 1992.

Authors Larry P. Tilley and Craig E. McInnis

Consulting Editors Larry P. Tilley and Francis W.K. Smith, Jr.

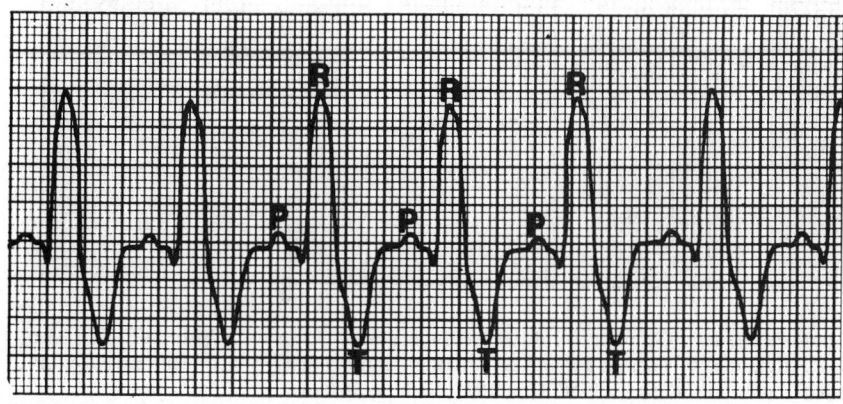

Left bundle branch block and a sinus rhythm. Heart rate is 175 beats/min. (From Tilley LP. Essentials of canine and feline electrocardiography, 3rd ed. Baltimore: Williams & Wilkins, 1992, with permission.)

RIGHT BUNDLE BRANCH BLOCK

BASICS

OVERVIEW
Conduction delay or block in the right bundle branch resulting in late activation of the right ventricle. The block can be complete or incomplete.

ECG FEATURES
• A right axis deviation and wide QRS (≥ 0.08 sec in dogs; ≥ 0.06 in cats) in most animals
• Large, wide, S-waves in leads I, II, III, and aVF

SIGNALMENT
• Occasionally seen in normal and healthy dogs and cats • In beagles, incomplete right bundle branch block can be a genetically determined localized variation in right ventricular wall thickness.

SIGNS

Historical Findings
• Usually an incidental ECG finding • Does not cause hemodynamic abnormalities • Any signs are usually associated with the underlying condition.

Physical Examination Findings
• Splitting of heart sounds because of asynchronous activation of ventricles in some animals • Does not cause signs or hemodynamic compromise

Causes and Risk Factors
• Occasionally seen in normal and healthy dogs and cats • Congenital heart disease
• Chronic valvular fibrosis • After surgical correction of a cardiac defect • Trauma caused by cardiac needle puncture to obtain blood sample. • Trauma from other causes
• Chronic infection with Trypanosoma cruzi (Chagas' disease) • Neoplasia • Heartworm disease • Acute thromboembolism • Cardiomyopathy • Hyperkalemia (most commonly in cats with urethral obstruction)

DIAGNOSIS

DIFFERENTIAL DIAGNOSIS
• Right ventricular enlargement. Absence of right ventricular enlargement on thoracic radiographs or cardiac ultrasonogram lends support to a diagnosis of right bundle branch block. • It can also be confused with ventricular ectopic beats (especially if the block is intermittent), but the PR intervals would be consistent and there would be no pulse deficits with right bundle branch block.

CBC/BIOCHEMISTRY/URINALYSIS
• None specifically for right bundle branch block • Serum potassium may be extremely high in cats with urethral obstruction.

OTHER LABORATORY TESTS
• Occult heartworm test may be positive in dogs or cats • Chagas indirect fluorescent antibody test, direct hemagglutination, and complement fixation test may be positive in dogs.

IMAGING
• Echocardiogram may show structural heart disease. Absence of right heart enlargement lends support to a diagnosis of right bundle branch block. • Thoracic and abdominal radiographs may show masses or pulmonary metastatic lesions. Traumatic injuries could cause localized or diffuse pulmonary densities.

OTHER DIAGNOSTIC PROCEDURES
N/A

TREATMENT
Directed toward the underlying cause

MEDICATIONS

DRUGS AND FLUIDS   N/A

CONTRAINDICATIONS/POSSIBLE INTERACTIONS   N/A

FOLLOW-UP
• The lesion causing the block could progress, leading to a more serious arrhythmia or complete heart block. • Serial ECG may show clearing of the lesion or progression to complete heart block.

MISCELLANEOUS

References
Tilley LP. Essentials of canine and feline electrocardiography. 3rd ed. Baltimore, Williams & Wilkins, 1992.
Authors Larry P. Tilley and Craig E. McInnis
Consulting Editors Larry P. Tilley and Francis W.K. Smith, Jr.

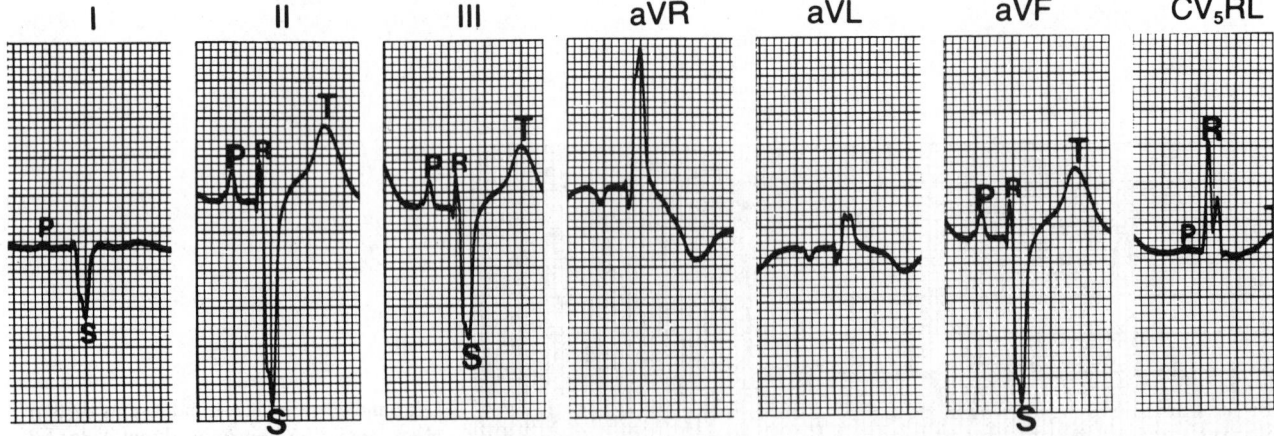

Right bundle branch block. The electrocardiographic features include QRS duration of 0.08 seconds; positive QRS complex in aVR, aVL, and CV₅RL (M shaped); and large wide S waves in leads I, II, III, and aVF. There is a right axis deviation (approximately – 110°). (From Tilley LP. Essentials of canine and feline electrocardiography, 3rd ed. Baltimore: Williams & Wilkins, 1992, with permission.)

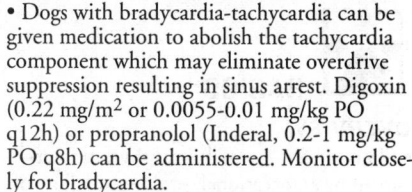

SICK SINUS SYNDROME

BASICS

OVERVIEW
• Clinical manifestations vary. • Episodic weakness, syncope, and Stokes-Adams seizures are common findings because of reduced cardiac output with resultant hypoperfusion and hypotension. • Sudden death is uncommon.

ECG FEATURES
• Cardiac rhythm disturbance that may include one or more of the following: sinus bradycardia (Figure), alternating bradycardia-tachycardia rhythm, sinus arrest, sinoatrial block, supraventricular tachycardias, transient asystole, supraventricular premature complexes, and, in many animals, atrioventricular nodal and intraventricular conduction disturbances. • The heart rate is rapid or slow with possible long pauses. • P waves and QRS complexes usually normal

SIGNALMENT
• Miniature schnauzers (especially female) genetically predisposed • Common in pugs, dachshunds, cocker spaniels • Most patients elderly but spares no age group • Not reported in cats

SIGNS
Historical Findings
• Lethargy • Weakness • Episodic ataxia • Syncope • Stokes-Adams seizures • Clinical manifestations range from none to infrequent to frequent occurrence of clinical signs

Physical Examination Findings
• Periods of bradycardia or tachycardia • Long pauses (of sinus arrest or block) auscultated in some animals • May be normal

CAUSES AND RISK FACTORS
• Idiopathic • Genetic inheritance, especially in female miniature schnauzers • Metastatic disease • Cardiomyopathy characterized by fibrous tissue replacing sinoatrial node tissue • Ischemic heart disease

DIAGNOSIS

DIFFERENTIAL DIAGNOSIS
• Asymptomatic bradycardia secondary to causes other than sick sinus syndrome • If syncope is present, differentiate from seizure disorder secondary to metabolic or neurologic disease

CBC/BIOCHEMISTRY/URINALYSIS
N/A

OTHER LABORATORY TESTS N/A

IMAGING N/A

OTHER DIAGNOSTIC PROCEDURES
• Atropine response test in dogs with sinus bradycardia or arrest. Administer atropine (0.04 mg/kg IM) and evaluate by ECG 30 minutes later. Animals with sick sinus syndrome generally show depressed response to atropine. • Electrophysiologic testing to evaluate sinus node function. • 24-hour Holter monitoring or event recorder to correlate signs with ECG • No definitive tests confirm sick sinus syndrome. Diagnosis is often elusive, especially if patient is asymptomatic or clinical signs occur infrequently • Atrial pacing can be used to demonstrate sinus node recovery time—a prolonged time supports sick sinus syndrome, but a normal time does not exclude it.

TREATMENT
• Treatment unnecessary in asymptomatic patients
• Symptomatic dogs can be subdivided into those that show primarily bradycardia or sinus arrest and those that have supraventricular tachycardia followed by sinus arrest.
• Clinical response to medical treatment often inconsistent
• Permanent artificial pacemaker insertion used to treat patients that fail to respond to medical treatment or who cannot tolerate side effects of anticholinergics
• Pacemaker also indicated in animal in which treatment of tachyarrhythmia t may aggravate bradyarrhythmia, or vice versa

MEDICATIONS

DRUGS AND FLUIDS
• Symptomatic dogs with bradycardia or sinus arrest that are atropine responsive are treated with anticholinergic drugs (propantheline [Probanthine]—small dogs, 3.75-7.5 mg PO q8h-q12h; medium dogs, 15 mg PO q8h; large dogs, 30 mg PO q8h)

• Dogs with bradycardia-tachycardia can be given medication to abolish the tachycardia component which may eliminate overdrive suppression resulting in sinus arrest. Digoxin (0.22 mg/m^2 or 0.0055-0.01 mg/kg PO q12h) or propranolol (Inderal, 0.2-1 mg/kg PO q8h) can be administered. Monitor closely for bradycardia.
• Long-acting forms of theophylline (Theo-Dur, 20 mg/kg PO q12h) in dogs with bradycardia and sinus arrest.

CONTRAINDICATIONS/POSSIBLE INTERACTIONS
• Caution should be taken when treating bradycardia-tachycardia syndrome. The drug treatment for supraventricular tachycardia may worsen the bradycardia/sinus arrest and vice versa. These patients generally require an artificial pacemaker.
• Side effects with anticholinergic drugs are common and include constipation, dry mucous membranes, emesis, and keratoconjunctivitis sicca.

FOLLOW-UP
• If patient is asymptomatic, monitor with serial ECG for progression • Owner should watch for development of clinical signs including lethargy, weakness, and syncope. • If patient is treated medically or by insertion of pacemaker, monitor routinely by ECG. • In animals that have pacemaker inserted and no signs of CHF, prognosis is good. • Prognosis varies in animals treated medically; clinical response is often inconsistent and the disease may progress.

MISCELLANEOUS

SEE ALSO
• Sinus Arrest or Block • Atrial Tachycardia • Sinus Bradycardia

ABBREVIATIONS None

Reference
Tilley LP. Essentials of canine and feline electrocardiography. 3rd ed. Baltimore: Williams & Wilkins, 1992.
Author Deborah J. Hadlock
Consulting Editors Larry P. Tilley and Francis W. K. Smith, Jr.

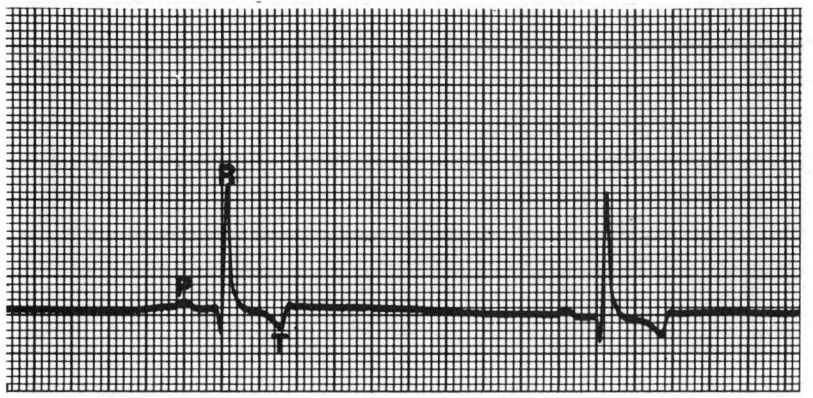

Sinus bradycardia (approx. 60 beats/min) in a miniature schnauzer with fainting. Peper speed = 50 mm/sec. (From Tilley LP. Essentials of canine and feline electrocardiography, 3rd ed. Baltimore: Williams & Wilkins, 1992, with permission.)

SINUS ARREST OR BLOCK

BASICS

OVERVIEW
• Sinus arrest—normal sinus rhythm interrupted by an occasional, prolonged failure of the sinoatrial node to initiate an impulse. • Sinus block—conduction disturbance in which normal sinus rhythm is interrupted by an occasional, prolonged failure of the impulse generated by the sinoatrial node to reach the atria. • With prolonged pauses, periods of low cardiac output may occur.

ECG Features
• Heart rate varies and is often correlated with bradycardia. • Rhythm is regularly irregular or irregular with pauses. • Normal P wave for each QRS complex • Pauses — two times the normal R-R interval

SIGNALMENT
• Normal incidental finding in brachycephalic breeds of dog • Seen in dog breeds predisposed to sick sinus syndrome (e.g., miniature schnauzers, dachshunds, and cocker spaniels). • Seen in purebred pugs with hereditary stenosis of the bundle of His. • Reported in dalmatian coach hounds that are born deaf. • Uncommon in cats.

SIGNS

Historical Findings
• Usually no signs • Signs of low cardiac output (e.g., weakness and syncope)

Physical Examination Findings
• May be normal • Extremely slow heart rate if arrest or block is prolonged or frequent • Signs of poor cardiac output if condition is serious

CAUSE AND RISK FACTORS
• Vagal stimulation • Coughing • Pharyngeal irritation • Carotid sinus massage • Degenerative heart disease • Sick sinus syndrome • Irritation of vagus nerve secondary to thoracic or cervical neoplasia • Neoplastic heart disease, e.g., hemangiosarcoma • Electrolyte imbalance • Drug toxicity (e.g., digitalis, quinidine, and propranolol)

DIAGNOSIS

DIFFERENTIAL DIAGNOSIS
To distinguish sinus arrest from sinus block—sinus block is suggested by pauses that are double the duration of the dominant beat interval.

CBC/BIOCHEMISTRY/URINALYSIS
Serum electrolyte abnormalities in some animals

OTHER LABORATORY TESTS N/A

IMAGING
Thoracic radiographs should be taken if neoplastic or cardiac cause is suspected. Cardiac ultrasound should be done if structural heart disease or neoplasia is suspected.

OTHER DIAGNOSTIC PROCEDURES
• Provocative atropine test to assess sinus node function. Administer 0.04 mg/kg atropine IM; assess ECG lead-II rhythm strip 30 minutes later. • Holter monitoring may reveal prolonged periods of a failure of impulses from the sinoatrial node if signs of weakness or syncope present

TREATMENT
• None if animal is asymptomatic
• Treat underlying cause
• An artificial demand pacemaker can be considered in animals unresponsive to treatment.

MEDICATIONS

DRUGS AND FLUIDS
• Discontinue any causative drugs.
• Correct any electrolyte abnormalities.

• If animal is symptomatic, consider atropine (0.02 mg/kg IV, 0.04 mg/kg IM), glycopyrrolate (0.005-0.01 mg/kg IV, IM), or isoproterenol (0.04-0.09 ug/kg/minute IV, titrate to effect, or 0.1-0.2 mg q 4-6 hour IM, SQ). • Congestive heart failure may develop, in which case diuretics and vasodilators must be considered.

CONTRAINDICATIONS/POSSIBLE INTERACTIONS
Avoid drugs that may further depress sinoatrial node function (e.g., digitalis, beta blockers, calcium channel blockers, and quinidine)

FOLLOW-UP
• Monitor with serial ECG for progression to more serious dysrhythmia • If condition is associated with primary cardiac disease or neoplasia, long-term prognosis is poor. • If cause is sick sinus syndrome, symptomatic animal may respond well to medical intervention. If poorly responsive, permanent pacemaker would improve prognosis markedly.

MISCELLANEOUS

SEE ALSO Sick Sinus Syndrome

Reference

Tilley LP. Essentials of canine and feline electrocardiography. 3rd ed. Baltimore: Williams & Wilkins 1992.
Author Deborah J. Hadlock
Consulting Editors Larry P. Tilley and Francis W.K. Smith, Jr.

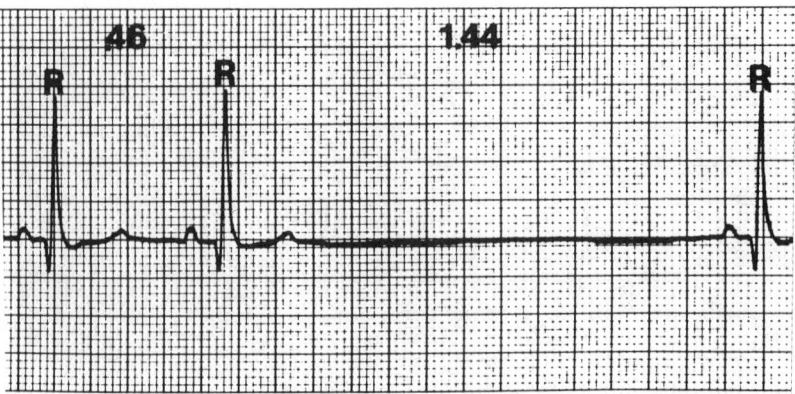

Intermittent sinus arrest in a brachycephalic breed with an upper respiratory disorder and episodes of fainting. The pauses (1 and 1.44 sec) are greater than twice the normal R-R interval (0.46). (From Tilley LP. Essentials of canine and feline electrocardiography, 3rd ed. Baltimore: Williams & Wilkins, 1992, with permission.)

SINUS ARRHYTHMIA

BASICS

OVERVIEW
• Normal variation in sinus rhythm related to respiratory rate and resulting from vagal tone inhibition • Heart rate increases with inspiration and decreases with expiration. • Not an abnormal rhythm • Can be nonrespiratory in origin with no relationship to the phases of respiration. • May be exacerbated by labored respiratory effort, i.e., respiratory disease or underlying conditions that increase vagal tone.

ECG Features
• P wave for every QRS • R-R internals vary in a regular pattern (respiratory sinus arrhythmia) or irregular pattern. • P-wave morphology may vary as P-P intervals vary (wandering pacemaker).

SIGNALMENT
• Normal finding in dogs • Common in brachycephalic breeds. • Uncommon and usually abnormal finding in cats

SIGNS

Historical Findings
• Usually none • Possibly, signs of the underlying cause if there is one

Physical Examination Findings
• None if arrythmia is physiologic • Irregular rhythm on auscultation • Signs of respiratory disease if present

CAUSES AND RISK FACTORS
• Chronic respiratory disease • Underlying conditions that increase vagal tone (e.g., digitalis toxicity, high intracranial pressure, gastrointestinal disease, and cerebral disorders)

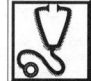

DIAGNOSIS

DIFFERENTIAL DIAGNOSIS
• Auscultation of sinus arrythmia is often confusing; ECG helpful in differentiating normal sinus arrythmia from true pathologic arrhythmia. • Wandering sinus pacemaker often associated with sinus arrythmia. Site of impulse formation shifts within the SA node or to an atrial focus or atrioventricular node, changing the configuration of the P-wave. • Important to differentiate this normal finding from other pathologic arrhythmias such as atrial premature complexes

CBC/BIOCHEMISTRY/URINALYSIS
N/A

OTHER LABORATORY TESTS
• Measure serum digoxin concentration if applicable—may be too high • Feline leukemia or feline immunodeficiency virus test in cats with chronic respiratory disease may be positive.

IMAGING N/A

OTHER DIAGNOSTIC PROCEDURES
N/A

TREATMENT
• No specific treatment required
• Underlying cause is treated if arrhythmia is not related to respiration.

MEDICATIONS

DRUGS AND FLUIDS
• Appropriate antibiotic management of respiratory infection
• Stop digoxin if toxicity a problem

CONTRAINDICATIONS/POSSIBLE INTERACTIONS N/A

FOLLOW-UP
None unless underlying problem is being treated

MISCELLANEOUS

References
Tilley LP. Essentials of canine and feline electrocardiography. 3rd ed. Baltimore: Williams & Wilkins, 1992.
Author Deborah J. Hadlock
Consulting Editor Larry P. Tilley and Francis W.K. Smith, Jr.

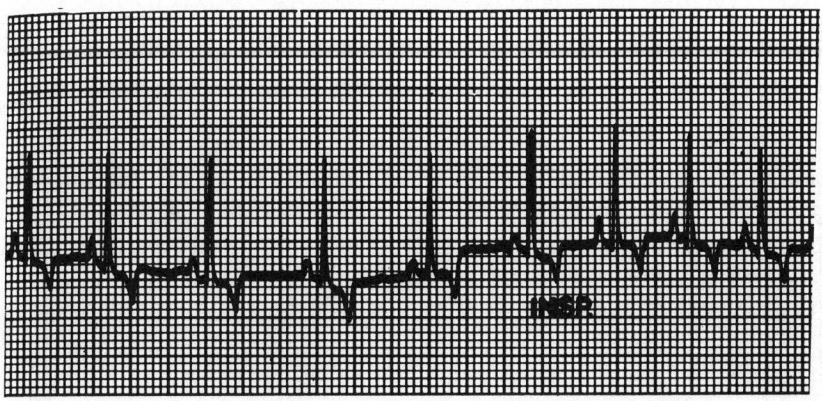

Sinus arrhythmia. Heart rate increases with inspiration (Insp.) secondary to decreased vagal tone. (From Tilley LP. Essentials of canine and feline electrocardiography, 3rd ed. Baltimore: Williams & Wilkins, 1992, with permission.)

SINUS BRADYCARDIA

BASICS

OVERVIEW
• Importance depends on cause. May be normal or serious depending upon signs and underlying cause. • Marked sinus bradycardia may severely impair cardiac output. • Caused by decreased sympathetic tone (e.g., beta-blocking agent) or enhanced cardiac parasympathetic tone (e.g., Valsalva maneuver).

ECG Features
• Sinus rhythm with impulses arising from the sinoatrial node where sinus rate is < 70 beats/minute in dogs (< 60 in giant breeds) and < 120 bpm in cats • Rhythm regular, with a slight variation in R-R interval. • Normal P wave for each QRS complex. • PR interval is constant.

SIGNALMENT
• Heart rates of 60-70 bpm often normal in large-breed dogs • In cats, often associated with serious underlying disorder which warrants attention and treatment.

SIGNS

Historical Findings
• May be none • Lethargy • Exercise intolerance • Syncope

Physical Examination Findings
• Pulse rate slow (dogs, < 60-70 bpm; cats, < 120 bpm) • Hypothermia may be present

CAUSES AND RISK FACTORS
• Physiologic secondary to increased vagal tone due to vomiting, intubation, hypothyroidism, hypothermia, good conditioning, or respiratory disease • High intracranial pressure • Hyperkalemia • May precede cardiac arrest • Hypothyroidism • Drugs including phenothiazines, beta-blockers, digitalis, quinidine, anesthetics, and calcium channel blockers

DIAGNOSIS

DIFFERENTIAL DIAGNOSIS N/A

CBC/BIOCHEMISTRY/URINALYSIS
• Hyperkalemia (serum K^+ > 5.7 to 6.0 mEq/l) predisposes to bradycardia • CBC and serum chemistry profile may reveal changes associated with metabolic disease such as renal failure

OTHER LABORATORY TESTS
Baseline T_3, T_4 values if hypothyroidism is suspected

IMAGING N/A

OTHER DIAGNOSTIC PROCEDURES
N/A

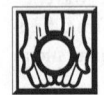

TREATMENT
• No treatment if patient is asymptomatic.
• Treat underlying cause.
• If patient has clinical signs and medical intervention is ineffective, increase heart rate with drugs or pacemaker.

MEDICATIONS

DRUGS AND FLUIDS
• Correct hyperkalemia if present.
• If patient is hypothyroid, supplement with thyroxine.
• If patient has acute signs of collapse, administer atropine (0.02 mg/kg IV) or glycopyrrolate (0.005 mg-0.01 mg/kg IV).
• If helpful, atropine (0.04 mg/kg IM, SQ q6h-q8h) or glycopyrrolate (0.01-0.02 mg/kg IM or SQ q6h-q8h) can be continued short term.
• Continuous IV infusion of isoproterenol (0.04-0.09 µg/kg/minute) or dobutamine (dogs, 2.5-10 µg/kg/minute; cats, 1-5 µg/kg/minute) can be considered as short-

term management if the patient is unresponsive to atropine.
• Pro-Banthine (small dogs, 7.5 mg PO q8h; medium dogs, 15 mg PO q8h; large dogs, 30 mg PO q8h; cats, 7.5 mg PO q8h to q24h) for long-term management
• Xanthine bronchodilators (theophylline) or terbutaline (dogs 0.2 mg/kg PO q8h-q12h; cats, 0.625 mg PO q12h) may help to speed up heart rate.

CONTRAINDICATIONS/POSSIBLE INTERACTIONS
Initially, dosage of thyroid supplementation should be divided in half for old dogs and dogs with cardiac problems.

FOLLOW-UP
• Signs, if present, should resolve with correction of causative metabolic or endocrine problem. • Measure serum thyroxine concentration 4-6 hours after administering medication, at 30 and 60 days after starting treatment, and then every 6 months. • If arrythmia is secondary to hypoadrenocorticism, assess electrolytes every 3-4 months after patient is stable.

MISCELLANEOUS

Reference
Tilley LP. Essentials of canine and feline electrocardiography. 3rd ed. Baltimore: Williams & Wilkins, 1992.
Author Deborah J. Hadlock
Consulting Editors Larry P. Tilley and Francis W.K. Smith, Jr.

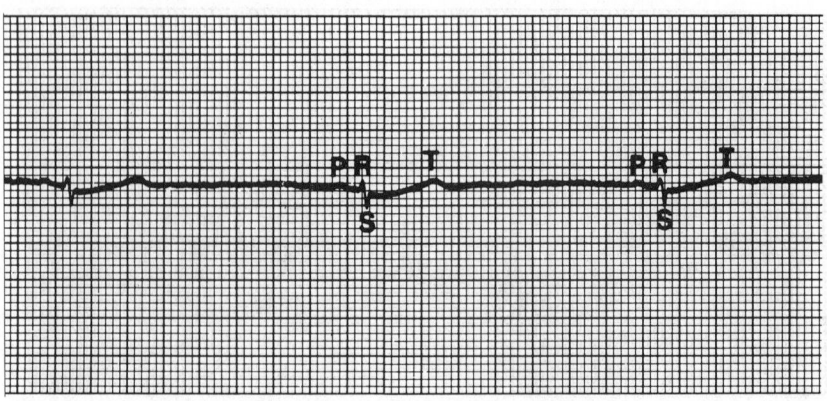

Sinus bradycardia at a rate of 75 beats/min in a cat during anesthetic complications during surgery. (From Tilley LP. Essentials of canine and feline electrocardiography, 3rd ed. Baltimore: Williams & Wilkins, 1992, with permission.)

BASICS

OVERVIEW
• Mechanism involves high rate of impulse formation because of enhanced adrenergic effect or cholinergic inhibition • A natural response to certain physiologic and pathologic factors—not actually an arrhythmia • If persistent, can be serious, leading to myocardial damage by increasing oxygen demands

ECG Features
• Acceleration of the sinoatrial node beyond its normal discharge rate, resulting in a heart rate > 160 bpm in dogs (180 in toy breeds, 220 in puppies, and > 140 in giant breeds) and > 240 bpm in cats • Rhythm regular, possibly with a slight variation in RR interval • PR interval is constant

SIGNALMENT
Most common arrhythmia in dogs and cats

SIGNS

Historical Findings
• None, if arrhythmia is physiologic response to stress • Weakness and exercise intolerance if arrhythmia is associated with primary cardiac disease or extracardiac disorder

Physical Examination Findings
• High heart rate • May otherwise be normal if arrhythmia not associated with pathologic condition • Pale mucous membranes if arrhythmia is associated with anemia or congestive heart failure (CHF) • Fever in some animals • Signs of CHF in some animals

CAUSES AND RISK FACTORS

Physiologic
• Exercise • Pain • Restraint

Pathologic
• Fever • Congestive heart failure • Hyperthyroidism • Shock • Anemia • Infection • Hypoxia • Pulmonary thromboembolism

Pharmacologic
• Atropine • Epinephrine • Ketamine • Quinidine • Xanthine bronchodilators • Beta agonists

DIAGNOSIS

DIFFERENTIAL DIAGNOSIS
• Important to differentiate sinus tachycardia from atrial tachycardia. As sinus rate increases, the P wave appears closer to the T wave of the previous beat, and at very rapid rates, it becomes hard to distinguish sinus from atrial tachycardia. • Consider vagal maneuver to differentiate atrial from sinus tachycardia. Atrial tachycardia may be terminated by carotid sinus or ocular pressure. With sinus tachycardia, vagal maneuvers usually produce only gradual, transient slowing of the heart rate, if at all. ECG monitoring is recommended while performing these vagal maneuvers.

CBC/BIOCHEMISTRY/URINALYSIS
• Low PCV if animal has anemia • Leukocytosis with left shift if cause of arrhythmia is secondary to infection

OTHER LABORATORY TESTS
• High T_4 (cats) if arrhythmia is secondary to hyperthyroidism • Consider T_3 suppression test or TRH response test if T_4 values are normal and hyperthyroidism is suspected

IMAGING N/A

OTHER DIAGNOSTIC PROCEDURES
N/A

TREATMENT
Treat underlying disease

MEDICATIONS

DRUGS AND FLUIDS
Administer appropriate antibiotics and fluids if animal has fever or infection

Dogs
If the dog has CHF, it may respond to administration of diuretic and vasodilator. If arrhythmia persists, then digoxin (.22 mg/m² or 0.007 mg/kg PO q12h) is the drug of

choice. If arrhythmia persists despite digoxin, consider adding beta blocker or calcium channel blocker.

Cats
• If arrhythmia is secondary to hyperthyroidism, administer propranolol (2.5-5 mg PO q12h-q8h) or atenolol (6.25 mg q212h). • Consider digoxin (0.01 mg/kg PO q48h, tablet preferred) if cat has chronic hyperthyroidism causing dilated cardiomyopathy or primary dilated cardiomyopathy. • If arrhythmia is associated with hypertrophic cardiomyopathy, administer diltiazem (01.0-2.5 mg/kg PO q12h-q8h).

CONTRAINDICATIONS/POSSIBLE INTERACTIONS
Avoid atropine and catecholamines (epinephrine) until arrhythmia resolves.

FOLLOW-UP
• Arrhythmia usually resolves with correction of the underlying cause. • If arrhythmia is associated with CHF, the prognosis is poor despite treatment. • Prognosis for remission of sinus tachycardia is favorable when hyperthyroidism is controlled medically, surgically, or by radioactive iodine.

MISCELLANEOUS

ABBREVIATIONS
CHF = Congestive heart failure

Reference
Miller MS, Tilley LP. Manual of canine and feline cardiology. 2nd ed. Philadelphia: WB Saunders, 1995.
Author Deborah J. Hadlock
Consulting Editors Larry P. Tilley and Francis W. K. Smith, Jr.

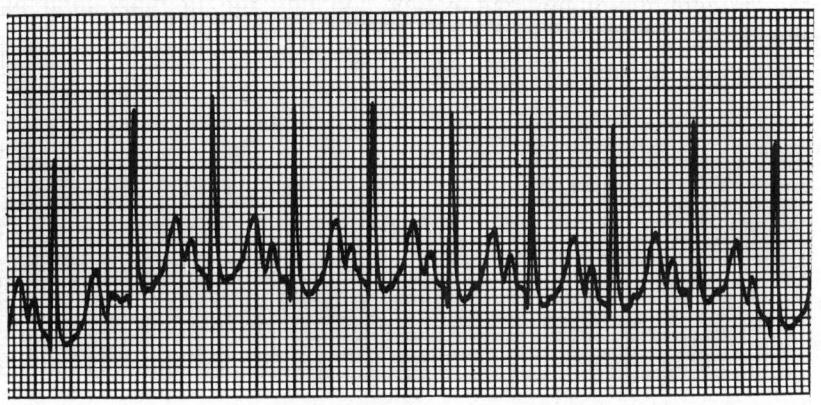

Sinus tachycardia at a rate of 272/min in a dog in shock. The rhythm is sinus because the P waves are normal, the P-R relationship is normal, and the rhythm is regular. (From Tilley LP. Essentials of canine and feline electrocardiography, 3rd ed. Baltimore: Williams & Wilkins, 1992, with permission.)

VENTRICULAR FIBRILLATION

BASICS

OVERVIEW
Cardiac output approaches zero, making this a life-threatening and generally terminal rhythm

ECG features
• Rapid, chaotic, irregular rhythm with bizarre waves or oscillations • No P waves • No QRS complexes • Oscillations may be large (coarse fibrillation) or small (fine fibrillation)

SIGNALMENT N/A

SIGNS

Historical Findings
• History of severe systemic illness or cardiac disease in many animals. • Previous history of other cardiac arrhythmias in some animals.

Physical Examination Findings
• Cardiac arrest • Collapse • Death

CAUSES AND RISK FACTORS
Any severe systemic illness or heart disease

DIAGNOSIS

DIFFERENTIAL DIAGNOSIS
Rule-out ECG artifact. Re-apply ECG clips and make sure of good skin contact and adequate alcohol applied to leads.

CBC/BIOCHEMISTRY/URINALYSIS
N/A

OTHER LABORATORY TESTS N/A

IMAGING N/A

OTHER DIAGNOSTIC PROCEDURES
N/A

TREATMENT

• Rapidly fatal rhythm requiring immediate, aggressive treatment
• Patient will probably die without electrical cardioversion.

TECHNIQUE FOR CARDIOVERSION
• External Countershock—1-10 ws/kg
• Internal Countershock—0.1-1 ws/kg
• Repeat twice if first attempts fail.
• Start at the low end and increase power with each shock.
• If no access to electrical defibrillator, administer a precordial thump. Apply a sharp blow with your open fist to the chest wall over the heart. Rarely successful, but you have nothing to lose.
• Treat any problems such as hypothermia, hyperkalemia, and acid-base disorders.

MEDICATIONS

DRUGS AND FLUIDS
• Institute CPCR
• Epinephrine (0.2 mg/kg IV, IT, IL; double the dose and dilute with equal volume of saline for IT administration) may change fine fibrillation to coarse fibrillation and increase the chances of electrical cardioversion.
• Once animal is successfully converted, administer lidocaine to lower the risk of refibrillation or development of ventricular tachycardia.
• Chemical conversion can be attempted if no access to electrical defibrillator. Administer 1.0 mEq potassium/kg and 6.0 mg acetylcholine/kg IC. Rarely successful.

CONTRAINDICATIONS/POSSIBLE INTERACTIONS
• Bretylium is recommended in humans to treat recurrent ventricular fibrillation, but in dogs and cats this drug may precipitate ventricular arrhythmias, including ventricular fibrillation.
• Lidocaine raises the fibrillation threshold, but makes defibrillation more difficult.

FOLLOW-UP
• CBC, urinalysis, and biochemistry profile.
• If primary cardiac disease is suspected, an echocardiogram and thoracic radiographs are indicated. • Monitor ECG closely and frequently.

MISCELLANEOUS

SEE ALSO
• Cardiopulmonary arrest

ABBREVIATIONS
IC = intracardiac
IL = intralingual
IT = intratracheal
ws = watts/sec

Reference
Tilley LP. Essentials of canine and feline electrocardiography, 3rd Ed. Baltimore: Williams & Wilkins. 1992.
Author Francis W. K. Smith, Jr.
Consulting Editors Larry P. Tilley and Francis W.K. Smith, Jr.

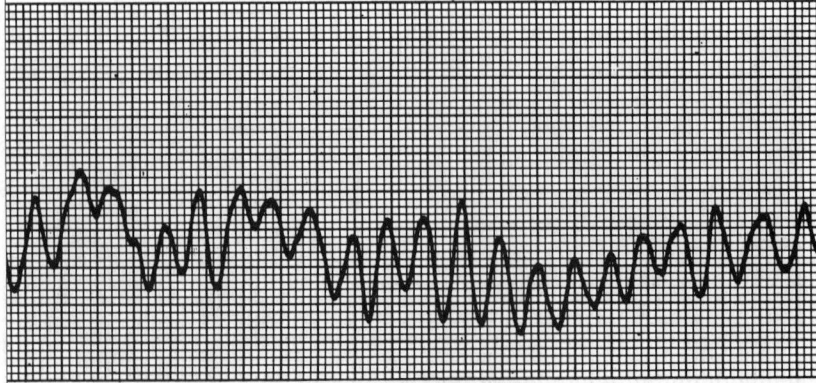

Coarse ventricular fibrillation. (From Tilley LP. Essentials of canine and feline electrocardiography, 3rd ed. Baltimore: Williams & Wilkins, 1992, with permission.)

VENTRICULAR PREMATURE COMPLEXES

BASICS

OVERVIEW
• Cardiac impulses initiated within the ventricles instead of the sinus node • Mechanisms include increased automaticity and reentry • Direct effects on the cardiovascular system with secondary effects on other systems because of poor perfusion.

ECG Features
• QRS complexes typically wide and bizarre • P waves dissociated from the QRS complexes

SIGNALMENT
• Commonly seen in large-breed dogs with cardiomyopathy, especially boxers and Doberman pinschers. • Common in cats with cardiomyopathy; occasionally seen in cats with hyperthyroidism.

SIGNS

Historical Findings
• Weakness • Exercise intolerance • Syncope • Sudden death

Physical Examination Findings
• Irregular rhythm associated with pulse deficits; may auscult splitting of the first or second heart sound • May be normal if arrhythmia is intermittent and absent during examination • Signs of congestive heart failure or murmur may be observed depending on the cause of arrhythmia

CAUSES AND RISK FACTORS
• Cardiomyopathy • Congenital defects (especially subaortic stenosis) • Chronic valve disease • Gastric torsion/volvulus • Traumatic myocarditis (dogs) • Digitalis toxicity • Hyperthyroidism (cats) • Cardiac neoplasia • Myocarditis

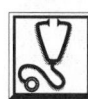

DIAGNOSIS

DIFFERENTIAL DIAGNOSIS
Supraventricular premature beats with bundle branch block

• Look for P waves associated with the wide QRS complexes. An atrial premature complex with abberant conduction has an associated P wave. • An atrial premature complex is usually followed by a noncompensatory pause. • A ventricular premature complex is usually followed by a compensatory pause.

CBC/BIOCHEMISTRY/URINALYSIS
• Hypokalemia and hypomagnesemia predispose animals to ventricular tachycardia and blunt the response to class 1 antiarrhythmic drugs (e.g., lidocaine, procainamide, and quinidine) • High amylase and lipase if condition is secondary to pancreatitis

OTHER LABORATORY TESTS
High T_4 (cats) if condition is secondary to hyperthyroidism

IMAGING
Echocardiography may reveal structural heart disease.

OTHER DIAGNOSTIC PROCEDURES
Long-term ambulatory (Holter) recording of the ECG is indicated for detection of transient ventricular arrhythmias in animals with unexplained syncope or weakness.

TREATMENT
• Symptomatic patient—treat as inpatient and restrict activity until arrhythmia is controlled.
• Treatment of the asymptomatic patient is controversial.
• Alert owner to potential for the arrhythmia worsening and sudden death.

MEDICATIONS

DRUGS AND FLUIDS
Correct hypokalemia or hypomagnesemia, if present

Dogs
• Start procainamide (8-20 mg/kg PO q8h-q6h), quinidine (6-20 mg/kg PO q8h-q6h), tocainide (10-20 mg/kg PO q8h), or mexiletine (5-8 mg/kg PO q8h).

• Combine previous drugs with a beta blocker (propranolol or atenolol) if important arrhythmia persists.
• Consider sotalol or amiodarone as last resorts.

Cats
Propranolol (2.5-5 mg PO q8h) or atenolol (6.25 mg PO q12h) are preferred drugs in cats.

CONTRAINDICATIONS/ POSSIBLE INTERACTIONS
• Avoid atropine, catecholamines (e.g., epinephrine and dopamine), and digoxin until arrhythmia is controlled
• Use beta blockers cautiously in animals with congestive heart failure

FOLLOW-UP
• Monitor with serial ECG or telemetry • If cause is metabolic, condition may resolve with good prognosis. • If condition is associated with cardiac disease, prognosis is guarded.

MISCELLANEOUS

SEE ALSO
• Ventricular Tachycardia • Myocarditis

Reference
Tilley LP. Essentials of canine and feline electrocardiography. 3rd ed. Baltimore: Williams & Wilkins, 1992.
Author Francis W. K. Smith Jr.
Consulting Editor Larry P. Tilley and Francis W. K. Smith Jr.

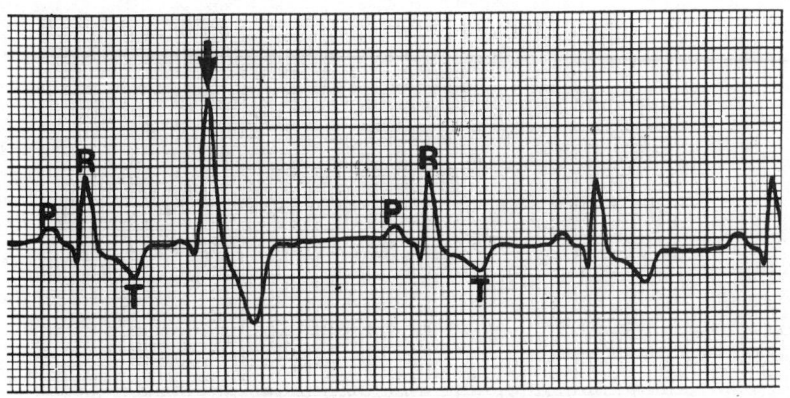

One ventricular premature beat (arrow). Heart rate is 30 beats/min. (From Tilley LP. Essentials of canine and feline electrocardiography, 3rd ed. Baltimore: Williams & Wilkins, 1992, with permission.)

VENTRICULAR STANDSTILL (ASYSTOLE)

BASICS

OVERVIEW
• Cardiac output approaches zero, making this a life-threatening and generally terminal rhythm

ECG Features
• P waves present if animal has complete atrioventricular (AV) block • No QRS complexes • Severe sinoatrial block or arrest

SIGNALMENT N/A

SIGNS

Historical Findings
• History of severe systemic illness or cardiac disease in many animals • History of other cardiac arrhythmias in some animals

Physical Examination Findings
• A ventricular pulse connot be palpated
• Cardiac arrest • Collapse • Death

CAUSES AND RISK FACTORS
• Any severe systemic illness (e.g., severe acidosis and hyperkalemia) or heart disease
• Ventricular fibrillation and complete AV block • Electrical-mechanical dissociation represents a recorded ECG and no effective cardiac output.

DIAGNOSIS

DIFFERENTIAL DIAGNOSIS
Rule out ECG artifact. Reapply ECG clips and make sure skin contact is good and adequate alcohol applied to leads.

CBC/BIOCHEMISTRY/URINALYSIS
N/A

OTHER LABORATORY TESTS N/A

IMAGING N/A

OTHER DIAGNOSTIC PROCEDURES
Systemic blood pressure—readable pressure absent

TREATMENT
• Rapidly fatal rhythm requiring immediate aggressive treatment
• Treat any treatable problems such as hypothermia, hyperkalemia, and acid-base disorders.
• Artificial pacing with a transvenous pacemaker may be successful if myocardium is mechanically responsive.
• DC electrical conversion is not effective unless the rhythm can first be converted to ventricular fibrillation with medications.

MEDICATIONS

DRUGS AND FLUIDS
• Institute CPR
• Epinephrine 0.2 mg/kg IV, IT, or IL (double the dose for IT administration and deliver with equal volume of saline)
• Atropine 0.05 mg/kg IV, IT, or IL (Double the dose for IT administration and deliver with equal volume of saline)
• Sodium bicarbonate 1 mEq/kg IV for each 10 minutes of cardiac arrest

CONTRAINDICATIONS/POSSIBLE INTERACTIONS N/A

FOLLOW-UP
• If animal is resuscitated, evaluate CBC, biochemical anaysis, and urinalysis • If animal survives and you suspect primary cardiac disease, an echocardiogram and thoracic radiographs are indicated. • Monitor ECG closely and frequently. Animals that arrest frequently have recurrent arrest.

MISCELLANEOUS

SEE ALSO
• Cardiopulmonary Arrest • Atrioventricular Block, Complete • Sinus Arrest or Block

ABBREVIATIONS
CPR = cardiopulmonary resuscitation
DC = direct current
IT = intratracheal
IL = intralingual

Reference
Tilley LP. Essentials of canine and feline electrocardiography 3rd ed. Baltimore: Williams & Wilkins, 1992.
Author Francis W. K. Smith, Jr.
Consulting Editors Larry P. Tilley and Francis W. K. Smith, Jr.

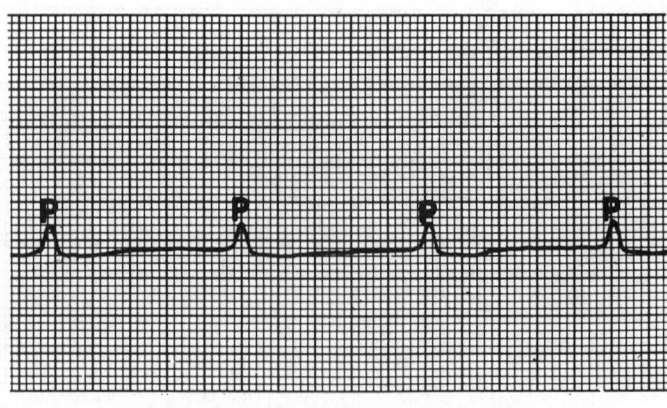

Ventricular standstill. Third degree AV block is present with no QRS complexes. (From Tilley LP. Essentials of canine and feline electrocardiography, 3rd ed. Baltimore: Williams & Wilkins, 1992, with permission.)

VENTRICULAR TACHYCARDIA

BASICS

OVERVIEW

ECG Features
• Three or more ventricular premature contractions in a row • May be intermittent (paroxysmal) or sustained. Heart rate is > 150 bpm with a regular rhythm. • QRS complexes are typically wide and bizarre. • If P waves are seen, they are dissociated from the QRS complexes (figure). • Mechanisms include increased automaticity and reentry. • Potentially life-threatening arrhythmia, usually signifying important myocardial disease or metabolic derangement. • Direct effects are on the cardiovascular system, with secondary effects on other systems because of poor perfusion.

SIGNALMENT
• Commonly seen in large-breed dogs with cardiomyopathy, especially boxers and doberman pinschers • Uncommon in cats

SIGNS

Historical Findings
• Weakness • Exercise intolerance • Syncope • Sudden death

Physical Examination Findings
• Paroxysmal or sustained tachycardia • May be normal if arrhythmia is intermittent and absent during examination • Signs of CHF or murmur may be present, depending on cause of arrhythmia

CAUSES AND RISK FACTORS
• Cardiomyopathy • Congenital defects (especially subaortic stenosis) • Chronic valve disease • Gastric dilation volvulus/torsion • Traumatic myocarditis (dogs) • Digitalis toxicity • Hyperthyroidism (cats) • Cardiac neoplasia • Myocarditis • Pancreatitis

DIAGNOSIS

DIFFERENTIAL DIAGNOSIS
• Supraventricular tachycardia with bundle branch block. Use response to lidocaine to differentiate. • Termination of arrhythmia after administration of lidocaine supports ventricular tachycardia.

CBC/BIOCHEMISTRY/URINALYSIS
• Hypokalemia and hypomagnesemia predispose animal to ventricular tachycardia and blunt response to class 1 antiarrhythmic drugs (e.g., lidocaine, procainamide, and quinidine) • High amylase and lipase if arrythimia is secondary to pancreatitis

OTHER LABORATORY TESTS
High T4 (cats) if arrythmia is secondary to hyperthyroidism.

IMAGING
Echocardiography may reveal structural heart disease.

OTHER DIAGNOSTIC PROCEDURES
Long-term ambulatory (Holter) recording of the ECG is indicated for detection of transient ventricular arrhythmias in animals with unexplained syncope or weakness.

TREATMENT
• Treat the animal as an inpatient and restrict activity until arrhythmia is controlled.
• Alert the owner to the potential for sudden death.

MEDICATIONS

DRUGS AND FLUIDS
Correct hypokalemia or hypomagnesemia, if present.

Dogs
• Administer lidocaine slowly in 2 mg/kg IV boluses (up to 8 mg/kg total) to convert to sinus rhythm. Follow with lidocaine infusion at 25-75 µg/kg/min.
• If lidocaine fails, administer procainamide slowly in 2 mg/kg IV boluses (up to 20 mg/kg total) to convert to sinus rhythm. Follow with procainamide infusion at 20-50 µg/kg/min or 8-20 mg/kg IM q6h.
• When the animal is stable, start procainamide (8-20 mg/kg PO q8h-q6h), quinidine (6-20 mg/kg PO q8h-q6h), tocainide (10-20 mg/kg PO q8h), or mexiletine (5-8 mg/kg PO q8h).
• Combine previous drugs with a beta blocker (e.g., propranolol or atenolol) if arrhythmia persists.
• Consider sotalol or amiodarone for refractory arrhythmias.

Cats
• Use lidocaine cautiously and only for sustained ventricular tachycardia. Neurotoxicity is common in cats. Use one-tenth of the dosage for dogs.
• Propranolol (2.5-5 mg PO q8h) or atenolol (6.25-12.5 mg PO q12h) is preferred in cats.

CONTRAINDICATIONS/POSSIBLE INTERACTIONS
• Avoid atropine, catecholamines (epinephrine, dopamine), and digoxin until arrhythmia is controlled.
• Use beta blockers cautiously in animals with CHF.

FOLLOW-UP
• Monitor the animal with serial ECG or Holter monitoring. • If the cause is metabolic or traumatic, arrythmia may resolve and then the prognosis is good. • If the cause is cardiac disease, the prognosis is guarded.

MISCELLANEOUS

SEE ALSO
• Ventricular premature complexes • Myocarditis

ABBREVIATION
BPM = beats per minute
CHF = congestive heart failure
ECG = electrocardiogram

Reference
Tilley LP. Essentials of canine and feline electrocardiograph. 3rd ed. Baltimore: Williams & Wilkins, 1992.

Author Francis W. K. Smith, Jr.
Consulting Editors Larry P. Tilley and Francis W. K. Smith, Jr.

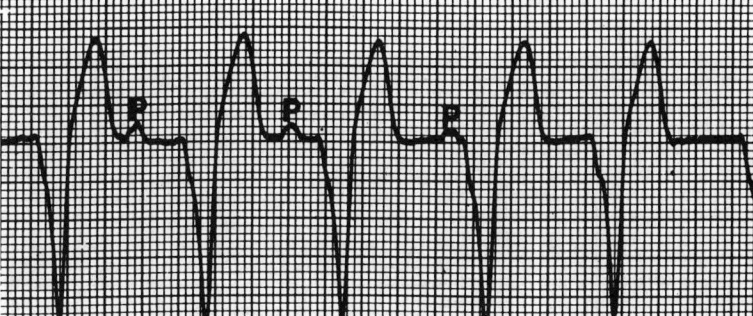

Ventricular tachycardia. The wide and bizarre QRS complexes occur at a rate of 160 beats/min, with no relationship to the P waves. There are more QRS complexes than P waves. (From Tilley LP. Essentials of canine and feline electrocardiography. 3rd ed. Baltimore: Williams & Wilkins, 1992, with permission).

WOLFF-PARKINSON-WHITE SYNDROME AND VENTRICULAR PREEXCITATION

BASICS

OVERVIEW
• Ventricular preexcitation occurs when impulses originating in the sinoatrial node or atrium activate a portion of the ventricles prematurely through an accessory pathway without going through the atrioventricular (AV) node. The remainder of the ventricles are activated normally through the usual conduction system. • Wolff-Parkinson-White (WPW) syndrome consists of ventricular preexcitation with episodes of paroxysmal supraventricular tachycardia.

ECG Features of Ventricular Preexcitation
• Normal heart rate and rhythm (figure)
• Normal P waves • Short P-R interval (dogs, < 0.06 sec; cats, < 0.05 sec) • Widened QRS (small dogs, > 0.05 sec; large dogs, > 0.06 sec; cats, > 0.04 sec), often with a slurring or notching of the upstroke of the R wave (delta wave)

ECG Features of Ventricular Preexcitation with WPW Syndrome
• Extremely rapid heart rate (dogs, often > 300 bpm; cats, approaching 400-500 bpm)
• P waves may be difficult to recognize.
• QRS complexes may be normal, wide with delta wave, or very wide and bizarre depending on the circuit • Conduction is usually 1:1 (ie, 1 P wave for every QRS complex).

SIGNALMENT
• Can be associated with congenital or acquired cardiac defects in dogs or cats • May be associated with hypertrophic cardiomyopathy in cats

SIGNS
Historical Findings
• None in animals with ventricular preexcitation
• Syncope in animals with WPW syndrome

Physical Examination Findings
• None in animals with ventricular preexcitation • Rapid heart rate in animals with WPW syndrome

CAUSES AND RISK FACTORS
• Congenital defect limited to the conduction system • Atrial septal defect in dogs or cats • Tricuspid valvular dysplasia in dogs • Hypertrophic cardiomyopathy in cats

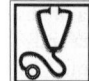

DIAGNOSIS

DIFFERENTIAL DIAGNOSIS
• Ventricular preexcition must be differentiated from other causes of short P-R intervals (e.g., fever, hyperthyroidism, and anemia). These conditions do not cause delta waves.
• Narrow complex WPW syndrome must be differentiated from supraventricular arrhythmias (e.g., atrial tachycardia, atrial flutter, and atrial fibrillation). WPW syndrome is most easily recognized after conversion to normal heart rate and rhythm. • Alternating WPW syndrome should not be confused with ventricular bigeminy. • Wide complex WPW syndrome must be differentiated from ventricular tachycardia. • Short PR interval may be correlated with a normal QRS complex if the anomalous pathway bypasses the AV node to the area of His bundle (i.e., Lown-Ganong-Levine syndrome).

CBC/BIOCHEMISTRY/URINALYSIS
N/A

OTHER LABORATORY TESTS N/A

IMAGING
Echocardiography may show structural heart disease.

OTHER DIAGNOSTIC PROCEDURES
N/A

TREATMENT
• Ventricular preexcitation without tachycardia does not require treatment.
• WPW syndrome requires conversion by ocular or carotid sinus pressure, direct current shock (the most effective treatment), or drugs.

MEDICATIONS

DRUGS AND FLUIDS
• A variety of drugs are used in humans, and opinions differ on agents of choice.
• Lidocaine IV bolus (2 mg/kg) followed by IV drip (25-75 µg/kg/min CRI—dogs only)
• Procainamide (8-20 mg/kg q8h—dogs only)
• Propranolol (cats, 2.5-5 mg PO q8h-q12h; dogs, 0.2-1.0 mg/kg PO q8h), or atenolol (cats, 6.2-12.5 mg PO q24h; dogs, 0.25-1.0 mg/kg PO q12h)
• Diltiazem may be effective (cats, 1-2.5 mg/kg PO q8h; dogs, 0.5-1.5 mg/kg PO q8h).

CONTRAINDICATIONS/POSSIBLE INTERACTIONS
• Digitalis, verapamil, and propranolol may be contraindicated because by slowing conduction through the AV node, these drugs may favor conduction through the anomalous pathways.
• In cats, however, propranolol and atenolol are the drugs of choice.

FOLLOW-UP
Monitor with serial ECG

MISCELLANEOUS

ABBREVIATIONS
AV = atrioventricular
bpm = beats per minute
WPW = Wolff-Parkinson-White

References
Tilley LP. Essentials of canine and feline electrocardiography. 3rd ed. Baltimore: Williams & Wilkins, 1992.
Hill BL, Tilley LP. Ventricular preexcitation in seven dogs and nine cats. J Am Vet Med Assoc 1985;187:1026-1031.
Atkins CE, Wright KN. Supraventricular tachycardia associated with accessory atrioventricular pathways in dogs. In: Kirk RW, Bonagura JD, eds. Current veterinary therapy XII. Philadelphia: WB Saunders, 1995.

Authors Larry P. Tilley and Craig E. McInnis
Consulting Editors Larry P. Tilley and Francis W. K. Smith, Jr.

CV₆LU

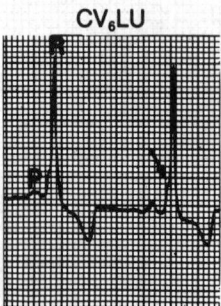

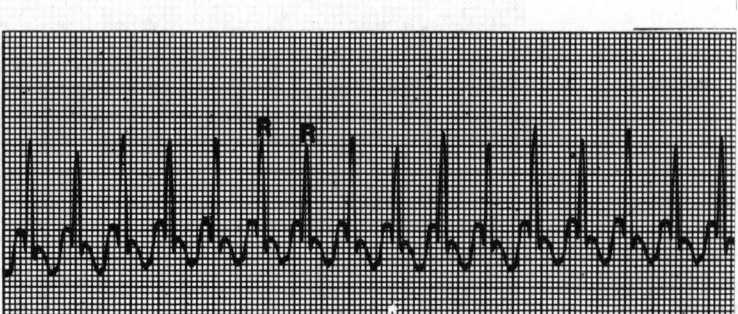

Wolff-Parkinson-White syndrome (canine). Ventricular pre-excitation is represented by the short P-R interval, wide QRS complex, and delta wave (arrow) in CV₆LU. Paroxysms of supraventricular tachycardia in this same case are represneted in the long lead II rhythm strip. (From Tilley LP. Essentials of canine and feline elctrocardiography. 3rd ed. Baltimore: Williams & Wilkins, 1992, with permission).

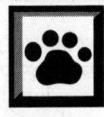

DISEASES AND
CLINICAL SYNDROMES

ABSCESSATION

BASICS

DEFINITION
An abscess is a localized collection of purulent exudate (a cloudy, variably-colored exudate composed primarily of degenerate or toxic neutrophils with lesser numbers of macrophages and lymphocytes, serum, and liquified necrotic tissue) contained within a cavity.

Pathophysiology
Pyogenic organisms or foreign bodies persisting in tissue lead to the formation of purulent exudate. If not quickly cleared by the body or discharged to an external surface, accumulation stimulates the formation of a fibrin capsule. Progressive increase of intracavitary pressure may eventually lead to abscess rupture, but prolonged delay of evacuation prompts the formation of a rigid, fibrous abscess wall. In the latter situation, healing requires filling of the cavity by granulation tissue from which the inciting agent may not be totally eliminated; chronic or intermittent discharge of exudate from a draining sinus tract is a potential sequela.

Systems Affected
• Skin/exocrine—percutaneous (cats > dogs) • Anal sac—dogs > cats • Reproductive—prostate gland (dogs > cats), mammary gland • Ophthalmic—orbit

Genetics N/A

Incidence/Prevalence N/A

Geographic Distribution N/A

SIGNALMENT

Species Dogs and cats

Breed Predilections N/A

Mean Age and Range N/A

Predominant Sex
Mammary glands (female), prostate gland (male)

SIGNS

General Comments
• Clinical signs determined by organ system affected • Associated with a combination of inflammation (pain, swelling, redness, heat, and loss of function), tissue destruction, and/or organ system dysfunction caused by pressure from the abscess mass

Historical Findings
A history of trauma or previous infection often precedes abscessation. If the affected area is visible externally, owners may report a rapidly appearing painful swelling with or without discharge.

Physical Examination Findings
• Determined by the organ system affected • A mass may be detectable. • Inflammation and discharge from a fistulous tract may be visible if the abscess is superficial and has ruptured to an external surface. • A variably-sized, painful mass of fluctuant to firm consistency attached to surrounding tissues may be palpable. • Fever occasionally • Sepsis occasionally, especially if abscess ruptures internally

CAUSES
• Foreign bodies
Pyogenic organisms, including • Staphylococcus spp. • Escherichia coli • Streptococcus spp. • Pseudomonas • Mycoplasma and Mycoplasma-like organisms (L-forms) • Pasteurella multocida • Corynebacterium • Actinomyces • Nocardia • Obligate anaerobes, including Bacteroides, Clostridium spp., Eubacterium, Fusobacterium, and Peptostreptococcus • A presently unnamed bacterium causing migrating subcutaneous abscesses in cats

RISK FACTORS
• Anal sac—impaction and anal sacculitis • Brain—otitis interna, sinusitis, oral infection • Liver—omphalophlebitis • Lung—foreign body aspiration, bacterial pneumonia • Mammary gland—mastitis • Orbital—dental disease, chewing of wood or other plant material • Percutaneous—fighting • Prostatic—bacterial prostatitis • Immunosuppression (FeLV/FIV infection, immunosuppressive chemotherapy, acquired or inherited immune system dysfunctions, underlying predisposing disease [diabetes mellitus, hyperadrenocorticism])

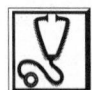

DIAGNOSIS

DIFFERENTIAL DIAGNOSIS

Mass Lesions
• Cyst—less or only transiently painful, slower growing • Fibrous scar tissue—firm and nonpainful • Granuloma—less painful and slower growing, generally firmer without fluctuant center • Hematoma/seroma—variable pain depending on cause, nonencapsulated, rapid initial growth but slow increase once full size is attained, unattached to surrounding tissues. Fluctuant and fluid-filled initially, but more firm with organization. • Neoplasia—variable growth, consistency, and pain

Draining Tracts
• Mycobacterial disease • Mycetoma (botryomycosis, actinomycotic mycetoma, eumycotic mycetoma) • Neoplasia • Phaeohyphomycosis • Sporotrichosis • Systemic fungal infection (blastomycosis, coccidioidomycosis, cryptococcosis, histoplasmosis, trichosporosis)

CBC/BIOCHEMISTRY/URINALYSIS
• CBC—normal or neutrophilia with or without regenerative left shift. Neutropenia and degenerative left shift if septicemic • Urinalysis and serum chemistry results dependent upon system affected • Pyuria with prostatic abscess • High liver enzymes and/or bilirubin with liver abscess and/or pancreatic abscess • High amylase/lipase with pancreatic abscess • Persistent hyperglycemia and glucosuria with diabetes mellitus

OTHER LABORATORY TESTS
• FeLV/FIV testing for cats with recurrent or nonhealing abscesses • CSF evaluation—increase in WBC and protein expected with brain abscess • Adrenal function testing • Special culture techniques to isolate a novel unnamed bacterium responsible for migrating, recurrent subcutaneous abscesses in cats; negative culture results using routine methods

IMAGING

Radiography
Soft tissue density mass in affected area. May reveal foreign body if causative.

Ultrasonography
Determines if mass is fluid-filled or solid, and organ system affected. Flocculent-appearing fluid characteristic of pus. A foreign object may be demonstrated if causative.

Echocardiography
Helpful for diagnosis of pericardial abscess

CT Scan/MRI
Helpful for diagnosis of brain abscess

OTHER DIAGNOSTIC PROCEDURES
• Aspiration reveals a red, white, yellow, or green liquid with protein content > 2.5-3.0 g/dl, a nucleated cell count of 3000 to > 100,000 cells/microliter (primarily degenerative neutrophils with lesser numbers of macrophages and lymphocytes). Pyogenic bacteria may be present in cells and free within the fluid. If the causative agent is not readily identified with a Romanovsky-type stain, specimens should be stained with an acid-fast stain (mycobacteria, Nocardia) and PAS stain (fungus). • Biopsy should contain both normal and abnormal tissue in the same specimen. Impression smears should be stained and examined, and tissue submitted for histopathologic examination and culture. Contact the lab for specific instructions. • Culture of affected tissue and/or exudate for aerobic and anaerobic bacteria and fungus • Bacterial sensitivity testing

GROSS AND HISTOPATHOLOGIC FINDINGS

Gross Findings
Pus-containing mass lesion accompanied by inflammation. If palpable, variably firm or fluctuant, painful mass. If ruptured, pus may be seen draining directly from the mass or an adjoining tract.

Histopathologic Findings
• Exudate consists of large numbers of neutrophils in various stages of degeneration, other inflammatory cells, serum, and necrotic tissue. • Surrounding tissue is congested and contains fibrin, serum, large numbers of neutrophils, variable numbers of lymphocytes, plasma cells, and macrophages. The etiologic agent is variably detectable.

TREATMENT

Basic treatment principles include establishment and maintenance of adequate drainage, surgical removal of nidus of infection or foreign material if necessary, and institution of appropriate antimicrobial therapy.

INPATIENT VERSUS OUTPATIENT

Dependent upon location of abscess and treatment required. Most patients with bite-induced abscesses are treated as outpatients; those with septicemia or requiring more extensive surgical procedures or treatment require extended hospitalization.

ACTIVITY

Should be restricted until the infection has resolved and adequate healing of tissues has taken place.

DIET

• No changes usually necessary
• Dependent upon location of abscess and treatment required

CLIENT EDUCATION

• Discuss necessity to correct or prevent predisposing conditions.
• Discuss need for adequate drainage and continuation of antimicrobial therapy for an adequate period of time.

SURGICAL CONSIDERATIONS

Appropriate debridement and drainage is crucial and may require leaving wound open to an external surface or placement of surgical drains. Early drainage is necessary to prevent further tissue damage and formation of a rigid abscess wall. Foreign material, necrotic tissue, or any nidus of infection must be removed.

MEDICATIONS

DRUGS AND FLUIDS

• Antimicrobial drugs effective against the infectious agent and that gain access to the site of infection are chosen. Until culture sensitive results are known, a broad-spectrum agent, preferably one that is bactericidal and possesses both aerobic and anaerobic activity, may be used empirically. Suggestions include amoxicillin (11-22 mg/kg PO q8-12h), amoxicillin/ clavulanic acid (12.5-25 mg/kg PO q12h), and trimethoprim/sulfadiazine (15 mg/kg PO IM q12h). Doxycycline (3-5 mg/kg PO q12h) for cat abscesses caused by Mycoplasma, L-forms, and the presently unnamed bacterium. • Resulting sepsis or peritonitis requires aggressive fluid and antimicrobial therapy and support.

CONTRAINDICATIONS N/A

PRECAUTIONS N/A

POSSIBLE INTERACTIONS N/A

ALTERNATE DRUGS N/A

FOLLOW-UP

PATIENT MONITORING

Progressive decrease in drainage, resolution of inflammation, and improvement of clinical signs should be seen.

PREVENTION/AVOIDANCE

• Percutaneous abscesses—prevent fighting
• Anal sac abscesses—prevent impaction, consider anal saculectomy for recurrent cases
• Prostatic abscesses—castration possibly helpful • Mastitis—prevent lactation (spaying) • Orbital abscesses—disallow chewing of foreign material

POSSIBLE COMPLICATIONS

• Sepsis • Peritonitis/pleuritis if intraabdominal or intrathoracic abscess ruptures
• Compromise of organ function • Delayed evacuation may lead to chronically draining fistulous tracts.

EXPECTED COURSE AND PROGNOSIS

Dependent on organ system involved and amount of tissue destruction

MISCELLANEOUS

ASSOCIATED CONDITIONS

• FeLV/FIV infections • Immunosuppression

AGE RELATED FACTORS N/A

ZOONOTIC POTENTIAL

• Minimal for pyogenic bacteria
• Mycobacteria and systemic fungal infections carry some potential for zoonotic infection.

PREGNANCY

Avoid use of teratogenic agents in pregnant animals.

SYNONYM

Pus = purulent exudate

SEE ALSO

See causes

ABBREVIATIONS N/A

References

McCaw D. Lumps, bumps, masses, and lymphadenopathy. In: Ettinger SJ, Feldman EC, eds. Textbook of veterinary internal medicine. 4th ed. Philadelphia: WB Saunders, 1995.

DeBoer DJ. Nonhealing cutaneous wounds. In: August JR, ed. Consultations in feline internal medicine. Philadelphia: WB Saunders, 1991.

Birchard SJ, Sherding RG, eds. Saunders manual of small animal practice. Philadelphia: WB Saunders, 1994.

Author James R. Richards
Consulting Editor Fred W. Scott

ACETAMINOPHEN TOXICITY

BASICS

DEFINITION
Toxicity caused by overdosing dogs or cats with over-the-counter acetaminophen-containing analgesic or antipyretic medication.

Pathophysiology
In animals in which the normal biotransformation mechanisms for acetaminophen detoxification (ie, glucuronidation and sulfation) are diminished, cytochrome P-450-mediated oxidation produces a toxic metabolite, N-acetyl benzoquinoneimine, that is electrophilic, conjugates with glutathione, and toxicologically binds to liver proteins.
Dogs receiving 150-200 or more mg acetaminophen/kg body weight generate sufficient electrophilic metabolite 1) to cause RBC glutathione binding, which produces methemoglobinemia, and 2) to attack liver proteins causing hepatotoxicity in a dose-dependent fashion.
Cats, having less ability to glucuronidate and more limited capacity for acetaminophen elimination than dogs, saturate the glucuronidation and sulfation biotransformation routes and develop the toxic cytochrome P-450 metabolite at much lower doses of acetaminophen than dogs. Cats are poisoned by as little as 50-60 mg acetaminophen/kg body weight (often as little as one-half tablet). The drug causes rapid depletion of RBC glutathione concentration. The hemoglobin molecule in cats is unique; it contains eight sulfhydryl groups, making it sensitive to oxidation. As a result, methemoglobulinemia rapidly develops when glutathione levels are low. Hepatotoxicosis develops more slowly and may not be fully expressed before the development of fatal methemoglobinemia.

Systems Affected
• Hemic/lymphatic/immune—methemoglobin develops after glutathione depletion
• Heptobiliary—liver necrosis • Cardiovascular—edema of the face, paws and, to a lesser degree, the forelimbs of cats; mechanism undefined

Genetics
The genetic deficiency in the glucuronide conjugation pathway in cats makes them more vulnerable to acetaminophen toxicity than dogs.

Incidence/Prevalence
• Over-the-counter medications are the fourth most common cause of poisoning in small animals. • Acetaminophen toxicity is relatively common because of the increasing use of acetaminophen in human beings.
• Acetaminophen toxicity is the most common drug toxicity in cats; it is considerably less frequently observed in dogs.

Geographic Distribution N/A

SIGNALMENT N/A
Species Cats more common than dogs
Breed Predilections N/A
Mean Age and Range N/A
Predominant Sex N/A

SIGNS
General Comments
Signs may develop 1-4 hours after administration.

Historical Findings
• Owners develop concern because of animal's depression and rapid breathing; some observe darkened mucous membranes.
• Owner may recall warnings about acetaminophen in cats after dosing their pet.

Physical Examination Findings
• Progressive depression • Salivation
• Vomiting • Abdominal pain • Tachypnea and cyanosis reflect methemoglobinemia • Edema of the face, paws, and possibly forelimbs develops after several hours.
• Cats are particularly prone to voiding chocolate-colored urine (hematuria or hemaglobinuria). • Death in dogs may occur within a few days as a result of liver necrosis.
• Death in cats caused by methemoglobinemia occurs 18-36 hours after ingestion.

CAUSES Acetaminophen overdosing

RISK FACTORS
• Nutritional deficiencies of glucose or sulfate • Simultaneous administration of other glutathione-depressing drugs

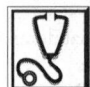

DIAGNOSIS

DIFFERENTIAL DIAGNOSIS
Must differentiate from other drug toxicites that cause methemoglobinemia:
• Nitrites • Phenacetin • Nitrobenzene
• Phenol and cresol compounds • Sulfites
• History of exposure is important in differentiating these methemoglobin-forming drugs from acetaminophen

CBC/BIOCHEMISTRY/URINALYSIS
• Methemoglobinemia with progressively rising serum activities of liver enzymes • Heinz bodies prominent in RBC of cats • Hematuria or hemoglobinuria

OTHER LABORATORY TESTS
• Acetaminophen serum concentration is maximally elevated 1-3 hours after ingestion; elimination rate is dose-dependent with cats having approximately 10% the plasma elimination rate of dogs. • Blood glutathione is markedly depressed.

IMAGING N/A

OTHER DIAGNOSTIC PROCEDURES
N/A

GROSS AND HISTOPATHOLOGIC FINDINGS
• Methemoglobinemia • Pulmonary edema
• Liver and kidney congestion • In dogs, centrilobular necrosis of the liver and icterus in chronic cases

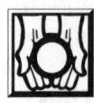

TREATMENT

INPATIENT VS OUTPATIENT
• Patients with methemoglobinemia must be evaluated promptly. • Dark or bloody colored urine or the presence of icterus requires hospitalization.

ACTIVITY
Restricted physical activity and gentle handling is imperative in clinically-affected animals.

DIET N/A

CLIENT EDUCATION
• Treatment in clinically affected animals may be prolonged and expensive. • Animals exhibiting liver injury may require prolonged and costly management.

SURGICAL CONSIDERATIONS N/A

MEDICATIONS

DRUGS AND FLUIDS
• Emesis and gastric lavage useful within 4-6 hours of ingestion • Activated charcoal (2 g/kg PO) immediately after completion of emesis or gastric lavage • N-acetylcysteine (Mucomyst, 140 mg/kg PO, IV loading dose; thereafter, 70 mg/kg PO, IV, q6h for 5-7 treatments) • Anemia, hematuria, or hemoglobinuria may require whole blood transfusion. • Fluids and electrolytes (IV) to maintain hydration and electrolyte balance
• Drinking water available at all times, and food offered 24 hours after initiation of treatment

CONTRAINDICATIONS
Drugs that contribute to methemoglobinemia or offer the risk of liver damage

PRECAUTIONS
Drugs requiring extensive liver metabolism or biotransformation should be used with caution; expect their half-lives to be extended.

POSSIBLE INTERACTIONS
Drugs requiring activation or metabolism by the liver may be reduced in effectiveness.

ALTERNATE DRUGS
• Other sulfur donor drugs (eg, sodium sulfate 50 mg of 1.6% solution/kg IV, q4h for 6 treatments) are alternatives if N-acetylcysteine is not available. Their effective use requires conscientious management. • A 1% methylene blue solution (8.8 mg/kg IV q2h-q3h for 2-3 treatments) combats the methemoglobinemia in dogs and cats without inducing a hemolytic crisis. • Ascorbic acid (125 mg/kg PO q6h for 6 treatments) only slowly reduces methemoglobinemia.

FOLLOW-UP

PATIENT MONITORING

• Continual clinical monitoring of methemoglobinemia is vital for effective management. Laboratory determination of methemoglobin percentage should be done every 2-3 hours. • Liver enzyme activities in serum (ie, ALP and ALT) should be determined q12h to monitor liver damage. • Measurement of blood glutathione provides evidence of the effectiveness of sulfhydryl replacement.

PREVENTION/AVOIDANCE

• Acetaminophen medication never should be given to cats. • Careful attention to the dose of acetaminophen given to dogs prevents toxicity.

POSSIBLE COMPLICATIONS

Liver necrosis and resulting fibrosis may compromise long-term liver function in recovered patients.

EXPECTED COURSE AND PROGNOSIS

• Rapidly progressive methemoglobinemia is a serious sign, and methemoglobin concentration in excess of 50% warrants a grave prognosis. • Progressively high serum liver enzymes 12-24 hours after ingestion warrants serious concern. • Clinical signs may be expected to persist for 12-48 hours, with death due to methemoglobinemia possible at any time. • Dogs or cats promptly treated by reversing methemoglobinemia and preventing excessive liver necrosis can recover fully.

MISCELLANEOUS

ASSOCIATED CONDITIONS N/A

AGE RELATED FACTORS

Young and small-sized dogs or cats are more adversely affected than other animals by single-dose acetaminophen medications.

ZOONOTIC POTENTIAL N/A

PREGNANCY

Pregnancy imposes additional stress and higher risk on acetaminophen-poisoned animals.

SYNONYMS

• Paracetamol • Tylenol

SEE ALSO

Poisoning (Intoxication)

ABBREVIATIONS

ALP = alkaline phosphatase
ALT = alanine transaminase
RBC = red blood cells

References

Savides MC, Oehme FW, Nash SL, Leipold HW. The toxicity and biotransformation of single doses of acetaminophen in dogs and cats. Toxicol Appl Pharmacol 1984;74:26-34.

Savides MC, Oehme FW, Leipold HW. Effects of various antidotal treatments on acetaminophen toxicosis and biotransformation in cats. Am J Vet Res 1985;46: 1485-1489.

Oehme FW. Aspirin and Acetaminophen. In: Kirk RW, ed. Current veterinary therapy IX: small animal practices. Philadelphia: WB Saunders, 1986:188-189.

Hjelle JJ, Grauer GF. Acetaminophen-induced toxicosis in dogs and cats. J Am Vet Med Assoc 1986;188:742-746.

Rumbeiha WK, Oehme FW. Methylene blue can be used to treat methemoglobinemia in cats without inducing Heinz body hemolytic anemia. veterinary and human toxicology 1992;34:120-122.

Author Frederick W. Oehme
Consulting Editor Gary D. Osweiler

ACNE—CATS

BASICS

OVERVIEW
Affects the chin and lower lips of cats of any sex and any age – the cause is unknown.

SIGNALMENT N/A

SIGNS
• Comedones and mild erythematous papules and serous crusts develop on the chin and less commonly on the lips. • Some cats develop swelling of the chin. • More severe cases have nodules, hemorrhagic crusts, pustules, severe erythema, alopecia, and pain. This latter presentation indicates the presence of furunculosis.

CAUSES AND RISK FACTORS
• Poor grooming • Abnormalities of keratinization, sebum production, or immune barrier function

DIAGNOSIS

DIFFERENTIAL DIAGNOSIS
• Demodicosis • Malassezia infection • Feline leprosy • Dermatophytosis • Neoplasia of the sebaceous glands, and other follicular and epidermal neoplasia

CBC/BIOCHEMISTRY/URINALYSIS
N/A

OTHER LABORATORY TESTS N/A

IMAGING N/A

OTHER DIAGNOSTIC PROCEDURES
• Biopsies are rarely needed but are sometimes necessary in selected cats • Histopathologic examination allows one to differentiate acne from other disease such as demodicosis, dermatophytosis and, rarely, neoplasia.

GROSS AND HISTOPATHOLOGIC FINDINGS
• In the mild disease, there is follicular distention with keratin (comedo), hyperkeratosis, and follicular plugging. • In the more severe disease, the findings vary from mild to severe folliculitis and perifolliculitis with follicular pustule formation. • Follicular rupture of keratin and hair into the dermis leads to furunculosis, which is manifested by neutrophils and numerous macrophages surrounding the keratin debris. • Bacteria and Malassezia seen in these lesions are considered secondary invaders and not causative agents.

TREATMENT
• Some cats have one episode but in many cats this condition is a lifelong, recurrent problem. The frequency and the severity of each occurrence varies with each cat.
• In a few cats, the disease process is continual and lifelong treatment twice per week is necessary.
• For the initial treatment, use one or a combination of the medications listed below until all lesions have resolved. Then treatment should be discontinued by tapering over a 2-3 week period. Once the recurrence rate is determined, an appropriate maintenance protocol can be designed for each individual cat.

MEDICATIONS

DRUGS AND FLUIDS

• Systemic antibiotics – amoxicillin with clavulanate, enrofloxacin, or cephalosporin
• Shampoo – weekly to twice weekly with antiseborrheic (sulfur–salicylic acid, benzoyl peroxide, or ethyl lactate) products
• Topical cleansing agents – benzoyl peroxide or salicylic acid products
• Other topicals – clindamycin or erythromycin solution or ointment
• Combination topicals – benzoyl peroxide/antibiotic gels (e.g. benzamycin)
• Topical retinoids (Retin-A) (0.01 gel);, tretinoin (vitamin A acid, retinoic acid

CONTRAINDICATIONS/POSSIBLE INTERACTIONS

• Benzoyl peroxide and salicylic acids can be irritating to some cats.
• Systemic isotretinoin (2mg/kg/day) can be used with caution, if cats will not allow application of topical medications. People should be cautioned that this drug can have potentially deleterious side effects in humans (drug interactions and teratogenic) if taken by mistake. When isotretinoin is prescribed for pets, it should be labeled for animal use only and should be kept separate from human medications to avoid accidental use by humans.

 FOLLOW-UP

After discontinuing medication, monitor the cat for relapses. Maintenance cleansing programs can be used in between relapses to extend the time between episodes.

 MISCELLANEOUS

Systemic isotretinoin should not be used on breeding animals.

References

Scott DW. Feline dermatology 1900–1978. A monograph. J Am Anim Hosp Assoc 1980;6:331-459.

Author David Duclos
Consulting Editor Lowell Ackerman

ACNE—DOGS

BASICS

OVERVIEW
• Chronic inflammatory disorder of the chin and lips of young dogs • Characterized by folliculitis and furunculosis • Recognized almost exclusively in short-coated breeds • The initial lesions are hairless follicular papules which are characterized histopathologically by marked follicular keratosis, plugging, dilatation, and perifolliculitis. • Bacteria are not seen and cannot be isolated from the lesions in the early stages of the condition. As the disease progresses, the papules enlarge and rupture promoting a suppurative folliculitis and furunculosis. It was previously felt that hormones played a triggering role in this dermatosis. It is speculated that genetic predisposition plays a more important role than hormone fluctuations.

SIGNALMENT
Predisposed short coated-breeds: boxers, Doberman pinschers, English bulldogs, great Danes, weimaraners, mastiffs, rottweilers, and German shorthaired pointers

SIGNS
• The area may be minimally to markedly swollen with numerous erythematous papules • In advanced stages, the lesions may be exudative and indicate a secondary deep bacterial infection • The lesions may be painful on palpation • Chronic resolved lesions may be scarred and lichenified

CAUSES AND RISK FACTORS
Some short-coated breeds appear to be genetically predisposed to follicular keratosis and secondary bacterial infection

DIAGNOSIS

DIFFERENTIAL DIAGNOSIS
• Dermatophytosis • Demodecosis • Foreign body • Contact dermatitis

CBC/BIOCHEMISTRY/URINALYSIS
N/A

OTHER LABORATORY TESTS N/A

IMAGING N/A

OTHER DIAGNOSTIC PROCEDURES
N/A

GROSS AND HISTOPATHOLOGICAL FINDINGS
Clinical signs and histopathologic confirmation are diagnostic

TREATMENT
• Depends on the severity and chronicity of the disease
• Reduce behavioral trauma to the chin (rubbing on the carpet, chewing bones that increase salivation, etc.)
• Frequent cleaning to reduce the bacterial numbers on the surface of the skin with benzoyl peroxide shampoo or gel or mupirocin ointment
• Owners should be instructed to avoid expressing the lesions which may cause internal rupture of the papule with massive inflammation

MEDICATIONS

DRUGS AND FLUIDS

Topical
- Benzoyl peroxide shampoo or gel (antibacterial)
- Mupirocin ointment (antibacterial-Staph)
- Isotretinoin (Retin-A) tretinoin (vitamin A acid, retinoic acid gel) may reduce follicular keratosis
- Corticosteroids may be necessary to reduce inflammation

Systemic
- Antibiotics appropriate for deep bacterial infection; cephalosporins are an excellent choice (Cephalexin - 10mg/lb PO q8h for 6-8 weeks)
- May need to perform bacterial culture and sensitivity test.

CONTRAINDICATION/POSSIBLE INTERACTIONS
- Benzoyl peroxide may bleach carpets and fabrics and may be irritating
- Mupirocin ointments are greasy
- Topical retinoids may be drying and irritating
- Topical steroids may cause adrenal suppression with repeated use

FOLLOW-UP
Long-term topical treatment required.

MISCELLANEOUS

Reference
Scott DW, Miller WH, Griffin CE. Miller and Kirk's small animal dermatology. 5th ed. Philadelphia: WB Saunders, 1995;304-305.

Author Karen Helton Rhodes
Consulting Editor Lowell Ackerman

ACROMEGALY—CATS

 ## BASICS

OVERVIEW
• Clinical syndrome caused by chronic hypersecretion of growth hormone (i.e., somatotropin). Growth hormone has both anabolic and catabolic effects which are mediated by somatomedins or insulin-like growth factors synthesized and released from the liver in response to growth hormone. • Anabolic effects include overgrowth of connective tissue, bone, muscle, and viscera. Hypertrophic cardiomyopathy is commonly associated with acromegaly in cats. • Catabolic effects of growth hormone include increased lipolysis, hyperglycemia, and restricted glucose transport, which eventually causes clinical diabetes mellitus. Growth hormone has strong antiinsulin and diabetogenic activities, and the vast majority of feline acromegalics are also insulin resistant diabetics.

SIGNALMENT
• Most affected cats are middle- to old-aged (mean, 10 years; range, 8-14 years), mixed breed males; appears to be uncommon in females • No apparent breed predilection

SIGNS

Historical Findings
• Polyuria and polydipsia (most affected cats are diabetic) • Insulin resistant diabetes mellitus

Physical Examination Findings
• Altered facial appearance (i.e., primarily mandibular enlargement; broad, blunt facial structure) • Overweight • Abdominal enlargement or pot-bellied appearance • Hepatomegaly • Cardiac murmurs • Evidence of congestive cardiac failure (i.e., pulmonary edema, pleural effusion, or ascites).

CAUSES AND RISK FACTORS
In cats, acromegaly usually results from excessive secretion of growth hormone by a pituitary adenoma.

 ## DIAGNOSIS

DIFFERENTIAL DIAGNOSIS
•Simple diabetes mellitus • Hyperadrenocorticism

CBC/BIOCHEMISTRY/URINALYSIS
Routine laboratory abnormalities are nonspecific:
• Mild erythrocytosis • Marked hyperglycemia and glucosuria associated with diabetes mellitus • Mild hypercholesterolemia • Mild hyperproteinemia • Hyperphosphatemia
• Moderately high ALT and ALP activity.

OTHER LABORATORY TESTS
Definitive diagnosis requires demonstration of high circulating somatotropin concentration or evaluation of pituitary somatotropin responsiveness to a glucose load. Unfortunately, a validated assay for somatotropin in cats is not currently available.

IMAGING
• CT scanning of the pituitary region may identify a mass lesion supporting the clinical diagnosis of acromegaly. • CT may aid in characterizing tumor location and size which is important for selecting treatment.

OTHER DIAGNOSTIC PROCEDURES
N/A

 ## TREATMENT

• Treat associated conditions (e.g., diabetes mellitus and congestive heart failure).
• Therapeutic options for pituitary neoplasms include surgical excision, radiotherapy, and medical treatment with dopamine agonists or somatostatin analogues. Surgical excision of pituitary adenoma has not been sufficiently evaluated in the cats, and large pituitary tumors may not be amenable to surgery. Pituitary directed cobalt radiation has limited availability in veterinary medicine but is recommended as the primary treatment in cats with signs of acromegaly and evidence of a pituitary mass on CT.

MEDICATIONS

DRUGS AND FLUIDS

Dopaminergic agonists (e.g., bromocriptine and levodopa), estrogens, and long-acting somatostatin analogs are used in humans, but experience is limited in veterinary patients. The somatostatin analog SMS 201-995 was used to treat four acromegalic cats with little appreciable effect on serum growth hormone concentration.

CONTRAINDICATIONS/POSSIBLE INTERACTIONS Unknown

 FOLLOW-UP

• The prognosis for acromegaly in cats caused by pituitary neoplasia is guarded to poor since the effect of treatment varies and has not been fully evaluated. • Death can be caused by rapid tumor growth, cardiac failure due to hypertrophic cardiomyopathy, or uncontrolled diabetes mellitus.

 MISCELLANEOUS

SEE ALSO

Diabetes Mellitus, Uncomplicated

ABBREVIATIONS

GH = growth hormone
ALP = alkaline phosphatase
ALT = alanine aminotransferase
CT = Computed tomography

Reference

Peterson ME, Taylor RS, Greco DS, et al. Acromegaly in 14 cats. J Vet Intern Med 1990;4:192-200.
Author Leland Thompson
Consulting Editor Rhett Nichols

ACTINOMYCOSIS

 BASICS

OVERVIEW
• Actinomycosis is an infectious disease caused by gram-positive, branching, pleomorphic, rod-shaped bacteria of the genus Actinomyces. Actinomyces viscosus is most commonly identified. The organism survives in microaerophilic or anaerobic conditions.
• It is rarely found as the single bacterial agent in a lesion; more commonly, it is a component of a polymicrobial infection. There may be synergism between Actinomyces and other organisms.

SIGNALMENT
Dogs and cats; especially common in young male dogs of sporting breeds

SIGNS
Infections usually are localized but may be disseminated. The cervicofacial area is commonly involved.

Physical Examination Findings
• Cutaneous swellings or abscesses with draining tracts—yellow granules (so-called "sulfur granules") may be seen in associated exudates • Pain and fever • Exudative pleural or peritoneal effusions • Retroperitonitis—in one study, Actinomyces was identified in 3 of 34 dogs with retroperitonitis • Osteomyelitis of vertebrae or long bones probably occurs secondary to extension of cutaneous infection. Lameness or a swollen extremity may develop with osteomyelitis. • Motor and sensory deficits are reported with spinal cord compression by granulomas.

CAUSES AND RISK FACTORS
• Actinomyces spp are normal inhabitants of the oral cavity in dogs and cats. Loss of normal protective barriers (mucosa, skin), immunosuppression, or change in the bacterial microenvironment could predispose to actinomycosis. It is thought to occur as an opportunistic infection. • Specific risk factors include trauma (bite wound), migrating foreign body (foxtail in the western United States), and periodontal disease.

 DIAGNOSIS

DIFFERENTIAL DIAGNOSIS
• Nocardiosis represents the primary differential diagnosis. Actinomyces is not reliably distinguished from Nocardia spp. by Gram's staining, cytology, or clinical signs. • Other causes of chronic draining tracts and pleural or peritoneal effusions must be addressed.

CBC/BIOCHEMISTRY/URINALYSIS
No abnormalities are specific for actinomycosis; however, common findings include leukocytosis with a left shift, monocytosis, hypoglycemia, and hyperglobulinemia. Nonregenerative anemia may develop.

OTHER LABORATORY TESTS
N/A

IMAGING
Radiographs of infected bone reveal periosteal new bone production, reactive osteosclerosis, and osteolysis.

OTHER DIAGNOSTIC PROCEDURES
• Pus or osteolytic bone fragments should be submitted in anaerobic specimen containers for culture (see Anaerobic Infections). This provides the only definitive diagnosis. It is helpful to inform the lab that actinomycosis is a rule-out for the patient. • Fresh smears should be made for Gram's staining, cytology, and acid-fast staining (however, these do not preclude the need for culture). Actinomyces does not stain acid-fast; Nocardia is variable.

GROSS AND HISTOPATHOLOGIC FINDINGS
• Histopathologic examination does not reliably distinguish actinomycosis from nocardiosis, although it is still a useful diagnostic tool, especially if sulfur granules are present.
• Histopathologic study may demonstrate pyogranulomatous or granulomatous cellulitis with colonies of filamentous bacteria.

 TREATMENT

• Abscesses should be drained and lavaged for several days. Such lesions should be left open for continued drainage; Penrose drains may be needed.
• If bony involvement is present, the bone may need to be debrided or removed.
• Surgical resection of tissue may not be needed in all cases.

MEDICATIONS

DRUGS AND FLUIDS

• It is important to distinguish between Actinomyces and Nocardia spp for appropriate antimicrobial selection.

• One retrospective study suggested that antibiotics should be administered for a minimum of 3-4 months beyond resolution of all signs. Therapy may also need to be directed against other microbes associated with actinomycosis.

• Penicillin G is considered to have the most reliable activity against Actinomyces, although specific recommendations for duration of therapy are yet to be determined. Recommended dosaging is 65,000 U/kg q 8 h.

• Metronidazole is a drug commonly used to treat anaerobic infections. It should be noted that actinomycosis is unlikely to respond and metronidazole should be avoided.

• Aminoglycosides should not be used because they are ineffective in treating anaerobic infections.

• Actinomyces hordeovulneris is a cell-wall deficient variant (L-phase) that does not usually respond well to penicillin. Clindamycin, erythromycin, and chloramphenicol are better choices in this situation.

CONTRAINDICATIONS/POSSIBLE INTERACTIONS N/A

 FOLLOW-UP

Redevelopment of infection at the initial site may be expected in about half of all patients. Patients should be closely monitored for recurrence of disease in the months after discontinuation of therapy.

 MISCELLANEOUS

Reference

Hardie EM. Actinomycosis and nocardiosis. In: Greene CE, ed. Infectious diseases of the dog and cat. Philadelphia: WB Saunders, 1990:585-591.

Author Sharon K. Fooshee

Consulting Editor Fred W. Scott

ADENOCARCINOMA, ANAL SAC/PERIANAL/RECTAL

BASICS

DEFINITION

Anal sac carcinoma is a malignant neoplasm derived from apocrine glands of the anal sac. Perianal gland tumors arise from modified sebaceous glands of the skin. They are often benign (adenoma) but may be malignant (adenocarcinoma).

Pathophysiology

• Anal sac carcinoma may be hormonally influenced since it occurs primarily in females.
• Perianal gland tumors may be caused by androgen stimulation since they occur predominantly in males. Combined androgenic and estrogenic influences may be involved because when they do occur in females, spayed females are more commonly affected than sexually intact females.

Systems Affected

• Skin/Exocrine—anal sac carcinoma invades surrounding tissues and metastasizes to the regional lymph nodes; perianal tumors (i.e., adenoma) affect the skin at the site of origin, around the anus; adenocarcinoma invades locally and causes distant metastasis. • Renal/Urologic—hypercalcemia (paraneoplastic syndrome) adversely affects renal function in some patients

Genetics N/A

Incidence/Prevalence

Tumors of the perianal region compose 4.8% of all tumors in dogs.

Geographic Distribution N/A

SIGNALMENT

Species Dogs

Breed Predilections

• Anal sac carcinoma N/A • Perianal tumors—dachshund, cocker spaniel, German shepherd dog, beagle, English bulldog, and samoyed.

Mean Age and Range

Dogs greater than 8 years old most commonly affected

Predominant Sex

• Anal sac carcinoma—females (either intact or spayed) • Perianal tumors—intact males

SIGNS

Historical Findings

• Anal sac carcinoma—presence of a mass, difficult defecation, anorexia, polyuria and polydipsia • Perianal tumors—presence of a mass (often multiple), licking at the anal region, and scooting

Physical Examination Findings

• Anal sac carcinoma—mass originating in the anal sac. Sublumbar lymphadenopathy (metastasis) is common. • Perianal tumor—adenomas are usually nonfixed, encapsulated masses in the skin around the anus. May be present along dorsal midline beginning at the neck, tail, and ventral midline, especially on the prepuce, ending at the umbilicus. They may become ulcerated secondary to self-trauma. Adenocarcinomas are fixed to the underlying tissues and will metastasize, often to sublumbar lymph nodes and distant organs.

CAUSES

Hormonal role hypothesized

RISK FACTORS N/A

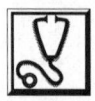

DIAGNOSIS

DIFFERENTIAL DIAGNOSIS

• Tumors of other glands in the perineum including dermal sebaceous and apocrine glands as well as merocrine anal glands
• Cutaneous malignant lymphoma • Squamous cell carcinoma • Mast cell tumor • Anal sac abscess • Perineal hernias.

CBC/BIOCHEMISTRY/URINALYSIS

• Anal sac carcinoma—high serum calcium and occasionally concurrent hypophosphatemia; secondary renal failure may occur with hypercalcemia. • Perianal tumors—results usually normal

OTHER LABORATORY TESTS N/A

IMAGING

• Abdominal radiography to evaluate sublumbar lymph nodes • Thoracic radiography should be done, but pulmonary metastasis is not common.

OTHER DIAGNOSTIC PROCEDURES

• Cytologic examination of fine-needle aspirate to rule out conditions other than anal sac or perianal tumors; however, differentiation of benign versus malignant is seldom possible. • Surgical biopsy required for a definitive diagnosis • Whenever possible, excisional biopsy should be done.

GROSS AND HISTOPATHOLOGIC FINDINGS

Gross

• Anal sac carcinoma—infiltrative tumor, ranging from 0.5-10 cm in diameter. May be unilateral or bilateral. • Perianal tumors—often multiple. Adenomas are encapsulated, often ulcerated, and confined to the skin, ranging from 0.5-5 cm in diameter. Adenocarcinomas are frequently fixed to the underlying tissues and ulcerated.

Histopathology

• Anal sac tumors—areas of both acinar formation and solid lobules of carcinoma cells
• Perianal tumors—adenomas characterized by cells that resemble hepatocytes. Malignant tumors may have characteristic morphology of either adenocarcinoma or carcinoma.

TREATMENT

INPATIENT VERSUS OUTPATIENT

• Outpatient for diagnosis unless hypercalcemia and resultant renal failure dictates hospitalization.
• Biopsy or surgical resection requires hospitalization until the postoperative status of the patient is stable.

ACTIVITY

• Unrestricted
• May need a side brace or Elizabethan collar to prevent licking

DIET

Normal unless patient has hypercalcemia-induced renal failure

CLIENT EDUCATION

• Anal sac carcinoma—poor prognosis
• Perianal tumors—prognosis good in patient with adenomas after castration. Estrogen administration may be complicated by pancytopenia. Adenomas also respond well to radiotherapy. Adenocarcinomas have a poor prognosis and are not likely to respond to hormonal manipulation. If resection is impossible, consider radiotherapy.

SURGICAL CONSIDERATIONS

• Excisional biopsy when possible
• If metastasis has occurred to the sublumbar lymph nodes, consider abdominal surgery and resection of affected nodes.
• In males with multiple or large perianal adenomas, castration and observation for 4-6 weeks is recommended before attempting aggressive surgery. Orchiectomy alone often causes the tumors to go into complete remission.
• Cryosurgery offers no advantage over conventional surgery.
• Fecal incontinence may develop if more than 50% of the anal sphincter is resected or destroyed by freezing. If fewer than 50% is resected or frozen, transient (approximately 1 week) of fecal incontinence is likely.

MEDICATIONS

DRUGS AND FLUIDS

• Anal sac carcinoma—if patient is hypercalcemic, saline diuresis (200 ml/kg/day if possible) and furosemide (1-2 mg/kg PO q6h-q12h) should be given to reduce serum calcium. If inoperable, consider cisplatin (60 mg/m^2 IV q21days).
• Perianal adenomas—if orchiectomy is rejected in males, consider treatment with estrogen.

CONTRAINDICATIONS None

PRECAUTIONS

• Use estrogen with caution because of risk of bone marrow suppression and pancytopenia.

• Cisplatin can cause acute gastrointestinal disturbances, bone marrow suppression, and renal failure.

• Chemotherapy can be toxic. Seek advice if you are unfamiliar with cytotoxic drugs.

POSSIBLE INTERACTIONS None

ALTERNATE DRUGS N/A

FOLLOW-UP

PATIENT MONITORING

• Anal sac carcinoma—if completely resected, physical examination, abdominal radiography and biochemical analysis 1, 3, 6, 9 and 12 months after surgery. If incomplete resection, tumor measurements to determine if the neoplasm is responding to treatment. Careful monitoring of serum calcium and renal function necessary. • Perianal tumors—evaluation 4 weeks after castration. If orchiectomy has not been performed in males, monitor additional tumor development. If estrogen is administered, CBC and platelet count monthly

PREVENTION/AVOIDANCE

• Anal sac carcinoma—N/A • Perianal tumors—castration in males

POSSIBLE COMPLICATIONS

• Metastasis of malignant tumors • Fecal incontinence after surgery

EXPECTED COURSE AND PROGNOSIS

• Anal sac carcinoma—prognosis for cure is poor. Local progression and metastasis to sublumbar lymph nodes common. Life expectancy is seldom more than 1 year without treatment, but quality of life may be good if hypercalcemia does not cause renal failure. Cisplatin may be very useful in selected patients. • Perianal tumors—patients with adenomas have a good prognosis after castration.

• Adenocarcinomas—prognosis guarded to poor. Progressive disease and metastasis to sublumbar lymph nodes and other organs are likely.

MISCELLANEOUS

ASSOCIATED CONDITIONS

If perianal adenomas recur in castrated males or in females, consider adrenal glands (i.e., hyperadrenaocorticism) as a possible source of testosterone.

AGE-RELATED FACTORS

Old dogs more than 8 years old

ZOONOTIC POTENTIAL N/A

PREGNANCY N/A

SYNONYMS

• Anal sac carcinoma—anal sac tumor, anal sac adenocarcinoma, and apocrine gland tumor of the anal sac • Perianal tumor—perianal adenoma, circumanal gland adenoma, hepatoid gland tumor, and perianal adenocarcinoma

SEE ALSO N/A

ABBREVIATIONS NONE

References

Madewell BR, Theilen GH. Tumors and tumor-like conditions of epithelial origin. In: Theilen GH, Madewell BR, eds. Veterinary cancer medicine. 2nd ed. Philadelphia: Lea & Febiger, 1987.

Withrow SJ. Perianal tumors. In: Withrow SJ, MacEwen EG, eds. Clinical veterinary oncology. Philadelphia: JB Lippincott, 1989.

Weiss E, Frese K. Tumors of the skin. Bull WHO, 1974;50:79.

Meuten DJ, et al. Hypercalcemia associated with adenocarcinoma derived from the apocrine glands of the anal sac. Vet Pathol 1981;18:454.

Author Ralph C. Richardson

Consulting Editor Wallace B. Morrison

ADENOCARCINOMA, LUNG

BASICS

OVERVIEW
• Primary pulmonary neoplasms are rare in dogs and cats. Adenocarcinoma is the most common histologic type, representing 75% of all primary malignant lung tumors.

SIGNALMENT
• Mean ages in dogs and cats are 10 and 12 years, respectively • A few investigators report predisposition in the boxer breed, whereas others report no breed prevalence. • No sex predilection in dogs or cats

SIGNS

Historical Findings
• Nonproductive cough • Exercise intolerance • Dyspnea and tachypnea • Anorexia • Weight loss • Hemoptysis • Pain (caused by pleural involvement) • Lameness (caused by metastases or hypertrophic osteopathy) • Polyuria and polydipsia (caused by hypercalcemia) • Weakness or muscle wasting (caused by polyneuropathy and polymyopathy)

Physical Examination Findings
• Fever • Ascites • Limb swelling

CAUSES AND RISK FACTORS
No evidence to date correlates urban environment and passive cigarette smoke inhalation with lung cancer in dogs.

DIAGNOSIS

DIFFERENTIAL DIAGNOSIS
• Granulomatous lesion • Pulmonary abscess • Primary lung tumor (e.g., squamous cell carcinoma) • Metastatic lung tumor • Pneumonia • Asthma • Congenital cysts • Parasitic lesion

CBC/BIOCHEMISTRY/URINALYSIS
• Results usually normal • Normocytic, normochromic nonregenerative anemia in some patients with advanced metastatic disease

OTHER LABORATORY TESTS N/A

IMAGING
• Abdominal radiography or ultrasonography if clinically warranted. • Thoracic radiography usually demonstrate a focal, solitary, well-circumscribed mass.

OTHER DIAGNOSTIC PROCEDURES
• Thoracocentesis and cytologic examination if patient has pleural effusion • Transtracheal lavage for cytologic evaluation is rarely of diagnostic value • Cytologic examination of transthoracic, fine-needle aspirate • Tissue biopsy via percutaneous cutting-needle biopsy, transbronchoscopic lung biopsy, or open lung biopsy (i.e., thoracotomy).

GROSS AND HISTOPATHOLOGIC FINDINGS
• Adenocarcinoma is classified according to its location (i.e., bronchial, bronchiolar, bronchiolar-alveolar, or alveolar) and degree of differentiation. • Undifferentiated adenocarcinoma tends to be more highly invasive and more likely to metastasize than others.

TREATMENT
Surgery (partial or complete lobectomy)

MEDICATIONS

DRUGS AND FLUIDS

Cisplatin

• Cisplatin (dogs only)—prediuresis with 0.9% NaCl (18.3 ml/kg/hr for 4 hours by IV infusion); premedicate with metoclopramide (0.2-0.4 mg/kg IV) and dexamethasone sodium phosphate (0.25 mg/kg IV); administer cisplatin (50-70 mg/m2 in 100 ml 0.9% NaCl over 20 minutes); postdiuresis with 0.9% NaCl (18.3 ml/kg/hr for 2 hours by IV infusion). Another antiemetic (e.g., butorphanol, 0.4 mg/kg SQ) can be substituted if necessary.

• Malignant pleural effusion can be palliated by intrathoracic administration of cisplatin (50 mg/m2 q4 wk). Dogs should be diuresed with 0.9% NaCl before and after cisplatin administration.

Doxorubicin

• Dogs—pretreat with diphenhydramine (Benadryl—1 mg/kg SQ or IM). Do not use heparinized saline; administer doxorubicin (30 mg/m2 slowly IV over 20-30 min; repeat q3wk).

• Cats—pretreat with dexamethasone sodium phosphate (0.5 mg/kg IV) before doxorubicin administration; administer doxorubicin (20-25 mg/m2 q3-4wk).

Vincristine, doxorubicin, and 5-fluorouracil (dogs only)

• Vincristine (0.75 mg/M2 IV) days 8 and 15; doxorubicin (30 mg/m2 IV) day 1; 5-fluorouracil (150 mg/m2 IV) days 1, 8, 15; repeat cycle on day 22.

CONTRAINDICATIONS/POSSIBLE INTERACTIONS

• Cisplatin is contraindicated in cats because of potentially fatal pulmonary edema. Nephrotoxicity is a major concern in dogs, although myelosuppression, gastrointestinal toxicity, ototoxicity, neurotoxicity, and anaphylactoid reactions are other potential consequences.

• Doxorubicin causes dose-dependent, cumulative cardiotoxicity (usually > 250 mg/m2). Dogs with heart disease should be monitored by ECG and echocardiography. Gastrointestinal toxicity, myelosuppression, and anaphylaxis are other potential consequences. Nephrotoxicity develops in some cats at dosages x100 mg/m2.

• 5-fluorouracil is contraindicated in cats because of potentially fatal cerebellar neurotoxicity.

• Vincristine: Toxicities include vomiting, constipation, peripheral neuropathy, and anorexia. Perivascular injection is associated with pain, erythema, moist dermatitis, and necrosis of the affected area.

• Seek advice before starting treatment if you are unfamiliar with cytotoxic drugs.

FOLLOW-UP

PROGNOSIS

• Identification of lymph node involvement during surgery is the best single prognostic indicator. Other prognostic factors after surgery include ability to achieve complete cytoreduction, the size of the primary tumor, and evidence of distant metastases. • Patients with T1 tumors have a median survival of 224 days, whereas those with T3 tumors have a median survival of 45 days after surgery. Dogs with lymph node involvement have a median survival of 14 days in contrast to dogs with negative nodal involvement (180 days).

• Patients with differentiated adenocarcinoma have a better prognosis than those with undifferentiated carcinoma.

PATIENT MONITORING

• Thoracic radiography at monthly intervals during chemotherapy • Biochemical analysis (especially BUN and creatinine) and urinalysis before repeat treatment with cisplatin

• A minimum of two cycles of chemotherapy should be administered before evaluating response to treatment.

POSSIBLE COMPLICATIONS

Caused by disease—anemia, DIC, hemoptysis, spontaneous pneumothorax, hypercalcemia, and hypertrophic osteopathy.

MISCELLANEOUS

PREGNANCY

Chemotherapy is not advised in pregnant animals.

Reference

Ogilvie GK, Weigel RM, Haschek WM, et al. Prognostic factors for tumor remission and survival in dogs after surgery for primary lung tumor: 76 cases (1975-1985). J Am Vet Med Assoc 1989;195:109-112.

Author Stanley L. Marks

Consulting Editor Wallace B. Morrison

ADENOCARCINOMA, NASAL

 BASICS

OVERVIEW
Nasal adenocarcinoma causes slow, progressive, local invasion of neoplastic epithelial and glandular epithelial cells within the nasal and paranasal sinuses.

SIGNALMENT
• Median age in dogs, 10 years (range, 18 months to 18 years) • Medium to large breeds are more commonly affected than small

SIGNS

Historical Findings
• Intermittent and progressive history of unilateral to bilateral epistaxis • Sneezing • Halitosis • Anorexia • Seizures secondary to cranial invasion

Physical Examination Findings
• Noninfectious nasal discaharge • Facial deformity or exophthalmia • Pain with nasal or paranasal sinus examination • Obstructed nares (unilateral or bilateral)

CAUSES AND RISK FACTORS N/A

 DIAGNOSIS

DIFFERENTIAL DIAGNOSIS
• Bacterial sinusitis (uncommon) • Viral infection (cats) • Aspergillosis • Cryptococcosis (cats) • Foreign body • Trauma • Tooth root abscess • Oronasal fistula • Coagulopathy

CBC/BIOCHEMISTRY/URINALYSIS
N/A

OTHER LABORATORY TESTS N/A

IMAGING
• Survey skull radiography shows typical pattern of asymmetrical destruction of turbinates with superimposition of a soft tissue mass. Fluid density in the frontal sinuses secondary to outflow obstruction is observed in some animals. • Thoracic radiography—to evaluate for lung metastasis (uncommon) • Computed tomography or magnetic resonance imaging—best method to observe integrity of cribiform plate or orbital invasion

OTHER DIAGNOSTIC PROCEDURES
• Rhinoscopy • Tissue biopsy necessary for definitive diagnosis • Bacterial culture often positive

 TREATMENT

• Surgery alone is ineffective.
• Turbinectomy may be done before external (teletherapy) or internal (brachytherapy) irradiation.
• Inpatient radiotherapy, with or without surgery, provides the best clinical control in dogs. Median disease-free intervals range from 8 to 25 months in dogs. Median disease-free intervals range from 1–36 months in cats. With radiotherapy, 38–57% of dogs and cats have 1-year survival rate, and 30–48% have 2-year survival rate.

MEDICATIONS

DRUGS AND FLUIDS

• Chemotherapy is a good option in some animals. Median survival after cisplatin chemotherapy (60–70 mg/m^2 IV once q3wk) in dogs is 22 weeks.
• Chemotherapuetic management in cats is unreported.

CONTRAINDICATIONS/POSSIBLE INTERACTIONS

Chemotherapy can be toxic. Seek advice before initiating treatment if you are unfamiliar with cytotoxic drugs.

FOLLOW-UP

PROGNOSIS

• Physical examination with survey thoracic radiography at 1, 2, 3, 6, 9, 12, 15, 18, and 24 months after treatment • Survey skull radiography, computed tomography, magnetic resonance imaging when clinical signs recur

MISCELLANEOUS

Reference

Hahn KA, Knapp DW, Richardson RC, Matlock CL. Clinical response of nasal adenocarcinoma to cisplastin chemotherapy in 11 dogs. J Am Vet Med Assoc 1992;200:355–357.

Author Kevin A. Hahn
Consulting Editor Wallace B. Morrison

ADENOCARCINOMA, PANCREAS

BASICS

OVERVIEW
Pancreatic adenocarcinoma is a malignant tumor of ductal or acinar origin and is usually metastatic by the time of diagnosis.

SIGNALMENT
• Rare in dogs (0.5-1.8% off all tumors in dogs) and cats (2.8% of all tumors in cats) • Older female dogs and Airedale terriers at higher risk • Median age in dogs, 9.2 years

SIGNS
• Nonspecific—fever, vomiting, weakness, anorexia, icterus, maldigestion, and weight loss • Abdominal pain variable • Metastasis to bone and soft tissue common • Pathologic fractures secondary to metastasis reported • Diabetes insipidus secondary to pituitary metastasis reported in one dog • Abdominal mass

CAUSES AND RISK FACTORS
Unknown

DIAGNOSIS

DIFFERENTIAL DIAGNOSIS
• Must distinguish from primary pancreatitis and other causes of vomiting and icterus • Pancreatitis may be concurrent and complicate or delay early diagnosis

CBC/BIOCHEMISTRY/URINALYSIS
• Usually nonspecific changes such as mild anemia and neutrophilia • Hyperamylasemia less reliable than hyperlipasemia. Lipase concentration often markedly high

OTHER LABORATORY TESTS N/A

IMAGING
• Abdominal radiographs may reveal a mass or loss of contrast associated with concurrent pancreatitis. • Ultrasonography may reveal a mass or concurrent pancreatitis by findings of mixed echogenicity or large pancreas and hyperechoic peripancreatic fat.

OTHER DIAGNOSTIC PROCEDURES
Definitive diagnosis based on surgical biopsy

TREATMENT
• No successful curative treatment reported • Palliation of pain and intestinal and biliary obstruction • Partial or total pancreatectomy

MEDICATIONS N/A

DRUGS AND FLUIDS N/A

CONTRAINDICATIONS/POSSIBLE INTERACTIONS N/A

FOLLOW-UP
Palliation of pain and intestinal obstruction unless more successful treatment becomes available

POSSIBLE COMPLICATIONS
• Intestinal obstruction • Biliary obstruction • Pancreatic abscess • Peritonitis

EXPECTED COURSE AND PROGNOSIS
Usually a rapid progression to death since no successful curative treatment is available

MISCELLANEOUS

ASSOCIATED CONDITIONS
Gastrin secreting pancreatic carcinoma has been reported in dogs and cats. Clinical signs in these animals are also caused by hypergastrinemia, which results in inappropriate HCI secretion by the stomach leading to gastroduodenitis.

Reference
Harari J, Lincoln J. Surgery of the exocrine pancreas. In: Slatter D, ed. Textbook of small animal surgery. Philadelphia: WB Saunders Co., 1993:678-691.

Author Wallace B. Morrison
Consulting Editor Wallace B. Morrison

BASICS

OVERVIEW
Prostate adenocarcinoma is a malignant tumor occurring with equal frequency in castrated and intact male dogs. It is highly metastatic to the regional lymph nodes, lungs, and skeleton (lumbosacral area and pelvis most often).

SIGNALMENT
• Primarily medium-to large-breed, intact or neutered male dogs • Median age on examination, 9-10 years • Rare in cats

SIGNS
• None in some animals • Tenesmus and ribbonlike feces • Stranguria, dysuria, and urinary incontinence • Hind limb lameness, lethargy, and exercise intolerance • Anorexia • Prostatomegaly— firm, asymmetrical, and immobile • Pain in some animals • Sublumbar lymphadenomegaly in some animals

CAUSES AND RISK FACTORS
None identified

DIAGNOSIS

DIFFERENTIAL DIAGNOSIS
• Other primary or metastatic neoplasm • Acute or chronic prostatitis • Benign prostatic hypertrophy • Prostatic cysts

CBC/BIOCHEMISTRY/URINALYSIS
• Inflammatory leukogram • High ALP activity • Hematuria, pyuria, and malignant epithelial cells

OTHER LABORATORY TESTS N/A

IMAGING
• Thoracic and abdominal radiography—pulmonary nodules or diffuse increase in interstitial markings indicate metastatic disease. Sublumbar lymphadenomegaly, mineralization within the prostate, and lytic lesions to the lumbar vertebrae or pelvis are common signs. • Prostatic ultrasonography—focal to multifocal hyperechogenicity with asymmetry and irregular outline of the prostate; intraprostatic mineralization in some animals • Contrast cystography—may help differentiate prostatic disease from urinary bladder disease

OTHER DIAGNOSTIC PROCEDURES
• Prostatic biopsy • Prostatic wash or aspirate—may recover cells with criteria of malignancy. Interpret with caution if inflammation is observed.

TREATMENT
• Prostatectomy if local disease only. Success of prostatectomy depends on the skill of the surgeon and extent of disease.
• Castration may provide temporary decrease in rate of growth or partial remission. Most tumors are not androgen responsive.
• Radiotherapy may palliate bone pain.

MEDICATIONS N/A

DRUGS AND FLUIDS
• Pain relief and supportive care are the main thrust of treatment.
• Stool softeners and high-fiber diet may decrease tenesmus.
• Carboplatin, cisplatin, and doxorubicin are potentially beneficial.

CONTRAINDICATIONS/POSSIBLE INTERACTIONS N/A

FOLLOW-UP

PATIENT MONITORING
Ability to urinate and defecate, pain secondary to skeletal metastases, and quality of life

PREVENTION/AVOIDANCE
Castration does not prevent disease

POSSIBLE COMPLICATIONS
• Urethral obstruction • Metastatic spread to skeleton (lumbar vertebral bodies), lungs, and lymph nodes

EXPECTED COURSE AND PROGNOSIS
• Grave prognosis • Survival, 1-3 months

MISCELLANEOUS

ASSOCIATED CONDITIONS N/A

AGE RELATED FACTORS N/A

ZOONOTIC POTENTIAL N/A

PREGNANCY N/A

ABBREVIATION
ALP = alkaline phosphatase

Reference
Bell FW, et al. Clinical and pathologic features of prostatic adenocarcinoma in sexually intact and castrated dogs: 31 cases (1970 - 1987). J Am Vet Med Assoc 1991:1623-1630
Author Ruthanne Chun
Consulting Editor Wallace B. Morrison

ADENOCARCINOMA, RENAL

BASICS

OVERVIEW
Uncommon (approximately 1% of all reported neoplasms in dogs), highly metastatic, locally invasive, and often bilateral malignant tumor, accounting for most primary renal tumors. Female German shepherd dogs are prone to renal cystadenocarcinoma, a less aggressive disease with a better long-term prognosis than renal adenocarcinoma.

SIGNALMENT
• Renal adenocarcinoma—older dogs; 1.5:1 male to female ratio • Renal cystadenocarcinoma—female German shepherd dogs predominates

SIGNS
• Renal adenocarcinoma—primarily insidious, nonspecific signs such as weight loss, inappetance, lethargy, hematuria, and anemia.
• Renal cystadenocarcinoma—physical examination findings include painless, firm, fibrous lesions of the skin and subcutaneous tissues (nodular dermatofibrosis) and uterine polyps in some animals

CAUSES AND RISK FACTORS
Unknown for both diseases

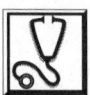

DIAGNOSIS

DIFFERENTIAL DIAGNOSIS
• Other primary neoplasia • Renal adenoma or cyst • Pyelonephritis

CBC/BIOCHEMISTRY/URINALYSIS
• Polycythemia • Anemia • Biochemistry normal or reveals evidence of renal failure
• Proteinuria and microscopic or gross hematuria; findings nonspecific in many animals

OTHER LABORATORY TESTS N/A

IMAGING
• Thoracic radiographs—metastatic disease up to 30% of patients • Abdominal radiographs, intravenous pyelography, ultrasonographic examination of abdomen—to assess extent of local disease and regional lymph nodes

OTHER DIAGNOSTIC PROCEDURES
Renal biopsy for definitive diagnosis

TREATMENT
• Renal adenocarcinoma is often a bilateral disease.
• In a patient with unilateral disease, survival is approximately 6-10 months after nephrectomy.
• Renal cystadenocarcinoma has a much better prognosis, with affected dogs surviving 12 months or longer with no definitive treatment.

MEDICATIONS N/A

DRUGS AND FLUIDS
• Definitive drug therapy for renal adenocarcinoma has not been reported.
• Supportive treatment to patients with renal failure.

CONTRAINDICATIONS/POSSIBLE INTERACTIONS N/A

FOLLOW-UP

PATIENT MONITORING
• Renal failure • Quality of life if bilateral or otherwise nonsurgical disease

PREVENTION/AVOIDANCE N/A

POSSIBLE COMPLICATIONS
Renal failure if bilateral disease

EXPECTED COURSE AND PROGNOSIS
Even if disease is localized, long-term prognosis is poor.

MISCELLANEOUS

ASSOCIATED CONDITIONS
• Hypertrophic osteopathy in some animals
• Renal failure concurrent in some animals
• Nodular dermatofibrosis in some animals with renal cystadenocarcinoma

AGE RELATED FACTORS N/A

ZOONOTIC POTENTIAL N/A

PREGNANCY N/A

Reference
Crow SE. Urinary tract neoplasms in dogs and cats. Compend Cont Ed Small Anim Pract 1985;7:607-617.
Author Ruthanne Chun
Consulting Editor Wallace B. Morrison

ADENOCARCINOMA, SALIVARY GLAND

BASICS

OVERVIEW
Adenocarcinoma of the salivary gland may arise from major (i.e., parotid, mandibular, sublingual, or zygomatic) or minor glands. The parotid gland is most frequently affected. Tumors are locally invasive and regional lymph node metastasis is common; distant metastasis has been reported but may be slow to develop.

SIGNALMENT
• Mean age of affected dogs and cats, 10-12 years • Spaniel dogs may be at relatively higher risk; no additional breeds or sex predilection has been determined.

SIGNS
Physical Examination Findings
Unilateral, firm, painless swelling of the upper neck (mandibular and sublingual), ear base (parotid), upper lip or maxilla (zygomatic), or mucous membrane of lip (accessory or minor salivary tissue)

CAUSES AND RISK FACTORS
Unknown

DIAGNOSIS

DIFFERENTIAL DIAGNOSIS
• Mucocele • Abscess • Lymphosarcoma

CBC/BIOCHEMISTRY/URINALYSIS
Results normal

OTHER LABORATORY TESTS N/A

IMAGING
Regional radiographs are usually normal, but periosteal reaction on adjacent bones or displacement of surrounding structures are observed in some animals.

OTHER DIAGNOSTIC PROCEDURES
• Cytologic examination of aspirate should allow differentiation of salivary adenocarcinoma from mucocele and abscess. • Needle core or wedge biopsy necessary for definitive diagnosis

TREATMENT

• Aggressive surgical resection should be done when possible. Most tumors are, unfortunately, invasive and difficult to excise.
• Radiotherapy resulted in good local control and prolonged survival in three reported cases.
• Chemotherapy for salivary gland adenocarcinoma is largely unreported.
• Clinical experience in a limited number of patients suggests that aggressive local resection (usually histologically incomplete) followed by adjuvant radiation can attain permanent local control and long term survival.

MEDICATIONS

DRUGS AND FLUIDS N/A

CONTRAINDICATIONS/POSSIBLE INTERACTIONS N/A

FOLLOW-UP
Evaluations dictated by tumor growth characteristics, but 3-6 month intervals are reasonable.

MISCELLANEOUS

ASSOCIATED CONDITIONS
The long-term prognosis for salivary gland adenocarcinoma is unknown.

Reference
Carberry CA, Flanders JA, Harvey HJ, et al. Salivary gland tumors in dogs and cats: a literature and case review. J Am Anim Hosp Assoc 1988;24:561-567.
Author James P. Thompson
Consulting Editor Wallace B. Morrison

ADENOCARCINOMA, SKIN (SWEAT GLANDS, SEBACEOUS)

BASICS

OVERVIEW
Malignant growth originating from sebaceous and apocrine sweat glands within the skin

SIGNALMENT
• Sebaceous gland adenocarcinoma occurs rarely in dogs and cats. • Apocrine sweat gland adenocarcinoma is also rare in dogs and cats, but it occurs more frequently in cats than sebaceous gland adenocarcinoma.
• Both tumor types are more common in older patients.

SIGNS
• Sebaceous and apocrine sweat gland tumors appear as a solid, firm raised lesions. They may be ulcerated and bleeding, and inflammation of the surrounding tissue may be seen. • Apocrine sweat gland tumors are often poorly circumscribed and very invasive into underlying tissue.

CAUSES AND RISK FACTORS
Unknown

DIAGNOSIS

DIFFERENTIAL DIAGNOSIS
Any other skin tumor; cellulitis

CBC/BIOCHEMISTRY/URINALYSIS
Normal

OTHER LABORATORY TESTS N/A

IMAGING
Thoracic radiographs and cytologic examination or biopsy of regional lymph nodes at the time of diagnosis required to rule out metastatic disease

OTHER DIAGNOSTIC PROCEDURES
• Histopathologic examination of the tumor essential to confirm the diagnosis • Apocrine sweat gland adenocarcinoma is typically invasive into the underlying stroma and blood vessels. The tumor has poorly demarcated borders and a high mitotic index.

TREATMENT

• Aggressive surgical excision required for treatment of both sebaceous and apocrine sweat gland adenocarcinoma
• It is critical that the entire tissue specimen be evaluated histologically to assess completeness of resection.
• Radiotherapy recommended for local control when complete surgical excision is not possible

MEDICATIONS

DRUGS AND FLUIDS
• Chemotherapy after surgery recommended for apocrine sweat gland adenocarcinoma, particularly in cats.

• Chemotherapuetic agents such as doxorubicin, cyclophosphamide, carboplatin and taxol have been used with variable success.

FOLLOW-UP
• Little is known about the metastatic potential of sebaceous gland adenocarcinoma. Prognosis is good if complete surgical excision is achieved. • Apocrine sweat gland adenocarcinoma is associated with a very guarded prognosis; aggressive surgical resection required for local tumor control; postoperative chemotherapy recommended to delay or prevent development of metastasis.

MISCELLANEOUS

Reference
Carpenter JL, Andrews LK, Holzworth J. Tumors and tumor like lesions. In: Holzworth J, ed. Diseases of the cat. Medicine and surgery.. Philadelphia: WB Saunders, 1987;406-596.
Author Robyn Elmslie
Consulting Editor Wallace B. Morrison

ADENOCARCINOMA, STOMACH, SMALL AND LARGE INTESTINE, RECTAL

BASICS

OVERVIEW
Adenocarcinoma of the stomach, small and large intestine and rectal region is an uncommon tumor arising from the epithelial lining of the gastrointestinal tract. Prognosis is usually poor.

SIGNALMENT
• Middle-aged to old (> 6 years) dogs and cats • Dogs more commonly affected than cats • No breed predisposition

SIGNS

Historical Findings
• Stomach—anorexia, weight loss, vomiting, hematemesis, and melena • Small intestine—vomiting, weight loss, borborygmus, flatulence, and melena • Large intestine and rectum—mucous and blood-tinged feces and tenesmus

Physical Examination Findings
• Stomach—nonspecific • Small intestine—midabdominal mass and in some animals, distended, painful loops of small bowel • Large intestine and rectum—palpable mass per rectum, forming a "napkin ring," or multiple nodular lesions protruding into the colon; bright red blood on feces

CAUSES AND RISK FACTORS
Unknown

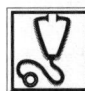

DIAGNOSIS

DIFFERENTIAL DIAGNOSIS
• Foreign body, lymphosarcoma, leiomyoma, leiomyosarcoma, and pancreatitis

CBC/BIOCHEMISTRY/URINALYSIS
• Stomach and small intestine—microcytic, hypochromic anemia • Large intestine and rectum—N/A

OTHER LABORATORY TESTS N/A

IMAGING
• Ultrasound may reveal a thickened stomach or bowel wall or a mass. • Positive contrast radiography may reveal a filling defect (stomach) or intraluminal space-occupying or annular constriction (small bowel). • Large intestine and rectum—double contrast radiography may reveal polypoid or annular space-occupying masses.

OTHER DIAGNOSTIC PROCEDURES
Endoscopic biopsy may be nondiagnostic because the tumors are frequently deep in the mucosal surface; surgical biopsy is frequently required.

TREATMENT
• Surgical resection is the treatment of choice, but surgery is seldom curative.
• Gastric carcinoma is usually nonresectable.
• Small intestinal adenocarcinoma can be removed by resection and anastomosis, but metastasis to regional lymph nodes and the liver is common.
• Large intestine and rectal tumors may occasionally be resected by a pull-through surgical procedure, but metastasis is common. Transcolonic debulking may provide palliation of obstruction.

MEDICATIONS

DRUGS AND FLUIDS
Chemotherapy is usually unsuccessful. This author has observed partial remission in a dog receiving 5-Fluorouracil (200 mg/m^2 IV q7days).

CONTRAINDICATIONS/POSSIBLE INTERACTIONS
• 5-Fluorouracil (5-FU) is lethal to cats and should not be used. Dogs occasionally have seizures.

• Seek advice before initiating treatment if you are unfamiliar with cytotoxic drugs.

CONTRAINDICATIONS/ POSSIBLE INTERACTIONS N/A

FOLLOW-UP
Physical examination and abdominal and thoracic radiographs at 1, 3, 6, 9 and 12 months after surgery

MISCELLANEOUS

ASSOCIATED CONDITIONS N/A

Reference
Theilen GH, Madewell BR. Tumors of the digestive tract. In: Theilen GH, Madewell BR, eds. Veterinary Cancer Medicine. 2nd ed. Philadelphia: Lea & Febiger, 1987.
Author Ralph C. Richardson
Consulting Editor Wallace B. Morrison

ADENOCARCINOMA, THYROID—DOGS

BASICS

DEFINITION
Thyroid adenocarcinoma is a malignant neoplasm arising from the thyroid gland.

Pathophysiology
Usually not functional but highly invasive and metastatic

Systems Affected
• Endocrine/metabolic—thyroid gland and surrounding soft tissue (e.g., esophagus and trachea) • Respiratory—common metastatic sites are lungs and regional lymph nodes • Cardiovascular

Genetics
Unknown

Incidence/Prevalence
• 10-15% of all primary tumors in the head and neck • Reported prevalence up to 1.2-3.7% of all tumors in dogs

Geographic Distribution
More common in areas of endemic goiter secondary to iodine deficiency

SIGNALMENT

Species Dogs

Breed Predilections
Boxers, golden retriever, and beagle reported to be at relatively higher risk

Mean Age and Range
Median age and range variably reported 0-9.6 years (range, 4-18 years)

Predominant Sex None

SIGNS

General Comments
• Characterized by rapid invasive growth and usually diagnosed when disease is advanced • Most tumors (65-70%) unilateral

Historical Findings
• Cervical mass dyspnea, dysphagia, or dysphonia • Less frequently, regurgitation, precaval syndrome, weight loss, and excessive hemorrhage secondary to disseminated intravascular coagulation (DIC) • Hyperthyroidism characterized by polyuria, polydipsia, and weight loss despite a normal-to-high food intake • Hypothyroidism characterized by weakness, lethargy, and poor hair coat

Physical Examination Findings
• Firm, nonpainful, movable or fixed neck mass • About 2/3 of thyroid carcinomas are unilateral.

CAUSES Unknown

RISK FACTORS
• Breed predilection • Geographic areas of endemic goiter caused by iodine deficiency

DIAGNOSIS

DIFFERENTIAL DIAGNOSIS
• Abscess • Granuloma • Salivary mucocele • Metastatic tonsillar squamous cell carcinoma • Lymphosarcoma • Carotid body tumor • Other soft tissue sarcoma

CBC/BIOCHEMISTRY/URINALYSIS
• Results usually normal • Normocytic, normochromic, nonregenerative anemia, and DIC in some animals with advanced disease.

OTHER LABORATORY TESTS
• Measurement of T_4 and T_3 • TSH stimulation if warranted

IMAGING
• Thoracic radiographs to check for metastasis • Cervical radiographs to identify location of the mass, proximal airway, and esophagus before performing a biopsy • Thyroid gland scintigraphy (^{99m}Tc-pertechnetate) imaging to delineate location of the tumor(s), including ectopic tumors and metastases. Radioiodine studies with ^{131}I or ^{125}I provide similar information and can also determine functional status of the tumor.

OTHER DIAGNOSTIC PROCEDURES
• Cytologic examination of fine-needle aspirate of mass to rule out nonthyroid disease; blood contamination is a relatively constant feature because of the vascular nature of thyroid tumors. • Cytologic examination of the regional lymph nodes is done for staging purposes. • Biopsy and histologic evaluation is required for definitive diagnosis. Bleeding can be a problem during biopsy.

GROSS AND HISTOPATHOLOGIC FINDINGS

Gross
• Coarsely multinodular, often with large areas of hemorrhage and necrosis near the center • Poorly encapsulated and local invasion into the wall of the trachea, esophagus, larynx, surrounding lymphatic vessels, and blood vessels

Histopathology
• Subdivided into follicular, papillary, and compact cellular (i.e., solid) types • Mixed patterns (i.e., follicular and solid) most common in dogs • Undifferentiated carcinoma and medullary carcinoma (i.e., malignant neoplasms arising from the parafollicular cells [C cells]) uncommon in dogs

TREATMENT

INPATIENT VERSUS OUTPATIENT
Stable patients can be discharged after surgery or chemotherapy.

ACTIVITY N/A

DIET N/A

CLIENT EDUCATION
Discuss importance of early thyroid tumor detection to improve the prognosis.

SURGICAL CONSIDERATIONS
• Complete surgical excision treatment of choice for freely moveable carcinoma • Examine cervical lymph nodes closely and remove or biopsy if indicated • Carefully inspect the contralateral gland because approximately 33% of thyroid carcinomas are bilateral • Invasive thyroid carcinoma impossible to remove completely but may be debulked and biopsied • Invasive tumor amenable to surgical removal after external beam radiotherapy or systemic chemotherapy in some patients

MEDICATIONS

DRUGS AND FLUIDS
• Doxorubicin (30 mg/M² IV over 20-30 min q3wk for a total of 5 treatments) reported to effect partial regression in about 50% of patients • Maintenance concentration of thyroxin (20-40 mg/kg q24h) has been recommended to suppress pituitary production and release of thyroid stimulating hormone. The theoretical benefit derived from this treatment has not been evaluated in dogs.

CONTRAINDICATIONS
• Compromised myocardial function • Severe myelosuppression

PRECAUTIONS
• Do not exceed doxorubicin cumulative dose of 200 mg/M²—causes hepatic disease and renal insufficiency. • Chemotherapy can be toxic. Seek advice before initiating treatment if you are unfamiliar with cytotoxic drugs.

POSSIBLE INTERACTIONS
Verapamil can potentiate doxorubicin-induced cardiotoxicity; concurrent use should be avoided.

ALTERNATE DRUGS
• Cisplatin (60 mg/M²) has had limited use for managing thyroid carcinoma; further study is warranted. • Radiotherapy has been used for treatment of nonresectable tumors. The efficacy of preoperative versus postoperative radiotherapy has not been determined. • Radioactive iodine (^{131}I) has been used in dogs with hyperfunctioning tumors. The efficacy of this treatment has not been determined.

FOLLOW-UP

PATIENT MONITORING
• Serum calcium concentration is monitored

after bilateral thyroidectomy. Patient with signs of hypocalcemia (i.e., nervousness, irritability, panting, high body temperature, muscle tremors, tetany, pruritis, and convulsions) should receive 10% calcium gluconate IV (1.0-1.5 ml/kg IV over 10-20 min).
• heart by auscultation or ECG • Vitamin D administered orally (dihydrotachysterol) after emergency treatment • Thyroid hormone replacement (i.e., L-thyroxine or sodium levothyroxine) usually required after bilateral thyroidectomy

PREVENTION/AVOIDANCE Unknown

POSSIBLE COMPLICATIONS

From Tumor
Anemia, hypercalcemia, and DIC

From Chemotherapy
• Dilated cardiomyopathy • Nephrotoxicity • Hepatopathy • Myelosuppression • Anorexia • Gastrointestinal toxicity

From Surgery
• Intraoperative hemorrhage • Hypothyroidism • Hypoparathyroidism • Laryngeal paralysis

EXPECTED COURSE AND PROGNOSIS
Factors that have the biggest influence on prognosis include the total tumor volume of the primary tumor, the degree of local invasion, the number and extent of regional lymph node involvement, and the presence of distant metastases. Of dogs with thyroid carcinoma < 20 cm^3, < 20% have metastatasis; of dogs with tumor > 21 cm^3, 75% have metastasis.

MISCELLANEOUS

ASSOCIATED CONDITIONS
Many dogs with thyroid adenocarcinoma develop other primary tumors. Most common are chemodectoma, perianal gland adenoma, mast cell tumor, lipoma, and adrenal adenoma. The syndrome of multiple endocrine neoplasia consisting of medullary carcinoma, pheochromocytoma, and parathyroid hyperplasia has also been reported in dogs.

AGE RELATED FACTORS
See Signalment

ZOONOTIC POTENTIAL None

PREGNANCY
Chemotherapy should not be used in pregnant animals.

SYNONYMS N/A

SEE ALSO N/A

ABBREVIATIONS
DIC = disseminated intravascular coagulation
ECG = electrocardiography
FNA = fine needle aspiration

References

Capen CC. Tumors of the endocrine glands. In: Moulton JE, ed. Tumors in domestic animals. 3rd ed. Berkeley, CA: University of California Press, 1990;583-602.

Loar AS. Canine thyroid tumors. In: Kirk RW, ed. Current veterinary therapy XI, Philadelphia: WB Saunders, 1986;1033-1039,.

Susaneck, SJ. Thyroid tumors in the dog. Compend Contin Ed Pract Vet 1983;5:35-40.

Jeglum KA, Whereat A. Chemotherapy of canine thyroid carcinoma. Compend Contin Ed Pract Vet 1983;5:96-98.

Author Stanley L. Marks
Consulting Editor Wallace B. Morrison

AFLATOXIN TOXICITY

BASICS

OVERVIEW

Aflatoxicosis occurs in dogs as a result of exposure to aflatoxin produced by Aspergillus flavus, Aspergillus parasiticus, or Penicillium puberulum. The liver is the target organ. The toxicity is rarely reported but possible in hot, humid climates where grain-based dog foods are exposed to moisture, or when contaminated grains are used in the production of feeds.

SIGNALMENT

• Dogs—young males and pregnant females probably more susceptible • Not reported in cats

SIGNS

• Clinical signs and lesions are dose- and time-dependent. • Sudden death • Anorexia • Weight loss • Icterus • Ascites • Hemorrhage

CAUSES AND RISK FACTORS

• Grain-based feeds contaminated with Aspergillus flavus, Aspergillus parasiticus, or Penicillium puberulum • Feeds exposed to elements with obvious mold spoilage • Outside dogs more at risk

DIAGNOSIS

DIFFERENTIAL DIAGNOSIS

Other causes of subacute to chronic liver disease and associated disseminated intravascular coagulopathy. No differentiating tests.

CBC/BIOCHEMISTRY/URINALYSIS

• High ALT • High SAP • Hypoalbu-minemia • High blood ammonia • Hyper-bilirubinemia • Bilirubinuria

OTHER LABORATORY TESTS

• Coagulation profile—PT and PTT prolonged (reduction in absolute concentration or reduction in activated liver produced clotting factors) • Thrombocytopenia • High FDP • Hyperfibrinogenemia

IMAGING N/A

OTHER DIAGNOSTIC PROCEDURES

Liver biopsy not definitive

GROSS AND HISTOPATHOLOGIC FINDINGS

• Fatty change • Icterus • Ascites • Mottled liver • Biliary proliferation • Hepatocellular necrosis • Cholestasis • Cholecystic edema

TREATMENT

• Aim treatment to reduce stress to liver. • Feed high quality protein diet. • Include dietary source of glucose (eg, Karyo syrup).

MEDICATIONS

DRUGS AND FLUIDS

Heparin if animal has disseminated intravascular coagulation

CONTRAINDICATIONS/ POSSIBLE INTERACTIONS

• Avoid drugs metabolized by the liver for activation. • Avoid exposure to organophosphates or strong pyrethroid insecticides.

FOLLOW-UP

PREVENTION/AVOIDANCE

• Avoid feed that is obviously moldy. • Store feed in clean, dry area before using. • Clean feed dispensers and feed bowls regularly.

POSSIBLE COMPLICATIONS

Impaired liver function or failure

EXPECTED COURSE AND PROGNOSIS

Poor prognosis even with treatment

MISCELLANEOUS

ASSOCIATED CONDITIONS

Nephropathy (liver-Induced)

PREGNANCY

Indirect effects on uterus

SEE ALSO

• Hepatorenal Syndrome • Poisoning (Intoxication)

ABBREVIATIONS

• ALP = alkaline phosphatase • ALT = alanine transaminase • FDP = fibrin degradation products • PTT = partial thromboplastin time • PT = prothrombin time

Reference

Nicholson SS. Mycotoxicosis. In: Kirk RW, ed. Current veterinary therapy IX. small animal practice. Philadephia: WB Saunders, 1986:225-226.

Author George H. D'Andrea
Consulting Editor Gary Osweiler

BASICS

OVERVIEW
Ameloblastoma is an oral tumor of odonto-genic (i.e., tooth structure) origin and known as adamantinoma in old literature. Most are benign, but malignant (i.e., highly invasive) forms occur rarely.

SIGNALMENT
• Middle-aged and old dogs • Uncommon in dogs compared with epulides • Rare in cats

SIGNS N/A

CAUSES AND RISK FACTORS N/A

DIAGNOSIS

DIFFERENTIAL DIAGNOSIS
• Epilus • Malignant oral tumor • Gingival hyperplasia

CBC/BIOCHEMISTRY/URINALYSIS
Results normal

OTHER LABORATORY TESTS N/A

IMAGING
Radiography of the skull often shows bone Iysis deep to the superficial mass.

OTHER DIAGNOSTIC PROCEDURES
Deep tissue biopsy necessary for definitive diagnosis

TREATMENT
Radical surgical excision with at least 1-2 cm margins to insure complete excision

MEDICATIONS

DRUGS AND FLUIDS N/A

CONTRAINDICATIONS/POSSIBLE/ INTERACTIONS N/A

FOLLOW-UP
Careful oral examination at 1, 3, 6, 9, and 12 months after definitive treatment

MISCELLANEOUS
Many histologic subtypes exist and all have similar invasive behavior

Reference
Richardson RC, Jones MA, Elliott GS. Oral neoplasms in the dog: a diagnostic and therapeutic dilemma. Comp Cont Ed Pract Vet 1983;5:441-446.

Author Wallace B. Morrison
Consulting Editor Wallace B. Morrison

AMYLOIDOSIS

 BASICS

DEFINITION

Amyloidosis is a group of conditions of diverse cause that are characterized by extracellular deposition of insoluble fibrillar proteins (amyloid) in organs and tissues compromising their normal function.

Pathophysiology

Patients usually are affected by systemic reactive amyloidosis. Tissue deposits contain amyloid A protein (AA), which is a fragment of an acute phase reactant called serum amyloid A protein (SAA).

Phases of Amyloid Deposition
• Predeposition phase—SAA concentration is high but without amyloid deposits. Colchicine administration may prevent development of the disease.
• Deposition phase (rapid portion)—Amyloid deposits increase rapidly. Colchicine administration delays but does not prevent tissue deposition of amyloid. Dimethylsulfoxide (DMSO) may promote resolution of amyloid deposits and a persistent decrease in SAA concentration.
• Deposition phase (plateau portion)—net deposition of amyloid changes little. Neither DMSO or colchicine is beneficial.
• Clinical signs usually are associated with amyloid deposition in the kidneys. In dogs, amyloid deposits usually are found in the glomeruli leading to proteinuria and nephrotic syndrome. In cats, amyloid deposits usually are found in the medullary interstitium, but may occur in glomeruli. Some Chinese shar pei dogs with familial amyloidosis have medullary amyloidosis without glomerular involvement.

Systems Affected
• Renal/urologic—predilection for renal AA deposition. Liver, spleen, adrenal glands, pancreas, and gastrointestinal tract may be affected.

Genetics

No genetic involvement has been clearly established, but familial amyloidosis occurs in Chinese shar pei dogs and in Abyssinian, Oriental shorthair, and Siamese cats.

Incidence/Prevalence

Uncommon disease in domestic animals occurring most commonly in dogs. Rare in cats, with the exception of the Abyssinian breed.

Geographic Distribution N/A

SIGNALMENT

Species Dogs and cats

Breed Predilections
• Dogs—Chinese shar pei, beagle, collie, pointer, and walker hound. German shepherd dog and mixed breeds are at lower risk.
• Cats—Abyssinian, Oriental shorthair, and Siamese

Mean Age and Range
• Most affected dogs and cats are more than 5 years old
• Dogs—mean age at diagnosis 9 years, range 1-15 years
• Cats—mean age at diagnosis 7 years, range 1-17 years
• Prevalence increases with age
• Abyssinian cats—range, less than 1 to 17 years
• Chinese Shar pei dogs are usually less than 6 years of age when signs of renal failure develop; range, 1.5 to 6 years
• Siamese cats with familial amyloidosis of the liver and thyroid gland usually develop signs of liver disease 1-4 years old.

Predominant Sex

For dogs and Abyssinian cats, females appear to be at a slightly higher risk (< 2:1)

SIGNS

General Comments
• Clinical signs depend on the organs affected, the amount of amyloid present, and the reaction of the affected organs to amyloid deposits.
• Clinical signs usually caused by renal involvement. Occasionally, hepatic involvement may cause signs in Chinese shar pei dogs and Oriental shorthair and Siamese cats.

Historical Findings
• No clear history of a predisposing disorder in most (~ 75%) cases
• Anorexia, lethargy, polyuria and polydipsia, weight loss, vomiting, and diarrhea (uncommon)
• Ascites and peripheral edema in animals with nephrotic syndrome
• Chinese shar pei dogs may have a history of previous episodic joint swelling and high fever that resolves spontaneously within a few days.

Physical Examination Findings
• Signs related to renal failure—oral ulceration, emaciation, vomiting, and dehydration. Kidneys usually small, firm, and irregular in affected cats. They may be small, normal-sized, or slightly large in affected dogs.
• Signs of nephrotic syndrome (e.g,. ascites and subcutaneous edema)
• Signs related to the primary inflammatory or neoplastic disease process
• Thromboembolic phenomena up to 40% of affected dogs. Signs vary with the location of the thrombus. Patients may develop pulmonary thromboembolism (dyspnea) or iliac or femoral artery thromboembolism (caudal paresis).
• Chinese shar pei dogs and Oriental shorthair and Siamese cats may have signs of hepatic disease (e.g., jaundice, cachexia, and spontaneous hepatic rupture with intraperitoneal bleeding).

CAUSES
• Chronic inflammation—systemic mycoses (e.g., blastomycosis and coccidioidomycosis),

chronic bacterial infection (e.g., osteomyelitis, bronchopneumonia, pleuritis, steatitis, pyometra, pyelonephritis, chronic suppurative dermatitis, chronic suppurative arthritis, chronic peritonitis, nocardiosis, and chronic stomatitis), dirofilariasis, and immune-mediated disease (e.g., systemic lupus erythematosus)
• Neoplasia (e.g., lymphosarcoma, plasmacytoma, multiple myeloma, mammary tumor, and testicular tumor)
• Familial (e.g., Chinese shar pei and beagle; Abyssinian, Siamese, and Oriental shorthair cats).
• Others—cyclic hematopoiesis in gray collie breed

RISK FACTORS
• Chronic inflammation or neoplasia
• Family history in certain breeds

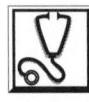 **DIAGNOSIS**

DIFFERENTIAL DIAGNOSIS
• In dogs, glomerulonephritis is the main differential diagnosis. Proteinuria tends to be more severe in dogs with glomerular amyloidosis than those with glomerulonephritis (see below).
• In cats and Chinese shar pei dogs with medullary amyloidosis, consider other causes of medullary renal disease (e.g., pyelonephritis and chronic interstitial disease)
Renal biopsy necessary for definitive diagnosis

CBC/BIOCHEMISTRY/URINALYSIS
• Nonregenerative anemia is found in some dogs with amyloid-induced renal failure
• Hypercholesterolemia (> 85% of dogs), azotemia (> 70% of dogs), hypoalbuminemia (70% of dogs), hyperphosphatemia (> 60% of dogs), hypocalcemia (50% of dogs), and metabolic acidosis may be observed. Hypercholesterolemia is a common finding in cats with renal disorders (> 70% of cats with renal disease in one study) and does not reliably predict glomerular disease.
• Hypoproteinemia is more common than hyperproteinemia (24% versus 8.5%) in dogs. Hyperproteinemia resulting from hyperglobulinemia is common in cats.
• Proteinuria with an inactive sediment is common in dogs. Proteinuria mild or absent in animals with medullary amyloidosis without glomerular involvement (most mixed-breed cats, at least 25 % of Abyssinian cats, and at least 33 % of Chinese shar pei dogs). Isosthenuria, and hyaline, granular, and waxy casts are found in some patients.

OTHER LABORATORY TESTS
• Proteinuria can be quantified by 24-hour urinary protein excretion or urine protein:creatinine ratio.
• Proteinuria tends to be more severe in patients with amyloidosis than those with glomerulonephritis.

IMAGING

Abdominal Radiographic Findings
• Kidneys usually small in affected cats.
• Kidneys small, normal-sized or large in affected dogs

Abdominal Ultrasonographic Findings
Kidneys usually hyperechoic and small in affected cats, but may be small, normal-sized, or large in affected dogs.

OTHER DIAGNOSTIC PROCEDURES
• Renal biopsy is necessary to differentiate amyloidosis from glomerulonephritis. In dogs other than the Chinese shar pei, amyloidosis is primarily a glomerular disease and diagnosis can be obtained by renal cortical biopsy. In most domestic cats, some Abyssinian cats, and some Chinese shar pei dogs, medullary amyloidosis can occur without glomerular involvement. In this setting, renal cortical biopsy does not reveal amyloidosis, and the diagnosis cannot be made unless sufficient medullary tissue is obtained.

GROSS AND HISTOPATHOLOGIC FINDINGS
• Small kidneys are found in cats. Kidneys are small, normal, or large in dogs.
• Amyloid deposits have a homogeneous, eosinophilic appearance when stained by hematoxylin and eosin and viewed by conventional light microscopy. They demonstrate green birefringence after Congo red staining when viewed under polarized light. Evaluation of Congo red-stained sections before and after permanganate oxidation permits a presumptive diagnosis of AA amyloidosis versus other types because AA amyloidosis loses its Congo red affinity after permanganate oxidation.

TREATMENT

INPATIENT VERSUS OUTPATIENT
• Patients with chronic renal failure and dehydration should be hospitalized for initial medical management.
• Stable patients and patients with asymptomatic proteinuria can be managed as outpatients.

ACTIVITY
• Normal

DIET
• Patients with chronic renal failure have a diet restricted in phosphorus and moderately restricted in protein.
• Patients with hypertension should be fed a sodium-restricted diet.

CLIENT EDUCATION
• Discuss progression of the disease.
• Discuss familial predisposition in susceptible breeds.
• Discuss potential complications (eg, hypertension and thromboembolism).

SURGICAL CONSIDERATIONS N/A

MEDICATIONS

DRUG AND FLUIDS
• Underlying inflammatory and neoplastic processes should be identified and treated if possible.
• Dehydration should be corrected with 0.9% NaCl solution or lactated Ringer's solution. Patients with severe metabolic acidosis may require bicarbonate supplementation (see Acidosis, Metabolic).
• Renal failure should be managed according to the principles of conservative medical treatment (see Renal Failure, Acute and Chronic).
• Patients with hypertension should have blood pressure normalized (see Hypertension, Systemic).
• Patients with thromboembolic syndrome or nephrotic syndrome caused by glomerular amyloidosis usually have a low plasma concentration of antithrombin III. Heparin therefore is relatively ineffective in these patients. A low dosage of aspirin (0.5 mg/kg q12h) has been suggested for dogs with glomerular disease. This low dosage is as effective in preventing platelet aggregation as is 10 mg/kg q24h.
• DMSO helps amyloidosis by solubilizing amyloid fibrils, reducing serum concentration of SAA, and reducing interstitial inflammation and fibrosis in the affected kidneys. DMSO may cause lens opacification in dogs. Perivascular inflammation and local thrombosis can occur if undiluted DMSO is administered intravenously. Subcutaneous administration of undiluted DMSO may be painful. The authors have used 90% DMSO diluted 1:4 with sterile water subcutaneously at a dosage of 90 mg/kg three times per week in dogs. Whether DMSO is beneficial in the treatment of renal amyloidosis in dogs remains controversial..
• Colchicine impairs the release of SAA from hepatocytes. Colchicine prevents development of amyloidosis in humans with familial Mediterranean fever (a familial amyloidosis) and stabilizes renal function in patients with nephrotic syndrome but without overt renal failure. There is no evidence that it is beneficial once the patient develops renal failure. Colchicine may cause vomiting, diarrhea, and idiosyncratic neutropenia in dogs.

CONTRAINDICATIONS
• Avoid use of nephrotoxic drugs (e.g., aminoglycosides).

PRECAUTIONS
• The dosage of drugs excreted by the kidneys may need to be adjusted in patients with renal failure.
• Nonsteroidal antiinflammatory drugs should be used cautiously in patients with medullary amyloidosis because they can decrease renal blood flow when used in presence of dehydration.

POSSIBLE INTERACTIONS None

ALTERNATE DRUGS None

FOLLOW-UP

PATIENT MONITORING
Appetite and activity level daily by the owner; body weight weekly
• Serum albumin, creatinine, and BUN concentrations every 2-6 months in stable patients
• Degree of proteinuria can be serially assessed by urine protein/creatinine ratio

PREVENTION/AVOIDANCE
• Affected animals should not be used for breeding.

POSSIBLE COMPLICATIONS
• Renal failure
• Nephrotic syndrome
• Systemic hypertension
• Hepatic rupture causing hemorrhage
• Thromboembolic disease

EXPECTED COURSE AND PROGNOSIS
• Amyloidosis is a progressive disease and it is usually advanced at the time of diagnosis. Survival for dogs with glomerular amyloidosis varied from 3 to 20 months in one study, although some dogs may occasionally live longer. Cats with renal failure because of amyloidosis usually survive less than a year. Mildly affected cats, however, may not develop renal failure and have an almost normal life expectancy.

MISCELLANEOUS

ASSOCIATED CONDITIONS
• Urinary tract infection
• Polyarthritis in Chinese shar pei

AGE- RELATED FACTORS N/A

ZOONOTIC POTENTIAL N/A

PREGNANCY
• High risk in affected animals

SYNONYMS
• None

SEE ALSO
• Renal Failure, Acute and Chronic
• Glomerulonephritis
• Nephrotic Syndrome
• Proteinuria

ABBREVIATIONS
AA = amyloid A protein
SAA = serum amyloid A protein
DMSO = dimethylsulfoxide

References
DiBartola SP. Renal amyloidosis. In Canine and feline urology. Osborne CA, Low D, Finco DR, editors. 2nd ed. Philadelphia, WB Saunders. In press.
DiBartola SP, Tarr MJ, Webb DM et al. Renal Amyloidosis in related Chinese shar pei dogs. J Am Vet Med Assoc 1990, 197:483-487.
Authors Helio Autran de Morais and Stephen P. DiBartola
Consulting Editors Larry G. Adams and Carl A. Osborne

ANAL SAC DISORDERS

BASICS

OVERVIEW
• Anal sac disorders of dogs can be divided into three types: impaction, sacculitis, and abscesses. All probably represent various stages of the same disease process. • Anal sac disorders are rare in cats. Impaction is noted on occasion.

SIGNALMENT
• No age or sex predispositions. • Small breed dogs, including miniature poodles, toy poodles, and chihuahuas are reportedly predisposed.

SIGNS
• Scooting • Tenesmus • Perianal pruritus • Tail chasing • Perianal discharge if abscess ruptures • Behavioral changes • Pyotraumatic dermatitis

CAUSES AND RISK FACTORS
• Unknown, but possible predisposing factors include chronically soft feces, recent diarrhea, excessive glandular secretions, and poor muscle tone. • Retained secretions may lead to infection and abscessation.

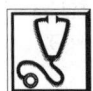

DIAGNOSIS

DIFFERENTIAL DIAGNOSIS
• Anal sac neoplasia may also cause erythema and swelling of the perineum. • Perianal pruritus may be caused by food hypersensitivity, flea allergy dermatitis, atopy, tapeworms, tail fold pyoderma, and seborrheic skin disorders affecting the perineum. • Anal sac abscesses need to be differentiated from perianal fistulas.

CBC/BIOCHEMISTRY/URINALYSIS
N/A

OTHER LABORATORY TESTS N/A

IMAGING N/A

OTHER DIAGNOSTIC PROCEDURES
• The history and examination of the anal sacs by digital palpation will establish the diagnosis. If easily palpated through the skin, they are considered enlarged. • On expression, normal anal sacs fluid is clear or pale yellow-brown. Thick, pasty brown secretion is characteristic of impaction, and creamy yellow or thin green-yellow secretion is often seen in animals with anal sacculitis.
• Abscessed anal sacs are often associated with a red-brown exudate, fever, swelling, and erythema over the anal sacs. Ruptured anal sacs will have a discharging sinus.
• Cytology of anal sac contents can help establish whether infection is present based on the number of leukocytes and bacteria.
• Bacterial culture and sensitivity may be helpful in animals with chronic or recurrent anal sac infections.

TREATMENT
• Expressing the contents is indicated to treat anal sac impaction or sacculitis.
• Instilling an antibiotic/corticosteroid ointment into infected anal sacs is helpful.

• If not already present, drainage should be established in abscessed anal sacs. These should be cleaned and flushed.
• If anal sacs abscess recurrently, anal sac excision should be considered.

MEDICATIONS

DRUGS AND FLUIDS
Systemic and topical antibiotics are indicated to treat anal sac abscesses.

CONTRAINDICATIONS/POSSIBLE INTERACTIONS N/A

FOLLOW-UP
Anal sac abscesses should be examined after three to seven days of therapy.

MISCELLANEOUS

Reference
Burrows CF, Ellison GW. Recto-anal diseases. In: Textbook of veterinary internal medicine. 3rd ed. Ettinger SJ, ed. Philadelphia: WB Saunders, 1989;1570-1572.
Author Jon D. Plant
Consulting Editor Lowell Ackerman

ANEMIA, APLASTIC (APLASTIC PANCYTOPENIA)

BASICS

OVERVIEW
• Also called aplastic pancytopenia • Uncommon cause of pancytopenia in dogs and cats • Mechanisms unknown, but immune mechanisms are often suspected • May be caused or exacerbated by hormonal imbalance, previous bone marrow injury, or genetic predisposition

SIGNALMENT
Occurs in dogs and cats

SIGNS
• Lethargy or pallor due to anemia • Petechial hemorrhage or mucosal bleeding, hematuria, hemoptysis, melena due to thrombocytopenia • Repeated febrile episodes, or frequent or persistent infections due to leukopenia

CAUSES AND RISK FACTORS N/A

DIAGNOSIS

DIFFERENTIAL DIAGNOSIS
• Infectious and toxic agents • Proliferative and infiltrative diseases of the bone marrow • Differentiation of these conditions is discussed in greater detail in the "Pancytopenia" chapter.

CBC/BIOCHEMISTRY/URINALYSIS
• Pancytopenia with mature erythrocytes, neutrophils, and platelets • Severe, normocytic, normochromic anemia with little or no polychromasia and anisocytosis • Reticulocyte count is usually low. • Severe leukopenia and fully segmented or hypersegmented neutrophils • Variable thrombocytopenia with small or normal-sized platelets

OTHER LABORATORY TESTS
• Tests to eliminate causes of pancytopenia (e.g., ehrlichiosis, feline leukemia virus • Tests for antibodies against RBC (e.g., Coombs' test), WBC, and platelets • Tests for other immune-mediated diseases (e.g., antinuclear antibody [ANA] titer for systemic lupus erythematosus)

IMAGING N/A

OTHER DIAGNOSTIC PROCEDURES
Bone marrow aspiration is difficult to perform. Bone marrow aspirate and punch biopsies reveal hypocellularity with few hematopoietic elements and abundant fat.

TREATMENT
Provide supportive therapy appropriate to the clinical situation. This may include aggressive antibiotic therapy, blood transfusion, or transfusion of platelet-rich plasma.

MEDICATIONS

DRUGS AND FLUIDS
• Treatment has been characterized by a variety of treatment approaches and responses. Glucocorticoids and other immunosuppressive agents, anabolic steroids, and colony-stimulating factors have been used alone or in combination.
• Therapy is often unsuccessful. When it is successful, therapy often must be prolonged and response is sometimes transient.

CONTRAINDICATIONS/POSSIBLE INTERACTIONS
Patients' compromised immune status precludes the use of glucocorticoids and other immunosuppressive drugs in most cases.

When their use is absolutely necessary, they should be administered with extreme care.

FOLLOW-UP
• Monitor patients for development of lethargy, fever, and hemorrhage. These may represent recurrence of anemia, leukopenia, and thrombocytopenia, respectively. • Perform daily physical examinations, with special attention to lymph node palpation and body temperature, and periodic CBC.
• Obtain CBC on a daily, biweekly, or weekly basis. Frequency depends on the degree to which different cell types and platelets are decreased, the age and general physical condition of the patient, and the underlying cause of the pancytopenia. • Recovery, if it occurs, may be noted within one month, or it may take several months.

MISCELLANEOUS

SEE ALSO Pancytopenia

ABBREVIATIONS
RBC = red blood cells
WBC = white blood cells

Reference

Tvedten H. Erythrocyte disorders. In: Willard MD, Tvedten H, Turnwald GH, eds. Small animal clinical diagnosis by laboratory methods. 2nd ed. Philadelphia: WB Saunders, 1994:31-51.

Author Ronald D. Tyler
Consulting Editor Alan H. Rebar

ANEMIA, HEINZ BODY

 BASICS

OVERVIEW
• Hemolytic anemia resulting from RBC inclusions called Heinz bodies, which are clumps of oxidized, denatured hemoglobin that cause splenic entrapment or lysis of RBC • Caused by ingestion or administration of chemical or dietary oxidants • New methylene blue stain used to identify Heinz bodies • Condition sometimes accompanied by methemoglobinemia • Treatment includes removing the offending oxidant and providing supportive care.

SIGNALMENT
• More common in cats, which have oxidant-sensitive hemoglobin • No sex, breed, or age disposition

SIGNS

Historical Findings
• Exposure to oxidant drug, plant, or chemical • Sudden onset of weakness, anorexia, and fever • Reddish brown urine (hemoglobinuria), if anemia severe

Physical Examination Findings
• Pale or icteric mucous membranes • Hemoglobinemia and hemoglobinuria, if anemia severe • Cyanosis, if concurrent methemoglobinemia

CAUSES AND RISK FACTORS
• Acetaminophen (cats) • Phenacetin (cats) • Phenazopyridine • Methylene blue • Onions (raw, cooked, or dehydrated) • Vitamin K_3 (not vitamin K_1) • Zinc toxicity • D, L-methionine (cats) • Benzocaine (topical) • Propylene glycol, some diets, diabetes, and other systemic diseases can cause Heinz bodies in cats, but oxidation is not severe enough to cause hemolytic anemia.

 DIAGNOSIS

DIFFERENTIAL DIAGNOSIS
Other causes of regenerative, hemolytic anemia (e.g., immune-mediated, RBC organisms)

CBC/BIOCHEMISTRY/URINALYSIS
• PCV and reticulocyte counts indicate regenerative, mild to severe anemia. (Remember, not all cats with Heinz bodies have hemolytic anemia.) • Blood smear—Heinz bodies may be visible as pale, spherical inclusions that protrude from RBC. • Dogs have fragmented RBC and eccentrocytes. • Supravital new methylene blue stain—Heinz bodies stain blue for easy visibility and quantitation. Heinz bodies can be present in up to 100% of RBC. In dogs, Heinz bodies usually appear small and multiple. In cats, they are single and large. Normal cats have Heinz bodies in < 5% of RBC.

OTHER LABORATORY TESTS
• Serum zinc concentration, if indicated • Methemoglobin test, if animal is cyanotic

IMAGING N/A

OTHER DIAGNOSTIC PROCEDURES
N/A

 TREATMENT

• Identify and remove the source of the oxidant (may be enough for recovery).
• Provide supportive care for anemia (e.g., transfusion, oxygen, and quiet).

MEDICATIONS

DRUGS AND FLUIDS

• For acetaminophen toxicity—N-acetylcysteine (140 mg/kg q8h PO or IV)
• For acetaminophen toxicity—sodium sulfate (50 mg/kg q8h IV)
• For methemoglobinemia—methylene blue (1 mg/kg IV once)

CONTRAINDICATIONS/POSSIBLE INTERACTIONS

Methylene blue is an oxidant in high doses. Use with caution.

FOLLOW-UP

• Monitor PCV, reticulocytes, and percentage of Heinz bodies. • Document disappearance of Heinz bodies and regeneration of RBC. • Counsel clients on potential causes of the disorder and how to avoid exposing their pets. • Prognosis is good, once the hemolytic crisis is over.

MISCELLANEOUS

ABBREVIATIONS

RBC = red blood cells
PCV = packed cell volume

Reference

Weiser MG. Erythrocyte responses and disorders. In: Ettinger SJ, ed. Textbook of veterinary internal medicine. Philadelphia: WB Saunders, 1989:2145-2180.
Author Mary M. Christopher
Consulting Editor Alan H. Rebar

ANEMIA, IMMUNE MEDIATED

BASICS

DEFINITION
Accelerated destruction/removal of RBCs due to anti-RBC antibodies with or without complement.

Pathophysiology
• Anti-RBC antibodies are formed against normal (primary IMHA) or altered (secondary IMHA) RBC membrane antigens. Infectious organisms, exposure of previously unexposed antigens, or adsorption of preformed antigen-antibody complexes to the RBC membrane can alter RBC membrane antigens. Antibodies can be warm type (reactive at body temperature, usually IgG) or cold type (reactive at subnormal body temperature, usually IgM). • Immunoglobulin (IgG or IgM, with or without complement) is deposited on the RBC membrane, causing either direct intravascular hemolysis, intravascular agglutination of RBC, or accelerated removal by the reticuloendothelial system in the spleen and/or liver (extravascular hemolysis). Intravascular hemolysis occurs when adsorbed antibodies (usually IgG) activate complement. In vivo agglutination of RBC occurs when IgM or high titers of IgG molecules cause bridging of RBC; the removal of the RBC occurs in the spleen and/or liver, and is considered a type of extravascular hemolysis. • There is a form of nonregenerative IMHA believed to be caused by immune-mediated destruction of RBC precursors in the bone marrow.

Systems Affected
• Hemic/Lymphatic/Immune • Hepatobiliary—hemolysis leads to hyperbilirubinemia and icterus when hepatic function is overwhelmed; hypoxia may result in centrilobular necrosis • Cardiovascular—hypoxia leads to tachycardia; low blood viscosity and turbulent blood flow cause low grade heart murmurs. High output heart failure with chronic anemia • Respiratory—hypoxia causes tachypnea • Renal/urologic—hypoxia causes renal tubular necrosis • Skin/Exocrine—cold-type IMHA may cause necrosis of extremeties and ear tips due to capillary sludging

Genetics
Isolated families of dogs have been documented to be affected (Viszla, Scottish terrier), but no genetic basis has been established.

Incidence/Prevalence
Unknown

Geographic Distribution
Secondary IMHA may have an increased prevalence in areas endemic to associated infectious diseases.

SIGNALMENT
Species Dogs affected more than cats.

Breed Predilections
Old English sheepdog, cocker spaniel, poodle, Irish setter, English springer spaniel, collie

Mean Age and Range
Mean age 6.4 years; range 1-13 years.

Predominant Sex Females

SIGNS

General Comments
• The remaining discussion will focus on primary IMHA. • Aspects of the secondary causes of IMHA are covered in their respective chapters.

Historical Findings
Collapse, weakness, lethargy, anorexia, exercise intolerance, dyspnea, tachypnea, vomiting, diarrhea, occasionally polyuria/polydipsia.

Physical Examination Findings
• Pale mucous membranes, tachycardia, tachypnea • Splenomegaly, hepatomegaly • Icterus, pigmenturia (hemoglobin or bilirubin) • Fever, lymphadenomegaly • Systolic murmur, S3 gallop • Petechia, ecchymoses, or melena may be present with concurrent thrombocytopenia or DIC. • Skin lesions may be present with cold type IMHA. • Other systemic signs may be present (e.g., joint pain, glomerulonephritis) if IMHA is part of SLE.

CAUSES

Primary IMHA (normal RBC membrane antigens)
• Autoimmune hemolytic anemia • Systemic lupus erythematosus • Neonatal isoerytholysis • Dysregulated immune system (e.g., depressed suppressor T cell activity, high production of immunoglobulins) • Shared antigenic determinants (e.g., infectious agents, drugs) • Idiopathic

Secondary IMHA (altered RBC membrane antigens)
• Infectious causes (e.g., Hemobartonella, Babesia, Leptospirosis, Ehrlichia, feline leukemia virus, other viral agents) • Exposure of previously unexposed antigens • Microangiopathic hemolytic anemia (e.g., heartworm diease, vascular or gastrointestinal neoplasia, vasculitis, DIC) • Adsorption of antigen-antibody complexes to RBC Membrane • Drugs (e.g., sulfa drugs, cephalosporins, heparin, quinidine, propylthiouracil, methimazole) • Type III hypersensitvity reactions (Arthus reaction)

RISK FACTORS N/A

DIAGNOSIS

DIFFERENTIAL DIAGNOSIS

Dogs
• Hemorrhage • Pyruvate kinase deficiency • Phosphofructokinase deficiency • Heinz body anemia (onions, toxins) • Zinc toxicity (pennies) • Splenic torsion • Chronic progressive hepatitis in Bedlington terriers

Cats
• Hemorrhage • Heinz body anemia (propylene glycol, methylene blue, topical benzocaine) • Acetaminophen toxicity • Severe hypophosphatemia • Methermoglobin reductase deficiency • congenital feline porphyria • Cytauxzoonosis

CBC/BIOCHEMISTRY/URINALYSIS
•CBC: anemia, high MCV (3-5 days post hemolytic episode), spherocytes, anisocytosis, polychromasia, nucleated red blood cells, leukocytosis with neutrophilic left shift • Serum Biochemistry: hyperbilirubinemia, hemoglobinemia, elevated ALT • Urinalysis: hemoglobinuria, bilirubinuria

OTHER LABORATORY TEST
• Positive direct antiglobulin (Coombs) test (titer >/= 1:64)—positive in 60% of IMHA cases • In-saline spontaneous autoagglutination • Reticulocytosis-absolute count > 60,000 (dogs), > 50,000 (cats) • Thrombocytopenia with Evan's syndrome • Elevated partial thromboplastin and prothrombin time with DIC • Positive anti-nuclear antibody titer with SLE • Positive serologic titers for infectious causes • Evidence of hematologic parasites on capillary blood smears • Increased RBC distribution width • Increased RBC osmotic fragility (may be useful in cats)

IMAGING
• Radiographs: Hepatomegaly, splenomegaly. Thorax usually within normal limits; may see evidence of pulmonary thromboembolism, cardiomegaly or evidence of heart failure if chronic anemia. • Echocardiography: Generalized cardiomegaly, eccentric hypertrophy and hyperdynamic state with chronic anemia • Abdominal Ultrasonography: Hepatomegaly, splenomegaly; liver and spleen can be mottled and hyper- or hypoechoic

OTHER DIAGNOSTIC PROCEDURES
• Bone marrow aspirate usually reveals hyperplasia of the erythroid seres; with nonregenerative IMHA may see maturation arrest or decreased erythroid precursors; with chronic IMHA, may see myelofibrosis

GROSS AND HISTOPATHOLOGIC FINDINGS
• Hepatosplenomegaly • Splenic and hepatic extramedullary hematopoeisis • Reactive lymphadenomegaly • Signs of congestive heart failure (e.g., pulmonary edema, cardiomegaly, hepatic congestion), pulmonary embolism, DIC

TREATMENT

INPATIENT VS. OUTPATIENT
• Inpatient during the acute hemolytic crisis. Outpatient when the PCV has stabilized,

ongoing hemolysis has been controlled, and clinical signs of anemia have resolved.
• Complications such as DIC, PTE, thrombocytopenia, gastrointestinal bleeding, heart failure, and the need for multiple transfusions indicate the need for hospitalization.
• Chronic, low grade, extrvascular hemolysis can be treated on an outpatient basis if the patient is not exhibiting clinical signs secondary to anemia

ACTIVITY
Cage rest until stable

DIET N/A

CLIENT EDUCATION
• IMHA and its complications (e.g., DIC, PTE) can be fatal.
• Life-long therapy may be needed; and the disease may recur
• Side effects of therapy may be severe

SURGICAL CONSIDERATIONS
• Splenectomy can be considered if medical management fails to control the disease after 4-6 weeks of therapy.

MEDICATIONS

DRUGS AND FLUIDS
• Address underlying cause (e.g., infection, drugs) if secondary IMHA
• Crossmatched, packed RBCs (6-10 ml/kg) for severe anemia
• IV fluids to maintain vascular volume
• Supportive therapy for DIC (see DIC chapter)
• Corticosteroids
• Prednisone 2 mg/kg/day divided bid for 2-4 weeks
• If PCV stable, decrease to 1 mg/kg/day for 2-4 weeks
• Then, if PCV stable, decrease to 1 mg/kg every other day for 2-4 weeks
• Then, if PCV stable, gradually discontinue over another 2-4 weeks
• Cytotoxic drugs if autogglutination or peracute hemolysis is present, or if there is a poor response to prednisone after 14-21 days.
• Cyclophosphamide 50 mg/M^2/day (2 mg/kg/day) for 4 consecutive days, then skip 3 days; repeat for up to 6-8 weeks
• Azathioprine 50 mg/M^2 (2 mg/kg/day) for 1-2 weeks, then every other day. Do not use in cats
• Chlorambucil 2 mg every other to every third day (cats)

CONTRAINDICATIONS
Azathioprine should NOT be used in cats.

PRECAUTIONS
• Check blood type prior to any transfusion in cats
• Prednisone may cause Cushing's syndrome, PTE, pancreatitis (with azathioprine), secondary infection, gastric ulcers (consider misoprostol (2-5 mcg/kg PO bid-tid) or sucralfate to prevent ulcers)

• Cytotoxic drugs may cause bone marrow suppression, secondary infection, pancreatitis (azathioprine), cystitis (cyclophosphamide).

POSSIBLE INTERACTIONS N/A

ALTERNATE DRUGS
• Dexamethasone (0.3-0.9 mg/kg/day) can be used instead of prednisone. Follow similar tapering schedule
• Danazol (5-10 mg/kg PO bid) taper to 5 mg/kg/day when in remission, then gradually discontinue over 3-4 months
• Human gamma globulin (0.5-1.5 g/kg over 12 hours, single IV infusion)
• Cyclosporine (10-20 mg/kg/day IM or PO)
• Eicosapentanoic acid
• Plasmapheresis

FOLLOW-UP

PATIENT MONITORING
• During the acute crisis, monitor the PCV at least daily, to assess the effectiveness of medical therapy and the need for transfusion
• The heart and respiratory rates should be monitored several times daily during hospitalization. • If PTE is suspected, monitor chest radiographs and arterial blood gases frequently • During the first month of outpatient therapy, check the PCV weekly until stable. Then recheck PCV every two weeks for two months. If still stable, recheck PCV monthly for 6 months and then 2-4 times per year. Rechecks may need to be more frequent if patient is on long-term medication.
• A complete CBC should be rechecked at least once monthly during outpatient therapy, especially if using cytotoxic drugs. If the neutrophil count decreases below 3000 cells/ml, discontinue cytotoxic drugs until the count recovers; reinstitute at a lower dose.
• Reticulocyte counts and Coombs' tests can be monitored if the PCV is not rising as expected.

PREVENTION/AVOIDANCE N/A

POSSIBLE COMPLICATIONS
• Pulmonary and multiorgan thromboembolism (up to 44% of all cases) • Portal vein thrombosis • DIC • Cardiac arrhythmias, centrilobular hepatic necrosis and renal tubular necrosis secondary to hypoxia • Secondary infection, endocarditis • Splenic infarcts

EXPECTED COURSE AND PROGNOSIS
• Peracute disease is usually due to autogglutination or intravascular hemolysis. Acute disease is usually due to intravascular or extravascular hemolysis. Chronic disease is usually due to extravascular hemolysis or cold reacting antibodies • Hyperbilirubinemia > 10 mg/dl and low reticulocyte counts are associated with a poor prognosis. • Overall mortality is 33.3%. Autoagglutination is associated with up to 50% mortality. Peracute,

fulminating hemolytic disease is associated with up to 80% mortality. • Warm type IMHA has a guarded prognosis; of patients survive hospitalization (up to 71% will do so), long term prognosis is relatively good. Cold type IMHA is more resistant to immunosuppressive therapy • Response to therapy may take weeks to months. Nonregenerative IMHA may have a more gradual onset and may be slower to respond to therapy. • Hemolysis may recur despite prior or current therapy.

MISCELLANEOUS

ASSOCIATED CONDITIONS
Evan's syndrome, SLE

AGE RELATED FACTORS N/A

ZOONOTIC POTENTIAL N/A

PREGNANCY
Cytotoxic drugs should not be used in pregnant animals.

SYNONYMS
Autoimmune hemolytic anemia, immune mediated hemolytic disease

SEE ALSO
• Anemia • Chapters on various causes of secondary IMHA

ABBREVIATIONS
CHF = congestive heart failure
DIC = disseminated intravascular coagulation
GI = gastrointestinal
IMHA = immune mediated hemolytic anemia
PTE = pulmonary thromboembolism
RBC = red blood cell
SLE = systemic lupus erythematosus

REFERENCES
Bucheler J, Cotter S. Canine immune-mediated hemolytic anemia. In: Bonagura J, Kirk R, eds. Current veterinary therapy XII. Philadelphia: WB Saunders, 1995.
Cotter S. Autoimmune hemolytic anemia in dogs. Comp Cont Ed 1992;14:53-59.
Klag A, Giger U, Shofer F. Idiopathic immune-mediated hemolytic anemia in dogs: 42 cases (1986-1990). J Am Vet Med Assoc 1993;202:783-788.
Stewart A, Feldman B. Immune-mediated hemolytic anemia. Part I. An overview. Comp Cont Ed 1993; 15:372-381.
Stewart A, Feldman B. Immune-mediated hemolytic anemia. Part II. Clinical entity, diagnosis, and treatment theory. Comp Cont Ed 1993; 15:1479-1491.
Author Cathryn M. Calia
Consulting Editor Alan H. Rebar

ANEMIA, IRON DEFICIENCY

BASICS

OVERVIEW
• Specific form of anemia in adult animals caused by hemorrhage • Develops when erythrocytes are produced under the condition of limited iron availability • Characteristic changes include erythrocyte microcytosis and hypochromic appearance caused by thin cell geometry. • Importance of recognizing—leads the clinician to the underlying problem, which is chronic external blood loss. Most common site of blood loss is the gastrointestinal tract.

SIGNALMENT
• Fairly common in adult dogs • Rare in adult cats • Transient, neonatal, iron deficiency anemia occurs at 5-10 weeks of age in about 50% of kittens.

SIGNS
• Nonspecific signs of anemia (e.g., lethargy, depression, weakness, anorexia, and tachypnea) • Melena with gastrointestinal blood loss • Heavy blood-sucking parasite load (e.g., fleas)

CAUSES AND RISK FACTORS
• Any form of chronic external blood loss. Blood loss most often occurs through the gastrointestinal tract. • Lymphoma • Intestinal carcinoma • Hookworm infestation • Other, less common sites (causes) of blood loss • Skin (flea infestation) • Urinary tract • Overuse of blood donors

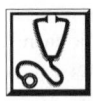

DIAGNOSIS

DIFFERENTIAL DIAGNOSIS
• Any cause of anemia, especially a hemorrhage pattern • Specific features in the hemogram are used to identify iron deficiency.

CBC/BIOCHEMISTRY/URINALYSIS
• Microcytosis, indicated by a low normal or low mean cell volume, is accompanied by increased volume heterogeneity, detected by erythrocyte histogram widening or an increased red cell distribution width value. • PCV usually low; generally ranges from 10-40% in dogs • Changes in erythrocytes seen on blood film include hypochromia, indicated by marked central pallor, oxidative lesions such as keratocytes, and fragmentation. • Anemia, either regenerative or nonregenerative • Hypoproteinemia a consistent finding if blood loss is sustained • Both albumin and globulin fractions usually low normal or low

OTHER LABORATORY TESTS
• Hypoferremia (serum iron < 70 µg/dl) and low transferrin saturation (< 15%) support the diagnosis. Serum iron value may be normal, even in animals with hematologic features of iron deficiency, if blood loss has ceased and the animal is undergoing iron repletion. • Fecal flotation to rule out hookworms

IMAGING
Radiographic or ultrasonographic studies may reveal evidence of gastrointestinal disease that accounts for blood loss.

OTHER DIAGNOSTIC PROCEDURES
• Cytologic examination of bone marrow specimen stained with Prussian blue for iron particles should reveal absence of hemosiderin. This examination is useful only when documentation of the problem is difficult. It is best performed on a core biopsy specimen of marrow. • The histopathology laboratory and pathologist can evaluate the section using the Prussian blue stain for iron particles.

TREATMENT
• Identify and correct cause of chronic external blood loss.
• Administer iron therapy to continue treatment.

MEDICATIONS

DRUGS AND FLUIDS
If anemia is unusually severe (i.e., PCV < 12%), transfusion may be required to treat life-threatening anemia. Whole blood at a rate of 10-20 ml/kg IV is appropriate.

Iron Supplementation
• Animals with severe iron deficiency have impaired intestinal absorption of iron. Thus, oral supplementation is of little or no value until partial iron repletion has been accomplished. Parenterally injected iron should be followed by oral iron supplementation for 1-2 months or until features of iron deficiency have resolved.
• In kittens, neonatal iron deficiency can be prevented by a single, 50-mg iron injection at 1-2 weeks of age. Kittens undergo spontaneous recovery and iron repletion beginning at 5-6 weeks of age, coinciding with intake of solid food.
Parenteral iron supplement:
• Iron dextran (Imferon), 10-20 mg/kg IM once. This is a slowly released form of injectable iron. One injection is followed by oral supplementation.
Oral iron supplements:
• Ferrous sulfate (various; 100-300 mg PO q24h)—powder placed in food or drinking water
• Ferrous gluconate (Fergon; one 325-mg tablet PO q24h)
• Iron and vitamins (Visorbin; 1 tsp PO q24h)—liquid iron and multiple vitamin supplement

CONTRAINDICATIONS/POSSIBLE INTERACTIONS
Oral iron supplementation has been associated with unexplained death in kittens and should be avoided.

FOLLOW-UP
• The most useful approach is hematologic monitoring every 1-4 weeks. If the anemia is severe, monitor more frequently to follow the animal through recovery from a life-threatening illness. The effectiveness of iron supplementation can be monitored less frequently.
• Effective treatment is associated with an increase in mean corpuscular volume and movement of the erythrocyte histogram to the right as new, normal cells are produced. The subpopulation of microcytes produced under conditions of iron deficiency slowly disappear from the histogram as these cells complete their survival time. It may take a few months in some animals to establish a normal erythrocyte volume distribution histogram.

MISCELLANEOUS

Reference
Weiser MG. Erythrocyte responses and disorders. In: Ettinger SJ, Feldman EC, eds. Textbook of veterinary internal medicine. 4th ed. Philadelphia: WB Saunders, 1994:1864-1891.
Author M. Glade Weiser
Consulting Editor Alan H. Rebar

ANEMIA, METABOLIC (ANEMIAS WITH SPICULATED RED CELLS)

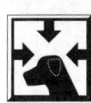

BASICS

OVERVIEW
• Occurs in some animals concomitantly with diffuse diseases of the liver and kidney. In most animals with liver disease, these spiculated cells have 2-10 elongated, blunt, finger-like projections from their surfaces and are classified as acanthocytes. • Acanthocytic anemias can be associated with renal disease, but, more often, anemias of renal disease have oval red cells with irregular or ruffled membranes. These latter cells have been referred to as burr cells. • Pathogenesis not entirely clear. Abnormal lipid metabolism with free cholesterol loading of red cell membranes has been implicated most frequently as the cause of acanthocyte formation. Pathogenesis of burr cell formation is unknown.

SIGNALMENT
• Occurs more frequently in dogs • Occurs infrequently in cats. (It has been observed in cats with fatty liver syndrome.)

SIGNS
• None in most animals (usually mild to moderate condition) • Detection of spiculated red cells on peripheral blood film can be first marker for liver or kidney disease

CAUSES AND RISK FACTORS
• Any disease of the liver or kidneys • Increased severity of organ involvement indicates increased likelihood of red cell morphologic abnormalities.

DIAGNOSIS

DIFFERENTIAL DIAGNOSIS
Determination of renal or hepatic causes based on results of the biochemistry profile and urinalysis

CBC/BIOCHEMISTRY/URINALYSIS
• Mild to moderate decreases in PCV, RBC count, and hemoglobin • Normal mean corpuscular volume and mean corpuscular hemoglobin concentration—in most animals, condition is normocytic, normochromic, and nonregenerative • Evidence of polychromasia and poikilocytosis on blood films only if there is accompanying blood loss (as with hepatic hemangiosarcoma) • White cell changes variable based on underlying cause of hepatic or renal pathology. Inflammatory conditions are likely to be accompanied by inflammatory leukograms. • Variable serum chemistry changes in liver and kidney. The most common changes are listed below.

Hepatic Diseases
• High ALT • High ALP • High GGT • High bile acids • Possible low albumin • Possible low urea nitrogen • Urinalysis findings include elevated urine bilirubin.

Renal Diseases
• High urea nitrogen and creatinine • High phosphorus
Highly variable urinalysis findings. Below is a list of possibilities:
• Isosthenuric urine specific gravity (1.008-1.025 in dogs, 1.008-1.035 in cats) • Tubular and/or protein casts • Leukocytes and/or red cells in urine • Protein positive on reagent strip • Occult blood positive on reagent strip

OTHER LABORATORY TESTS N/A

IMAGING N/A

OTHER DIAGNOSTIC PROCEDURES
N/A

TREATMENT

Focus treatment on diagnosis and treatment of underlying hepatic or renal disease.

MEDICATIONS

DRUGS AND FLUIDS
Variable according to underlying cause

CONTRAINDICATIONS/POSSIBLE INTERACTIONS
Variable according to underlying cause

FOLLOW-UP

Monitor CBC periodically while treating the underlying condition.

MISCELLANEOUS

SEE ALSO
Anemia of Chronic Renal Disease

ABBREVIATIONS
ALP = alkaline phosphatase
ALT = alanine transaminase
GGT = gamma glutamyl transferase
PCV = packed cell volume
RBC = red blood cells

References
Weiser EG. Erythrocyte responses and disorders. In: Ettinger SJ, Feldman EC, eds. Textbook of veterinary internal medicine. Philadelphia: WB Saunders, 1995:1870.
Rebar AH, Lewis HB, DeNicola DB, Halliwell WH, Boon GD. Red blood cell fragmentation in the dog: an editorial review. Vet Pathol 1981;18(4):415-426.

Author Alan H. Rebar
Consulting Editor Alan H. Rebar

ANEMIA, NUCLEAR MATURATION DEFECT (ANEMIA, MEGALOBLASTIC)

BASICS

OVERVIEW
• Nonregenerative anemia characterized by arrested development of the nuclei of RBC precursors (as a result of interference with DNA synthesis) while the cytoplasm develops normally (nuclear-cytoplasmic asynchrony) • Affected RBC precursors fail to divide normally and thus are larger than corresponding normal precursors with the same degree of cytoplasmic maturity (hemoglobinization). Because their nuclei are deficient in chromatin (DNA), they have a distinctive open and stippled appearance. These giant precursors with atypical, immature nuclei are known as megaloblasts. • Although these asynchronous changes are most prominent in RBC precursors, WBC and platelet precursors are similarly affected.

SIGNALMENT
• Dogs and cats • Spontaneous, clinically unimportant occurrence in toy poodles (occasional) • No breed or sex predilections—essentially acquired events

SIGNS
• Generally mild and usually not clinically important • In cats with FeLV-associated, nuclear maturation anemia, FeLV-related signs can be anticipated.

CAUSES AND RISK FACTORS

Infectious FeLV in cats

Nutritional
• Folic acid deficiency • Vitamin B_{12} deficiency

Toxic
• Dilantin toxicity • Methotrexate toxicity (folate antagonist)

Congenital Toy poodles

DIAGNOSIS

DIFFERENTIAL DIAGNOSIS
• All the other mild to moderate nonregenerative anemias including the anemia of inflammatory disease, renal disease, and lead poisoning • Differentiation is based on the distinctive CBC and bone marrow findings listed.

CBC/BIOCHEMISTRY/URINALYSIS
• Mild to moderate anemia (PCV in dogs, 30-40%; PCV in cats, 25-38%) • Large, fully hemoglobinized RBC; occasional to numerous megaloblasts, particularly at the feather edge; no polychromasia • Anemia classically macrocytic (high mean corpuscular volume) and normochromic (normal mean corpuscular hemoglobin concentration) • Mild panleukopenia in many animals • Mild thrombocytopenia in many animals • In cats with FeLV, anemia may occur in association with a myelodysplastic syndrome or in conjunction with leukemia of a different cell line.

OTHER LABORATORY TESTS
FeLV/FIV test—retroviral infection is the most common cause of megaloblastic anemia in cats

IMAGING N/A

OTHER DIAGNOSTIC PROCEDURES
Bone Marrow Findings
• Hyperplastic bone marrow, often in all cell lines • Maturation arrest with nuclear and cytoplasmic asynchrony in all cell lines. Many megaloblastic RBC precursors may be observed. • Macrophagic hyperplasia with active phagocytosis of nucleated RBC and megaloblasts in many animals

TREATMENT
• Treat by targeting the underlying cause, if possible. (Except for those occurring with FeLV in cats, megaloblastic anemias are relatively mild conditions.)
• Treat most patients on an outpatient basis.

ANEMIA, NUCLEAR MATURATION DEFECT (ANEMIA, MEGALOBLASTIC)

MEDICATIONS

DRUGS AND FLUIDS
• In animals with drug toxicity, discontinue the offending drug.
• In all animals, folic acid or vitamin B_{12} supplementation should be considered.

CONTRAINDICATIONS/POSSIBLE INTERACTIONS
Drugs known to cause megaloblastic anemia (e.g., methotrexate and Dilantin) should be avoided in patients whose condition results from other causes.

FOLLOW-UP

• Monitor response to treatment by the CBC (weekly) and occasional bone marrow collection and evaluation. • Closely monitor cats that are also FeLV-positive for evidence of onset of other signs of hematopoietic dyscrasia in the peripheral blood and marrow.
• Prognosis depends on underlying cause. In FeLV-positive cats, prognosis is guarded. In contrast, animals with drug-associated anemia have a good prognosis when use of the offending drug is interrupted.

MISCELLANEOUS

SEE ALSO
• Anemia, Nonregenerative • Feline Immunodeficiency Virus • Feline Leukemia Virus Infection

ABBREVIATIONS
FeLV = feline leukemia virus
FIV = feline immunodeficiency virus
RBC = red blood cells
WBC = white blood cells

Reference

Weiser MG. Erythrocyte responses and disorders. In: Ettinger SJ, Feldman EC, eds. Textbook of veterinary internal medicine. Philadelphia: WB Saunders, 1995:1888-1890.

Author Alan H. Rebar
Consulting Editor Alan H. Rebar

ANEMIA OF CHRONIC RENAL DISEASE

BASICS

DEFINITION
Low PCV, RBC count, and hemoglobin and hypoplasia of erythroid elements of the bone marrow are associated with progressive or end-stage renal failure. Anemia is normocytic, normochromic, nonregenerative, and proportional to the severity of the azotemia. Principal cause is bone marrow failure secondary to inadequate production of erythropoietin by the diseased kidneys. Shortened RBC lifespan, uremic inhibitors of erythropoiesis, blood loss, nutritional deficiencies, and marrow fibrosis may contribute.

SIGNALMENT
Middle-aged to old dogs and cats are mostly affected but is seen in young animals with heritable, congenital, or acquired chronic renal failure.

SIGNS
• Anemia contributes to development of anorexia, weight loss, fatigue, lethargy, depression, weakness, apathy, cold intolerance, behavior and personality changes characterizing chronic renal failure.
• Syncope and seizures (rare)
• Pallor of the mucous membranes
• Tachycardia
• Systolic murmur

CAUSES AND RISK FACTORS
• Inherited, congenital, and acquired forms of chronic renal failure (eg, pyelonephritis, glomerulonephritis, amyloidosis, and lymphoma)
• Exacerbated by iron deficiency, inflammatory or neoplastic disease, gastrointestinal blood loss, hemolysis, and myeloproliferative disorder

DIAGNOSIS

DIFFERENTIAL DIAGNOSIS
• Anemia of chronic infectious, inflammatory, or neoplastic disease, myeloproliferative disease, chronic blood loss, aplastic anemia, endocrine disease, drug reaction, and immune-mediated or parasitic hemolytic anemia.
• Regenerative anemia excludes diagnosis of anemia of chronic renal failure.

CBC/BIOCHEMISTRY/URINALYSIS
• Normocytic, normochromic, nonregenerative anemia (anemia may be masked by dehydration).
• Reticulocytes—low corrected indices and absolute counts
• High BUN, creatinine, and phosphorus; variably high calcium; variably low bicarbonate and potassium.
• High BUN:creatinine ratio may predict concurrent gastrointestinal blood loss.
• Impaired urine concentrating ability, mild to moderate proteinuria, and variably active sediment

OTHER LABORATORY TESTS
• Serum iron normal or variably low ($\leq$ 60 mg/dl).
• Transferrin saturation normal or variably low ($\leq$ 15%).
• FeLV and FIV testing (cats) to exclude viral-induced myelodyscrasia
• Serum erythropoietin normal (inappropriately) or low

IMAGING
Small, irregular kidneys with loss or disruption of renal architecture on radiographs

OTHER DIAGNOSTIC PROCEDURES
Cytologic examination of bone marrow—erythroid hypoplasia, myeloid:erythroid ratio normal or high, and stainable iron normal or variably low.

TREATMENT
• Increase RBC mass if patient is symptomatic for anemia (dogs, PCV $\leq$ 25%; cats, $\leq$ 20)
• Stabilize azotemia in patients in uremic crisis (ie, acute decompensation).
• Establish appropriate nitrogen, caloric, vitamin, and iron intake to reduce uremic inhibitors and bleeding tendency and lengthen lifespan of RBC
• Ensure that iron is not deficient.
• Correct gastrointestinal ulceration and blood loss by administrating cimetidine, ranitidine, or sucralfate.
• Correct systemic hypertension.

MEDICATIONS

DRUG AND FLUIDS
Erythropoietin Replacement
• Recombinant human errythropoietin (r-HuEPO) is a replica of human erythropoietin available as epoetin alfa (brands, EPOGEN® and PROCRIT®) and epoetin beta (brand, MAROGEN®). It provides consistent, rapid, and long-term correction of anemia in dogs and cats with chronic renal failure.
• Target PCV—dogs, 37-45%; cats, 30-40%.
• Initial dosage—50-100 U/kg SC thrice weekly until PCV reaches 37% in dogs or 30% in cats (2 to 8 weeks), then decrease to twice weekly.
• Maintenance dosage—50-100 U/kg SQ once or twice weekly to maintain target PCV; individualize to each patient; life-long treatment required.
• If PCV exceeds target, discontinue until upper target range achieved, then decrease previous dosage by 25-50% or increase dosage interval.
• Serum iron and transferrin saturation should be normalized before initiating and during r-HuEPO administration. Give ferrous sulfate (dogs, 100 to 300 mg PO q24h; cats, 50 to 100 mg PO q24h) if deficiencies are documented.

Blood Transfusion
• For short-term or rapid correction (PCV $\leq$ 20%), give compatible whole blood or packed RBC.
• Target PCV 25-30%.
• May be given intermittently for prolonged management.

Anabolic Steroids
Little or no efficacy or indication for use.

FOLLOW-UP

PATIENT MONITORING
• PCV weekly-semimonthly for 3 months, then monthly to bimonthly
• Blood pressure semimonthly to monthly
• Iron and transferrin saturation at 1, 3, and 6 months, then semiannually
• Discontinue erythropoietin if animal develops evidence of polycythemia, local or systemic sensitivity, anti-r-HuEPO antibody formation, or refractory hypertension.

POSSIBLE COMPLICATIONS
Erythropoietin related complications:
• Development of anti-r-HuEPO antibodies, polycythemia, seizures, hypertension, iron depletion, injection pain, and mucocutaneous reactions
• Anti-r-HuEPO antibodies neutralize r-HuEPO and native erythropoietin causing severe anemia in 20-30% of animals; reversible with cessation of treatment.
• Signs associated with production of anti-r-HuEPO antibodies while the patient is receiving erythropoietin include decreasing PCV, erythroid hypoplasia, and myeloid:erythroid ratio $\leq$ 8.
• Use r-HuEPO cautiously or withhold if hypertension or iron deficiency develops. Treatment can be reinstituted once hypertension and iron deficiency are corrected

Transfusion related complication:
• Incompatibility reaction
• Circulatory or iron overload
• Transmissible infection

EXPECTED COURSE AND PROGNOSIS
• Correction of disease increases appetite, activity, grooming, affection and playfulness,

weight gain, and cold tolerance, and decreases sleeping.

• Although highly effective, use of r-HuEPO in dogs and cats requires careful assessment of the risks versus benefits in individual patients.

• Short-term prognosis depends on the severity of the renal failure. Long-term prognosis is guarded to poor because of the underlying chronic renal failure.

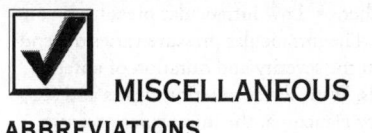

MISCELLANEOUS

ABBREVIATIONS

r-HuEPO = recombinant human erythropoietin

Reference

Cowgill LD. Pathophysiology and management of anemia in chronic progressive renal failure. Sem Vet Med Surg 1992;7:175-182.

Author Larry D. Cowgill

Consulting Editors Larry G. Adams and Carl A. Osborne

ANTERIOR UVEITIS—CATS

BASICS

DEFINITION
Inflammation of the iris and/or ciliary body

Pathophysiology
The common theme to anterior uveitis from all causes is tissue destruction secondary to breakdown of the blood-aqueous barrier. Increased vascular permeability mediated by histamine, serotonin, prostaglandins, and leukotrienes results in the extravasation of fluids, plasma proteins, and cells. Together with cellular infiltration, the clinical signs of iridal congestion, aqueous flare, hypopyon, keratic precipitates, and corneal edema develop.

Systems Affected
• Ophthalmic—the eye • Other organ systems potentially affected if uveitis results from systemic disease process

Genetics N/A

Incidence/Prevalence
Common, although the true incidence is unknown

Geographic Distribution N/A

SIGNALMENT

Species Cats

Breed Predilections None

Mean Age and Range
The mean age is 8-9 years with a range of several weeks to 21 years.

Predominant Sex
• Marked predilection for males among cats with idiopathic anterior uveitis • Even sex distribution in cats in which a definitive diagnosis is made • Strong predilection in older male cats with feline immunodeficiency virus (FIV) infection

SIGNS

General Comments
Clinical signs are related to the severity of anterior uveitis and range from low intraocular pressure to hyphema with blindness.

Historical Findings
Most owners complain of a change in appearance of the affected eye(s). In general, pain and conjunctival hyperemia secondary to anterior uveitis are less pronounced in cats than in dogs.

Physical Examination Findings
• Photophobia, blepharospasm, and epiphora suggest ocular discomfort. • Conjunctival hyperemia is a common but nonspecific sign of ocular irritation. • Aqueous flare, an increased turbidity of aqueous humor, is common in cats with anterior uveitis. Light scattering from particles causes a continuous beam of light to be seen in the anterior chamber (Tyndall phenomenon). In cats with severe disease, fibrinous exudation can cause fibrin clot formation within the anterior

chamber. • Low intraocular pressure is common. The intraocular pressure varies depending on the severity and duration of anterior uveitis. With severe anterior uveitis and secondary glaucoma, the intraocular pressure can be high. • Miosis, or pupillary constriction. Subtle miosis is best observed in a darkened room by simultaneously examining both eyes with retroillumination. • Iridal swelling, nodules, and congestion can be observed, and the pupil is often slow to dilate after installation of a short acting mydriatic (1% Tropicamide). • Keratic precipitates are seen on the corneal endothelial surface. Their presence always indicates active or previous anterior uveitis. • Ciliary flush can be observed in the limbal region as a result of hyperemia of the perilimbal anterior ciliary vessels. Along with conjunctival hyperemia, this may contribute to the "red eye" seen in cats with anterior uveitis. • Corneal edema is not present in cats as much as in dogs. • Hyphema, an accumulation of RBC in the anterior chamber, and hypopyon, an accumulation of WBC in the anterior chamber, develop in cats with extreme breakdown of blood-aqueous barrier. In both instances, the cellular components typically settle homogeneously in the ventral anterior chamber. Hyphema is common in cats with intraocular tumors and systemic hypertension.

CAUSES
• Metabolic—Systemic hypertension
• Neoplastic—Primary (melanoma most common), secondary (lymphoma most common), post-traumatic sarcoma • Immune-mediated—Lens trauma (rupture of lens capsule), immune-mediated vasculitis, immune-mediated thrombocytopenia
• Infectious—Bacterial (due to any systemic bacterial disease), fungal (Blastomyces dermatitidis, Candida albicans, Coccidioides immitis, Cryptococcus neoformans, Histoplasma capsulatum), protozoan (Toxoplasma gondii), viral (Coronavirus of FIP, FeLV, and FIV) • Traumatic—Blunt or penetrating injuries • Idiopathic
• Miscellaneous—Coagulopathy, ulcerative keratitis of any cause, periarteritis nodosa

RISK FACTORS None

DIAGNOSIS

DIFFERENTIAL DIAGNOSIS
• Must differentiate from other cause of red eye (see red eye chapter). • Conjunctivitis. Clinical signs such as hyperemia, chemosis, follicles, ocular discharge, and pain vary with the duration and severity of the process. However, the intraocular pressure and results of intraocular examination are normal. • In cats with glaucoma, the pupil is usually dilated; however, the clinical signs of glaucoma can be identical to those of anterior uveitis. It

is imperative to measure the intraocular to distinguish between these two diseases. • In most cats with nonulcerative keratitis, results of the intraocular examination are normal. Ulcerative keratitis can be accompanied by anterior uveitis. • Horner's syndrome may give the appearance of anterior uveitis because the pupil is miotic and upper lid ptosis creates the impression of blepharospasm; however, unlike in cats with anterior uveitis, the intraocular pressure is normal, aqueous flare is not present, and the conjunctiva is not injected or only mildly so.

CBC/BIOCHEMISTRY/URINALYSIS
• Results of CBC and urinalysis are usually unremarkable. • Serum biochemistry analysis reveals high concentration of plasma proteins caused by high globulin concentration in many cats. This elevation is usually lower than that observed in cats with feline infectious peritonitis (FIP).

OTHER LABORATORY TESTS
If standard laboratory tests fail to reveal abnormalities, serologic testing for feline infectious diseases is indicated. These include detection of antigen for feline leukemia (FeLV) virus or cryptococcus, antibody titre FIP, Toxoplasma gondii (both IgM and IgG concentration), and FIV. A high or rising titre for FIP supports a diagnosis of FIP, but this test lacks specificity because of cross reactivity with the enteric coronavirus. High titers in animals with clinical signs of anterior uveitis are important.

IMAGING
• Thoracic radiographs are indicated to rule out neoplastic and fungal diseases. • Abdominal radiographs and ultrasound are indicated if an abdominal mass is palpated. • Ocular ultrasonography is indicated in cats that have had trauma to rule out penetrating wounds and foreign bodies not obviously visible, and, when the ocular media are too opaque, to allow complete examination of the eye.

OTHER DIAGNOSTIC PROCEDURES
• Blood pressure measurements are high in cats with systemic hypertension. • Aqueous humor paracentesis is seldom helpful.
• Tonometry usually demonstrates low intraocular pressure unless secondary glaucoma has developed.

GROSS AND HISTOPATHOLOGIC FINDINGS
• The eye is inflamed with conjunctival hyperemia, ciliary flush, aqueous flare, miosis, and variable vision. • The iris and ciliary body are diffusely infiltrated with primarily lymphocytes and plasma cells in cats with idiopathic anterior uveitis. Iridal nodules are composed of accumulations of lymphocytes and plasma cells.

TREATMENT

INPATIENT VERSUS OUTPATIENT
Patients with severe anterior uveitis should be hospitalized for initial diagnostic work-up and medical management. Patients with mild to moderate disease may be managed as outpatients unless the intraocular pressure is high.

ACTIVITY No restrictions

DIET No restrictions

CLIENT EDUCATION
• Discuss the need for early aggressive medical management and a thorough diagnostic work-up to identify the cause. Also discuss adverse sequelae of anterior uveitis, including blindness, cataracts, endophthalmitis/ panophthalmitis, lens luxation, phthisis bulbi, posterior synechiae with iris bombé, and secondary glaucoma. • Cats with infectious causes of uveitis (e.g., FeLV, FIV, and FIP) may be contagious to other cats.

SURGICAL CONSIDERATIONS None

MEDICATIONS

DRUGS AND FLUIDS
Frequency of treatment with topical medication depends on the severity of disease.

Topically Applied Corticosteroids
• 1% prednisolone acetate or 0.1% dexamethasone
• Administer q 1-2h initially, then q4h-q8h in cats with severe disease

Topically Applied Nonsteroidal Antiinflammatory Drugs
• 0.03% flurbiprofen (Ocufen) or 1% suprofen (Profenal)
• Administer q6h daily in cats with severe disease

Subconjunctivally Applied Corticosteroids
• Administer as an adjunct to topical administration
• Betamethasone 0.75-1.5 mg/eye
• Dexamethasone 4.0-8.0 mg/eye
• Methylprednisolone acetate 4.0-8.0 mg/eye
• Triamcinolone acetonide 4.0-8.0 mg/eye

Systemically Administered Corticosteroids
• Indicated in cats with moderate to severe disease when the presence of a systemic infectious disease has been eliminated
• Prednisone 1.0-2.0 mg/kg/day for 7 days, then gradually decrease dosage

Topically Applied Mydriatic-Cycloplegic Drugs
• Indicated in the acute stages of disease
• 1% atropine q6h-q12h (ointment may produce less salivation than solution)

Antibiotics
Clindamycin HCL 25 mg/kg PO divided twice daily for 14 to 21 days is indicated in affected cats with high Toxoplasma gondii titers.

CONTRAINDICATIONS
Topical or subconjunctival administration of steroids should be avoided in cats with a corneal ulcer.

PRECAUTIONS
• Topical atropine may cause salivation and occasionally vomiting in cats.
• The safety of topical NSAIDs in cats has not been determined.

POSSIBLE INTERACTIONS N/A

ALTERNATE DRUGS N/A

FOLLOW-UP

PATIENT MONITORING
A complete ocular examination should be repeated in 5-7 days after the initiation of treatment in cats with severe anterior uveitis. The intraocular pressure should be measured to monitor for secondary glaucoma. Reevaluations can be done every 2-3 weeks depending upon the response to treatment.

PREVENTION/AVOIDANCE N/A

POSSIBLE COMPLICATIONS
• Adverse sequelae include blindness, cataracts, endophthalmitis/panophthalmitis, iris atrophy, lens luxation, phthisis bulbi, rubeosis iridis, posterior synechiae with iris bombé, and secondary glaucoma.
• Secondary glaucoma is a frequent complication in cats with idiopathic uveitis and tends to be recalcitrant to medical treatment.
• Idiopathic uveitis can be so insidious that buphthalmia may be the presenting complaint.

EXPECTED COURSE AND PROGNOSIS
• In cats with anterior uveitis secondary to a systemic disease, the prognosis is usually determined by the systemic disease rather than by the anterior uveitis. The prognosis for resolution of the inflammation without deleterious sequelae depends on the severity of the disease at initial examination and on the response to aggressive medical treatment.

• Regardless of the initial response to treatment, anterior uveitis should be treated for at least 2 months with decreasing frequency because the blood-aqueous barrier remains disrupted for about 8 weeks after an insult.

MISCELLANEOUS

ASSOCIATED CONDITIONS N/A

AGE RELATED FACTORS
Cats with serologically confirmed infectious disease tend to be younger (mean, 5.0 years) than cats with idiopathic anterior uveitis (mean, 9.3 years) or ocular melanoma (mean, 9.0 years).

ZOONOTIC POTENTIAL None

PREGNANCY
Systemic steroids should not be used in pregnant cats if at all avoidable, and topical steroids should be used with caution because systemic absorption will occur with more than twice-a-day treatment.

SYNONYMS Iridocyclitis

SEE ALSO Red eye

ABBREVIATIONS N/A

References

Nasisse MP. Feline ophthalmology. In: Gelatt KN, ed. Veterinary ophthalmology. 2nd ed. Philadelphia: Lea & Febiger, 1991:527–575.

Slatter D. Fundamentals of veterinary ophthalmology. 2nd ed. Philadelphia: WB Saunders, 1990:304–337.

Davidson MG, Nasisse MP, English RV, Wilcock BP, Jamieson VE. Feline anterior uveitis: A study of 53 cases. J Am Anim Hosp Assoc 1991;27:77–83.

Author Michael J. Ringle
Consulting Editor Paul E. Miller

ANTERIOR UVEITIS—DOGS

BASICS

DEFINITION
Inflammation of the iris and/or ciliary body

Pathophysiology
Anterior uveitis from all causes is tissue destruction secondary to a breakdown of the blood-aqueous barrier. Increased vascular permeability mediated by histamine, serotonin, prostaglandins, and leukotrienes results in the extravasation of fluids, plasma proteins, and cells. Together with cellular infiltration, the clinical signs of iridal congestion, aqueous flare, aqueous fibrin, hypopyon, keratic precipitates, and corneal edema develop.

Systems Affected
• Ophthalmic—the eye • Other organ systems potentially affected if uveitis results from systemic disease

Genetics N/A

Incidence/Prevalence
Common although true prevalence is unknown

Geographic Distribution
Prevalence of some causes varies with geographic location in the United States (e.g., the deep fungals and Ehrlichia canis).

SIGNALMENT

Species Dogs

Breed Predilections None

Mean Age and Range Any

Predominant Sex None

SIGNS

General Comments
Clinical signs are related to the severity of anterior uveitis and may range from low intraocular pressure to hyphema with blindness.

Historical Findings
• Pain exhibited as photophobia, blepharospasm, or epiphora • Redness due to conjunctival hyperemia or hyphema • Blue/white cornea from edema • Blindness

Physical Examination Findings
• Photophobia, blepharospasm, and epiphora suggest ocular discomfort. These clinical signs are not specific for anterior uveitis. • Conjunctival hyperemia is common. • Low intraocular pressure is common. The intraocular pressure varies depending on the severity and duration of anterior uveitis. With severe disease and secondary glaucoma, the intraocular pressure can be high. • Miosis, or pupillary constriction. Subtle miosis is best observed in a darkened room by simultaneously examining both eyes with retroillumination. • Iridal swelling can be seen, and the pupil is often slow to dilate after installation of a short acting mydriatic (1% Tropicamide). • Corneal edema is of-

ten present. • Ciliary flush may be observed in the limbal region as a result of hyperemia of the perilimbal anterior ciliary vessels. Along with conjunctival hyperemia, this may contribute to the "red eye" seen in dogs with anterior uveitis. • Aqueous flare is excess turbidity of aqueous humor. Light scattering from particles causes a continuous beam of light to be seen in the anterior chamber (Tyndall phenomenon). In dogs with severe disease, fibrinous exudation can cause fibrin clot formation within the anterior chamber. • Hyphema, an accumulation of RBC in the anterior chamber, and hypopyon, an accumulation of WBC in the anterior chamber, occur in dogs with extreme breakdown of blood-aqueous barrier. In both instances, the cellular components typically settle homogeneously in the ventral anterior chamber. Hyphema is common in dogs with intraocular tumors. • Keratic precipitates are seen on the corneal endothelial surface. Their presence always indicates active or previous anterior uveitis.

CAUSES
• Metabolic—diabetes mellitus (lens-induced uveitis), hyperlipidemia, systemic hypertension • Neoplastic—primary (melanoma most common), secondary (lymphoma most common), hyperviscosity syndrome • Immune-mediated—cataracts (lens-induced uveitis), lens trauma (rupture of lens capsule), Vogt-Koyanagi-Harada-like syndrome, immune-mediated vasculitis, immune-mediated thrombocytopenia • Infectious—algal (Prototheca spp.), bacterial (Brucella canis, Borrelia burgdorferi, Leptospira spp., or any systemic bacterial disease), fungal (Blastomyces dermatitidis, Coccidioides immitis, Cryptococcus neoformans, Histoplasma capsulatum), parasitic (Baylisascaris spp., Diptera spp., Dirofilaria immitis, Toxocara spp.), protozoan (Leishmania donovani, Toxoplasma gondii), rickettsial (Ehrlichia canis, Ehrlichia platys, Rickettsia rickettsii), viral (Adenovirus, distemper virus) • Traumatic—blunt or penetrating injuries • Miscellaneous—coagulopathy, secondary to episcleritis/scleritis, idiopathic, radiation therapy, ulcerative keratitis from any cause

RISK FACTORS
Exposure to causative organisms

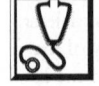

DIAGNOSIS

DIFFERENTIAL DIAGNOSIS
• Must differentiate from other causes of red eye (see red eye topic). • Conjunctivitis. Clinical signs such as hyperemia, chemosis, ocular discharge, and pain vary with the duration and severity of the process. However, the intraocular pressure and results of intraocular examination are normal.

• Episcleritis and scleritis can be nodular, diffuse and infiltrative, or necrotizing. In uncomplicated cases, only the fibrous tunic of the globe is involved. However, in some dogs, anterior uveitis may also be present because of extension of the inflammation to adjacent tissues. • In dogs with glaucoma, the pupil is usually dilated; however, the clinical signs of glaucoma can be identical to those of anterior uveitis. It is imperative to measure the intraocular pressure to distinguish between these two diseases. • In most dogs with nonulcerative keratitis, results of the intraocular examination are normal. Ulcerative keratitis can be accompanied by anterior uveitis. • Horner's syndrome may give the appearance of anterior uveitis because with this disease, the pupil is miotic and upper lid ptosis creates the false impression of blepharospasm; however, unlike in dogs with anterior uveitis, the intraocular pressure is normal, aqueous flare is not present, and the conjunctiva is not injected or only mildly so.

CBC/BIOCHEMISTRY/URINALYSIS
• Results of a CBC, biochemistry profile, and urinalysis are usually normal.
• Abnormalities, if present, reflect the systemic disease causing or associated with anterior uveitis. Examples include neutropenia or neutrophilia with systemic bacterial or fungal disease, high serum glucose concentration with diabetes mellitus, thrombocytopenia with hyphema, and high triglycerides with hyperlipidemia.

OTHER LABORATORY TESTS
• Serum titers for infectious agents (e.g., toxoplasmosis, ehrlichiosis, and the deep fungals) can be done if appropriate for the geographic location. High titers in dogs with clinical signs of anterior uveitis are usually important.
• A clotting profile is indicated if hyphema of undetermined cause is observed.

IMAGING
• Thoracic radiographs are indicated to rule out neoplastic and fungal disease. • Abdominal radiographs and ultrasound are indicated if an abdominal mass is palpated. • Ocular ultrasonography is indicated in dogs with trauma to rule out penetrating wounds and radiolucent foreign bodies not obviously visible and, when the ocular media are too opaque, to completely examine the eye.

OTHER DIAGNOSTIC PROCEDURES
• Blood pressure measurements are high in dogs with systemic hypertension. • Aqueous humor paracentesis is seldom helpful. • Tonometry usually demonstrates low intraocular pressure unless secondary glaucoma has developed.

GROSS AND HISTOPATHOLOGIC FINDINGS
• The eye is inflamed with conjunctival hyperemia, ciliary flush, corneal edema, aqueous flare, miosis, and variable vision. • The iris and ciliary body are infiltrated with a mixture of in-

flammatory or neoplastic cell types, depending on the cause and chronicity of the disease.

TREATMENT

INPATIENT VERSUS OUTPATIENT
Patients with severe anterior uveitis should be hospitalized for initial diagnostic work-up and medical management. Mild to moderate disease can be managed with the dog as outpatient unless the intraocular pressure is high.

ACTIVITY No restrictions

DIET N/A

CLIENT EDUCATION
• Discuss the need for early aggressive medical management and a thorough diagnostic work-up to identify the cause. • Discuss adverse sequelae of anterior uveitis, including blindness, cataracts, endophthalmitis and panophthalmitis, lens luxation, phthisis bulbi, posterior synechia with iris bombe, and secondary glaucoma.

SURGICAL CONSIDERATIONS None

MEDICATIONS

DRUGS AND FLUIDS
The frequency of treatment with topical medication depends on the severity of disease.

Topically Applied Corticosteroids
• 1% prednisolone acetate or 0.1% dexamethasone.
• Administer q 1-2 h initially, then q4h-q8h in dogs with severe disease.

Topically Applied Nonsteroidal Antiinflammatory Drugs
• 0.03% flurbiprofen (Ocufen) or 1% suprofen (Profenal)
• Administer q6h in dogs with severe disease

Subconjunctivally Applied Corticosteroids
• Administer as an adjunct to topical therapy
• Betamethasone 0.75-1.5 mg/eye
• Dexamethasone 4.0-8.0 mg/eye
• Methylprednisolone acetate 4.0-8.0 mg/eye
• Triamcinolone acetonide 4.0-8.0 mg/eye

Systemically Administered Corticosteroids
• Indicated in dogs with moderate to severe disease when the presence of a systemic infectious disease has been eliminated.
• Prednisone 1.0-2.0 mg/kg/day for 7 days, then gradually decrease dosage.

Immunosuppressive Drugs
• Can be used in dogs unresponsive to conventional therapy
• Azathioprine (Imuran) 2mg/kg/day for 5 days, then decrease dosage

Topically Applied Mydriatic-Cycloplegic Drugs
• Indicated to dilate the pupil and minimize the occurrence of posterior synechia, and to paralyze the ciliary muscle (cycloplegia), reducing ocular pain
• 1% atropine q4h-q6h initially in dogs with severe disease, then q6h-q12h times daily

Systemicaly Administered Antibiotics or Antifungal Drugs
Rarely indicated unless a susceptible infectious agent (e.g., Ehrlichia spp, Toxoplasma gondii, and deep fungals) has been identified

CONTRAINDICATIONS
• Topical or subconjunctival steroids should not be used in a dog with a corneal ulcer.
• Systemic steroids are contraindicated in dogs with diabetes mellitus, and topical steroids should be used with caution because they may alter insulin requirements. Alternatively, topical nonsteroidals can be used.

PRECAUTIONS
Azathioprine should be used with extreme caution. Frequent blood cell and platelet counts and liver enzyme determinations are recommended because of potential myelosuppressive and hepatotoxic effects.

POSSIBLE INTERACTIONS N/A

ALTERNATE DRUGS N/A

FOLLOW-UP

PATIENT MONITORING
A complete ocular examination should be repeated in 5-7 days after initiation of treatment in dogs with severe anterior uveitis. The intraocular pressure should be measured to monitor for secondary glaucoma. Reevaluations can be done every 2-3 weeks depending on response to treatment.

PREVENTION/AVOIDANCE N/A

POSSIBLE COMPLICATIONS
Adverse sequelae include blindness, cataracts, endophthalmitis and panophthalmitis, iris atrophy, lens luxation, phthisis bulbi, rubeosis iridis, posterior synechia with iris bombe, and secondary glaucoma.

EXPECTED COURSE AND PROGNOSIS
• The prognosis in dogs with anterior uveitis secondary to a systemic disease (e.g., blastomycosis and lymphosarcoma) is usually determined by the systemic disease. • The prognosis for resolution of the inflammation without deleterious sequelae depends on the severity of the disease at initial examination and on the response to aggressive medical treatment. • Regardless of the initial response to treatment, anterior uveitis should be treated for at least 2 months with decreasing frequency because the blood-aqueous barrier remains disrupted for about 8 weeks after an insult.

MISCELLANEOUS

ASSOCIATED CONDITIONS None

AGE RELATED FACTORS None

ZOONOTIC POTENTIAL
Although anterior uveitis itself is not transmissible to human beings, some of the infectious agents that cause canine anterior uveitis may be (e.g., Brucella canis and Blastomyces dermatitidis—rare) in certain circumstances.

PREGNANCY
Systemic steroids should not be used in pregnant dogs if at all avoidable, and topical steroids should be used with caution because systemic absorption occurs with more than twice-a-day treatment.

SYNONYMS Iridocyclitis

SEE ALSO Red eye

ABBREVIATIONS N/A

References
Collins BK, Moore CP. Canine anterior uvea. In: Gelatt KN, ed. Veterinary ophthalmology. 2nd ed. Philadelphia: Lea & Febiger, 1991:357–395.
Slatter D. Fundamentals of veterinary ophthalmology. 2nd ed. Philadelphia: WB Saunders, 1990:304–337.
Author Michael J. Ringle
Consulting Editor Paul E. Miller

AORTIC STENOSIS

BASICS

DEFINITION
Narrowing of the left ventricular outflow tract of the heart, most commonly seen as a congenital or perinatal disease. Defect can be valvular, subvalvular (most common in dogs), or supravalvular (most common in cats). As a congenital anomaly in dogs, the obstruction is usually caused by fibrous tissue proximal to the valve, and the disease is referred to as subaortic stenosis (SAS).

Pathophysiology
Marked aortic obstruction compels the left ventricle to increase intraventricular pressure to maintain forward blood flow and systemic blood pressure. The myocardium compensates by hypertrophy of myocytes leading to thickening of the heart walls. Coronary artery disease, relative cardiac ischemia, arrhythmias, aortic or mitral regurgitation, left-sided congestive heart failure (CHF), and diminished systemic blood flow may result.

Systems Affected
• Cardiovascular because of pressure overload of the left ventricle • Pulmonary if CHF develops • Multisystemic signs may develop secondary to CHF or low cardiac output. If bacterial endocarditis is the cause of the stenosis, the animal may have signs of septic embolization.

Genetics
Inherited trait in Newfoundland dogs. Polygenic transmission exhibiting pseudo-dominance; a major dominant gene with modifiers may be involved.

Incidence/Prevalence
• Approximately 1.5 to 2.0 per 1000 dogs admitted to veterinary teaching institutions; SAS is probably the second most common congenital heart defect in dogs. • Approximately 0.2 per 1000 cats admitted to veterinary teaching institutions. In one study, aortic stenosis accounted for 6% of congenital cardiac defects in cats.

Geographic Distribution N/A

SIGNALMENT

Species Dogs and cats

Breed Predilections
• Common in Newfoundland, German shepherd, golden retriever, rottweiler, and boxer • Samoyed, English bulldog, and Great Dane also at higher risk than other breeds

Mean Age and Range
• Develops postnatally over the first weeks to months of life • Onset of clinical signs can occur at any age depending on the severity of obstruction • Signs may be seen on physical examination without any historical evidence of disease.

Predominant Sex None

SIGNS

Historical Findings
Related to the severity of obstruction; range from none to CHF, syncope, and sudden death

Physical Examination Findings
• Systolic ejection murmur loudest near the left, fourth intercostal space at the heart base to costochondral junction, which may radiate to the thoracic inlet, carotid arteries, and, if very loud, even to the cranium. Radiation to the left apex and right cranial thorax is common. Some animals have an associated thrill at the left heart base to costochondral junction. • If aortic regurgitation develops, a diastolic murmur may be heard at the left apex. If mitral regurgitation develops, a left apical holosystolic murmur may be present.
• Dyspnea, tachypnea, and crackles with the onset of left-sided CHF • Femoral pulses typically weakened and late rising (pulsus tardus) in animals with disease severe enough to affect hemodynamics. • A left ventricular "heave" (i.e., prolonged and pronounced cardiac impulse palpated on the thorax) in animals with left ventricular hypertrophy
• Arrhythmias

CAUSES
• Congenital disease • Secondary to bacterial endocarditis of the aortic valve in some dogs
• In cats with hypertrophic cardiomyopathy, functional stenosis (e.g., muscular or subvalvular) is common . "Dynamic" subaortic stenosis reported in dogs in which muscular hypertrophy can contribute to narrowing of the aortic outflow tract.

RISK FACTORS
Familial history of subaortic stenosis

DIAGNOSIS

DIFFERENTIAL DIAGNOSIS
• Systolic ejection murmur may represent an innocent murmur in a young animal, anemia, pain, fever, and excitement. • Systolic murmurs on the left thorax are commonly caused by patent ductus arteriosus (usually a continuous murmur, but diastolic component may be localized), pulmonic stenosis, mitral regurgitation, ventricular septal defect, atrial septal defect, and tetralogy of Fallot in dogs.
• Weakened pulses may occur in animals with other cardiac conditions in which stroke volume is limited (e.g., pulmonic stenosis and cardiomyopathy) or in animals with aortic obstruction distal to the outflow tract (e.g., aortic coarctation, aortic interruption, and aortic thromboembolism).

CBC/BIOCHEMISTRY/URINALYSIS
Typically normal

OTHER LABORATORY TESTS
N/A

IMAGING

Thoracic Radiographic Findings
• May be subtle because myocardial hypertrophy from pressure overload may not increase the size of the cardiac silhouette.
• Left-sided heart enlargement, which may appear on lateral radiographs as straightening of the caudal border of the heart • Normal lung fields unless CHF develops causing pulmonary venous distention and interstitial or alveolar pulmonary infiltrates • Mediastinum may be widened and cranial waist of the cardiac silhouette filled as a result of post-stenotic dilation of the aorta.

Echocardiographic Findings
• Spectrum of findings depending on the severity of disease • Thickening of the left ventricular wall and interventricular septum
• Echogenic ridge and gross narrowing of the left ventricular outflow tract may be visible proximal to the aortic valve. The mitral valve is adjacent to the outflow tract, and its anterior leaflet may also be thickened and echogenic. • Post-stenotic dilation of the aorta in some animals • Increased echogenicity of the myocardium in some animals, particularly the subendocardial zone and papillary muscles. • "Premature closure" of the aortic valve often seen on M-mode echocardiography
• Doppler echocardiography. Stenosis leads to high peak ejection velocity (> 2 m/s), which may be delayed to a later time in ejection, and a jet of turbulent blood flow distal to the valve recognized as a wide range of measured velocities ("spectral broadening").
• Transvalvular pressure gradient can be estimated from the flow velocity (pressure gradient = $4 \times$ flow velocity squared) with variable accuracy. • Color-flow Doppler allows direct visualization of the jet.

Angiocardiographic Findings/Cardiac Catheterization
• Contrast radiography shows thickening of the left ventricular wall and septum, narrowing of the left ventricular outflow tract, and post-stenotic dilation of the aorta. • Cardiac catheterization allows determination of the transvalvular pressure gradient. Pressure gradients < 50 mm Hg indicates mild disease;, 50–75 mm Hg, moderate;, 75–100 mm Hg, severe; and > 100 mm Hg, very severe disease. Anesthesia depresses myocardial function, so these gradients may underestimate the actual ones (unanesthetized).
• Angiocardiography and cardiac catheterization allow characterization of uncommon types of stenosis including valvular, supravalvular, and "tunnel outflow tract" and evaluation of concurrent defects.

OTHER DIAGNOSTIC PROCEDURES

Electrocardiographic Findings
• ECG may show signs of left ventricular hypertrophy such as a tall R wave in lead II (> 3.0 mv in dogs), CV6LL (> 3.0 mv in dogs), and others (leads I, III, aVF, CV6LU).

• Widening of the QRS complex (> 0.06 sec in dogs) may also be evident. • Mean electrical axis may be shifted to the left (< 40° in dogs) but is typically normal. • Slurring of ST segment consistent with left ventricular hypertrophy ischemia; ST-segment deviation after mild exercise strongly suggests coronary insufficiency

GROSS AND HISTOPATHOLOGIC FINDINGS See Pathophysiology.

TREATMENT

Management recommendations for small animals are controversial and vary among experts.

INPATIENT VERSUS OUTPATIENT

Inpatient management appropriate for complications including arrhythmias, episodes of collapse or syncope, and CHF

ACTIVITY

Restricted in animals with more than mild disease. Syncope, collapse, and sudden death may be brought on by exertion in animals with severe disease.

DIET

Restricted sodium in animals with overt or impending CHF

CLIENT EDUCATION

• Affected animals should be neutered or otherwise not permitted to breed.
• Related animals are suspected and should be examined for evidence of clinical disease.
• Alert owners to potential complications (e.g., sudden death and CHF) in severely affected animals.

SURGICAL CONSIDERATIONS

• Definitive treatment requires open heart surgery and is rarely practical in small animals for economic and technical reasons.
• Balloon dilation of the outflow tract during cardiac catheterization results in acute reduction of transvalvular gradients and improvement of clinical signs in some symptomatic dogs. Long-term benefits have not been adequately studied in animals.

MEDICATIONS

DRUGS AND FLUIDS

• Medical management is, at best, palliative and empirical; no data have been published supporting a specific treatment.
• Beta adrenergic blockers have been advocated for dogs with subaortic stenosis with a history of syncope, a transvalvular pressure gradient > 100 mm Hg, or when ventricular arrhythmias or ST-segment changes are evident on a postexercise ECG. Potential benefits include limitation of myocardial oxygen requirements, protection from ventricular arrhythmias, and slowing of the heart rate. Beta

blockers are always given to effect which depends on the state of the autonomic system of the individual.
• They should be initiated with caution. Propranolol (dogs, 0.2-1.0 mg/kg PO q8h; cats, 2.5-5.0 mg/cat PO q8h-q12h) is the prototype beta blocker.
• Specific treatment for ventricular arrhythmias, atrial fibrillation, or left-sided CHF may also be required. Requires careful monitoring (see precautions).
• Affected animals are at risk of developing bacterial endocarditis. Meticulous treatment of infections is recommended as is chemoprophylaxis for dental or genitourinary procedures.

CONTRAINDICATIONS

Beta blockers in animals with CHF and bronchoconstrictive disorders; discontinue if these complications develop

PRECAUTIONS

• Beta blockers limit the ability of the dysfunctional heart to increase cardiac output, which occurs primarily by an increase in heart rate.
• The incompliant myocardium is dependent on adequate filling pressure (preload), and overzealous use of diuretics or venodilators in animals with CHF may cause a precipitous drop in cardiac output.
• Marked reduction of systemic blood pressure by ACE inhibitors, calcium channel blockers, or arteriolar dilators may worsen outflow obstruction or coronary insufficiency.
• Digitalis glycosides and positive inotropes may exacerbate outflow obstruction or ventricular arrhythmias.
• Anesthetic agents and sedatives with marked hypotensive, arrhythmogenic, or cardiac depressant side effects should be avoided. A narcotic (e.g., butorphanol or oxymorphone) with diazepam for sedation can be combined with low inspired concentrations of isofluorane for anesthesia if necessary.

POSSIBLE INTERACTIONS N/A

ALTERNATE DRUGS

• Metoprolol tartrate (5-60 mg/dog PO q8h; 2-15 mg/cat PO q8h), nadolol (0.25-0.5 mg/kg PO q12h), and atenolol (6.25-12.5 mg/dog PO q12h; 6.25-12.5 mg/cat PO q24h) are alternate beta blockers.
• Diltiazem (dogs, 0.5-2.0 mg/kg PO q8h; 7.5-15.0 mg/cat PO q8h) may have similar theoretical benefits in this disease.

FOLLOW-UP

PATIENT MONITORING

• Monitor by ECG, thoracic radiography, two-dimensional and Doppler echocardiography. • Treatment of complications (e.g., CHF and arrhythmias) necessitates careful monitoring to detect renal/electrolyte, proarrhythmic, negative inotropic, and hypotensive side effects of drugs.

PREVENTION/AVOIDANCE

See client education

POSSIBLE COMPLICATIONS

CHF, arrhythmias, myocardial infarction, aortic regurgitation, mitral regurgitation, and bacterial endocarditis

EXPECTED COURSE AND PROGNOSIS

• Mildly affected dogs may live a normal life span without treatment. • Severe disease typically limits longevity. • CHF suggests severe disease and an ominous prognosis.

MISCELLANEOUS

ASSOCIATED CONDITIONS

Other cardiac defects

AGE RELATED FACTORS

Murmur typically not present at birth; develops in the first weeks to months postnatally along with development of stenotic lesion

ZOONOTIC POTENTIAL N/A

PREGNANCY Contraindicated

SYNONYMS N/A

SEE ALSO

• Endocarditis • CHF, Left-Sided • Cardiomyopathy, Hypertrophic—Cats and Dogs

ABBREVIATIONS

CHF = congestive heart failure
ACE = angiotensin converting enzyme
SAS = subaortic stenosis

References

Bonagura JD, Darke PGG. Congenital heart disease. In: Ettinger SJ, Feldman EC, eds. Textbook of veterinary internal medicine. 4th ed. Philadelphia: WB Saunders, 1995.
Sisson D. Fixed and dynamic subvalvular aortic stenosis in dogs. In: Kirk RW, Bonagura JD, eds. Current veterinary therapy XI. Philadelphia: WB Saunders, 1992.
Author Donald J. Brown
Consulting Editors Larry P. Tilley and Francis W. K. Smith, Jr.

AORTIC THROMBOEMBOLISM

BASICS

DEFINITION
Aortic thromboembolism (ATE) results from a thrombus or blood clot that is dislodged within the aorta, causing severe ischemia to the tissues served by that segment of aorta. It is one of the most devastating complications associated with myocardial diseases in cats.

Pathophysiology
• ATE is most commonly associated with myocardial disease in cats, including hypertrophic, restrictive, and dilated cardiomyopathy. • Although the exact etiology of ATE has not been determined, it is theorized that abnormal blood flow (stasis) and a hypercoaguable state contribute to the formation of the thrombus within the left atrium. The blood clot is then embolized distally to the aorta. • The most common site of embolization is the caudal aorta trifurcation (hindlegs). Other less common sites include the front leg, kidneys, gastrointestinal tract, or cerebrum. • Rarely, aortic thromboembolism occurs in dogs. ATE in dogs typically is associated with neoplasia, sepsis, Cushing's disease, protein-losing nephropathy, or other hypercoaguable states.

Systems Affected
• Cardiovascular—the majority of affected cats will experience left heart failure and advanced heart disease • Nervous/musculoskeletal—severe ischemia to the muscles and nerves served by the segment of occluded aorta causes variable pain and paresis • Gait abnormalities or paralysis results in the leg or legs involved

Genetics N/A

Incidence/Prevalence
• Although ATE is a well-recognized complication of myocardial disease in cats, the exact prevalence of ATE is not known in the general population of cats. In one study of cats with hypertrophic cardiomyopathy, 12% presented with signs of ATE. • In a retrospective study of 100 cats with ATE, only 11% of cats had previous evidence of heart disease. Therefore, it is usually the initial sign of cardiovascular disease in most cases. • Rare in dogs.

GEOGRAPHIC DISTRIBUTION N/A

SIGNALMENT

Species Cats, rarely dogs

Breed Predilections
No breed predilection is described.

Mean Age and Range
Age distribution is 1-20 years. The median age is 10.5 years; the mean age is 7.7 years.

Predominant Sex
Males are more commonly affected than females (2:1).

SIGNS

Historical Findings
• Acute onset paralysis and pain are the most common complaints. • Lameness or a gait abnormality • Tachypnea or respiratory distress is common. • Vocalization and anxiety are common.

Physical Examination Findings
• Usually paraparesis or paralysis of the rear legs. Less commonly, monoparesis of a front leg. • Pain upon palpation of the legs. Gastrocnemius muscle often becomes firm several hours after embolization. • Absent or diminished femoral pulses • Cyanotic or pale nail beds and foot pads • Cardiac murmur or gallop sound • Tachypnea or dyspnea • Cardiac arrhythmias

CAUSES
• Hypertrophic cardiomyopathy • Restrictive cardiomyopathy • Dilated cardiomyopathy

RISK FACTORS
Although clear risk factors have not been defined, it is theorized that an enlarged left atrium or spontaneous echo contrast (smoke) may be risk factors.

DIAGNOSIS

DIFFERENTIAL DIAGNOSIS
Hind limb paresis secondary to other causes such as spinal neoplasia, trauma, myelitis, fibrocartilaginous infarction, or intervertebral disk protrusion

CBC/BIOCHEMISTRY/URINALYSIS
• Increased creatine phosphokinase as a result of muscle injury • Increased aspartate aminotransferase and alanine aminotransferase as a result of muscle and liver injury • Increased blood glucose secondary to stress • Mild increases in blood urea nitrogen and creatinine as a result of possible dehydration and renal emboli • CBC and urinalysis changes are nonspecific.

OTHER LABORATORY TESTS
• Coagulation profile typically does not reveal significant abnormalities because the hypercoagulability results from hyperaggregable platelets. • Coagulation profile may be helpful to titrate heparin and possibly warfarin dosages.

IMAGING

Radiography
• Cardiomegaly is seen in 85-90% of cats. • Pulmonary edema and/or pleural effusion is seen in approximately 66% of cats.

Echocardiography
• The majority of cats will have hypertrophic cardiomyopathy characterized by left ventricular hypertrophy, nondilated left ventricular lumen, enlarged left atrium, and hypercontractility. • The second most common echocardiographic diagnosis is restrictive cardiomyopathy. • Dilated cardiomyopathy also can be seen. • Regardless of the type of myocardial disease present, the majority (> 50%) have severe left atrial enlargement, i.e., a left atrial to aortic ratio of 2.0 or greater. • Occasionally, a left atrial thrombus or spontaneous echo contrast (smoke) may be seen.

Abdominal Ultrasonography
An experienced sonographer may be able to identify the thrombus in the caudal aorta. However, this imaging modality typically is not necessary to reach a diagnosis.

Angiography
Nonselective angiography should identify a negative filling defect in the caudal aorta representing the thrombus. As with abdominal sonography, this test may not be necessary to reach a diagnosis.

OTHER DIAGNOSTIC PROCEDURES

Electrocardiography
• The most common rhythm diagnoses are sinus rhythm and sinus tachycardia. • Less common rhythm disturbances include atrial fibrillation, ventricular arrhythmias, supraventricular arrhythmias, and sinus bradycardia. • Left ventricular enlargement pattern and left ventricular conduction disturbances (left anterior fascicular block) are commonly noted.

GROSS AND HISTOPATHOLOGIC FINDINGS
• Thrombus typically is identified at the aortic trifurcation. Occasionally, a left atrial thrombus is seen. • Emboli of the kidneys, gastrointestinal tract, cerebrum, and other organs also may be seen.

TREATMENT

INPATIENT VERSUS OUTPATIENT
Initially, cats with ATE should be treated as inpatients because most have concurrent congestive heart failure and require injectable drugs.

ACTIVITY
Activity should be restricted and the cat should be kept quiet and stress-free.

DIET
• Initially, most cats are anorexic. Tempt these cats with any type of diet. It is important to keep these cats eating to avoid hepatic lipodosis.
• Chronic dietary management usually involves sodium restriction.

CLIENT EDUCATION
• Owners should be aware of the poor short- and long-term prognosis.
• Most cats will reembolize. • Most cats that survive an initial episode will be on some type of anticoagulant therapy that may require frequent reevaluations and an indoor lifestyle.

• Typically, most cats that survive an initial episode will recover complete function to the legs; however, neurologic deficits may persist.

SURGICAL CONSIDERATIONS

Surgical embolectomy typically is not recommended because these patients are high risks for surgery as a result of their heart disease.

MEDICATIONS

DRUGS AND FLUIDS

• Thrombolytic therapy such as streptokinase and tissue plasminogen activator is used extensively in humans and infrequently in cats. These drugs are prohibitively expensive and carry a significant risk for bleeding complications and thus are rarely used in general practice.

• Heparin is the preferred drug in general practice. It has no effect on the established clot; however, it prevents further activation of the coagulation cascade. The initial dose typically is given intravenously then followed with subcutaneous administrations every 8 hours. The initial IV dose is 200-300 units/kg and the subsequent SQ dose is 100-300 units/kg. The dose is then titrated to prolong the activated partial thromboplastin time (APTT) approximately twofold.

• Aspirin is theoretically beneficial during and after an episode of thromboembolism by its antiplatelet effects. The dose is an 81 mg tablet PO every second or third day.

• Butorphenol may be used for its analgesic effects at a dose of 0.5-1.0 mg SQ or IV q6h-q8h.

• Acepromazine may be used for its sedative and vasodilatory properties at a dose of 0.1-0.5 mg SQ tid.

• Warfarin, a vitamin K antagonist, is the anticoagulant most widely used in humans and has recently been proposed for prevention of reembolization in cats surviving an initial episode. The initial dose is 0.25-0.5 mg PO once daily. It should be overlapped with heparin therapy for 3 days. The dose is then adjusted to prolong the prothrombin time (PT)

approximately two times its baseline value or to attain an international normalized ratio (INR) of 2.0-4.0.

• Treatment of the patient's heart disease should be addressed.

• Fluid therapy is rarely necessary as most cats are in congestive heart failure.

CONTRAINDICATIONS N/A

PRECAUTIONS

• Anticoagulant therapy with heparin, warfarin, or the thrombolytic drugs may cause severe bleeding complications.

• Avoid a nonselective beta blocker such as propranolol as it may enhance peripheral vasoconstriction.

POSSIBLE INTERACTIONS

Warfarin may interact with other drugs, which may enhance its anticoagulant effects.

ALTERNATE DRUGS N/A

FOLLOW-UP

PATIENT MONITORING

• Daily examination of the legs should be performed to assess clinical response to therapy. • Initially, APTT should be performed once daily to titrate the heparin dose. • If warfarin is used, PT or INR is measured approximately 3 days after initiation then weekly until adequate anticoagulant effect is reached. Thereafter, it could be measured 3-4 times yearly or when drug regimen is altered.

PREVENTION/AVOIDANCE

Venapuncture and urine scald should be avoided in the hind legs.

POSSIBLE COMPLICATIONS

• Bleeding complications may arise with the anticoagulant therapy. • Urinary retention is possible, thus these patients may require periodic bladder expression. • Permanent neurological deficits or muscular abnormalities in the hindlimbs may arise in severe cats with prolonged ischemia.

EXPECTED COURSE AND PROGNOSIS

• Expected course is days to weeks for full recovery of function to the legs. • Prognosis in general is poor. In one study of 100 cats, approximately 60-70% of cats were euthanized or died during the initial thromboembolic episode. Long-term prognosis varies between 2 months to several years; however, the average is approximately 11 months with treatment.

MISCELLANEOUS

ASSOCIATED CONDITIONS

See causes and risk factors.

AGE RELATED FACTORS N/A

ZOONOTIC POTENTIAL N/A

PREGNANCY N/A

SYNONYMS

• Saddle thromboembolism • Systemic thromboembolism

SEE ALSO

• Hypertrophic Cardiomyopathy—Cats
• Restrictive Cardiomyopathy • Dilated Cardiomyopathy

ABBREVIATIONS

APTT = activated partial thromboplastic time
ATE = aortic thromboembolism
PT = prothrombin time

References

Laste NJ, Harpster NK. A retrospective study of 100 cats with feline distal aortic thromboembolism: 1977-1993. J Am An Hosp Assoc 1995;31492-500.

Flanders JA. Feline aortic thromboembolism. Compend Cont Ed Pract Ved 1986;8:473-484.

Miller WP, Sisson DD. Myocardial diseases. In: Ettinger SJ, Feldman EC, eds. Textbook of Veterinary Internal Medicine. 4th ed. Philadelphia: WB Saunders, 1995.

Author Terri C. deFrancesco

Consulting Editors Larry P. Tilley and Francis W. K. Smith, Jr.

APUDOMA

BASICS

OVERVIEW
• Tumors of endocrine cells that are capable of amine precursor uptake and decarboxylation (APUD) and secretion of peptide hormones. The tumors are named after the hormone they secrete. APUD cells generally are found in the gastrointestinal tract and CNS. Gastrin and pancreatic polypeptide-secreting tumors are discussed here. Insulinoma and glucagonoma are discussed separately.
• Hypergastrinemia from gastrin-secreting tumors causes gastric and duodenal hyperacidity which can cause gastric ulceration, esophageal dysfunction from chronic reflux, and intestinal villous atrophy. • High concentration of pancreatic polypeptide also causes gastric hyperacidity and its consequences.

SIGNALMENT
• Gastrinoma—rare in dogs and cats. Age range 3-12 years; mean, 7.5 years (dogs)
• Pancreatic polypeptide—extremely rare in dogs

SIGNS
• Vomiting • Weight loss • Anorexia
• Diarrhea • Lethargy depression • Polydipsia
• Melena • Abdominal pain • Hematemesis
• Hematochezia • Fever

CAUSES AND RISK FACTORS
Unknown

DIAGNOSIS

DIFFERENTIAL DIAGNOSIS
Other conditions associated with hypergastrinemia, gastric hyperacidity, and gastrointestinal ulceration:
• Uremia • Hepatic failure • Drug-induced ulceration (e.g., NSAIDS or steroids) inflammatory gastritis • Stress-induced ulceration
• Mast cell disease

CBC/BIOCHEMISTRY/URINALYSIS
• Results are normal or reflect the chronic effects of general disease. • Iron deficiency anemia secondary to gastrointestinal bleeding

• Hypoproteinemia • Electrolyte abnormalities with chronic vomiting

OTHER LABORATORY TESTS
• Serum gastrin concentration normal or high in patients with gastrinoma • Provocative test of gastrin secretion—an increase in gastrin after IV calcium gluconate or secretin administration suggests gastrinoma. See appendix for protocol and interpretation.

IMAGING
Abdominal ultrasound sometimes demonstrates a pancreatic mass.

OTHER DIAGNOSTIC PROCEDURES
• Endoscopy with gastric and duodenal biopsy • Any detectable masses should be aspirated because of the suspicion of mast cell disease. In animals with no detectable masses, a buffy coat smear should be examined for mast cells.

TREATMENT
• Medical management to treat gastric hyperacidity
• Surgical exploration and excisional biopsy of a pancreatic mass is important both diagnostically and therapeutically.
• Owners should be aware that most apudomas are malignant and have metastasized by the time of diagnosis, and long-term control is often difficult. Aggressive medical management can sometimes palliate signs for months to years.

MEDICATIONS

DRUGS AND FLUIDS
• Histamine-2 receptor antagonists—cimetidine, ranitidine, and famotidine decrease acid secretion by parietal cells.
• Omeprazole—a proton pump inhibitor and the most potent inhibitor of gastric acid secretion available. The drug is highly effective and very expensive.
• Sucralfate—this drug adheres to ulcerated gastric mucosa and protects it from acid and promotes healing by binding pepsin and bile acids and stimulating local prostaglandins.

CONTRAINDICATIONS/POSSIBLE INTERACTIONS N/A

FOLLOW-UP
• Physical examination and clinical signs are the most useful measures of effectiveness of treatment and progression of disease. Gastroscopy can be used to monitor progression of gastritis, but is not necessary. Abdominal radiography or ultrasound may detect the development of abdominal masses.
• The course of the disease is difficult to predict. Patients with gastrinoma have been controlled on medical management for months to years.

MISCELLANEOUS

SEE ALSO
Gastric Erosions and Ulcers

ABBREVIATIONS
CNS = central nervous system
NSAID = nonsteoridal antiinflammatory drugs

Reference
Zerbe CA. Islet cell tumors secreting insulin, pancreatic polypeptide, gastrin, or glucagon. In: Kirk RW, Bonagura JD, eds. Current veterinary therapy XI. Philadelphia: WB Saunders, 1992.
Author Thomas K. Graves
Consulting Editor Rhett Nichols

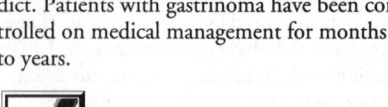

BASICS

OVERVIEW
Caused by herbicides, insecticides, wood preservatives, and treatments for blood parasites

SIGNALMENT
Cats are more commonly poisoned than dogs.

SIGNS

Acute Exposure
• Abdominal pain • Vomiting • Weakness • Diarrhea • Hematochezia • Rapid, weak pulse • Prostration • Subnormal temperature • Collapse • Death

Subchronic to Chronic Oral Exposure
Anorexia

CAUSES AND RISK FACTORS
• Ingestion of arsenic-containing compounds
• Lethal dose varies greatly.

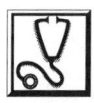

DIAGNOSIS

DIFFERENTIAL DIAGNOSIS
• Heavy metals toxicity • Ingestion of caustic agents • Ingestion of irritating plants • Canine parvovirus

CBC/BIOCHEMISTRY/URINALYSIS
Results of serum biochemical analysis reflect liver and renal damage.

OTHER LABORATORY TESTS
• Measurement of arsenic concentration in urine (acute), kidney, liver, hair (chronic), vomitus or stomach. • Arsenic concentration in urine, kidneys, and liver decreases dramatically 1-2 days after exposure.
• Measurement of arsenic concentration in blood is unreliable.

IMAGING N/A

OTHER DIAGNOSTIC PROCEDURES
N/A

GROSS AND HISTOPATHOLOGIC FINDINGS
• Peracute poisoning causes death without lesions. • Lesions in the gastrointestinal tract are common and severe—reddening of the gastric mucosa and proximal small intestine, watery gastrointestinal content, and blood and sloughed mucosa in feces. • Soft, yellow liver • Edematous lungs

TREATMENT
• Remove arsenic source. • Gastric lavage if vomiting has not occurred • Promote excretion. • Dialysis for renal failure

MEDICATIONS

DRUGS AND FLUIDS
• Dimercaprol (British anti-Lewisite [BAL] 2.5 to 5 mg/kg in oil by deep IM injection q4h for 2 days, q8h on day 3, and then q12h for up to 10 days. Use higher dosage in acutely affected animals first day.) • Signs of BAL toxicity include vomiting, tremors, and convulsions. • BAL releases arsenic which may worsen signs; additional BAL should be given. • DMSA (2,3-dimercapto succinic acid, succimer) is less toxic than BAL. Dosage in children is 10 mg/kg q8h . Effective in laboratory animals and humans. • Appropriate fluid therapy to treat dehydration. • Kaolin-pectin to soothe the gastrointestinal tract.

CONTRAINDICATIONS/POSSIBLE INTERACTIONS
• Emetics • Strong cathartics • Parasympathomimetic drugs

FOLLOW-UP
Monitor closely for signs of BAL toxicity during treatment.

MISCELLANEOUS

SEE ALSO
Poisoning (Intoxication)

ABBREVIATIONS
• BAL = British anti-Lewisite
• DMSA = 2,3-dimercapto succinic acid, succimer

Reference
Hatch RC. Poisons causing abdominal distress of liver or kidney damage. In: Booth NH and McDonald LE ed. Veterinary pharmacology and therapeutics. 6th Ed. Ames IA: Iowa State Press, 1988: 1102-1125.

Author Regg D. Neiger
Consulting Editor Gary Osweiler

ARTERIOVENOUS FISTULA

BASICS

OVERVIEW
• An abnormal, low resistance connection between an artery and vein • A large arteriovenous fistula allows a large fraction of the total cardiac output to bypass the capillary bed. The resulting increase in cardiac output may lead to "high output" congestive heart failure (CHF). • Location of arteriovenous fistula varies. Reported sites include the head, neck, ear, tongue, limbs, flank, spinal cord, cerebrum, lung, liver, vena cava, and gastrointestinal tract. • Usually seen as an acquired lesion

SIGNALMENT
• Dogs and cats. (rare in both). • No specific age, breed, or sex predilections known

SIGNS

Historical Findings
• Animals with acquired disease often have a history of trauma to the affected area. • Owner may notice a warm, nonpainful swelling at the site. • History consistent with impending or overt CHF is possible depending on shunt size and duration. • Other historical findings depend on the location of the lesion.

Physical Examination Findings
• Vary and depend on location of the arteriovenous fistula. • Signs of CHF (e.g., coughing, dyspnea, tachypnea, and exercise intolerance) may develop in animals with longstanding disease and high blood flow. • Bounding pulses are present in some animals because of high ejection volume and rapid runoff through the arteriovenous fistula. • Continuous murmur (bruit) at the site caused by blood flow through the lesion. Cautious compression of the artery proximal to the lesion abolishes the bruit. When blood flow is high, this compression may also elicit an immediate reflex decrease in heart rate (Branham's sign). • Edema, ischemia, and congestion of organs and tissues caused by high venous pressure in the proximity of the lesion. If the lesion is on a limb, pitting edema, lameness, ulceration, scabbing, and gangrene may result. • Lesion near vital organs may cause signs associated with organ failure such as ascites (liver), seizures (brain), paresis (spinal cord), and dyspnea (lung).

CAUSES AND RISK FACTORS
• Rarely, a congenital lesion • Acquired arteriovenous fistula is more common. Lesion typically results from local damage to vasculature secondary to trauma, surgery, venipuncture, perivascular injection (e.g., barbiturates), or tumor.

DIAGNOSIS

DIFFERENTIAL DIAGNOSIS
• The lesion may look like an aneurysm or false aneurysm. • Bizarre clinical findings, depending on location of arteriovenous fistula, may suggest other disease processes; arteriovenous fistula may be a late consideration.

CBC/BIOCHEMISTRY/URINALYSIS
May reflect damage to systems proximal to the lesion

OTHER LABORATORY TESTS N/A

IMAGING

Thoracic Radiographic Findings
Cardiac enlargement and pulmonary overcirculation in some animals with hemodynamically important arteriovenous fistula

Echocardiography
• Allows imaging of the arteriovenous fistula depicting its cavernous nature • Doppler ultrasound demonstrates high velocity, turbulent flow within the lesion.

Angiography
Selective angiography outlines the lesion, may be necessary for definitive diagnosis, and is highly desirable for surgical evaluation. Placement of the catheter close to the lesion and rapid injection is necessary; high volume blood flow dilutes the contrast medium quickly.

OTHER DIAGNOSTIC TESTS N/A

TREATMENT
• Definitive treatment requires surgery to divide and remove abnormal vascular connections—recommended in animals with clinical arteriovenous fistula since lesions may increase in size.
• Surgery can be difficult and labor intensive and may require blood transfusion; delineation of lesion before surgery by angiography is advised.
• Although surgery is often successful, arteriovenous fistula may recur. In some animals, amputation of the affected part may be necessary.

MEDICATIONS

DRUGS AND FLUIDS

• Concurrent medical treatment depends on the site of the arteriovenous fistula and secondary clinical features.
• Medical treatment for congestive heart failure may be required before surgery.

CONTRAINDICATIONS / POSSIBLE INTERACTIONS

• Avoid excessive fluid administration; animals with arteriovenous fistula are volume overloaded.

FOLLOW-UP

• Postoperative reevaluation is needed to determine whether arteriovenous fistula recurred.

MISCELLANEOUS

SEE ALSO

• Congestive Heart Failure, Left-sided

ABBREVIATION

CHF = congestive heart failure

References

Suter PF, Fox PR. Peripheral vascular disease. In: Ettinger SJ, Feldman EC, eds. Textbook of veterinary internal medicine. 4th ed. Philadelphia: WB Saunders, 1995.

Author Donald J. Brown
Consulting Editors Larry P. Tilley and Francis W. K. Smith, Jr.

ARTHRITIS (OSTEOARTHRITIS)

BASICS

DEFINITION
Arthritis (osteoarthritis) is a progressive deterioration of articular cartilage found in diarthrodial joints. Degenerative joint disease (DJD) is a more appropriate term used to describe this condition in veterinary medicine. The two broad classes of DJD are primary (idiopathic) and secondary.

Pathophysiology
Although DJD is usually categorized as non-inflammatory, mild inflammation plays an important role. Adverse stimuli cause release of inflammatory mediators from leukocytes, chondrocytes and synoviocytes, which leads to loss of proteoglycans from the extracellular matrix of articular cartilage due to excess destruction and reduced production. The breakdown and loss of collagen and chondrocytes follow as the disease progresses, leading to irreversible change.

Systems Affected
Musculoskeletal—diarthrodial joints

Genetics
Generally DJD is not assumed to be associated with hereditary factors, although primary DJD has been associated with a colony of Beagles. Secondary causes of DJD may be hereditary such as hip dysplasia and osteochondrosis.

Incidence/Prevalence
Degenerative joint disease is probably the most common skeletal disease encountered in dogs. The actual incidence, however, is unknown.

Geographic Distribution   N/A

SIGNALMENT

Species Dogs and cats

Breed Predilections
Any breed is susceptible.

Mean Age And Range
Many immature dogs develop DJD due to hereditary or developmental disorders such as osteochondrosis, elbow dysplasia, or hip dysplasia. Trauma-induced DJD can occur at any age.

Predominant Sex None

SIGNS

General Comments
Clinical signs vary greatly among affected animals. The severity of signs seen radiographically often does not correlate with those seen clinically.

Historical Findings
• Dogs suffering from DJD often show intermittent lameness that slowly becomes more severe and frequent with time. • Clinical signs may be exacerbated by exercise, long periods of recumbency, and weather changes

(cold weather). • Some dogs have a stiff gait, rather than lameness. • Dogs may have a history of previous joint trauma (fracture, ligament injury, dislocation), osteochondral disease or developmental disorders (patellar luxation, fragmented medical coronoid process, ununited anconeal process, hip dysplasia).

Physical Examination Findings
Clinical signs include stiffness of gait, lameness, reduced range of motion, crepitus, and joint swelling and pain. Depending on the duration of disease, joint instability may be present (ligament tear, subluxation).

CAUSES
• Primary DJD is thought to be due to long term exercise combined with aging. Primary DJD is not associated with a known predisposing cause. • Secondary DJD is much more common and results from an initiating cause such as joint instability, trauma, osteochondral defects, or joint incongruity.

RISK FACTORS
• Working dogs, athletic dogs and obese animals place more stress on their joints, thus are more likely to incur injury and DJD. • Dogs with Cushing's disease or diabetes mellitus may also be more prone to DJD due to catabolic processes.

DIAGNOSIS

DIFFERENTIAL DIAGNOSIS
• Immune-mediated arthritis • Infectious arthritis • Neoplasia

CBC/BIOCHEMISTRY/URINALYSIS
N/A

OTHER LABORATORY TESTS
Coombs, antinuclear antibody (ANA) and rheumatoid factor tests help rule out immune-mediated arthritis. Serum titers for Borrelia, Ehrlichia and Rickettsia evaluate for infectious arthritis.

IMAGING
Radiographic changes include joint capsular distension, osteophytosis, soft tissue thickening, narrowed joint spaces, and subchondral sclerosis in severely affected patients.

OTHER DIAGNOSTIC PROCEDURES
• Arthrocentesis and synovial fluid analysis can be used to support a diagnosis of DJD. A slightly high number of mononuclear cells is seen, generally less than 2000 cells/ml. Cell counts having large numbers of neutrophils are likely due to underlying immune-mediated or infectious arthritis. • Synovial fluid can be submitted for bacterial culture and sensitivity. • Biopsy of the synovial tissue is helpful in ruling out other arthritides or neoplasia.

GROSS AND HISTOPATHOLOGIC FINDINGS
Erosion of articular cartilage is present. Eburnation and sclerosis of subchondral bone appears with full thickness cartilage loss in

chronic cases. Thickening and fibrosis of the joint capsule is evident. Synovial fluid appears grossly normal, but is usually increased in volume. Osteophytes and enthesiophytes are found at joint capsular attachments and adjacent to the joint.

TREATMENT

INPATIENT VERSUS OUTPATIENT
• Treatment of DJD may include medical or surgical options. Most patients are initially treated medically. • Medical management of DJD includes a wide variety of pharmaceuticals that inhibit prostaglandins, leukotrienes, serine proteases, metalloproteases, interleukins, and tumor necrosis factor. • Other drugs, such as the chondroprotective agents not only inhibit inflammatory mediators, but also stimulate metabolic activity of synoviocytes and chondrocytes. • If an inadequate response is obtained, surgical options should be considered.

ACTIVITY
Exercise should be limited to a level that minimizes aggravation of clinical signs.

DIET
• Weight reduction in obese pets will reduce the stress placed on affected joints. • Reduced caloric intake is recommended as activity diminishes due to DJD and as the patient ages.

CLIENT EDUCATION
• Clients should be informed that medical therapy is palliative and DJD is likely to progress. • Treatment options, activity level, and diet should be discussed.

SURGICAL CONSIDERATIONS
• Arthrotomy is often used to treat underlying causes of DJD such as fragmented medical coronoid process, osteochondral diseases, or ununited anconeal process • Reconstructive procedures are used to eliminate joint instability or correct anatomic deficiences • Arthroplasty procedures are commonly performed to treat DJD of the hip. Total hip replacement (THR) can give excellent results and is recommended in dogs that can accomodate the implants. Femoral head ostectomy is performed in smaller dogs and cats, or select patients that can not afford total hip. • Arthrodesis is used in selective patients with chronic DJD and joint instability. Complete or partial arthrodesis can be performed based on the location of DJD or instability. Arthrodesis of the carpus generally yields excellent results, while arthrodesis of the shoulder, elbow, stifle or hock gives less predictable results.

MEDICATIONS

DRUGS AND FLUIDS

• Nonsteroidal Anti-inflammatory Drugs (NSAIDs)—these agents work by inhibiting prostaglandin synthesis. Aspirin (25 mg/kg PO q12h) and phenylbutazone (3-7 mg/kg PO q8h) are the most commonly used agents in dogs. Meclofenemic acid can also be given (0.5 mg/kg PO q12h). Carprofen (2.2 mg/kg PO q12h), a new NSAIDs which is less ulcerogenic, is presently not available in the United States. Use of NSAIDs in cats should be limited to aspirin (10 mg/kg PO every 3 days).

• Chondroprotective agents—a drug (Adequan®) which is gaining popularity for use in dogs is a glycosaminoglycan polysulfate ester (GAGPS). Chondroprotection is achieved due to the inhibition of various destructive enzymes and prostaglandins. Chondrostimulation is associated with increased production of proteoglycan, hyaluronate, and collagen. A recent clinical study in hip dysplastic dogs found the greatest improvement in orthopedic scores at a dosage of 4.4 mg/kg (2 mg/lb), im, every 3 to 5 days for 8 injections.

CONTRAINDICATIONS

• Drugs in both classes listed above should be avoided or used cautiously in dogs having disorders of hemostasis due to their ability to inhibit platelets and coagulation.

• Simultaneous use of NSAIDs and GAGPS is not recommended due to potential additive inhibition of hemostasis.

PRECAUTIONS

Due to the potential for gastric ulceration, NSAIDs should be used cautiously. Although many references have suggested dosages for naproxen, piroxicam, flunixin meglumine and ibuprofen, they appear to have ulcerogenic potential, and therefore their use is discouraged.

POSSIBLE INTERACTIONS

None known

ALTERNATE DRUGS

• Nutraceuticals—these products are classified as nutritional supplements, rather than pharmaceuticals. Little controlled experimental or clinical research substantiate their efficacy in dogs. Manufacturer recommendations

should be followed. Glycosaminoglycan products contain varying amounts of chondroitin sulfates. Cosequin® provides raw materials needed for glycosaminoglycan synthesis. Cosequin contains glucosamine, chondroitin sulfate, mixed glycosaminoglycans, and manganese ascorbate. Methyl sulfonyl methane (MSM) is a derivative of dimethyl sulfoxide (DMSO) that is promoted as an agent to reduce pain, inflammation and free radicals.

• Free-radical scavengers—the use of oral superoxide dismutase (SD) is controversial due to lack of controlled clinical studies evaluating its efficacy and questions regarding its bioavailability following ingestion. The efficacy of subcutaneously administered SD is unproven. Topical DMSO may provide short term relief in some dogs.

• Corticosteroids—the use of glucocorticoids (GCC) for treatment of DJD would appear to be ideal due to inhibition of inflammatory mediators and cytokines; however, chronic use of these drugs has been found to delay healing and initiate damage to articular cartilage. If used, prednisone is given orally at an initial dose of 1-2 mg/kg PO q24h in dogs and 4 mg/kg PO q24h in cats. The potential systemic side effects of GCC are documented; therefore, low dose (0.5-2.0 mg/kg in dogs), alternate day therapy is the goal. Intraarticular injection of 5 mg triamcinolone hexacetonide in dogs showed a protective and therapeutic effect in one DJD model.

FOLLOW-UP

PATIENT MONITORING

Clinical deterioration indicates the need for a change in drug selection, or dosage or surgical intervention.

PREVENTION/AVOIDANCE

Early identification of predisposing causes and prompt treatment will help reduce progression of secondary DJD.

POSSIBLE COMPLICATIONS N/A

EXPECTED COURSE AND PROGNOSIS

• Slow progression of disease is likely. • Some form of medical or surgical treatment will usually allow a good quality of life.

MISCELLANEOUS

ASSOCIATED CONDITIONS N/A

AGE RELATED FACTORS N/A

ZOONOTIC POTENTIAL N/A

PREGNANCY N/A

SYNONYMS

• Osteoarthritis • Degenerative joint disease

SEE ALSO N/A

ABBREVIATIONS

ANA = antinuclear antibody
DJD = degenerative joint disease
DMSO = dimethyl sulfoxide
GAGPS = glycosaminglycan polysulfate ester
GCC = glucocorticoid
MSM = methyl sulfonyl methane
NSAIDs = nonsteroidal anti-inflammatory drugs
SD = superoxide dismutase

References

Beale BS, Goring RL. Degenerative joint disease. In: Bojrab MJ, ed. Disease mechanisms in small animal surgery. Philadelphia: Lea and Febiger, 1993;727–736.

Beale BS. Arthropathies. In: Bloomberg MS, Taylor RT, Dee J, eds. Canine sports medicine and surgery. Philadelphia: WB Saunders, in press.

Pedersen NC. Joint diseases of dogs and cats. In: Ettinger SJ, ed. Textbook of veterinary internal medicine. 3rd ed. Philadelphia: WB Saunders, 1989;2329-2377.

Todhunter RJ, Lust G. Polysulfated glycosaminoglycan in the treatment of osteoarthritis. J Am Vet Med Assoc 1994;204:1245-1251.

Author Brian S. Beale
Consulting Editor Peter D. Schwarz

ARTHRITIS, SEPTIC

BASICS

DEFINITION
The presence of pathogenic microorganisms within the closed space of one or more synovial joints.

Pathophysiology
In most patients, septic arthritis is caused by hematogenous spread of the microorganisms from a distant septic foci, or from contamination associated with traumatic injury such as a direct penetrating injury (bite wounds, gunshot wounds), and extension of a primary osteomyelitis or contaminated surgery. The absence of a basement membrane may predispose the synovium to bacterial seeding. Sources of infection have included skin, severe dental disease, gastrointestinal, prostate and anal sacs.

Systems Affected
Musculoskeletal system—most often one joint is infected.

Genetics N/A

Incidence/Prevalence
Septic arthritis is a relatively uncommon cause of monoarticular arthritis in the dog and cat.

Geographic Distribution
There may be a high incidence of septic arthritis in Lyme disease endemic areas.

SIGNALMENT

Species
Most common in the dog; rare in cat.

Breed Predilections
Medium to large breeds with German shepherds, Dobermans, and Labrador retrievers most commonly affected.

Mean Age and Range
Any age, but most cases occurring between 4 and 7 years.

Predominant Sex Male

SIGNS

General Comments
Bacterial arthritis must always be considered in cases of monoarticular lameness associated with soft tissue swelling and pain.

Historical Findings
Most often the owner reports acute onset of lameness. The animal may be lethargic and anorexic. Previous trauma such as dog bites, injuries, etc. may be reported. Some patients have a mild lameness with a gradual onset.

Physical Examination Findings
• Monoarticular lameness • Joint pain and swelling • Reduced range of motion • Fever
• Common joints infected include the carpus, stifle, hock, shoulder, and cubital joints

CAUSES
• Most common aerobic bacterial agents—staphylococci, streptococci, coliforms, and pasteurella • Most common anaerobic organisms—propioni bacterium, peptostreptococcus, fusobacterium, and bacteroides • Borrelia burgdorferi (spirochete) • Mycoplasma
• Fungal agents: blastomyces, cryptococcus, coccidiodes • Ehrlichia • Leishmania

RISK FACTORS
• Predisposing factors for hematogenous infection include diabetes, chronic Addison's disease, and immunosuppression. • Penetrating trauma to the joint.

DIAGNOSIS

DIFFERENTIAL DIAGNOSIS
• Immune-mediated arthropathy • Post vaccine transient polyarthritis • Greyhound polyarthritis • Crystal induced joint disease

CBC/BIOCHEMISTRY/URINALYSIS
• Hemogram—inflammatory left shift
• Serum chemistry profile and urinalysis normal

OTHER LABORATORY TESTS
Serologic testing for specific pathogens

IMAGING
Radiographs—early patients may have increased thickness and density of periarticular tissues. Evidence of synovial effusion may be present. Evidence of bone destruction, osteolysis, irregular joint space, discreet erosions, and periarticular osteophytosis becomes evident later.

OTHER DIAGNOSTIC PROCEDURES

Synovial Fluid Analysis
• Increased volume • Turbid fluid • Low mucin clot reaction • High WBC count (predominate neutrophils <40,000/mm^3) (normal joint fluid <10% neutrophils) • Bacteria in the synovial fluid or within neutrophils show chromatolysis, nuclear swelling, and loss of segmentation.

Synovial Fluid Culture
• Fluid must be collected aseptically and this procedure often requires general anesthesia.
• Synovial fluid is placed in an aerobic and anaerobic culturette and also in blood culture medium. Samples from the culturettes are immediately cultured upon arrival to the laboratory. • The blood culture medium should be recultured after 24 hours of incubation (increases accuracy by 50%).

Synovial Fluid Glucose Level
A level that is below a paired serum glucose level is very suggestive of sepsis

Synovial Biopsy
• May be done to rule out immune mediated joint disease. • Synovial biopsy is no more effective than culturing incubated blood culture medium for diagnosing bacterial arthritis.

GROSS AND HISTOPATHOLOGIC FINDINGS
• Thickened, discolored synovium often very proliferative • Histologic evidence of hyperplastic synviotocytes • High numbers of neutrophils and macrophages fibrinous debris.

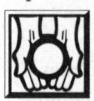

TREATMENT

INPATIENT VERSUS OUTPATIENT
Patients with septic arthritis should be hospitalized for initial stabilization and then discharged for long-term management.

ACTIVITY Restricted

DIET N/A

CLIENT EDUCATION
• Discuss probable cause
• Discuss need for long-term antibiotics
• Discuss possible need for corticosteroid usage and residual degenerative joint disease

SURGICAL CONSIDERATIONS
Open arthrotomy or placement of irrigation catheter (ingress/egress) to lavage joint

MEDICATIONS

DRUGS AND FLUIDS
• Administration of a first generation cephalosporin and ampicillin/clavulonic acid pending culture and susceptibility data.
• Choice of antimicrobial drugs primarily depends on in vitro determination of susceptibility of microorganisms. Consider also possible toxicity, frequency and route of administration, and expense. Most antimicrobials penetrate the synovium well, but need to be given for 4 to 8 weeks minimum.
• Nonsteroidal anti-inflammatory drugs (NSAIDs) may be helpful for analgesia and to reduce inflammation..

CONTRAINDICATIONS
Avoid use of quinolones in pediatric patients because experimentally they induced cartilage lesions.

PRECAUTIONS
Failure to respond to conventional antibiotic therapy may indicate anaerobic septic arthritis or other unusual causes (fungal, spirochete, etc.)

POSSIBLE INTERACTIONS N/A

ALTERNATE DRUGS N/A

FOLLOW-UP

PATIENT MONITORING
• Drainage and irrigation catheters may be pulled after 4-6 days or following reassessment of synovial fluid cytology. • Antibiotic therapy is continued for 4-8 weeks or longer depending on clinical signs and pathogenic organism. • Some dogs show persistent synovial inflammation in the absence of viable

bacterial organisms. Antigenic bacterial fragments or antigen antibody deposition may be the cause. • Systemic corticosteroid therapy and aggressive physical therapy may be needed to maximize normal joint dynamics.

PREVENTION/AVOIDANCE N/A

POSSIBLE COMPLICATIONS

• Severe degenerative joint disease in chronically affected patients • Recurrence of infection • Limited joint range-of-motion • Generalized sepsis • Osteomyelitis

EXPECTED COURSE AND PROGNOSIS

• Patients diagnosed quickly respond well to antibiotic therapy • Patients in which there is a delayed diagnosis or the presence of resistant or highly virulent organisms have a guarded to poor prognosis

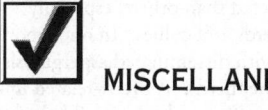

MISCELLANEOUS

ASSOCIATED CONDITIONS N/A

AGE RELATED FACTORS N/A

ZOONOTIC POTENTIAL N/A

PREGNANCY N/A

SYNONYMS

• Infectious arthritis • Joint ill

SEE ALSO

• Polyarthritis • Immune-Mediated Joint Disease • Osteomyelitis

ABBREVIATIONS

NSAIDs = nonsteroidal anti-inflammatory drugs

References

Hodgin EC, Michaelson F, Howerth EW. Anaerobic bacterial infections causing osteomyelitis/arthritis in a dog. J Am Vet Med Assoc 1992;201:886-888.

Montgomery RD, Long IR, Milton JL. Comparison of aerobic culturette, synovial membrane biopsy, and blood culture medium in detection of canine bacterial arthritis. Vet Surg 1989;18:300-303.

Ellison RS. The cytologic examination of synovial fluid. Sem Vet Med Surg (Small Anim) 1988;3:133-139.

Bennett D, Taylor DJ. Bacterial infective arthritis in the dog. J Small Anim Pract 1988;29:207-230.

Author Robert A. Taylor
Consulting Editor Peter D. Schwarz

ASPERGILLOSIS

BASICS

OVERVIEW
• Aspergillosis is an opportunistic fungal infection caused by the Aspergillus genus of common molds. A. fumigatus is the most frequent isolate; A. terreus occurs less commonly but is likely to be involved when disease is disseminated. • The organism is ubiquitous in the environment and is abundant in air, soil, water, and decaying vegetation. • The organism forms numerous spores in dust, straw, grass clippings, and hay.

SIGNALMENT
Primarily dogs; a limited number of incidences in cats have been reported

SIGNS
• Aspergillosis most commonly presents with rhinitis and sinusitis; varying degrees of turbinate invasion and destruction are present. • Chronic unilateral or bilateral nasal discharge is the primary sign; the discharge may be serous, mucopurulent, or hemorrhagic. History indicates lack of response to antimicrobial therapy. Nasal swelling is uncommon, although there may be discomfort on palpation. The external nares may be ulcerated. • Less commonly, invasion of the cribriform plate leads to signs of CNS involvement. • Disseminated infection in dogs is reported but is less common than localized disease.

Physical Examination Findings
• Lameness or spinal pain • Diskospondylitis plus involvement of other parts of the skeletal system • Inflammatory ocular disease • Nonspecific signs such as fever, weight loss, vomiting, and anorexia • Disseminated disease is more common in cats, with pulmonary involvement most frequently reported.

CAUSES AND RISK FACTORS
• More common in outdoor and farm dogs • Immune deficiency may contribute to establishment of infection as the organism is widespread, but the disease is infrequent. In some dogs, deficient cell-mediated immunity has been recognized. However, it has not been established whether potential immune deficiency is a primary or secondary abnormality. • Dolichocephalic breeds are more

commonly infected than others, especially German shepherds and collies. In one report, 13 of 15 dogs with disseminated aspergillosis were German shepherds. A breed-related immune defect was proposed as a possible cause.

DIAGNOSIS

DIFFERENTIAL DIAGNOSIS
• Nasal neoplasia • Bacterial rhinitis/sinusitis • Penicilliosis • Foreign body • Nasal mites

CBC/BIOCHEMISTRY/URINALYSIS
• The CBC, chemistry profile, and urinalysis are nondiagnostic. • Dogs often have a neutrophilic leukocytosis and lymphopenia; hyperglobulinemia and azotemia are reported in disseminated disease. • Cats have a nonregenerative anemia and leukopenia.

OTHER LABORATORY TESTS
• Fungal serology is useful as an aid in the diagnosis of aspergillosis. Positive results of the agar gel double diffusion, counterimmunoeletrophoresis, and enzyme-linked immunosorbent assay support a diagnosis; however, false-positives and cross-reactivity with Penicillium spp are reported. • Cats should be tested for FeLV and FIV because these diseases impact on prognosis.

IMAGING
Sinus radiographs will often show increased soft tissue density but findings are nondiagnostic. Radiography is helpful in the basic workup of nasal and sinus disease and may help delineate the extent of disease.

OTHER DIAGNOSTIC PROCEDURES
• Cytology of nasal swabs and flushes is usually nondiagnostic. Cytologic findings reflect an inflammatory process; hyphae may be recognized. • Rhinoscopy with biopsy provides an extremely useful tool for diagnosis. • Fungal cultures of nasal exudate may give false-positive or false-negative results; the organism is a common laboratory contaminant. If a positive culture is obtained, it is desirable to search for the organism in histopathologic specimens to help secure the diagnosis.

GROSS AND HISTOPATHOLOGIC FINDINGS
• Histopathologic examination of tissue is most likely to render a definitive diagnosis.

Special stains may sometimes be required to visualize the organism. • Granulomas and multiple organ infarcts are noted with disseminated disease. In particular, the kidneys, spleen, and vertebrae are involved.

TREATMENT

For dogs with localized disease, administration of enilconazole or clotrimazole through surgically implanted nasal tubes has met with success.

MEDICATIONS

DRUGS AND FLUIDS
• Itraconazole is more effective than ketoconazole in animals with systemic disease. One protocol suggests 5 mg/kg twice daily for 2-3 months; another recommends 10 mg/kg once daily. • Thiabendazole at 10 mg/kg twice daily has achieved cure in up to 50% of cases. • Amphotericin B is also effective but resistance may develop; nephrotoxicity is a limiting factor in its use. • Dogs with disseminated disease caused by A. terreus are unlikely to be cured although they may be maintained with intraconazole.

CONTRAINDICATIONS/POSSIBLE INTERACTIONS N/A

MISCELLANEOUS

There is no public health significance to this disease because it is not spread from animal to animal or animal to human.

Reference
Sharp NJH. Aspergillosis. In: Greene CE, ed. Infectious diseases of the dog and cat. Philadelphia: WB Saunders, 1990:714-722.
Author Sharon K. Fooshee
Consulting Editor Fred W. Scott

BASICS

OVERVIEW
• Administered to animals to relieve minor pain and discomfort. • Less commonly used than previously due to increasing popularity of other over-the-counter pain-relieving drugs.

SIGNALMENT
Toxicity occurs more in cats than dogs; longer biological half-life in cats (44.6 hours) than dogs (7.5 hours).

SIGNS
• Depression • Vomiting; may be blood-tinged • Tachypnea • High body temperature • Muscular weakness • Ataxia • Coma and death in 1 or more days

CAUSES AND RISK FACTORS
• Employing human dosage guidelines to cats. • Deficiency in glucuronide conjugation capability in cats causes a higher risk than in dogs.

DIAGNOSIS

DIFFERENTIAL DIAGNOSIS
• Clinical signs are uncharacteristic.
• History of aspirin ingestion or medication is important. • History of medication within 5 days of development of signs should raise concern. • History of musculoskeletal injury calls for questioning owner about giving aspirin to their pet.

CBC/BIOCHEMISTRY/URINALYSIS
• Heinz body formation in cats • Suppression of bone marrow activity and anemia, especially in cats • Hyponatremia • Hypokalemia

OTHER LABORATORY TESTS
• High ketones and pyruvic, lactic, and amino acid concentrations • Low sulfuric and phosphoric acid renal clearance • Respiratory alkalosis followed by metabolic acidosis • Salicylic acid concentration in serum or urine

IMAGING N/A

OTHER DIAGNOSTIC PROCEDURES
N/A

GROSS AND HISTOPATHOLOGIC FINDINGS
• Gastric irritation and hemorrhage in 10-20% of affected animals • Repeated aspirin administration may cause ulceration and perforation • Toxic hepatitis

TREATMENT
• Specific antidote not available • Treat as inpatient with general principles of poisoning management • Induce gastric emptying by gastric lavage or induced emesis • Heroic procedures—peritoneal or hemodialysis or hemoperfusion

MEDICATIONS

DRUGS AND FLUIDS
• Activated charcoal (2 g/kg PO) • Continuous intravenous administration of fluids to correct acid-base imbalance • Sodium bicarbonate (1 mEq/kg IV) to alkalinize urine

CONTRAINDICATIONS/POSSIBLE INTERACTIONS N/A

FOLLOW-UP
• Maintaining renal function and acid-base balance is vital. • Severe acid-base disturbances, severe dehydration, toxic hepatitis, bone marrow depression, and coma are poor prognostic indicators.

MISCELLANEOUS
Ascertain that history of "aspirin medication" does not refer to other, more recently available pain medications.

SEE ALSO
Poisoning (Intoxication)

Reference

Oehme FW. Aspirin and acetaminophen. In: Kirk RW, ed. Current veterinary therapy IX: small animal practice. Philadelphia: WB Saunders, 1986: 188-189.

Author Frederick W. Oehme
Consulting Editor Gary D. Osweiler

ASTHMA, BRONCHITIS—CATS

BASICS

DEFINITION
• Chronic bronchitis is a condition that causes a chronic cough, in which other causes of cough (pneumonia, heartworm infestation, bronchopulmonary neoplasia, heart failure) have been excluded. • Asthma is a disorder characterized by spontaneous bronchoconstriction, which may resolve spontaneously or in response to therapy.

Pathophysiology
• Although the potential causes of chronic bronchial disease are numerous, the airways are capable of responding to noxious stimuli in a limited number of ways. Airway epithelium may hypertrophy, undergo metaplastic change, erode, or ulcerate. Airway goblet cells and submucosal glands may hypertrophy and produce excessive amounts of viscid mucus. Bronchial mucosa and submucosa are usually infiltrated with variable numbers and types of inflammatory cells and may become edematous. Bronchial smooth muscle may remain unaffected, become hypertrophied, or spasm. • The resulting clinical signs of cough, wheeze, and lethargy are a result of airflow limitation from excessive mucus secretions, airway edema, airway narrowing from cellular infiltrates, and airway smooth muscle constriction. Cough also may result from stimulation of mechanoreceptors located in inflamed and contracted airway smooth muscle. • Eosinophils specifically have been implicated as primary effector cells in the development of asthmatic airways. Toxic eosinophil granular proteins such as major basic protein and eosinophilic cationic protein can cause epithelial sloughing, ciliary stasis, and augment airway smooth contraction. Interleukin-5, a cytokine produced from activated T lymphocytes, may play a critical role in the development of asthma by recruiting and activating eosinophils in airways.

Systems Affected
• Respiratory • Cardiovascular—chronic airway disease may cause right ventricular pressure overload and cor pulmonale in dogs, humans, and, potentially, cats.

Genetics
The Siamese breed may have an increased incidence of lower airway disease.

Incidence/Prevalence
The prevalence of lower airway disease in the general adult cat population is estimated to be approximately 1%; prevalence in the Siamese breed may be 5%.

Geographic Distribution N/A

SIGNALMENT

Species Cats

Breed Predilections
Siamese, Himalayan

Mean Age and Range
Asthma and chronic bronchitis are diagnosed in cats of all ages.

Predominant Sex N/A

SIGNS

General Comments
• Clinical signs include cough, wheeze and decreased activity. • In mild cases symptoms may be limited to occasional and brief episodes of coughing. • All cats with chronic bronchitis, by definition, have symptoms of cough on most days throughout the year. • Some cats with asthma may be asymptomatic in between occasional episodes of acute airway obstruction. • Severely affected cats may have persistent daily cough and many episodes of life-threatening acute bronchoconstriction.

Historical Findings
• Chronic cough is the defining feature of chronic bronchitis. • Acute bronchoconstriction manifested as respiratory distress is a defining feature of asthma.

Physical Examination Findings
• Cats with bronchitis or asthma may have a normal physical examination at rest. • Respiratory distress primarily during the expiratory phase of breathing is the hallmark of chronic bronchial disease. • Wheezing is more commonly found in cats with asthma although it can be heard in cats with both conditions. Adventitious sounds, including crackles, are commonly heard.

CAUSES
Unknown. (See pathophysiology)

RISK FACTORS
Air pollution, dust, or cigar or cigarette smoke may exacerbate already established airway disease.

DIAGNOSIS

DIFFERENTIAL DIAGNOSIS
• Congestive heart failure • Pulmonary parasitism (heartworm, aelurostrongylus, capillariasis) • Foreign body aspiration • Pleural space disorders • Bronchopulmonary malignancy • Noninfectious pneumonitis • Infectious pneumonia/acute bronchitis

CBC/BIOCHEMISTRY/URINALYSIS
• Hemograms often demonstrate both relative and absolute increases in eosinophils. However, peripheral eosinophilia is found in many non–respiratory-related disorders in cats. Additionally, normal peripheral eosinophilia does not exclude a diagnosis of chronic bronchitis or asthma. • Analyze stool samples to help rule out pulmonary parasitism.

OTHER LABORATORY TESTS N/A

IMAGING

Radiography
• Routine survey chest radiographs may be normal and should not cause the practitioner to abandon the diagnosis of lower airway disease. • Radiographs often reveal diffuse, prominent bronchial markings consistent with inflammatory airways. • Approximately 10% of cats with bronchial disease have air bronchograms within the right middle lung lobe associated with a mediastinal shift to the right. This is evidence of atelectasis. • Cats with asthma commonly have radiographic signs of increased lung lucency and flattening and caudal displacement of the diaphragm. These changes are evidence of hyperinflation and suggest air trapping.

Echocardiography
Echocardiography is helpful in selected cats to determine the presence or absence of cardiac disease, and also to determine the presence and degree of cor pulmonale; a finding that suggests a poor prognosis.

OTHER DIAGNOSTIC PROCEDURES
• Transtracheal wash, bronchial wash, or bronchoalveolar lavage may all be used to collect samples for cytologic examination and culture. • Large numbers of neutrophils are frequently recovered from the airways of cats with chronic bronchitis. • Eosinophils are commonly found in airway washings from cats with asthma. However, eosinophils are found in airway washings from normal cats and thus may not be a reliable marker for asthma. • Bronchoscopy may suggest lower airway disease by the finding of excessive bronchial secretions. Irregular airway outlines and collapsing bronchi are features of lower airway disease in dogs but are not commonly found in cats with bronchitis or asthma. • Pulmonary function studies are available at certain universities and can assist in differentiating cats with asthma from cats with chronic bronchitis.

GROSS AND HISTOPATHOLOGIC FINDINGS
• Epithelial erosion • Goblet cell hypertrophy and hyperplasia • Submucosal gland hyperplasia • Smooth muscle hyperplasia and contraction generally are features of asthma. • Inflammatory cellular infiltrate of submucosa that extends through lamina propria to airway lumen • The predominant inflammatory cell in asthma usually is the eosinophil. • Relatively more neutrophils are found in tissues from cats with chronic bronchitis.

TREATMENT

INPATIENT VERSUS OUTPATIENT
• The decision to hospitalize an individual cat is determined on an individual basis. • Cats with asthma more commonly require hospitalization than cats with chronic bronchitis.

ACTIVITY
• Cats with chronic bronchial disease usually will limit their own activity.
• If a particular activity is associated with an increase in signs of lower airway obstruction, this activity should be prevented.

DIET N/A

CLIENT EDUCATION
• Chronic bronchitis and asthma are progressive syndromes that are rarely cured.
• Client education should stress realistic expectations regarding the extent of the pet's improvement while on medication. The frequency of cough can usually be reduced but not eliminated.
• Obese cats benefit from weight reduction.
• Owners of cats with asthma should be instructed to report early signs of wheezing or cough immediately, and should be instructed in the subcutaneous administration of terbutaline.

SURGICAL CONSIDERATIONS N/A

MEDICATIONS

DRUGS AND FLUIDS
• Corticosteroids are the primary method of chronic treatment. Cats initially should be treated with 1 mg/kg prednisone orally twice daily for 5 days, followed by prednisone 0.5 mg/kg orally twice a day for 5 more days. As the symptoms decrease in severity, the dose and frequency of drug administration are gradually reduced over a 2 to 4-month period.
• Many cats can be effectively maintained on 2.5 mg prednisone orally every other day.
• Individual cases will require careful and sometimes frequent readjustment of this basic regimen.
• In cats that cannot be treated orally, methylprednisolone can be given IM starting at 10-20 mg every 2 weeks, gradually reducing the dosage over 2-4 months.
• Terbutaline 0.1 mg/kg orally twice daily, or theophylline (Theodur, Shering, Kenilworth, NJ) 50-100 mg orally once a day at night is given concurrently with prednisone to cats that require more than 10 mg prednisone daily to control clinical signs, or to cats that experience an unacceptable number of bouts of acute onset respiratory distress.
• Cats with acute onset of respiratory distress should be treated with terbutaline (0.01 mg/kg parenterally SC), followed by dexamethasone (1 mg/kg, IV or IM) plus oxygen support. If an oxygen cage is not available, an oxygen mask can be placed in close proximity to the cat's face if it does not cause further distress.
• If mycoplasma or other aerobic bacteria are cultured from airway secretions, antibiotic treatment should be instituted for 10-14 days. Choice of antibiotic is based on sensitivity testing.

CONTRAINDICATIONS
Beta agonists are contraindicated in the presence of cardiac disorders in cats with left ventricular outflow tract obstruction (hypertrophic cardiomyopathy, subaortic stenosis).

PRECAUTIONS
• Chronic daily prophylactic use of bronchodilators may mask the signs of worsening airway inflammation and should be avoided.
• Chronic daily use of corticosteroids is associated with well-recognized complications. Diabetes mellitus, congestive heart failure, hepatic lipidosis, and urinary tract infections can occur in predisposed individuals. The dosage and frequency of administration of corticosteroids should be titrated to the lowest effective dosage needed to control clinical signs.

POSSIBLE INTERACTIONS
Corticosteroids and beta agonists may act synergistically. When these drugs are administered at the same time it may be possible to lower the usual dosage of each drug.

ALTERNATE DRUGS
• Cyproheptadine (Periactin, Merck Co.; 1-2 mg PO q12h) has been used to control clinical signs in an experimental model of asthma in cats.
• Cyclosporine A may be used in severe life threatening cases that are unresponsive to high doses of corticosteroids.

FOLLOW-UP

PATIENT MONITORING
• Cats should be reevaluated every 3-6 months for signs of worsening symptoms at rest. • Clients should be instructed to call at the first sign of acute wheezing or other evidence of respiratory distress.

PREVENTION/AVOIDANCE
Precipitating or aggravating factors have not been well characterized. Anecdotal reports have implicated house dust and feathers. Aggravating situations or environments should be avoided if identified.

POSSIBLE COMPLICATIONS
Acute bronchoconstriction is a feature of asthma. This may be life-threatening and should be identified, reported, and treated promptly.

EXPECTED COURSE AND PROGNOSIS
• Many cats with bronchitis or asthma do fairly well for long periods with steroid therapy.
• The chronic prophylactic use of beta-2 agonists (such as terbutaline or albuterol) has been associated with an increase in morbidity and mortality in asthmatic humans.

MISCELLANEOUS

ASSOCIATED CONDITIONS
None recognized

AGE RELATED FACTORS
Young cats are at increased risk for upper respiratory viral infections. These infections may exacerbate signs of preexisting lower airway disease.

ZOONOTIC POTENTIAL
None recognized

PREGNANCY
Corticosteroids should be used with caution in pregnant animals.

SYNONYMS
Chronic obstructive pulmonary disease
• Asthmatic bronchitis • Allergic bronchitis
• Allergic asthma • Eosinophilic bronchitis
• Bronchitis with emphysema

SEE ALSO N/A

ABBREVIATIONS N/A

References

Boothe DM, McKiernan B. Respiratory therapeutics. In: Update on respiratory diseases. Vet Clin N Amer 1992;22:1231-1259.

Moise NS, Wiedenkeller D, Yeager AC, et al. Clinical, radiographic, and bronchial cytologic features of cats with bronchial disease: 65 cases (1980-1986). J Am Vet Med Ass 1989;194:1467-1473.

Padrid PA. Chronic lower airway disease in the dog and cat. In: Spaulding GL, ed. Problems in veterinary medicine. Philadelphia: JB Lippincott, 1992;4:320-345.

Author Philip Padrid
Consulting Editors Lynelle Johnson and Bradley L. Moses

ASTROCYTOMA

BASICS

OVERVIEW
Astrocytoma is a glial cell neoplasm that develops most often within the piriform lobe in dogs and the parietal region in cats. Onset of signs is insidious in some animals, who may compensate initially to gradual increases in intracranial pressure and peritumoral edema.

SIGNALMENT
• Dogs—brachycephalic breeds; most dogs 6-11 years old; no sex predilection • Cats—generally old (> 9 years); no strong sex or breed predilection • Less common in cats than dogs

SIGNS
• Signs on examination depend on tumor location • Seizures • Behavioral changes • Disorientation or wandering in wide circling pattern • Loss of conscious proprioception, cranial nerve abnormalities, upper motor neuron tetraparesis

CAUSES AND RISK FACTORS
Unknown

DIAGNOSIS

DIFFERENTIAL DIAGNOSIS
• Other primary or metastatic neoplasm • Granulomatous meningoencephalitis • Trauma • Cerebrovascular accident • Aberrant parasite migration • Meningitis

CBC/BIOCHEMISTRY/URINALYSIS
Results usually normal

OTHER LABORATORY TESTS N/A

IMAGING
• Computerized tomography • Magnetic resonance imaging • Radiography of the calvarium rarely aids in detecting brain tumor

OTHER DIAGNOSTIC PROCEDURES
• Cerebrospinal fluid analysis—normal to mild increase in protein with or without WBC pleomorphism • Electroencephalography may indicate location of a lesion.

TREATMENT
• Symptomatic
• Control clinical signs
• Control seizures
• Chemotherapy indicated
• Surgery not indicated
• Excellent tumor remission and control achieved by radiotherapy in some animals
• Ultimate prognosis is poor

MEDICATIONS

DRUGS AND FLUIDS

Seizure Control
Status epilepticus (emergency):
• Mannitol—2 g/kg IV with a second dose 12 hours later
• Dexamethasone—2.2 mg/kg IV with a second dose 12 hours later

Long-term Management:
• Prednisone (0.5 - 1 mg/kg PO q12h) to reduce associated inflammation and edema
• Phenobarbital (1-4 mg/kg PO q12h)

Tumor Control
Carmustine (50 mg/m^2 IV q6wk)

CONTRAINDICATIONS/POSSIBLE INTERACTIONS
• Prednisone and phenobarbital cause polyphagia, polydipsia, and polyuria.
• Sedation for up to 2 weeks after initiation of phenobarbital

FOLLOW-UP

PATIENT MONITORING
• Modify phenobarbital dosage according to serum concentrations 5-7 days after initiating treatment. • Dose-limiting side effect of carmustine administration is myelosuppression; a CBC and platelet count should be performed in 10-14 days • Cumulative dose of 1400 mg/m^2 can cause pulmonary toxicity. • Seek advice before initiating treatment if unfamiliar with cytotoxic drugs.

EXPECTED COURSE AND PROGNOSIS
• Guarded prognosis • Survival time with no treatment reportedly 2 months • Median survival time for carmustine plus prednisone, and phenobarbital as needed, 218 days

MISCELLANEOUS

SEE ALSO
Seizures

ABBREVIATION
WBC = white blood cells

Reference
Frenier SL, et al. Canine intracranial astrocytomas and comparison with the human counterpart. Compend Cont Ed Pract Vet 1990;12:1422-1433.
Author Ruth Ann Chun
Consulting Editor Wallace B. Morriso

BASICS

OVERVIEW
An uncommon intestinal viral infection characterized by enteritis and diarrhea

SIGNALMENT
• Cats • No known breed, sex, or age predilection

SIGNS Enteritis with diarrhea

CAUSES AND RISK FACTORS
A small, nonenveloped, RNA virus of the genus Astrovirus. Details of the incidence, prevalence, and predisposing factors are unknown.

DIAGNOSIS

DIFFERENTIAL DIAGNOSIS
Many causes of gastroenteritis, including intestinal parasites, viral infections (panleukopenia, rotavirus, enteric coronavirus, enteric calicivirus), bacterial infections (salmonellosis, coliforms), and protozoal infections (giardia)

CBC/BIOCHEMISTRY/URINALYSIS
N/A

OTHER LABORATORY TESTS
None specific for astrovirus infections

IMAGING N/A

OTHER DIAGNOSTIC PROCEDURES
• Electron microscopy of feces to identify astrovirus particles • Astroviruses are difficult to isolate in the laboratory.

TREATMENT
• Control diarrhea.
• Reestablish fluid and electrolyte balance.

MEDICATIONS

DRUGS AND FLUIDS
• Symptomatic
• There are no antiviral drugs specific for astroviruses.

CONTRAINDICATIONS/POSSIBLE INTERACTIONS
None known

FOLLOW-UP

PATIENT MONITORING
Monitor fluid and electrolytes.

PREVENTION
Isolate infected cats during acute disease.

POSSIBLE COMPLICATIONS
Secondary intestinal viral and bacterial infections

EXPECTED COURSE AND PROGNOSIS
• Usually less than 1 week • Mortality appears to be low. • Prognosis is good.

MISCELLANEOUS
• Zoonotic potential of feline astrovirus infection is unknown. • Astroviruses produce enteritis in many species, including sheep and humans.

References

Barr MC, Olsen CW, Scott FW. Feline viral diseases. In: Ettinger SJ, Feldman EC, eds. Veterinary internal medicine. Philadelphia: WB Saunders, 1995;409-439.

Harbour DA, Greene CE. Feline astroviral and rotaviral infections. In: Greene CE, ed. Infectious diseases of the dog and cat. Philadelphia: WB Saunders, 1990;313-314.

Hoshino Y, Zimmer JF, Moise NS, Scott FW. Detection of astroviruses in feces of a cat with diarrhea. Arch Virol 1981;70:373-376.

Todd KS, Paul AJ. Metazoal and protozoal parasites of the alimentary system. In: Pratt PW, ed. Feline medicine. Santa Barbara: American Veterinary Publications, 1983;226-247.

Pedersen NC. Feline astrovirus infection. In: Pratt PW, ed. Feline infectious diseases. Goleta, CA: American Veterinary Publications, 1988;71-73.

Author Fred W. Scott

Consulting Editor Fred W. Scott

ATHEROSCLEROSIS

BASICS

OVERVIEW
• Thickening of the inner arterial wall in association with lipid deposits • Chronic arterial change characterized by loss of elasticity, luminal narrowing, and proliferating and degenerative lesions of the intima and media

SIGNALMENT
• Rare in dogs • Not described in cats • Geriatric patients (> 9 years) • Higher prevalence in miniature schnauzer, Doberman pinscher, poodle, and Labrador retriever

SIGNS

Historical Findings
• None in some animals • Lethargy • Anorexia • Weakness • Dyspnea • Collapse • Vomiting/diarrhea

Physical Examination Findings
• Dyspnea • Irregular rhythm • Heart failure • Disorientation • Blindness • Circling • Coma

CAUSES AND RISK FACTORS
• Severe hypothyroidism • Increasing age • Hyperlipidemia in miniature schnauzers • Male gender (male dogs may have predisposition) • High total cholesterol

DIAGNOSIS

DIFFERENTIAL DIAGNOSIS
Arteriosclerosis

CBC/BIOCHEMISTRY/URINALYSIS
• Hypercholesterolemia • Hyperlipidemia • High BUN and liver enzymes

OTHER LABORATORY TESTS
• Low T_3 and T_4 • High values for alpha-2 and beta fractions on protein electrophoresis

IMAGING

Radiography
Thoracic and abdominal radiographs may reveal cardiomegaly and hepatomegaly.

OTHER DIAGNOSTIC PROCEDURES

Electrocardiography
• Conduction abnormalities and myocardial infarction • Atrial fibrillation, notched QRS complexes, and ST segment elevation or depression

TREATMENT

Treat the underlying disorder and clinical signs (e.g., CHF).

MEDICATIONS

DRUGS AND FLUIDS
• Treat conduction disturbances and arrhythmias in-hospital until controlled.
• Thyroid replacement
• Antihypertensive therapy
• Enalapril—0.5 mg/kg PO q24h-q12h
• Lotensin—0.5 mg/kg PO q24h-q12h
• Blood cholesterol reducing medications (e.g., Niacin, Lopid)
• Diet—low-fat diet, weight loss program, and high soluable fiber intake

CONTRAINDICATIONS/POSSIBLE INTERACTIONS N/A

FOLLOW-UP
• Monitor T_4 concentration 4-6 hours postadministration after the first 6 weeks of treatment and adjust dosage accordingly.
• Monitor blood triglyceride and cholesterol.
• Monitor ECG for conduction disturbances and ST segment changes.

MISCELLANEOUS

ASSOCIATED CONDITIONS
Hypothyroidism

AGE RELATED FACTORS
Geriatric patients (> 9 years)

SEE ALSO
Myocardial Infarction

ABBREVIATION
CHF = Congestive heart failure

References
Ettinger SJ, ed. Textbook of veterinary internal medicine. 3rd ed. Philadelphia: WB Saunders, 1993.
Smith FWK, Cali JV, Fox PF. In: Miller M, Tilley LP, eds. Manual of canine and feline cardiology. 2nd ed. Philadelphia: WB Saunders, 1995.
Liu S-k, Tilley LP, Tappe JP, Fox PR. Clinical and pathologic findings in dogs with artheriosclerosis: 21 cases (1970-1983). J Am Vet Med Assoc 1986;189:227-232.
Hamlen HJ. Sinoatrial node arteriosclerosis in two young dogs. J Am Vet Med Assoc 1994;204:751.

Authors T. Arch Robertson and Larry P. Tilley
Consulting Editors Larry P. Tilley and Francis W. K. Smith, Jr.

BASICS

OVERVIEW

• Atlantoaxial instability is a congenital anomaly involving the first two cervical vertebrae (atlas and axis), which causes spinal cord compression. • Spinal cord compression at this location can cause neck pain and/or upper motor neuron tetraparesis to paralysis • Stability between the atlas and axis is largely dependent on the odontial process of the axis (dens) and how the dens attaches to the ventral floor of the atlas. The dens forms between 9 and 12 weeks of age and fuses to the body of the axis between 7 and 9 months. Abnormalities in fusion can result in aplasia, hypoplasia, or deviation of the dens and lead to atlantoaxial instability

SIGNALMENT

• Congenital atlantoaxial instability affects toy breed dogs including toy poodle, chihuahua and Pekingese. • Most affected dogs exhibit clinical signs prior to 12 months of age. • There is no gender predilection.

SIGNS

Historical Findings
Neck pain is the mildest clinical sign associated with atlantoaxial instability.

Physical Examination Findings
• Depending on the degree of spinal cord compression, affected dogs may also have proprioception deficits to complete paralysis. • Because the location of spinal cord compression causes upper motor neuron signs, spinal reflexes are normal to exaggerated in all four limbs. • Atlantoaxial instability may lead to catastrophic, acute spinal cord trauma, respiratory arrest and death.

CAUSES AND RISK FACTORS

• Atlantoaxial instability is caused by abnormal formation of the dens. • Clinical signs may be exacerbated by activity, especially flexion of the neck. • Toy breed dogs are at risk.

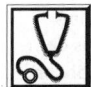

DIAGNOSIS

DIFFERENTIAL DIAGNOSIS

Differential diagnoses include disk herniation, neoplasia, and trauma. However, disk herniation and neoplasia affect older dogs.

CBC/BIOCHEMISTRY/URINALYSIS

• Hemogram—normal • Serum chemistry profile—normal • Urinalysis—normal

OTHER LABORATORY TESTS N/A

IMAGING

• Cervical spinal radiographs under general anesthesia usually confirm the diagnosis.
• Lateral spinal radiographs reveal an increase in the dorsal atlantoaxial space. During radiography, care must be taken not to hyperflex the neck, resulting in severe spinal cord trauma. • Myelography is seldom, if ever, needed

OTHER DIAGNOSTIC PROCEDURES N/A

TREATMENT

• Conservative and surgical treatments have been advocated for dogs with atlantoaxial instability. Conservative treatment is reserved for dogs with neck pain only and includes the use of a neck brace and cage confinement for several weeks. Recurrence is common after conservative treatment.
• Surgery is a more definitive treatment for atlantoaxial instability, but is not without possible complications.
• The use of a dorsal approach followed by wire or suture stabilization of the dorsal spinous process of the axis to the dorsal arch of the atlas has been advocated. A common postoperative complication with this technique is the suture or wire breaking through the dorsal arch of the atlas resulting in recurrence of clinical signs.
• A ventral approach followed by cancellous bone grafting and pinning the atlantoaxial joints has also been described. A common postoperative complication with this technique is pin migration resulting in recurrence of clinical signs. To avoid this problem, a small amount of polymethyl methacrylate (bone cement) can be used to lock the diverging pins together ventrally and prevent pin migration.

MEDICATIONS

DRUGS AND FLUIDS

Methylprednisolone (30 mg/kg) should be used in animals with acute paralysis and perioperatively in animals undergoing surgery.

CONTRAINDICATIONS/POSSIBLE INTERACTIONS

• Glucocorticoids can be used in conjunction with conservative treatment; however, glucocorticoids can reduce pain resulting in more activty and potentially more spinal cord trauma. Because of this, caution should be used when glucocorticoids are given in conjunction with conservative treatment.
• The use of nonsteroidal anti-inflammatory drugs (NSAIDs) in combination with glucocorticoid increases the risk of life-threatening gastrointestinal hemorrhage. This combination of drugs should be avoided in all patients.

FOLLOW-UP

• Conservatively treated dogs with diagnosed atlantoaxial instability should be reevaluated weekly for worsening neurologic signs until clinical signs have resolved. • Many animals treated conservatively have recurrences and ultimately require surgery. • Recurrence of neck pain with or without neurologic deficits is possible. • Most animals treated surgically do not have recurrent episodes. • Success of surgery is influenced by the expertise and experience of the surgeon. • Atlantoaxial instability may lead to catastrophic, acute spinal cord trauma, respiratory arrest, and death.
• Atlantoaxial instability is unavoidable in certain breeds

MISCELLANEOUS

ASSOCIATED CONDITIONS N/A

SYNONYMS
A-A Luxation

Reference
Shires PK. Atlantoaxial instability. In: Slatter DH, ed. Textbook of small animal surgery. 2nd ed. Philadelphia: WB Saunders, 1993;1048.

Author Michael S. Bauer
Consulting Editor Peter D. Schwarz

ATOPY

BASICS

DEFINITION
Predisposition in the development of cutaneous hypersensitivity to environmental allergens.

Pathophysiology
Susceptible animals may become sensitized to multiple pollens (grass, tree, and weed), mold spores, house dust mites, and animal epithelial allergens. Allergen specific IgE binds to cutaneous mast cells, which may degranulate upon subsequent exposure, releasing pruritogenic molecules, including histamine. Whether allergens reach cutaneous mast cells percutaneously or through inhalation has not been established in the dog or cat. An IgG subclass (IgG(d)) has been shown to mediate some cases of atopy in the dog.

Systems Affected
• Skin/Exocrine—due to self-inflicted damage caused by pruritus. • Ears—due to predisposition to otitis externa caused by chronic inflammation. • Reproductive, gastrointestinal disorders, and internal ocular disorders have been attributed to atopy with much less certainty.

Genetics
• Probably inherited as a polygenic trait with environmental factors also important in the dog. • Uncertain that genetics are important in the cat

Incidence/Prevalence
Atopy is reported to account for 8- 30 % of canine skin diseases, and may occur in as many as 10–15 % of the canine population. The prevalence in the cat population is much lower.

Geographic Distribution
Local environmental factors, which influence the seasonality of allergens (temperature, humidity, flora), will influence the severity and duration of signs in an individual.

SIGNALMENT
Species Dogs and cats

Breed Predilections
• Beagles, Boston terriers, Cairn terriers, Chinese shar peis, dalmatians, English bulldogs, English setters, golden retrievers, Lhasa apsos, miniature schnauzers, Scottish terriers, West Highland white terriers, and wirehaired fox terriers. Those breeds found to be predisposed may vary geographically. • Breed predilections have not been reported in cats.

Mean Age and Range
The mean age for first developing signs of atopy is one to two years in the dog, with a range of three months to seven years. Signs usually worsen with age, and a seasonal condition may become nonseasonal.

Predominant Sex
Both sexes, but females reported to be more commonly affected in dogs.

SIGNS
General
Pruritus may be the only sign in some dogs. Most of the lesions observed are secondary to self-trauma. The pruritus in cats is often limited to the head.

Historical Findings
• Pruritus, which is usually initially seasonal. Manifested by interdigital licking and biting, muzzle scratching and rubbing, and groin and axillary licking and scratching. • Has usually responded well to corticosteroid therapy, if previously administered. • Sneezing is sometimes noted. • Recurrent pyoderma and otitis externa have often occurred in the past.

Physical Examination Findings
• Areas most commonly affected include interdigital spaces, carpal and tarsal areas, muzzle, periocular region, axillae, groin, and pinnae. • Cutaneous lesions affecting these areas may include erythema, partial to complete alopecia, scaling, crusts, salivary staining, hyperpigmentation, and lichenification.
• Follicular papules, pustules, round crusts and epidermal collarettes are signs of possible secondary pyoderma, usually caused by Staphylococcus intermedius. • Otitis externa, often complicated by Malassezia pachydermatis. • Concurrent signs of fleas and flea allergy dermatitis are present in many patients.
• Excessively oily coats and hyperhidrosis are sometimes observed. • Chronic affected animals with scaling, crusting, lichenification and secondary pyoderma may appear seborrheic.
• Conjunctivitis may accompany cutaneous findings.

CAUSES
• Airborne pollens: grasses, trees, and weeds. • Fungal spores: both indoor and outdoor genuses. • Indoor allergens: animal dander, natural fibers, and house dust mites.

RISK FACTORS
• Temperate environments with long allergy seasons and high pollen and mold spore levels. • Concurrent pruritic dermatoses, such as flea allergy dermatitis and food hypersensitivity (summation effect).

DIAGNOSIS

DIFFERENTIAL DIAGNOSIS
• Food hypersensitivity may cause identical lesion distribution and physical examination findings but should be nonseasonal. May occur concurrently with atopy. • Flea allergy dermatitis is the most common cause of seasonal pruritus in many geographical regions and may occur concurrently with atopy. Differentiation is made by noting lesion distribution and flea burden, response to flea

control, and results of intradermal skin testing. • Sarcoptic mange often occurs in young, or recently stray dogs, and often causes severe pruritus of the ventral chest, lateral elbows, lateral hocks, and pinnal margins. Multiple skin scrapings and/or complete response to a trial of miticidal therapy are indicated to rule out sarcoptic mange. • Contact dermatitis, either allergic or irritant, may affect the feet and thinly haired areas of the ventral abdomen, causing pruritus. A history of exposure to a known contact sensitizer or irritant, response to a change of environment, and patch testing may be used to explore the possibility of contact dermatitis, although it is thought to be rare in the dog and cat.
• Malassezia dermatitis, either primary or as a secondary problem to seborrheic disorders, can cause intense pruritus of the feet, perioral region, ventral neck, and axillae. Demonstration of numerous yeast organisms by skin cytology and obtaining a favorable response to antifungal therapy is diagnostic.

CBC/BIOCHEMISTRY/URINALYSIS
Eosinophilia is rare in the dog without concurrent flea infestation, but common in the cat.

OTHER LABORATORY TESTS
Serum allergy testing to detect allergen-specific IgE is commercially available, with the same indications as intradermal skin testing (IDST). Advantages over IDST relate to the availability of the test to practitioners. Disadvantages include frequent false positive reactions, limitations on the number of allergens tested, and inconsistent assay validation and quality control, which may vary with the laboratory used.

IMAGING N/A

OTHER DIAGNOSTIC PROCEDURES
• Intradermal skin testing (IDST), in which small amounts of test allergens are injected intradermally and wheal formation is measured, is the most accurate method of identifying offending allergens for possible avoidance or inclusion in an immunotherapy prescription. IDST and subsequent immunotherapy are indicated when it is desirable to avoid or reduce the amount of corticosteroids required to control the atopy, when pruritus lasts longer than 4-6 months per year, or when non-steroidal forms of therapy are ineffective. • Test results are sometimes difficult to interpret in cats due to the relatively small wheals produced.
• Skin biopsy may prove helpful in narrowing the list of differential diagnoses, but findings are not pathognomonic.

GROSS AND HISTOPATHOLOGIC FINDINGS
• Gross findings are as described in physical examination findings. • Dermatohistopathological findings include acanthosis, mixed mononuclear superficial perivascular

dermatitis, and sebaceous gland metaplasia. Findings consistent with pyoderma are often present as secondary findings.

TREATMENT

INPATIENT VERSUS OUTPATIENT
Outpatient

ACTIVITY
Avoid offending allergens that have been identified when possible.

DIET
Essential fatty acid supplementation may be beneficial.

CLIENT EDUCATION
Clients should be advised that atopy cannot be cured once and for all, and some form of therapy may be necessary for life.

SURGICAL CONSIDERATIONS N/A

MEDICATIONS

DRUGS AND FLUIDS
• Immunotherapy (hyposensitization), in which allergens for inclusion are selected based on allergy test results, patient history, and knowledge of local flora are administered subcutaneously, in gradually increasing amounts. Immunotherapy successfully reduces pruritus in 60-70% of patients. The response is slow, often requiring three to six months.
• Prednisolone suspension (0.5 - 1.0 mg/kg SQ or IM) may be given for short term relief and to break the itch-scratch cycle.
• Hydroxyzine (1-2 mg/kg PO q8h) is an antihistamine commonly used to treat atopy in dogs. Efficacy as a sole treatment is probably only in the 10-20% range.
• Chlorpheniramine (0.5 mg/kg PO q12h) is the antihistamine most commonly given to atopic cats. Estimates on efficacy vary from 10 to 50%.

CONTRAINDICATIONS N/A

PRECAUTIONS
• Antihistamines should be used with caution in patients with cardiac arrhythmias.
• Corticosteroids should be used judiciously in atopic dogs to prevent iatrogenic hyperglucocorticism and associated problems, aggra-

vating pyoderma, and inducing demodicosis.

POSSIBLE INTERACTIONS
The antihistamines terfenidine and astemazole have been associated with life-threatening cardiac arrhythmias in man when administered concomitantly with imidazole antifungal drugs.

ALTERNATE DRUGS
• Corticosteroids should be tapered to the lowest dosage that adequately controls pruritus: Prednisone or methylprednisolone (0.2 - 0.5 mg/kg PO q48h).
• Antihistamines are less effective than corticosteroids. They may act synergistically with essential fatty acid supplements. Corticosteroid therapy can often be avoided or given at a reduced dosage when used concurrently. Antihistamines commonly prescribed for dogs: hydroxyzine (1–2 mg/kg PO q8h), chlorpheniramine (0.2–0.4 mg/kg PO q12h), diphenhydramine (2.2 mg/kg PO q8h), and clemastine (0.04–0.10 mg/kg PO q12h). Chlorpheniramine (0.4 mg/kg PO q12h) is the most commonly prescribed antihistamine for cats.
• Tricyclic antidepressants may be given for their H1-blocking activity: doxepin (1.02.0 mg/kg PO q12h) or amitriptyline (1.0–2.0 mg/kg PO q12h).
• Repository injectable corticosteroids should be avoided in dogs. The pruritus of atopic cats may require methylprednisolone acetate treatment (4 mg/kg SQ or IM).

FOLLOW-UP

PATIENT MONITORING
• Follow-up examinations should be scheduled every two to eight weeks when a new course of therapy is started. Pruritus, signs of self-trauma, signs of pyoderma, and possible adverse drug reactions should be monitored.
• Once an acceptable level of control is achieved, follow-up examinations should be done every 3-12 months.
A CBC, serum chemistry profile, and urinalysis is recommended every 6-12 months for patients on chronic corticosteroid therapy.

PREVENTION/AVOIDANCE
• If the offending allergens have been identified through allergy testing, the owner should undertake to reduce the pet's exposure to those for which it is possible (e.g. house dust, animal

epithelia, indoor mold spores). • Minimizing other sources of pruritus such as fleas, food hypersensitivity, and a dirty or unkept coat may reduce the level of pruritus below the threshold that is tolerated by the animal.

POSSIBLE COMPLICATIONS
Secondary pyoderma and concurrent flea allergy dermatitis are the most common complications of atopy.

EXPECTED COURSE AND PROGNOSIS
• Not life-threatening unless intractable pruritus results in euthanasia • Untreated, the degree of pruritus worsens and the duration of signs last longer each year of the pet's life. • Only rare cases spontaneously resolve.

MISCELLANEOUS

ASSOCIATED CONDITIONS
• Flea allergy dermatitis • Food hypersensitivity • Pyoderma • Otitis externa

AGE RELATED FACTORS
Severity worsens with age.

ZOONOTIC POTENTIAL N/A

PREGNANCY
• Corticosteroids are contraindicated during pregnancy. • The safety of antihistamines during pregnancy has not been established.

SYNONYMS
• Canine atopic dermatitis • Canine allergic inhalant dermatitis • Canine atopic disease

SEE ALSO
• Flea and Flea Control • Food Reactions • Pyoderma • Otitis Externa

ABBREVIATIONS
IDST = Intradermal skin test

References

Griffin CE. Canine atopic disease. In: Griffin CE, Kwochka KW, MacDonald JM, ed. Current veterinary dermatology. St. Louis: Mosby Year Book, 1993;99-120.

Muller GH, Kirk RW, Scott DW. Small animal dermatology. 4th ed. Philadelphia: WB Saunders, 1989;450.

Author Jon D. Plant
Consulting Editor Lowell Ackerman

ATRIAL SEPTAL DEFECT

BASICS

OVERVIEW
• Congenital cardiac anomaly allowing communication between the atria through a defect in the interatrial septum (figure). Defects occur in one of three locations: ostium primun defect—lower atrial septum, ostium secundum defect—near fossa ovalis, and sinus venous defect—craniodorsal to fossa ovalis. • Blood usually shunts into the right atrium causing volume overload to the right side of the heart. • If right-sided pressures are high, shunting may occur right to left causing generalized cyanosis.

SIGNALMENT
• Dogs and cats • Genetic basis suggested for Old English sheepdog • Doberman pinscher, boxer, and Samoyed may be overrepresented.

SIGNS

General
If defect is small, maybe none

Historical Findings
Variable degrees of exercise intolerance, syncope, and dyspnea the first year of life

Physical Examination Findings
• Soft systolic murmur over the pulmonic valve and tricuspid valve • Splitting of the second heart sound • Dyspnea

CAUSES AND RISK FACTORS
Unknown; genetic basis not documented

DIAGNOSIS

DIFFERENTIAL DIAGNOSIS
Pulmonic stenosis—murmur of pulmonic stenosis usually harsh and loud

CBC/BIOCHEMISTRY/URINALYSIS
Polycythemia in some animals with right to left shunt

OTHER BLOOD TESTS N/A

IMAGING

Radiographic Findings
• None in animals with small defects
• Right-sided heart and pulmonary vessel enlargement in animals with large defects

Echocardiographic Findings
• Right atrial and right ventricular dilation
• May reveal the defect • Doppler useful in documenting flow through the defect and high ejection velocity through the pulmonary artery

OTHER DIAGNOSTIC PROCEDURES
Right ventricular enlargement pattern on ECG in some animals with large defects

TREATMENT
• Animals with congestive heart failure (CHF) should be hospitalized until stable.
• Activity should be restricted.
• A low- sodium diet may be of value.
• Surgical correction is prohibitively expensive for most owners.
• Pulmonary artery banding may be palliative in animals with severe disease.

MEDICATIONS

DRUGS AND FLUIDS
• Diuretics when CHF is present; aggressiveness of diuretic therapy proportional to the degree of pulmonary edema (furosemide, 1-2 mg/kg PO q6h-q12h)

• Vasodilators may be beneficial in reducing clinical signs (enalapril, 0.5 mg/kg PO q12h-q24h).

CONTRAINDICATIONS/POSSIBLE INTERACTIONS N/A

FOLLOW-UP

PATIENT MONITORING
Recheck when decompensation or other clinical signs develop

EXPECTED COURSE AND PROGNOSIS
• Depend on size of the defect and coexisting abnormalities; small, isolated defects unlikely to cause signs or to progress • Progressive, right-sided CHF expected if the defect is large

MISCELLANEOUS

ASSOCIATED CONDITIONS
Pulmonic stenosis and tricuspid dysplasia

SEE ALSO
Congestive Heart Failure, Right-Sided

ABBREVIATIONS
CHF = congestive heart failure

Reference
Bonagura JD, Darke P. Congenital heart disease. In: Ettinger SJ, Feldman EC, eds. Textbook of veterinary internal medicine. 4th ed. Philadelphia: WB Saunders, 1995.
Author John-Karl Goodwin
Consulting Editors Larry P. Tilley and Francis W. K. Smith, Jr.

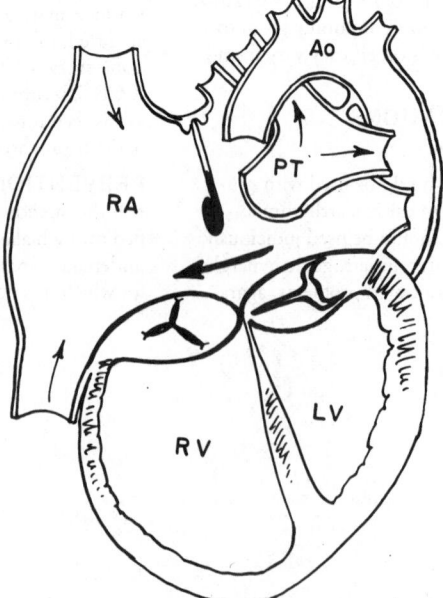

Atrial septal defect. Defect involves the lowermost part of the atrial septum, known as ostium primum defect. Note the dominant left-to-right shunt. RV = right ventricle, LV = left ventricle, RA = right atrium, Ao = aorta, PT = pulmonary trunk. From Roberts W. Adult congenital heart disease. Philadelphia: FA Davis Co., 1987, with permission.

BASICS

OVERVIEW

• Split in the endocardial surface or complete tear (rupture) in the atrial wall when the left atrium is distended beyond its elastic limits. If the split is incomplete, fibrin may seal the defect temporarily. This either heals as a depression in the atrial surface or subsequently ruptures completely. • Once a tear is complete, bleeding occurs into the pericardial sac and cardiac tamponade quickly ensues. If the interatrial wall is affected, an acquired atrial septal defect may form. • Death occurs quickly in most animals.

SIGNALMENT

• Since atrial tears are secondary to several cardiac disorders that cause the atrium to enlarge, both large- and small-breed dogs are affected. Similarly, tears can be secondary to congenital heart disease, and thus both young and old dogs are affected. • Rare in cats

SIGNS

Historical Findings

• Acute onset of weakness and collapse that may progress quickly to death • Long-standing cardiac disease in most animals, so other signs of congestive heart failure may have been observed

Physical Examination Findings

• Pale mucous membranes • Tachycardia • Weak arterial pulses • Collapse • Signs of right heart failure (e.g., ascites and jugular venous distension) in some animals • Other signs of cardiac disease (e.g., murmur, gallop rhythm, arrhythmia, and dyspnea) in some animals • If a murmur was heard before the atrial wall tear occurred, it may not be as loud.

CAUSES AND RISK FACTORS

• Mitral valve endocardiosis (chronic valvular heart disease) • Dilated cardiomyopathy • Patent ductus arteriosus • Cardiac neoplasia • Chest trauma

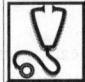

DIAGNOSIS

DIFFERENTIAL DIAGNOSIS

Other diseases that cause acute cardiovascular collapse:
• Pericardial effusion from other causes (e.g., neoplastic and idiopathic) • Severe cardiac arrhythmias • Myocardial infarction • Pulmonary thromboembolism • Other causes of hypotension

CBC/BIOCHEMISTRY/URINALYSIS

Prerenal azotemia in some animals

OTHER BLOOD TESTS N/A

IMAGING

Radiographic Findings

• Comparison with previous thoracic radiographs may show rounding of cardiac silhouette; however, the spherical cardiac silhouette seen in animals with pericardial effusion is often not observed. • Ascites and large caudal vena cava in some animals

Echocardiographic Findings

• Pericardial effusion is seen as an echo-free space between the heart and pericardial sac; the heart may swing in the pericardial sac. • Left atrium often remains large and a clot may be observed in the left atrium or pericardial sac.

OTHER DIAGNOSTIC PROCEDURES

Electrocardiographic Findings

• Arrhythmias • Tachycardia • Dampening of the QRS complex • Electrical alternans • ST-segment abnormalities • May reveal underlying cardiac disease

TREATMENT

• If a left atrial tear is highly suspected, pericardiocentesis should be performed only if the effusion is felt to be life-threatening, since further hemorrhage into the pericardial sac or exsanguination may occur. If a fibrin clot forms over the defect, the animal may stabilize. If pericardiocentesis is performed, remove only enough fluid to improve clinical signs.

• Strict cage rest
• Surgical exploration may be considered if hemorrhage persists or recurs.

MEDICATIONS

DRUGS AND FLUIDS

• Administer fluids intravenously to expand the intravascular space and maintain cardiac output.
• Combination of fluids and dobutamine has been useful in improving hemodynamic status in models of cardiac rupture.

CONTRAINDICATIONS/POSSIBLE INTERACTIONS

Preload (e.g., diuretics and venous dilators) and afterload reducers (e.g., arterial vasodilators) are not indicated in the treatment of left atrial rupture, since they may further diminish cardiac output. If necessary for treating concomitant congestive heart failure, use sparingly.

FOLLOW-UP

• Prognosis is poor. Even if the tear seals, the animal is prone to further tears because of underlying cardiac disease.
• If the animal survives, follow-up examination with echocardiography is helpful to determine resolution of pericardial effusion and resorption of an atrial or pericardial clot.

MISCELLANEOUS

SEE ALSO Pericardial Effusion

Reference

Allen DG. Small animal medicine. Philadelphia: JB Lippincott, 1991.
Author Patti S. Snyder
Consulting Editors Larry P. Tilley and Francis W. K. Smith, Jr.

ATRIOVENTRICULAR VALVE DYSPLASIA

 BASICS

DEFINITION

A congenital malformation of either the mitral valve apparatus or the tricuspid valve apparatus

Pathophysiology

• Atrioventricular valve dysplasia (AVD) causes insufficiency of the affected valve. Depending on the type of malformation, various degrees of valvular stenosis may be present as well. • In animals with mitral valve dysplasia, mild to severe mitral regurgitation is present, with corresponding dilation of the left atrium and rise in pulmonary venous pressure. Left-sided congestive heart failure (CHF) may develop. • Tricuspid valve dysplasia causes right atrial dilation subsequent to tricuspid regurgitation, which may lead to signs of right-sided CHF. High right atrial pressure may maintain a patent foramen ovale, allowing right-to-left shunting of blood at the atrial level. • Cardiac arrhythmias (especially atrial fibrillation) may occur secondary to atrial dilation.

Systems Affected

• Cardiovascular because of volume overload
• Pulmonary, if pulmonary edema or cyanosis is present

Genetics

A genetic basis is likely in some breeds but has not been confirmed.

Incidence/Prevalence

One of the most common cardiac congenital anomalies in cats; infrequently diagnosed in dogs

Geographic Distribution N/A

SIGNALMENT

Species Dogs and cats

Breed Predilections

• Great Dane, German shepherd, Afghan hound (mitral valve dysplasia) • Labrador retriever, Old English sheepdog (tricuspid valve dysplasia)

Mean Age and Range

Most affected animals develop clinical signs within the first year of life.

Predominant Sex Male

SIGNS

General Comments

Progression and severity of clinical signs correlates with severity of the valvular insufficiency.

Historical Findings

• Classic signs of left-sided CHF (i.e., cough, dyspnea, and exercise intolerance) are usually present in animals with moderate to severe mitral valve dysplasia. • Stunted growth, exercise intolerance, and ascites are usually present in animals with moderate to severe tricuspid valve dysplasia.

Physical Examination Findings

Mitral valve dysplasia
• Prominent holosystolic murmur heard over the mitral valve area (left apex), often associated with a precordial thrill; an S3 in some animals with severe disease • Tachypnea and abnormally loud respiratory sounds in animals with left-sided heart failure

Tricuspid valve dysplasia
• Prominent holosystolic murmur heard over the tricuspid valve area (right apex), often associated with a precordial thrill. • Prominent jugular pulsations in most animals • Ascites in animals with right-sided heart failure; peripheral edema in some animals • Variable degrees of generalized cyanosis in animals with right-to-left shunting through a patent foramen ovale or coexisting atrial septal defect

CAUSES

Unknown; possible genetic basis

RISK FACTORS N/A

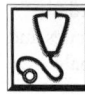 DIAGNOSIS

DIFFERENTIAL DIAGNOSIS

• Degenerative valve disease (especially If AVD is present in an old dog) • Other defects causing a systolic murmur, especially ventricular septal defect • Tricuspid dysplasia may be a variant of Ebstein's anomaly • Mitral and tricuspid stenosis have some features in common with mitral and tricuspid dysplasia. They differ in that the stenotic valve lesions cause a diastolic murmur.

CBC/BIOCHEMISTRY/URINALYSIS

Usually normal

OTHER LABORATORY TESTS N/A

IMAGING

Thoracic Radiographic Findings

Mitral valve dysplasia
• Left-sided cardiomegaly, with a prominent left atrium on both lateral and ventrodorsal views • An alveolar-interstitial pattern in animals with left-sided failure

Tricuspid valve dysplasia
• Severe right-sided cardiomegaly (right atrial enlargement) in most animals • Enlargement of the caudal vena cava in some animals

Echocardiographic Findings

Mitral valve dysplasia
• Moderate to severe left atrial dilation with abnormal appearing mitral valve leaflets—hallmark findings; malposition of the leaflets or chordae tendineae in some animals
• Moderate to severe left ventricular dilation in most animals • Fractional shortening usually normal, but may be reduced if myocardial failure develops • Doppler echocardiography demonstrates mitral regurgitation; high transmitral flow in animals with valvular stenosis

Tricuspid valve dysplasia
• Moderate to severe right atrial dilation with abnormal appearing tricuspid valve leaflets—hallmark findings; malposition of the leaflets or chordae tendineae in some animals • Right ventricle diminished in size and may be hypoplastic • Doppler echocardiography demonstrates tricuspid regurgitation; high transtricuspid flow in animals with valvular stenosis.

Cardiac Catheterization

• Can be used to confirm the diagnosis • Infrequently employed because of invasiveness and the ability of echocardiography to confirm the diagnosis

Mitral valve dysplasia
• Left ventriculogram demonstrates various degrees (usually severe) of mitral insufficiency and severe left atrial dilation. • Selective catheterization of the left ventricle required
• Pressure measurements demonstrate high left atrial pressure.

Tricuspid valve dysplasia
• Right ventriculogram demonstrates various degrees (usually severe) of tricuspid insufficiency and severe right atrial dilation.
• Contrast within the left atrium immediately after a right-sided injection indicates the presence of a patent foramen ovale or coexisting atrial septal defect. • Selective catheterization of the right ventricle required. • Pressure measurements demonstrate high right atrial pressure.

OTHER DIAGNOSTIC PROCEDURES

Electrocardiographic Findings

• Evidence of atrial enlargement in some animals—P-pulmonale (tall P waves) for right atrial enlargement, and P-mitrale (widened P waves) for left atrial enlargement
• Chamber enlargement in some animals—right bundle branch block often present in animals with tricuspid valve dysplasia
• Arrhythmias common, especially atrial premature complexes or atrial fibrillation

GROSS AND HISTOPATHOLOGIC FINDINGS

• Valvular abnormalities may include leaflet thickening, notching, rolling, and shortening; fusion, thickening, or aplasia of the chordae tendineae; dysplastic and malpositioned papillary muscles. • Dilation of the affected chambers • Evidence of congestion—pulmonary (mitral dysplasia) or systemic (tricuspid dysplasia)

 TREATMENT

INPATIENT VERSUS OUTPATIENT

Inpatient if animal has CHF

ACTIVITY Restricted

DIET

Sodium restriction in animals with CHF

CLIENT EDUCATION
• This defect may be inherited—advise against breeding.
• Signs of CHF probably progressive

SURGICAL CONSIDERATIONS
Impractical because of by-pass requirement and remarkable expense

MEDICATIONS

DRUGS AND FLUIDS
• Diuretics indicated in animals with CHF; aggressiveness of diuretic therapy proportional to the degree of pulmonary edema-furosemide (1-3 mg/kg PO q6h-q8h)
• Vasodilators may be beneficial in reducing clinical signs—enalapril, (0.5mg/kg PO q12h-q24h).
• Specific antiarrhythmic therapy may be warranted—digoxin is most often used in the management of atrial arrhythmias.

CONTRAINDICATIONS
Fluids contraindicated in animals with severe CHF

PRECAUTIONS
Standard patient monitoring for cardiac medication side effects is necessary (e.g., digitalis toxicity and azotemia).

POSSIBLE INTERACTIONS N/A
ALTERNATE DRUGS N/A

FOLLOW-UP

PATIENT MONITORING
Recheck when decompensation or other clinical signs occur.

PREVENTION/AVOIDANCE
Do not breed affected animals.

POSSIBLE COMPLICATIONS
• Left heart failure (mitral) • Right heart failure (tricuspid) • Arrhythmias

EXPECTED COURSE AND PROGNOSIS
• Prognosis guarded to poor depending on severity of defect • Refractory heart failure develops in most animals.

MISCELLANEOUS

ASSOCIATED CONDITIONS
May accompany other cardiac defects, especially endocardial cushion defects (cats) and atrial septal defect (dogs)

AGE RELATED FACTORS
Clinical signs usually evident in young animals; however, onset of signs may be delayed until maturity

ZOONOTIC POTENTIAL N/A

PREGNANCY
Likely to cause CHF

SYNONYMS N/A

SEE ALSO
• Congestive Heart Failure, Left-Sided
• Congestive Heart Failure, Right-Sided

ABBREVIATIONS
AVD = atrioventricular valve dysplasia
CHF = congestive heart failure

References

Bonagura JD. Cardiovascular diseases. In: Sherding RG, ed. The cat—diseases and clinical management. New York: Churchill Livingstone, 1989.

Bonagura JD, Darke P. Congenital heart disease. In: Ettinger SJ, Feldman J, eds. Textbook of veterinary internal medicine. 4th ed. Philadelphia: WB Saunders, 1995.

Author John-Karl Goodwin
Consulting Editors Larry P. Tilley and Francis W. K. Smith, Jr.

ATRIOVENTRICULAR VALVE ENDOCARDIOSIS

BASICS

DEFINITION
A chronic degenerative disease affecting the mitral and tricuspid valves leading to valvular insufficiency and heart failure.

Pathophysiology
• Proliferation and deposition of mucopolysaccharide within the subendothelial spongiosa layer leads to thickening, distortion, and stiffening of the atrioventricular (AV) valves. Initially, swellings are nodular, but coalescence occurs until the entire valve and often the attached chordae are involved. • AV valve incompetence cause regurgitation, high atrial pressure, reduced cardiac output, activation of compensatory mechanisms (sympathetic nervous system, renin-angiotensin-aldosterone system, and atrial naturetic factor), and congestive heart failure. • Volume overload leads to progressive ventricular dilation, advancing ventricular stiffness, and impaired ventricular function. Congestive and low output (forward) failure result. • With atrial tear, acute cardiac tamponade may result. • Degenerative changes in the chordae tendineae lead to distortion, weakening, and rupture causing valvular instability and increased regurgitation.

Systems Affected
• Cardiovascular—both AV valves are affected but Buchanan (1979) showed the distribution in necropsy specimens to be mitral alone, 62%, tricuspid alone, 1%, and both, 33%. • Respiratory—if edema develops • Renal/Urologic—prerenal azotemia • Hepatobiliary—passive congestion of the liver

Genetics Not established

Incidence/Prevalence
Chronic valvular disease increases from about 5% in middle-aged dogs (5-7 years) to > 35% in older dogs (≥ 12 years).

Geographic Distribution N/A

SIGNALMENT

Species
Predominantly dogs, but may be seen in older cats

Breed Predilections
• Typically small breeds • Prevalence highest in cavalier King Charles spaniel, Chihuahua, miniature poodle, miniature pinscher, and whippet

Mean Age and Range
Manifestation of heart failure is 10-12 years, although a murmur may have been noticed for several years. Cavalier King Charles spaniels are typically affected much earlier (6-8 years).

Predominant Sex
More prevalent in males (male/female ratio 1.5:1)

SIGNS

General Comments
The International Small Animal Cardiac Health Council (ISACHC) divides patients into those with mild to moderate heart failure and those with severe heart failure for treatment purposes.

Asymptomatic Valve Disease
Systolic murmur heard best at the left fifth intercostal space (mitral) or right fourth intercostal space (tricuspid). Murmurs may vary in character from a low frequency, holosystolic, band-shaped sound to a shorter, high frequency, midsystolic murmur. Occasionally, only a midsystolic click is detected. As the disease progresses, the murmur typically gets louder and radiates more widely. With severe disease, the volume of regurgitation becomes so large that the murmur may decrease in frequency and loudness.

Mild Heart Failure
Coughing, exercise intolerance, and dyspnea with exercise

Moderate Heart Failure
Coughing, exercise intolerance, and dyspnea at all times

Severe Heart Failure
Severe dyspnea, profound weakness, abdominal distension, productive coughing (i.e., pink, frothy fluid), orthopnea, cyanosis, and syncope develop. Occasionally, syncope may be the only owner complaint.

CAUSES

Idiopathic

RISK FACTORS N/A

DIAGNOSIS

DIFFERENTIAL DIAGNOSIS
• Dilated cardiomyopathy • Congenital heart disease • Chronic airway or interstitial lung diseasem • Pneumonia • Pulmonary embolism • Pulmonary neoplasia • Heartworm disease

CBC/BIOCHEMISTRY/URINALYSIS
• Prerenal azotemia secondary to impaired renal perfusion. Urine specific gravity is high unless complicated by underlying renal disease or previous diuretic administration. • High liver enzyme in many animals with passive congestion

OTHER LABORATORY TESTS N/A

IMAGING

Radiography
• Heart size ranges from normal to left-sided or generalized cardiomegaly. • Left atrial enlargement in the lateral projection is characterized by elevation of the distal fourth of the trachea and splitting of the mainstem bronchi. Dorsoventral projection shows accentuation of the angle between the main-stem bronchi, a double shadow at the six o'-clock position where the caudal edge of the atrium extends beyond the left ventricle, and bulging of the left atrial appendage in the one to three o'clock position. • With left-sided heart failure, the pulmonary vein is larger than the associated pulmonary artery. Air bronchograms are typical of, but not pathognomic for, cardiogenic pulmonary edema. Initially, congestion and edema are perihilar, with all lung fields eventually showing changes. The right lung may be affected before the left.

Echocardiography
• Thickening and distortion of the mitral valve; septal leaflet is most severely affected • Elongation and rupture of the chordae tendineae causing mitral valve prolapse • Large left atrium • The left ventricle may be distended and is hyperdynamic if the regurgitant flow is high and myocardial function intact. As the ventricle becomes more grossly distended, it may become hypodynamic due to myocardial failure. • Pericardial effusion in some animals • Doppler studies document a jet of regurgitation into the left atrium and the area of the regurgitant jet on color flow. • Doppler has been used to assess severity.

OTHER DIAGNOSTIC PROCEDURES
• Abdominocentesis/pleurocentesis—a modified transudate is characteristic of congestive heart failure. • Arterial/venous blood gases—measurement has been used to quantify hypoxemia and monitor the response to treatment.

Electrocardiography
• Sinus tachycardia is common in animals with CHF. • May show evidence of left atrial enlargement (P mitrale) or left ventricular enlargement (tall and wide R waves) • Atrial arrhythmias (e.g., atrial premature complexes, atrial tachycardia, and atrial fibrillation) or ventricular arrhythmias may develop.

GROSS AND HISTOPATHOLOGIC FINDINGS
• Gross valvular changes are divided into four types—type I showing only a few discrete nodules at the line of closure, and type IV showing gross distortion of the valve by gray-white nodules and plaques causing contraction of the cusps and rolling of the free edge. The chordae are irregularly thickened with regions of tapering and rupture. • Jet lesions (i.e., irregular thickening and opacity of the atrial endocardium) • Recent and healed left atrium splits or tears in some animals. Full-thickness tears lead to hemopericardium (free wall) or acquired atrial septal defect (septum). • Left atrium and left ventricle dilation in many animals • The degree of left ventricular hypertrophy may only be apparent on weighing the heart. • Small thrombi in the left atrium are rare in dogs—more common and extensive in cats. • Histopathologic examination reveals thickening of the valve spongiosa due

to fibroblast proliferation, deposition of mucopolysaccharide and edema (myxomatous degeneration), and degeneration of the fibrosa.

TREATMENT

INPATIENT VERSUS OUTPATIENT
Patients needing oxygen support should be treated as inpatients. If stable, patients may be less stressed at home.

ACTIVITY
• Absolute exercise restriction is recommended in symptomatic patients.
• In stable patients receiving medical treatment, exercise should be restricted to leash walking, avoiding sudden, explosive exercise.

DIET
A salt-restricted diet is recommended if tolerated by a patient in heart failure. Close monitoring of sodium concentration is recommended. Hyponatremia may develop as CHF progresses and with patients in which severely sodium-restricted diets are used in conjunction with loop diuretics and ACE inhibitors. Signs of hyponatremia include weakness. If hyponatremia develops, switch to a less sodium-restricted diet (i.e., diet prepared for the management of renal disease or the geriatric patient).

CLIENT EDUCATION
• Discuss the progressive nature of the disease.
• Emphasize the importance of consistent dosaging of all medications and diet and exercise management.
• Signs of digoxin toxicity should be highlighted and the owner advised to stop treatment and notify the veterinarian immediately should signs develop.

SURGICAL CONSIDERATIONS
Surgical valve replacement and purse-string suture techniques to reduce the area of the mitral valve orifice have been used. Experience with these techniques is limited, and they are unlikely to become a practical alternative to medical management.

MEDICATIONS

DRUGS AND FLUIDS
Recommended treatment depends on the stage of the disease. These recommendations follow the guidelines set by the ISACHC.

Asymptomatic Patients
• If patient has no cardiac enlargement, no treatment is recommended.
• Administration of ACE inhibitors to asymptomatic patients showing progressive cardiomegaly *may* slow progression. This hypothesis is, as yet, unsubstantiated.

Mild or Moderate Congestive Heart Failure
• Diuretics—furosemide (1-2 mg/kg q8h-q12h)

• ACE inhibitors (vasodilators)—enalapril ([Enacard] 0.5 mg/kg q12h-q24h)
• Nitroglycerine (venodilator)—2% percutaneous ointment (0.125-1″ q6h until patient is stable)
• Digoxin—especially if supraventricular arrhythmias, including atrial fibrillation, are documented (0.005 mg/kg or 0.22 mg/m^2 q12h)
• Sodium restriction if tolerated
• Antiarrhythmics (as needed)
• Calcium channel blockers (to treat atrial arrhythmias)
• Beta blockers (to treat atrial and ventricular arrhythmias)
• Class 1 antiarrhythmics—procainamide, quinidine, mexelitine, and tocainide (to treat ventricular arrhythmias)

Severe Congestive Heart Failure
• Oxygen—40% in O_2 cage (can go as high as 100%) up to 24h. Use nasal O_2 in large-breed dogs, 50-100 ml/kg/min through humidifier.
• Diuretics—furosemide (Lasix, 2-4 mg/kg IV q4h-q8h)
Vasodilators:
• Benasepril—Lotensin (0.25-0.5 mg/kg q12h-q24h)
• Enalapril—Enacard (0.5 mg/kg q12h-q24h)
• Hydralazine—Apresoline (0.5 mg/kg q12h titrated up to 2mg/kg if necessary). Used in the acute stages to decrease afterload rapidly. May cause hypotension.
• Nitroglycerine—ointment (1/4 in/5 kg up to 2 in percutaneously) or 1-5 mcg/kg/min CRI
• Sodium nitroprusside—1-10 mcg/kg/min; monitor blood pressure
Positive inotropes:
• Digoxin (0.005mg/kg [0.22 mg/m^2]q12h)
• Dobutamine (dogs, 1-10 mcg/kg/min; cats, 1-5 mg/kg/min [may cause seizures])
• Dopamine (1-10 mcg/kg/min)

CONTRAINDICATIONS N/A

PRECAUTIONS
Use digoxin, diuretics, and ACE inhibitors with caution in patients with renal disease.

POSSIBLE INTERACTIONS
Monitor digoxin concentration in patients receiving concurrent calcium channel blockers or quinidine.

ALTERNATE DRUGS
• Diuretics—add thiazide and potassium sparing diuretic in refractory animals.
• Bumetanide is an alternative to furosemide.
• Vasodilators—other ACE inhibitors include lisinopril. Isosorbide dinitrate can be used in place of nitroglycerin ointment in patients requiring long-term nitrate administration.

FOLLOW-UP

PATIENT MONITORING
• A baseline radiograph should be taken when a murmur is first detected and every 6-12

months thereafter to document progressive cardiomegaly. • After an episode of congestive failure, patients should be checked weekly during the first month of treatment. Thoracic radiographs and an ECG may be repeated at the first weekly checkup and then on subsequent visits if any changes are seen on physical examination. • Monitor BUN and creatinine when diuretics and ACE inhibitors are used in combination.

PREVENTION/AVOIDANCE N/A

POSSIBLE COMPLICATIONS
Endocarditis because of bacterial colonization of the diseased mitral valve

EXPECTED COURSE AND PROGNOSIS
Progressive degeneration of both valve changes and myocardial function occurs, necessitating increasing drug dosages. Long-term prognosis depends on response to treatment and stage of heart failure.

MISCELLANEOUS

ASSOCIATED CONDITIONS N/A

AGE RELATED FACTORS N/A

ZOONOTIC POTENTIAL N/A

PREGNANCY N/A

SYNONYMS
Degenerative valve disease, chronic valve disease, acquired valvular insufficiency, and valve fibrosis

SEE ALSO
• Congestive Heart Failure, Left-Sided and Right-Sided • Atrial Wall Tear

ABBREVIATIONS
ACE = angiotensin converting enzyme
BUN = blood urea nitrogen
ECG = electrocardiogram
ISACHC = International Small Animal Cardiac Health Council

References
Keene BW. Chronic valvular disease in the dog. In: Fox PR, ed. Canine and feline cardiology. New York: Churchill Livingstone, 1988:409-418.
Atkins CE. Acquired valvular insufficiency. In: Miller MS, Tilley LP, eds. Manual of canine and feline cardiology. Philadelphia: WB Saunders, 1995:129-143.
Author Andrew Beardow
Consulting Editors Larry P. Tilley and Francis W. K. Smith, Jr.

ATRIOVENTRICULAR VALVE STENOSIS

BASICS

OVERVIEW
• Congenital or acquired narrowing of the mitral or tricuspid valve orifice leading to obstruction of transvalvular inflow • Obstruction creates a diastolic pressure gradient across the atrioventricular (AV) orifice during ventricular filling, which causes high atrial pressure. In animals with mitral stenosis, high left atrial pressure may lead to left-sided CHF. In animals with tricuspid stenosis, high right atrial pressure may lead to right-sided CHF or right-to-left shunting of blood through a patent foramen ovale or atrial septal defect. • Stenosis is usually accompanied by regurgitation of the affected valve, making the individual contributions of insufficiency and stenosis to the overall pathophysiology and clinical findings difficult to assess.

SIGNALMENT
• Rare in dogs and cats. • Usually seen in young to middle-aged animals, although there are exceptions • Mitral stenosis overrepresented in bull terriers, Newfoundlands, and maybe Siamese cats; tricuspid stenosis has been reported in a litter of Old English sheepdogs.

SIGNS

Historical Findings
• Weakness, exercise intolerance • Cough (mitral stenosis) • Tachypnea, dyspnea • Syncope • Cyanosis • Abdominal distension (ascites; tricuspid stenosis)

Physical Examination Findings
• Soft, diastolic murmur over the left apex (mitral stenosis) or right hemithorax (tricuspid stenosis) • Holosystolic murmur of mitral regurgitation over the left apex or holosystolic murmur of tricuspid regurgitation over the right hemithorax • Dyspnea, crackles (mitral stenosis) • Ascites, jugular distension, hepatomegaly (tricuspid stenosis) • Cyanosis

CAUSES AND RISK FACTORS
• Congenital malformation of the AV valve most likely • Intracardiac neoplasia • Endocarditis

DIAGNOSIS

DIFFERENTIAL DIAGNOSIS
Must differentiate from the more common causes of mitral and tricuspid regurgitation (e.g., AV valve endocardiosis and AV valve dysplasia). Unlike AV valve stenosis, AV valve endocardiosis and AV valve dysplasia are not associated with a diastolic murmur.

CBC/BIOCHEMISTRY/URINALYSIS
Normal

OTHER LABORATORY TESTS N/A

IMAGING

Thoracic Radiographic Findings
• Evidence of atrial and possibly ventricular enlargement of the affected side of the heart • Pulmonary edema and pulmonary venous congestion in some animals with mitral stenosis • Right-to-left shunt, underperfusion of the lungs in some animals with tricuspid stenosis

Echocardiographic Findings
• Atrial and ventricular enlargement, thickened valve leaflets, abnormal diastolic motion of the valve, and high transvalvular inflow velocities • Echocardiography, including Doppler, important for diagnosis and assessment

OTHER DIAGNOSTIC PROCEDURES

Electrocardiographic Findings
• Atrial and ventricular enlargement patterns • Atrial and ventricular arrhythmias.

Pathologic Findings
• Narrowing of the AV valve orifice and structural changes in the AV valves compatible with mitral and tricuspid valve dysplasia • Supramitral membranes have been reported.

TREATMENT
• Treat as an inpatient if the animals has moderate to severe CHF.
• Restrict activity and dietary sodium intake.
• Suppress tachyarrhythmias.
• Ideally, surgical repair; however, this is not economically or technically feasible in most animals. Balloon dilation is another invasive management option that is rarely done.

MEDICATIONS

DRUGS AND FLUIDS
Management of CHF
• Furosemide (dogs, 2-6 mg/kg IV, IM, SC, or PO q8h-q24h; cats, 1-4 mg/kg IV, IM, SC, or PO q8h-q24h).
• Digoxin (dogs, 0.22 mg/m^2 PO q12h; cats, 0.007 mg/kg PO q48h)

CONTRAINDICATIONS/POSSIBLE INTERACTIONS
• Treatment with arterial vasodilator (low dose enalapril) may be done cautiously in animals with mitral stenosis and marked mitral regurgitation. Excessive vasodilation may lead to arterial hypotension.

FOLLOW-UP
• Monitor for hypokalemia, azotemia, and arterial hypotension related to overdiuresis.
• Morbidity high, related to mitral valve stenosis, tricuspid valve stenosis, or a combination of one of these abnormalities and other congenital cardiac defects. Except for mild cases, prognosis is poor.

MISCELLANEOUS

ASSOCIATED CONDITIONS
Concomitant congenital defects common (e.g., subvalvular aortic stenosis with mitral stenosis)

SEE ALSO
• AV valve dysplasia • AV valve endocardiosis

ABBREVIATIONS
AV = atrioventricular
CHF = congestive heart failure

References
Lehmkuhl LB, Ware WA, Bonagura JD. Mitral stenosis in 15 dogs. J Vet Intern Med 1994;8:2-17.

Stamoulis ME, Fox PR. Mitral valve stenosis in three cats. J Small Anim Pract 1993;34: 452-456.

Ljunggren F, Nilsson O, Olsson SE, Pennock P, Persson S, Sateri H. Four cases of congenital malformation of the heart on a litter of eleven dogs. J Small Anim Pract 1966;6:611-623.

Author Linda B. Lehmkuhl
Consulting Editors Larry P. Tilley and Francis W. K. Smith, Jr.

BASICS

OVERVIEW

• Red blood cell destruction and anemia caused by Babesia species of intracellular protozoa • *Babesia canis*—a large (4-7 μm in length), pear-shaped parasite of canine RBCs. In the U.S., strains generally cause mild or inapparent disease in adult dogs (unless immunosuppressed), but severe disease in pups. South African strains cause severe disease and death in some adult dogs. • Babesia gibsoni—a small (2.5 μm), ring-shaped organism that causes severe disease in most infected adult dogs. It is rare in the U.S. and occurs commonly in Africa and Asia. Organism can be difficult to see in stained blood films.

SIGNALMENT

• Occurs in dogs in many countries, including the U.S. • Occurs in cats in Africa and southern Asia • Clinical signs and laboratory findings similar in cats and dogs

SIGNS

• Vary with age of the animal and the species and strain of Babesia • Course of disease may be acute and fulminating, subclinical, or chronic • In dogs, signs include lethargy, anorexia, pale mucous membranes, fever, emesis, amber to brown urine, splenomegaly, icterus, weight loss, rapid respiration, and rapid heart rate.

CAUSES AND RISK FACTORS

• Caused by Babesia canis and Babesia gibsoni • Can be transmitted by ticks and blood transfusions • Risk of infection increased by immunosuppression

DIAGNOSIS

DIFFERENTIAL DIAGNOSIS

• Other causes of hemolytic anemia, including autoimmune hemolytic anemia, haemobartonellosis, cytauxzoonosis (in cats only), Heinz body hemolytic anemia, microangiopathic hemolytic anemia, pyruvate kinase deficiency, and phosphofructokinase deficiency (in dogs only) • Difficult to differentiate from autoimmune hemolytic anemia if parasites are not recognized in blood—both may be Coombs' positive. • New methylene blue stains used to identify Heinz bodies • Enzyme assays or specialized DNA tests used to identify pyruvate kinase or phosphofructokinase deficiencies

CBC/BIOCHEMISTRY/URINALYSIS

• Precipitous decrease in packed cell volume early in the disease indicative of poorly regenerative anemia. A peracute form of disease, resulting in disseminated intravascular coagulation and death before anemia is severe, has been reported in dogs in South Africa.
• Differential leukocyte counts are variable and provide little diagnostic assistance—mild lymphocytosis may occur. • Mild to severe thrombocytopenia present in many animals • Bilirubinemia and anemic hypoxia demonstrated in clinical chemical profiles of some animals; normal profiles seen in other animals • Bilirubinuria in many animals; prominent hemoglobinuria rarely recognized in dogs in the U.S.

OTHER LABORATORY TESTS

• Definitive diagnosis made by identification of protozoal organisms in stained blood films • Indirect fluorescent antibody tests for *B. canis* and *B. gibsoni* demonstrate antibodies in serum directed against these organisms, but some cross-reactivity occurs between babesial species. High titers suggest infection. IFA tests may be negative in acutely infected animals, especially pups. • Direct Coombs' test positive in some animals • Prolonged coagulation times (APTT, PT, ACT) and positive fibrin degradation product test in some animals with severe disseminated intravascular coagulation • Metabolic acidosis in some severely affected animals secondary to tissue hypoxia and shock

IMAGING N/A

OTHER DIAGNOSTIC PROCEDURES N/A

TREATMENT

None required in adult dogs with mild anemia and clinical signs, although these dogs can be reservoirs of infection for other animals.

MEDICATIONS

DRUGS AND FLUIDS

• For treatment— diminazene aceturate (3.5 mg/kg SQ or IM, single injection) OR imidocarb dipropionate (5 mg/kg SQ, single injection) OR phenamidine (15 mg/kg SQ on 2 consecutive days) is efficacious. Unfortunately, these drugs are not approved for use in the U.S.; therefore, an Investigational New Animal Drug (INAD) number from the Food and Drug Administration is required before drugs can be obtained from suppliers.
• For life-threatening anemia—blood transfusions are necessary.
• For shock—use Intravenous fluids with added bicarbonate.

CONTRAINDICATIONS/POSSIBLE INTERACTIONS

Antibabesial drugs are potentially dangerous and can cause neuromuscular signs and liver or kidney injury.

FOLLOW-UP

Animals may relapse after completion of therapy—more likely to occur in dogs with B. gibsoni than in those with B. canis infections. Many treated and untreated dogs remain carriers. • Organisms not usually seen in blood films of recovered carrier animals

MISCELLANEOUS

Reference

Breitschwerdt E. Babesiosis. In: Greene CE, ed. Infectious diseases of the dog and cat. Philadelphia: WB Saunders Company, 1990:796—805.

Author John W. Harvey
Consulting Editor Alan H. Rebar

BACTERIAL INFECTIONS, ANAEROBIC

BASICS

OVERVIEW
• Anaerobic infections are caused by bacteria requiring reduced oxygen tension. • The genera most commonly found in anaerobic infections are Bacteroides, Fusobacterium, Actinomyces, Clostridium, and Peptostreptococcus. • Individual organisms will vary in their potential to withstand oxygen exposure. • A number of injurious toxins and enzymes may be elaborated by the organisms, leading to extension of the infection into adjacent, healthy tissue.

SIGNALMENT
Dogs and cats

SIGNS

General Comments
• Certain areas of the body are more commonly associated with anaerobic infection, perhaps because of proximity to mucosal surfaces. Specific signs of infection would be determined by the body system that is involved. • In most cases, the practitioner will readily recognize the infectious process. What may be overlooked is the potential for anaerobes to be involved in the process. This may lead to confusion in interpreting culture results and the selection of inappropriate antimicrobials.

Physical Examination Findings
• A foul odor associated with a wound or exudative discharge • Gas in the tissue or associated exudate • Peritonitis, pyothorax, or pyometra • Severe dental disease • Wounds or deep abscesses that do not heal as anticipated

CAUSES AND RISK FACTORS
Anaerobic infections are usually caused by normal flora of the body; a break in protective barriers allows bacterial invasion. Bite wounds, dental disease, open fractures, abdominal surgery, and foreign bodies may be predisposing factors.

DIAGNOSIS

DIFFERENTIAL DIAGNOSIS
• Anaerobic infection should be suspected when wounds are nonhealing and fail to respond to appropriate medical therapy. If only aerobic cultures are submitted, the lab may report a negative culture. • Cats with non-healing wounds should be tested for FeLV and FIV. • In middle-aged and older patients, tumor invasion (such as in the GI tract) may be responsible for establishing infection.

CBC/BIOCHEMISTRY/URINALYSIS
• None specific • Neutrophilic leukocytosis and monocytosis are common. • Biochemical abnormalities depend upon specific organ involvement.

OTHER LABORATORY TESTS N/A

IMAGING
N/A, except perhaps with bone infection

OTHER DIAGNOSTIC PROCEDURES
• Sample exposure to air should be minimized when collecting and transporting clinical specimens. Appropriate transport devices should be available before sample collection. Such devices may include screw-top glass vials containing media that accepts a culturette swab, as well as syringes evacuated of all air and capped with a rubber stopper. • Appropriate samples for submission include pus (1-2 ml in stoppered syringe) and tissue samples (minimum 1g sample).

GROSS AND HISTOPATHOLOGIC FINDINGS N/A

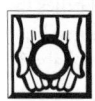

TREATMENT
• Surgery generally is indicated for all except pyothorax and CNS infections. The combination of surgery and systemic antimicrobial therapy usually offers the best chance of a positive outcome. • Surgery usually is indicated when anaerobic organisms complicate pyometra, osteomyelitis, and peritonitis. • Surgery helps to cleanse the wound of toxins and devitalized tissue, enhance drainage of pus, improve local blood flow, and increase oxygen tension; it should not be delayed when the presence of anaerobes is suspected. • Hyperbaric oxygen has some potential use but may be limited in availability.

MEDICATIONS

DRUGS AND FLUIDS
• Antimicrobial therapy alone is unlikely to be successful because of poor drug penetration into exudates. • Antibiotic selection is largely empiric as a result of the difficulty in isolating anaerobes and the delay in return of culture results. Cytology and Gram's staining of exudates may aid in selecting the initial antibiotic. • Even though most anaerobic infections are polymicrobial, antibiotic therapy targeted against the anaerobes is more likely to be successful than selecting multiple antibiotics because of the symbiotic nature of the infection. • Penicillin G is considered the antibiotic of choice for anaerobic infections except for those complicated by Bacteroides strains. Amoxicillin is comparable to penicillin G in spectrum of activity and is more convenient and accessible in routine veterinary practice. When Bacteroides is suspected, amoxicillin combined with clavulanic acid may be useful. • Cefoxitin is the only cephalosporin with reliable activity against anaerobes. The expense of this drug may prohibit its use. • Clindamycin especially may be useful when the respiratory tract is infected. • Chloramphenicol has good tissue penetration but is bacteriostatic. • Metronidazole is useful against all clinically significant anaerobes (except Actinomyces). • Aminoglycoside is uniformly ineffective against anaerobes; trimethoprim-sulfa combinations are ineffective because of poor penetration into purulent exudates.

CONTRAINDICATIONS/POSSIBLE INTERACTIONS N/A

FOLLOW-UP
Antibiotic therapy may be long-term.

MISCELLANEOUS

Reference
Dow SW. Anaerobic infections. In: Greene CE, ed. Infectious diseases of the dog and cat. Philadelphia: WB Saunders, 1990:530-537

Author Sharon K. Fooshee

Consulting Editor Fred W. Scott

BASICS

OVERVIEW

Basal cell tumor originates from the basal epithelium of the skin. This category of tumor includes benign (ie, basal cell epithehelioma and basiloid tumor) and malignant tumors (ie, basal cell carcinoma).

SIGNALMENT

• Common skin tumor; 3-12% and 15-18% of all skin tumors in dogs and cats, respectively. • Occurs in dogs 6-9 years of age and cats 5-18 years of age (mean, 10.8 years) • Cocker spaniels, poodles, and Siamese cats are more commonly affected than other breeds

SIGNS

• Animals have a solitary, well-circumscribed, form, hairless, intradermal raised mass on examination, typically located on the head, neck, or shoulders. • Variable in size, from 0.2-10 cm in diameter. • In cats, masses are often heavily pigmented, cystic, and occasionally ulcerated.

CAUSES AND RISK FACTORS

Unknown

 DIAGNOSIS

DIFFERENTIAL DIAGNOSIS

Other skin tumors (e.g., mast cell tumor, melanoma, hemangioma, and hemangiosarcoma) and intradermal cysts.

CBC/BIOCHEMISTRY/URINALYSIS

Results normal

OTHER LABORATORY TESTS N/A

IMAGING N/A

OTHER DIAGNOSTIC PROCEDURES

Histopathologic examination of tumor is required for definitve diagnosis.

GROSS AND HISTOPATHOLOGIC FINDINGS

• Histologic cellular patterns vary from solid to cystic to ribbon appearance. • Some tumor cells contain melanin pigmentation or have a fine eosinophilic stroma.

 TREATMENT

Surgical excision is the treatment of choice and is generally curative.

 MEDICATIONS

None

 FOLLOW-UP

• Less than 10% of basal cell tumors are malignant • Complete surgical excision is usually curative.

 MISCELLANEOUS N/A

Reference

Holzworth J. Dieases of the cat: Medicine and surgery. Philadelphia: WB Saunders, 1987.

Author Robyn Elmslie
Consulting Editor Wallace B. Morrison

BEAGLE PAIN SYNDROME (NECROTIZING VASCULITIS)

BASICS

OVERVIEW
Meningitis and polyarteritis causing cervical pain in young beagles

SIGNALMENT
• Most often seen in colonies of beagles bred for research, occasionally in pet beagles
• Most affected dogs 4-10 months old
• Males and females equally affected

SIGNS
• Fever, anorexia, and cervical pain are the hallmarks of the disease. The animals have a hunched stance and are reluctant to move.
• If untreated, the disease has a remitting and relapsing course (a few days to 2 weeks), with intervals of a few weeks to a few months between episodes. • Occasional forelimb proprioceptive deficits

CAUSES AND RISK FACTORS
• Probably hereditary • Immunologic basis suspected

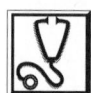

DIAGNOSIS

DIFFERENTIAL DIAGNOSIS
• Aseptic meningitis is a similar disease that can only be differentiated on the basis of breed. • Bacterial meningitis is differentiated by the waxing and waning nature of the untreated disease. • Infectious meningoencephalomyelitis and granulomatous meningoencephalomyelitis are differentiated by signalment, CSF analysis, and appropriate culturing and serologic testing. • Cervical disk disease causes cervical pain, but the dogs are usually older and there is no fever, leucocytosis, or pleocytosis on examination of CSF. • Polyarthritis can cause cervical pain with a stiff gait in dogs, but results of CSF analysis are normal and cytologic examination of joint fluid reveals inflammation.
• Affected beagles can have polyarthritis. Examination of CSF and joint fluid should be done. • Diskospondylitis can cause cervical pain and fever, but results of CSF analysis are usually normal and radiography of the affected vertebrae is diagnostic.

CBC/BIOCHEMISTRY/URINALYSIS
• Leucocytosis with neutrophilia • Mild nonregenerative anemia common • Hypoalbuminemia during the episodes common
• Results of urinalysis usually normal

OTHER LABORATORY TESTS
• Antinuclear antibody tests are negative.
• Serologic tests for infectious agents are negative.

IMAGING N/A

OTHER DIAGNOSTIC PROCEDURES
• CSF analysis—neutrophilic pleocytosis and mildly high protein concentration during the episodes • Occasionally, cytologic examination of joint fluid reveals inflammation.
• Bacterial cultures of CSF, blood, and urine are negative. • Histopathologic findings are those of severe necrotizing vasculitis and thrombosis of the small and medium-sized arteries of the meninges and coronary vessels.

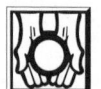

TREATMENT
• Hospitalize the patient for initial medical management.
• Restrict activity.

MEDICATIONS

DRUGS AND FLUIDS
• Administer prednisone at 2-4mg/kg/day. Dogs should respond within 48 hours. Gradually decrease prednisone dosage, but maintain on at least 1 mg/kg every 48 hours.
• Medication can be discontinued in some dogs after 2-6 months.
• Other immunosuppressive drugs (eg, cyclophosphamide and azathioprine) may be effective in dogs that do not respond completely to prednisone.

CONTRAINDICATIONS/POSSIBLE INTERACTIONS N/A

FOLLOW-UP
• Monitor for the presence of neck pain.
• Continue prednisone medication for at least 4 months or until patient is 18 months old to decrease the likelihood of relapse. • Some dogs relapse in spite of appropriate treatment.
• Episodes of pain often become less frequent as dogs mature. • The disorder may resolve spontaneously at 18-24 months of age in some dogs.

MISCELLANEOUS

ABBREVIATION
CSF = cerebrospinal fluid

Reference

Scott-Moncrieff JCR, Snyder PW, Glickman LT, Davis EL, Felsburg PJ. Systemic necrotizing vasculitis in nine young beagles. J Am Vet Med Assoc 1992;201:1553-1558.
Author Susan M. Taylor
Consulting Editor Joane M. Parent

BASICS

DEFINITION

Benign prostatic hyterplasia has the following characteristics:

• Age related pathologic change in the prostate gland causing it to be nonpainfully large • Occurs in 2 phases, glandular and complex • Glandular phase characterized by high number and large size of prostatic cells and a symmetrically large prostate gland • Complex phase characterized by glandular hyperplasia, glandular atrophy, small cyst formation, chronic inflammation, and squamous metaplasia of epithelium

SIGNALMENT

• Observed initially in intact male dogs 1-2 years old • Prevalence increases linearly so that 60% of male dogs are affected by 6 years of age and 95% of male dogs are affected by 9 years of age

SIGNS

Historical Findings
• None in most dogs • Bloody urethral discharge • Hematuria • Blood in ejaculate • Straining to defecate • Ribbon-like stools • Dysuria

PHYSICAL EXAMINATION FINDINGS

• Symmetric, nonpainfully large prostate gland • Prostatic pain in dogs with complication of bacterial infection or prostatic carcinoma

CAUSES AND RISK FACTORS

• Testosterone and 5-alpha dihydrotestosterone • Estrogens • Prostatic stroma • Aging process • Risk eliminated by castration

DIAGNOSIS

DIFFERENTIAL DIAGNOSIS

• Acute bacterial prostatitis—typically associated with fever, depression, pain on rectal palpation, neutrophilia, pyuria, and bacteriuria. It may occur concurrently with benign prostatic hyperplasia. • Chronic bacterial prostatitis—typically associated with recurrent lower urinary tract infections it may occur concurrently with benign prostatic hyperplasia. • Prostatic adenocarcinoma—typically associated with poor appetite, weight loss, hind limb weakness, dysuria, hematuria, and dyschezia. Carcinoma cells may be seen in urine sediment. • Prostatic and paraprostatic cysts—can cause palpable abdominal cystic mass filled with yellow to orange fluid.

CBC/BIOCHEMISTRY/URINALYSIS

• Results of CBC and biochemistry normal • Urinalysis may be normal or reveal hematuria. Pyuria and bacteriuria are absent unless dog has concurrent bacterial infection.

OTHER LABORATORY TESTS

• Prostatic fluid obtained by ejaculation or prostatic massage is clear or hemorrhagic. RBC count high. WBC count normal. Culture reveals < 10,000 bacteria/ml unless the dog has concurrent bacterial infection. • Serum concentration of prostatic esterase is high in some dogs.

IMAGING

Radiography

• Abdominal radiographs reveal prostatomegaly • Retrograde urethrocystography may be normal or reveal narrowing of prostatic urethra or reflux of contrast media into the prostate gland

Ultrasonography

Reveals large prostate gland with uniform prostatic parenchymal echogenicity; small, fluid-filled cysts in some dogs

OTHER DIAGNOSTIC PROCEDURES

N/A

TREATMENT

• Frequently not required • Castration the most effective treatment and prevents recurrence. If benign prostatic hyperplasia is complicated by acute bacterial prostatitis, delay castration until the infection is resolved

MEDICATIONS

DRUG AND FLUIDS

• If castration is not acceptable, the following drugs may temporarily shrink the prostate gland:
• Finasteride (5mg/day)
• Megestrol acetate (0.11 mg/kg PO daily for 3 weeks)
• Medroxyprogesterone (3mg/kg SQ)

CONTRAINDICATIONS/POSSIBLE INTERACTIONS

• Avoid estrogens because of possible hematologic toxicity
• Chronic administration of megestrol acetate or medroxyprogesterone may result in development of diabetes mellitus.

FOLLOW-UP

• Castration results in rapid involution of the large prostate gland

MISCELLANEOUS

ASSOCIATED CONDITIONS

• Bacterial prostatitis and prostatic carcinoma (in intact dogs) • Prostatomegaly in a castrated dog strongly suggests prostatic carcinoma

SEE ALSO

• Prostatic Cysts • Prostatitis and Prostatic Abscess • Prostatomegaly

Reference

Barsanti JA, Finco DR. Canine prostatic diseases. In: Ettinger SJ, ed. Textbook of veterinary internal medicine. Philadelphia: WB Saunders, 1989;662-1685.

Author Jeffrey S. Klausner
Consulting Editors Larry G. Adams and Carl A. Osborne

BERNESE MOUNTAIN DOG STEROID RESPONSIVE MENINGITIS-POLYARTERITIS

BASICS

OVERVIEW
Meningitis and polyarteritis causing severe cervical/spinal pain in young Bernese mountain dogs

SIGNALMENT
• Most affected dogs 3-18 months old; occasionally seen in older dogs • Males and females equally affected

SIGNS
• Severe neck pain and cervical rigidity • Stiff and stilted gait • Reluctance to move • Spinal pain with arched back—not as consistently observed as the neck pain • Depression and fever common in the acute phase • In patients with this typical form of the disease, no neurologic deficits • In patients with the more protracted form, signs may be intermittent initially and progress to neurologic deficits such as weakness, paralysis, blindness, and seizures.

CAUSES AND RISK FACTORS
• 1-2% of the Bernese mountain dogs are affected. Littermates and closely related dogs often are affected. • Probably hereditary • Immunopathologic basis suspected

DIAGNOSIS

DIFFERENTIAL DIAGNOSIS
• Aseptic meningitis is a very similar disease that can only be differentiated on the basis of breed. • Bacterial meningitis cannot be differentiated from the acute form on the basis of clinical signs. However, the high prevalence of aseptic meningitis compared with septic disease in Bernese mountain dogs facilitates the diagnosis. Serum IgA concentration may help rule out bacterial infection. • Patients with infectious meningoencephalomyelitis and granulomatous meningoencephalomyelitis often have neurologic deficits on examination. These diseases can be further differentiated on the basis of signalment, CSF analysis, and appropriate culturing and serologic testing.
• Large-breed dogs with disk disease are comparatively older, do not have fever, leucocytosis, or pleocytosis on examination of CSF.
• Idiopathic polyarthritis can cause cervical pain and lameness, but results of CSF analysis are normal and cytologic examination of joint fluid cytology reveals inflammation. Dogs with the Bernese syndrome may have polyarthritis. Examination of CSF and joint fluid should be performed. • Cervical diskospondylitis causes cervical pain and possibly fever, but results of CSF analysis are usually normal, and the survey radiography of the affected vertebrae is diagnostic.

CBC/BIOCHEMISTRY/URINALYSIS
• Leucocytosis with neutrophilia common, especially in animals with the acute form
• Results of biochemical analysis and urinalysis normal

OTHER LABORATORY TESTS
• High serum and CSF IgA concentrations
• Results of serologic tests for infectious agents negative

IMAGING N/A

OTHER DIAGNOSTIC PROCEDURES
• CSF analysis—marked neutrophilic pleocytosis and high protein concentration in animals with the acute form. In patients with more protracted disease, the protein concentration is normal or slightly high. Pleocytosis is mild to moderate with a mixed or mononuclear cell population. • Cytologic examination of joint fluid shows inflammation in some animals. • Bacterial culture of CSF, blood, and urine negative • Histopathologic findings are those of severe necrotizing vasculitis and thrombosis of the small and medium-sized arteries of the meninges.

TREATMENT
• Hospitalize the patient for initial treatment.
• Restrict activity.

MEDICATIONS

DRUGS AND FLUIDS
• Administer prednisone at 2-4 mg/kg/day. Dogs should respond within 48 hours.
• Gradually decrease prednisone dosage after 2 weeks, but maintain at least 1 mg/kg every 48 hours.
• Continue prednisone medication for at least 4-6 months after signs have resolved to decrease the likelihood of relapse.
• Medication can be discontinued in some dogs after 4-6 months.
• Azathioprine (Imuran) has been used with success in some dogs (2mg/kg/q24h) that do not respond to prednisone.

CONTRAINDICATIONS/POSSIBLE INTERACTIONS N/A

FOLLOW-UP
• Monitor for presence of neck pain and leucocytosis. • Some dogs relapse in spite of appropriate treatment; try azathioprine. • 10% of dogs require lifelong treatment. • The disorder may resolve spontaneously when patient is 18-24 months old.

MISCELLANEOUS

ABBREVIATION
CSF = cerebrospinal fluid

Reference

Tipold A, Jaggy A. Steroid responsive meningitis-arteritis in dogs: long-term study of 32 cases. J Small Anim Practice 1994;35:311-316.

Author Susan M. Taylor
Consulting Editor Joane M. Parent

BASICS

OVERVIEW

Bile duct carcinoma (also, cholangiocellular carcinoma and cholangiocarcinoma) is the most frequently reported malignant liver tumor in cats, and the second most common primary malignant liver tumor in dogs. Bile duct carcinoma arises from the intrahepatic (most common in dogs) or extrahepatic bile duct or the gallbladder.

SIGNALMENT

• Dogs and cats > 10 years old • More common in females in both dogs and cats • No breed predilection identified

SIGNS

Historical Findings

• Highly variable • Anorexia • Weight loss • Vomiting • Lethargy • Abdominal swelling • Signs associated with advanced disease: icterus, ascites, and CNS abnormalities (e.g., seizures and behavioral changes)

Physical Examination Findings

• Hepatomegaly • Ascites • Abdominal pain • Abdominal distention • Icterus • Hepatocellular carcinoma easier to detect by abdominal palpation than bile duct carcinoma

CAUSES AND RISK FACTORS

Unknown

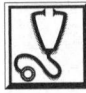

DIAGNOSIS

DIFFERENTIAL DIAGNOSIS

Gross Differentials

• Hepatocellular adenoma • Hepatocellular carcinoma • Nodular hyperplasia • Cirrhosis • Chronic active hepatitis • Bile duct carcinoma easily distinguished histologically from hepatocellular carcinoma

CBC/BIOCHEMISTRY/URINALYSIS

• Changes in hematologic and biochemical values common but are nonspecific in patients with liver cancer • High serum enzyme activities (i.e., ALP, ALT, and AST) , hypoalbuminemia, hypergammaglobulinemia, hypoglycemia, and high direct and indirect bilirubin—support a diagnosis of liver disease • Leukocytosis in many patients

OTHER LABORATORY TESTS

A coagulogram should be performed before biopsy or surgery.

IMAGING

• Abdominal radiography to help localize the abdominal mass to the liver • Thoracic radiography to identify pulmonary metastases • Abdominal ultrasound to assess parenchymal integrity, confirm the organ of origin, and guide fine needle aspiration or biopsy of the mass.

OTHER DIAGNOSTIC PROCEDURES

• Abdominocentesis and cytologic examination in animals with ascites • Examination of neoplastic tissue obtained by percutaneous biopsy, laparoscopy, or laparotomy for definitive diagnosis

GROSS AND HISTOPATHOLOGIC FINDINGS

• The tumor is either large and diffuse or small and nodular. • Frequently solid but may be cystic • Location any lobe of the liver • Several histologic types of bile duct carcinoma are seen, but all show similar biologic behavior.

TREATMENT

• Surgical excision the treatment of choice • Up to 75% of the liver can be resected without clinically important hepatic dysfunction.

MEDICATIONS

DRUGS AND FLUIDS

No successful chemotherapy has been reported in dogs or cats.

CONTRAINDICATIONS/POSSIBLE INTERACTIONS

• Medications requiring metabolism by the liver should be used with caution in patients with hepatopathy.
• Hepatotoxicity from anticancer drugs appears to be of little or no clinical importance in small animals.

FOLLOW-UP

EXPECTED COURSE AND PROGNOSIS

• Bile duct carcinoma is an aggressive neoplasm with a high rate of metastases (87.5%). • Most common sites of metastasis are the lungs, hepatic lymph nodes, and peritoneum. • The prognosis is poor, even when resection is possible and no metastases are seen during surgery. • The degree of invasiveness, presence of metastases, and tumor resectability are the most reliable indicators of survival.

MISCELLANEOUS

ASSOCIATED CONDITIONS

• Cirrhosis or other primary hepatic disease does not appear to be a prerequisite for bile duct carcinoma in dogs and cats. • Hepatic neoplasms are commonly diagnosed in geriatric, debilitated animals that require concurrent management of cardiac, renal, metabolic, and electrolyte abnormalities.

PREGNANCY

Chemotherapy drugs may be carcinogenic and mutagenic.

ABBREVIATIONS

ALP = alkaline phosphatase
ALT = alanine transaminase
AST = aspartate transaminase

Reference

Popp, JA. Tumors of the liver, gall bladder, and pancreas. In: Moulton JE, ed. Tumors in domestic animals. 3rd ed. Berkeley, CA: University of California Press, 1990;436-449.

Author Stanley L. Marks
Consulting Editor Wallace B. Morrison

BILOUS VOMITING SYNDROME

 **BASICS**

OVERVIEW
• Clinical entity associated with chronic intermittent vomiting of bile caused by bile reflux into the stomach • Normal gastric motility and pressure gradients generally prevent or quickly remove any refluxed bile before gastric mucosal irritation occurs. Bile reflux is suspected to be secondary to alterations in normal gastrointestinal motility. The presence of bile in the gastric lumen subsequently causes gastric mucosal damage.
• Clinical signs usually occur early in the morning suggesting that fasting or inactivity may modify normal motility patterns resulting in duodenal reflux.

SIGNALMENT
• Commonly observed in dogs and occasionally in cats. • Most animals are middle-aged to old. • No breed, age or sex predisposition

SIGNS
• Chronic intermittent vomiting of bile associated with an empty stomach • Signs generally occur late at night or early in the morning. • Signs may occur daily but are usually more intermittent. Between episodes, the animal appears normal in all other respects.
• Results of physical examination are usually unremarkable.

CAUSES AND RISK FACTORS
• Cause unknown • Primary gastric hypomotility is suspected as the underlying cause.
• Conditions causing gastritis or duodenitis are also responsible for altered motility and may cause bile reflux.

 DIAGNOSIS

DIFFERENTIAL DIAGNOSIS
• Any number of gastrointestinal and nongastrointestinal disorders can cause chronic vomiting. • Giardia should be excluded since the signs of this disease may mimic those of bilious vomiting. • Intestinal obstruction or partial obstruction should be ruled out.

CBC/BIOCHEMISTRY/URINALYSIS
Results usually normal

OTHER LABORATORY TESTS
Fecal examination to detect giardia or other parasites

IMAGING
Liquid barium contrast study may reveal delayed gastric emptying or depressed gastric contractions.

OTHER DIAGNOSTIC PROCEDURES
• Endoscopic findings are frequently normal. Evidence of bile in the stomach or gastritis in the antral region seen in some patients. • Endoscopy useful to rule out structural disease of the stomach and inflammatory changes in the duodenum

 TREATMENT

• Not a serious debilitating disorder and the patient should be treated symptomatically.
• Feeding the animal a late evening meals often resolves clinical signs. Possibly food acts as a buffer to the refluxed bile or enhances gastric motility.
• If diet modification fails, medical treatment should be considered.

MEDICATIONS

DRUGS AND FLUIDS

• Choices include agents for gastric mucosal protection from the refluxed bile and gastric prokinetic agents for improving motility. Often a single evening dose of medication is all that is required to prevent clinical signs.
• Drugs for gastric mucosal protection include cimetidine (5 mg/kg), ranitidine (2 mg/kg), and carafate (1 gm/ 25 kg).
• Gastric prokenetic agents include metoclopramide (0.2 to 0.4 mg/kg) and cisapride (0.1 mg/kg).
• Erythromycin (1 to 5 mg/kg) promotes gastric motility and may resolve signs. A benefit of this drug is that it is inexpensive.

CONTRAINDICATIONS/POSSIBLE INTERACTIONS

• Gastric prokenetic agents should not be administered in patients with gastrointestinal obstruction.
• Metoclopramide is contraindicated with concurrent phenothiazine and narcotic administration and in animals with epilepsy.
• Metoclopramide can cause nervousness, anxiety, or depression.
• Cisapride can cause vomiting, diarrhea, or abdominal cramping
• Erythromycin can cause vomiting.

 ## FOLLOW-UP

• Most patients respond to one of the above treatments and a clinical response supports the diagnosis. • Failure to respond suggests other underlying or causative factor.

 ## MISCELLANEOUS

ASSOCIATED CONDITIONS

Gastroesophageal reflux

SEE ALSO

• Gastric Motility Disorders • Gastroesophageal Reflux

Reference

Hall JA, Twedt DC, Burrows CF. Gastric motility in dogs. Part 2. Disorders of gastric motility. Compend Small Anim Med Pract Vet 1990;12:1373-1390.
Author David C. Twedt
Consulting Editor Brent D. Jones

BLASTOMYCOSIS

BASICS

DEFINITION
A systemic mycosis caused by the dimorphic fungus Blastomyces dermatitidis

Pathophysiology
After inhalation (or rarely, inoculation through the skin) of infective spores of the filamentous mold form of the organism, the parasitic yeast form arises and spreads through the lungs, from where it can disseminate to other tissues of the body. The fungus causes a pyogranulomatous inflammation that results in pneumonia, skin and bone lesions, ocular disease, and CNS abnormalities. Unlike histoplasmosis and coccidioidomycosis, extrapulmonary dissemination in blastomycosis is very common.

Systems Affected
• Respiratory—by far the most commonly affected • Skin, eyes, bone, CNS, lymph nodes, and testes may be involved when extrapulmonary dissemination occurs.

Genetics
Unknown, but possibly there are inherited or acquired defects in host immune defenses that favor growth of the parasitic yeast form of Blastomyces in tissues.

Incidence/Prevalence
Dogs are highly susceptible to blastomycosis. In endemic areas they may exhibit an infection rate 10 times greater than that of cohabitant humans. The disease is at least 100 times less common in cats than in dogs.

Geographic Distribution
Primarily the mid-Atlantic seaboard, north-central states, and Ohio/Mississippi/Missouri river valley regions

SIGNALMENT

Species
Much more common in dogs than in either cats or humans

Breed Predilections
• Dogs—larger (often sporting) breeds, especially Labrador retrievers and doberman pinschers • Cats—none recognized

Mean Age and Range
• Dogs—ages 1-5 years • Cats—ages 2-7 years

Predominant Sex
• Dogs—male • Cats—none recognized

SIGNS

Historical Findings
Exercise intolerance, anorexia, weight loss, chronic cough, neurologic dysfunction, and ocular abnormalities are commonly reported signs.

Physical Examination Findings
Dogs
• The respiratory form is characterized by pneumonia, coughing, dyspnea, fever, weight loss, and lymph node enlargement. • Lameness may be seen when bone invasion (osteomyelitis) occurs. • Skin lesions can occur alone or in combination with lesions in other organs. They are most common on the face, planum nasale, limbs, nail beds, and sometimes the tongue. Lesions usually appear as abscesses or as thickened, ulcerated areas that exude fluid. • Most common ocular lesion is uveitis. • Painful testicular and/or prostatic enlargement may be present in some male dogs.
Cats
Dyspnea, weight loss, fever, ocular signs (ranging from conjunctivitis to blindness), skin lesions, lameness, and posterior paresis have been reported.

CAUSE
Blastomyces dermatitidis, a presumed soil fungus with a geographically restricted distribution that requires high humidity. It usually is associated with moist, rotting organic debris, often enriched with bird droppings and protected from direct sunlight. Infection of dogs, cats, or humans occurs when they encroach unknowingly upon one of these isolated areas of fungal growth.

RISK FACTORS
Aggressive nosing about in soil and underbrush, as in the sporting and hunting breeds of dogs, may expose susceptible animals to large doses of the causative fungus.

DIAGNOSIS

DIFFERENTIAL DIAGNOSIS
• Pulmonary lesions may resemble those of other systemic mycoses. Such lesions should be differentiated from metastatic tumors and canine distemper. • Lymphadenopathy may be seen in lymphosarcoma, in other systemic mycoses, and in localized bacterial infections. • Skin lesions should be differentiated from routine abscesses or other bacterial disease processes. • Bone lesions may resemble those caused by primary or metastatic bone tumors or bacterial osteomyelitis.

CBC/BIOCHEMISTRY/URINALYSIS
• Hemogram—mild nonregenerative anemia, moderate leukocytosis with a mild left shift, lymphopenia, and monocytosis (all nonspecific) • Serum chemistry profile—hyperglobulinemia, hypoalbuminemia, sometimes hypercalcemia (all nonspecific) • Urinalysis—few abnormalities recognized

OTHER LABORATORY TESTS
• Detection of a positive serum antibody titer, usually by the agar gel immunodiffusion (AGID) test, may provide a presumptive diagnosis but is not definitive. As a general rule, the more disseminated the infection the higher the antibody titer. • Feline blastomycosis does not appear to be associated with feline leukemia virus infection.

IMAGING
Radiography of lung (nodular or diffuse interstitial infiltrate) and bone (osteolysis)

OTHER DIAGNOSTIC PROCEDURES
• Biopsy or cytology may reveal infiltrating Blastomyces organisms.• Microscopic identification of the thick-walled, budding Blastomyces yeast forms in biopsy/cytology or other lesion material is the recommended method of diagnosis. Lymph node aspirates and impression smears of skin lesions or draining exudate are good sources of material. Patients with primarily lung involvement may require a tracheal wash or pulmonary aspirate. In most patients with blastomycosis, fungal organisms are present in large numbers and can be readily recognized.

GROSS AND HISTOPATHOLOGIC FINDINGS
• Pyogranulomatous inflammation present in many tissues • Lymph node hyperplasia
• Presence of characteristic yeast form (and occasionally filamentous mold form) of the fungus in affected tissues

TREATMENT

INPATIENT VERSUS OUTPATIENT
Because treatment of blastomycosis requires long-term therapy, the patient should be treated as an outpatient. Patients treated with amphotericin B (AMB), however, will need to be hospitalized several times a week during their initial treatment period.

ACTIVITY
Activity levels should be restricted during the period of antifungal therapy.

DIET
Because affected animals have often experienced weight loss, provision should be made for feeding a high-quality diet. Protein levels may need to be restricted, however, owing to the nephrotoxic effects of AMB.

CLIENT EDUCATION
• The necessity and expense of long-term therapy of a potentially fatal illness, in addition to the possible side effects of such therapy, need to be thoroughly discussed with the client.
• The quality of life for the patient should be balanced against the likelihood of successful therapy, based upon the physical condition of the animal at the time of diagnosis.

SURGICAL CONSIDERATIONS N/A

MEDICATIONS

DRUGS AND FLUIDS

Dog
• Amphotericin B remains the primary drug of choice for the treatment of blastomycosis,

and can be administered either alone or in combination. When used alone it can be administered at a dosage of 0.5 mg/kg, 3 times a week, for a total cumulative dosage of 8-10 mg/kg. It is given IV either as a slow infusion (in dogs that are gravely ill or are in kidney failure) or as a rapid bolus (in fairly healthy dogs without renal impairment). For slow infusion, add AMB to 250-500 ml of 5% dextrose solution and administer as a drip over a period of 4-6 hours. For a rapid bolus, add AMB to 30 ml of 5% dextrose solution and administer over a period of 5 minutes through a butterfly catheter.
• To lessen the adverse renal effects of AMB, give 0.9% NaCl (2 ml/kg/hr) for several hours before initiating AMB therapy.
• Ketoconazole (KTZ) represents an alternative to AMB in dogs that are not gravely ill. It may also be given in sequential fashion after AMB therapy has been completed, depending on the clinical response. In general, KTZ is not as effective as AMB when given alone and the response to therapy is much slower. KTZ can be administered at 10-30 mg/kg PO, divided 2 or 3 times daily for 2-3 months. The medication should be given in the food. Higher dosages (40 mg/kg) may be needed in dogs with bone or CNS involvement.
• A combination of AMB and KTZ has been used in dogs that have not responded to either drug alone or that have exhibited significant toxicity. It may also be a useful alternative to therapy with AMB alone. For combination chemotherapy, administer AMB as described to a total cumulative dosage of 4-6 mg/kg, together with KTZ at 10 mg/kg PO divided daily for at least 2-3 months.
• A newer azole derivative, itraconazole (ITZ), is reportedly more effective than KTZ and may be curative at a dosage of 5 mg/kg PO q12h over a period of 2-3 months. The medication should be given in the food.

Cat
• AMB should be administered by rapid IV bolus at a dosage of 0.25 mg/kg, 3 times a week, for a total cumulative dosage of 4 mg/kg. This can be followed by KTZ therapy, depending on the clinical response.
• KTZ should be administered at 10-20 mg/kg PO, divided 2 or 3 times daily, to cats that are not gravely ill. If side effects occur, reduce to alternate-day therapy. The medication should be given in the food.

• ITZ may be curative at a dosage of 5 mg/kg PO q12h over a period of 2-3 months. It should be given in the food.

CONTRAINDICATIONS
• Drugs metabolized primarily by the kidneys should not be administered along with AMB.
• Drugs metabolized primarily by the liver should not be administered along with KTZ or ITZ.

PRECAUTIONS
• Side effects of AMB therapy can be severe and include renal dysfunction, fever, inappetence, vomiting, and phlebitis.
• Side effects of KTZ or ITZ therapy include inappetence, vomiting, and hepatotoxicity. Side effects are much less common with ITZ.

POSSIBLE INTERACTIONS N/A

ALTERNATE DRUGS N/A

FOLLOW-UP

PATIENT MONITORING
• BUN should be monitored in all animals treated with AMB. Treatment should be temporarily discontinued if the BUN rises above 50 mg/dl. • Liver enzymes should be monitored in animals receiving KTZ or ITZ.

PREVENTION/AVOIDANCE
There is no available vaccine. Restrict hunting and roaming in geographical areas where the organism is suspected of persisting.

POSSIBLE COMPLICATIONS
• Pulmonary disease may temporarily worsen soon after therapy is inititated, owing to the inflammation resulting from the death of fungal cells in the lungs. • Nephrotoxicity may result from AMB therapy. • Hepatotoxicity may result from KTZ or ITZ therapy.

EXPECTED COURSE AND PROGNOSIS
• The prognosis is always guarded except in an animal with the rarer superficial skin infections, which often responds favorably to treatment. • Many dogs can be cured if they receive aggressive treatment and if the disease has not progressed beyond a critical point.
• Relapses after treatment may occur, most often in animals exhibiting severe lung involvement. The relapse rate for dogs treated with AMB has been reported to be about 17%. Reinitiation of a complete course of

therapy is usually necessary. • In most cases, animals that are still healthy one year after completion of therapy will remain free of the disease. • Spontaneous recovery from severe disseminated blastomycosis without treatment is considered extremely rare.

MISCELLANEOUS

ASSOCIATED CONDITIONS N/A

AGE RELATED FACTORS N/A

ZOONOTIC POTENTIAL
The parasitic yeast form of the fungus, as found in animal tissues, is not directly transmissible to people or other animals. Under certain rare circumstances, however, there may be reversion to growth of the infective mold form of the fungus on or within bandages placed over a draining lesion or in contaminated bedding. This author recommends that prudent care be exercised whenever handling an infected dog or cat.

PREGNANCY
• AMB—no teratogenic effects have been identified • KTZ and ITZ should be used in pregnant animals only if the potential benefit justifies the potential risk to offspring.

SYNONYMS
Gilchrist's disease, Chicago disease (in humans).

SEE ALSO N/A

ABBREVIATIONS
AGID = agar gel immunodiffusion
AMB = amphotericin B
KTZ = ketoconazole
ITZ = itraconazole

References
Rudmann DG, Coolman BR, Perez CM, Glickman LT. Evaluation of risk factors for blastomycosis in dogs: 857 cases (1980-1990). J Am Vet Med Assoc 1992;201: 1754-1759.
Sherding RG. Systemic mycoses. In: Birchard SJ, Sherding RG, eds. Saunders manual of small animal practice. Philadelphia: WB Saunders, 1994;133-140.
Author Jeffrey E. Barlough
Consulting Editor Fred W. Scott

BLEPHARITIS

BASICS

DEFINITION
Inflammation of the outer (skin) and middle portion (muscle, connective tissue, and glands) of the eyelid, usually with secondary inflammation of the palpebral conjunctiva

Pathophysiology
The eyelid is capable of duplicating virtually every condition that affects the skin in general. Mechanisms of inflammation include immune-mediated, infectious, endocrine-mediated, self- and external trauma, parasitic, radiation, and nutritional. Because eyelid conjunctiva is exceptionally rich in mast cells and eyelid tissue is densely vascularized, inflammatory response is often exaggerated compared to that of other cutaneous tissues.

Systems Affected
Ophthalmic—usually bilateral, diffuse involvement of the eyelids, but it can be unilateral (upper and lower) or affect only one eyelid. Adjacent tissues (e.g., conjunctiva and cornea) can be inflamed secondarily or the blepharitis may itself be secondary to self-trauma from ocular pain or irritation, such as anterior uveitis, conjunctivitis, or keratitis.

Genetics N/A

Incidence/Prevalence N/A

Geographic Distribution N/A

SIGNALMENT See causes

SIGNS
Dependent on the cause and include • Serous, mucoid, or mucopurulent ocular discharge
• Dark brown, mucoid or granular discharge (cats) • Blepharospasm • Eyelid diffuse or marginal hyperemia, edema, and thickening
• Pruritus • Depigmentation of skin or (in Siamese and Himalayan cats) hair • Swollen, cream-colored meibomian glands • Elevated, "pinpoint" meibomian gland orifices (cats)
• Excoriation • Abscesses • Alopecia
• Scales and crusts • Papules/ pustules
• Single or multiple nodular swellings
• Concurrent conjunctivitis or keratitis

CAUSES
Congenital
Congenital eyelid and periocular abnormalities can promote eyelid self trauma or moist palpebral dermatitis: prominent nasal folds and medial lower lid entropion (shih tzu, Pekingese, English bulldog, lhasa apso, pug, Persian and Himalayan cat); medial trichiasis (same breeds); distichia (shih tzu, Shetland sheepdog, pug, golden retriever, Labrador retriever, English bulldog); ectopic cilia; lateral lid entropion (various dog breeds such as shar pei and chow chow; adult cats [rare]); lagophthalmos (brachycephalic dogs; Persian, Himalayan, and Burmese cats); deep medial canthal pockets (dolichocephalic dogs); dermoids (rottweiler,

dachshund, and other breeds; Burmese cat); and eyelid agenesis (cats).

External Trauma
Eyelid lacerations, thermal or chemical burns, and cat claw or bite injuries

Allergic
Type I immediate hypersensitivity reactions (e.g., atopy, food allergy, insect bite, inhalant allergy, Staph hypersensitivity); type II cytotoxic hypersensitivity reactions (e.g., pemphigus, pemphigoid, and drug eruption); type III immune complex hypersensitivity reactions (e.g., systemic lupus erythematosus, Staph hypersensitivity, drug eruption); and type IV cell-mediated hypersensitivity (e.g., contact and flea bite hypersensitivity, drug eruption)

Bacterial
Hordeolum (localized abscess of eyelid glands, usually staphylococcal) which can be external ("sty" in young dogs, involving glands of Zeis) or internal (in older dogs, involving one or multiple meibomian glands); generalized bacterial blepharitis and meibomianitis (usually Staph or Strep); pyogranulomas; Staph hypersensitivity (in young and older dogs)

Mycotic
Dermatophytosis; granulomas in cats with systemic histoplasmosis

Parasitic
Demodicosis (dogs and cats); sarcoptic mange (dogs); Cuterebra and Notoedres cati in cats

Granulomatous
Halations are usually sterile, yellow-white, painless eyelid swellings caused by a granulomatous inflammatory response to escape of meibum into the surrounding eyelid tissue.

Neoplastic
Sebaceous adenomas originate from the meibomian gland; squamous cell carcinoma in cats with white-haired eyelids.

Nutritional
Zinc-responsive dermatosis (Siberian huskies, Alaskan malamutes, puppies); fatty acid deficiency

Endocrine
Hypothyroidism in dogs; hyperadrenocorticism in dogs; diabetic dermatosis

Viral
Chronic blepharitis secondary to feline herpesvirus (FHV-I) keratoconjunctivitis

Irritant
Topical ocular drug reaction; nicotine smoke in environment; after parotid duct transposition

Miscellaneous
Familial canine dermatomyositis (collies and Shetland sheepdogs); nodular granulomatous episclerokeratitis (i.e., fibrous histiocytoma and collie granuloma) in collies sometimes affects the eyelids in conjunction with corneal or conjunctival disease; eosinophilic granuloma in cats can sometimes affect the eyelids in

conjunction with corneal or conjunctival disease; blepharitis secondary to eyelid contact with purulent exudate; blepharitis secondary to conjunctivitis, keratitis, dry eye, dacryocystitis, orbital disease, and after radiotherapy

Idiopathic
Chronic blepharitis often occurs with no underlying identifiable cause, particularly secondarily in cats with chronic idiopathic conjunctivitis

RISK FACTORS
Breeds prone to congenital eyelid abnormalities (see previous section), acquired entropion (rottweiler, Labrador retriever and adult cats); outdoor animals are more prone to traumatic injuries; hypothyroidism can promote chronic bacterial blepharitis in dogs; canine seborrhea can promote chronic generalized meibomianitis.

DIAGNOSIS

DIFFERENTIAL DIAGNOSIS
The clinical signs are diagnostic.

CBC/BIOCHEMISTRY/URINALYSIS
Usually nondiagnostic unless metabolic causes of blepharitis are present (e.g., high serum glucose concentration in animal with diabetic dermatosis)

OTHER LABORATORY TESTS
Indicated if a systemic disorder is suspected. Consider tests for hypothyroidism.

IMAGING N/A

OTHER DIAGNOSTIC PROCEDURES
• Cytologic examination of deep skin scraping, conjunctival scraping, and expressed exudate from meibomian glands and pustules
• Dermatophyte culture of deep skin scrapings; Wood's light evaluation of skin; KOH preparation of skin scrapings • Bacterial culture and sensitivity testing of exudate from skin, conjunctiva, and expressed exudate from meibomian glands and pustules. In animal with chronic meibomianitis and suspected Staph hypersensitivity, Staph is often not recovered. • Fluorescent antibody testing of conjunctival scrapings In cats in which conjunctivitis or keratitis is the primary disease may aid in diagnosis of FHV-I or chlamydial infection. • Examine eye for potential inciting cause such as corneal ulcer, foreign body, distichiasis, and dry eye. Ancillary ocular tests include fluorescein application and Schirmer tear test. Do not apply topical anesthetic or fluorescein before obtaining samples for culture. • A thorough medical history and dermatologic examination are helpful in identifying generalized dermatologic disease.
• Full-thickness wedge biopsy of eyelid for histologic evaluation. Special tests can be performed on tissue, such as direct immunofluorescence testing for autoimmune disease.
• Tests for hypersensitivity-induced disease: intradermal skin testing, RAST and ELISA testing for atopy, food elimination diet for food allergy.

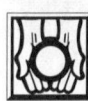

TREATMENT

• Treat primary disease condition if blepharitis is secondary. • If self-trauma is the suspected cause, apply neck restraint collar to prevent rubbing by paw or against other surfaces; collar must be of sufficient length to prevent rubbing against other objects.
• Rarely, an irritant blepharoconjunctivitis may occur with ocular application of gentamicin, neomycin, terramycin, antiviral medication (i.e., viroptic), and most ointments. Withdrawal of these medications may resolve of the blepharitis. • Cleanse eyelids: warm compresses, applying for 5-15 minutes 3-4 times daily. Use saline, lactated Ringer's solution, or an ocular cleansing agent such as Eye Scrub (CIBA), sold in individual packets in most pharmacies over the counter or in a bottle as a veterinary product, to remove crusts, avoiding ocular surfaces. Periocular hair must be clipped short.

INPATIENT VERSUS OUTPATIENT
Outpatient

ACTIVITY N/A

DIET N/A

CLIENT EDUCATION
Most cats and many dogs with chronic blepharitis cannot be cured, but they often can be controlled medically. If FHV-I conjunctivitis is the underlying cause, the client must understand that cure is impossible, and that clinical signs often recur when the animal is stressed. If a restraint collar is prescribed, the owner must keep it on the animal at all times.

SURGICAL CONSIDERATIONS
• Place temporary everting eyelid sutures if spastic entropion has occurred; also used in some patients with primary entropion before performing permanent corrective surgery. • Surgically repair eyelid lacerations. • Lance only large abscesses. Hordeola usually do not require lancing and curettage unless resistant to medical treatment, or if chalazia have hardened and "come to a point," causing keratitis. Manually express infected meibomian secretions.

MEDICATIONS

DRUGS AND FLUIDS
In general, systemic antibiotics are required to effectively treat bacterial eyelid infections. Good empirical choices include amoxicillin/clavulanic acid, oxacillin, or cephalexin at 20 mg/kg q8h. Topically, neomycin, polymyxin B, and bacitracin or chloramphenicol are reasonable first choices for use in the eye.

Congenital
To prevent frictional rubbing of eyelid hairs or cilia on the ocular surface, apply a topical ophthalmic antibiotic ointment q6h-q12h un-til surgery is performed. Regularly flush deep medial canthal pocket debris with saline, lactated Ringer's solution, or ocular irrigant.

External Trauma
If spastic entropion is present secondary to pain and blepharospasm, apply a topical ophthalmic antibiotic ointment q6h-q12h to reduce friction until entropion is relieved. Systemic antibiotics are indicated.

Allergic
Treat Staph hypersensitivity blepharitis with systemic, broad-spectrum antibiotics and systemic corticosteroids (prednisolone, 0.5mg/kg q12h for 3-5 days then taper). Many animals respond to systemic corticosteroids alone. Also use topical polymyxin B and neomycin with 0.1% dexamethasone (Dexacidin) q6h-q8h to the eye. If treatment fails, injections of homologous or commercial Staphylococcus aureus bacterin (Staphage Lysate) may aid in disease control. Propionibacterium acnes immunotherapy is investigational and of unknown value. Eyelid lesions associated with puppy strangles usually benefit from treatment of the generalized condition.

Bacterial
Based on results of culture and sensitivity testing. While tests are pending, use topical polymyxin B and neomycin with 0.1% dexamethasone ointment q4-6 hrs, in addition to one of the systemic broad spectrum antibiotics listed.

Mycotic
Most Microsporum canis infections are self-limiting, but treatment includes 2% miconazole cream, 1% clotrimazole cream, and diluted povidone-iodine solution (1 part to 300 parts saline), applied q12h-q24h for at least 6 weeks. Do not use lotions.

Parasitic
Demodicosis (see demodicosis topic)—for localized disease, diluted amitraz (1 part amitraz to 9 parts mineral oil; Mitaban) once every 3 days for 4-8 weeks is fairly safe around the eyes. Notoedres infection—lime sulfur dips. Sarcoptic mange— treat same as for generalized disease.

Idiopathic
Topical polymyxin B and neomycin with 0.1% dexamethasone q8h-q24h or as needed will often control clinical signs. Occasionally, systemic prednisolone (0.5mg/kg q12h for 3-5 days then taper) and/or one of the above systemic antibiotics are also needed.

CONTRAINDICATIONS
Topical corticosteroids should not be used if corneal ulceration is present. Many cats with idiopathic blepharoconjunctivitis actually have FHV-I infection, and topical and systemic corticosteroids exacerbate the infection.

PRECAUTIONS
When treating ectoparasitism, wear gloves and do not contact ocular surfaces with the drug. Apply artificial tear ointment to the eye for protection.

POSSIBLE INTERACTIONS
If staphylococcal bacterin is used in treatment of Staph hypersensitivity, anaphylactic reactions are rarely encountered.

ALTERNATE DRUGS N/A

FOLLOW-UP

PATIENT MONITORING
Varies with cause. An animal with bacterial blepharitis should be given systemic and topical treatment for at least 3 weeks, and improvement should be noticed within 3-7 days. The most common causes of treatment failure are use of subinhibitory antibiotic concentrations, not correcting the myriad of potential predisposing factors, and stopping medications too soon.

PREVENTION/AVOIDANCE
Varies with the cause

POSSIBLE COMPLICATIONS
• Cicatricial lid contracture resulting in trichiasis, ectropion, or lagophthalmos
• Spastic entropion because of blepharospasm and pain • Inability to open eyelids due to matting of discharge and hair • Qualitative tear film deficiency due to loss of proper meibum secretion • Recurrence of bacterial infection or FHV-I blepharo-conjunctivitis

EXPECTED COURSE AND PROGNOSIS
Varies with the cause

MISCELLANEOUS

ASSOCIATED CONDITIONS See causes

AGE-RELATED FACTORS See causes

ZOONOTIC POTENTIAL
Dermatophytosis and sarcoptic mange

PREGNANCY N/A

SYNONYMS N/A

SEE ALSO
• Conjunctivitis • Epiphora • Keratitis, ulcerative and nonulcerative • Red eye

ABBREVIATIONS
• FHV-I = feline herpesvirus I
• Staph = staphylococcal/staphylococcus
• Strep = streptococcal/streptococcus

References
Muller GH, Kirk RW, Scott DW. Small animal dermatology. 4th ed. Philadelphia: WB Saunders, 1989.
Pentlarge VW. Blepharitis. In: Lorenz MD et al, eds. Small animal medical therapeutics. New York: JB Lippincott, 1992:398–406.
Gelatt KN. Veterinary ophthalmology. 2nd ed. Philadelphia: Lea & Febiger, 1991:263–271.
Author Terri L. McCalla
Consulting Editor Paul E. Miller

BLOOD TRANSFUSION REACTIONS

BASICS

OVERVIEW
• Classified as acute, delayed, immune-mediated, or not immune-mediated reactions
• Severe reactions usually occur during or shortly after transfusion.

SIGNALMENT Dogs and cats

SIGNS

Acute Hemolytic Reaction
• Restlessness, fever, tachycardia, vomiting, tremors, weakness, incontinence, collapse, shock, oliguria, loss of transfusion benefits

Delayed Hemolytic Reaction
• Loss of transfusion efficacy, usually no clinical signs

Acute Non-Hemolytic Reaction
• Anaphylactic reaction: fever, urticaria, erythema, pruritus • Transfusion of contaminated blood: acute septicemia, fever, shock
• Circulatory overload / rapid transfusion: vomiting, distended jugular veins, dyspnea, cough, cyanosis, congestive heart failure
• Citrate toxicity: hypocalcemia, myocardial depression, weakness • Hyperammonemia: encephalopathy • Hypothermia: shivering, decreased platelet function

CAUSES AND RISK FACTORS

Acute Hemolysis
• Blood group mismatch • Transfusion of damaged and hemolyzed red blood cells (after excessive heating, freezing, or mechanical damage)

Delayed Hemolysis
Immune reaction to minor red cell antigens; hemolysis occurs after 3-14 days.

Acute Non-Hemolytic Reactions
• Anaphylaxis and immune reaction to donor leukocyte, major histocompatibility antigens, or plasma antigens: release of inflammatory mediators and pyrogens • Transfusion of contaminated blood: lack of aseptic collection and storage conditions • Circulatory overload: rapid transfusions, excessive volumes of blood in small animals or animals with heart failure
• Citrate toxicity: after circulatory overload, particularly in small animals or animals with hepatopathies • Hyperammonemia: high ammonia levels in stored blood, important only in animals with hepatopathies • Hypothermia: rapid transfusion of refrigerated blood to small or already hypothermic animals

Delayed Non-Hemolytic Reactions
Transmission of bloodborne disease: use of infected donors

DIAGNOSIS

DIFFERENTIAL DIAGNOSIS
• Hemolysis: Rule-out ongoing fulminant hemolytic disease, use of hemolyzed blood.
• Fever, hypotension: Rule out underlying infectious or inflammatory diseases.

CBC/BIOCHEMISTRY/URINALYSIS
Hemoglobinemia, leukocytosis, bilirubinemia, hemoglobinuria, and bilirubinuria

OTHER LABORATORY TESTS
• Repeat crossmatch to confirm incompatibility • Culture or gram staining of contaminated blood may reveal organism.

IMAGING N/A

OTHER DIAGNOSTIC PROCEDURES
N/A

TREATMENT
• Immediately discontinue transfusion.
• Provide fluid therapy to maintain blood pressure and renal blood flow.

MEDICATIONS

DRUGS AND FLUIDS
• For hypotension—LRS (50-90 ml/kg/hr to effect)
• For hemolysis—prednisolone (4 mg/kg), heparin (75 U/kg SC q6h)—not for use in bleeding animals
• For urticaria, fever—diphenhydramine (1-2 mg/kg), prednisolone. Continue transfusion afterward, if clinically indicated.
• For septicemia—IV antibiotics, fluid therapy, heparin

CONTRAINDICATIONS/POSSIBLE INTERACTIONS N/A

FOLLOW-UP

PATIENT MONITORING
Check attitude, temperature, vital signs, PCV/TS, and plasma color before, during, and after transfusion.

PREVENTION/AVOIDANCE
Adhere to standard transfusion protocols (e.g,. blood typing, crossmatching, use of healthy donors, and appropriate collection, storage, and administration techniques).

POSSIBLE COMPLICATIONS
• Fulminant hemolysis causes acute renal failure, pulmonary thromboembolism, and disseminated intravascular coagulation in some animals. • Volume overload may cause heart failure.

EXPECTED COURSE AND PROGNOSIS
• An acute course in most animals • Prognosis good in stable animals, guarded in severely ill animals or when not recognized early

MISCELLANEOUS

References

Stone MS, Cotter SM. Practical guidelines for transfusion therapy. In: Kirk RW, Bonagura JD, eds. Textbook of veterinary therapy., 11th ed. Philadelphia,: W.B. Saunders Company,1992:475-479.

Giger U. Feline transfusion medicine. In: Hohenhaus AE, ed. Transfusion medicine, problems in veterinary medicine. Philadelphia:, J.B. Lippincott, 1992:600-611 .

Hohenhaus AE. Canine blood transfusions. In: Hohenhaus AE, ed. Transfusion medicine, problems in veterinary medicine. Philadelphia,: J.B. Lippincott, 1992:612-624 .

Author Jorg Bhucheler
Consulting Editor Alan H. Rebar

BRACHYCEPHALIC AIRWAY SYNDROME

BASICS

DEFINITION
Brachycephalic airway syndrome is partial upper airway obstruction resulting from the conformation of shorthead breeds of dogs and cats. Obstruction may include any of the following airway passages: nasal (stenotic nares), pharyngeal (overlong soft palate), laryngeal (everted laryngeal ventricles, laryngeal collapse), and tracheal (hypoplastic trachea). Both stertor and stridor typically are present.

Pathophysiology
Compressed, narrowed air passages occur in animals that are selectively bred for a flat face, round head, and short, thick neck. To produce airflow through these narrowed passages, the respiratory muscles must generate more force than in normal animals. This force can result in barotrauma to the soft tissues lining the airways, causing edema, inflammation, and even inward collapse that further narrows the airways. In extreme cases, the respiratory muscles will become fatigued and ventilatory failure can result.

Systems Affected
• Respiratory—only system directly affected by brachycephalic airway syndrome • Gastrointestinal—secondary effects can result from aerophagia and the high forces used to breathe that compress abdominal contents • If the animal becomes hypoxic, all organ systems sensitive to hypoxia will be affected.

Genetics
While the condition appears to be linked to anatomic features that result from selective breeding, no experimental data exist to identify the underlying genetics.

Incidence/Prevalence
Within the affected breeds, this syndrome is common. For example, some authors assert that virtually all English bulldogs suffer from some degree of upper airway obstruction.

Geographic Distribution N/A

SIGNALMENT

Species
Both dogs and cats of brachycephalic breeds can exhibit signs of upper airway obstruction. However, cats rarely present with clinical signs so severe that surgery is recommended.

Breed Predilections
English bulldogs have been noted to be the breed that most commonly requires surgery. Other breeds affected include other bulldogs, Lhasa apsos, Pekingese, shar-peis, shih tzus, and boxers. Among cats, Persians and Himalayans have the most extreme conformation.

Mean Age and Range
The majority of the animals that require surgery are recognized as having difficulty as young adults (i.e., at 1-2 years of age).

However, animals as old as 9-10 years have been presented for surgery. In older animals, the search for an exacerbating cause that has led a subclinical obstruction to manifest should be particularly important.

Predominant Sex None

SIGNS

Historical Findings
Virtually all brachycephalic animals have some degree of stertorous or stridorous breathing. To relieve the high upper airway resistance, many dogs will breathe with their mouths open, panting even at cool ambient temperatures. The vast majority also snore during rest or sleep. Because these signs are present most of the time, the owner may not consider the noisy or rapid breathing as abnormal unless there has been a sudden or dramatic increase in severity. Rather, the presenting complaint may be collapse, exercise intolerance, and gastrointestinal signs such as vomiting, regurgitation, or dysphagia.

Physical Examination Findings
Stertor arising from the pharynx and stridor arising from the nasal and laryngeal areas are present in most, if not all, animals with brachycephalic conformation. These sounds usually are audible without the use of a stethoscope. However, careful auscultation can be helpful in locating the point of origin. Stenotic nares, if present, are readily noted by an external examination. If abnormally increased force is required to overcome the increased upper airway resistance, accessory muscles (e.g., nasolabial elevators, strap muscles of the ventral neck during inspiration, abdominal muscles during expiration) will be recruited and this effort is readily seen or felt during the physical examination. Another result of breathing against a partial obstruction is paradoxical respiratory movements. The soft tissues surrounding the chest cavity (thoracic inlet, intercostal spaces, abdomen) will collapse inward during inspiration, and may also puff outward during expiration. These movements give the appearance of "increased effort" or "abdominal breathing" and represent wasted work for the respiratory muscles. If aerophagia is present, the stomach may be grossly dilated with air.

CAUSES
Brachycephalic head and neck conformation. An underlying congenital obstruction may become clinical as a result of a number of exacerbating factors.

RISK FACTORS
In addition to the underlying conformation, risk factors that may result in signs of upper airway obstruction include the following: • Environmental factors—exercise; ambient temperature; stimuli causing excitement, anxiety, or fear • Respiratory factors—pulmonary disease (infections, edema, etc.); conditions that further narrow the airway (foreign body, tumor, fat accumulation)

• Metabolic factors—any condition that increases metabolic rate such as fever or hyperthyroidism • Neuromuscular conditions that affect upper airway muscles—myasthenia gravis; polyneuropathy; polymyopathy • State of consciousness—sleep can trigger severe snoring and obstruction; sedation or anesthesia • Endocrine—acromegaly

DIAGNOSIS

DIFFERENTIAL DIAGNOSIS
In brachycephalic animals exhibiting stertor or stridor and paradoxical movements, the diagnosis of brachycephalic airway syndrome can be made. However, a careful search for additional contributing factors and risk factors should be undertaken so that complications can be anticipated and prevented or treated.

CBC/BIOCHEMISTRY/URINALYSIS
N/A

OTHER LABORATORY TESTS N/A

IMAGING
• Lateral radiographs of the head and neck are useful for suggesting an overlong soft palate and are diagnostic for hypoplastic trachea. • Hypoplastic trachea—lateral radiograph and measurement of the ratio of the tracheal diameter at the thoracic inlet to the distance from the sternum to the ventral surface of T1. In normal dogs, the ratio is > 0.16; in brachycephalics it averages 0.13. However, the ratio does not correlate well with clinical signs.

OTHER DIAGNOSTIC PROCEDURES
• Stenotic nares—physical examination • Overlong soft palate, laryngeal collapse, and everted laryngeal ventricles—direct pharyngoscopy/laryngoscopy

GROSS AND HISTOPATHOLOGIC FINDINGS
The tracheal cartilages may be thick and noncompliant, with only a narrow strip of dorsal tracheal membrane at necropsy. When palate tissue resected for a "palate clip" is submitted for biopsy, edema has been noted.

TREATMENT

INPATIENT VERSUS OUTPATIENT
Animals that are suffering respiratory distress as a result of obstruction should be evaluated as candidates for surgery. Animals whose owners believe they are not compromised may be allowed to continue their usual lives, with appropriate owner education.

ACTIVITY
Brachycephalic animals often limit their own activity; however, owners should be instructed not to force their pets to exercise, and es-

pecially to limit exertion in high ambient temperatures to the absolute minimum.

DIET

Obesity can worsen the condition because fat accumulation may further narrow the airway and also compromise chest wall movements. Therefore, every effort must be made to keep brachycephalic animals lean.

CLIENT EDUCATION

It can be difficult to communicate to owners that their pet's congenital conformation is a risk factor for serious, even fatal, respiratory distress. Individuals who own a brachycephalic pet, and most especially those whose pets are exhibiting signs of obstruction, must be educated so that they are aware of the risk factors that may trigger a serious episode. They should avoid allowing their pets to become overweight; should limit exercise, especially in high ambient temperatures; and should be cautious when considering sedation or anesthesia. They should be alert to exacerbating factors such as infectious respiratory disease. All of these precautions apply even if surgical correction has been attempted because resection of the soft tissue cannot alleviate the bony or cartilaginous abnormalities that narrow the nasal turbinates, larynx, and trachea.

SURGICAL CONSIDERATIONS

Surgical resection of the soft tissues that narrow the airway is the most appropriate treatment for uncomplicated brachycephalic airway syndrome. These procedures can open up the stenotic nares, remove the excessive tissue at the caudal edge of the soft palate, and remove the everted laryngeal ventricles. However, these procedures will not relieve a collapsed larynx or hypoplastic trachea. Obviously, pulmonary or cardiovascular factors cannot be relieved by the surgery, and may dramatically increase the risk of the anesthesia. Careful postoperative monitoring is required both short- and long-term.

MEDICATIONS

DRUGS AND FLUIDS N/A

CONTRAINDICATIONS N/A

PRECAUTIONS

Although anxiety or fear may be present in brachycephalic animals, sedatives must be used with extreme caution. Atropine should be avoided because it will dehydrate the respiratory secretions.

POSSIBLE INTERACTIONS N/A

ALTERNATE DRUGS N/A

FOLLOW-UP

PATIENT MONITORING

During the postoperative period, the animal must be observed continuously until completely recovered from anesthesia. Subsequently, close observation for airway obstruction resulting from postoperative inflammation or edema is necessary. For several days, the animal must be observed while eating to ensure that aspiration does not occur. Finally, lifelong avoidance of all risk factors is necessary.

PREVENTION/AVOIDANCE

The prevention of brachycephalic airway syndrome would presumably require that breeders refrain from selecting animals with this conformation for breeding. As there is no evidence at present that families within the breeds vary in the severity of the syndrome, no other rational advice can be given regarding prevention. To avoid severe obstruction, avoidance of the risk factors is required.

POSSIBLE COMPLICATIONS

Animals who have been through an obstructive event may aspirate. Airway obstruction can lead to noncardiogenic pulmonary edema, which may progress to adult (acute) respiratory distress syndrome, a condition with a high mortality rate.

EXPECTED COURSE AND PROGNOSIS

Animals who have signs of upper airway obstruction and do not have surgery will often adjust their behavior so that they reduce their activity. They may thus survive for several years, but will not be able to have a normal life. If additional factors are introduced, these animals usually will decompensate and become severely obstructed. Animals who have surgery to resect the obstructing soft tissue

usually will improve, according to their owners, even if they are still far from normal. Long-term outcome studies have not been conducted in pets who have had surgery.

MISCELLANEOUS

ASSOCIATED CONDITIONS N/A

AGE RELATED FACTORS

It appears that brachycephalic animals compensate for the chronic insult to the airways by increasing the activity of their upper airway dilating muscles. However, decompensation appears to occur after a prolonged period of compensation. This might be a result of further narrowing of the airways caused by inward collapse or inflammation and edema, respiratory muscle fatigue leading to ventilatory failure, or myopathy of the chronically hyperactive upper airway dilating muscles.

ZOONOTIC POTENTIAL N/A

PREGNANCY

As is the case for obesity, the presence of large additional abdominal contents tends to compromise the movement of the diaphragm. Thus, some dams become noticeably worse during the late stages of pregnancy. Whether the chronic or intermittent respiratory distress also plays a role in the small litter sizes typical of brachycephalics is a matter for speculation.

SYNONYMS N/A

SEE ALSO Stertor and Stridor

ABBREVIATIONS

References

Hendricks JC. Brachycephalic airway syndrome. Vet Clin N Am (Small Anim Pract) 1992;22:1145-1153.

Petrof BJ, Pack AI, Kelly AM, Eby J, Hendricks JC. Pharyngeal myopathy of loaded upper airway in dogs with sleep apnea. J Appl Physiol 1994;76:1746-1752.

Harvey CE. Soft palate resection of brachycephalic dogs. J Am Animal Hosp Assoc 1982;18:535-537.

Author Joan C. Hendricks
Consulting Editors Lynelle Johnson and Bradley L. Moses

BRAIN INJURY (HEAD TRAUMA AND HYPOXIA)

BASICS

DEFINITION
Primary brain injury is a direct result of the initial insult, is complete at the time of presentation, and cannot be altered. Secondary brain injury is an alteration of brain tissue, either anatomic or physiologic, occuring after the primary injury, and can be prevented or ameliorated with optimal supportive care.

Pathophysiology
Secondary injury can result from bleeding, cerebral edema, or vasospasms and causes an elevation in intracranial pressure (ICP). A vicious cycle occurs when high ICP leads to low cerebral perfusion and blood flow, leading to further ischemia and brain swelling. A brain shift or herniation can result. A slow, progressive rise in ICP is better tolerated than a small, acute increase. Hypotension and hypoxia are the major contributors to ICP elevation and secondary brain injury. At the cellular level, high energy substrates are depleted and anaerobic glycolysis results in lactic acid production and intracellular acidosis.

Systems Affected
• Nervous—as a result of secondary brain injury and interruption of function
• Ophthalmic—as a result of potential changes in eye position, eye movements, pupillary light reflexes, and vision
• Cardiovascular—as a result of arrhythmias caused by dysfunction of the central cardiovascular centers • Respiratory—as a result of abnormal breathing patterns from dysfunction of the respiratory regulatory centers
• Musculoskeletal—as a result of possible postural and/or gait abnormalities that result from lesions of the central motor pathways

Genetics N/A

Incidence/Prevalence N/A

Geographic Distribution N/A

SIGNALMENT

Species Dogs and cats

Breed Predilections N/A

Mean Age and Range N/A

Predominant Sex N/A

SIGNS

General Comments
• Clinical signs are related to the degree of secondary brain injury. The absence of focal or lateralizing signs is more suggestive of diffuse cerebrocortical involvement.
• Trauma-induced brain injury can worsen dramatically during resuscitative efforts as a result of hypertension and intracranial bleeds.
• The brain has high oxygen and glucose requirements, minimal storage of oxygen, few recruitable capillaries, and consumes oxygen

at a constant rate, setting the stage for hypoxic injury.

Historical Findings
• Ascertain past history of inciting causes of hypoxia or ischemic brain injury, including trauma, cardiac arrest, prolonged syncopal episodes, severe heart failure, thromboembolic episodes, coagulopathies with intracranial bleeding, and prolonged severe respiratory compromise. • A decline in the level of consciousness implies progression of secondary brain injury resulting from intracranial bleeding or cerebral edema. • Whether the animal had seizure activity aids in localizing the brain lesion to the cerebral cortex or diencephalon.
• Traumatic injuries are associated with secondary brain injury from either bleeding or cerebral edema. • Ischemic etiologies found in the history are most likely associated with secondary brain injury from cerebral edema.

Physical Examination Findings
• Look for external and internal evidence of trauma. • Evidence of hypoxia or cyanosis, ecchymosis or petechiations, or cardiac or respiratory insufficiency warrants investigation for metabolic etiologies. • Retinal hemorrhages or distended vessels suggest hypertension or coagulopathy; papilledema suggests cerebral edema; retinal detachment suggests infectious, neoplastic, or hypertensive causes.
• Bradycardia reflects midbrain, pontine, or medullary lesion. • Evidence of blood from the ears or nose suggests trauma severe enough to cause intracranial bleeding.
• Palpation of the skull can reveal fractures that require surgical decompression.
• Ischemic etiologies require careful examination for cardiovascular, respiratory, or hemorrhagic problems.

Neurologic Examination Findings
• Determine level of consciousness and whether the animal is arousable. • Evaluate pupillary light reflexes—normal or miotic responsive pupils reflect cerebral or diencephalic lesion; dilated unresponsive pupils (unilateral or bilateral) or midpoint fixed unresponsive pupils reflect midbrain lesion; miotic or normal pupils reflect pontine or medullary lesion • Perform oculocephalic reflex (if cervical manipulation is possible)—loss of normal vestibular nystagmus reflects midbrain, pons, or medullary involvement
• Observe respiratory patterns—Cheyne-Stokes respiration reflects severe, diffuse, cerebral or diencephalic pathology; hyperventilation reflects midbrain pathology; ataxic or apneustic breathing reflects pontine or medullary pathology • Evaluate cranial nerves—the exam is normal with lesions of cerebrum-diencephalon; deficits of cranial nerve III with the midbrain; deficits of CN V-XII associated with the pons or medulla
• Examine for postural changes—decerebrate rigidity is a result of midbrain lesion

CAUSES
• Head trauma • Prolonged hypoxia or ischemia

RISK FACTORS
• Free roaming animals—trauma
• Coexisting cardiac or respiratory disease

DIAGNOSIS

DIFFERENTIAL DIAGNOSIS
• Differentiate from other causes of brain diseases, including neoplasia, inflammation, immune-mediated processes, infection, and congenital problems. • Differentiate from systemic causes of altered states of consciousness, including narcolepsy, syncope, metabolic diseases, toxins, drugs, infection, and nutritional causes. • Brainstem signs are caused by bleeding, thrombosis, trauma, and, frequently, tentorial herniation after cerebral edema.

CBC/BIOCHEMISTRY/URINALYSIS
Hemogram, serum chemistry profile, and urinalysis changes reflect the systemic effects of trauma or hypoxemia, with no specific changes attributable to the brain injury.

OTHER LABORATORY TESTS
• Arterial blood gases are evaluated for evidence of hypoxemia, severe pH changes, or hypercarbia. • When intracranial bleeding or thrombosis may be responsible for the neurologic signs, a coagulogram is performed.

IMAGING
• Skull radiographs are evaluated for fractures in trauma patients. • Computed tomography scanning is an excellent imaging modality for detection of acute hemorrhage within the calveria. It is also the method of choice for imaging the skull bones, looking for depressed fractures or penetrating foreign bodies.

OTHER DIAGNOSTIC PROCEDURES
• Intracranial pressure measurements are evaluated to determine the severity of ICP elevation and the response to therapy. • Brain stem auditory evoked potentials are evaluated to determine brain stem function. • Electrocardiographic evaluation aids in determining cardiac dysfunction.

GROSS AND HISTOPATHOLOGIC FINDINGS
Brain edema, herniation, hemorrhage, laceration, contusion, hematomas, skull fracture

TREATMENT
• The head should be leveled with the body or elevated to a 20° angle. It should never be lower than the body to avoid significant elevations in ICP.
• The arterial pCO_2 should be maintained between 35-45 mm Hg. If ICP elevations are suspected, hyperventilating to arterial pCO_2

of 25-30 mm Hg may reduce cerebral blood flow and ICP.

• Arterial pO_2 must be above 50 mm Hg to maintain cerebral blood flow autoregulation. A cough or sneeze reflex must be avoided during intubation or oxygen supplementation by nasal cannula since this can severely elevate ICP.

• Lidocaine (dogs, 0.75 mg/kg IV) given before intubation can blunt the gag and cough reflex.

• Utilize peripheral veins, leaving the jugular vein blood flow unobstructed. Shifting of blood volume into the jugular veins is an important compensatory mechanism during ICP elevation.

• Meticulous nursing care prevents secondary complications of recumbency—maintain unobstructed airways; use suction and humidify if intubated; lubricate the eyes; turn the animal q2h to avoid hypostatic pulmonary congestion; prevent fecal or urine soiling; maintain the core body temperature normal or mildly hypothermic; avoid hyperthermia.

INPATIENT VERSUS OUTPATIENT
All should be treated as inpatients.

ACTIVITY
All activity is to be restricted.

DIET
Nutrition must be maintained during recovery with requirements adjusted to compensate for elevated metabolic demands of brain injury.

CLIENT EDUCATION
• The extent of neurologic recovery may not be evident for several days in the acute phase, and possibly longer than 6 months for residual neurologic deficits.

• There may be serious systemic abnormalities that could contribute to the instability of the nervous system.

SURGICAL CONSIDERATIONS
Serious consideration for surgical decompression and exploration must be given when there is worsening of neurologic signs, increased ICP not responsive to medical therapy, midbrain signs with history of cerebral trauma or bleed, depressed skull fracture, or penetrating foreign body.

MEDICATIONS

DRUGS AND FLUIDS
• Poor perfusion—resuscitation should be done with a minimal amount of crystalloids because these contribute to brain edema. A combination of large molecular weight colloids (i.e. hetastarch) with crystalloids allows small fluid volume resuscitation. However, colloids should not be used if there is intracranial hemorrhage.

• Hydration is maintained with a balanced electrolyte crystalloid solution.

• Mean arterial blood pressure is maintained around 80 mm Hg using crystalloids and/or colloids. Avoid hypertension.

• Intracranial pressure elevations can be treated by hyperventilation and drug therapy. Furosemide (0.75 mg/kg IV) decreases CSF production and lowers ICP. Mannitol (0.1-0.5 gm/kg IV followed by a 10% mannitol infusion) improves brain blood flow and lowers ICP, and should be given after furosemide. These are most commonly used in patients with hypoxic or ischemic brain injury or traumatic injury if there is decline in neurologic status or if surgical decompression is imminent.

• Reduce inflammation—glucocorticosteroids (methylprednisolone sodium succinate 30mg/kg IV slowly after fluids) can be given soon after brain trauma to reduce brain inflammation and prevent brain edema. Methylprednisolone (12.5 mg/kg IV) is given 2 and 6 hours after the initial dosage. A constant rate of infusion of glucocorticosteroids is given (2.5 microgram/kg/hour of methylprednisolone) 8-42 hours after the initial dosage. Misoprostil (2-5 microgram/kg q8-12h PO) should be given during glucocorticosteroid administration. Glucose supplementation is given as required for hypoglycemia.

• Thrashing, seizures, or other uncontrolled motor activity is to be prevented since it can elevate ICP. Diazepam infusion (0.5-1 mg/kg/hour for 4-6 hours) may succeed in controlling the seizures. If not, phenobarbital is added at 4 mg/kg as an initial IV bolus. Boluses can be repeated if needed, for a maximum of 16 mg/kg (with at least a 20-minute interval between boluses).

CONTRAINDICATIONS
• Drugs that cause hypertension
• Drugs that cause hyperexcitability

PRECAUTIONS
• Avoid hypertension.
• Avoid intravascular volume overload.
• Do not allow head to lie below plane of body.
• Do not use the jugular veins.
• Do not use colloids when there is intracranial hemorrhage.
• Mannitol and hypertonic saline can worsen neurologic status when there is intracranial hemorrhage.
• When hyperventilating, maintain $pCO_2 > 25$ mm Hg. Do not hyperventilate for extended periods (> 48 hours).

POSSIBLE INTERACTIONS N/A
ALTERNATE DRUGS N/A

FOLLOW-UP

PATIENT MONITORING
• Repeat neurologic exams to detect deterioration of function that warrants aggressive

therapeutic intervention. • Blood pressure to keep fluid therapy adequate for perfusion but avoiding hypertension • Blood gases to assess need for oxygen supplementation or ventilation; to monitor pCO_2 when hyperventilation is required • Blood glucose to ensure an adequate blood level to maintain brain functions and avoid hyperosmolality from high amounts • ECG to detect arrhythmias that may affect perfusion, oxygenation, and cerebral blood flow • ICP monitoring to detect significant elevations and monitor success of therapeutics

PREVENTION/AVOIDANCE
• Keep pets in a confined area with supervised activity. • Avoid hypoxic or ischemic episodes.

POSSIBLE COMPLICATIONS
Increasing ICP, brain herniation, intracranial hemorrhage, progression from cerebro-cortical to midbrain signs, seizures, malnutrition, hypostatic pulmonary congestion, corneal desiccation, urine scalding, airway obstruction from mucus, cardiac arrhythmias (usually bradyarrhythmias), respiratory failure, death

EXPECTED COURSE AND PROGNOSIS
• Best prognosis is with minimal primary brain injury and secondary injury consisting of cerebral edema. • Animals without deterioration of neurologic status for 48 hours have a better prognosis.

MISCELLANEOUS

ASSOCIATED CONDITIONS N/A
AGE RELATED FACTORS N/A
ZOONOTIC POTENTIAL N/A
PREGNANCY N/A
SYNONYMS
• Head trauma • Traumatic brain injury

SEE ALSO
Stupor and Coma

ABBREVIATIONS
ECG = electrocardiogram
ICP = intracranial pressure

Reference
Hayek DA, Veremakis C. Therapeutic options in brain resuscitation. In: Veremakis C, ed. Problems in critical care: resuscitation following acute brain injury. Philadelphia: JB Lippincott, 1991:156-186.
Author Rebecca Kirby
Consulting Editor Joane M. Parent

BRONCHIECTASIS—DOGS

BASICS

OVERVIEW
Bronchiectasis is characterized by an irreversible dilatation of the bronchi associated with inflammation and/or infection. In dogs, it is seen in association with primary ciliary dyskinesia (PCD) as a sequella to long-standing chronic pulmonary disease and, rarely, as a complication of radiation-induced pneumonitis.

SIGNALMENT
• This disorder affects dogs primarily. Young animals (< 1 year) may present with bronchiectasis secondary to PCD. • Middle-aged to older dogs with chronic pulmonary disease may develop bronchiectasis, although the pathogenesis is unknown. • Cocker spaniels seem to be predisposed in the author's opinion, and an increased incidence in large-breed dogs has been reported in England.

SIGNS
• Chronic cough, usually productive and moist • Tachypnea or dyspnea • Exercise intolerance • Fever • Chronic nasal discharge or sinusitis • Crackles and moist rales, increased expiratory lung sounds • Tracheal hypersensitivity • Cyanosis

CAUSES AND RISK FACTORS
• PCD • Smoldering infectious or inflammatory bronchitis that is inadequately cleared may result in irreversible lung disease caused by severe pulmonary inflammation and tissue destruction.

DIAGNOSIS

DIFFERENTIAL DIAGNOSIS
• Recurrent bacterial bronchopneumonia • Chronic bronchitis • Infectious or parasitic tracheobronchitis • Congestive heart failure • Tracheal collapse

CBC/BIOCHEMISTRY/URINALYSIS
• CBC—neutrophilia • Chemistry profile—high globulin fraction • Urinalysis—proteinuria with a greatly increased urine protein-creatinine ratio may be seen if secondary amyloidosis develops

OTHER LABORATORY TESTS
Arterial blood gas—hypoxemia, increased alveolar-arterial gradient (see Tracheal Collapse)

IMAGING
Radiography—dilatation of the lobar bronchi; a mixed bronchial, interstitial, and alveolar pattern; diffuse bronchial wall thickening

OTHER DIAGNOSTIC PROCEDURES
• Bronchoscopy—saccular or tubular dilatation of the airways; blunting of airway bifurcations and loss of the cylindrical shape to the lumen; increased mucus and airway edema • Transtracheal wash or bronchoalveolar lavage—samples should be submitted for bacterial culture and sensitivity, cytology, and Mycoplasma culture. Fungal cultures should be considered. Typical findings include suppurative inflammation with increased neutrophils and monocytes. Bacteria are usually present in a mixed population, although some cases are sterile.

TREATMENT
• Severe hypoxemia necessitates hospitalization for oxygen therapy.
• Intravenous, broad spectrum antibiotics should be given based on airway culture results whenever possible. If unavailable, antibiotics effective against Streptococcus, Pseudomonas, and Mycoplasma should be chosen. Antibiotics are usually required in animals in which airway cultures are sterile also.
• Long-term antibiotic therapy should be expected (2- 6 months, potentially for life). A rotating schedule of antibiotics may be required.
• Nebulization and physiotherapy may enhance resolution of disease.
• Moderate exercise restriction and weight control are important in disease management.
• Lobar excision should be considered for focal bronchiectasis.

MEDICATIONS

DRUGS AND FLUIDS
• Bronchodilators
• Theophylline tablets (long-acting forms)—Theo-Dur tablets (20 mg/kg PO q12h)
• Beta agonists—terbutaline (1.25-5 mg/dog PO q12h), albuterol (0.03-0.05 mg/kg PO q8h)
• Antibiotics—amoxicillin-clavulanic acid, trimethoprim-sulfa, fluoroquinolones, cephalexin, chloramphenicol, and tetracycline
• Hydration status should be carefully maintained to prevent inspissation of bronchial secretions.
• Lasix should be avoided despite auscultation of crackles.

CONTRAINDICATIONS/POSSIBLE INTERACTIONS
Fluoroquinolones should not be used with theophylline.

FOLLOW-UP

• The patient may be followed by measurement of arterial blood gases, CBC to document inflammation, temperature monitoring at home, and radiographs to detect recurrent pneumonia. • Aggressive, long-term therapy is recommended. • Possible complications include recurrent pulmonary infection, pulmonary hypertension, and cor pulmonale.
• Owners should be advised of the potential for chronicity.

MISCELLANEOUS

ASSOCIATED CONDITIONS
• Primary ciliary dyskinesia • Sinusitis
• Chronic bronchitis

AGE RELATED FACTORS N/A

ZOONOTIC POTENTIAL N/A

PREGNANCY N/A

SEE ALSO
• Tracheal Collapse • Bronchitis, Chronic
• Ciliary Dyskinesia, Primary

ABBREVIATION
PCD = primary ciliary dyskinesia

Reference
Barker AF, Bardana EJ. Bronchiectasis: update of an orphan disease. Am Rev Respir Dis 1988;137:969.
Author Lynelle Johnson
Consulting Editors Lynelle Johnson and Bradley L. Moses

BRONCHITIS, CHRONIC (COPD)

BASICS

DEFINITION
Chronic bronchitis in dogs and cats is used to describe chronic coughing occurring for 2 consecutive months that is not attributable to another cause (e.g., neoplasia, congestive heart failure). Because of the pathologic changes accompanying the process, it also implies a nonreversible and often slowly progressive condition.

Pathophysiology
• The specific etiology of chronic bronchitis is rarely determined. Recurrent airway inflammation (e.g., infections, inhaled irritants) is suspected. • Persistent tracheobronchial irritation causes chronic coughing and changes in the tracheobronchial epithelium and wall. Airway inflammation, epithelial edema, thickening, and metaplasia are prominent. Mucus production is increased. • The net effect of these changes is to narrow airways, increase lung resistance, and decrease expiratory air flow rates.

Systems Affected
• Respiratory • Cardiovascular—pulmonary hypertension, cor pulmonale • Nervous—syncope

Genetics N/A

Incidence/Prevalence N/A

Geographic Distribution N/A

SIGNALMENT

Species Dogs and cats

Breed Predilections
• Chronic bronchitis is common in small/toy breed dogs, but is also observed in large dogs. • West Highland white terriers have been noted to develop a progressive disorder characterized by chronic coughing, dyspnea, and crackles. Bronchiectasis has frequently been observed in young to middle-aged cocker spaniels after a long history of chronic bronchitis.

Mean Age and Range
Chronic bronchitis most often affects middle-aged and older animals.

Predominant Sex N/A

SIGNS

Historical Findings
• Coughing is the hallmark of tracheobronchial irritation. The cough usually is dry but posttussive gagging is common (owners may misinterpret this as "vomiting"). • Exercise intolerance, exertional dyspnea, cyanosis, and even syncope may be noted.

Physical Examination Findings
• Animals usually are bright, alert, and afebrile. Tracheal palpation typically results in coughing (increased tracheal sensitivity). Small airway disease may be assumed when an expiratory abdominal push (during quiet breathing) and/or end-expiratory wheezing are detected. • Bronchovesicular lung sounds, end-inspiratory crackles, and wheezing as a result of airways obstructed by secretions may be heard. • Cardiac auscultation is important in differentiating chronic heart from bronchial disease. Murmurs secondary to valvular insufficiency are common but are not always associated with congestive heart failure. Heart rate, taken at rest, is a helpful method of determining whether congestive heart failure or chronic bronchitis is present; congestive heart failure commonly is associated with an elevated heart rate, while chronic bronchitis typically results in a normal/ slower than normal heart rate. • Obesity is a common, significant factor in chronic bronchitis in dogs.

CAUSES
Chronic airway inflammation results in chronic bronchitis. Multiple etiologies may start the inflammation or initiate an acute episode of coughing.

RISK FACTORS
• Recurrent bacterial infections • Long-term exposure to inhaled irritants • Obesity • Dental disease and laryngeal disease (bacterial showering of airways)

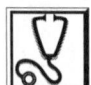

DIAGNOSIS

DIFFERENTIAL DIAGNOSIS
• Bacterial or fungal pneumonia • Bronchiectasis • Allergic lung disease • Foreign bodies • Heartworm disease • Neoplasia (metastatic more common than primary) • Pulmonary parasites or parasitic larval migration • Pulmonary fibrosis • Pulmonary granulomatosis

CBC/BIOCHEMISTRY/URINALYSIS
• Routine laboratory tests are rarely diagnostic. • An absolute eosinophilia is suggestive but not diagnostic of allergic bronchitis (present in less than 50% of confirmed cases). • Polycythemia secondary to chronic hypoxia may be noted. • SAP and ALT may be increased as a result of passive congestion.

OTHER LABORATORY TESTS
• Routine fecal and heartworm tests should be run. • Arterial blood gas is the only pulmonary function test widely available; it documents gas exchange impairment and quantitate changes over time. • Arterial blood gases may be collected, iced, and analyzed at local hospitals; decreased PaO_2, but not increased $PaCO_2$, is commonly found with severe chronic bronchitis.

IMAGING
Thoracic radiographs are extremely important in the diagnosis of chronic bronchitis. Commonly reported radiographic patterns of chronic bronchitis in dogs and cats include (in descending order of frequency) bronchial (classically "doughnuts" and "tram lines"), interstitial, middle lobe consolidation, atelectasis, and hyperinflation/diaphragmatic flattening.

OTHER DIAGNOSTIC PROCEDURES
• A complete cardiac evaluation is indicated to rule-out congestive heart failure and determine whether cor pulmonale is present. Common ECG findings in chronic bronchitis in dogs include wandering atrial pacemaker, marked sinus arrhythmia, P pulmonale, and, occasionally, evidence of right ventricular hypertrophy. Pulmonary hypertension may be estimated using color flow Doppler echocardiography. • Secretions from the lower airways must be evaluated to establish underlying etiologies. "Throat swab" cultures are not representative of lower airway flora. Either transtracheal aspiration biopsy or bronchoscopy aspiration lavage may be used to collect specimens for cytology and culture. • Inflammation is the primary cytology from animals with chronic bronchitis. The majority of cells may be neutrophils, eosinophils, or macrophages. Specimens also should be evaluated for bacteria, parasites, and neoplastic cells. • Although recurrent infections are implicated in the pathogenesis of chronic bronchitis, positive cultures are not frequently reported (two recent studies revealed 24% of cats and 17% of dogs had positive aerobic cultures). Mycoplasma is discussed but rarely confirmed as a cause of chronic bronchitis. • Bronchoscopy is the preferred diagnostic test for assessing the lower airways. It allows direct visualization of the structural and functional (dynamic) changes of the disease process and allows selected airway sampling (biopsy, washings). • Gross bronchoscopic changes of chronic bronchitis include excess mucoid to mucopurulent secretions, epithelial edema/thickening and blunting of bronchial bifurcations, irregular/granular mucosa, and (pathognomonic) mucosal polypoid proliferations. • Large airway caliber changes (e.g., dynamic airway collapse and bronchiectasis) may be detected as complicating problems.

GROSS AND HISTOPATHOLOGIC FINDINGS
• Excess airway mucus, epithelial roughening/granularity and hyperemia, nodules or mucosal polypoid projections (especially at bifurcations), and areas of pneumonia are observed grossly in most cases of chronic bronchitis.

TREATMENT

INPATIENT VERSUS OUTPATIENT
Most cases may be treated as outpatients. Exceptions are those requiring O_2 therapy, parenteral medication, or aerosolization, or instances where the owners are unable to keep the animal calm at home during recovery.

ACTIVITY
Moderate exercise (not forced) is useful in facilitating secretion clearance and in assisting

with weight loss in overweight animals. Exercise should be limited if exertion is a significant cause of coughing. A harness should be used.

DIET
Weight loss has resulted in significant improvement in PaO_2, cough frequency, attitude, and exercise tolerance in obese dogs with chronic bronchitis.

CLIENT EDUCATION
• It is important that owners understand that chronic bronchitis is, by definition, an incurable disease, and complete suppression of all coughing is an unattainable goal.
• Aggressive treatment, including weight control, avoidance of risk factors (see above), and medical therapy (bronchodilators and corticosteroids), in most instances, will minimize the severity of the coughing episodes.

SURGICAL CONSIDERATIONS
Severe dental disease should be aggressively treated to minimize secondary bacterial complications.

MEDICATIONS

DRUGS AND FLUIDS
• Antitissives are indicated when the cough is nonproductive, paroxysmal, continuous, and/or debilitating. Butorphanol (0.55 mg/kg PO q6h-q12h; 0.055-0.11 mg/kg SQ), hydrocodone (2.5-5 mg/dog q6h-q24h PO), and codeine (0.1-0.3mg/kg q6h-q8h PO) are most commonly used in dogs.
• Antibiotics are selected based on sensitivity results. If culture results are unavailable, antibiotic choice should be toward products with good gram-negative spectrum, tissue and secretion penetration, and those that are bactericidal with minimal toxicity, (e.g., enrofloxacilin, potentiated sulfa/trimethoprim or amoxicillin/clavulanic acid). Anaerobic and gram-positive spectrum antibiotics might be preferred when faced with chronic aspiration or dental associated chronic bronchitis.
• Corticosteroids will decrease airway inflammation and coughing regardless of the underlying etiology. Short-term administration is indicated in chronic bronchitis cases that are not infectious in nature. Allergic or hypersensitivity cases may require long-term administration, although attempts to wean off steroids should be made or the lowest effective dosage determined.
• Different families of bronchodilators may be used in the treatment of chronic bronchitis in dogs and cats. Beneficial effects of bronchodilators include bronchodilation, increased mucociliary clearance, improvement in diaphragmatic contractility, decreased pulmonary artery pressure, increased CNS sensitivity to $PaCO_2$, and stabilization of mast cells (depending on drug).
• The beta agonists terbutaline (1.25-5

mg/dog q8-12h) and albuterol (20-50 µg/kg q8h in dogs) have been recommended in treating chronic obstructive airway disease.
• Oral sustained release theophylline is recommended for long-term bronchodilator therapy; recommended drug dosages are product- and species-specific. Theo-Dur tablets (not capsules) and Slo-Bid gyrocaps are recommended at 20 and 25 mg/kg, respectively, q12h in dogs. Dosing recommendations are designed to achieve theophylline therapeutic plasma concentrations between 5-20 µg/ml.

CONTRAINDICATIONS
Lasix and atropine should not be used because of their drying effects on tracheobronchial secretions.

PRECAUTIONS
• Beta agonists (e.g., terbutaline and albuterol) may cause tachycardia, nervousness, and muscle tremors; side effects are typically transient.
• Potential side effects of methylxanthines (e.g., aminophylline and theophylline) include tachycardia, restlessness, excitability, vomiting, and diarrhea; side effects are unlikely using oral sustained release theophylline. EDTA plasma samples (drawn 4-5 hours post-sustained release theophylline administration) may be run to evaluate peak plasma theophylline concentrations.

POSSIBLE INTERACTIONS
Theophylline metabolism in people is affected by drugs that inhibit P450 hepatic enzymes, including erythromycin, cimetidine (but not ranitidine), fluoroquinolones, and phenobarbital.

ALTERNATE DRUGS
Many sustained release theophylline products are available; unfortunately differences in bioavailability between products makes sustained release theophylline dosages product-specific (do not allow generic substitution).

FOLLOW-UP

PATIENT MONITORING
Abnormalities from history and physical and selected diagnostic tests should be followed to determine response to therapy. Weight should be monitored. Arterial blood gases improve after weight loss.

PREVENTION/AVOIDANCE
Avoid and address risk factors (see above).

POSSIBLE COMPLICATIONS
• Syncope is a frequent complication of chronic coughing, particularly in toy breed dogs.
• The most serious complication of chronic bronchitis is the development of pulmonary hypertension.

EXPECTED COURSE AND PROGNOSIS
Chronic bronchitis implies irreversibility, and airway changes often progress to syncopal episodes, chronic hypoxia, right ventricular hypertrophy, and, possibly, pulmonary hypertension. Acute exacerbations are common seasonally, with changes in air quality, or with the development of secondary infections.

MISCELLANEOUS

ASSOCIATED CONDITIONS
Syncope secondary to chronic coughing, increased susceptibility to airway infections, chronic hypoxia, pulmonary hypertension, and cor pulmonale may develop.

AGE RELATED FACTORS N/A

ZOONOTIC POTENTIAL N/A

PREGNANCY
The safety of most drugs recommended for treatment of chronic bronchitis has not been established in pregnant animals.

SYNONYMS
Chronic obstructive pulmonary/lung disease (COPD/COLD), bronchiolitis, small airway disease

SEE ALSO
• See causes. • Cough • Hypoxia • Asthma, Bronchitis • Tracheal Collapse • Tracheobronchitis, Infectious • Bronchiectasis

ABBREVIATIONS
CHF = congestive heart failure
SRT = sustained release theophylline

References

Bonagura JD. Bronchopulmonary disorders. In: Birchard SJ, Sherding RG, eds. Saunders manual of small animal practice. Philadelphia: WB Saunders, 1994;561-573.
Padrid PA, Hornoff WJ, Kurpershoek CJ, Cross CE. Canine chronic bronchitis. J Vet Int Med 1990;4:172-180.
Author Brendan C. McKiernan
Consulting Editors Lynelle Johnson and Bradley L. Moses

BRUCELLOSIS—DOGS

BASICS

DEFINITION
• A contagious disease of dogs caused by Brucella canis (B. canis), a small, intracellular, gram-negative organism in the genus Brucella • Characterized by abortions in females, epididymitis, testicular atrophy, and infertility in females. It is often insidious; many dogs, especially females, do not have prominent signs.

Pathophysiology
B. canis is an intracellular parasite that has a propensity for growth in lymphatic, placental, and male genital (epididymis and prostate) tissues.

Systems Affected
• Reproductive—target tissues of gonadal steroids (gravid uterus, fetus, testes [epididymides], prostate gland) • Hemic/lymphatic/immune—lymph nodes and spleen; bone marrow; mononuclear leukocytes • Other tissues—intervertebral disks, anterior uvea, meninges (uncommon)

Genetics
No known genetic predisposition, although the disease is most common in beagles

Incidence/Prevalence
• Incidence is unknown. Seroprevalence rates have not been accurately defined. False-positive results are common with agglutination tests. • Relatively low prevalence rates (1-18%) have been reported in the United States and Japan. In the United States, prevalence rates are higher in rural areas of the southern states. Rates of 25-30% have been reported in stray dogs in Mexico and Peru.

Geographic Distribution
Diagnosed in stray dogs, pets, and kennels in the United States, Mexico, Japan, and several South American countries. Also recognized in Spain, Tunisia, and China. Individual outbreaks have occurred in Germany and Czechoslovakia; some have been traced to the importation of dogs, mostly beagles from the United States.

SIGNALMENT

Species
Dogs; infrequently, human

Breed Predilections
• Exceptionally high prevalence in beagles; there is no evidence of breed susceptibility • Recently, several kennels of Labrador retrievers have been found infected.

Mean Age and Range
No age preference. Most common in sexually mature dogs.

Predominant Sex
Both sexes are affected; more common in females.

SIGNS

General Comments
Suspect brucellosis whenever female dogs experience abortions or reproductive failures, or males have genital disease.

HISTORICAL FINDINGS
• Dogs, especially females, may appear healthy or have vague signs of illness. They may show lethargy, loss of libido, swollen lymph nodes, or back pain. A frequent sign is an abortion, commonly 6-8 weeks after conception, although pregnancy may terminate at any stage. Signs in males include swollen scrotal sacs, often with scrotal dermatitis; enlarged and firm epididymides; unilateral or bilateral testicular atrophy in chronically infected dogs. • Chronically infected dogs may have cloudy eyes (anterior uveitis with corneal edema), spinal pain, posterior weakness, or ataxia.

PHYSICAL EXAMINATION FINDINGS
Most infections are not diagnosed by routine physical examinations. Fever is rare; hematological and urinalysis values are normal. Enlarged superficial lymph nodes (e.g., retropharyneal, external inguinal) are common. The vaginal discharge after an abortion may last for several weeks and contain an abundance of bacteria. Suspect males should always be examined for testicular abnormalities.

CAUSES
Brucella canis is a gram-negative coccobacillus, morphologically indistinguishable from other members of the genus Brucella. The canine organism, unlike the classic Brucella species (e.g., B. abortus, B. suis or B. melitensis), can result in a high rate (50%) of false-positive reactions with the commonly used tests.

RISK FACTORS
Breeding kennels and pack hounds appear to be at highest risk. Risk increases when popular breeding animals become infected. Dogs in contact with strays in endemic areas are at higher risk.

DIAGNOSIS

DIFFERENTIAL DIAGNOSIS
• Abortions resulting from maternal, fetal, or placental abnormalities • Systemic infections—canine distemper, canine herpesvirus, B. abortus, Escherichia coli, leptospirosis, and toxoplasmosis • Inguinal hernias may provoke epididymitis and scrotal edema, blastomycosis and other granulomatous infections, and Rocky Mountain spotted fever. • Discospondylitis resulting from fungal infections, actinomycosis, staphylococcal infections, nocardiosis, streptococci, and Corynebacterium diphtheroides

CBC/BIOCHEMISTRY/URINALYSIS
Biochemical and hematologic tests are of little significance, except to rule out other infec-

tions. Values are generally normal in uncomplicated cases.

OTHER LABORATORY TESTS
• Serologic testing is the most commonly used method. Most tests are subject to error. False-positive reactions to lipopolysaccharide antigens of several species of bacteria are common with the rapid 2-mercaptoethanol (2-ME) slide or tube agglutination tests. The three commonly used serologic tests include the following:
• Rapid 2-ME slide agglutination test (RSAT)—this commercially available test is simple and rapid. It detects infected dogs 3-4 weeks postinfection and is accurate in identifying noninfected ("negative") dogs. However, it suffers a high rate (50%) of false-positive reactions. RSAT results must be confirmed by other tests. • Mercaptoethanol tube agglutination test—a semiquantitative test, generally performed by commercial diagnostic laboratories. This test provides information similar to the RSAT and suffers comparable lack of specificity.
• Agar gel immunodiffusion (AGID) tests—two AGID tests are commonly used. One test employs a lipopolysaccharide antigen derived from the cell walls of B. canis (cell wall antigen) and is highly sensitive. Test conditions have not been standardized and results of tests on sera from noninfected dogs are frequently interpreted as "positive." A second AGID test employs soluble antigens (SA) that consist of proteins extracted from the bacterial cytoplasm. Such antigens are highly specific for antibodies against members of the genus Brucella. Antibodies that react with the soluble antigen appear 4-12 weeks after infection and they persist for long periods of time; they may give precipitin lines after other tests become equivocal or negative. Use of the soluble antigen also detects infection by other brucella (e.g., B. abortus or B. suis).

IMAGING
Dogs should be tested for brucellosis if there is radiographic evidence of diskospondylitis.

OTHER DIAGNOSTIC PROCEDURES
• Isolation of the organism. Blood cultures should always be done when clinical and serologic findings suggest brucellosis. Brucella are readily isolated from the blood of infected dogs, provided that the animals had not received antibiotic treatment. • The onset of bacteremia occurs 2-4 weeks after oral-nasal exposure and may persist for periods of 8 months to 5.5 years postinfection. • After an abortion, cultures of vaginal fluids usually give positive results. Cultures of semen or urine may be done, but they are not practical for routine diagnosis because overgrowth of contaminants is common. Use of media that contains antibiotics (e.g., Thayer-Martin medium) has proved useful with contaminated samples. • Examination for semen quality—sperm motility, immature sperm, pres-

ence of inflammatory cells (neutrophils)—is indicated in males with evidence of epididymitis. Sperm abnormalities are usually evident by 5-8 weeks postinfection and are conspicuous by 20 weeks. Aspermia without inflammatory cells is a common finding in dogs with bilateral testicular atrophy.
• Lymph node biopsies reveal lymphoid hyperplasia with large numbers of plasma cells. Intracellular bacteria may be observed in macrophages with special stains (e.g., Brown-Brenn stain). If biopsies are done in a sterile manner, tissues should be cultured on appropriate media.

GROSS AND HISTOPATHOLOGIC FINDINGS
• Gross findings include lymph node enlargement. Splenomegaly is typical. Males commonly have enlarged and firm epididymides, scrotal edema, or atrophy of one or both testes. Anterior uveitis and discospondylitis may occur in chronically infected dogs.
• Microscopic changes are relatively consistent. Prominent changes include diffuse lymphoreticular hyperplasia. Lymph node sinusoids of chronically infected dogs have abundant plasma cells and macrophages that contain bacteria. There is diffuse lymphocytic infiltration and granulomatous lesions in all genitourinary organs, especially the prostate gland, epididymis, uterus, and scrotum. There may be extensive inflammatory cell infiltration and necrosis of the prostate parenchyma and seminiferous tubules. Ocular changes include granulomatous iridocyclitis, exudative retinitis, and leukocytic exudates in the anterior chamber.

TREATMENT

INPATIENT VERSUS OUTPATIENT
Patients should be treated as outpatients if treatment is decided upon.

ACTIVITY Restrict in working dogs

DIET N/A

CLIENT EDUCATION
• Eradication of B. canis from the animal is the goal of treatment. Successful treatment is indicated by the return of dogs to seronegative status and the absence of bacteremia for at least 3 months. In some instances, treatment results in persistent low antibody titers in the absence of systemic infection (bacteremia). • Antibiotic treatment, especially with minocycline and doxycycline, is expensive, time-consuming and highly controversial because outcomes are uncertain.

Treatment is not recommended in breeding or commercial kennels. Treatment is recommended only for nonbreeding dogs or those who have been spayed or castrated. In exceptional cases, treatment of intact household pets or breeding stock may be attempted, but only if the owner and veterinarian reach clear agreement to neuter or destroy the animal if treatment is unsuccessful.

SURGICAL CONSIDERATIONS
Neutering/spaying, plus treatment, is recommended in cases in which euthanasia is unacceptable to an owner.

MEDICATIONS

DRUGS AND FLUIDS
Several therapeutic regimens have been evaluated, but results have been equivocal. The most successful treatment has been a combination of a tetracycline (e.g., tetracycline hydrochloride, chlortetracycline, minocycline, or doxycycline) given per os at 25 mg/kg q8h for 4 weeks, plus streptomycin. Gentamicin is a possible substitute for streptomycin (see below), but data are limited and, unlike streptomycin treatment, renal function must be monitored.

CONTRAINDICATIONS
• Tetracyclines should not be used in immature pups.
• Gentamicin (see below) may cause renal damage and is contraindicated in dogs with kidney disease. Dogs that receive gentamicin should be monitored closely for renal function.

PRECAUTIONS N/A

POSSIBLE INTERACTIONS N/A

ALTERNATE DRUGS
One drug that may substitute for streptomycin is gentamicin at 3 mg/kg q12h. However, there are insufficient data on the efficacy of gentamicin plus tetracycline.

FOLLOW-UP

PATIENT MONITORING
• Serologic tests should be performed at monthly intervals for at least 3 months after completion of a course of treatment. A continuous and persistent decline in antibodies to negative status indicates successful treatment. • Dogs that have recrudescent infections (i.e., a rise in antibody levels and a recurrence of bacteremia after a course of therapy) should be re-treated, neutered, and treated again, or euthanatized. • Negative

blood cultures should be obtained for at least 3 months after cessation of treatment.

PREVENTION/AVOIDANCE
• There is no vaccine. A vaccine would further complicate serologic testing. • Test all brood bitches before they come into estrus if a breeding is planned. Male dogs used for breeding should be tested at frequent intervals. • Newly acquired dogs must not be allowed to enter a breeding kennel. Quarantine and test all new dogs twice at monthly intervals before being allowed to enter a breeding kennel.

POSSIBLE COMPLICATIONS
Owners may be reluctant to neuter or destroy valuable dogs, regardless of treatment failure. Owners should be reminded of ethical considerations and their obligation not to sell or distribute infected dogs.

EXPECTED COURSE AND PROGNOSIS
• The prognosis is guarded. • Dogs infected for periods less than 3-4 months are most likely to respond to treatment; chronically infected males have been more unyielding to therapy.

MISCELLANEOUS

ASSOCIATED CONDITIONS N/A

AGE RELATED FACTORS N/A

ZOONOTIC POTENTIAL
Human infections have been reported. Most are mild and respond readily to tetracyclines.

PREGNANCY
Abortions at 45-60 days of gestation are typical. Pups from infected bitches may be infected or normal.

SYNONYM
Contagious canine abortion

ABBREVIATIONS
RSAT = rapid 2-ME slide agglutination test
AGID = agar gel immunodiffusion

Reference

Carmichael LE, Greene CE. Canine brucellosis. In: Greene CE, ed. Infectious diseases of the dog and cat. Philadelphia: WB Saunders, 1990:573-585.
Author Leland Carmichael
Consulting Editor Fred W. Scott

CALICIVIRUS—CATS

BASICS

DEFINITION
A common viral respiratory disease of domestic and exotic cats characterized by upper respiratory signs, oral ulceration, pneumonia, and occasionally arthritis

Pathophysiology
Infection with the causative virus results in rapid cytolysis of infected cells with resulting tissue pathology and clinical disease.

Affected
• Respiratory— rhinitis, interstitial pneumonia, ulceration of the tip of the nose • Oral cavity—ulceration of the tongue is common and also occasionally occurs on the hard palate and lips • Musculoskeletal—acute arthritis • Gastrointestinal—infection occurs in intestines usually without clinical disease

Genetics None

Incidence/Prevalence
Persistent infection with feline calicivirus (FCV) is common. Clinical disease in multicat facilities and breeding catteries also is common. While routine vaccination has reduced the incidence of clinical disease, it has not decreased the prevalence of the virus.

Geographic Distribution Worldwide

SIGNALMENT

Species Cats

Breed Predilections None

Mean Age and Range
Young kittens more than 6 weeks are most commonly affected, but cats of any age may show clinical disease.

Predominant Sex No sex predilection

SIGNS

Historical Findings
• Sudden onset • Ocular or nasal discharge • Ulcers on the tongue, hard palate, lips, tip of nose, or around claws • Dyspnea from pneumonia • Acute, painful lameness

Physical Examination Findings
• Generally alert and in good condition upon presentation • Fever • Ocular and/or nasal discharge, usually serous and mild • Dyspnea from pneumonia may occur in some cats.
• Ulcerations are common on the tongue, hard palate, lips, and occasionally the tip of the nose and around the claws.

CAUSES
Feline calicivirus is a small, nonenveloped single-stranded RNA virus. Numerous strains of virus exist in nature, with varying degrees of cross-reactivity antigenically. More than one serotype of virus exists. FCV is relatively stable and resistant to many disinfectants.

RISK FACTORS
• Lack of vaccination or improper vaccination • Multicat facilities • Concurrent infections with other pathogens, such as FHV-1 or FPV • Poor ventilation

DIAGNOSIS

DIFFERENTIAL DIAGNOSIS
See Rhinotracheitis—Cats

CBC/BIOCHEMISTRY/URINALYSIS
There are no characteristic or consistent findings on routine laboratory tests in cats with acute FCV infection.

OTHER LABORATORY TESTS
Serologic testing on paired serum samples will detect a rise in neutralizing antibody titers against FCV.

IMAGING
Radiographs of the lungs will show a condensation of lung tissue in cats with pneumonia.

OTHER DIAGNOSTIC PROCEDURES
• Virus can be readily isolated in cell cultures from samples taken from the oral pharynx, lung tissue, feces, blood, and secretions from the nose and conjunctiva. • Immunofluorescent assays of lung tissue will detect viral antigen.

GROSS AND HISTOPATHOLOGIC FINDINGS
• Gross findings may include evidence of upper respiratory infection including ocular and nasal discharge, pneumonia with consolidation of large portions of individual lung lobes, and possibly ulcerations on the tongue, lips, and hard palate. Mortality is rare with FCV infection unless severe pneumonia is present.
• Histopathologic findings include interstitial pneumonia of large portions of individual lung lobes, ulcerations on epithelium of the tongue, lips, and hard palate, and mild inflammatory reactions in the nose and conjunctiva.

TREATMENT

INPATIENT VERSUS OUTPATIENT
Unless severe pneumonia is present, FCV-infected cats can be treated as outpatients whenever possible.

ACTIVITY
Infected cats should be restricted from contact with other cats to prevent transmission of the disease.

DIET
Diet does not need to be restricted, but special diets may be indicated in order to entice anorectic cats to resume eating.

CLIENT EDUCATION
Clients should be educated about the need for proper vaccination, and the need to modify the vaccination protocol in breeding catter-

ies to include kittens before they become infected from the carrier queen, often at 6-8 weeks of age.

SURGICAL CONSIDERATIONS
None

MEDICATIONS

DRUGS AND FLUIDS
• There are no specific antiviral drugs that are effective against FCV.
• Broad-spectrum antibiotics such as amoxicillin (22 mg/kg PO q12h) are usually indicated, although secondary bacterial infections in cats with FCV infection are not nearly as important as with FHV-1 infections.
• Oxygen may be indicated in cats with severe pneumonia.
• Antibiotic eye ointments may be given to reduce secondary bacterial infections of the conjunctiva.
• General supportive care should be given as indicated.
• Appropriate pain medication can be given for transient arthritis pain.

CONTRAINDICATIONS None

PRECAUTIONS None

POSSIBLE INTERACTIONS None

ALTERNATE DRUGS None

FOLLOW-UP

PATIENT MONITORING
Patients should be monitored for the sudden development of dyspnea associated with pneumonia. There are no specific laboratory tests to monitor this disease.

PREVENTION/AVOIDANCE
• All cats should be vaccinated against FCV at the same time they are vaccinated against FHV-1. Routine vaccination with either MLV or inactivated vaccines should be done at 8-10 weeks of age and repeated 3-4 weeks later. In breeding catteries where respiratory disease is a problem, kittens must be vaccinated at an earlier age, either with an additional vaccination at 4-5 weeks of age, or by giving a vaccine approved for intranasal administration when the kittens are 10-14 days of age with follow-up vaccinations at 6, 10, and 14 weeks of age. Although annual vaccines are recommended, immunity undoubtedly lasts longer than one year. • Vaccination will not eliminate infection subsequent exposure, but vaccination by prevent clinical disease caused by most strains of FCV.

POSSIBLE COMPLICATIONS
• The most serious complication of FCV infection is the development of interstitial pneumonia, which can be life-threatening.

• Secondary bacterial infections of the lungs or upper airways may complicate recovery.
• Oral ulcers and the acute arthritis usually heal without complications.

EXPECTED COURSE AND PROGNOSIS

• Clinical disease usually appears 3-4 days after exposure, and once neutralizing antibodies appear about 7 days after exposure, recovery is usually rapid. • Unless severe pneumonia occurs, the prognosis is excellent for complete recovery. • Recovered cats are persistently infected for long periods of time and will continuously shed small quantities of virus in oral secretions.

 MISCELLANEOUS

ASSOCIATED CONDITIONS

Cats with FCV infection may also be infected concurrently with FHV-1, especially in multicat and breeding facilities.

AGE RELATED FACTORS

FCV infection usually occurs in young kittens whose maternally derived immunity has waned, although unvaccinated cats of any age may be affected.

ZOONOTIC POTENTIAL None

PREGNANCY

Generally there is not a problem with pregnancy because most cats have either been exposed or vaccinated before becoming pregnant.

SYNONYMS

Feline picornavirus infection. This virus was originally classified as a picornavirus and older literature refers to the infection by this name. At the time of this writing, there is no known picornavirus that infects cats.

SEE ALSO

Rhinotracheitis—Cats

ABBREVIATIONS

FCV = feline calicivirus
FHV = feline herpesvirus
FVR = feline viral rhinotracheitis
FPV = feline parvovirus

References

Barr MC, Olsen CW, Scott FW. Feline viral diseases. In: Ettinger SJ, Feldman EC, eds. Veterinary internal medicine. 4th ed. Philadelphia: WB Saunders, 1995:409-439.

Ford RB. Role of infectious agents in respiratory disease. Vet Clin North Am (Small Anim Pract) 1993;23:17-35.

Ford RB, Levy JK. Infectious diseases of the respiratory tract. In: Sherding RG, ed. The cat: diseases and clinical management. New York: Churchill Livingstone, 1994:489-500.

Pedersen NC. Feline calicivirus infection. In: Pratt PW, ed. Feline infectious diseases. Goleta, CA: American Veterinary Publicatons, 1988:61-67.

Povey RC. Feline respiratory diseases. In: Greene CE, ed. Infectious diseases of the dog and cat. Philadelphia: WB Saunders, 1990:346-357.

Author Fred W. Scott
Consulting Editor Fred W. Scott

CAMPYLOBACTERIOSIS

BASICS

OVERVIEW
• Campylobacter jejuni is a fastidious, microaerophilic, gram-negative curved bacteria found in the GI tract of mammals. • C. jejuni is a commensal in the GI tract of dogs, cats, and other mammals. • Causes a superficial erosive enterocolitis • Localizes in mucus-filled crypts of the intestine; darting motility (flagella) essential for colonization; produces enterotoxin, cytotoxin, cytolethal distending toxin, invasin

SIGNALMENT
• Some studies indicate up to 49% of normal, nondiarrheic dogs and 45% of normal cats carry C. jejuni as a commensal and shed it in their feces. • Prevalence is higher in puppies from birth up to 6 months (less frequently cats up to 6 months of age—both with and without diarrhea), in kennel/pound dogs and cats, and in dogs and cats in other types of close confinement. • Fecal-oral route of infection results from contamination of food, water, fresh meat (poultry, beef) and the environment with feces.

SIGNS
• Young animals (up to 6 months of age)—clinical signs are most severe and are attributable to enterocolitis/diarrhea • Diarrhea (mucous, watery, bile-streaked, with and without blood and leukocytes)—tenesmus, fever (mild or absent), 3-15 days duration, leukocytosis, anorexia, vomiting, Campylobacter shed in feces for weeks to months • Invasion of mucosa of GI tract causes—hematochezia, leukocytes in feces, ulceration, edema, congestion of intestine along with bacteremia and occasionally septicemia • Adult dogs and cats—most harbor Campylobacter without clinical signs

CAUSES AND RISK FACTORS
• Campylobacter jejuni is the causative agent • Confined animals (kennels, pounds)—exposed to poor sanitation and hygiene, fecal buildup in the environment • Young animals that are debilitated, immunosuppressed, or parasitized are more susceptible • Adults with concurrent infections (Salmonella, parvovirus, hookworms) more likely to become clinically affected.

DIAGNOSIS

DIFFERENTIAL DIAGNOSIS
Bacterial culture, viral serologic and fluorescent antibody tests and isolation will differentiate causes of diarrhea:

• Viral gastroenteritis—feline panleukopenia, FeLV, FIV, enteric coronavirus, rotavirus, and canine distemper • Bacterial gastroenteritis—Salmonella, Yersinia enterocolitica, Clostridium difficile, and Clostridium perfringens • Parasites—helminths and protozoa • Dietary • Drug or toxin induced • Extraintestinal disease • Functional/mechanical ileus • Neurological disorder

CBC/BIOCHEMISTRY/URINALYSIS
CBC—if the Campylobacter strain is invasive and bacteremia develops, leukocytosis results • Chemistry profile—likely to show effects of diarrhea and dehydration on the host

OTHER LABORATORY TESTS N/A

IMAGING N/A

OTHER DIAGNOSTIC PROCEDURES
• Fecal leukocytes are present in GI tract and stool. • Fecal culture positive for Campylobacter (culture-microaerophilic approximately 42C, 48hr, on special Campy blood agar plates). • Fecal Gram's stain—make a smear of watery stool on glass slide, heat fix, and Gram's stain, leaving counterstain (safranin) on for longer than usual • Fecal wet mount—drop small amount of stool (if not watery mix with a small amount of saline or broth) on slide, coverslip, view on phase or darkfield objective (40X), see large numbers of curved bacteria, highly motile (characteristic darting motility)

GROSS AND HISTOPATHOLOGIC FINDINGS
• Gross pathology—diffuse colon thickening and congestion/edema; hyperemia of small intestine; enlarged mesenteric lymph nodes • Histopathology—colon-mucosal thickening, exfoliation of brush border and goblet cells; epithelium becomes cuboidal, crypt height reduced; crypt abscesses present; RBC and neutrophils in lamina propria and intestinal lumen

TREATMENT
• If enteritis/colitis—treat as outpatient; disease usually self-limiting
• If severely dehydrated or prolonged bloody diarrhea—treat as inpatient for fluid and electrolyte replacement, especially neonatal and immature patients
• Isolate and confine to cage with monitoring and rest if neonatal disease is severe

MEDICATIONS

DRUGS AND FLUIDS
Neonatal/immature Patients
• Treat signs/supportive care/fluid and electrolyte replacement

• Balanced polyionic isotonic solution (lactated ringers)
• Oral fluids—hypertonic glucose solutions (for secretory diarrhea)
• Plasma transfusions if serum albumin < 2.0 g/dl
• Locally acting intestinal adsorbents and protectants

All Patients Regardless of Age
• If high fever is present, bloody diarrhea, massive diarrhea, persistent signs > 7 days, worsening signs, immune suppression of host, antimicrobial therapy recommended
• Erythromycin (10-20 mg/kg PO q8h for 5 days) drug of choice
• Chloramphenicol—dogs, 35-55 mg/kg PO q8h, 16-22 mg/kg IM, or SQ q8h; cats, 50 mg/kg total PO, IV, IM, SQ q12h
• Gentamicin (dogs and cats)—2.4-4.4 mg/kg IV (only in acute sepsis) or IM q8h

CONTRAINDICATIONS/POSSIBLE INTERACTIONS N/A

FOLLOW-UP

PATIENT MONITORING
Repeat fecal culture after treatment completed

PREVENTION/AVOIDANCE
• Good hygiene (hand washing) • Routinely clean and disinfect runs, food and water bowls, etc.

POSSIBLE COMPLICATIONS
Animal may become bacteremic/septicemic

EXPECTED COURSE AND PROGNOSIS
• Disease usually self-limiting in adult dogs and cats • Puppies/kittens with enterocolitis—treat with antibiotics

MISCELLANEOUS

ASSOCIATED CONDITIONS N/A

AGE RELATED FACTORS
Young animals at greatest rick of infection

ZOONOTIC POTENTIAL
High potential to infect humans

PREGNANCY
Erythromycin safe to use in early pregnancy; chloramphenicol and gentamicin should not be used in pregnant animal

Reference

Greene CE. Enteric bacterial infections. In: Clinical microbiology and infectious diseases of the dog and cat. Philadelphia: WB Saunders, 1984:617-632.
Author Patrick L. McDonough
Consulting Editor Fred W. Scott

BASICS

OVERVIEW
• Candida is a genus of fungi that normally inhabit the alimentary, nasal, and genital mucosa in mammalian species. • Opportunistic infections can occur in patients whose normal endogenous microflora has been disturbed by prolonged antibiotic therapy or who have diminished cell-mediated immunocompetence. • Signs vary with site of overgrowth or dissemination. Lesions secondary to Candida spp. overgrowth have been found in the oral cavity, intestinal tract, ear canal, genitourinary tract, and skin as generalized dermatitis. Embolic colonization and microabscess formation after dissemination via the blood stream has been shown to produce lesions at sites including the lung, skin, kidneys, liver, brain, myocardium, eyes and skeletal muscle.

SIGNALMENT
• Dogs and cats. Rare in both as a pathogen.
• No specific age, breed, or sex predilections known.

SIGNS
Historical Findings
• A history of prolonged antibiotic usage or immunosuppressive therapy may be found.
• Previous burns, surgery, trauma, or indwelling vascular or urinary catheters may be noted in the history.

Physical Examination Findings
• Oral—creamy, white plaquelike lesions on tongue, oral mucosa, lips, and mucocutaneous junctions • Intestinal—chronic diarrhea, weight loss • Aural—ear canal inflammation, pinnal inflammation, and/or otitis media • Genital—white vaginal or prepucial discharge • Skin—nonhealing, erythematous, moist, exuding, and crusting lesions of the skin and nail beds • Esophageal—fever, depression, ptyalism, regurgitation, anorexia, and pain upon palpation of the cervical esophagus. • Signs of systemic candidiasis vary with site of microabscess formation and may include fever, dermatitis, anterior uveitis, pleural effusion, osteomyelitis with fistulous tracts, diarrhea, and brainstem or cerebellar dysfunction.

CAUSES AND RISK FACTORS
• Normal flora. Usually opportunistic infections. • Prolonged antibiotic usage • Immunosuppressive therapy • Diminished cell-mediated immunity of any cause • FIV or FeLV (cats) • Neutropenia (dogs) • Diabetes mellitus • Parvoviral infection • Long-term glucocorticoid treatment • Disruption of cutaneous or mucosal barriers

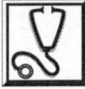 DIAGNOSIS

DIFFERENTIAL DIAGNOSIS
Must differentiate from other infectious causes of oral lesions (e.g., Leptospirosis, viral diseases [cats], Blastomyces spp., Histoplasma spp.)
• Esophagitis, acute or chronic vomiting/reflux, or trauma/foreign body • Differentiate systemic candidiasis from bacterial sepsis/toxemia, other systemic mycoses, autoimmune disease, drug eruption, nonseptic thromboembolic disease, viral disease (e.g., FIP), protozoal disease (e.g., toxoplasmosis), neoplasia, severe metabolic disease, and anaphlylaxis.

CBC/BIOCHEMISTRY/URINALYSIS
• Usually normal in localized infection • May see leukopenia or thrombocytopenia with disseminated disease • Muscle or liver enzymes may be elevated, depending on what tissues are affected.

OTHER LABORATORY TESTS N/A

IMAGING N/A

OTHER DIAGNOSTIC PROCEDURES
• Skin scrapings may be useful. May require skin biopsy to confirm. • Fecal cultures are generally unreliable. • Urine culture may isolate Candida spp. more readily than blood culture because renal embolization occurs consistently in disseminated infection. • If blood cultures are obtained, arterial samples are recommended because tissues filter out organisms before they reach the systemic venous circulation.

GROSS AND HISTOPATHOLOGIC FINDINGS
• Disseminated candidasis produces gross lesions that consist of multiple white foci in the heart, liver, spleen, lymph nodes, CNS, kidneys, and other organs, depending on the pattern of embolization. • Microscopically, these white foci appear as multifocal abscesses or areas of necrosis. Foci may contain blastoconidia, pseudohyphae, and true hyphae.

 TREATMENT

• Drying of superficial Candida lesions is recommended.
• Systemic candidiasis patients should be treated as inpatients.
• Because underlying immunosuppresion is often documented or suspected, these patients are best treated in isolation from other animals.
• Patients with severe ulceration of the oral, esophageal, or intestinal mucosa may require feeding tube placement.

 MEDICATIONS

DRUGS AND FLUIDS
Topical Treatments
• Nystatin 100,000 U/g applied q8h-q12h x 1-2 weeks • Clotrimazole 1% applied q6h-q8h x 1 week • Amphotericin B 3% applied q6h-q8h x 1 week

Oral Treatments
• Ketoconazole 5-11 mg/kg PO q12h x 4 weeks (dog) • Ketoconazole 50-100 mg/cat PO q12h-q24h x 4 weeks (cat)
• Itraconazole 5-7 mg/kg PO q12h x 4 weeks (dog or cat)
• Oral vitamin A supplementation may be of benefit.

CONTRAINDICATIONS/POSSIBLE INTERACTIONS
• Potential toxic side effects limit the usefulness of intravenous antifungals currently available to treat candidiasis.
• Some ongoing clinical work suggests that blood dyscrasias may develop in FIV positive cats that are treated with ketoconazole.
• Ketoconazole and itraconazole should be used cautiously in patients with documented hepatic disease or thrombocytopenia.

 FOLLOW-UP

PATIENT MONITORING
• If adverse gastrointestinal side effects or ALT elevations are seen in cats while on itraconazole, it is recommended that the drug be discontinued until signs or enzyme elevations resolve and then restarted at a lower dosage.
• If previous blood or urine cultures were positive for Candida spp. then follow-up cultures are advised. • Monitor for liver enzyme elevations and hypokalemia during treatment.

EXPECTED COURSE AND PROGNOSIS
• Superficial, cutaneous, or mucocutaneous candidiasis carries a fair prognosis.
• Prognosis for animals with generalized or disseminated candidiasis is grave.

 MISCELLANEOUS

Reference
Greene CE, Chandler FW. Candidiasis. In: Greene CE, ed. Infectious diseases of the dog and cat. Philadelphia: WB Saunders, 1990:723-727.
Author Matthew S. Mellema
Consulting Editor Fred W. Scott

CAPILLARIASIS

BASICS

DEFINITION
Capillaria plica is a parasite that invades the mucosa or submucosa of the bladder or (rarely) the renal pelvis and ureter, causing a mild inflammatory response. *C. plica* in dogs and *C. feliscati* in cats have been uncommonly associated with signs of lower urinary tract disease. First stage in life cycle of *C. plica* is passage of bipolar ova in urine. After ingestion of embryonated ova by earthworms, the parasite develops into the infective stage. Ingestion of infective earthworm results in a patent infection in dogs in 61-88 days. Details of life cycle of *C. feliscati* are poorly understood.

SIGNALMENT
• Dogs—no predilection reported • Cat—affected cats almost always > 8 months old

SIGNS
• Usually none • Pollakiuria, hematuria, stranguria, and dysuria in some animals, particularly those heavily infected

CAUSES AND RISK FACTORS
• In dogs—High prevalence of infection (up to 50%) in the natural hosts, raccoons and foxes, in the southeastern United States may predispose animals in this geographic region. • In kennels, high infection rates are associated with the use of soil surfaces. • In cats—Rare in the United States; prevalence of infection of 18-34% reported in Australia

DIAGNOSIS

DIFFERENTIAL DIAGNOSIS
Other more common causes of lower urinary tract disease, such as urolithiasis, urinary tract infection, trauma, and neoplasia

CBC/BIOCHEMISTRY/URINALYSIS
• Bipolar ova in the urine is diagnostic. • The possibility of fecal contamination of urine with *Trichuris vulpis* ova should be considered if free-catch urine specimens are used for testing or if inadvertent rectal puncture occurs during cystocentesis. • Alternatively, urine contamination of feces in an affected animal can result in false fecal examination findings.

OTHER LABORATORY TESTS N/A

IMAGING N/A

OTHER DIAGNOSTIC PROCEDURES N/A

TREATMENT

• Infection is usually self-limiting in both species, with dogs developing negative ova counts in 10-12 weeks if kept isolated. • The replacement of soil surfaces with sand, gravel, or concrete may reduce prevalence of infection in kennels.

MEDICATIONS

• Anthelmintic administration can be considered if animal has clinical signs. Success of treatment is monitored by urine ova counts and observation of clinical signs. • Fenbendazole (25 mg/kg PO q12h 3-10 days) has been reported to result in negative ova counts in dogs and cats. • Ivermectin has been suggested as an alternative but objective information on its efficacy in this disease is limited.

CONTRAINDICATIONS/POSSIBLE INTERACTIONS N/A

FOLLOW-UP

Success of treatment monitored by urine ova counts and observation of clinical signs

MISCELLANEOUS

Reference

Brown SA, Prestwood KA. Parasites of the urinary tract. In: Kirk RW, ed. Current veterinary therapy IX. Philadelphia, WB Saunders. 1986:1153-1155.

Author Scott A. Brown
Consulting Editor Larry G. Adams and Carl A. Osborne

BASICS

OVERVIEW
Carbon monoxide is an odorless, colorless, nonirritating gas produced by the inefficient combustion of carbonaceous fuels. Carbon monoxide is absorbed into the blood, forming carboxyhemoglobin (COHb) and reducing oxygen, which causes hypoxia of the brain and heart.

SIGNALMENT
All animals are susceptible.

SIGNS

History
Exposure to automobile exhaust or supplemental heating devices

Acute Signs
• Drowsiness • Lethargy • Weakness • Incoordination • Reduced heart excitability • Cherry-red color to skin and mucous membranes • Dyspnea • Coma • Terminal clonic spasms • Acute death

Chronic Signs
• Low exercise tolerance • Disturbance of postural and position reflexes, and gait

CAUSES AND RISK FACTORS
• Incomplete combustion • Automobile exhaust in a closed garage, or faulty exhaust system • Unvented or faulty furnace, gas water heater, or gas or kerosene space heater • Fires and carbon monoxide can reach 10% in the atmosphere of a burning building. • Animals with impaired cardiac or pulmonary function at higher risk than clinically normal animals

 ## DIAGNOSIS

DIFFERENTIAL DIAGNOSIS
Similar clinical signs observed in animals with barbiturate, ethanol, cyanide, or hydrogen sulfide gas toxicity

CBC/BIOCHEMISTRY/URINALYSIS
Creatine kinase high because of muscle ischemia

OTHER LABORATORY TESTS
Carboxyhemoglobin (expressed as % of Hb in the COHb brrn) in whole blood • Low blood pH secondary to metabolic acidosis • PAO_2 normal, but percent oxygen saturation low

IMAGING N/A

OTHER DIAGNOSTIC PROCEDURES
ECG consistent with anoxia and necrosis of single heart muscle fibers

 ## TREATMENT
• Restore adequate oxygen to brain and heart. • Provide fresh air, maintain patient airway, and provide artificial respiration if necessary. • Hyperbaric oxygen promotes recovery.

 ## MEDICATIONS

DRUGS AND FLUIDS
Supportive fluids

CONTRAINDICATIONS/POSSIBLE INTERACTIONS
Avoid respiratory depressants.

 ## FOLLOW-UP
• Response to treatment should occur in 1 to 4 hours depending on cellular hypoxia and damage. • Monitor cardiac, pulmonary, and neurologic functions and limit physical activity for 2 weeks. • Neurologic signs may appear from within a few days to as long as 6 weeks after apparent recovery. • Eliminate the source of carbon monoxide and prevent reexposure by using carbon monoxide detectors available at hardware stores.

 ## MISCELLANEOUS

PREGNANCY
Carbon monoxide reduces oxygen carrying ability of maternal blood and crosses the placenta, producing fetal hypoxia, abortion, or neurologic impairment of the fetus, even when the dam is asymptomatic.

ZOONOTIC POTENTIAL
People in the same carbon monoxide-contaminated environment are at risk.

SEE ALSO
Poisoning (Intoxication)

ABBREVIATIONS
ECG = electrocardiogram

Reference
Ellenhom MJ and Barceloux DG. Medical toxicology: diagnosis and treatment of human poisoning. New York: Elsevier, 1988.
Author Thomas L. Carson
Consulting Editor Gary D. Osweiler

CARDIOMYOPATHY, DILATED–CATS

 BASICS

OVERVIEW
• Dilated cardiomyopathy is a disease of the ventricular muscle characterized by systolic myocardial failure and an enlarged, volume overloaded heart that leads to signs of congestive heart failure or low cardiac output.
• Before 1987, dilated cardiomyopathy was one of the most commonly diagnosed heart diseases in cats. Most cats probably had secondary cardiomyopathy as a result of taurine deficiency. • Primary idiopathic dilated cardiomyopathy is now an uncommon cause of heart disease in cats.

SIGNALMENT
• Various breeds have a reported increased incidence (Siamese, Abyssinian, and Burmese breeds). • Familial patterns have been identified in some families of cats.

SIGNS
Historical Findings
• Signs related to low cardiac output (anorexia, weakness, depression) • Signs related to congestive heart failure (dyspnea, tachypnea) • Signs related to thromboembolism (sudden-onset painful paraparesis)

Physical Examination Findings
• Soft systolic heart murmur • Weak left cardiac impulse • Gallop rhythm (an extra heart sound as a result of passive ventricular filling) • Hypothermia • Prolonged capillary refill time • Quiet lung sounds (pleural effusion) • Crackles (pulmonary edema) • Hypokinetic femoral pulses • Possibly posterior pararesis as a result of aortic thromboembolism

CAUSES AND RISK FACTORS
• The underlying etiology of idiopathic dilated cardiomyopathy remains unknown, although a genetic predisposition has been identified in some families of cats. • Taurine deficiency was a common cause of secondary myocardial failure before 1987.

 DIAGNOSIS

DIFFERENTIAL DIAGNOSIS
• Taurine deficiency dilated cardiomyopathy. Because primary idiopathic dilated cardiomyopathy and taurine deficiency have similar clinical presentations, cats with myocardial failure should be assumed to be taurine deficient until shown to be unresponsive to taurine. • Myocardial failure secondary to long-standing congenital or acquired left ventricular volume overload diseases

CBC/BIOCHEMISTRY/URINALYSIS
Many cats will have prerenal azotemia related to low cardiac output.

OTHER LABORATORY TESTS
Plasma or whole blood taurine concentrations less than 25 nmoles/ml is considered too low in cats. This assay is performed at a limited number of institutions.

IMAGING
Radiography
Radiography often shows pleural effusion or pulmonary edema. The cardiac silhouette typically is enlarged in a globoid manner.

Echocardiography
Echocardiography is the diagnostic modality of choice. Characteristic findings include thin ventricular walls, enlarged left ventricular end systolic and end diastolic dimensions, left atrial enlargement, and low fractional shortening.

OTHER DIAGNOSTIC TESTS
Electrocardiography
Electrocardiography may be normal or may show left atrial or ventricular enlargement patterns. Both ventricular and supraventricular arrhythmias can be seen.

Pleural Effusion Analysis
Pleural effusion typically is a modified transudate with total protein less than 4.0 g/dl and nucleated cell counts of less than 2500/ml. Analysis of the pleural effusion is important to rule out other causes of pleural effusion such as pyothorax, infectious peritonitis, or lymphosarcoma.

GROSS AND HISTOPATHOLOGIC FINDINGS
• Heart to body ratio is increased. Ventricle walls are thin and the lumen is enlarged.
• Valve anatomy is normal. Histopathology shows myocyte atrophy and myocardial fibrosis.

 TREATMENT

• These cats usually are in congestive heart failure and should be treated as inpatients.
• Thoracocentesis is both therapeutic and diagnostic.
• These cats have a poor prognosis despite intensive therapy.
• These cats typically are anorexic, thus tempting their appetite with many types of food may be necessary. Eventually, a low-sodium diet could be considered.

MEDICATIONS

DRUGS AND FLUIDS

• Furosemide is recommended at the lowest effective dose to eliminate pulmonary edema and pleural effusion. Recommended dose range is 1-3 mg/kg q8-12h. Initially, furosemide should be administered parenterally.

• Nitroglycerin (2% ointment) 0.25-0.5 inch applied topically can be used in conjunction with diurectics in the acute management of congestive heart failure to further reduce preload. Nitroglycerin will lower the dose of furosemide and is particularly useful in a patients with hypothermia or dehydration.

• Enalapril at a dose of 0.5 mg/kg PO q24h is recommended to reduce afterload and preload.

• Digoxin is recommended to strengthen contractility at a dose of 0.3125 mg (one quarter of a 0.125 mg tablet) PO q48h.

• Taurine supplementation is recommended in all cats with myocardial failure at 250 mg PO q12h until it is demonstrated that the patient is unresponsive to taurine.

• Dobutamine at extremely low dosages can be given to a patient with severe signs of congestive heart failure and low cardiac output. Dose varies from 1-5 mcg/kg/min.

• See aortic thromboembolism chapter for therapeutic recommendations.

CONTRAINDICATIONS/POSSIBLE INTERACTIONS

• Unless needed for cardiac rhythm control, avoid drugs that reduce contractility such as calcium channel blockers or beta adrenergic blockers. • Overzealous diuretic therapy may cause dehydration and hypokalemia.

• Digoxin dose should be reduced if renal insufficiency is documented or suspected.

• Dobutamine may cause seizures.

 FOLLOW-UP

• Repeat thoracic radiographs within 1 week to determine efficacy of therapy. • Periodically monitor electrolyte and renal parameters.• Digoxin concentrations should be measured 2 weeks after initiating therapy. Therapeutic range is between 1-2 ng/dl 8-12 hours postpill. • Repeat echocardiogram in 3-6 months after initiating taurine supplementation to determine response to therapy.

 MISCELLANEOUS

Reference

Ware WA. Myocardial diseases of the cat. In: Essential of small animal internal medicine. Mosby, 1992.

Author Terri C. DeFrancesco

Consulting Editors

Larry P. Tilley and Francis W. K. Smith, Jr.

CARDIOMYOPATHY, DILATED—DOGS

BASICS

DEFINITION
• Left- and right-sided dilation, normal coronary arteries, normal (or minimally diseased) atrioventricular valves, low contractility, and myocardial dysfunction occurring primarily during systole

Pathophysiology
• Myocardial failure leads to reduced cardiac output and congestive heart failure (CHF).
• Atrioventricular annulus dilation and altered papillary muscle function promote valvular insufficiency.

Systems Affected
• Cardiovascular • Pulmonary if edema develops • Renal/urologic (prerenal azotemia) • All organ systems affected by reductions in cardiac output

Genetics
• Genetic cause or heritable susceptibility strongly suspected but as yet unproven

Incidence/Prevalence
Estimated at 0.5-1.1%

Geographic Distribution
N/A with the exception of Chagas' cardiomyopathy which is limited to the Southern United States

SIGNALMENT

Species Dogs

Breed Predilections
• Doberman pinscher, boxer • "Giant" breeds—Scottish deerhound, Irish wolfhound, Great Dane • Cocker spaniels

Mean Age and Range 4-10 years.

Predominant Sex
Males > females in most but not all breeds

SIGNS

Historical Findings
• Respiratory—tachypnea, dyspnea, coughing
• Weight loss • Weakness, lethargy, anorexia
• Abdominal distension • Syncope • Some dogs are asymptomatic.

Physical Examination Findings
• Weakness • Depression • Possibly cardiogenic shock • Hypokinetic femoral pulse from low cardiac output • Pulse deficits in anmials with atrial fibrillation, ventricular premature complex, paroxysmal ventricular tachycardia • Jugular pulses from tricuspid regurgitation, arrhythmias, or right-sided CHF • Muffled breath sounds and heart sounds in animals with pleural effusion.
• Crackles in animals with pulmonary edema
• S3 or summation gallops • Systolic murmur of mitral regurgitation and/or tricuspid regurgitation is common but usually soft
• Auscultatory evidence of cardiac arrhythmia
• Slow capillary refill time • Possible cyanosis
• Hepatomegaly with or without ascites

CAUSES
• Primary mechanism yet to be identified—idiopathic in the vast majority of animals
• Proposed—viral, protozoal, immune-mediated, and nutritional

RISK FACTORS N/A

DIAGNOSIS

DIFFERENTIAL DIAGNOSIS
• Endocardiosis • Congenital heart disease
• Heartworm disease • Bacterial endocarditis
• Cardiac tumors and pericardial effusion
• Airway obstruction—foreign body, neoplasm, laryngeal paralysis • Primary pulmonary disease—bronchial disease, pneumonia, neoplasia, aspiration, and vascular disease (heartworms) • Pleural effusions (e.g., pyothorax, hemothorax, and chylothorax)
• Trauma —diaphragmatic hernia, pulmonary hemorrhage, and pneumothorax

CBC/BIOCHEMISTRY/URINALYSIS
• Results usually normal unless altered by severe heart failure (e.g., prerenal azotemia, high alanine transaminase, low Na+), treatment for heart failure (e.g., hypokalemia, hypochloremia, and metabolic alkalosis from diuresis) or concurrent disease

OTHER LABORATORY TESTS N/A

IMAGING

Thoracic Radiographic Findings
• Generalized cardiomegaly and signs of CHF are common. • Left ventricular and left atrial enlargement most evident early in course of disease • Doberman pinschers—marked LAE is the main finding; pulmonary edema is often patchy and diffuse • Pleural effusion
• Hepatomegaly • Splenomegaly • Ascites

Echocardiography
• "Gold standard" for diagnosis • Ventricular and atrial dilation • Myocardial systolic dysfunction (low % fractional shortening)
• Doppler studies may document mitral or tricuspid regurgitation.

OTHER DIAGNOSTIC PROCEDURES

Electrocardiographic Findings
• Sinus rhythm or sinus tachycardia with isolated atrial or ventricular premature complexes • Atrial fibrillation is common • Ventricular tachycardia is very common in Doberman pinschers and boxers (Figure).
• Prolonged QRS (> 0.06 sec), possible high voltages (R > 3.0 mV lead II) suggesting left ventricular enlargement (figure) • "Sloppy" R wave descent with ST-T coving suggesting myocardial disease or left ventricular ischemia in some animals • Low voltages in animals with pleural effusion, pericardial effusion, or hypothyroidism)

Biopsy
• Percutaneous endomyocardial biopsy with histopathologic examination and quantitative carnitine assay

GROSS AND HISTOPATHOLOGIC FINDINGS
• Dilation and thinning of all chambers
• Slightly thickened endocardium with pale areas within the myocardium (i.e., necrosis, fibrosis) • Histopathologic (light microscopic) changes are minimal—small areas of myocyte atrophy, myocytolysis, myocardial necrosis, and fibrosis

TREATMENT

INPATIENT VERSUS OUTPATIENT
• With the exception of severely atrial fibrillation affected dogs, most treatment can be administered on an outpatient basis.

ACTIVITY
Allow the dog to choose its own level of activity.

DIET
• Goal to reduce dietary Na+ intake to < 12-15 mg/kg/day in heart failure patients
• Severe Na+ restriction is not necessary when potent vasodilators and diuretics are used.
• Best to use commercially prepared diets

CLIENT EDUCATION
• Emphasize potential signs associated with disease progression (e.g., CHF and sudden death) and adverse side effects of medications.

SURGICAL CONSIDERATIONS
• Dynamic cardiomyoplasty—information regarding surgical success and long-term follow-up is unavailable

MEDICATIONS

DRUGS AND FLUIDS OF CHOICE
First identify problems—CHF (left- or right-sided), arrhythmia, hypothermia, renal failure, and shock

Initial Stabilization
• Treat hypoxemia with O₂ administration.
• Prevent heat loss if the animal is hypothermic (warm environment).
• Administer fluids IV or SQ (D5W or 0.45% NaCl with 2.5% dextrose) only after pulmonary edema is controlled or pleural effusion has been aspirated.
• For pulmonary edema:
• Furosemide (2-4 mg/kg then 1-2 mg/kg IM or IV q8h-q12h for the first 2-3 days)
• 2% topically applied nitroglycerin for the first 24-48 hours; apply 1-2 inches q8h (for large- and giant-breed dogs)
• Aminophylline (initial 24 h) to treat bronchodilation and to strengthen the muscles of respiration (4-6 mg/kg slowly IV q8h)
• For marked pleural effusion, drain each hemithorax with an 18-20 g butterfly catheter.
• For severe heart failure and cardiogenic shock:

• Digoxin—oral administration (see below)
• Dobutamine (5-10 mcg/kg/min infused for 24-72 hours with care)
• Digoxin and dobutamine may predispose to malignant arrhythmias, particularly in hypoxic dogs.
• If animal has paroxysmal ventricular tachycardia, administer lidocaine slowly in 2 mg/kg boluses (up to 8 mg/kg total) to convert to sinus rhythm. Follow with lidocaine infusion (40-75 mcg/kg/min). If lidocaine is ineffective, administer procainamide slowly in 2 mg/kg /IV boluses (up to 20 mg/kg total) to convert to sinus rhythm. Follow with a 20-50 mcg/kg/min infusion or 8-20 mg/kg IM q6h.

Maintenance Therapy
• Vasodilators, especially the ACE inhibitors, are considered the cornerstone of treatment for dilated cardiomyopathy. Enalapril (0.25-0.5 mg/kg PO q12h-q24h) should be initiated early in the therapeutic regimen.
• A daily maintenance dosage of digoxin (0.187-0.375 mg q12h) is given to most giant-breed dogs. In large-breed dogs, do not exceed 0.015 mg/kg/day of digoxin, and do not exceed 0.375 mg of digoxin per day in Doberman pinschers.
• If necessary, an oral loading dose of digoxin (2 x maintenance dose) can be given the first 24-48 hours to dogs with atrial fibrillation or cardiogenic shock.
• Furosemide (0.5-1 mg/kg q8h-q24h) is used to control pulmonary edema, pleural effusion, or ascites.

Arrhythmias
• In dogs with atrial fibrillation, slowing the ventricular rate response is achieved by chronic administration of digitalis combined with atenolol (0.75-1.5 mg/kg PO q12h) or diltiazem (1-1.5 mg/kg PO q8h).
• Therapeutic goal is a ventricular rate of 100-140 bpm at rest.
• The above treatment merely controls the ventricular rate by depressing atrioventricular node conduction; it generally does not convert the rhythm from atrial fibrillation to sinus rhythm.

• Chronic treatment for ventricular tachycardia includes procainamide (8-20 mg/kg PO q6h-q8h), tocainide (10-20 mg/kg PO q8h) or mexiletine (5-8 mg/kg PO q8h). These drugs can be combined with a beta blocker if necessary.
• The role of carnitine and taurine in the treatment of dilated cardiomyopathy is controversial.

CONTRAINDICATIONS
Digoxin should be avoided in animals with severe uncontrolled paroxysmal ventricular tachycardia.

PRECAUTIONS
• Beta blockers and calcium channel blockers are negative inotropes and may adversely affect myocardial function.
• The combination of diuretics and ACE inhibitors may cause azotemia, especially in patients with severe heart failure or preexistent renal dysfunction.

POSSIBLE INTERACTIONS
• Both quinidine and verapamil will raise serum digoxin concentration and predispose the patient to digitalis intoxication.
• Propranolol will lower lidocaine excretion and predispose the patient to toxicity.
• Renal dysfunction, hypothyroidism, and hypokalemia predispose the patient to digitalis intoxication.

ALTERNATE DRUGS
• Other vasodilators, including hydralazine and prazosin, may be used instead of an ACE inhibitor.
• Propranolol (0.2-1 mg/kg q8h) can be used instead of diltiazem or atenolol to help control ventricular response rate in animals with atrial fibrillation.

FOLLOW-UP

PATIENT MONITORING
• Serial clinical examinations, thoracic radiographs, and ECG most helpful • Repeat echocardiography rarely informative • Serial

evaluation of serum digoxin concentration (therapeutic range, 1.0-2.5 ng/ml 8-10 h after administration) and serum biochemistry analysis may help prevent iatrogenic problems.

PREVENTION/AVOIDANCE N/A

POSSIBLE COMPLICATIONS
• Sudden death (arrhythmia) • Iatrogenic problems associated with medical management (see above)

EXPECTED COURSE AND PROGNOSIS
• Always fatal 6-24 month after atrial fibrillationtioner diagnosis • Doberman pinscher typically has a worse prognosis (< 6-month survival)
• Atrial fibrillation, paroxysmal ventricular tachycardia, and markedly low % fractional shortening are probably markers for short survival and sudden death.

MISCELLANEOUS

ASSOCIATED CONDITIONS N/A

AGE RELATED FACTORS
Prevalence increases with age

ZOONOTIC POTENTIAL N/A

PREGNANCY N/A

SYNONYMS
• Congestive cardiomyopathy • Giant- breed cardiomyopathy

SEE ALSO
• Carnitine Deficiency • Taurine Deficiency
• Ventricular Tachycardia • Atrial Fibrillation

ABBREVIATIONS
ACE = angiotensin converting enzyme
CHF = congestive heart failure

References
Sisson DD, Thomas WP. Myocardial diseases. In: Ettinger SJ, Feldman EC, eds. Textbook of veterinary internal medicine. 4th ed. Philadelphia: WB Saunders, 1995.
Author Matthew W. Miller
Consulting Editors Larry P. Tilley and Francis W. K. Smith, Jr.

A

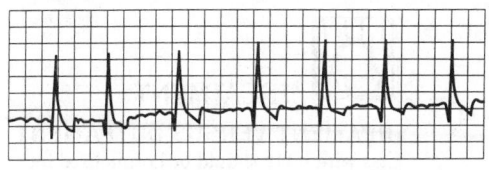

B

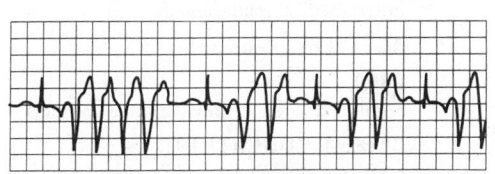

C

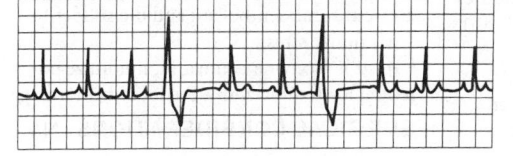

Figure A. Atrial fibrillation, typical of cardiomyopathy in giant breeds.

Figure B. Ventricular premature complexes and unsustained ventricular tachycardia in a Doberman pinscher with dilated cardiomyopathy.

Figure C. Right ventricular premature complexes, typical of dilated cardiomyopathy in boxer dogs.

CARDIOMYOPATHY, HYPERTROPHIC—CATS

BASICS

DEFINITION
Hypertrophic cardiomyopathy is characterized by inappropriate concentric hypertrophy of the ventricular free wall or the intraventricular septum of the nondilated left ventricle. The disease occurs independently of other cardiac or systemic disorders.

PATHOPHYSIOLOGY
• Diastolic dysfunction results from a thickened, noncompliant left ventricle. • High left ventricular filling pressure develops, causing left atrial enlargement. • Pulmonary venous hypertension causes pulmonary edema. Some cats have evidence of biventricular failure (i.e., pulmonary edema, pleural effusion, and rarely ascites) on examination. • Stasis of blood in the large left atrium predisposes the patient to aortic thromboembolism. • Dynamic aortic outflow obstruction occurs in some cats.

Systems Affected
• Cardiovascular—congestive heart failure (CHF), aortic thromboembolism, and arrhythmias • Pulmonary—dyspnea if pulmonary edema or pleural effusion develops • Renal/urologic—azotemia due to poor perfusion

Genetics
Some families of cats have been identified with a high prevalence of the disease, but the genetics have not been determined.

Incidence/Prevalence
Unknown, but relatively common

Geographic Distribution N/A

SIGNALMENT

Species
Cats (see cardiomyopathy, hypertrophic—dogs)

Breed Predilections
A familial association has been documented in Maine coon cats.

Mean Age and Range
5-7 years with reported ages of 6 months to 16 years

Predominant Sex
Male > female

SIGNS

Historical Findings
• Dyspnea • Anorexia • Exercise intolerance • Vomiting • Collapse • Sudden death • Coughing is uncommon in cats with cardiomyopathy and usually suggests pulmonary disease.

Physical Examination Findings
• Gallop rhythm (S3 or S4) heard best with the bell of the stethoscope in most animals • Systolic murmur in many animals • Apex heart beat may be exaggerated. • Muffled heart sounds, lack of chest compliance, and dyspnea characterized by rapid shallow respirations may be associated with pleural effusion. • Dyspnea and louder than normal lung sounds and crackles if pulmonary edema is present • Weak femoral pulse in many animals • Acute pelvic limb paralysis with cyanotic pads and nailbeds, cold limbs, and absence of femoral pulse in animals with aortic thromboembolism • Arrhythmia in some animals

CAUSES
Unknown—probably multiple causes exist

Possible causes:
• Abnormality affecting catecholamine influenced excitation-contraction coupling • Abnormal myocardial calcium metabolism • Collagen or other intercellular matrix abnormality • Growth hormone excess • Abnormality of the contractile protein myosin

RISK FACTORS
Offspring of animals with familial HCM

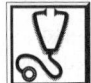

DIAGNOSIS

DIFFERENTIAL DIAGNOSIS
• Hyperthyroidism • Aortic stenosis • Systemic hypertension • Acromegaly • Noncardiac causes of pleural effusion (e.g., pyothorax, chylothorax, neoplasia, diaphragmatic hernia)

CBC/BIOCHEMISTRY/URINALYSIS
• Results usually normal • Prerenal azotemia in some animals

OTHER LABORATORY TESTS
• In cats over 6 years old, check thyroid concentration to rule out hyperthyroidism. Hyperthyroidism causes myocardial hypertrophy that might be confused with HCM (hyperthyroidism does not cause HCM). • A validated growth hormone assay for cats is not currently available. Some cats with HCM have high growth hormone concentration.

IMAGING

Radiography
• Dorsal ventral radiographs often reveal a valentine-appearing heart because of biatrial enlargement and a left ventricle that comes to a point. • Radiographs are not sensitive enough to differentiate the different forms of cardiomyopathy. • Pulmonary edema or pleural effusion or both in some animals • Radiographs may be normal in asymptomatic cats.

Echocardiography
• Hypertrophy of the interventricular septum (IVS, diameter > 6 mm) • Hypertrophy of the left ventricular posterior wall (diameter > 6 mm) • Hypertrophy may be symmetric (affecting IVS and posterior wall) or asymmetric (affecting IVS or posterior wall, but not both) • Hypertrophy of the papillary muscles • Normal or high fractional shortening • Normal or reduced left ventricular lumen • Left atrial enlargement • Systolic anterior motion of the mitral valve (some animals) • Left ventricular outflow obstruction (some animals) • Thrombus in the left atrium (rare) • Note: There is some overlap between normal cats (especially ketaminized and dehydrated) and cats with mild HCM. Correlate echocardiographic findings with physical examination findings. Presence of left atrial enlargement favors HCM.

Angiography
Since the advent of echocardiography, angiography is rarely used to diagnose cardiomyopathy.

OTHER DIAGNOSTIC PROCEDURES

Electrocardiography
• ECG is the procedure of choice for documenting arrhythmias and conduction disturbances but can not differentiate different forms of cardiomyopathy or distinguish cardiomyopathy from hyperthyroidism. • Cats with HCM may have a normal ECG. • A left axis deviation is seen in many cats. • Sinus tachycardia (HR > 240) is common in patients in heart failure; however, some cats with severe heart failure and hypothermia are bradycardic. • Atrial premature complexes and ventricular premature complexes occasionally seen • Atrial fibrillation is uncommon in cats; when it occurs, it is often associated with HCM or restrictive cardiomyopathy.

Systemic Blood Pressure
• Patients are normotensive or hypotensive. • Evaluate blood pressure in all patients with myocardial hypertrophy to rule out systemic hypertension as the cause or contributing factor.

GROSS AND HISTOPATHOLOGIC FINDINGS
• Nondilated left ventricle with hypertrophy of intraventricular septum or left ventricular free wall • Hypertrophy of papillary muscles • Left atrial enlargement • Mitral valve thickening • Myocardial hypertrophy with disorganized alignment of myocytes • Interstitial fibrosis • Myocardial scarring • Hypertrophy and lumenal narrowing of intramural coronary arteries

TREATMENT

INPATIENT VERSUS OUTPATIENT
Cats with CHF should be hospitalized for initial medical management.

ACTIVITY Restricted

DIET
Sodium restriction only if animal has CHF

CLIENT EDUCATION
• Many cats diagnosed while asymptomatic eventually develop CHF and may develop aortic thromboembolism and die suddenly. • Minimize stress. • If cat is receiving coumadin, minimize potential for trauma and subsequent hemorrhage.

SURGICAL CONSIDERATIONS N/A

MEDICATIONS

DRUGS AND FLUIDS

Diltiazem
• Dosage—7.5-15 mg/cat PO q8h or 10 mg/kg PO q24h (Cardizem CD)
• Beneficial effects may include slower sinus rate, resolution of supraventricular arrhythmias, improved diastolic relaxation, coronary vasodilation, peripheral vasodilation, platelet inhibition.
• Reduces hypertrophy and left atrial dimensions in some cats with HCM
• Superior to propranolol and verapamil according to one small study
• Role in asymptomatic patients unresolved

Beta Blockers
• Dosage—propranolol (2.5-10 mg/cat PO q8h-q12h) or atenolol (6.25-12.5 mg/cat PO q12h-q24h)
• Beneficial effects may include slowing of sinus rate, correcting atrial and ventricular arrhythmias, platelet inhibition.
• More effective than diltiazem in controlling sinus tachycardia
• Role in asymptomatic patients unresolved

Aspirin
• Dosage—80 mg/cat q 2-3 days
• Depresses platelet aggregation, hopefully minimizing the risk of thromboembolism
• Warn owners that thrombi can still develop despite aspirin administration.

Furosemide
• Dosage—1-2 mg/kg PO IM IV q8h-q24h
• Critically dyspneic animals often require high dosage (4 mg/kg IV) to stabilize. This dose can be repeated in 1 hour if the cat is still severely dyspneic. Indicated to treat pulmonary edema, pleural effusion, and ascites.
• Cats are sensitive to furosemide and prone to dehydration, prerenal azotemia, and hypokalemia.
• Once pulmonary edema resolves, taper the dosage to the lowest that controls edema.
• Not indicated in asymptomatic patients

Nitroglycerin Ointment
• Dosage—0.25-0.5 in/cat topically applied q6h-q8h or 2.5 mg/24-hr patch
• Apply to a hairless area in the inguinal or axillary region or the inside of the pinna. If the pinna are cold, choose an alternate site.
• Tolerance develops with frequent dosing, so use intermittently and with 12-hour dose-free interval between the last dose of one day and the first dose of the next day.
• Causes venodilation, low atrial filling pressures, pulmonary edema, and pleural effusion
• Often used in the acute stabilization of cats with severe pulmonary edema or pleural effusion
• When used intermittently, it may be useful for long-term management.

CONTRAINDICATIONS
Avoid beta blockers in cats with HCM with

emboli; these agents cause peripheral vasoconstriction. If beta blockers must be used in this setting for arrhythmia control, choose a beta-1 selective blocker like atenolol.

PRECAUTIONS
• Arterial vasodilators such as hydralazine may worsen or cause aortic outflow tract obstruction.
• Use ACE inhibitors cautiously if the cat has renal disease.

POSSIBLE INTERACTIONS N/A

ALTERNATE DRUGS

Enalapril
• Dosage—0.5 mg/kg PO q24h-q48h
• Indications in cats with HCM not well-defined—authors currently use for repeat bouts of CHF or pleural effusion
• Potential benefits include lowered angiotensin II concentration, lowered catecholamine concentration, minimizing of diuretic-induced potassium depletion.
• Angiotensin II is a potent stimulator of myocardial hypertrophy.
• Potential deleterious effects are arterial vasodilator induced aortic outflow tract obstruction and hypotension.

Warfarin
• Dosage—0.5 mg/cat PO q24h and then titrate to effect
• Lowers risk of aortic thromboembolism
• A procoagulant effect precedes the anticoagulant effect by several days. Use heparin (50-100 IU/kg SQ q8h) along with warfarin for the first 3-4 days of treatment.
• Raises risk of spontaneous hemorrhage, so requires careful and frequent monitoring

Beta Blocker Plus Diltiazem
Cats that remain tachycardic on a single agent can be treated cautiously with a combination of a beta blocker and diltiazem.
• Monitor closely for bradycardia and hypotension.

FOLLOW-UP

PATIENT MONITORING
• Observe closely for signs of dyspnea, lethargy, weakness, anorexia, and posterior paralysis. • If treating with warfarin, monitor prothrombin time (PT) frequently to avoid bleeding complications. Adjust warfarin dose to achieve a PT value that is 1.5-2 times the baseline value. International normalization ratios (INR) are recommended to minimize the effects of test kit variability on PT results.
• If treating with enalapril, monitor renal function frequently at first. • Repeat echocardiogram in 4 months to assess efficacy of treatment for hypertrophy. If a beta blocker or diltiazem was prescribed in an asymptomatic animal and there is no evidence of improvement, consider discontinuing treatment or switch to another class of medications and recheck the patient 4 months later.

PREVENTION/AVOIDANCE
Avoid stressful situations that might precipitate CHF.

POSSIBLE COMPLICATIONS
• Left heart failure • Aortic thromboembolism and paralysis • Cardiac arrhythmias (e.g., atrial fibrillation and ventricular arrhythmias)

EXPECTED COURSE AND PROGNOSIS
• Prognosis varies considerably, probably because there are multiple causes. Some animals have complete resolution and remain normal after medications are withdrawn. Others show poor response to medications and die shortly after examination. • In one study, cats that were asymptomatic at the time of diagnosis lived from 1 day to 6 years:
    median survival for cats with aortic thromboembolism was 61 days
    median survival for cats with heart failure was 92 days
    cats with a resting heart rate < 200 live longer than cats with rates > 200.

MISCELLANEOUS

ASSOCIATED CONDITIONS
Aortic thromboembolism

AGE RELATED FACTORS N/A

ZOONOTIC POTENTIAL N/A

PREGNANCY
• High risk of complications • Avoid aspirin

SYNONYMS N/A

SEE ALSO
• Acromegaly • Congestive Heart Failure, Left-Sided • Murmurs • Aortic Thromboembolism • Hypertension, Systemic • Hyperthyroidism

ABBREVIATIONS
CHF = congestive heart failure
HCM = hypertrophic cardiomyopathy
IVS = intraventricular septum
PT = prothrombin time
PW = posterior wall

References
Atkins CE, Gallo AM, Kurman ID. A retrospective study of risk factors, presenting signs, and survival in 74 cases of feline idiopathic hypertrophic cardiomyopathy. J Vet Intern Med 1991;5:122.
Medinger TL, Bruyette DS. Feline hypertrophic cardiomyopathy. Compend Small Anim Med Pract Vet 1992;14:479-492.
Pion PD, Kienle RD. Feline cardiomyopathy. In: Miller MS, Tilley LP, eds. Manual of canine and feline cardiology. 2nd ed. Philadelphia: WB Saunders, 1995.
Authors Francis W. K. Smith, Jr and Bruce W. Keene.
Consulting Editors Larry P. Tilley and Francis W. K. Smith, Jr.

CARDIOMYOPATHY, HYPERTROPHIC—DOGS

 BASICS

OVERVIEW
• A rare disease of unknown cause, characterized by interventricular septal and left ventricular free wall hypertrophy • The primary disease process is confined to the heart.
• Causes diastolic heart dysfunction characterized by inadequate filling of a stiff, noncompliant left ventricle. The left atrium dilates in response to high left ventricular diastolic pressures. Mitral valve insufficiency may result from the distortional changes of the mitral valve apparatus imposed by the hypertrophy.

SIGNALMENT
• Has been described in dogs of all ages (10 weeks to 13 years) • Many breeds have been identified, but German shepherds may be overrepresented. • May be more common in males

SIGNS
Historical Findings
• Asymptomatic • Heart failure • Sudden death (especially during anesthesia)

Physical Examination Findings
• Systolic heart murmur • Signs of congestive heart failure (CHF; e.g., dyspnea, coughing, and exercise intolerance) • Cardiac gallop rhythm

CAUSES AND RISK FACTORS
Unknown

 DIAGNOSIS

DIFFERENTIAL DIAGNOSIS
• Hypertensive heart disease • Congenital aortic stenosis • Physiologic hypertrophy (working and athletic dogs) • Hyperthyroid heart disease

CBC/BIOCHEMISTRY/URINALYSIS
Results generally normal

OTHER LABORATORY TESTS N/A

IMAGING
Radiographic Findings
• May be normal • Left atrial and left ventricular enlargement in some animals • Pulmonary edema and venous congestion in some animals

Echocardiographic Findings
• Abnormal thickness of the interventricular septum (most common) and left ventricular free wall • Dilated left atrium in many animals • Reduced diameter of the left ventricular cavity

OTHER DIAGNOSTIC PROCEDURES
Electocardiography
• May be normal • Conduction disturbances (i.e., AV block and bundle branch block) in some animals • ST-T segment abnormalities have been reported.

Blood Pressure
Arterial blood pressure should be measured to exclude systemic hypertension as a cause of hypertrophy.

GROSS AND HISTOPATHOLOGIC FINDINGS
• Abnormal heart/body weight ratio on gross examination • Disproportionately thick septum in many animals • Histopathologic findings reveal various degrees of myofiber disarray and fibrosis. Excessive connective tissue between the intramural coronary arteries has been observed.

 TREATMENT
• Unless there is evidence of heart failure, treat the animal as an outpatient.
• Consider altering the diet to reduce sodium intake if the animal has CHF.
• Restrict exercise.
• The risk of arterial thromboembolism appears to be less in dogs than in cats.
• Warn owners of the risk of sudden death.

MEDICATIONS

DRUGS AND FLUIDS
• Treatment regimens are not well described for dogs; treatment usually similar to that for cats and humans
• Preload reducers (diuretics, venodilators) used to reduce pulmonary edema
• Beta adrenergic blockers (propranolol or atenolol) or calcium channel blockers (diltiazem) can be used to improve myocardial oxygenation, reduce heart rate, improve ventricular filling, and control arrhythmias. The negative inotropic effects of the beta adrenergic blockers and calcium channel blockers may help reduce left ventricular outflow obstruction caused by interventricular septal hypertrophy.
• Since arterial dilation may potentially worsen outflow obstruction by the hypertrophied interventricular septum, afterload reducers (arterial vasodilators) should be used cautiously in dogs with predominant septal hypertrophy. Primary indications for these drugs include improvement in tissue perfusion and reduction in AV valvular regurgitation.

CONTRAINDICATIONS/POSSIBLE INTERACTIONS
• Avoid positive inotropic drugs such as the cardiac glycosides, dobutamine, and dopamine.
• Avoid concurrent use of beta adrenergic blockers and calcium channel blockers, since both classes are negative inotropic agents. They also slow conduction through the AV node, so use with caution in dogs with AV conduction abnormalities.
• When the hypertrophied interventricular septum is obstructing the left ventricular outflow tract, arterial vasodilators should be used cautiously and aggressive diuretic administration should be avoided.

FOLLOW-UP
• Reevaluation of the patient depends on the severity of the history and clinical signs.
• Since this condition is rare in dogs, little information on prognosis is available. If the hypertrophy is severe and the animal has arrhythmias, ST-T segment changes on the ECG, and collapsing/weakness episodes, the prognosis is guarded. • Reevaluation by echocardiography may be useful, since the rate of disease progression may be useful as an indicator of prognosis.

MISCELLANEOUS

ABBREVIATIONS
CHF = congestive heart failure
AV = atrioventricular

Reference
Allen DG. Small animal medicine. Philadelphia: JB Lippincott, 1991.
Author Patti S. Snyder
Consulting Editors Larry P. Tilley and Francis W. K. Smith, Jr.

CARDIOMYOPATHY, RESTRICTIVE—CATS

BASICS

OVERVIEW
• A poorly defined feline myocardial disease caused by regional or diffuse ventricular myocardial or subendocardial fibrosis, sometimes referred to as "intermediate" or "intergrade" cardiomyopathy • Myocardial fibrosis results in both systolic (pumping) and diastolic (filling) dysfunction, leading to congestive heart failure (CHF), arrhythmias, and arterial thromboembolism • May be "final common pathway" of more than one myocardial disease • Usually diagnosed by recognition of "typical" clinical, radiographic, and echocardiographic finding

SIGNALMENT   Cats

SIGNS

Historical Findings:
If cat does not have CHF:
• Lethargy • Poor appetite and weight loss
• Syncope (rare; usually indicates serious arrhythmia) • Paresis or paralysis (i.e., signs of arterial thromboembolism) • Some cats asymptomatic
If cat has CHF, above signs plus the following:
• Dyspnea • Tachypnea • Open mouth breathing • Cyanosis • Abdominal distention

Physical Examination Findings:
If cat does not have CHF:
• Depression • Cachexia • Tachycardia
• Arrhythmias • Gallop rhythm +/- systolic heart murmur
If cat does have CHF, above signs plus the following:
• Tachypnea • Dyspnea • Panting • Cyanosis
• Hepatomegaly or ascites with jugular venous distention • Pulmonary crackles
• Muffled cardiac or respiratory sounds if cat has pleural effusion • Paralysis or paresis with loss of femoral pulses; cold and painful extremities (arterial thromboembolism)

CAUSES AND RISK FACTORS
• True cause(s) unknown; often no "predisposing" disease can be documented • Suspected initiating causes include myocarditis, endomyocarditis, eosinophilic myocardial infiltration, hypertrophic cardiomyopathy with myocardial infarction, diffuse "small vessel disease," and other causes of myocardial ischemia

DIAGNOSIS

DIFFERENTIAL DIAGNOSIS
Other causes of CHF (e.g., pulmonary edema, ascites, exercise intolerance):
• Hypertrophic cardiomyopathy • Dilated cardiomyopathy • Decompensated congenital cardiac abnormalities (e.g., aortic stenosis,

ventricular septal defect, atrioventricular canal defect, and excessive left ventricular moderator bands) • CHF secondary to thyrotoxicosis or hypertensive heart disease
Other causes of syncope, collapse, weakness, and lethargy:
• Arrhythmias associated with any other form of cardiac disease • Arrhythmias associated with metabolic or neurologic disease • Neurologic or musculoskeletal abnormality • Metabolic disease or electrolyte disturbance
Other causes of paralysis or paresis (arterial thromboembolism):
• Any form of cardiac disease • Neurologic or musculoskeletal abnormality

CBC/BIOCHEMISTRY/URINALYSIS
• Most laboratory testing does not contribute to diagnosis of restrictive cardiomyopathy
• Routine chemistry panel (with electrolytes) and urinalysis helpful to document concurrent or complicating conditions (e.g., prerenal azotemia and potassium abnormality)

OTHER LABORATORY TESTS
• Plasma taurine concentration low in some cats

IMAGING

Thoracic Radiographic Findings
• Cardiomegaly with disproportionate atrial enlargement • Interstitial or alveolar infiltrates or pleural effusion with pulmonary venous distention if cat has CHF

Echocardiographic Findings
Note—"Typical" findings controversial; diagnosis of restrictive cardiomyopathy usually based on the following echocardiographic findings (see references):
• Mild or moderate right atrial and ventricular enlargement • Left atrial enlargement inappropriate to the magnitude of left ventricular hypertrophy, myocardial failure, or mitral insufficiency • Normal to slightly thickened left ventricular wall • Small left ventricular lumen size or narrowing in midventricle caused by fibrosis or fibrous bands • Dilation of the left ventricle immediately distal to the mitral valve • Regional wall motion abnormalities or hypertrophy, hyperechoic subendocardial foci, and moderator bands • Normal to slightly decreased shortening fraction
• No or mild atrioventricular valve insufficiency detected by Doppler-echocardiography • Pericardial effusion of variable severity
• Echodense intracardiac thrombi in atria or attached to atrial or ventricular wall in some cats

OTHER DIAGNOSTIC PROCEDURES

Electrocardiographic Findings
• Sinus tachycardia common • Intraventricular conduction defects, including bundle branch blocks • Isolated ectopy, paroxysmal or sustained supraventricular or ventricular tachycardias, and atrial fibrillation • Atrial or ventricular enlargement patterns

TREATMENT
• Patients with acute, severe CHF are hospitalized for emergency care
• Severely dyspneic animals should be given oxygen
• Life-threatening pleural effusions are reduced by thoracocentesis
• Low stress environment important
• Heating pad may be necessary for hypothermic patients
• Low salt diet may decrease fluid retention

MEDICATIONS

DRUGS AND FLUIDS

Acute CHF
• Parenteral administration of furosemide (0.5 - 2 mg/kg IV, IM, SC q8h-q24h)
• Dermal application of nitroglycerine ointment (2%, 1/8-1/4 inch q12h)
• Oxygen delivered by cage, mask, nasal tube (beware of stress to patient)
• Thoracocentesis as necessary to relieve dyspnea due to pleural effusion
• Low sodium fluids administered cautiously if dehydration occurs (beware of worsening CHF)
• Severe supraventricular arrhythmias may be treated with diltiazem (1.5-2.5 mg/kg PO q8h)
• Ventricular tachycardia may resolve with resolution of CHF
• Acute treatment of ventricular tachycardia may include lidocaine (0.25-0.5 mg/kg IV SLOWLY); monitor closely for neurologic signs of toxicity
• Beta blockers (propranolol [2.5-7.5 mg PO q8h], atenolol [6.25-12.5 mg PO q24h]) may be used to treat ventricular arrhythmias but not until CHF is treated (see contraindications)

Chronic CHF
• Furosemide gradually decreased to lowest effective dosage
• Chronic treatment with diltiazem improves diastolic function, decreases heart rate, and improves supraventricular arrhythmias
• Beta blockers may be used to slow heart rate and treat supraventricular or ventricular arrhythmias
• Enalapril (0.25-0.5 mg/kg PO q 24h-q48h) may reduce fluid retention and lessen need for diuretics
• Digoxin (0.01 mg/kg PO q48h) may be used if systolic function is impaired or atrial fibrillation is present
• Treat associated conditions (e.g., dehydration and hypothermia)
• Aspirin (80 mg PO q72h) may be administered to prevent thromboembolism, but efficacy is questionable
• Warfarin (0.5 mg PO q24h) may be administered to prevent thromboembolism but is not recommended unless close monitoring and repeated measurement of PT are feasible

CONTRAINDICATIONS/POSSIBLE INTERACTIONS

Contraindications:

• Beta-blocking drugs—atrioventricular block, untreated CHF, bradycardia, myocardial failure, and asthma

• Diltiazem—bradycardia, atrioventricular block, myocardial failure, and hypotension

• Digoxin—azotemia, atrioventricular block, and severe ventricular arrhythmias

• Furosemide—dehydration, hypokalemia, and azotemia

• Nitroglycerine ointment—hypotension

• Enalapril—azotemia, hypotension, and hyperkalemia

Possible Interactions:

• Beta blockers and diltiazem should rarely be used together; combination may lead to bradycardia, hypotension, or severe atrioventricular block

• Use of enalapril in dehydrated or hyponatremic animals may result in hypotension, azotemia, and hyperkalemia

• Chronic aspirin administration may increase risk of renal side effects of enalapril

FOLLOW-UP

PATIENT MONITORING

• Frequent serial physical examinations (minimal stress to patient) to assess response to treatment and resolution of pulmonary edema and effusions • Frequent assessment of hydration and renal function important in first few days of treatment to avoid overdiuresis and azotemia • Repeated thoracocentesis may be necessary to maintain effusions at level compatible with comfort. • Radiographs may be repeated in 12-24 hours to monitor pulmonary infiltrate resolution. • Electrolytes (especially creatinine and potassium) should be monitored closely during first 3-5 days of treatment to detect dehydration, renal failure, and hypokalemia (caused by diuretic administration and anorexia) or hyperkalemia (if enalapril is administered) • Do not apply strict dietary changes during acute CHF; encourage appetite by hand feeding, if necessary. • Perform physical examination and electrolyte analysis after approximately 10-14 days of treatment. • ECG and radiographs are repeated at clinician's discretion. • Stable patients are reevaluated every 2-4 months or more frequently if problems develop.

EXPECTED COURSE AND PROGNOSIS

Most cats with restrictive cardiomyopathy and CHF live 3-12 months, some to 2 years

MISCELLANEOUS

ASSOCIATED CONDTIONS

Aortic thromboembolism

SEE ALSO

• Aortic thromboembolism
• Congestive heart failure, left-sided
• Congestive heart failure, right-sided

SYNONYMS

• Intermediate cardiomyopathy
• Intergrade cardiomyopathy

ABBREVIATIONS

CHF = congestive heart failure
PT = prothrombin time

Reference

Bonagura JD. Cardiovascular diseases. In: Sherding RG, ed. The cat. Diseases and clinical management. 2nd ed. New York: Churchill Livingstone, 1994.

Pion PD, Kienle RD. Feline cardiomyopathy. In: Miller MS, Tilley LP, eds. Manual of canine and feline cardiology. 2nd ed. Philadelphia: WB Saunders, 1995.

Author Rebecca L. Stepien

Consulting Editors Larry P. Tilley and Francis W. K. Smith Jr.

CARNITINE DEFICIENCY

BASICS

OVERVIEW

• The diagnosis of l-carnitine deficiency has been limited to dogs with dilated cardiomyopathy (DCM). • Probably represents a myocardial, l-carnitine membrane transport defect. • Evidence suggests (with 95% confidence) that from 17–60% of dogs with DCM have associated myocardial l-carnitine deficiency, but this does not prove that l-carnitine deficiency causes DCM.

SIGNALMENT

• Large-breed dogs: boxers, Doberman pinschers, Great Danes • Cocker spaniels • Has not been reported in cats

SIGNS

Historical Findings
• See Cardiomyopathy, Dilated—Dogs

Physical Examination Findings
• See Cardiomyopathy, Dilated—Dogs

CAUSES AND RISK FACTORS N/A

DIAGNOSIS

DIFFERENTIAL DIAGNOSIS
See Cardiomyopathy, Dilated—Dogs

CBC/BIOCHEMISTRY/URINALYSIS
Normal

OTHER LABORATORY TESTS
• Plasma carnitine concentration is often normal or high, and thus it is a poor indicator of myocardial carnitine concentration.

IMAGING
See Cardiomyopathy, Dilated—Dogs

OTHER DIAGNOSTIC TESTS
• Endomyocardial biopsy with quantitative carnitine analysis is the only way to confirm myocardial carnitine deficiency.

TREATMENT

• Treatment with l-carnitine does not replace conventional treatment for DCM.
• The efficacy of this therapy is not known.
• Dogs with l-carnitine deficiency should be treated the same as those with DCM.

MEDICATIONS

DRUGS AND FLUIDS
Carnitine supplementation:
• Large-breed dogs, 2 g PO q8h-q12h
• Cocker spaniel,1 g PO q8h-q12h

CONTRAINDICATIONS/POSSIBLE INTERACTIONS
• None have been identified
• Mild diarrhea has been associated with supraphysiologic doses of carnitine

FOLLOW-UP

Repeat echocardiogram 4-6 months after initiating l-carnitine supplementation to assess the efficacy of treatment

MISCELLANEOUS

• With the exception of one study (two boxers), little information is available to support the efficacy of l-carnitine supplementation in dogs with DCM. • Available over-the-counter in health food stores

ABBREVIATIONS
DCM = dilated cardiomyopathy

Reference

Keene BW. L-carnitine supplementation in the therapy of canine dilated cardiomyopathy. Vet Clin North Am (Small Anim Prac) 1991;21:1005-1010.

Author Matthew W. Miller
Consulting Editors Larry P. Tilley and Francis W. K. Smith, Jr.

BASICS

OVERVIEW
• Syndrome in people typified by regional lymphadenopathy after a cat scratch or bite distal to the involved lymph node • Agents—small, curved, argyrophilic, gram-negative rod Bartonella henselae (formerly Rochalimaea henselae) in majority of cases, Afipia felis reported in some cases • World-wide occurrence • Estimated 24,000 cases/year in United States, with over 2000 cases requiring hospitalization but almost no fatalities

SIGNALMENT
• More males than females (1.2:1) • Majority of cases (80%) under the age of 21 years • Seasonal, with more cases reported between July and January

SIGNS
• Human—erythematous papule at inoculation site (scratch, bite), then unilateral regional lymphadenopathy (painful often suppurative) in 3-10 days (> 90%). Mild fever, infrequent chills, malaise, anorexia, myalgia, and nausea. Atypical manifestations—encephalopathy (7%), palpebral conjunctivitis (3-5%), meningitis, osteolytic lesions, granulomatous hepatitis, and pneumonia • Cats—no signs of illness; high percentage of cats are seropositive (5-60%, depending on geographical area). May cause lymphoid hyperplasia in some cats.

CAUSES AND RISK FACTORS
• Contact with domestic kittens and cats (> 90%), particularly young cats with fleas • Scratched by cat (up to 83%) • 95% of cats residing in households of people with cat scratch disease are seropositive • Members of patients' families are more likely to have been exposed to B. henselae

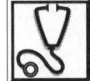

DIAGNOSIS

DIFFERENTIAL DIAGNOSIS
• Most common cause of chronic, benign adenopathy in children and young adults • Diagnosis based on several criteria—history of contact with a cat; formation of a papule at the site of primary inoculation (scratch or bite); compatible clinical picture, usually with unilateral regional lymphadenitis; exclusion of other identifiable causes; characteristic histopathological findings; serologic test (indirect fluorescent antibody) for B. henselae; positive skin test no longer used • Other causes of lymphadenopathy are lymphogranuloma venereum, syphilis, typical or atypical tuberculosis, other forms of bacterial adenitis, sporotrichosis, tularemia, brucellosis, histoplasmosis, sarcoidosis, toxoplasmosis, infectious mononucleosis, and benign or malignant tumors.

CBC/BIOCHEMISTRY/URINALYSIS
Noncontributory

OTHER LABORATORY TESTS
• Indirect fluorescent-antibody test • Enzyme immunoassay for IgG antibodies to B. henselae (Specialty Laboratories, Santa Monica, CA)

IMAGING N/A

OTHER DIAGNOSTIC PROCEDURES
N/A

TREATMENT
• Supportive treatment (bed rest, application of heat to swollen lymph nodes, needle aspiration of suppurative nodes) • Thoroughly cleanse all cat scratches or bites • Prevent cats from contacting open wounds • Immunocompromised persons should avoid young cats

MEDICATIONS

DRUGS AND FLUIDS
• Specific antimicrobials have not been proven to be efficacious. • Most cases spontaneously resolve in a few weeks or months. • In more severely affected patients, antibiotic therapy (gentamicin, doxycycline, erythromycin) based on the antimicrobial susceptibility of B. henselae may be appropriate.

CONTRAINDICATIONS/POSSIBLE INTERACTIONS N/A

FOLLOW-UP
• Complications and sequelae in typical cases are uncommon. • One episode appears to confer lifelong immunity.

MISCELLANEOUS
• Bacillary angiomatosis (a vascular proliferative disease of the skin), which may also be caused by B. henselae, responds to antimicrobial drugs, whereas cat scratch disease rarely does. • Natural host of B. henselae is unknown but a related species, Bartonella quintana, is spread by lice and causes trench fever in humans. • Zoonotic implications of bartonella infections in dogs and cats uncertain

Reference

Groves MG, Harrington KS. Rochalimaea henselae infections: newly recognized zoonoses transmitted by domestic cats. J Am Vet Med Assoc 1994;204:267-271.
Author J. Paul Woods
Consulting Editor Fred W. Scott

CATARACTS

BASICS

DEFINITION
Opacification of the lens. The term can be used to refer to an entire lens that is opaque or to an opacity within the lens.

Pathophysiology
The basic mechanism of cataract formation is thought to be cross-linking of lens protein. The specific causes are numerous and include genetic defects, nutritional deficiency, focal disruption of normal lens metabolism by adhesion to uveal tissue (synechia), radiation, high blood glucose, hypocalcemia, toxins, faulty embryogenesis, and altered composition of the aqueous humor caused by uveitis. Traditionally, cataracts have been referred to as "immature" if only part of the lens is involved, "mature" if the entire lens is opaque, and "hypermature" if lens liquefaction has occurred. The problem with this nomenclature is that it implies that a cataract will progress serially from one stage to the next, and that each stage is mutually exclusive. In reality, an affected lens may contain lens protein that is in each of these stages. Although the lenses of young animals liquefy more readily than those of older animals, some degree of liquefaction will eventually occur if the cataract is present long enough.

Systems Affected
Ophthalmic—the lens

Genetics
Most cataracts are inherited, and the most common mode of inheritance is simple autosomal recessive. Cataracts in some breeds, however, are inherited dominantly.

Incidence/Prevalence
• Although the exact prevalence is unknown, cataracts are common in dogs, representing one of the most important causes of vision loss. • They are uncommon in cats.

Geographic Distribution N/A

SIGNALMENT

Species Dogs and cats

Breed Predilections
• Because so many dog breeds are affected by hereditary cataracts, the reader is referred to general reference texts for a comprehensive listing. Breeds that are affected with hereditary cataracts that typically progress to blindness are miniature poodle, American cocker spaniel, and miniature schnauzer. Other commonly affected breeds are golden retriever, Boston terrier, and Siberian husky.
• Hereditary cataracts have been reported in the Persian, Birman, and Himalayan cats.

Mean Age and Range
Varies depending on the cause. Hereditary cataracts may be congenital or acquired at anywhere from several months to many years of age depending on the breed. In cats, all hereditary cataracts reported to date have been congenital.

Predominant Sex
The sexes are equally affected.

SIGNS

Historical Findings
• Whether signs are noticed by owners is related to the degree of vision impairment. If cataracts occupy less than 30% of the lens, or if they affect only one eye, they often go unnoticed. Owners rarely fail to detect visions problems when cataracts occupy more than 60% of the lens. If caused by diabetes mellitus, polyuria, polydipsia, and weight loss are usually noticed. When owners notice "cloudiness" before vision impairment, most often the condition is sclerosis rather than cataracts.
• Cataracts may be associated with progressive retinal degeneration. If so, most owners will notice their dog having difficulty seeing in dimly lighted conditions (nyctalopia).

Physical Examination Findings
• Opacification of the lens. Cataracts are detected most easily by carefully examining the tapetal reflection for obstruction of light by lenticular opacities (retroillumination). Cataracts appear as a black or grey spots over the bright tapetal reflection. If the lens cloudiness is caused by normal sclerosis, discreet foci of tapetal obstruction will not be seen. A slit lamp biomicroscope is used to determine exactly where in the lens the cataract is located (e.g., nuclear, cortical). • Cataracts that are hypermature have minute crystals within the lens. If the liquefied lens material leaks from the lens, wrinkling of the lens capsule can also be seen. • If cataracts are associated with uveitis, other clinical signs such as aqueous flare, synechia, and low intraocular pressure typically are observed.

CAUSES
• Heredity • Diabetes mellitus • Spontaneous (age related) • Advanced retinal degeneration (response to toxic dyaldehydes) • Uveitis (secondary to synechia formation or altered aqueous humor composition) • Toxic substances (e.g., dinitrophenol and naphthalene) • Nutrition (milk replacer diets) • Hypocalcemia • Radiation • Electric shock

RISK FACTORS
• Faulty heredity • Multiple congenital ocular defects • Disease capable of causing uveitis • Advanced retinal degeneration • Systemic metabolic diseases (e.g., diabetes and diseases capable of causing hypocalcemia)

DIAGNOSIS

DIFFERENTIAL DIAGNOSIS
• The normal aging phenomenon referred to as lenticular sclerosis is often mistaken for cataracts. Lenticular sclerosis does not cause vision loss, and it is distinguished easily from cataracts by retroillumination (see physical examination findings). Sclerosis is not associated with vision loss. • Cataracts may be either the cause or effect of uveitis. Normally, this distinction is made on the basis of signalment, history, extent of cataract formation, and appearance of the cataract. In pure breed dogs with complete cataracts and uveitis, the uveitis is assumed to be lens induced until proven otherwise. Incomplete cataracts associated with uveitis, especially in nonpure breed dogs, are assumed to be secondary to the inflammation. Focal cataracts in cats are frequent sequelae to chronic uveitis.

CBC/BIOCHEMISTRY/URINALYSIS
• Laboratory tests are not usually necessary because most cataracts are hereditary.
• Routine hematologic testing is used to screen for infectious diseases when cataracts are associated with uveitis. • Blood chemistry profiles are evaluated to rule out systemic metabolic disease such as diabetes mellitus and hypocalcemia.

OTHER LABORATORY TESTS
• If cataracts are associated with uveitis that is thought not to be lens induced, serologic testing is routinely done. • In dogs, use serologic tests to rule out systemic mycoses (e.g., histoplasmosis, coccidiomycosis, blastomycosis, and cryptococcosis), rickettsial disease (e.g., Ehrlichia canis, Borrelia burgdorferi, Rickettsia rickettsii), and brucellosis. • In cats with chronic uveitis and secondary cataracts, use serologic testing to rule out toxoplasmosis, feline leukemia virus infection, and feline immunodeficiency virus infection.

IMAGING
• Ophthalmic ultrasonography is indicated when cataracts are hypermature and surgery is anticipated because hypermature cataracts are associated with retinal detachment.
• Ultrasonographic evaluation of the eye is also indicated when complete cataracts are present congenitally to rule out other intraocular defects (e.g., persistent hyaloid artery, persistent primary vitreous, and lenticonus).

OTHER DIAGNOSTIC PROCEDURES
Electroretinography should always be done to evaluate the retina when cataract surgery is anticipated to rule out concurrent retinal degeneration.

GROSS AND HISTOPATHOLOGIC FINDINGS
Lens fiber swelling, posterior migration of lens epithelium, liquefaction of lens material, lens epithelial fibrous metaplasia, and lens mineralization

TREATMENT

INPATIENT VERSUS OUTPATIENT
Dogs undergoing cataract surgery may be managed as either inpatients or outpatients. Rarely is hospitalization required for longer than 48 hours.

ACTIVITY N/A

DIET N/A

CLIENT EDUCATION
• Surgery can normally be done on any hereditary cataract that is causing or is anticipated to cause vision loss. Inform clients that the prognosis for cataract surgery is better if surgery is done early in the course of cataract development, before hypermaturity, lens induced uveitis, and retinal detachment occur. It is not advisable to delay surgery until the animal is blind in both eyes.
• Surgery may or may not be indicated to treat nonhereditary cataracts.
• Because of the high success rate of surgery by phacoemulsification, it is no longer appropriate to observe cataracts for possible resorption, even in young dogs.

SURGICAL CONSIDERATIONS
The procedure of choice for cataract removal is phacoemulsification (ultrasonic lens fragmentation). The prognosis for successful surgery should be > 90%, depending on the stage of the cataract and other concurrent findings. Intraocular lenses can safely be implanted at the time of surgery so that the animal does not suffer extreme farsightedness.

MEDICATIONS

DRUGS AND FLUIDS
Animals with progressing cataracts for which surgery is planned should be treated q6h with 1% prednisolone acetate to prevent lens induced uveitis. The same treatment is normally effective in controlling lens-induced uveitis after it has developed.

CONTRAINDICATIONS
Chronic topical atropine administration should be avoided in dogs that will be undergoing surgery because it causes parasympathetic receptor hyperplasia, thereby contributing to intraoperative miosis.

PRECAUTIONS N/A

POSSIBLE INTERACTIONS N/A

ALTERNATE DRUGS N/A

FOLLOW-UP

PATIENT MONITORING
Animals with cataracts of all types should be monitored carefully for cataract progression. Hereditary cataracts in young dogs can progress quickly.

PREVENTION/AVOIDANCE
Animals with cataracts that are known or suspected to be inherited should not be bred.

POSSIBLE COMPLICATIONS
Cataracts that become complete, regardless of the underlying cause, can potentially cause lens induced uveitis, secondary glaucoma, and retinal detachment.

EXPECTED COURSE AND PROGNOSIS
• Once a cataract develops, its rate of progression varies depending on its location within the lens and the age of the animal. Cataracts that are nuclear in location, because the nucleus is compressed with age, may appear to become smaller. Cortical cataracts almost always progress, except for specific hereditary cataracts such as the posterior cortical triangular cataracts seen in the golden retriever. As the normal lens ages, lens protein becomes insoluble and sclerotic, conditions which inhibit cataract progression. As a result, a small cataract in a 1-year-old cocker spaniel may enlarge to cause blindness within several months, whereas a cataract of the same size in a 10-year-old poodle may require years to cause blindness. Cataracts caused by diabetes mellitus usually progress rapidly. • With appro-

priate surgical intervention, the prognosis for good vision should be excellent after removal of hereditary or diabetic cataracts. The prognosis after removal of other types of cataracts varies with the cause.

MISCELLANEOUS

ASSOCIATED CONDITIONS
See causes

AGE RELATED FACTORS
Although the subject of debate, cataracts can develop as a spontaneous, nonhereditary problem in senile dogs. Age by itself is not a factor in considering whether to do cataract surgery.

ZOONOTIC POTENTIAL N/A

PREGNANCY N/A

SYNONYMS N/A

SEE ALSO
• Anterior Uveitis, dogs and cats • Blind quiet eye • Diabetes mellitus • Retinal degeneration

ABBREVIATIONS N/A

References

Gelatt KN. The canine lens. In: Gelatt KN, ed. Veterinary ophthalmology. 2nd Ed. Philadelphia: Lea & Febiger, 1992: 429–460.

Nasisse MP. Innovations in cataract surgery. In: Kirk RW, ed. Current veterinary therapy XII. Philadelphia: WB Saunders, 1994.

Nasisse MP, Davidson MG, Jamieson VE, English RV, Olivero DK. Phacoemulsification and intraocular lens implantation: a study of technique in 182 dogs. Prog Vet Comp Ophthalmol 1991;1:225–232.

Author Mark P. Nasisse
Consulting Editor Paul E. Miller

CECAL INVERSION

BASICS

OVERVIEW
Cecal inversion or cecocolic intussusception causes partial to complete, intermittent obstruction of the ileocolic junction.

SIGNALMENT
• Reported more frequently in dogs but has been reported in one cat • No age, sex, or breed predilection • Age range: 1-15 years

SIGNS

Historical Findings
• Possibly weight loss • Chronic intermittent hematochezia and soft stools • Non-responsive to administration of anthelmintics, protectants, and antibiotics, dietary adjustment, and motility modification

Physical Examination Findings
• Usually unremarkable • Acute vomiting, depression, dehydration in patients with complete obstruction • Painful midabdominal mass may be palpable.

CAUSES/RISK FACTORS
Cause unknown. Possiblities include parasitism (whipworms) and neoplasia. Intestinal lymphosarcoma has been seen in patients with intussusception.

DIAGNOSIS

DIFFERENTIAL DIAGNOSIS
Any disease characterized by hematochezia and intermittent soft stool must be considered. Rule out parasitism, neoplasia, inflammatory bowel disease, ileocolic intussusception, and infectious bowel disease.

CBC/BIOCHEMISTRY/URINALYSIS
Results normal or nonspecific. Some reports have recorded anemia or hypoalbuminemia associated with chronic blood loss.

OTHER LABORATORY TESTS N/A

IMAGING

Abdominal Radiography
Usually nonspecific unless the patient has gastrointestinal obstruction.

Contrast Radiography
• Upper or lower gastrointestinal positive contrast study—the inverted cecum may be seen in the proximal colon surrounded by contrast material. • Pneumocolon (negative lower contrast study—the inverted cecum may be seen in the proximal colon.

Other Diagnostic Procedures
• Endoscopy allows visualization of a finger-like projection protruding into the colon through the ileocolic junction. • Surgical exploration on the basis of radiologic findings

TREATMENT
Surgical exploration and typhlectomy are recommended. If reduction can be achieved, the typhlectomy is performed from the serosal surface. If the cecal inversion cannot be reduced, then an incision is made opposite the lesion on the antimesenteric border of the colon and the cecum removed from the mucosal surface. In general, a two-layer closure is recommended for the colotomy and typhlectomy.

MEDICATIONS

DRUGS AND FLUIDS
• Standard anesthetic protocols should be adequate.
• Perioperative antibiotics appropriate for colonic surgery can be used as prophylaxis (during surgery and 12 hours postoperatively).

CONTRAINDICATIONS/POSSIBLE INTERACTIONS N/A

FOLLOW-UP

PATIENT MONITORING
• Standard care for abdominal surgery
• Suture removal in 10-14 days

POSSIBLE COMPLICATIONS
• Potential for fecal staining with blood from typhlectomy site for 10-14 days • Potential for colonic stricture if colotomy is required

MISCELLANEOUS

Reference
Aronsohn M. Large intestine. In: Slatter DH, ed. Textbook of small animal surgery. 2nd ed. Philadelphia: WB Saunders, 1993:613-627.

Author Michelle Waschak
Consulting Editor Brent D. Jones

CEREBELLAR DEGENERATION

BASICS

OVERVIEW
• Acquired nonprogressive cerebellar degeneration occurs after in utero or neonatal viral infection in cats (feline panleukopenia) and dogs (canine herpesvirus). • Cerebellar abiotrophy is a progressive, breed-specific, and, apparently, genetically-induced defect of unknown cause and pathogenesis with neonatal, postnatal, and rarely adult onset of signs. Premature aging and death of cerebellar cortical neurons ensue.

SIGNALMENT
• Nonprogressive cerebellar dysfunction—signs appear when patient is 3-5 weeks old; breeds include Irish setter, wirehaired fox terrier, Samoyed, chow chow, rough-coated collie, Border collie, bullmastiff, Labrador retriever, beagle, and other breeds of dogs and cats • Progressive cerebellar dysfunction—signs appear when patient is 6-16 weeks old; breeds include Kerry blue terrier, rough-coated collie in Australia, Finnish harrier, Bern running dog, Irish setter, and English pointer. In the Gordon setter and Brittany spaniel, signs appear when dogs are 6-36 months and 7-13 years, respectively. The progression of signs varies. • An autosomal recessive mode of inheritance is probable in the Gordon setter, Kerry blue terrier, and rough-coated collie; in the English pointer, the disease appears to be X-linked because only males are affected.

SIGNS
• Dysmetria (frequently hypermetria), broad-based stance, swaying of the body, and intention tremor • Menace responses absent in the presence of normal vision and facial muscle strength • Head tilt and episodes of vestibular ataxia with resting or positional nystagmus • Decerebellate posture (opisthotonos with extensor rigidity of the forelimbs and flexed hind limbs) • Alterations of mentation, proprioceptive deficits, and paresis are not features of cerebellar dysfunction

CAUSES AND RISK FACTORS
• Feline panleukopenia or canine herpesvirus infection in utero or neonatally • Poor vaccination history or exposure to a modified live virus during gestation • Breeding affected animals or those with a familial history and predisposition to cerebellar degeneration

DIAGNOSIS

DIFFERENTIAL DIAGNOSIS
• Lysosomal storage diseases are diffuse diseases of the CNS and can be differentiated by the presence of signs related to other parts of the CNS in addition to the cerebellar deficits. • Toxicity (eg, hexachlorophene) differentiated by history of exposure • Inflammatory diseases such as canine distemper and FIP frequently accompanied or preceded by systemic signs of illness and are differentiated by CSF analysis • Medulloblastoma (cerebellar tumor) reported in dogs and cats < 1 year old and is differentiated by imaging (ie, MRI and CT) and CSF analysis. Other primary and metastatic tumors in adult dogs similarly differentiated from late-onset cerebellar degeneration.

CBC/BIOCHEMISTRY/URINALYSIS
Results usually normal

OTHER LABORATORY TESTS N/A

IMAGING N/A

OTHER DIAGNOSTIC PROCEDURES
• CSF analysis—normal in patients with nonprogressive disease; normal or high protein concentration and normal cell counts in patients with progressive disease • MRI—the cerebellum may be smaller than normal • Cerebellar biopsy may be the only definitive means of antemortem diagnosis.

TREATMENT
• Generally as an outpatient unless severe deficits preclude nursing care at home • Restrict activity to areas where a fall and injury can be avoided (eg, avoid stairs, swimming pools, etc).

• Feed regular diet. Restrict intake if vestibular episodes are accompanied by emesis to avoid aspiration pneumonia.
• No treatment available that will alter the course of the disease. Patients with nonprogressive causes of cerebellar degeneration may show some improvement with time as the animal learns to compensate for the disability.

MEDICATIONS

DRUGS AND FLUIDS N/A

CONTRAINDICATIONS/POSSIBLE INTERACTIONS N/A

FOLLOW-UP
• Evaluate neurologic status by serial examinations at weekly to monthly intervals if progression of signs is uncertain. Consider evaluating serial videotapes of the animal to more objectively determine progression. • Cerebellar degeneration has a variable rate of progression of signs, from days to years, depending on signalment. • Do not vaccinate pregnant animals with modified live vaccines. • Do not breed animals with a familial history of cerebellar disease.

MISCELLANEOUS

ABBREVIATIONS
CNS = central nervous system
CSF = cerebrospinal fluid
CT = computed tomography
FIP = feline infectious peritonitis
MRI = magnetic resonance imaging

Reference
de Lahunta A. Comparative cerebellar disease in domestic animals. Compend Cont Educ Pract Vet 1980;8:8-19.
Author Richard J. Joseph
Consulting Editor Joane M. Parent

CERUMINOUS GLAND ADENOCARCINOMA, EAR

BASICS

OVERVIEW
Ceruminous gland adenocarcinoma of the ear is a primary malignant tumor of the external auditory meatus arising from coiled tubular apocrine sweat glands (i.e., ceruminous glands). It may be invasive and capable of distant metastasis.

SIGNALMENT
• Rare but the most common malignant tumor of the ear canal in dogs and cats • No known sex predisposition • Cocker spaniel may be predisposed • Mean age—dogs, 8-10 years; cats, 10.5-13 years

SIGNS
• Similar to those in animals with otitis externa • Early appearance—pale pink, friable, ulcerative, bleeding, nodular mass(es) • Late appearance—large mass(es) filling the canal and invading through canal wall into surrounding structures • Local lymphadenomegaly • Vestibular signs in some animals

CAUSES AND RISK FACTORS
Chronic inflammation may play a role in tumor development.

DIAGNOSIS

DIFFERENTIAL DIAGNOSIS
Nodular hyperplasia, pedunculated inflammatory polyps (cats), squamous cell carcinoma, basal cell tumor, papilloma, sebaceous gland tumor, and ceruminous gland adenoma

CBC/BIOCHEMISTRY/URINALYSIS
Results usually normal

OTHER LABORATORY TESTS N/A

IMAGING
• Skull radiography to determine involvement of tympanic bulla • Thoracic radiography to evaluate for lung metastasis • CT scan useful before radiotherapy

OTHER DIAGNOSTIC PROCEDURES
Cytologic examination of large lymph nodes

GROSS AND HISTOPATHOLOGIC FINDINGS
Histopathologic characteristics—apocrine type differentiation from ceruminous glands and local invasion into stroma

TREATMENT
• Ear canal ablation and lateral bulla osteotomy preferred over lateral ear resection • Radiotherapy for large or incompletely excised masses

MEDICATIONS

DRUGS AND FLUIDS
Chemotherapy not evaluated

CONTRAINDICATIONS/POSSIBLE INTERACTIONS N/A

FOLLOW-UP

PATIENT MONITORING
Physical examination and thoracic radiography at 1, 3, 6, and 12 months after treatment

POSSIBLE COMPLICATIONS
Permanent or transient Horner's syndrome

EXPECTED COURSE AND PROGNOSIS
Median survival for cats after lateral ear resection, 10 months (33.3% have 1 year survival) versus 42 months (75% have 1 year survival) after ear ablation and lateral bulla osteotomy and 39.5 months (56% have 1 year survival) after radiotherapy

MISCELLANEOUS

ASSOCIATED CONDITIONS
Otitis externa and peripheral vestibular disease

AGE RELATED FACTORS None

ZOONOTIC POTENTIAL None

Reference

Marino DJ, MacDonald JM, Matthisen DT, et al. Results of surgery in cats with ceruminous gland adenocarcinoma. J Am Anim Hosp Assoc 1994;30:54-58.

Author Joanne C. Graham

Consulting Editor Wallace B. Morrison

BASICS

OVERVIEW
• Caused by the zoonotic hemoflagellate protozoan parasite Trypanosoma cruzi • Infection occurs when infected feces of a vector (Triatominae, commonly called kissing or assassin bugs) are deposited in a wound (bite site of vector) or mucous membrane, or when a dog eats an infected vector or another infected host (opossum, raccoon, armadillo) in which the organism is sequestered in muscle. Transmission by contaminated blood transfusion also occurs. • Endemic (in both humans and pets) in South and Central America. Most cases seen in Texas, but also Louisiana, Oklahoma, South Carolina, and Virginia. Infected vectors and reservoir hosts also reported in the western (California, New Mexico), southern (Florida, Georgia) and southeastern (North Carolina, Maryland) states. • After local multiplication at site of entry (5 days postinfection), hematogenous spread occurs to most organs but mainly the heart and brain. Organisms become intracellular, multiply, then rupture out into the circulation to produce maximal parasitemias (14 days postinfection) associated particularly with acute myocarditis and, less commonly, diffuse encephalitis. • Parasitemias wane (subpatent by 30 days postinfection), antibody titers rise (detectable by 26 days postinfection), and the dog enters a protracted asymptomatic period (can last for months to years) if he survives the acute myocarditis. During this time, there is progressive and insidious development of myocardial degeneration and eventual dilative cardiomyopathy of unknown pathogenesis.

SIGNALMENT
• Commonly seen in young (acute form—usually under 2 years) but reported in old dogs (chronic form), hunting breeds, more often in males (dogs likely to contact vectors or reservoir hosts) • Cats can become infected, but no case has been reported in North America.

SIGNS
Two syndromes—acute (myocarditis or encephalitis in young dogs) or chronic (dilative cardiomyopathy in older dogs)

Historical Findings
Acute
• Sudden death • Lethargy, depression, anorexia • Diarrhea • Weakness • Exercise intolerance • Mild to severe CNS dysfunction (like distemper) • Ataxia, seizures
Chronic
• Weakness • Exercise intolerance • Syncope • Sudden death

Physical Examination Findings
Acute
• Generalized lymphadenopathy • Signs of both left and right heart failure • Tachycardia with or without arrhythmias • Neurologic signs, weakness, ataxia, chorea, seizures (indistinguishable from distemper)
Chronic
Sustained or paroxysmal tachycardia

CAUSES AND RISK FACTORS N/A

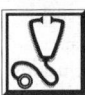

DIAGNOSIS

DIFFERENTIAL DIAGNOSIS
• Cardiomyopathy • Congenital cardiac defects • Traumatic myocarditis • Distemper • Toxoplasmosis • Neosporosis

CBC/BIOCHEMISTRY/URINALYSIS
CBC, biochemical panel, and urinalysis unremarkable.

OTHER LABORATORY TESTS
• Serology (available at Texas Veterinary Medical Diagnostic Laboratory, Drawer 3040, College Station, TX 77840 or CDC, Parasitology Unit, US Dept. of Health and Human Services, Atlanta, GA 30333). Positive titer confirms infection. • Organism isolation into LIT culture (collect 50 ml heparinized blood) • Using the 40 X microscope objective, examination above the buffy coat in a microhematocrit tube (spun down to read PCV) will reveal organisms during period of high parasitemia.

IMAGING
Radiography
Acute
Dilated cardiac silhouette, pulmonary edema (rarely, mild pleural effusion)
Chronic
Cardiomegaly

Echocardiography
Acute
Rarely shows chamber or wall abnormalities
Chronic
Reduced ejection fraction and fractional shortening, thinning of right and left ventricular free wall

OTHER DIAGNOSTIC PROCEDURES
Electrocardiography
Acute
First- and second-degree heart block, atrioventricular block, depression of R wave and QRS amplitude, right bundle branch block
Chronic
Depression of R wave and QRS amplitude, right bundle branch block, ventricular arrhythmias (initially unifocal VPC becoming multiform, then degenerating into various forms of ventricular tachycardia)

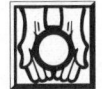

TREATMENT
• Alert owner to possible zoonotic risk and potential for sudden death.

• The acute form invariably develops into the chronic form, which is usually fatal.
• The infected intact female could transfer infection to offspring.

MEDICATIONS

DRUGS AND FLUIDS
• Several drugs have limited efficacy against the parasite during the acute stage, but none produces a clinical cure. Even treated animals progress to chronic disease.
• Nifurtimox (Lampit, Bayer 2502)—investigational drug available only from the Communicable Disease Center (dosage: 30 mg/kg PO q12h, for 90-120 days)
• Allopurinol has some efficacy in humans (use not reported in dogs); try 30 mg/kg PO q12h for 100 days.
• Benznidazole (Radamil, Roche 7-1051, NJ) at 5 mg/kg PO q24h for 60 days markedly improves acute disease in humans.
• The use of ketoconazole has been described but with little efficacy.
• Verapamil (calcium channel blocker) improves acute cardiac pathology and survival of T. cruzi-infected mice. Authors experience of use of the drug in dogs has not been as successful.
• Cythioate (Proban, Cyanamid, NY) at 3.3 mg/kg PO every other day is effective in reducing vector populations.
• Supportive treatment of dilative cardiomyopathy (right and left cardiac failure) and ventricular arrhythmias

CONTRAINDICATIONS/POSSIBLE INTERACTIONS N/A

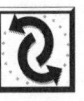

FOLLOW-UP
• Cardiac disease—prognosis is always guarded • Neurologic disease—prognosis is guarded to hopeless

MISCELLANEOUS
Chagas' disease has zoonotic potential, and because it is essentially incurable in humans, euthanasia of infected dogs is an option.

ABBREVIATIONS
CDC = Center for Disease Control
CHF = congestive heart failure
CNS = central nervous system
LIT = liver infusion tryptose
VPC = ventricular premature complex

Reference
Barr SC. American trypanosomiasis in dogs. Compendium Continuing Practice Education 1991;13:745.
Author Stephen C. Barr
Consulting Editor Fred W. Scott

CHEDIAK-HIGASHI SYNDROME

 BASICS

OVERVIEW
• Autosomal recessive inherited disorder of Persian cats characterized by abnormalities in cellular morphology and pigment formation • Enlarged intracytoplasmic granules in circulating leukocytes and melanocytes formed by fusion of preexisting granules • Storage pool deficiency of ADP, ATP, magnesium, and serotonin results from lack of platelet-dense granules. • Prolonged bleeding from trauma, venipuncture, or minor surgery occurs because of impaired platelet aggregation and release reactions. • Normal coagulation times, depressed chemotaxis, no change in rates of infection • Mildly depressed neutrophil counts but within clinical laboratory reference intervals

SIGNALMENT
• Persian cats with dilute smoke blue coat color and yellow-green irises (and white tigers) • Does not occur in dogs • Some Arctic foxes with blue or pearl hair coat color

SIGNS
Historical Findings
• Dilute smoke blue coat color and yellow-green irises • Photophobia (blepharospasm and epiphora) in bright light

Physical Examination Findings
Red fundic reflex (lack of choroidal pigment).

CAUSES AND RISK FACTORS
Genetic disease

 DIAGNOSIS

DIFFERENTIAL DIAGNOSIS
Dilute hair coat color

CBC/BIOCHEMISTRY/URINALYSIS
Romanowsky-stained blood smear reveals leukocytes, especially neutrophils, that contain pink to magenta cytoplasmic inclusions 2 mm in diameter

OTHER LABORATORY TESTS N/A

IMAGING N/A

OTHER DIAGNOSTIC PROCEDURES N/A

 TREATMENT

Provide ascorbic acid (vitamin C) to increase cyclic guanosine monophosphate concentration, and to improve cell and platelet function (no controlled studies in cats).

 MEDICATIONS

DRUGS AND FLUIDS
Ascorbic acid (100 mg PO q8hr)

CONTRAINDICATIONS/POSSIBLE INTERACTIONS N/A

 FOLLOW-UP

PATIENT MONITORING N/A

PREVENTION/AVOIDANCE
• Advise owner of potential for prolonged bleeding following trauma, venipuncture, or minor surgery. • Provide genetic counseling to eliminate Chediak-Higashi syndrome from breeding animals. • Neuter affected and carrier animals, or advise owner not to breed.

POSSIBLE COMPLICATIONS
Prolonged bleeding time

EXPECTED COURSE AND PROGNOSIS
Normal lifespan

 MISCELLANEOUS

ASSOCIATED CONDITIONS None

AGE-RELATED FACTORS None

ZOONOTIC POTENTIAL None

PREGNANCY None

SYNONYMS None

ABBREVIATIONS
ADP = Adenosine diphosphate
ATP = Adenosine triphosphate

Reference
August JR. Consultations in feline internal medicine. 2nd ed. Philadelphia: WB Saunders, 1994.

Author Kenneth S. Latimer
Contributing Editor Alan H. Rebar

BASICS

OVERVIEW
Two most common types of chemodectoma are aortic body tumor in the heart-base region and carotid body tumor in the neck.

SIGNALMENT
• Rare in cats • Uncommon in dogs • 80-90% of chemodectomas in dogs are aortic body tumors. • Affected dogs are 10-15 years old • Boxers and Boston terriers most commonly affected • Males predisposed to aortic body tumors, but no sex predilection for carotid body tumors

SIGNS

Aortic Body Tumor
• Signs of congestive heart failure • Coughing • Dyspnea

Carotid Body Tumor
• Regurgitation • Dysphagia • Neck mass • Arteriovenous fistula in the neck

Aortic and Carotid Body Tumors
• Sudden death if acute hemorrhage from invaded blood vessels • Distant metastasis with associated signs of organ dysfunction in up to 20% of patients • Local invasion of blood vessels in up to 50% of patients

CAUSES AND RISK FACTORS
• Chronic hypoxemia is a suspected risk factor. This may explain the predisposition of the brachycephalic breeds.

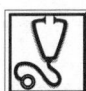

DIAGNOSIS

DIFFERENTIAL DIAGNOSIS
• Congestive heart failure • Megaesophagus • Thyroid carcinoma

CBC/BIOCHEMISTRY/URINALYSIS
• Anemia from bleeding • Nucleated RBC without anemia in some animals • High liver enzymes, BUN, and creatinine with metastasis to liver or kidneys

IMAGING
Thoracic radiography to identify heart-base mass, lung metastasis, or vertebral invasion in animals with aortic body tumor

OTHER DIAGNOSTIC PROCEDURES
Histopathologic examination to differentiate chemodectoma from other tumors

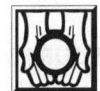

TREATMENT
• Surgical removal difficult because the tumors are highly invasive. Debulking may be the treatment of choice, especially if the masses are somewhat freely movable.
• Radiotherapy has been used successfully as adjuvant treatment to surgery in two dogs with carotid body tumor.

MEDICATIONS

DRUGS AND FLUIDS
• Treatment with chemotherapy has not been reported.
• This author treated one dog with a metastatic carotid body tumor with doxorubicin and cyclophosphamide. Partial remission was achieved and the dog lived 15 months.

CONTRAINDICATIONS/POSSIBLE INTERACTIONS
Doxorubicin should not be used in animals with congestive heart failure.

FOLLOW-UP
• Thoracic radiography and physical examination every 3 months to monitor for recurrence and metastasis.
• Median survival time in dogs with carotid body tumors after surgery, 23 months
• Survival of two dogs treated by surgery and radiotherapy were 6 and 27 months, respectively

MISCELLANEOUS N/A

Reference

Obradovich JE, Withrow SJ, Powers BE, et al. Carotid body tumors in the dog: eleven cases (1978-1988). J Vet Intern Med 1992;6:96-101.

Author Terrance A. Hamilton
Consulting Editor Wallace B. Morrison

CHEYLETIELLOSIS

BASICS

OVERVIEW
• A highly contagious parasitic skin disease of dogs, cats, and rabbits caused by infestation with Cheyletiella spp. mites • Clinical signs of scaling and pruritus can mimic other, more common diseases. • Often referred to as "walking dandruff" due to the large mite size and excessive scaling • Prevalence varies by geographic region due to variation of mite susceptibility to common flea control insecticides • Human (zoonotic) lesions can occur.

SIGNALMENT
• Young animals, and those frequently in contact with others, are most at risk.
• Common sources of infestation include animal shelters, breeders, and grooming establishments.

SIGNS
• Scaling is the most important clinical sign of disease and is most severe in the chronically infested and debilitated animal. • A dorsal orientation to lesions is commonly noted, and scaling may be diffuse or plaque-like. Underlying skin irritation may be minimal. Cats may exhibit bizarre behavioral signs or excessive grooming as well as bilaterally symmetrical alopecia. • Pruritus can vary from none to severe depending upon the individual's response to infestation. • Cocker spaniels, poodles, and long-haired cats are common asymptomatic carriers. • Infestation may be suspected only after lesions in humans have developed. In humans, pruritic papular rash may develop in areas of contact with the pet.

CAUSES AND RISK FACTORS N/A

DIAGNOSIS

DIFFERENTIAL DIAGNOSIS
• Cheyletiellosis should be considered in every case of scaling with or without pruritus.
• Seborrhea, flea allergic dermatitis, Sarcoptes spp. mite infestation, atopy, food hypersensitivity, and idiopathic pruritus are common differentials.

CBC/BIOCHEMISTRY/URINALYSIS
N/A

OTHER LABORATORY TESTS N/A

IMAGING N/A

OTHER DIAGNOSTIC PROCEDURES
• Examination of epidermal debris is very effective in diagnosing infestation. Cheyletiella mites are large and can be visualized using a simple, handheld magnifying lens. • Debris may be collected using flea combing (most effective), skin scraping, and acetate tape preparation techniques. Scales and hair may be examined under low magnification; staining is not necessary. • Response to the use of insecticide preparations may be required to definitively diagnose suspicious cases in which mites cannot be identified.

TREATMENT
• All animals in the household must be treated.
• Long coats should be clipped to facilitate treatment.
• Six to eight weekly baths to remove scale, followed by rinses with an insecticide, is the mainstay of treatment.
• Lime-sulfur and pyrethrin rinses are recommended for cats, kittens, puppies, and rabbits.
• Pyrethrin or organophosphates are recommended for dogs.
• Routine flea sprays and powders are not always effective.
• Environmental treatment with frequent cleanings and insecticide sprays is important to eliminate infestation.
• Combs, brushes, and grooming utensils should be discarded or thoroughly disinfected prior to reuse.

MEDICATIONS

DRUGS AND FLUIDS
• Alternatives (or additions) to topical therapy include the use of amitraz or ivermectin.
• Amitraz can be used on dogs at two-week intervals for four rinses.
• Ivermectin is highly effective against Cheyletiella mites. Three subcutaneous injections of 300 μg/kg are administered at two-week intervals. Dogs, cats, and rabbits over three months of age may be safely treated. Topical therapy should also be performed on these animals.

CONTRAINDICATIONS/POSSIBLE INTERACTIONS
Ivermectin is not FDA-approved for this use in dogs, cats, or rabbits. Therefore, client disclosure and consent is paramount prior to administration of ivermectin. In addition, several breeds of dogs have shown high sensitivity to this medication and should not be treated.

FOLLOW-UP

• Treatment failure necessitates re-evaluation for other causes of pruritus and scaling.
• Re-infestation may indicate contact with an asymptomatic carrier or the presence of an unidentified source of mites (e.g., untreated bedding).

MISCELLANEOUS

Reference

Moriello KA. Cheyletiellosis. In: Griffin CE, Kwochka KW, MacDonald JM, eds. Current veterinary dermatology: the science and art of therapy. St. Louis: Mosby Year Book, 1993.

Author Alexander H. Werner
Consulting Editor Lowell Ackerman

CHLAMYDIOSIS—CATS

BASICS

DEFINITION
A chronic respiratory infection of cats caused by an intracellular bacterium, characterized by conjunctivitis with mild upper respiratory signs, and mild pneumonitis

Pathophysiology
The bacterium replicates on the mucosa of the upper and lower respiratory epithelium, producing a persistent commensal flora that causes a local irritation with resulting mild upper and lower respiratory signs. C. psittaci can also colonize the mucosa of the gastrointestinal tract and the reproductive tract. The incubation period of 7-10 days is longer than that for other common respiratory pathogens of the cat.

Systems Affected
• Respiratory—mild rhinitis, bronchitis, and bronchiolitis • Ophthalmic—chronic conjunctivitis, often unilateral, but may be bilateral • Gastrointestinal—infection without clinical disease usually occurs in the cat. Other species infected with chlamydia may have clinical gastroenteritis. • Reproductive—infection may occur in the cat but without clinical disease. Other species, such as sheep, infected with other strains of the organism may experience outbreaks of abortion.

Genetics None

Incidence/Prevalence
The prevalence of Chlamydia psittaci in the feline population is not uncommon, with various studies indicating that 5-10% of the cat population is chronically infected. The incidence of clinical disease is sporadic, but outbreaks of respiratory disease may occur, especially in multicat facilities.

Geographic Distribution Worldwide

SIGNALMENT
Species Cats, humans

Breed Predilections None

Mean Age and Range
Kittens 2-6 months of age usually are affected, although the organism can produce disease in any age cat.

Predominant Sex None

SIGNS
General Comments
Infection in the cat is often subclinical, with clinical disease only occurring as a coinfection by other organisms.

Historical Findings
• Upper respiratory infection, with some sneezing, watery eyes, and coughing • Some cats exhibit difficult breathing. • Varying degrees of anorexia

Physical Examination Findings
• Conjunctivitis, often granular and starting unilateral but sometimes becoming bilateral. • Lacrimation, photophobia, and blepharospasm may occur. • Rhinitis with nasal discharge may occur but is usually mild. • Pneumonitis may occur with the inflammatory process in the alveoli and bronchiolar tubes and airways giving audible rales.

CAUSES
Chlamydia psittaci, an obligate intracellular bacterium

RISK FACTORS
• Concurrent infections with other respiratory pathogens • Lack of vaccination against C. psittaci • Multicat facilities, especially adoption shelters and breeding catteries

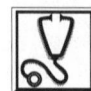

DIAGNOSIS

DIFFERENTIAL DIAGNOSIS
• Feline viral rhinotracheitis—shorter incubation period of 4-5 days, rapid bilateral conjunctivitis, severe sneezing, and ulcerative keratitis • Feline calicivirus infection—short incubation period of 3-5 days, ulcerative stomatitis, and severe pneumonia • Feline reovirus infection—very mild upper respiratory infection with a short incubation and duration of disease • Bronchial pneumonia caused by bacteria such as Bordetella bronchiseptica—localized areas of density within the lungs on radiographs

CBC/BIOCHEMISTRY/URINALYSIS
Routine laboratory tests reveal bacterial infection indicated by leukocytosis.

OTHER LABORATORY TESTS
None

IMAGING
Radiographs of lungs may be helpful in cats with pneumonitis.

OTHER DIAGNOSTIC PROCEDURES
• Conjunctival scrapings stained with Giemsa stain may reveal intracytoplasmic inclusions characteristic of chlamydia. • Swab samples taken from conjunctiva can be submitted for isolation of the causative organism in cell cultures. • Immunofluorescence assay can be applied to smears of infected cells taken from the conjunctiva to detect chlamydial antigen.

GROSS AND HISTOPATHOLOGIC FINDINGS
• Gross findings include evidence of chronic conjunctivitis with mucopurulent ocular discharge, minor rhinitis with nasal discharge, and, in some cats, lung changes indicative of pneumonitis. • Histopathologic findings in conjunctiva include an early intense infiltration of neutrophils, with the inflammatory response changing to lymphocytes and plasma cells. While chlamydial inclusions can be detected within conjunctival cells stained with special stains, inclusions are invisible in routine hematoxylin and eosin (H & E) stained sections.

TREATMENT

INPATIENT VERSUS OUTPATIENT
Generally, affected cats should be treated as outpatients.

ACTIVITY
Infected cats should be quarantined from contact with other cats, and not allowed to go outside.

DIET
Regular diets

CLIENT EDUCATION
Clients should be informed of the causative organism, the anticipated chronic course of disease, and the need to vaccinate other cats before exposure.

SURGICAL CONSIDERATIONS
None

MEDICATIONS

DRUGS AND FLUIDS
• Tetracycline is the drug of choice for treating C. psittaci infections. Systemic infections respond to dosage of 22 mg/kg q8h PO for 3-4 weeks. Ocular infections should be treated with ophthalmic ointments containing tetracycline applied tid.
• Infections generally do not require other supportive therapy, such as fluids, unless complicated by concurrent infections.

CONTRAINDICATIONS None

PRECAUTIONS
In colony situations, the entire colony may have to be treated, and the treatment may have to be continued for as long as 6 weeks.

POSSIBLE INTERACTIONS None

ALTERNATE DRUGS
Other antibiotics are generally less effective than tetracycline.

FOLLOW-UP

PATIENT MONITORING
General monitoring for improved health as treatment proceeds

PREVENTION/AVOIDANCE
Both inactivated and modified live vaccines are available to reduce the severity of infection by C. psittaci. None of the vaccines will prevent infection but will reduce the clinical disease to a mild disease of short duration. In endemic or high risk areas, cats should be vaccinated twice at 8-10 and 12-14 weeks of age, with booster vaccinations given annually.

POSSIBLE COMPLICATIONS

Adverse vaccine reactions, including mild clinical disease, have occurred in a small percentage of vaccinated cats.

EXPECTED COURSE AND PROGNOSIS

Chlamydiosis tends to be a chronic disease, lasting for several weeks or months, unless successful antibiotic treatment is applied. The prognosis is good for eventual recovery.

 MISCELLANEOUS

ASSOCIATED CONDITIONS None

AGE RELATED FACTORS

Chlamydiosis tends to be primarily a disease of young cats. Cats of all ages can be affected.

ZOONOTIC POTENTIAL

C. psittaci can infect humans, with several reports of mild conjunctivitis in humans resulting from transmission of the organism from infected cats to their owners.

PREGNANCY

The role of C. psittaci as a pathogen during pregnancy is not clear. The organism can colonize the reproductive mucosa, and severe conjunctivitis neonatorum can occur in neonatal kittens infected at or shortly after birth.

SYNONYMS

Feline pneumonitis

SEE ALSO   N/A

References

Ford RB. Role of infectious agents in respiratory disease. Vet Clin North Am (Small Anim Pract) 1993;23:17-35.

Ford RB, Levy JK. Infectious diseases of the respiratory tract. In: Sherding RG, ed. The cat: diseases and clinical management. New York: Churchill Livingstone, 1994:489-500.

Gaskell RM. Upper respiratory disease in the cat (including chlamydia): control and prevention. Feline Pract 1993;21(2):29-34.

Greene CE. Chlamydial infections. In: Greene CE, ed. Infectious diseases of the dog and cat. Philadelphia: WB Saunders, 1990:443-449.

Hoover EA. Viral respiratory diseases and chlamydiosis. In: Holzworth J, ed. Diseases of the cat. Philadelphia: WB Saunders, 1987:214-237.

Author Fred W. Scott

Consulting Editor Fred W. Scott

CHOCOLATE TOXICITY

 **BASICS**

DEFINITION

Acute gastroenteric, neurologic, and cardiac toxicosis caused by excessive intake of methylxanthine alkaloids present in chocolate.

Pathophysiology

Methylxanthine alkaloids (primarily theobromine and caffeine) inhibit adenosine receptors, which leads to vasoconstriction, tachycardia, and CNS stimulation. Also, inhibition of phosphodiesterase increases cyclic AMP which potentiates catecholamine effects, causing catecholamine release to increase. Combined effects of these pathways results in cerebral vasoconstriction, cardiac muscle contraction, and CNS stimulation and seizures.

Systems Affected

• Gastrointestinal—early onset of vomiting and diarrhea which may be mediated centrally and result even from parenteral administration of methylxanthine alkaloids. • Nervous —stimulation with enhanced alertness and reflex hyperactivity, tremors, and seizures. • Cardiovascular—increased myocardial contractility and tachyarrhythmias.

Genetics N/A

Incidence/Prevalence

• Excessive and inadvertent chocolate ingestion by dogs is among the 20 most common poisonings reported in recent literature and by the National Animal Poison Control Center and the Hennepin County (Minneapolis) Poison Control Center. • Poisoning is more common at holiday times when chocolate products and candies are readily available. • Caffeine-containing stimulant tablets are an occasional source of methylxanthine poisoning.

Geographic Distribution

Urban and indoor dogs may be more at risk due to their close proximity to chocolate products.

SIGNALMENT

Species

Predominantly dogs

Breed Predilections

Small dogs may be more at risk because of amount of chocolate available relative to body weight.

Mean Age and Range

Puppies and young dogs may be more likely to ingest large amounts of unusual foods.

Predominant Sex N/A

SIGNS

Historical Findings

• History of recent chocolate ingestion • Vomiting and diarrhea are often the first signs reported (2-4 hours after ingestion). • Affected dogs show early restlessness and

enhanced activity. • Polyuria may result from diuretic action of methylxanthines. • Advanced signs include stiffness, excitement, seizures, and hyperreflexia.

Physical Examination Findings

• Hyperthermia • Hyperreflexia • Muscle rigidity • Tachypnea • Tachycardia • Hypotension. • Advanced signs lead to cardiac failure, weakness, coma, and death. • Death occurs 12-36 hours after ingestion.

CAUSES

Most toxic ingestions are of different forms of processed chocolate used in candies and baking, since these contain high concentrations of theobromine and caffeine. Examples of products with high methylxanthine concentrations:

Product:	Methylxanthines (mg/ounce)
Cacao bean	400-1500
Baking chocolate	450
Semi-sweet chocolate	260
Milk chocolate	60
Hot chocolate	12
White chocolate	1

Minimum lethal dosage of caffeine and theobromine in dogs ranges from 100-200 mg/kg. One-quarter ounce of baking chocolate or 2 ounces of milk chocolate per kilogram of body weight is a potential lethal dosage in dogs. Thus, 1 pound of milk chocolate or four ounces of baking chocolate could be lethal to a 16-lb dog.

RISK FACTORS

• Dogs most commonly affected because they consume large amounts of unusual foods quickly. • Chocolate is highly palatable and attractive, and often readily available and unprotected in homes and kitchens. • Methylxanthine alkaloids are readily and rapidly absorbed and only slightly bound (20%) to plasma proteins.

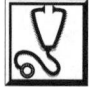 **DIAGNOSIS**

DIFFERENTIAL DIAGNOSES

• Convulsant or excitatory alkaloids (e.g., strychnine, amphetamine, nicotine, and 4-aminopyridine) • Convulsant pesticides, ie, cyclodiene chlorinated hydrocarbons (e.g., chlordane, toxaphene, and lindane) • Tremorgenic mycotoxins (e.g., penitrem A and aflatrem) • Acute psychogenic drugs (e.g., LSD and morning glory) • Fluoroacetate toxicosis • Cardioactive glycosides (Digitalis spp, Nerium oleander) • Hypomagnesemia and hypocalcemia

CBC/BIOCHEMISTRY/URINALYSIS

• No changes specific to methylxanthine • Hypoglycemia in some animals secondary to increased muscular activity • Diuretic action leading to low specific gravity • Proteinuria from renal damage in some animals

OTHER LABORATORY TESTS

• Stomach contents, plasma, and urine can be analyzed chemically for methylxanthines. • Elimination half-life in dogs is 17.5 hours (Hooser and Beasley (1986); detectable plasma or serum concentration should persist for 3-4 days).

IMAGING N/A

OTHER DIAGNOSTIC PROCEDURES

ECG can be used to confirm tachycardia and ventricular tachyrhythmia.

GROSS AND HISTOPATHOLOGIC FINDINGS

• Small or large amounts of chocolate may be found in stomach contents. • Microscopic renal lesions characterized by hyaline droplets degeneration, pyknosis, and karyorrhexis have been reported

 TREATMENT

INPATIENT VS OUTPATIENT

If reported by phone, attempt to determine type and amount of exposure. If this is not possible, recommend referral to hospital as a potential toxicologic emergency.

ACTIVITY

Avoid stress and excitement that could precipitate hyperreflexia or seizures.

DIET

Do not feed the acutely affected animal. In convalescence, a bland diet for several days allows recovery from gastroenteritis.

CLIENT EDUCATION

Inform client of the hazards of chocolate ingestion.

SURGICAL CONSIDERATIONS N/A

 MEDICATIONS

DRUGS AND FLUIDS

• Induce emesis ONLY IF THE ANIMAL IS NOT ALREADY SEIZING. Apomorphine (0.03 mg/kg IV) is effective; syrup of ipecac (1-2 ml/kg PO) or hydrogen peroxide (1-5 ml/kg PO) can also be used. • Gastric lavage should only be used before onset of vomiting and other clinical signs, and if emetics are not effective. • If vomiting is controlled, use activated charcoal (0.5-1.0 gm/kg PO) to adsorb remaining alkaloids in the gastrointestinal tract. • An osmotic cathartic (sodium sulfate, 1 gm/kg PO) promotes gastrointestinal elimination of chocolate. • Fluid therapy to correct electrolyte disturbances caused by vomiting may be indicated. • Hyperactivity and seizures are controlled with diazepam (0.5 mg/kg IV every 10 - 20 minutes up to 4 times) • Premature ventricular contractions in dogs should be treated with lidocaine (without epinephrine)

at (1-2 mg/kg IV followed by IV drip 0.03-0.05 mg/kg/min; (Drolet et al. 1984)
• Metoprolol or propranolol can be used (0.04 - 0.06 mg/kg IV) to control serious or refractory premature ventricular contractions at a rate not greater than 1 mg/min. Metoprolol is preferred but may be difficult to obtain. Continue to monitor the ECG and watch for hypotension as a sequela to this treatment.

CONTRAINDICATIONS
• Do not use epinephrine concurrent with lidocaine. • Erythromycin and corticosteroids reduce the excretion of methylxanthines and should be avoided. • Do not use lidocaine in cats with methylxanthine toxicity.

PRECAUTIONS
• Effects of methylxanthines may persist longer than the effective life of therapeutic drugs. Keep animals under observation until drug administration is no longer needed.
• Methylxanthines cross the placenta and are also excreted in milk.

POSSIBLE INTERACTIONS N/A
ALTERNATE DRUGS
If response to diazepam is inadequate, consider phenobarbital (30 mg/kg IV) administered over a 5 to 10- minute period. For refractory seizures, use pentobarbital (3 to 15 mg/kg IV slowly as needed).

FOLLOW-UP
PATIENT MONITORING
• Successfully treated animals usually recover completely. • Watch for mild to moderate nephrosis in convalescent animals.

PREVENTION/AVOIDANCE
Educate owners regarding the toxicologic hazards of chocolate.

POSSIBLE COMPLICATIONS
Pregnant or nursing animals may be at risk for teratogenesis of newborns or stimulation of nursing neonates

EXPECTED COURSE AND PROGNOSIS
• Expected course is 12-36 hours depending on dosage and effectiveness of decontamination and treatment. • Prognosis is good if oral decontamination occurs within 2-4 hours of ingestion. • Prognosis may be guarded in animals with advanced signs of seizures and arrhythmias.

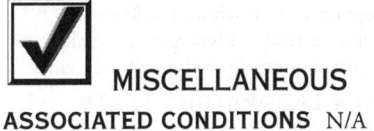

MISCELLANEOUS
ASSOCIATED CONDITIONS N/A

AGE RELATED FACTORS N/A
ZOONOTIC POTENTIAL N/A
PREGNANCY
Methylxanthines are teratogens in laboratory animals.

SYNONYMS N/A
SEE ALSO
• Strychnine Poisoning • Metaldehyde Toxicity • Poisoning (Intoxication)

ABBREVIATIONS
CNS = central nervous system
ECG = electrocardiogram

References
Drolet R, Arendt TD, Stowe CM. Cacao bean shell poisoning in a dog. J Am Vet Med Assoc 1984;185:902-904.
Glauberg A, Blumenthal HP. Chocolate toxicosis in a dog. J Am Anim Hosp Assoc 1983; 19:246.
Hooser SB, Beasley VR. Methylxanthine poisoning (chocolate and caffeine toxicosis) In: Kirk RW, ed. Current veterinary therapy IX. Philadelphia: WB Saunders; 1986.
Author Gary D. Osweiler
Consulting Editor Gary D. Osweiler

CHOLANGITIS/CHOLANGIOHEPATITIS

 BASICS

DEFINITION
Inflammation of the biliary ducts, especially the intrahepatic ducts. Cholangiohepatitis is inflammation of the biliary ducts and liver. Three histopathologic types are recognized: suppurative, lymphocytic, and lymphoplasmacytic.

PATHOPHYSIOLOGY
General Comments
• Concurrent cholecystitis, pancreatitis, extrahepatic bile duct obstruction, and inflammatory bowel disease are common. • Most cats have sludged or inspissated bile which causes partial or complete biliary obstruction.
• Biliary stasis allows migration of bacteria into the biliary system. • Bile duct hyperplasia occurs secondary to bile stasis.
Suppurative
• Bacteria infection possible (15% of affected animals have positive culture) • Escherichia coli most commonly isolated but anaerobes also possible
Lymphocytic-plasmacytic
• Immunologic mechanism proposed as cause; may be preceded by suppurative form
Lymphocytic
• Immunologic mechanism proposed as cause; may be preceded by suppurative form

SYSTEMS AFFECTED
Hepatobiliary—bile ducts, gall bladder, and liver

GENETICS
Persian cats may have genetic predisposition.

INCIDENCE/PREVALENCE
• Estimated to be 4/1000 cats
• Rare in dogs

GEOGRAPHIC DISTRIBUTION N/A

SIGNALMENT
SPECIES Cats and dogs (rare)

BREED PREDILECTIONS Persian

MEAN AGE AND RANGE
• 3 months to 16 years • Most animals middle aged to older

PREDOMINANT SEX N/A

SIGNS
General Comments
• Some cats have mild disease, and clinical signs resolve with administration of antibiotics. • Signs can be acute, intermittent, or chronic. • Suppurative—signs tend to be acute, lasting a few days. • Lymphocytic-plasmacytic—signs usually last at least 3 weeks. • Lymphocytic—signs usually last > 2 months.

Historical Findings
• Anorexia • Depression • Weight loss
• Intermittent vomiting • Diarrhea • Some have good appetites

Physical Examination Findings
• Icterus • Hepatomegaly • Sometimes fever. • Animals with chronic severe disease may have ascites.

CAUSES
• Bacterial migration from intestinal tract is presumed. • Immune response: may be triggered by bacteria. • Bile sludging or stasis

RISK FACTORS
• Pancreatitis • Extrahepatic bile duct obstruction • Inflammatory bowel disease

 DIAGNOSIS

DIFFERENTIAL DIAGNOSIS
• Hepatic lipidosis • Feline infectious peritonitis • Feline leukemia virus • Liver flukes • Neoplasia • Drug induced hepatopathy

CBC/BIOCHEMISTRY/URINALYSIS
Consistent Findings
• Bilirubinuria • Bilirubinemia • High ALP • High ALT • High GGT

Variable Findings
• Nonregenerative anemia • Left shifted leukogram with or without leukocytosis • Lymphocytosis • Hyperglobulinemia • Hyperammonemia • Hypoalbuminemia

OTHER LABORATORY TESTS
• High resting and postprandial bile acids
• Prolonged clotting times

IMAGING
Radiography and ultrasonography may indicate hepatomegaly, choleliths, or biliary sludge with biliary obstruction.

OTHER DIAGNOSTIC PROCEDURES
Liver biopsy is necessary to diagnose the specific disease and is indicated for treatment and to determine prognosis. Clotting times must be performed and abnormalities corrected before liver biopsy.

Laparotomy
• Allows for gross visualization of the gall bladder, common bile duct, and pancreas to assess for involvement. • Specimens for bacterial culture of the liver and bile can be obtained.

Percutaneous biopsy
• Less invasive • Adequate for diagnosis

GROSS AND HISTOPATHOLOGIC FINDINGS
• In most cats, sludged or inspissated bile which causes partial or complete biliary obstruction. • Bile duct hyperplasia secondary to bile stasis.

Suppurative
Suppurative exudate within the biliary lumen

Lymphocytic-plasmacytic
Mixture of lymphocytes and plasma cells surrounding and invading the portal triads.

Lymphocytic
Lymphocytic infiltrate in the periportal region.

 TREATMENT

INPATIENT VS OUTPATIENT
• Initial hospitalization is required for sick and malnourished patients.
• Assuming adequate nutrition and medication can be administered, these animals can be treated as outpatients.

ACTIVITY N/A

DIET
• Highly digestible, protein-restricted (but high biologic value of protein) diet is recommended. Higher protein diets may be fed to cats that do not have signs of encephalopathy.

CLIENT EDUCATION
• Proper diagnosis by biopsy is important.
• Treatment is long-term.
• Some cats have progression of disease despite appropriate treatment.

SURGICAL CONSIDERATIONS
• If the animal is not eating, a gastrostomy tube should be placed.
• Hepatic biopsy is required for diagnosis.
• Surgical relief of biliary obstruction if present. Early relief of obstruction is vital to prevent or control septicemia.

 MEDICATIONS

DRUGS AND FLUIDS
Antibiotics
• Bacterial infection has been associated with all forms of cholangiohepatitis. Aerobic, gram-negative and anaerobic bacteria are most commonly involved.
• Amoxicillin (11-22 mg/kg q8h) has some activity against gram-negative aerobes and good activity against anaerobes.
• Aminoglycosides (gentamicin 2.2 mg/kg q8h or kanamycin 5 mg/kg q8h-q12h) have good activity against gram-negative organisms. They should be combined with amoxicillin in animals with signs of systemic infection.
• Metronidazole (Flagyl) (10-15 mg/kg q8h-q12h) is an excellent drug for treating anaerobic infections; it can be given with amoxicillin and aminoglycosides.

Immunomodulation
• Lymphocytic and lymphocytic/plasmacytic cholangitis are thought to be the result of an immune-mediated process.
• Prednisolone 1-2 mg/kg/day
• Metronidazole (Flagyl) has been reported to modulate cell-mediated immune mechanisms. A reduced dosage (7.5 mg/kg PO q12h) to avoid toxicity due to impaired hepatic metabolism is recommended for long-term treatment.
• Ursodeoxycholic acid (Actigal, Ciba Geigy) 10-15 mg/kg PO q24h has been shown to reduce the expression of self antigens on the surface of hepatocytes and bile ducts.

Other treatment
• Ursodeoxycholic acid (Actigal)10-15 mg/kg PO q24h appears to be beneficial to "thin" bile and reduce sludging. It must not be given until underlying extrahepatic obstruction is corrected. The 300 mg capsules can be repackaged into 30 mg capsules.
• Administer injectable vitamin K_1 if coagulation times are prolonged.

CONTRAINDICATIONS
• Tetracycline—potentially hepatotoxic.
• Chloramphenicol—requires hepatic metabolism and causes anorexia
• Ursodeoxycholic acid (Actigal, Ciba Geigy) if extrahepatic obstruction is present.
• Surgery or liver biopsy before evaluating and correcting clotting abnormalities.
• Aminoglycosides in dehydrated animals.

PRECAUTIONS
• Drugs that are hepatically excreted should be used with caution.

POSSIBLE INTERACTIONS

Metronidazole
• Seizures possible with high dosage; impaired hepatic function may result in high serum concentration
• Carcinogenic with long-term administration
• Cimetidine increases serum metronidazole concentration

Ursodeoxycholic acid
Lithocholic acid, a metabolite of ursodeoxycholic acid, is known to be hepatotoxic. Monitor ALT every 1-3 months during long-term treatment.

ALTERNATE DRUGS
• Immune altering drugs—methotrexate has been used in humans. None have been documented to be efficacious in cats, but they have potential.

FOLLOW-UP

PATIENT MONITORING
• Liver enzymes should be monitored every 2 weeks. If patient with suppurative cholangiohepatitis does not return to normal in 4 weeks, the bile should be recultured. • If no response to treatment occurs in 4-6 weeks, re-biopsy of the liver is indicated to identify new problems. Current thinking suggests suppurative may progress to lymphocytic cholangiohepatitis. • Treatment should extend 2-3 months after liver enzymes return to normal. • Serum ALP and GGT should be monitored for cholestasis and possible cholelithiasis. • If patient is receiving ursodeoxycholic acid, monitor ALT every 1-3 months during long-term therapy for hepatotoxicity.

PREVENTION/AVOIDANCE
Treat gastrointestinal disease aggressively.

POSSIBLE COMPLICATIONS
• Ascites • Hepatic encephalopathy

EXPECTED COURSE AND PROGNOSIS
• Suppurative has best prognosis, but treatment must continue for 4 months. • Lymphocytic and lymphocytic-plasmacytic have poor prognosis. Progression to cirrhosis may occur.

MISCELLANEOUS

ASSOCIATED CONDITIONS
• Cholelithiasis • Hepatic encephalopathy
• Inflammatory bowel disease • Pancreatitis

AGE RELATED FACTORS N/A

ZOONOTIC POTENTIAL N/A

PREGNANCY
Metronidazole should not be used during pregnancy and lactation.

SYNONYMS N/A

SEE ALSO N/A

ABBREVIATIONS
ALP = alkaline phosphatase
ALT = alanine aminotransferase
GGT = gamma–glutamyl transferase

References

Johnson SE, Sherding RG. Diseases of the liver and biliary tract. In: Birchard SJ, Sherding RG, eds. Saunders manual of small animal practice. Philadelphia: WB Saunders, 1994;722-767.

Bunch SE. Hepatobiliary diseases of the cat. In: Nelson RW, Couto CG, eds. Essentials of small animal internal medicine. St. Louis: Mosby Year Book, 1992;398-411.

Center SA, Rowland PH. The cholangitis/ cholangiohepatitis complex in the cat. Proceedings 12th Annu Forum Am Col Vet Int Med 1994;766–771.

Author Dudley L. McCaw
Consulting Editor Albert E. Jergens

CHOLECYSTITIS

BASICS

OVERVIEW
• Inflammation of the gallbladder • May be accompanied by inflammation of the common bile duct (choledochitis), hepatic ducts (cholangitis), or hepatic parenchyma (cholangiohepatitis) • Usually of bacterial origin

SIGNALMENT
• Dogs and cats • In cats it may be associated with the cholangiohepatitis complex.

SIGNS
• Acute onset anorexia and depression
• Vomiting • Icterus • Fever (variable)
• Abdominal pain (variable)

CAUSES AND RISK FACTORS
• Previous biliary surgery, obstructive biliary disease, and bile sludging • Escherichia coli and anaerobic bacterial organisms are the most common causes. • Hematogenous spread of bacteria or local extension from the bile duct • Liver flukes in cats • Biliary coccidiosis • Toxoplasmosis

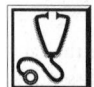

DIAGNOSIS

DIFFERENTIAL DIAGNOSIS
• Pancreatitis • Peritonitis • Gastroenteritis
• Cholangiohepatitis • Hepatic abscess

CBC/BIOCHEMISTRY/URINALYSIS
• Leukocytosis, neutrophilia with or without a left shift. • Hyperbilirubinemia and high alanine and aspartate aminotransferase, serum alkaline phosphatase, and gamma glutamyl-transferase

OTHER LABORATORY TESTS N/A

IMAGING
• Abdominal radiographs are normal unless radiodense choleliths or emphysematous cholecystitis are present. • Ultrasound may reveal a hypoechoic border around the gallbladder wall or irregular hyperechoic densities within the gallbladder lumen.

OTHER DIAGNOSTIC PROCEDURES
Cholecystocentesis and hepatic biopsy should be performed so that aerobic and anaerobic bacterial culture and sensitivity testing can be done.

TREATMENT
• Severely ill patients should be hospitalized and given fluids IV and antibiotics.
• Antibiotic choice should be based on results of bacterial culture and sensitivity if possible.

MEDICATIONS

DRUGS AND FLUIDS
• Initial antibiotic choice should include B-lactam antibiotics (e.g., ampicillin and cephalosporins), potentiated B-lactams (e.g., amoxicillin/clavulanate), fluorinated quinolones (e.g., enrofloxacin), metronidazole, or clindamycin.

• Combination therapy should be initiated in severely ill patients.

CONTRAINDICATIONS/POSSIBLE INTERACTIONS N/A

FOLLOW-UP
• Bilirubin and liver enzymes should be monitored. • Possible acute complications include septicemia and necrotizing cholecystitis, resulting in gall bladder or bile duct rupture and septic bile peritonitis. • Chronic complications can include cholangiohepatitis.
• Prognosis is fair to good if diagnosis is made and appropriate treatment initiated early. It is guarded if obstructive biliary disease or biliary rupture and septic peritonitis develop.

MISCELLANEOUS

ABBREVIATIONS N/A

Reference
Fossum TW, Willard MD. Diseases of the gallbladder and extrahepatic biliary system. In: Ettinger SJ, ed. Textbook of veterinary internal medicine., Philadelphia:. WB Saunders, 1994.
Author Joseph Taboada
Consulting Editor Albert E. Jergens

BASICS

OVERVIEW
The presence of radioopaque or radiolucent calculi in the gallbladder. The pathophysiology is not well understood in animals. Less cholesterol is found in gallstones from dogs than those from humans; cholesterol-containing choleliths are more frequent in cats. Most gallstones consist of insoluble bile salts, calcium, magnesium, phosphorus, and other components including cholesterol. Most are incidental findings not associated with clinical signs. Choleliths associated with disease may cause cholecystitis due to concurrent bacterial infection, cholangitis, or obstruction of the common bile duct or bile ductules.

SIGNALMENT
• Both dogs and cats, but the disease is rare.
• No breed predilection or genetic basis is known. • Disorder occurs primarily in adults. • Females are affected more frequently than males.

SIGNS

General Comments
Choleliths often asymtomatic. Clinical signs most common when choleliths are complicated by bacterial infection, bile duct obstruction, or secondary hepatic involvement (cholangiohepatitis).

Historical Findings
• Severe depression • Lethargy • Anorexia • Vomiting • Diarrhea • Fever

Physical Examination Findings
• Fever • Ascites • Abdominal pain • Acholic feces • Icterus • Hepatomegaly • Depression • Excessive bleeding

CAUSES AND RISK FACTORS
Specific cause(s) unknown. Theoretically, bile stasis, inflammation of the common bile duct, pancreas, or liver parenchyma near the biliary system, and changes in bile composition predispose an animal to cholelithiasis.

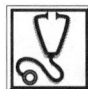

DIAGNOSIS

DIFFERENTIAL DIAGNOSIS
Any disease, disorder, or toxin causing cholestasis or hepatobiliary disease should be included in the differential diagnosis.

CBC/BIOCHEMISTRY/URINALYSIS
• Neutrophilic leukocytosis (inflammatory leukogram), left shift in some patients, and nonregenerative anemia associated with chronic disease. • Very high ALP and GGT, high ALT and AST in some animals; high bilirubin (both conjugated and unconjugated) and cholesterol, low albumin, glucose, and BUN (chronic). Cats may only have high ALP and bilirubin. • Bilirubinuria.

OTHER LABORATORY TESTS
• Moderately high bile acid assay • High BSP retention in some animals • Coagulation assays—high PT due to poor vitamin K absorption if patient has a long-standing extrahepatic obstruction; PTT and ACT are usually normal.

IMAGING
• Radiology—hepatomegaly, calculi if enough calcium is present to make them radioopaque, and loss of abdominal detail (peritonitis)
• Cholecystography used if other imaging methods are not available, but requires general anesthesia and may not be diagnostic. • Scintigraphy used to differentiate extrahepatic biliary obstruction from hepatocellular disease.
• Ultrasonography often the most definitive method of visualizing calculi in the gallbladder or common bile duct; also useful to evaluate the hepatic parenchyma, hepatobiliary system, and surrounding structures.

OTHER DIAGNOSTIC PROCEDURES
• Exploratory laparotomy diagnostic and often necessary to remove choleliths • Once choleliths are removed, they should be analyzed to help determine their cause.

GROSS AND HISTOPATHOLOGIC FINDINGS
Mild cholangitis and cholecystitis are common. Suppurative cholangitis associated with bacterial infection is a relatively common finding in dogs. With chronic cholelithiasis, the bile ducts, ductules, and gallbladder become thickened and contain fibrous connective tissue, which may extend to adjacent portal areas resulting in biliary cirrhosis.

TREATMENT
Depends on the clinical findings —if the cholecystoliths are not causing clinical disease, then a wait-and-see approach is best; if the patient has signs of hepatitis, obstructive hepatopathy, or peritonitis due to gallbladder rupture, aggressive, supportive, symptomatic, and surgical treatment are required. The prognosis for these two extremes are quite different, and the owners should be notified. Diet is not a proven cause of cholelith formation;, it is unknown whether diet will alter the course of disease .

MEDICATIONS

DRUGS AND FLUIDS
• Lactated Ringer's solution with potassium (10-20 mEq/L) at a rate to correct fluid, electrolyte, and acid/base imbalances before surgery; add 5% dextrose if patient is hypoglycemic due to hepatic failure or sepsis.
• Use broad spectrum, bacteriocidal, antibiotics directed at enteric pathogens; best if choice is based on results of culture and sensitivity testing; use amoxicillin/aminoglycoside, cephalosporins, clindamycin, and metronidazole.
• Antiemetics or H2 blockers are used if indicated to control vomiting or treat gastrointestinal ulceration secondary to hepatic disease.
• Vitamin K_1 supplementation—for acute bleeding, administer 3-5 mg/kg/day SC or IM and monitor with coagulation assays. For prevention of bleeding before an invasive procedure, administer 0.5 mg/kg SC or IM q12h starting 24 hours before the procedure. For chronic use, administer 0.5 mg/kg SC or IM q7-q10 days with monitoring of coagulation assays and adjustment of dosage if necessary. Oral absorption of vitamin K_1 is poor due to poor absorption of lipids.
• Bile acid supplementation (dehydrocholic acid is best; chenodeoxycholic acid is less effective) may be tried to reduce bile sludging but should not be relied upon to dissolve choleliths, and is contraindicated if animal has bile duct obstruction.

CONTRAINDICATIONS / POSSIBLE INTERACTIONS N/A

FOLLOW-UP

PATIENT MONITORING:
Monitoring postoperative recovery, fluid balance, and acid/base status may include biochemical analysis, coagulation assays, and ultrasound examination.

COMPLICATIONS/PROGNOSIS
Bile peritonitis due to ruptured gallbladder; abnormal digestion due to lack of bile salts to emulsify fat.

EXPECTED COURSE AND PROGNOSIS
Prognosis good if patient is asymptomatic, guarded in patient with signs of obstructive hepatobiliary disease, and poor if biliary cirrhosis is diagnosed on histopathologic examination of the affected liver and biliary system.

MISCELLANEOUS

ABBREVIATIONS
ACT = activated clotting time
ALP = alkaline phosphatase
ALT = alanine aminotransferase
AST = aspartate aminotransferase
BSP = sulfobromophthalein
BUN = blood urea nitrogen
GGT = gamma-glutamyl transferase
PT = prothrombin time
PTT = partial thromboplastin time

References

Neer, TM. A review of disorders of the gallbladder and extrahepatic biliary tract in the dog and cat. J Vet Int Med. 1992;6:186-92.
Johnson, SE. Cholelithiasis and cholangitis. In: Kirk RW. Current veterinary therapy X. Philadelphia: WB Saunders, 1989;884-887.

Author Debra L. Zoran
Consulting Editor Albert E. Jergens

CHONDROSARCOMA, BONE

BASICS

OVERVIEW
• Malignant neoplasm arising from cartilage characterized histologically by malignant cartilage • Second most common primary bone tumor in dogs, but represents less than 10% of all primary bone tumors • More common in the axial skeleton • Most common primary rib tumor • Must differentiate from chondroblastic osteosarcoma • Histologic grade helpful in predicting survival in patients with long-bone chondrosarcoma • High-grade tumors behave similarly to osteosarcoma in respect to metastatic potential • Metastasizes to any tissue, but lung is the most common site

SIGNALMENT
• Most common in large (not giant) breeds of dog • Uncommon in cats

SIGNS

Historical Findings
• Lameness • Pain in affected limb • Visible swelling at tumor site

Physical Examination Findings
Long-bone tumors
• Monostotic swelling, typically in metaphyseal site • Pain on palpation of tumor site • Pathologic fracture in some patients
Rib tumors
• Asymptomatic palpable mass in thoracic wall • Pleural effusion secondary to intrathoracic extension of tumor in some patients

CAUSES AND RISK FACTORS
Unknown

DIAGNOSIS

DIFFERENTIAL DIAGNOSIS
• Other primary bone neoplasm, including osteosarcoma, fibrosarcoma, and hemangiosarcoma, can be clinically indistinguishable from chondrosarcoma. • Metastatic bone lesion from another primary site • Osteomyelitis (i.e., fungal or bacterial)

CBC/BIOCHEMISTRY/URINALYSIS
Results usually normal

OTHER LABORATORY TESTS N/A

OTHER DIAGNOSTIC PROCEDURES
Biopsy and histopathologic examination of suspected tumor as described for osteosarcoma. Small specimens of osteosarcoma may be misdiagnosed as chondrosarcoma.

IMAGING
• Findings on radiographs of primary lesion may be impossible to differentiate from those of other primary bone tumors—lytic or productive lesions, or both. Lesions in long bones usually located in metaphyseal sites. • Thoracic radiography to detect metastasis • CT may be helpful to determine local extent of disease, especially in patient with rib tumor • Nuclear bone scan or radiographic scan of entire skeleton useful for staging

TREATMENT
• Surgical resection (amputation or limb salvage) to remove primary tumor
• Chest wall resection (and reconstruction if necessary) in patient with rib tumor
• Hemipelvectomy in patient with tumor involving bones of the pelvis
• Consider radiotherapy for palliation in patient with inoperable tumor

MEDICATIONS

DRUGS AND FLUIDS
• For dogs with high-grade tumors, surgery as described followed by chemotherapy with cisplatin as recommended for osteosarcoma
• Chemotherapy for inoperable tumors of little value

CONTRAINDICATIONS/POSSIBLE INTERACTIONS
Cisplatin contraindicated in cats and should not be used in patients with compromised renal function
Doxorubicin should not be used in animals with congestive heart failure.

FOLLOW-UP
• Thoracic radiography monthly for 3 months followed by every third month thereafter
• Prognosis in patients with low-grade tumor of long bones, excellent; cure possible
• Prognosis for patients with high-grade tumors of long bones, guarded to poor; survival statistics similar to those for patients with osteosarcoma

MISCELLANEOUS

ABBREVIATION
CT = computed tomography

Reference
Withrow SJ, MacEwen EG. Clinical veterinary oncology. Philadelphia: JB Lippincott, 1989.

Author Joyce E. Obradovich
Consulting Editor Wallace B. Morrison

CHONDROSARCOMA, LARYNX AND TRACHEA

BASICS

OVERVIEW
• Chondrosarcoma of the larynx and trachea are malignant, cartilage-producing tumors with progressive local invasion of the surrounding tissues. These slowly progressive (weeks) tumors are uncommon in dogs and cats.

SIGNALMENT
• Middle-aged to older animals (5-15 years)
• Males affected slightly more than females

SIGNS

Historical Findings
• Change in voice, loss of bark or purr, or harsh, noisy breath • Exercise intolerance
• Severe respiratory distress, open-mouth breathing, cyanosis, and acute collapse

Physical Examination Findings
• Inspiratory stridor • Laryngeal mass
• Aspiration pneumonia secondary to laryngeal dysfunction

CAUSES AND RISK FACTORS N/A

DIAGNOSIS

DIFFERENTIAL DIAGNOSIS
Laryngeal paralysis • Laryngeal spasm and collapse • Laryngeal trauma and secondary inflammation • Other neoplastic conditions

CBC/BIOCHEMISTRY/URINALYSIS
N/A

OTHER LABORATORY TESTS N/A

IMAGING
• Survey radiography often not helpful
• Thoracic radiography to detect pulmonary metastasis

OTHER DIAGNOSTIC PROCEDURES
• Deep tissue biopsy • Cytologic examination of tumor or lymph node usually nondiagnostic • Bacterial culture and sensitivity rarely helpful

TREATMENT
• Treat as inpatient
• Complete laryngectomy with a permanent tracheostomy has rarely been done in animals but is the treatment of choice.
• Inpatient radiotherapy—rarely reported but not very helpful in humans
• Guarded prognosis because of advanced infiltrative disease at the time of diagnosis.

MEDICATIONS

DRUGS AND FLUIDS N/A

CONTRAINDICATIONS/POSSIBLE INTERACTIONS N/A

FOLLOW-UP
• Repeat head and neck examination with survey thoracic radiography at 1, 2, 3, 6, 9, 12, 15, 18, and 24 months after definitive treatment. • Guarded prognosis because of advanced infiltrative disease at the time of diagnosis • Local recurrence common with extension to regional lymph nodes • Aspiration pneumonia can occur secondary to laryngeal dysfunction or via tracheostomy site

MISCELLANEOUS

Reference
Flanders JA, Castleman W, Carberry CA, et al. Laryngeal chondrosarcoma in a dog. J Am Vet Med Assoc 1987;190:68-70.
Author Kevin A. Hahn
Consulting Editor Wallace B. Morrison

CHONDROSARCOMA, NASAL AND PARANASAL SINUS

BASICS

OVERVIEW
Nasal and paranasal sinus chondrosarcoma is a local invasion of neoplastic mesenchymal cells within the nasal and paranasal sinuses. The disease progresses slowly (months), and most begin unilaterally but progress to bilateral.

SIGNALMENT
• More common in dogs than cats • Median age, 7 years (range, 2-11 years). • Tendency to occur at a younger age than other nasal tumors (64% occur in dogs < 8 years old) • Prevalence of nonepithelial nasal neoplasia in the dogs and cats, 0.3-4.7% of all tumors • Rare in cats

SIGNS

Historical Findings
• Most common signs are epistaxis, purilent discharge, and swelling • Epiphora • Sneezing • Halitosis • Anorexia • Asphyxia during swallowing • Seizures secondary to cranial invasion

Physical Examination Findings
• Noninfectious nasal discharge • Facial deformity or exophthalmia

CAUSES AND RISK FACTORS N/A

DIAGNOSIS

DIFFERENTIAL DIAGNOSIS
• Primary bacterial rhinitis (rare) • Viral infection (cats) • Aspergillosis (dogs) • Crypto-coccosis (cats) • Foreign body • Trauma • Parasitic infection • Tooth root abscess • Oronasal fistula • Coagulopathy • Rickettsial infection • Immune-mediated thrombocytopenia • Hyperviscosity syndrome (e.g., myeloma and polycythemia) • Von Willebrand's disease

CBC/BIOCHEMISTRY/URINALYSIS
Results usually normal

OTHER LABORATORY TESTS N/A

IMAGING N/A

OTHER DIAGNOSTIC PROCEDURES
• Results of cytologic examination rarely helpful • Bacterial culture often positive • Deep tissue biopsy necessary for diagnosis

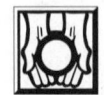

TREATMENT
Radiotherapy

MEDICATIONS

DRUGS AND FLUIDS N/A

CONTRAINDICATIONS/POSSIBLE INTERACTIONS N/A

FOLLOW-UP
• Repeat a head and neck examination with survey thoracic radiography at 1, 2, 3, 6, 9, 12, 15, 18, and 24 months after definitive treatment. • Median survival if left untreated ranges from 3-5 months. • With radiotherapy, 1-year survival rate in 38-57% of dogs and cats; 2-year survival rate in 30-48% of dogs and cats. Median survival 1-36 months, although some report a shorter survival time (< 8 months) in patient with nonepithelial nasal tumor compared with epithelial nasal tumor. • Local recurrence is common with extension to brain. Brain (31%), lung (11% to 19%), lymph nodes (0% to 18%), and liver (0.8%) are reported metastatic sites. • Secondary fungal rhinitis may occur following turbinectomy.

MISCELLANEOUS

Reference
Patnaik AK. Canine sinonasal neoplasms: soft tissue tumors. J Am Anim Hosp Assoc 1989;25:491-497.
Author Kevin A. Hahn
Consulting Editor Wallace B. Morrison

BASICS

OVERVIEW
Oral chondrosarcoma is a malignant, cartilage-producing tumor with progressive local invasion of the surrounding tissues and has the following characteristics:
• Slowly progressive (months) • Uncommon in dogs and cats • Highly invasive to surrounding bone • Metastasis rare; however, lung is a more common site than regional lymph node. • Death usually secondary to local recurrence and cachexia

SIGNALMENT
• Patients usually middle aged • More common in large-breed dogs • Most common location, maxilla

SIGNS

Historical Findings
• Excessive salivation • Halitosis • Bloody oral discharge • Dysphagia • Weight loss

Physical Examination Findings
• Cervical lymphadenopathy in a few patients • Facial deformity

CAUSES AND RISK FACTORS N/A

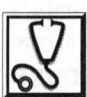

DIAGNOSIS

DIFFERENTIAL DIAGNOSIS
• Osteosarcoma • Squamous cell carcinoma • Melanoma • Epulis • Abscess • Multilobular osteoma (i.e., chondroma rodens; appears radiographically as an osteoma arising from flat bones of the skull; highly metastatic; complete surgical excision uncommon) • Osteoma • Multiple cartilaginous exostoses (i.e., osteochondromatosis; condition of growing dogs; cartilage-capped bony growths from the surface of flat bones; growth stops with skeletal maturity) • Undifferentiated oral malignancy

CBC/BIOCHEMISTRY/URINALYSIS
N/A

OTHER LABORATORY TESTS N/A

IMAGING
• Skull radiography to reveal bony lysis and proliferative changes • Survey thoracic radiography to detect pulmonary metastasis

OTHER DIAGNOSTIC PROCEDURES
• A large, deep tissue biopsy (down to bone) required to sufficiently differentiate from osteosarcoma • Examination of cytologic preparations rarely diagnostic • Careful palpation of regional lymph nodes (i.e., mandibular and retropharyngeal) important

TREATMENT
• Radical excision required (e.g., hemimaxillectomy) and well-tolerated by patient; margins of at least 2 cm necessary
• Metastatic behavior of most chondrosarcomas is low (< 15%); survival improves when excisional margins are free of neoplastic cells.
• Soft foods recommended to prevent tumor ulceration and after radical oral excision.
• Inpatient radiotherapy results are unreported; most chondrosarcomas poorly responsive.
• Chemotherapy results are unreported; most chondrosarcomas poorly responsive.
• Death related to local recurrence and secondary anorexia and cachexia.

MEDICATIONS

DRUGS AND FLUIDS N/A

CONTRAINDICATIONS/POSSIBLE INTERACTIONS N/A

FOLLOW-UP
• Repeat head and neck examination with survey thoracic radiography at 1, 2, 3, 6, 9, 12, 15, 18, and 24 months after definitive treatment.
• Most oral chondrosarcomas are locally invasive, but metastasis is low (< 15%).

MISCELLANEOUS

Reference
Oakes MG, Lewis DD, Hedlund CS, et al. Canine oral neoplasia. Comp Cont Ed Pract Vet 1993;15:15-31.
Author Kevin A. Hahn
Consulting Editor Wallace B. Morrison

CHYLOTHORAX

BASICS

DEFINITION
• Chylothorax is a collection of chyle in the pleural space. • "Chyle" is the term used to denote lymphatic fluid that arises from the intestine and therefore contains a high quantity of fat.

Pathophysiology
• In most affected animals, abnormal flows or pressures within the thoracic duct are thought to lead to exudation of chyle from intact but dilated thoracic lymphatic vessels (known as thoracic lymphangiectasia). • Lymphangiectasia may occur as a result of high lymphatic flows, low lymphatic drainage into the venous system because of high venous pressures, or both factors acting simultaneously. • Any disease or process that increases systemic venous pressures (e.g., right heart failure, mediastinal neoplasia, cranial vena cava thrombi, or granulomas) may cause chylothorax. • Trauma is an uncommon cause of chylothorax in the dog and cat.

Systems Affected
• Respiratory—chylothorax affects the respiratory system by preventing normal expansion of the lungs as a result of fluid accumulation in the pleural space • Chronic chylothorax causes fibrosing pleuritis, which interferes with the ability of the lungs to expand.

Genetics Unknown

Incidence/Prevalence Unknown

Geographic Distribution
Chylothorax has been diagnosed throughout the United States and occurs worldwide.

SIGNALMENT

Species
• Both dogs and cats are affected. • Chylothorax occurs in humans and commonly results from surgical trauma or neoplasia.

Breed Predilections
• A breed predisposition has been suspected in the Afghan hound for a number of years. • More recently, it appears that the Shiba Inu breed may also be predisposed to this disease. • Among cats, Oriental breeds (i.e., Siamese and Himalayan) appear to have a relatively high prevalence.

Mean Age and Range
• Animals of any age may be affected. • Old cats may be more likely to develop chylothorax than young cats. (This may be indicative of an association between chylothorax and neoplasia). • Afghan hounds develop this disease in middle age. • Affected Shiba Inus have been < 1 year of age.

Predominant Sex N/A

SIGNS

General Comments
• Clinical signs vary depending on the underlying etiology, rapidity of fluid accumulation, and volume of fluid. • Most animals do not exhibit clinical signs until there is significant impairment of ventilation.

Physical Examination Findings
• Coughing • Muffled heart and lung sounds • Loud bronchovesicular sounds • Dyspnea • Tachypnea • Cyanosis • Depression • Anorexia • Weight loss • Pale mucous membranes • Arrhythmias • Murmurs • Pericardial effusion

CAUSES
• Anterior mediastinal masses (mediastinal lymphosarcoma, thymoma) • Heart disease (cardiomyopathy, pericardial effusion, heartworm infection, tetralogy of Fallot, tricuspid dysplasia, or cor triatriatum) • Fungal granulomas • Venous thrombi • Congenital abnormalities of the thoracic duct • In a majority of animals, despite extensive diagnostic workups, the underlying etiology is undetermined (idiopathic chylothorax).

RISK FACTORS N/A

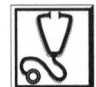

DIAGNOSIS

DIFFERENTIAL DIAGNOSIS
• Any cause of respiratory distress or coughing should be considered a differential diagnosis. • Once pleural effusion has been identified, differentials include diseases that cause exudative pleural effusion such as pyothorax. • "Pseudochylous effusion" is a term that has been misused in the veterinary literature to describe effusions that look like chyle, but in which a ruptured thoracic duct is not found.

CBC/BIOCHEMISTRY/URINALYSIS
• Fluid cholesterol > serum cholesterol • Fluid triglyceride > serum triglyceride

OTHER LABORATORY TESTS
• Comparison of fluid and serum triglyceride levels. If the effusion is truly chylous, it will contain a higher level of triglycerides than serum collected simultaneously. • Sudan III stain for lipid droplets • Ether clearance test

Fluid Analysis
• Characteristics—usually milky white and opaque, but can range from yellow to pink, depending on diet and the presence of concurrent hemorrhage • Protein content—inaccurate because of interference of the refractive index by the high lipid content of the fluid • Total nucleated cell count is usually <10,000 cells/dl

Cytology
Primarily small lymphocytes or neutrophils. Nondegenerative neutrophils may predominate with prolonged loss of lymphocytes, and if multiple therapeutic thoracocentesis, may have induced inflammation.

IMAGING

Radiography
• If the animal is overtly dyspneic, take dorsoventral (rather than ventrodorsal views) and "standing lateral" thoracic radiographic views. • If the animal is not dyspneic, take ventrodorsal and expiratory views. • Radiographic signs associated with pleural effusion include blurring of the cardiac silhouette, interlobar fissure lines, rounding of lung margins at the costophrenic angles, widening of the mediastinum, separation of the lung borders from the thoracic wall, and scalloping of the lung margins at the sternal border (may be the earliest radiographic sign of pleural effusion). • Radiographs should be repeated after removal of most of the pleural fluid. • Animals that have collapsed lung lobes that do not appear to reexpand after removal of pleural fluid should be suspected of having underlying pulmonary parenchymal or pleural disease such as fibrosing pleuritis. • Fibrosing pleuritis also should be considered in animals with persistent dyspnea in the face of minimal pleural fluid.

Ultrasonography
• Perform ultrasonography before fluid removal because the fluid acts as an "acoustic window," enhancing visualization of thoracic structures. • Ultrasonography is used to evaluate cardiac function, valvular lesions and function, congenital cardiac abnormalities, pericardial effusion, and mediastinal masses.

OTHER DIAGNOSTIC PROCEDURES
• Chest compression should be performed in all cats with suspected pleural effusion. A noticeably impaired ability to compress the anterior chest is present in many cats with cranial mediastinal masses and pleural effusion. • Thoracic auscultation may reveal muffled heart and lung sounds, particularly ventrally. • Cardiovascular abnormalities such as murmurs or arrhythmias may be present. • Loud bronchovesicular sounds may be heard, particularly in the dorsal lung fields. • Jugular pulses or jugular venous distension may be detected in association with right-sided heart failure (e.g., pericardial effusion). • Thoracentesis should be performed before taking radiographs in dyspneic animals in which pleural effusion is suspected and asthma, diaphragmatic hernia, and bleeding disorders are unlikely. Removal of even small amounts of pleural effusion may improve the ventilation.

GROSS AND HISTOPATHOLOGIC FINDINGS
• Lymphatics (including the thoracic duct) are difficult to identify at necropsy. • If fibrosing pleuritis is present, the lungs will appear shrunken and the pleura (visceral and parietal) will be diffusely thickened. • Fibrosing pleuritis is characterized histologically by a diffuse, moderate to marked, thickening of the pleura by fibrous connective tissue with moderate infiltrates of lymphocytes, macrophages, and plasma cells.

TREATMENT

INPATIENT VERSUS OUTPATIENT

• It is imperative that the underlying etiology be determined, if possible.
• If medical management is elected (versus surgery), most animals can be treated as outpatients with intermittent thoracentesis as necessary to prevent dyspnea.
• Chest tubes should only be placed in those animals with suspected chylothorax secondary to trauma (rare), with rapid fluid accumulation, or after surgery.

ACTIVITY

• Animals with chylothorax should be observed closely for dyspnea.
• Most animals will restrict their own exercise as their pleural fluid volume increases or as fibrosing pleuritis develops.

DIET

• A low-fat diet may decrease the amount of fat in the effusion, which may improve the animal's ability to reabsorb fluid from the thoracic cavity.
• In dogs, medium chain triglycerides (once thought to be absorbed directly into the portal system, bypassing the thoracic duct) are transported via the thoracic duct. Thus, they may be less useful than previously believed. It is unlikely that dietary therapy will "cure" this disease, but it may help in the management of animals with chronic chylothorax.

CLIENT EDUCATION

Clients should be informed that with the idiopathic form of this disease, there is no effective treatment that will stop the effusion in all animals. However, the condition may spontaneously resolve in some animals after several weeks or months.

SURGICAL CONSIDERATIONS

• Thoracic duct ligation with mesenteric lymphangiography, or placement of a pleuroperitoneal or pleurovenous shunt, should be considered in animals that do not respond to medical management.
• Animals with extensive fibrosing pleuritis are poor surgical candidates and should be given a grave prognosis.
• The reader is referred to other sources for detailed descriptions of surgical techniques for the treatment of chylothorax.

MEDICATIONS

DRUGS AND FLUIDS

• The author has been experimenting with a drug from the benzopyrone family for the treatment of chylothorax in animals in which surgery is not an option.
• Benzopyrone drugs have been used for the treatment of lymphedema in humans for years. Whether these drugs are effective in decreasing the pleural effusion in animals with chylothorax is not known; however, preliminary findings suggest that at least 25% of animals treated with this drug had complete resolution of their effusion at 2 months after the initiation of therapy. Determination of whether the effusion resolved spontaneously in these animals, or was associated with the drug therapy, will require further study.

CONTRAINDICATIONS

Animals with severe fibrosing pleuritis should be given a poor prognosis. Medical or surgical therapy is unlikely to benefit these patients.

PRECAUTIONS N/A

POSSIBLE INTERACTIONS N/A

ALTERNATE DRUGS N/A

FOLLOW-UP

PATIENT MONITORING

• These patients should be monitored closely for the dyspnea and thoracentesis performed as necessary. • If chylothorax resolves spontaneously or after surgery, periodic reevaluations for several years are warranted to detect recurrence.

PREVENTION/AVOIDANCE N/A

POSSIBLE COMPLICATIONS

• Fibrosing pleuritis is the most common, serious complication of chronic chylothorax.
• Immunosuppression may occur in patients undergoing repeated and frequent thoracentesis as a result of lymphocyte depletion.
• Hyponatremia and hyperkalemia have been documented in dogs with chylothorax undergoing multiple thoracentesis.

EXPECTED COURSE AND PROGNOSIS

• This condition may resolve spontaneously or after surgery. • Untreated or chronic chylothorax may result in severe fibrosing pleuritis and persistent dyspnea. • Euthanasia frequently is performed in animals that do not respond to surgery or medical management.

MISCELLANEOUS

ASSOCIATED CONDITIONS

Diffuse lymphatic abnormalities (e.g., intestinal lymphangiectasia, hepatic lymphangiectasia, pulmonary lymphangiectasia, and chylous ascites) may worsen the prognosis.

AGE RELATED FACTORS

Young animals may have a better prognosis than older animals because of the association of neoplasia and advanced age.

ZOONOTIC POTENTIAL N/A

PREGNANCY N/A

SYNONYMS N/A

SEE ALSO N/A

ABBREVIATION N/A

References

Fossum TW, Birchard SJ, Jacobs RM. Chylothorax in thirty-four dogs. J Am Vet Med Assoc 1986;188:1315-1318.

Fossum TW, Jacobs RM, Birchard SJ. Evaluation of chylous and nonchylous pleural effusions using serum and pleural fluid cholesterol and triglyceride concentrations. J Am Vet Med Assoc 1986;188:49-51.

Fossum TW, Evering WN, Miller MW, et al. Severe bilateral fibrosing pleuritis associated with chronic chylothorax in dogs and cats. J Am Vet Med Assoc 1992;201:317-324.

Fossum TW, Miller MW, Rogers KS, et al. Chylothorax associated with right-sided heart failure in 5 cats. J Am Vet Med Assoc 1994;204:84-89.

Kerpsack SJ, McLoughlin MA, Birchard SJ, et al. Evaluation of mesenteric lymphangiography and thoracic duct ligation in cats with chylothorax: 19 cases (1987-1992). J Am Vet Med Assoc 1994;205:711-715.

Author Theresa W. Fossum
Consulting Editors Lynelle Johnson and Bradley L. Moses

CILIARY DYSKINESIA, PRIMARY

 BASICS

OVERVIEW

• Primary ciliary dyskinesia (PCD) is a disorder in dogs and humans in which defective development of ciliary ultrastructure causes ineffective ciliary beat and dyskinetic ciliary movement. • In dogs with PCD, ciliary ultrastructural abnormalities include dynein arm defects, radial spoke defects, translocated microtubules, and random orientation of the central pair of microtubules. • Any organ system that contains cilia can be affected (respiratory, reproductive, auditory tubes, central nervous system, renal tubules), but clinical signs in dogs are primarily referable to the respiratory system. • Normal respiratory cilia beat in a uniplanar, coordinated fashion, carrying the overlying mucous blanket craniad from the lungs (mucociliary escalator). • In dogs with PCD, mucociliary clearance of foreign material and mucus from the respiratory tract by the mucociliary escalator is impaired, causing chronic, recurring, respiratory abnormalities.

SIGNALMENT

• Most commonly in young, purebred dogs; not reported in cats or mongrel dogs • Familial tendencies have been reported in English springer spaniels, shar-peis, and Old English sheepdogs. Other reported breeds include pointers, golden retriever, chow chow, rottweiler, doberman pinscher, Gordon setter, bichon frise, border collie, and dalmatian. • Believed to be an autosomal recessive disorder in dogs and humans

SIGNS

Historical Findings

• Recurring chronic respiratory signs beginning at a young age, although some dogs with PCD develop clinical signs as adults • Good response to symptomatic therapy (antibiotics, rest, fluid administration) • Male dogs may have a history of sterility if sperm are affected (sperm flagella are modified cilia).

Physical Examination Findings

• Respiratory findings are most common and include tachypnea, dyspnea, cough, nasal discharge, and fever associated with bronchopneumonia, bronchiectasis, and/or rhinosinusitis. • Central nervous system findings may include seizures and depressed mentation associated with hydrocephalus (caused by dysfunctional ciliated ependymal cells of the lateral ventricles and impaired cerebrospinal fluid circulation).• Hearing may be impaired (caused by otitis media from chronic obstruction of the ciliated auditory tube).

CAUSES AND RISK FACTORS

• Familial tendency as stated above • Purebred dogs

 DIAGNOSIS

DIFFERENTIAL DIAGNOSIS

• Acquired respiratory tract diseases such as chronic bronchitis, recurrent respiratory infections, and bronchopneumonia • Selective immunoglobulin A deficiency • Host-defense failure syndromes involving cell-mediated immunity, neutrophil release, cell function, or complement deficiency

CBC/BIOCHEMISTRY/URINALYSIS

• CBC may reveal systemic inflammation associated with bronchopneumonia. • Biochemical profile and urinalysis often are normal.

OTHER LABORATORY TESTS N/A

IMAGING

• Radiographic examination of the thorax may reveal a peribronchial lung pattern, bronchiectasis, bronchopneumonia (alveolar lung pattern), and, in 50% of patients, situs inversus (lateral transposition of viscera). • Radionuclide mucociliary clearance studies reveal no cranial movement of radionuclide (e.g., technetium Tc 99m albumin macroaggregated) deposited at the tracheal bifurcation.

OTHER DIAGNOSTIC PROCEDURES

• Less than or equal to 2% of normal respiratory cilia in dogs have ultrastructural abnormalities. In dogs with PCD, electron microscopic examination of cilia of caudal nasal or tracheal mucosal epithelial tissue samples reveals that much greater than 2% of the cilia have abnormal ultrastructure. Transient ciliary ultrastructural abnormalities may be present in dogs with acquired disease unrelated to PCD. If transient ciliary ultrastructural abnormalities are suspected, mucosal biopsies should be repeated or delayed until completion of treatment of the primary respiratory abnormality. • Male dogs may have abnormal sperm motility, and sperm evaluation may be a good screening test for PCD. Confirmatory diagnostic testing should then be performed.

 TREATMENT

• Therapy is based on treatment of secondary bacterial infections caused by ineffective respiratory clearance mechanisms.
• Alert owner to the high incidence of recurrent bacterial infections and that cure of PCD is not possible.

MEDICATIONS

DRUGS AND FLUIDS

• Treat secondary infections with appropriate antibiotics based on microbial culture and sensitivity results (from transtracheal wash, endotracheal wash, or bronchoalveolar lavage samples in the case of bronchopneumonia). The most common organisms isolated are Streptococcus and Mycoplasma. Special media is required for isolation of Mycoplasma spp.
• Intravenous fluid administration, intravenous antibiotic administration, and coupage are recommended for treatment of bronchopneumonia.

CONTRAINDICATIONS/POSSIBLE INTERACTIONS

• Cough suppressants are contraindicated because normal mucociliary transport is dysfunctional.
• Oxygen treatment should be used conservatively because high oxygen concentration may further depress mucociliary clearance.

 FOLLOW-UP

• Prognosis is generally good provided recurring infections are treated appropriately. • Life-threatening bronchopneumonia and sepsis may be sequelae to resistant bacterial organisms from inappropriate antibiotic therapy (therapy not based on culture and sensitivity, inappropriate length of antibiotic therapy, etc.).

 MISCELLANEOUS

ASSOCIATED CONDITIONS

• Kartagener's syndrome, a subcategory of PCD, is characterized by the triad of rhinosinusitis, bronchiectasis, and situs inversus. The incidence of Kartagener's syndrome in dogs with PCD is unknown. • Neutrophil migratory abnormalities have been documented in humans and dogs with PCD, implying abnormal assembly and function of neutrophil microtubules; however, this may not be clinically significant. • Less frequent clinical findings reported in dogs with PCD include dilated distal renal tubules and renal fibrosis.

ABBREVIATION

PCD = primary ciliary dyskinesia

Reference

Crager CS. Canine primary ciliary dyskinesia. Comp Cont Ed Pract Vet 1992;14:1440-1445.
Author Cynthia Crager Ramsey
Consulting Editors Lynelle Johnson and Bradley L. Moses

CIRRHOSIS/FIBROSIS OF THE LIVER

BASICS

DEFINITION
Hepatic fibrosis is accumulation of extracellular collagen and connective tissue within the liver. Hepatic cirrhosis is fibrosis with regenerative nodules.

Pathophysiology
Fibrosis develops as a sequela to hepatic parenchymal damage and inflammation or as an idiopathic event. Cirrhosis is an irreversible sequela to chronic liver disease such as hepatic copper accumulation, anticonvulsant drug or other toxin-induced hepatitis, chronic inflammatory liver disease, immunologic injury to the liver, chronic cholestasis, and chronic hypoxia. A single episode of massive hepatic necrosis can also cause cirrhosis (i.e., postnecrotic cirrhosis). In most animals, the cause of cirrhosis is not apparent. Fibrosis and regenerative nodules impair hepatic blood and bile flow, thus perpetuating hepatocellular injury. Hepatic vascular resistance increases, resulting in the consequences of cirrhosis: portal hypertension, ascites, multiple acquired portosystemic vascular shunts, and hepatic encephalopathy.

Systems Affected
• Gastrointestinal—liver failure, portal hypertension leading to ascites, altered gastrointestinal blood flow leading to gastric and duodenal erosive or ulcer disease, and cholestasis leading to jaundice, and possibly to fat malabsorption and steatorrhea
• Nervous—hepatic encephalopathy
• Respiratory—tachypnea in some animals secondary to pleural effusion or CNS induced respiratory changes; pulmonary edema secondary to hypoalbuminemia (rare)
• Skin/Exocrine—necrolytic migratory erythema, a severe ulcerative epidermal disease
• Renal/Urologic—renal failure as part of the hepatorenal syndrome (rare).

Genetics
• Familial type breed susceptibilities to chronic hepatitis in Bedlington, West Highland white, and Skye terrier, doberman pinschers, and American and English cocker spaniel • Idiopathic hepatic fibrosis—young dog predisposition, especially German shepherd, suggests a congenital or genetic basis.

Incidence/Prevalence
Highest in populations of dogs with known predisposition to chronic liver disease

Geographic Distribution N/A

SIGNALMENT

Species
Dogs and cats (less common in cats)

Breed Predilection
Any breed can be affected but certain breeds are predisposed.
Cirrhosis

• Bedlington, West Highland white, and Skye terrier—secondary to hepatic copper toxicosis • Doberman pinscher—chronic active hepatitis of dobermans • American and English cocker spaniel, standard poodle, Labrador retriever, Scottish terrier—idiopathic. • Cats—biliary cirrhosis is a sequela to the cholangiohepatitis complex.
Idiopathic Hepatic Fibrosis
German shepherd

Mean Age and Range
Cirrhosis
• Dogs of any age are affected, but signs most commonly develop in middle-aged to older dogs. • Bedlington and West Highland white terrier and cocker spaniel tend to be younger (1.5-5 years) when signs first occur.

Idiopathic Hepatic Fibrosis
• Dogs usually < 2 years old (i.e., 4 months to 7 years)

Predominant Sex
• Cocker spaniel—males affected 2 to 8 times more often than females • Doberman pinscher and Labrador retriever—females affected more commonly than males.

SIGNS

General comments
• Signs related to hepatic dysfunction and the underlying hepatic disease. • Signs initially vague and nonspecific with later signs related to portal hypertension and hepatic encephalopathy.

Historical Findings
• Most patients have a chronic history of waxing and waning lethargy, depression, anorexia, and weight loss. Vomiting, diarrhea, melena, and polydipsia and polyuria may be observed. • Later signs may include abdominal distension, jaundice, spontaneous bleeding, and neurologic signs such as personality changes, stupor, pacing, circling, staggering, ataxia, blindness, weakness, collapse, seizures, head pressing, hyperactivity, cervical ventroflexion, head and muscle tremors, deafness, and coma. • Vomiting, hypersalivation, and abdominal distension are prominent findings in cats with biliary cirrhosis or fibrosis.

Physical Examination Findings
• Depression and evidence of weight loss are primary. • Ascites, icterus, and hepatic encephalopathy strongly suggest cirrhosis.
• Microhepatica is typically seen in dogs, whereas normal to large liver size is typical in cats. • Melena or petechial or ecchymotic hemorrhages may be seen. • Necrolytic migratory erythema—bilaterally symmetrical skin lesions characterized by erythema, erosion, ulceration, and crusting. The muzzle, mucocutaneous junctions of the face, and distal extremities are typically affected, and the external genitalia, edges of the pinnas, and ventral abdomen are affected in more than 50% of affected animals. Digital hyper-

keratosis is a consistent finding.

CAUSES
• Hepatic copper toxicosis • Chronic inflammatory or immune-mediated hepatitis • Drug- and toxin-induced liver disease (e.g., anticonvulsant, azole antifungal, mebendazole, oxibendazole-diethylcarbamazine, trimethoprim-sulfa, and phenolic disinfectant) • Viral hepatitis—end stage of acidophil cell hepatitis and, possibly, infectious canine hepatitis. • Leptospirosis (serogroup grippotyphosa) • Cholangiohepatitis complex in cats

RISK FACTORS
• Hepatic copper accumulation. • Chronic hepatobiliary inflammation.

DIAGNOSIS

DIFFERENTIAL DIAGNOSIS

Dogs
• Chronic hepatitis or cholangiohepatitis that has not yet progressed to cirrhosis • Chronic obstructive biliary disease • Chronic fibrosing pancreatitis • Congenital portosystemic shunt • Hepatic neoplasia • Metastatic neoplasia or carcinomatosis • Right-sided heart failure • Hemolytic anemia

Cats
• Cholangiohepatitis • Chronic pancreatitis • Feline infectious peritonitis • Hepatic lipidosis • Chronic obstructive biliary disease • Metastatic neoplasia or carcinomatosis • Hepatic neoplasia • Congenital portosystemic shunts • Right-sided heart failure • Hemolytic anemia

CBC/BIOCHEMISTRY/URINALYSIS
• Microcytic or normocytic, normochromic nonregenerative anemia • Thrombocytopenia (mild) in some animals • Hyperbilirubinemia • Liver enzyme activities are high before clinical signs develop, mostly ALP and ALT. They may be only slightly high or normal in animals with end-stage disease (rare). • Hypoalbuminemia • Hyperglobulinemia • BUN low in some animals • Hypoglycemia.
• Hypokalemia—may predispose animal to hepatic encephalopathy • Isosthenuria in some animals • Ammonium biurate crystalluria

OTHER LABORATORY TESTS
• Ascitic fluid analysis—transudate or modified transudate with low cellularity. • Hyperammonemia • High fasting and postprandial bile acid concentration • Prolonged PT, PTT, ACT, and buccal mucosal bleeding time.

IMAGING

Radiographic Findings
• Small liver in dogs • Normal to large liver in cats • Ascites may result in poor abdominal detail • Urate calculi are radiolucent but

may become apparent if combined with calcium stones

Ultrasonographic Findings
• The liver may have a hyperechoic to mixed echogenicity • Nodular pattern, abdominal effusion, and splenomegaly in some animals • Multiple portosystemic vascular shunt in some animals

OTHER DIAGNOSTIC PROCEDURES
• Examination of fine needle aspirate—hyperplastic or reactive hepatocytes and bile ductule epithelial cells • Laparoscopy—small nodular liver • Biopsy is needed for definitive diagnosis. Needle biopsy is not always sufficient.

GROSS AND HISTOPATHOLOGIC FINDINGS

Gross appearance
In animals with hepatic fibrosis or cirrhosis, the liver appears small and firm with irregular to nodular proliferations observed throughout. Nodules are more prominent in animals with cirrhosis.

Histopathology
• Hepatic fibrosis—noninflammatory fibrosis characterized as central perivenous, diffuse pericellular, or periportal. • Cirrhosis—necrosis and fibrosis with hepatocyte degeneration and nodular regeneration. Marked architectural distortion.

TREATMENT

INPATIENT VS OUTPATIENT
Dogs and cats that are still eating can usually be treated as outpatients. Inpatient evaluation and treatment is needed for dehydrated, anorectic, or neurologically affected animals.

ACTIVITY Limit activity

DIET
A normal to low-protein diet should be fed. Protein content should be geared toward feeding an amount that will limit neurologic complications while maintaining weight. A geriatric diet is probably best for an animal not showing neurologic signs, whereas a low-protein diet should be used if neurologic signs are observed. Fiber may be beneficial in controlling hepatic encephalopathy.

CLIENT EDUCATION
• Treatment is only symptomatic once animal has cirrhosis .
• Dehydration, infection, hypokalemia, and high-protein meals may predispose animal to hepatic encephalopathy.

SURGICAL CONSIDERATIONS
• Animals with hepatic failure are anesthetic risks. Barbiturates should be avoided and benzodiazepines should be used with care. Isoflurane is the gas anesthetic of choice.

• Coagulation abnormalities associated with hepatic failure may lead to hemorrhagic complications. Strict attention to hemostasis is important.
• Animals with hepatic failure are predisposed to bacterial infection. Strict attention to sterile procedure is important.
• Postoperative intensive care is critical, because anesthesia and surgery predispose animals with cirrhosis to development of a hepatic encephalopathic crisis. Hydration should be maintained, and perioperative antibiotics and lactulose should be administered.

MEDICATIONS

DRUGS AND FLUIDS
Lactated Ringer's solution or 0.9% NaCl with KCl (20-30 mEq/L) and B-complex vitamins (2 ml/L) added. Glucose should be added if hypoglycemia is present.

For Hepatic Encephalopathy
• Lactulose (1 ml/kg PO q8h)
• Antibiotics–metronidazole (7.5 mg/kg PO q8h), ampicillin (20 mg/kg PO q8h), or neomycin (20 mg/kg PO q8h)

For Ascites
• Sodium-restricted diet
• Diuretics—spironolactone (1-2 mg/kg PO q12h) or furosemide (1-2 mg/kg PO q12h)
• Repeated abdominocentesis in patients refractory to diet and diuretics

For Hemorrhage
Fresh whole blood transfusion.

For Fibrosis (questionable value)
• Prednisone (1 mg/kg PO q24h-q48h)
• Colchicine (0.03 mg/kg PO q24h)
• d-penicillamine (10-15 mg/kg PO q12h)

Altered Bile Acid Dynamics
Ursodiol (10-15 mg/kg PO q24h)

CONTRAINDICATIONS
• Diuretics may worsen hepatoencephalopathy if prerenal azotemia results.
• Prednisone should not be used in animals with secondary infection.
• The following drugs should be avoided if possible: chloramphenicol, tetracycline, clindamycin, meperidine, pentazocine, aspirin, and azathioprine.

PRECAUTIONS
Care should be taken when the following drugs are administered to patients with hepatic failure: doxycycline, some of the cephalosporins, some of the sulfa drugs, azole antifungals, NSAIDs, barbiturates including phenobarbital, propranolol, captopril, lidocaine, procainamide, and theophylline.

POSSIBLE INTERACTION N/A

ALTERNATE DRUGS N/A

FOLLOW-UP

PATIENT MONITORING
• Liver enzymes, albumin, BUN, and bile acids monthly • Body weight the most important prognostic indicator

PREVENTION/AVOIDANCE N/A

POSSIBLE COMPLICATIONS
• Worsening of signs mentioned. • Hepatic encephalopathy, septicemia, and bleeding complications can be life-threatening.

EXPECTED COURSE AND PROGNOSIS
• The short-term prognosis is fair but the long-term prognosis is very poor. • Survival of up to 4 years has been reported in dogs with idiopathic hepatic fibrosis.

MISCELLANEOUS

ASSOCIATED CONDITIONS
End stage of many types of liver disease.

AGE RELATED FACTORS
Young animals are predisposed to idiopathic hepatic fibrosis.

ZOONOTIC POTENTIAL N/A

PREGNANCY N/A

SYNONYMS NA

SEE ALSO Hepatic encephalopathy

ABBREVIATIONS
ACT = activated clotting time
ALP = serum alkaline phosphatase
ALT = alanine aminotransferase
BUN = blood urea nitrogen
CNS = central nervous system
NSAID = nonsteroidal antiinflammatory drugs
PT = prothrombin time
PTT = partial thromboplastin time

References
Rutgers HC, Haywood S, Kelly DF. Idiopathic hepatic fibrosis in dogs. Vet Rec 1993;133:115-118.
Twedt DC. Cirrhosis: a consequence of chronic liver disease. Vet Clin Am Small Anim Pract 1985;15:151-176.
Johnson SE. Diseases of the liver. In: Ettinger SJ, Feldman EC, eds. Textbook of veterinary internal medicine. Philadelphia: WB Saunders, 1994.
Bunch SE. Specific and symptomatic medical management of diseases of the liver. In: Ettinger SJ, Feldman EC, eds. Textbook of veterinary internal medicine. Philadelphia: WB Saunders, 1994.

Author Joseph Taboada
Consulting Editor Albert E. Jergens

CLOSTRIDIAL ENTEROTOXICOSIS

BASICS

DEFINITION
A syndrome characterized by large bowel diarrhea due to enterotoxin production by certain strains of enteric Clostridium perfringens (CP).

Pathophysiology
Clostridium perfringens is a common enteric inhabitant generally found in the vegetative form living in a symbiotic relationship with the host. Certain strains of CP are capable of producing enterotoxin which binds to the enteric mucosa and alters cell permeability and results in cell damage and or subsequent cell death. Enterotoxin production is a by-product of enteric sporulation of CP. There are a number of intrinsic factors that appear to influence enterotoxin production and pathogenicity of CP.

Systems Affected
Gastrointestinal

Genetics N/A

Incidence and Prevalence
Incidence is unknown, but it is suspected to be associated with up to 15-20% of cases of chronic large bowel diarrhea in dogs. Less common in cats.

Geographical Distribution N/A

SIGNALMENT

Species Dogs and cats

Breed Predilections N/A

Mean Age and Range
• Disease may occur in any age animal. • Most animals that develop clinical signs are middle aged or older.

Predominant Sex N/A

SIGNS

General Comments
• Clinical syndromes are associated with either an acquired acute self-limiting large bowel diarrhea lasting for 5-7 days, chronic intermittent large bowel diarrhea or signs associated in conjunction with other gastrointestinal or non-gastrointestinal disease.
• Chronic signs are often characterized by intermittent episodes occurring every 2-4 weeks that may persists for months to years. • The syndrome may result as a nosocomial (hospital acquired) disease with signs precipitated during or shortly following hospitalization or boarding at a kennel.

Historical Findings
• The most common sign is large bowel diarrhea which is associated with fecal mucus, small amounts of fresh blood, small scant stools, tenesmus with an increased frequency of stools. • Occasionally dogs will have signs of small bowel diarrhea characterized by large volumes of watery stools. • Other signs include vomiting, flatulence, abdominal discomfort or a generalized unthriftyness.

Physical Examination Findings
• Fever, evidence of systemic illness or debilitation is uncommon. • Abdominal discomfort may be detected on palpation. • There may be evidence of blood or mucus in the feces.

CAUSES
It is unknown if enterotoxigenic CP is a true acquired infection or an opportunistic pathogen. It appears that only certain strains of CP are capable of producing enterotoxin and only certain animals affected clinically.

RISK FACTORS
• Stress factors to the gastrointestinal tract, dietary change, concurrent disease or hospitalization may precipitate signs. • The pathogenicity of CP may depend on the metabolic, mucosal and immunologic integrity of the colon. • IgA deficiency • Alkaline intestinal luminal environment

DIAGNOSIS

Cases having chronic intermittent clinical signs should always be evaluated during the onset of clinical episodes.

DIFFERENTIAL DIAGNOSIS
• All causes of large bowel diarrhea including systemic or metabolic disease as well as specific intestinal disorders should be considered.
• Gastrointestinal parasites, inflammatory bowel disease, chronic idiopathic colitis and nervous or irritable bowel syndrome may resemble CP enterotoxicosis.

CBC/BIOCHEMISTRY/URINALYSIS
Usually normal.

OTHER LABORATORY TESTS
Fecal floatation should be performed to rule out intestinal parasites.

Microbiology
• Anaerobic fecal cultures will generally identify high concentrations of CP organisms but occasionally will be negative. • Specific fecal spore cultures will detect high concentrations of Clostridial spores in affected animals ($> 10^6$ spores per gram of feces).

Enterotoxin Assay
• Identification of fecal CP enterotoxin in conjunction with clinical signs supports CP as a contributing pathogen. • Enterotoxin analysis is performed using a fecal ELISA or reverse passive latex agglutination assay (RPLA, Oxoid USA, Columbia, MO). Enterotoxin is not species specific and these tests are valid for use in the dog and cat. The assay requires one gram (small pea-size sample) of feces. The enterotoxin is quite stable and feces can be refrigerated or frozen prior to analysis. • False positive results have been observed in a number of asymptomatic dogs suggesting inherent resistance to pathogenicity of the entertoxin. • False negative results may occur from interfering substances in the feces or from samples taken during the recovery period.

Fecal Cytology
• Identification of high numbers of CP spores in the feces in a patient with evidence of clinical disease correlates well with fecal enterotoxin assay. Greater than 5 spores per high power oil immersion is considered abnormal
• Cytology involves making a thin fecal smear on a microscope slide, air drying or heat fixing and staining with Diff-Quick or Wright's stain. Specific spore stain Malachite green can also be used to identify spores. • CP spores will have a "safety-pin" appearance with a dense body at one end of the cell wall.

IMAGING N/A

OTHER DIAGNOSTIC PROCEDURES
Colonoscopy will help rule out concurrent intestinal disease.

GROSS AND HISTOPATHOLOGIC FINDINGS.
• Colon biopsies taken during asymptomatic periods are usually normal. • Patients with CP enterotoxicosis may have colonoscopic evidence of hyperemic or ulcerated mucosa.
• Histology may show catarrhal or suppurative colitis. Occasionally mild inflammatory bowel disease is present.

TREATMENT

INPATIENT VERSUS OUTPATIENT
• Most treated as outpatients.
• When diarrhea or vomiting is severe, resulting in dehydration and electrolyte imbalance, hospitalization may be required.

ACTIVITY
Restricted during acute disease.

DIET
• Dietary manipulation plays an important role in the treatment and management of cases with chronic reoccurring disease. Diets formulated high in both soluble and insoluble fiber result in clinical improvement by reducing enteric clostridial numbers and by acidifying the distal intestine, thus limiting CP sporulation and enterotoxin production.
• Commercial high fiber diets should be prescribed and supplemented with psyllium (1/2-2 tsp./day) as a source of soluble fiber.
• Diets low in fiber should be supplemented with course bran (1-3 tbs./day) as a source of insoluble fiber with psyllium added as a source of soluble fiber.

CLIENT EDUCATION
• Acute disease is often self-limiting while chronic cases may require lifelong therapy.

SURGICAL CONSIDERATIONS N/A

MEDICATIONS
DRUGS AND FLUIDS
Antibiotics
• Acute self-limiting disease usually requires a 5-7 day antibiotic course. Most patients respond well to appropriate antibiotic therapy (e.g., oral ampicillin or amoxicillin, clindamycin, metronidazole or tylosin)
• Chronic cases often require prolonged antibiotic therapy. Tylosin (Tylan Soluble® Elanco) given at a dose of 10-20 mg/kg q12h-q24h (approximately 1/8 tsp. per 25 kg) mixed with the food is suggested for long term management.
• Administration of oral antibiotics at submicrobial inhibitory concentrations appears to be effective in chronic cases. Low antibiotic levels may not reduce enteric CP numbers but may change the ecological microenvironment preventing sporulation and enterotoxin production.

CONTRAINDICATIONS N/A
PRECAUTIONS N/A
POSSIBLE INTERACTIONS N/A
ALTERNATE DRUGS
• Chronic cases may respond well to high fiber diets (see Diet) and dietary manipulation should be attempted as the sole therapy.

FOLLOW-UP
PATIENT MONITORING
Patient's response to therapy supports the diagnosis and rarely are repeated diagnostics necessary.

PREVENTION/AVOIDANCE
• Infection is associated with environmental contamination and disinfection is difficult.
• Feeding high fiber diets may decrease the incidence of nosocomial acquired diarrhea.

POSSIBLE COMPLICATIONS N/A
EXPECTED COURSE AND PROGNOSIS
• Most animals respond well to therapy. Chronic cases may require lifelong therapy to control clinical signs. • A failure in response suggests concurrent disease and further diagnostic evaluation is indicated.

MISCELLANEOUS
ASSOCIATED CONDITIONS
CP enterotoxicosis is frequently associated with other enteric disease such as parvovirus or inflammatory bowel disease.

AGE RELATED FACTORS N/A

ZOONOTIC POTENTIAL Unknown.
PREGNANCY
Antibiotic therapy may be contraindicated.
SYNONYMS
Idiopathic chronic colitis
SEE ALSO
• Colitis and Proctitis • Small Intestinal Bacterial Overgrowth
ABBREVIATIONS
CP = Clostridium perfringens
tbs = tablespoon
tsp = teaspoon

References
McClane BA, Hanna PC, Wnek AP. Clostridium Perfringens enterotoxin. Microb Pathog 1988;4:317.
Kirth SA, Prescott JF, Welch MK, et al. Nosocomial diarrhea associated with enterotoxegenic Clostridium perfringens infection in dogs. J Am Vet Med Assoc 1989;195:331.
Twedt DC. Clostridium perfringens associated enterotoxicosis in dogs. In: Kirk RW, Bonagura JD. Current veterinary therapy XI. Philadelphia: WB Saunders, 1992:602-604.
Author David C. Twedt
Consulting Editor Brent D. Jones

COAGULOPATHY OF LIVER DISEASE

BASICS

OVERVIEW
• Most patients (90%) with liver disease have some measurable hemostatic defect, but few exhibit clinical bleeding. • The liver is the primary site of synthesis and posttranslational modification of all the coagulation factors except factor VIII, as well as most of the major inhibitors of the activated coagulation cascade. • Hemostasis can be adversely affected in patients with hepatobiliary disease because of reduced synthesis of clotting factors, synthesis of abnormal clotting proteins, vitamin K deficiency, high concentration of FDP and other anticoagulants, low platelet numbers, impaired platelet function, reduced synthesis of normal inhibitors of coagulation, enhanced fibrinolytic activity, and disseminated intravascular coagulation (DIC).

SIGNALMENT
• Dogs and cats

SIGNS
• No obvious signs of bleeding in most animals with liver disease • Gastrointestinal blood loss manifested as melena, hematemesis, hematochezia, or anemia. • Prolonged bleeding from venipuncture, biopsy sites, or surgical wounds • Spontaneous petechia, ecchymoses, or hematomas (uncommon)

CAUSES AND RISK FACTORS
• Fulminant hepatic failure • Acute viral liver disease • Cirrhosis • Portosystemic vascular anomalies • Bile duct obstruction • Chronic liver disease does not usually cause clinically important bleeding until cirrhosis has developed. • Concurrent small intestinal disease, often seen in cats with the cholangiohepatitis complex, may predispose patient to vitamin K deficiency.

DIAGNOSIS

DIFFERENTIAL DIAGNOSIS
• Vitamin K antagonist rodenticide toxicity • Primary coagulation defect • Other causes of DIC • Immune-mediated thrombocytopenia

CBC/BIOCHEMISTRY/URINALYSIS
Thrombocytopenia (rarely severe unless caused by DIC).

OTHER LABORATORY TESTS
• Prolonged PT, aPTT, and ACT • Prolonged bleeding time • Impaired platelet aggregation • High FDP because of impaired hepatic clearance or DIC. • Concentrations of most individual clotting factors are low. • Proteins indicative of vitamin K antagonism may be increased if patient has poor vitamin K absorption.

IMAGING N/A

OTHER DIAGNOSTIC PROCEDURES
N/A

TREATMENT
• Treat underlying liver disease. • Treat actively bleeding lesions (such as gastric ulcers) if possible. • Treatment of coagulopathy not usually necessary unless invasive procedures are planned. Coagulopathy does not contraindicate fine needle aspiration of liver for cytologic examination. • Prolongation of bleeding time, PT, aPTT, or ACT by more than 50% or thrombocytopenia (< 50,000/ml) increases the likelihood of bleeding during biopsy procedure. • Spontaneous bleeding indicates severe liver dysfunction and treatment should be initiated.

MEDICATIONS

DRUGS AND FLUIDS
• Fresh whole blood should be given to patients with anemia and those undergoing an invasive procedure. • Fresh frozen plasma (5-10 ml/kg) or cryoprecipitate supplies enough clotting factors and ATIII for immediate use. • Transfusion of platelets rarely beneficial • Parenteral vitamin K1 (3-5 mg/kg/day) should be given to patients with clinically important cholestasis or concurrent malabsorptive disease. • Desomopressin acetate (0.3 mg/kg IV in saline) may prolong factors VII, VIII, IX, and XII and shorten the PT and aPTT. • Heparin and ATIII may be necessary in patients with DIC.

CONTRAINDICATIONS/POSSIBLE INTERACTIONS
• Whole blood transfusion may precipitate hepatoencephalopathy, especially if stored blood is used.

FOLLOW-UP
• Follow-up assessment of PT and bleeding time are the best tests to monitor response to treatment. • If improvement in PT and aPTT is not seen 24 hours after vitamin K injection, subsequent injections are not useful. • Spontaneous hemorrhage is a poor prognostic sign in animals with liver disease.

MISCELLANEOUS

SEE ALSO
• Blood transfusion reactions • Clotting factor deficiencies

ABBREVIATIONS
ACT = activated clotting time
aPTT = activated partial thromboplastin time
ATIII = antithrombin III
DIC = disseminated intravascular coagulation
FDP = fibrin degradation products
PT = prothrombin time

Reference
Strombeck DR, Guilford WG, eds. Small animal gastroenterology. 2nd ed. Davis, CA: Stonegate, 1990.
Author Joseph Taboada
Consulting Editor Albert E. Jergens

BASICS

OVERVIEW
Congenital anomaly in which there is selective malabsorption of cobalamin (vitamin B_{12}) secondary to absence of the receptor for intrinsic factor-cobalamin complex in the ileal brush border. Very rare.

SIGNALMENT
Only reported in the Giant Schnauzer breed. Inherited as a simple autosomal recessive trait. Signs appear at 6–12 weeks of age.

SIGNS
• Anorexia • Lethargy • Failure to gain weight

CAUSES AND RISK FACTORS
The disease is inherited.

DIAGNOSIS

DIFFERENTIAL DIAGNOSIS
• Other congenital metabolic diseases. • Gastrointestinal parasite infection.

CBC/BIOCHEMISTRY/URINALYSIS
• Mild to severe neutropenia (1,760–4,440/mm³) • Chronic nonregenerative anemia (PCV 21–33%)

OTHER LABORATORY TESTS
• Serum cobalamin concentrations are very low (<50 ng/L; normal >225 ng/L). • Serum and urine methylmalonic acid concentrations are above normal.

IMAGING N/A

OTHER DIAGNOSTIC PROCEDURES
N/A

TREATMENT
Long term parenteral replacement of cobalamin.

MEDICATIONS

DRUGS AND FLUIDS
Cobalamin (0.5-1.0 mg IM q24h for 7 days then every 3-6 months).

CONTRAINDICATIONS/POSSIBLE INTERACTIONS N/A

FOLLOW-UP
Periodic parenteral administration of cobalamin

MISCELLANEOUS

Reference

Fyfe JC, Giger U, Hall CA, et al. Inherited selective intestinal cobalamin malabsorption and cobalamin deficiency in dogs. Pediatric Research 1991;29:24–31.
Author David A. Williams
Consulting Editor Brent D. Jones

COCCIDIODOMYCOSIS

BASICS

DEFINITION
A systemic mycosis caused by the dimorphic fungus Coccidioides immitis

Pathophysiology
• After inhalation of infective arthrospores (the infective units of the mold form of the fungus), mild signs of fever, lethargy, partial inappetence, coughing, and sometimes joint pain or stiffness may develop; alternatively, the infection may be asymptomatic. The majority of animals become solidly immune after initial infection. • Fewer than 10 inhaled arthrospores are sufficient to cause disease in susceptible animals. "Susceptible" refers to the small percentage of animals in which extrapulmonary dissemination occurs. Signs of dissemination may not be evident for several months after the initial infection.

Systems Affected
• Respiratory—the site of initial infection • Extrapulmonary spread may occur to long bones and joints, eyes, skin, liver, kidneys, CNS, and testes.

Genetics
Unknown, but possibly there are inherited or acquired defects in host immune defenses that favor growth of the spherule form of Coccidioides in tissues

Incidence/Prevalence
Coccidioidomycosis is considered an uncommon disease, even in endemic areas. It is only rarely diagnosed in cats.

Geographic Distribution
This fungus resides in soil of the dry cactus country of the southwestern United States from California to central Texas.

SIGNALMENT

Species
At least 100 times more common in dogs than in cats.

Breed Predilections
• Dogs—boxers and doberman pinschers may be more susceptible to disseminated coccidioidomycosis • Cats—none recognized

Mean Age and Range
Most patients are young animals < 4 years of age.

Predominant Sex
• Dogs—male • Cats—none recognized

SIGNS

Historical Findings
Anorexia, weight loss, weakness, coughing, and lameness may be reported.

Physical Examination Findings
Dogs
• Affected dogs may exhibit signs of chronic fever nonresponsive to antibiotics, dyspnea, lymphadenopathy, inappetence, lethargy, and

wasting. • Other signs of disseminated coccidioidomycosis include bone swelling and joint enlargement that may give rise to lameness; ulcers and draining tracts usually located over areas of infected bone; neurologic dysfunction caused by impingement of the disease process on the local nerve supply or by direct extension into the nervous system; ocular disease (uveitis, keratitis). Liver or kidney dysfunction may occur in some animals. • The fungus may also be introduced into the body through a penetrating wound. After this mode of inoculation the infection usually remains localized. • In some dogs, clinical signs may be restricted to the lungs and include coughing and dyspnea.
Cats
Wasting, dyspnea, draining skin lesions, uveitis, and lameness caused by bone involvement have been observed.

CAUSE
Coccidioides immitis is a dimorphic soil fungus with a geographically restricted distribution. It is found in the southwestern United States from California to central Texas, particularly in areas where the creosote bush is common, in an ecological niche known as the Lower Sonoran life zone. The fungus grows several inches deep in the soil, where it is aided in its spread by the activities of burrowing rodents. After a period of wet weather, wind and dust storms whipping up the surface soil may spread the filamentous mold forms across great distances. The fungus is normally dormant in the summer and is killed by freezing temperatures.

RISK FACTORS
• Aggressive nosing about in soil and underbrush, as in the sporting breeds of dogs, may expose susceptible animals to large doses of the fungus in contaminated soil. • The risk of infection may be higher during dust storms after the rainy season.

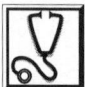

DIAGNOSIS

DIFFERENTIAL DIAGNOSIS
• Pulmonary lesions may resemble those of other systemic mycoses. Such lesions should be differentiated from metastatic tumors and canine distemper. • Lymphadenopathy may be seen in lymphosarcoma, other systemic mycoses, and localized bacterial infections. • Bone lesions may resemble those caused by primary or metastatic bone tumors or bacterial osteomyelitis. • Skin lesions must be differentiated from routine abscesses or other bacterial disease processes.

CBC/BIOCHEMISTRY/URINALYSIS
• Hemogram—mild nonregenerative anemia, neutrophilic leukocytosis, monocytosis (all nonspecific) • Serum chemistry profile—hyperglobulinemia, hypoalbuminemia (nonspecific) • Urinalysis—azotemia and proteinuria with renal involvement

OTHER LABORATORY TESTS
Immunologic tests for antibody to C. immitis may provide a presumptive diagnosis, particularly if spherules cannot be located in lesion material.

IMAGING
Radiography of lung (interstitial infiltrates) and bone (osteolysis) lesions may aid in diagnosis.

OTHER DIAGNOSTIC PROCEDURES
Microscopic identification of the large spherule form of C. immitis in lesion or biopsy material is the recommended method of diagnosis. Lymph-node aspirates and impression smears of skin lesions or draining exudate may, in some patients, yield organisms. Biopsy of infected tissue often is preferred to avoid false-negatives. A diligent search of available material may be necessary to locate organisms.

GROSS AND HISTOPATHOLOGIC FINDINGS
• Granulomatous, suppurative, or pyogranulomatous inflammation present in many tissues. • Presence of the characteristic spherule forms in affected tissues. In some patients, the numbers of spherules present may be small.

TREATMENT

INPATIENT VERSUS OUTPATIENT
Because treatment of coccidioidomycosis requires long-term therapy, the patient should be treated as an outpatient. Patients treated with amphotericin B, however, will need to be hospitalized several times a week during their initial treatment period (see below).

ACTIVITY
Activity levels should be restricted during the period of antifungal therapy.

DIET
Because affected animals often have experienced weight loss, provision should be made for feeding a high-quality diet. Protein levels may need to be restricted, however, owing to the nephrotoxic effects of amphotericin B.

CLIENT EDUCATION
• The necessity and expense of long-term therapy of a potentially fatal illness, in addition to the possible side effects of such therapy, need to be thoroughly discussed with the client. • The quality of life for the patient should be balanced against the likelihood of successful therapy, based upon the physical condition of the animal at the time of diagnosis.

SURGICAL CONSIDERATIONS   N/A

MEDICATIONS

DRUGS AND FLUIDS
Coccidioidomycosis is considered the most severe and life-threatening of the systemic

mycoses. Aggressive, long-term antifungal therapy is required to effect a remission.

Dogs

• Ketoconazole (KTZ) is considered the current drug of choice for treatment. It can be administered at 10-30 mg/kg PO, divided 2 or 3 times daily, for at least 8-12 months (extremely long-term therapy is required). The medication should be given in the food.

• Amphotericin B (AMB) can be given as an alternative at a dosage of 0.5 mg/kg, 3 times a week, for a total cumulative dosage of 8-10 mg/kg. It is given IV either as a slow infusion (in dogs that are gravely ill) or as a rapid bolus (in fairly healthy dogs). For slow infusion, add AMB to 250-500 ml of 5% dextrose solution and administer as a drip over a period of 4-6 hours. For a rapid bolus, add AMB to 30 ml of 5% dextrose solution and administer over a period of 5 minutes through a butterfly catheter.

• To lessen the adverse renal effects of AMB, give 0.9% NaCl (2 ml/kg/hr) for several hours before initiating AMB therapy.

• A combination of AMB and KTZ may be used in dogs that have not responded to either drug alone or have exhibited significant toxicity. For combination chemotherapy, administer AMB as described to a total cumulative dosage of 4-6 mg/kg, together with KTZ at 10 mg/kg PO divided daily for at least 8-12 months.

Cats

• Little information is available regarding treatment of coccidioidomycosis in cats. As a general recommendation, KTZ can be administered at 10 mg/kg PO q12h for at least 8-12 months. It should be given in the food.

• Alternatively, AMB can be administered by rapid IV bolus at a dosage of 0.25 mg/kg, 3 times a week, for a total cumulative dosage of 4 mg/kg. This can then be followed by long-term KTZ therapy, depending on the clinical response.

CONTRAINDICATIONS

• Drugs metabolized primarily by the liver should not be administered along with KTZ.
• Drugs metabolized primarily by the kidneys should not be administered along with AMB.

PRECAUTIONS

• Side effects of KTZ therapy include inappetence, vomiting, and hepatotoxicity.

• Side effects of AMB therapy can be severe and include renal dysfunction, fever, inappetence, vomiting, and phlebitis.

POSSIBLE INTERACTIONS N/A

ALTERNATE DRUGS N/A

FOLLOW-UP

PATIENT MONITORING

• Liver enzymes should be monitored in animals receiving KTZ. • BUN should be monitored in all animals treated with AMB. Treatment should be temporarily discontinued if the BUN rises above 50 mg/dl.

PREVENTION/AVOIDANCE

• There is no available vaccine for dogs or cats. • Exposure to Coccidioides—contaminated soil in endemic areas should be avoided, particularly during dust storms after the rainy season

POSSIBLE COMPLICATIONS

• Pulmonary disease may temporarily worsen soon after therapy is begun, owing to inflammation resulting from the death of fungal cells in the lungs. • Hepatotoxicity may result from KTZ or itraconazole therapy. • Nephrotoxicity may result from AMB therapy.

EXPECTED COURSE AND PROGNOSIS

• The prognosis is guarded to grave. Many dogs will improve following KTZ therapy; however, a much smaller number will be completely cured. The overall recovery rate has been estimated at 60%. • Little information is available regarding the prognosis for cats. • Relapses after treatment may occur. • Spontaneous recovery from disseminated coccidioidomycosis without treatment is extremely rare

MISCELLANEOUS

ASSOCIATED CONDITIONS N/A

AGE RELATED FACTORS N/A

ZOONOTIC POTENTIAL

The spherule form of the fungus, as found in animal tissues, is not directly transmissible to people or other animals. Under certain rare circumstances, however, there could be reversion to growth of the infective mold form of the fungus on or within bandages placed over a draining lesion or in contaminated bedding. This author recommends that prudent care be exercised whenever handling an infected dog or cat.

PREGNANCY

• KTZ should be used in pregnant animals only if the potential benefit justifies the potential risk to offspring. • Teratogenic effects of AMB have not been identified.

SYNONYMS

San Joaquin Valley fever, valley fever, desert rheumatism (in humans)

SEE ALSO N/A

ABBREVIATIONS

KTZ = ketoconazole
AMB = amphotericin B

References

Armstrong PJ, DiBartola SP. Canine coccidioidomycosis: a literature review and report of eight cases. J Am Anim Hosp Assoc 1983;19:937-945.

Barsanti JA, Jeffery KL. Coccidioidomycosis. In: Greene CE, ed. Infectious diseases of the dog and cat. Philadelphia: WB Saunders, 1990:696-706.

Legendre AM. Coccidioidomycosis. In: Sherding RG, ed. The cat: diseases and clinical management. 2nd ed. New York: Churchill Livingstone, 1994:561-562.

Stevens DA. Coccidioidomycosis. N Engl J Med 1995;332:1077-1082.

Wolf AM. Coccidioidomycosis. In: Barlough JE, ed. Manual of small animal infectious diseases. New York: Churchill Livingstone, 1988:309-318.

Author Jeffrey E. Barlough
Consulting Editor Fred W. Scott

COCCIDIOSIS

 BASICS

OVERVIEW
• Coccidiosis is an enteric infection, traditionally associated with Isospora canis (dogs) and Isospora felis (cats) as potential pathogens. Other species of Isospora may be present. Strictly host specific, i.e., no cross-transmission. Eimeria spp are not parasitic for dogs, cats. Disease with a watery to mucoid diarrhea. • Toxoplasma gondii in cats and Cryptosporidium parvum in neonatal pups and kittens are coccidians in a nontraditional sense. • Toxoplasma in cats may cause clinical signs similar to Isospora with oocysts shed in the environment that may potentially cause a public health problem. • Cryptosporidium is still being assessed as an acute life-threatening coccidiosis (cryptosporidiosis) of neonatal pups and kittens. Voluminous watery diarrhea is characteristic; autoinfection and continuing recycling within the lower intestinal tract results in a rapid loss of the mucosal lining.

SIGNALMENT
Dogs and cats

SIGNS
• Watery to mucoid, occasionally blood-tinged diarrhea • Weak pups and kittens

CAUSES AND RISK FACTORS
• Infected dogs or cats contaminating environment with oocysts of Isospora spp or Cryptosporidium • Stress

 DIAGNOSIS

DIFFERENTIAL DIAGNOSIS
Enteric viral infections

CBC/BIOCHEMISTRY/URINALYSIS
Usually normal. May be hemoconcentrated if dehydrated.

OTHER LABORATORY TESTS
• Fecal examination for oocysts; special staining such as acid fast for Cryptosporidium
• Isospora oocysts ovoid at 40 μm length; cysts of Toxoplasma 15 μm length; cysts of Cryptosporidium ~ 5 μm length

IMAGING N/A

OTHER DIAGNOSTIC PROCEDURES
N/A

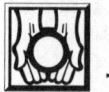 **TREATMENT**

Inpatient if debilitated

MEDICATIONS

DRUGS AND FLUIDS

• Sulfadimethoxine at 55mg/kg PO on the first day, then 27.5mg/kg for 4 days or until dog is asymptomatic for Isospora
• On an extra-label use basis, albendazole (Valbazen) at 25 mg/kg PO q12h for 2 days or fenbendazole (Panacur) at 50 mg/kg PO q24h for 3 days for Isospora
• None known for Cryptosporidium although pyrimethamine has been used experimentally
• Fluid therapy usually necessary

CONTRAINDICATIONS/POSSIBLE INTERACTIONS None known

FOLLOW-UP

Fecal examination for oocysts 1–2 weeks after treatment

MISCELLANEOUS

AGE RELATED FACTORS

More severe disease in young animals

SEE ALSO

Toxoplasmosis, Cryptosporidiosis

Reference

Bowman DD. Georgi's parasitology for veterinarians. 6th ed. Philadelphia: WB Saunders, 1994.
Author Robert M. Corwin
Consulting Editor Brent D. Jones

COLIBACILLOSIS

BASICS

DEFINITION

Escherichia coli is a gram-negative member of the Enterobacteriaceae and a normal inhabitant of the intestine of most mammals. It can cause an acute infection of young puppies and kittens in the first week of life and is characterized by septicemia and multiple organ involvement. Mere isolation of E. coli from stool of young animals is inconclusive evidence of its pathogenic potential because it is normal flora; however, isolation from blood cultures or internal organs constitutes good evidence of causality. E. coli infections in older dogs and cats have been documented but individual strains of E. coli are poorly characterized with regard to virulence attributes. E. coli, along with other infectious agents, may increase the severity of parvovirus infections.

Pathophysiology

The virulence factors of E. coli strains from dogs and cats have not been well defined. It is likely that E. coli as a cause of septicemia in neonatal dogs and cats has more to do with the immunologic immaturity of the host than with the virulence of a particular E. coli strain. ETEC (enterotoxigenic E. coli), EPEC (enteropathogenic E. coli), uropathogenic, CNF (cytotoxic necrotizing factor)+ E. coli's strains have been recovered from dogs, and EPEC, VTEC (verocytotoxigenic E. coli), and uropathogenic strains from cats. Intestinal strains colonize and multiply in the small intestine; ETEC then elaborates K99 or other uncharacterized adhesins and enterotoxins, while EPEC's attaching and effacing factor (eae+) or VTEC (eae +) produces Shiga-like toxin (SLT); also many strains of E. coli from dogs and cats are hemolytic.

Systems Affected

• Neonatal animals—small intestine (enteritis); multiple body systems (septicemia)
• Older puppies/kittens and adults—small intestine (enteritis); urogenital (cystitis, endometritis, pyelonephritis, prostatitis); mammary gland (mastitis)

Genetics N/A

Incidence/Prevalence

• Few statistics available • More common in neonatal puppies and kittens under 1 week of age who have not received colostrum or have not received adequate colostrum; problem in overpopulated kennels and catteries • Sporadic accounts in older dogs and cats—diarrhea and urogenital problems

Dogs

• Prevalence of ETEC in diarrheic dogs—2.7-29.5%: K99+/-, Sta/STb+/- • CNF + E. coli isolated from diarrheic dogs along with hemolysin • E. Coli major cause of septicemia in newborn puppies; often beta-he-

molytic; infection arising from exposure in utero, during birth, or from mastitic milk

Cats

EPEC/VTEC found in diarrheic cats (strains are eae+, SLT+, hemolytic, aerobactin +, serum resistant, CNF+)

Geographic Distribution

Worldwide occurrence

SIGNALMENT

Species Dogs and cats

Breed Predilections N/A

Mean Age and Range

• Neonatal infections common (diarrhea, septicemia) up to 2 weeks of age • Older puppies/kittens and adult animals have sporadic disease often associated with other infectious agents.

SIGNS

General Comments

E. coli is one of the most common causes of septicemia and death in puppies and kitttens.

Historical Findings

• Neonates—sudden onset of vomiting, weakness/lethargy, diarrhea, cold skin
• Older puppies/kittens and adults—vomiting and diarrhea

Physical Examination Findings

• Neonates—acute depression, anorexia, vomiting, tachycardia, weakness, hypothermia, cyanosis, watery diarrhea, high mortality; 1 or more animals affected in a litter • Older ages—ETEC associated with acute vomiting, diarrhea, anorexia, rapid dehydration, fever

CAUSES

• E. coli is a member of the endogenous microbial flora of the adult dog's and cat's GI tract, prepuce, and vagina. • Many E.coli strains isolated from case material are poorly characterized with regard to virulence factors.
• Often found in older dogs and cats concurrently with other infectious agents

RISK FACTORS

Neonates

• Bitch/queen in poor health and nutritional status (unable to provide good care and colostrum to offspring) • Lack of colostrum/insufficient colostrum • Dirty birthing environment • Difficult/prolonged labor and birth • Puppies/kittens in crowded facilities (build up of feces in environment, greater chance for fecal-oral spread of infection)

Immature Ages and Adults

• Concurrent disease/parvovirus/heavy parasitism • Upset of GI tract's microbial flora with antimicrobial drugs • Immunosuppression

DIAGNOSIS

DIFFERENTIAL DIAGNOSIS

Adult Enteritis

GI inflammation • Infectious enteritis—need serologic testing and/or bacterial culture to differentiate etiologies:

Viral Gastroenteritis

• Feline panleukopenia • FeLV • FIV • Feline enteric coronavirus • Canine enteric coronairus • Canine parvovirus • Rotavirus
• Canine distemper

Bacterial Gastroenteritis

• Salmonellae • E. coli • Campylobacter jejuni • Yersinia enterocolitica • Bacterial overgrowth syndrome • Clostridium difficile, Cl. perfringens

Parasites

• Helminths (hookworms, ascarids, whipworms, Strongyloides) • Protozoa (Giardia, coccidia, Cryptosporidia) • Rickettsiae
• Salmon poisoning

Dietary Induced

• Overeating • Abrupt changes/starvation/thirst • Allergy or food intolerance
• Indiscretions (foreign material, garbage)

Drug or Toxin Induced

• Antimicrobial agents • Antineoplastic agents (cytotoxic drugs) • Anthelminthic
• Heavy metal or organophosphates

Extraintestinal Disorders/Metabolic Disease

• Acute pancreatitis • Hypoadrenocorticism
• Liver/kidney disease • Pyometra • Peritonitis

Neurological Disorders

• Vestibular disease • Psychogenic (fear, excitement, pain)

Functional/Mechanical Ileus

• Gastric-dilatation volvulus • Intussusception
• Electrolyte disorder • GI foreign body

Fading Neonates

• Canine distemper • Canine herpesvirus
• Canine brucellosis • Feline herpesvirus
• Salmonellae • Toxoplasma • Feline panleukopenia • FeLV • FIP

CBC/BIOCHEMISTRY/URINALYSIS

• Few abnormalities noted as a result of rapidity of death in puppies • Older animals with enteritis may show chemistry abnormality, depending on the state of dehydration

OTHER LABORATORY TESTS N/A

IMAGING N/A

OTHER DIAGNOSTIC PROCEDURES

• The use of antimicrobials before obtaining bacterial cultures may produce false-negative results. • Routine bacterial culture and identification of E. coli from blood (antemortem) or necropsy tissue (bone marrow, heart blood, liver/spleen, brain, mesenteric lymph node) is required; appropriate testing of E. coli strains is needed to identify adhesins and toxins (by DNA colony hybridization, PCR) in ETEC and VTEC strains.

GROSS AND HISTOPATHOLOGIC FINDINGS

Acute Enteritis

Mucosal inflammation of small intestine

Septicemias

• Petechia and hemorrhagic lesions on serosa surface of GI mucosae and all body cavities

• Fibrin on abdominal wall • Necrosis of liver/spleen

TREATMENT

INPATIENT VERSUS OUTPATIENT

Acutely ill puppies/kittens need inpatient care and good nursing care.

ACTIVITY

Acutely ill immature puppies/kittens (bacteremic/septicemic) need restricted activity, cage rest, monitoring, and warmth.

DIET

Puppies likely to still be nursing when affected with colibacillosis; good nursing care needed with bottle-feeding and/or IV nutrients

CLIENT EDUCATION

Neonatal E. coli infections are life-threatening with poor prognosis.

SURGICAL CONSIDERATIONS N/A

MEDICATIONS

DRUGS AND FLUIDS

• Balanced parenteral polyionic isotonic solution (lactated Ringer's) to restore fluids
• Oral hypertonic glucose solution (for secretory diarrhea) as required
• Antimicrobial therapy needed if septicemic
• Treatment must be guided by culture and susceptibility (MIC) testing of E. coli
• Empiric therapy until bacterial susceptibility (MIC) results available
• Trimethoprim-sulfa—dogs (30 mg/kg PO or once daily); cats (30 mg/kg PO or SQ q12-24h)
• Chloramphenicol—dogs (50 mg/kg PO, IM, IV, SQ q8h); cats (50 mg/kg total PO, IV, IM, SQ q12h)
• Amoxicillin—dogs and cats (10-20 mg/kg PO q8-12h)

CONTRAINDICATIONS

Do not use fluoroquinolones in immature dogs and cats.

PRECAUTIONS

Caution using chloramphenicol and trimethoprim/sulfa in neonatal animals; monitoring needed

POSSIBLE INTERACTIONS N/A

ALTERNATE DRUGS

Adult Patients

Fluoroquinolones—use in dogs only (enrofloxacin, 2.5-5 mg/kg PO q12h); *avoid* use in pregnant, neonatal, or growing animals (medium-sized dogs less than 8 months of age; large or giant breeds less than 12-18 months of age) because of cartilage lesions

Immature Patients

Third-generation cephalosporin class drugs may be used

FOLLOW-UP

PATIENT MONITORING

• Blood culture of puppies/kittens if fever and/or diarrhea develop • Monitor temperature if signs of lethargy and/or depression develop • Monitor behavior to assure eating/drinking/nursing are normal. • Ensure adequate weight gain.

PREVENTION/AVOIDANCE

• Make sure bitch/queen in good health, vaccinated, good nutritional status • Clean and disinfect parturition environment (1:32 dilution of bleach); frequently clean bedding after birth • Ensure adequate colostrum intake of all litter mates. • Separate queen with nursing kittens or bitch with nursing puppies from other cats or dogs. • Keep kennel or cattery rooms low density. • Wash hands, change clothes/shoes after handling other cats/dogs and before dealing with neonates

POSSIBLE COMPLICATIONS

Neonatal infections are life-threatening. Prognosis often is poor.

EXPECTED COURSE AND PROGNOSIS

The bacteremic/septicemic neonate may rapidly succumb to infection; quick treatment with supportive care is essential for s urvival; adult enteritis should be self-limiting with supportive care depending on the degree of dehydration and whether or not other disease agents are present

MISCELLANEOUS

ASSOCIATED CONDITIONS N/A

AGE RELATED FACTORS

Neonatal puppies and kittens are at greatest risk of infection and subsequent septicemia.

ZOONOTIC POTENTIAL

• There is little documented information of the virulence potential of E. coli strains from dogs or cats for humans. • Always wash hands after handling animals (especially diarrheic cases) because of the risk of acquiring other infectious agents (e.g., salmonellae, Giardia) • Caution: keep children and immunosuppressed persons away from diarrheic pets

PREGNANCY N/A

SYNONYMS

Neonatal enteritis/E. coli septicemia

SEE ALSO N/A

ABBREVIATIONS

CNF = cytotoxic necrotizing factor
EPEC = enteropathogenic E. coli
eae = attaching and effacing factor (an adhesin)
ETEC = enterotoxigenic E. coli
SLT = Shiga-like toxin
Sta = heat stable toxin
VTEC = verocytotoxigenic E. coli

References

Greene CE. Enteric bacterial infections. In: Clinical microbiology and infectious diseases of the dog and cat. Philadelphia: WB Saunders, 1984:617-632.

Peeters JE. Escherichia coli infections in rabbits, cats, dogs, goats and horses. In: Gyles CL, ed. Escherichia coli in domestic animals and humans. Wallingford: CAB International, 1994:261-283.

Gyles CL. Escherichia coli. In: Gyles CL, Thoen CO, eds. Pathogenesis of bacterial infections in animals. 2nd ed. Ames: Iowa State University Press, 1993:164-187.

Author Patrick L. McDonough
Consulting Editor Fred W. Scott

COLITIS AND PROCTITIS

BASICS

DEFINITION
Colitis is inflammation of the colon. Proctitis is inflammation of the rectum.

Pathophysiology
Inflammation of the colon causes accumulation of inflammatory cytokines, disrupts tight junctions between epithelial cells, stimulates colonic secretion, stimulates goblet cell secretion of mucus, and disrupts motility. These mechanisms reduce the ability of the colon to absorb water and store feces. This causes infrequent diarrhea, often with mucus and blood.

Systems Affected
Gastrointestinal

Genetics
Breed predisposition to histiocytic ulcerative colitis in young boxers.

Incidence/Prevalence
Approximately 30% of dogs with chronic diarrhea examined at the University of Florida Veterinary Medical Teaching Hospital; prevalence not well documented.

Geographic Distribution N/A

SIGNALMENT

Species Dogs and cats

Breed Predilections
Boxer (histiocytic ulcerative colitis)

Mean Age and Range
Any age; boxers usually symptomatic by 2 years old

Predominant Sex None

SIGNS
• Chronic diarrhea often with mucus or blood • Feces vary from semiformed to liquid • High frequency of defecation with small volume of feces • Prolonged tenesmus after defecation • Vomiting in some dogs • Weight loss is uncommon. • Results of physical examination usually normal

CAUSES
• Infectious: Trichuris vulpis, Ancylostoma caninum, Entamoeba histolytica, Balantidium coli, Giardia spp, Trichomonas spp, Salmonella spp, Clostridium spp, Campylobacter spp, Yersinia enterocolitica, Escherichia coli, Prototheca, Histoplasma capsulatum, and Phycomycosis • Traumatic: Foreign body and abrasive material • Uremic: Segmental; secondary to chronic pancreatitis • Allergic: Dietary protein and possibly bacterial protein • Rectocolonic polyps • Cecal inversion • Ileocecocolic intussusception • Inflammatory: Lymphoplasmacytic, eosinophilic, granulomatous, and histiocytic • Neoplasia: Lymphosarcoma and adenocarcinoma • Irritable bowel syndrome

RISK FACTORS N/A

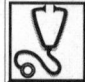

DIAGNOSIS

DIFFERENTIAL DIAGNOSIS
Must differentiate from small bowel diarrhea

CBC/BIOCHEMISTRY/URINALYSIS
• Results usually normal; possibly neutrophilia with a left shift is possible • Mild microcytic, hypochromic anemia in some patients with persistent and chronic bleeding • Hyperglobulinemia in some patients with chronic disease

OTHER LABORATORY TESTS
• Examination of fecal floatation and direct smear and bacterial culture may reveal an infectious cause. • Serologic testing—histoplasma titer may be positive in patients with fungal colitis. (Editor's note: this is not usually a useful diagnostic tool.) • Test of feces for Clostridium perfringens may be positive.

IMAGING
Abdominal radiography usually normal but may reveal foreign material in the colon Barium enema may reveal mucosal irregularities or filling defects in severely affected patients, but this procedure is time consuming and not cost-effective.

OTHER DIAGNOSTIC PROCEDURES
• Colonoscopy with biopsy is the technique of choice for diagnosis—may see disappearance of submucosal blood vessels, granular appearance of mucosa, hyperemia, excessive mucus, ulceration, pinpoint hemmorhage (small ulcerations), or mass • Biopsy should always be done, because extent of mucosal change does not necessarily reflect severity or absence of disease

GROSS AND HISTOPATHOLOGIC FINDINGS
• Gross findings as described • Histopathologic findings depend on type of colitis: lymphoplasmacytic, eosinopholic, granulomatous, or histiocytic; hyperplastic mucosa may be seen in patients with irritable bowel syndrome; various infectious agents may be seen with the use of special stains.

TREATMENT

INPATIENT VERSUS OUTPATIENT
Outpatient unless diarrhea is severe enough to cause dehydration

ACTIVITY N/A

DIET
• Patients with acute colitis can be fasted for 24-48 hours
• A nonallergenic diet should be tried in patients with inflammatory colitis; use a commercial or home prepared diet that contains a protein to which the dog has not been exposed

• Fiber supplementation with a poorly fermented fiber (e.g., bran and a cellulose) is recommended to increase fecal bulk, improve colonic muscle's contractility, and bind fecal water to produce formed feces.
• Some fermentable fiber (e.g., psyllium) may be beneficial (short chain fatty acids may help the colon heal).

CLIENT EDUCATION
• Treatment may be intermittent and long-term in patients with inflammatory colitis and repeated recurrence, especially those with the histiocytic and granulomatous forms • Granulomatous, histiocytic, fungal, protothecal colitis, and lymphosarcoma of the colon respond poorly to medical treatment; surgery may indicated.

SURGICAL CONSIDERATIONS
Segments of colon that are severely affected by fibrosis caused by chronic inflammation and subsequent stricture formation may need to be surgically removed, especially in patients with the granulomatous form of the disease; cecal inversion, ileocecocolic intussusception, and neoplastic processes require surgical intervention

MEDICATIONS

DRUGS AND FLUIDS
Balanced electrolyte solution with potassium supplementation in dehydrated patients

Antimicrobial Drugs
• Trichuris, Ancylostoma, and Giardia—fenbendazole (50mg/kg q24h for 3 days, repeat in 3 months)
• Entamoeba, Balantidium, Giardia, and Trichomonas—metronidazole (25mg/kg q12h for 5-7 days)
• Salmonella—treatment is controversial because a carrier state can be induced; in patients with systemic involvement, choose antibiotic on the basis of bacterial culture and sensitivity testing (e.g., chloramphenicol, trimethoprim-sulfa, and enrofloxacin)
• Clostridium—metronidazole (25 mg/kg q12h for 5-7 days), tylosin (45 mg/kg q24h for 7 days), or penicillin antibiotic
• Campylobacter—erythromycin (30-40 mg/kg q24h for 5 days) or tylosin (45 mg/kg q24h for 5 days)
• Yersinia and E. coli—choose drug on the basis of bacterial culture and sensitivity testing
• Prototheca—no known treatment
• Histoplasma and phycomycosis—ketaconazole (dogs, 10-30 mg/kg q24h in divided doses; cats, 5-10mg/kg q8h-q12h), itraconazole (5mg/kg q12h), amphotericin B (0.25-0.5mg/kg IV q48h up to cumulative dose of 4-8mg /kg)
• Metronidazole and tylosin may have more than just antimicrobial properties

Anti-inflammatory and Immunosupprssive Drugs for Inflammatory Colitis
• Sulfasalazine (25-40mg/kg q8h for 2-6 weeks)
• Corticosteroids—prednisone (dogs, 1-2mg/kg q24h; cats, 2-4mg/kg q24h; dosage is tapered once clinical remission is achieved)
• Azathioprine (dogs, 1mg/kg q24h for 2 weeks followed by alternate-day administration; cats, 0.3mg/kg q24h for 3-4 months)

Motility Modifiers (for symptomatic relief only)
• Loperamide (0.1mg/kg q8h-q12h)
• Diphenoxylate (0.1-0.2mg/kg q8h)
• Paregoric (0.06mg/kg q8h-q12h)
• Propantheline bromide (0.25-0.5mg/kg q8h) if colonic spasm is contributing to clinical signs

CONTRAINDICATIONS
• Anticholinergics

PRECAUTIONS
• Monitor patients on sulfasalazine for signs of keratoconjunctivitis sicca
• Monitor patients on azathioprine for bone marrow suppression (i.e., CBC every 2-3 weeks; stop treatment or go to alternate-day if WBC count falls below 4000 cells/μL)

POSSIBLE INTERACTIONS N/A

ALTERNATE DRUGS
Albendazole (25 mg/kg q12h for 2 days) to treat giardiasis if metronidazole is ineffective

FOLLOW-UP

PATIENT MONITORING
Clinical signs every 2-3 weeks initially then every 3-4 months

PREVENTION/AVOIDANCE
• Avoid exposure to infectious agents (e.g., other dogs, contaminated foods, and moist environments) • Avoid abrupt diet changes

POSSIBLE COMPLICATIONS
• Recurrence of signs without treatment, when treatment is tapered, and with progression of disease • Stricture formation due to chronic inflammation

EXPECTED COURSE AND PROGNOSIS
• Most infections—prognosis excellent with treatment (cure) • Prototheca—no known treatment except excision; prognosis grave • Histoplasma and phycomycosis—poorly responsive to treatment; prognosis guarded • Traumatic, uremic, and segmental—prognosis good if underlying cause is treatable • Cecal inversion, ileocecocolic intussusception, and polyps—prognosis good with surgical removal • Inflammatory—prognosis in patients with lymphoplasmacytic and eosinophlic disease good with treatment; prognosis poor in patients with granulomatous and histiocytic disease in the short term and worsens with recurrence or poor response to treatment • Neoplasia—prognosis fair to good in patients with adenocarcinoma if surgically resectable and no metastasis; prognosis poor with lymphosarcoma

MISCELLANEOUS

ASSOCIATED CONDITIONS
Small intestines may also be affected by inflammatory disease, infectious agents, and neoplasia

AGE RELATED FACTORS N/A

ZOONOTIC POTENTIAL
Entamoeba, Balantidium, Giardia, Salmonella, Clostridium, Campylobacter, Yersinia, and E. coli; Prototheca, Histoplasma in immunosuppressed individuals

PREGNANCY
Caution with drug use—corticosteroids, azathioprine, and antibiotics

SYNONYMS
Large bowel diarrhea
Inflammatory bowel disease

SEE ALSO
• Inflammatory Bowel Disease • Colitis, Histiocytic Ulcerative

ABBREVIATIONS N/A

References
Burrows CF. Canine colitis. Comp Cont Ed Pract Vet 1992;10:1347-1354.
Sherding RG, Burrows CF. Diarrhea. In: Veterinary gastroenterology. Anderson NV, ed. Philadelphia: Lea and Febiger, 1992;455-477.
Leib MS, Matz ME. Diseases of the large intestine. In: Textbook of veterinary internal medicine. Ettinger SJ, Feldman EC, eds. Philadelphia: WB Saunders, 1995;1232-1260.

Author Colin F. Burrows and Lisa E. Moore

Consulting Editor Brent D. Jones

COLITIS, HISTIOCYTIC ULCERATIVE

BASICS

OVERVIEW
Rare disease characterized by colonic mucosal ulceration and inflammation with periodic acid-Schiff (PAS) positive histiocytes; breed predisposition in young boxer dogs. Etiologic and pathogenic mechanism unknown.

SIGNALMENT
• Dogs • Primarily affects young boxers, usually < 2 years old • Reported in a French bulldog • Possible genetic basis but unknown

SIGNS
• Bloody, mucoid diarrhea with increasing frequency • Tenesmus • Weight loss and debilitation may develop late in the disease process.

CAUSES AND RISK FACTORS
No known cause or predisposing factors

DIAGNOSIS

DIFFERENTIAL DIAGNOSIS
• Must differentiate from other causes of colitis, cecal inversion, ileocecocolic intussusception, other inflammatory disease, neoplasia, and foreign body. • Differentiation made by examination of fecal flotations and direct smears, bacterial culture (infectious disease), and colonoscopy and biopsy (inflammatory disease and neoplasia)

CBC/BIOCHEMISTRY/URINALYSIS
Results usually normal; neutrophilia and mild anemia in some patients

OTHER LABORATORY TESTS N/A

IMAGING N/A

OTHER DIAGNOSTIC PROCEDURES
Colonoscopy reveals patchy red foci (pinpoint ulcerations), overt ulceration, thick mucosal folds, areas of granulation tissue, and strictures.

GROSS AND HISTOPATHOLOGIC FINDINGS
Biopsy reveals thickening of the lamina propria and histiocytes, lymphocytes, and plasma cells in the submucosa; ulceration with neutrophil infiltration in some animals. Histiocytes are PAS positive.

TREATMENT
• Outpatient
• Diet should be changed to include fiber supplementation
• Advise owner of progressive nature and possibility of recurrence and ultimate inability to control disease

MEDICATIONS

DRUGS AND FLUIDS

Anti-inflammatory/Immunosuppressive Drugs
• Corticosteroids—prednisone (1-2mg/kg q24h until clinical remmission then taper slowly)
• Sulfasalazine (25-40mg/kg PO q8h)
• Azathioprine (1mg/kg q24h for 2 weeks followed by alternate-day administration)

Antimicrobials
• Metronidazole (25mg/kg PO q12h)
• Tylosin (45mg/kg PO q24h)

CONTRAINDICATIONS/POSSIBLE INTERACTIONS
Avoid anticholinergic drugs

FOLLOW-UP

PATIENT MONITORING
Clinical signs and body weight

POSSIBLE COMPLICATIONS
• Progressive, uncontrollable disease
• Colonic stricture

EXPECTED COURSE AND PROGNOSIS
Patient may initially respond to treatment if begun early in course of disease; eventually disease progresses and prognosis is guarded.

MISCELLANEOUS

PREGNANCY
Caution with drug use (e.g., corticosteroids and azathioprine)

SEE ALSO
Colitis and Proctitis

ABBREVIATIONS
PAS = periodic acid-Schiff

References
Sherding RG, Burrows CF. Diarrhea. In: Veterinary Gastroenterology. Anderson NV, ed. Philadelphia: Lea and Febiger, 1992;465-466.
Hall EJ, Rutgers HC, et.al. Histiocytic ulcerative colitis in boxer dogs in the U.K. J Small Anim Pract 1994;35:509-515.
Authors Lisa E. Moore and Colin F. Burrows
Consulting Editor Brent D. Jones

BASICS

OVERVIEW
A congenital, autosomal recessive condition minimally consisting of temporal to superiotemporal choroidal hypoplasia and excessive tortuosity of primary retinal vessels. Possible accompanying defects indicating more severe manifestations of the condition include optic nerve coloboma, staphylomas, retinal detachment, and intraocular hemorrhage. It is always bilateral, although the severity may be disparate between eyes. There is potential for blindness because of retinal detachment. Associated anomalies not directly part of the syndrome include enophthalmia, microphthalmia, retinal folds, and mineralization of the anterior corneal stroma.

SIGNALMENT
• Present at birth • Occurs in both smooth and rough-coated collies • Similar condition affects Shetland sheepdog and border collie

SIGNS
• None to various degrees of partial or complete blindness. • The minimal ophthalmoscopic findings necessary for a diagnosis are increased retinal vessel tortuosity and choroidal hypoplasia. The latter is defined as a focal to diffuse area of anomalous choroidal vasculature. The number of choroidal vessels is reduced and, rather than being present in the normal radiating pattern, they are tortuous and disorganized. The overlying tapetum is usually focally absent (which allows for the visualization of the underlying choroid), and the underlying sclera may be seen between choroidal vessels. Choroidal hypoplasia is present temporal or superior-temporal to the optic disc and may extend nasally more in dogs with severe disease. • Optic nerve coloboma (pitting of the optic nerve head), retinal detachment, and intraocular hemorrhage occur in some animals.

CAUSES AND RISK FACTORS
• Because the anomaly is an autosomal recessive trait, it can only occur by breeding two affected or carrier animals to each other.
• Approximately 85% of collies in North America are homozygous affected or heterozygous carriers of the condition. • Less than 10% of collies in Europe are affected or carrier animals.

DIAGNOSIS

DIFFERENTIAL DIAGNOSIS
• Excessive tortuosity of retinal vessels in the absence of choroidal hypoplasia does not classify as collie eye anomaly. • Lack of pigment in the pigmented epithelial layer of the retina may allow visualization of normal choroidal vasculature. This is usually associated with merling of the coat, and it is differentiated from collie eye anomaly by the presence of normal, regular, radiating choroidal vessels, not reduced numbers or anomalous ones.
• Optic nerve colobomata and retinal detachments may occur independent of choroidal hypoplasia and, as such, do not indicate collie eye anomaly.

CBC/BIOCHEMISTRY/URINALYSIS
N/A

OTHER LABORATORY TESTS N/A

IMAGING N/A

OTHER DIAGNOSTIC PROCEDURES
N/A

TREATMENT
• There is no treatment to reverse the condition. • Cryosurgery or laser around the area of the optic nerve coloboma may prevent retinal detachment or may be used to assist in reattachment of an already detached retina.

MEDICATIONS
DRUGS AND FLUIDS None

CONTRAINDICATIONS/POSSIBLE INTERACTIONS N/A

FOLLOW-UP

PATIENT MONITORING
Dogs with colobomata should be monitored in the first year of life for occurrence of secondary retinal detachments. After this time, retinal detachments rarely occur.

PREVENTION/AVOIDANCE
Because the anomaly is caused by a recessive trait, breeding of only genotypically normal dogs will prevent occurrence of the condition. Breeding of minimally affected dogs to other minimally-affected or carrier dogs may result in minimally affected offspring. However, any level of severity can be produced by breeding affected or carrier dogs to other affected or carrier dogs.

EXPECTED COURSE AND PROGNOSIS
With the exception of colobomata potentially leading to retinal detachment after birth, the condition does not progress. Occasionally, animals with minor areas of choroidal hypoplasia will develop pigment across this area with time and will appear to be phenotypically normal. For this reason, early examination (in the first 6-8 weeks of life) is highly recommended.

MISCELLANEOUS

ASSOCIATED CONDITIONS
• Microphthalmia • Enophthalmia • Retinal folds • Anterior corneal stromal mineralization

SYNONYM Scleral ectasia syndrome

Reference
Roberts SR. The collie eye anomaly. J Am Vet Med Assoc 1969:155:859–864.
Author Stephanie L. Smedes
Consulting Editor Paul E. Miller

CONGESTIVE HEART FAILURE, LEFT-SIDED

BASICS

DEFINITION
• Failure of the left side of the heart to advance blood at a sufficient rate to meet the metabolic needs of the patient or to prevent blood from pooling within the pulmonary venous circulation

Pathophysiology
Mechanisms
• Pump failure (muscle failure) of the left ventricle • Pressure overload to the left heart • Volume overload of the left heart • Impediment to filling of left heart • Rhythm disturbances
Consequences
• Low cardiac output causes lethargy, exercise intolerance , syncope, and prerenal azotemia. • High hydrostatic pressure causes leakage of fluid from pulmonary venous circulation into pulmonary interstitium and alveoli. • When fluid leakage exceeds ability of lymphatics to drain the affected areas, pulmonary edema develops.

Systems Affected
• All organ systems can be affected by poor delivery of blood. • Respiratory because of edema • Cardiovascular

Genetics
• Vary with cause; some congenital defects have a genetic basis in certain breeds.

Incidence/Prevalence
• Common syndrome in clinical practice

Geographic Distribution
• Seen everywhere, but prevalence of causes varies with location.

SIGNALMENT
Species Dogs and cats

Breed Predilections Varies with cause

Mean Age and Range Varies with cause

Predominant Sex
Males, except for animals with patent ductus arteriosus (PDA)

SIGNS
General Comments
• Signs vary with underlying cause and between species

Historical Findings
• Weakness, lethargy, exercise intolerance. • Coughing (dogs) and dyspnea. Respiratory signs often worsen at night and can be relieved by assuming a standing, sternal, or "elbows abducted" position (orthopnea). • Cats rarely cough.

Physical Examination Findings
• Tachypnea • Coughing, often soft in conjunction with tachypnea • Inspiratory and expiratory dyspnea when animal has pulmonary edema • Pulmonary crackles and wheezes • Prolonged capillary refill time

• Possible murmur (eg, mitral insufficiency) or gallop (e.g., S3 or S4, a sign of excess ventricular stiffness) • Weak femoral pulses

CAUSES
Pump (Muscle) Failure
• Idiopathic dilated cardiomyopathy (DCM) • Trypanosomiasis (rare) • Doxorubicin cardiotoxicity (dogs) • Hypothyroidism (rare) • Hyperthyroidism (rarely causes pump failure; more commonly causes high output failure)

Pressure Overload
• Systemic hypertension • Subaortic stenosis • Coarctation of the aorta (rare; airdales predisposed) • Left ventricular tumors (rare)

Volume Overload of the Left Heart
• Mitral valve endocardiosis • Mitral valve dysplasia • PDA • Ventral septal defect

Impediment to Filling of Left Heart
• Pericardial effusion with tamponade • Restrictive pericarditis • Restrictive cardiomyopathy • Hypertrophic cardiomyopathy • Left atrial masses (e.g., tumors and thrombus) • Pulmonary thromboembolism • Mitral stenosis (rare)

Rhythm Disturbances
• Bradycardia (AV block) • Tachycardia (e.g., atrial fibrillation, atrial tachycardia, and ventricular tachycardia)

RISK FACTORS
Diseases that magnify demand for cardiac output (eg, hyperthyroidism, anemia, and pregnancy)

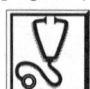

DIAGNOSIS

DIFFERENTIAL DIAGNOSIS
Must differentiate from other causes of coughing, dyspnea, and weakness; generally requires a complete diagnostic work-up.

CBC/BIOCHEMISTRY/URINALYSIS
• CBC usually normal; may be stress leukogram • Mild to moderately high alanine transaminase, aspartate transaminase, and serum alkaline phosphatase; Bilirubin generally normal. • Prenatal azotemia (high BUN +/- high creatinine with normal urine concentrating ability) in some animals

OTHER LABORATORY TESTS
Thyroid disorders may be detected.

IMAGING
Radiographic Findings
• Left heart enlargement; and pulmonary venous enlargement • Pulmonary edema, often hilar, initially; may be patchy, especially in cats; usually symetrical, but may begin in right caudal lung lobe

Echocardiography
• Findings vary markedly with cause, but left atrial enlargement a relatively consistent finding • Diagnostic test of choice for documenting congenital defects, cardiac masses, and pericardial effusion

OTHER DIAGNOSTIC PROCEDURES
Electrocardiographic Findings
• Atrial or ventricular arrhythmias • Evidence of left heart enlargement (eg, wide P waves, tall and wide QRS complexes, and left axis orientation) • May be normal

GROSS AND HISTOPATHOLOGIC FINDINGS
• Cardiac findings vary with disease

TREATMENT
• Identify and correct underlying cause whenever possible.
• Minimize handling of critically dyspneic animals. Stress can kill!

INPATIENT VERSUS OUTPATIENT
• Usually treat as outpatient unless animal is dyspneic or severely hypotensive

ACTIVITY
Restrict activity

DIET
Initiate moderately sodium-restricted diet. Severe sodium restriction indicated in animals with advanced disease.

CLIENT EDUCATION
• With few exceptions (ie, animals with thyroid disorders, arrhythmias, idiopathic and pericardial effusion); left congestive heart failure (L-CHF) is not curable.

SURGICAL CONSIDERATIONS
• Surgical intervention or balloon valvuloplasty may benefit selected patients with congenital defects such as PDA and aortic stenosis. Response to these interventions varies.
• Pericardiocentesis in animals with pericardial effusion

MEDICATIONS
DRUGS AND FLUIDS
Oxygen
• Oxygen is life saving in critically dyspneic patients; administer in an oxygen cage, by oxygen mask, or by nasal catheter.

Diuretics
• Furosemide (1-2 mg/kg q8h-q24h) or other loop diuretic is the initial diuretic of choice; diuretics indicated to remove pulmonary edema
• Critically dyspneic animals often require high doses (4-8 mg/kg) given IV to stabilize; this dose can be repeated in 1 hour if animal is still severely dyspneic.
• Predisposes the patient to dehydration, prerenal azotemia, and electrolyte disturbances.
• Once pulmonary edema resolves, always taper the diuretic to the lowest dosage that controls edema.

Digoxin
• Digoxin (dogs, 0.22 mg/M^2 q12h; cats, 0.01 mg/kg q48h) is used in animals with

CONGESTIVE HEART FAILURE, LEFT-SIDED

myocardial failure (e.g., dilated cardiomyopathy and cyclophosphamide cardiotoxicity).
• Digoxin also indicated to treat supraventricular arrhythmias (e.g., sinus tachycardia, atrial fibrillation, and atrial or junctional tachycardia) in patients with CHF

Venodilators
• Nitroglycerin ointment (0.25 in/5 kg q6h-q8h) causes venodilation, lowering left atrial filling pressures and the forces that cause pulmonary edema.
• Often used for acute stabilization of patients with severe pulmonary edema and dyspnea. Apply directly to the gums, a hairless area in the inguinal or axillary region, or the inside of the pinna. If the pinna are cold, choose an alternate site.
• When used intermittently, it may be useful in animals with chronic L-CHF.
• Tolerance will develop with frequent administration, so best to use intermittently and with 12-hour, dose-free interval between the last dose of one day and the first dose of the next day.

ACE Inhibitors
• ACE inhibitor such as enalapril (0.5 mg/kg q12h-q24h) indicated in animal with L-CHF secondary to degenerative mitral valve disease and in dog with DCM. In such patients, ACE inhibitor improves survival and quality of life.
• ACE inhibitor may also be of benefit in selected animals with congenital defects (eg, mitral valve dysplasia and ventral septal defect).
• Indications in cats with cardiomyopathy nothave yet to be defined.

Positive Inotropes
• Dopamine (dogs, 2.5-10 mcg/kg/min; cats, 1-5 mcg/kg/min) and dobutamine (dogs, 2.5-10 mcg/kg/min; cats, 2-10 mcg/kg/min) are potent positive inotropic agents that may provide valuable short-term support of a heart failure patient with poor cardiac contractility.
• These agents are arrhythmogenic, and dopamine can cause hypertension at high infusion rates. Careful monitoring is required.

Antiarrhythmic Agents
Treat arrhythmias if clinically indicated.

CONTRAINDICATIONS
• Avoid vasodilators in patients with pericardial effusion or fixed outflow obstruction.

PRECAUTIONS
• ACE inhibitor and arterial dilators must be used with caution in patients with possible outflow obstruction.
• Patients with pulmonary hypertension and hypoxia are at high risk for digoxin toxicity.
• ACE inhibitor and digoxin must be used cautiously in patients with renal disease.
• Use dobutamine cautiously in cats.
• Hypothyroidism predisposes animal to digoxin toxicity, while hyperthyroidism diminishes effects of digoxin.

POSSIBLE INTERACTIONS
• Combination of high-dose diuretics and ACE inhibitor may alter renal perfusion, and

cause azotemia, especially in animals with severe sodium restriction.
• Combination diuretic therapy adds to risk of dehydration and electrolyte disturbances.
• Combination vasodilator therapy predisposes animal to hypotension.

ALTERNATE DRUGS

Arterial Dilators
• Hydralazine (1-2 mg/kg PO q12h) can be substituted for an ACE inhibitor in patients that do not tolerate the drug or have advanced renal failure, or if the cost is prohibitive. Monitor for hypotension and reflex tachycardia. Add digoxin if sinus tachycardia develops. Can be used with an ACE inhibitor in animals with refractory L-CHF.
• Nitroprusside (1-10 mcg/kg/min) is a potent arterial dilator. Usually reserved for short-term support of patients with life-threatening edema.

Calcium Channel Blockers
• Diltiazem (0.5-1.5 mg/kg PO q8h) is frequently used in L-CHF patients for rate control in animals with supraventricular arrhythmias not controlled by digoxin and in cats with hypertrophic cardiomyopathy.

Beta Blockers
• Propranolol, atenolol, and metoprolol are used for rate control in animals with supraventricular tachycardia, hypertrophic cardiomyopathy, and hyperthyroidism.
• Used alone or with a class 1 antiarrhythmic drug for control of ventricular arrhythmias. These drugs depress contractility (negative inotropes), so use cautiously in patients with myocardial failure.
• On basis of human studies, may enhance survival in animals with idiopathic DCM. Treatment best initiated under the guidance of a cardiologist, starting with very low dosage and gradually increasing the dosage.
• Patients unresponsive to furosemide, vasodilator, and digoxin (if indicated) may benefit from combination diuretic therapy by adding spironolactone (1-2 mg/kg PO q12h) and/or a thiazide diuretic to furosemide.

Supplements
• Potassium supplementation if hypokalemia is documented. Use potassium supplements cautiously in animals receiving ACE inhibitor or spironolactone.
• Taurine supplementation in cats with DCM and dogs with DCM and taurine deficiency
• L-carnitine supplementation may help some dogs with DCM.

FOLLOW-UP

PATIENT MONITORING
• Monitor renal status, electrolytes, hydration, respiratory rate and effort, heart rate, body weight, and abdominal girth (dogs).

• If azotemia develops, reduce the dosage of diuretic. If azotemia persists and the animal is also on an ACE inhibitor, reduce or discontinue the ACE inhibitor. Use digoxin with caution if azotemia develops. • Monitor ECG if arrhythmias are suspected. • Check digoxin concentration if concerned about digoxin toxicity or lack of improvement on medication. Normal range is 1-2 ng/ml, 8-10 hours after a dose.

PREVENTION/AVOIDANCE
• Minimize stress, exercise, and sodium intake in patients with heart disease.
• Prescribing an ACE inhibitor early in the course of heart disease in patients with mitral valve disease and DCM may slow the progression of heart disease and delay onset of CHF. Consider this in asymptomatic animals if they have DCM or if they have mitral valve disease and radiographic or echocardiographic evidence of left heart enlargement.

POSSIBLE COMPLICATIONS
• Syncope • Aortic thromboembolism (cats) • Arrhythmias • Electrolyte imbalances • Digoxin toxicity • Azotemia and renal failure

EXPECTED COURSE AND PROGNOSIS
Prognosis varies with underlying cause

MISCELLANEOUS

ASSOCIATED CONDITIONS N/A

AGE RELATED FACTORS
• Congenital causes seen in young animals
• Degenerative heart conditions and neoplasia generally seen in old animals

ZOONOTIC POTENTIAL N/A

PREGNANCY N/A

SYNONYMS N/A

SEE ALSO
• Diseases Causing L-CHF • Pulmonary Edema

ABBREVIATIONS
ACE = angiotensin converting enzyme
DCM = dilated cardiomyopathy
CHF = congestive heart failure
L-CHF = left-sided congestive heart failure
PDA = patent ductus arteriosus

References
Kittleson MD. Pathophysiology and treatment of heart failure. In: Miller MS, Tilley LP, eds. Manual of canine and feline cardiology. 2nd ed. Philadelphia: WB Saunders, 1995.
Authors Francis W. K. Smith, Jr. and Bruce W. Keene
Consulting Editors Larry P. Tilley and Francis W. K. Smith, Jr.

CONGESTIVE HEART FAILURE, RIGHT-SIDED

BASICS

DEFINITION
• Failure of the right side of the heart to advance blood at a sufficient rate to meet the metabolic needs of the patient or to prevent blood from pooling within the systemic venous circulation

Pathophysiology
Mechanisms
• Pump (muscle) failure of the right ventricle
• Pressure overload to the right heart • Volume overload of the right heart • Impediment to filling of the right heart • Rhythm disturbances
Consequences
• High hydrostatic pressure leads to leakage of fluid from venous circulation into the pleural and peritoneal space and interstitium of peripheral tissue. • When fluid leakage exceeds ability of lymphatics to drain the affected areas, pleural effusion, ascites, and peripheral edema develop.

Systems Affected
• All organ systems can be affected by either poor delivery of blood or the effects of passive congestion from backup of venous blood.

Genetics
• Vary with cause; some congenital defects have a genetic basis in certain breeds.

Incidence/Prevalence
• Common syndrome in clinical practice

Geographic Distribution
• Syndrome seen everywhere, but prevalence of various causes varies with location

SIGNALMENT

Species Dogs and cats

Breed Predilections Vary with cause

Mean Age and Range Vary with cause

Predominant Sex Varies with cause

SIGNS

General Comments
• Signs vary with underlying cause and between species • Pleural effusion without ascites and hepatomegaly is rare in dogs with R-CHF (right-sided congestive heart failure). • Ascites without pleural effusion is rare in cats with R-CHF.

Historical Findings
• Weakness • Lethargy • Exercise intolerance. • Abdominal distension • Dyspnea, tachypnea

Physical Examination Findings
• Jugular venous distention • Hepatojugular reflex • Jugular pulse in some animals • Hepatomegaly • Ascites common in dogs and rare in cats with R-CHF • Possible regurgitant murmur in tricuspid valve region or ejection murmur at left heart base (pulmonic stenosis) • Muffled heart sounds if animal has pleural or pericardial effusion • Weak femoral pulses

• Rapid, shallow respiration if animal has pleural effusion or severe ascites • Peripheral edema (infrequent) from R-CHF in dogs and cats

CAUSES

Pump (Myocardial) Failure
• Idiopathic dilated cardiomyopathy (DCM) • Trypanosomiasis • Doxorubicin cardiotoxicity

Pressure Overload
• Heartworm disease • Chronic obstructive pulmonary disease • Pulmonary thromboembolism • Pulmonic stenosis • Tetralogy of Fallot • Right ventricular tumors • Primary pulmonary hypertension

Impediment to Right Ventricular Filling
• Pericardial effusion • Restrictive pericarditis • Right atrial or caval masses (caval syndrome and tumors) • Tricuspid stenosis • Cortiriatriatum dexter

Rhythm Disturbances
• Bradycardia, generally atrioventricular block • Tachyarrhythmias, generally supraventricular tachycardia

RISK FACTORS
• No heartworm prophylaxis • Offspring of animal with right-sided congenital cardiac defect • Diseases that augment demand for cardiac output (e.g., hyperthyroidism, anemia, pregnancy)

DIAGNOSIS

DIFFERENTIAL DIAGNOSIS
• Must differentiate from other causes of pleural effusion and ascites; generally requires a complete diagnostic work-up to include CBC, biochemistry profile, heartworm test, thoracentesis or abdominocentesis with fluid analysis and cytologic examination and, sometimes, thoracic and abdominal ultrasound • Animals with ascites or pleural effusion due to heart failure should have jugular venous distension.

CBC/BIOCHEMISTRY/URINALYSIS
• CBC usually normal; animal with heartworm disease may have eosinophilia • Mild to moderately high alanine transaminase, aspartate transaminase, serum alkaline phosphatase because of passive congestion of the liver; bilirubin generally normal • Prerenal azotemia (i.e., high BUN +/- high creatinine with normal urine concentrating ability) in some animals

OTHER LABORATORY TESTS
Heartworm test may be positive

IMAGING

Thoracic Radiographic Findings
• Right heart enlargement in some animals • Dilated caudal vena cava (diameter greater than the length of the vertebra directly above the heart) • Pleural effusion (especially cats)

• Hepatosplenomegaly and possible ascites (especially dogs)

Echocardiography
• Recommended when cardiac cause is suspected but the nature of the disease is uncertain. • Findings vary with underlying cause. Especially useful for documenting congenital defect, cardiac mass, and pericardial effusion. • Abdominal ultrasound reveals hepatomegaly with hepatic vein dilation and, possibly, ascites.

OTHER DIAGNOSTIC PROCEDURES

Electrocardiographic Findings
• Small complexes if animal has pericardial or pleural effusion • Electrical alternans or elevated ST segment in animal with pericardial effusion • Evidence of right heart enlargement (i.e., tall P waves in lead II, deep S waves in leads I, II, aVF) • Right axis deviation • Atrial or ventricular arrhythmias
Note: ECG may be normal in patients with R-CHF

Abdomenocentesis
• Analysis of ascitic fluid in patients with R-CHF generally reveals modified transudate with a TP>2.5 mg/dl.

Thoracentesis
• Cats with pleural effusion associated with R-CHF may have transudate, modified transudate, pseudochylous, or chylous effusion. • Dogs with pleural effusion and R-CHF may have transudate or modified transudate.

Central Venous Pressure
Central venous pressure is high (> 9 cm H_2O)

GROSS AND HISTOPATHOLOGIC FINDINGS
• Cardiac findings vary with disease • Hepatomegaly in animals with centrolobular necrosis (chronic condition)

TREATMENT
Identify and correct underlying cause whenever possible.

INPATIENT VERSUS OUTPATIENT
Most animals treated as outpatient unless dyspneic

ACTIVITY Restrict activity.

DIET
Restrict sodium moderately; severe sodium restriction is indicated for animals with advanced disease.

CLIENT EDUCATION
• With few exceptions (e.g., heartworm disease, arrhythmias, and idiopathic pericardial effusion), R-CHF is not curable. • Most patients improve with initial treatment but often have recurrent failure. • High risk for sudden death

SURGICAL CONSIDERATIONS
• Surgical intervention or balloon valvulo-

plasty indicated to treat certain congenital defects such as pulmonic stenosis.
• Thoracentesis and abdomenocentesis may be required periodically for patients no longer responsive to medical management or for those with severe dyspnea due to pleural effusion or ascites.
• Pericardiocentesis if animal has perciardial effusion.

MEDICATIONS

DRUGS AND FLUIDS
Drugs should be administered only after a definitive diagnosis is made.

Diuretics
• Furosemide (1-2 mg/kg q8h-q24h) or other loop diuretic is the initial diuretic of choice. Diuretics are indicated to remove excess fluid accumulation (i.e., ascites or pleural effusion).
• Predisposes the patient to dehydration, pre-renal azotemia, and electrolyte disturbances.
• Contraindicated in animals with pericardial disease

Digoxin
• Digoxin (dogs, 0.22 mg/M² q12h; cats, 0.01 mg/kg q48h) is used in animals with myocardial failure (eg, dilated cardiomyopathy and cyclophosphamide cardiotoxicity).
• Digoxin is also indicated in animals with CHF that have supraventricular arrhythmias (e.g., sinus tachycardia, atrial fibrillation, and atrial or junctional tachycardia).

ACE Inhibitors
ACE inhibitors such as enalapril (0.5 mg/kg q12h-q24h) may be helpful, especially if R-CHF results from L-CHF.

CONTRAINDICATIONS
Avoid vasodilators in patients with pericardial effusion or fixed outflow obstructions.

PRECAUTIONS
• ACE inhibitors and arterial dilators must be used with caution in patients with possible outflow obstructions.
• Patients with pulmonary hypertension and hypoxia are at higher risk than others for digoxin toxicity.
• ACE inhibitors and digoxin must be used cautiously in patients with renal disease.
• Animals with hypothyroidism are predisposed to digoxin toxicity, while hyperthyroidism diminishes digoxin effects.

POSSIBLE INTERACTIONS
• Combination of high-dose diuretics and ACE inhibitor may alter renal perfusion and cause azotemia.
• Combination diuretic therapy promotes risk of dehydration and electrolyte disturbances.
• Combination vasodilator therapy predisposes animal to hypotension—monitor closely in hospital when initiating treatment with a second vasodilator

ALTERNATE DRUGS
• Patients unresponsive to furosemide, vasodilator, and digoxin (if indicated) may benefit from combination diuretic therapy by adding spironolactone or a thiazide diuretic to furosemide.
• Potassium supplementation if animal has hypokalemia; use potassium supplements cautiously in animals receiving ACE inhibitor or spironolactone. These drugs cause potassium retention.
• Treat arrhythmias if clinically indicated.
• Taurine supplementation in cats with DCM and dogs with DCM and taurine deficiency
• Carnitine supplementation may help some dogs with DCM.

FOLLOW-UP

PATIENT MONITORING
• Monitor renal status, electrolytes, hydration, respiratory rate and effort, body weight, and abdominal girth (dogs). • If azotemia develops, reduce the diuretic dosage. If azotemia persists and the animal is also on an ACE inhibitor, reduce or discontinue this drug. If azotemia develops, reduce the digoxin dosage to avoid toxicity. • Monitor ECG periodically to detect arrhythmias.
• Check digoxin concentration if concerned about digoxin toxicity or lack of improvement on medication. Normal values are 1-2 ng/ml for a serum sample obtained 8-10 hours after a dose is administered.

PREVENTION/AVOIDANCE N/A

POSSIBLE COMPLICATIONS
• Pulmonary thromboembolism • Arrhythmias • Electrolyte imbalances • Digoxin toxicity • Azotemia and renal failure

EXPECTED COURSE AND PROGNOSIS
Prognosis varies with underlying cause.

MISCELLANEOUS

ASSOCIATED CONDITIONS N/A

AGE RELATED FACTORS
• Congenital causes seen in young animals
• Degenerative heart conditions and neoplasia generally seen in old animals

ZOONOTIC POTENTIAL N/A

PREGNANCY N/A

SYNONYMS N/A

SEE ALSO
• Diseases causing R-CHF • Ascites • Pleural Effusion • Chylothorax

ABBREVIATIONS
ACE = angiotensin converting enzyme
DCM = dilated cardiomyopathy
L-CHF = left-sided congestive heart failure
R-CHF = right-sided congestive heart failure

References

Kittleson MD. Pathophysiology and treatment of heart failure. In: Miller MS, Tilley LP, eds. Manual of canine and feline cardiology. 2nd ed. Philadelphia: WB Saunders, 1995.

Smith TW, Braunwald E, Kelly RA. The management of heart failure. In: Braunwald E, ed. Heart disease. A textbook of cardiovascular medicine. 4th ed. Philadelphia: WB Saunders, 1992.

International Small Animal Cardiac Health Council. Recommendations for the diagnosis of heart disease and the treatment of heart failure in small animals. In: Miller MS, Tilley LP, eds. Manual of canine and feline cardiology. 2nd ed. Philadelphia: WB Saunders, 1995.

Authors Francis W. K. Smith, Jr. and Bruce W. Keene

Consulting Editors Larry P. Tilley and Francis W. K. Smith, Jr.

CONJUNCTIVITIS

BASICS

DEFINITION
Inflammation of the conjunctiva, the vascularized mucous membrane that covers the anterior portion of the globe (bulbar portion) and lines the lids and third eyelid (palpebral portion)

Pathophysiology
Can be primary (e.g., allergic, infectious, environmental, and keratoconjunctivitis sicca) or secondary to an underlying ocular or systemic disease (e.g., glaucoma, uveitis, immune-mediated disease, neoplasia)

Systems Affected
Ophthalmic—ocular with occasional lid involvement (e.g., blepharoconjunctivitis)

Genetics N/A

Incidence/Prevalence Common

Geographic Distribution N/A

SIGNALMENT

Species Dogs and cats

Breed Predilections
• Dog breeds predisposed to allergic or immune-mediated skin diseases (e.g., atopy) tend to have more problems with allergic conjunctivitis or dry eye. • Purebred cats seem predisposed to infectious conjunctivitis.

Mean Age and Range N/A

Predominant Sex N/A

SIGNS
• Blepharospasm • Conjunctival hyperemia • Ocular discharge (serous, mucoid or mucopurulent) • Chemosis • Follicle formation • Bulbar or palpebral conjunctiva may be primarily involved • Upper respiratory infection in cats possible

CAUSES

Bacterial
• Bacterial infection as a primary condition (i.e., not secondary to other condition such as keratoconjunctivitis sicca) is rare in dogs and cats, with the exception of chlamydial and mycoplasma conjunctivitis in cats.
• Neonatal conjunctivitis is an accumulation of exudates, often with a bacterial or viral component, seen before lid separation.

Viral
• Canine distemper virus • Feline herpes virus—may cause corneal changes (e.g., dendritic or geographic ulcers) • Calicivirus in cats

Immune Mediated
• Allergic, especially in atopic dogs • Follicular conjunctivitis • Plasma cell conjunctivitis, especially in German shepherds • Eosinophilic conjunctivitis in cats • Related to systemic immune-mediated diseases (e.g., pemphigus)

Neoplastic, Pseudoneoplastic
• Tumors reported to involve the conjunctiva in dogs and cats are rare and include melanoma,

hemangioma, hemangiosarcomas, lymphosarcoma, papilloma, and mast cell tumors. • A pseudoneoplastic condition most commonly seen in Collies and mixed collies is nodular episcleritis (also called fibrous histiocytoma, ocular nodular granuloma, and conjunctival pseudotumor). The condition is believed to be immune-mediated, and appears as a flesh colored mass, most commonly located at the temporal limbus.

Secondary to Adnexal Disease
• Aqueous tear film deficiency—see keratoconjunctivitis sicca. • Lid diseases such as entropion, ectropion, exaggerated cul-de-sac, and lash diseases such as distichiasis and ectopic cilia may lead to clinical signs of conjunctivitis.
• Secondary to obstruction of the outflow portion of the nasolacrimal system (e.g., obstructed nasolacrimal duct and imperforate punctum).

Secondary to Trauma or Environmental Causes
• Conjunctival foreign body • Irritation from dust, chemicals, or ophthalmic medications

Secondary to Other Ocular Diseases
• Ulcerative keratitis • Anterior uveitis
• Glaucoma

RISK FACTORS N/A

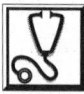

DIAGNOSIS

DIFFERENTIAL DIAGNOSIS
• Primary conjunctivitis should be distinguished from conjunctivitis secondary to other ocular diseases. • Involvement of the bulbar conjunctiva with minimal or no involvement of the palpebral conjunctiva generally indicates intraocular disease. Involvement of mainly the palpebral conjunctiva sparing the bulbar conjunctiva is usually seen in animals with primary or allergic conjunctivitis. If both surfaces are involved, primary and secondary causes should be considered. • Differentiating between conjunctival vessels (freely mobile and will blanch with sympathomimetic) and episcleral (deep) vessels (immobile and do not blanch with sympathomimetics) is important, because episcleral congestion indicates intraocular disease, whereas conjunctival hyperemia may be a sign of primary conjunctivitis or intraocular disease.

CBC/BIOCHEMISTRY/URINALYSIS
Normal unless the animal has a systemic disease

Other Laboratory Tests
Serologic test for FeLV and FIV should be considered in cats with infectious conjunctivitis to rule out underlying immunocompromise.

IMAGING N/A

OTHER DIAGNOSTIC PROCEDURES
• Complete ophthalmic examination, includ-

ing Schirmer tear test (to rule out keratoconjunctivitis sicca), fluorescein stain (to rule out ulcerative keratitis), intraocular pressures (to rule out glaucoma), and examining for signs of anterior uveitis (e.g., hypotony, aqueous flare, and miosis). • Thorough adnexal examination to rule out lid abnormalities, lash abnormalities, and foreign bodies in cul-de-sacs or under nictitans. • Consider a nasolacrimal flush to rule out nasolacrimal disease. • If a mucopurulent discharge is present, an aerobic bacterial culture and sensitivity test should be considered. Specimens should ideally be taken before anything is placed in the eye (e.g., topical anesthetic, fluorescein, and flush) because some believe that these may inhibit or dilute bacterial growth. If the animal has keratoconjunctivitis sicca and a mucopurulent discharge, then secondary bacterial overgrowth is almost certain, and culture is not routinely indicated. • Conjunctival cytology. Eosinophils and basophils can help diagnose allergic and eosinophilic conjunctivitis, but these are rarely seen in animals with allergic conjunctivitis except on biopsy. Degenerate neutrophils and intracytoplasmic bacteria indicate bacterial infection. Inclusion bodies can occasionally be found—intracytoplasmic in dogs with distemper virus and cats with chlamydial or mycoplasmal infection. Feline herpes virus inclusions are very rarely seen.
• Conjunctival scrapings can be obtained from cats, and the material tested for feline herpes virus or Chlamydia by an immunofluorescent antibody (IFA) technique or for Chlamydia with special stains. Fluorescein staining done the previous week can give a false-positive result of IFA testing. Stains for Chlamydia are fairly reliable; however, IFA test for feline herpesvirus is often falsely negative in animals with chronic disease. • Viral culture, if available, may help diagnose feline herpes virus, calicivirus, and canine distemper infection. • Conjunctival biopsy may be useful in animals with mass lesions, immune-mediated disease, or in chronic conjunctivitis in which a definitive diagnosis has not been made.

GROSS AND HISTOPATHOLOGIC FINDINGS
Histopathologic features of mass lesions are consistent with similar lesions elsewhere.

TREATMENT

INPATIENT VERSUS OUTPATIENT
Primary conjunctivitis can often be treated on an outpatient basis. Animals with conjunctivitis secondary to other diseases (e.g., uveitis and ulcerative keratitis) may need hospitalization while the underlying problem is diagnosed and treated.

ACTIVITY
No restriction of activity is required in most

animals with primary conjunctivitis. If contact irritant or acute allergic conjunctivitis is suspected, the animal should not (if possible) be allowed contact with the offending agent. If feline herpes virus is suspected, minimizing stress is recommended. Animals with infectious conjunctivitis should not be exposed to susceptible animals.

DIET

If underlying skin disease is suspected and food allergy is a consideration, then adherence to a food allergy elimination diet is recommended.

CLIENT EDUCATION

If copious discharge is present, the eyes should be cleaned before treatment. If solutions and ointments are both prescribed, the solution(s) should be used before the ointment(s). If several solutions are used, the owner should wait several minutes between treatments. If the conditions worsens, the owners should call for instructions. The condition may not be responsive, may be progressing, or the animal may be having an adverse reaction to a prescribed medication. The owner should be informed that an Elizabethan collar should be placed on the animal if evidence of self trauma is observed.

SURGICAL CONSIDERATIONS

Treatment of a nasolacrimal duct obstruction is difficult and often not recommended. See epiphora chapter. Treatment of conjunctival neoplasia may require only local resection, or may involve excision followed by beta-irradiation, cryotherapy, radiofrequency hyperthermia, enucleation, or exenteration depending on the type of tumor and the extent of involvement.

MEDICATIONS

DRUGS AND FLUIDS

Bacterial Conjunctivitis

Treatment is based on bacterial culture and sensitivity results. Initial treatment with a broad-spectrum topical antibiotic or based on results of cytologic examination may be indicated while awaiting culture results. In general, if cocci are seen on cytologic examination, topical treatment with triple antibiotic or chloramphenicol is best. If rods are seen, gentamicin or tobramycin are usually effective. Treat q6h-q12h depending on severity of disease. Empirical treatment may be elected initially and culture performed only if animal is refractory to treatment. Systemic antibiotics are occasionally indicated, especially if more generalized disease (e.g., pyoderma) is present.

Neonatal Conjunctivitis

Carefully open the lid margins (medial to temporal), establish drainage, and treat with topical antibiotic and an antiviral if feline herpesvirus is suspected.

Chlamydia or Mycoplasmal Conjunctivitis

Treat with topical tetracycline q6h. Continue therapy for several days past resolution of all clinical signs. Recurrence or reinfection is common, and some advocate systemic tetracycline in difficult cases.

Herpetic Conjunctivitis

An antiviral is indicated in animals with herpetic keratitis, before keratectomy for corneal sequestrums suspected to be related to feline herpes virus, and in animals with severe intractable conjunctivitis. Herpesvirus conjunctivitis in cats is usually mild and self-limiting, and antiviral drug penetration is poor. Antiviral treatment in these cats is optional, and treatment may be directed at only controlling secondary bacterial infection. The drug of choice is trifluridine, and recommended treatment frequency is hourly the first day and then 5 times a day.

Immune-Mediated Conjunctivitis

Treatment depends on the severity. Corticosteroids administered topically (e.g., 0.1% dexamethasone) improve clinical signs of allergic conjunctivitis, follicular conjunctivitis, and plasma cell conjunctivitis, but the improvement is often temporary. Treating an underlying disease, if present (e.g., atopy), often improves clinical signs.

CONTRAINDICATIONS

• Topically administered corticosteroids should be avoided in animals with known or suspected herpetic conjunctivitis because some evidence exists that this predisposes to corneal sequestrum formation. They should also be avoided if corneal ulceration is present. • Topically administered cyclosporine should probably be avoided in animals with known or suspected herpetic conjunctivitis, unless a topically administered antiviral is used concurrently.

PRECAUTIONS

• Topically applied aminoglycosides and antiviral medication may be irritating. • Any animal being treated with corticosteroids topically should be monitored carefully for signs of corneal ulceration. If corneal ulceration occurs, corticosteroids should be discontinued immediately.

POSSIBLE INTERACTIONS N/A

ALTERNATE DRUGS

• Other antiviral medications include adenine arabinoside and idoxuridine. • Other corticosteroids include 1% prednisolone acetate, betamethasone, and hydrocortisone.

FOLLOW-UP

PATIENT MONITORING

Recheck shortly after beginning treatment (i.e., 5-7 days). Thereafter, recheck as needed.

PREVENTION/AVOIDANCE

• Treat any underlying disease that may be exacerbating the ocular disease, such as allergic or immune-mediated skin disease or keratoconjunctivitis sicca. • Prevent reexposure of animal to source of infection. • In an animal with herpetic conjunctivitis, minimize stress. • Cats with infectious conjunctivitis should ideally be isolated to prevent spread. • Vaccination against viral causes of conjunctivitis is recommended, but infection is still possible. Animals may be exposed to an infectious agent before vaccination (e.g., feline herpes virus infection of a kitten from an infected queen).

POSSIBLE COMPLICATIONS N/A

EXPECTED COURSE AND PROGNOSIS

• Bacterial conjunctivitis resolves in most animals with appropriate administration of antibiotics. If an underlying disease is found (e.g., keratoconjunctivitis sicca), resolution of bacterial conjunctivitis may depend on appropriate treatment and resolution of the disease. • Most cats infected with feline herpesvirus become chronic carriers. Episodes tend to lessen as the cat matures; however, in some cats, repeated exacerbations occur. Cats tend to have more severe clinical signs at times of stress or immunocompromise. • Immune-mediated diseases such as plasma cell conjunctivitis and eosinophilic conjunctivitis are diseases that tend to be controlled and not cured, and chronic treatment at the lowest level possible may be necessary.

MISCELLANEOUS

ASSOCIATED CONDITIONS

FeLV and FIV may predispose a cat to the chronic carrier state of feline herpesvirus conjunctivitis.

AGE RELATED FACTORS

Feline herpes virus tends to be more severe in kittens and in old cats in which immunity is waning.

ZOONOTIC POTENTIAL

Chlamydia psittaci has a low zoonotic potential.

PREGNANCY

Systemic antibiotics and corticosteroids should be used with caution, if at all, in pregnant animals. Absorption of topically applied medications should be considered a possibility, and the benefits of treatment should be weighed against the possible complications.

SYNONYMS N/A

SEE ALSO Keratoconjunctivitis sicca

ABBREVIATIONS N/A

References

Gelatt KN. Veterinary ophthalmology. 2nd ed. Philadelphia: Lea & Febiger, 1991.
Nasisse MP. Manifestations, diagnosis, and treatment of ocular herpesvirus infection in the cat. Compend Contin Educ Pract Vet 1982;4:962–971.

Author Erin S. Champagne
Consulting Editor Paul E. Miller

COONHOUND PARALYSIS (POLYRADICULONEURITIS, IDIOPATHIC)

BASICS

DEFINITION
• Acute inflammation of multiple nerve roots and peripheral nerves in dogs, with or without a previous history of contact with a raccoon • A proposed animal model for Guillain-Barré syndrome in humans

Pathophysiology
• Largely unknown • Suspected immune-mediated disease

Systems Affected
Nervous
• Peripheral nervous system with the most severe involvement occurring in the ventral nerve roots and the ventral root components of the spinal nerves • Cranial nerves involved in some patients, primarily cranial nerve VII and X • Respiratory paralysis secondary to intercostal and phrenic nerve involvement in some patients

Genetics
No proven genetic basis

Incidence/Prevalence
Most commonly recognized polyneuropathy in dogs in North America, although incidence is still low

Geographic Distribution
• Coonhound paralysis—relative to the distribution of raccoons (ie, North, Central, and parts of South America) • Acute canine idiopathic polyradiculoneuritis (ACIP)—worldwide

SIGNALMENT

Breed Predilections
• Coonhound, although any breed in contact with raccoons is susceptible • ACIP—none

Mean Age and Range N/A

Predominant Sex N/A

SIGNS

Historical Findings
• Signs appear 7-14 days after contact with a raccoon. • Initially, a stiff-stilted gait in all 4 limbs, with rapid progression to a flaccid, lower motor neuron tetraparesis to tetraplegia

Physical Examination Findings
• Generalized hyporeflexia to areflexia, hypoatonia to atonia, and severe neurogenic muscle atrophy. Pelvic limbs more severely affected than thoracic limbs in a few patients, and signs are usually symmetrical. • Labored respiration common in severely affected dogs, with occasional progression to respiratory paralysis. Aphonia or dysphonia in most dogs. • Facial paresis in a few dogs • Pain sensation is intact; many dogs have evidence of hyperesthesia because of variable dorsal nerve root involvement. However, motor dysfunction always predominates. Even tetraplegic dogs usually can wag their tail. • Appetite and water consumption usually normal • Urina-

tion and defecation normal • Initial progression of signs usually occurs over 4-5 days, although maximum progression can take up to 10 days. • The duration of the neurologic dysfunction ranges from several weeks up to 3-4 months and somewhat depends on the initial severity of neurologic involvement.
• Neurologic signs and progression of disease are the same for dogs with ACIP and disease progression, although without the initial history of a raccoon encounter.

CAUSES
• Contact with a raccoon, and perhaps more importantly, raccoon saliva • ACIP—no proven etiologic agents. Possibilities include previous respiratory or gastrointestinal viral or bacterial infection and vaccination.

RISK FACTORS
• Coonhounds tend to be a predisposed breed, primarily because of the nature of their activities. • Previous development of coonhound paralysis does not confer immunity, and it even appears that previously affected dogs are at greater risk of redeveloping the disease than the general population. It is not uncommon for dogs to have multiple bouts of the disease. • No known risk factors for ACIP

DIAGNOSIS

DIFFERENTIAL DIAGNOSIS
• Other acute polyneuropathy • Distal denervating disease • Botulism • Tick paralysis • Generalized (diffuse) or multifocal myelopathy (involving both the cervical and lumbosacral intumescences)

CBC/BIOCHEMISTRY/URINALYSIS
Results usually normal

OTHER LABORATORY TESTS
• Serum immunoglobulins—high serum IgG but not IgM in some patients • Immunologic studies—affected dogs have a strong positive serum reaction to raccoon saliva on ELISA assay, which decreases in intensity over time. Dogs that have been exposed to raccoon saliva but do not have the disease also have a strong positive reaction. Dogs with ACIP without raccoon contact are negative.

IMAGING N/A

OTHER DIAGNOSTIC PROCEDURES
• CSF analysis—high lumbar protein without an increase in leukocytes at all stages of the disease. Cerebellomedullary CSF may have mildly high protein in dogs examined after the acute stages of the disease. Albumin leakage across a suspected disrupted blood brain barrier is the primary cause of the protein increase. Most dogs have no intrathecal production of immunoglobulin. • Electrodiagnostics—electromyography reveals generalized spontaneous activity, the severity of which depends on the time of examination

after disease onset and the severity of neurologic signs. Other abnormalities include markedly low compound muscle action potential (CMAP) amplitudes after motor nerve stimulation, high minimum F wave latencies, high F ratio, and low F wave amplitudes (F waves represent late waves that evaluate proximal motor nerve and ventral nerve root function). Motor nerve conduction velocities are usually within normal range except in the most severely affected dogs, which may have mildly low values. Sensory nerve function is usually normal. These abnormalities indicate evidence of severe peripheral axonopathy, along with both axonal involvement and demyelination occurring in the ventral nerve roots.

GROSS AND HISTOPATHOLOGIC FINDINGS
The ventral nerve roots and the ventral root components of the spinal nerves develop the most severe lesions, consisting of various degrees of axonal degeneration, paranodal and segmental demyelination, and leukocyte infiltration (predominantly monocytes and macrophages, with scattered groups of lymphocytes and plasma cells). The peripheral nerves are similarly affected, although to a lesser degree. Dorsal nerve roots are much less severely affected than ventral roots.

TREATMENT

INPATIENT VERSUS OUTPATIENT
• Dogs in the progressive stage of the disease (especially during the first 4 days) should be closely monitored in-hospital for respiratory problems.
• Animals showing signs of severe respiratory compromise should be placed in intensive care.
• Ventilatory support may be required.
• Dogs that have stabilized can return home after initial diagnostic confirmation of their disease.

ACTIVITY
Encourage as much movement as possible. However, many dogs are tetraplegic.

DIET
• No restrictions
• Ensure dog is able to reach food and water
• Dogs with cervical weakness need to be hand-fed.

CLIENT EDUCATION
• Good nursing care essential
• Primary goals to prevent pressure sores and urine scalding and to limit the degree of muscle atrophy by diligent physiotherapy (e.g., passive limb movement and swimming as the dog's strength begins to improve)
• The dog needs soft and resilient bedding (straw is excellent), which must be kept clean and free of urine and feces, frequent turning

COONHOUND PARALYSIS (POLYRADICULONEURITIS, IDIOPATHIC)

(every 3-4 hours), frequent bathing, and an adequate nutritional status.

SURGICAL CONSIDERATIONS N/A

MEDICATIONS

DRUGS AND FLUIDS
• No specific treatment available
• Intravenous fluid therapy with lactated Ringer's solution is necessary only if the dog is dehydrated on examination because of an inability to reach water.

CONTRAINDICATIONS
• Corticosteroids do not improve clinical signs or shorten the course of disease.
• Corticosterioids may reduce survival in humans with Guillain-Barré syndrome.

PRECAUTIONS N/A

POSSIBLE INTERACTIONS N/A

ALTERNATE DRUGS N/A

FOLLOW-UP

PATIENT MONITORING
• If the owners are caring for the dog at home, keep in close contact regarding complications or changes in the dog's condition.
• Perform urinalysis periodically to check for cystitis in tetraplegic or severely tetraparetic dogs. • Ideally, reevaluate the patient every 2-3 weeks.

PREVENTION/AVOIDANCE
• Coonhound paralysis—avoid contact with raccoons. However, this is often not feasible because of these dogs' environment and their primary use as raccoon hunters. • ACIP—none

POSSIBLE COMPLICATIONS
• In the initial progressive stage of the disease, respiratory paralysis • Pressure sores, urine scalding, and cystitis common in chronically recumbent dogs

EXPECTED COURSE AND PROGNOSIS
• Most dogs recover fully. • The most severely affected dogs may be left with mild residual neurologic deficits. The duration of these abnormalities ranges from several weeks, in mildly to moderately affected dogs, up to 3-4 months in dogs with severe disease.

MISCELLANEOUS

ASSOCIATED CONDITIONS N/A
AGE RELATED FACTORS N/A
ZOONOTIC POTENTIAL N/A
PREGNANCY
Unknown effect of coonhound paralysis and ACIP on the fetus of an affected bitch

SYNONYMS
• Coondog paralysis • Idiopathic polyradiculoneuritis

SEE ALSO
• Peripheral Neuropathies (Polyneuropathies)
• Tick Bite Paralysis

ABBREVIATIONS
CSF = cerebrospinal fluid
ACIP = acute canine idiopathic polyradiculoneuritis

References
Cummings JF, Hass DC. Coonhound paralysis: an acute idiopathic polyradiculoneuritis resembling the Landry-Guillain-Barré syndrome. J Neurol Sci 1967;4:51-81.
Northington JW, Brown MJ. Acute canine idiopathic polyneuropathy: a Guillain-Barré-like syndrome in dogs. J Neurol Sci 1982;56:259-273.
Cummings JF, de Lahunta A, Holmes DF, Schultz RD. Coonhound paralysis: further clinical studies and electron microscopic observations. Acta Neuropathol 1982;56:167-178.
Cuddon PA. Acute canine idiopathic polyradiculoneuropathy—electrophysiology, CSF analysis, and immunology. In: Proceedings, 8th Annu Symp Euro Soc Vet Neurol. Limoges, France, 1994:34-36.
Author Paul A. Cuddon
Consulting Editor Joane M. Parent

COPPER HEPATOPATHY

BASICS

DEFINITION
Hepatic accumulation of copper causing chronic hepatitis and eventually cirrhosis

Pathophysiology
• Most commercial diets are high in copper. Copper is normally absorbed from the small intestine, stored in the liver, and excreted by the biliary system. • Copper accumulates in the liver of animals with abnormal copper binding proteins (Bedlington terrier) or abnormal bile metabolism (Skye terrier and, possibly, Doberman pinscher). Inflammation occurs once hepatic copper concentrations exceed 2000 mg/gm dry weight (DW).
• Chronic hepatitis eventually results in cirrhosis and hepatic failure. • Episode of acute hepatic necrosis may cause release of hepatic copper causing hemolysis.

Systems Affected
• Hepatobiliary—focal hepatitis leading to diffuse chronic hepatitis and eventually cirrhosis • Hemic/lymphatic/immune—hemolytic anemia occurs as a rare sequela to hepatic copper toxicosis in dogs

Genetics
• Autosomal recessive trait in Bedlington terriers • The mode of inheritance in West Highland white and Skye terriers is unknown. • Doberman pinschers have breed-related hepatic copper accumulation; the importance of which is controversial.

Incidence/Prevalence
• Bedlington terrier—as many as two-thirds of Bedlingtons in the United States may be affected • The prevalence of high hepatic copper concentration is high in the West Highland white terrier but the incidence of clinical disease is low.

Geographic Distribution None

SIGNALMENT

Species Dogs

Breed Predilection
• Bedlington terrier • West Highland white terrier • Skye terrier • Doberman pinschers, cocker spaniels, keeshonds, and Labrador retrievers often have hepatic copper concentrations higher than other breeds; the origin (primary or secondary) is unknown.

Mean Age and Range
• Bedlington terrier—copper accumulates over time to a maximum at about 6 years of age. Dogs can be clinically affected at any age. Young dogs can be clinically normal or have acute or recurring episodes of hepatic necrosis, whereas middle-aged to older dogs have progressive chronic hepatitis. • West Highland white terrier—maximum copper accumulation is observed by 6 months of age but clinical disease can occur at any age • Skye terrier—all ages can be affected

• Doberman pinscher—middle age

Predominant Sex
Doberman pinscher—female

SIGNS

General Comments
Clinically affected dogs usually fall into one of three clinical categories:
• Category 1-Young adult dogs with acute onset of severe clinical signs • Category 2-Middle-aged to older dogs with progressive clinical signs • Category 3-Subclinically affected dogs. • Bedlington terriers may fall into all three categories, whereas other breeds tend to fall into the second or third category.

Historical Findings
Category 1
• Acute onset of lethargy, anorexia, depression, and vomiting • Most of these dogs die despite intensive supportive treatment.
Category 2
• A more chronic history of waxing and waning lethargy, depression, anorexia, and weight loss • Vomiting, diarrhea, and polydipsia and polyuria may be seen. • Later signs may include abdominal distension, jaundice, spontaneous bleeding, and hepatic encephalopathy.

Physical Examination Findings
Category 1
• Depression, dehydration, and hepatomegaly
• Jaundice in many dogs • Hemoglobinuria in some dogs
Category 2
• Evidence of weight loss, ascites, and jaundice • Microhepatica is characteristic.
• Melena or petechial or ecchymotic hemorrhages in some dogs

CAUSES
• Abnormal copper binding protein, metallothionein • Abnormal biliary excretion of copper • Zinc deficiency

RISK FACTORS
• A diet high in copper may increase hepatic copper accumulation. • Chronic hepatobiliary disease

DIAGNOSIS

DIFFERENTIAL DIAGNOSIS

Acute Disease
• Infectious diseases (e.g., infectious canine hepatitis, Tyzzer's disease, leptospirosis, and bacterial septicemia) • Acute hepatic necrosis • Hepatic abscessation • Drug or toxin-induced hepatic injury • Acute pancreatitis • Hepatic lymphosarcoma • Autoimmune hemolytic anemia • Zinc intoxication

Chronic Disease
• Chronic hepatitis of inflammatory or immune-mediated origin • Drug or toxin-induced hepatic injury • Infectious hepatitis • Idiopathic chronic hepatitis • Cholangiohepatitis • Chronic obstructive biliary disease • Chronic fibrosing pancreatitis • Congenital portosystemic shunt • Hepatic neoplasia • Metastatic neoplasia or carcinomatosis • Lobular dissecting hepatitis

CBC/BIOCHEMISTRY/URINALYSIS

CBC
• Results may be normal. • Regenerative anemia, leukocytosis, neutrophilia, and left shift in some animals with acute crisis • Microcytic or normocytic, normochromic nonregenerative anemia in some dogs with chronic progressive disease

Biochemistry
High liver enzyme activities (i.e., ALT, AST, and SAP) before onset of clinical signs should raise a high index of suspicion for copper toxicity in predisposed breeds. However, up to one-third of affected asymptomatic dogs have normal liver enzyme activity.
Chronically Affected Dogs
• Hypoalbuminemia • Hyperglobulinemia—beta and gamma globulins • Low BUN in some • Hypoglycemia • Hypokalemia

Urinalysis
Results usually normal

OTHER LABORATORY TESTS
• High fasting and postprandial bile acid concentration • Prolonged PT, APTT, ACT, and buccal mucosal bleeding time • Blood copper concentration is not of value—generally normal • Hepatic copper determination with histopathologic examination of liver is diagnostic. Hepatic copper concentrations range from 850-12,000 mg/gm DW in affected Bedlington terriers and up to 3,500 mg/gm DW in affected West Highland white terriers.

IMAGING

Radiography
• Hepatomegaly in some acutely affected Bedlington terriers • Small liver in some chronically affected dogs • Poor abdominal detail if dog has ascites • Abdominal radiographs unremarkable in most dogs

Ultrasonography
• Early, the sonographic appearance of the liver is normal. • Later, the liver may have a hyperechoic to mixed echogenic pattern.

OTHER DIAGNOSTIC PROCEDURES
• Hepatic copper determination can be performed on fresh or formalin-fixed liver tissue. Most labs need 1 g or less of tissue. Copper concentrations < 400 mg/gm DW are considered normal, whereas concentrations in the 400-2000 mg/gm DW range may be either a cause or an effect of chronic liver disease. Generally, a copper concentration > 850 mg/gm DW is considered diagnostic for hepatic copper toxicity. • Both biopsy and copper determination should be performed on any liver specimen from a breed predisposed to hepatic copper toxicosis. • Examination of fine needle aspirate—hepatocytes may appear hyperplastic or reactive. Rhodanine stains copper within the cells. • Analysis of stool ra-

dioactivity after IV administration of copper-64. Affected dogs do not properly excrete the labeled copper, thus reducing stool radioactivity relative to normal dogs.

GROSS AND HISTOPATHOLOGIC FINDINGS

• In dogs with end-stage disease the liver grossly appears nodular and cirrhotic.
• Histologically, most dogs < 6 years have few degenerative or inflammatory changes. The first observed change is the accumulation of lysosomal granules containing copper.
• Inflammatory changes—initially, focal hepatic necrosis that progresses over time to chronic active hepatitis and finally to cirrhosis. • Histochemical staining—semiquantitative evaluation for copper can be performed by special copper stains such as rhodanine, rubeanic acid, and Timm's silver sulfide.

TREATMENT

INPATIENT VERSUS OUTPATIENT

Most dogs treated as outpatients. Inpatient evaluation and treatment is needed for dogs with signs of hepatic failure.

ACTIVITY Normal

DIET

• A normal protein diet should be fed until signs of protein intolerance are noticed, and then a low protein diet should be fed.
• Protein content should be geared toward maintaining body weight.
• Ideally, low copper diets should be used before clinical signs become apparent; however, commercially available diets are all very high in copper.
• Avoid copper rich foods (e.g., organ meats) whenever possible.

CLIENT EDUCATION

• Copper chelation is needed for life.
• Affected animals should not be bred.

SURGICAL CONSIDERATIONS

• High risk dogs should have a liver biopsy at 6 and 15 months, especially if the dog is going to be used for breeding.
• Animals with hepatic failure are surgical and anesthetic risks.

MEDICATIONS

DRUGS AND FLUIDS

• Severely affected dogs should be treated symptomatically with lactated Ringer's solution or 0.9% NaCl with KCl (20-30 mEq/L) and B complex vitamins (2 ml/L) added. Glucose should be added if dog has hypoglycemia.
• Lactulose (1 ml/kg PO q8h) and antibiotics (metronidazole [7.5 mg/kg PO q8h], ampicillin [20 mg/kg q8h], or neomycin [20 mg/kg PO q8h]) should be added if signs of

hepatic encephalopathy are observed.
• Copper chelation should be started but is not usually effective in severely affected animals.
• d-penicillamine (10-15 mg/kg PO q12h) chelates copper and promotes urinary excretion. Reductions of only about 1000 mg/gm DW per year of treatment can be expected. Treatment should be initiated in affected Bedlington terriers and affected West Highland white and Skye terriers with hepatic copper concentrations > 2000 mg/gm DW.
• Zinc (100 mg of elemental zinc PO q12h given as zinc acetate) should be administered 1 hour before feeding to reduce intestinal absorption of copper.

CONTRAINDICATIONS

The following drugs should be avoided if possible—chloramphenicol, tetracycline, clindamycin, meperidine, pentazocine, aspirin, and azathioprine.

PRECAUTIONS N/A

POSSIBLE INTERACTIONS None

ALTERNATE DRUGS

• Trientine hydrochloride (2,2,2 tetramine; 10-15 mg/kg PO q12h) equally effective as d-penicillamine
• 2,3,2 tetramine (7.5 mg/kg PO q12h) a more potent chelator but not commercially available
• Ascorbic acid (500-1000 mg PO daily) may reduce intestinal absorption of copper, but this is unproven.

FOLLOW-UP

PATIENT MONITORING

• Liver enzymes every 4-6 months • Body weight • Measure hepatic copper concentration within 1 year and thereafter as required by clinical findings. • Assess serum zinc concentration every 2 weeks until stable in desired range (200-600 mcg/dl) and then every 4-6 months. Discontinue if > 1000 mcg/dl to avoid hemolytic crisis.

PREVENTION/AVOIDANCE

Only breed dogs that do not carry the gene causing the disease. A liver registry is available for Bedlington terriers that are unaffected on the basis of hepatic copper concentration < 400 mg/gm DW at 1 year of age or older (Canine Liver Registry, Veterinary Medical Data Base, 1235 SCC-A, Purdue University, West Lafayette, IN 47907-1235).

POSSIBLE COMPLICATIONS

• d-penicillamine can cause anorexia and vomiting. Starting at the low end of the dosage for the first week may reduce adverse effects. Give 1 hour before meals. A small amount of meat may be included, but drug effect is reduced 50% when given with meals.
• d-penicillamine may, in rare cases, cause an autoimmune-like vesicular disease of the mu-

cocutaneous junctions that resolves on withdrawal of the drug. • Excess zinc (oral dose of >200 mg/day or blood concentration of > 1000 mcg/dl) can cause hemolytic anemia.

EXPECTED COURSE AND PROGNOSIS

• The prognosis is poor in acutely affected young dogs with fulminant hepatic failure and older dogs with cirrhosis. • Young dogs with mild to moderate acute hepatic failure usually respond to symptomatic treatment and can be started on chelation. The prognosis is fair for these animals. • The prognosis is good if the disease is detected before clinically important inflammatory changes are noticed, and the dog is started on chelation therapy and zinc acetate.

MISCELLANEOUS

ASSOCIATED CONDITIONS None

AGE RELATED FACTORS

• Determining copper concentrations at 6 and 15 months of age aids in determining which animals should be treated and which animals should not be bred. Homozygously affected dogs have high copper (> 400 mg/gm DW) at 6 months and higher concentrations at 15 months. Heterozygously affected dogs have high concentrations at 6 months that decrease to normal at 15 months. • Affected West Highland white terriers have the highest concentration at 6 months of age.

ZOONOTIC POTENTIAL None

PREGNANCY

Do not breed affected animals and carriers.

SYNONYMS

• Bedlington hepatitis • Chronic active hepatitis • Chronic copper toxicity • Copper toxicosis

SEE ALSO

Hepatitis, Chronic Active

ABBREVIATIONS

DW = dry weight

References

Johnson SE. Diseases of the liver. In: Ettinger SJ, Feldman EC, eds. Textbook of veterinary internal medicine. Philadelphia: WB Saunders, 1994.
Twedt DC, Whitney EL. Management of hepatic copper toxicosis in dogs. In: Kirk RW, ed. Current veterinary therapy X: small animal practice. Philadelphia: WB Saunders, 1989.

Authors Joseph Taboada and Larry J. Thompson
Consulting Editor Albert E. Jergens

CORNEAL DEGENERATIONS AND INFILTRATIONS

BASICS

OVERVIEW
• Corneal degeneration is a secondary, non-inhrited, unilateral or bilateral condition characterized by lipid or calcareous deposition within the corneal stroma and sometimes the epithelium. • Arcus lipoides corneae is a bilateral but not necessarily symmetrical infiltration of lipid in the cornea associated with systemic hyperlipoproteinemia.

SIGNALMENT
• Corneal degeneration occurs most often in dogs, and uncommon in cats. • Corneal degeneration can occur in any dog or cat breed of any age. • Arcus lipoides corneae occurs most often in dogs that are hyperlipoproteinemic secondary to hypothyroidism. It usually occurs in middle-aged or older dogs and is rare in cats.

SIGNS
• Corneal degeneration or infiltration causes variable opacity of the cornea. • Animals with corneal degeneration usually have some degree of corneal inflammation, neovascularization, or pigmentation concurrent with the lipid and calcium deposits. Deposits are grey or white and may be circular, band-shaped, irregular, or any combination thereof. Affected cornea may appear roughened. Ocular conditions often associated with corneal degeneration include corneal scars, keratoconjunctivitis sicca, exposure keratitis, chronic uveitis, and phthisis bulbi. • Arcus lipoides corneae appears as a bilateral, silvery or blue-grey, and usually complete annulus (or ring) around the peripheral cornea. Corneal vascularization varies. There is often a clear area (or lucid interval) between the affected cornea and the limbus.

CAUSES & RISK FACTORS
• Hyperlipoproteinemia secondary to hypothyroidism increases the risk for arcus lipoides corneae. • Consider also hyperlipoproteinemia of other causes, including primary hyperlipidemia of miniature schnauzers and secondary hyperlipoproteinemia caused by diabetes mellitus, pancreatitis, nephrotic syndrome, or liver disease. • German shepherds with hypothyroidism may have a breed predilection for arcus lipoides cornea. • Hyperlipoproteinemia may modify the course of corneal degeneration once it has developed, possibly increasing the severity, but hyperlipoproteinemia alone is not sufficient to cause corneal deposits. • Dogs with external eye disease, commonly seen in brachycephalic breeds, may be at higher than average risk of developing corneal degeneration.

DIAGNOSIS

DIFFERENTIAL DIAGNOSIS
• Rule out other causes of corneal opacity, including stromal lipid dystrophies, ulcers, edema, scars, and inflammatory cell infiltrates. • A corneal ulcer retains fluorescein stain. • An uncomplicated scar is variably opaque with negative fluorescein stain retention and a relatively smooth corneal surface. • Stromal lipid dystrophies are fluorescein negative, bilateral, often symmetrical foci of corneal lipid deposition which are familial and not associated with ocular inflammation. • Edema is usually more homogenous and bluish-white. • Cytologic examination of a corneal scraping may help rule out inflammatory cell infiltrates.

CBC/BIOCHEMISTRY/URINALYSIS
• Hyperlipoproteinemia with high serum cholesterol and triglyceride concentrations are seen in animals with arcus lipoides corneae. • Fasting cholesterol, triglyceride, and calcium concentrations should be checked in animals with corneal degeneration because high concentrations may modify the corneal deposits although they do not usually cause the degeneration.

OTHER LABORATORY TESTS
Low thyroid hormone concentration and depressed response to TSH in animals with arcus lipoides cornea secondary to hypothyroidism.

IMAGING N/A

OTHER DIAGNOSTIC PROCEDURES
Eyes with corneal degeneration of arcus lipoides corneae may retain fluorescein stain if epithelial deposits are excessive.

TREATMENT
• The primary ocular disease or systemic condition should be treated in animals with corneal degeneration and arcus lipoides corneae, respectively. • Dogs with sufficient lipid and calcium deposits to impair vision, disrupt the corneal epithelium, or cause ulceration and ocular discomfort may benefit from vigorous corneal scraping or superficial keratectomy followed by medical treatment (see medications). • Animals with arcus lipoides corneae and possibly other lipid degenerations may benefit from low-fat diet.

MEDICATIONS

DRUGS AND FLUIDS
• Antibiotics adminstered topically (e.g., triple antibiotic) are indicated if the cornea is ulcerated. • 1% atropine applied topically may reduce pain associated with corneal ulceration when used to effect (i.e., q8h-q24h). • EDTA solution applied topically (0.4%-1.38% q6h) may be beneficial in minimizing corneal degeneration but only if calcium deposits are present. Treatment is usually combined with a procedure to first remove most of the deposits and the epithelium to improve efficacy (i.e., corneal scraping). • Lubrication with an artificial tear ointment (q6h-q12h) may prevent or reduce the frequency of recurrent corneal ulceration.

CONTRAINDICATIONS/POSSIBLE INTERACTIONS
• Topically applied corticosteroids are of questionable benefit for treating corneal degenerations or infiltrations and should not be used if corneal ulceration is present. • Topically applied atropine is contraindicated in animals with glaucoma and lens luxation and is a relative contraindication for animals with keratoconjunctivitis sicca.

FOLLOW-UP
• Corneal ulceration may accompany progression of corneal degeneration or arcus lipoides corneae. • Vision is not substantially affected except in animals with advanced corneal degeneration or in animals in which the primary disease has caused irreparable damage to the globe (e.g., chronic uveitis). • In animals with arcus lipoides cornea, serum cholesterol and triglycerides can be monitored to assess efficacy of dietary management or treatment of the primary systemic disease. • Lipid and calcium deposits may recur in animals that have undergone keratectomy surgery.

MISCELLANEOUS

SEE ALSO
• Keratitis (Ulcerative) • Corneal Dystrophies

Reference

Crispin SM, Barnett KC. Dystrophy, degeneration and infiltration of the canine cornea. J Small Anim Pract 1983;24:63–83.
Author B. Keith Collins
Consulting Editor Paul E. Miller

BASICS

OVERVIEW
A primary, inherited (or familial), bilateral and often symmetrical condition of the cornea that is not associated with other ocular or systemic diseases. Three types are recognized on the basis of anatomic location: 1) that associated with abnormality of the epithelium or basement membrane; 2) that caused by lipid deposition within the corneal stroma; and 3) that which occurs as a degenerative change of the corneal endothelium.

SIGNALMENT
Most often in dogs; rare in cats

Epithelial Dystrophy
• Develops in the Shetland sheepdog sometimes before 1 year of age with slow progression throughout life. • Boxers develop corneal erosions (see ulcerative keratitis).

Lipid Corneal Dystrophy
• Usually a disease of young adult dogs.
• Higher prevalence in females suggested for some breeds. • Affected breeds include the Siberian husky, Alaskan malamute, samoyed, bearded collie, bichon frise, German shepherd, Ihasa apso, mastiff, miniature pinscher, weimaraner, whippet, Cavalier King Charles spaniel, American cocker spaniel, beagle, rough collie, Afghan hound, and airedale terrier. • The inheritance pattern has been identified in only a few breeds of dog.

Endothelial Corneal Dystrophy
• Primarily affects the Boston terrier and chihuahua but may affect other breeds; typically occurs in middle-aged or older dogs, and a female predilection is suggested. • Rare in cats, occurs at a young age, and is described most often in the domestic shorthair. A condition that appears similar but occurs in the absence of endothelial disease is inherited in the Manx cat as an autosomal recessive disorder.

SIGNS
All corneal dystrophies cause variable opacity of the cornea.

Epithelial Dystrophy
Asymptomatic or blepharospasm associated with corneal erosions.

Stromal Lipid Corneal Dystrophies
• Usually asymptomatic with no associated ocular inflammation. • Vision is usually not affected, but visual deficit is possible in animals with advanced, diffuse, or annular dystrophy. • Central dystrophy is most common and usually appears as a grey, white, or silver, oval to circular opacity of the central or paracentral cornea. Magnification may reveal multiple fibrillar to coalescing opacities that impart a crystalline or ground-glass appearance to the cornea, and thus the term, crystalline corneal dystrophy. • Diffuse dystrophy occurs in the airedale and appears as a

more diffuse corneal opacity than central dystrophy. • Annular dystrophy occurs in the Siberian husky and appears as a doughnut-shaped opacity of the paracentral or peripheral cornea.

Endothelial Corneal Dystrophy
• Asymptomatic in the early stages. • Initial findings include corneal edema of the lateral or ventrolateral cornea that usually progresses to involve the entire cornea over a period of months to years. Corneal epithelial bullae (or bullous keratopathy) and subsequent corneal erosion or ulceration may develop. • Pain caused by corneal ulceration and impaired visual acuity are observed in animals with advanced disease.

CAUSES AND RISK FACTORS
• Epithelial dystrophy is the result of degenerative or innate abnormalities of the corneal epithelium or basement membrane. • Lipid dystrophy is the result of an innate abnormality or localized error in corneal lipid metabolism. Hyperlipoproteinemia may modify the course of lipid dystrophy, possibly increasing the opacity. • Endothelial dystrophy is the result of degeneration of the endothelial cell layer, with corresponding loss of endothelial cell pump function and subsequent corneal edema.

DIAGNOSIS

DIFFERENTIAL DIAGNOSIS
• Rule out other causes of corneal opacity, including corneal degenerations, ulcers, scars, and inflammatory cell infiltrates. • Endothelial dystrophy must be distinguished from other causes of diffuse corneal edema, notably uveitis and glaucoma.

CBC/BIOCHEMISTRY/URINALYSIS
Check cholesterol and triglyceride concentrations in dogs with lipid dystrophy. High concentrations may modify the course of disease but are not the cause.

OTHER LABORATORY TESTS N/A

IMAGING N/A

OTHER DIAGNOSTIC PROCEDURES
• Eyes with lipid dystrophy usually do not retain fluorescein stain. • Eyes with epithelial or endothelial dystrophy may retain fluorescein stain, particularly in animals with advanced disease.

TREATMENT
• Dogs with advanced epithelial or endothelial dystrophy and ulceration may require treatment for ulcerative keratitis.
• Most dogs with lipid dystrophy require no treatment. Superficial keratectomy can be performed to remove lipid deposits, but this is usually unnecessary, and deposits may re-

cur after surgery. Inform breeders that some corneal dystrophies are inherited.
• Animals with advanced endothelial dystrophy may benefit from penetrating keratoplasty surgery (i.e., corneal transplant), but success rates vary. Other treatments include debriding redundant corneal epithelial tags, using therapeutic soft contact lenses, creating conjunctival flaps, and thermokeratoplasty.

MEDICATIONS

DRUGS AND FLUIDS
• Topical antibiotics and possibly atropine if the cornea is ulcerated (see ulcerative keratitis).
• Topical 5% sodium chloride ointment (Muro-128) q6h for animals with endothelial dystrophy. Treatment is palliative and does not clear cornea markedly but may prevent progression and rupture of corneal epithelial bullae.

CONTRAINDICATIONS/POSSIBLE INTERACTIONS
Topical corticosteroids are of no benefit to animals with lipid dystrophy and are of questionable benefit to those with other forms of dystrophy.

FOLLOW-UP
• Rechecks are necessary only if signs of ocular pain or corneal ulceration develop. Corneal opacity may "wax and wane" in animals with lipid dystrophy but is unlikely to resolve. Corneal ulceration may accompany progression of epithelial or endothelial dystrophy. Vision is not substantially affected except in animals with advance dystrophy.

MISCELLANEOUS

SEE ALSO
• Keratitis (Ulcerative) • Corneal Degenerations and Infiltrations

Reference
Crispin SM, Barnett KC. Dystrophy, degeneration and infiltration of the canine cornea. J Small Anim Pract 1983;24:63–83.
Author B. Keith Collins
Consulting Editor Paul E. Miller

CORONAVIRUS INFECTION—DOGS

 BASICS

OVERVIEW

• Canine coronavirus (CCV) was first isolated from military dogs in Germany with enteric illness. Subsequently, it has been the cause of sporadic outbreaks of vomiting and diarrheal disease in dogs in several countries. Inapparent infections are usual, but mild to severe enteritis may occur, from which most dogs recover. Deaths, however, have been reported in young pups. CCV is widely distributed in the world dog population, including wild canids. • Simultaneous infections with CCV and canine parvovirus type 2 (CPV-2) may occur. In such instances the disease is more severe, often fatal. • As with several other animal coronaviruses, infection with CCV is restricted to the upper two thirds of the small intestine and associated lymph nodes. Unlike in dogs with canine parvovirus type 2 infection, crypt cells are spared. There is no viremia or other manifestations of systemic disease.

SIGNALMENT

• Only wild and domestic dogs are known to be susceptible to disease; however, the virus may cause inapparent infections in cats.
• Dogs of all ages and breeds are susceptible.

SIGNS

• Signs vary greatly. Most infections in adult dogs are inapparent. Pups, however, may develop severe, fatal enteritis. • The incubation period ranges from 1-3 days. In animals that become ill, signs include sudden onset of vomiting, usually only once, and loose or liquid diarrhea. The diarrhea may be explosive. Anorexia and depression also are common signs. Typically, dogs do not become febrile and there is no leukopenia or lymphopenia.
• In affected dogs, the feces is loose or liquid, yellow-green or orange in color, and, typically, exceptionally malodorous. The foul odor is claimed to be "characteristic." The diarrhea may persist for a few days, or it may last for more than 3 weeks in some dogs. Pups with severe, protracted diarrhea often become dehydrated. • Mortality rates from CCV infections are low. As noted, mortality in pups with concurrent infections (e.g., CCV plus CPV-2) is exceptionally high.

CAUSES AND RISK FACTORS

• CCV is closely related to feline infectious peritonitis virus (FIPV), feline enteric coronavirus, and transmissible gastroenteritis virus of swine. The pig and cat viruses, however, are not known to cause illness in dogs.
• Puppies and dogs under stress appear to be at greatest risk. Sporadic outbreaks have occurred in dogs attending shows and in kennels where introductions of new dogs are frequent. Crowding and unsanitary conditions appear to promote clinical illness. • The feces is the primary source of infection. Virus is shed for about 2 weeks. Unlike CPV-2, CCV is readily inactivated by common disinfectants.

 DIAGNOSIS

DIFFERENTIAL DIAGNOSIS

Infections caused by enteric bacteria, protozoa or other viruses (e.g., parvovirus) • Food intoxication or intolerance

CBC/BIOCHEMISTRY/URINALYSIS

Hemograms are normal.

OTHER LABORATORY TESTS

Serologic tests are available, but they are not standardized. The presence of antibodies may not indicate recent CCV infection because the seroprevalence is high in some populations.

IMAGING N/A

OTHER DIAGNOSTIC PROCEDURES

• Viral isolation in cell cultures at onset of diarrhea in cats. • Immunofluorescent staining of frozen sections of the small intestine. • Electron microscopy may reveal typical CCV particles, but interpretation of electron micrographs requires expertise and is subject to error. • Histopathology may reveal atrophy and fusion of small intestinal villi. Crypt cells are normal, but crypts may be deepened by increased cellularity of the lamina propria. Lesions are often obscured by postmortem autolysis.

 TREATMENT

• Most affected dogs recover without treatment. Supportive fluid and electrolyte treatment is indicated in severe infections.
• Antibiotics are not indicated unless enteritis persists or there is evidence of sepsis.

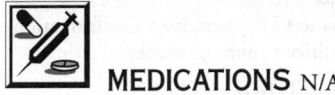

MEDICATIONS N/A

FOLLOW-UP
• Follow-up is not usually required. A rise (> fourfold) in antibody titers done at the onset of disease and 3 weeks later may provide a retrospective diagnosis. • The prognosis is good, except in young pups with severe infections. The majority of cases recover after a few days of illness. As noted, fluid or soft stools may persist in some animals for several weeks.

MISCELLANEOUS
• Infections by CCV, canine parvovirus, or other agents may occur concurrently. • No zoonotic potential is known. • Inactivated vaccines are available commercially. A live, attenuated CCV vaccine that appears safe is licensed in California. Both vaccines appear to be safe, but efficacy data are lacking. A licensed vaccine that contained live "CCV," later shown to be similar to FIPV, was recalled after several hundred dogs developed severe or fatal postvaccinal meningoencephalitis.

ABBREVIATIONS
CCV = canine coronavirus
CPV-2 = canine parvovirus type 2
FIPV = feline infectious peritonitis virus

Reference
Pollock RHV, Carmichael LE. Canine viral enteritis. In: Greene CE, ed. Infectious diseases of the dog and cat. Philadelphia: WB Saunders, 1990:281-283.
Author Leland E. Carmichael
Consulting Editor Fred W. Scott

CRUCIATE DISEASE, CRANIAL

 BASICS

DEFINITION
The acute or degenerative injury of the cranial cruciate ligament (CrCL) that results in partial to complete instability of the stifle joint.

Pathophysiology
• The function of the CrCL is to constrain the stifle joint by limiting internal rotation, cranial displacement of the tibia relative to the femur, and to prevent hyperextension.
• CrCL injury can result from traumatic (acute) or degenerative (chronic) causes. Breaking strength of the CrCL is approximately equal to 4 times the body weight of the dog. Acute rupture due to exceeding the strength of the ligament accounts for less than 20% of canine patients with CrCL rupture.
• The most common modes of acute rupture of the CrCL are hyperextension and excessive internal rotation with the stifle in partial flexion (20 to 50 degrees). • Traumatic rupture of the CrCL is the most common cause in cats. A ligament weakened by degeneration can be ruptured more easily than a normal ligament. • Various causes of ligament degeneration have been identified: aging, conformational abnormalities, disuse related to sedentary habits or limb immobilization, and immune mediated. Degeneration related to aging has been shown to be related to size, with dogs > 15 kg showing the most changes. Degenerative changes and a decrease in material properties have consistently been shown in dogs > 5 years of age. • Dogs weighing < 15 kg have less change in CrCL strength than do larger dogs. • Conformational abnormalities such as genu varum (bowlegged), genu valgum (knock-knee), straight stifles and hock, caudal sloping of the tibial plateau, patella luxation, and narrowing of the intercondylar notch may predispose toward rupture of the CrCL.
• Immune-mediated arthritis, lymphocytic-plasmocytic synovitis, and septic arthritis may predispose the CrCL to rupture. Immune complexes have been found in dogs with unilateral and bilateral CrCL rupture; however, whether these immune complexes are a cause or a result of the rupture is unknown.
• Partial rupture of the CrCL accounts for a high percentage (25% to 30%) of patients presented for stifle lameness. • Untreated patients with CrCL rupture show degenerative joint disease (DJD) changes within a few weeks and severe changes within a few months. • Due to abnormal joint mechanics following CrCL injury, medial meniscal (caudal horn) damage occurs in >50% of the patients. • Cranial tibial thrust may play an important role in the acute or degenerative rupture of the CrCL. A cranially directed force is theoretically generated during weight bearing based on the caudal slope of the tibial plateau and the tibial compression mechanism.

Systems Affected Musculoskeletal
Genetics
• Unknown • May be important in predisposing an animal to DJD, degeneration of the CrCL or developing conformation abnormalities.

Incidence/Prevalence
CrCL ruptures are one of the most common causes of lameness in the dog and the major cause of DJD in the stifle joint.

Geographic Distribution N/A

SIGNALMENT
Species
• Dogs • Uncommon in cats
Breed Predilections
• All breeds are susceptible • Rottweilers and Labrador retrievers have an increased incidence of CrCL rupture when younger than 4 years of age.
Mean Age and Range
• Dogs > 5 years of age • Between 1-2 years of age in large-breed dogs.
Predominant Sex
Possibly female dogs

SIGNS
General Comments
Clinical signs are related to the degree of rupture (partial versus complete), the mode of rupture (acute versus chronic), the presence of meniscal injury, and the severity of inflammation and DJD.

Historical Findings
• Athletic or traumatic events generally precede acute CrCL injuries that result in non-weight bearing lameness with the affected limb held in flexion. • Normal activity resulting in acute lameness should make one suspicious of degenerative CrCL rupture. • Subtle to marked intermittent lameness that has been going on for weeks to months is consistent with partial tears of the CrCL progressing towards complete rupture.

Physical Examination Findings
• Demonstration of cranial drawer motion is diagnostic for CrCL rupture. It is often dramatic following acute injuries. Subtle, almost imperceptible motion that ends gradually as a result of tissue stretching is consistent with chronic rupture or partial tears of the CrCL. Drawer motion should be tested in both flexion, normal standing angle, and extension.
• Cranial movement of the tibia relative to the femur during the tibial compression test.
• Joint effusion • Palpable thickening of the joint capsule especially on the medial aspect (medial "buttress"). • Hindlimb muscle atrophy—especially the quadriceps muscle group. • Absence of cranial drawer sign (or tibial compression test) does not rule out CrCL rupture. • False negative results may occur with chronic or partial tears of the CrCL and in painful or anxious animals that are not sedated or anesthetized.

CAUSES
• Traumatic • Degenerative • Conformation abnormalities • Immune mediated

RISK FACTORS
• Obesity • Patella luxation • Poor conformation

 DIAGNOSIS

DIFFERENTIAL DIAGNOSIS
• Skeletally immature dogs and dogs with muscle atrophy, commonly have slight drawer motion, but such motion stops abruptly as the CrCL is stretched taut. • Caudal cruciate ligament rupture is uncommon as an isolated occurrence. Palpation can distinguish cranial from caudal cruciate ligament ruptures.
• Patella luxation (medial or lateral) either by itself or concurrent with CrCL rupture.
• Stifle joint trauma • Osteochondritis dissecans of the femoral condyle or patella.
• Neoplasia (i.e., synovial cell sarcoma) is generally more painful than CrCL rupture.

CBC/BIOCHEMISTRY/URINALYSIS
N/A

OTHER LABORATORY TESTS N/A
IMAGING
• Radiographs rarely are diagnostic for CrCL rupture, but they help confirm the presence of intra-articular disease findings including: joint effusion with capsular distention and compression of the infrapatellar fat pad, periarticular osteophytes, enthesiophytes, CrCL avulsion fractures, and calcification of the CrCL. • Magnetic resonance imaging can graphically show cruciate ligament and meniscal pathology.

OTHER DIAGNOSTIC PROCEDURES
• Arthrocentesis—joint cytology can be used to identify the presence of intra-articular disease and to rule out sepsis and immune mediated disease. • Arthroscopy can be used to directly visualize the cruciate ligaments, menisci, and other intra-articular structures.

GROSS AND HISTOPATHOLOGIC FINDINGS
• Varying degrees of cartilage fibrillation and erosion, periarticular osteophyte formation, meniscal damage and synovitis. • Ruptured fibers of the CrCL undergo hyalinization, fibrous tissue invasion, necrosis, and loss of the parallel orientation of ligament bundles.

 TREATMENT

INPATIENT VERSUS OUTPATIENT
• Dogs <15 kg can be treated conservatively as outpatients with 85% being improved or normal by 6 months. • Only 20% of dogs >15 kg are improved by 6 months when treated conservatively; therefore, medium-to

large-breed dogs should have surgery. • Surgery should be recommended for all dogs to speed the rate of recovery and to prevent degenerative changes and to enhance function.

ACTIVITY
Restricted activity whether treated conservatively or following surgical stabilization. Duration dependent on method of treatment and progress of animal.

DIET
Weight control is important to reduce the load and therefore the stress on the stifle joint.

CLIENT EDUCATION
• Regardless of method of treatment, DJD is common. • Return to complete athletic function is uncommon following CrCL injury. • 20% to 40% of dogs with unilateral CrCL rupture will rupture their contralateral ligament within 17 months.

SURGICAL CONSIDERATIONS
• No surgical technique has been shown to be superior when compared to the others. • Extra-articular methods: Embrace a wide variety of stabilization techniques that utilize a heavy gauge implant to imbricate the joint and restore stability. The implant material is placed in the approximate plane of the CrCL origin and insertion. • Intra-articular methods—these techniques are designed to replace the CrCL anatomically. Autografts (patella ligament, fascia), allografts (bone-tendon-bone) and synthetic materials (Gore-tex) are commonly used. • Modiified extra-articular techniques—fibular head transposition and popliteal tendon transposition are procedures that realign the tension of the lateral collateral ligament or popliteal tendon, respectively, to restrict internal rotation and cranial drawer. • Tibial plateau leveling osteotomy: A rotational osteotomy of the proximal tibia is performed to level the tibial plateau and neutralize cranial tibial thrust.

MEDICATIONS

DRUGS AND FLUIDS
Nonsteroidal anti-inflammatory drugs (NSAIDs) and analgesics can be used to symptomatically treat associated synovitis and DJD

CONTRAINDICATIONS
Corticosteroids should be avoided because of the potential side effects and the articular cartilage damage associated with long-term usage.

PRECAUTIONS
Gastrointestinal irritation may occur with the use of NSAIDs and may preclude their use in individual animals.

POSSIBLE INTERACTIONS N/A

ALTERNATIVE DRUGS
Chondroprotective drugs such as polysulfated glycosaminoglycans may be of benefit in limiting cartilage damage and degeneration.

FOLLOW-UP

PATIENT MONITORING
Dependent on method of treatment.

PREVENTION/AVOIDANCE
Avoid breeding animals with conformation abnormalities.

POSSIBLE COMPLICATIONS
A second surgery is required in 10% to 15% of patients because of meniscal damage.

EXPECTED COURSE AND PROGNOSIS
Regardless of surgical technique, success rate is approximately 85%.

MISCELLANEOUS

ASSOCIATED CONDITIONS
Always look for associated meniscal damage.

AGE RELATED FACTORS
See pathophysiology section

ZOONOTIC POTENTIAL N/A

PREGNANCY N/A

SYNONYMS N/A

SEE ALSO
• Arthritis (Osteoarthritis) • Patellar Luxation

ABBREVIATIONS
CrCL = cranial cruciate ligament
DJD = degenerative joint disease
NSAIDs: Nonsteroidal anti-inflammatory drugs

References

Johnson JM, Johnson AL. Cranial cruciate ligament rupture: pathogenesis, diagnosis, and postoperative rehabilitation. Vet Clin North Am 1993;23:717-733.
Author Peter D. Schwarz
Consulting Editor Peter D. Schwarz

CRANIOMANDIBULAR OSTEOPATHY

 **BASICS**

OVERVIEW
• Craniomandibular osteopathy (CMO) is a nonneoplastic, noninflammatory proliferative disease of the bones of the head. • The primary bones affected are mandibular rami, occipital and parietal bones, tympanic bullae, and the zygomatic portion of the temporal bone. • Bilateral symmetric involvement is most common

SIGNALMENT
• Most commonly seen in Scottish, Cairn, and West Highland white terrier breeds. • Other affected breeds include Labrador retriever, great Dane, Boston terrier, Doberman pinscher, Irish setters, English bulldogs, and boxers. • Usually affects growing puppies 4-8 months of age. • No gender predilection, but neutering may increase incidence.

SIGNS

Historical Findings
• Signs usually relate to pain around the mouth and difficulty in eating. • If the angular processus of the mandible is involved, jaw movement is progressively restricted. • Difficulty in prehension, mastication, and swallowing can lead to starvation. • Lameness or limb swelling can precede cranial involvement.

Physical Examination Findings
• Temporal and masseter muscle atrophy. • Palpable irregular thickening of the mandibular rami and/or temporomandibular joint (TMJ) region. • Inability to fully open jaw, even under general anesthesia. • Intermittent pyrexia (104° F) • Bilateral exopthalmos

CAUSES AND RISK FACTORS
• Believed to be hereditary because of its occurrence in certain breeds and families. • An autosomal recessive trait in West Highland white terriers. • Possible predispostion in Scottish terriers • Possible link to infection due to pyrexia and histologic evidence of inflammation only at the periphery of the lesion. • Presentation of a young terrier with periosteal long bone disease should prompt monitoring for CMO.

 DIAGNOSIS

DIFFERENTIAL DIAGNOSIS
• Osteomyelitis: bones not symmetrically affected; generally not as extensive; presence of lysis; lack of breed predilection; and history of penetrating wound. • Traumatic periostitis: bones not symmetrically affected; generally not as extensive; history of trauma. • Neoplasia: older age; not symmetrically affected; more lytic bone reaction; presence of metastatic disease.

CBC/BIOCHEMISTRY/URINALYSIS
• Serum alkaline phosphatase and serum inorganic phosphate may be high. • Hypogammaglobulinemia or α-2 hyperglobulinemia may be present.

OTHER LABORATORY TESTS N/A

IMAGING
• Radiographs of the skull show uneven, bead-like osseous proliferation of the mandible or tympanic bullae (bilateral); extensive, periosteal new bone formation (exostoses) affecting one or more bones around the TMJ. Fusion of the tympanic bullae and angular process of the mandible may occur.
• CT scan may be useful in evaluating the osseous involvement of the TMJ.

OTHER DIAGNOSTIC PROCEDURES
• Biopsy necessary only in atypical patients.
• Bone biopsy reveals normal lamellar bone being replaced by an enlarged coarse fiber bone and osteoclastic osteolysis of the periosteal/subperiosteal region. The bone marrow is replaced by a vascular, fibrous-type stroma. Inflammatory cells occasionally can be seen at the periphery of the bony lesion.

 TREATMENT

• Treatment is only palliative.
• Surgical excision of exostoses has resulted in regrowth within weeks.
• Feeding a high caloric, protein enriched gruel diet will help maintain nutritional balance.
• Surgical placement of a pharyngostomy, esophagostomy, or gastrostomy tube should be considered to help maintain nutritional balance.

MEDICATIONS

DRUGS AND FLUIDS
Palliative use of analgesics and anti-inflammatory drugs is warranted.

CONTRAINDICATIONS/POSSIBLE INTERACTIONS N/A

FOLLOW-UP
• Prognosis dependent on involvement of bones surrounding the TMJ. • Frequent rechecks are mandatory to ensure adequate nutritional balance and pain control. • Pain and discomfort may diminish at skeletal maturity (10-12 months of age), and the exostoses may regress. • Elective euthanasia may be necessary. • Dam/sire breedings that result in offspring with CMO should not be repeated. • Breeding of affected animals is to be discouraged.

MISCELLANEOUS

SYNONYMS
Lion jaw

ABBREVIATIONS
CMO = Craniomandibular osteopathy
TMJ = Temporomandibular joint

Reference
Watson ADJ, Adams WM, Thomas CB. Craniomandibular osteopathy in dogs. Compend Contin Educ Pract Vet 1995;17:911-921.

Author Peter D. Schwarz
Consulting Editor Peter D. Schwarz

CRYPTOCOCCOSIS

BASICS

DEFINITION
A systemic mycosis caused by the dimorphic fungus Cryptococcus neoformans

Pathophysiology
In contrast to the other systemic mycoses, inhalation of the yeastlike form of the organism, rather than mycelial spores, is responsible for initiation of infection. Cryptococcus usually colonizes the upper respiratory tract (nasal cavity and sinuses) rather than the lungs, although pulmonary infection can occur. In susceptible animals, the organism can disseminate from the respiratory tract to the CNS, eyes, lymph nodes, skin of the head, and elsewhere.

Systems Affected
• Nervous • Skin/exocrine • Respiratory • Ophthalmic

Genetics
Unknown, but possibly there are inherited defects in host immune defenses that favor growth of Cryptococcus

Incidence/Prevalence
Cryptococcosis is a relatively rare disease in dogs, but is more common in cats.

Geographic Distribution
Commonly present in soil and bird droppings in warm, humid climates throughout the world

Signalment

SPECIES
Occurs more commonly in cats than in dogs

Breed Predilections
• Cats—none recognized • Dogs—more common in the larger breeds

Mean Age and Range
• Cats—all ages • Dogs—primarily younger dogs

Predominant Sex None recognized

SIGNS

Historical Findings
Cats most often are presented for nasal discharge and chronic rhinitis, while neurologic and ocular abnormalities are common presenting complaints in dogs.

Physical Examination Findings
Cats
• Upper respiratory signs predominate. These can include a nasal discharge (unilateral or bilateral), sneezing, and a firm swelling over the bridge of the nose. Submandibular lymphadenopathy may also be present.
• Papules and nodules may be present on the skin of the head or elsewhere on the body. These lesions usually drain or ulcerate.
• Neurologic signs can occur as a result of cryptococcal meningitis. They can include depression, disorientation, seizures, head

pressing, ataxia, and posterior paresis. Cranial-nerve deficits and upper motor neuron lesions may be evident. • Ocular abnormalities may occur, either in conjunction with CNS disease or as a result of severe systemic dissemination. They can include pupillary dilation, chorioretinitis, optic neuritis, and retinal detachment.
Dogs
• Canine cryptococcosis is characterized most often by CNS and ocular disease. Dissemination of cryptococci to other organs is more widespread in dogs than in cats. • Neurologic signs that may be observed include a head tilt, nystagmus, circling, disorientation, head pressing, varying degrees of paresis or paralysis, incoordination, and seizures. • Chorioretinitis and optic neuritis are the most common ocular signs. • Skin lesions with ulcerations have also been reported.

CAUSES
Cryptococcus neoformans is an encapsulated, yeastlike fungus that exhibits a preference for tissues of the CNS. Unlike other dimorphic fungi, such as Blastomyces and Histoplasma, C. neoformans retains its yeastlike appearance even when cultured outside an infected host (although a filamentous mold form of the organism has been identified in nature). The organism is found commonly in bird droppings, particularly those of pigeons, and in the soil. If protected from sunlight and drying, cryptococci may remain viable in contaminated droppings for as long as two years. Warm, humid climates are the most favorable for growth and proliferation of C. neoformans.

RISK FACTORS
• Excessive nosing about in contaminated soil or droppings may increase exposure to large numbers of infective cryptococci. • Infection of cats with feline leukemia virus (FeLV) or feline immunodeficiency virus (FIV) may facilitate subsequent infection with C. neoformans. Cryptococcosis associated with FIV may be particularly severe and widespread. • Immunosuppressive conditions in dogs, such as canine ehrlichiosis, may predispose to cryptococcosis.

DIAGNOSIS

DIFFERENTIAL DIAGNOSIS
Cats
• Chronic rhinitis, lymphosarcoma, toxoplasmosis, feline infectious peritonitis, granulomatous meningoencephalitis, intracranial neoplasia, and other systemic mycoses are all potential diagnoses. • Skin lesions should be differentiated from routine abscesses or other bacterial disease processes.

Dogs
Canine distemper, intracranial neoplasia, and rabies are potential diagnoses in dogs with CNS signs.

CBC/BIOCHEMISTRY/URINALYSIS
• Hemogram—often normal • Serum chemistry profile—often normal • Urinalysis—rarely, cryptococci may be found in urine when the kidneys are involved in widely disseminated disease

OTHER LABORATORY TESTS
• Latex agglutination test for Cryptococcus capsular antigen in serum, CSF, or urine can provide a presumptive diagnosis. Negative results do not rule out a diagnosis of cryptococcosis, especially with localized disease.
• Many cats with cryptococcosis are positive for FeLV and/or FIV.

IMAGING
Radiography of the nasal cavity may reveal bone lysis or abnormal soft-tissue densities associated with growth of the fungus.

OTHER DIAGNOSTIC PROCEDURES
• Biopsy or cytologic examinations may reveal Cryptococcus organisms in tissues or exudates. • Microscopic identification of the yeastlike Cryptococci, usually by means of an India ink, new methylene blue, or Gram's stain preparation, in smears of nasal discharge, tissue aspirates, CSF, ulcerated skin scrapings, or biopsy samples. Organisms are often present in considerable numbers; visualization of the characteristic budding yeast forms with their huge capsules is usually sufficient to make the diagnosis. In some samples (e.g., CSF), the organisms may be more difficult to locate.

GROSS AND HISTOPATHOLOGIC FINDINGS
Cats
• Granulomatous lesions may be found in the nasal cavity and lungs. • Meningitis, peripheral neuritis, and granulomatous chorioretinitis are found in cats with CNS and ocular involvement. • Granulomas also may be found in the lymph nodes, kidneys, and spleen.

Dogs
• The disease usually is more disseminated than in the cat. • Meningoencephalitis, peripheral neuritis, and granulomatous chorioretinitis are common. • Lesions also may be found in the lungs, kidneys, lymph nodes, spleen, and elsewhere.

TREATMENT
Because treatment of cryptococcosis requires long-term therapy, the patient should be treated as an outpatient.

ACTIVITY N/A

DIET
Provision should be made for feeding a high-quality diet.

CLIENT EDUCATION
• The necessity and expense of long-term therapy of a potentially fatal illness, in addi-

tion to the possible side effects of such therapy, need to be thoroughly discussed with the client. Attention should be paid to the particularly unfavorable prognosis for dogs with cryptococcosis.
• The quality of life for the patient should be balanced against the likelihood of successful therapy, based upon the physical condition of the animal at the time of diagnosis.

SURGICAL CONSIDERATIONS N/A

MEDICATIONS

In general, treatment of cryptococcosis is more likely to be successful in cats than in dogs.

Cats
• Itraconazole (ITZ) and fluconazole (FCZ) are considered the drugs of choice for treatment.
• ITZ can be admininstered at 50 mg PO q24h in cats weighing < 3.2 kg, and at 100 mg PO q24h in cats weighing > 3.2 kg. An alternative regimen is 5 mg/kg PO q12h. The medication should be given in the food. Treatment should be continued for 1-2 months past resolution of clinical signs.
• FCZ can be administered at 50 mg PO q12h for 2-6 months. The medication should be given in the food.

Dogs
• Treatment of cryptococcosis in dogs is not as successful as it is in cats. The inability of amphotericin B and flucytosine to cross the blood-brain barrier limits the utility of these antifungal compounds in treating canine cryptococcosis, which often involves the CNS.
• Ketoconazole (KTZ) has been tried, but the response is usually erratic. It can be administered at 10-30 mg/kg PO, divided 2 or 3 times daily for 3-6 months.
• The usefulness of ITZ or FCZ in the dog has not been evaluated.

CONTRAINDICATIONS
Drugs metabolized primarily by the liver should not be administered along with ITZ, FCZ, or KTZ.

PRECAUTIONS
Side effects of ITZ or FCZ therapy are uncommon but can include inappetence, vomiting, and hepatotoxicity. Hepatotoxicity is more common with KTZ.

POSSIBLE INTERACTIONS N/A

ALTERNATE DRUGS N/A

FOLLOW-UP

PATIENT MONITORING
Liver enzymes should be monitored in animals receiving ITZ, FCZ, or KTZ.

PREVENTION/AVOIDANCE
• There is no available vaccine. • Exposure to Cryptococcus-contaminated soil in endemic areas should be avoided.

POSSIBLE COMPLICATIONS
Hepatotoxicity may possibly result from ITZ, FCZ, or KTZ therapy.

EXPECTED COURSE AND PROGNOSIS
• The prognosis in cats is usually good. A more guarded prognosis is reserved for those with widely disseminated disease involving the CNS and eyes. • Relapses after apparently successful treatment may occur in cats treated with ITZ or FCZ. • The prognosis in dogs is guarded to poor.

MISCELLANEOUS

ASSOCIATED CONDITIONS N/A

AGE RELATED FACTORS N/A

ZOONOTIC POTENTIAL
Cryptococcosis differs from the other systemic mycoses in that the tissue (yeastlike) form of the organism also appears to be the infective form (i.e., it is potentially transmissible from an infected animal to humans), although it does not aerosolize. Although there has never been a documented case of trans-

mission of cryptococcosis from an affected cat or dog to a human, it is this author's belief that prudence dictates caution whenever handling an animal with cryptococcosis.

PREGNANCY
ITZ, FCZ, and KTZ should be used in pregnant animals only if the potential benefit justifies the potential risk to offspring.

SYNONYM
European blastomycosis (in humans)

SEE ALSO N/A

ABBREVIATIONS
CNS = central nervous system
CSF = cerebral spinal fluid
KTZ = ketoconazole
ITZ = itraconazole
FCZ = fluconazole

References
Legendre AM. Cryptococcosis. In: Sherding RG, ed. The cat: diseases and clinical management. 2nd ed. New York: Churchill Livingstone, 1994:554-557.
Malik R, Wigney DI, Muir DB, Gregory DJ, Love DN. Cryptococcosis in cats: clinical and mycological assessment of 29 cases and evaluation of treatment using orally administered fluconazole. J Med Vet Mycol 1992;30:133-144.
Medleau L, Jacobs GJ, Marks MA. Itraconazole for the treatment of cryptococcosis in cats. J Vet Int Med 1995;9:39-42.
Sherding RG. Systemic mycoses. In: Birchard SJ, Sherding RG, eds. Saunders manual of small animal practice. Philadelphia: WB Saunders, 1994:133-140.
Wilkinson GT. Cryptococcosis. In: Barlough JE, ed. Manual of small animal infectious diseases. New York: Churchill Livingstone, 1988:319-326.
Author Jeffrey E. Barlough
Consulting Editor Fred W. Scott

CRYPTORCHIDISM

BASICS

OVERVIEW
• The incomplete descent of one or both testes into the scrotum • May be inguinal, in which case the retained testis is often palpable. • When abdominal, the testis is difficult to palpate or identify by radiology. • Can be imaged with ultrasound • Descent to final scrotal position is expected to be complete by 2 months postpartum. • In the beagle, the testes are at the exterior inguinal ring day 5 postpartum, between the inguinal ring and scrotum day 15, and in the scrotum day 40. • Testicular descent may occur later in some breeds, but rarely after 4 months in any individual. Absence of palpable testes at 2 months is presumptive evidence of cryptorchidism.

SIGNALMENT
Reported in almost all breeds, but toy poodle, Pomeranian, Yorkshire terrier, (especially toy and miniature breeds) are at significantly higher risk. • Unilateral cryptorchidism is more common than bilateral (75:25) and the right testis is retained twice as often as the left. Prevalence in dogs is 1.2%, in cats 1.7%.

SIGNS
• Rarely associated with pain or other signs of disease • Has been associated with other congenital defects such as patellar subluxation

CAUSES AND RISK FACTORS
• Thought to be an inherited trait; a single autosomal recessive gene is often assumed when owners of affected dogs are counseled, although more than one gene is probably involved. • Nonhereditary predisposing factors (such as birth weight) have been identified in humans but not reported in dogs. Removal of cryptorchid males from breeding lines is believed to cause a reduction in the frequency of the defect.

DIAGNOSIS

DIFFERENTIAL DIAGNOSIS
• The only concern is differentiating bilateral cryptorchidism from castration. • Bilaterally cryptorchid cats can have the urine odor and behavior of intact cats.

CBC/BIOCHEMISTRY/URINALYSIS
N/A

OTHER LABORATORY TESTS
Human chorionic gonadotropin stimulation causes doubling of blood testosterone in animals with bilateral cryptorchidism and in those with unilateral cryptorchidism in which the scrotal testis has been removed without concurrent removal of the retained testis. This test differentiates between cryptorchidism and castration.

IMAGING
The testes can be located by ultrasound.

OTHER DIAGNOSTIC PROCEDURES
N/A

TREATMENT

• No treatment other than castration of both retained and scrotal testes is generally recommended.
• Orchiopexy, surgical placement of a retained testis into the scrotum, is considered unethical.
• Anecdotal evidence reported of human chorionic gonadotropin or gonadotropin releasing hormone (GnRH) causing descent when given to dogs less than 4 months old.

MEDICATIONS

DRUGS
Human chorionic gonadotropin—100-1000 IU IM 4 times in a 2-week period before16 weeks of age (dogs). After 16 weeks, treatment is generally unsuccessful.

CONTRAINDICATIONS/POSSIBLE INTERACTIONS N/A

FOLLOW-UP

• Descent after 4 months is rare; after 6 months, unlikely • Owners should be warned of the increased risk of testicular neoplasia in dogs with retained testes and encouraged to have their pet castrated by 4 years of age; 53% of sertoli cell tumors and 36% of seminomas are found in cryptorchid dogs. • Risk of testicular neoplasia is thought to be approximately 10 times greater in cryptorchid than normal dogs.

MISCELLANEOUS

ABBREVIATIONS
GnRH = gonadotropin releasing hormone

Reference

Romagnoli SE. Canine cryptorchidism. Vet Clin North Am Small Anim Pract 1991;21.
Author Rolf E. Larsen
Consulting Editor Sara K. Lyle

BASICS

OVERVIEW
• Infection with a protozoan of the genus Cryptosporidium • Small intestine

SIGNALMENT
A rare disease of immunocompetent dogs and cats. No breed predilection.

Incidence/Prevalence
Common in some hosts (e.g., calves), but rare in dogs and cats

Mean Age and Range All ages

PREDOMINANT SEX N/A

SIGNS
Diarrhea with no polysystemic signs

CAUSES AND RISK FACTORS
• Ingestion of oocyst by ingesting feces or water contamination • Immunosuppression

DIAGNOSIS

DIFFERENTIAL DIAGNOSIS
• Diet • Giardiasis • Trichuriasis • Chronic inflammatory bowel disease • Lactose intolerance • Histoplasmosis

CBC/BIOCHEMISTRY/URINALYSIS
N/A

OTHER LABORATORY TESTS N/A

IMAGING   Not contributory

OTHER DIAGNOSTIC PROCEDURES
• Fecal antigen detection tests • Fecal analysis by sugar flotation, oocysts are acid-fast positive • fluorescent antibody tests

GROSS AND HISTOPATHOLOGICAL FINDINGS
Malabsorption, blunting, and shortening of intestinal villi

TREATMENT
• The owner should be advised of potential zoonotic transmission from organisms in contaminated feces.
• It is also important to be aware of the immune status (eg, HIV infection, chemotherapy, systemic steroids) of the client and the client's family members.

MEDICATIONS

DRUGS AND FLUIDS
• In asymptomatic animals, no treatment is required.
• In dogs and cats with signs, treatment with paromomycin has resulted in the resolution of signs and the cessation of oocyst shedding.
• Parenteral fluid replacement

CONTRAINDICATIONS/POSSIBLE INTERACTIONS

FOLLOW-UP

PATIENT MONITORING
Fecal exam 2 weeks posttreatment or if signs persist

EXPECTED COURSE AND PROGNOSIS
• If the animal is otherwise healthy, the infection is transient and self-limiting.
• Immunocompromised animals may be severely affected with prolonged signs of infection.
• Treatment must be directed towards the underlying immunodeficiency.

MISCELLANEOUS

Reference
Barr SC, Jamrosz GF, Hornbuckle WE, Bowman DD, Fayer R. Use of paromomycin for treatment of cryptosporidiosis in a cat. JAm Vet Med Assoc 1994;205:1742-1743.

Author Dwight Bowman

Consulting Editor Edward Pearce

CUTANEOUS ASTHENIA

BASICS

OVERVIEW
• A group of hereditary diseases characterized by abnormal skin hyperextensibility and fragility. • Also known as Ehlers-Danlos syndrome and dermatosparaxis. • Abnormal collagen synthesis or fiber formation is responsible for the skin fragility in most syndromes, however, the biochemical defects have been elucidated in only few canine and feline patients.
• Varying modes of inheritance have been suspected.

SIGNALMENT
• As a congenital syndrome, patients are usually presented quite young. • Dogs reported to be affected include the beagle, dachshund, boxer, St.Bernard, German shepherd dog, English springer spaniel, greyhound, Manchester terrier, Welsh corgi, red kelpie, soft-coated wheaten terrier, Irish setter, Keeshond, English setter, and mongrels.
• Cats affected include domestic shorthair, domestic longhair, and Himalayan.

SIGNS
• Skin hyperextensibility • Easily torn skin • Diminished skin elasticity • Scars from previous trauma • Widening of the bridge of the nose • Joint laxity • Elbow hygromas • Lens luxation • Cataracts

CAUSES AND RISK FACTORS
Even minor trauma to the skin can produce large skin tears.

DIAGNOSIS

DIFFERENTIAL DIAGNOSIS
This is a clinically characteristic syndrome.

CBC/BIOCHEMISTRY/URINALYSIS
N/A

OTHER LABORATORY TESTS N/A

IMAGING N/A

OTHER DIAGNOSTIC PROCEDURES
The skin extensibility index can be useful for identifying affected animals. It is calculated by dividing the maximal height of a dorsal lumbar skin fold by the body length (from the base of the tail to the occipital crest) and converting to a percentage. Affected dogs and cats will have values above 14.5 per cent and 19 per cent, respectively

GROSS AND HISTOPATHOLOGIC FINDINGS
• Histopathologic examination of the skin may show either normal dermal architecture or collagen abnormalities (disoriented, fragmented, abnormal tinctorial properties or abnormal organization). • Electron microscopy can be used to ascertain collagen abnormalities more precisely.

TREATMENT
• Because of the poor prognosis, affected animals may be euthanatized.

• If an owner chooses to keep the animal, it should be kept in an environment free of sharp corners and other animals. They must be handled and restrained carefully to prevent large tears in their skin. Resting areas should be well padded to prevent elbow hygromas.

MEDICATIONS

DRUGS AND FLUIDS
No proven medical therapy.

CONTRAINDICATIONS/POSSIBLE INTERACTIONS N/A

FOLLOW-UP
Lacerations should be surgically repaired as they occur.

MISCELLANEOUS

Reference
Scott DW, Miller WH, Griffin CE. Muller and Kirk's small animal dermatology. 5th ed. Philadelphia: WB Saunders, 1995:351.
Author Jon D. Plant
Consulting Editor Lowell Ackerman

BASICS

OVERVIEW

• Disease in color-dilute (gray) collie pups characterized by diarrhea, conjunctivitis, gingivitis, pneumonia, skin infections accompanied by fever and, occasionally, intussusception • Episodes of illness, varying from inactivity accompanied by fever to life-threatening infection, repeat at 11-14 day intervals. • The pups are smaller than normal at birth, weak, and often abandoned by the bitch. • The condition has been observed in many collie bloodlines throughout the United States. However, experienced collie breeders do not attempt to raise gray pups and, therefore, gray collies are rare.

SIGNALMENT

• Cyclic neutropenia has been observed only in color-dilute collies. The condition is inherited as an autosomal recessive trait. However, because it is a recessive trait, it is possible to observe similar color-dilute pups in any mongrel litter from parents with collie parentage in their background. • Clinical signs usually are apparent by 8-12 weeks of age.

SIGNS

Historical Findings

• Weakness • Failure to thrive • Conjunctivitis • Gingivitis • Diarrhea • Pneumonia • Swollen and moist skin lesions

Physical Examination Findings

• Dilute coat color (gray) • Smaller and weaker than normal-colored littermates • Fever • Watery eyes, reddened gums, and diarrhea are nearly always present during the phase of the hematopoietic cycle when clinical signs are evident. Other signs vary depending on the site of sepsis. • Painful carpal joints during the recovery portion of the disease cycle

CAUSES AND RISK FACTORS

Inherited disease

DIAGNOSIS

DIFFERENTIAL DIAGNOSIS

• Coat color dilution is pathognomonic for the disease. A transient color dilution in collie pups has been observed that is not associated with cyclic neutropenia. Pups with this color variant do not develop frequent infection and attain normal coat color intensity by 6 months of age. The pups can be differentiated from the gray pups by normal color intensity of the nose.

CBC/BIOCHEMISTRY/URINALYSIS

Severe neutropenia, lasting from 2-5 days and occurring at 11 to 12-day intervals with marginal normocytic to microcytic anemia. It is important to recognize that signs of infection often are minimal during the neutropenic episodes. Local swelling, redness, and systemic signs of infection usually occur during the initial neutrophilic phase of the cycle and, therefore, on initial examination, neutrophilia with mild to moderate monocytosis is observed. The CBC should be repeated at 2 to 3-day intervals to confirm the diagnosis.

OTHER LABORATORY TESTS N/A

IMAGING N/A

OTHER DIAGNOSTIC PROCEDURES
N/A

TREATMENT

• Advise clients not to attempt to raise the pup(s).
• Antibiotics and supportive treatment may extend the life of the gray pups for several years but at considerable cost.

• The disease cycle has been interrupted experimentally by bone marrow transplantation from normal littermates and daily treatment with endotoxin, lithium carbonate, or recombinant human granulocyte colony-stimulating factor (rH G-CSF).

MEDICATIONS

DRUGS AND FLUIDS

Antibiotics and fluids as required

CONTRAINDICATIONS/POSSIBLE INTERACTIONS

None

FOLLOW-UP

• Guarded prognosis • Antibiotic and supportive therapy required for the life of the dog

MISCELLANEOUS

ABBREVIATION

rH G-CSF = recombinant human granulocyte colony-stimulating factor

Reference

Lund JE, Padgett GA, Ott RL. Cyclic neutropenia in grey collie dogs. Blood 1967;29:452-461.

Author John E. Lund

Consulting Editor Alan H. Rebar

CYTAUXZOONOSIS

BASICS

OVERVIEW
• Infection with a protozoan of the genus Cytauxzoon • Affects vascular system of lungs, liver, spleen, kidneys, and brain; also in bone marrow, and stages in red blood cells.

SIGNALMENT
• A disease of cats • No breed predilection

Incidence/Prevalence
Rare; a disease of cats in southcentral and southeastern United States

Mean Age and Range All ages

Predominant Sex N/A

SIGNS
• Severe illness at presentation • Anemia • Depression • High fever • Dehydration • Icterus • Splenomegaly • Hepatomegaly

CAUSES AND RISK FACTORS
• Bite of infected tick • Roaming in areas shared by the reservoir host, the bobcat, Lynx rufus

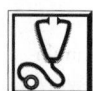

DIAGNOSIS

DIFFERENTIAL DIAGNOSIS
Anemia, marked decrease in packed red cell volume beginning 6 days after infection

CBC/BIOCHEMISTRY/URINALYSIS
N/A

IMAGING Not contributory

OTHER DIAGNOSTIC PROCEDURES
N/A

GROSS AND HISTOPATHOLOGIC FINDINGS
• Lymphocyte and eosinophil counts are decreased significantly within 8 days of infection. • Parasites inside mononuclear cells in bone marrow aspirates and in dramatically enlarged endothelial cells of venules of lung, liver, spleen, kidney, and brain.

TREATMENT
• Inpatient with supportive therapy or euthanasia • No known risk to humans; cannot be directly transmitted to another cat except by blood or tissue inoculation

MEDICATIONS

DRUGS AND FLUIDS
No known chemotherapy; suggest supportive therapy or euthanasia

CONTRAINDICATIONS/POSSIBLE INTERACTIONS N/A

FOLLOW-UP

PATIENT MONITORING N/A

EXPECTED COURSE AND PROGNOSIS
• All infected cats have died within 2 weeks of inoculation. • Consider euthanasia.

MISCELLANEOUS
Unfortunately, diagnosis usually is postmortem.

Authors Dwight Bowman and Edward Pearce

Consulting Editor Fred W. Scott

DANCING DOBERMAN DISEASE (DISTAL POLYNEUROPATHY)

BASICS

OVERVIEW
Syndrome characterized by the flexion of one rear limb when standing, progressing over months to years to involve the opposite pelvic limb. The animal flexes and extends the limbs alternately as in a dancing motion. A primary myopathy is suspected but not proven.

SIGNALMENT
• Doberman pinscher • Age of onset 6 months-7 years • Males and females

SIGNS
• Typical complaint is that affected dog holds one pelvic limb flexed while standing. In most patients, the alternate limb also becomes affected in 3-6 months. • Hyperactive tendon and muscle reflexes with gastrocnemius muscle atrophy are early clinical signs, followed by more extensive pelvic limb muscle atrophy as the disease progresses. • Proprioceptive deficits are seen occasionally.

CAUSES AND RISK FACTORS
• Unknown • Possible genetic predisposition

DIAGNOSIS

DIFFERENTIAL DIAGNOSIS
• Lumbosacral stenosis, intervertebral disc disease, and discospondylitis of the lower lumbar spine are usually painful. • Neoplasia of the lumbar spinal cord or nerve roots progresses more rapidly and can be painful.

CBC/BIOCHEMISTRY/URINALYSIS
Results usually normal

OTHER LABORATORY TESTS N/A

IMAGING N/A

OTHER DIAGNOSTIC PROCEDURES
• Electromyography—prolonged insertion activity, positive sharp waves, and fibrillations • Motor and sensory nerve conduction velocity—normal • Biopsy of gastrocnemius muscles—findings vary; some consistent with primary muscle disease, others more suggestive of denervation

TREATMENT

No treatment has been effective at controlling clinical signs or altering the progression of the disease.

MEDICATIONS

DRUGS AND FLUIDS N/A

CONTRAINDICATIONS/POSSIBLE INTERACTIONS N/A

FOLLOW-UP

Several patients have been followed for more than 5 years and all remain acceptable pets.

MISCELLANEOUS

ABBREVIATIONS None

Reference

Chrisman CL. Dancing doberman disease: clinical findings and prognosis. Prog Vet Neurol 1990;1:83-90.

Author Karen R. Dyer

Consulting Editor Joane M. Parent

DEMODECOSIS

BASICS

OVERVIEW
Canine demodecosis is an inflammatory parasitic disease of dogs characterized by the presence of a high number of mites in the hair follicles which often leads to furunculosis and secondary bacterial infection. The mite, Demodex canis, is part of the normal fauna of canine skin and is normally present in small numbers. The mite resides in the hair follicles and sebaceous glands of the skin. Dead and degenerate mites may be found in extracutaneous sites: lymph node, intestinal wall, spleen, liver, kidney, urinary bladder, lung, thyroid gland, blood, urine, and feces, and are considered to represent drainage to these areas by blood and/or lymph.
Pathologic changes develop from mite infestation when numbers exceed that tolerated by the immune system. The initial proliferation of mites may be due to a genetic or immunologic disorder.

SIGNALMENT
Localized Demodecosis
Most cases occur in young dogs with a median age of 3-6 months. There are no recognized breed or sex predilections.

Generalized Demodecosis
The generalized form of the disease can occur in both the young and old. Adult onset demodecosis is often a severe canine skin disease that is refractory to treatment.

SIGNS
Localized Demodecosis
Clinical lesions are usually mild and consist of erythema and a light scale. One to several patches may be present, and the most common site is the face, especially around the perioral and periocular areas. Patches may also be seen on the trunk and limbs. Most cases heal spontaneously with less than 10% progressing to generalized demodecosis.

Generalized Demodecosis
The disease can be widespread from the onset with multiple, poorly circumscribed patches of erythema, alopecia, and scale. As hair follicles become distended with large numbers of mites, secondary bacterial infections are common, often with rupturing of the follicle (furunculosis). As the condition progresses, the skin can become severly inflamed, exudative, and granulomatous. The sudden occurrence of adult onset demodecosis is often associated with internal disease, malignant neoplasia, or immunosuppressive disease. Approximately 25% of the adult onset cases are idiopathic over a follow-up period of 1-2 years.

CAUSES AND RISK FACTORS
• The exact immunopathomechanism of canine demodecosis is unknown. • Recent studies have indicated that dogs with generalized demodecosis have a subnormal percentage of interleukin-2 receptors on their lymphocytes and subnormal interleukin-2 production.

DIAGNOSIS

DIFFERENTIAL DIAGNOSIS
• Bacterial folliculitis/furunculosis
• Dermatophytosis • Contact dermatitis
• Pemphigus complex • Dermatomyositis
• Systemic lupus erythematosus

CBC/BIOCHEMISTRY/URINALYSIS
Nondiagnostic

OTHER LABORATORY TESTS N/A

IMAGING N/A

OTHER DIAGNOSTIC PROCEDURES
Skin scrapings are diagnostic - large numbers of mites in the majority of cases. Exceptions are lesions that are chronic, granulomatous, and fibrotic (especially on the paw), and diagnosis may necessitate a cutaneous biopsy.

TREATMENT

Localized Demodecosis
Treatment of the localized form of the disease should be conservative. Most cases (90%) resolve spontaneously with no treatment.

Generalized Demodecosis
• Demodecosis in the adult dog is a frequent management problem for the owner. Expense and frustration with the chronicity of the problem are an issue. Many of these patients are medically controlled rather than cured. The prognosis for canine demodecosis depends heavily on genetic, immunologic, and underlying diseases.
• The general health status of dogs with the localized or the generalized form of the disease should be evaluated.

MEDICATIONS

DRUGS AND FLUIDS
Amitraz
• Amitraz (Mitaban-Upjohn; Taktic-EC-Hoechst-Roussel Agri-Vet, Somerville, NJ) is a formamidine, which inhibits monamine oxidase and prostaglandin synthesis, and is an alpha 2 adrenergic agonist.
• Dosage and regimen: use weekly (the label reads every other week) 1/2 vial (5mls)/gallon of water until resolution of clinical signs and no mites are found on skin scrapings (do not rinse off the dip, let air dry).
• Apply a benzoyl peroxide shampoo prior to the application of the dip as a bactericidal therapy and to increase exposure of the mites to the miticide through follicular flushing activity.
• The efficacy of amitraz is proportional to the frequency and concentration of the dip.
• Amitraz may be mixed with mineral oil (3 ml amitraz to 30ml mineral oil) for application to focal areas such as pododemodecosis.
• Success with the 9% amitraz collar has not been established.
• 11-30% of patients will not be cured with Amitraz; may need to choose an alternate therapy or control the case with maintenance amitraz dips every 2-8 weeks.

Ivermectin
• Ivermectin (Ivomec, Eqvalan Liquid-MSD AgVet, Rahway, NJ) is a macrocyclic lactone.
• Dosage and regimen: daily oral administration of 300-600 micrograms/kg/day is very effective, even in amitraz failures.
• Treatment is continued for 60 days beyond negative skin scrapings (3-8 months).

Milbemycin
• Milbemycin (Interceptor-Ciba Geigy Health, NC) is a macrocyclic lactone.
• Dosage and regimen: 1 mg/kg orally q24h for a cure rate of 50%; 2 mg/kg orally q24h for a cure rate of 85%
• Treatment should be continued for 60 days beyond multiple negative skin scrapings

CONTRAINDICATIONS/POSSIBLE INTERACTIONS
Amitraz
• Adverse drug interactions are possible with heterocyclic antidepressants, xylazine, benzodiazepines, and macrocyclic lactones.
• Most common side effects include somnolence, lethargy, depression, anorexia seen in 30% of patients for 12-36 hrs. post treatment
• Other side effects include vomiting, diarrhea, pruritus, polyuria, mydriasis, bradycardia, hypoventilation, hypotension, hypothermia, ataxia, ileus, bloat, hyperglycemia, convulsions, and death
• The incidence and severity of the side effects do not appear to be proportional to the dosage or frequency of use
• Humans can develop dermatitis, headaches, and respiratory difficulty after exposure
• Yohimbine 0.11mg/kg IV is an antidote

Ivermectin
• Causes elevated levels of monoamine neurotransmitter metabolites, which could result in adverse drug interactions with amitraz and benzodiazepines.
• Contraindicated in collies, shetland sheepdogs, Old English sheepdogs, other herding breeds, and crosses with these breeds
• Signs of toxicity include salivation, vomiting, mydriasis, confusion, ataxia, hypersensitivity to sound, weakness, recumbancy, coma, and death

Milbemycin

- Adverse drug interaction with amitraz and benzodiazepines
- Signs of toxicosis are as for ivermectin.
- Ivermectin-sensitive breeds appear to tolerate the acaricidal dosages given.

FOLLOW-UP

Examination of multiple skin scrapings and evidence of clinical resolution are used to monitor progress.

MISCELLANEOUS

Reference
Scott, Miller, Griffin. Muller and Kirk's
  small animal dermatology. 5th Ed.
  Philadelphia: WB Saunders, 1995;417-432

Author Karen Helton-Rhodes

Consulting Editor Lowell Ackerman

DERMATITIS, ACRAL LICK

BASICS

OVERVIEW
This disease is defined as a firm, raised, ulcerative or thickened plaque that is usually located on the dorsal aspect of the carpus, metacarpus, tarsus or metatarsus.

SIGNALMENT
• This disease is primarily seen in dogs. It is most common in large-breed dogs, especially doberman pinschers, Labrador retrievers, great Danes, Irish and English setters, golden retrievers, akitas, dalmatians, shar peis, and weimaraners. • Age is dependent on the cause. • Some sources suggest this is more common in males. Others indicate that there is no sex predilection.

SIGNS
• Historical findings include excessive licking and chewing of the affected area. Occasionally there is history of trauma to the affected area. • Physical examination findings include alopecic, ulcerative, thickened and raised firm plaques. The lesions are usually located on the areas indicated in the overview. Often the lesions occur singly, although they may affect more than one location.

CAUSES AND RISK FACTORS
Diseases that have been associated with acral lick dermatitis (ALD) include staphylococcal furunculosis, allergy, endocrinopathy, demodicosis, dermatophytosis, foreign body reaction, neoplasia, trauma, and psychogenic and sensory nerve dysfunction.

DIAGNOSIS

DIFFERENTIAL DIAGNOSIS
• Allergic animals often have multiple lick granulomas and other areas of pruritus compatible with the specific allergy. • Endocrinopathies, demodicosis and dermatophytosis are determined on the basis of laboratory test results.

CBC/BIOCHEMISTRY/URINALYSIS
Complete blood count and serum chemistry profiles are normal except in cases of hyperadrenocorticism.

OTHER LABORATORY TESTS
Low thyroid levels would be suggestive of hypothyroidism. An abnormal ACTH stimulation test or abnormal low-dose dexamethasone suppression test would be suggestive of hyperadrenocorticism.

IMAGING
Radiology determines if neoplasia and some forms of trauma or radiopaque foreign bodies are present.

OTHER DIAGNOSTIC PROCEDURES
• Examination of skin scrapings, dermatophyte culture and Tzanck preparations should be done to determine if demodicosis, dermatophytosis or a bacterial infection is present. If a bacterial infection is present, a bacterial culture and sensitivity should be performed to determine the appropriate antibiotics. • A food elimination diet can be done to determine if food allergy is present.

GROSS AND HISTOPATHOLOGIC FINDINGS
Histopathologic reveals ulcerative, hyperplastic epidermis with mild perivascular dermatitis. Varying degrees of fibroplasia are present.

TREATMENT

• Be sure the pet is getting plenty of attention and exercise.
• No modification of diet is necessary unless a food allergy is suspected.
• This can be a difficult condition to treat especially if no underlying cause is found. The owner should be warned that patience and time are necessary.
• Surgery should not be considered in these patients unless absolutely necessary (i.e. after all other therapies have been exhausted). This often causes increased licking and attention to the affected area with resultant poor wound closure.

MEDICATIONS

DRUGS AND FLUIDS
• Antibiotics based on bacterial culture and sensitivity should be given until infection is completely resolved.
• After all other underlying diseases have been ruled out or treated, then therapies for psychogenic dermatoses may be tried.
• Systemic medications include hydroxyzine HCl (1-2 mg/kg PO q8h), chlorpheniramine 4-8 mg/dog q12h PO (maximum of .5 mg/kg q12h), naltrexone (2.2 mg/kg PO q12h-q24h) and amitriptyline HCl (1.1-2.2 mg/kg q12h). Amitriptyline should be used at the lower dosage for 10 days. If no improvement, then it can be used at the higher dosage for 10 days. Doxepin may also be tried at 3-5 mg/kg q12h. Maximum dosage for doxepin is 150 mg q12h. None of these medications should be used concurrently.
• Topicals that may be tried include flunixin meglumine and fluocinolone in dimethyl sulfoxide (combined), mupirocin, topical 5% benzoyl peroxide, Heet (analgesic) and Bitter Apple (1:1). Do not use the Heet and Bitter Apple combination if owners or animals have respiratory conditions. Intralesional corticosteroids may be used in early or very small lesions. These are rarely of any use in chronic lesions. Any topicals should be applied with gloves. The animals should be kept from licking the area for 10-15 minutes.

CONTRAINDICATIONS/POSSIBLE INTERACTIONS
• Do not use any of the oral medications in animals that have had previous amitriptyline
• Doxepin should not be used with monoamine oxidase inhibitors, clonidine, anticonvulsants, oral anticoagulants, steroid hormones, antihistamines, or aspirin.
• More than 1 antihistamine should not be used at a time. Antihistamines should not be used in prostatic hypertrophy, angle closure glaucoma, or pyloroduodenal or bladder neck obstruction. They should be used cautiously in hyperthyroidism, cardiovascular disease, or hypertension.

FOLLOW-UP

• The level of licking and chewing should be monitored closely. • Underlying disease should be treated to prevent recurrence. • If no underlying disease is detected, the ALD may be psychogenic (obsessive-compulsive or self-mutilation disorder). The prognosis is then guarded. • Every 1-2 months a complete blood count, chemistry profile, and electrocardiogram should be done when patients are receiving tricyclic antidepressants since there is potential for cardiotoxicity and hepatotoxicity.

MISCELLANEOUS

• If dog is less than 5 years old, allergy as an etiology should be strongly considered.
• This may only be transmitted to humans if dermatophytosis is the underlying cause.

ABBREVIATIONS
ALD = acral lick dermatitis
ACTH = adrenocorticotropic hormone

References
Shanley K, Overall K. Psychogenic dermatoses. In: Kirk RW, Bonagura JD, eds. Current veterinary therapy XI. Philadelphia: WB Saunders, 1992:552-557.

Author Karen A. Kuhl
Consulting Editor Lowell Ackerman

BASICS

OVERVIEW

• Irritant and allergic contact dermatitis are two rare and distinctly different pathophysiologic syndromes with similar clinical signs.
• Irritant contact dermatitis (ICD) results from direct damage to keratinocytes by exposure to a particular compound. Damaged keratinocytes induce an inflammatory response directed at the skin. • Allergic contact dermatitis (ACD) is an immunologic event requiring sensitization, memory, and elicitation. • In patients with ACD, Langerhans cells process antigens that penetrate the skin and present them to naive T-cells within lymph nodes. Sensitized T-cell clones (memory cells) then proliferate and circulate throughout the body. When a Langerhans cell encounters the antigen again, it presents the antigen to sensitized T-cells, resulting in an immunologic response.

SIGNALMENT

• ICD occurs at any age as a direct result of the irritant nature of the offending compound. • ACD is rare in young animals; most are chronically exposed to the antigen. • German shepherd dogs are predisposed to ACD. French poodles, terriers, and golden retrievers are considered at increased risk. • ACD is extremely rare in cats, except due to exposure to d-limonene-containing insecticides. • Breed predilection has not been substantiated; although wire-haired fox terriers, Scottish terriers, West Highland white terriers, French poodles, golden retrievers, and Danish German shepherd dogs may be at increased risk.

SIGNS

• Lesion location depends upon the way in which the antigen is contacted. The thick hair coat of dogs is an effective barrier against contact. • Most lesions are limited to glabrous skin or regions frequently in contact with the ground such as the chin, ventral neck, sternum, ventral abdomen, inguinum, perineum, scrotum, and ventral contact regions of the tail and interdigital areas. • Reactions to topical medications (most often otic preparations) are usually localized; generalized reactions, resulting from shampoos or insecticide sprays, are least common. • Initial lesions consist of erythema and swelling leading to papules and plaques: vesicles are uncommon. • Pruritus varies from moderate to severe, although severe pruritus is most common. • A seasonal incidence may indicate that the offending antigen is a plant or outdoor compound.

CAUSES AND RISK FACTORS

• Inflamed skin may increase the penetration of antigens through the skin. Therefore, any inflammatory dermatitis may facilitate ACD.
• Substances which can cause contact dermatitis: plants, carpet and litter deodorizers, plastics or rubber, leather, soaps, detergents, floor waxes, rugs, carpets, herbicides, fertilizer, mulch, insecticides (including topical flea treatments), leather and flea collars, concrete, topical preparations, fabrics, concrete, and rubber or plastic food dishes and toys

DIAGNOSIS

DIFFERENTIAL DIAGNOSIS

Atopy, food allergy, drug eruptions, parasite hypersensitivity, parasite infestation, insect bites, pyoderma, Malassezia dermatitis, dermatophytosis, demodicosis, lupus erythematosus, seborrheic dermatitis, solar dermatitis, thermal injuries, and trauma from rough surfaces.

CBC/BIOCHEMISTRY/URINALYSIS

No abnormalities on routine CBC, serum chemistries, or urinalysis.

OTHER LABORATORY TESTS N/A

IMAGING N/A

OTHER DIAGNOSTIC PROCEDURES

• Skin biopsies demonstrate intraepidermal vesiculation and spongiosis and superficial dermal edema with mononuclear cell infiltrate in ICD and ACD; ICD also has polymorphonuclear cell infiltrate. • Closed patch testing can sometimes be helpful (corticosteroids and nonsteroidal anti-inflammatory drugs must be stopped 3-6 weeks prior to testing), either using materials directly from the environment or by using a standard patch test kit for humans (Hermal Pharmaceutical Laboratories, Inc., Oak Hill, NY) applied to the skin under a bandage for 48 hours.
• Best diagnostic test is elimination of contact irritant or antigen, followed by provocative exposure testing. Perform bacterial cultures to define secondary pyoderma.

GROSS AND HISTOPATHOLOGIC FINDINGS

Histologic findings vary with the duration of antigen contact. The most frequent findings include a perivascular pattern of dermal infiltrate in addition to exocytosis of leukocytes.

TREATMENT

• Eliminate offending substance(s)
• Baths with hypoallergenic shampoos.
• Mechanical barriers: socks, T-shirts.

MEDICATIONS

DRUGS AND FLUIDS

• Systemic corticosteroids: prednisone 0.25-0.5 mg/kg PO q24h for 3-5 days, then every 48 hours for two weeks.
• Topical corticosteroids.

CONTRAINDICATIONS/POSSIBLE INTERACTIONS N/A

FOLLOW-UP

PREVENTION/AVOIDANCE

Remove offending substances from the environment.

EXPECTED COURSE AND PROGNOSIS

• ICD is often an acute condition which may occur after only one exposure and can be manifested within 24 hours of exposure.
• Steroids rarely helpful. Lesions resolve 1-2 days after irritant removal.
• ACD requires months to years of exposure for the hypersensitivity to develop.
• Reexposure results in the development of clinical signs 3-5 days following exposure, and the signs may persist for several weeks. This type of contact dermatitis responds well to corticosteroids, but the pruritus returns upon discontinuation if the antigenic stimulation has not been removed. Hyposensitization is disappointing.
• Prognosis is good if allergen is identified and removed but is poor if the allergen is not identified. In the latter circumstance, treatment may be life-long.

MISCELLANEOUS

ABBREVIATIONS

ICD = irritant contact dermatitis
ACD = allergic contact dermatitis

Reference

Walder EJ, Conroy JD. Contact dermatitis in dogs and cats: pathogenesis, histopathology, experimental induction, and case reports. Vet Dermatol, in press.

Authors Margaret S. Swartout and Alexander H. Werner
Consulting Editor Lowell Ackerman

DERMATITIS, INTERDIGITAL

 BASICS

OVERVIEW
This is a disease with several possible known causes as well as unknown (idiopathic) causes. Interdigital dermatitis is a disease of the feet of dogs and is also known as pododermatitis, interdigital pyoderma, or pedal folliculitis and furunculosis

SIGNALMENT
• Interdigital dermatitis affects dogs of any age, sex, or breed. • Short–coated male dogs may be predisposed. Short–coated breeds possibly predisposed include the English bulldog, great Dane, bassett hound, mastiff, bull terrier, boxer, dachshund, dalmatian, German shorthaired pointer and weimaraner. • Long coated breeds possibly predisposed are the German shepherd, Labrador retriever, golden retriever, Irish setter and Pekinese.

SIGNS
• One foot and one interdigital space or multiple interdigital spaces and feet may be involved. • The diseased tissue is usually erythematous, swollen, and has either intact bullae or ruptured draining tracts or a combination of these. • Some dogs will have mild to severe swelling of the affected feet. Mild to severe lameness may also be present.

CAUSES AND RISK FACTORS

One Foot Involved
• Foreign bodies (e.g., grass awns, wood slivers, suture material) • Osteomyelitis
• Neoplasia

More Than One Foot Involved
• Hypersensitivity reactions (food, atopy, contact dermatitis) • Infections (bacterial, fungal) • Trauma (clipper burns, cuts)
• Chemical (contact irritant dermatitis)
• Metabolic (hypothyroidism, hyperadrenocorticism) • Parasitic (demodicosis, pelodera, hookworm, heartworm) • Demodicosis is often complicated by the presence of furunculosis and draining tracts. Heartworm, hookworm, and pelodera are seen on the feet as erythematous, pruritic, patchy alopecic lesions. Pelodera also affects the limbs and the ventral abdomen.

Idiopathic
• Recurrent pododermatitis • Clinically important footpad involvement with the interdigital dermatitis • Immune-mediated (pemphigus, pemphigoid, systemic lupus erythromatosis) • Zinc deficiency or zinc responsive • Superficial necrolytic dermatitis

 DIAGNOSIS

DIFFERENTIAL DIAGNOSIS
Adult onset demodicosis — underlying hypothyroidism, hyperadrenocorticism, allergic disease, or neoplasia

CBC/BIOCHEMISTRY/URINALYSIS
• Most cases will not have any diagnostic changes. • In cases of superficial necrolytic dermatitis changes in liver and pancreatic enzymes may be seen.

OTHER LABORATORY TESTS
• Blood tests for heartworm microfilaria
• T_4 tests confirm or deny a diagnosis of hypothyroidism • Adrenal response tests (low-dose dexamethasone suppression, urine cortisol:creatinine ratios, and ACTH stimulation) to confirm or deny the presence of hyperadrenocorticism.

IMAGING
Radiographs are useful if underlying osteomyelitis is suspected.

OTHER DIAGNOSTIC PROCEDURES
• Biopsies — helpful in the diagnosis of foreign bodies, demodicosis, neoplasia, infectious agents such as fungi, and bacteria parasites such as heartworm and, rarely, hookworm. • Skin scrapings helpful in identification of parasites, demodicosis, pelodera, or fungi (dermatophytosis) • Fecal flotation — helpful in identification of hookworm
• Cytologic examination of the exudate stained with Wright–Giemsa staining technique is helpful in identification of yeast, bacteria, and rarely, parasites. Cytologic examination of the exudate also allows the evaluation of the type of inflammatory response.(e.g., eosinophils may suggest parasites or hypersensitivity).

GROSS AND HISTOPATHOLOGIC FINDINGS
Other than causal findings listed above (e.g., parasites, and bacteria), the reaction pattern is a folliculitis, perifolliculitis, and pyogranulomatous dermatitis if the follicles have ruptured.

 TREATMENT

• Treatment of the underlying cause if found and antibacterial treatment if bacteria are present.
• Antibiotics must be used until the deep tissues have healed. Culture and sensitivity is very important in deep pyoderma for the selection of an appropriate antibiotic at the beginning of treatment. Usually, several months of antibiotics are necessary so it is important to begin as soon as possible with the right antibiotic.
• If draining lesions are present, daily foot soaks (10 minutes twice daily) are helpful until draining stops.
• Restricting the animal's activity or protection of the feet may be beneficial
• In severe refractory cases complete surgical debridement and removal of the interdigital tissue and joining the digits together (fusion podoplasty) can be helpful.

MEDICATIONS

DRUGS AND FLUIDS

• For the deep bacterial infection (furunculosis) use a broad spectrum antibiotic that is effective against the staphylococcal organisms based on culture and sensitivity.

• Amoxicillin with clavulanate, enrofloxacin or cephalosporin antibiotics are good for the long term 6–8 week therapy needed in these cases.

CONTRAINDICATIONS/POSSIBLE INTERACTIONS

Rifampin can be used with caution for short periods at 5–10 mg/kg q24h. Due to its lipid solubility, rifampin penetrates deep lesions well. It must be accompanied by a good antibiotic because bacteria rapidly develop resistance to rifampin. The liver enzymes and CBC must be monitored every 2 weeks. Animals with liver disease should not be given rifampin.

FOLLOW-UP

• While treating this disease, follow–ups are essential for the careful consideration of the various possible underlying causes. • Finding the cause of the interdigital dermatitis in these cases can be tedious and frustrating, but identification is essential for complete resolution and healing. • Medication for the bacterial infection should be continued 2 weeks after all palpable dermal lesions are resolved.

MISCELLANEOUS

Reference

Scott DW. Canine pododermatitis. In: Kirk RW, ed. Current veterinary therapy VII. Philadelphia: WB Saunders, 1980;467.

Author David Duclos

Consulting Editor Lowell Ackerman

DERMATOMYOSITIS

BASICS

DEFINITION
Dermatomyositis in dogs is an inherited inflammatory condition that involves the skin and muscle and, occasionally, the blood vessels. This disease occurs primarily in collies, shetland sheepdogs, and their related crossbreeds.

Pathophysiology
The exact pathogenesis of dermatomyositis is unknown. Although it is well-accepted that there is a genetic predisposition for this disease, some suspect that an infectious agent (i.e., virus) triggers the clinical signs. Others feel that an immune-mediated or autoimmune process may be involved.

Systems Affected
• Skin/exocrine—variable dermatitis on the face, ears, tail tip, and over the bony prominences of the distal extremities develops first • Musculoskeletal—myositis, which can be subtle to severe, develops after the dermatitis. Usually the temporal and masseter muscles are involved. In more severe cases, there may be generalized muscle disease and involvement of the esophageal muscles. In general, the more severe the dermatitis, the more severe the myositis.

Genetics
In collies and shetland sheepdogs, dermatomyositis is thought to be inherited as an autosomal dominant with variable expressivity.

Incidence/Prevalence
The exact prevalence is unknown.

Geographic Distribution
Probably worldwide

SIGNALMENT

Species Dogs

Breed Predilection
• Collies, shetland sheepdogs, and their crossbreeds. • Also isolated reports for an Australian cattle dog, Welsh corgi, chow chow, German shepherd, and kuvasz.

Mean Age and Range
• Cutaneous lesions usually develop when the dog is between 7 weeks and 6 months of age. In mildly affected dogs, the lesions may resolve in 3 months. In moderately affected dogs, lesions may persist for 6 months or more. In severely affected dogs, lesions usually persist throughout life. • Adult-onset dermatomyositis can occur, but is much less common.

Predominant Sex
None (affects both equally)

SIGNS

General Comments
The clinical signs vary from subtle skin lesions and subclinical myositis to severe skin lesions and generalized muscle atrophy.

Historical Findings
• Waxing and waning skin lesions around the eyes, lips, face, inner ear pinnae, tip of the tail, and bony prominences of distal extremities usually are seen in affected dogs before they are 6 months old. When the lesions heal, residual scarring may occur. • Muscle atrophy of the masseter and/or temporal muscles may be evident in some dogs. More severely affected dogs may have difficulty eating, drinking, and swallowing. Severely affected dogs may have stunted growth, be lame, have widespread muscle atrophy, and be infertile. • Several littermates may be affected, but the severity of the disease often varies significantly among the affected dogs.

Physical Examination Findings
• Skin lesions are characterized by papules and vesicles (rare) and variable degrees of erythema, alopecia, scaling, crusting, ulceration, and scarring on the face, around the lips and eyes, in the inner ear pinnae, on the tip of the tail, and over bony prominences on the distal extremities. Rarely, foot pad and oral ulcers are seen. • Signs of myositis may vary from none to a bilateral symmetric decrease in the mass of the temporalis muscles to generalized symmetric muscle atrophy. Dogs with megaesophagus may present with aspiration pneumonia, and dogs with generalized myositis may be lame.

CAUSES
• Hereditary • Infectious agents • Immune-mediated

RISK FACTORS
• Trauma • Sunlight • Estrus, parturition, and lactation

DIAGNOSIS

DIFFERENTIAL DIAGNOSIS
• Demodicosis • Dermatophytosis • Bacterial folliculitis • Juvenile cellulitis • Discoid lupus erythematosus • Systemic lupus erythematosus • Polymyositis

CBC/BIOCHEMISTRY/URINALYSIS
• Nonregenerative anemia may be seen in severely affected dogs. • Serum creatine kinase may be normal or slightly high.

OTHER LABORATORY TESTS
Antinuclear antibody titers and lupus erythematosus tests are negative.

IMAGING N/A

OTHER DIAGNOSTIC PROCEDURES
• Electromyographic (EMG) abnormalities are present in affected muscles. Findings include fibrillation potentials, bizarre high frequency discharges, and positive sharp waves. • For skin biopsies, papules, vesicles, or lesions that show alopecia and erythema should be chosen. Infected and scarred lesions should be avoided. • Proper muscle selection for muscle biopsy can be difficult because pathologic changes may be mild, mutifocal, or, in early cases, absent. Ideally, electromyography is used to select affected muscles for biopsy. If EMG is not available, atrophied muscles should be biopsied. If the muscles appear clinically normal, random muscle biopsies may not be diagnostic.

GROSS AND HISTOPATHOLOGIC FINDINGS

Skin Biopsy
• Scattered necrosis or vacuolation of individual basal cells may be seen. Necrotic basal cells are called colloid bodies. • Vesicles that contain small amounts of RBC occasionally are found. • Superficial, mild, diffuse dermal inflammatory infiltrates composed of lymphocytes and histiocytes with variable numbers of mast cells and neutrophils are seen, especially perifollicularly. • Follicular basal cell degeneration and follicular atrophy are usually seen. • Secondary epidermal ulceration and dermal scarring may be present. • The combination of perifollicular inflammation, epidermal and follicular cell degeneration, and follicular atrophy are highly suggestive of dermatomyositis.

Muscle Biopsy
• Variable multifocal accumulations of inflammatory cells, including lymphocytes, macrophages, plasma cells, neutrophils, and eosinophils • Myofibril degeneration characterized by fragmentation, vacuolation, and increased eosinophilia of the myofibrils • Myofiber atrophy and regeneration

TREATMENT

INPATIENT VERSUS OUTPATIENT
Most dogs can be treated as outpatients. Dogs with severe myositis may need to be hospitalized for supportive care.

ACTIVITY
Avoid activities that may traumatize the skin. Keep indoors during the day to avoid exposure to intense sunlight.

DIET N/A

CLIENT EDUCATION
• Discuss the hereditary nature of the disease. • Advise that affected dogs should not be bred. • The disease is not curable, although spontaneous resolution can occur. • Discuss prognosis and possible complications especially in severely affected dogs. • Advise that medications may or may not help.

SURGICAL CONSIDERATIONS N/A

MEDICATIONS

DRUGS AND FLUIDS

• Nonspecific symptomatic therapy includes hypoallergenic shampoo baths, treating secondary pyoderma and demodicosis, and avoiding trauma and intense sunlight. Because estrus exacerbates the disease, neutering intact female dogs is recommended.
• The therapeutic efficacy of medical treatment can be difficult to assess because the disease tends to be cyclic in nature and is often self-limiting.
Drugs that have been used to treat dermatomyositis include:
• Vitamin E, 100-400 IU PO q12-24h
• Prednisone, 1-2 mg/kg PO q12h until remission, then alternate-day administration using the lowest dosage possible for long-term control
• Pentoxifylline (Trental; Hoechst-Roussel, Somerville, NJ) is a human drug that increases microvascular blood flow and tissue oxygenation by lowering blood viscosity, inhibiting platelet aggregation, increasing RBC deformability, and reducing serum fibrinogen levels. It is sold as 400-mg tablets that should not be divided. This drug has been found beneficial in some dogs with dermatomyositis, but improvement may not be seen for 1 or 2 months. The dosage is 400 mg PO with food every 24 hours.

CONTRAINDICATIONS

Pentoxifylline should not be used in dogs that are sensitive to methylxanthine derivatives.

PRECAUTIONS

• Pentoxifylline can cause gastric irritation. Dogs with prolonged clotting times and dogs receiving anticoagulant therapy should be monitored carefully when treated with this drug.
• When glucocorticoids are used, their possible side effects should be discussed with the owner.

POSSIBLE INTERACTIONS

See precautions.

ALTERNATE DRUGS N/A

FOLLOW-UP

PATIENT MONITORING N/A

PREVENTION/AVOIDANCE

• Minimize trauma and exposure to sunlight. Spay intact female dogs to prevent estrus, parturition, and lactation (all precipitating causes of active dermatomyositis). • Do not breed affected animals.

POSSIBLE COMPLICATIONS

• Secondary pyoderma and demodicosis can be complicating factors. • Mildly to moderately affected dogs may have residual foci of alopecia, hypopigmentation, and hyperpigmentation in areas of previously active skin lesions. These areas of mild scarring occur most frequently on the bridge of the nose and around the eyes. • In more severely affected dogs, scarring tends to be extensive. Because the degree of myositis correlates with the severity of the dermatitis, severely affected dogs may have trouble chewing, drinking, and swallowing if the masticatory and esophageal muscles are involved. Megaesophagus may develop, predisposing the dog to aspiration pneumonia. If the myositis is generalized, the dog's growth may be stunted.

EXPECTED COURSE AND PROGNOSIS

The long-term prognosis is variable depending on the severity of the disease. The prognosis for minimally affected dogs is good because these dogs tend to spontaneously resolve with no evidence of scarring. Mildly to moderately affected dogs tend to eventually spontaneously resolve, but residual scarring is usually present. For severely affected dogs, the prognosis for long-term survival is poor. In these dogs, the dermatitis and myositis are severe and life-long.

MISCELLANEOUS

ASSOCIATED CONDITIONS

Ulcerative dermatosis is a poorly understood disease that has been described in collies and Shetland sheepdogs. This disease is characterized by well-demarcated serpiginous ulcers in the intertriginous areas of the groin and axillae. Ulcerative dermatosis may occur alone or it can occur concurrently with dermatomyositis. Possibly, ulcerative dermatosis represents a subgroup of dermatomyositis.

AGE RELATED FACTORS

Clinical signs usually are seen first in dogs less than 6 months old. Adult-onset dermatomyositis is rare and is more commonly seen in dogs that had subtle lesions as puppies yet developed more noticeable lesions as adults because of some precipitating event (i.e., trauma, estrus).

ZOONOTIC POTENTIAL N/A

PREGNANCY

Affected dogs should not be bred because the disease is inherited. Pregnancy will also exacerbate the clinical symptoms of dermatomyositis in affected bitches.

SYNONYMS

• Familial canine dermatomyositis • Canine familial dermatomyositis

SEE ALSO

• Systemic Lupus Erythematosus • Lupus Erythematosus, Discoid

ABBREVIATIONS

EMG = Electromyographic

References

Hargis AM, Prieur DJ, Haupt KH, Collier LI, Evermann JF, Ladiges WC. Postmortem findings in four litters of dogs with familial canine dermatomyositis. Am J Pathol 1986;123:480-496.

Hargis AM, Mundell AC. Familial canine dermatomyositis. Comp Cont Ed 1992;14:855-864.

White SD, Shelton GD, Sisson A, McPherron M, Rosychuk RAW, Olson PJ. Dermatomyositis in an adult Pembroke Welsh corgi. J Am Anim Hosp Assoc 1992;28:398-401.

Gross TL, Ihrke PJ, Walder E. Veterinary dermatopathology: a macroscopic and microscopic evaluation of canine and feline skin disease. St. Louis: Mosby, 1992:34-36.

Author Linda Medleau

Consulting Editor Lowell Ackerman

DERMATOPHILOSIS

BASICS

OVERVIEW
• Dermatophilus congolensis is a gram-positive, branching, filamentous Actinomycete that is part of the normal dermal flora of several domestic species, including horses, sheep, goats, and cattle. It is aerobic, non–spore-forming, and not acid-fast. • Dogs, cats, or humans can become secondary hosts. Exposure typically involves contamination of wounds or traumatic implantation of the organism (especially in cats). • Lesions in dogs are usually limited to the skin and produce few signs of systemic illness. Dogs may, however, appear systemically ill secondary to an underlying disease process that predisposed them to developing dermatophilosis. • Cats typically have deeper infections and the skin becomes secondarily involved by extension. Lesions occur in four forms: lingual and tonsillar crypt granulomas, granulomatous lymphadenitis with fistulation, cutaneous dermatophilosis, and miscellaneous lesions (e.g., the bladder).

SIGNALMENT
• Dogs and cats. Rare in both. • No specific age, sex, or breed predilections known.

SIGNS
Historical Findings
• Cats often have a history of exposure to barnyard animals although cases have been reported with no known history of exposure to primary carrier species. • History of ectoparasites, minor trauma, inflammation, or other skin infections may be noted.

Physical Examination Findings
Dogs
Lesion typically found on haired regions of skin. Classic lesion is a crust with imbedded hairs. When crust is removed underlying skin is typically erythematous and ulcerated and a green purulent exudate may be noted. Lesions are usually distributed over caudal dorsum, lateral thighs, and scapulae.
Cats
• Varies with site of infection • Oral—proliferative masses on the dorsum of the tongue extending into tonsillar crypts. Drooling, difficulty swallowing, and respiratory difficulties may be noted. • Lymph nodes (especially popliteal)—localized lymphadenitis and fistualtion. Firm subcutaneous nodules may be palpated. Fistulous tracts may extend to the overlying skin. • Cutaneous—abscessation extending from subcutaneous lesions • Miscellaneous—a large solitary granuloma has been reported involving the serosal layer of the bladder

CAUSES AND RISK FACTORS
• Infection is thought to occur through minor abrasions and wounds to the mucous membranes, epithelium of the tongue, and the skin. • Ectoparasite infestation may increase risk. • Moist conditions are likely to promote dissemination. • Direct implantation likely plays a major role in infections in cats.

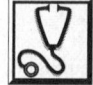

DIAGNOSIS

DIFFERENTIAL DIAGNOSIS
• Staphylococcal pyodermas • Acute moist dermatitis • Dermatophytosis • Keratinization disorders • Zinc-responsive dermatitis • Pemphigus foliaceus • Atypical mycobacterial infections • Other causes of lymphadenitis

CBC/BIOCHEMISTRY/URINALYSIS
• Usually normal in cutaneous infections
• Leukocytosis may be seen.

OTHER LABORATORY TESTS N/A

IMAGING N/A

OTHER DIAGNOSTIC PROCEDURES
• Cultures of crusts or biopsies may allow identification.
• Minced preparations of crusts can be prepared as wet mounts and stained with new methylene blue. • Heat fixed preparations can be stained by Giemsa methods, Wright, or Gram's stains. Biopsy of deep lesions is diagnostic. • Monoclonal antibodies have been used with indirect immunoflourescent staining.

GROSS AND HISTOPATHOLOGIC FINDINGS
Dogs
Histopathologic examination a suppurative dermatitis characterized by a palisading crust with orthokeratotic-parakeratotic hyperkeratosis and underlying dermal edema and hemorrhage. Neutrophils and branching chains of organisms are seen. There is little involvement of the hair follicles.

Cats
Pyogranulomas of the subcutaneous tissues and lymph nodes.

TREATMENT
• Drying and clipping of affected areas is recommended.
• Remove crusts.
• Bathe with lime sulfur 2% preparations or an organic iodine preparation.
• Crust removal and baths should continue for a minimum of 2 weeks.
• Patients generally can be treated as outpatients.
• Owners should wear gloves to avoid developing exudative pustular dermatitis.

MEDICATIONS

DRUGS AND FLUIDS
- Penicillin V 10 mg/kg PO q12h × 10 days
- Gentamicin 2 mg/kg IM q12h × 7 days
- Ampicillin 10-20 mg/kg PO q12h × 10 days
- Amoxicillin 10-20 mg/kg PO q12h × 10 days

CONTRAINDICATIONS/POSSIBLE INTERACTIONS
Gentamicin is not recommended in patients with known renal insufficiency.

 FOLLOW-UP

PATIENT MONITORING N/A
Positive cultures may be obtained from the skin of healed cases for up to 15 months.
- Owners should be instructed to monitor for lesions and return for examination if new lesions develop.

PREVENTION/AVOIDANCE
Infection is best avoided by minimizing contact with carrier species, keeping skin dry, and minimizing trauma and external parasite burden.

EXPECTED COURSE AND PROGNOSIS
Prognosis with treatment is generally good.

 MISCELLANEOUS

ZOONOTIC POTENTIAL
Humans can become accidentally infected but are not primary carriers.

References

Greene CE. Dermatophilosis. In: Greene CE, ed. Infectious diseases of the dog and cat. Philadelphia: WB Saunders, 1990:592-594.

Pedersen NC. Dermatophilosis. In Pratt PW, ed. Feline infectious diseases. Goleta, CA: American Veterinary Publications, 1988:187-188.

Author Matthew S. Mellema
Consulting Editor Fred W. Scott

DERMATOPHYTOSIS

BASICS

DEFINITION
A cutaneous fungal infection affecting the cornified regions of hair, nails, and occasionally the superficial layers of the skin. The most commonly isolated organisms are Microsporum canis, Trichophyton mentagrophytes, and Microsporum gypseum.

Pathophysiology
Exposure to or contact with a dermatophyte does not necessarily result in an infection. Infection may not result in clinical signs. Dermatophytes grow in the keratinized layers of hair, nail and skin. They do not thrive in living tissue or persist in the presence of severe inflammation. The incubation period is 1-4 weeks. An infected animal which is not showing signs may remain in this inapparent carrier state for a prolonged period of time. Some may never become symptomatic. Corticosteroids can modulate inflammation and prolong the infection.

Systems Affected
Skin/Exocrine — Keratinized layers of the hair, nails, and skin may harbor the hyphae and spores.

Genetics N/A

Incidence/Prevalence
Diagnosis of dermatophytosis based on clinical signs and incorrectly interpreted Wood's lamp examination results in overdiagnosis of this disease. Infection rates vary widely depending on the population studied.

Geographic Distribution
Although infections are ubiquitous, a higher incidence of dermatophytosis is observed in regions with a hot and humid climate.

SIGNALMENT

Species
Dogs, cats and other mammals

Breed Predilections
In cats, infections are more commonly seen in long-haired breeds.

Mean Age and Range
Clinical signs are more commonly seen in young animals.

Predominant Sex N/A

SIGNS

Historical Findings
Lesions may begin as alopecia or poor haircoat. A history of previously confirmed infection or exposure to an infected animal or an environment such as a cattery is useful but not a consistent finding in patients with dermatophytosis.

Physical Examination Findings
Signs may range from an inapparent carrier state to alopecia which may be patchy or circular. The classic sign of circular alopecia is more common in cats but often misinterpreted in dogs. Scales, erythema, hyperpigmenta-

tion, and pruritus are variable. Paronychitis, granulomatous lesions, or kerions may also be seen. In cats, dermatophytosis should be considered as a differential diagnosis for miliary dermatitis and almost any other dermatitis. In dogs, it should be considered as a differential diagnosis for folliculitis, furunculosis, and most cases of alopecia.

CAUSES
Microsporum canis is by far the most common cause of dermatophytosis in cats. In dogs, the three most common etiologic agents include M. canis, M. gypseum, and T. mentagrophytes. The incidence of each agent varies geographically. Less common species of dermatophytes can also cause dermatophytosis.

RISK FACTORS
Immunocompromising diseases or immunosuppressive medications predispose an animal to dermatophytosis and increase the potential for a more clinically severe infection. A high population density, poor nutrition, poor management practices, and a lack of an adequate quarantine period increase the risks of infection.

DIAGNOSIS

DIFFERENTIAL DIAGNOSIS
The most common differential diagnoses for patients exhibiting classic signs of dermatophytosis include demodicosis and bacterial skin infection. The presence of epidermal collarettes is more typical of a bacterial infection while grossly enlarged follicular ostia with furunculosis are more suggestive of demodicosis. However, these characteristics are not consistently true, and concurrent bacterial or mite infections can be seen with dermatophytosis. All three diseases can cause focal hyperpigmentation. In patients with severe inflammation associated with dermatophytosis affecting the face or feet, immune-mediated skin diseases should also be considered as differential diagnoses. In cats, the differential diagnosis for miliary dermatitis and granulomatous lesions must also be considered if either of these signs are present.

CBC/BIOCHEMISTRY/URINALYSIS
Not useful for diagnosis. May help identify an underlying problem which could be a contributing factor in the development of the disease.

OTHER LABORATORY TESTS N/A

IMAGING N/A

OTHER DIAGNOSTIC PROCEDURES
• A fungal culture with macroconidia identification is the best means of confirming the diagnosis of dermatophytosis. Site selection for sample collection is extremely important. If hairs exhibit a positive apple green florescence with Wood's lamp examination, these are considered ideal candidates for culture. It is preferable to pluck hairs from the periphery of an alopecic area rather than using a ran-

dom pattern. Utilizing a sterile toothbrush to brush the hair coat of an asymptomatic animal yields better results. Dermatophyte test media changes to a red color when the pH becomes alkaline associated with protein metabolism. Most dermatophytes typically produce this color change during the early and growing phase of their culture. Saphrophytes can also produce this color change, but generally not until after they have utilized the carbohydrates in the medium and begin to use the proteins. Consequently, it is important to examine the media on a daily basis in order to gain accurate information. Microscopic examination of the macroconidia formed by the growing fungus is necessary to confirm the presence of a pathogenic dermatophyte and to identify the genus and species. This information is helpful when trying to identify the source of infection. • Microscopic examination of hair after using a clearing solution can help provide a more rapid diagnosis. However, this process is time consuming and often produces false-negative results. Use of hairs that fluoresce under Wood's lamp illumination increases the likelihood of identifying the fungal hyphae associated with the hair shaft. Wood's lamp examinations are not very useful as a screening tool. Many pathogenic dermatophytes do not fluoresce and false fluorescence is common. The Wood's lamp should "warm up" for a minimum of 5 minutes and then be exposed to suspicious lesions for up to 5 minutes. A true positive reaction associated withe M. canis consists of apple green florescence affecting the hair shaft. Keratin associated with epidermal scales and sebum will often produce a false-positive fluorescence. • A skin biopsy is not usually needed but can be helpful in confirming true invasion and infection. A positive culture indicates that a dermatophyte was present, but it may only have been transiently present on the surface of the haircoat. This situation is more common when the culture is obtained from the feet which are more likely to come in contact with a geophilic dermatophyte.

GROSS AND HISTOPATHOLOGIC FINDINGS
The most common histopathologic finding is some degree of folliculitis, perifolliculitis, or furunculosis. However, hyperkeratosis, intraepidermal pustules, and pyogranulomatous reaction pattern may be observed. Fungal hyphae may be observed in H & E stained sections, but special stains allow the organism to be more easily visualized.

TREATMENT

INPATIENT VERSUS OUTPATIENT
Most animals are treated as outpatients but due to the infective and zoonotic nature of the disease, quarantine procedures should be considered.

ACTIVITY

Within the limits of quarantine, physical activity can remain as normal as possible.

DIET

Depending on the drug used, the diet should remain normal. If Griseofulvin PO is used as treatment, a fatty meal improves absorption.

CLIENT EDUCATION

• Many dogs and short-haired cats in a single cat environment will undergo spontaneous remission. The treatment of dermatophytosis can be both frustrating and expensive, especially in multianimal households or recurrent cases. Environmental treatment, including fomites, is not pursued as often as it probably should be, especially in recurrent cases.

• Studies by Moriello and DeBoer have shown that dilute bleach (1:10) is a practical and relatively effective means of providing environmental decontamination. Concentrated bleach and formalin (1%) are more effective at killing spores, but their use is not as practical in many situations. Chlorhexidine was ineffective in pilot studies.

• In a multianimal environment or cattery situation, treatment and control of this disease can be very complicated. The option of referral to a veterinarian with expertise in dealing with this type of situation should be discussed with the client. Several excellent discussions concerning this topic are listed in the reference list.

MEDICATIONS

DRUGS AND FLUIDS

• Griseofulvin is the most widely prescribed systemic drug for the treatment of dermatophytosis. The dose for microsized formulations is 25-60 mg/kg q12h for 4-6 weeks and the dose for the ultramicrosized formulation is 2.5-5.0 mg/kg q12h-q24h. Griseofulvin pediatric suspension is available and the recommended dose is 20-50 mg/kg divided twice per day. Griseofulvin's absorption is enhanced by dividing the dose twice per day or giving it with a fatty meal. Gastrointestinal upset is the most likely side effect. This can be alleviated by reducing the dose or dividing the dose for more frequent administration. Bone marrow suppression (anemia, pancytopenia, and neutropenia) can also occur as an idiosyncratic reaction or with prolonged therapy. Neutropenia is the most common fatal reaction in cats and can persist after discontinuation of the drug. Weekly or biweekly CBC is recommended. Cats with feline immunodeficiency virus (FIV) infections should not receive griseofulvin due to the likelihood of a life-threatening neutropenia. Neurologic side effects have also been reported. This drug should not be used during the first two trimesters of pregnancy because it is teratogenic.

• Ketoconazole has also shown to be effective in the treatment of dermatophytosis. It is not labeled for use in dogs or cats in the United

States. The dose is 10 mg/kg q24h or divided twice per day for 3-4 weeks. Anorexia is the most common side effect. Hepatopathy has also been reported and can be quite severe. Ketoconazole also inhibits endogenous production of steroidal hormones.

• Itraconazole is similar to ketoconazole, but has fewer side effects and is probally more effective. It is expensive and must usually be reformulated from 100-mg capsules for use in cats. The recommended dose is 10 mg/kg q24h.

• Vaccination for dermatophytosis in cats has received a great deal of publicity. However, the product literature claims are based upon clinical signs and Wood's lamp findings. Asymptomatic carriers can be frustrating to both the client and the veterinarian, as well as complicate the diagnosis and management of this disease. Studies involving dermatophyte cultures as a measure of achieving a cure or prevention of the disease are necessary to ensure true efficacy. The vaccine may be useful as adjuvant to systemic therapy in the treatment of dermatophytosis.

• Topical therapy and clipping of infected animals was once strongly advocated in treating animals with of dermatophytosis. These measures may be helpful in preventing environmental contamination, but are often associated with an initial exacerbation of signs after the procedures are initiated. Studies indicate that lime sulfur (1:16), enilconazole (bottle dilution) and miconazole shampoo were the most effective agents. Lime sulfur is odiferous and can stain, Enilconazole is not available in the United States.

CONTRAINDICATIONS

Corticosteroids are contraindicated in patients with this disease.

PRECAUTIONS

Use of griseofulvin should be avoided in patients infected with FIV. Testing all feline patients for FIV prior to initiating griseofulvin therapy should be performed. Periodic CBC should also be considered because fatal bone marrow suppression can occur in FIV negative animals. Teratogenicity is also a factor with this drug. The hepatotoxicity associated with ketoconazole appears to be idiosyncratic.

POSSIBLE INTERACTIONS N/A

ALTERNATE DRUGS

Therapeutic recommendations and drugs utilized to treat dermatophytosis are evolving. Several new drugs are on the horizon and may alter the current treatment recommendations.

FOLLOW-UP

PATIENT MONITORING

Dermatophyte culture is the only means of truly monitoring response to therapy. Many animals will clinically improve, but remain culture positive. It is advisable to repeat fungal cultures toward the end of the treatment regimen and continue treatment until at least

one culture result is negative. In resistant cases, the culture may be repeated on a weekly basis utilizing the toothbrush technique and the treatment continued until 2-3 consecutive negative results are obtained.

PREVENTION/AVOIDANCE

The use of a quarantine period and dermatophyte cultures of all animals entering the household is necessary to prevent reinfection from other animals. The possibility of rodents aiding in the spread of the disease should be considered. If a geophillic dermatophyte was involved, avoidance of the infective soil environment is necessary. Prophylactic treatment of exposed animals with griseofulvin for 10-14 days can be utilized.

POSSIBLE COMPLICATIONS

Falsely negative dermatophyte cultures complicate the management of this disease.

EXPECTED COURSE AND PROGNOSIS

Many animals will self clear a dermatophyte infection over a period of a few months. Treatment for the disease hastens clinical cure and helps reduce environmental contamination. Some infections, particularly in long-haired cats or multianimal situations, can be very persistent.

MISCELLANEOUS

ASSOCIATED CONDITIONS N/A

AGE RELATED FACTORS N/A

ZOONOTIC POTENTIAL

Dermatophytosis is a zoonotic disease.

PREGNANCY

The reproductive state of the female patient is important to consider when griseofulvin therapy is being considered. Ketoconazole can affect steroidal hormone, especially testosterone synthesis.

SYNONYMS Ringworm

SEE ALSO N/A

ABBREVIATIONS

FIV = feline immunodeficiency virus

References

Moriello KA, DeBoer DJ. Dermatophytosis. In: August JR, ed. Consultations in feline internal medicine 2. Philadelphia: WB Saunders, 1994;219-225.

Veterinary Dermatology. CE Griffin, KW Kwochka, JM MacDonald, eds. St. Louis: Mosby Year Book, 1993;22-33.

Scott DW, Miller WH, Griffin CE. Muller and Kirk's small animal dermatology. 5th ed. Philadelphia: WB Saunders, 1995;332-350.

Author W. Dunbar Gram
Consulting Editor Lowell Ackerman

DERMATOSES, GROWTH HORMONE

BASICS

OVERVIEW
• Uncommon dermatoses resulting from a growth hormone deficiency, or dermatoses responding to growth hormone therapy.
• Pituitary dwarfism is due to a primary growth hormone deficiency. • Adult-onset growth hormone-responsive dermatosis is defined as a clinical syndrome that responds to growth hormone therapy; and patients may or may not be strictly growth hormone deficient.

SIGNALMENT
• Pituitary dwarfism is most commonly seen in the German shepherd dog, but also reported in the spitz, toy pinscher, and Carnelian bear dog. Noted at 2-3 months of age. • Adult-onset growth hormone-responsive dermatosis is reported in the chow chow, pomeranian, poodle, keeshond, samoyed, and American water spaniel. Generally patients are 1-2 years of age, and primarily males; although the disease is reported in adults of both sexes (neutered and intact) and of all ages.

SIGNS

Pituitary Dwarfism
• Dogs appear normal at birth, but by 2-3 months bilaterally symmetrical alopecia begins to be apparent; with trunk, neck and caudal thighs severely affected. • Primary hair growth present over face and distal extremities only. Retained puppy coat is easily-epilated. • Skin is thin, hypotonic, scaly, hyperpigmented, and comedones present.

Adult-Onset Growth Hormone Responsive Dermatosis
• Alopecia is bilaterally symmetrical and involves the trunk, neck, caudomedial thighs, tail, ventral abdomen, perineum, and pinnae; while the head and legs are spared. • Primary hairs are lost first, with subsequent loss of secondary hairs in the affected areas. Hair readily epilated, with tufts of regrowth at trauma or biopsy sites. • Skin is thin and hyperpigmented. Secondary seborrhea and pyoderma are uncommon

CAUSES AND RISK FACTORS
• Pituitary Dwarfism is mediated by an autosomal recessive trait, which results in a developmental abnormality of the pituitary and lack of growth hormone production. • The cause of adult-onset growth hormone-responsive dermatosis is unknown, though breed predisposition suggests a hereditary influence; pituitary neoplasia has also been suggested as a cause • An absolute growth hormone deficiency may be present. It may also be that there are multiple causes which demonstrate a similar clinical syndrome and respond to growth hormone supplementation (i.e. castration-responsive dermatosis, insufficient adrenal 21-hydroxylase resulting in androgen accumulation, and others).

DIAGNOSIS

DIFFERENTIAL DIAGNOSIS
• Pituitary dwarfism: hypothyroidism, malnutrition, and metabolic disorders. • Adult-onset growth hormone responsive dermatosis: hypothyroidism, hyperadrenocorticism, castration-responsive dermatosis, estrogen/testosterone responsive dermatosis, follicular dysplasia, and adrenal enzyme (21-hydroxylase) deficiency.

CBC/BIOCHEMISTRY/URINALYSIS
Routine laboratory evaluation usually unremarkable.

OTHER LABORATORY TESTS
• Growth hormone stimulation testing: administer clonidine 10 μg/kg or xylazine 100-300 μg/kg IV, collecting serum prior to testing, and at 15, 30, 45, 60 and 90 minutes after stimulation. Little stimulation is noted in patients affected by pituitary dwarfism and by adult-onset growth hormone-responsive dermatosis. It is critical that hyperadrenocorticism, hypothyroidism, and sex hormone abnormalities (especially castration-responsive dermatosis and adrenal 21-hydroxylase deficiency) be ruled out before this test is performed because these conditions can inhibit release of growth hormone. Assay for growth hormone not now available. • Somatomedin C (insulin-like growth factor-1) is growth hormone dependent. Concentrations parallel body size, and their release may be impaired by glucocorticoids and estrogens. As an indirect assay of growth hormone levels, they are expected to be low in growth hormone deficient states. • Pituitary dwarfs also demonstrate low thyroid stimulating hormone (TSH), adrenocorticotropin (ACTH), gonadotropin releasing hormone (GnRH), and human chorionic gonadotropin (HCG) response test results. • Insulin response test may aid diagnosis but cause severe hypoglycemia. • Adrenal reproductive hormone test

IMAGING N/A

OTHER DIAGNOSTIC PROCEDURES
• Skin biopsy findings are compatible with general endocrinopathy: orthokeratotic hyperkeratosis; epidermal atrophy; follicular keratosis, dilation, and atrophy; telogenization of hair follicles; atrophy of sebaceous glands. Amounts and sizes of dermal elastin fibers are small. • In dogs with castration-responsive or growth hormone-responsive dermatoses, hypereosinophilic tricholemmal keratinization of hair follicles ("flame follicles") is present.

TREATMENT
• Treat as out-patient with monitoring at recheck visits.

MEDICATIONS

DRUGS AND FLUIDS
Bovine, porcine, or synthetic human growth hormone: 0.1 IU/kg SQ three times per week for 4-6 weeks; may repeat if no response.

CONTRAINDICATIONS/POSSIBLE INTERACTIONS
• Neuter intact males to rule out castration-responsive dermatosis. Sometimes, intact male dogs with low growth hormone response to xylazine will respond to castration as the only therapy.

FOLLOW-UP

PATIENT MONITORING
Blood glucose determination prior to each growth hormone treatment.

PREVENTION/AVOIDANCE N/A

POSSIBLE COMPLICATIONS
Growth hormone therapy can result in diabetes mellitus (transient or permanent) since growth hormone is diabetogenic.

EXPECTED COURSE AND PROGNOSIS
• Pituitary Dwarfism: hair regrowth will begin within 4-8 weeks of beginning therapy, and will last for 6 months to 2 years; retreatment usually necessary. • Adult Onset Growth Hormone Responsive Dermatosis: following growth hormone therapy, hair regrowth is usually observed in 2-12 weeks, and lasts from 6 months to 3 years. Retreatment is possible. • Signs are confined to skin, so treatment is not mandatory; owners may decline therapy based on possible side effects of treatment.

MISCELLANEOUS

Reference
Schmeitzel LP. Sex hormone-related and growth hormone-related alopecias. Vet Clin North Am Small Anim Pract 1990;20: 1579-1601.
Author Margaret S. Swartout
Consulting Editor Lowell Ackerman

DERMATOSES, NUTRITIONALLY RESPONSIVE

BASICS

DEFINITION
• Nutritionally-responsive dermatoses represent a diverse group of disorders in which clinical signs improve following specific supplementation. • These conditions do not necessarily represent deficiency syndromes. Various nutrients have been shown to exert pharmacologic properties distinct from their nutritional status. • The nutrients that have been best studied in this regard are vitamin A, zinc, vitamin E, fatty acids, and enzymes.

Pathophysiology
• Most beneficial nutrients exert their effects on the immune system or directly on the skin. • Zinc is a cofactor in many enzyme systems, is essential for DNA/RNA polymerase, stabilizes cells and lysosomes and is involved in several immune mechanisms. • Vitamin A has a normalizing effect on keratinization, suppresses sebaceous gland secretion, modulates immune response and alters prostaglandin synthesis. • Vitamin E is a natural antioxidant and mild antagonist of leukotriene formation. • Eicosapentaenoic acid, an omega-3-fatty acid, competes for enzymes (5-lipoxygenase and 15-lipoxygenase) with arachidonic acid, inhibits inflammatory leukotrienes (LTB4), limits production of pro-inflammatory prostaglandins (PGE2) and inhibits the cyclooxygenase pathway. • Gamma-linolenic acid, an omega-6 fatty acid, competes for enzymes with arachidonic acid, decreases levels of inflammatory eicosanoids, increases anti-inflammatory eicosanoids (PGE1, 15-HETrE), blocks pro-inflammatory leukotrienes (LTB4) and inhibits release of arachidonic acid. • Certain enzyme supplements containing phytase and proteases such as bromelain and papain seem to increase circulating levels of zinc, selenium, and cis-linoleic acid.

Systems Affected
• Skin / exocrine • Beneficial effects sometimes extend to the oral cavity, gastrointestinal tract, cardiovascular system, and musculoskeletal system.

Genetics N/A

SIGNALMENT
• Vitamin A-responsive dermatosis most commonly first appears in dogs less than 3 years of age. Breed predisposition for cocker spaniels, Labrador retrievers, miniature schnauzers, and Chinese shar-peis. No sex predilection. • Zinc-responsive dermatosis most commonly first appears in dogs less than 3 years of age. Breed predisposition for Siberian huskies, Alaskan malamutes, doberman pinschers, and great Danes. No sex predilection. • No age, breed, or sex predisposition for conditions that might benefit from supplementation with fatty acids although most commonly used for inhalant allergies in dogs and cats, keratinization disorders in dogs, and eosinophilic granuloma complex in cats. • No age, breed or sex predisposition for conditions that might benefit from vitamin E supplementation although most commonly used for demodicosis, lupus erythematosus and dermatomyositis. • No age, breed or sex predisposition for conditions that might benefit from enzyme supplementation although most commonly used for keratinization disorders.

SIGNS
• Zinc-responsive dermatosis appears as a primary keratinization disorder affecting the face, footpads, elbows, and hocks. Tenacious crusts evident. • Vitamin A-responsive dermatosis is also a keratinization disorder but the crusting has a follicular orientation. Appears as multifocal proliferative crusts; usually involves face, back and ventrum. • No consistent clinical signs for conditions that respond to vitamin E, fatty acids or enzymes. See descriptions for individual conditions.

CAUSES
• Vitamin A affects cells on a molecular level. The synthetic retinoids act similarly but with more profound effects and less toxicity. • Zinc absorption can be reduced by high-fiber diets and supplements that include calcium, iron, tin, and copper. In addition, an inherited malabsorptive defect has been documented in Siberian huskies. • Vitamin E requirements are increased when antioxidant activity is required and when the diet is rich in polyunsaturated fatty acids. • Omega-3 and omega-6 fatty acids may be required when animals have enzyme deficits, the diet is deficient in precursors, or when conditions result in imbalance of the arachidonic acid cascade. Skin lacks desaturase enzymes and can't convert cis-linoleic and alpha-linolenic acids to their active forms; requires preformed, polyunsaturated fatty acids. • Enzyme supplements of phytase and protease likely work by liberating nutrients trapped in dietary fiber.

RISK FACTORS
Zinc-responsive dermatosis predisposed in animal fed high-cereal diets or oversupplemented with calcium.

DIAGNOSIS

DIFFERENTIAL DIAGNOSIS
• Vitamin A-responsive dermatosis: bacterial pyoderma, demodicosis, dermatophytosis, adverse food reactions, and other keratinization disorders. • Zinc-responsive dermatosis: pemphigus erythematosus, pemphigus foliaceus, lupus erythematosus, demodicosis, dermatophytosis, dermatomyositis, pyoderma, demodicosis, other keratinization disorders.

CBC/BIOCHEMISTRY/URINALYSIS
Routine hematology and biochemistry usually normal or negative.

OTHER LABORATORY TESTS N/A

IMAGING N/A

OTHER DIAGNOSTIC PROCEDURES
Biopsies for histopathology most useful test to determine underlying cause.

TREATMENT

• Nutritionally-responsive dermatoses invariably treated on an outpatient basis. • Diet modification or supplementation is the basis of treatment. • Zinc supplementation has been used for treatment of the following: Zinc-responsive dermatosis; Zinc deficiency; any chronic degenerative process; to encourage wound healing; to encourage immune responsiveness. • Vitamin A supplementation has been used to treat vitamin A-responsive dermatosis and other keratinization disorders, certain ophthalmic disorders and some malabsorptive disorders. • Vitamin E has been used as adjunctive treatment for lupus erythematosus, demodicosis, acanthosis nigricans, steatitis and for poor wound healing. • Omega-3 and Omega-6 fatty acid supplements have been used as adjunctive treatments for inhalant allergies, eosinophilic granuloma complex, keratinization disorders, hyperlipidemia and some forms of arthritis. • Enzyme supplements are typically used for keratinization disorders, some alopecic conditions and some forms of arthritis.

MEDICATIONS

DRUGS AND FLUIDS
Zinc sulfate 10 mg/kg q24h or divided q12h PO with food; or Zinc Methionine 2 mg/kg q24h PO. • Vitamin A dosage: 500-1,000 IU/kg q24h-q12h • Vitamin E dosage: 20 IU/KG q12h-q8h • Follow label recommendations when using fatty acids and enzyme supplements.

CONTRAINDICATIONS N/A

PRECAUTIONS
• Fatty acids should be used cautiously in animals with pancreatitis or malabsorptive disorders. • Vitamin A should be used cautiously in animals with KCS or liver disease.

POSSIBLE INTERACTIONS
• Excessive fatty acid suppplementation increases vitamin E requirements. • Excessive zinc supplementation decreases absorption of copper, iron and tin.

ALTERNATE DRUGS

Synthetic retinoids such as etretinate, isotretinoin and etretin are sometimes used in place of high doses of vitamin A.

FOLLOW-UP

PATIENT MONITORING

• Zinc: watch for vomiting, diarrhea and other gastrointestinal upset. • Vitamin A: CBC, biochemical profile, lipid profile, urinalysis, Schirmer tear test - initially monthly, then q3-6 months. • Vitamin E: coagulation profile q6 months. • Enzymes: watch for vomiting, diarrhea and other gastrointestinal upset.

POSSIBLE COMPLICATIONS

• Vitamin A overdose can cause conjunctivitis, hypertriglyceridemia, hypercholesterolemia, bone pain and serum elevations of ALT. • Zinc overdose can cause gastrointestinal upset. • Possible side effect with vitamin E toxicity is decreased coagulability of blood. • Enzyme overdose can cause gastrointestinal upset.

MISCELLANEOUS

ASSOCIATED CONDITIONS N/A

AGE RELATED FACTORS N/A

ZOONOTIC POTENTIAL N/A

PREGNANCY

Vitamin A and all the retinoids are teratogenic and should not be used in pregnant animals.

SYNONYMS N/A

SEE ALSO

• Exfoliative Skin Disorders • Nasal Dermatoses • Atopy

ABBREVIATIONS

ALT = alanine aminotransferase
KCS = keratoconjunctivitis sicca

References

Ackerman L, Enzyme therapy in veterinary practice. Adv Nutr 1993;1:9-11.

Codner EC, Thatcher CD. Nutritional management of skin disease. Compend Contin Educ Pract Vet 1993;15:411-423.

Kwochka KW. Retinoids and vitamin A therapy. In: Griffin CE, Kwochka KW, MacDonald JM, eds. Current veterinary dermatology. St. Louis: Mosby Year Book, 1993;203-214.

Author Lowell Ackerman
Consulting Editor Lowell Ackerman

DERMATOSES, SEX HORMONE

BASICS

OVERVIEW
Uncommon alopecias and dermatoses suspected to result from an imbalance of sex hormones; often defined on the basis of response to sex hormone therapy.

SIGNALMENT
See causes and risk factors

SIGNS
• Alopecia initially involves the perineum, ventrum, thighs, pericervical and later, the caudodorsal back, and flanks. Flank alopecia may present as the first or as the only sign in some patients with hyperestrogenism and may be seasonal in some spayed females.
• Fur may be soft or dry and brittle.
• Often nipples, mammary glands, vulva, and prepuce, testicles, ovaries, and prostate have associated abnormalities. • Variable secondary seborrhea, pruritus, pyoderma, comedones, ceruminous otitis externa, and hyperpigmentation. • Urinary incontinence may occur in estrogen and testosterone-responsive conditions.

CAUSES AND RISK FACTORS

Estrogen-Responsive Dermatosis of Female Dogs (Ovarian Imbalance II)
• Deficiency of sex hormones, commonly estradiol • Following ovariohysterectomy in noncycling intact females, and occasionally during pseudopregnancy • Possible inadequate production of adrenal sex hormones • Possible cutaneous defect in the sex hormone receptor/metabolism system • Dachshunds and boxers are predisposed. • Variant with cyclical flank alopecia and hyperpigmentation only: airedales, boxers, English bulldogs. Worsens in winter.

Hyperestrogenism in Female Dogs (Ovarian Imbalance I)
• Estrogen excess due to cystic ovaries, ovarian tumors (rare), or exogenous estrogen overdose. • Middle-aged and older intact female dogs.

Hyperestrogenism in Male Dogs with Testicular Tumors
• Estrogen excess (or rarely hyperprogesteronism) due to sertoli cell tumor (most common), seminoma, or interstitial cell tumor (rarely) • Intact males—usually middle-aged or older • Cryptorchidism predisposes to the formation of testicular tumors. • Boxers, shetland sheepdogs, weimaraners, German shepherd dogs, Cairn terriers, Pekingese, and collies predisposed; associated with male pseudohermaphrodism in miniature schnauzers.

Hyperandrogenism Associated with Testicular Tumors
Androgen producing testicular tumors (especially interstitial cell tumors) in intact male dog.

Idiopathic Male Feminizing Syndrome
• Cause undetermined. Serum sex hormone concentrations normal; blockage of androgen receptors in the skin may prevent attachment of testosterone. • Intact, middle-aged male dogs.

Testosterone-Responsive Dermatosis of Male Dogs
• Suspected hypoandrogenism or a possible defect in the skin sex hormone receptor system • Older males, intact males with atrophied testicles, testicular neoplasia, or asymmetrical cryptorchidism, and males castrated at a very young age.

Castration-Responsive Dermatosis
• Variably high (or low) estradiol, testosterone, or progesterone. • Intact males with normal testicles. • Onset 1-3 years.
• Predisposed breeds: chow chow, samoyed, keeshond, pomeranian, husky, malamute, and miniature poodles.

Adrenal Sex Hormone Imbalance
• Adrenal enzyme (21-hydroxylase) deficiency resulting in excessive adrenal androgen or progesterone secretion. • Males and females, intact or neutered. • Onset 1-5 years of age.
• Pomeranians predisposed.

DIAGNOSIS

DIFFERENTIAL DIAGNOSIS
• Critical to rule out hypothyroidism and hyperadrenocorticism first; note that these diseases generally cause trunkal alopecia first.
• Growth hormone responsive dermatosis
• Dachshunds—pattern baldness • Keratinization disorders • Allergic skin disease

CBC/BIOCHEMISTRY/URINALYSIS
• Routine CBC, serum biochemistries and urinalysis unremarkable. • Bone marrow hypoplasia/aplasia noted occasionally in states of estrogen excess due to testicular tumors and hyperestrogenism in female dogs.

OTHER LABORATORY TESTS
• Serum estrogen/estradiol concentrations are sometimes high (30-40% of patients) with hyperestrogenism of female dogs, hyperestrogenism in male dogs with testicular tumors, and castration-responsive dermatosis. Rarely helpful in estrogen-responsive dermatosis, because serum estradiol 17B concentrations in spayed females are similar to intact females.
• Serum testosterone and progesterone sometimes increased in animals with castration-responsive dermatosis, and occasionally in hyperestrogenism (ovarian imbalance) in female dogs • Often serum sex hormone concentrations are normal, and one must treat according to the suspected diagnosis based on clinical signs, ruling out other disorders, and response to therapy. • Combined ACTH stimulation and adrenal reproductive hormone test: administer ACTH (cosyntropin 0.5 IU/kg IV, or ACTH gel 0.22 USP

unit/kg IM), obtaining plasma and serum samples pre-injection and at 1 hour post-injection (also a 2-hour sample if ACTH gel is used). A partial deficiency of 21-hydroxylase enzyme results in accumulation of steroid precursors such as progesterone, 17-hydroxyprogesterone, androstenedione, and DHEAS, resulting in dermatosis of pomeranians and other breeds that is clinically similar to growth hormone responsive dermatosis.
• Gonadotropin-releasing hormone (GnRH; cystorelin) response test is used to demonstrate response of gonads to stimulation, and is especially useful when basal hormones are normal. Baseline serum estradiol, testosterone, and progesterone determinations are made; GnRH injected at 0.22 mg/kg IV, and serum samples obtained 1-2 hours later for analysis of the three sex hormones above. Values vary with lab.

IMAGING
Radiography, ultrasonography, and laparoscopy can be used to detect cystic ovaries, ovarian tumors, testicular tumors (scrotal and abdominal), sublumbar lymphadenopathy, and possible thoracic metastases of malignant tumors.

OTHER DIAGNOSTIC PROCEDURES
• Preputial cytology may demonstrate cornification of cells (similar to bitch in estrus) in advanced patients with testicular feminizing tumors. • Skin biopsies reflects general endocrinopathy findings (see above) in all syndromes (exception is hyperandrogenism due to testicular tumors). Perivascular dermatitis may be noted in pruritic animals (male feminizing syndrome, hyperestrogenism of female dogs). Sebaceous glands relatively spared in estrogen-responsive dermatosis of female dogs and in testosterone-responsive dermatosis of male dogs. Castration-responsive dermatosis may demonstrate hypereosinophilic tricholemmal keratinization of hair follicles ("flame follicles").

TREATMENT
• Exploratory laparotomy can diagnose and be a means of treatment (i.e. ovariohysterectomy or castration) for ovarian cysts and tumors and abdominal testicular tumors.
• Castration for castration-responsive dermatosis and for scrotal testicular tumors.
• Discontinuation of excessive exogenous estrogen administration.

MEDICATIONS

DRUGS AND FLUIDS

Estrogen-Responsive Dermatosis
• For spayed females: DES 0.02 mg/kg (max = 1 mg) PO q24h for 14-21 days, stop for one week, repeat cycle till hair regrowth, then

give 2-3 times weekly to maintain hair coat. Occurrence of estrus indicates discontinuation until estrus subsides, then continuation of maintenance dose. If treatment fails, try testosterone or milbolerone.

• For intact females: DES 5 mg PO q24h till bloody discharge. If no response after 7 days, double the dose; give until proestrus day 2 (maximum 14 days total) until sanguineous vaginal discharge and vulvar edema noted and for 2 days following, then LH 5 mg IM on day 5 of proestrus; then FSH on day 9 and day 11 of proestrus.

• Alternative treatment: FSH at 0.75 mg/kg/day IM till signs of estrus appear.

• For testosterone-responsive dermatosis of male dogs, and for some estrogen-responsive dermatoses of female dogs: methyltestosterone 0.5-1.0 mg/kg (max=30 mg) PO q48h until response (takes 1-3 months), with maintenance 2-3 times/week once regrowth of hair is completed. Repositol testosterone 2 mg/kg IM (max=30 mg) q1-4 months as needed to maintain normal hair coat.

• Hyperestrogenism of female dogs: GnRH or HCG are alternative treatments.

• Adrenal 21-hydroxylase enzyme deficiency: lysodren (o,p'-DDD) is used if adrenal sex hormones are high, beginning dose of 15-25 mg/kg PO q24h for 7 days, then using a maintenance dose of 15-25 mg/kg PO q5-14 days as maintenance.

• Maintenance doses titrated to maintain post ACTH-stimulation cortisol within the baseline range. • Topical antiseborrheic therapy for conditions with associated flakiness.

• For pruritus, (assuming infections and bone marrow suppression have been ruled out), prednisone may be administered 0.5 mg/kg

PO q12h 5-7 days, 0.5 mg q24h 5-7 days, the 0.5 mg/kg q48h for 7 days.

CONTRAINDICATIONS/POSSIBLE INTERACTIONS N/A

FOLLOW-UP

PATIENT MONITORING

• DES supplementation: monitor CBC for bone marrow hypoplasia/aplasia every 2 weeks for the first month, then every 3-6 months thereafter. • Testosterone supplementation: monitor serum biochemistry with an emphasis on liver enzymes every 3-4 weeks for the first 1-3 months then every 4-6 months. • Lysodren therapy indicates electrolyte monitoring with ACTH stimulation testing every 3 months.

POSSIBLE COMPLICATIONS

• Estrogen therapy can uncommonly result in bone marrow hypoplasia/aplasia. It can rarely result in signs of estrus. • Cholangiohepatitis (rare), behavior changes (uncommon), and seborrhea oleosa have been associated with methyltestosterone administration. • Lysodren therapy can be associated with potential toxicities: vomiting, diarrhea, collapse, and iatrogenic hypoadrenocorticism.

EXPECTED COURSE AND PROGNOSIS

• With estrogen responsive dermatosis, regrowth of hair may take about 3 months; it may be transient. • Following OVH for female hyperestrogenism, improvement should occur within 3-6 months. • Following castration for estrogen-secreting testicular tumors,

regrowth of hair may be noted in 3-6 weeks. Resolution of signs noted within 3-6 months of castration for both estrogen and androgen secreting tumors. Note that bone marrow aplasia associated with hyperestrogenism usually does not respond to castration, and the prognosis for recovery is grave. Relapse of signs following a positive response after castration of a malignant testicular tumor can indicate metastases; if confirmed, the prognosis is poor. • Following castration for castration-responsive dermatosis, response is observed in 2-3 months. • Testosterone therapy may result in hair regrowth in 4-12 weeks.

MISCELLANEOUS

Do not breed cryptorchid animals; neuter cryptorchid animals when young.

ABBREVIATIONS

ACTH = adrenocorticotropin
DES = diethylstilbestrol
DHEAS = dehydroepiandrosterone sulfate
FSH = follicle stimulating hormone
GnRH = gonadotropin releasing hormone
HCG = human chorionic gonadotropin
LH = luteinizing hormone
TSH = thyrotropin

Reference

Schmeitzel LP: Sex hormone-related and growth hormone-related alopecias. Vet Clin North Am (Small Anim Pract) 1990;20: 1579-1601.

Author Margaret S. Swartout
Consulting Editor Lowell Ackerman

DIABETES INSIPIDUS

BASICS

DEFINITION
Disorder of water balance characterized by polyuria, urine of low specific gravity or osmolality, and polydipsia

Pathophysiology
• Central diabetes insipidus—deficiency in the secretion of antidiuretic hormone (ADH) • Nephrogenic diabetes insipidus—renal insensitivity to ADH

Systems Affected:
• Endocrine/Metabolic • Renal/Urologic

Genetics N/A

Incidence/Prevalence
• Central diabetes insipidus—rare • Nephrogenic diabetes insipidus—rare

Geographic Distribution N/A

SIGNALMENT

Species Dogs and cats

Breed Predilection
None

Mean Age and Range
• Congenital forms of central and nephrogenic diabetes insipidus, < 1 year • Acquired forms of central diabetes insipidus (e.g., neoplastic, traumatic, and idiopathic)—any age

Predominant Sex None

SIGNS
• Polyuria • Polydipsia • Incontinence (occasional)

CAUSES

Inadequate Secretion Of ADH
• Congenital defect • Idiopathic cause • Trauma • Pituitary gland neoplasia

Renal Insensitivity to ADH
• Congenital defect • Secondary to drugs (e.g., lithium, demeclocycline, and methoxyfluorane) • Secondary to endocrine and metabolic disorders (e.g., hyperadrenocorticism, hypokalemia, pyometra, and hypercalcemia)

RISK FACTORS N/A

DIAGNOSIS

DIFFERENTIAL DIAGNOSIS

Polyuric Disorders
• Hyperadrenocorticism • Diabetes mellitus • Hypercalcemia • Pyometra • Renal failure • Liver disease • Pyelonephritis • Hyperthyroidism (cats) • Psychogenic polydipsia

CBC/BIOCHEMISTRY/URINALYSIS
• Results usually normal hypernatremia in some patients • Urine specific gravity low (usually < 1.012 and often < 1.008)

OTHER LABORATORY TESTS
•Plasma ADH concentration (not routinely performed)

Imaging
MRI or CT scan if a pituitary tumor is suspected

Other Diagnostic Procedures
• Modified water deprivation test (see appendix for protocol) • ADH trial—therapeutic trial with synthetic ADH product (DDAVP®); a positive response (water intake decreases by 50% in 3-5 days) is diagnostic for central diabetes insipidus. Note: all other causes of polyuria and polydipsia (PU/PD)should be ruled out before conducting an ADH trial

GROSS AND HISTOPATHOLOGIC FINDINGS
Degeneration and death of neurosecretory neurons in the neurohypophysis patients.

TREATMENT

INPATIENT VERSUS OUTPATIENT
Patients should be hospitalized for the modified water deprivation test, whereas the ADH trial is often performed as an outpatient procedure.

ACTIVITY Not restricted

DIET
Normal with free access to water

CLIENT EDUCATION
• Review dosage of DDAVP and administration technique • Importance of access to water at all times

SURGICAL CONSIDERATIONS N/A

MEDICATIONS

DRUGS OF CHOICE
• Central diabetes insipidus—DDAVP.(1-2 drops of the intranasal preparation in the conjunctival sac q12h-q24h to control polyuria and polydipsia). Alternatively, the intranasal preparation may be given subcutaneously (2 to 5 mcg q12h-q24h).
• Nephrogenic diabetes insipidus—chlorothiazide (10-40 mg/kg PO q12h)

CONTRAINDICATIONS None

PRECAUTIONS
Overdose of DDAVP can cause water intoxication in patients with excessive water intake.

ALTERNATIVE DRUGS
Chlorpropamide (Diabinese; 125-250 mg/day may reduce PU/PD)

FOLLOW-UP

PATIENT MONITORING
• Treatment adjusted according to the patient's signs. The ideal dosage and frequency of DDAVP administration is based on water intake. •Laboratory tests such as PCV, total solids, and serum sodium concentration to detect dehydration (inadequate DDAVP replacement); usually not necessary.

PREVENTION/AVOIDANCE
Circumstances that might cause marked increase in water loss

POSSIBLE COMPLICATIONS
Complications of primary disease (pituitary tumor) should be anticipated

EXPECTED COURSE AND PROGNOSIS
• The condition is usually permanant, exept in rare patients in which the condition was trauma induced • In general, the prognosis is good depending on the underlying disorder.
• Without treatment, dehydration can lead to stupor, coma, and death

MISCELLANEOUS

ASSOCIATED CONDITIONS N/A

AGE RELATED FACTORS
• Congenital central and nephrogenic diabetes insipidus is usually manifest before 6 months of age. • Central diabetes insipidus related to pituitary tumors is usually seen in dogs > 5 years old.

PREGNANCY N/A

SYNONYMS
• Central diabetes insipidus • Cranial diabetes insipidus • Neurogenic diabetes insipidus • ADH responsive diabetes insipidus

SEE ALSO
Hyposthenuria

ABBREVIATIONS
ADH = antidiuretic hormone
CT = computed tomography
DDAVP = brand name of desmopressin
MRI = magnetic resonance imaging
PCV = packed cell volume
PU/PD = polyuria/polydipsia

Reference
Feldman EC, Nelson RW. Canine and feline endocrinology and reproduction. Philadelphia: WB Saunders, 1987
Author Rhett Nichols
Consulting Editor Rhett Nichols

DIABETES MELLITUS, KETOACIDOTIC

BASICS

DEFINITION
A true medical emergency secondary to absolute or relative insulin deficiency characterized by hyperglycemia, ketonemia, metabolic acidosis, dehydration, and electrolyte depletion

Pathophysiology
• Insulin deficiency causes an increase in lipolysis, which results in excessive ketone body production and acidosis. An inability to maintain fluid and electrolyte homeostasis causes dehydration, prerenal azotemia, electrolyte disorders, obtundation, and death.
• Many diabetic ketoacidosis patients have underlying conditions such as infection, inflammation, or heart disease that cause stress hormone (e.g., glucagon, cortisol, growth hormone, and epinephrine) secretion, and this probably contributes to the development of diabetic ketoacidosis.

Systems Affected
Endocrine/metabolic

Genetics N/A

Incidence/Prevalence Unknown

Geopgraphic Distribution N/A

Breed Predilections
• Dogs—miniature poodle and dachshund
• Cats—none

Mean Age and Range
• Dogs—mean age, 8.4 years • Cats—median age, 11 years (range, 1-19 years)

Predominant Sex
• Dogs—females 1.5 times > males • Cats—males 2 times > females

SIGNS
• Polyuria • Polydipsia • Diminished activity • Anorexia • Weakness • Vomiting • Lethargy and depression • Muscle wasting • Unkempt haircoat • Dehydration • Thin body condition • Hypothermia • Dandruff • Thickened bowel loops • Hepatomegaly

CAUSES
• Insulin dependent diabetes mellitus
• Infection (e.g., skin, respiratory, urinary tract, and prostate gland) • Concurrent disease (e.g., heart failure, renal failure, and pancreatitis) • Idiopathic • Medication noncompliance • Stress • Surgery

RISK FACTORS
• Any condition that leads to an absolute or relative insulin deficiency • History of corticosteroid or beta-blocker administration

DIAGNOSIS

DIFFERENTIAL DIAGNOSIS
• Hyperosmolar nonketotic coma • Acute hypoglycemic coma • Uremia • Lactic acidosis

CBC/BIOCHEMISTRY/URINALYSIS
• Leukocytosis with mature neutrophilia
• Hyperglycemia (blood glucose usually > 250 mg/dl) • High liver enzyme activity
• Hypercholesterolemia • Azotemia • Hypochloremia • Hypokalemia • Hyponatremia
• Hypophosphatemia • High anion gap—anion gap = (sodium + potassium) - (chloride + bicarbonate); normal is 16 +/- 4 • Glucosuria and ketonuria • Variable urine specific gravity with active or inactive sediment

OTHER LABORATORY TESTS
• Metabolic acidosis (venous TCO_2 < 15 mEq/L) caused by ketosis • Hyperosmolarity
• Bacterial culture of urine and blood

IMAGING N/A

OTHER DIAGNOSTIC PROCEDURES
ECG may help evaluate potassium status; prolonged Q-T interval in some patients with hypokalemia; tall tented T waves in some patients with hyperkalemia

GROSS AND HISTOPATHOLOGIC FINDINGS
Pancreatic islet cell atrophy

TREATMENT

INPATIENT VERSUS OUTPATIENT
• If the animal is bright, alert, and well-hydrated, intensive care and intravenous fluid administration is not required. Start subcutaneous administration of insulin (short- or intermediate-acting insulin), offer food and supply constant access to water, monitor closely for signs of illness (e.g., anorexia, lethargy, vomiting).
• Treatment of "sick" diabetic ketoacidotic dog or cat requires inpatient intensive care. This is a life-threatening emergency. Goals are to correct the depletion of water and electrolytes, reverse ketonemia and acidosis, and increase the rate of glucose utilization by insulin-dependent tissues.

ACTIVITY N/A

DIET
A low fat, high fiber, high complex carbohydrates diet recommended once the patient is stabilized

CLIENT EDUCATION
Serious medical condition requiring lifelong insulin administration in most patients

SURGICAL CONSIDERATIONS N/A

MEDICATIONS

DRUGS AND FLUIDS

Fluids
• Necessary to ensure adequate cardiac output and tissue perfusion and to maintain vascular volume; also reduces blood glucose concentration

• IV administration of 0.9% saline supplemented with potassium is the initial fluid of choice.
• Volume determined by dehydration deficit plus maintenance requirements. Replace over 24-48 hours

Insulin
• Necessary to inhibit lipolysis, inhibit hepatic gluconeogenesis, and promote peripheral glucose uptake
• Regular insulin is the insulin of choice
• Initial dosage—0.2 U/kg IM (or SC if hydration is normal)
• Subsequent dosage—0.1-0.2 U/kg given 3-6 hours later (may be given hourly if patient is closely monitored); response to previous insulin dosage should be considered when calculating subsequent dosages. Ideally, glucose concentration should drop to 50-100 mg/dl/h.
• Monitor blood glucose every 1-3 hours by use of Chemstrip BG reagent strips and an automated test strip analyzer (Accu-Chek III by Boehringer Mannheim).
• Monitor urine glucose and ketones daily.
• Administration of longer-acting insulin (e.g., NPH, lente, and ultralente) is initiated when the patient is eating, drinking, and no longer receiving IV fluids and ketosis is resolved or greatly diminished. The dosage is based on that for short-acting insulin given in hospital.

Potassium Supplementation
• These patients are total body potassium depleted and treatment (e.g., fluids and insulin) will further lower serum potassium; thus, potassium supplementation is always necessary.
• If possible, check potassium concentration before initiation of insulin therapy to guide supplementation dosage. If it is extremely low, insulin therapy may need to be delayed (hours) until serum potassium concentration increases.
• If potassium concentration is unknown, add potassium (40 mEq/L) to the IV fluids, obtain results of pretreatment biochemical analysis ASAP, and draw blood for follow-up biochemical analysis 24 hours after treatment is initiated.

Dextrose Supplementation
• Insulin must be given regardless of the blood glucose concentration to correct the ketoacidotic state.
• Whenever blood glucose is < 200-250 mg/dl, 50% dextrose should be added to the fluids to produce a 2.5% dextrose solution (increase to 5% dextrose if needed). Discontinue dextrose once glucose is maintained above 250 mg/dl.
• Do not stop insulin therapy!

Bicarbonate Supplementation
• Controversial. If patient's venous blood pH is < 7.0 or total CO_2 is < 11 mEq/L, consider bicarbonate administration (bicarbonate is of no benefit if the pH is > 7.0).

• Dosage—body weight (kg) x 0.3 x base deficit (base deficit = normal serum bicarbonate - patient's serum bicarbonate). *Slowly* administer one quarter to half the dosage intravenously and the remainder in fluids to be given over 3-6 hours.

• Recheck blood gas or serum TCO_2 before further supplementation.

Phosphorus Supplementation

• Pretreatment serum phosphorus usually is normal; however, treatment of ketoacidosis reduces phosphorus, and serum concentrations should be monitored every 12-24 hours once supplementation is initiated.

• Dosage—0.01-0.03 mmole/kg/hour for 6-12 hours in IV fluids (may need to increase dosage to 0.03-0.06)

CONTRAINDICATIONS

If the patient is anuric or oliguric or if potassium is > 5 mEq/L, do not supplement potassium until urine flow is established or until potassium concentration decreases.

PRECAUTIONS

Use bicarbonate with caution in patients without normal ventilation because of their inability to excrete carbon dioxide created during treatment.

POSSIBLE INTERACTIONS N/A

ALTERNATE DRUGS N/A

FOLLOW-UP

PATIENT MONITORING

• Attitude, hydration, cardiopulmonary status, urine output, and body weight • Blood sugar q1-3h initially, then q6h once stable • Electrolytes q4-8h initially, then q24h once stable • Acid-base status q8-12h initially, then q24h once stable

PREVENTION AVOIDANCE

Appropriate insulin administration

POSSIBLE COMPLICATIONS

• Hypokalemia • Hypoglycemia • Hypophosphatemia • Cerebral edema • Pulmonary edema • Renal failure • Heart failure

EXPECTED COURSE AND PROGNOSIS Guarded

MISCELLANEOUS

ASSOCIATED CONDITIONS

• Pancreatitis • Hyperadrenocorticism • Diestrus • Bacterial infection • Electrolyte depletion

AGE RELATED FACTORS N/A

ZOONOTIC POTENTIAL N/A

PREGNANCY

• Risk of fetal death may be relatively high.

• Glucose regulation is often difficult.

SYNONYMS N/A

SEE ALSO

Diabetes Mellitus—Uncomplicated

ABBREVIATIONS

None

References

Feldman EC, Nelson RW. Diabetic ketoacidosis. Canine and feline endocrinology and reproduction. 2nd ed. Philadelphia: WB Saunders, 1996.

Nichols R, Crenshaw KL. Complications and concurrent disease associated with diabetic ketoacidosis and other severe forms of diabetes mellitus. In: Bonagura JB, ed. Small animal practice current veterinary therapy XII. Philadelphia: WB Saunders, 1995.

MacIntire DK. Emergency treatment of diabetic crisis: insulin overdose, diabetic ketoacidosis and hyperosmolar coma. Vet Clin North Am Small Anim Pract 1995;25:639.

Author Kathy L. Crenshaw
Consulting Editor Rhett Nichols

DIABETES MELLITUS, NONKETOTIC HYPERMOLAR SYNDROME

BASICS

DEFINITION

Disease characterized by severe hyperglycemia, hyperosmolarity, severe dehydration, lack of urine or serum ketones, lack of or mild to moderate metabolic acidosis, and CNS depression.

Pathophysiology

• Insulin deficiency causes reduced utilization of glucose and excessive glucose production. The resultant high, extracellular blood glucose causes a hyperosmolar state with a reduction in extracellular fluid volume. Intracellular dehydration, azotemia, and uremia develop and the intracellular dehydration becomes more pronounced as the glomerular filtration rate decreases and tissue hypoxia ensues. Azotemia, hyperglycemia, and hyperosmolarity worsen as a result of glucose retention and glucose-induced osmotic diuresis.
• Although ketonemia and ketonuria usually are not features of this syndrome, anorexia (especially when prolonged) may cause mild ketoacidosis in some patients. However, high lactic acid is a major contributor to the metabolic acidosis that may develop in these patients.

Systems Affected

• Renal/urologic—prerenal and primary renal azotemia because of reduced extracellular fluid volume, reduced tissue perfusion, or diabetic glomerulonephropathy • Urine specific gravity is low because of osmotic diuresis, diabetic glomerulonephropathy, or concurrent renal insufficiency • Cardiovascular—hypotension because of low extracellular fluid volume, vascular collapse, and depressed myocardial contractility • Nervous—depression, disorientation or mental confusion, seizures, and coma are caused by intracellular dehydration and hyperosmolarity. CNS dysfunction worsens as serum osmolarity rises.

Genetics N/A

Incidence/Prevalence Uncommon

Geographic Distribution N/A

SIGNALMENT

Species Dogs and cats

Breed Predilections N/A

Mean Age and Range

• Dogs—peak prevalence, 7-9 years old
• Cats—any age; most > 6 years old

Predominant Sex

• Dogs—female • Cats—neutered males

SIGNS

Historical Findings

• Early signs—polydipsia, polyuria, polyphagia, and weight loss • Late signs—weakness, vomiting, anorexia, depression, stupor, and coma

Physical Examination Findings

• Dehydration • Hypothermia • Prolonged capillary refill time • Cataracts • Lethargy • Depression • Seizures (severe hyperosmolarity) • Stupor or coma (severe hyperosmolarity)

CAUSES

Diabetes mellitus associated with severe hyperosmolarity, severe hyperglycemia, and severe dehydration

RISK FACTORS

• Concurrent problems such as heart disease, renal insufficiency, pneumonia, acute pancreatitis, and other severe diseases • Drugs—anticonvulsants, glucocorticoids, and thiazide diuretics may precipitate or aggravate this syndrome.

DIAGNOSIS

DIFFERENTIAL DIAGNOSIS

• Uncomplicated diagnosis mellitus—mentally alert with fasting hyperglycemia and glucosuria • Ketoacidotic diabetes mellitus—fasting hyperglycemia with glucosuria, ketonuria, and metabolic acidosis • Extreme lethargy and depression with severe hyperosmolarity, severe hyperglycemia, severe dehydration without ketonemia and ketonuria usually differentiate diabetes mellitus nonketotic hyperosmolar syndrome from uncomplicated and ketoacidotic diabetes mellitus.

CBC/BIOCHEMISTRY/URINALYSIS

• Severe hyperglycemia (usually > 600 mg/dl)
• High BUN and creatinine concentration
• Normokalemia (despite total body potassium depletion) or hypokalemia • Hyperkalemia is expected in patients with anuric or oliguric renal failure. • Low TCO_2 • High anion gap • Glucosuria • Low urine specific gravity

OTHER LABORATORY TESTS

• Severe hyperosmolarity (usually > 350 mOsm/L) • High plasma lactate concentration may help confirm metabolic lactic acidosis in the absence of ketonemia and ketonuria.

IMAGING N/A

OTHER DIAGNOSTIC PROCEDURES N/A

GROSS AND HISTOPATHOLOGIC FINDINGS

Pancreatic islet cell atrophy patients.

TREATMENT

INPATIENT VERSUS OUTPATIENT

Nonketotic hyperosmolar diabetes mellitus is a life-threatening medical emergency requiring inpatient treatment.

ACTIVITY N/A

DIET

A low fat, high fiber, high complex carbohydrates diet is recommended once the patient is stabilized.

CLIENT EDUCATION

• Poor to guarded prognosis
• Intensive care and frequent monitoring are required during hospitalization.

SURGICAL CONSIDERATION N/A

MEDICATIONS

DRUGS AND FLUIDS

Fluids

• Fluid therapy is a major component of medical management.
• Replace one half the fluid deficit in the first 12 hours and the remainder during the next 24 hours.
• IV administration of normal saline (0.9%) if the patient is hypotensive or hyponatremic.
• Add potassium (20 mEq/L) to the initial fluids unless the patient has hyperkalemia.
• Switch to IV administration of 0.45% saline after restoration of normal blood pressure and normal urine output.
• Switch to 5% dextrose plus 0.45% saline when blood glucose is < 250 mg/dl and continue until the patient is eating and drinking on its own.

Insulin

• Regular insulin for patients < 10 kg—initial dosage is 2 units IM followed by 1 unit IM hourly until blood glucose is < 250 mg/dl
• Regular insulin for patients > 10 kg—initial dosage is 0.25 units/kg IM followed by 0.1 unit/kg IM hourly until blood glucose is < 250 mg/dl
• Monitor blood glucose hourly. Aim is to drop blood glucose concentration by 50-100 mg/dl/hr. Adjust insulin dosage accordingly.
• Discontinue hourly IM regular insulin when blood glucose is < 250 mg/dl. Switch to regular insulin (0.5 units/kg) IM q4-6h or SC q6-8h if blood glucose concentration remains between 150-250 mg/dl.
• Once the patient is stabilized (eating and drinking on its own without vomiting), discontinue fluids and regular insulin. NPH or Lente insulin can then be administered SC in a routine manner.
• Other concurrent diseases must be treated appropriately.

CONTRAINDICATIONS N/A

PRECAUTIONS

Avoid rapid reduction of serum osmolarity and glucose because the brain will become hyperosmolar compared to serum. Fluid may then shift from extracellular to intracellular spaces, resulting in cerebral edema and worsening of neurologic status.

DIABETES MELLITUS, NONKETOTIC HYPERMOLAR SYNDROME

POSSIBLE INTERACTIONS N/A

ALTERNATE DRUGS

Once stable, oral administration of hypoglycemics (e.g., glipizide, Glucotrol) may be tried. These agents are more likely to be efficacious in cats with type II (noninsulin dependent diabetes mellitus) than in dogs.

FOLLOW-UP

PATIENT MONITORING

• Blood glucose concentration closely to avoid hypoglycemia and abrupt, preciptous decrease. Ideally, the blood glucose drops 50-100 mg/dl/hr until a concentration of 250 mg/dl is reached. • Blood glucose hourly before administering the next dose of regular insulin IM during initial stabilization • Urine output for early detection of acute renal failure • Urine output, hydration status, ECG, CVP, serum electrolytes, BUN, and urine glucose every 2 hours during the initial stabilization period • Long-term glucose control by determining serum glycosylated hemoglobin and serum fructosamine concentrations • For return of clinical signs such as polydipsia, polyuria, and polyphagia

PREVENTION/AVOIDANCE

Appropriate insulin therapy

POSSIBLE COMPLICATIONS

• Irreversible coma and death are possible, especially in patients with renal insufficiency.
• Acute renal failure

EXPECTED COURSE AND PROGNOSIS

Although improvement in clinical signs and laboratory values may be seen within the initial 24 hours of treatment, these patients have a guarded prognosis.

MISCELLANEOUS

ASSOCIATED CONDITIONS

Congestive heart failure, renal disease, infection, gastrointestinal hemorrhage, and other serious illnesses

AGE RELATED FACTORS N/A

ZOONOTIC POTENTIAL N/A

PREGNANCY

Insulin resistance and, thus, poor glycemic control may be encountered in pregnant animals.

SYNONYMS

• Diabetic coma • Hyperosmolar coma

SEE ALSO

• Diabetes Mellitus, Uncomplicated
• Diabetes Mellitus, Ketoacidotic
• Osmolarity, Hyperosmolarity • Glucose, Hyperglycemia

ABBREVIATIONS

BUN = blood urea nitrogen
CVP = central venous pressure
ECG = electrocardiogram

References

Carlson RA. Hyperosmolar nonketotic diabetes mellitus in a cat. Feline Pract 1994;22:20-24.

Chastain CB, Ganjam VK. Diabetes mellitus. In: Clinical endocrinology of companion animals. Philadephia: Lea & Febiger, 1986:257-302.

Nelson RW. Diabetes mellitus. In: Ettinger SJ, Feldman EC, eds. Textbook of veterinary internal medicine. 4th ed. Philadelphia: WB Saunders, 1995:1510-1537.

Murtaugh RJ, Kaplan PM. Veterinary emergency and critical care medicine. St. Louis: Mosby, 1992:253-254.

Brody GM. Diabetic ketoacidosis and hyperosmolar hyperglycemic nonketotic coma. Topics Emerg Med 1992;14:12-22.

Author Margaret R. Kern
Consulting Editor Rhett Nichols

DIABETES MELLITUS, UNCOMPLICATED

BASICS

DEFINITION
Disorder of carbohydrate, fat, and protein metabolism caused by an absolute or relative insulin deficiency. Type I (insulin-dependent diabetes mellitus [DM]) is characterized by very low to absent insulin secretory ability. These patients die if not treated with insulin and are prone to ketoacidosis. Type II (non–insulin-dependent DM) is characterized by inadequate or delayed insulin secretion relative to the needs of the patient. Many of these patients live without exogenous insulin and are less prone to ketoacidosis.

Pathophysiology
Insulin deficiency causes an impaired ability of tissues, especially muscle, adipose tissue, and liver, to utilize carbohydrates, fats, and proteins. Impaired glucose utilization and ongoing gluconeogenesis cause hyperglycemia. Glucosuria develops, causing osmotic diuresis, polyuria, and compensatory weight loss. Mobilization of free fatty acids to the liver causes both hepatic lipidosis and ketogenesis.

Systems Affected
• Endocrine/metabolic—electrolyte depletion and metabolic acidosis • Hepatobiliary—hepatic lipidosis. Liver failure may develop, particularly in cats. • Ophthalmic—cataracts in dogs • Renal/urologic—urinary tract infection and osmotic diuresis • Nervous—peripheral neuropathy in cats

Genetics
Familial associations in some breeds of dog

Incidence/Prevalence
Prevalence in both dogs and cats varies between 1:400 and 1:500.

Geographic Distribution N/A

SIGNALMENT

Species Dogs and cats

Breed Predilections
• Higher risk than other breeds—keeshond, puli, miniature pinscher, and cairn terrier • Possible higher risk than other breeds— poodle, dachshund, miniature schnauzer, and beagle • No breed predilections in cats

Mean Age and Range
• Dogs—mean about 8 years; range, 4-14 years (excluding rare juvenile form) • Cats— 75% are 8-13 years; range, 1-19 years

Predominant Sex
• Dogs—female predisposition • Cats—male predisposition

SIGNS
• Signs are more often noticed in the early stages of disease in dogs than in cats.
• Early signs—polyuria and polydipsia (PU/PD), polyphagia, and weight loss • Later signs—anorexia, lethargy, depression, and vomiting • Obesity with recent weight loss is typical. • Dorsal muscle wasting and an oily coat with dandruff common in cats • Hepatomegaly in both species, but jaundice more prevalent in cats • Less common findings— cataracts in dogs and a plantigrade stance in cats (diabetic neuropathy)

CAUSES
• Genetic susceptibility • Infectious (viral) diseases • Immune-mediated beta cell destruction • Pancreatitis • Predisposing diseases (e.g., hyperadrenocorticism and acromegaly) • Drugs (e.g., glucocorticoids and progestagens)

RISK FACTORS
• Obesity for type II DM • Diestrus in the bitch • See causes.

DIAGNOSIS

DIFFERENTIAL DIAGNOSIS
• Renal glucosuria—usually does not cause PU/PD, weight loss, or hyperglycemia
• Stress hyperglycemia in cats—no PU/PD or weight loss. Blood glucose concentration normal if sample taken when cat is not stressed.

CBC/BIOCHEMISTRY/URINALYSIS
• Results of hemogram usually normal
• Glucose > 200 mg% in dogs; > 250 mg% in cats • High SAP, ALT, and AST activities and hypercholesterolemia and lipemia common • Electrolytes vary, but hypernatremia, hypokalemia, and hypophosphatemia indicate severe decompensation. • Total CO_2 or HCO_3 are low if the patient has ketoacidosis or severe dehydration. • Glucosuria is a consistent finding. • Ketonuria is common.
• Urine specific gravity often is low.

OTHER LABORATORY TESTS
• Anion gap—high in patients with ketoacidosis • Plasma insulin—may be helpful in differentiating type I from type II DM. Normal or high insulin concentration with hyperglycemia found in patients with type II DM. Low insulin concentration suggests type I DM but may be an incorrect diagnosis because persistent hyperglycemia can impair insulin secretory activity, even if functional beta cells are present. • Glucose tolerance test— best way to differentiate types of DM but impractical

IMAGING
• Radiography—useful to evaluate for concurrent or underlying disease (e.g., cystic or renal calculi, emphysematous cystitis or cholecystitis, and pancreatitis) • Ultrasonography—indicated in selected patients, particularly those with jaundice, to evaluate for hepatic lipidosis, cholangiohepatitis, and pancreatitis

OTHER DIAGNOSTIC PROCEDURES
Liver biopsy (percutaneous)—indicated in some jaundiced patients

GROSS AND HISTOPATHOLOGIC FINDINGS
• Usually no gross necropsy changes
• Histopathologic findings may be normal or reveal vacuolar degeneration of the islets of Langerhans or low numbers of islet cells. Immunohistochemical staining is necessary to show low numbers of beta cells. In cats, amyloid deposits in the islets are usually seen.

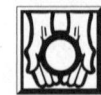

TREATMENT

INPATIENT VERSUS OUTPATIENT
Compensated dogs and cats can be managed as outpatients. They are alert, hydrated, and eating and drinking without vomiting. For management of decompensated patients, see Diabetes Mellitus, Ketoacidotic.

ACTIVITY
Strenuous activity may lower insulin requirement. Consistent amount of activity each day is helpful.

DIET
• Avoid soft, moist foods because they cause severe postprandial hyperglycemia.
• Nonobese dogs and cats—feed a consistent diet that the pet will reliably eat. Keep daily calorie intake constant.
• Obese dogs and cats—gradual weight reduction improves insulin sensitivity and reverses diabetes in some cats with type II DM. Technique 1—reduce the calorie intake to 70% (cats) or 60% (dogs) of the caloric requirement for the animal's ideal body weight. Technique 2—feed a high-fiber, low-calorie food in a quantity similar to what the pet is accustomed. Try to achieve the target weight over 2-4 months. Rapid weight loss is inadvisable, especially in obese cats with DM because they are prone to hepatic lipidosis.
• Thin dogs and cats—avoid reduced calorie diet. Starvation exacerbates ketoacidosis and poor immune function.
• Role of fiber—key role is in weight loss and obesity prevention. Another beneficial effect may be improved glycemic control. Recommended diet is high in fiber, low in fat, and high in complex carbohydrates.
• Feed the pet half its daily food every 12 hours to coincide with twice-daily insulin injections or orally administered hypoglycemic agent. For animals on once-daily insulin injections, half the food is given with the injection and the remainder in 8-10 hours or at the time of peak insulin activity, if that has been determined. For nibblers, dry food can be fed ad libitum, and two small meals of canned food given as described.

CLIENT EDUCATION
Discuss daily feeding and medication schedule, home monitoring, signs of hypoglycemia and what to do, and when to call or visit veterinarian. Clients are encouraged to keep a chart of pertinent information about the pet,

such as urine dipstick results, daily insulin dose, and weekly body weight.

SURGICAL CONSIDERATIONS

Intact females should have an ovariohysterectomy when stable. Progesterone secreted during diestrus makes management of DM difficult.

MEDICATIONS

DRUGS AND FLUIDS

• Fluid therapy—see Diabetes Mellitus, Ketoacidotic
• Insulin—treatment of choice for all dogs and most cats
• Regular crystalline insulin has rapid bioavailability, short duration of action, and can be given by any parenteral route. Used for patients with anorexia, vomiting, or ketoacidosis. Can be mixed with other insulins.
• NPH (Isophane) insulin—intermediate in duration; given SQ q12h in all cats and most dogs; initial dosage—dogs, 0.5 unit/kg; cats, 0.25-0.5 unit/kg; adjust the dosage according to individual response
• Lente insulin—intermediate in duration; given SQ; initial dosage same as for NPH. Often given q12h but may be suitable q24h in some animals.
• Ultralente insulin—long acting insulin; given SQ, usually q24h. Some animals require injections q12h.
• Insulin mixtures add rapid bioavailability to longer duration insulins. The lente series can be mixed in any combination. NPH and regular insulin mixtures are commercially available. A combination of 25% regular and 75% ultralente can be used after it equilibrates in the vial for 24 hours. Most animals can be managed without insulin mixtures.
• Species of origin of the insulin may affect pharmacokinetics. Beef, pork, beef/pork, and human recombinant insulin are options. Animal-origin insulins are being phased out. Keep the pet on the same type and species of insulin if possible. When changing from an animal origin to human recombinant insulin, lower the dosage and reregulate the animal.
• Oral administration of hypoglycemic agent—glipizide is useful with dietary therapy in some cats with type II DM. The cat should have uncomplicated DM and no history of ketoacidosis. Initial dosage, 2.5 mg PO q12h. Monitoring is the same as for patients on insulin. If hyperglycemia is not controlled, 5 mg q12h may be tried. Potential side effects are hypoglycemia, hepatic enzyme alterations, icterus, and vomiting.

CONTRAINDICATIONS N/A

PRECAUTIONS

• Glucocorticoids, megestrol acetate, and progesterone cause insulin resistance.
• Hyperosmotic agents (e.g., mannitol and radiographic contrast agents) if the patient is already hyperosmolar from hyperglycemia

POSSIBLE INTERACTIONS

Many drugs (e.g., NSAIDs, sulfonamides, miconazole, chloramphenicol, monoamine oxidase inhibitors, and beta blockers) potentiate the effect of hypoglycemic agents given orally. Consult the product insert.

ALTERNATE DRUGS

Dietary therapy or oral administration of hypoglycemic agents or both can be tried if owners are unwilling or unable to give insulin. This is more successful in cats than dogs.

FOLLOW-UP

PATIENT MONITORING

• Glucose curve—the best method of monitoring. The owner feeds the pet, injects the insulin, and then brings the patient to the hospital for serial blood glucose testing every 1-2 hours, beginning about an hour after the injection. Animals receiving insulin q12h are followed for 12 hours, and those on insulin q24h are followed for 24 hours. The goal is to maintain blood glucose between 100 and 200 mg% for at least 20-22 hours per day in dogs, and between 100 and 300 mg% in cats. The curve is performed every few weeks until the disease is regulated, and then every few months or whenever a problem arises.
• Urine glucose monitoring—urine is tested for glucose and ketones before the meal and insulin injection. To use this as a regulatory method, the pet must be allowed to have trace to 1/4% glucosuria to avoid hypoglycemia. Animals regulated by urine alone may be more hyperglycemic than ideal, and insulin overdose with rebound hyperglycemia is an inherent risk with this method. It is most useful to combine urine monitoring with intermittent glucose curves. Owners should seek veterinary attention if ketonuria is detected. • Clinical signs—owner can assess degree of PU/PD, appetite, and body weight. If these are normal, the disease is well regulated.

PREVENTION/AVOIDANCE

Prevent or correct obesity. Avoid unnecessary use of glucocorticoids or megestrol acetate.

POSSIBLE COMPLICATIONS

• Cataracts (dogs) and diabetic neuropathy (cats) with poor glycemic control • Seizure or coma with insulin overdose • Anemia and hemoglobinemia with severe hypophosphatemia, which can occur after initial insulin therapy

EXPECTED COURSE AND PROGNOSIS

Some cats recover but may relapse at a later time. Dogs have permanent disease. Prognosis with treatment is good. Most animals have a normal life span.

MISCELLANEOUS

ASSOCIATED CONDITIONS

Urinary tract infection

AGE RELATED FACTORS

Juvenile DM is rare and may be more difficult to manage.

ZOONOTIC POTENTIAL N/A

PREGNANCY

Diabetes mellitus can develop during pregnancy, in which case the pregnancy is difficult to maintain. Exogenous insulin administration may cause fetal oversize and dystocia. Insulin resistance develops, making hyperglycemia difficult to control. The pregnant bitch is prone to ketoacidosis. An emergency ovariohysterectomy may be necessary. Dogs with DM should not be used for breeding.

SYNONYMS N/A

SEE ALSO

Diabetes Mellitus, Ketoacidotic

ABBREVIATIONS

ALP = alkaline phosphatase
ALT = alanine aminotransferase
AST = aspartate aminotransferase
NSAID = nonsteroidal antiinflammatory drug
PU/PD = polyuria and polydypsia
DM = diabetes mellitus

References

Nelson RW. Diabetes mellitus. In: Ettinger SJ, Feldman EC, eds. Textbook of veterinary internal medicine. Philadelphia: WB Saunders, 1995:1510-1537.
Wallace MS, Kirk CA. The diagnosis and treatment of insulin-dependent and non-insulin-dependent DM in the dog and the cat. Prob Vet Med 1990;2:573-590.
Author Melissa S. Wallace
Consulting Editor Rhett Nichols

DIAPHRAGMATIC HERNIA

BASICS

OVERVIEW
• The protrusion of an abdominal organ through an abnormal opening in the diaphragm either as an acquired injury or a congenital defect. • Traumatic diaphragmatic hernia (TDH) is most common, usually the result of automobile trauma, although any forceful blow may be a cause. A sudden increase of pressure results in an abdominal-thoracic pressure gradient, causing a tear in the diaphragm usually at a muscular portion. • Congenital diaphragmatic hernia (CDH) may be either pleuroperitoneal or peritoneopericardial. Other congenital defects may be present (i.e., ventricular septal defect, aortic stenosis, portal caval shunt, cranioventral abdominal wall defects). • A number of mechanical and organic factors contribute to the clinical signs. Normal lung expansion is impaired because of lack of lung contact with parietal pleura. Rib fractures may contribute because of pain or mechanical (flail chest) factors. These result in hypoventilation. • Accumulation of fluid and/or air or organ entrapment prevents lung expansion and contributes to hypoventilation. Fluid may be hemothorax from lung laceration or intercostal vessel tear, chylothorax from thoracic duct trauma, or hydrothorax from abdominal organ entrapment with transudation of fluid from venous stasis and increased hydrostatic pressures. • Intrapulmonary changes such as lung contusion, atelectasis, and capillary permeability changes causing edema contribute to poor gas exchange. • Myocardial trauma may result in various dysrhythmias, most commonly ventricular tachyarrhythmias. These may result in decreased cardiac output and tissue hypoxia. They are most commonly seen within 24-72 hours after trauma, are difficult to control with conventional therapy, and commonly resolve within 5 days. • Various stages of shock may results in multiple organ system failure.

SIGNALMENT
• Both dogs and cats are affected. • No breed predilection (younger animals at higher risk) • Weimeraners and cocker spaniels may be predisposed to CDH, which can be diagnosed at any age because clinical signs are variable and intermittent.

SIGNS
TDH
• May present as an acute, subacute, or chronic disorder (with no history of trauma) • Low grade respiratory signs may be seen; vague history of gastrointestinal problems may be mentioned; signs may be progressive. • Dyspnea most common; acutely affected animals frequently in shock • Arrhythmias may be detected; muffled heart and lung sounds along with intestinal sounds may be auscultated in the thorax. • The abdomen may feel "empty" on palpation; acute incarceration of bowel may result in vomiting, diarrhea, retching, bloating, pain, and acute collapse.

CDH
• May be asymptomatic or may become symptomatic late in life • Signs may be referable to the respiratory, cardiac, or gastrointestinal systems. • Dyspnea, muffled heart sounds, murmurs, and concurrent ventral abdominal wall defects are most commonly found. • Signs can be acute from strangulation of incarcerated bowel, liver, or spleen or rapid formation of pericardial effusions.

CAUSES AND RISK FACTORS
TDH-lack of confinement and exposure to automobiles; any blunt trauma; roaming animals and male dogs are at increased risk

DIAGNOSIS

DIFFERENTIAL DIAGNOSIS
See Dyspnea and Pleural effusion

CBC/BIOCHEMISTRY/URINALYSIS
Nonspecific changes may be noted as a result of isehemia or shock.

OTHER LABORATORY TESTS N/A
IMAGING
• Radiography is the most useful diagnostic test. • Significant pleural effusion may necessitate thoracentesis before radiographs. • If a definitive diagnosis cannot be made, perform positive-contrast celiography and/or ultrasonography.

OTHER DIAGNOSTIC PROCEDURES
N/A

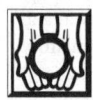

TREATMENT

TDH
• Patients are hospitalized and therapy is directed at treating shock, improving ventilation and cardiac output, and management of concurrent injury; the goal is to stabilize the patient before surgery.
• Surgical intervention in the first 24 hours historically has resulted in a higher mortality rate.
• The inability to stabilize the patient does not mean that surgical repair of the DH will improve the patient's cardiovascular and respiratory status.
• Early surgical intervention is indicated when persistent hypotension occurs despite adequate fluid therapy (including transfusion when needed), severe respiratory failure from excessive lung compression is present, severe liver failure secondary to organ entrapment is detected, bowel rupture is found, or an enlarging, gas-filled bowel is noted radiographically.

• Intrathoracic gastric dilation requires immediate decompression, but methods other than immediate surgery should be used.

CDH
• Surgical repair is performed as early as possible to avoid adhesion formation and organ entrapment. • If clinical signs are present, the patient should be stablized before surgery.

MEDICATIONS

DRUGS AND FLUIDS
• Shock is treated according to standard acceptable procedures.
• Oxygen administration can be a critical factor in managing these patients.
• Cardiac arrhythmias often are difficult to control.

CONTRAINDICATIONS/POSSIBLE INTERACTIONS
Care must be taken when treating for shock in the presence of concurrent, severe, pulmonary contusion; administration of products such as Hespan may be beneficial.

FOLLOW-UP
• Pneumothorax from excessive pressure on damaged lung tissue during anesthetic bagging or from failure to remove air from the chest cavity after diaphragmatic closure may occur. • Pulmonary edema may occur as a result of excessive fluid administration in the face of decreased oncotic pressure from blood loss, capillary permeability changes secondary to inflammation in response to pulmonary contusion, or reexpansion pulmonary edema. • Frequent electrocardiographic monitoring is advised to evaluate for the presence of arrhythmias. • Always initially give a guarded prognosis. The prognosis after the successful control of shock, the elimination of any cardiac arrhythmias, a successful surgical procedure, and the lack of reexpansion pulmonary edema is favorable.

MISCELLANEOUS

ABBREVIATIONS
TDH = traumatic diaphragmatic hernia
CDH = congenital diaphragmatic hernia

Reference
Boudrieau RJ, Muir WW. Pathophysiology of traumatic diaphragmatic hernia in dogs. Compend Cont Ed Pract Vet 1987;9:379-385.

Author Justin H. Straus
Consulting Editors Lynelle Johnson and Bradley L. Moses

BASICS

OVERVIEW
Common in veterinary practice because of digoxin's narrow therapeutic index and prevalence of renal impairment in elderly patients with cardiac disease

SIGNALMENT
• Dogs and cats • More common in geriatric patients

SIGNS

Historical Findings
• Anorexia • Vomiting • Diarrhea • Lethargy • Depression

Physical Examination Findings
Heart rate may range from severe bradycardia to severe tachycardia.

CAUSES AND RISK FACTORS
• Renal disease, which impairs elimination • Chronic pulmonary disease, resulting in hypoxia and acid-base disturbances • Obesity increases risk if dosage is not based on lean body weight • Hypokalemia, hypercalcemia, hypomagnesemia, and hypoxia, which predispose to digitalis induced arrhythmias • Drugs and conditions that alter digoxin metabolism and elimination (e.g., quinidine and hypothyroidism) • Rapid IV digitalization • Administration of diuretic leading to hypokalemia

DIAGNOSIS

DIFFERENTIAL DIAGNOSIS
• Arrhythmias and conduction disturbances may reflect structural heart disease and not digoxin toxicity.
• Anorexia is common in animals with heart failure.

CBC/BIOCHEMISTRY/URINALYSIS
• Animals with hypokalemia, hypercalcemia, hypomagnesemia, and renal failure are predisposed to toxicity.

OTHER LABORATORY TESTS
• Consider checking thyroid status.

• Obtain digoxin serum concentration 8-10 hours after an oral dose— therapeutic range is between 1-2 ng/ml. Not all animals with concentrations > 2 ng/ml have signs of toxicity, and some animals with values in the normal range have signs of toxicity, especially if hypokalemic.

IMAGING N/A

OTHER DIAGNOSTIC PROCEDURES

Electrocardiographic Findings
• Conduction disturbances (atrioventricular [AV] block), arrhythmias, and ST segment depression in some animals • Digoxin can cause any arrhythmia.

TREATMENT
• If signs are mild, discontinuing digoxin for 24-72 hours may be sufficient.
• Severe arrhythmias (ventricular tachycardia) and conduction disturbances can be life-threatening and require hospitalization and aggressive treatment.

MEDICATIONS

DRUGS AND FLUIDS
• Treat arrhythmias or conduction disturbances if present and indicated.
• Treat bradyarrhythmias with atropine or temporary transvenous pacemaker.
• Treat ventricular arrhythmias with lidocaine or phenytoin. Phenytoin also reverses high-degree AV block.
• Maintain hydration and correct any electrolyte disturbance (especially hypokalemia) with parenteral fluid administration.
• Digoxin binding antibodies (Digibind) can be used to rapidly drop digoxin concentration in critically ill animals. The use of these products is limited in veterinary practice by their exorbitant cost.
• Discontinue digoxin until signs of toxicity resolve (24-72 hours). Reevaluate the need for the medication. If necessary, resume treatment at a dosage based on the serum digoxin concentration.

• Thyroxin supplementation necessary if hypothyroidism confirmed

CONTRAINDICATIONS/POSSIBLE INTERACTIONS
• Avoid or discontinue drugs that slow digoxin elimination or metabolism (e.g., quinidine, verapamil, and diltiazem).
• Avoid drugs that could worsen conduction disturbances (e.g., beta blockers and calcium channel blockers).
• Class 1A antiarrhythmic drugs (e.g., quinidine and procainamide) may enhance AV block.

FOLLOW-UP

PATIENT MONITORING
• Monitor renal function and electrolytes carefully and frequently in animals receiving digoxin. • Monitor serum digoxin concentration periodically if there is concern about toxicity recurring. • Monitor ECG periodically to assess for arrhythmia or conduction disturbances that may suggest digoxin toxicity.
• Monitor body weight frequently and alter dosage accordingly. Animals with CHF may lose a lot of weight.

MISCELLANEOUS
Use digoxin cautiously in animals with renal or pulmonary disease.

SEE ALSO Ventricular tachycardia

ABBREVIATIONS
AV = atrioventricular
CHF = congestive heart failure

Reference
Marcus FI, Opie LH, Sonnenblick EH. Digitalis and other inotropes. In: Opie LH, ed. Drugs for the heart. 3rd ed. Philadelphia: WB Saunders, 1991:129-154.
Author Francis W. K. Smith, Jr.
Consulting Editors Larry P. Tilley and Francis W. K. Smith, Jr.

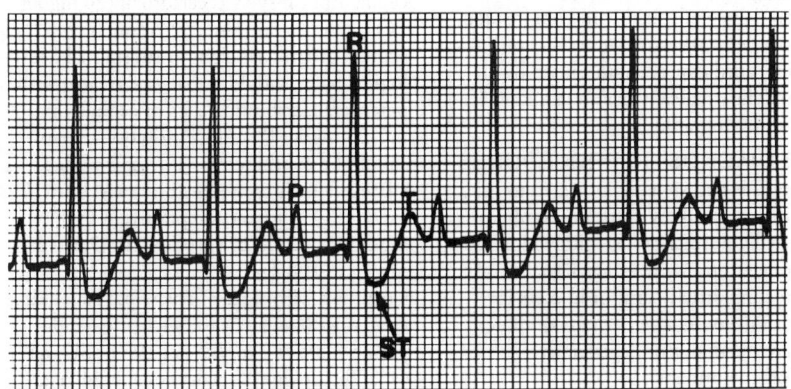

"Sagging" type of S-T segment depression in a dog with digitalis toxicity. This concavity to the S-T segment is most often correlated with digitalis. The long P-R interval is also compatible with digitalis toxicity. (From Tilley LP. Essentials of canine and feline electrocardiography. 3rd ed. Baltimore: Williams & Wilkins, 1992, with permission).

DISKOSPONDYLITIS

BASICS

DEFINITION
Diskospondylitis is a bacterial or fungal infection of the intervertebral disks and adjacent vertebral bodies

Pathophysiology
Hematogenous spread of bacterial or fungal organisms is the most common cause. Occasionally the cause is foreign body migration, surgery or, in cats, local soft tissue infection caused by bite wounds. Neurologic dysfunction, if it occurs, is usually due to spinal cord compression caused by proliferation of bone and fibrous tissue. Less commonly, spinal cord damage is due to luxation or pathologic fracture of the spine or extension of infection to the meninges and spinal cord.

Systems Affected
• Musculoskeletal system—due to infection and inflammation of the spine • Nervous system—due to compression of the spinal cord

Genetics
Although an inherited immunodeficiency has been detected in a few cases, a definite genetic predisposition has not been identified.

Incidence and Prevalence
Approximately 0.2% of dog hospital admissions

Geographic Distribution   N/A

SIGNALMENT

Species   Dogs, rare in cats

Breed Predilections
Large and giant breeds, especially German shepherds and great Danes

Mean Age and Range
• 4 to 5 years • Range of 5 months to 12 years

Predominant Sex
Males outnumber females by ~ 2:1

SIGNS

Historical Findings
• Onset is usually relatively acute but some animals have mild signs for several months before examination • Signs of pain such as difficulty rising, reluctance to jump, or stilted gait are most common • Ataxia or paresis • Weight loss/anorexia • Lameness • Draining tracts

Physical Examination Findings
• Focal or multifocal areas of spinal pain • Any disk space can be affected—lumbosacral space most commonly involved • Paresis or paralysis • Fever • Lameness

CAUSES
• Bacterial—Staphylococcus aureus and Staphylococcus intermedius are most commonly isolated. Other bacteria include Brucella canis, Streptococcus spp, Corynebacterium spp, Escherichia coli,

Proteus spp, Pasteurella spp, and Bactericides spp. • Fungal—Aspergillus spp and Coccidioides immitis

RISK FACTORS
• Urinary tract infection • Periodontal disease • Bacterial endocarditis • Dermatitis • Immunodeficiency

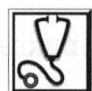

DIAGNOSIS

DIFFERENTIAL DIAGNOSIS
• Intervertebral disk protrusion may cause similar clinical signs but can be differentiated on the basis of radiography and myelography • Vertebral fracture/luxation can be detected on radiographs • Vertebral neoplasia usually does not affect adjacent vertebral end-plates • Spondylosis deformans rarely causes clinical signs but has similar radiographic features, including sclerosis, ventral spur formation, and collapse of the disk space. However, spondylosis rarely causes lysis of the vertebral end-plates. • Focal meningomyelitis

CBC/BIOCHEMISTRY/URINALYSIS
• Hemogram is often normal but leukocytosis can occur. • Urinalysis may reveal pyuria and/or bacteriuria in cases with concurrent urinary tract infections

OTHER LABORATORY TESTS
• Aerobic, anaerobic and fungal cultures of blood identify the causative organism in up to 75% of cases and should be performed if available. • Sensitivity testing is indicated if cultures are positive. • Urine cultures are indicated and are positive in about 25% of patients. • Organisms other than Staphylococcus spp may not be the cause of the diskospondylitis. • Serologic testing for Brucella canis is indicated in any dog with diskospondylitis.

IMAGING
• Spinal radiographs usually reveal lysis of vertebral endplates adjacent to the affected disk, collapse of the disk space, and varying degrees of sclerosis of the endplates and ventral spur formation. These lesions may not be seen until 3-4 weeks after infection. • Myelography is indicated in animals with substantial neurological deficits to determine the location and degree of spinal cord compression, especially if decompressive surgery is considered. Spinal cord compression caused by diskospondylitis typically has an extradural pattern on myelography.

OTHER DIAGNOSTIC PROCEDURES
CSF analysis is occasionally indicated to rule out meningomyelitis. With diskospondylitis, CSF is usually normal or has mildly high protein. • Bone scintigraphy is occasionally useful in detecting early lesions or in cases in which it is uncertain whether radiographic changes are infectious or degenerative (spondylosis deformans).

GROSS AND HISTOPATHOLOGIC FINDINGS
• Grossly loss of the normal disk space and bony proliferation of adjacent vertebrae. • Microscopically, fibrosing pyogranulomatous destruction of the disk and vertebral bodies

TREATMENT

INPATIENT VERSUS OUTPATIENT
• Patients with mild pain can be managed as outpatients. • Patients with severe pain or progressive neurologic deficits should be hospitalized for treatment.

ACTIVITY   Restricted

DIET   Normal

CLIENT EDUCATION
• Observation of response to treatment very important in determining the need for further diagnostic or therapeutic procedures. • Owner should be instructed to immediately contact the veterinarian if clinical signs progress or recur, or if neurologic deficits develop

SURGICAL CONSIDERATIONS
• Curettage of a single affected disk space is occasionally necessary in patients refractory to antibiotic therapy. The goal of surgery is to remove infected tissue and obtain tissue for culture and histologic evaluation. • Decompression of the spinal cord by hemilaminectomy or dorsal laminectomy is indicated if substantial spinal cord compression is evident on myelography. Curettage of the infected disk space is also performed. Surgical stabilization may be necessary if more than one articular facet is removed.

MEDICATIONS

DRUGS AND FLUIDS
• Selection of an antibiotic is based on results of blood cultures and serology. If these results are negative, the causative organism is assumed to be Staphylococcus spp and a cephalosporin such as cefadroxil (20 mg/kg PO q12h) is administered. Animals with acutely progressive signs or substantial neurologic deficits should initially be treated with parenteral antibiotics, such as cephalothin (20-35 mg/kg IV q6h). Antibiotic therapy should be continued for at least 6 weeks. • Brucellosis is treated with tetracycline (10 mg/kg PO q8h) and streptomycin (3.4 mg/kg IM q24h) or enrofloxacin (2.5-5.0 mg/kg PO q12h). • Animals with signs of severe pain should be treated with an analgesic such as oxymorphone (0.05-0.2 mg/kg IV, IM, or SQ, q4-6h). The dosage of analgesics should be ta-

pered after 3-5 days to gauge effectiveness of antibiotic therapy.

CONTRAINDICATIONS
Glucocorticoids

PRECAUTIONS
Nonsteroidal anti-inflammatory drugs (NSAIDs) or other analgesics should be used cautiously because they may cause a temporary resolution of clinical signs even if the infection is progressing. If analgesics are necessary, they should be discontinued after 3-5 days to assess efficacy of antibiotic therapy.

POSSIBLE INTERACTIONS None

ALTERNATE DRUGS
Cephradine (20 mg/kg PO q8h) and cloxacillin (10 mg/kg PO q8h) are other good choices for initial therapy. Clindamycin (11 mg/kg PO q12h) or enrofloxacin (2.5-5.0 mg/kg PO q12h) may be effective in refractory patients.

 FOLLOW-UP

PATIENT MONITORING
• Patients should be reevaluated after 5 days of therapy. If there is no improvement in clinical signs (decrease in pain, resolution of fever, improvement of appetite) therapy should be reassessed. Use of a different antibiotic or surgery should be considered.
• Patients that improve with antibiotic therapy should be evaluated clinically and radiographically every 2-4 weeks.

PREVENTION/AVOIDANCE
Recurrence is common if antibiotic therapy is stopped prematurely (before 6 weeks of therapy).

POSSIBLE COMPLICATIONS
• Spinal cord compression due to proliferative bony and fibrous tissue • Vertebral fracture/luxation • Meningitis or meningomyelitis • Epidural abscess

EXPECTED COURSE AND PROGNOSIS
• Prognosis depends on the causative organism and the degree of spinal cord damage.
• Dogs with mild or no neurologic dysfunction usually respond within 5 days of starting antibiotic therapy. • Although the prognosis for dogs with substantial paresis or paralysis is guarded, the neurologic dysfunction may gradually resolve after several weeks of therapy so treatment is still warranted. • The clinical signs of diskospondylitis due to Brucella canis usually resolve with therapy, although the infection may not be eradicated, so recurrence is common.

 MISCELLANEOUS

ASSOCIATED CONDITIONS
See risk factors

AGE-RELATED FACTORS N/A

ZOONOTIC POTENTIAL
Although human infection with Brucella canis is uncommon, this organism does have zoonotic potential

PREGNANCY N/A

SYNONYMS
• Intradiskal osteomyelitis • Intervertebral disk infection • Vertebral osteomyelitis • Diskitis

SEE ALSO Brucellosis

ABBREVIATIONS
CSF = cerebrospinal fluid
NSAID = nonsteroidal anti-inflammatory drugs

References
Hurov L, Troy G, Turnwald G. Diskospondylitis in the dog: 27 cases. J Am Vet Med Assoc 1978;173:275-281.
Kerwin SC, Lewis DD, Hribernik TN, et al. Diskospondylitis associated with Brucella canis infection in dogs: 14 cases (1989-1991). J Am Vet Med Assoc 1992;201:1253-1257.
Kornegay JN, Barber DL. Diskospondylitis in dogs. J Am Vet Med Assoc 1980;177:337-341.
Kornegay JN. Diskospondylitis. In: Kirk RW, ed. Current veterinary therapy IX. Philadelphia: WB Saunders, 1986;810-814.
Johnson RG, Prata RG. Intradiskal osteomyelitis: a conservative approach. J Am Anim Hosp Assoc 1983;19:743-750.
Author William B. Thomas
Consulting Editor Peter D. Schwarz

DISSEMINATED INTRAVASCULAR COAGULATION (DIC)

BASICS

DEFINITION
A complex hemostatic defect with enhanced coagulation and fibrinolysis secondary to severe systemic disease

Pathophysiology
DIC occurs secondary to activation of coagulation and fibrinolysis. These changes are induced in patients with diseases characterized by stasis of blood flow, vascular damage, activation and consumption of coagulation factors, reduced clearance of activated clotting factors by the liver, or release of tissue factors from damaged cells, tumors, or other tissues. Activation of fibrinolysis is a secondary response to clear fibrin thrombi in capillaries. The bleeding defect is complicated by thrombocytopenia related to consumption at sites of damaged endothelium and thrombi, and by a platelet function defect induced by coating of platelets with FDP from the action of the fibrinolytic mechanism on fibrin or fibrinogen.

Systems Affected
DIC is a multisystemic disease with hemorrhages in many tissues and organ dysfunction related to obstruction of capillaries.

Genetics N/A

Incidence/Prevalence
DIC is associated with severe systemic disease and is common in the terminal stages of a variety of fatal diseases.

Geographic Distribution N/A

SIGNALMENT

Species
Dogs and cats, but more commonly recognized in dogs

Breed Predilections
None

Mean Age and Range
Correlates with those of the severe systemic disease

Predominant Sex
None

SIGNS
• Clinical signs and history usually relate to the primary disease. • Findings that raise concern about DIC include petechiae, abnormal bleeding from venipuncture sites, and other abnormal bleeding.

CAUSES
Malignancies, shock, pancreatitis, heatstroke, infectious canine hepatitis, other systemic infectious diseases, including gram-negative septicemia, heart failure, hemorrhagic gastroenteritis, chronic active liver disease, splenic torsion, heartworm disease, snake venom, hemolysis, and gastric dilatation-volvulus

RISK FACTORS
See causes.

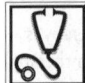

DIAGNOSIS

DIFFERENTIAL DIAGNOSIS
• Immune-mediated or idiopathic thrombocytopenia • Anticoagulant toxicity • Coagulation factor deficiency • Deficient production of clotting factors in severe liver disease • Paraproteinemia

CBC/BIOCHEMISTRY/URINALYSIS
• Thrombocytopenia is common and macroplatelets provide evidence of enhanced thrombopoiesis. • Schistocytes are caused by mechanical fragmentation of erythrocytes on intraluminal fibrin strands. • Biochemistry analysis may reveal azotemia, acidosis, and high enzyme activities related to the primary disease and organ dysfunction, or necrosis related to capillary obstruction.

OTHER LABORATORY TESTS
• PT and APTT may show various degrees of prolongation secondary to the anticoagulant effects of FDP and consumption of coagulation factors, especially factor VIII and fibrinogen. • The latex agglutination test for FDP (Thrombo-Wellcotest, Burroughs-Wellcome Company, Research Triangle Park, NC) reveals a high concentration. • Practical assays to demonstrate depletion of clotting factors include fibrinogen and antithrombin III.

IMAGING N/A

OTHER DIAGNOSTIC PROCEDURES
Because DIC is a syndrome characterized by significant variation, diagnosis is usually based on the combination of at least three of the following: petechiae or abnormal bleeding from venipuncture sites, thrombocytopenia, prolonged PT, prolonged APTT, and high FDP.

GROSS AND HISTOPATHOLOGIC FINDINGS
• These usually relate to the primary disease. • Petechiae are common. • Fibrin thrombi may be dissolved by fibrinolysis during the postmortem interval.

TREATMENT

INPATIENT VERSUS OUTPATIENT
DIC is associated with severe disease, requiring intensive, inpatient treatment.

ACTIVITY
Not an issue because of the severity of the primary disease

DIET N/A

CLIENT EDUCATION
The owner should be informed of the life-threatening nature of the processes associated with DIC. The prognosis usually is that associated with the primary disease.

SURGICAL CONSIDERATIONS
Relate to primary disease

MEDICATIONS

DRUGS AND FLUIDS
• The most important element of therapy is intensive treatment of the primary disease. • Fluid therapy to correct deficits in plasma volume or acid-base imbalance is an important part of treatment to reduce the potential for activation of clotting factors and enhance clearance of activated clotting factors by the mononuclear phagocyte system. • Heparin administration is controversial but may be used to inhibit proteolytic activation of coagulation, preferably by continuous intravenous infusion sufficient to prolong the APTT to one and a half to two times normal. Low-dose heparin is safer and has been reported to produce beneficial results in some dogs when intravenously infused at 5–10 iu/kg/hour or subcutaneously at 75 iu/kg q8h. • The anticoagulant effect of heparin is achieved by binding to antithrombin III, which may be depleted in patients with DIC. Therefore, it may be beneficial to transfuse with heparinized blood or heparinized plasma.

CONTRAINDICATIONS
• Although use of a high dosage of corticosteroids may be indicated to treat shock, the long-term use of corticosteroids should be considered carefully because of the inhibition of mononuclear phagocyte function, which might be important in clearance of activated coagulation factors. • Inhibitors of fibrinolysis should not be used because fibrinolysis is important in the clearance of thrombi.

PRECAUTIONS
High doses of heparin may cause bleeding episodes that could be life-threatening.

POSSIBLE INTERACTIONS N/A

ALTERNATE DRUGS N/A

FOLLOW-UP

PATIENT MONITORING
• Clinical improvement and the arrest of bleeding are positive indications of a response to treatment. • Low to undetectable concentration of FDP is a positive sign. • Platelet counts usually increase slowly over a period of days.

PREVENTION/AVOIDANCE
Related to primary disease

EXPECTED COURSE AND PROGNOSIS
Because of the serious nature of the primary diseases, animals with DIC have a high rate of mortality.

DISSEMINATED INTRAVASCULAR COAGULATION (DIC)

MISCELLANEOUS

ASSOCIATED CONDITIONS
See causes.

AGE RELATED FACTORS N/A

ZOONOTIC POTENTIAL N/A

PREGNANCY
Obstetric complications have been associated with DIC in human beings but are not as well-documented in dogs or cats. They include dystocia, eclampsia, and retained fetuses.

SYNONYMS
• Consumption coagulopathy • Intravascular coagulation-fibrinolysis syndrome

SEE ALSO
Clotting Factor Deficiencies

ABBREVIATIONS
APTT = activated partial thromboplastin time
DIC = disseminated intravascular coagulation
FDP = fibrin degradation products
PT = prothrombin time

References
Dodds WJ. Hemostasis. In: Kaneko JJ, ed. Clinical biochemistry of domestic animals. New York: Academic Press, 1989:310-312.

Feldman BF, Madewell BR, O'Neil S. Disseminated intravascular coagulation: antithrombin, plasminogen, and coagulation abnormalities in 41 dogs. J Am Vet Med Assoc 1981;179:151-154.

Slappendel RJ. Disseminated intravascular coagulation. In: Kirk RW, Bonagura JD, eds. Current veterinary therapy X. Philadelphia: WB Saunders, 1989:451-457.

Slappendel RJ. Disseminated intravascular coagulation. In: Feldman BF, ed. Hemostasis. Vet Clin North Am 1988;18:169-184.

Author Gary J. Kociba
Consulting Editor Alan H. Rebar

DISTEMPER—DOGS

BASICS

DEFINITION

Canine distemper is an acute to subacute contagious febrile and often fatal disease with respiratory, gastrointestinal, and central nervous system (CNS) manifestations. The disease is caused by canine distemper virus (CDV), a morbillivirus in the Paramyxoviridae family. The disease affects many different species of the order Carnivora and the mortality rate varies greatly between species.

Pathophysiology

The natural route of infection is by airborne and droplet exposure. From the nasal cavity, pharynx, and lungs, macrophages carry the virus to local lymph nodes, where virus replication occurs. Within one week, virtually all lymphatic tissues become infected. Elevated body temperature for 1 or 2 days and lymphopenia may be the only clinical signs during this period. Further developments depend upon the virus strain involved and the immune response. If a strong cellular and humoral immune response occurs, the infection may remain subclinical as virus is eliminated by lysis of infected cells and neutralization of virus. Failure of immune responses leads to acute death within 2-4 weeks after infection. Animals with a weak immune response may survive longer with a subacute infection. The virus spreads from lymphatic tissues via viremia to the surface epithelium of respiratory, gastrointestinal, and urogenital tracts and to the CNS. Convulsions and other CNS disturbances are frequently the cause of death.

Systems Affected

• Multisystemic—all lymphatic tissues, surface epithelium in the respiratory, alimentary, and urogenital tracts, and endocrine and exocrine glands • Nervous—the skin and cells of gray and white matter in the CNS

Genetics N/A

Incidence/Prevalence

• Common among dogs and other carnivores before modified live virus (MLV) vaccines became available in the early 1960s. It is now restricted to sporadic outbreaks. • Distemper in wildlife (e.g., raccoon, skunk, fox) is still fairly common.

Geographic Distribution Worldwide

SIGNALMENT

Most species of the order Carnivora are susceptible to CDV infection, including members of the Canidae, Hyaenidae, Mustelidae, Procyonidae, Viverridae, and, more recently, the Felidae families. There is no specific breed or sex predilection. Young animals are more susceptible than adults.

SIGNS

• The first fever 3-6 days after infection may pass unnoticed; the second temperature peak (several days later and intermittent thereafter) is usually associated with nasal and ocular discharge, depression, and anorexia. Gastrointestinal and/or respiratory signs may follow, often enhanced by secondary bacterial infection. • Many infected dogs develop CNS signs, often, but not always, after systemic disease. Depending on the virus strain, the signs may be more related to acute gray matter or subacute white matter disease. Seizures and myoclonus with depression predominate in dogs with gray matter disease; incoordination ataxia, paresis, paralysis and muscle tremors in those with white matter disease. Meningeal signs of hyperesthesia and cervical rigidity may be seen in both. Optic neuritis and retinal lesions in dogs with CDV are not uncommon. Some dogs have infected scleral blood vessels from anterior uveitis. Hardening of the foot pads (hyperkeratosis) and nose is caused by some virus strains but is now much less common in dogs with CDV than in the past. In growing dogs, enamel hypoplasia of the teeth after neonatal CDV infection is a common observation.

CAUSES

Canine distemper is caused by CDV, a morbillivirus within the Peramyxoviridae family. The virus is closely related to measles virus, rinderpest virus of cattle, and phocine (seal) and dolphin distemper viruses. Secondary bacterial infections frequently involve the respiratory and gastrointestinal systems.

RISK FACTORS

Contact of nonimmunized animals with CDV infected dogs or wildlife carnivores is the main source of infection.

DIAGNOSIS

DIFFERENTIAL DIAGNOSIS

Agents that cause kennel cough in dogs can mimic the respiratory disease of canine distemper. The enteric disease of canine distemper should be differentiated from canine parvovirus and coronavirus infections and possibly bacterial or protozoal infections such as giardia. The CNS forms of canine distemper can be confused with granulomatous meningoencephalomyelitis, protozoal encephalitis (toxoplasmosis, neosporosis), cryptococcosis, pug encephalitis, and lead poisoning.

CBC/BIOCHEMISTRY/URINALYSIS

Lymphopenia during early infection

OTHER LABORATORY TESTS

Serology is of limited value. Positive antibody tests do not differentiate between vaccination and exposure to virulent virus. Dogs may die from acute disease before antibody can be produced.

IMAGING

Radiographs are only helpful in determining the extent of pneumonia. Brain changes typically are not detected by CT or MRI scans.

OTHER DIAGNOSTIC PROCEDURES

• Viral antigen or viral inclusions can be found in buffy coat cells and conjunctival or vaginal imprints. However, negative results do not rule out distemper. • Cerebrospinal fluid (CSF) can be tested for cell and protein content, CDV specific antibody, and viral antigen early in the disease course. • Postmortem diagnosis is by histopathology, immunofluorescence and/or immunocytochemistry, and virus isolation. Preferred tissues are from the lungs, stomach, urinary bladder, lymphs, and brain.

GROSS AND HISTOPATHOLOGIC FINDINGS

• On gross inspection, only few changes can be expected in dogs or other carnivores with uncomplicated distemper. In young animals, the thymus is greatly reduced in size and sometimes gelatinous. The lungs may be patchily consolidated as a result of interstitial pneumonia. Rarely hyperkeratosis of footpads and nose may be present. Mucopurulent discharges from eyes and nose, bronchopneumonia, catarrhal enteritis, and skin pustules are probably caused by secondary bacterial infections but are commonly seen in cases of natural distemper. • Histological changes may be seen in many tissues. Intracytoplasmic eosinophilic inclusion bodies are frequently found in epithelium of the bronchi, stomach, and urinary bladder. They can also be seen in reticulum cells and leukocytes in lymphatic tissues. Inclusion bodies in the CNS in glial cells and neurons are frequently intranuclear but can also be found in cytoplasm. Staining by fluorescent antibody or immunoperoxydase may detect viral antigen where inclusion bodies are not seen.

TREATMENT

INPATIENT VERSUS OUTPATIENT

Dogs with distemper should be kept as inpatients in isolation to prevent infection of other dogs.

ACTIVITY Should be limited

DIET

Any change in diet depends on the extent of gastrointestinal involvement.

CLIENT EDUCATION

Clients should understand that the mortality rate in dogs with distemper is about 50%. Dogs that appear to recover from early catarrhal signs may later develop fatal CNS signs.

SURGICAL CONSIDERATIONS N/A

MEDICATIONS

DRUGS AND FLUIDS

No antiviral drugs are known to be effective. Because canine distemper is highly immunosuppressive, antibiotics should always be given to reduce secondary bacterial infections. Treatment of respiratory and alimentary signs and conjunctivitis is symptomatic. The possibilities for treatment of CNS signs are limited.

CONTRAINDICATIONS

Corticosteroids may ameliorate signs for a short period; however, they should not be given because they add to the immunosuppression induced by CDV and may enhance viral dissemination.

PRECAUTIONS

Young and growing animals should not be treated with tetracyclines or fluorinated quinolones.

POSSIBLE INTERACTIONS N/A

ALTERNATE DRUGS N/A

FOLLOW-UP

PATIENT MONITORING

• Dogs should be constantly observed for several reasons. Pneumonia or dehydration from diarrhea in the acute phase could cause a crisis. Once CNS signs are present, convulsions are expected. • Euthanasia may be indicated when repeated convulsions occur.

PREVENTION/AVOIDANCE

• Vaccination of dogs with MLV-CD vaccines prevents infection and disease. Inactivated (killed) vaccines that were on the market before MLV became available in the early 1960s did not significantly reduce canine distemper. There are two types of MLV-CD vaccines on the market today; both have advantages and disadvantages. • The canine tissue culture adapted vaccines (e.g., Rockborn strain) induce complete immunity in virtually 100% of susceptible dogs. However, on rare occasions, a postvaccinal fatal encephalitis may be seen 7-14 days after vaccination. • The chick embryo adapted vaccines (e.g., Onderstepoort, Lederle strain) are safer, and postvaccinal encephalitis is not known to occur. However, it has been estimated that only about 80% of susceptible pups seroconvert. • Chick embryo adapted vaccines can safely be used in a variety of zoo and wildlife species such as the gray fox. The

Rockborn-type vaccine was found to be fatal in these animals. Other species such as the red panda or black-footed ferret can be vaccinated only with killed vaccines; any MLV-CD would be fatal. • The role of maternal antibody in canine distemper is important. Most pups lose protection from maternal antibody between 6 and 12 weeks of age. Two or three vaccinations should be given during this period. Heterotypic (measles virus) vaccination of pups that have maternal antibody is recommended. However, it induces protection from disease but not from infection. • Infection of pups with CDV can be avoided by isolation to prevent infection from wildlife (e.g., raccoons, foxes, skunks) or from CDV-infected dogs. Recovered dogs are not carriers of CDV infection.

POSSIBLE COMPLICATIONS

The occurrence of CNS signs for up to 2-3 months after catarrhal signs have subsided is always a possibility.

EXPECTED COURSE AND PROGNOSIS

• Depending on the CDV strain and the individual host response, canine distemper may range from subclinical to acute or subacute to fatal or nonfatal infection. • Death may occur from 2 weeks to 3 months after infection. In general, the mortality rate in dogs is approximately 50%. In other species (e.g., mustelidae) it may reach 100%. • Dogs with mild CNS signs (e.g., myoclonus) may recover with myoclonus continuing for several months. Once dogs are fully recovered, they do not shed CDV.

MISCELLANEOUS

ASSOCIATED CONDITIONS

Because of the immunosuppressive nature of canine distemper, persistent or latent toxoplasma infections can be reactivated. Also, respiratory infections with Bordetella bronchiseptica (a major cause of kennel cough) is frequently seen in dogs with canine distemper.

AGE RELATED FACTORS

Although susceptible dogs of any age may become infected with CDV, young pups are

more susceptible to disease and the mortality rate is higher. Nonimmunized older dogs are highly susceptible to infection and disease.

ZOONOTIC POTENTIAL

• Because CDV has a wide host range, it is possible that humans may become subclinically infected with CDV. However, most humans are immunized against measles virus, which would also protect against CDV infection. • It has been speculated that CDV may be the cause of multiple sclerosis (MS). Several studies have refuted this proposition. The most compelling evidence against the hypothesis is that canine distemper became rare in dogs after the introduction of MLV-CD vaccines in the early 1960s, although the incidence of MS remained unchanged. Because the incubation period of MS is usually less than 30 years, CDV cannot be a factor.

PREGNANCY

• In utero infection of fetuses with CDV may lead to abortion or persistent infection. Infected pups may appear normal at birth but may develop fatal disease by 4-6 weeks of age. • In utero infection occurs in antibody-negative bitches and is rare.

SYNONYMS

Canine distemper, maladie de Carré, hard pad disease, hundestaupe

SEE ALSO N/A

ABBREVIATIONS

CDV = canine distemper virus
MLV = modified live virus
MV = measles virus
MS = multiple sclerosis

References

Greene CE, Appel MJ. Canine distemper. In: Greene CE, ed. Infectious diseases of the dog and cat. Philadelphia: WB Saunders, 1990:226-241.

Krakowka S, Olsen R, Confer A, Koestner A, McCullough B. Serologic response to canine distemper viral antigens in gnotobiotic dogs infected with canine distemper virus. J Infect Dis 1975;132:384-392.

Author Max J. G. Appel
Consulting Editor Fred W. Scott

DOUBLE AORTIC ARCH

BASICS

OVERVIEW
• A vascular ring anomaly caused by persistence of both sides of the fourth aortic arch
• The ascending aorta divides into a left branch (left and ventral to the esophagus) and a right branch (right and dorsal to the esophagus) which reunite to form the descending aorta. • The two arches may cause constriction of the esophagus. • Both left and right branches are usually patent.

SIGNALMENT
German shepherd

SIGNS

Historical Findings
• Regurgitation secondary to esophageal obstruction • Failure to thrive

Physical Examination Findings
Stunted growth

CAUSES AND RISK FACTORS
Unknown; genetic basis not documented

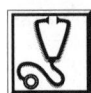

DIAGNOSIS

DIFFERENTIAL DIAGNOSIS
Persistent right aortic arch—exploratory surgery required to differentiate

CBC/BIOCHEMISTRY/URINALYSIS
No consistent abnormalities

OTHER LABORATORY TESTS N/A

IMAGING

Radiographic Findings
Esophageal dilatation cranial to heart

Echocardiographic Findings
Not reported

Angiographic Findings
Diagnostic outline of double aortic arch

OTHER DIAGNOSTIC TESTS

Electrocardiographic Findings
No consistent abnormalities

TREATMENT
• Patients with aspiration pneumonia should be hospitalized until stable.
• Surgical correction indicated; the procedure is similar to correction of persistent right aortic arch. The branch with the least blood flow is removed.

MEDICATIONS

DRUGS AND FLUIDS
• Broad-spectrum antibiotics indicated if animal has aspiration pneumonia
• No cardiac medications indicated

CONTRAINDICATIONS/POSSIBLE INTERACTIONS N/A

FOLLOW-UP
• Clinical signs resolve after successful surgery
• Very poor prognosis unless corrected
• Serious postoperative complications occurred in one reported case (acute left heart failure).

MISCELLANEOUS

ASSOCIATED CONDITIONS
Pulmonic stenosis and tricuspid dysplasia

SEE ALSO
Persistent right aortic arch

Reference
Bonagura JD, Darke P. Congenital heart disease. In: Ettinger SJ, Feldman EC, eds. Textbook of veterinary internal medicine. 4th ed. Philadelphia: WB Saunders, 1995.
Author John-Karl Goodwin
Consulting Editors Larry P. Tilley and Francis W. K. Smith, Jr.

BASICS

OVERVIEW
• Dysfunction of the autonomous nervous system • Etiopathogenesis unknown

SIGNALMENT
• Mainly cats in Great Britain. Rare in dogs and cats worldwide. • Most affected dogs and cats < 3 years old • No breed or sex predilection and no genetic basis

SIGNS
• Generally acute • Most common signs—depression, anorexia, constipation, dry external nares and mouth, reduced tear production, regurgitation due to megaesophagus, dilated pupils with absent or depressed pupillary light responses, prolapsed third eyelids, and bradycardia • Less common signs—anal areflexia, fecal incontinence, and dysuria or urinary incontinence • In dogs, diarrhea is more common than constipation.

CAUSES AND RISK FACTORS
Unknown

DIAGNOSIS

DIFFERENTIAL DIAGNOSIS
• Dehydration secondary to a primary gastrointestinal disorder is the most likely differential. • Dilated, poorly responsive pupils, absence of tear production on Schirmer tear test, and poor esophageal motility on contrast radiography differentiate dysautonomia from most primary gastrointestinal diseases.

CBC/BIOCHEMISTRY/URINALYSIS
• Results normal or indicate dehydration
• Heinz body anemia in some cats

OTHER LABORATORY TESTS N/A

IMAGING
• Survey radiography of the thorax often reveals megaesophagus. • Barium contrast radiography or fluoroscopy best demonstrate esophageal dysfunction. Delayed gastric emptying and contrast retention in the colon seen in many affected animals.

OTHER DIAGNOSTIC PROCEDURES
• Schirmer tear test value < 5 mm/minute in most affected animals • Ophthalmic pharmacologic testing—phospholine iodide 0.06% has no miotic effect; pilocarpine 0.1% has an exaggerated miotic effect because of denervation hypersensitivity. Testing is not 100% reliable. Some animals with dysautonomia do not respond as expected. • Low plasma or urinary catecholamine concentration confirms sympathetic insufficiency. • Intradermal histamine (1:1000) response test fails to demonstrate the normal weal and flare reaction because of the defect in sympathetic innervation of blood vessels.

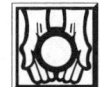

TREATMENT
• Patients are hospitalized for initial treatment.
• Oral intake is temporarily withheld, especially in dogs, to prevent aspiration pneumonia secondary to regurgitation.
• Extensive nursing care at home necessary for several months to a year for recovery to take place. Even in the best managed patients, relapse and death are common.

MEDICATIONS

DRUGS AND FLUIDS
• Intravenously administer warm isotonic fluids initially to correct hypovolemia, hypothermia, hypoglycemia and other electrolyte abnormalities.

• Metoclopromide may reduce vomiting and improve gastric emptying.
• In almost all patients, nutrition must be provided by nasogastric tube, percutaneous gastrostomy tube, or total parenteral nutrition for weeks to months until regurgitation has subsided. The percutaneous gastrostomy tube is generally the best method, since it permits the owner to easily feed the animal at home for a long period.
• Parasympathomimetic eye drops such as pilocarpine (0.1-1%) q8h-q12h improve lacrimation.
• Bethanechol (2.5-7.5 mg PO divided q8h-q12h) may improve gastrointestinal motility and bladder emptying.

CONTRAINDICATIONS/POSSIBLE INTERACTIONS
Pilocarpine and bethanechol should be used carefully, starting with the lowest possible dosage, since denervation hypersensitivity can cause arrhythmias and bradycardia.

FOLLOW-UP
• Prognosis poor. Only 20-50% of affected animals survive after several months to 1 year of slow recovery. • Megaesophagus, constipation, fecal incontinence, and pupil dilation may persist. • Aspiration pneumonia may cause death.

MISCELLANEOUS

Reference
Sharp NJH. Feline dysautonomia. Sem Vet Med Surg (Small Anim) 1990;5:67-71.
Author Allen Sisson
Consulting Editor Joane M. Parent

DYSRAPHISM, SPINAL

BASICS

OVERVIEW
Abnormal spinal cord development along the median plane leading to a variety of structural anomalies such as hydromyelia, duplicated or absent central canal, syringomyelia, and aberrations in the dorsal median septum and ventral medial fissure. The thoracic and lumbar spinal segments are most commonly affected.

SIGNALMENT
• Hereditary in weimaraners • Also described in English bulldog, Samoyed, dalmatian, English setter, golden retriever, mixed-breed dogs, and cats • No sex predilection

SIGNS
• Apparent by 3-6 weeks of age and do not progress • Vary in severity • Simultaneous flexion and extension of pelvic limbs ("bunny hopping") • Proprioceptive deficits, base wide stance, and crouched pelvic limb posture

CAUSES AND RISK FACTORS
• Genetic in weimaraners. The homozygous condition is lethal. Clinically affected dogs are heterozygote. • In utero spinal cord damage caused by infection, trauma, and vascular compromise may cause syringomyelia (cavitation of the spinal cord). • Idiopathic in isolated patients

DIAGNOSIS

DIFFERENTIAL DIAGNOSIS
• The disease is easily differentiated from the common spinal cord diseases, because it is present at birth and nonprogressive. • The diagnostic challenge is to define the malformations.

CBC/BIOCHEMISTRY/URINALYSIS
Results usually normal

OTHER LABORATORY TESTS N/A

IMAGING
• Survey and contrast spinal radiography reveals associated vertebral column anomalies and spinal cord compression in some patients. • Without sophisticated imaging techniques, an antemortem diagnosis may be impossible to make in dogs other than weimaraners.

OTHER DIAGNOSTIC PROCEDURES
N/A

TREATMENT
• None available
• Mildly affected animals can be acceptable pets.
• Severely affected animals may benefit from a canine cart. Euthanasia is a consideration.

MEDICATIONS

DRUGS AND FLUIDS
Antibiotics are chosen on the basis of bacterial culture of urine and sensitivity test if the patient has secondary urinary tract infection.

CONTRAINDICATIONS/POSSIBLE INTERACTIONS N/A

FOLLOW-UP
• Because of the hind limb gait disturbance, affected animals are more prone than normal animals to temporary or permanent exacerbation of signs along with the development of metabolic, degenerative joint, or spinal column disease. • Secondary urinary tract infection develops in severely affected animals because of disorders of micturition. • Decubitus ulcers and urine and faecal scalds in recumbent animals can be avoided by proper care.

MISCELLANEOUS
Congenital vertebral arch (ie, spina bifida) and vertebral body-disk malformation (eg, hemivertebra and block vertebra) may be associated with myelodysplasia but alone often do not cause clinical signs.

ABBREVIATIONS
CT = computed tomography
MRI = magnetic resonance imaging

Reference
Bailey CS, Morgan JP. Congenital malformations. In: Moore MP, ed. Diseases of the spine. Philadelphia: WB Saunders. Vet Clin North Am (Small Anim Pract) 1992;22:985-1015.

Author Richard J. Joseph
Consulting Editor Joane M. Parent

BASICS

OVERVIEW
These mites (Otodectes cynotis) cause a hypersensitivity reaction which results in intense irritation of the external ear of dogs and cats.

SIGNALMENT
• This is a common disease in young dogs and cats although it may occur at any age.
• No breed or sex predilection exists.

SIGNS
• This disease is characterized by pruritus primarily located around the ears, head and neck. • Occasionally, the pruritus may be generalized. • Thick, red-brown or black crusts are usually present in the outer ear.
• Crusting and scales may also be present on the neck, rump, and tail. • Excoriations on the convex surface of the pinnae are often present due to the intense pruritus.

CASES AND RISK FACTORS N/A

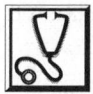

DIAGNOSIS

DIFFERENTIAL DIAGNOSIS
• Flea bite hypersensitivity • Pediculosis
• Pelodera dermatitis • Sarcoptic mange
• Chiggers • Allergic dermatitis

CBC/BIOCHEMISTRY/URINALYSIS
Complete blood counts, serum chemistry profiles, and urinalysis are normal in this process.

OTHER LABORATORY TESTS N/A

IMAGING N/A

OTHER DIAGNOSTIC PROCEDURES
• Skin scrapings may reveal mites if signs are generalized. • Ear swabs placed in mineral oil are usually a very effective means of identifying this mite.

TREATMENT
• The patient should be treated as an outpatient.
• No alteration of diet or activity is necessary.
• This is a very contagious disease. Therefore, all in-contact animals must be treated.
• The environment should also be thoroughly cleaned and treated.

MEDICATIONS

DRUGS AND FLUIDS
• First, the ears should cleaned thoroughly with mineral oil or a commercial ear cleaner to remove debris.
• Then the ears can be treated with rotenone-based products twice per week initially, then decreased to weekly. This should be continued until 2 weeks post clinical cure.
• Alternatively, ivermectin can be used systemically or topically. Systemic treatment with ivermectin (bovine 1%) (300 mcg/kg subcutaneously) every 1-2 weeks for approximately 4 treatments was found to be effective in one recent study. Topical treatment with 500 mcg of ivermectin directly placed in the ears was necessary every 1-2 weeks for approximately 5 weeks and was associated with a higher incidence of recurrence. This dosage of ivermectin is not approved for use in dogs or cats in the United States. Additionally, heartworm positive dogs may exhibit a shock-like reaction, probably due to dying microfilaria.
• Amitraz (1 ml in 33 ml mineral oil) has also been applied as a topical directly into the ear. Amitraz is not approved for this usage.
• The entire animal should be treated with pyrethrin-based flea spray weekly for 4-6 weeks if not using systemic ivermectin.
• The environment should also be treated with a flea type preparation two times, 2-4 weeks apart.

CONTRAINDICATIONS/POSSIBLE INTERACTIONS
• Ivermectin should not be used in collies, shelties, their crosses, or other herding breeds.
• It should be used only if absolutely necessary in animals less than 6 months of age since an increasing number of toxic reactions have recently been reported in kittens.
• Amitraz used topically for generalized mite infestations has been reported to cause adverse reactions in cats and thus is not recommended.

FOLLOW-UP
• An ear swab and physical examination should be done 1 month after therapy commences. • In most patients, the prognosis is good. Rarely, the ear mites will be cleared only to find an underlying allergy that keeps the otitis externa active.

MISCELLANEOUS

ZOONOTIC POTENTIAL
The mites will also bite humans (rare).

Reference
Mueller GH, Kirk RW, Scott DW, eds. Small animal dermatology. 4th ed. Philadelphia:WB Saunders, 1989:367-369.
Author Karen A. Kuhl
Consulting Editor Lowell Ackerman

EBSTEIN'S ANOMALY

BASICS

OVERVIEW
• Atrialization of the right ventricle—an apical displacement of the tricuspid valve complex into the right ventricle • Accompanied by various degrees of tricuspid insufficiency • Major pathophysiology related to the degree of tricuspid insufficiency • An abnormal accessory pathway may lead to supraventricular tachycardias.

SIGNALMENT
A very rare lesion, occasionally encountered in dogs and cats. No breed or sex predilection. Murmur ausculted at a young age.

SIGNS
• Animals with mild tricuspid insufficiency are asymptomatic. • Animals with severe insufficiency have right-sided congestive heart failure (R-CHF) with pleural effusion and/or ascites .

CAUSES AND RISK FACTORS N/A

DIAGNOSIS

DIFFERENTIAL DIAGNOSIS
Tricuspid dysplasia

CBC/BIOCHEMISTRY/URINALYSIS
Results usually normal

OTHER LABORATORY TESTS N/A

IMAGING
Thoracic Radiographic Findings
• Right atrial and ventricular enlargement
• Hepatomegaly

Echocardiography
Two-dimensional echocardiography reveals apically displaced tricuspid valve.

OTHER DIAGNOSTIC PROCEDURES
Electrocardiography
• Simultaneous intracardiac pressure and ECG tracings may be needed to verify the diagnosis. • Accessory conduction pathway (ventricular pre-excitation) or supraventricular tachycardia

TREATMENT

• Medical management currently the only practical approach
• Restrict sodium intake if right heart failure develops

MEDICATIONS

DRUGS AND FLUIDS
• In animals with R-CHF, treatment with furosemide (2-4 mg/kg q6h-q12h) and enalapril (0.5 mg/kg q12h) should be instituted.
• In animals with supraventricular tachycardia (WPW), procainamide (15 mg/kg q8h) can be started.
• If the tachycardia (WPW) persists, consider a calcium channel blocker (verapamil or diltiazem) or a beta blocker (propranolol or atenolol).

CONTRAINDICATIONS/POSSIBLE INTERACTIONS
Do not use calcium channel blockers and beta blockers concurrently.

FOLLOW-UP
• Monitor with serial echocardiograms, ECG, and radiographs.

MISCELLANEOUS

SEE ALSO
Tricuspid valve dysplasia

ABBREVIATIONS
WPW = Wolff-Parkinson-White syndrome
R-CHF = right-sided congestive heart failure

References
Zipes DP. Specific arrhythmias. In: Braunwald E, ed. Heart disease. 4th ed. Philadelphia: WB Saunders, 1992.
Friedman WF. Congenital heart disease in infancy and childhood. In: Braunwald E, ed. Heart disease. 4th ed. Philadelphia: WB Saunders, 1992.
Bonagura JD. Congenital heart disease. In: Ettinger SJ, ed. Textbook of veterinary internal medicine. 3rd ed. Philadelphia: WB Saunders, 1989.

Author Carroll Loyer
Consulting Editors Larry P. Tilley and Francis W. K. Smith, Jr.

BASICS

OVERVIEW
• Postparturient hypocalcemia • Usually develops 1-4 weeks postpartum but can happen at term, prepartum, or late lactation • Alters cell membrane potentials causing spontaneous discharge of nerve fibers and tonoclonic contraction of skeletal muscles • Life-threatening tetany and convulsions leading to hyperthermia • Cerebral edema possible

SIGNALMENT
• Postpartum bitch • Most common in toy breeds • Higher incidence with first litter • Rare in the queen

SIGNS

Historical Findings
• Restlessness, nervousness • Panting, whining • Ataxia, stiff gait • Muscle tremors, tetany, convulsions • Recumbency, extensor rigidity usually seen 8-12 hours after onset of signs

Physical Examination Findings
• Hyperthermia • Rapid respiratory rate • Dilated pupils, sluggish pupillary light responses • Muscle tremors, muscular rigidity, convulsions

CAUSES AND RISK FACTORS
• Calcium supplementation during gestation • Large litter size • Poor prenatal nutrition

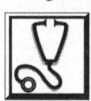

DIAGNOSIS

DIFFERENTIAL DIAGNOSIS
• Hypoglycemia—may be concurrent; muscular rigidity does not occur with hypoglycemia alone • Toxicosis—signalment and history differentiate • Epilepsy or other neurologic disorder—signalment helps to differentiate. Calcium concentration diagnostic.

CBC/BIOCHEMISTRY/URINALYSIS
• Serum calcium < 7 mg/dl • Hypoglycemia may be concurrent.

IMAGING OTHER LABORATORY TESTS N/A

OTHER DIAGNOSTIC PROCEDURES N/A

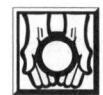

TREATMENT
• Emergency inpatient treatment
• Cool hyperthermic patient with cool water soak and fans. Cool water enemas used with caution.
• Puppies removed from dam to hand raise. If owner refuses to hand raise pups, remove them for a minimum of 24 hours to spare the dam, and provide her with food supplementation.

MEDICATIONS

DRUGS AND FLUIDS
• Calcium gluconate—10% solution 1 ml/kg IV given slowly to effect over 5 minutes; monitor heart rate or ECG during administration; additional calcium gluconate can be given IM or SQ
• Correct hypoglycemia.
• Diazepam (5 mg IV) if seizures unresponsive
• Treat cerebral edema if indicated.
• Calcium lactate, carbonate, or gluconate at 30-100 mg/kg/day PO until lactation ends
• Feed balanced diet

CONTRAINDICATIONS/POSSIBLE INTERACTIONS
Avoid corticosteroids because they decrease intestinal absorption and increase renal excretion of calcium.

FOLLOW-UP
• Monitor serum calcium concentration until it stabilizes in the normal range. • Avoid calcium supplementation during gestation.
• Feed diet with calcium-phosphorus ratio of 1:1 or 1.2:1 • Avoid diet high in phytates (e.g., soybeans) • Supplement feeding of the pups in large litters. • Probably will recur with subsequent litters

POSSIBLE COMPLICATIONS
• Cerebral edema • Death • Hand-raising of puppies

EXPECTED COURSE AND PROGNOSIS
• Good with immediate treatment • Poor if treatment delayed

MISCELLANEOUS

Reference
Kaufman J. Eclampsia in the bitch. In: Morrow DA, ed. Current therapy in theriogenology. 2nd ed. Philadelphia: WB Saunders, 1986:511-512.

Author Joni L. Freshman

Consulting Editor Sara K. Lyle

ECTOPIC URETERS

BASICS

DEFINITION
Ectopic ureters have the following characteristics:
- Congenital abnormality in which the ureter opens into urethra or vagina. One or both ureters can be affected.
- In dogs, the ureter may enter the bladder in the normal location, tunnel through the bladder wall, and bypass the trigone.
- Less frequently, the ureter opens into the trigone and continues as a trough into the urethra.
- In cats, the ureter completely bypasses the bladder and enters the urethra. This rarely occurs in dogs.

SIGNALMENT
- The following dog breeds are predisposed— Siberian husky, Newfoundland, bulldog, West Highland white terrier, fox terrier, and miniature and toy poodle.
- Infrequently diagnosed in cats and male dogs

SIGNS
- Intermittent or continuous incontinence
- Normal voiding in some animals
- Vaginitis from urine scalding

CAUSES AND RISK FACTORS
- Apparent breed predisposition
- Unknown mode of inheritance; bitches with ectopic ureters have had litters of puppies with no observed incontinence.

DIAGNOSIS

DIFFERENTIAL DIAGNOSIS
- Inappropriate urination, i.e., wrong place or time, but under voluntary control
- Urethral sphincter mechanism incompetence. (Use excretory urogram to exclude possibility of ectopic ureter.)
- Patent urachus. Moist abdomen.

Radiographic contrast studies identify opening in ventral abdomen.
- Paradoxical incontinence. Occurs secondary to urethral obstruction. Pass catheter to identify calculi, stricture, or mass.
- Urinary tract infection. Can cause pollakiuria mimicking incontinence.
- Severe polyuria associated with renal failure caused by either congenital kidney disease or severe pyelonephritis. Measure urine specific gravity to determine ability to concentrate urine. Polyuria and polydipsia associated with low urine specific gravity.

CBC/BIOCHEMISTRY/URINALYSIS
Urine specific gravity and serum creatinine or urea nitrogen concentration should be normal.

OTHER LABORATORY TESTS
Urine bacteriologic culture, collected by cystocentesis, often reveals concurrent urinary tract infection.

IMAGING
Excretory urography and a pneumocystogram, followed by a vaginourethrogram (female) or urethrogram (male) used to identify ectopic ureter. May also diagnose hydroureter, absent, small or misshapen kidneys, hydronephrosis, and tortuous or obstructed ureters.

OTHER DIAGNOSTIC PROCEDURES
None

TREATMENT
- Surgical creation of a new ureteral opening into the bladder or excision of a hydronephrotic or infected kidney
- Warn owners that incontinence may continue if dog also has urethral sphincter mechanism incompetence.

MEDICATIONS

DRUGS AND FLUIDS N/A

CONTRAINDICATIONS/POSSIBLE INTERACTIONS N/A

FOLLOW-UP
- Incontinence may persist after surgery.
- Incontinent dogs need repeat evaluation including excretory urogram, pneumocystogram, and vaginourethrogram.
- An intrapelvic bladder neck may contribute to urinary incontinence in dogs with urethral sphincter mechanism incompetence. Moving the bladder neck to an intra–abdominal position by colposuspension may correct the incontinence.
- If incontinence persists, try phenylpropanolamine (1.5 mg/kg PO q8h), an alpha–blocker drug, or imipramine (0.5 to 1 mg/kg PO q8h), a tricyclic antidepressor agent.

MISCELLANEOUS

Reference
Stone EA, Barsanti JA. Urologic Surgery of the Dog and Cat. Philadelphia. Lea & Febiger. 1992. 201-211.
Author Elizabeth Arnold Stone
Consulting Editor Larry G. Adams and Carl A. Osborne

BASICS

OVERVIEW

Ectropion is the eversion or rolling out of the eyelid margin resulting in exposure of the palpebral conjunctiva. Exposure and poor tear distribution may predispose affected individuals to sight-threatening corneal disease.

SIGNALMENT

• Seldom seen in cats. • Canine breeds with higher than average prevalence include sporting breeds (i.e., spaniels, hounds, and retrievers), giant breeds (i.e., St. Bernard and Mastiff), and any breed with loose facial skin (especially bloodhound). • Developmental ectropion is genetically predisposed in the above-mentioned breeds and may be noticed in dogs less than 1 year old. • Acquired ectropion may be seen in other breeds and occurs later in life secondary to age-related loss of facial musculature and developing skin laxity. • Intermittent ectropion caused by fatigue may be observed in animals after strenuous exercise or when drowsy.

SIGNS

• Eversion of the lower eyelid with lack of contact of the lower lid to the globe and exposure of the palpebral conjunctiva and third eyelid is usually obvious. • Common owner complaints include facial staining caused by poor tear drainage (tears spill over onto the face instead of passing from the eye to the nose via the nasolacrimal ducts) and history of mucoid to mucopurulent discharge due to conjunctival exposure, recurrent foreign body irritation, or bacterial conjunctivitis.

CAUSES AND RISK FACTORS

• Disease in most animals is secondary to breed associated alterations in facial conformation and eyelid support. • Marked weight loss or muscle mass loss about the head and orbits may result in acquired ectropion.
• The tragic facial expression in hypothyroid dogs may lead to ectropion. • Scarring of the eyelids secondary to injury or after overcorrection of entropion may result in cicatricial ectropion.

DIAGNOSIS

DIFFERENTIAL DIAGNOSIS

• Ectropion is usually clinically obvious, but in nonpredisposed breeds and animals with late-age onset ectropion, patients should be scrutinized to determine if there is an underlying disorder. • Loss of orbital or periorbital mass may cause ectropion in patients with masticatory myositis. • Animals with palpebral nerve paralysis may have ectropion associated with lack of muscle tone of the orbicularis oculi muscles.

CBC/BIOCHEMISTRY/URINALYSIS

N/A

OTHER LABORATORY TESTS

• Animals with possible masticatory myositis should be tested for autoantibodies against type 2M muscle fibers. • Consider testing for hypothyroidism in animals with palpebral nerve paralysis or tragic facial expression.

IMAGING N/A

OTHER DIAGNOSTIC PROCEDURES

• Animals with palpebral nerve paralysis should have full neurologic evaluation and potentially be tested for hypothyroidism.
• Consider bacterial culture or cytologic examination of conjunctiva if secondary conjunctivitis is present to help select an appropriate topical antibiotic. • Fluorescein or Rose Bengal staining of the cornea and conjunctiva may document corneal ulcerations and the severity of the exposure problem.

TREATMENT

• Supportive care and good ocular and facial hygiene is sufficient to medically manage most mildly affected patients.
• Surgical treatment in the form of eyelid shortening or radical facelift is necessary in more severely affected patients that have chronic ocular irritation.
• Intermittent, fatigue-induced ectropion should not be treated surgically.

MEDICATIONS

DRUGS AND FLUIDS

• Supportive treatment in the form of topically administered, broad-spectrum ophthalmic antibiotics for bacterial conjunctivitis or corneal ulceration is indicated.
• Lubricant eye drops and ointments are indicated to reduce conjunctival and corneal desiccation secondary to exposure.
• Patients with hypothyroid and masticatory myositis-induced ectropion may respond well to appropriate medical treatment of the underlying disease.

CONTRAINDICATIONS/POSSIBLE INTERACTIONS N/A

FOLLOW-UP

• As patients age, ectropion may become more severe. • Nonsurgically treated animals should be monitored for signs of infectious conjunctivitis, exposure keratopathy and corneal ulceration, and facial dermatitis.

MISCELLANEOUS

SEE ALSO

• Hypothyroidism • Myopathy, masticatory muscle myositis

Reference

Slatter D. Eyelids. In: Fundamentals of veterinary ophthalmology. 2nd ed. Philadelphia: WB Saunders, 1990.

Author J. Phillip Pickett

Consulting Editor Paul E. Miller

EHRLICHIOSIS

BASICS

DEFINITION
• Ehrlichiosis is a tick-borne rickettsial disease of which the main clinically important organisms include Ehrlichia canis (causing canine ehrlichiosis and is found intracytoplasmically in circulating leukocytes) and E. platys (causing infectious cyclic thrombocytopenia and is found in platelets). • E. equi (found in neutrophils) may infect dogs. • Cats can be infected with E. risticii, and there is serologic evidence to suggest that a species similar to E. canis can cause illness in cats.

Pathophysiology
E. canis

Ticks (Rhipicephalus sanguineus—brown dog tick) transmit the disease to dogs in saliva. Following a 1-3 week incubation period, three stages of disease may occur.

Acute

Spread from the bite site to the spleen, liver, and lymph nodes occurs (causing organomegaly). Infects mainly endothelial cells producing vasculitis resulting in a reduction in platelet survival time causing thrombocytopenia, leukopenia variable, and mild anemia.

Subclinical

Organism persists and antibody response increases (hyperglobulinemia). Thrombocytopenia persists.

Chronic

Impaired bone marrow production (platelets, erythroid suppression) as bone marrow becomes hypercellular with plasma cells.

Systems Affected
Multisystemic Involvement

• Bleeding tendencies from thrombocytopenia and vasculitis • Lymphadenopathy • Splenomegaly • CNS, eyes (anterior uveitis), and lungs rarely affected by vasculitis.

Genetics N/A

Incidence/Prevalence
• Occurs throughout the year mainly because of the insidious nature of the disease.
• Average duration of illness from onset of illness to presentation is usually over 2 months.
• Prevalence varies between geographic localities.

Geographic Distribution
Worldwide. Within North America, mainly the Gulf coast and eastern seaboard, but also the Midwest and California.

SIGNALMENT
• Dogs are infected with E. canis and E. platys. Cats can be infected with E. risticii and there is serologic evidence to suggest that a species similar to E. canis can cause illness in cats. • Chronic form of E. canis seems to be more severe in doberman pinschers and German shepherds. • Average age of animals is 5.22 years, with a range of 2 months to 14

years. The duration of clinical signs from initial acute illness until presentation is usually more than 2 months.

SIGNS

Historical Findings
• Lethargy, depression, and anorexia
• Weight loss • Fever • Spontaneous bleeding (sneezing, epistaxis) • Respiratory distress
• Neurologic signs (ataxia, head tilt)
• Ocular pain

Physical Examination Findings
Acute

• Bleeding diathesis (petechiation of mucous membranes as a result of thrombocytopenia) in association with fever (associated with depression, anorexia, weight loss) and generalized lymphadenopathy should raise suspicions.
• Ticks present in acute stage 40% of time.
• Respiratory signs, including dyspnea (even cyanosis), and increased bronchovesicular sounds • Diffuse central nervous disease, ataxia with upper motor neuron dysfunction, vestibular dysfunction, and generalized or local hyperesthesia • Most dogs recover from acute stage without treatment to enter subclinical state.

Chronic

• In nonendemic areas, ehrlichiosis is usually chronic. • Spontaneous bleeding • Anemia
• Generalized lymphadenopathy • Scrotal and limb edema • Splenomegaly, and hepatomegaly • Uveitis, hyphema, retinal hemorrhages and detachment with blindness, and corneal edema. • Rarely, arthritis (both poly and mono) and seizures

CAUSES N/A

RISK FACTORS
Concurrent infection with Babesia, Haemobartonella, E. platys, and Hepatozoon canis will worsen the clinical syndrome.

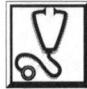

DIAGNOSIS

DIFFERENTIAL DIAGNOSIS
• Rocky Mountain spotted fever (Rickettsia rickettsii)—usually occurs seasonally between March and October. Serologic testing for diagnosis. Both RMSF and ehrlichiosis respond to same treatment. • Immune-mediated thrombocytopenia—not usually associated with fever or lymphadenopathy. Serologic testing used to best distinguish from ehrlichiosis. Often treat for both until titers back. • Systemic lupus erythematosus—antinuclear antibody test usually negative in animals with ehrlichiosis. Serology for diagnosis.
• Multiple myeloma—differentiated from chronic ehrlichiosis by serology to distinguish cause of hyperglobulinemia. • Chronic lymphocytic leukemia (CLL)—differentiated from chronic ehrlichiosis by lymphocytosis, and cytology of bone marrow • Brucellosis as a cause of scrotal edema—serology for diagnosis

CBC/BIOCHEMISTRY/URINALYSIS

Acute
• Thrombocytopenia • Anemia • Leukopenia (mainly resulting from lymphopenia, eosinopenia) • Leukocytosis (and monocytosis) as disease becomes more chronic
• Morulae (intracytoplasmic inclusions in leukocytes) are rare. • Usually nonspecific changes, including mild increases in ALT, ALP, BUN, creatinine, and total bilirubin (rare). • Hyperglobulinemia progressively increases from 1-3 weeks postinfection.
• Hypoalbuminemia (usually from renal loss)
• Proteinuria (with or without azotemia) occurs in about half of dogs with ehrlichiosis.
• The rest of the urinalysis is nonspecific.

Chronic
• Typically, pancytopenia, although monocytosis and lymphocytosis may be present.
• Hyperglobulinemia—magnitude of globulin increases correlates with duration of infection. Usually polyclonal gammopathy, but monoclonal (IgG) gammopathies occur.
• Hypoalbuminemia • Elevations in BUN and creatinine may occur from primary renal disease (resulting from glomerulonephritis and renal interstitial plasmacytosis).

OTHER LABORATORY TESTS
• Serologic testing is the most clinically useful and reliable method to diagnose ehrlichiosis. IFA is highly sensitive, although a low level of cross-reactivity with other ehrlichia can occur.
• Titers > 1:10 are diagnostic (titers reliable after 3 weeks postinfection). • Coombs' positive anemia may be present, confusing the diagnosis.

IMAGING N/A

OTHER DIAGNOSTIC PROCEDURES
Bone marrow aspirate—in acute disease, hypercellularity of megakaryocytic and myeloid series. In chronic disease, erythroid hypoplasia with increased M:E ratios and plasmacytosis often occurs. Occasionally, increased numbers of mast cells are seen on marrow smears.

GROSS AND HISTOPATHOLOGIC FINDINGS

Acute
Petechial hemorrhages on serosal and mucosal surfaces of most organs. Generalized lymphadenopathy (brownish discoloration), splenomegaly, hepatomegaly, and red bone marrow (hypercellularity).

Chronic
• Marrow is pale (hypoplastic). Subcutaneous edema. • Histologically, perivascular plasma cell infiltrate in numerous organs is the most characteristic finding. • Multifocal nonsuppurative meningoencephalitis with lymphoplasmacytic cell infiltrate into the meninges is common.

TREATMENT

INPATIENT VERSUS OUTPATIENT

• Patient with anemia and/or hemorrhagic tendency resulting from thrombocytopenia should be hospitalized for initial medical stabilization.

• Stable patients can be treated as outpatients with frequent monitoring of blood picture and response to medication.

ACTIVITY Restricted

DIET N/A

CLIENT EDUCATION

• Excellent prognosis is expected in acute cases with appropriate therapy. Response may take a month in chronic cases, unless the bone marrow is severely hypoplastic, in which case the prognosis is poor.

• Progression of disease from acute to chronic form can be easily prevented by early, effective treatment.

• Other pathogens may accompany E. canis infection (Babesiosis, Haemobartonellosis, E. platys, and Hepatozoon canis) and should be tested.

• German shepherds and doberman pinschers display a more chronic and severe form of the disease.

SURGICAL CONSIDERATIONS

If surgery is needed for other reasons, blood transfusion may be needed to correct anemia and/or thrombocytopenia.

MEDICATIONS

DRUGS AND FLUIDS

• Doxycycline, a synthetic derivative of tetracycline, is the drug of choice (5 mg/kg q12h PO for 14 days) and can be given intravenously for 5 days if the dog is vomiting. Oxytetracycline and tetracycline (22 mg/kg, q8h PO for 21 days) are also effective and less expensive.

• In puppies under 6 months of age, chloramphenicol (20 mg/kg q8h PO for 14 days) is recommended to avoid yellow discoloration of erupting teeth caused by tetracyclines. However, owners should be warned of chloramphenicol's public health risks because it directly interferes with heme and bone marrow synthesis. Similarly, its use should be avoided in dogs with thrombocytopenia, pancytopenia, or anemia.

• Glucocorticoids (prednisolone/prednisone 1-2 mg/kg q12h PO for 5 days) may be indicated in acute cases in which thrombocytopenia is life-threatening (thought to be a result of immune-mediated mechanisms). Also, because immune-mediated thrombocytopenia is the main other differential diagnosis, glucocorticoid therapy may be indicated until results of serologic tests are available.

• Balanced electrolyte solution is indicated in dehydrated animals.

• Blood transfusion is indicated in anemic animals.

• Platelet-rich plasma or a blood transfusion is indicated in animals with hemorrhage resulting from thrombocytopenia.

• Androgenic steroids can be used to stimulate bone marrow production in chronically affected dogs with hypoplastic marrows. Oxymetholone (2 mg/kg q24h PO until response) and nandrolone decanoate (1.5 mg/kg/wk, IM) are the drugs of choice.

CONTRAINDICATIONS

• Do not use tetracyclines (or derivatives) in dogs under 6 months of age because permanent yellowing of the teeth will occur.

• Do not use tetracyclines in dogs with renal insufficiency. Doxycycline may be used as it can be excreted via the gastrointestinal tract.

PRECAUTIONS

Prolonged use of glucocorticoids at immunosuppressive levels may interfere with the clearance and elimination of E. canis after therapy with tetracycline.

POSSIBLE INTERACTIONS N/A

ALTERNATE DRUGS

Imidocarb dipropionate (5 mg/kg, q24h, IM once) is effective against both E. canis and Babesiosis but is unavailable in the United States.

FOLLOW-UP

PATIENT MONITORING N/A

• Repeat platelet count every 3 days after initiating antirickettsial agent until showing an increase into normal range. Should be rapid improvement in acute cases. • Repeat serology in 9 months. If treatment has been successful, most dogs will be seronegative. A positive titer suggests reinfection (prior infection does not imply protective immunity) or ineffective first treatment, and a subsequent treatment regimen should be instituted.

PREVENTION/AVOIDANCE

• Control tick infestation on dogs using dips or sprays containing dichlorvos, chlorfenvinphos, dioxathion, propoxur, or carbaryl. Flea and tick collars may reduce reinfestation but their reliability is unproven. Avoid tick-infested areas. • When removing ticks from dogs by hand, use gloves (see zoonosis) and ensure tick mouth parts are removed, because a foreign body reaction is likely to result if they are left in place.

POSSIBLE COMPLICATIONS N/A

EXPECTED COURSE AND PROGNOSIS

Acute cases have an excellent prognosis with appropriate treatment. Chronic forms may take 4 weeks for a clinical response. If the marrow is hypoplastic, the prognosis is poor.

MISCELLANEOUS

ASSOCIATED CONDITIONS

Babesia, Haemobartonella, and E. platys may all occur with Ehrlichiosis.

AGE RELATED FACTORS N/A

ZOONOTIC POTENTIAL

• Serologic evidence indicates that E. canis (or possibly a related species) occurs in people (most cases in the southern and south central United States. People probably do not become infected directly from dogs; a tick exposure is thought to be necessary. However, Rhipicephalus sanguineus is probably not the vector in humans. • Major clinical signs in humans include fever, headaches, myalgia, ocular pain, and gastrointestinal upsets. Treatment with tetracyclines results in rapid recovery.

PREGNANCY N/A

SYNONYMS

• Tropical canine pancytopenia • Canine rickettsiosis • Canine hemorrhagic fever • Lahore canine fever • Canine typhus • Tracker dog disease • Nairobi bleeding disease

SEE ALSO N/A

ABBREVIATIONS

CNS = central nervous system
CLL = chronic lymphocytic leukemia

References

Troy GC, Forrester SD. Canine ehrlichiosis. In: Greene CE, ed. Infectious diseases of the dog and cat. Philadelphia: WB Saunders, 1990:404-414.

Perille AL, Matus RE. Canine ehrlichiosis in six dogs with persistently increased antibody titers. J Vet Int Med 1991;5:195-198.

Author Stephen C. Barr
Consulting Editor Fred W. Scott

ELBOW DYSPLASIA

BASICS

DEFINITION

Elbow dysplasia is a general term that describes a series of four developmental abnormalities that lead to malformation and degeneration of the elbow joint.

Pathophysiology

• Elbow dysplasia includes: (1) ununited anconeal process (UAP); (2) osteochondritis dissecans (OCD); (3) fragmented medial coronoid process (FMCP); and (4) incongruity. One or more of these developmental anomalies may occur alone or in combination within one or both elbows of an affected animal. Bilateral disease is common (50%). • UAP is characterized by failure of the anconeus process, which contains a separate ossification center, to unite with the proximal ulnar metaphysis (olecranon) by 5 months of age. • OCD affects the medial trochlear ridge of the distal humerus. Retention of articular cartilage due to a disturbance in endochondral ossification and mechanical stress lead to the formation of a cartilage flap lesion. • FMCP is the chondral or osteochondral fragmentation or fissure of the medial coronoid process of the ulna. It is not considered a traumatic injury but a manifestation of osteochondrosis of the coronoid process. This differs from the related pathology of the anconeal process since the coronoid does not have a separate ossification center. • Incongruity is the manifestation of malalignment and malformation of the elbow joint. Asynchronous proximal growth between the radius and ulna can lead to abnormal load and wear and erosion of cartilage in the humeroulnar compartment of the elbow joint. Incongruity may also be the result of malformation of the trochlear notch of the ulna. A slightly elliptical trochlear notch with a decreased arc of curvature would be too small to articulate with the humeral trochlea. This would result in major points of contact in areas of the anconeal process, coronoid process, and medial humeral condyle and little or no contact in other areas of the trochlea. • Abnormal mechanical stress on the anconeal process, medial coronoid, and medial humeral condyle may also result in UAP, FMCP, and OCD, respectively.

Systems Affected Musculoskeletal

Genetics

• Elbow dysplasia is an inherited disease and the heritability is high. • Heritability index range between 0.25 to 0.45.

Incidence/Prevalence

The most common cause for elbow pain and lameness. One of the most common causes for forelimb lameness in large-breed dogs.

Geographic Distribution N/A

SIGNALMENT

Species Dogs

Breed Predilection

• Large and giant breeds. • Labrador retrievers, Rottweilers, golden retrievers, German shepherds, Bernese mountain dogs, chow, bearded collie, and Newfoundlands

Mean Age And Range

• Age of onset of clinical signs is typically 4-10 months. • Age of diagnosis is generally between 4-18 months. • Signs related to degenerative joint disease (DJD) can occur at any age.

Predominant Sex

• Predisposition for males (FMCP) • None established for UAP, OCD or incongruity

SIGNS

General Comments

• If no distinct abnormalities are noted on physical exam or radiographs when a dog presents for lameness, repeat the examination 4-8 weeks later. • Not all animals are symptomatic at an early age; older animals often present with an acute episode of elbow lameness due to advanced DJD changes.

Historical Findings

Usually examined at 8-10 months of age because of forelimb lameness having progressed from a stiffness that initially was present only after rest to an intermittent or persistent lameness that is exacerbated by exercise.

Physical Examination Findings

• Pain elicited on elbow hyperflexion/extension. • Pain elicited while holding the elbow and carpus at 90° and then pronating and supinating the carpus. • Affected limb has a tendency to be held in abduction and supination. • Joint effusion and capsular distension especially noted between lateral epicondyle and olecranon. • Crepitus can be palpated with advanced DJD • Diminshed range of motion

CAUSES

• Developmental • Nutritional

RISK FACTORS

• Rapid growth and weight gain • Feeding high caloric diet

DIAGNOSIS

DIFFERENTIAL DIAGNOSIS

• Trauma • Septic arthritis • Panosteitis
• Avulsion/calcification of the flexor muscles

CBC/BIOCHEMISTRY/URINALYSIS
N/A

OTHER LABORATORY TESTS N/A

IMAGING

• Four radiographic views may be necessary to diagnose elbow dysplasia. The most common views are a) mediolateral; b) mediolateral hyperflexed; c) 25° craniocaudal-lateromedial oblique; and d) craniocaudal. • Radiograph both elbows because of the high incidence of bilateral disease. • UAP is best diagnosed by the mediolateral hyperflexed view. Lack of bony union is easily seen on this view.
• OCD is best diagnosed by the craniocaudal and oblique views. A radiolucent "defect" or flattening of the medial humeral condyle can be seen. • FMCP is seldom visualized radiographically. Diagnosis is presumptive based on DJD and the absence of UAP or OCD lesions. Common changes include osteophyte formation on the proximal rim of the anconeal process, medial coronoid process, cranial margin of the radial head, and epicondyles (medial and lateral); sclerosis of the ulna caudal to the coronoid process and trochlear notch; and a "stair-step" between the joint surface of the radius and lateral coronoid. These changes are not unique to FMCP and will occur with UAP, OCD, and incongruity. • CAT scan and linear tomography have been shown to be accurate in diagnosing FMCP.

OTHER DIAGNOSTIC PROCEDURES

• Joint tap with analysis of synovial fluid is useful to confirm involvement of joint. Grossly, it should be straw colored with normal to low viscosity. Cytologic evaluation demonstrates <10,000 nucleated cells/microl with more than 90% being mononuclear cells. • Arthroscopy can be used to diagnose UAP, FMCP, and OCD.

GROSS AND HISTOPATHOLOGIC FINDINGS

• UAP-fibrous union between anconeal process and proximal ulnar metaphysis; fibrous tissue invasion and degeneration of the anconeal process; DJD. • OCD-chondral flap on medial humeral condyle; sclerosis of underlying subchondral bone with fibrous tissue invasion; erosive lesion on apposing coronoid cartilage; DJD. • FMCP-chondral or osteochondral fragmentation of the cranial tip or lateral margin of the medial coronoid; erosive lesion on opposing medial humeral condyle cartilage; DJD.

TREATMENT

INPATIENT VERSUS OUTPATIENT

• Surgery is recommended for UAP, OCD, and FMCP.
• Surgery for incongruity is controversial; type of incongruity dictates method of treatment.
• Severity of DJD and age of animal influence surgical outcome.

ACTIVITY

Restricted activity after surgery for all forms of dysplasia.

DIET

• Weight control is important to reduce the load and stress on the affected joint(s).

• Restricted weight gain and growth in young dogs may reduce the incidence and severity.

CLIENT EDUCATION
• Discuss the hereditability of the disease
• Discuss the potential for DJD progression
• Discuss the influence of excessive intake of nutrients that promote rapid growth

SURGICAL CONSIDERATIONS
• UAP—options include: a) removal; b) lag screw fixation; c) dynamic proximal ulnar osteotomy; and d) lag screw fixation plus dynamic proximal ulnar osteotomy. Decision is based on DJD present, age of animal and surgical expertise.
• OCD/FMCP—medial approach to elbow is needed; therefore, diagnostic differentiation is not necessary. Removal of loose fragment(s) is goal.
• Incongruity—surgical treatment is controversial; options include a) no surgery; b) coronoidectomy; c) dynamic proximal ulnar osteotomy; and d) intra-articular osteotomy. Decision is based on: type of incongruity, DJD, age of animal and surgical expertise.

MEDICATIONS

DRUGS AND FLUIDS
• Analgesic and nonsteroidal anti-inflammatory drugs(NSAIDs) can be used to symptomatically treat associated DJD.
• There are no drugs that promote healing of the osteo/chondral fragments.

CONTRAINDICATIONS
Corticosteroids should be avoided because of the potential side effects and the articular cartilage damage associated with long-term usage.

PRECAUTIONS
Gastrointestinal irritation may occur with the use of NSAIDs and may preclude their use in individual animals.

POSSIBLE INTERACTIONS N/A

ALTERNATE DRUGS
Chondroprotective drugs such as polysulfated glycosaminoglycans may be of benefit in patients with limiting cartilage damage and degeneration. They may also help alleviate pain and inflammation.

FOLLOW-UP

PATIENT MONITORING
• If surgery is performed, activity should be limited for a minimum of 4 weeks. • Early, active movement of the affected joint(s) is to be encouraged. • Yearly examinations are recommended to evaluate progression of DJD.

PREVENTION/AVOIDANCE
• Breeding of affected animals is to be discouraged • Dam/sire breedings that result in offspring with elbow dysplasia should not be repeated.

POSSIBLE COMPLICATIONS N/A

EXPECTED COURSE AND PROGNOSIS
• Prognosis is good to fair for all forms of elbow dysplasia. • Progression of DJD is expected.

MISCELLANEOUS

ASSOCIATED CONDITIONS N/A

AGE RELATED FACTORS
Middle to older aged dogs with advanced DJD are not candidates for surgical intervention.

ZOONOTIC POTENTIAL N/A

PREGNANCY N/A

SYNONYMS
Elbow Osteochondrosis

SEE ALSO
Osteochondrosis

ABBREVIATIONS
UAP = ununited anconeal process
OCD = osteochondritis dissecans
FMCP = fragmented medial coronoid process
DJD = degenerative joint disease
NSAID = nonsteroidal anti-inflammatory drug

References

Olsson SE. Pathophysiology, morphology, and clinical signs of osteochondrosis in the dog. In: MJ Bojrab, ed. Disease mechanisms in small animal surgery. Philadelphia: Lea & Febiger, 1993;777-779.

Wind AP. Elbow incongruity and developmental elbow diseases in the dog: Part I & II. J Am Anim Hosp Assoc 1986;22:711-724.

Author Peter D. Schwarz
Consulting Editor Peter D. Schwarz

EOSINOPHILIC GRANULOMA COMPLEX

BASICS

DEFINITION
•The eosinophilic granuloma complex (EGC) of cats is an often confusing term for three distinct syndromes: eosinophilic plaque, eosinophilic granuloma, and indolent ulcer. • These syndromes are grouped primarily due to their clinical similarities, their frequent concurrent development, and their positive response to corticosteroids.

Pathophysiology
• Eosinophilic plaque is a hypersensitivity reaction, most often to insects (fleas, mosquitos), and less often to food or environmental allergens. • Eosinphilic granuloma may have multiple etiologies, including hypersensitivity and genetic predisposition. • Indolent ulcer, like eosinophilic granuloma, may have both hypersensitivity and genetic causes. • In all three syndromes, the eosinophil is the major infiltrative cell. Eosinophils are leukocytes located in greatest number in epithelial tissues. Although most often associated with allergic or parasitic conditions, the eosinophil has a more general role in the inflammatory reaction.

Systems Affected
•Skin/exocrine - the integument is most affected. • Oral cavity - eosinophilic granuloma can affect the tongue, palatine arches, and palate.

Genetics
•The genetic basis for these diseases is unknown. However, several reports of related affected individuals and a study of disease development in a colony of specific pathogen-free cats indicates that, in at least some individuals, genetic predisposition (perhaps resulting in a heritable dysfunction of eosinophilic regulation) is an important component of the disease.

Incidence/Prevalence N/A

Geographic Distribution
Seasonal incidence in some geographical locations may be indicative of insect or environmental allergen exposure.

SIGNALMENT

Species
The eosinophilic granuloma complex is restricted to cats; eosinophilic granulomas occur in dogs and other species, but are not considered part of this disease complex.

Breed Predilections None reported

Mean Age and Range
• The eosinophilic plaque is a disorder of the young cat (ages 2-6 years). • The genetically-initiated eosinophilic granuloma usually occurs in cats under two years of age. The allergic disorder may occur at older ages. • No age predisposition has been reported for the indolent ulcer.

Predominant Sex
A predilection for females has been reported only for the indolent ulcer.

SIGNS

General Comments
•Distinguishing between the three EGC syndromes is dependent on both clinical signs and histopathologic findings. • Frequently, lesions of more than one syndrome may occur simultaneously.

Historical Findings
• Lesions of all three syndromes may develop spontaneous and acutely. • Development of eosinophilic plaques can be preceded by periods of lethargy. • A seasonal incidence is common. • Waxing and waning of clinical signs is frequent in all three syndromes.

Physical Examination Findings
•Eosinophilic plaques are alopecic, erythematous, erosive patches and plaques most often occuring in the inguinal, perineal, lateral thigh, and axillary regions. They are frequently moist or glistening in appearance. • Eosinophilic granulomas may occur in a distinctly linear orientation (linear granuloma) on the caudal thigh, or as individual or coalescing plaques located anywhere on the body. Lesions are often ulcerated with a "cobblestone" or coarse pattern and white or yellow in color, possibly representing collagen degeneration. Common signs include lip margin and chin swelling ("pouting"); foot pad swelling, pain, and lameness; and oral cavity ulcerations, especially on the tongue, palate, and palatine arches. Cats with oral lesions may be dysphagic, have halitosis, and may drool. • Lesion development may stop spontaneously in some cats, especially with the heritable form of eosinophilic plaque. • Indolent ulcers are classically raised and indurated ulcerations confined to the upper lips adjacent to the philtrum.

CAUSES
• Allergic causes include flea or insect allergy, food hypersensitivity, and atopy. • A heritable dysfunction of eosinophil regulation has been proposed because of clinical disease seen in related individuals and in a colony of specific pathogen-free cats. No relationship to estrus cycle, hormone levels, or photoperiod has been identified in these cats.

RISK FACTORS N/A

DIAGNOSIS

DIFFERENTIAL DIAGNOSIS
• Differential diagnoses for each of these syndromes include the other diseases of the EGC. • Unresponsive lesions should be pursued in order to exclude pemphigus foliaceus, dermatophytosis and deep fungal infection, demodicosis, pyoderma, and neoplasia (especially metastatic adenocarcinoma and cutaneous lymphosarcoma).

CBC/BIOCHEMISTRY/URINALYSIS
• Serum chemistry profile and urinalysis are usually normal. • Hemograms may reveal mild to moderate eosinophilia.

OTHER LABORATORY TESTS
Testing for FeLV and FIV is warranted, because pruritic diseases have been associated with these viruses.

IMAGING N/A

OTHER DIAGNOSTIC PROCEDURES
•Impression smears from lesions may reveal large numbers of eosinophils. • Comprehensive flea and insect control should assist in excluding flea or mosquito bite hypersensitivity as causes. • A food elimination trial should be initiated for all patients. Food elimination trials should consist of the feeding of a protein source, such as lamb or pork, to which the cat has never been exposed. This protein source is fed exclusively for eight to ten weeks. At the conclusion of the trial, the previous diet is re-instituted and the cat is observed for development of new lesions. • Environmental allergy (atopy) is diagnosed by intradermal skin testing. In this test, small amounts of dilute allergens are injected intradermally. A positive reaction (allergy) is indicated by the development of a hive or wheal at the injection site. • In vitro serum tests are available for the diagnosis of atopy in the cat. However, these tests have not been validated, and are not recommended.

GROSS AND HISTOPATHOLOGIC FINDINGS
• Histopathologic diagnosis is required to distinguish the syndromes of EGC. • Eosinophilic plaque: severe epidermal and follicular acanthosis with eosinophilic exocytosis and spongiosis. An intense eosinophilic dermal infiltrate is common. The epidermis is commonly eroded or ulcerated. • Eosinophilic granuloma: distinct foci of eosinophilic degranulation and collagen degeneration similar to granuloma formation. The epidermis may be eroded or ulcerated. • Indolent ulcer: early lesions may be indistinguishable from those of eosinophilic granuloma, i.e., eosinophilic infiltration and collagen degeneration. Late-stage lesions are characterized by fibrosis with perivascular neutrophilic and mononuclear infiltration.

TREATMENT
• Identification and elimination of the offending allergen(s) should be attempted prior to medical intervention.
• All three syndromes of the EGC may respond to corticosteroids, with the eosinophilic plaque being the most responsive.
• The damaging of lesions by excessive grooming should be discouraged.

INPATIENT VERSUS OUTPATIENT
Most patients can be treated as outpatients

unless severe oral disease prevents adequate fluid intake.

ACTIVITY No restrictions

DIET
No restrictions unless a food allergy is suspected.

CLIENT EDUCATION
Clients should be informed about the possible allergic or heritable causes, and the waxing and waning nature of these diseases. Responsible clients may choose to postpone medical intervention unless severe lesions develop.

SURGICAL CONSIDERATIONS N/A

MEDICATIONS

DRUGS AND FLUIDS

Eosinophilic Plaque
• Injectable methylprednisone (20 mg/cat), repeated in two weeks (as needed) is the most common treatment.
• Ongoing treatment with prednisone (3-5mg/kg q48h) is rarely required to control lesions. Steroid tachyphylaxis may occur and may be specific to the form of corticosteroid administered. Changing the steroid formulation may be useful.
• Other corticosteroids used include dexamethasone (0.1-0.2mg/kg q24-72h) and triamcinolone (0.1-0.2mg/kg q24-72h). Higher induction dosages may be required, but should be tapered as quickly as possible.

Eosinophilic Granuloma
• Injectable or oral corticosteroids, as listed above, are most commonly used.
• Severe lesions may be managed with a combination of oral corticosteroids and selective immunosuppressive agents, such as chlorambucil (0.1-0.2mg/kg q24-48h).
• Chrysotherapy with aurothioglucose (1mg/kg IM q7days) has been administered with mixed results. Cyclophosphamide (1mg/kg q24h for 4 out of every 7 days) is another alternative. Antibiotics may be beneficial if oral lesions are secondarily infected.

Indolent Ulcer
Lesions respond to corticosteroids at the above dosages. Antibiotic therapy has also been effective in some cats, and is preferable to long-term corticosteroid administration. Antibiotic response may be due to the anti-inflammatory activity of these medications, rather than to a primary bacteriacidal property. Commonly used antibiotics include trimethoprim-sulfadiazine (15 mg/kg q12h), cephalexin (22 mg/kg q12h), and amoxicillin trihydrate-clavulanate (12.5 mg/kg q12h).

CONTRAINDICATIONS N/A

PRECAUTIONS N/A

POSSIBLE INTERACTIONS N/A

ALTERNATE DRUGS
Megestrol acetate (2.5-5 mg q48 to 7 days) can be effective in rare cases of EGC. However, this drug is not recommended due to the severity of possible side effects.

FOLLOW-UP

PATIENT MONITORING
• Baseline and frequent hemograms, serum chemistry profiles, and urinalyses are recommended for any animal receiving corticosteroids regularly. • If selective immunosuppressant drugs are utilized, frequent hemograms (biweekly at first, then monthly or bimonthly as therapy continues) must be performed to monitor for bone marrow suppression. In addition, routine serum chemistry profiles and urinalyses are recommended (monthly at first, then every three months) to monitor for complications including renal disease, diabetes mellitus, and urinary tract infection.

PREVENTION/AVOIDANCE N/A

POSSIBLE COMPLICATIONS N/A

EXPECTED COURSE AND PROGNOSIS
• If a primary cause (allergy) can be determined and controlled, lesions should resolve permanently unless the animal re-encounters

the offending allergen. • Most lesions wax and wane, with or without therapy; therefore, an unpredictable schedule of recurrence should be anticipated. • Drug dosages should be tapered, and discontinued if possible, to the lowest possible level once lesions have resolved.

MISCELLANEOUS

ASSOCIATED CONDITIONS N/A

AGE RELATED FACTORS N/A

ZOONOTIC POTENTIAL N/A

PREGNANCY
Systemic glucocorticoids and immunosuppressive drugs should not be used during pregnancy.

SYNONYMS
•Eosinophilic granuloma: feline collagenolytic granuloma; feline linear granuloma.
• Indolent ulcer: eosinophilic ulcer; rodent ulcer; feline upper lip ulcerative dermatitis.

SEE ALSO
• Fleas • Food reactions • Atopy

ABBREVIATIONS
EGC = Eosinophilic granuloma complex

References

Power HT, Ihrke PJ. Selected feline eosinophilic skin diseases (eosinophilic granuloma complex). Vet Clin North Am (Small Anim Prac) Philadelphia: WB Saunders Company, 1995;25:833-850.
Rosenkrantz WS. Feline eosinophilic granuloma complex. In: Griffin CE, Kwochka KW, MacDonald JM. Current veterinary dermatology: the science and art of therapy. St. Louis: Mosby Year Book, 1993.

Author Alexander H. Werner

Consulting Editor Lowell Ackerman

ENCEPHALITIS

BASICS

DEFINITION
Inflammation of the brain. May be accompanied by spinal cord and/or meningeal involvement.

Pathophysiology
The inflammation is caused by an infectious agent or by the patient's own immune system. In immune-mediated encephalitis, the etiology of the immune system derangement generally is not known.

Systems Affected
• Nervous • Multisystemic signs may be present in patients with infectious diseases.

Genetics N/A

Incidence/Prevalence Unknown

Geographic Distribution
Varies with the cause or agent implicated

SIGNALMENT

Species
Dogs and cats

Breed Predilections
• Granulomatous meningoencephalomyelitis (GME)—mostly small-breed dogs, especially terriers and miniature poodles, but large-breed dogs also affected • Pugs with pug encephalitis (PE), German shorthaired pointer dogs with pyogranulomatous meningoencephalomyelitis (PME), and Maltese dogs with Maltese encephalitis (ME)

MEAN AGE AND RANGE N/A

Predominant Sex N/A

SIGNS

Historical Findings
In most patients, a peracute to acute onset of clinical signs that rapidly progresses. In some patients with GME, fungal and protozoal encephalitis; the signs may have a more chronic progressive history.

Physical Examination Findings
• Most, but not all, of the infectious encephalitis have systemic signs such as fever, lung disease, and/or gastrointestinal signs preceding the encephalitis. • Physical exam findings are generally normal in primary diseases of the brain. • Animals with mycotic, rickettsial, viral, and protothecal organisms frequently have fundic lesions.

Neurologic Examination Findings
• The portion of the brain most affected determines the clinical signs. If the rostral fossa is affected; seizures, circling, pacing, personality change, and decreasing level of responsiveness are reported. If the caudal fossa is affected, abnormalities related to the brainstem (i.e., depression, head tilt, facial paresis/paralysis, incoordination) may be observed.

• Progression of clinical signs, including anisocoria, pinpoint pupils, decreasing level of consciousness, and poor physiologic nystagmus, is suggestive of tentorial herniation.

CAUSES

Dogs
• Idiopathic, immune-mediated—GME, PE, ME, and eosinophilic meningoencephalitis (EME) • Viral—canine distemper virus (CDV), rabies, herpes, parvovirus, adenovirus, pseudorabies • Postvaccinal encephalomyelitis—CDV, rabies, canine coronavirus-parvovirus • Rickettsial—Rocky Mountain spotted fever (RMSF), ehrlichiosis • Mycotic—cryptococcosis, blastomycosis, histoplasmosis, coccidioidomycosis, aspergillosis, phaeohyphomycosis • Bacterial (anaerobic and aerobic) • Protozoal—toxoplasmosis, neosporosis, encephalitozoonosis • Spirochetes—borreliosis • Parasite migration—Dirofilaria immitis, Toxocara canis, Ancylostoma caninum, cuterebriasis, cysticercosis • Migrating foreign body—plant awn, others • Prototheca • PME

Cats
• Idiopathic, immune-mediated—GME, EME • Idiopathic polioencephalomyelitis • Viral—feline infectious peritonitis (FIP), rabies, feline immunodeficiency virus (FIV), pseudorabies, panleukopenia, rhinotracheitis • Mycotic—cryptococcosis, blastomycosis, phaeohyphomycoses • Bacterial (anaerobic and aerobic) • Protozoal—toxoplasmosis • Parasite migration—Dirofilaria immitis, cuterebriasis

RISK FACTORS
• Immunosuppressive drugs and FIV or FeLV infection predispose to infectious encephalitides. • Tick-infected areas for rickettsial and Borrelia infections • Travel history increases the risk of mycotic infections.

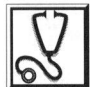

DIAGNOSIS

DIFFERENTIAL DIAGNOSIS
• Fungal encephalitides are frequently accompanied by systemic signs. • Protozoal diseases are systemic diseases and may have a chronic history. • Rickettsial diseases commonly have hemogram abnormalities. • Feline infectious peritonitis (FIP), usually seen in cats less than 3 years of age, has a protracted course and characteristic CSF analysis. • Canine distemper virus (CDV) commonly is seen as acute encephalitis with systemic signs in dogs less than 1 year. It can be difficult to confirm CDV in the live dog. • Primary CNS neoplasia may have signs similar to encephalitis. • Degenerative disorders usually have a slow, insidiously progressive onset. • Metabolic or toxic encephalopathy causes bilateral, symmetrical neurologic abnormalities that relate to the cerebrum. Laboratory tests or serum assay for specific toxins confirm the diagnosis.

CBC/BIOCHEMISTRY/URINALYSIS
• Hemogram results frequently are normal in encephalitis. Leukocytosis may be seen in diseases that produce systemic signs. There may be lymphopenia in the early stages of CDV and rickettsial infection. Rickettsial encephalitis may be accompanied by thrombocytopenia and anemia. • Serum chemistry profile results are also frequently normal in encephalitis. Hyperproteinemia with polyclonal gammopathy often is present in cats with FIP and in animals with chronic systemic infections.

OTHER LABORATORY TESTS
• Serology is available for the fungal, protozoal, rickettsial, and viral diseases. Although helpful, the results must be interpreted with caution as a positive titer is not always indicative of an active disease (e.g., toxoplasma in cats), and a negative titer does not rule out presence of an active disease (e.g., FIP in cats). • Ehrlichiosis can be diagnosed from a single positive indirect fluorescent antibody (IFA) titer of 1:10 or greater. A fourfold rise between acute and convalescent immunoglobulin G (IgG) enzyme-linked immunosorbent assay (ELISA) titers with the first titer > 1:128 is diagnostic for RMSF. • The presence of an IgM titer of > 1:256 suggests infection within the previous 16 weeks by Toxoplasma gondii and may indicate exacerbation of chronic infection. • Cryptococcus is diagnosed from a single positive latex agglutination antigen titer performed on serum or CSF. Agar-gel immunodiffusion can be used to diagnose blastomycosis with a high degree of accuracy. • Local production of CDV-specific antibody (IgG and IgM) can be detected in CSF after CNS distemper virus infection. • A positive FIP titer only indicates infection with a coronavirus, some of which are not pathogenic. • Positive serology for Borrelia burgdorferi indicates exposure to the organism, not necessarily an active disease.

IMAGING
• Thoracic radiographs may confirm lung abnormalities. • Skull radiographs may confirm sinusitis/rhinitis in some cats with cryptococcosis. • Computed tomography (CT) or MRI of the brain may detect multifocal or single mass lesions in many forms of encephalitis.

OTHER DIAGNOSTIC PROCEDURES
• CSF analysis should be done in all animals with clinical signs suggestive of encephalitis. • In almost all patients, the CSF will be abnormal. Normal CSF analysis does not rule out the presence of a viral encephalitis that is acute and limited to the parenchyma. • The predominance of a particular cell type indicates the type of CNS reaction. Neutrophils are indicative of acute active inflammatory process. Lymphocytes (small) indicate an antigenic response.

Eosinophils indicate an allergic response or a reaction to foreign material (tumor, parasite). • If there is a pleocytosis, the CSF should be cultured for bacteria, aerobically and anaerobically.

GROSS AND HISTOPATHOLOGIC FINDINGS
The pathologic lesions are a function of the brain response to the infectious agent or other cause.

TREATMENT

INPATIENT VERSUS OUTPATIENT
Hospitalization is necessary for both diagnosis and initial therapy of animals with encephalitis.

ACTIVITY
As tolerated.

DIET
Animals with severe depression or vomiting should have nothing per os until their condition improves to prevent aspiration.

CLIENT EDUCATION
• In most patients, the condition is life-threatening if left untreated. • If an idiopathic or immune-mediated encephalitis is present, relapse is possible when therapy is discontinued.

SURGICAL CONSIDERATIONS
Brain biopsy may be needed in some patients for specific diagnosis.

MEDICATIONS

DRUGS AND FLUIDS
• Symptomatic treatment may be necessary to control brain edema and seizure activity.
• Specific therapy is applied once the diagnosis is reached or highly suspected. • Idiopathic and immune-mediated diseases respond to immunosuppressive dosage of prednisone. • Rickettsial diseases and borreliosis are treated with doxycycline.
• Protozoal diseases are treated with clindamycin. • Mycotic encephalitis requires treatment for 1-2 years. • Itraconazole 5 mg/kg PO q12h with food or fluconazole 6.25-12.5 mg/kg PO or IV q12h may be used. Corticosteroids often are needed in the first 4-6 weeks of treatment to control cerebral edema. • Viral and postvaccinal encephalitis have no definitive treatment and are treated symptomatically. • Bacterial encephalitis is treated with broad-spectrum antibiotics that penetrate the blood-brain barrier. A combination of enrofloxacin (5 mg/kg PO q12h) and metronidazole (10 mg/kg PO q8h) is advised if the bacterial agent is unknown.

CONTRAINDICATIONS
• Corticosteroids are contraindicated in bacterial and RMSF encephalitis. • In puppies less than 6 months of age and suffering from a rickettsial disease, chloramphenicol should be used to avoid doxycycline-induced teeth discoloration. • Aminoglycosides and most cephalosporines should not be used in the treatment of CNS infections because CNS penetration is poor.

PRECAUTIONS
• It may be helpful to administer one dose IV of dexamethasone 0.25 mg/kg 10 minutes before anesthesia for CSF collection to decrease the ICP. • If corticosteroids are used, the patient should be closely observed for worsening signs that suggest an infectious etiology.

POSSIBLE INTERACTIONS
• Chloramphenicol, cimetidine, and ranitidine should not be used concurrently with phenobarbital to avoid toxic serum phenobarbital levels secondary to interference with liver metabolism. • Corticosteroids given 12 hours or more before CSF collection alter the CSF.

ALTERNATE DRUGS
Cyclosporine at a dosage of 15 mg/kg PO q24h may be effective in maintaining remission in patients with immune-mediated diseases that repeatedly relapse when prednisone is withdrawn.

FOLLOW-UP

PATIENT MONITORING
• Frequent neurologic evaluations in the first 48-72 hours to monitor the patient's progress
• If a relapse occurs as medication is withdrawn, a repeat CSF analysis should be done.
• The serum titer of cryptococcus capsular antigen should be measured every 3 months until it is negative.

PREVENTION/AVOIDANCE
Regularly look for the presence of ticks on animals that live in endemic areas.

POSSIBLE COMPLICATIONS
• Signs of iatrogenic hyperadrenocorticism may develop from long-term corticosteroid therapy. • CSF collection or the natural course of the disease may lead to tentorial herniation and death of the animal.

EXPECTED COURSE AND PROGNOSIS
• Resolution of signs generally is gradual (2-8 weeks). • Viral and protothecal encephalitis almost always progress to death. • Immune-mediated encephalitides will have a fair prognosis for complete remission if aggressive immunosuppresion is used. Rickettsial, mycotic, bacterial, protozoal, and spirochete infections have a fair chance of survival. • Parasite migration, migrating foreign bodies, PME, PE, ME, and polioencephalomyelitis are generally

fatal. • Postvaccinal encephalomyelitis may resolve on its own, but permanent damage or death often result.

MISCELLANEOUS

ASSOCIATED CONDITIONS N/A

AGE RELATED FACTORS
• Young (< 2 years) and older (> 8 years) animals are more at risk for infectious diseases.
• Immune-mediated and idiopathic encephalitides usually occur in dogs less than 6 years of age.

ZOONOTIC POTENTIAL
• In endemic area, rabies should be kept in mind if the patient is an outdoor animal that has rapidly progressive encephalitis.
• Humans may be infected by the same vector tick that affects the pet. • Exudates from animals with mycosis can revert to the spore forming, infectious mycelial stage. Cultures are highly contagious and should be handled with great care.

PREGNANCY N/A

SYNONYMS N/A

SEE ALSO
• See causes. • Seizures—Cats • Seizures—Dogs • Stupor and Coma

ABBREVIATIONS
CDV = canine distemper virus
CK = creatine kinas
CNS = central nervous system
CSF = cerebrospinal fluid
EME = eosinophilic meningoencephalitis
FIP = feline infectious peritonitis
FIV = feline immunodeficiency virus
GME = granulomatous meningoencephalitis
ICP = intracranial pressure
ME = maltese encephalitis
PE = pug encephalitis
PME = pyogranulomatous meningoencephalitis

References

Braund KG. Clinical syndromes in veterinary neurology. 2nd ed. Baltimore: Mosby, 1994.
Greene CE, ed. Infectious diseases of the dog and cat. Philadelphia: WB Saunders, 1990.
Author Allen Sisson
Consulting Editor Joane M. Parent

ENCEPHALITOZOONOSIS

BASICS

OVERVIEW
• Infection with a protozoan of the genus Encephalitozoon • Involvement of kidneys, brain, heart, lungs

Incidence/Prevalence
Unusual in the United States

SIGNALMENT

Species
An occasional disease of dogs; rarely seen in cats.

Breed Predilection None

Mean Age and Range All ages

Predominant Sex N/A

SIGNS

Neonates
• Appear a few weeks postpartum • Stunted growth • Unthriftiness • Progressing to renal failure • Neurologic abnormalities

Adults
Same signs and may manifest as aggressive behavior, convulsion, or blindness

CAUSES AND RISK FACTORS
• Most likely route is oranasal from contaminated urine • Kennel housing

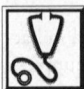

DIAGNOSIS

DIFFERENTIAL DIAGNOSIS
• Rabies • Distemper • Neosporosis • Toxoplasmosis

CBC/BIOCHEMISTRY/URINALYSIS

Dogs
Nonspecific, normochromic, normocytic anemia, increased lymphocytes and monocytes. High ALT and serum ALP expected.

Cats N/A

OTHER LABORATORY TESTS
Serology on blood and testing of cerebrospinal fluid (CSF)

IMAGING
May be contributory but not diagnostic

OTHER DIAGNOSTIC PROCEDURES
Urinalysis, sediment stained with Gram's or Ziehl-Neelsen; spores are gram-positive, birefringent; and positive identification requires immunologic procedures.

GROSS AND HISTOPATHOLOGIC FINDINGS
• Nonsuppurative interstitial nephritis is a consistent finding. • Hepatomegaly and petechiae throughout surfaces of multiple organs • Swollen kidneys, hemorrhagic cystitis, renal cortical cysts, or infarcts • Brain—if lesions present, thrombosis and encephalomalacia, cystic spaces in brain parenchyma

TREATMENT
• Inpatient with supportive therapy or euthanasia
• Potential risk to humans, especially those who are immunosuppressed.
• Sanitation is important and can be accomplished with 70% ethanol.

MEDICATIONS

DRUGS AND FLUIDS
• No known chemotherapy for dogs and cats, but work in mice and humans is highly suggestive of efficacy with benzimidazoles, particularly albendazole (suggest 50 mg/kg q8h for 3 days).
• Maintain supportive therapy and suggest euthanasia when severe neurologic signs manifest.

CONTRAINDICATIONS/POSSIBLE INTERACTIONS N/A

FOLLOW-UP

PATIENT MONITORING N/A
EXPECTED COURSE AND PROGNOSIS
A number of animals recover without further signs if neither the renal nor the cerebral manifestation becomes severe.

MISCELLANEOUS

Reference
Szabo JR, Pang V, Shadduck JA. Encephalitozoonosis. In: Infectious disease of the dog and cat. CE Greene, ed. Philadelphia: WB Saunders, 1990:786-791.
Authors Dwight Bowman and Edward Pearce
Consulting Editor Fred W. Scott

ENCEPHALOPATHY, ISCHEMIC—CATS

BASICS

DEFINITION
Naturally occurring neurologic syndrome characterized by acute ischemic necrosis of brain tissue

Pathophysiology
• The underlying cause is unknown. In many patients, the main lesion involves the middle cerebral artery on one side of the brain. • Unilateral lesions near the frontal lobe or rostral thalamus often cause the patient to circle or turn toward the affected side, referred to as the adversive syndrome. Involvement of the limbic system may cause behavioral changes. Vascular abnormalities, such as venous thrombosis and vasculitis, have not been consistently found. • Lesions have not consistently been found elsewhere, including in the heart.

Systems Affected
Nervous—specifically the cerebrum or brainstem

Genetics N/A

Incidence/Prevalence Unknown

Geographic Distribution N/A

SIGNALMENT
Species Cats

Breed Predilections N/A

Mean Age and Range Any age

Predominant Sex N/A

SIGNS
General Comments
Clinical signs related to the severity and location of the ischemia

Historical Findings
• Signs are acute in onset. • Generalized or partial seizures commonly reported • Behavioral changes can include aggression, depression, dementia, polyphagia, and stupor. • Many cats are ambulatory but ataxic and may circle toward the side of the lesion (adversive syndrome). • Blindness may occur.

Physical Examination Findings
No major changes

Neurologic Examination Findings
• Signs consistent with a unilateral cerebral lesion—circling to the side of the lesion and contralateral deficits (i.e., reduced facial movements—eyelid closure and lip retraction), facial sensation, and menace response, impaired hemiwalking and hopping, and proprioceptive deficits • Changes in the cat's behavior may be evident during the examination. • Blindness with normal pupillary light reflexes implies a cerebral lesion, whereas blindness with dilated, unresponsive pupils suggests a lesion at the optic chiasm or midbrain area.

CAUSES Unknown

RISK FACTORS
• A history of recent upper respiratory infec-

tion has been observed in a few cats. • The disease is seen throughout the year, but one author noticed a higher prevalence in summer.

DIAGNOSIS

DIFFERENTIAL DIAGNOSIS
• For young to middle-aged cats—trauma and encephalitis • For old cats—neoplasia, trauma, and encephalitis • The only way to distinguish between these diseases is to perform skull radiography (to rule in trauma), spinal fluid analysis (to rule in encephalitis), and CT or MRI (to rule in neoplasia, trauma, and vascular disease). • If such tests are unavailable or nondiagnostic, keep in mind that clinical signs are usually nonprogressive in cats with ischemia and trauma, but progressive in cats with neoplasia or encephalitis.

CBC/BIOCHEMISTRY/URINALYSIS
• Results usually normal • FeLV and FIV tests usually negative

OTHER LABORATORY TESTS N/A

IMAGING
Skull Radiography
• Results normal; useful to rule in patients with trauma and bony neoplasia • CT and MRI • Edema and disruption of the blood-brain barrier in the acute stage of disease in some cats • Asymmetry of cerebral hemispheres and excessive CSF filling of subarachnoid space in the chronic stages of disease

OTHER DIAGNOSTIC PROCEDURES
CSF Analysis
• Results normal or high protein or high WBC count • Primary cell type often mononuclear (i.e., lymphocytes and macrophages). Xanthochromia or erythrophagocytosis in some patients. • Cytologic findings may differ according to time of sampling in relation to onset of signs

Electroencephalogram
May confirm brain dysfunction or help confirm a specific location. However, results cannot distinguish between vascular disease, neoplasia, trauma, and infection.

GROSS AND HISTOPATHOLOGIC FINDINGS
• Gross changes include widened sulci and atrophy of the affected area. • Histologic changes include atrophy, degeneration and necrosis, astrocytosis, gliosis, and phagocytic macrophages.

TREATMENT

INPATIENT VERSUS OUTPATIENT
• Cats should be observed and treated as inpatients for at least 2 days. • If seizures are controlled and the cat is able to eat and drink, most owners can manage follow-up care at home.

ACTIVITY N/A

DIET N/A

CLIENT EDUCATION
• About one-half of cats that the author has observed remained functional pets. • Some cats develop secondary epilepsy.

SURGICAL CONSIDERATIONS N/A

MEDICATIONS

DRUGS AND FLUIDS
• Edema and inflammation treated with dexamethasone (0.5-1 mg/kg IV) or methylprednisolone sodium succinate (30 mg/kg IV bolus followed by 15 mg/kg IV 2-6 hours after initial dose). • Hyperventilation (oxygen therapy) may be beneficial in reducing cerebral edema associated with ischemia. • Intravenous diazepam (0.5-1.0 mg/kg) to stop seizure activity • Intravenous administration of fluids should be done conservatively to reduce risk of overhydration and worsening cerebral edema. • Because acquired epilepsy is a potential sequela, chronic oral administration of phenobarbital or diazepam is recommended for cats with seizures. If the cat remains seizure-free for 6 months, it can be weaned from the drug slowly (over 12 weeks).

CONTRAINDICATIONS
• Drugs that raise the intracranial pressure • Drugs that can lower the seizure threshold (e.g., acepromazine and amphetamines)

PRECAUTIONS
Overhydration with fluids can contribute to cerebral edema and worsen the clinical signs.

POSSIBLE INTERACTIONS N/A

ALTERNATE DRUGS N/A

FOLLOW-UP

PATIENT MONITORING
Daily neurologic examination to determine if signs are stabilizing or improving

PREVENTION/AVOIDANCE N/A

POSSIBLE COMPLICATIONS
• Status epilepticus • Death (uncommon)

EXPECTED COURSE AND PROGNOSIS
• Prognosis guarded until it can be determined that the clinical signs are not progressive • Steadily improving signs over 1-2 weeks associated with a favorable prognosis • Permanent behavioral changes (especially aggressive behavior) and seizures are common sequelae.

✓ **MISCELLANEOUS**

ASSOCIATED CONDITIONS N/A

AGE RELATED FACTORS N/A

ZOONOTIC POTENTIAL N/A

PREGNANCY N/A

SYNONYMS
• Feline cerebral infarct • Feline stroke • FIE

SEE ALSO
• Seizures—Cats • Brain Injury (Head Trauma and Hypoxia)

ABBREVIATIONS
CSF = cerebrospinal fluid
CT = computerized tomography
FeLV = feline leukemia virus
FIV = feline immunodeficiency virus
MRI = magnetic resonance imaging

References

Zaki FA, Nafe LA. Ischemic encephalopathy and focal granulomatous meningoencephalitis in the cat. J Small Anim Pract 1980;21:429-438.

Bernstein NM, Fiske RA. Feline ischemic encephalopathy in a cat. J Am Anim Hosp Assoc 1986;22:205-206.

de Lahunta A. Upper motor neuron system. In: Veterinary neuroanatomy and clinical neurology. 2nd ed. Philadelphia: WB Saunders, 1983:130-155.

Author Linda G. Shell
Consulting Editor Joane M. Parent

ENDOCARDITIS, BACTERIAL

BASICS

DEFINITION
An infection of the heart valves or mural endocardium

Pathophysiology
Bacteremia develops from various portals of entry, and bacteria invade and colonize the heart valves. Ulceration of the endocardium exposes collagen, causing platelet aggregation and clot formation. Any valve can be affected, but the aortic and mitral valves are the most common. Vegetations that develop on the heart valves vary in size, may affect more than one valve, and are covered by a layer of clotted blood. Valvular insufficiency develops in virtually all patients. Aortic insufficiency almost invariably leads to intractable, left-sided congestive heart failure (CHF) within weeks to several months. CHF is less frequent and latent when only the mitral valve is affected.

Systems Affected
• Cardiovascular and pulmonary because of CHF • Cardiovascular, renal/urologic, gastrointestinal, and nervous because of embolization

Genetics
Genetic predisposition unlikely

Incidence/Prevalence
• Varies by geographic region and habitus. • Necropsy records vary tremendously and are probably not accurate. At the author's hospital, 20% of dogs with dilated cardiomyopathy are affected.

Geographic Distribution
No well-documented patterns have been published. Bacteremia, and hence bacterial endocarditis, may be more common in tropical and semitropical regions.

SIGNALMENT

Species Dogs and cats (rare in cats)

Breed Predilections
• Middle to large breeds • Breeds predisposed to subaortic stenosis

Mean Age and Range
Most affected dogs are 4 – 6 years of age, although infection can occur at any age.

Predominant Sex
Most studies report a male predominance which may be as great as 2:1 (i.e., bacterial prostatitis).

SIGNS

General Comments
• Clinical signs depend on whether the infection is subacute or chronic and whether CHF, renal failure, metastatic abscessation, or secondary immune complications are present. • Signs associated with sepsis and CHF most prevalent

Historical Findings
• History of infectious disease at the time of examination or within the past weeks to several months in some animals • Signs of CHF (e.g., coughing, dyspnea, and exercise intolerance)

Physical Examination Findings
• Fever and general malaise • Dyspnea caused by CHF • Multiple, single, or shifting leg lameness in some animals • Systolic heart murmur • Diastolic heart murmur associated with aortic insufficiency. This murmur is difficult to detect unless careful auscultation of the right, cranioventral precordium is employed. • Hyperdynamic femoral arterial pulses strongly suggest aortic valve endocarditis. Volume overload produces high systolic arterial pressure followed by a rapid, accentuated drop in diastolic pressure associated with blood "run-off" back into the left ventricle.

CAUSES
• Bacterial infection associated with the oral cavity, bone, prostate, and other sites • Invasive diagnostic or surgical procedures forcing bacteria into the bloodstream

RISK FACTORS
• Congenital subaortic stenosis • Immunosuppresion from chronic or high-dose corticosteroid administration

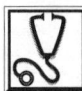

DIAGNOSIS

DIFFERENTIAL DIAGNOSIS
• Bacteremia of any cause produces identical hematologic abnormalities and similar clinical signs. • Specific infections • Polysystemic, immune-mediated disorders often difficult to differentiate from bacteremia and rickettsemia • Left-sided CHF caused by dilated cardiomyopathy or congenital subaortic stenosis

CBC/BIOCHEMISTY/URINALYSIS
• Active, severe infection associated with an inflammatory leukogram (i.e., neutrophilia, left-shift, and monocytosis). Animals with chronic, relatively inactive, or walled-off infection may have normal or nearly normal leukogram. Animals with chronic infection may have mature neutrophilia with monocytosis. • Thrombocytopenia of variable severity develops depending on the duration and severity of infection, vasculitis, and DIC. • Serum biochemistry abnormalities inconsistently associated with sepsis are low-normal or low albumin, low-normal or low glucose, and high SAP activity. • Proteinuria caused by bacteremia and septic embolization or infarction of the kidneys. Hematuria, pyuria, and casts associated with pyelonephritis and glomerulonephritis.

OTHER LABORATORY TESTS
• Blood culturing—three samples taken over a 24-hour period. Two should yield the same

microbe. Both aerobic and anaerobic cultures recommended. Antibiotic removal systems available for diagnosis in animals that have been given antibiotics. • Catheter tips should be cultured when appropriate. • Urine cultures are easy to perform, often yield positive results, and do not necessarily incriminate the urinary tract as the source of infection, but they are not a substitute for blood cultures. • Tests for prostate, kidney, and bone infection may be warranted. • Positive antinuclear antibody, lupus erythematosus, rheumatoid factor, and Coombs' test results occasionally are encountered but are nonspecific and tend to confound the diagnosis.

IMAGING

Thoracic Radiographic Findings
Cardiac chamber enlargement and, rarely, calcification of one or more heart valves

Echocardiography
Cardiac ultrasound invaluable for diagnosis. Vegetative endocarditis of the aortic valve is easily discerned, while mitral valve infection is difficult to differentiate from endocardiosis.

OTHER DIAGNOSTIC PROCEDURES
Joint taps for cytologic examination and culture. Unfortunately, cytologic examination may not differentiate septic from immune-mediated arthritis, and either can exist with bacterial endocarditis. Very high cell counts favor septic arthritis, the neutrophils are usually nondegenerate regardless of cause, and bacterial culture is often negative.

Electrocardiographic Findings
• The ECG may be normal, occasionally reflects left heart enlargement, often detects ventricular tachyarrhythmias, and occasionally reveals heart block of variable severity. • Heart block suggests aortic valve involvement with infection or infarction of the adjacent septum. • Intermittent heart rhythm disturbances often require extended ECG monitoring (Holter or cage) for detection.

GROSS AND HISTOPATHOLOGIC FINDINGS
• Cardiac enlargement • Vegetative lesions and blood clot on one or more valves • Infection, hemorrhage, and infarction of adjacent myocardium • Renal infarcts • Primary or secondary sites of infection • Pulmonary hemorrhage or edema

TREATMENT

INPATIENT VERSUS OUTPATIENT
Virtually all animals with suspected bacterial endocarditis should be hospitalized.

ACTIVITY
In-hospital only and variable depending on whether or not CHF is present or imminent

DIET
Sodium restriction if CHF is present or imminent.

CLIENT EDUCATION
• Guarded prognosis if mitral valve only involved and grave prognosis if aortic valve involved
• Even in the absence of CHF, caution is advised before committing to treatment if the aortic valve has an obvious vegetation indicated by ultrasound.

SURGICAL CONSIDERATIONS
Aortic valve endocarditis almost always results in intractable left-sided CHF; therefore, aortic valve replacement is indicated. This procedure is routine in human medicine but rarely attempted in veterinary medicine because of lack of expertise and facilities and high cost.

MEDICATIONS

DRUGS AND FLUIDS
Treatment invariably dependent on the severity of sepsis and presence or absence of CHF

Antibiotics
• The backbone of treatment but may not eradicate infection before irreversible and severe valve damage occurs. Anything more than minimal damage to the aortic valve is life-threatening, because AV insufficiency tends to be a lethal complication.
• High-dose, intravenous administration of bactericidal antibiotics imperative; choice determined by both the urgency of septic complications and results of bacterial culture.
• Long-term (2-4 months) treatment required to eradicate the infection from sanctuary sites, principally the vegetations.
• Bactericidal antibiotics required because the bacteria are sequestered from the bloodstream.
• Drugs that cannot penetrate fibrin such as sulfas should be avoided.
• Since coagulase positive staphylococci and streptococci are most often incriminated, antibiotic choices can be logically made before culture results obtained
• Coagulase positive staphylococci usually resistant to penicillin and ampicillin
• Streptococci often resistant to aminoglycocides and quinalones
• Gram-negative bacteria often sensitive to cephalosporins, quinalones, and aminoglycocides
• First generation cephalosporin a reasonable choice for stable patients until culture results are obtained. Cephalothin or cephadrine can be administered at a dosage of 20-40 mg/kg q6h-q8h. To avoid vomiting, give slowly.
• Treat immediately life-threatening sepsis with drug combinations. Pending culture results, one of two regimens is recommended:
   1) Either a penicillin, ampicillin, or cephalosporin is combined with an aminoglycocide. High doses of the latter cannot be ad-

ministered, and good hydration with monitoring for nephrotoxity is required. Thus, aminoglycocides are not good choices for animals with overt or impending CHF. Gentamicin recommended (2 mg/kg q8h).
   2) Clindamycin (5 to 10 mg/kg IV q8h) plus Baytril (5 mg/kg q8h given slowly IV diluted 1:4 in D5W)
• Advanced generation cephalosporins such as cefatoxime or cephapirin, at high dosages, are recommended for animals with resistant infections and, at normal dosages, for animals with renal failure.
• IV antibiotic administration is recommended for as long as feasible, followed by SQ administration. Aminoglycocides, when used, are recommended for 5-14 days only. Orally administered antibiotics are recommended only after at least 4 weeks of injectable therapy and at least 1 week after hematologic and clinical signs of infection and inflammation have disappeared.

Treatment of CHF
• Digoxin, enalapril, and furosemide indicated for animals with chronic CHF
• Oxygen, nitroglycerin, high-dose furosemide (2-8 mg/kg IV) and, possibly, dobutamine (4-5 mcg/kg/min CRI) are indicated for animals with acute, severe, pulmonary edema associated with aortic valve endocarditis.

Fluid Therapy
• Good hydration for septic patients, particularly those receiving aminoglycosides
• Aggressive therapy (at least twice maintenance) required in animals with renal failure
• Overt or impending CHF complicates treatment by limiting fluid volumes that can be administered. This problem is virtually insurmountable in animals with concomitant renal failure.
• When CHF is imminent, fluid therapy is minimized, no more than maintenance volumes are provided, D5W is alternated with LRS (or 2.5% dextrose in half-strength LRS), and potassium supplementation may be required.

CONTRAINDICATIONS N/A
PRECAUTIONS
• Renal disease and digoxin, enalapril, and aminoglycoside administration

POSSIBLE INTERACTIONS
• Concurrent use of aminoglycoside and furosemide raises the risk of nephrotoxicity and ototoxicity.

ALTERNATE DRUGS N/A

FOLLOW-UP

PATIENT MONITORING
• Vigilance for the emergence of antibiotic re-

sistance (i.e., relapsing fever and inflammatory leukogram) is imperative with treatment adjustments on the basis of culture results.
• Weekly examination and CBC after discharge • Repeat blood cultures 1 week after antibiotics are discontinued or if fever recurs.

PREVENTION/AVOIDANCE
• Restrict indwelling catheters to appropriate indications and aseptic placement; replace within 3-5 days. • Administer antibiotics to animals undergoing dentistry (controversial except in animals with congenital heart defects and oral infections). • Avoid careless use of corticosteroids.

POSSIBLE COMPLICATIONS
• CHF • Renal failure • Septic embolization of many tissues and organs • Persistent or latent, immune-mediated polyarthropathy.

EXPECTED COURSE AND PROGNOSIS
• Best prognosis associated with short history of bacteremia, rapid diagnosis, and aggressive treatment. • Mortality relatively higher in animals that have recently been given corticosteroids. • Grave prognosis for most animals with aortic valve endocarditis • Latent CHF may develop (months to years later) with mitral valve endocarditis.

MISCELLANEOUS

ASSOCIATED CONDITIONS
Congenital heart defects (usually subaortic stenosis) in some animals

AGE RELATED FACTORS N/A

ZOONOTIC POTENTIAL N/A

PREGNANCY N/A

SYNONYMS Infective endocarditis

SEE ALSO
• CHF, Left-sided • Bacteremia • Discospondylitis • Prostatitis • Renal Failure, Acute

ABBREVIATIONS
CHF = congestive heart failure
CRI = constant rate infusion

References

Woodfield J, Sisson D. Infective endocarditis. In: Ettinger .SJ, ed. Textbook of veterinary internal medicine. 3rd ed. Philadelphia: WB.Saunders, 1989.
Thomas WP. Update: infective endocarditis. In: Kirk RW, Bonagura J, eds. Current veterinary therapy XI. Philadelphia: WB Saunders, 1992.

Author Clay A. Calvert
Consulting Editors Larry P. Tilley and Francis W. K. Smith, Jr.

ENTERITIS, EOSINOPHILIC

BASICS

DEFINITION
An inflammatory disease of the small intestine characterized by an infiltration of eosinophils usually into the lamina propria, but occasionally involving the submucosa and muscularis.

Pathophysiology
Antigens bind to IgE on the surface of mast cells resulting in mast cell degranulation. Some of the products released are potent eosinophil chemotactants. Eosinophils contain granules which contain substances which damage surrounding tissues. Eosinophils also stimulate mast cells directly, setting up a viscious cycle of degranulation and tissue destruction.

Systems Affected
• Gastrointestinal—the intestine is seldom the only portion of the gastrointestinal tract affected. • In cats, hypereosinophilic syndrome can involve gastrointestinal tract, liver, spleen, kidney, adrenal glands and the heart

Genetics N/A

Incidence/Prevalence
Eosinophilic gastroenteritis is reported to be more common in dogs than cats. It is less common than lymphocytic-plasmacytic enteritis.

Geographic Distribution N/A

SIGNALMENT

Species Dogs and cats

Breed Predilections
German shepherd, rottweiller, shar pei may be predisposed

Mean Age and Range
• In dogs, most common in young animals less than five years of age, although any age may be affected. • In cats, a median age of 8 years with a range of 1.5–11 years has been reported.

Predominant Sex None reported

SIGNS

Historical Findings
• Intermittent vomiting (even if only the intestine is involved) • Small bowel diarrhea • Anorexia • Weight loss • Hematochezia or melena reported in 50% of cats with eosinophilic gastroenteritis

Physical Examination Findings
• Thickened bowel loops may be palpated in cats • Evidence of weight loss • If hypereosinophilic syndrome is the cause of the gastrointestinal disease, enlarged peripheral lymph nodes, mesenteric lymphadenopathy, hepatomegaly and splenomegaly may be noted.

CAUSES
• Idiopathic eosinophilic gastroenteritis • Parasitic • Trichuris • Visceral larval migrans • Giardia • Immune-mediated • Food allergy • Adverse drug reaction • Systemic mastocytosis • Hypereosinophilic syndrome (commonly associated with eosinophilic enteritis in cats) • Eosinophilic granuloma

RISK FACTORS N/A

DIAGNOSIS

DIFFERENTIAL DIAGNOSIS
• All of the above listed causes are included in the differential of eosinophilic intestinal infiltrates. • Idiopathic eosinophilic gastroenteritis is a diagnosis of exclusion. • Multiple fecal flotations and direct smears are imperative to rule in or out intestinal parasitism. • Intestinal biopsy will differentiate among the other causes of inflammatory bowel disease and eosinophilic gastroenteritis. • A dietary trial will rule in or out food allergy or hypersensitivity.

CBC/BIOCHEMISTRY/URINALYSIS
• Peripheral eosinophilia (more common in cats than dogs). • Panhypoproteinemia, or hypoalbuminemia may be present if a protein losing enteropathy is also present. • Urinalysis is usually normal.

OTHER LABORATORY TESTS
A buffy coat smear is indicated to rule out systemic mastocytosis.

IMAGING
• Plain abdominal radiographs provide little information. • Barium contrast radiography may demonstrate thick intestinal walls and mucosal irregularities but does not provide any information regarding etiology or specifics regarding the nature of the thickening. • Ultrasonography may be used to examine the liver, spleen and mesenteric lymph nodes in cats with hypereosinophilic syndrome.

OTHER DIAGNOSTIC PROCEDURES
• Definitive diagnosis can only be established by endoscopic examination and biopsy. • Bone marrow aspirates are recommended if systemic mastocytosis is suspected. • Exploratory laparotomy may be indicated in cases where other portions of the gastrointestinal tract, unapproachable by endoscopy, are involved, and if abdominal organomegaly is present.

GROSS AND HISTOPATHOLOGIC FINDINGS
• Endoscopically, thickened rugal folds, erosions, ulcers and increased mucosal friability may be present in the stomach, although grossly the stomach can appear normal. Ulcerations and erosions may also be seen in the intestine. Eosinophilic infiltrates can be patchy in the intestine, so multiple biopsies may be necessary in order to obtain a diagnostic sample. • Histopathology reveals a diffuse infiltrate of eosinophils into the lamina propria, although the submucosa and muscu-laris can also be involved (reportedly more common in cats than in dogs).

TREATMENT

INPATIENT VERSUS OUTPATIENT
• Patients with idiopathic eosinophilic enteritis can generally be treated as outpatients. • In patients with systemic mastocytosis, hypereosinophilic syndrome, protein-losing enteropathies or other concurrent illnesses, hospitalization may be required until they are stabilized.

ACTIVITY
No restriction in stable patients treated on an outpatient basis. Activity may be restricted in individuals who have concurrent illnesses or are significantly debilitated by this disease.

DIET
• In most cases, dietary manipulation is a critical component of therapy. In patients with severe intestinal involvement and protein losing enteropathy, total parenteral nutrition may be indicated until remission is obtained.
• Monomeric diets such as elemental diets, which have non-allergenic components, can be used in patients who are not vomiting but have moderate to severe gastrointestinal inflammation, and are useful if a food allergy is suspected.
• A highly digestible diet with limited nutrient sources (For dogs: Hill's prescription diets d/d and l/d, IAMS chunks and eukanuba, ANF, Hill's Science Diets Maximum Stress and Canine Growth or homemade diets; For cats: IAMS feline, Tender Vittles, Hill's prescription diet c/d) is extremely useful in getting the patients into remission and can be used once the patient is stabilized as a maintenance diet.
• Once the patient is stabilized, an elimination diet or food trial may be instituted if food allergy or intolerance is the suspected cause of the eosinophilic enteritis.

CLIENT EDUCATION
• Owners need to be educated regarding the waxing and waning nature of the disease, and the necessity of life-long vigilance regarding inciting factors.
• Owners need to be counseled about the potential for long-term therapy.

SURGICAL CONSIDERATIONS
N/A

MEDICATIONS

DRUGS AND FLUIDS
• Any balanced fluid such as Lactated Ringer's or Normosol-R is adequate for a patient with no other concurrent disease. Otherwise, fluids should be selected based on secondary diseases.

• Corticosteroids are the mainstay of treatment for idiopathic eosinophilic enteritis, with prednisone used most frequently (1-2 mg/kg PO q12h in the dog and 2-3mg/kg PO q12h in the cat). Cats may require a higher dose in order to control their disease. Corticosteroids should be gradually tapered; relapses are more common in individuals who are taken off corticosteroids too quickly.
• Occassionally other immunosuppressive drugs can be used to allow a reduction in corticosteroid dose and avoid some of the adverse effects of steroid therapy. Azathioprine (1-1.5 mg/kg q24h PO in the dog and 0.3 mg/kg q48h in the cat) is the most common adjunctive immunosuppressive therapy utilized.
• The vast majority of dogs with eosinophilic enteritis will respond to a combination of dietary manipulation and prednisone therapy. Cats often require higher doses of prednisone for longer periods of time to bring them into remission.

CONTRAINDICATIONS None

PRECAUTIONS

Azathioprine rarely causes bone marrow suppression, usually more of a problem in cats than dogs. All individuals placed on azathioprine should have a complete blood count performed 10-14 days after the start of treatment, with rechecks monthly and then bimonthly thereafter. Usually the condition is reversible when the drug is discontinued. Pancreatitis, hepatic damage and anorexia are other potential side-effects of this drug.

POSSIBLE INTERACTIONS N/A

ALTERNATE DRUGS N/A

FOLLOW-UP

PATIENT MONITORING

• Initially, some more severely affected patients may require frequent monitoring; peripheral eosinophil counts can be helpful in monitoring therapy, (especially in cats). The dose of corticosteroid therapy is usually adjusted during these visits. • Patients with less severe disease may be checked 2-3 weeks after their initial evaluation; and then monthly to bimonthly thereafter until prednisone is discontinued. • Patients receiving azathioprine should be monitored as mentioned above.
• Patients usually do not require long term follow-up unless the problem recurs.

PREVENTION/AVOIDANCE

In cases where a food intolerance or allergy is suspected or documented, avoidance of that particular item with strict adherence to dietary changes is required.

POSSIBLE COMPLICATIONS

• Weight loss, debilitation in refractory cases.
• Unacceptable side effects of prednisone therapy. • Bone marrow suppression, pancreatitis, hepatitis or anorexia caused by azathioprine.

EXPECTED COURSE AND PROGNOSIS

• Dogs have an excellent prognosis, although dietary therapy and possibly prednisone therapy may need to be continued indefinitely.
• Cats often have a more severe form of the disease, carrying a poorer prognosis than in dogs.

MISCELLANEOUS

ASSOCIATED CONDITIONS N/A

AGE RELATED FACTORS N/A

ZOONOTIC POTENTIAL

Only a consideration in cases of eosinophilic infiltrates secondary to parasites such as Ancyclostoma, Giardia and Ascarids.

PREGNANCY

• Prednisolone has been used safely in pregnant women, but corticosteroids have been associated with increased incidence of congenital defects, abortion and fetal death.
• Azathioprine has been used safely in pregnant women, and may be a good substitute for corticosteroids in pregnant animals.

SYNONYMS N/A

SEE ALSO

• Gastritis, Eosinophilic • Gastritis, Lymphocytic-Plasmacytic • Enteritis, LymphocyticæPlasmacytic • Inflammatory Bowel Disease • Mast Cell Tumor

References

Strombeck DR, Gullford WG. Idiopathic inflammatory bowel diseases. In: Strombeck DR, Gullford WG, eds. Small animal gastroenterology. 2nd ed. Davis, CA: Stonegate, 1990.
Author Kelly J. Diehl
Consulting Editor Brent D. Jones

ENTERITIS, LYMPHOCYTIC-PLASMACYTIC

BASICS

DEFINITION
A form of inflammatory bowel disease (IBD) characterized by a lymphocyte and/or plasma cell infiltration into the lamina propria of the intestine. Less commonly the infiltrates may extend into the submucosa and muscularis.

Pathophysiology
An abnormal immune response to environmental stimuli is most likely responsible for the initiation of gastrointestinal inflammation. Continued exposure to antigen, coupled with self-perpetuating inflammation, results in disease. The exact mechanisms, antigens and patient factors involved in initiation and progression remain unknown.

Systems Affected
• Gastrointestinal—the small intestine may be the only region affected, although concurrent lymphocytic-plasmacytic gastritis and colitis are frequently present as well.
• Hemic/ Lymphatic/Immune, Ophthalmic, Skin/ Exocrine—other immune mediated diseases affecting the hematopoietic system (AIHA, coagulopathies), ocular (uveitis) and integument are frequently detected in humans with inflammatory bowel diseases. Animals may also develop these complications although to date they are not as well characterized.

Genetics
Basenjis and Ludenhunds have particular familial forms of inflammatory bowel disease.

Incidence/Prevalence
Common problem in cats and dogs, representing most of the cases of inflammatory bowel disease.

Geographic Distribution N/A

SIGNALMENT

Species Dog and cat

Breed Predilections
Ludenhunds and basenjis have particular forms of IBD and wheat sensitive enteropathy affects Irish setters. German shepherds and shar peis have been reported to be predisposed to lymphocytic-plasmacytic gastroenteritis. There is no reported breed predilection in cats.

Mean Age and Range
Most common in middle-aged to older animals. Dogs as young as 8 months and cats as young as 5 months of age have been noted with IBD

Predominant Sex None reported

SIGNS

General Comments
Signs associated vary greatly between individuals in type, severity and frequency. Signs often intermittent, but eventually increase in frequency over time.

Historical Findings
• Cats: Intermittent, chronic vomiting is the most common sign. Chronic small bowel diarrhea is the second most common sign.
• Dogs: Chronic small bowel diarrhea is the most common sign. Vomiting is also common. • Both dogs and cats: Anorexia, sometimes alternating with periods of revenous appetite, coupled with chronic weight loss is common. Hematochezia, hematemesis and melena are occasionally noted.

Physical Examination Findings
• Vary from a perfectly normal animal to a dehydrated, cachectic and depressed patient.
• Thickened bowel loops and mesenteric lymphadenopathy can sometimes be palpated, especially in cats.

CAUSES
Pathogenesis is most likely multi-factorial. Several causative factors have been identified

Infectious Agents
Giardia, Salmonella, Campylobacter, and normal resident gastrointestinal flora have been implicated but are not documented causes

Dietary Agents
Meat proteins, food additives, artificial coloring, preservatives, milk proteins, and gluten (wheat) have all been proposed as causative agents.

Genetic Factors
• Certain forms of IBD are more common in some breeds of dogs (see above). • Certain major histocompatibility genes, which are important components of normal immune responses, may render an individual susceptible to the development of IBD.

RISK FACTORS See Causes

DIAGNOSIS

DIFFERENTIAL DIAGNOSIS
• Other infiltrative inflammatory bowel conditions (e.g., eosinophilic enteritis, granulomatous IBD) • Neoplastic conditions
• Infectious diseases like histoplasmosis, giardiasis, salmonellosis, Camphylobacter sp., and bacterial overgrowth. • Miscellaneous diseases like lymphangiectasia, gastrointestinal motility disorders, and exocrine pancreatic insufficiency. • In the cat, hyperthyroidism, FIP and FIV infection should be considered as well.

CBC/BIOCHEMISTRY/URINALYSIS
• Test results are often normal. • A mild non-regenerative anemia and mild leukocytosis without a left shift is sometimes seen in cats.
• Neutrophilic leukocytosis with a left shift frequently seen in dogs • Hypoproteinemia is more common in dogs than cats with IBD

OTHER LABORATORY TESTS
• Tests to eliminate other differentials (e.g.,

T_4 in cats, FIV/FeLV serology, fecal examinations) are recommended • In dogs, tests to evaluate other differentials include serum trypsin-like immunoreactivity, fecal proteolytic activity using an azocasein substrate, microscopic examination of the feces and serum cobalamin and folate assays. • Breath hydrogen test is useful in the diagnosis of bacterial overgrowth and malassimilation in dogs. • In cats, microscopic examination of the stool may be helpful. Most of the tests listed above have not been validated in the cat.

IMAGING
• Survey abdominal radiographs are usually normal. Barium contrast studies occasionally reveal mucosal abnormalities, and thickened bowel loops, but are generally not helpful in establishing a definitive diagnosis. They can be normal in individuals with even severe disease.

OTHER DIAGNOSTIC PROCEDURES
• A hypoallergenic diet trial may be initiated first in order to rule in or out dietary allergy or intolerance. Occasionally, certain forms of IBD will respond to dietary manipulations. However, if signs completely resolve, a diagnosis of dietary allergy or intolerance is likely, and no further work-up is necessary. • Intestinal biopsy is the only way to confirm lymphocytic-plasmacytic enteritis and eliminate other infiltrative diseases. • Collect duodenal aspirates for Giardia sp. during endoscopy. • Intestinal fluid can be submitted for quantitative culture if bacterial overgrowth is suspected.

GROSS AND HISTOPATHOLOGIC FINDINGS
• Grossly, the intestine may appear normal (even if severely affected) but can appear edematous, thickened and ulcerated. • Histopathology reveals an infiltrate of lymphocytes and plasma cells in the lamina propria. The distribution may be patchy, so several biopsy specimens should be taken. In severe cases villus clubbing, atrophy and fusion can be seen on biopsy.

TREATMENT

INPATIENT VERSUS OUTPATIENT
Outpatient, unless the patient is debilitated from dehydration, hypoproteinemia, or cachexia.

ACTIVITY No restrictions

DIET
• Dietary therapy is an essential component of patient management.
• Patients with severe intestinal involvement and protein losing enteropathy may require total parenteral nutrition until in remission.
• Monomeric diets such as elemental diets, which have non-allergenic components, can be used in patients who are not vomiting but have moderate to severe gastrointestinal inflammation, and are useful if a food allergy is suspected.

• A highly digestible diet with limited nutrient sources (For dogs: Hill's prescription diets d/d and i/d, IAMS chunks and eukanuba, AMF, Hill's Science diets Maximum Stress and Canine Growth or homemade diets; For cats: IAMS feline, Tender Vittles, Hill's prescription diet c/d) is extremely useful in getting patients into remission and can be used once the patient is stabilized as a maintenance diet.

• Once the patient is stabilized, an elimination diet or food trial may be instituted if food allergy or intolerance is the suspected cause.

CLIENT EDUCATION

Inflammatory bowel disease is not necessarily cured as much as controlled. Relapses are common. Patience is required during the various food and medication trials that are often necessary.

SURGICAL CONSIDERATIONS

There are no surgical procedures available in veterinary patients for relief of IBD.

MEDICATIONS

DRUGS AND FLUIDS

• Any balanced fluid such as Lactated Ringer's or Normosol-R is adequate for a patient with no other concurrent disease. Otherwise, fluids should be selected based on secondary diseases.

• Corticosteroids are the mainstay of treatment for idiopathic lymphocytic-plasmacytic enteritis, with prednisone used most frequently (1-2 mg/kg PO q12h in dogs and 2-3 mg/kg PO q12h in cats). Cats may require a higher dose in order to control their disease. When signs resolve, gradually taper the corticosteroid dose. Relapses are more common in individuals who are taken off corticosteroids too quickly.

• Azathioprine (1-1.5 mg/kg q 24h PO in dogs and 0.3 mg/kg q 48 h in cats) is an immunosuppressive drug that can be used to allow a reduction in corticosteroid dose and avoid some of the adverse effects of chronic steroid therapy.

• Metronidazole has antibacterial and antiprotozoal properties, and there is some evidence that it also has immune-modulating effects. The dose used for IBD in dogs and cats is 10 mg/kg PO q8h.

CONTRAINDICATIONS N/A

PRECAUTIONS

• Azathioprine rarely causes bone marrow suppression, usually more of a problem in cats than dogs. Evaluate a complete blood count 10-14 days after starting azathioprine, with rechecks monthly and then bimonthly thereafter. Usually the hematologic changes are reversible when the drug is discontinued. Pancreatitis, hepatic damage and anorexia are other potential side-effects.

• Metronidazole can cause reversible neurotoxicity and is carcinogenic and mutagenic in laboratory animals. Discontinuation of the drug usually reverses the neurologic signs.

• Cyclophosphamide side effects include bone marrow suppression in dogs and cats and hemorrhagic cystitis (especially in dogs). A CBC every two weeks is recommended, as side effects can occur months after initiating therapy.

• Cyclosporine can cause gastrointestinal irritation, gingival hyperplasia and papillomatosis.

POSSIBLE INTERACTIONS

Cyclosporine can interfere with the metabolism of phenobarbital and phenytoin, and ketaconazole, erythromycin and cimetidine can decrease hepatic metabolism of cyclosporine. Any drugs which are potentially nephrotoxic should be used with caution in conjunction with cyclosporine.

ALTERNATE DRUGS

• Cyclophosphamide and cyclosporine can be used in place of azathioprine.

• Cyclophosphamide dose for cats and dogs is 50 mg/M_2 PO four times a week.

• Cyclosporine is currently undergoing evaluation for the treatment of inflammatory bowel disease in humans. It may be useful in the therapy of refractory cases of lymphocytic-plasmacytic gastroenteritis. A wide dose range, from 0.5 - 8.5 mg/kg PO q12h has been reported. Initiate therapy at a high dose and taper the dose as signs resolve. Cost prohibits routine use of this drug.

FOLLOW-UP

PATIENT MONITORING

Monitor for resolution of clinical signs. Severely affected patients require frequent monitoring. Patients with less severe disease may be checked 2-3 weeks after their initial evaluation; and then monthly to bimonthly until immunosuppressive therapy is discontinued. • Patients receiving azathioprine or cyclophosphamide should be monitored as mentioned above.

PREVENTION/AVOIDANCE

In cases where a food intolerance or allergy is suspected or documented, avoidance of that particular item, with strict adherence to dietary changes is required.

POSSIBLE COMPLICATIONS

• Weight loss, debilitation in refractory cases.
• Unacceptable side effects of prednisone therapy. • Bone marrow suppression, pancreatitis, hepatitis or anorexia caused by azathioprine.
• One author reports 4 cases of cats that developed gastrointestinal lymphosarcoma subsequent to their inflammatory bowel disease.

EXPECTED COURSE AND PROGNOSIS

Dogs and cats with mild inflammation have a good to excellent prognosis for full recovery. Patients with severe infiltrates, particularly if other portions of the GI tract are involved, carry a more guarded prognosis. Often the initial response to therapy sets the tone for a given individual's ability to recover.

MISCELLANEOUS

ASSOCIATED CONDITIONS N/A

AGE RELATED FACTORS N/A

ZOONOTIC POTENTIAL N/A

PREGNANCY

• Corticosteroids have been associated with increased incidence of congenital defects, abortion and fetal death. • Azathioprine has been used safely in pregnant women, and may be a good substitute for corticosteroids in pregnant animals. • Metronidazole is mutagenic in laboratory animals. Avoid during pregnancy.

SYNONYMS N/A

SEE ALSO

• Gastritis, Eosinophilic • Enteritis, Eosinophilic • Gastritis, Lymphocytic-Plasmacytic • Inflammatory Bowel Disease

ABBREVIATIONS

IBD = inflammatory bowel disease

References

Strombeck DR, Gullford WG. Idiopathic inflammatory bowel diseases. In: Strombeck DR, Gullford WG, eds. Small animal gastroenterology. 2nd ed. Davis, CA: Stonegate, 1990.

Author Kelly J. Diehl
Section Editor Brent D. Jones

ENTROPION

BASICS

OVERVIEW
Entropion is the inversion of part or all of the eyelid margin. Frictional irritation of the cornea results because of contact by the eyelash or eyelid hair, which may result in corneal ulceration or perforation or pigmentary keratitis. Vision may be threatened.

SIGNALMENT
• Commonly seen in dogs, occasionally in cats. • In cats, primary entropion is usually seen in brachycephalic breeds (i.e., Persian and Himalayan). • In dogs, primary entropion is seen in chow chow, shar pei, Norwegian elkhound, sporting breeds (e.g., spaniels and retrievers), brachycephalic breeds (e.g., English bulldog, pug, and Pekingese), toy breeds (e.g., poodle and Yorkshire terrier), and giant breeds (i.e., mastiff, St. Bernard, and Newfoundland). • Entropion may be seen in puppies 2-6 weeks old, especially chow and shar pei, and is usually identified in dogs less than 1 year old.

SIGNS
• Vary depending on the type and amount of entropion. • Chronic epiphora and medial pigmentary keratitis may be seen in toy dogs and brachycephalic dogs and cats with mild medial entropion. • Chronic mucoid to mucopurulent ocular discharge may be seen in giant-breed dogs with mild lateral entropion. • Severe blepharospasm, purulent discharge, pigmentary or ulcerative keratitis, and potential cornea rupture may be seen in chow chow, shar pei, and sporting breeds with upper lid, lower lid, or lateral canthal entropion.

CAUSES AND RISK FACTORS
• Genetic predisposition in facial conformation and eyelid support is the primary cause of entropion in the listed breeds. • In brachycephalic dogs and cats, excessive tension on the ligamentous structures of the medial canthus coupled with nasal folds and facial conformation defects results in rolling inward of the medial canthus and upper and lower lids medially. • In giant breeds and breeds with heavy facial skin (e.g., bloodhound) or excessive facial folds (e.g., chow and shar pei), laxity of the lateral canthal ligamentous structures allows for upper eyelid entropion as well as lateral entropion and lower eyelid involvement. • In cats, chronic infectious conjunctivitis or keratitis may lead

to functional entropion caused by chronic blepharospasm (spastic entropion). • In dogs, spastic entropion may be seen in entropion predisposed breeds if ocular irritation (e.g., distichia, ectopic cilia, trichiasis, foreign body, and irritant conjunctivitis) leads to excessive blepharospasm. Entropion in non-predisposed breeds may be the result of a primary irritant causing secondary spastic entropion. • Loss of orbital fat or periorbital musculature may lead to enophthalmos and entropion in dogs with severe weight loss or muscle atrophy caused by masticatory muscle myositis.

DIAGNOSIS

DIFFERENTIAL DIAGNOSIS
• Many first-time breeders of chows and shar peis may mistakenly think that the puppy's eyelids have not opened at 4-5 weeks of age, when actually the puppy has severe blepharospasm and entropion. • Entropion is usually obvious clinically, but underlying causes of spastic entropion (as mentioned previously) should be ruled out and corrected if possible before an attempt at surgical correction of entropion is made.

CBC/BIOCHEMISTRY/URINALYSIS
N/A

OTHER LABORATORY TESTS N/A

IMAGING N/A

OTHER DIAGNOSTIC PROCEDURES
N/A

TREATMENT
• Young puppies (especially shar pei and chows) should not initially have skin resection surgery performed to correct entropion. Instead, an eyelid eversion suture technique should be used to evert the eyelid margins temporarily to break the spasm-irritation-spasm cycle seen in these puppies. Some puppies may not require a permanent procedure if temporary suture eversion is successful. Postponement of skin resection technique will allow the puppy's facial conformation to mature, thus making a permanent skin resection technique more likely to be successful. • Toy dog breeds and brachycephalic dogs and cats may need a medial canthal recon-

struction, if medial entropion and trichiasis is causing pigmentary keratitis.
• Mature dogs with chronic entropion need some type of eyelid margin everting surgery, either in the form of a simple Hotz-Celsus type procedure or a more radical lateral canthoplasty type procedure.
• Mature dogs with no history of previous entropion and clinical signs of acute entropion should be examined meticulously for a cause of spastic entropion. If a cause of spastic entropion is detected, it should be corrected, and a temporary eversion suture technique may be used before performing a more permanent skin resection entropion correction technique if it becomes necessary.

MEDICATIONS

DRUGS AND FLUIDS
Although permanent or temporary surgical intervention is the treatment of choice, topically applied triple antibiotic ophthalmic ointment or other appropriate antibiotic chosen on the basis of culture and sensitivity testing may be used postoperatively or as an ocular lubricant before surgery (q12-q24h).

CONTRAINDICATIONS/POSSIBLE INTERACTIONS NA

FOLLOW-UP
Puppy that has had a temporary eversion suture technique may revert to an entropic state when everting sutures are removed or loosened. Suture eversion may be repeated as necessary until the puppy is old or mature enough to undergo a more permanent form of skin resection entropion repair (approximately 6 months of age).

MISCELLANEOUS

Reference

Slatter D. Eyelids. In: Fundamentals of veterinary ophthalmology. 2nd ed. Philadelphia: WB Saunders, 1990.

Author J. Phillip Pickett
Consulting Editor Paul E. Miller

BASICS

OVERVIEW
• Inflammation of the epididymis/inflammation of a testis • Can be acute or chronic; direct trauma to the scrotum is most common cause of the acute form.

SIGNALMENT
• More common in dogs than cats • No genetic basis

SIGNS
• Swollen testis • Pain • Licking of the scrotum that may lead to dermatitis • Listlessness • Anorexia • Reluctance to walk • Open wound or abscess

CAUSES AND RISK FACTORS
• Brucella canis—has a predilection for infecting the tail of the epididymis. • Distemper with ascending infection associated with prostatitis and cystitis • Retrograde urine contamination of the ductus deferens as a sequel to high intra-abdominal pressure as caused by automobile trauma • Bite wounds and other puncture wounds—Staphylococcus, Streptococcus, Escherichia coli, and Mycoplasma have all been isolated from infected testes. • Lymphocytic autoimmune thyroiditis and orchitis (familial in the beagle)

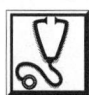

DIAGNOSIS

DIFFERENTIAL DIAGNOSIS
• Inguinoscrotal hernia • Scrotal dermatitis • Testicular neoplasia • Prostatitis • Cystitis

CBC/BIOCHEMISTRY/URINALYSIS
Leukocytosis

OTHER LABORATORY TESTS
Immediate testing for B. canis antibodies should be performed.

IMAGING
Ultrasonographic evaluation of the prostate: (guided aspiration for cytologic examination and bacterial culture) as well as evaluation of the testes and epididymis (appearance and measurements) for future comparison

OTHER DIAGNOSTIC PROCEDURES
• Semen should be collected if possible, evaluated cytologically, and cultured.
• Microscopic examination of semen reveals leukocytes, bacteria, and spermatozoa with coiled tails, detached heads, and retained proximal and distal cytoplasmic droplets; head-to-head agglutination (B. canis)
• Prostatic massage for cytologic examination and bacterial culture of material collected aseptically by urethral catheter • Bacterial culture of open wounds

TREATMENT

• If fertility is of no concern, culture appropriate specimen, administer appropriate antibiotics, stabilize medically, and castrate
• Unilateral orchitis can be treated by unilateral castration when the patient's future as a sire must be maintained

MEDICATIONS

DRUGS AND FLUIDS
Continue antibiotics for at least 3 weeks. Choose oxacillin, trimethoprim-sulfonamide, aminoglycoside, or enrofloxacin for initial antibiotic and change after results of culture and sensitivity testing are available

FOLLOW-UP

• Prognosis for fertility is guarded to poor, especially in patients with bilateral orchitis.
• Testicular heating causes degeneration, and trauma or inflammation can cause obstruction of the efferent tubules or epididymal duct leading to spermatoceles or sperm granuloma. • Evaluate semen characteristics in dogs 3 months after treatment for orchitis is completed.

MISCELLANEOUS

Reference
Feldman EC, Nelson RW. Canine and feline endocrinology and reproduction. Philadelphia: WB Saunders, 1987.
Author Rolf E. Larsen
Consulting Editor Sara K. Lyle

EPILEPSY, IDIOPATHIC, GENETIC, PRIMARY

BASICS

DEFINITION
Primary epilepsy is a primary brain disorder characterized by recurrent seizures in the absence of morphologic brain lesion. The brain is structurally normal but not functionally normal.

Pathophysiology
The exact mechanism is unknown. The dysfunction may be biochemical or an intrinsic propensity to have seizures.

Systems Affected
Nervous

Genetics
Genetic in many breeds but the mode of inheritance is unknown. Different modes have been suggested.

Incidence/Prevalence
• 0.5 to 2.3% of all dogs and higher for dogs in research colonies • Highly prevalent, representing 40-80% of dogs with seizure activity • Rare in cats and poorly documented

Geographic Distribution
Widespread

SIGNALMENT

Species Dogs

Breed Predilections
• Beagle, Belgian Tervuren, border collie, boxer, cocker spaniel, collie, dachshund, German shepherd, golden retriever, Irish setter, keeshond, Labrador retriever, poodle, Saint Bernard, shetland, Siberian husky, springer spaniel, Welsh corgi, wirehaired fox terrier • Not in Doberman and sight hound

Mean Age and Range
6 months to 5 years with a prevalence between 6 months and 3 years of age

Predominant Sex Male

SIGNS

General Comments
The seizures are generalized (bilateral and symmetrical) and usually convulsive. Clinical seizures may be mild with no loss of consciousness but include altered mentation, incoordination, and subtle motor signs.

Historical Findings
• Most seizures occur while the animal is resting or asleep. • Most seizures occur at night or early morning. • The animal becomes stiff, chomping his jaw, salivating profusely, urinating, defecating, vocalizing, and paddling with all four limbs in varying combinations. • Periods of confusion and disorientation follow with the animal pacing aimlessly, compulsively, and blindly. Frequent polydipsia, polyphagia. • Recovery may be immediate or take up to 24 hours. • Seizure frequency tends to increase with time if the animal is left untreated. • Dogs with established epilep-

sy experience cluster seizures at regular intervals of 1-4 weeks; particularly prevalent in large breed dogs.

Physical Examination Findings
No findings, the animal has often recovered by the time he is presented . May be in the postictal phase of the seizure.

CAUSES
Likely genetic in some breeds, idiopathic in others

RISK FACTORS
Ketamine and acepromazine may cause seizures in otherwise normal dogs by lowering a subclinical threshold.

DIAGNOSIS

DIFFERENTIAL DIAGNOSIS
• Age at onset and pattern of seizures (type and frequency) are the two most important factors to consider in diagnosis. • The onset of the first seizure when the animal is between 6 months and 5 years means the younger the animal, the more severe the epilepsy. As a rule, a dog with an onset before the age of 2 has greater chance to become refractory to medication. • Acute onset of cluster seizure or status epilepticus is unusual and is more indicative of toxicity or structural brain disease. If there are more than two seizures within the first week at onset, a diagnosis other than idiopathic/genetic epilepsy should be sought. • Seizures that occur at less than 6 months or more than 5 years may be metabolic or intracranial. • Partial seizures or presence of neurologic deficits are indicative of a structural intracranial disease.

CBC/BIOCHEMISTRY/URINALYSIS
Hemogram, serum chemistry profile, and urinalysis usually are normal. These should be done as a baseline before initiation of antiepileptic medication.

OTHER LABORATORY TESTS N/A

IMAGING
Use MRI and CT scans only for suspected structural intracranial diseases.

OTHER DIAGNOSTIC PROCEDURES
CSF analysis if structural intracranial diseases are suspected.

GROSS AND HISTOPATHOLOGIC FINDINGS
No primary lesion but secondary neuronal loss and gliosis from prolonged or repeated seizures.

TREATMENT

INPATIENT VERSUS OUTPATIENT
• Dogs experiencing moderate to severe cluster seizures or status epilepticus should be hospitalized and treated rapidly and aggres-

sively. • Dogs with recurrence of isolated seizures should be treated as outpatients.

ACTIVITY
Avoid swimming to prevent drowning.

DIET
• Most dogs on chronic antiepileptic drugs become overweight. Closely monitor and add a weight-reducing program. • Dogs treated with potassium bromide should have steady levels of salt in their diet. An increase in salt causes an increase in bromide excretion preferentially over chloride, with subsequent decreased serum KBr levels. S/D prescription diets have higher chloride contents than most diets.

CLIENT EDUCATION
• Animals do not die after a seizure. However, severe cluster seizures and status epilepticus are life-threatening emergencies that require immediate and aggressive medical attention. • During a seizure, prevent the animal from injuring itself on surrounding objects. • Keep a calendar of the seizures as it is the only objective way to assess response to treatment. • Once treatment is instituted, the animal requires medication for life.

SURGICAL CONSIDERATIONS
In selected refractory patients, corpus callosotomy may be applicable.

MEDICATIONS

• Treatment is initiated if there is more than one seizure per 6-8 weeks, cluster seizures, or status epilepticus.
• Phenobarbital (PB) and potassium bromide (KBr) are drugs of choice in the dog, requiring, respectively, 12-15 days and 3-4 months to reach steady-state. Seizures may continue until steady-state is reached.
• PB is the first-line antiepileptic drug (AED). The initial oral dosage is 2-5 mg/kg divided twice daily. Optimal serum levels are 100-120 micromol/L or 23-28 µg/ml. The oral dosage is increased and the serum levels remeasured until these levels are reached. The serum levels are evaluated at steady-state (i.e., 12-15 days after onset of treatment and after a new increment).
• If seizures continue at a frequency of more than one per 6-8 weeks, KBr is added to PB at an oral dosage of 10-20 mg/kg twice daily. The optimal serum levels are 15-20 mmol/L or 1.2-1.6 mg/ml.
• Dogs presented with moderate to severe cluster seizures or status epilepticus are treated with diazepam (DZ) IV bolus 0.5-1.0 mg/kg. Repeat safely in 5 minutes if gross motor seizure activity persists. Immediately follow with a constant-rate infusion of DZ, 0.5-1.0 mg/kg added to the maintenance fluids in an inline burette (prepare only 1-2 hours of infusion at a time to avoid adsorption of DZ to the plastic tubing). If seizures

continue, PB is added to the DZ infusion at a rate of 2-6 mg/dog/hour. Once the seizures have been controlled for at least 4-6 hours, slowly decrease the infusion rate over many hours (4-12). Reinstate oral medications as soon as possible, increasing the oral dosage to optimal ranges if the serum drug level before emergency treatment is found inadequate.
• If the patient's seizure calendar demonstrates cluster seizures, on the seizing day in-home injectable DZ may be administered rectally. A dosage of 0.5-1.0 mg/kg is inserted in the rectum via a teat cannula as soon as a seizure occurs and is repeated 20 and 40 minutes later for a total of three insertions within 40 minutes. This mimics a DZ infusion and has the advantage of being given early in the course of ongoing seizures, increasing the chances to abort subsequent seizures.

CONTRAINDICATIONS
Do not administer acepromazine, ketamine, or xylazine. May result in seizure activity.

PRECAUTIONS
• In the treatment of status epilepticus, PB must be added cautiously to DZ because they act synergistically. Cardiac and respiratory depression may ensue.
• PB may cause polyphagia or polydipsia, which may disappear in a few weeks.

POSSIBLE INTERACTIONS
• Cimetidine, ranitidine, and chloramphenicol interfere with the metabolism of PB, potentially toxic level of PB.
• Epileptics are on lifetime medication. If other drugs must be given, refer to the manufacturer's drug profile or a pharmacist for interactions.

ALTERNATE DRUGS
Many of the human antiepileptic drugs including phenytoin, valproic acid, and carbamazepine cannot be used in dogs with epilepsy because of unsuitable pharmacokinetics in the dog, . If PB and KBr have failed, contact a veterinary neurologist.

 FOLLOW-UP

PATIENT MONITORING
• Monitoring of serum drug levels is essential

in the treatment of epilepsy. Blood is usually drawn at trough and if possible at the same time for each sampling. • The serum PB level is measured 2 weeks after onset of medication (when steady-state is reached) and the oral dose adjusted accordingly. Repeat the PB levels until the optimal serum levels have been reached (i.e., 100-120 umol/L or 23-28 µg/ml). At these levels, hepatotoxicity is unlikely and the dogs that are going to respond to PB will.
• Because of varying concentration of salt in dog foods, dogs have different elimination rates for Kbr. The serum levels for PB and KBr are measured 4-6 weeks after KBr has been added to PB. KBr seems to enhance the excretion or metabolism of PB and frequently the serum PB levels drop after KBr is introduced. Early measurements of KBr levels help avoid over- or underdose at steady-state. Kbr serum levels at 4-6 weeks should be between 8-12 mmol/L or 0.5-1.0 mg/ml. At steady-state, the optimal serum levels are 15-20 mmol/L or 1.2-1.6 mg/ml
• Dogs on chronic antiepileptic treatment should have hemogram, serum chemistry profile, and drug levels performed every 6-12 months to monitor drug-related side effects. A flow chart of the albumin, liver enzymes, and PB serum levels should be kept.

PREVENTION/AVOIDANCE
• The possibility of inheritance should be discussed. For this reason and because estrogen decreases seizure threshold, neutering should be considered, especially in females. • Abrupt discontinuation of oral medication may precipitate seizures.

POSSIBLE COMPLICATIONS
• PB-induced high SAP (isoenzyme—steroid band) occurs frequently and although may be an early sign of hepatotoxicity, is of less concern if ALT is within reference range.
• PB-induced hepatotoxicity may occur after chronic treatment at serum PB levels in the upper therapeutic range (> 140 µmol/L or 33ug/ml). Hepatotoxicity can be insidious in onset.
• Rare neutropenia may develop after onset of PB. These patients must be taken off PB.
• With Kbr levels above 22 mmol/L or 1.8 mg/ml, the owner frequently complains of the dog's unsteadiness while managing stairs.

EXPECTED COURSE AND PROGNOSIS
• Antiepileptic treatment decreases the frequency, severity, and length of the seizures. Perfect control is rarely achieved. Treatment goal is to have less than one seizure per 6-8 weeks. • In many young, large-breed dogs, seizures may continue despite adequate treatment. Refractoriness may develop. • The animal may develop status epilepticus and die.

 MISCELLANEOUS

ASSOCIATED CONDITIONS N/A

AGE RELATED FACTORS
The dog that develops idiopathic epilepsy before the age of 2 years has seizures that are more likely to be difficult to control. Dogs with onset after age 2 generally are adequately controlled or may not require treatment.

ZOONOTIC POTENTIAL N/A

PREGNANCY
Avoid breeding these animals.

SYNONYMS
Primary generalized epilepsy

SEE ALSO
Seizures—Dogs

ABBREVIATIONS
ALT = alanine aminotransferase
CSF = cerebrospinal fluid
CT = computed tomography
DZ = diazepam
KBr = potassium bromide
PB = phenobarbital
SAP = serum alkaline phosphatase

References
LeCouteur RA, Child G. Clinical management of epilepsy of dogs and cats. In: Indrieri RJ, ed. Epilepsy. Prob Vet Med. Philadelphia: JB Lippincott, 1989;1:578-595.
Parent JM. Seizures. In: Allen DG, Kruth SA, Garvey MS, eds. Small animal medicine. Philadelphia: JB Lippincott, 1991:735-741.
Author Joane M. Parent
Consulting Editor Joane M. Parent

EPISCLERITIS

BASICS

OVERVIEW
Episcleritis is focal or diffuse infiltration of the episclera/scleral stroma by a varying mix of inflammatory cells and fibroblasts. Primary episcleritis affects only the eye and is probably immune-mediated. It appears either as a perilimbal episcleral/scleral nodule (nodular episcleritis) or as diffuse thickening of the episclera (diffuse episcleritis). The cornea and third eyelid may also be affected by similarly appearing nodules in the nodular form. Secondary episcleritis is usually diffuse and results from the "spill over" of inflammatory cells into the episclera from other ocular disorders, such as endophthalmitis and panophthalmitis. In animals with secondary episcleritis, virtually any other organ system in addition to the eye may also be involved.

SIGNALMENT
Dogs, especially young to middle-aged collies and shetland sheepdogs

SIGNS
• Nodular episcleritis typically appears as a smooth, painless, localized, raised, pink-tan, firm episcleral/scleral mass. • Diffuse episcleritis is less common and appears as a diffuse reddening and thickening of the entire episclera/sclera and is accompanied by variable amounts of ocular pain. In animals with secondary episcleritis, uveitis is often pronounced. • The conjunctiva usually moves freely over the surface of the lesion, and the nodules tend to be slowly progressive, bilateral, and prone to recurrence.

CAUSES AND RISK FACTORS
• Nodular or diffuse primary episcleritis is idiopathic but believed to be immune-mediated. • Secondary episcleritis may be caused by deep fungal or bacterial ocular infection, lymphosarcoma, systemic histiocytosis in the Bernese mountain dog, chronic glaucoma, and ocular trauma.

DIAGNOSIS

DIFFERENTIAL DIAGNOSIS
• Other causes of a red eye—differentiate by careful ophthalmic examination and tonometry • Other mass-like lesions—differentiate by biopsy or cytologic examination • Neoplasia—lymphosarcoma, squamous cell carcinoma, extension of an intraocular mass, or other tumor • Granuloma—deep fungal or retained foreign body • Granulation tissue following trauma, healing corneal ulcer, or globe perforation with uveal prolapse

CBC/BIOCHEMISTRY/URINALYSIS
• Usually normal if the lesion is confined to eye or adnexa • Abnormalities consistent with other systemic diseases (i.e., deep fungal or systemic histiocytosis may be present in animals with secondary episcleritis)

OTHER LABORATORY TESTS
• Rheumatoid factor, antinuclear antibody, and lupus erythematosus cell preparations are usually not helpful. • Serologic testing may help rule out deep fungal infection.

IMAGING
• Thoracic and abdominal radiographs may help rule out deep fungal infection or disseminated neoplasia. • Abdominal ultrasound may help rule out deep fungal infection or disseminated neoplasia. • Ocular ultrasound may help determine whether other ocular abnormalities are present if media opacities prevent a thorough ocular examination.

OTHER DIAGNOSTIC PROCEDURES
• Incisional biopsy and histopathologic examination of tissue. Nodular episcleritis is typified by varying numbers of histiocytes, lymphocytes, plasma cells, and fibroblasts. • Perform a uveitis work-up if uveitis is prominent.

TREATMENT
• Try to verify the diagnosis histologically or cytologically before treatment.
• Primary nodular episcleritis tends to have a benign course and observation alone may be appropriate in animals with mild disease.
• Initiate treatment if animal has ocular pain, diffuse scleral involvement, disruption of eyelid function, corneal encroachment, or a threat to vision.
• Treat animal as an out-patient.

MEDICATIONS

DRUGS AND FLUIDS
• Progress down the list only if the previous modality was ineffective.
• Topically applied 1% prednisolone acetate q4h for 1 week then q6h for 2 weeks, then taper.
• Systemically administered prednisolone 1-2 mg/kg/day; taper as animal improves.
• Systemically administered azathioprine 1-2 mg/kg/day for 3-7 days; taper to as low a dosage as possible.
• Cryosurgery or attempt excision.

CONTRAINDICATIONS/POSSIBLE INTERACTIONS
• Avoid systemic immunosuppressive drugs in animal with deep fungal infection.
• Systemically administered prednisolone and azathioprine may precipitate pancreatitis and are potentially hepatotoxic.
• Azathioprine may induce potentially fatal myelosuppression.

FOLLOW-UP
• Monitor primary episcleritis for nodule regression or reduction in episcleral thickening and reddening every 2-3 weeks for 6-9 weeks, and then as needed. Although the prognosis is usually good, treatment may be required for months to life. • Follow-up, prognosis, and complications in animals with secondary episcleritis are usually the function of the primary disease rather than episcleritis itself.
• If animal is given azathioprine, repeat CBC, platelet count, and measurement of liver enzymes q1-2 weeks for the first 8 weeks, then periodically. • Vision loss, chronic ocular pain, uveitis, and secondary glaucoma may develop.

MISCELLANEOUS

SYNONYMS
• Collie granuloma • Nodular granulomatous episcleritis • Nodular fasciitis • Fibrous histiocytoma • Necrogranulomatous sclerouveitis • Proliferative keratoconjunctivitis • Limbal granuloma

Reference
Murphy CJ. Disorders of the cornea and sclera. In Kirk RW, ed. Current veterinary therapy XI. Philadelphia: WB Saunders, 1992:1101–1111.
Author Paul E. Miller
Consulting Editor Paul E. Miller

BASICS

OVERVIEW
• Categories of epulides are fibromatous, ossifying , and acanthomatous • Tumors of non-odontogenic origin that arise from periodontal squamous cell epithelial cell residues and surface epithelium • Usually solitary and most frequently located in the molar region, especially around the carnassial teeth and least commonly around the incisors • Fourth most common oral malignancy in dogs • Rare oral malignancy in cats • Most tumors adhere to bone and are nonencapsulated with a smooth to slightly nodular surface.

SIGNALMENT
• May have a familial distribution in the boxer breed • Mean age, 7 years • Most commonly occurs in brachycephalic breeds

SIGNS

Historical Findings
• Often none (i.e., incidental finding) • Excessive salivation • Halitosis • Bloody oral discharge

Physical Examination Findings
• Oral or gingival mass • May be ulcerated and infected • Possible facial deformity

CAUSES AND RISK FACTORS N/A

DIAGNOSIS

DIFFERENTIAL DIAGNOSIS
• Fibroma • Benign polyp • Ameloblastoma • Malignant oral tumor • Abscess

CBC/BIOCHEMISTRY/URINALYSIS
Results usually normal

OTHER LABORATORY TESTS
A large, deep tissue biopsy (down to bone) required for definitive diagnosis

IMAGING
• Skull radiography to evaluate for bone involvement • Thoracic radiography to detect evidence of pulmonary metastasis

OTHER DIAGNOSTIC PROCEDURES
N/A

TREATMENT
• Radical excision the treatment of choice (e.g., hemimandibulectomy)
• Mean survival time after surgery, 43 months (range, 6-134 months) • Mean survival times for patients with acanthomatous, ossifying, and fibromatous epulides are 52, 29, and 47 months, respectively.
• Most epulides are cured when excisional margins are free of neoplastic cells.
• Recurrence is likely if excision is incomplete.
• Radiotherapy also offers long-term control in dogs with an acanthomatous epulis that is deemed inoperable. Mean survival after treatment, 37 months (range, 1-102 months). The 1-year survival rate is 85%; the 2-year survival rate is 67%.
• Malignant transformation of an acanthomatous epulis has been reported in up to 20% of irradiated patients years after treatment, suggesting that an acanthomatous epulis may be a precancerous lesion.

MEDICATIONS

DRUGS AND FLUIDS N/A.

CONTRAINDICATIONS/POSSIBLE INTERACTIONS N/A

FOLLOW-UP
• Thorough oral, head, and neck examination at 1, 2, 3, 6, 9, 12, 15, 18, and 24 months after treatment • These tumors do not metastasize. • The long-term prognosis after excision is good. • Acanthomatous epulides are highly invasive to bone.

MISCELLANEOUS

References
Verstraete FJM, Ligthelm AJ, Weber A. The histological nature of epulides in dogs. J Comp Pathol 1992;106:169-182.
Bjorling DE, Chambers JN, Mahaffey EA. Surgical treatment of epulides in dogs: 25 cases (1974-1984). J Amer Vet Med Assoc 1987;190:1315-1318.
Author Kevin A. Hahn
Consulting Editor Wallace B. Morrison

ESOPHAGEAL AND GASTROINTESTINAL FOREIGN BODIES

 BASICS

DEFINITION
A non-food item located in the esophagus, stomach, or intestine.

Pathophysiology
Some foreign bodies will pass through the gastrointestinal tract with the ingesta and will subsequently be eliminated from the body in the feces. Others may cause an obstruction, most commonly of the esophagus or of the small intestine. Rarely foreign bodies will perforate the intestinal tract.

Systems Affected
Gastrointestinal - If an obstruction has occurred, the patient may become dehydrated from fluid loss via vomiting. If a perforation has occurred they may develop mediastinitis or peritonitis.

Genetics N/A

Incidence/Prevalence Not known

Geographic Distribution N/A

SIGNALMENT

Species
Because of indiscriminate eating habits and inadequate mastication, dogs have a higher incidence of foreign bodies compared to cats.

Breed Predilections N/A

Mean Age and Range
Younger animals ingest foreign bodies more frequently than older animals.

Predominate Sex N/A

SIGNS

General Comments
Many times the owner will see their pet ingest a foreign body.

Historical Findings
Esophageal
• The most common acute signs are regurgitation and persistent gulping. Painful dysphagia, ptyalism, and anorexia may also be seen in the acute stage. • Chronic signs include depression, weight loss, and signs of complications which include severe esophagitis, mucosal lacerations, esophageal stricture, diverticula, perforated esophagus, pleuritis, mediastinitis and pyothorax. • Liquids and semi-solids may bypass partial obstructions and regurgitation may only be evident after eating solid foods. • Respiratory distress secondary to airway impingement may occur if the ingested object is very large.
Gastric
• Nausea and vomiting are common.
• Anorexia may be the presenting clinical sign.
• Hematemesis and/or melena may be present if the foreign body has caused a gastric erosion or ulcer.

Intestinal
Vomiting is the classical sign of intestinal obstruction. With high small intestinal obstruction the vomiting is usually of acute onset, however it can be delayed for 24-72 hours after the onset of the obstruction. Vomiting with low small intestinal obstruction frequently starts two to fours days after the obstruction and it may be intermittent. With incomplete obstructions the patient may not vomit or may vomit infrequently.

Physical Examination Findings
• Abdominal palpation may reveal a mass in the small intestine or may elicit signs of abdominal pain. • In the cat, carefully observe the base of the tongue for the presence of linear foreign objects that may extend further into the gastrointestinal tract. A linear foreign body may cause bunching of the intestines.

CAUSES
Intestinal foreign bodies usually pass through the intestine. When they do not, it usually implies an underlying disease such as a tumor and requires surgery for the removal of the foreign body and the primary disease.

RISK FACTORS N/A

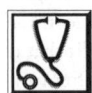 **DIAGNOSIS**

DIFFERENTIAL DIAGNOSIS
Any disease that can cause vomiting or regurgitation is included in the differential diagnosis.

CBC/BIOCHEMISTRY/URINALYSIS
• These tests are usually normal. • If there has been a perforation there may be an inflammatory leukogram and anemia if gastric bleeding is significant. • Hemoconcentration may be present if the patient is dehydrated from vomiting.

OTHER LABORATORY TESTS N/A

IMAGING
• Radiographs are extremely valuable in elucidating the type and location of a radiopaque foreign body. If a foreign body is causing an obstruction of the esophagus air may be visualized cranial to the foreign body. If gas is visualized in the adjacent mediastinal or pleural space, perforation of the esophagus by a foreign body should be considered. A mechanical ileus or displacement of bowel loops may be present with an intestinal foreign body. Plication of the bowel may be evident with a linear foreign body. • A positive contrast study will reveal a delay in the intestinal transit time and will document the presence of a radiolucent foreign body. • Abdominal ultrasound is useful in documenting a gastric or intestinal foreign body.

OTHER DIAGNOSTIC PROCEDURES
Upper gastrointestinal endoscopy is the best method of diagnosing esophageal and gastric foreign bodies. In addition, it allows one to access the extent of esophageal and/or gastric injury. Endoscopy is superior to radiography in recognizing inflammation, punctures, lacerations, erosions and ulcers.

GROSS AND HISTOPATHOLOGIC FINDINGS N/A

 TREATMENT

INPATIENT VERSUS OUTPATIENT
• Treat as inpatient. If endoscopy is utilized and is successful in removing the foreign body the patient can go home the same day.
• Esophageal foreign bodies must be considered an emergency since the incidence of complications increases with the length of time the foreign body is present.
• Gastric foreign bodies are considered an urgency rather than an emergency, unless the patient has evidence of a gastric erosion or gastric ulcer.
• Intestinal foreign bodies are considered an urgency unless there are systemic clinical signs or evidence that the patient is deteriorating at which time treatment becomes an emergency.

ACTIVITY
The patient may resume normal activity after the foreign body is removed.

DIET
The diet does not need to be modified.

CLIENT EDUCATION
Discuss possible complications.

SURGICAL CONSIDERATIONS
• Foreign bodies may be removed via endoscopy or by surgery. Endoscopy is less traumatic than surgery and most patients undergoing endoscopic removal of a foreign body are able to go home within a few hours of the procedure. In the author's experience most esophageal and gastric foreign bodies can be removed by endoscopy (85-90%) with embedded fish hooks being, by far, the most difficult to remove (66% success rate). Therefore, surgery should only be considered if esophagoscopy has failed or if it is not available. If after 35-45 minutes of "endoscopy time" the foreign body has not been removed, consider sending the patient to surgery for removal of the foreign body.
• Occasionally surgery and endoscopy can be compliment each other. An example would be a fishhook that has perforated through the wall of the esophagus or stomach. The surgeon can remove the barb of the hook and the endoscopist can then remove the shank of the fishhook and a surgical incision of that organ is avoided. Intestinal foreign bodies must be managed surgically.

ESOPHAGEAL AND GASTROINTESTINAL FOREIGN BODIES

MEDICATIONS

DRUGS AND FLUIDS
If the patient is dehydrated from vomiting, balanced electrolyte solutions should be administered.

CONTRAINDICATIONS N/A

PRECAUTIONS N/A

POSSIBLE INTERACTIONS N/A

ALTERNATE DRUGS N/A

FOLLOW-UP

PATIENT MONITORING
After the foreign body has been removed, assess mucosal damage. Usually, the degree of mucosal injury is directly proportional to the length of time the foreign body is within the esophagus and the texture of the foreign body in the stomach. Erythema and mild ulceration at the site of entrapment within the esophagus are common. Special attention should be given to any evidence of tears, lacerations, or perforations of the esophageal wall. Obtain survey thoracic radiographs after the removal of all esophageal foreign bodies, as pneumothorax or pneumomediastinum may be present if the esophagus was perforated. • Monitor the patient for at least 2 months after foreign body removal, for evidence of stricture formation at the site of the foreign body. The main clinical sign of an esophageal stricture is regurgitation.

PREVENTION/AVOIDANCE
Monitoring the environment of the pet is the best preventive measure. The owner should not feed bone scraps to dogs and should monitor the pet while fishing.

POSSIBLE COMPLICATIONS
Approximately 1/3 of the animals with esophageal foreign bodies will develop complications after the foreign body has been removed. Most complications are relatively minor and include esophagitis and mucosal lacerations. Serious complications such as esophageal perforation, mediastinitis and pleuritis are rare. The incidence of complications appears greatest when foreign objects become lodged between the heart and diaphragm. This may, however, just be a reflection of the increased frequency of foreign bodies in this area. Stricture, diverticulum formation, and local deficits in motility may occur several weeks following the successful removal of an esophageal foreign body. • Complications are very rare after the removal of a gastric foreign bodies. Gastric erosions and/or ulcers, if present, quickly heal with routine medical therapy after the foreign body has been removed.

EXPECTED COURSE AND PROGNOSIS
See Possible Complications

MISCELLANEOUS

ASSOCIATED CONDITIONS N/A

AGE RELATED FACTORS
There is a higher incidence of foreign bodies in younger animals.

ZOONOTIC POTENTIAL N/A

PREGNANCY N/A

SYNONYMS N/A

SEE ALSO N/A

ABBREVIATIONS N/A

Reference
Burrows CF, Batt RM, Sherding RG. Diseases of the small intestine. In: Ettinger SJ, Feldman EC, eds. Textbook of veterinary internal medicine. 4th ed. Philadelphia: WB Saunders, 1995;1169-1232.
Author Brent D. Jones
Consulting Editor Brent D. Jones

ESOPHAGEAL DIVERTICULA

 BASICS

OVERVIEW
An abnormal, circumscribed, enlargement or dilatation of the esophagus producing a region for accumulation of ingesta. It can be separated into two categories depending on the cause. Pulsion (true) diverticuli are associated with high intraluminal pressure leading to mucosal herniation through the muscularis. Histologically, the cellular remnants are epithelium and connective tissue. Traction (false) diverticuli are caused by the outward pull of connective tissue on the esophagus, and all four cell layers (i.e., mucosa, submucosa, muscularis, and adventitia) remain intact. 50-70% of diverticuli (especially epiphrenic pulsion types) are associated with other lesions of the esophagus or diaphragm.

SIGNALMENT
• Rare in small animals, but more common in dogs than cats • Congenital or acquired
• No important breed or sex predisposition

SIGNS
• Postprandial regurgitation • Dysphagia
• Weight loss • Coughing or respiratory distress • Anorexia

CAUSES AND RISK FACTORS
Congenital (Pulsion)
Inherent weakness of the esophageal wall, an abnormality of embryonic separation, or eccentric vacuole formation in the esophageal wall

Acquired
Pulsion
• Caused by high intraluminal pressure and abnormal regional peristalsis • Esophagitis
• Stricture • Foreign body • Neoplasia
• Vascular ring anomaly • Megaesophagus or motility disturbance
Traction
Inflammatory process associated with the trachea, lungs, hilar lymph nodes, or pericardium causing fibrous tissue formation around the esophagus

 DIAGNOSIS

DIFFERENTIAL DIAGNOSIS
• Esophageal redundancy—contrast accumulation in the region of the thoracic inlet can occur normally in young dogs (especially brachycephalic breeds). Extension of the neck during esophagram eliminates the lesion.
• Megaesophagus—endoscopy or contrast esophagram should differentiate

CBC/BIOCHEMISTRY/URINALYSIS
Results normal

OTHER LABORATORY TESTS N/A

IMAGING
• Thoracic radiography may show an air or soft tissue mass located cranial to the diaphragm (i.e., epiphrenic; most common) or cranial to the thoracic inlet (occasional).
• Contrast esophagram displays a focal dilated region of the esophagus. • Fluoroscopy is useful to evaluate concurrent motility disorders.

OTHER DIAGNOSTIC PROCEDURES
Esophagoscopy to remove impacted ingesta and evaluate the mucosal surface

 TREATMENT

• If the diverticula is small and not causing clinical signs, the patient can be treated conservatively with elevated feedings of a soft bland diet followed by copious amounts of liquids.
• If the diverticula is large or associated with important clinical signs, surgical intervention is recommended.

MEDICATIONS

DRUGS AND FLUIDS

- No medication for esophageal diverticula
- An H_2 histamine antagonist (e.g., cimetidine and ranitidine) is indicated if the patient has concurrent esophagitis.
- Antibiotics are indicated if the patient has concurrent aspiration pneumonia.

CONTRAINDICATIONS/POSSIBLE INTERACTIONS

Unless the patient has evidence of esophageal ulceration and esophagitis, avoid metoclopromide because of its effects on the lower esophageal sphincter.

 FOLLOW-UP

- Patients with diverticuli and associated impaction are predisposed to developing perforation, fistula, stricture, and postoperative incisional dehiscence. • Evaluate for evidence of high body temperature, dyspnea, tachypnea, inflammatory leukogram, and sepsis
- Prognosis is guarded in patients with lesions that cause clinically important clinical signs.

 MISCELLANEOUS

SEE ALSO

- Esophagitis • Megaesophagus

References

Fingeroth J. Surgical diseases of the esophagus. In: Slatter D, ed. Textbook of small animal surgery. 2nd ed. Philadelphia: WB Saunders, 1993.

Author James E. Williams
Consulting Editor Brent Jones

ESOPHAGEAL STRICTURE

BASICS

DEFINITION
An abnormal narrowing of the esophageal lumen

Pathophysiology
Esophageal stricture is most often caused by fibrosis secondary to severe ulcerative inflammatory changes in the esophageal mucosa, submucosa, and muscularis. Gastroesophageal reflux, injury from swallowed chemicals, and esophageal foreign body are the most important causes of esophageal inflammation (see Esophagitis). Esophageal stricture can also be caused by esophageal surgery and by intraluminal or extraluminal mass lesions (e.g., neoplasia or abscess). Spirocerca lupi granuloma is occasionally associated with esophageal stricture.

Systems Affected
• Gastrointestinal—esophagus affected segmentally or diffusely • Respiratory—aspiration pneumonia may develop secondary to regurgitation

Genetics
No apparent genetic basis

Incidence/Prevalence
Unknown but believed to be low

Geographic Distribution
Spirocerca lupi granulomatous strictures are occasionally seen in the Southeastern United States. No specific geographic distribution for other causes.

SIGNALMENT
Species Dogs and cats

Breed Predilections None reported

MEAN AGE AND RANGE
Any age, but neoplastic strictures tend to occur in middle-aged to old animals

PREDOMINANT SEX None

SIGNS
General Comments
• Clinical signs related to the severity and extent of esophageal stricture. • Stricture can occur in any segment or over any length of the esophagus.

Historical Findings
• Regurgitation—usually observed shortly after feeding, and affected animals may reingest the regurgitated meal. Liquid meals often tolerated better than solid meals • Dysphagia
• Good appetite initially, but eventually anorexia with progressive esophageal narrowing and inflammation • Weight loss and malnutrition as the disease progresses
• Aspiration pneumonia with progressive regurgitation and dysphagia

Physical Examination Findings
• Aside from cachexia and malnutrition, the physical examination is often nonremarkable

• Salivation may be observed in animals that have concurrent esophagitis. • Pulmonary wheezes and coughing may also be detected in animals with aspiration pneumonia.

CAUSES
• Ingestion of chemical irritants • Gastroesophageal reflux of gastric and intestinal juice • Esophageal foreign body • Esophageal surgery • Malignancies—intramural and extramural • Spirocerca lupi granuloma

RISK FACTORS
Anesthesia—poor patient preparation and poor patient positioning during anesthesia place some animals at risk for gastroesophageal reflux, esophagitis, and subsequent stricture formation.

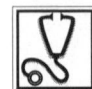

DIAGNOSIS

DIFFERENTIAL DIAGNOSIS
• Vascular ring anomaly—an important differential diagnosis in a young animal with midesophageal body stricture and proximal esophageal dilation. These animals are usually examined shortly after weaning. • Esophagitis —patient may have identical clinical signs as those of esophageal stricture. Differentiation requires barium contrast radiography or endoscopy. • Intraluminal mass—often detected by radiography, but some may require endoscopy. Leiomyoma, squamous cell carcinoma, fibrosarcoma, and osteosarcoma are the most common esophageal malignancies.
• Extraluminal periesophageal mass—often detected by radiography, but may require thoracic ultrasonography. Lymphosarcoma, heart base tumor, and mediastinal abscessation are the most common causes of extraluminal esophageal compression.

CBC/BIOCHEMISTRY/URINALYSIS
Results usually normal. Animals with ulcerative esophagitis or aspiration pneumonia may have leukocytosis and neutrophilia.

OTHER LABORATORY TESTS N/A

IMAGING
• Survey thoracic radiographs are usually normal. An intraluminal or extraluminal mass lesion may occasionally be seen. Aspiration pneumonia may also be evident in animals with dysphagia and frequent regurgitation. • Barium contrast radiography is usually diagnostic for the disorder. Segmental or diffuse narrowing is observed with liquid barium and barium meal. Some dilation proximal to the stricture may be seen. • Ultrasonography has not proved useful in diagnosing this disorder, unless an extramural compressive mass lesion is suspected.

OTHER DIAGNOSTIC PROCEDURES
Endoscopy should be performed in all patients to confirm the site and severity of stricture and to exclude the possibility of intraluminal malignancy.

GROSS AND HISTOPATHOLOGIC FINDINGS
• Esophageal stricture • Esophagitis in some patients • Dilation and muscular hypertrophy proximal to the stricture • Aspiration pneumonia

TREATMENT

INPATIENT VERSUS OUTPATIENT
Initially inpatient. Animals may be discharged from the hospital after adequate rehydration, dilation of the affected segment, and appropriate treatment for aspiration pneumonia.

ACTIVITY Regular

DIET
Oral feedings should be withheld in animals with severe esophagitis. In such patients, a temporary gastrostomy tube may be placed at the time of esophageal dilation as a means of providing continual nutritional support. Liquid meals should be used when reinstituting oral feedings.

CLIENT EDUCATION
• Animals do not recover from untreated esophageal stricture.
• Benign strictures are best treated by esophageal dilation.
• Animals with malignant stricture have a poor prognosis.
• Discuss probability of recurrence.

SURGICAL CONSIDERATIONS
• Esophageal stricture is probably best managed by mechanical dilation with bougienage tube or balloon dilation catheter. Balloon dilation is probably safer and more effective than by bougienage tube. Balloon dilation applies radial forces to expand the stricture site. A greater risk of perforation is associated with the use of bougienage tubes because of shearing forces applied by the instrument. Redilation at 1-2 week intervals may be necessary with either approach until the stricture is resolved.
• Surgical resection of esophageal stricture has been reported, but surgical failure and stricture recurrence are common. Jejunal and colonic interposition surgeries have been described but they are technically difficult to perform.

MEDICATIONS

DRUGS AND FLUIDS
• Animals with concurrent esophagitis should be given sucralfate suspension (0.5-1.0 grams PO q8h) and a gastric acid antisecretory agent (cimetidine 5-10 mg/kg PO q8h; ranitidine 0.5 mg/kg PO q12h; or omeprazole 0.7 mg/kg PO q24h).

• Anti-inflammatory dosage of corticosteroids (e.g., prednisone 0.5-1.0 mg/kg PO q12h) has also been advocated to prevent fibrosis and restricture during the healing phase.

CONTRAINDICATIONS None

PRECAUTIONS None

POSSIBLE INTERACTIONS
Sucralfate may inhibit the gastrointestinal absorption of other drugs (e.g., cimetidine, ranitidine, and omeprazole)

ALTERNATE DRUGS N/A

 FOLLOW-UP

PATIENT MONITORING
Repeat barium contrast studies or endoscopy every 2-3 weeks until clinical signs have resolved and adequate esophageal lumen has been achieved.

PREVENTION/AVOIDANCE
Prevent animals from ingesting caustic substances and foreign bodies.

POSSIBLE COMPLICATIONS
Esophageal perforation is a potentially life-threatening complication of esophageal stricture dilation. This usually occurs at the time of esophageal dilation, although it have been observed several days to weeks after dilation.

EXPECTED COURSE AND PROGNOSIS
Animals with fibrosing esophageal stricture generally have a fair to guarded prognosis. Many of these strictures recur despite repeated esophageal dilation. Animals with malignant stricture have a poor prognosis.

 **MISCELLANEOUS**

ASSOCIATED CONDITIONS N/A

AGE RELATED FACTORS N/A

ZOONOTIC POTENTIAL None

PREGNANCY
Animals with esophageal stricture may have difficulty with pregnancy because of the anesthesia required and because malnutrition may develop.

SYNONYMS
• Esophageal narrowing • Esophageal obstruction

SEE ALSO
• Esophagitis • Gastroesophageal Reflux
• Megaesophagus

ABBREVIATIONS N/A

References

Burk RL, Zawie DA, Garvey MS. Balloon catheter dilation of intramural esophageal strictures in the dog and cat: a description of the procedure and a report of six cases. Sem Vet Med Surg 1987;2:241-247.

Twedt DC. Diseases of the esophagus. In: Ettinger SJ, Feldman EC, eds. Textbook of veterinary internal medicine. Philadelphia: WB Saunders, 1994:1124-1142.

Author Robert J. Washabau
Consulting Editor Brent Jones

ESOPHAGITIS

 BASICS

DEFINITION
Inflammation of the esophagus, typically the esophageal body, but it may also involve the cricopharyngeal and gastroesophageal sphincters. Esophagitis varies from mild inflammation of the superficial mucosa to severe ulceration involving the submucosa and muscularis.

Pathophysiology
Esophagitis is most often caused by gastroesophageal reflux of gastric or intestinal juice, chemical injury from swallowed substances, or esophageal foreign body. The esophageal mucosa has several important barrier mechanisms to withstand caustic substances, including stratified squamous epithelium with tight intracellular junctions, mucus gel, and surface bicarbonate ions. Disruption of these barrier mechanisms causes inflammation, erosion, or ulceration of the underlying structures.

Systems Affected
• Gastrointestinal—esophageal body most commonly and occasionally the gastroesophageal sphincter. • Respiratory—aspiration pneumonia may develop if regurgitation is severe.

Genetics
No apparent genetic basis

Incidence/Prevalence
Unknown but believed to be low

Geographic Distribution N/A

SIGNALMENT

Species Dogs and cats

Breed Predilections None reported

Mean Age and Range
Any age, but young animals with congenital esophageal hiatal hernia may be at higher risk than others for reflux esophagitis. Affected animals generally have a normal life span if the disorder is recognized and treated before the development of strictures.

Predominant Sex None

SIGNS

General Comments
Clinical signs are related to the type of chemical injury, the severity of inflammation, and the involvement of structures underlying the esophageal mucosa (e.g., muscularis).

Historical Findings
• Regurgitation • Salivation • Howling/crying during swallowing (odynophagia) • Extension of the head and neck during swallowing • Avoidance of food • Coughing in animals with concurrent aspiration pneumonia

Physical Examination Findings
• Often unremarkable • Fever and excessive salivation in some patients with severe ulcerative esophagitis • Pulmonary wheezes and coughing in patients with aspiration pneumonia

CAUSES
• Gastroesophageal reflux of gastric and intestinal juice • Ingestion of chemical irritants • Esophageal foreign body

RISK FACTORS
Anesthesia—poor patient preparation and poor patient positioning during anesthesia places some animals at risk for gastroesophageal reflux and esophagitis.

 DIAGNOSIS

DIFFERENTIAL DIAGNOSIS
• Esophageal foreign body—usually detected by survey radiography or esophagoscopy • Esophageal stricture—segmental narrowing revealed by barium contrast radiography or esophagoscopy. • Hiatal hernia—the congenital form is usually recognized as a caudodorsal gas-filled opacity in the thoracic cavity. Contrast studies may be required to document acquired hiatal hernia. • Megaesophagus—survey radiography usually reveals diffuse dilation of the esophageal body. • Esophageal diverticula—focal pouches are detected by survey or contrast radiography or esophagoscopy. • Vascular ring anomaly—usually revealed by barium contrast radiography as a focal dilation of the proximal esophageal body.

CBC/BIOCHEMISTRY/URINALYSIS
Results usually normal. Animals with severe ulcerative esophagitis or aspiration pneumonia may have leukocytosis and neutrophilia.

OTHER LABORATORY TESTS N/A

IMAGING
• Survey thoracic radiographs are usually unremarkable. Aspiration pneumonia may be evident in the dependent portions of the lung. • Barium contrast radiography may reveal an irregular mucosal surface, segmental narrowing, esophageal dilation, or diffuse esophageal hypomotility. Stricture formation may be apparent in severely affected animals. • Ultrasonography not useful with this disorder

OTHER DIAGNOSTIC PROCEDURES
Endoscopy and biopsy are the most reliable means of diagnosing the disorder. In patients with severe esophagitis, the mucosa appears hyperemic and edematous with areas of ulceration and active bleeding. More mildly affected patients may appear endoscopically normal and require mucosal biopsy for confirmation of the diagnosis.

GROSS AND HISTOPATHOLOGIC FINDINGS
• Esophageal inflammation or ulceration • Aspiration pneumonia

 TREATMENT

INPATIENT VERSUS OUTPATIENT
Mildly affected animals can be managed as outpatients. Animals with more severe esophagitis (e.g., complete anorexia, dehydration, and aspiration pneumonia) may require hospitalization.

ACTIVITY No restrictions

DIET
Oral intake of food should be withheld for 2-3 days in animals with mild esophagitis. Food and water should be withheld in animals with severe esophagits, and these animals should be maintained either by gastrostomy tube feedings or total parenteral nutrition.

CLIENT EDUCATION
• Discuss need to restrict food intake in animals with severe esophagitis. • Discuss possibility of aspiration pneumonia.

SURGICAL CONSIDERATIONS
The disorder is best managed medically.

 MEDICATIONS

DRUGS AND FLUIDS
• Specific treatment for esophagitis should include sucralfate suspension (0.5-1.0 grams PO q8h). Intact sucralfate tablets are not as therapeutic as liquid suspensions. • Gastric acid antisecretory agent (e.g., cimetidine 5-10 mg/kg PO q8h; ranitidine 0.5 mg/kg PO q12h; and omeprazole 0.7 mg/kg PO q24h) might be useful in animals with suspected gastroesophageal reflux esophagitis.

CONTRAINDICATIONS None

PRECAUTIONS None

POSSIBLE INTERACTIONS
Sucralfate may inhibit the gastrointestinal absorption of other drugs (e.g., cimetidine, ranitidine, and omeprazole)

ALTERNATE DRUGS
Indomethacin might be useful in refractory cases. However, this drug should be used for only short periods because of its potential to cause gastrointestinal ulcers.

 FOLLOW-UP

PATIENT MONITORING
Animals with mild esophagitis do not necessarily require follow-up endoscopy. It may be sufficient to simply follow clinical signs in these animals. Endoscopy should be considered in animals with ulcerative esophagitis and animals at risk for esophageal stricture.

PREVENTION/AVOIDANCE
Prevent animals from ingesting caustic sub-

stances and foreign bodies. If gastroesophageal reflux is the pathogenesis of esophagitis, pet owners should avoid late night feedings as this tends to diminish gastroesophageal sphincter pressure during the animal's sleep.

POSSIBLE COMPLICATIONS

Stricture formation causing progressive regurgitation, weight loss, and malnutrition. Esophagitis and stricture also place animals at risk for aspiration pneumonia.

EXPECTED COURSE AND PROGNOSIS

Best results are obtained if affected animals are treated with a diffusion barrier (e.g., sucralfate) and gastric acid secretory inhibitor (e.g., cimetidine, ranitidine, and omeprazole). Animals with mild esophagitis have a generally favorable prognosis. Animals affected with severe or ulcerative esophagitis have a guarded prognosis.

MISCELLANEOUS

ASSOCIATED CONDITIONS N/A

AGE RELATED FACTORS N/A

ZOONOTIC POTENTIAL None

PREGNANCY

Animals with ulcerative esophagitis and aspiration pneumonia may have difficulty with pregnancy.

SYNONYMS

Esophageal inflammation

SEE ALSO

• Esophageal Stricture • Gastroesophageal Diverticulum Reflux • Esophageal • Megaesophagus

ABBREVIATIONS None

References

Eastwood CL, Castell DO, Higgs RH. Experimental esophagitis in cats impairs lower esophageal sphincter pressure. Gastroenterology 1975;69:146-153.

Eastwood CL, Beck BD, Castell DO, et al. Beneficial effect of indomethacin on acid-induced esophagitis in cats. Digest Dis Sci 1981;26:601-608.

Higgs RH, Castell DO, Eastwood GL. Studies on the mechanism of esophagitis-induced lower esophageal sphincter hypotension in cats. Gastroenterology 1976;71:51-57.

Katz PD, et al. Acid-induced esophagitis in cats is prevented by sucralfate but not synthetic prostaglandins. Digest Dis Sci 1988;33:217-224.

Author Robert J. Washabau
Consulting Editor Brent Jones

ESTROGEN TOXICITY

BASICS

OVERVIEW
• In dogs, a well-documented cause of pancytopenia (less well-documented in cats)
• Mechanism(s) by which estrogen toxicity causes pancytopenia unknown • Wide individual variability in susceptibility to estrogen toxicity • Estrogen-induced pancytopenia may take 1 to 3 weeks to develop. • Condition may begin with variable leukocytosis (total white blood cell count may be in excess of 100,000/ml; decreased RBC and platelet counts). • Severe pancytopenia then follows and may persist for several weeks or months before recovery occurs.

SIGNALMENT
Greatest risk: reproductive-age females and aged males—these groups commonly receive estrogenic compounds and may develop estrogen-producing tumors.

SIGNS
• Lethargy and/or pallor due to anemia
• Petechial hemorrhage and/or mucosal bleeding, hematuria, hemoptysis, melena due to thrombocytopenia • Repeated febrile episodes, or frequent or persistent infections due to leukopenia • Thin hair coat, evidence of estrus in females, and feminization in males may also be noted.

CAUSES AND RISK FACTORS
• Estrogen-producing tumors • Administration of estrogen to induce abortion or treat prostatic hyperplasia/neoplasms, circumanal gland neoplasms, or urinary incontinence

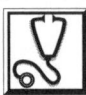

DIAGNOSIS

DIFFERENTIAL DIAGNOSIS
• Other causes of pancytopenia, including infectious and toxic agents, proliferative and infiltrative diseases, immune-mediated diseases, and idiopathic conditions • Important factors in diagnosis include history of administration of an estrogenic compound, presence of a testicular or ovarian tumor, thin hair coat, evidence of estrus, and/or signs of feminization.

CBC/BIOCHEMISTRY/URINALYSIS
• Early in disease course: decreased RBC and platelet counts (bicytopenia); normal or increased total white blood cell count • Pancytopenia develops later.

OTHER LABORATORY TESTS
Reticulocyte count and/or bone marrow biopsy—to investigate bicytopenia or pancytopenia. Pancytopenia phase: Hypocellular bone marrow; no increase in reticulocyte count.

IMAGING
Radiography and ultrasonography—to locate and identify potential estrogen-producing tumors

OTHER DIAGNOSTIC PROCEDURES
Abdominal laparoscopy or laparotomy and/or biopsy—to locate and identify potential estrogen-producing tumors

TREATMENT
• Remove source of estrogen and provide supportive care.
• Supportive therapy includes aggressive antibiotic therapy, blood transfusion, and/or transfusion of platelet-rich plasma, according to the clinical situation.

MEDICATIONS

DRUGS AND FLUIDS
• Therapy should be appropriate for the clinical situation (e.g., the degree to which each cell population is decreased, the presence of a fever or infection, and the identified source of estrogen).
• Develop an appropriate therapeutic plan by reviewing the sections that discuss therapy for the specific cytopenias and sources of hyperestrogenism.

CONTRAINDICATIONS/POSSIBLE INTERACTIONS
Use glucocorticoids and other immunosuppressive drugs only when absolutely necessary and with extreme care (because the patient's immune status is compromised).

FOLLOW-UP
• Perform daily physical examinations, with special attention to lymph node palpation and body temperature, and periodic complete blood counts (CBCs) to monitor patient's status. The frequency at which CBCs are performed depends upon the severity and cause of the cytopenia and the age and general physical condition of the patient. Generally, CBCs are performed daily, biweekly, or weekly. • Monitor patients for development of lethargy, fever, and hemorrhage because these may represent recurrence of anemia, leukopenia, and thrombocytopenia, respectively. Recovery may occur within a month, but may take several months.

MISCELLANEOUS

SEE ALSO
• Leukopenia • Pancytopenia • Thrombocytopenia

ABBREVIATIONS
RBC = red blood cell

Reference

Tvedten H. Erythrocyte disorders. In: Willard MD, Tvedten H, Turnwald GH, eds. Small animal clinical diagnosis by laboratory methods. 2nd ed. Philadelphia: WB Saunders 1994:31-51.

Author Ronald D. Tyler

Consulting Editor Alan H. Rebar

BASICS

OVERVIEW

Ethanol is a short-chain, aliphatic alcohol that is highly miscible with water and soluble in aqueous systems. The chemical formula is CH_2OH. Its volatility is less than that for comparable hydrocarbons (e.g., methane). It is used as a solvent in medications and is a major component of alcoholic beverages (beer, 5%; wines, 9-12%; whisky, 50-90%). The alcohol concentration is expressed as a "proof" number which is twice the percentage concentration. Ethanol is metabolized to acetaldehyde. Acute toxicity occurs after ingestion of 5-8 ml/kg. The mechanism of action is related to ethanol's effect on the lipids and proteins of cell membranes, the result of which is reduced sodium and potassium conduction in nerve membranes.

SIGNALMENT

• Most common in dogs • No breed or gender predilections

SIGNS

General comments

• CNS signs predominate and develop within 15-30 minutes (empty stomach) or 1-2 hours (full stomach) after ingestion.
• Recovery from clinical signs is usually within 8-12 hours.

Physical Examination Findings

• Odor of alcohol on breath or from stomach contents • High dosages cause ataxia, impaired reflexes, behavioral changes, and excitement or depression • Polyuria or incontinence • Signs of severe toxicity include depression or narcosis, slowed respiratory rate, cardiac arrest, and death.

CAUSES AND RISK FACTORS

• Accidental access of pets to spilled medications or alcoholic beverages • Intentional administration by owners or others. Dogs may readily consume beer if offered.
• Ingestions of fermented products (e.g., bread dough) • Dermal exposure to alcohol containing products

DIAGNOSIS

DIFFERENTIAL DIAGNOSIS

• Exposure to other alcohols (e.g., methane isopropand and butane) • Exposure to abused drugs (e.g., marijuana) • Early stages of ethylene glycol (ie, antifreeze) toxicosis
• Toxicosis by halogenated or aliphatic hydrocarbon solvent

CBC/BIOCHEMISTRY/URINALYSIS

Monitor for hypoglycemia

OTHER LABORATORY TESTS

• High osmolality (determined by freezing point depression method) and high osmolal gap • Blood ethanol determination is definitive for diagnosis, and available at most human laboratories. • Blood ethanol concentration > 0.6 mg/ml in puppies, > 1-4 mg/ml in adults is toxic. • Measure blood gases and anion gap to evaluate potential acidosis.

IMAGING N/A

OTHER DIAGNOSTIC PROCEDURES

Neurologic examination to rule out other CNS diseases

TREATMENT

• Gastrointestinal detoxication with activated charcoal • Artificial ventilation if respiratory function is depressed • Cardiopulmonary resuscitation if cardiac arrest occurs

MEDICATIONS

DRUGS AND FLUIDS

• Activated charcoal (2 gm/kg, PO) as soon as possible after exposure • Possible inhibition of alcohol metabolism with 4-methylpyrazole (see Ethylene Glycol)
• Sodium bicarbonate (0.3 mEq x kg body weight x bicarbonate deficit) to treat acidosis; give half of the dose as a slow IV bolus over 20 minutes and the remaining half in crystalloid fluids over 4 hours. • Epinephrine, atropine, and bicarbonate to treat cardiac arrest

CONTRAINDICATIONS/POSSIBLE INTERACTIONS N/A

FOLLOW-UP

Monitor blood pH, blood gases, urine pH, and anion gap for evidence of acidosis.

MISCELLANEOUS

SEE ALSO

• Acidosis, Metabolic • Cardiopulmonary Arrest • Ethylene Glycol Toxicity
• Poisoning (Intoxication)

ABBREVIATIONS

CNS = central nervous system

Refereces

Valentine WM. Short-chain alcohols. Vet Clin North Am Small Anim Pract 20:515-523.

Author Gary D. Osweiler
Consulting Editor Gary D. Osweiler

ETHYLENE GLYCOL POISONING

BASICS

DEFINITION
Consequence of ingestion of ethylene glycol-containing substances such as antifreeze. Minimum lethal dose is 1.4 ml/kg in cats, and 4.4-6.6 ml/kg in dogs.

Pathophysiology
Ethylene glycol is rapidly absorbed from gastrointestinal tract. Absorption is delayed if food is in the stomach. Ethylene glycol is rapidly metabolized by the liver enzyme alcohol dehydrogenase to glycoaldehyde, glycolic acid, glyoxalic acid, and oxalic acid, substances which cause severe metabolic acidosis and renal epithelial damage.

Systems Affected
• Nervous—direct effect of ethylene glycol and glycoaldehyde on the CNS. Metabolic acidosis and high plasma osmolality contribute to the CNS signs. • Gastrointestinal—mucosal irritation • Endocrine/metabolic—metabolic acidosis • Renal/urologic—ethylene glycol causes osmotic diuresis and stimulates thirst center by increasing serum osmolality. Metabolites of ethylene glycol damage renal tubular epithelium by direct cytotoxicity, causing renal failure. Calcium oxalate crystals form within the lumina of tubules, causing minor renal tubular damage.

Genetics N/A

Incidence/Prevalence
• Common toxicosis • Highest fatality rate of all poisons • Fatality rates higher for cats than dogs

Geographic Distribution
Prevalence higher in cold areas where antifreeze is more commonly used

SIGNALMENT

Species Dogs and cats

Breed Predilections N/A

MEAN AGE AND RANGE
• Any age • In one study, mean age, 3 years; range, 3 months-13 years

Predominant Sex N/A

SIGNS

General Comments
Clinical signs are dose-dependent and can be divided into those caused by unmetabolized ethylene glycol, observed from 30 minutes-12 hours after ingestion, and those caused by the toxic metabolites of ethylene glycol, which are frequently fatal. Onset of clinical signs is almost always acute.

Early Clinical Signs
• Mild to severe depression, nausea, vomiting, ataxia, knuckling, muscle fasciculations, nystagmus, head tremors, impaired withdrawal reflexes and righting ability, PU/PD (dogs), PU without PD (cats), severe hypo-

thermia (cats) • As depression increases, dogs drink less but polyuria continues, causing dehydration. • In dogs, CNS signs abate after approximately 12 hours, and patients may briefly appear to have recovered. Cats usually remain markedly depressed.

Late Clinical Signs (Renal Stage)
Oliguric renal failure develops from 36-72 hours in dogs and 12-24 hours in cats. Signs include severe lethargy or coma, seizures, anorexia, vomiting, oral ulcers, salivation, and oliguria with isosthenuria. Anuria often develops by 72-96 hours after ingestion. Kidneys are often swollen and painful, particularly in cats.

CAUSES
Ingestion of ethylene glycol, the principal component of most antifreeze solutions

RISK FACTORS
Widespread availability, somewhat pleasant taste, small minimum lethal dose, and lack of public awareness of the toxicity of the compound

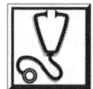

DIAGNOSIS

DIFFERENTIAL DIAGNOSIS

Acute Stage (30 minutes-12 Hours after Ingestion)
• Ethanol toxicosis can cause metabolic acidosis and similar gastrointestinal and CNS signs, but it is rare in dogs and cats. • Ketoacidotic diabetes mellitus, pancreatitis, and gastroenteritis can cause similar gastrointestinal signs and metabolic acidosis. • Primary CNS disorders and hepatic encephalopathy cause CNS signs.

Renal Stage
Acute renal failure in dogs and cats is most commonly caused by nephrotoxins (e.g., ethylene glycol [most common], aminoglycoside antibiotics, amphotericin B, cancer chemotherapeutic drugs, cyclosporin, and heavy metals). Nontoxic causes include tubulointerstitial nephritis, glomerular and vascular disease, and renal ischemia (i.e., hypoperfusion).

CBC/BIOCHEMISTRY/URINALYSIS
• PCV and total protein are often high because of dehydration. • Stress leukograms (e.g., mature neutrophilia and lymphopenia) are common. • High serum urea nitrogen and creatinine concentrations 36-48 hours (dogs) and 12 hours (cats) after ingestion • High phosphorus concentration. May increase 3-6 hours after ingestion because of phosphate rust inhibitors in the antifreeze. Phosphorus then returns to normal and increases again with the onset of azotemia. • Hyperkalemia with oliguria and anuria • Hypocalcemia (50% of cases) is usually subclinical because acidosis causes a shift to the ionized, physiologically active form of calcium. • Hyperglycemia (50% of cases).

Glucose may be >350 mg/dl in cats. • Isosthenuria by 3 hours after ingestion • Calcium oxalate crystalluria is a consistent finding and may be observed as early as 3 and 6 hours after ingestion in cats and dogs, respectively. • Urine pH consistently low • Inconsistent findings include hematuria, proteinuria, and glucosuria; granular and cellular casts, WBC, RBC, and renal epithelial cells in some patients.

OTHER LABORATORY TESTS
• Severe metabolic acidosis develops within 3 hours after ingestion. • Total CO_2, plasma bicarbonate concentration, and blood pH are low. • The $PaCO_2$ often decreases because of partial respiratory compensation. • The anion gap is high by 3 hours after ingestion, peaks at 6 hours, and remains high for approximately 48 hours. • Serum osmolality is markedly high by 1 hour after ingestion and usually remains high for approximately 18 hours after ingestion. Ethylene glycol toxicosis is the most common cause of a high osmolal gap. To estimate serum ethylene glycol concentration, multiply the osmolal gap by 6.2. • Serum and urine ethylene glycol concentrations peak between 1 and 6 hours after ingestion and are usually not detectable in the serum or urine by 72 hours. Commercial kits (Ethylene Glycol Test Kit, PRN Pharmacal, Inc., 5830 McAllister Ave, Pensacola, Florida 32504) measure blood ethylene glycol concentration at > 50 mg/dl.

IMAGING
Ultrasound—renal cortices can be hyperechoic because of the presence of crystals

OTHER DIAGNOSTIC PROCEDURES
If the animal is anuric, kidney biopsy may be necessary to confirm the diagnosis. Cytologic examination of kidney imprints reveals calcium oxalate crystals.

GROSS AND HISTOPATHOLOGIC FINDINGS
• Kidneys often swollen • Intratubular calcium oxalate crystals are diagnostic; renal tubular epithelial cells are usually necrotic and disrupted.

TREATMENT

INPATIENT VERSUS OUTPATIENT
Inpatient

ACTIVITY N/A

DIET N/A

CLIENT EDUCATION N/A

SURGICAL CONSIDERATIONS N/A

MEDICATIONS

DRUGS AND FLUIDS
• Induction of vomiting and gastric lavage

with activated charcoal indicated within 1-2 hours after ingestion; beyond this time, the procedure is of little benefit.

• To prevent metabolism of ethylene glycol, inhibit liver alcohol dehydrogenase (ADH) by direct inactivation or by giving competitive substrates such as ethanol. A very effective and nontoxic ADH inhibitor in dogs is 4-methylpyrazole (4-MP). Dosage of 5% (50 mg/ml) 4-MP—20 mg/kg IV initially, followed by 15 mg/kg IV at 12 and 24 hours, and 5 mg/kg IV at 36 hours. To make 100 ml of a 5% solution, 5g of 4-MP (Aldrich Chemical Company) is added to 50 ml of polyethylene glycol (400) and 46 ml of bacteriostatic water. The solution should be filtered with a 0.22 mm filter before use. The refrigerated solution is stable for at least 2 years. 4-MP is not approved by the FDA for use in animals, but veterinarians can now purchase it without obtaining an investigational new animal drug (INAD) number from the FDA.

• 4-MP is ineffective in cats. Ethanol is the drug of choice in cats. Recommended dosage—5 ml of 20% ethanol/kg diluted in fluids and given as IV drip over 6 hours for 5 treatments and then over 8 hours for 4 more treatments.

• Fluids should be given (IV) to correct dehydration, increase tissue perfusion, and promote diuresis.

• Bicarbonate should be given slowly IV to correct metabolic acidosis.

• In dogs that have azotemia and oliguric renal failure, almost all of the ethylene glycol will have been metabolized, and treatment to inhibit alcohol dehydrogenase is of little benefit. Fluid, electrolyte, and acid-base disorders should be corrected, and establishment of diuresis is desirable. Diuretics, particularly mannitol, and peritoneal dialysis may be helpful.

CONTRAINDICATIONS
Drugs that cause CNS depression

PRECAUTIONS
• Cats usually become hypothermic, necessitating an external heat source. • Ethanol con-

tributes to CNS depression and further increases serum osmolality.

POSSIBLE INTERACTIONS
4-MP does not interact with other drugs.

ALTERNATE DRUGS
Ethanol, propylene glycol, and 1,3-butanediol have a higher affinity for alcohol dehydrogenase than does ethylene glycol and can be used effectively to inhibit ethylene glycol metabolism. Disadvantages include CNS depression and a tendency to further increase serum osmolality. Ethanol is commonly used, but patients often become comatose from the additive effects of ethylene glycol and ethanol, and ethanol is metabolized rapidly, necessitating frequent or constant treatment. The dosage for dogs is 5.5 ml of 20% ethanol/kg diluted in fluids and given as an IV drip over 4 hours for 5 treatments, then over 6 hours for 4 more treatments. Constant serum ethanol concentration of 100 mg/dl inhibits most ethylene glycol metabolism.

FOLLOW-UP

PATIENT MONITORING
BUN, acid/base status, and urine output daily during the first few days after ingestion

PREVENTION/AVOIDANCE
• Increasing client awareness of the toxicity of ethylene glycol • Use of an antifreeze product containing propylene glycol, which is relatively nontoxic

POSSIBLE COMPLICATIONS
• If patient does not become azotemic, usually none • Urine concentrating ability may be impaired in animals that become azotemic but recover.

EXPECTED COURSE AND PROGNOSIS
• Prognosis is excellent in dogs treated with 4-MP within 5 hours after ethylene glycol ingestion. • Most dogs recover if treatment is initiated as late as 8 hours after ingestion. • In animals examined up to 36 hours after inges-

tion, preventing metabolism of any remaining unmetabolized ethylene glycol may be of benefit. • Prognosis for cats is good if treatment with ethanol is instituted within 3 hours after ingestion. • Prognosis is poor in dogs and cats with azotemia and oliguric renal failure on examination.

MISCELLANEOUS

ASSOCIATED CONDITIONS N/A

AGE RELATED FACTORS
Animals < 6 months old with oliguric renal failure sometimes recover fully, unlike older animals. It is possible that the regenerative capacity of the kidneys is greater in young animals.

ZOONOTIC POTENTIAL N/A

PREGNANCY N/A

SYNONYMS
Antifreeze poisoning

SEE ALSO
Poisoning (Intoxication) • Osmolality • Renal Failure, Acute

ABBREVIATIONS
4-MP = 4 methyl pyrazole
ADH = alcohol dehydrogenase

References

Dial SM, Thrall MA, Hamar DW. Efficacy of 4-methylpyrazole for treatment of ethylene glycol intoxication in dogs. Am J Vet Res 1994;55:1762-1770.

Dial SM, Thrall MA, Hamar DW. Comparison of ethanol and 4-methylpyrazole as therapies for ethylene glycol intoxication in the cat. Am J Vet Res 1994;55:1771-1782.

Thrall MA, Grauer GF, Mero KN. Clinicopathologic findings in dogs and cats with ethylene glycol intoxication. J Am Vet Med Assoc 1984;184:37-41.

Authors Mary Anna Thrall, Gregory F. Grauer, and Sharon M. Dial
Editor Gary Osweiler

EXOCRINE PANCREATIC INSUFFICIENCY

 BASICS

DEFINITION

Progressive loss of exocrine pancreatic acinar cells causing failure to absorb nutrients because of inadequate production of digestive enzymes.

Pathophysiology

Idiopathic pancreatic acinar atrophy is the most common cause of exocrine pancreatic insufficiency in dogs. Chronic pancreatitis with resulting destruction of pancreatic tissue is much less common in dogs, but is the most common cause in cats. Rarely, exocrine pancreatic insufficiency develops with adenocarcinoma and pancreatic duct obstruction. Deficient exocrine pancreatic secretion results in maldigestion, nutrient malabsorption, and osmotic diarrhea. Malabsorption contributes to bacterial overgrowth, which may cause secretory diarrhea.

Systems Affected

• Gastrointestinal—duodenal mucosal disease (e.g., villus atrophy, inflammatory cellular infiltrates, and abnormal mucosal enzyme activities) and bacterial overgrowth. • Endocrine/metabolism—dogs may be protein-caloric malnourished for a considerable period before diagnosis.

Genetics

Assumed to be hereditary in the German shepherd dog and transmitted by an autosomal recessive trait

Incidence/Prevalence

Relatively common in the German shepherd dog but may be seen in all breeds; rare in cats.

Geographic Distribution

• None for dogs • Cats with pancreatic fluke infection living in southeast United States.

SIGNALMENT

Species Dogs and cats

Breed Predilections
German shepherd dog

Mean Age and Range
• Signs typically occur as a consequence of pancreatic acinar atrophy in young dogs. Chronic pancreatitis is a likely cause in older dogs. • Cats— middle-aged to older

Predominant Sex N/A

SIGNS

General Comments

• Consider exocrine pancreatic insufficiency in young German shepherd dogs with a history of chronic diarrhea suggestive of malassimilation. • Severity of clinical signs varies, and depends on the time elapsed before diagnosis and treatment.

Historical Findings

• Weight loss accompanied by a normal to increased appetite • Chronic watery diarrhea of small bowel origin in many animals. Diarrhea is continuous or intermittent. Fecal volumes larger than normal and steatorrhea is present. Diarrhea generally lessens in severity when a low–fat, highly digestible diet is fed.
• Flatulence and borborygmus common
• Coprophagia and pica in some animals
• Polyuria and polydipsia may be seen in animals with diabetes mellitus caused by chronic pancreatitis.

Physical Examination Findings

• Thinness • Reduced muscle mass
• "Unthrifty" appearance with a poor quality haircoat

CAUSES

• Pancreatic acinar atrophy • Chronic relapsing pancreatitis • Pancreatic adenocarcinoma • Duodenal mucosal disease • Pancreatic fluke (Eurytrema procyonis) infection in cats

RISK FACTORS

• German shepherd dogs • Any condition predisposing patients to recurrent pancreatitis

 DIAGNOSIS

DIFFERENTIAL DIAGNOSIS

• Exocrine pancreatic insufficiency should be differentiated from all other causes of malabsorption. • Common causes of malabsorption include small intestinal mucosal diseases which are best diagnosed by intestinal mucosal biopsy. • Rule out chronic parasitism by performing multiple fecal examinations. • Rule out diabetes mellitus and hyperthyroidism in cats.

CBC/BIOCHEMISTRY/URINALYSIS

Results usually normal.

OTHER LABORATORY TESTS

Screening Tests for Malassimilation

Microscopic examination of feces for undigested food, assessment of fecal proteolytic activity by X-ray film digestion, and the plasma turbidity test are unreliable and not recommended.

Assay for Serum Trypsin-like Immunoreactivity (TLI)

• Diagnostic test of choice for exocrine pancreatic insufficiency in dogs • Theory of test—serum TLI can be detected by a species–specific assay that measures trypsinogen leaked directly into the blood from pancreatic acinar tissue. Serum TLI is detected in all normal dogs with a functional exocrine pancreatic mass. Dramatically reduced serum TLI concentration is observed in dogs with exocrine pancreatic insufficiency. Assay not commercially available for cats • Advantages —simple, quick, highly sensitive, and requires single serum specimen

Other Tests

• The bentiromide (BT–PABA) absorption test indirectly assesses pancreatic enzyme activity in the small intestine. Disadvantages include the technical constraints of the test, need for multiple sampling, and absence of proven benefit over TLI assay. • Assays of fecal proteolytic activity by use of casein-based substrates are accurate means of diagnosing exocrine pancreatic insufficiency in both dogs and cats. Disadvantages include the need for collecting multiple fecal specimens and the lack of availability for clinicians. • Typically, serum folate concentration is high and cobalamine concentration is low in animals with concurrent bacterial overgrowth.

IMAGING

Abdominal radiographs and ultrasound unremarkable

OTHER DIAGNOSTIC PROCEDURES

N/A

GROSS AND HISTOPATHOLOGIC FINDINGS

• Marked atrophy and absence of pancreatic acinar tissue on gross inspection. • Microscopically, acini and possibly islets depleted and replaced by fibrous tissue in animals with chronic pancreatitis

 TREATMENT

INPATIENT VS OUTPATIENT

• The vast majority of patients are readily treated as outpatients.
• Patients with exocrine pancreatic insufficiency and concurrent diabetes mellitus require an initial period of hospitalization for insulin regulation of hyperglycemia.

ACTIVITY Normal

DIET

• Dietary modification is a cornerstone of treatment in dogs.
• Characteristics of the ideal diet include highly digestible, low–fat, low–fiber, and nutritionally balanced.
• High digestibility reduces nutrient availability for bacterial overgrowth.
• Avoid high fat diets since fat absorption remains impaired despite appropriate administration of enzymes.
• Avoid high-fiber diets since fiber inhibits the activity of pancreatic enzymes.
• Severely malnourished dogs may require supplementation with cobalamin, tocopherol, and fat-soluble vitamins A, D, E, and K.

CLIENT EDUCATION

• Discuss hereditary nature of disease in German shepherd dogs.
• Discuss expense of pancreatic enzymes and need for lifelong treatment.
• Discuss the possibility of diabetes mellitus in patients with recurrent pancreatitis.

SURGICAL CONSIDERATIONS

Mesenteric torsion in German shepherd dogs with exocrine pancreatic insufficiency has been reported in Scandinavia but not in North America.

MEDICATIONS

DRUGS AND FLUIDS

Pancreatic Enzyme Replacement

• Administration of pancreatic enzyme concentrates is the treatment of choice. Powdered nonenteric coated preparations are most ideal.

• Enzyme powder is initially mixed in food (2 teaspoons/20 kg with each meal). Feed two meals daily at first to promote weight gain.

• Preincubation of enzymes with food does not improve the effectiveness of oral administration of enzymes.

• The administration of bicarbonate or histamine blockers (cimetidine) does not improve the effectiveness of enzymes.

• Most dogs show a rapid response to treatment within 5–7 days. At this time, the amount of daily pancreatic enzyme supplement may be gradually reduced to a dosage that prevents return of clinical signs.

Antibiotics

Antibiotics (e.g., metronidazole and oxytetracycline) may be required for 5–7 days in dogs with concurrent bacterial overgrowth.

CONTRAINDICATIONS

Avoid the use of enteric coated tablets since the dissolution of their enteric protective coating is unpredictable.

PRECAUTIONS N/A

POSSIBLE INTERACTIONS N/A

ALTERNATE DRUGS N/A

FOLLOW-UP

PATIENT MONITORING

• Monitor patients weekly for first month of treatment. • Diarrhea usually resolves within one week. • Gain in body weight will be observed. • Dogs that fail to respond after one week of enzyme administration should be placed on antibiotics for bacterial overgrowth. • Once body weight and conditioning normalize, the daily dosage of enzyme supplements may be gradually reduced to a level that maintains normal body weight.

PREVENTION/AVOIDANCE

Do not breed affected animals.

POSSIBLE COMPLICATIONS

• Failed response to pancreatic enzymes—20% of dogs. • Small intestinal bacterial overgrowth

EXPECTED COURSE AND PROGNOSIS

• Most causes of exocrine pancreatic insufficiency are irreversible and lifelong treatment is required. • Prognosis in dogs with exocrine pancreatic insufficiency alone is good with appropriate enzyme and dietary management. • Prognosis is more guarded in patients with exocrine pancreatic insufficiency and diabetes mellitus caused by chronic pancreatitis.

MISCELLANEOUS

ASSOCIATED CONDITIONS

• Small intestinal bacterial overgrowth
• Diabetes mellitus • Exocrine pancreatic insufficiency and associated vitamin K-responsive coagulopathy has been reported in a cat.

AGE RELATED FACTORS

Consider exocrine pancreatic insufficiency in young adult dogs with chronic diarrhea.

ZOONOTIC POTENTIAL N/A

PREGNANCY N/A

SYNONYMS

• Juvenile pancreatic atrophy • Pancreatic acinar atrophy

SEE ALSO

• Diarrhea, Chronic—Dogs • Small Intestinal Bacterial Overgrowth
• Pancreatitis

ABBREVIATIONS

TLI = trypsin–like immunoreactivity

References

Williams DA Exocrine pancreatic disease. In: Ettinger SJ, Feldman EC, eds . Textbook of veterinary internal medicine. 4th. ed. Philadelphia: WB Saunders, Philadelphia, 1995.

Williams DA New tests of pancreatic and small intestinal function. Compend Contin Educ Pract Vet 1987; 9:1167–1174.

Williams DA Sensitivity and specificity of serum trypsin–like immunoreactivity for the diagnosis of canine exocrine pancreatic insufficiency. J Am Vet Med Assoc 1988;192;195–201.

Simpson JW, Maskell IE Quigg J, et al. Long term management of canine exocrine pancreatic insufficiency. J Small Anim Pract 1994; 35:133–138.

Strombeck, DR, Guilford WG Small animal gastroenterology. Davis, Calif: Stonegate Publishing, 1990.

Author Albert E. Jergens
Consulting Editor Albert E. Jergens

EYELASH DISORDERS (TRICHIASIS/DISTICHIASIS/ECTOPIC CILIA)

 ## BASICS

OVERVIEW
Trichiasis develops when hair arising from normal sites contacts the corneal or conjunctival surfaces. Distichiasis develops when cilia emerge from or near the meibomian gland orifices on the lid margin. These cilia may or may not contact the cornea. Ectopic cilia are single or multiple hairs that arise from the palpebral conjunctival surface several millimeters from the lid margin, most commonly near the middle of the superior lid.

SIGNALMENT
• Eyelash disorders are common in dogs and rare in cats. • Problems tend to occur most commonly in young dogs. • Any breed can be affected; however, some breeds are predisposed—breeds with prominent facial folds such as the pekingese, pug, and bulldog frequently have facial fold trichiasis; most cocker spaniels have distichiasis to some degree; ectopic cilia are more common than average in the dachshund, lhasa apso, and shetland sheepdog, among other breeds.

SIGNS

Trichiasis From Facial Folds
• Nasal corneal vascularization and pigmentation • Blepharospasm • Epiphora

Distichiasis
• Asymptomatic in most animals. • If stiff, stout distichia are contacting the cornea, blepharospasm, epiphora, corneal vascularization, pigmentation, and ulceration may develop.

Ectopic Cilia
• Ocular pain • Severe blepharospasm • Epiphora • Often cause superficial corneal ulcers with a linear appearance (corresponding to lid movement) on the superior cornea. These ulcers are resistant to healing until the underlying problem is diagnosed and corrected.

CAUSES AND RISK FACTORS
In most dogs, the disorder is related to facial conformation to breed predisposition, or it is idiopathic.

 ## DIAGNOSIS

DIFFERENTIAL DIAGNOSIS
Other adnexal abnormalities (e.g., entropion), keratoconjunctivitis sicca, conjunctival foreign body, and infectious conjunctivitis should be ruled out. Diagnosis is made on the basis of direct observation of the abnormal cilia.

CBC/BIOCHEMISTRY/URINALYSIS
N/A

OTHER LABORATORY TESTS N/A

IMAGING N/A

OTHER DIAGNOSTIC PROCEDURES
N/A

 ## TREATMENT

• Trichiasis can be managed conservatively in some animals. Keeping the periocular hair short may help; however, clipping the hair on facial folds may make it stiffer and more irritating. Surgical correction of adnexal abnormalities is indicated, such as entropion correction. Facial folds can be resected; however, a medial canthal closure is often a better procedure because it eliminates lagophthalmos and medial entropion as well as facial fold trichiasis.
• Distichiasis is asymptomatic in most animals, and no treatment is indicated. When symptomatic, distichia can be treated surgically by cryotherapy, electrocautery or electroepilation, or resection from the conjunctival surface. Lid splitting techniques should be avoided because postoperative scarring can predispose to cicatricial entropion and impaired lid function.
• Ectopic cilia should be treated surgically with an en-bloc resection of the cilia and associated meibomian gland. Cryotherapy can be used as the sole treatment method or as an adjunct after surgical resection.

EYELASH DISORDERS (TRICHIASIS/DISTICHIASIS/ECTOPIC CILIA)

MEDICATIONS

DRUGS AND FLUIDS

• Medical treatment is rarely indicated; however, lubricant ointments are sometimes valuable when used to soften cilia and lessen irritation before surgical correction. • Perioperative, topically applied antibiotics are recommended in animals undergoing surgery in an effort to minimize conjunctival flora in the surgical sites.

CONTRAINDICATIONS/POSSIBLE INTERACTIONS N/A

FOLLOW-UP

• Regrowth of distichia is common because destructive procedures such as cryotherapy and electroepilation have to be done conservatively to minimize lid damage. • Animals that develop ectopic cilia are at risk for developing ectopic cilia at other locations.
• Owners should be advised to have their animal rechecked if clinical signs recur.

MISCELLANEOUS

Reference

Gelatt KN. Veterinary ophthalmology. 2nd ed. Philadelphia: Lea & Febiger, 1991.
Author Erin S. Champagne
Consulting Editor Paul E. Miller

FACIAL NERVE PARESIS/PARALYSIS

 BASICS

DEFINITION
Dysfunction of the facial or seventh cranial nerve, causing paralysis or weakness of the muscles of the ears, lids, lips, and nostrils

Pathophysiology
Weakness and paralysis are caused by impairment of the facial nerve or the neuromuscular junction peripherally or its nucleus in the brainstem.

Systems Affected
• Nervous— facial nerve peripherally or its nucleus in the brainstem • Ophthalmic—if parasympathetic preganglionic neurons that supply the lacrimal glands and course with the facial nerve are involved, conjunctivitis and keratitis develop because of the inability to close the lids and lack of tear secretion

Genetics N/A

Incidence/Prevalence
More common in dogs than cats

Geographic Distribution N/A

SIGNALMENT
Species Dogs and cats

Breed Predilections
For idiopathic facial nerve paralysis—cocker spaniel, Pembroke Welsh corgi, boxer, English setter, and domestic longhair cats

Mean Age and Range Adult animals

Predominant Sex N/A

SIGNS
General Comments
• Paresis is unilateral and idiopathic in most animals. • Not infrequently, unaffected facial nerves become affected within a few weeks to months. • Idiopathic paresis occurs bilaterally but rarely; most patients have signs of systemic disease and facial weakness is often missed. • In most patients, facial paresis and paralysis accompany other clinical signs and indicate focal or systemic disease.

Historical Findings
• Messy eating; food left around mouth
• Excessive drooling • Facial asymmetry, inability to close the eye • Rubbing of the eye; discharge from the eye; cloudy eye

Physical Examination Findings
• Unilateral paresis and paralysis are characterized by ipsilateral ear and lip drooping, excessive drooling, food falling from the side of mouth, collapse of the nostril, inability to close the eyelids, wide palpebral fissure, decreased or absent menace response, and palpebral reflex. • Chronically affected animals may have deviation of the face toward the affected side. • Some patients have mucopurulent discharge from the affected eye and exposure conjunctivitis or keratitis.

CAUSES
Unilateral Peripheral
• Idiopathic and metabolic (e.g., hypothyroidism) • Other causes of impairment or destruction of the middle ear • Inflammatory—otitis media and interna; nasopharyngeal polyps in cats • Neoplasia • Trauma—fracture of the petrous temporal bone; trauma to the facial nerve external to the stylomastoid foramen or secondary to surgical ablation of external ear canal

Bilateral Peripheral
• Idiopathic—rare • Inflammatory and immune-mediated—polyradiculoneuritis including coonhound paralysis, polyneuropathies, and myasthenia gravis • Metabolic—paraneoplastic polyneuropathy (e.g., insulinoma) • Botulism • Pituitary neoplasm • CNS (most cases unilateral)—brainstem signs such as altered mentation, other cranial nerve deficits, and gait abnormalities predominate

RISK FACTORS Chronic ear disease

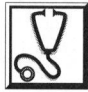 **DIAGNOSIS**

DIFFERENTIAL DIAGNOSIS
• Important to differentiate unilateral from bilateral and whether there are other neurologic deficits • Likely idiopathic if patient has no historical or physical signs of ear disease and no other neurologic deficits • Check for hypothyroidism if clinical evidence of this disease exists (e.g., lethargy and poor hair coat) • If patient also has head tilt or Horner's syndrome, diagnostic workup for middle/inner ear disease indicated • If the patient is depressed and displays neurologic signs related to the brainstem, CNS disease should be suspected.

CBC/BIOCHEMISTRY/URINALYSIS
• Results usually normal in patients with idiopathic facial paralysis • Hypercholesterolemia or nonregenerative anemia in some patients with hypothyroidism-associated facial paralysis • Hypoglycemia if patient has insulinoma

OTHER LABORATORY TESTS
• Mainly indicated in animals with bilateral weakness • Amended insulin-glucose ratio to detect insulinoma, acetylcholine receptor antibodies to detect myasthenia gravis, ELISA test to detect coonhound paralysis • TSH stimulation to detect hypothyroidism

IMAGING
• Radiographs of bullae (ie, oblique, open-mouthed) useful for defining middle ear disease and fractures • CT and MRI can be used to define brainstem disease.

OTHER DIAGNOSTIC PROCEDURES
• Schirmer tear test to evaluate tear production
• Electromyography and evaluation of motor nerve conduction velocity to rule in polyradiculoneuritis and polyneuropathy • CSF examination to detect brainstem disease

GROSS AND HISTOPATHOLOGIC FINDINGS
In some patients with idiopathic disease, degeneration of large and small myelinated fibers without evidence of inflammation

 TREATMENT

INPATIENT VERSUS OUTPATIENT
• Patients with idiopathic facial paralysis are treated as outpatients.
• Animals that are systemically ill or have CNS disease should be hospitalized for initial medical workup and management.

ACTIVITY N/A

DIET No change required

CLIENT EDUCATION
• Although most animals have idiopathic disease, middle ear disease should be ruled out.
• Affects are usually permanent, but as muscle fibrosis develops, there is a natural "tuck up" which reduces asymmetry. Drooling usually stops within 2-4 weeks.
• The other side can become affected.
• The cornea on the affected side may need lubrication.
• Most animals tolerate this nerve deficit well.
• Extra care for the eye if the animal is of a breed with natural exophthalmos. Check for corneal ulcer regularly.

SURGICAL CONSIDERATIONS
Bulla osteotomy may be useful in patients with disorders of the middle ear.

 MEDICATIONS

DRUGS AND FLUIDS
• Treat specific disease if possible
• In patients with idiopathic disease, no specific treatment applicable. Efficacy of steroids unknown.
• Tear replacement required if Schirmer tear test value is low and in patients with ectropion or exophthalmic globes

CONTRAINDICATIONS N/A

PRECAUTIONS N/A

POSSIBLE INTERACTIONS N/A

ALTERNATE DRUGS N/A

 FOLLOW-UP

PATIENT MONITORING
• Early reevaluation, looking for evidence of corneal ulcers • Although damage is permanent in most patients, monthly assessment of menace responses, palpebral reflexes, and lip and ear movements helpful to evaluate if facial nerve function returns and also to reassess the condition of the affected eye

PREVENTION/AVOIDANCE N/A

POSSIBLE COMPLICATIONS
• Keratoconjunctivitis sicca • Corneal ulcers
• Severe contracture on side of lesion

EXPECTED COURSE AND PROGNOSIS
• Depends on cause • In patients with idiopathic disease, prognosis for recovery is guarded. • Improvement may take weeks or months or may never occur. • Lip contracture develops in some patients.

 **MISCELLANEOUS**

ASSOCIATED CONDITIONS N/A

AGE RELATED FACTORS N/A

ZOONOTIC POTENTIAL N/A

PREGNANCY N/A

SYNONYMS
Idiopathic facial paresis and paralysis

SEE ALSO
• Otitis Media and Interna • Hypothyroidism
• Keratoconjunctivitis Sicca

ABBREVIATIONS
CNS = central nervous system
CSF = cerebrospinal fluid
CT = computerized tomography
MRI = magnetic resonance imaging

References
Kern TJ, Hollis NE. Facial neuropathy in dogs and cats: 95 cases (1975-1985). J Am Vet Med Assoc 1987;191:1604-1609.
Braund KG, et al. Idiopathic facial paralysis in the dog. Vet Rec 1979;105:297-299.
de Lahunta A. Veterinary neuroanatomy and clinical neurology. 2nd ed. Philadelphia: WB Saunders, 1983:110.

Author T. Mark Neer
Consulting Editor Joane M. Parent

FALSE PREGNANCY

BASICS

DEFINITION
Display of maternal behavior and physical signs of pregnancy in mid to late diestrus by a nonpregnant bitch

Pathophysiology
• The underlying endocrinologic mechanism is poorly understood. It is known that all bitches that ovulate produce functional corpora lutea and remain under progesterone influence for approximately 2-3 months. Serum progesterone concentrations are similar in pregnant, nonpregnant, and false pregnant animals, except for a sharp decline 1-2 days before parturition. It is thought that the falling serum progesterone concentration causes an increase in the serum prolactin concentration, which may be responsible for initiating the changes seen in false pregnant animals. • Mating during the preceding estrus has no influence on the occurrence of false pregnancy. Future fertility is not affected.

Systems Affected Reproductive

Genetics N/A

Incidence/Prevalence Unknown

Geographic Distribution N/A

SIGNALMENT
Nonpregnant females that were in estrus 2-3 months ago and are experiencing a decline in serum progesterone concentration.

Species
• Common in dogs • Rare in cats

Breed Predilections None

Mean Age and Range
Signs can occur at any age

Predominant Sex Female

SIGNS

General Comments
Severity of clinical signs varies between individuals and from one occurrence to the next within the same individual.

Historical Findings
• Behavior changes—nesting, mothering activity, restlessness, and self-nursing • Abdominal distention and mammary gland enlargement • Vomiting, depression, and anorexia • Signs of labor (rare)

Physical Examination Findings
Large mammary glands with secretion of a brownish serous fluid or milk

CAUSES
• There is an inverse relationship between progesterone and prolactin, and a drop in progesterone concentration in late diestrus causes the prolactin concentration to rise.
• Animals treated with progestin for conditions not related to false pregnancy may have signs of false pregnancy on withdrawal of the progestin. • Animals oophorectomized or ovariohysterectomized in diestrus when progesterone is high may have signs of false pregnancy after surgery. • Hypothyroid animals with high thyroid releasing hormone (TRH) concentration, which stimulates prolactin secretion, have some of the clinical signs associated with false pregnancy.

RISK FACTORS
It is thought that false pregnancy is not influenced by previous pregnancy and that false pregnancy does not cause predisposition to other reproductive diseases.

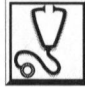

DIAGNOSIS

DIFFERENTIAL DIAGNOSIS
• Must differentiate from other causes of mammary gland enlargement (e.g., neoplasia and mastitis) and abdominal enlargement (e.g., ascites and organomegaly). • Closed pyometra—usually associated with more severe systemic signs than false pregnancy
• Pregnancy

CBC/BIOCHEMISTRY/URINALYSIS
Results usually normal; if not, suspect other reproductive tract or systemic disease
Diagnosis is made by a history of estrus within the preceding 2-3 months and clinical signs.

OTHER LABORATORY TESTS N/A

IMAGING
Radiography or ultrasonography recommended to rule out pyometra and normal pregnancy

OTHER DIAGNOSTIC PROCEDURES N/A

GROSS AND HISTOPATHOLOGIC FINDINGS N/A

TREATMENT
• Since all pregnant, nonpregnant, and false pregnant, ovulating dogs go through a similar diestrus stage, treatment is usually not necessary.
• Minimize stimuli to the mammary glands that promote lactation, such as cold and warm packs. Self nursing or licking the mammary glands can be prevented by use of an Elizabethan collar, but even rubbing of the Elizabethan collar on the mammary glands may be a sufficient stimulus to prolong lactation.
• Progestins and androgens suppress prolactin secretion.
• Recurrence of false pregnancy is prevented by ovariohysterectomy (OHE) during anestrus.

INPATIENT VERSUS OUTPATIENT
Patients can be discharged immediately if medical treatment is tried. However, if surgery is planned, inpatient care is required.

ACTIVITY N/A

DIET
Reduction of food over 3-4 days may reduce lactation.

CLIENT EDUCATION
• False pregnancy is a normal phenomenon in ovulatory bitches.
• No association between false pregnancy and reproductive abnormalities
• Attempt to have the bitch become pregnant during the next estrous cycle if she is to be bred

SURGICAL CONSIDERATIONS
If the bitch is not intended for breeding, advise OHE during the next anestrus. It is not advisable to perform OHE while the animal has clinical signs of false pregnancy, because doing so does not alleviate clinical signs, and medical treatment may be required.

MEDICATIONS

DRUGS AND FLUIDS
Bromocryptine (Parlodel, Sandoz, US); 10 ug/kg PO q12h for 5 days. This drug is not approved for veterinary use in U.S. and Canada but will reduce lactation.

CONTRAINDICATIONS
The use of bromocryptine induces abortion in pregnant animals.

PRECAUTIONS
If the drug causes vomiting, give half the dosage for the next 2 doses and then the full dosage again.

POSSIBLE INTERACTIONS
The concomitant use of erythromycin may increase bromocryptine plasma concentration.

ALTERNATE DRUGS
• Testosterone (1 mg/kg IM once)—may cause virilizing effects such as clitoral hypertrophy. Contraindicated in animals with hepatic or nephritic conditions. Causes masculinization of female fetus in the pregnant animal.
• Mibolerone (Cheque, 40 mcg/kg PO q24h for 5 days)—for side effects, see testosterone.
• Megestrol acetate (Ovaban, 1-2 mg/kg PO q24h for 8 days)—can cause mammary hyperplasia, pyometra, diabetes mellitus, increased appetite, weight gain, and atrophy of the adrenal cortex. Signs may recur after the drug is discontinued.
Mild tranquilizers may reduce behavioral signs, except for phenothiazines which cause prolactin concentrations to rise

FOLLOW-UP

PATIENT MONITORING N/A

PREVENTION/AVOIDANCE
OHE during anestrus prevents recurrence.

POSSIBLE COMPLICATIONS N/A

EXPECTED COURSE AND PROGNOSIS

• In most animals the condition resolves in 2-3 weeks without treatment. • The use of bromocryptine may reduce the time period of clinical signs to 1 week. • False pregnancy can develop during subsequent estrous cycles.

✓ **MISCELLANEOUS**

ASSOCIATED CONDITIONS N/A

AGE RELATED FACTORS N/A

ZOONOTIC POTENTIAL N/A

PREGNANCY

Do not treat pregnant animals.

SYNONYMS

Pseudopregnancy
Pseudocyesis
Phantom pregnancy

SEE ALSO N/A

ABBREVIATIONS

OHE = ovariohysterectomy
TRH = thyroid releasing hormone.

References

Allen WE. Pseudopregnancy in the bitch: The current view on aetiology and treatment. J Small Anim Pract 1986;27;419-424.

Arbeiter K, Brass W, Ballabio R, et al. Treatment of pseudopregnancy in the bitch with cabergoline, an ergoline derivative. J Small Anim Pract 1988;29:781-788.

Johnson CA. False pregnancy, disorders of pregnancy, parturition. In: Nelson RW, Couto CG, eds. Essentials of small animal internal medicine. St. Louis: Mosby, 1992;669-683.

Johnston SD. Pseudopregnancy in the bitch. In: DA Morrow, ed. Current therapy in theriogenology 2. Philadelphia: WB Saunders, 1986;490-491.

Author Klass Post
Consulting Editor Sara K. Lyle

FANCONI'S SYNDROME

 BASICS

DEFINITION

Fanconi's syndrome is a collection of abnormalities arising from defective renal tubular transport of water, sodium, potassium, glucose, phosphate, bicarbonate and amino acids. Impaired tubular reabsorption causes excessive urinary excretion of these solutes.

SIGNALMENT

• Documented in several breeds of dogs but not in cats
• Approximately 75% of the reported cases have occurred in the Basenji breed. Estimates of the prevalence within the Basenji breed in North America range from 10-30%. It is presumed to be inherited in this breed, but the mode of inheritance is unknown.
• No sex predilection
• Age at diagnosis ranged from 1-8 years, with most developing clinical signs from 2-4 years

SIGNS

General Comments

• Vary depending on the severity of specific solute losses and whether renal failure has developed.
• The losses of amino acids and glucose usually not associated with clinical signs

Historical Findings

• Polyuria
• Polydipsia
• Weight loss

Physical Examination Findings

• Muscle weakness in animals with hypokalemia results from severe renal potassium loss.
• Osteomalacia in adults or rickets in juveniles with severe phosphate and calcium losses

CAUSES AND RISK FACTORS

• Inherited (or idiopathic) in most cases; particularly true in the Basenji, Norwegian elkhound, Shetland sheepdog, and schnauzer breeds of dog
• Acquired Fanconi's syndrome has been reported in dogs treated with gentamicin and streptozotocin.

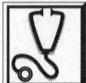 **DIAGNOSIS**

DIFFERENTIAL DIAGNOSIS

Primary renal glucosuria may be confused with Fanconi's syndrome; both cause glucosuria in the absence of hyperglycemia. The documentation of amino aciduria, mild proteinuria, or a normal anion gap metabolic acidosis (indicative of bicarbonate loss) suggests Fanconi's syndrome.

CBC/BIOCHEMISTRY/URINALYSIS

• Results of CBC usually normal
• Hypokalemia in about one third
• Azotemia if animal has renal failure
• Urine specific gravity usually low (1.005 to 1.018) and mild proteinuria common
• Glucosuria in the absence of hyperglycemia a frequent finding and often the first suggestive finding of Fanconi's syndrome

OTHER LABORATORY TESTS

• Blood gas analysis may reveal normal anion gap metabolic acidosis. This develops because of urinary bicarbonate loss (referred to as proximal renal tubular acidosis). However, urine pH remains acidic and bicarbonate does not appear in the urine unless a bicarbonate load is administered.
• Urinary clearance studies to document excessive excretion of solutes such as amino acids may be needed to confirm Fanconi's syndrome.

IMAGING N/A

OTHER DIAGNOSTIC PROCEDURES

None

GROSS AND HISTOPATHOLOGIC FINDINGS

Papillary necrosis in many animals

 TREATMENT

• Discontinue any drug that may cause Fanconi's syndrome or treat for a specific intoxication if present.
• No treatment will reverse the transport defects in dogs with inherited or idiopathic disease.
• Because there is marked variability in the number and severity of transport defects among animals, treatment for hypokalemia, metabolic acidosis, azotemia, and polyuria needs to be individualized. The treatment of hypokalemia and renal failure are discussed elsewhere in this publication.
• Treatment for metabolic acidosis is instituted if the patient's blood bicarbonate concentration is < 12 mEq/L. Large doses of bicarbonate may be required because reduced tubular reabsorptive capacity causes marked urinary bicarbonate loss. The goal of bicarbonate administration is to maintain a blood concentration from 12-18 mEq/L. Because bicarbonate administration may aggravate renal potassium loss, serum potassium should be monitored regularly.

MEDICATIONS

DRUGS AND FLUIDS

Sodium bicarbonate or potassium citrate—1 to 9 mEq/kg PO q24h in patients with metabolic acidosis.

CONTRAINDICATIONS/POSSIBLE INTERACTIONS

Avoid drugs that are nephrotoxic or have the potential to cause Fanconi's syndrome (see Causes and Risk Factors)

 FOLLOW-UP

• Serum biochemical analysis at 10- to 14-day intervals to assess the effect of treatment and any change in values (especially BUN and creatinine concentration). Because bicarbonate administration may aggravate renal potassium loss, serum potassium should be monitored regularly. Once stable, biochemical values should be monitored at 2- to 4-month intervals.

• The clinical course of the disease varies. Some dogs remain stable for years, whereas others develop rapidly progressive renal failure over a few months. The cause of death is usually acute renal failure, often associated with severe metabolic acidosis.

 MISCELLANEOUS

SEE ALSO

• Potassium, Hypokalemia
• Renal Failure, Chronic—Dogs
• Renal Failure, Acute—Dogs

Reference

Brown SA. Fanconi's syndrome. In: Kirk RW, ed. Current veterinary therapy X. Philadelphia: WB Saunders, 1989:1163-1165.

Author Darcy H. Shaw
Consulting Editors Larry G. Adams and Carl A. Osborne

FELINE IMMUNODEFICIENCY VIRUS

 BASICS

DEFINITION

Feline immunodeficiency virus (FIV) is a retrovirus that causes an immunodeficiency disease in domestic cats. It is in the same subfamily (lentiviruses) as human immunodeficiency virus, the causitive agent of human AIDS.

Pathophysiology

• Immune system function is disrupted by FIV infection, with feline lymphocytes and macrophages serving as the main targets for virus replication. Both $CD4^+$ and $CD8^+$ subsets of T cells can be infected lytically in culture; however, FIV selectively and progressively decreases feline $CD4^+$ cells in the infected cat. Inversion of the $CD4^+:CD8^+$ ratio develops slowly, with an absolute decrease of $CD4^+$ T cells after several months of infection. The loss of T helper cells results in dysfunction of both humoral and cell-mediated immunity. • Macrophages are the main "reservoir" of virus in FIV-infected cats; infected macrophages have several defects in function including an increased production of tumor necrosis factor. Astrocytes and microglial cells in the brain and megakaryocytes and mononuclear bone marrow cells may be infected in some cats. Coinfection with FeLV extends the host cell range of FIV to include kidney, brain, and liver cells.

Systems Affected

• Hemic/lymphatic/immune—immune system initially a result of loss of $CD4^+$ T cells • All other body systems a result of immunosuppression and secondary infections

Genetics

No genetic predisposition for infection. Genetics may play some role in the progression and severity of disease.

Incidence/Prevalence

In the United States and Canada, the prevalence of FIV infection is estimated to be 1.5-3% in the healthy cat population and 9-15% in cats exhibiting signs of clinical illness.

Geographic Distribution

The distribution of FIV is worldwide, but seroprevalence rates vary greatly.

SIGNALMENT

Species Cats

Breed Predilections None

Mean Age and Range

The prevalence of FIV infection increases with age, with a mean age of about 5 years at the time of diagnosis.

Predominant Sex

Male, because of more aggression and roaming than female

SIGNS

GENERAL COMMENTS

Because of the immunosuppressive nature of FIV infection, clinical signs in domestic cats are diverse. Diseases associated with FIV infection cannot be distinguished clinically from FeLV-associated immunodeficiencies.

Historical Findings

• Cats allowed outdoors • Recurrent minor illnesses, especially with upper respiratory and gastrointestinal signs, may be reported.

Physical Examination Findings

• Physical exam findings will depend on whether or not secondary or opportunistic infections are present. • Mild to moderate lymphadenopathy • Gingivitis/stomatitis/periodontitis (in 25-50% of positive cats) • Upper respiratory tract signs of rhinitis, conjunctivitis, and keratitis (in about 30% of FIV-positive cats)—often associated with feline herpesvirus and calicivirus infections • Persistent diarrhea (in 10-20% of infected cats)—bacterial or fungal overgrowth, parasite-induced inflammation, or a direct effect of FIV infection on the GI epithelium • Chronic, nonresponsive, or recurrent infections of the external ear and skin often result from bacterial infections or dermatophytosis. • Fever and wasting, especially in the later stages of disease, result from possible high levels of tumor necrosis factor. • Ocular disease—anterior uveitis, pars planitis, and glaucoma • Lymphosarcoma/other neoplasia • Neurological abnormalities—aggression and peripheral neuropathies

CAUSES

• Cat-to-cat transmission of FIV, usually by bite wounds • Occasional perinatal transmission

RISK FACTORS

• Male • Free-roaming

 DIAGNOSIS

DIFFERENTIAL DIAGNOSIS

• Feline leukemia virus infection • Bacterial, parasitic, viral, or fungal infections • Toxoplasmosis—neurologic and ocular manifestations may be a result of primary Toxoplasma infection, FIV infection, or coinfection with both pathogens • Nonviral neoplastic diseases

CBC/BIOCHEMISTRY/URINALYSIS

Hemogram may be normal. Anemia, lymphopenia, or neutropenia may be present; however, neutrophils can be elevated in response to secondary infections. Urinalysis and serum chemistry profile are usually normal except for increased serum protein resulting from hypergammaglobulinemia.

OTHER LABORATORY TESTS

• Serologic testing to detect antibodies to FIV. Enzyme-linked immunosorbent assay (ELISA) is used for routine screening and the Western blot for confirmatory testing of ELISA-positive samples. The format of the ELISA varies from kits designed for "in-house" use to a microtiter plate format designed for diagnostic laboratory use. Positive results on ELISA should be confirmed by additional testing, especially in healthy, low-risk cats or when diagnosis of FIV may result in euthanasia of the cat. Kittens less than 6 months of age may test positive as a result of passive transfer of antibodies from the FIV-positive queen; thus a positive test in a kitten does not indicate virus infection. Retest kittens at 8-12 months of age to determine if they are FIV-infected. • Virus isolation or detection by other methods occasionally is available on an experimental basis. Virus antigen detection procedures usually are not sensitive enough to be useful for diagnostic purposes. $CD4^+:CD8^+$ evaluation is sometimes available.

IMAGING N/A

OTHER DIAGNOSTIC PROCEDURES N/A

GROSS AND HISTOPATHOLOGIC FINDINGS

• Lymphadenopathy is associated with follicular hyperplasia and massive paracortical infiltration of plasmacytes. Later, a mixture of follicular hyperplasia and follicular depletion or involution may be observed. In the terminal stage of disease, lymphoid depletion is the predominant finding. • Lymphocytic and plasmacytic infiltrates of the gingiva, lymph nodes and other lymphoid tissues, spleen, kidney, and liver of affected cats • Intestinal lesions similar to those seen with feline parvovirus infection (feline panleukopenia-like syndrome)

 TREATMENT

INPATIENT VERSUS OUTPATIENT

Cats with severe secondary infections may require hospitalization until their condition is stable.

ACTIVITY Normal

DIET

Normal. Cats with diarrhea, kidney disease, or chronic wasting may require special diets.

CLIENT EDUCATION

• FIV infection is slowly progressive. Healthy antibody-positive cats may remain healthy for years. Clients should expect cats with clinical signs of immunodeficiency disease to have recurrent or chronic health problems that will require medical attention.
• Discuss the importance of keeping cats indoors to protect them from exposure to secondary pathogens and to prevent spread of FIV to other cats.

SURGICAL CONSIDERATIONS

Oral treatment or surgery (dental cleaning, tooth extraction, gingival biopsy) is frequently required. Biopsy or removal of tumors also may be necessary.

MEDICATIONS

DRUGS AND FLUIDS

• Immunomodulatory drugs may allieviate some clinical signs. Human recombinant alpha interferon (Roferon, diluted in saline, 30 units/day PO for 7 days every other week) may increase survival rates and improve clinical status. Additional immunomodulatory drugs include Propionibacterium acnes (Immunoregulin, 0.5 ml/cat IV, once or twice weekly) and acemannan (Carrisyn, 100mg/cat/day PO).
• Management of secondary and opportunistic infections is a primary consideration. Additional supportive therapy, such as parenteral fluids and nutritional supplements, may be required. Yearly vaccination for respiratory and enteric viruses with inactivated vaccines is recommended.
• Gingivitis and stomatitis may be refractory to treatment. Antibacterial or antimycotic drugs are useful for overgrowth of bacteria or fungi, but prolonged therapy or increased dosages may be required. Anaerobic bacterial infections can be treated with metronidazole (Flagyl, 7-15 mg/kg PO q8h or q12h) or clindamycin (Antirobe, 11 mg/kg PO q12h). Judicious but aggressive use of corticosteroids or gold salts may help control immune-mediated inflammation.
• Anorexic cats may benefit from IV diazepam (Valium, 0.2mg/kg) or oral oxazepam (Serax, 2.5 mg/kg). Anabolic steroids or megestrol acetate may achieve more prolonged stimulation of appetite and reversal of cachexia; however, the efficacy of these drugs in FIV-infected cats is not known.
• Anterior uveitis is treated with application of topical corticosteroids, but long-term response to therapy may be incomplete or poor. Pars planitis often will regress spontaneously and may recur. Management of FIV-related glaucoma is the same as for glaucoma resulting from other causes.

CONTRAINDICATIONS

• Severe neutropenias have been induced in several FIV-infected cats treated with griseo-

fulvin. Although the neutropenia is reversible if the griseofulvin is withdrawn early enough, secondary infections associated with the condition can be life-threatening; therefore, this drug should be avoided or used with extreme caution in FIV-positive cats. • Modified live vaccines may cause disease in immunosuppressed cats.

PRECAUTIONS

Systemic corticosteroids should be used with caution because of the potential for further immunosuppression.

POSSIBLE INTERACTIONS

See Contraindications

ALTERNATE DRUGS N/A

FOLLOW-UP

PATIENT MONITORING

Varies according to the secondary infections and other manifestations of disease

PREVENTION/AVOIDANCE

Prevent contact of cats with FIV-positive cats. Quarantine and test incoming cats for FIV before introduction into multiple cat households.

POSSIBLE COMPLICATIONS N/A

EXPECTED COURSE AND PROGNOSIS

Variable disease progression—death occurs in about 20% of cats within the first 2 years after diagnosis (4.5-6 years after the estimated time of infection); however, more than 50% of the infected cats remain asymptomatic during the same time period. Once a cat is in the late stages of disease (wasting and frequent or severe opportunistic infections), life expectancy is 1 year or less.

MISCELLANEOUS

ASSOCIATED CONDITIONS

Secondary bacterial, viral, fungal and parasitic disease, lymphoid tumors, and immune-mediated disease

AGE RELATED FACTORS

• Most common in middle-aged and older cats (mean age of 5 years) • Kittens may test positive because of passive antibody transfer.

ZOONOTIC POTENTIAL

• None known (evidence against FIV transmission to humans is compelling but cannot be considered conclusive owing to the relatively short period of time the virus has been studied) • A more important consideration is the potential zoonotic transmission of secondary pathogens such as Toxoplasma gondii from FIV-positive cats to immunocompromised humans.

PREGNANCY

Abortions and stillbirths have been reported in FIV-positive queens. Transmission of FIV from queen to kittens is infrequent if the queen is antibody-positive before conception.

SYNONYMS

Feline immunodeficiency syndrome (FIS)

SEE ALSO N/A

ABBREVIATIONS

FIV = feline immunodeficiency virus
AIDS = acquired immunodeficiency syndrome
ELISA = enzyme-linked immunosorbent assay

References

Barr MC, Olsen CW, and Scott FW. Feline viral diseases. In: Ettinger SJ, Feldman EC, eds. Textbook of veterinary internal medicine. 4th ed. Philadelphia: WB Saunders, 1994.

English RV, Nelson P, Johnson CM, Nasisse M, Tompkins WA, Tompkins MB. Development of clinical disease in cats experimentally infected with feline immunodeficiency virus. J Inf Dis 1994;170:543-552.

Ishida T, Taniguchi A, Matsumura S, Washizu T, Tomoda I. Long-term clinical observations on feline immunodeficiency virus infected asymptomatic carriers. Vet Immunol Immunopathol 1992;35:15-22.

Sparger EE. Current thoughts on feline immunodeficiency virus infection. Vet Clin N Am (Small Anim Pract) 1993;23:173-191.

Author Margaret C. Barr
Consulting Editor Fred W. Scott

FELINE INFECTIOUS PERITONITIS

BASICS

DEFINITION
Feline infectious peritonitis (FIP) is a systemic, viral disease characterized by insidious onset, persistent nonresponsive fever, pyogranulomatous tissue reaction, accumulation of exudative effusions in body cavities, and high mortality.

Pathophysiology
Feline infectious peritonitis virus (FIPV) replicates locally in epithelial cells of the upper respiratory tract or oropharynx. Antiviral antibodies are produced, and the virus is taken up by macrophages. The virus is transported within monocytes/macrophages throughout the body, localizing at various vein wall and perivascular sites. The local perivascular viral replication and subsequent pyogranulomatous tissue reaction produce the classic FIP lesion.

Systems Affected
• Multisystemic—pyogranulomatous or granulomatous lesions occur in the omentum, on the serosal surface of abdominal organs such as the liver, kidney, and intestines, within abdominal lymph nodes, and in the submucosa of the intestinal tract • Respiratory—lesions on lung surfaces; pleural effusion in the wet form of FIP • Nervous—vascular lesions can occur throughout the CNS, especially in the meninges • Ophthalmic—lesions may include uveitis and chorioretinitis

Genetics N/A

Incidence/Prevalence
The prevalence of antibodies against feline coronavirus (FCoV) is high in most populations, especially in multicat facilities. The incidence of clinical disease is low in most populations, especially in single cat households. Because of the difficulty in diagnosis, control, and prevention, outbreaks of FIP within breeding catteries may be catastrophic. In endemic catteries, the risk of a FCoV-antibody–positive cat eventually developing FIP is usually less than 10%.

Geographic Distribution Worldwide

SIGNALMENT

Species
• Cats • Domestic and exotic cats are susceptible to FIPV infection.

Breed Predilections
Some families or lines of cats appear more susceptible to development of clinical disease after FCoV infection. Among exotics, the cheetah is particularly susceptible to developing fatal FIP.

Mean Age and Range
The highest incidence of FIP occurs in kittens 3 months to 3 years of age. The incidence decreases sharply after cats reach 3 years of age.

Predominant Sex N/A

SIGNS

General Comments
A wide range of signs may occur depending on the virulence of the strain of virus involved, the effectiveness of the host immune response, and the organ system affected. Two classic forms of disease occur, the wet or effusive form that targets the body cavities and the dry or noneffusive form that targets a variety of organs.

Historical Findings
• Insidious onset • Gradual weight loss and decrease in appetite • Stunting in kittens • Gradual increase in the size of the abdomen to give a "potbellied" appearance • Persistent fever that is fluctuating and antibiotic unresponsive

Physical Examination Findings
• Depression, stunted growth • Poor condition from weight loss and a dull, rough hair coat • Icterus • Abdominal and/or pleural effusion • Palpation of the abdomen may reveal abdominal masses (granulomas or pyogranulomas) within the omentum, on the surface of viscera (especially the kidney), and within the intestinal wall. The mesenteric lymph nodes may be enlarged. • Ocular findings can include anterior uveitis, keratic precipitated color change to the iris, and an irregularly shaped pupil. • Neurologic findings may include brain stem, cerebrocortical, or spinal cord signs.

CAUSES
FIP is caused by one of two genomic types of feline coronavirus. Most infections, perhaps 85%, are caused by type 1 virus (FCoV-1), with the balance caused by type 2 virus (FCoV-2). There has been great effort to distinguish between the two biotypes of virus, the low virulent or avirulent enteric strains of virus (feline enteric coronavirus or FECV), and the virulent strains that produce FIP. In reality, FECV and FIPV occur as both type 1 and type 2 viruses. Within each type there is a spectrum of virulence from avirulent viruses that produce asymptomatic infections to those that produce fatal FIP.

RISK FACTORS
• Feline leukemia virus • Introduction of a FCoV-antibody–positive cat into a population of FCoV-antibody–negative cats • Cats in breeding catteries or in multicat facilities

DIAGNOSIS

Wet FIP can be relatively easy to diagnose clinically, whereas dry FIP can be difficult to accurately diagnose. There is no one laboratory test that is diagnostic for FIP because of the variability from case to case.

DIFFERENTIAL DIAGNOSIS
• Fever of unknown origin. This diagnosis is made when other causes of fever are ruled out. • Cardiac disease causing pleural effusion. This effusion will have a low specific gravity and cell count compared to the characteristic high specific gravity and high cell count of FIP effusions. • Lesions of lymphoma, especially in the kidney, can be confused with FIP on palpation. CNS tumors may produce signs similar to those of FIP. Most cats will test positive on FeLV antigen assays. In cats that test negative, a biopsy of the lesion (if accessible) should be submitted for histopathology and immunohistochemistry for FCoV antigen assay. • Respiratory disease caused by FCV, FHV, chlamydiosis, or various bacteria • Pansteatitis (yellow fat disease). Classic feel and appearance of fat within the abdominal cavity, pain on abdominal palpation, and often a fish-only diet. • Panleukopenia producing enteritis; WBC count will be low.

CBC/BIOCHEMISTRY/URINALYSIS
• FIP cats tend to have a leukopenia early in infection, but later develop leukocytosis with neutrophilia and lymphopenia. • Mild to moderate anemia may occur. • High total plasma globulin is common. • There is often a hyperbilirubinemia and hyperbilirubinuria.

OTHER LABORATORY TESTS
• Serum antibody tests (immunoassays, viral neutralization assays) detect antibodies against feline coronavirus. Positive tests are not diagnostic, but rather only indicate previous FCoV infection. The correlation between the height of the titer and the eventual confirmation of FIP is not high. • Polymerase chain reaction (PCR) assays are available to detect viral antigen. The accuracy of positive tests correlating with clinical FIP is still being evaluated at the time of this writing. • An immunohistochemistry (immunoperoxidase) assay is available (Diagnostic Laboratory, College of Veterinary Medicine, Cornell University, Ithaca, NY 14853) to detect FCoV antigen within specific cells of histopathologic sections of tissues from cats with fatal diseases or biopsy samples. This test is excellent as a confirmatory test for FCoV as the cause of specific lesions.

IMAGING
Generally not required. Abdominal and peural effusions may be confirmed and granulomatous lesions may be detected.

OTHER DIAGNOSTIC PROCEDURES
• Fluid obtained via thoraco- and abdominocentesis will be pale to straw-colored, viscous, often will have flecks of white fibrin, and will clot upon standing. The specific gravity of this fluid is usually high (1.030-1.040). • Laparoscopy may be helpful to observe specific lesions of the peritoneal cavity and to obtain a biopsy sample for histopathology or immunohistochemistry confirmation. • Exploratory laparotomy may be indicated in difficult to diagnose cats if laparoscopy is not available.

GROSS AND HISTOPATHOLOGIC FINDINGS

• Gross findings will vary depending on the organs or tissues involved. The cat will be emaciated with a rough hair coat. In wet FIP, the abdomen and/or the thoracic cavity may contain a thick, viscous exudate. White, rough, pyogranulomatous plaques may be on the serosal surface of abdominal organs and the omentum. Granulomatous lumps may protrude from the surface of the kidney, and granulomas may be present in the wall of the intestine. Fibrous strands may extend between organs. The liver may have focal, pale lesions. The iris may be discolored, and keratic precipitates may be present on the inner side of the cornea. Cats with neurologic signs will have lesions in the brain and/or the spinal cord that may be visible grossly.

• Histopathologic findings include granulomatous or pyogranulomatous lesions in any affected tissue. Lesions start around veins, but increase in size to involve large portions of tissue. The microscopic appearance of these lesions is suggestive of FIP.

TREATMENT

INPATIENT VERSUS OUTPATIENT

Cats can be treated as inpatient or outpatient, depending on the stage and severity of the disease and the owners' willingness and ability to provide good supportive care.

ACTIVITY

Activity of cats should be restricted to prevent exposure of other cats.

DIET

Anorexia and weight loss are major problems with FIP. Any special diet that will entice the cat to eat is indicated.

CLIENT EDUCATION

Discuss the various aspects of FIP, including the grave prognosis once the disease is definitively diagnosed.

SURGICAL CONSIDERATIONS N/A

MEDICATIONS

DRUGS AND FLUIDS

• No treatment has been shown to be routinely effective in treating cats with FIP. Cats with generalized and typical signs of FIP al-

most invariably die, although many cats, probably the majority, infected with FCoV either have subclinical infections or mild, localized granulomatous disease that is not diagnosed as FIP. • Immunosuppressive drugs such as prednisolone and cyclophosphamide have been tried with limited success. Corticosteroids given by subconjunctival injection may be helpful in cats with ocular involvement only.

• Interferons, although effective in vitro, have had limited success in treating FIP. A recombinant interferon has been reported to have some success in treating FIP in Japan.

• Antibiotics are ineffective because secondary bacterial infections are not part of the clinical disease.

CONTRAINDICATIONS N/A

PRECAUTIONS N/A

POSSIBLE INTERACTIONS N/A

ALTERNATE DRUGS

There are no antiviral drugs that have been shown to be efficacious against FIPV.

FOLLOW-UP

PATIENT MONITORING

Cats with FIP should be monitored for the development of large quantities of pleural effusion.

PREVENTION/AVOIDANCE

• An MLV intranasal vaccine is available for vaccination of cats against FIPV. However, the efficacy of this vaccine is low, and therefore one cannot rely on vaccination alone to control FIP. • The main method of transmission of FIPV appears to be from asymptomatic carrier queens to their kittens at 5-7 weeks of age after maternally derived immunity has waned. Therefore, early weaning of kittens at 4-5 weeks of age, with kittens then reared isolated from direct contact with other cats including the queen, can block the cycle of transmission of virus from dam to kitten.

• Routine disinfection of premise, cages, and water/food dishes readily inactivates the virus and thus reduces transmission of virus from infected or carrier cats to uninfected cats.

• Only FCoV-antibody–negative cats should be introduced into catteries or colonies that are free of virus. Vaccination may produce antibody-positive cats and may complicate monitoring catteries for the presence of virus.

POSSIBLE COMPLICATIONS

Pleural effusion may require thoracocentesis to treat.

EXPECTED COURSE AND PROGNOSIS

FIP can run a clinical course of a few days to several months. The prognosis is grave once typical signs of FIP occur because the mortality is nearly 100%.

MISCELLANEOUS

ASSOCIATED CONDITIONS

Cats that are FeLV-positive are more prone to develop clinical FIP.

AGE RELATED FACTORS

Generally FIP is a disease of cats 3 months to 3 years of age, but cats of any age can be affected.

ZOONOTIC POTENTIAL None

PREGNANCY

FIPV can infect fetuses, resulting in fetal death or neonatal FIP.

SYNONYMS

Feline coronavirus infection

SEE ALSO N/A

ABBREVIATIONS

FIP = feline infectious peritonitis
FIPV = feline infectious peritonitis virus
FECV = feline enteric coronavirus
FCoV = feline coronavirus
MLV = Modified live virus

Reference

Barr MC, Olsen CW, Scott FW. Feline viral diseases. In: Ettinger SJ, Feldman EC, eds. Veterinary internal medicine. 4th ed. Philadelphia: WB Saunders, 1995:409-439.

Author Fred W. Scott

Consulting Editor Fred W. Scott

FELINE LEUKEMIA VIRUS INFECTION

BASICS

DEFINITION
Feline leukemia virus (FeLV) is a retrovirus (oncovirus subfamily) that causes immunodeficiency and neoplastic disease in domestic cats.

Pathophysiology
• The early pathogenesis of FeLV infection consists of five stages: 1) viral replication in tonsils and pharyngeal lymph nodes; 2) infection of a few circulating B lymphocytes and macrophages that disseminate the virus; 3) replication in lymphoid tissues, intestinal crypt epithelial cells, and bone marrow precursor cells; 4) release of infected neutrophils and platelets from the bone marrow into the circulatory system; and 5) infection of epithelial and glandular tissues, with subsequent shedding of virus into the saliva and urine. An adequate immune response stops progression at stage 2 or 3 (4-8 weeks after exposure) and forces the virus into latency. Persistent viremia (stages 4 and 5) usually develops 4-6 weeks after infection, but may take 12 weeks in some cats. • Tumor induction in FeLV-infected cats occurs when the DNA provirus integrates into cat chromasomal DNA in critical regions ("oncogenes"). FeLV integration near the cellular gene, c-myc, or near genes influencing the expression of c-myc often results in the induction of thymic lymphosarcoma. Changes in the *env* gene of FeLV, either resulting from mutations or recombinations with endogenous retroviral *env* sequences, also play a role in tumorigenesis. In fact, feline sarcoma viruses are mutants of FeLV that arise by recombination between the genes of FeLV and host cells. The resulting virus-host fusion proteins are responsible for the efficient induction of fibrosarcomas by these viruses.

Systems Affected
• Hemic/lymphatic/immune—immune system, possibly resulting from neuroendocrine dysfunction • All other body systems—immunosuppression with secondary infections or development of neoplastic disease.

Genetics
No genetic predisposition for infection.

Incidence/Prevalence
In the United States, the prevalence of FeLV infection is estimated to be 2-3% of the healthy cat population and three to four times greater in cats exhibiting signs of clinical illness.

Geographic Distribution Worldwide

SIGNALMENT
Species Cats

Breed Predilections None

Mean Age and Range
The prevalence of FeLV infection is highest in cats between 1 and 6 years of age, with a mean age of 3 years.

Predominant Sex
Male-female ratio is 1.7:1.

SIGNS
General Comments
In most cats, the onset of FeLV-associated disease occurs over a period of months to years after infection. The FeLV-associated diseases can be categorized as nonneoplastic or neoplastic, with most of the nonneoplastic or degenerative diseases resulting from immunosuppression. Clinical signs of FeLV-induced immunodeficiency cannot be distinguished from those of FIV-induced immunodeficiency.

Historical Findings
Cats allowed outdoors; members of multiple cat households

Physical Examination Findings
• Physical exam findings depend on the type of disease (neoplastic or nonneoplastic) and whether or not secondary infections are present. • Mild to severe lymphadenopathy • Upper respiratory tract signs of rhinitis, conjunctivitis, and keratitis • Persistent diarrhea—bacterial or fungal overgrowth, parasite-induced inflammation, or a direct effect of FeLV infection on crypt cells • Gingivitis/stomatitis/periodontitis • Chronic, nonresponsive, or recurrent infections of the external ear and skin • Fever and wasting • Lymphoma (lymphosarcoma) is the most common FeLV-associated neoplastic disease. Thymic and multicentric lymphomas are highly associated with FeLV infection in cats; miscellaneous lymphomas (extranodal origin) most frequently involve the eye and nervous system. Erythroid and myelomonocytic leukemias are the predominant nonlymphoid leukemias. Fibrosarcomas develop in cats that are coinfected with FeLV and the mutated sarcoma virus, and occur most frequently in young cats. • Immune complex diseases such as thrombocytopenia, immune-mediated hemolytic anemia, and glomerulonephritis • Thymic atrophy (fading kittens) • Peripheral neuropathies

CAUSES
• Cat-to-cat transmission, by bites, close casual contact (grooming), and shared dishes or litter pans • Perinatal transmission—fetal and neonatal death of kittens from 80% of affected queens; also, transplacental and transmammary transmission of FeLV in at least 20% of surviving kittens from infected queens

RISK FACTORS
• Male (as a result of behavior) • Free-roaming • Multiple cat households

DIAGNOSIS

DIFFERENTIAL DIAGNOSIS
• Feline immunodeficiency virus
• Bacterial, parasitic, viral, or fungal infections
• Nonviral neoplastic diseases

CBC/BIOCHEMISTRY/URINALYSIS
Anemia (often severe), lymphopenia, or neutropenia may be present; however, neutrophils can be elevated in response to secondary infections. Urinalysis and serum chemistry profile depend on system affected and type of disease.

OTHER LABORATORY TESTS
• Serology to detect FeLV antigen, p27. The IFA test, available through diagnostic laboratories, identifies p27 in leukocytes and platelets in fixed smears of whole blood or buffy coat preparations; a positive result indicates a productive FeLV infection in the bone marrow cells. Most (97%) IFA-positive cats remain persistently infected and viremic for life. The p27 antigen usually can be detected by IFA by 4 weeks after infection, but some cats may take up to 12 weeks to develop a positive test. When testing leukopenic cats, use buffy coat smears rather than whole blood smears. • Enzyme-linked immunosorbent assay (ELISA) for detection of soluble p27 FeLV antigen in whole blood, serum, plasma, saliva, or tears is more sensitive than the IFA at detecting early or transient FeLV infections; however, a single positive ELISA test cannot predict which cats will be persistently viremic. A second ELISA test is recommended in 12 weeks, and many veterinarians test with IFA at this point. False-positive ELISA results are more common when whole blood is used rather than serum or plasma, or with tests using saliva and tears; cats with positive results should be retested using whole blood (IFA) or serum (ELISA).

IMAGING N/A

OTHER DIAGNOSTIC PROCEDURES
With erythroblastopenia (nonregenerative anemia), the bone marrow is most often hypercellular as a result of an arrest in differentation of erythroid cells, although true aplastic anemia with hypocellular bone marrow may be present. Some cases of anemia also result from myeloproliferative disease.

GROSS AND HISTOPATHOLOGIC FINDINGS
• Lesions depend on type of disease—bone marrow hypercellularity often accompanies neoplastic disease • Lymphocytic and plasmacytic infiltrates of the gingiva, lymph nodes and other lymphoid tissues, spleen, kidney, and liver of affected cats • Intestinal lesions similar to those seen with feline parvovirus infection (feline panleukopenia-like syndrome)

TREATMENT

INPATIENT VERSUS OUTPATIENT
Cats with severe secondary infections, anemia, or cachexia may require hospitalization until their condition is stable.

ACTIVITY Normal

DIET
Normal. Cats with diarrhea, kidney disease, or chronic wasting may require special diets.

CLIENT EDUCATION
Discuss the importance of keeping cats indoors, separated from negative cats, to protect them from exposure to secondary pathogens and to prevent spread of FeLV to other cats.

SURGICAL CONSIDERATIONS
• Biopsy or removal of tumors
• Oral treatment or surgery (dental cleaning, tooth extraction, gingival biopsy)

MEDICATIONS

DRUGS AND FLUIDS
• Management of secondary or opportunistic infections and supportive therapy, such as parenteral fluids and nutritional supplements, may be required. Yearly vaccination for respiratory and enteric viruses with inactivated vaccines is recommended.
• Immunomodulatory drugs may allieviate some clinical signs. Human recombinant alpha interferon (Roferon, diluted in saline, 30 units/day PO for 7 days every other week) may increase survival rates and improve clinical status. Additional immunomodulatory drugs include Propionibacterium acnes (Immunoregulin, 0.5 ml/cat IV, once or twice weekly) and acemannan (Carrisyn, 100mg/cat/day PO).
• Haemobartonella infection should be suspected in all cats with regenerative hemolytic anemias; treatment consists of administration of oxytetracycline (Terramycin, 15 mg/kg PO q8h or Liquamycin, 7 mg/kg IM or IV, q12h) for 3 weeks with short-term use of oral glucocorticoids in severe cases.
• Blood transfusions can provide emergency support; multiple transfusions may be necessary. Passive antibody transfer reduces the level of FeLV antigenemia in some cats; thus, immunization of blood donor cats with FeLV vaccines is useful.
• Lymphosarcoma in FeLV-positive cats has been managed successfully with combination chemotherapy. Regimens using vincristine, cyclophosphamide, and prednisone are most commonly used. Periods of remission average

3-4 months, but some cats may remain in remission for a much longer time. Myeloproliferative disease and leukemias are more refractory to treatment.

CONTRAINDICATIONS
Modified live vaccines may cause disease in immunosuppressed cats.

PRECAUTIONS
Systemic corticosteroids should be used with caution because of the potential for further immunosuppression.

POSSIBLE INTERACTIONS N/A

ALTERNATE DRUGS N/A

FOLLOW-UP

PATIENT MONITORING
Varies according to the secondary infections and other manifestations of disease

PREVENTION/AVOIDANCE
• Prevent contact of cats with FeLV-positive cats. Quarantine and test incoming cats before introduction into multiple cat households. • Most commercial FeLV vaccines induce virus-neutralizing antibodies specific for gp70. The reported efficacies of FeLV vaccines range from below 20% to almost 100%, depending on the trial and challenge system. Cats should be tested for FeLV before initial vaccination; if prevaccination testing is not done, clients should be aware that their cats already may be infected with FeLV.

POSSIBLE COMPLICATIONS N/A

EXPECTED COURSE AND PROGNOSIS
More than 50% of persistently viremic cats will succumb to FeLV-related diseases within 2-3 years after infection.

MISCELLANEOUS

ASSOCIATED CONDITIONS
Secondary bacterial, viral, fungal and parasitic disease, lymphoid tumors, fibrosarcomas, and immune-mediated disease

AGE RELATED FACTORS
• Younger cats (mean age of 3 years)

• Neonatal kittens are most susceptible to persistent infection (70-100%), with less than 30% of kittens susceptible by 16 weeks of age.

ZOONOTIC POTENTIAL
Controversial—studies have reported conflicting results of correlation between certain human leukemias and exposure to cats and presence of antibodies to FeLV in humans

PREGNANCY
Abortions, stillbirths, and fetal resorptions are common in FeLV-positive queens. Transmission of FeLV from queen to kittens occurs in at least 20% of live births.

SYNONYMS
FeLV-AIDS refers to a mutated FeLV that causes immunodeficiency to develop rapidly.

SEE ALSO
Individual topics on neoplasia, secondary infectious diseases, ocular disease, gingivitis/stomatitis

ABBREVIATIONS
FeLV = feline leukemia virus
AIDS = acquired immunodeficiency syndrome
ELISA = enzyme-linked immunosorbent assay

References

Barr MC, Olsen CW, Scott FW. Feline viral diseases. In: Ettinger SJ, Feldman EC, eds. Textbook of veterinary internal medicine. 4th ed. Philadelphia: WB Saunders, 1994:409-439.

Loar AS. Feline leukemia virus: immunization and prevention. Vet Clinics North Am (Small Anim Pract) 1993;23:193-211.

Rojko JL, Hardy WD Jr. Feline leukemia virus and other retroviruses. In: Sherding RG, ed. The cat: diseases and clinical management. 2nd ed. New York: Churchill Livingstone, 1994:263-432.

Author Margaret C. Barr
Consulting Editor Fred W. Scott

FELINE LOWER URINARY TRACT DISEASE

 BASICS

DEFINITION

The terms "feline urologic syndrome" and "FUS" are being less commonly used by the veterinary profession as diagnostic terms to describe disorders of domestic cats characterized by hematuria, dysuria, pollakiuria, and partial or complete urethral obstruction, because various combinations of these signs can be associated with any cause of lower urinary tract disease in cats. The similarity of clinical signs caused by diverse causes is not surprising, since the feline urinary tract responds to various diseases in a limited and predictable fashion. When used, the term "FUS" should refer to urologic signs. In this context, FUS is not a diagnosis any more than vomiting or pruritus are diagnoses. Idiopathic feline urinary tract disease is an exclusion diagnosis established only after known causes have been excluded.

Pathophysiology

• Refer to the specific chapters describing diseases listed under causes. • Experimental and clinical studies have implicated calicivirus, feline syncytia-forming virus, and a gamma herpesvirus (bovine herpesvirus 4) as potential etiologic agents in some cats.
• Initial episodes of lower urinary tract disease usually occur in the absence of significant numbers of detectable bacteria. In a prospective diagnostic study of male and female obstructed and nonobstructed cats, bacterial urinary tract infection was identified in < 3% of patients. The infrequency of urinary tract infection in cats may be related to highly effective local host defense mechanisms in this species. • Although uncommon, fungal urinary tract infection has been reported in cats. • Capillaria spp are rarely recognized as a cause of lower urinary tract disease in cats in North America. • Some cats with lower urinary tract disease have findings similar to those observed in humans with interstitial cystitis. They include low urine concentrations of glycosaminoglycans and similar gross and light microscopic changes. These similarities have prompted the hypothesis that some forms of lower urinary tract disease in cats are analogous to interstitial cystitis in humans. However, further studies are needed to prove or disprove this hypothesis.

Systems Affected

Renal/Urologic—lower urinary tract. Persistent urethral outflow obstruction causes postrenal azotemia.

Genetics N/A

Incidence Prevalence

• Several dozen epidemiologic studies of feline urinary syndrome have been published. Although many contain useful data, almost all have used the nonspecific "FUS" concept as the common denominator for categorizing affected cats. • Although there have been no recent studies, the incidence of hematuria, dysuria, and/or urethral obstruction or a combination in domestic cats in the United States and Great Britain has been reported to be approximately 0.5-1.0% per year. • The incidence of naturally occurring hematuria, dysuria, and/or urethral obstruction in domestic cats should not be confused with the frequency with which such cats are seen in veterinary hospitals (so called proportional morbidity ratios). Although the proportional morbidity ratio of cats with lower urinary tract disorders has been reported to be as high as 10%, the most commonly reported frequency is 1-6%. • Data from 23 colleges of veterinary medicine in North America compiled by the Veterinary Data Base, Purdue University indicated that from 1980 to 1990, lower urinary tract disease was diagnosed in 13,511 of 184,983 hospital admissions (7.3%).

Geographic Distribution N/A

SIGNALMENT

Species Cats

Breed Predilections None

Mean Age And Range

• Refer to specific chapters describing diseases listed under causes. • Idiopathic lower urinary tract disease can occur at any age but is most commonly recognized in young to middle-aged adult cats.

Predominant Sex

• Males and females • Refer to specific chapters describing diseases listed under causes

SIGNS

Historical Findings

• Dysuria • Hematuria • Pollakiuria
• Urinating in inappropriate locations
• Outflow obstruction

Physical Examination Findings

• A thickened, firm, contracted bladder wall
• Urethral plugs or uroliths may be detected by examination of the distal penis and penile urethral.

CAUSES

• See pathophysiology • Metabolic disorders including uroliths and urethral plugs • Inflammatory disorders—infectious agents (e.g., viruses, bacteria, mycoplasma and ureaplasma, fungal agents, and parasites); noninfectious diseases including interstitial cystitis • Trauma • Neurogenic disorders including reflex dyssynergia, urethral spasm, and hypotonic or atonic bladder (primary or secondary) • Iatrogenic disease including reverse flushing solution, urethral catheter, indwelling urethral catheter (especially open system), postsurgical urethral catheter, and urethrostomy complications • Anatomic abnormalities including urachal anomaly and acquired urethral stricture • Neoplasia (benign and malignant) • Idiopathic disorder

RISK FACTORS

Refer to specific chapters describing diseases listed under causes.

 DIAGNOSIS

DIFFERENTIAL DIAGNOSIS

• See causes • Clinical signs of lower urinary tract disease in cats can be confused with constipation, which can be ruled out by abdominal palpation.

CBC/BIOCHEMISTRY/URINALYSIS

• Complete urinalysis including examination of sediment may reveal hematuria, proteinuria, pyuria, crystalluria and, uncommonly, bacteriuria, funguria, or ova of Capillaria.
• If urethral obstruction is persistent, serum biochemical analysis reveals azotemia, hyperphosphatemia, hyperkalemia, and low TCO_2.

OTHER LABORATORY TESTS

• A definite diagnosis of bacteriuria is based on quantitative urine culture. Urine specimens should be collected by cystocentesis to avoid contamination with organisms that normally inhabit the distal urinary tract.
• Immunofluorescent antibody test may reveal serum antibodies against bovine herpesvirus in some cats. • Transmission electron microscopy may reveal calicivirus-like particles in some urethral plugs. • A definite diagnosis of fungiuria is based on culture of organisms on Sabouraud's dextrose agar or cycloheximide free blood agar.

IMAGING

• Survey radiography may reveal radiodense uroliths or urethral plugs. • Positive contrast retrograde urethrocystography or antegrade cystourethrography may reveal urethral stricture, vesicourachal diverticula, or neoplasia.
• Double contrast cystography may reveal small or radiolucent uroliths, blood clots, and thickening of the bladder wall due to inflammation or neoplasia. • Ultrasonography may reveal uroliths or neoplasia.

DIAGNOSTIC PROCEDURES

• Biopsy with the specimen obtained by urinary catheter, cystoscope, or surgery may permit morphologic characterization of inflammatory or neoplastic lesions, but it is not routinely needed. • The mineral composition of uroliths and urethral plugs should be determined by quantitative methods.

GROSS AND HISTOPATHOLOGIC FINDINGS

Idiopathic lower urinary tract disease is characterized by mucosal ulceration, congestion, submucosal edema, hemorrhage, and fibrosis. Inflammatory cells may not be prominent, unless secondary bacterial urinary tract infection has developed as a sequela to catheterization or perineal urethrostomy.

TREATMENT

INPATIENT VS. OUTPATIENT

• Cats with nonobstructive lower urinary tract diseases are typically managed as outpatients. However, diagnostic evaluation may require brief hospitalization.
• Patients with obstructive lower urinary tract disease usually require hospitalization for diagnosis and management.

ACTIVITY

Refer to specific chapters describing diseases listed under causes.

DIET

• Dietary management may be useful in cats with urolithiasis.
• Refer to specific chapters describing diseases listed under causes.

CLIENT EDUCATION

• Refer to specific chapters describing diseases listed under causes.
• Hematuria, dysuria, and pollakiuria are often self-limiting in cats with idiopathic lower urinary tract disease, subsiding within 4-7 days. However, these signs are often unpredictably recurrent.
• Male cats with lower urinary tract disease should be monitored for signs of urethral obstruction.

SURGICAL CONSIDERATIONS

• Refer to specific chapters describing diseases listed under causes.
• We do not recommend cystotomy to lavage and debride the bladder mucosa as a form of treatment.
• Perineal urethrostomy to minimize recurrent urethral obstruction should not be performed without localization of obstructive disease to the penile urethra by contrast urethrography.

MEDICATIONS

DRUGS AND FLUIDS

• Refer to specific chapters describing diseases listed under causes.
• Propantheline can be considered as an anticholinergic to minimize hyperactivity of the bladder detrusor muscle and urge incontinence (7.5 mg PO every third day).
• Phenoxybenzamine may be used to minimize reflex dyssynergia and functional urethral outflow obstruction (0.5 mg/kg PO q12h).
• Corticosteroids have not been shown to have any detectable effect on remission of clinical signs, but they predispose to bacterial urinary tract infection, especially in cats with an indwelling transurethral catheter.

• DMSO (dimethyl-sulfoxide) has not been shown to have any detectable effect on remission of clinical signs.
• Antibiotics and methenamine have not been shown to have any detectable effect on remission of clinical signs in cats with idiopathic lower urinary tract disease.

CONTRAINDICATIONS

• Phenazopyridine, a urinary tract analgesic used alone or in combination with sulfa drugs, can cause methemoglobinemia and irreversible oxidative changes in hemoglobin resulting in formation of Heinz-bodies and anemia.
• Methylene blue, a weak antiseptic agent, can cause Heinz-bodies and severe anemia.
• Bethanacol, a cholinergic drug used to manage hypotonic urinary bladders, should not be used in patients with urethral obstruction.

PRECAUTIONS

• Cats with urethral obstruction and postrenal azotemia are at increased risk for adverse drug events, especially with drugs and anesthetics that are dependent on renal elimination or renal metabolism.
• Indwelling transurethral catheters, especially when associated with fluid-induced diuresis, predispose patients to bacterial urinary tract infection.

POSSIBLE INTERACTIONS

Refer to specific chapters describing diseases listed under causes.

ALTERNATE DRUGS

Refer to specific chapters describing diseases listed under causes.

FOLLOW-UP

PATIENT MONITORING

• Refer to specific chapters describing diseases listed under causes. • Status of hematuria, pyuria, urine pH, and crystalluria by urinalysis • Status of bacterial or fungal infection by urinalysis and appropriate urine culture.

PREVENTION/AVOIDANCE

Refer to specific chapters describing diseases listed under causes.

POSSIBLE COMPLICATIONS

• Indwelling transurethral catheters often cause trauma and predispose to ascending bacterial urinary tract infection. • Perineal urethrostomy can predispose to bacterial urinary tract infection and urethral stricture.
• Infection of the urinary tract with urease producing bacteria, especially staphylococci, can lead to the formation of struvite uroliths.
• Refer to specific chapters describing diseases listed under causes.

EXPECTED COURSE AND PROGNOSIS

• Refer to specific chapters describing diseases listed under causes. • Hematuria, dysuria, and pollakiuria often are self-limiting in cats with idiopathic lower urinary tract disease, subsiding within 4 to 7 days. However, these signs are often unpredictably recurrent.

MISCELLANEOUS

ASSOCIATED CONDITIONS

Refer to specific chapters describing diseases listed under causes

AGE RELATED FACTORS

Refer to specific chapters describing diseases listed under causes

ZOONOTIC POTENTIAL N/A

PREGNANCY N/A

SYNONYMS

FUS (see section on definition), feline urologic disease, feline interstitial cystitis

SEE ALSO

• Urolithiasis, Struvite—Cats • Dysuria and pollakiuria • Lower Urinary Tract Infection • Hematuria

ABBREVIATIONS None

References

Osborne CA, Kruger JM, Lulich JP, et al. Disorders of the feline lower urinary tract. In: Osborne CA, Finco DR, eds. Canine and feline nephrology and urology. Philadelphia: Williams and Wilkins, 1995.

Osborne, CA, Kruger, JM, Lulich JP, et al. Feline lower urinary tract diseases. In: Ettinger SJ, Feldman EC, eds. Textbook of veterinary internal medicine. 4th ed. Philadelphia: WB Saunders, 1995;1805-1832.

Kruger JM, Osborne CA. The role of viruses in feline lower urinary tract disease. J Vet Intern Med 1990;4:71-78.

Kruger JM, Osborne CA, Goyal SM, et al. Clinical evaluation of cats with lower urinary tract disease. J Am Vet Med Assoc 1991;199:211-216.

Osborne CA, Kruger JM, Lulich JP, et al. Feline matrix-crystalline urethral plugs: A unifying hypothesis of causes. J Small Anim Pract 1992;33:172-177.

Authors Carl A. Osborne, John M. Kruger, Jody P. Lulich, David J. Polzin
Consulting Editors Larry G. Adams and Carl A. Osborne

FELINE PANLEUKOPENIA

 BASICS

DEFINITION
An acute, enteric, viral infection of cats characterized by sudden onset, depression, vomiting and diarrhea, severe dehydration, and a high mortality

Pathophysiology
The causative virus, feline parvovirus (FPV), only infects mitotic cells, causing cytolysis during replication. Hence, the pathophysiology involved in feline panleukopenia (FP) is a result of acute cell cytolysis of these rapidly dividing cells.

Systems Affected
• Hemic/lymphatic/immune—loss of all types of white blood cells results in severe panleukopenia and atrophy of the thymus • Gastrointestinal—intestinal crypt cells of the jejunum and ileum are destroyed, causing acute enteritis with vomiting and diarrhea, shortened blunt villi with poor adsorption of nutrients, dehydration, and secondary bacteremia • Reproductive—in utero infection results in fetal death with fetal resorption, abortion, stillbirth, or fetal mummification • Nervous system and ophthalmic—in neonatal kittens, rapidly dividing granular cells of the cerebellum and retinal cells of the eye are destroyed, causing cerebellar hypoplasia with ataxia and retinal dysplasia

Genetics N/A

Incidence/Prevalence
In unvaccinated populations, FP is the most severe and important feline infectious disease. However, routine vaccination has resulted in almost total control of this disease. FP is extremely contagious, and the virus is extremely stable, lasting for years on contaminated premises.

Geographic Distribution
Worldwide in unvaccinated populations

SIGNALMENT

Species
• All Felidae, both domestic and exotic, are susceptible to infection. • Canidae are susceptible to the closely related canine parvovirus, and some exotic canids may be susceptible to FPV infection. • Mustilidae, especially mink, may be susceptible to FPV infection. • Members of the Procyonidae family are also susceptible, including the raccoon and coatimundi.

Breed Predilections
There are no known breed predilections to FP.

Mean Age and Range
Unvaccinated and previously unexposed cats of any age can become infected with FPV once passively transferred maternal immunity has been lost, but kittens 2-6 months of age are the most susceptible to develop severe dis-

ease. Adult cats often will have mild or subclinical infection.

Predominant Sex N/A

SIGNS

General Comments
Cats properly vaccinated against FPV are probably immune for life.

Historical Findings
• History of recent exposure (e.g., adoption shelter), a newly acquired kitten, or a 2-4 month old kitten from a premise with a history of FP • No vaccination history or last vaccinated against FP when less than 12 weeks of age • Sudden onset of disease, with vomiting and diarrhea, depression, and complete anorexia. Owner may suspect "poisoning." • Possible history of cat "disappearing" or "hiding" for one or more days before being found. • Owner may report cat "hangs head" over water bowl or food dish, but won't eat or drink.

Physical Examination Findings
• Depression—may be mild to severe. Cats with FP often assume a typical "panleukopenia posture" with sternum and chin resting on floor, feet tucked under body, and top of scapulae elevated above the back. • Dehydration appears rapidly and may be severe. • Gastroenteritis with vomiting and diarrhea may occur. • Fever is usually mild to moderate in the early stages of disease, but temperature becomes severely subnormal as the cat becomes moribund. • Abdominal pain may be elicited on palpation, and the small intestine may feel either turgid and "hoselike" or flaccid. • Subclinical or mild infections with few or no clinical signs are common, especially in adult cats. • Ataxia from cerebellar hypoplasia in kittens infected in utero or neonatally. Signs become evident at 10-14 days of age and persist for life, including ataxia, hypermetria, dysmetria, and incoordination with a base-wide stance and an elevated "rudder" tail. These cats are alert, afebrile, and otherwise normal. Retinal dysplasia may also be present.

CAUSES
Feline parvovirus (FPV), a small, single-stranded DNA virus. A single antigenic serotype occurs, which has considerable antigenic cross-reactivity with canine parvovirus type 2 and mink enteritis virus. FPV is extremely stable against environmental factors, temperature, and most disinfectants. This virus requires a mitotic cell for replication.

RISK FACTORS
• Anything that will increase the mitotic activity of the small intestinal crypt cells such as intestinal parasites or pathogenic bacteria • Secondary or coinfections such as viral upper respiratory infections • Age, because kittens 2-6 months of age tend to be more severely affected

 DIAGNOSIS

DIFFERENTIAL DIAGNOSIS
• Panleukopenia-like syndrome of feline leukemia virus (FeLV) infection. This is a chronic infection with chronic enteritis, chronic panleukopenia, and often anemia. Cat is positive for FeLV antigen in the blood and/or saliva. • Salmonellosis, usually a subclinical infection, can cause severe gastroenteritis that may appear similar to FP. Total WBC counts are usually high. • Acute poisoning may present similar to acute or fulminating FP with severe depression and subnormal temperature, but the total WBC count will not be severely depressed. • Many diseases of cats can cause mild clinical signs that are hard to differentiate from mild FP. The total WBC count is always low during the acute infection with FP, even in subclinical infections.

CBC/BIOCHEMISTRY/URINALYSIS
Panleukopenia is the most consistent finding with FP. Therefore, a CBC must be done. Leukocyte counts are usually between 500 and 3000 cells/microl during the acute disease. Biochemical findings are usually nonspecific.

OTHER LABORATORY TESTS
• Canine parvovirus antigen fecal immunoassay (CITE[R] Canine Parvovirus Test Kit, IDEXX Labs.), although not licensed for FP, will detect FPV antigen in feces. • Serologic testing on paired serum samples (acute and convalescent) to detect a rising antibody titer

IMAGING N/A

OTHER DIAGNOSTIC PROCEDURES
• Viral isolation from feces or affected tissues (thymus, small intestine, spleen) • Electron microscopy of feces to detect parvovirus particles

GROSS AND HISTOPATHOLOGIC FINDINGS
• Gross findings include rough hair coat, severe dehydration, evidence of vomiting and diarrhea, weight loss, edematous and turgid small intestine, petechial or ecchymotic hemorrhages on the serosal and/or mucosal surfaces of the jejunum and ilium, thymic atrophy, and gelatinous or liquid bone marrow. In utero infection results in gross hypoplasia of the cerebellum. • Microscopic findings include dilated small intestinal crypts with sloughing of epithelial cells, shortened and blunt intestinal villi, absence of lymphocytic infiltrates in all tissues, and lymphocytic depletion of follicles of lymph nodes, Peyer's patches, and spleen. In neonatal and fetal infection, there is disorientation and depletion of the granular and Purkinje's cells of the cerebellum. Eosinophilic intranuclear inclusions are present in affected tissues during early stages of infection, although they usual-

ly are not observed on routine histopathological examination of formalin-fixed tissues.

TREATMENT

The main principles of treatment of FP are (1) rehydration, (2) reestablishment of electrolyte balance, and (3) supportive care until the patient's immune system produces antiviral antibodies that will neutralize the virus.

INPATIENT VERSUS OUTPATIENT

Severe cases must be hospitalized to receive hydration and replacement electrolyte therapy. Mild cases can be treated as outpatients.

ACTIVITY

Cats should be restricted from going outside during the acute disease to prevent contamination of the environment with the virus, and to prevent the cat from going into hiding because of the illness.

DIET

Food should be temporarily withheld until the acute gastroenteritis is controlled.

CLIENT EDUCATION

The client should be informed that all present and future cats in this household must be vaccinated against FPV before exposure, and that the virus will remain infectious on the premise for years unless the premise can be adequately disinfected with household bleach.

SURGICAL CONSIDERATIONS None

MEDICATIONS

DRUGS AND FLUIDS

• Balanced fluid and electrolyte solutions should be given by continuous IV drip until signs of illness subside. • Whole blood transfusions should be given if plasma protein falls below 4 gm/dl, or if total WBC counts fall below 2000 cells/microl.
• Broad spectrum antibiotics to counter secondary bacteremia from intestinal bacteria

CONTRAINDICATIONS

Oral medications until gastroenteritis has been controlled

PRECAUTIONS

FP must be treated vigorously to prevent shock and other complications from the severe dehydration and electrolyte imbalance.

POSSIBLE INTERACTIONS

None known

ALTERNATE DRUGS

At this time, there are no available antiviral drugs effective against FPV.

FOLLOW-UP

PATIENT MONITORING

Hydration and electrolyte balance should be monitored closely. CBC should be monitored daily or at least every 2 days until recovery. Recovered cats will be immune against FPV infection for life and will not require future vaccination against FP.

PREVENTION/AVOIDANCE

• FP is completely preventable by routine vaccination of kittens with either modified live virus (MLV) or inactivated vaccines. Immunity from these vaccines is of long duration, perhaps even for life. However, current vaccines in the United States are licensed for only one year duration of immunity. Kittens should be vaccinated at 8-10 weeks of age, and a second vaccination given after 12 weeks of age when maternally derived immunity has waned. Booster vaccinations given after the first year, and repeated every 3 years will provide excellent immunity. • Contaminated environments such as cages, floors, food and water dishes should be disinfected with a 1:32 dilution of household bleach. FPV is resistant to most commercial disinfectants.

POSSIBLE COMPLICATIONS

• Chronic enteritis from fungal or other cause. • Teratogenic effects from virus infection of fetus, including cerebellar hypoplasia resulting in ataxia for life.

EXPECTED COURSE AND PROGNOSIS

Most cases of FP are acute and last for only 5-7 days. If death does not occur during the acute disease, recovery is usually rapid and uncomplicated, although it may take several weeks for the cat to regain weight and body condition. The prognosis must be guarded during the acute disease, especially if the total WBC count is below 2000 cells/microl.

MISCELLANEOUS

ASSOCIATED CONDITIONS

Viral upper respiratory diseases, including feline viral rhinotracheitis and feline calicivirus infection, may occur concurrently with FP.

AGE RELATED FACTORS

Clinical FP is generally a kitten disease. Adult cats more often develop subclinical infections.

ZOONOTIC POTENTIAL None

PREGNANCY

Unvaccinated pregnant cats are at great risk of FPV infection. Fetuses almost always become infected with fatal or teratogenic effects, even when the dam has a subclinical infection. Fetal resorption, abortion, fetal mummification, stillbirths, or birth of weak, fading kittens may occur. Kittens may show ataxia from cerebellar hypoplasia when they become ambulatory.

SYNONYMS

Feline distemper, feline viral enteritis, feline parvovirus infection, FPL, FeLV (feline leukemia virus), MLV (modified live virus)

SEE ALSO N/A

ABBREVIATIONS

FP = feline panleukopenia
FPV = feline parvovirus
FeLV = feline leukemia virus
MLV = modified live virus

References

Barr MC, Olsen CW, Scott FW. Feline viral diseases. In: Ettinger SJ, Feldman EC, eds. Veterinary internal medicine. Philadelphia: WB Saunders, 1995:409-439.

Greene CE, Scott FW. Feline panleukopenia. In: Greene CE, ed. Infectious diseases of the dog and cat. Philadelphia: WB Saunders, 1990:291-299.

Pedersen NC. Feline panleukopenia. In: Pratt PW, ed. Feline infectious diseases. Goleta, CA: American Veterinary Publications, 1988:15-20.

Pollock RVH, Postorino NC. Feline panleukopenia and other enteric viral diseases. In: Sherding RG, ed. The cat: diseases and clinical management. New York: Churchill Livingstone, 1994:479-487.

Scott FW. Panleukopenia. In: Holzworth J, ed. Diseases of the cat. Philadelphia: WB Saunders, 1987:182-193.

Author Fred W. Scott
Consulting Editor Fred W. Scott

FELINE SYMMETRICAL ALOPECIA

BASICS

OVERVIEW
This condition is defined as alopecia in a symmetrical pattern with no gross changes in the skin. It is a common clinical syndrome in the cat and is a manifestation of several underlying disorders.

SIGNALMENT
This disease in cats has no age, breed, or sex predilection.

SIGNS
• Total to partial hair loss most often symmetrical but can occur in a patchy distribution. • Areas of the trunk most commonly affected are the ventrum, caudal dorsum, lateral, and caudal thighs. • Some cats may have patchy areas of hair loss (unsymmetrical) on their distal extremities or on various truncal locations.

CAUSES AND RISK FACTORS
• Hypersensitivity reactions – fleas, food, and atopy • Parasites—fleas, cheyletiella • Infections—dermatophytosis • Neurologic / behavioral (psychogenic) • Stress/metabolic — telogen effluvium • Neoplasia—pancreatic neoplasia (paraneoplastic alopecia) • Hyperadrenocorticism • Alopecia areata

DIAGNOSIS

DIFFERENTIAL DIAGNOSIS
See causes and risk factors

CBC/BIOCHEMISTRY/URINALYSIS
May see eosinophilia is some allergic cats

OTHER LABORATORY TESTS N/A

IMAGING N/A

OTHER DIAGNOSTIC PROCEDURES
• Flea combing—to identify presence or absence of fleas or flea excrement or both. • Microscopic examination of hair—self induced hair loss will have broken hairs while all ends are tapered with endogenous hair loss • Fecal examination—excess hair in feces, (cheyletiella) mites and ova, tapeworm or fleas may be present. • Diet trial (food elimination diet trial) (see Food Reactions) • Intradermal skin test (See Atopy)

GROSS AND HISTOPATHOLOGIC FINDINGS
• Biopsies can be very helpful in confirming an underlying cause such as allergic dermatitis, psychogenic, or rarely, systemic disease. The histopathologic findings will vary depending on the cause. • In cases of feline psychogenic alopecia, the hair follicles and skin are normal. • Findings of high numbers of mast cells, eosinophils, lymphocytes, or macrophages are suggestive of allergic dermatitis. • Alopecia areata is characterized by lymphocytic inflammation that encircles the bulb portions of the hair follicles. This latter condition is very rare.

TREATMENT
• Effective management of the underlying cause is important.
• Discuss with owner the diagnostic plan and length of time it may take to see response (e.g., fleas 4–6 weeks, diet 3–12 weeks).

MEDICATIONS

DRUGS AND FLUIDS
• Antihistamines (e.g., chlorpheniramine 0.25 mg / lb q8h)
• Glucocorticoids (0.25 mg/lb alternate day therapy)
• Amitriptyline 1–2 mg /kg /day

CONTRAINDICATIONS/POSSIBLE INTERACTIONS
• Glucocorticoids can be the cause of the alopecia. Some cats can develop diabetes mellitus with administration of glucocorticoids. Other side effects of glucocorticoids can include polydypsia, polyuria, polyphagia, and weight gain. Use of glucocorticoids can cause confusion for the clinician and owner in making a correct assessment about the underlying cause because these drugs suppress the pruritus.
• Glucocorticoids and other antipruritic medications should be withdrawn as the diagnostic tests near completion (e.g., food hypersensitivity reactions).

FOLLOW-UP
• Frequent follow-up examinations are essential in confirming or denying the differential diagnoses. • Successful identification of the underlying cause offers the best prognosis if this cause can be controlled (e.g., flea bites or food hypersensitivity.)

MISCELLANEOUS

Reference
O'Dair HA, Foster AP. Focal and generalized alopecia. Vet Clin North Am (Small Anim Pract) 1995;25:851–870.
Author David Duclos
Consulting Editor Lowell Ackerman

FELINE SYNCYTIUM-FORMING VIRUS INFECTION

BASICS

OVERVIEW
• Feline syncytium-forming virus (FeSFV) is a retrovirus in the spumavirus subfamily that infects cats, apparently with little or no pathogenic effect. • The virus is found worldwide; estimated prevalences range from 10-70% or greater. • Chronic progressive polyarthritis (CPA) has been linked statistically with FeSFV infection, but the disease has not been reproduced by experimental infection.
• Although the disease potential is low, FeSFV infection is a nuisance to researchers using feline origin tissue culture cells. Cats used in research should be tested and removed from the project if positive.

SIGNALMENT
• The prevalence of FeSFV is low in kittens and increases with age. • Male cats are more likely than females to be infected, and CPA occurs predominantly in males aged 1.5-5 years.

SIGNS
• Most cats infected with FeSFV are healthy; however, coinfections with FIV and FeLV are fairly common. • Statistical links between FeSFV infection and myeloproliferative disease or CPA may actually result from coninfection with FIV. • The signs of CPA include swollen joints, abnormal gait, and lymphadenopathy.

CAUSES AND RISK FACTORS
• Transmission of FeSFV is primarily by biting, thus free-roaming cats are at greater risk of infection. • The virus is also transmitted efficiently from infected queens to their kittens, probably in utero. • The high prevalence of infection in some cat populations suggests that casual contact may also play a role in transmission; however, this route of infection has not been demonstrated experimentally.

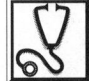

DIAGNOSIS

DIFFERENTIAL DIAGNOSIS
N/A except for cats with CPA. Cats with signs of CPA should be tested for FIV, FeLV, and septic joint disease.

CBC/BIOCHEMISTRY/URINALYSIS
Hemograms and serum chemistry profiles are usually normal.

OTHER LABORATORY TESTS
Serologic testing for FeSFV antibodies and virus isolation—on an experimental basis; testing is not particularly useful because the correlation between FeSFV infection and disease is so tenuous

IMAGING N/A

OTHER DIAGNOSTIC PROCEDURES
In cats with CPA, joint fluid cytology may reveal high numbers of neutrophils and large mononuclear cells.

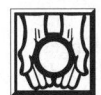

TREATMENT
N/A except for cats with CPA

MEDICATIONS

DRUGS AND FLUIDS
CPA may be treated with immunosuppressive dosages of prednisilone (10-15 mg/day) and cytoxan (7.5 mg/day for 4 days each week).

CONTRAINDICATIONS/POSSIBLE INTERACTIONS
Care must be taken when using immunosuppressive drugs in cats coinfected with FIV or FeLV.

FOLLOW-UP

PATIENT MONITORING N/A

EXPECTED COURSE AND PROGNOSIS N/A

MISCELLANEOUS

ABBREVIATIONS
FeSFV = feline syncytium-forming virus (also called feline syncytial virus)
CPA = chronic progressive polyarthritis

References

Pedersen NC. Feline Infectious diseases. Goleta, CA: American Veterinary Publications, 1988:77-82.
Greene CE. Syncytium-forming virus infection. In: Greene CE, ed. Infectious diseases of the dog and cat. Philadelphia: WB Saunders, 1990:358-359.

Author Margaret C. Barr
Consulting Editor Fred W. Scott

FIBROCARTILAGINOUS EMBOLIC MYELOPATHY

BASICS

DEFINITION
Acute ischemic necrosis of the spinal cord caused by fibrocartilaginous emboli

Pathophysiology
The emboli are found in spinal cord arteries or veins or both. The source of the emboli is possibly the intervertebral disc material. The exact mechanism of entry into the spinal vasculature is unknown.

Systems Affected Nervous

Genetics N/A

Incidence/Prevalence
• One of the common causes of spinal cord disease in nonchondrodystrophic breeds of dogs • It has not been reported in a chondrodystrophic breed. • Rare in cats

Geographic Distribution N/A

SIGNALMENT

Species Dogs and cats

Breed Predilections
Giant- and large-breed dogs have the highest prevalence. The miniature schnauzer and Shetland sheepdog are also overrepresented. It is suspected that the hyperlipoproteinemia and resultant hyperviscosity common in these two breeds could be causing spinal cord infarction without contribution of fibrocartilaginous emboli.

Mean Age and Range
Most patients are 3-5 years old but the range is 16 weeks-10 years.

Predominant Sex
Slight male predominance

SIGNS

Historical Findings
• Mild trauma or vigorous exercise at the onset of signs in many patients • Sudden onset. The dog typically cries in pain. The pain subsides in minutes to, at most, hours. Signs of paresis or paralysis develop over a matter of seconds, minutes, or hours. • The condition stabilizes within 12-24 hours.

Physical Examination Findings
• Neurologic deficits often lateralized. The limbs on the unaffected side are mildly affected or normal in many patients. Signs are symmetrically distributed in a few patients. • Although there is pain at the onset of signs, by the time the dog reaches a veterinarian, it has subsided. Spinal pain may be present for a few hours in severely affected patients. • Any level of the spinal cord can be affected depending on the distribution of the embolic material. • Signs range from mild ataxia to paralysis, upper motor neuron or lower motor neuron, with absence of pain perception. • Spinal cord injury may occur unilaterally to only the dorsal or ventral aspect of the spinal cord, causing an ip-

silateral limb with sensory loss but muscle tone and motor function preserved, or vice versa. Other odd combinations of signs are possible in patients with focal quadrant injuries. • If signs progress beyond 24 hours, other diseases that cause ascending and descending myelomalacia should be considered.

CAUSES Unknown

RISK FACTORS
• Vigorous exercise may trigger the incident.
• Hyperlipoproteinemia

DIAGNOSIS

DIFFERENTIAL DIAGNOSIS
• The acute, nonprogressive, asymmetric, and nonpainful nature of this disease is characteristic and greatly helps in the diagnosis. • Painful spinal diseases such as intervertebral disc disease, discospondylitis, vertebral tumor, and fracture and luxation are ruled out by the presence of back and neck pain and the rather symmetrical nature of the deficits. When in doubt, survey radiography and myelography help to confirm the diagnosis. • Parenchymal spinal cord hemorrhage secondary to a bleeding diathesis such as that caused by anticoagulant rodenticide ingestion, thrombocytopenia, or disseminated intravascular coagulation is ruled out by a careful physical examination for evidence of hemorrhage and by performing a platelet count and blood clotting times. • Focal myelitis is differentiated by a progressive history and CSF analysis.

CBC/BIOCHEMISTRY/URINALYSIS
Results usually normal

OTHER LABORATORY TESTS N/A

IMAGING
• Survey spinal radiography usually normal
• In the acute stage, myelography often demonstrates focal intramedullary swelling at the embolic site. Later on, the myelogram is often normal or shows an area of cord atrophy.

OTHER DIAGNOSTIC PROCEDURES
CSF analysis—results vary according to the location (ie, lumbar versus cerebellomedullary) and time of CSF collection in relation to the onset of clinical signs and location of the lesion. Patients in the acute stage may have high RBC count and mildly high neutrophil count. A few days later, the abnormalities may be limited to a mildly high protein. Results can also be normal.

GROSS AND HISTOPATHOLOGIC FINDINGS
• Grossly, focal spinal cord swelling with hemorrhage • Microscopically, emboli of fibrocartilage in both arteries and veins of the spinal cord and meninges and hemorrhagic necrosis and malacia of both gray and white matter

TREATMENT

INPATIENT VERSUS OUTPATIENT
Patients with suspected fibrocartilaginous embolic myelopathy are hospitalized for immediate medical treatment and diagnostic procedures.

ACTIVITY
Restricted until the diagnosis is made

DIET Regular

CLIENT EDUCATION
Recovery from paresis or paralysis is slow and gradual, when it occurs. Most patients need considerable supportive care at home during recovery.

SURGICAL CONSIDERATIONS N/A

MEDICATIONS

DRUGS AND FLUIDS
On the basis of research of acute spinal cord injury caused by spinal cord impact, methylprednisolone sodium succinate may be beneficial if given within the first 8 hours after the onset of signs. A first treatment of 30 mg/kg IV is given, followed by doses of 15 mg/kg at 2 and 6 hours and every 6 hours thereafter for a total treatment period of 24-48 hours. Each dose is given slowly over 10-15 minutes, because a too rapid injection can cause vomiting.

CONTRAINDICATIONS
Nonsteroidal analgesics should not be administered with methylprednisolone sodium succinate, because this increases the probability of gastrointestinal ulceration.

PRECAUTIONS
• Continuing methylprednisolone sodium succinate for longer than 24-48 hours is of no benefit and dramatically increases adverse effects such as gastrointestinal ulceration.
• Feeding a high-fiber diet during and after treatment reduces this adverse effect.

POSSIBLE INTERACTIONS N/A

ALTERNATE DRUGS N/A

FOLLOW-UP

PATIENT MONITORING
• Sequential neurologic evaluations during the first 12-24 hours after examination
• Once discharged, the patient's neurologic status should be evaluated at 2, 3, and 4 weeks after onset of clinical signs. • If the patient develops urinary incontinence, urinalysis and bacterial culture and sensitivity are done to detect urinary tract infection.
• Improvement such as return of pain percep-

tion or voluntary movements indicates a favorable prognosis. • Progression of clinical signs from upper to lower motor neuron and an enlarging area of sensory loss indicate ascending/descending myelomalacia and a hopeless prognosis. Euthanasia should be considered.

PREVENTION/AVOIDANCE
• Recurrence highly unlikely • No known method of prevention

POSSIBLE COMPLICATIONS
• Fecal and urinary incontinence • Urinary tract infection • Urine scalding and pressure sores

EXPECTED COURSE AND PROGNOSIS
• In most patients, the prognosis for marked improvement is good if pain perception remains and the signs are upper motor neuron. • The loss of pain perception is a poor prognostic sign, and patients with areflexia of limbs or sphincters have almost no chance of recovery. • Little change is seen in the neurologic status in the first 14 days after onset of

signs. Most of the improvement occurs between day 21 and 42. Improvement due to remyelination is complete in most patients within 6-12 weeks after the onset of signs. If improvement has not been detected after 21-30 days, recovery is highly unlikely. • Patients with lower motor neuron signs that have reduced purposeful movements and reflexes often make functional recoveries, but some degree of permanent deficit is likely.

MISCELLANEOUS

ASSOCIATED CONDITIONS
A disorder that leads to a compromise in circulatory function may predispose or mimic fibrocartilaginous embolic myelopathy. Such conditions include hyperadrenocorticism, hypothyroidism, high systemic blood pressure, hyperviscosity syndrome, hyperlipidemia, bleeding diathesis, and bacterial endocarditis.

AGE RELATED FACTORS N/A
ZOONOTIC POTENTIAL N/A

PREGNANCY
High-dose corticosteroid administration can cause premature delivery.

SYNONYMS
Ischemic myelopathy

SEE ALSO N/A

ABBREVIATION
CSF = cerebrospinal fluid
RBC = red blood cells

References
Braughler JM, Hall ED. Current application of "high-dose" steroid therapy for CNS injury: pharmacological perspective. J Neurosurg 1985;62:806-810.
Cauzinille L. Fibrocartilaginous embolism of the spinal cord. Proceedings 11th Annu Forum Am Col Vet Int Med, Washington, DC, 1993:713-716.
Cook JR. Fibrocartilaginous embolism. Vet Clin North Am Small Animal Pract 1988;18:581-592.
Author Allen Sisson
Consulting Editor Joane M. Parent

FIBROMATOUS PERIODONTAL HYPERPLASIA

BASICS

OVERVIEW
Also called gingival hyperplasia, the lesions appear as firm, nonpainful swellings of the attached gingiva. May occur as generalized or focal lesions. Focal lesions may be difficult to differentiate from fibromatous epulis (peripheral odontogenic tumor) because of the similar histologic appearance.

SIGNALMENT
• Large and giant breeds dogs primarily
• Rare in cats unless drug associated

SIGNS
Historical Findings
• Slowly enlarging mass or masses noticed along gingival margin • Bleeding from gums
Physical Examination Findings
• Diffuse or focal enlargement of gingivae
• Less than normal amount of tooth crown visible • Epithelium intact unless traumatized during chewing • Lesions are firm and not painful • Signs of periodontal disease (gingivitis and calculus deposits) usually not prominent

CAUSES AND RISK FACTORS
• Familial inheritance reported in boxer and suspected in Great Dane, collie, doberman pinscher, and dalmation • Chronic drug administration with diphenylhydantoin, nitrendipine, nifedipine, or cyclosporine

DIAGNOSIS

DIFFERENTIAL DIAGNOSIS
• Hyperplastic gingivitis resulting from plaque induced periodontitis. The lesions are usually not as severe and the gingiva is inflamed. Plaque and calculus accumulations are typically present on the teeth. • Oral neoplasia, especially epulides

CBC/BIOCHEMISTRY/URINALYSIS
None specific

OTHER LABORATORY TESTS N/A

IMAGING N/A

OTHER DIAGNOSTIC PROCEDURES
Biopsy

TREATMENT

• Discontinue drug administration, if possible
• If lesions are interfering with animal's ability to eat or if change in contour of gingiva predisposes to periodontal disease, gingivoplasty is indicated.

GINGIVOPLASTY
• Goal is to re-establish normal height and contour of gingival margin being sure to maintain adequate attached gingiva (at least 2mm).
• A periodontal probe should be used to assess the depth of the pocket and establish the amount of tissue to excise. A needle or dental explorer can be used to make bleeding points along the intended line of incision.
• The incision is beveled toward the tooth to re-establish a more normal gingival margin. The cut should begin apical to the line of bleeding points so that the gingival margin will be along the line of bleeding points. If the cuts begins at the marked line, excessive tissue will be left behind.
• The incisions can be made with a scalpel and Number 15C blade or an electroscalpel. Electrosurgery reduces blood loss but may cause excessive additional tissue loss if proper settings are not used. The lowest possible setting which will cut the tissue should be used. Test cuts can be made in tissue to be excised. A needle tip on a bendable shaft allows precise control of the cut. Since the the attached gingiva contains little elastic tissue, it will not retract from the cut edges. The cut tissue is removed with a sharp dental scaler or curette. Repeated passes with the electroscalpel will leave more devitalized tissue and can lead to thermal necrosis of the pulp chamber contents. The incised edge of the gingiva should be red but not bleeding. If the tissue is blanched, too high a setting was used.

• Hemorrhage is controlled with digital pressure.
• Dental prophylaxis should be performed.

POSTOPERATIVE CARE
• A soft diet should be fed until the re-epithelialization of the gingivae is complete. (typically 5-10 days)
• The application of chlorhexidine gluconate solution (CHX™, VRx Products™, Harbor City, CA) or oral hygiene gel (Maxi-Guard™ Gel, Addison Biological Laboratory, Inc., Fayette, MO) should be continued until healing is complete.

MEDICATIONS

DRUGS AND FLUIDS N/A

CONTRAINDICTIONS/POSSIBLE INTERACTIONS N/A

FOLLOW-UP

A thorough oral examination should be performed during routine check-ups to monitor for recurrence.

MISCELLANEOUS

References
Harvey CE, Emily PP. Small animal dentistry. St. Louis: Mosby-Year Book 1993.
Bojrab MJ, Tholen M. Small animal oral medicine and surgery. Philadelphia: Lea & Febiger. 1990.
Author Eric R. Pope
Consulting Editor Brent D. Jones

BASICS

OVERVIEW
• Osseous fibrosarcoma (fibrosarcoma) tends to develop in the axial skeleton more commonly than the appendicular skeleton.
• Fibrosarcoma is characterized histologically by well to poorly differentiated spindle-shaped cells. • Fibrosarcoma of the bone tends to be locally invasive but late to metastasize. • Primary bone fibrosarcoma is uncommon in cats.

SIGNALMENT
• More common in old dogs • Breed predilections not reported

SIGNS

Historical Findings
• Lameness • Visible or palpable mass • Same as for patients with other primary bone tumors

Physical Examination Findings
• Long bone tumor—monostotic swelling, typically at a metaphyseal site • Pain on palpation of the tumor site • Possibly, pathologic fracture • Axial tumor—palpable mass

CAUSES AND RISK FACTORS
• Unknown • Previous fracture repair with metallic implant may increase risk of tumor development.

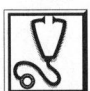

DIAGNOSIS

DIFFERENTIAL DIAGNOSIS
• Other primary bone neoplasms, including osteosarcoma, hemangiosarcoma, and chondrosarcoma, may be clinically indistinguishable from fibrosarcoma. • Metastatic neoplasia from another primary site • Osteomyelitis (i.e., fungal or bacterial)

CBC/BIOCHEMISTRY/URINALYSIS
Results usually normal

OTHER LABORATORY TESTS N/A

IMAGING
• On radiographs, the primary lesion may be impossible to differentiate from other primary bone tumors. Lesions are typically in metaphyseal sites of long bones and can be lytic, productive, or both (see osteosarcoma).
• Thoracic radiography to detect metastasis
• CT to determine extent of local disease in patients with an axial tumor

OTHER DIAGNOSTIC PROCEDURES
Biopsy and histopathologic examination of suspected tumor as described for osteosarcoma. Care must be taken to differentiate between fibrosarcoma and osteosarcoma and other bone sarcomas.

TREATMENT
• Surgical resection (e.g., amputation, limb-salvage, and hemipelvectomy for pelvic sites)
• Radiotherapy is palliative in patients with inoperable tumors.

MEDICATIONS

DRUGS AND FLUIDS
No evidence available to support the use of chemotherapy after surgery

CONTRAINDICATIONS/POSSIBLE INTERACTIONS N/A

FOLLOW-UP
• Thoracic radiography monthly for 3 months followed by every third month thereafter. • The biologic behavior of fibrosarcoma of the appendicular skeleton is believed to be less aggressive than that of osteosarcoma. Cures are possible with localized disease treated aggressively surgically, but survival data has not been published.

MISCELLANEOUS

ABBREVIATION
CT = computed tomography

Reference
Withrow SJ, MacEwen EG. Clinical veterinary oncology. Philadelphia: JB Lippincott, 1989.

Author Joyce E. Obradovich
Consulting Editor Wallace B. Morrison

FIBROSARCOMA, GINGIVA

BASICS

OVERVIEW
• Slowly progressive and locally invasive malignancy of dogs and cats • Third most common oral malignancy in dogs • Second most common oral malignancy in cats • May become ulcerated • Highly invasive to surrounding bone • Metastasis uncommon • A subset of histologically low-grade but biologically high-grade fibrosarcoma has been identified.

SIGNALMENT
• Mean age, 7.6 years (range, 0.5-15 years) • Slight male predilection • No known breed predilection • More common in medium to large breeds • Golden retrievers may be predisposed to histologically low-grade, biologically high-grade fibrosarcoma.

SIGNS

Historical Findings
• Excessive salivation • Halitosis • Bloody oral discharge • Dysphagia • Weight loss

Physical Examination Findings
• Facial deformity • Occasionally, cervical lymphadenopathy

CAUSES AND RISK FACTORS N/A

DIAGNOSIS

DIFFERENTIAL DIAGNOSIS
• Other oral malignant tumor • Epulis • Abscess • Benign polyp • Eosinophilic granuloma

CBC/BIOCHEMISTRY/URINALYSIS
N/A

OTHER LABORATORY TESTS N/A

IMAGING
• Skull radiography reveals a typical pattern of lysis. • Thoracic radiography to detect evidence of pulmonary metastasis

OTHER DIAGNOSTIC PROCEDURES
• A large, deep tissue biopsy (down to bone) required for diagnosis • Examination of cytologic preparation rarely diagnostic

TREATMENT
• Radical excision required (e.g., hemimandibulectomy) and generally well-tolerated. Margins of at least 2 cm are necessary; 1-year survival after excision ranges from 25-45%; 2-year survival after excision ranges form 20-35%. Median survival after excision ranges from 7-11 months in dogs. Survival improves when margins are free of neoplastic cells.
• Feed soft foods after oral excision
• Inpatient radiotherapy offers good long-term control if the tumor is deemed inoperable. Median survival after treatment, 7 months (range, 0-27 months).
• No effective chemotherapy protocol available for treating primary gingival fibrosarcoma. Other sarcomas are known to respond to adriamycin, vincristine, and cytoxan.
• Death related to local recurrence and secondary anorexia and cachexia

MEDICATIONS

DRUGS AND FLUIDS N/A.

CONTRAINDICATIONS/POSSIBLE INTERACTIONS N/A

FOLLOW-UP
• Head and neck examination with survey thoracic radiography at 1, 2, 3, 6, 9, 12, 15, 18, and 24 months after treatment • Some histologically low-grade fibrosarcomas have aggressive behavior. • Highly invasive of bone (> 70%) • Response to treatment is similar to that of patients with other fibrosarcomas. • A diagnosis of a low-grade fibrosarcoma does not warrant a conservative therapeutic approach.

MISCELLANEOUS

References
Oakes MG, Lewis DD, Hedlund CS, Hosgood G. Canine oral neoplasia. Comp Contin Ed Pract Vet 1993;15:15-31.
Author Kevin A. Hahn
Consulting Editor Wallace B. Morrison

FIBROSARCOMA, NASAL AND PARANASAL SINUS

BASICS

OVERVIEW
• Local invasion of neoplastic mesenchymal cells within the nasal and paranasal sinuses
• Fibrosarcoma is the second most common nonepithelial histologic tumor type in dogs.

SIGNALMENT
• No reported breed predilection in dogs
• Median age, 9-12 years (range, 1-16 years)
• Male predilection (2:1) • Prevalence of nonepithelial nasal neoplasia in dogs and cats, 0.3-4.7% of all tumors • Uncommon in cats

SIGNS

Historical Findings
• Progressive, intermittent to persistent unilateral becoming bilateral epistaxis (median duration, 3 months) • Sneezing • Halitosis
• Anorexia • Lethargy • Seizures secondary to cranial invasion

Physical Examination Findings
• Mucopurulent, purulent, or bloody nasal discharge • Facial deformity or exophthalmia

CAUSES AND RISK FACTORS N/A

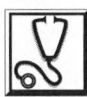

DIAGNOSIS

DIFFERENTIAL DIAGNOSIS
• Bacterial sinusitis • Viral infection (cats)
• Aspergillosis (dogs) • Cryptococcosis (cats)
• Foreign body • Trauma • Tooth root abscess

CBC/BIOCHEMISTRY/URINALYSIS
Results usually normal

OTHER LABORATORY TESTS N/A

IMAGING
• Skull radiography reveals typical pattern of asymmetrical destruction of caudal turbinates with superimposition of a soft tissue mass. Fluid density may be observed in the frontal sinuses secondary to outflow obstruction.
• Thoracic radiography to detect pulmonary metastasis • Rhinoscopy—visual observation often obscured by exudate • CT and MRI best methods of observing integrity of cribiform plate or orbital invasion

OTHER DIAGNOSTIC PROCEDURES
Deep tissue biopsy

TREATMENT
• Surgery alone is not curative.
• Turbinectomy before external (teletherapy) or internal (brachytherapy) irradiation
• Rhinitis developing after turbinectomy or radiotherapy rhinitis subsides in 1-2 months.
• Inpatient radiotherapy, with or without surgery, provides the best clinical control in dogs. Median disease-free interval in dogs, 8-25 months; median disease-free interval in cats, 1-36 months.
• Outpatient chemotherapy (doxorubicin), immunotherapy, and other treatment modalities may be palliative.

MEDICATIONS

DRUGS AND FLUIDS N/A

CONTRAINDICATIONS/POSSIBLE INTERACTIONS N/A

FOLLOW-UP
• Repeat examination with survey thoracic radiography at 1, 2, 3, 6, 9, 12, 15, 18, and 24 months after treatment. • Median survival if left untreated, 3-5 months • With radiotherapy, 1-year survival in dogs and cats (38-57%); 2-year survival rate (30-48%). Median survival, 1-36 months. • Local recurrence is common with extension to the brain.
• Secondary fungal rhinitis may occur after turbinectomy.

MISCELLANEOUS

Reference

Evans SM, Goldschmidt M, McKee LJ, Harvey CE. Prognostic factors and survival after radiotherapy for intranasal neoplasms in dogs: 70 cases (1974-1985). J Am Vet Med Assoc 1989;194:1460-1463.

Author Kevin A. Hahn

Consulting Editor Wallace B. Morrison

FLEAS AND FLEA CONTROL

 BASICS

DEFINITION

Flea allergy dermatitis is a hypersensitivity reaction to antigens in flea saliva with or without evidence of fleas and flea dirt. A flea infestation is the presence of a large number of fleas and a large amount of flea dirt with or without a flea allergy dermatitis.

Pathophysiology

• Flea bite hypersensitivity (FBH) is caused by both a low molecular weight hapten and two high molecular weight allergens that help initiate the allergic reaction. The high molecular weight allergens have increased binding to dermal collagen. When either type of allergen binds to collagen, this forms a complete antigen necessary for eliciting flea bite hypersensitivity. Flea saliva also contains histamine-like compounds that irritate skin. • Intermittent exposure to flea antigen favors a hypersensitivity reaction. Continuous exposure is less likely to result in flea bite hypersensitivity. Both IgE and IgG antiflea antibodies have been noted. Immediate and delayed hypersensitivity reactions have been noted. • More recently, late phase IgE-mediated response and cutaneous basophil hypersensitivity have been noted as part of this hypersensitivity reaction. Late phase IgE reactions occur 3-6 hours after exposure. With cutaneous basophil hypersensitivity, there is an infiltration of basophils into the dermis. This reaction is mediated either by IgE or IgG. Subsequent exposures cause the basophils to degranulate. This reaction manifests as immediate and delayed hypersensitivity.

Systems Affected

• Skin/Exocrine

Genetics

Flea bite hypersensitivity is the result of an unknown inheritance pattern, but is definitely more common in atopic breeds.

Incidence/Prevalence

The exact incidence/prevalence is unknown. This probably varies with climactic conditions and flea population.

Geographic Distribution

Flea bite hypersensitivity may occur anywhere. It usually only occurs nonseasonally in climates that are warm and humid year round.

SIGNALMENT

Species Dogs and cats

Breed Predilection

FBH may occur in any breed but most commonly occurs in atopic breeds.

Mean Age and Range

FBH is rare in animals less than 6 months of age. The average age range is 3-6 years.

Predominant Sex N/A

SIGNS

Historical Findings

• Somewhat dependent on the severity of the hypersensitivity and the amount of exposure to fleas (i.e. north = seasonal; south = year-round) • The most common clinical signs are compulsive biting, chewing ("corn-cob nibbling"), and licking primarily in the back half of the body but also including the antebrachial regions. Exposure to other animals and previous flea treatment should be ascertained. In cats, scratching around the head and neck may also be prominent. • Finding fleas and flea dirt is beneficial, although not essential, for the diagnosis of FBH.

Physical Examination Findings

• In dogs, the formation of lesions is concentrated in a triangular area of the caudal dorsal lumbosacral region. Additionally, the caudal aspect of the thighs, lower abdomen, inguinal region, and cranial forearms are usually involved. Papules are the primary lesions noted. Secondary lesions such as hyperpigmentation, lichenification, alopecia, and scaling are often observed in uncontrolled FBH. Secondary folliculitis and furunculosis may also be present. • In cats, several patterns of FBH are seen. Most commonly, cats develop a miliary crusting dermatitis in a wedge-shaped pattern over the caudal dorsal lumbosacral region. The miliary crusts are also often present around the head and neck. Another presentation is alopecia of the inguinal region with or without inflammation or eosinophilic plaques. Other forms of eosinophilic granuloma complex may also be seen.

CAUSES

See pathophysiology

RISK FACTORS

Intermittent exposure to fleas increases the likelihood of developing FBH. It is commonly seen in conjunction with atopy.

 DIAGNOSIS

DIFFERENTIAL DIAGNOSIS

The differential diagnoses include food allergy, atopy, sarcoptic mange, cheyletiellosis, and primary keratinization defects. The diagnosis is best based on the history and laboratory tests.

CBC/BIOCHEMISTRY/URINALYSIS

A complete blood count, serum chemistry profile, and urinalysis are usually normal. Hypereosinophilia may be detected in affected cats.

OTHER LABORATORY TESTS

• Skin scrapings are negative. Flea combings may detect fleas or flea dirt, but often none are found. • The radioallergosorbent test (RAST) and the enzyme linked immunosorbent assay (ELISA) techniques have variable accuracy with both false positives and false negatives.

IMAGING N/A

OTHER DIAGNOSTIC PROCEDURES

• Diagnosis of FBH is usually based on historical information and distribution of lesions. Finding fleas or flea dirt is supportive but is often quite difficult, especially in cats. • Identification of Dipylidium caninum segments is also supportive. • Intradermal allergy testing with flea antigen will reveal positive immediate reactions in 90% of flea allergic animals. Delayed reactions (24-48 hours) may be observed in some allergic animals who show no immediate reactions.

GROSS AND HISTOPATHOLOGIC FINDINGS

Superficial perivascular dermatitis. Eosinophilic intraepidermal microabscesses are strongly suggestive. If eosinophils are a major cellular component of the dermis, then this is also supportive.

 TREATMENT

INPATIENT VERSUS OUTPATIENT

Animals with FBH should be treated as outpatients.

ACTIVITY

No alteration of activity is necessary.

DIET

Diet does not need to be modified.

CLIENT EDUCATION

This is not a life-threatening disease, but it cannot be cured. Unfortunately, the flea allergic animals often become more sensitive to flea bites as they age. Controlling exposure to fleas is currently the only means of therapy. Hyposensitization has not worked satisfactorily.

SURGICAL CONSIDERATIONS N/A

 MEDICATIONS

DRUGS AND FLUIDS

• The pruritic component may be symptomatically controlled by anti-inflammatory dosages of corticosteroids while the fleas are being controlled
• Fleas are best treated on flea allergic animals by dips, sprays, powders, or foams. Organophosphates and synthetic pyrethrins are usually the chemicals found in dips. These should not be used more than once per week. Labels of each specific product should be followed for safest and best results. After repeated use, these agents can be drying or irritating.
• Sprays usually contain pyrethrins and pyrethroids (synthetic pyrethrins) with an insect growth regulator or synergist. Most of these products are effective less than 48-72 hours. Their advantages are low toxicity and repellent activity. Their disadvantages are

high frequency of application and increased expense. A permethrin spray is now available for use in dogs every 2 months. Finally, a new spray containing fipronil (GABA antagonist) has just come onto the market for cats and dogs.

• Powders usually contain organophosphates or carbamates. Their advantages include high residual effectiveness. Their disadvantages include drying of the skin and toxicity. Organophosphates and carbamates should be avoided in cats.

• Systemic flea treatments are of no benefit to flea allergic animals since these require a flea bite which has already initiated the FBH. In animals with flea infestation, these may be helpful. These are primarily licensed for use only in dogs. Cythioate (oral) and fenthion (spot-on) are 2 examples. Both are organophosphates. Lufenuron (program), a chitin inhibitor, has recently been marketed as an oral formulation in cats and dogs. Permethrin spot-ons currently available are reputed to have some repellant activity also. A new spot-on marketed imidacloprid (flea adulticide), is now available for use in dogs and cats.

• Indoor treatment should involve all areas of the house. Fogs and premise sprays can be applied by the owner. The advantage is that these are applied with weaker chemicals and are usually less costly to apply. The disadvantage is that they are more labor intensive. These products usually contain either organophosphates, pyrethrins, and/or insect growth regulators. Please follow manufacurers recommendations as these products are continuing to be developed.

Professional exterminators are less labor intensive, involve fewer applications, and are sometimes guaranteed. Disadvantages are strength of chemicals and cost. Their specific recommendations and guidelines must be followed.

• Inert substances are now available for "in home" use. These include boric acid, diatomaceous earth, and silica aerogel. Treatment must be done every 6-12 months. Follow manufacturer's recommendations. These products are very safe and effective if applied properly. The initial cost is somewhat more than previously discussed treatments.

• Outdoor treatment should be concentrated in shaded areas. Sprays usually contain pyrethroids or organophosphates and an insect growth regulator. Powders are usually organophosphates. A new product containing nematodes (Steinerma carpocapsae) is very safe and is not a chemical.

CONTRAINDICATIONS N/A

PRECAUTIONS

• Insecticidal sprays and dips should be used on dogs and cats three months of age or older unless otherwise specified on the label.

• Adverse reactions to pyrethrin/pyrethroid type flea products in dogs and cats may cause depression, hypersalivation, muscle tremors, vomiting, ataxia, dyspnea and anorexia. Adverse reactions to organophosphates in dogs and cats include hypersalivation, lacrimation, urination, defecation, vomiting, diarrhea, miosis, fever, muscle tremors, seizures, coma, and death. All pesticides must be applied according to label directions and if any signs of toxicity are noted, animals should be bathed thoroughly to remove any remaining chemical and treated appropriately.

• Rodents and fish are very sensitive to pyrethrins.

Using products beyond the label restrictions (extra label) is a violation of EPA regulations and is not legally permissible even if the practice is routinely followed by other veterinarians

POSSIBLE INTERACTIONS

More than 1 form of organophosphate treatment should not be used at one time. Topical organophosphates should be avoided in cats, very young animals (less than three months of age) and sick or debilitated animals. Straight permethrin sprays or spot-ons should not be used in cats. Cythioate is contraindicated in heartworm positive dogs and dogs of the greyhound breed. Piperonyl butoxide should not be used in concentrations of greater than 1% in cats.

ALTERNATE DRUGS N/A

FOLLOW-UP

PATIENT MONITORING

The level of pruritus should be monitored. If pruritus decreases, the FBH is being controlled. If fleas and flea dirt were originally present, then these should be monitored. Lack of fleas and flea dirt is not always a reliable indicator of treatment success in very sensitive animals.

PREVENTION/AVOIDANCE

See medications section. In dogs or cats in year-round warm climates, flea control should be done year round. In seasonal climates, the flea control should commence in May or June.

POSSIBLE COMPLICATIONS

Secondary bacterial infections, acute moist dermatitis and, occasionally, acral lick dermatitis may be seen with FBH.

EXPECTED COURSE AND PROGNOSIS

Prognosis is good if strict flea control is instituted.

MISCELLANEOUS

ASSOCIATED CONDITIONS

Eighty percent of atopic dogs are also allergic to flea bites.

AGE-RELATED FACTORS

Organophosphates should be used with utmost caution in old animals and are not recommended for use in very young animals (less than three months of age).

ZOONOTIC POTENTIAL

In areas of moderate to severe flea infestation, people can be bitten by fleas. These are usually papular lesions located on the wrists and ankles.

PREGNANCY

Corticosteroids and organophosphates should not be used in pregnant bitches and queens. Please follow the label directions of each individual product carefully to determine if safe to use in pregnancy.

SYNONYMS

• Flea bite allergy • Flea bite hypersensitivity

SEE ALSO N/A

ABBREVIATIONS

FBH = Flea bite hypersensitivity
RAST = radioallergosorbent test
ELISA = enzyme linked immunosorbent assay

References

Bevier-Tournay DE. Fleas and flea control. In: Kirk RW, Bonagura JD, eds. Current veterinary therapy X: Philadelphia: WB Saunders, 1989;586-591.

Griffin CE, Kwochka KW, MacDonald JM. Current veterinary dermatology. St. Louis: Mosby Year Book, 1993;57-71.

Author Karen A. Kuhl
Consulting Editor Lowell Ackerman

FLUKES, LIVER AND PANCREATIC

BASICS

OVERVIEW
Infections of domestic cats by Platynosomum concinnum or Eurytrema procyonis have been reported for many years. These flukes (trematodes) may be found in the biliary and pancreatic ducts. Geographic distribution particularly includes Florida, the Caribbean region, and Hawaii. The life cycle of the flukes depends upon ingestion by snails of ova passed in cat feces. The snail is then consumed by a second intermediate host, a toad or lizard. The cat then ingests this host. Adult flukes measure 1.1 mm wide by 2.7 mm long. They migrate from the intestine to the biliary or pancreatic ducts. The result is a variable degree of cholangitis, cholestasis, and uncommonly, pancreatic atrophy.

SIGNALMENT
• Cats are at risk if they are outside, predatory, and live in endemic areas. • Between 15 to 50% of cats at risk are reported to be infected.

SIGNS
• Few cats develop clinical signs. • Anorexia, icterus, and vomiting most common

CAUSES AND RISK FACTORS
• Platynosomum concinnum or Eurytrema procyonis • Risk factor: Living in an endemic area

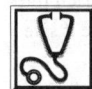

DIAGNOSIS

DIFFERENTIAL DIAGNOSIS
• Suppurative cholangitis • Lymphocytic cholangitis • Hepatic lipidosis • Pancreatitis

• Disorders causing cholestasis

CBC/BIOCHEMISTRY/URINALYSIS
• No consistant findings • Eosinophilia, hyperbilirubinemia, and high ALT and ALP activities in some patients

OTHER LABORATORY TESTS
• Fecal sedimentation techniques for detection of ova best for clinical diagnosis • Direct fecal-saline preparation may be useful. • Fecal flotation solution not as useful

IMAGING   N/A

OTHER DIAGNOSTIC PROCEDURES
Direct examination of bile obtained at surgery, necopsy, or by ultrasound guided aspiration usually reveals adult flukes and ova.

GROSS AND HISTOPATHOLOGIC FINDINGS
• A thick viscous bile in the obstructed ductules and gall bladder of heavily infected cats • Inflammation, hyperplasia, edema, and fibrosis of the ductules

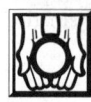

TREATMENT
• The level of treatment depends on the clinical status of the patient.
• Severely affected patients might need surgical cannulation of the common bile duct and drainage of the gall bladder.

MEDICATIONS

DRUGS AND FLUIDS
• Fenbendazole (50 mg/kg PO q24h for 5 to 10 days) is effective according to anecdotal reports.

• Praziquantel has been suggested (40 mg/kg q24h PO, IM, SC q24h for 3 consecutive days).
• A hydrocholoretic agent such as dehydrocholic acid or ursodeoxycholic acid may help to thin the bile, but should not be used if patient has marked biliary obstruction.

CONTRAINDICATIONS / POSSIBLE INTERACTIONS
• Avoid drugs that are potentially hepatotoxic and those excreted in the bile.
• The following drugs are not effective: diamphenethide, levamisole, mebendazole, rafoxanide, and thiabendazole.

FOLLOW-UP
Cats should be prevented from hunting the intermediate hosts.

MISCELLANEOUS

ABBREVIATIONS
ALP = alkaline phosphatase
ALT = alanine aminotransferase

Reference
Hitt, ME. Liver fluke infection in south Florida cats. Feline Pract 1981;11(3):26-28.
Author Mark E. Hitt
Consulting Editor Albert E. Jergens

BASICS

OVERVIEW
Canine follicular dysplasia refers to a group of hair and hair follicle abnormalities that often have a hereditary basis. The various clinical syndromes are still incompletely categorized and understood. They will be discussed here as color dilution alopecia (CDA), black hair follicular dysplasia (BHFD), and canine follicular dysplasia (CFD).

SIGNALMENT
• CDA affects dogs of an unusual color for their breed, ususally beginning between 4 and 6 months of age. • Blue color dilutions of doberman pinscher, great Dane, dachshund, whippet, Italian greyhound, chow chow, standard poodle, Yorkshire terrier, miniature pinscher, chihuahua, Bernese mountain dog, shetland sheepdog, and schipperke have been affected as well as fawn and red dobermans and fawn Irish setters. • BHFD affects some white dogs with dark spots by several weeks of age. • Beagle, basset hound, saluki, papillon, and bearded collies are predisposed. Mongrels can also be affected. • CFD usually begins at less than 3 years of age. Predisposed breeds include Siberian husky, Alaskan malamute, English springer spaniel, Irish water spaniel, Portuguese water dog, curly-coated retriever, Airedale terrier, boxer, English bulldog, French bulldog, and miniature schnauzer.

SIGNS
• CDA—unusual coat color (often lighter than normal), dry and brittle hair, patchy alopecia, follicular papules and pustules, and furunculosis. Areas with normal coloration are spared. • BHFD—areas of black hairs begin thinning by several weeks of age eventually resulting in alopecia and dry, scaly skin. • CFD—signs vary with coat type. Long-haired and curly-coated breeds often loose

primary hairs exposing a discolored (reddish-brown) undercoat that is brittle. Airedale terriers and short-coated breeds often develop complete alopecia in the flank areas. A cycle of complete hair loss and regrowth often occurs repeatedly in these dogs.

CAUSES AND RISK FACTORS
These syndromes have a genetic basis, although endocrine abnormalities may play some role as well.

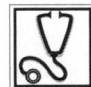

DIAGNOSIS

DIFFERENTIAL DIAGNOSIS
• Hypothyroidism • Hyperadrenocorticism • Reproductive hormone imbalances • Bacterial folliculitis • Demodicosis (follicular papules and pustules) • Malnutrition

CBC/BIOCHEMISTRY/URINALYSIS
N/A

OTHER LABORATORY TESTS N/A

IMAGING N/A

OTHER DIAGNOSTIC PROCEDURES
N/A

GROSS AND HISTOPATHOLOGIC FINDINGS
Dermatohistopathologic examination may reveal misshapen hair follicles, abnormal melanin deposition in the epidermis, hair shaft, and around the hair follicle, bacterial folliculitis and furunculosis, and exaggerated catagen hair follicles.

TREATMENT
The CFD syndromes are cosmetic diseases only. However, owners should be made aware that the prognosis for a full recovery is poor.

MEDICATIONS

DRUGS AND FLUIDS
• Antiseborrheic and follicular flushing shampoos containing benzoyl peroxide followed by emollient rinses are indicated every 3 to 14 days, depending on the severity of disease.
• Secondary bacterial folliculitis should be treated with appropriate antibiotics.
• Synthetic retinoid drugs (etretinate, 1-3 mg/kg q24h or isotretinoin 1-3 mg/kg q24h) have been used with success in some patients. Although responses are rarely complete, some hair growth, reduction in scaling, and reduced frequency of bacterial folliculitis may be noted.

CONTRAINDICATIONS/POSSIBLE INTERACTIONS N/A

FOLLOW-UP
• Physical examinations should be performed at least monthly until the condition stabilizes, then every 3-6 months. • Shampoo therapy can be modified based upon the response observed. • Monitoring for side effects of retinoid drugs can be done at these times.

MISCELLANEOUS

ABBREVIATIONS
CDA = color dilution alopecia
BHFD = black hair follicular dysplasia
CFD = canine follicular dysplasia

Reference
Gross TL, Ihrke PJ, Walder EJ. Veterinary dermatopathology. St. Louis: Mosby Yearbook, 1992.
Author Jon D. Plant
Consulting Editor Lowell Ackerman

FOOD REACTIONS (DERMATOLOGIC)

BASICS

DEFINITION
Food reactions (dermatologic) are pruritic, non-seasonal reactions associated with ingestion of one or more substances in the animal's food.

Pathophysiology
• The pathogenesis is not completely understood. Immediate reactions and delayed reactions to specific ingredients have been documented in the veterinary literature. • Immediate reactions are presumed to be Type I hypersensitivity reactions and the delayed reactions could be type III or IV hypersensitivity reactions. • Reactions to food may also be nonimmunologic and are referred to as food intolerances. Food intolerance refers to an idiosyncratic reaction involving metabolic, toxic or pharmacologic effects of offending ingredients. Food hypersensitivity is the most common term used because it not easy to distinguish between immunologic or idiosyncratic reactions.

Systems Affected
• Skin/Exocrine—pruritus in any location on the body, otitis externa • Gastrointestinal—vomiting, diarrhea, and more frequent bowel movements • Nervous—very rare; seizures have been documented with food hypersensitivity

Genetics N/A

Incidence/Prevalence
It is estimated that 5% of all skin disease and 10–15% of all allergic skin disease in dogs and cats is caused by food hypersensitivity. It is the third most common pruritic skin disease in the dog, second most common in the cat.

Geographic Distribution N/A

SIGNALMENT
• This disease is seen in the dog and cat, with no breed or sex predilection. • If a pruritic skin disorder first occurs at less than 6 months or over 6 years of age, then food hypersensitivity is more likely than inhalant allergy.

SIGNS

General Comments
Food hypersensitivity has a wide range of signs and can mimic any of the other hypersensitivity reactions.

Historical Findings
• Nonseasonal pruritus of any body location. • Poor response to antiinflammatory doses of glucocorticoids is suggestive of food hypersensitivity. • Less common signs that are associated with food hypersensitivity are vomiting, diarrhea, excessive borborygmus, flatulence, and more frequent bowel movements.

Physical Examination Findings
Malassezia dermatitis, pyoderma, and otitis externa can be associated with food hypersensitivity just as they are associated with other hypersensitivity reactions. These infections and the pruritus associated with food hypersensitivity can cause one or more of the following lesions: plaques, pustules, erythema, crusts, scale, self-induced alopecia, excoriation, lichenification, hyperpigmentation, urticaria, angioedema, and pyotraumatic dermatitis.

CAUSES
• Immune-mediated reactions are thought to occur as a result of the ingestion and subsequent presentation of one or more glycoproteins (allergens) either before or after digestion. The sensitization may occur at the level of the gastrointestinal mucosa or after it is absorbed or both. • Nonimmune (food intolerance) reactions are proposed to be due to foods that have high levels of histamine, or to substances that induce a release of histamine either directly or through histamine releasing factors.

RISK FACTORS
Unknown, but it has been speculated that in juvenile animals, intestinal parasites or intestinal infections may cause damage to the intestinal mucosa causing abnormal absorption of allergens with subsequent sensitization.

DIAGNOSIS

DIFFERENTIAL DIAGNOSIS
• Flea bite hypersensitivity, usually confined to the caudal half of the body and often seasonal. • Atopy, which is associated with pruritus on the face, ventrum, and feet, and often seasonal. • Drug reactions and scabies. The history of drug administration prior to the development of signs and improvement upon withdrawal from the suspect drug help to confirm or deny a drug reaction. Scabies is very specific in the location of the pruritus (ears, elbows and hocks). Finding mites in skin scrapings and the response to specific therapy confirms the diagnosis.

CBC/BIOCHEMISTRY/URINALYSIS
No important changes are seen

OTHER LABORATORY TESTS N/A

IMAGING N/A

OTHER DIAGNOSTIC PROCEDURES
• The definitive diagnostic test for food hypersensitivity is commonly referred to as a food elimination diet. This diet must be tailored to each individual patient. The ingredients in this diet must be restricted to one protein and one carbohydrate to which the animal has had limited or no previous exposure. The duration of this test diet may take up to 13 weeks for maximum improvement

of the clinical signs. If an animal is sensitive to a food ingredient or ingredients, it will begin to show some noticeable improvement by the 4th week of the diet trial. • Challenge and provocation diet trials: these are used if the animal improves on the elimination diet. The first test after a positive elimination test is to "challenge" the pet with the original diet. A return of the signs confirms that there is something in the diet that is causing these signs. The challenge period should last until the signs return but no longer than 10 days. The next step if the challenge confirms the presence of a food hypersensitivity is to provoke the signs by adding single ingredients to the elimination diet. The addition of single ingredients is called the "provocation diet trial." The period of provocation with each ingredient should last up to 10 days, less if signs develop sooner. In most dogs, signs will develop within 1-2 days of the addition of the test ingredient. The test ingredients should be all the major meat proteins (beef, chicken, fish, pork, lamb), grain proteins (corn, wheat, soybean, rice), and eggs and dairy products. From the results of the provocation diet, the clinician can recommend several commercial foods which do not contain the ingredient or ingredients that cause reactions in this pet.

GROSS AND HISTOPATHOLOGIC FINDINGS
Skin biopsies are not diagnostic but will help confirm or deny other differentials. The histopathologic findings are variable; the common findings are suggestive of hypersensitivity. Also, a secondary pyoderma or Malassezia infection may be present.

TREATMENT

INPATIENT VERSUS OUTPATIENT
These are usually outpatients since most animals do not improve for 3 to 4 weeks and many take several months before they are maximally improved.

ACTIVITY No activity change

DIET
Avoidance of any food substances that caused the clinical signs with reintroinduction during the provocation phase of the diagnosis.

CLIENT EDUCATION
The client must be thoroughly informed of the principles involved in each phase of the diagnostic test diets. It is also important to avoid treats, chewable toys, vitamins, and other chewable medications (heartworm, etc.) that may contain ingredients from the pet's previous diet. Handouts are very useful for clients to take home. All family members need to be made aware of the test protocol to help keep the test diet clean and free of any other food sources.

FOOD REACTIONS (DERMATOLOGIC)

SURGICAL CONSIDERATIONS N/A

MEDICATIONS

DRUGS AND FLUIDS
• Systemic antipruritic drugs may be useful during the first 2–3 weeks of diet trial to control self–mutilation. • Antibiotics or antifungal medications are useful to treat secondary pyodermas or Malassezia infections.

CONTRAINDICATIONS
• Avoidance of antibiotics that are known to have anti–inflammatory effects (e.g. tetracycline, erythromycin, trimethoprim–potentiated sulfas) • Glucocorticoids and antihistamines must be discontinued for at least 10–14 days while the animal is on diet trial to allow correct assessment of the animal's response.

PRECAUTIONS N/A

POSSIBLE INTERACTIONS
Chewable vitamins, heartworm medications, etc. may contain offending food substances.

ALTERNATE DRUGS N/A

FOLLOW-UP

PATIENT MONITORING
The patient should be examined and the pruritus and clinical signs should be evaluated and documented every 3- 4 weeks.

PREVENTION/AVOIDANCE
Avoid intake of any of the previous diet's food proteins. Treats and chewable toys should be limited to substances known to not cause hypersensitivity reactions.(e.g., apples, vegetables)

POSSIBLE COMPLICATIONS
Other causes of pruritus such as flea bite hypersensitivity, atopy, and external parasites like sarcoptic, notoedres, and cheyletiella mites can mask the response to the food elimination diet trial.

EXPECTED COURSE AND PROGNOSIS
Prognosis is good if food ingredients are the only cause of the pruritus. Avoidance of the offending ingredients have good prognosis. Rarely, a dog or cat may develop hypersensitivity to new substances. A new elimination diet trial may be necessary. If there are other hypersensitivities present (flea or atopy), these must be treated as well.

MISCELLANEOUS

ASSOCIATED CONDITIONS
• Superficial pyoderma • Malassezia dermatitis • Otitis externa

AGE RELATED FACTORS
• Food hypersensitivity reactions can occur at any age. • Animals who develop pruritus for the first time at less than 6 months and over 6 years of age are more likely to have food hypersensitivity than atopy.

ZOONOTIC POTENTIAL N/A

PREGNANCY N/A

SYNONYMS
• Food allergy • Food intolerance

SEE ALSO
• Flea and Flea Control • Atopy • Dermatitis, contact • Superficial Pyoderma • Malassezia Dermatitis • Otitis Externa

ABBREVIATIONS N/A

References

Jeffers JG, Shanley KJ. Diagnostic testing of dogs for food hypersensitivity. J Am Ved Med Assoc 1991;198:245.

MacDonald JM. Food allergy. In: Griffin CE, Kwochka KW, MacDonald JM, eds. Current veterinary dermatology. Mosby Year Book, 1993:121.

White SD. Food hypersensitivity in 30 dogs. J Am Ved Med Assoc 1986;188:695.

Rosser EJ. Diagnosis of food allergy in dogs. J Am Ved Med Assoc 1993;203:259.

Author David Duclos
Consulting Editor Lowell Ackerman

GASTRIC DILATION AND VOLVULUS SYNDROME (GDV)

BASICS

DEFINITION
A syndrome of dogs in which the stomach dilates and twists around its central axis which results in complex local and systemic pathologic and physiologic changes.

Pathophysiology
Fluid or ingesta accumulates in the stomach in conjunction with a mechanical or functional obstruction of the gastroesophageal and pyloric orifices. Dilation of the stomach may progress adding to functional obstruction and potentiating volvulus. Twisting of the stomach may occur without dilation. When viewing the dog in dorsal recumbency from caudal to cranial, the stomach may twist in a clockwise or counterclockwise direction. The most common presentation is clockwise with the duodenum passing ventrally from right to left. The rotation is around the long axis from the cardia to the pylorus. Rotation varies from 90° to 360°. Direct gastric damage and multiple systemic abnormalities occur secondary to ischemia and reperfusion injury. Ischemia results from rising intra-gastric pressures, decreased cardiac return as the stomach compresses the portal vein and caudal vena cava, direct outflow obstruction of gastric and splanchnic vessels due to twisting, infarction of the gastric mucosa due to neutrophil accumulation and margination, and edema due to multiple cell damage and inflammatory mediator release. These changes account for the acute clinical signs of GDV which include hypovolemic shock and cardiovascular failure. Reperfusion injury is a complex entity involving the formation of free radicals and multiple inflammatory mediators.

Systems Affected
• Gastrointestinal - fundus of the stomach is most severely compromised by the occlusion of its blood supply during torsion. • Cardiovascular - Low venous return to the right side of the heart results in severe hypoxia to other organ systems and hypovolemic shock. Arrhythmia secondarily due to the effects of hypoxia, inflammatory mediators and other cardiogenic factors. • Respiratory - Direct impedance of volume expansion due to gastric distension and secondly due to decreased cardiac output to the lungs. • Hemic/Lymphatic/Immune - Splenic infarction • Hepatobiliary - Multiple factors including inflammatory mediators, hypoxia, endotoxemia, and potentially reperfusion injury of the liver

Genetics
No direct genetic predisposition has been confirmed.

Incidence/Prevalence
Incidence and prevalence varies with geographic location and breed prevalence. Most metropolitan emergency clinics see these cases frequently.

Geographic Distribution
See Incidence/Prevalence

SIGNALMENT

Species Dog

Breed Predilections
German shepards, Great Danes, Saint Bernards, Rottweilers, Labrador retrievers, Alaskan malamutes, any large, deep, chested breeds, rarely reported in daschund and pekingese

Mean Age and Range
Symptom may occur at any age although most commonly in middle aged to older dogs.

Predominant Sex None

SIGNS

Historical Findings
• Non-productive retching • Ptyalism (hypersalivation) • Progressive abdominal distension • Weakness • Depression

Physical Examination Findings
• Tympanic cranial abdomen • Tachycardia • Tachypnea • Rectal body temperature may vary widely • Signs of hypovolemic shock (e.g., pale mucus membranes, decreased capillary refill time and weak pulses)

CAUSES
Theories of interest include pyloric outflow obstruction, gastric myoelectric abnormalities, dynamic movement of the stomach following ingestion of food or water, and aerophagia.

RISK FACTORS
• Activity following ingestion of large quantities of food or water • Any intense activity and stress

DIAGNOSIS

DIFFERENTIAL DIAGNOSIS
Gastric dilation without torsion due to overdistension usually from ingestion of excessive quantities of food. Other diseases including intestinal volvulus or splenic torsion which may result in abdominal distension.

CBC/BIOCHEMISTRY/URINALYSIS
• Generally not performed during acute treatment as will not change the treatment protocol. • Hemogram abnormalities consistent with acute inflammation may be expected. • Electrolyte abnormalities and acid/base alterations are common • Urinalysis generally reflects hypovolemia (high urine specific gravity due to prerenal azotemia).

OTHER LABORATORY TESTS N/A

IMAGING
If diagnosis is in doubt and the animal is stabilized, a right lateral abdominal radiograph is the imaging modality of choice. A "double bubble" compartmentalized stomach is considered pathognomonic. On a dorsoventral view the pylorus may be shifted towards or located in the left cranial abdomen.

OTHER DIAGNOSTIC PROCEDURES
N/A

GROSS AND HISTOPATHOLOGIC FINDINGS
Gastric distension with resultant gastric edema, hyperemia, congestion, infarction, and necrosis depending on duration of condition. Splenic torsion may also be present.

TREATMENT

INPATIENT VERSUS OUTPATIENT
Patients require immediate medical therapy with special attention to establishing improved cardiovascular function and then gastric decompression. Gastric decompression is first attempted by orogastric intubation. Light sedation with narcotics may facilitate this process. Decompression by other techniques such as trocarization and indwelling catheters is described. Maintenance of gastric decompression either by indwelling catheters or pharyngogastric tubes until definitive treatment or surgical derotation and gastropexy may necessitate hospitalization.

ACTIVITY
Severely restrict activity prior to surgery and for a minimum of 10-14 days post surgery.

DIET
Oral alimentation may be begun as soon as appropriate based on gastric integrity at surgery. Small multiple feedings of a high quality bland diet are recommended during surgical recovery to prevent gastric distension. Placement of a jejunostomy feeding tube at the time of surgery may allow for early enteral supplementation. Diet modification may be recommended permanently.

CLIENT EDUCATION
Potential risk factors and recurrence of the dilation should be discussed with owners. Explanation of signs so that the client may detect the condition in its early stages.

SURGICAL CONSIDERATIONS
Definitive treatment is exploratory celiotomy with gastric derotation and permanent right sided gastropexy. Timing of surgery is controversial and is based on the patient's cardiovascular condition, gastric decompression, and other physical parameters. Prolonged delay may result in gastric necrosis whereas premature surgery may result in death of the patient. Derotation without gastropexy results in an 80% recurrence rate. Multiple techniques for gastropexy are appropriate and de-

GASTRIC DILATION AND VOLVULUS SYNDROME (GDV)

scribed in detail in surgical texts. Partial gastrectomy may be required based on observation of gastric wall integrity especially in the fundic region. Supplemental alimentation may be indicated with partial gastrectomies depending on gastric integrity. A jejunostomy tube may be placed for enteral supplements. Splenic vasculature infarction is an indication for splenectomy. Surgical exploration should be thorough yet efficient. Decreased survival time is associated with prolonged surgery and anesthesia in a hemodynamically unstable patient.

MEDICATIONS

DRUGS AND FLUIDS

• Isotonic fluids at the rate of 90 ml/kg given within the first 30-60 minutes is the general treatment of choice for hypovolemic patients. Delivery of this volume in most cases requires the placement of two large bore intravenous catheters. Supportive fluids based on other physical parameters are recommended for animals not in shock. Postoperative fluid support is recommended until the animal is able to eat and drink.

• Corticosteroids are accepted as beneficial in these cases to stabilizes membranes, to aid in cardiovascular support, and as potential treatment of reperfusion injury (dexamethasone sodium phosphate 5 mg/kg slow IV, or prednisolone sodium succinate 11 mg/kg IV).

• Broad spectrum antibiotics effective against gastrointestinal flora are often recommended due to potential for endotoxemia associated with shock, gastric compromise and potential abdominal contamination at the time of surgery. Refer to drug spectrums for potential choices.

CONTRAINDICATIONS

Drugs which may exacerbate hypovolemia such as acepromazine should be avoided. Additional drugs for correction of acid base abnormalities should be reserved until the animal is stabilized.

PRECAUTIONS

Anesthetic agents should be chosen for their cardiovascular supportive effects. Special attention to maintenance of mean arterial pressure at or above 60 mmHg.

POSSIBLE INTERACTIONS N/A

ALTERNATE DRUGS N/A

FOLLOW-UP

PATIENT MONITORING

• Monitor cardiac function for at least 24 hours after surgery. Monitor blood pressure and perfusion. Electrocardiographic monitoring is indicated. Splenectomy frequently results in multifocal intermittent to continuous premature ventricular contractions. Antiarrhythmics should be administered only when deemed appropriate. • General supportive care with special attention to electrolyte and acid/base status should be instituted. Treatment should be prescribed as is deemed necessary based on serial lab work.

PREVENTION/AVOIDANCE

Avoid overingestion of foods or fluids, feed small meals multiple times during the day, and avoid exercise post-prandially.

POSSIBLE COMPLICATIONS

Gastric ulceration may occur within 5-7 days after surgery if severe mucosal defects remain. Rupture of gastric ulcers may result in septic peritonitis and it sequelae. Other complications reported following gastropexy include belching, and intermittent vomiting.

EXPECTED COURSE AND PROGNOSIS

Prognosis is based on surgical assessment and postoperative recovery. Animals still recovering well after seven days appears to have a good prognosis for complete recovery. Gastropexy appears to be the most significant factor preventing reoccurrence with reoccurrence rate as great as 80% without gastropexy as compared to the 3-5% with different gastropexy procedures.

MISCELLANEOUS

ASSOCIATED CONDITIONS N/A

AGE RELATED FACTORS N/A

ZOONOTIC POTENTIAL N/A

PREGNANCY

No specific considerations aside from hemodynamic support. Hypoxia may be detrimental to the fetuses.

SYNONYMS N/A

SEE ALSO N/A

ABBREVIATIONS

GDV - Gastric dilation and volvulus syndrome

References

Matthiesen DT. Gastric dilation-volvulus syndrome. In: Slatter D, ed. Textbook of small animal surgery. 2nd ed. Philadelphia: WB Saunders, 1993.

Matthiesen DT: Pathophysiology of gastric dilatation volvulus. In: Bojrab MJ, ed. Disease mechanisms in small animal surgery. 2nd ed. Philadelphia: Lea and Febiger, 1993.

Author Michelle Joy Waschak
Consulting Editor Brent D. Jones

GASTRIC EROSIONS AND ULCERS

BASICS

DEFINITION
Gastric erosions are superficial lesions involving the gastric mucosa; gastric ulcers extend through the mucosa and into the muscularis mucosa.

Pathophysiology
Gastric erosions and ulcers are the result of single or multiple factors altering, damaging, or overwhelming the normal defense and repair mechanisms of the "gastric mucosal barrier". Factors that comprise the "gastric mucosal barrier" and protect the stomach from erosion and ulcer formation include the mucus-bicarbonate layer over the epithelial cells, the gastric epithelial cells, gastric mucosal blood flow, epithelial cell restitution and repair, and prostaglandins produced by the gastrointestinal tract. Factors causing the mucosal barrier to be damaged, inhibiting the epithelial cells ability to repair, decreasing the mucosal blood supply, or increasing gastric acid secretion predispose to gastric erosion and ulcer formation. The risk of gastric erosion/ulcer formation increases with the number of insults to the "gastric mucosal barrier".

Systems Affected
Cardiovascular - acute hemorrhage
Respiratory - aspiration pneumonia secondary to vomiting

Genetics N/A

Incidence/Prevalence
True incidence unkown, but probably more common than clinically recognized

Geographic Distribution N/A

SIGNALMENT

Species
Dogs and less commonly cats

Breed Predilection N/A

Mean Age and Range All ages

Predominant Sex
Male dogs have increased incidence of gastric carcinoma.

SIGNS
• Asymptomatic in some patients • Hematemesis: blood may be fresh (flecks, clots) or digested (looks like coffee grounds). • Vomiting: with or without blood in vomitus. • Melena • Abdominal pain • Anorexia • Pale mucous membranes and weakness (if anemia) • Edema (if hypoproteinemia) • Acute depression, collapse, shock, abdominal pain, sudden death (if gastric ulcer perforates) • See signs and symptoms associated with primary problem

CAUSES
• Drugs: NSAIDs, glucocorticoids • Metabolic disease: Hepatic disease, Renal failure, Hypoadrenocorticism • Stress/Major Medical Illness: Shock, Severe illness, Hypotension,

Trauma, Major surgery, Sepsis, DIC • Gastric foreign objects • Gastric neoplasia • Gastritis: Lymphocytic/plasmacytic gastroenteritis, Eosinophilic gastroenteritis • Mast cell tumor • Gastrin secreting tumor • Helicobacter pylori: importance in dogs/cats unknown • Lead poisoning

RISK FACTORS
• Critically ill patients • Drugs: NSAIDs, glucocorticoids

DIAGNOSIS

DIFFERENTIAL DIAGNOSIS
• Blood from the oral cavity or respiratory system may be swallowed and result in hematemesis. • Confirm blood is in vomitus and not other fluids (i.e. urine, mucoid feces) • Pepto Bismol can turn feces dark and look like melena • Melena may be secondary to intestinal problems (e.g. hookworms, intestinal neoplasia) rather than gastric disease. • See Acute Gastritis and Chronic Gastritis

CBC/BIOCHEMISTRY/URINALYSIS
• Anemia may be present • Recent (3–5 days) blood loss: normochromic, normocytic, non-regenerative anemia. • Acute blood loss greater than 5 days in duration: normocytic, normochromic, regenerative anemia. • Chronic blood loss: iron deficiency anemia characterized by microcytic, hypochromic, non-regenerative anemia. • Thrombocytosis may be seen in association with iron deficiency • Mature neutrophilia may be present. • Low plasma proteins due to blood loss; evidence of dehydration may be present and mask decreases in plasma proteins • Urea nitrogen may be moderately high with gastrointestinal hemorrhage.

OTHER LABORATORY TESTS
• Fecal occult blood test may be positive. • ACTH stimulation if hyponatremia, hypochloremia, hyperkalemia present or lack of stress hemogram in systemically ill patient • Bile acids if suspect hepatic insufficiency • Gastrin levels if more common causes ruled out

IMAGING
• Radiographs will not demonstrate gastric erosions and rarely detect gastric ulcers. A positive contrast gastrogram may outline defects caused by gastric ulceration. • Ultrasonography is an insensitive method for detecting gastric erosions and ulcers. Occasionally focal deep gastric ulcers may alter the gastric wall and be detected on ultrasound examination.

OTHER DIAGNOSTIC PROCEDURES
• Search for mast cell tumor: Fine needle aspirate or biopsy of cutaneous masses that potentially are mast cell tumors; buffy coat examination or bone marrow biopsy; abdominal ultrasound; fine needle aspirate of spleen if abnormal. • If the history does not indicate

drug administration as a cause for hematemesis and the initial laboratory data does not indicate an underlying cause, gastroscopy is indicated to evaluate the stomach. Endoscopy may not always detect gastric erosions but ulcers will usually be visualized. Endoscopy is also indicated for foreign object removal and to obtain gastric biopsy samples for histopathology.

TREATMENT

INPATIENT VERSUS OUTPATIENT
Treat as outpatient if cause identified and removed, minimal signs, and no systemic effects. Treat as inpatient if cause undetermined, moderate to severe clinical signs, or systemic effects.

ACTIVITY N/A

DIET
Restrict oral intake if vomiting. When feeding is resumed, feed small amounts in multiple feedings, and feed a diet that is primarily an easily digested starch such as rice. The diet should be low in fiber and fat. Protein should be added gradually to the diet in small amounts and it is preferable that it be a vegetable (tofu) or milk protein (low fat cottage cheese).

CLIENT EDUCATION
Avoid gastric irritants (e.g. NSAIDs).

SURGICAL CONSIDERATIONS
Medical management and removal of initiating factors is attempted initially. Surgical treatment is indicated if hemorrhage is uncontrolled, ulceration or inflammation results in a gastric outlet obstruction, or gastric ulcer perforation occurs.

MEDICATIONS

DRUGS AND FLUIDS
• Histamine H-2 receptor antagonists (e.g. cimetidine or ranitidine) inhibit gastric acid secretion
• Sucralfate (Carafate) protects ulcerated tissue (cytoprotection) by binding to ulcer sites.
• Antibiotic(s) with spectrum of activity against enteric gram-negative and anaerobes are administered parenterally if a break in GI mucosal barrier allows for increased translocation of bacteria and potential sepsis.
• Antiemetics (e.g. chlorpromazine and metoclopramide) are administered if vomiting occurs frequently or results in significant fluid losses. Metoclopramide increases gastric emptying.
• Fluid therapy is indicated to correct hydration deficits, provide maintenance fluids if oral intake in restricted or inadequate, and to replace ongoing losses. Subcutaneous fluid administration is adequate if mild dehydration and no systemic signs are present.

Intravenous fluids are indicated if moderate to severe dehydration, hypovolemia, or systemic signs are present. A balanced electrolyte solution such as Ringer's solution is usually used initially until electrolyte and acid base status is determined. Maintenance potassium is usually added to the fluids unless a primary problem causing hyperkalemia (e.g. renal failure, hypoadrenocorticism) is suspected.
• Blood transfusion is indicated if severe blood loss occurs.

CONTRAINDICATIONS
• Phenothiazine derivatives should not be administered to hypovolemic patients or patients at risk for hypotension.
• Misoprostol—do not use in pregnant animals, causes abortion.

PRECAUTIONS N/A

POSSIBLE INTERACTIONS
• Cimetidine binds to hepatic cytochrome P450 enzyme and may interfere with metabolism of other drugs.
• Sucralfate may alter absorption of other drugs.

ALTERNATE DRUGS
• Omeprazol—potent inhibitor of gastric acid secretion
• Misoprostol—synthetic prostaglandin analog
• Antibiotics—if H. pylori suspected
• Bismuth-containing drug—if H. pylori suspected

FOLLOW-UP

PATIENT MONITORING
• Clinical signs: hematemesis, vomiting, melena, anorexia • Hematocrit and total protein

PREVENTION/AVOIDANCE
Avoid gastric irritants (e.g., NSAIDs, corticosteroids)

POSSIBLE COMPLICATIONS
• Gastric ulcer perforation • Severe blood loss requiring transfusion • Life-threatening blood loss • Sepsis • Signs of hepatic encephalopathy if hepatic failure present

EXPECTED COUSE AND PROGNOSIS
Varies with underlying cause

MISCELLANEOUS

ASSOCIATED CONDITIONS N/A

AGE RELATED FACTORS
Neoplasia more common in older animals

ZOONOTIC POTENTIAL N/A

PREGNANCY
Synthetic prostaglandins (e.g. misoprostol) cause abortion

SYNONYMS N/A

SEE ALSO
See Causes

ABBREVIATIONS N/A

References

DeNovo RC. Medical management of gastritis, ulcers, and erosions. In: Proceedings 17th annual Waltham/OSU Symposium. Columbus, OH:1993.

Stanton ME. Gastroduodenal ulceration in dogs. J Vet Int Med 1989;3:238.

Strombeck DR, Guilford WG. Acute gastritis. Strombeck DR, Guilford WG, eds. Small animal gastroenterology. 2nd ed. Davis, CA: Stonegate, 1990.

Author Linda J. DeBowes
Consulting Editor Brent D. Jones

GASTRIC MOTILITY DISORDERS

BASICS

DEFINITION
Gastric motility disorders result from conditions that directly or indirectly disrupt normal gastric emptying that results in gastric distention and subsequent gastric signs.

Pathophysiology
• The stomach has two distinct motor regions. The proximal region relaxes to accommodate food and regulates expulsion of liquids. Intrinsic slow sustained contractions of this region push liquids through the pylorus. The distal stomach mechanically breaks down and expels solids through strong peristaltic contractions. Distal gastric motility and emptying is regulated by a gastric pacemaker which is an area of intrinsic electrical activity found in the greater curvature. Gastric electrical activity, dietary composition and extrinsic factors influence emptying. • During fasting, nondigestible solids are expelled from the stomach by migrating myeoelectric complexes. These complexes produce strong contractions that sweep through the stomach and intestine occurring every 2 hours in the fasted state. This motility is under the regulation of the hormone motilin. • Dysrrhythmias in normal gastric electrical activity may be fundamental in the pathophysiology of disorders affecting gastric motility.

Systems Affected
Gastrointestinal

Genetics N/A

Incidence and Prevalence
Unknown. Many factors can alter gastric emptying though some may not result in clinical disease.

Geographical Distribution N/A

SIGNALMENT

Species Dogs and cats

Breed Predilections
Unknown

Mean Age and Range
Symptoms occur at any age though it is uncommon to observe primary motility disorders in young animals.

Predominant Sex N/A

SIGNS

General Comments
Clinical signs are often related to the cause of the gastric motility disorder and the motility disorder becomes a secondary complication.

Historical Findings
• The major clinical sign is chronic postprandial vomiting of food. The stomach should be empty of a meal by 8-10 hours after eating and vomiting of undigested food greater than that time suggests a gastric motility disorder or outflow obstruction. Vomiting can also oc-

cur anytime following eating. • Other signs include gastric distention, nausea, anorexia, belching, pica and weight loss.

Physical Examination Findings
• Normal or may reveal findings associated with the underlying cause of the disorder.
• Palpation of a large distended stomach.
• Decreased gastric sounds on abdominal auscultation.

CAUSES
• Primary idiopathic gastric motility disorders may arise from defects in normal myeoelectric activity. • Most motiltiy disorders occur secondary to primary conditions. • Metabolic disorders include hypokalemia, uremia, hepatic encephalopathy and hypothyroidism. • Nervous inhibition as the result of stress, fear, pain or trauma. • Drugs such as the anticholinergics, beta-adenergic agonists and narcotics. • Primary gastric disease such as outflow obstructions, gastritis, gastric ulcers, parvovirus and gastric surgery. • Gastric dilatation-volvulus syndrome (GDV) is suspected to result from a primary motility disorder of abnormal myeoelectric and mechanical activity. Dogs following surgical gastropexy may continue to have signs of gastric hypomotility. • Gastroesophageal reflux and enterogastric reflux syndromes may result from gastric hypomotility. • Dysautonomia syndromes.

RISK FACTORS
Any potential gastric disease may result in secondary hypomotility.

DIAGNOSIS

DIFFERENTIAL DIAGNOSIS
• The differential diagnosis is extensive and should include any condition causing vomiting. • Gastric outflow obstructions must always be ruled out.

CBC/BIOCHEMISTRY/URINALYSIS
• Routine hemogram, serum chemistry profile, urinalysis and fecal flotation must be performed to rule out the potential cause of gastric hypomotility. • Continued vomiting may result in dehydration, electrolyte abnormalities, or acid-base imbalance. • Hypokalemia is a common electrolyte abnormality associated with abnormal gastrointestinal motility.

OTHER LABORATORY TESTS
Specialized testing may be required to determine a specific cause of gastric hypomotility and is individualized for each patient.

IMAGING

Survey Radiographs
Abdominal radiographs may reveal a gas, fluid or an ingesta distended stomach.

Liquid Barium Contrast Study
May be evidence of delayed gastric emptying and decreased gastric contractions if evaluated

using fluoroscopy. Some cases may have normal emptying of liquids especially if the motility abnormality involves emptying of solids.

Food Barium Contrast Study
• Barium mixed with a standard meal will demonstrate delayed gastric emptying of solids. • Normal patients should empty their stomachs by 8-10 hours. Abnormal gastric retention is associated with longer gastric emptying times.

Food-Marker Contrast Study
Barium impregnated small markers or other radio-opaque markers mixed with a standard meal will demonstrate delayed gastric emptying similar to the food barium contrast study.

Radionuclide Emission Imaging
Radionuclide markers mixed with a meal gives the most clinically accurate measurement of emptying. Gastric emptying half times (time for half a standard meal to leave the stomach) ranges from 2-4 hours.

OTHER DIAGNOSTIC PROCEDURES

Endoscopy
• Endoscopic findings are frequently normal in idiopathic conditions. • Food may be found in the stomach when it should be empty following fasting. • Endoscopy is useful for ruling out structural diseases of the stomach.

GROSS AND HISTOPATHOLOGIC FINDINGS
• Idiopathic conditions have normal gastric mucosa. • Histology may identify inflammatory or neoplastic causes.

TREATMENT

INPATIENT VERSUS OUTPATIENT
Most patients are treated as an outpatient. With severe vomiting or dehydration and electrolyte imbalance hospitalization and specific therapy is required.

ACTIVITY
Restrictions are based on specific concurrent disease.

DIET
• Dietary manipulation is important in the management of primary gastric motility disorders.
• Diets should be formulated that are liquid or of a semi-liquid consistency and low in fat and fiber content. Small volumes with frequent feedings should be given.
• Often dietary manipulation alone is successful in managing patients with delayed gastric emptying from a motility disorder.

CLIENT EDUCATION
Discuss possible underlying etiologies of altered gastric motility and that the response to therapy will vary with individual case.

SURGICAL CONSIDERATIONS
• Dogs with chronic GDV syndrome and

gastric retention should have a surgical gastropexy.
• Patients with gastric outflow obstructions also require surgical correction.

MEDICATIONS

DRUGS AND FLUIDS

Gastric Prokinetic Agents
• Metoclopramide (Reglan®) increases the amplitude of antral contractions, inhibits fundic receptive relaxation and coordinates duodenal and gastric motility. It also has antiemetic effects blocking the chemoreceptor trigger zone in the brain stem. Oral dosage is 0.2-0.4 mg/kg q6h-q8h given 30 minutes before meals.
• Cisapride (Propulsid®) works directly by cholinergic neurotransmission of gastrointestinal smooth muscle stimulating motility. Cisapride increases lower esophageal sphincter pressure, improves gastric emptying and promotes increased motility of both the small and large intestine. A suggested dose is 0.1 mg/kg PO q8h-q12h given before meals Cisapride is reported to be more effective than metoclopramide.
• Erythromycin given at low sub-microbiological doses has a motolin hormone-like effect promoting gastric emptying. Suggested dose of erythromycin for specific motility effects is 1-5 mg/kg PO q8h-q12h, given 30 minutes before meals.

CONTRAINDICATIONS
• Gastric prokenetic agents should not be administered in patients having a gastric outflow obstruction.

• Metoclopramide is contraindicated with concurrent phenothiazine and narcotic administration or in animals with epilepsy.

PRECAUTIONS
• Metoclopramide may cause nervousness, anxiety or depression.
• Cisapride may cause depression, vomiting, diarrhea or abdominal cramping
• Erythromycin may cause vomiting.

POSSIBLE INTERACTIONS N/A

ALTERNATE DRUGS N/A

FOLLOW-UP

PATIENT MONITORING
• Response to therapy varies with the underlying cause. • Failure to respond medically necessitates further investigation for mechanical obstruction.

PREVENTION/AVOIDANCE N/A

POSSIBLE COMPLICATIONS N/A

EXPECTED COURSE AND PROGNOSIS
The length of treatment depends on ability to resolve the underlying disorder or on the response to therapy.

MISCELLANEOUS

ASSOCIATED CONDITIONS
• Gasrtic hypomotility may be associated with both reflux esophagitis and reflux gastritis (bile reflux).

AGE RELATED FACTORS N/A

ZOONOTIC POTENTIAL N/A

PREGNANCY
Avoid gastric prokinetic agents in pregnant animals.

SYNONYMS
• Gastric hypomotility • Gastric atony

SEE ALSO
• Gastroesophageal Reflux • Gastric Dilatation and Volvulus • Gastritis, Chronic

ABBREVIATIONS
GDV= Gastric dilatation volvulus syndrome

References

Hall JA, Burrows CF, Twedt DC. Gastric motility in dogs. Part 1. Normal gastric function. Compendium Small Animal. 1988;10:1282-1291.

Hall JA, Twedt DC, Burrows CF. Gastric motility in dogs. Part 2. Disorders of gastric motility. Compendium Small Animal. 1990;12:1373-1390.

Twedt DC. Diseases of the stomach. The cat diseases and clinical management. 2nd ed. New York: Churchill Livingstone, 1994;1181-1210.

Willard MD. Diseases of the stomach. In: Ettinger SJ, Feldamn EC, eds. Textbook of veterinary internal medicine. 4th ed. Philadelphia: WB Saunders, 1995.

Author David C. Twedt
Consulting Editor Brent D. Jones

GASTRINOMA

BASICS

OVERVIEW
• Pancreatic islet cell tumor that secretes gastrin • Gastrin stimulates hydrochloric acid secretion, which causes erosive gastritis and duodenitis, gastric mucosal hyperplasia, and gastrointestinal ulceration. • Excessive acid environment in the intestine interferes with fat absorption, which causes steatorrhea.
• Named Zollinger-Ellison syndrome in humans • Rare condition reported in 12 dogs and 3 cats

SIGNALMENT
• Middle-aged to old dogs; mean 7.5 years, range 3.5-12 years • Female dogs affected more than males • Cats reported > 10 years old

SIGNS

Common Findings
• Vomiting • Weight loss • Depression • Anorexia • Intermittent diarrhea

Less Common Findings
• Hematemesis • Melena • Polydypsia • Abdominal pain • Hematochezia • Obstipation

CAUSES AND RISK FACTORS N/A

DIAGNOSIS

DIFFERENTIAL DIAGNOSIS
• Inflammatory bowel disease • Hypoadrenocorticism • Intussusception • Foreign body • Renal failure • Hepatic disease • Gastrointestinal histoplasmosis • Gastrointestinal lymphosarcoma • Heartworm disease—cats • Hyperthyroidism—cats

CBC/BIOCHEMISTRY/URINALYSIS
• Regenerative anemia • Hyperglycemia • Hypoalbuminemia • Hypocalcemia • Hypokalemia • Hypochloremia

OTHER LABORATORY TESTS
• High basal gastrin concentration • Excessive release of gastrin in response to secretin or calcium stimulation test—supports diagnosis of gastrinoma

IMAGING
Contrast radiography may indicate thickened gastric rugal folds, gastric ulcer, or duodenal ulcer.

OTHER DIAGNOSTIC PROCEDURES
• Endoscopy provides same but superior information as radiography • Measurement of basal stomach acid reveals high concentration • Definitive diagnosis made by laparotomy and finding of tumor in the pancreas that is histopathologically confirmed to be a non-beta cell tumor

TREATMENT
• Long-term prognosis poor because of high malignancy of tumor
• Treatment of choice is surgical excision of the tumor
• Large peptic ulcers should also be resected
• Regional lymph nodes and liver should be examined for metastasis, which occurs early and is found in 76% of reported cases

MEDICATIONS

DRUGS AND FLUIDS

To Reduce Gastric Acid Secretion
• H$_2$ blockers—cimetidine (Tagamet) 5-10 mg/kg PO q4h-q6h or ranitidine (Zantac) 2 mg/kg PO q8h-q12h • Omeprazole (Losec) 0.7 mg/kg PO q24h

To Treat Gastric Ulcer
Sucralfate (Carafate) 1 gm q8h for large dogs; 0.5 gm q8h for small dogs; 0.25-0.5 gm q8h-q12h for cats

CONTRAINDICATIONS/POSSIBLE INTERACTIONS

Omeprazole
• High dosage causes gastric carcinoid in rats • High dosage causes abnormally high number of fetal resorptions in rabbits • Causes rise in serum concentrations of diazepam and phenytoin

Cimetidine
• Causes increase in serum concentrations of diazepam, metronidazole, phenytoin, and propanolol • Metoclopramide reduces absorption of cimetidine

Sucralfate
Reduces absorption of digoxin, phenytoin, ketoconazole, quinidine, and quinolone antibiotics

 FOLLOW-UP

Monitor for biochemical abnormalities and anemia every 2-3 weeks.

 MISCELLANEOUS

SEE ALSO Gastric Erosions and Ulcers

Reference

Zerbe CA, Washabau RJ. Gastrointestinal endocrine disease. In: Ettinger SJ, Feldman EC, eds. Textbook of veterinary internal medicine. 4th ed. Philadelphia: WB Saunders, 1995:1593-1602.

Author Dudley L. McCaw
Consulting Editor Albert E. Jergens

GASTRITIS, ACUTE

BASICS

DEFINITION
Acute onset of disease characterized by vomiting of less than 7 days duration with no other signs or mild signs of systemic involvement.

Pathophysiology
The gastric mucosa is injured leading to an inflammatory cell infiltrate into the lamina propria and potentially superficial gastric erosions.

Systems Affected
• Gastrointestinal • Respiratory - Aspiration pneumonia may occur, especially if profuse vomiting and patient becomes debilitated.

Genetics N/A

Incidence/Prevalence
Relatively common

Geographic Distribution N/A

SIGNALMENT

Species Dogs and cats

Breed Predilections N/A

Mean Age And Range
Ingestion of foreign objects is more likely to occur in young animals

Predominant Sex N/A

SIGNS
• Vomiting is the primary sign; usually resolves in 24-48 hours if inciting cause removed. • Inappetence, depression, and pain on abdominal palpation occur less frequently. • Physical examination is usually unremarkable. • Retching or vomiting may occur on abdominal palpation. • Degree of dehydration varies with the duration and frequency of vomition. • Systemic signs may be present if acute gastritis is secondary to a more serious disorder.

CAUSES

Gastric Causes
• Dietary indiscretion: spoiled food, bacterial toxins • Foreign object ingestion
• Ingestion of plant material • Dietary intolerance or allergy • Ingestion of diet with high osmolality or fat in young animal • Ingestion of chemical irritants or toxins: fertilizers, herbicides, cleaning agents, heavy metals
• Drugs: NSAIDs (aspirin, flunixin meglumate, phenylbutazone, ibuprofen), glucocorticoids, antibiotics (tetracycline) • Infectious agents: viral (parvovirus), bacterial, parasitic (Physaloptera spp)

Nongastric Causes
• Renal failure • Hepatic disease • Shock
• Sepsis • Stress • Hypoadrenocorticism
• Neurologic disease

RISK FACTORS
• Intentional or unintentional ingestion of inappropriate foods or materials. • See gastric erosions and ulcers.

DIAGNOSIS

Patients with acute onset of vomiting, no systemic signs, and the potential for acute gastritis may be treated symptomatically without diagnostic testing. If the history or physical examination indicates a more serious disorder, clinical signs worsen, or do not resolve within 2-3 days, diagnostic testing is indicated.

DIFFERENTIAL DIAGNOSIS
• Determine if the patient is vomiting or regurgitating. An animal may be both vomiting and regurgitating. • Vomiting is usually accompanied by signs of nausea (increased salivation, swallowing, licking lips), retching, and abdominal contractions. • See gastric erosions and ulcers. • Parvovirus gastroenteritis: acute onset of vomiting may occur 1-2 days prior to the development of additional signs

CBC/BIOCHEMISTRY/URINALYSIS
• These tests are usually normal. • Stress leukogram may be present. • Hematocrit and total protein may be elevated if dehydrated.
• Hypokalemia may be present if prolonged anorexia or profuse vomiting has occurred.
• Hypoglycemia may occur in young animals or toy breeds if anorexic. • Hypoproteinemia may be present if severe gastric inflammation is present. • Acid-base disorders may be present if vomiting is profuse.

OTHER LABORATORY TESTS
Fecal parvovirus antigen test in young puppy.

IMAGING
• Abdominal radiographs usually unremarkable unless radiodense foreign object present.
• Abdominal ultrasound may detect gastric foreign bodies or thickening of the gastric wall. • Positive or negative contrast studies may detect gastric foreign bodies

OTHER DIAGNOSTIC PROCEDURES
• Endoscopy for retrieval of known or suspected gastric foreign bodies. • Gastric biopsy collection not indicated in acute gastritis.

TREATMENT

INPATIENT VERSUS OUTPATIENT
Usually outpatient unless severely dehydrated

ACTIVITY N/A

DIET
• NPO (nothing per os) if vomiting frequently
• Introduce water 12-24 hours after vomiting has stopped.
• If vomiting infrequently allow small amounts of water.
• Introduce food 24-36 hours after vomiting has stopped.
• Feed diet high in starch (such as rice) and low in protein and fat

• Protein source ideally should be vegetable or milk based
• After 3-4 days gradually switch over to diet normally fed

CLIENT EDUCATION
Many cases resolve with short term symptomatic support. If signs persist, a more extensive diagnostic evaluation and aggressive therapeutic course may be required.

SURGICAL CONSIDERATIONS
Endoscopy or surgery to remove foreign bodies

MEDICATIONS

DRUGS AND FLUIDS

Drugs
• Antiemetics: Generally not necessary. If profuse, frequent vomiting occurs administer a phenothiazine derivative (e.g., chlorpromazine)
• Antibiotics: Generally not indicated, see gastric erosions and ulcers
• Gastric protectants: Generally do not work and may increase vomiting by local irritation or gastric distention.
• Antacids: Severe gastritis may warrant the use of histamine H-2 receptor antagonists.

Fluids
• Balanced electrolyte fluids (Ringer's solution) for replacement of hydration deficit.
• Subcutaneous fluids usually adequate. Do not administer hypertonic solutions subcutaneously.
• Intravenous fluids are indicated if systemic signs or moderate to severe dehydration is present.
• Potassium chloride supplementation if prolonged anorexia, profuse vomiting, or hypokalemic

CONTRAINDICATIONS
• Avoid oral administration of medication.
• Do not give phenothiazine derivative antiemetics if hypovolemic or at risk for hypotension

PRECAUTIONS N/A

POSSIBLE INTERACTIONS N/A

ALTERNATE DRUGS N/A

FOLLOW-UP

PATIENT MONITORING
• If signs last greater than 5-7 days consider continued exposure to inciting cause, chronic gastritis, or systemic disease. • If clinical signs progress, consider more aggressive treatment and diagnostic plan

PREVENTION/AVOIDANCE
Avoid ingestion of gastric irritants (e.g., NSAIDs and corticosteroids) and opportunities for dietary indiscretion

POSSIBLE COMPLICATIONS
• Chronic gastritis if not resolved • Fluid, electrolyte and acid-base disorders

EXPECTED COURSE AND PROGNOSIS
Many cases resolve with supportive care

 MISCELLANEOUS

ASSOCIATED CONDITIONS N/A

AGE RELATED FACTORS
Young animals more likely to ingest foreign objects

ZOONOTIC POTENTIAL N/A

PREGNANCY N/A

SYNONYMS N/A

SEE ALSO
Gastric Erosions and Ulcers

ABBREVIATIONS
NSAIDs = nonsteroidal anti-inflammatory drugs

References

Johnson SE. Fluid therapy for gastrointestinal, pancreatic, and hepatic disease. In: DiBartola SP, ed. Fluid therapy in small animal practice. Philadelphia: WB Saunders, 1992.

Johnson SE, Sherding RE, Bright RM. Diseases of the stomach. In: Birchard SJ, Sherding RG, eds. Saunders manual of small animal practice. Philadelphia: WB Saunders, 1994.

Strombeck DR, Guilford WG. Acute gastritis. In: Strombeck DR, Guilford WG, eds. Small Animal Gastroenterology. Davis, CA: Stonegate, 1990.

Author Linda J. DeBowes
Consulting Editor: Brent D. Jones

GASTRITIS, ATROPHIC

 BASICS

OVERVIEW
A class of chronic gastritis characterized histologically by a focal or diffuse reduction in size and depth of gastric glands.

SIGNALMENT
Probably highly variable. Not reported in cats.

SIGNS
Vomiting (usually intermittent), anorexia, lethargy, pica, weight loss.

CAUSES AND RISK FACTORS
Unknown. May reflect chronic gastritis due to any cause. Immunization of dogs with their own gastric juice can induce chronic gastritis. Helicobacter sp. may be important in the development of canine and feline gastritis.

 DIAGNOSIS

DIFFERENTIAL DIAGNOSIS
Other forms of chronic gastritis and chronic enteritis

CBC/BIOCHEMISTRY/URINALYSIS
Generally unremarkable.

OTHER LABORATORY TESTS N/A

IMAGING N/A

OTHER DIAGNOSTIC PROCEDURES
Gastroscopy may reveal prominent mucosal blood vessels due to mucosal thinning. Histologic examination of gastric biopsies reveals glandular atrophy. Urease activity in gastric biopsies indicates infection with Helicobacter sp.

 TREATMENT

Prevent progression of gastritis.

MEDICATIONS

DRUGS AND FLUIDS

• Histamine type 2 receptor antagonists to inhibit gastric acid secretion (e.g. famotidine).
• Antibiotic treatment if infection with Helicobacter sp. is confirmed.
• Dietary elimination studies are warranted if underlying dietary sensitivity is suspected.
• If vomiting persists, prokinetic agents such as metoclopramide, cisapride or low dose erythromycin may be beneficial.
• Immunosuppression (azathioprine, chlorambucil) may be helpful in refractory cases.

CONTRAINDICATIONS/POSSIBLE INTERACTIONS N/A

FOLLOW-UP

• Long-term intermittent antacid therapy may be required. • With severe atrophy gastric acid secretion may be impaired. This will likely be a subclinical abnormality.

MISCELLANEOUS

ASSOCIATED CONDITIONS

Gastritis,chronic

Reference

Twedt DC. Vomiting. In: Anderson NV, ed. Veterinary gastroenterology. Philadelphia: Lea and Febiger, 1992:336–367.
Author David A. Williams
Consulting Editor Brent D. Jones

GASTRITIS, CHRONIC

BASICS

DEFINITION
Intermittent vomiting of greater than 1-2 weeks duration secondary to gastric inflammation. Gastric erosions and ulcers may be present depending on the inciting cause and duration.

Pathophysiology
Chronic irritation of the gastric mucosa results in an inflammatory response in the mucosal surface which may extend to involve submucosal layers. Chronic gastritis secondary to immune-mediated or allergic response may occur with chronic antigenic stimulation.

Systems Affected
• Gastrointestinal—esophagitis may result from chronic vomiting, and gastroesophageal reflux. • Pulmonary—aspiration pneumonia infrequently seen secondary to chronic vomiting, more likely to occur if animal debilitated.

Genetics N/A

Incidence/Prevalence
Relatively common

Geographic Distribution N/A

SIGNALMENT

Species
Dogs and cats

Breed Predilections
Older, small-breed, male dogs (i.e., Lhasa Apso, Shih Tzu, Miniature Poodle). Antral mucosal hyperplasia and hypertrophy more common in dogs with this signalment.

Mean Age and Range
Varies with underlying cause

Predominant Sex
Varies with underlying cause

SIGNS
• Vomiting: Vomitus is frequently bile stained and may contain undigested food, flecks of blood, or digested blood ("coffee-grounds"). Frequency varies from daily to intermittently (every few days to weekly) with increasing frequency as gastritis progresses. • May be stimulated by eating or drinking. • Weight loss • Inappetence or anorexia • Melena • Diarrhea

CAUSES
• See Acute Gastritis, Gastric Erosions and Ulcers • Chronic exposure to causes of acute gastritis • Parasites: Ollulanus tricuspis, Physaloptera sp.

RISK FACTORS
• Medications: NSAIDs, glucocorticoids • Environmental: unsupervised/outside free-roaming pets more likely to have dietary indiscretion, foreign object ingestion. • Ingestion of a dietary antigen to which they have acquired an allergy or intolerance.

DIAGNOSIS

DIFFERENTIAL DIAGNOSIS
• See Acute Gastritis • Chronic vomiting must be differentiated from chronic regurgitation. • Chronic gastritis: superficial gastritis, chronic gastritis with lymphocytic, plasmacytic inflammatory infiltrate, eosinophilic gastritis, granulomatous gastritis, atrophic gastritis will have characteristic features on histologic evaluation of a gastric biopsy specimen. Atrophic gastritis differs on endoscopic examination with visualization of the submucosal vessels secondary to thinning of the gastric mucosa.

CBC/BIOCHEMISTRY/URINALYSIS
• Hemogram usually unremarkable unless systemic disease present • Hemoconcentration if severe dehydration present • Eosinophilia seen with eosinophilic gastroenteritis. • Hypoproteinemia (albumin and globulin) if severe protein loosing gastropathy. • Urinalysis usually normal.

OTHER LABORATORY TESTS
• Fecal flotation may reveal intestinal parasites.

IMAGING
• Radiographs are indicated if suspect radiodense foreign objects. • Radiographs may suggest/reveal gastric outlet obstruction or thickened gastric wall. • Positive contrast radiography may detect outlet obstruction, delayed gastric emptying, or gastric defects. • Ultrasonography may detect gastric wall thickening and gastric foreign objects.

OTHER DIAGNOSTIC PROCEDURES
• Gastric biopsy and histopathology is required for diagnosis. • Gastroscopy is usually adequate for visualization of the gastric mucosa and biopsy collection and often foreign objects can be identified and removed with use of the endoscope. Gastric biopsy should be performed even when gastric mucosa appears normal. • Exploratory celiotomy is indicated if a submucosal lesion of the gastric wall is suspected and a full thickness biopsy is required.

TREATMENT

INPATIENT VERSUS OUTPATIENT
Inpatient if fluid therapy is required

ACTIVITY N/A

DIET
• NPO for 12-36 hours if vomiting frequently • See Acute Gastritis and Gastric Erosions and Ulcers • Rice and cottage cheese (or tofu) • Restrict protein, low fat • Frequent, small meals • Maintain long term on "non-allergenic" diet if response observed

CLIENT EDUCATION
There are numerous causes of gastritis. Diagnostic work-up may be extensive and often requires a biopsy for a definitive diagnosis.

SURGICAL CONSIDERATIONS
• Surgical management if granulomatous mass or gastric outflow obstruction • Remove foreign objects by endoscopy or surgery

MEDICATIONS

DRUGS AND FLUIDS
• Treat gastric erosions and ulcers if present (see Gastric Erosions and Ulcers) • Glucocorticoids to treat chronic gastritis secondary to suspected immune-mediated mechanisms if clinical response not achieved with dietary management. • Fluid therapy as needed for replacement, maintenance, and to replace ongoing fluid losses. • Maintenance potassium if anorexia present and serum potassium normal; supplemental potassium should be administered with fluids if hypokalemia present. • Antiemetics when fluid and electrolyte disorders are caused by frequent or profuse vomiting (see Gastritis, Acute). • Metoclopramide (to increase gastric emptying) may be indicated if delayed gastric emptying, or duodenogastric reflux is present.

CONTRAINDICATIONS
• Metoclopramide: do not use if gastric outlet obstruction is present. • Antacids not indicated with atrophic gastritis and achlorhydria. • Do not administer misoprostol to pregnant animals

PRECAUTIONS N/A

POSSIBLE INTERACTIONS N/A

ALTERNATE DRUGS
• Synthetic PGE (misoprostol) to enhance gastric mucosal healing • Immunosuppressive drugs (Azathioprine) added if immune-mediated mechanism suspected and inadequate response to dietary management and glucocorticoid administration.

FOLLOW-UP

PATIENT MONITORING
• Resolution of presently clinical signs • Eosinophilic gastritis, monitor peripheral eosinophil count, should decrease with resolution of gastritis. • Hypoproteinemia associated with protein loosing gastropathy should resolve with resolution of the gastritis. • Electrolytes and acid-base status • Complete blood counts to monitor WBCs if on immunosuppressive drugs (i.e., Azathioprine)

PREVENTION/AVOIDANCE
• Avoid medications (e.g., steroids, NSAIDs) and foods that cause gastric irriation or aller-

gic response in the patient. • Prevent free roaming and potential for dietary indiscretion.

POSSIBLE COMPLICATIONS
• Chronic vomiting if chronic gastritis uncontrolled • Progression of gastritis from superficial to atrophic gastritis • Gastric erosions and ulcers

EXPECTED COURSE AND PROGNOSIS
Varies with underlying cause

 MISCELLANEOUS

ASSOCIATED CONDITIONS N/A

AGE RELATED FACTORS
Young animals are more likely to ingest foreign objects.

ZOONOTIC POTENTIAL N/A

PREGNANCY
Do not administer misoprostol to pregnant animal

SYNONYMS N/A

SEE ALSO
• Gastritis, Lymphocytic-Plasmacytic • Gastritis, Eosinophilic • Gastritis, Atrophic • Gastritis, Acute • Gastric Erosions and Ulcers • Physaloptera

ABBREVIATIONS
• NSAIDs - non-steroidal antiinflammatory drugs • NPO - nothing per os

References
DeNova RC. Medical management of gastritis, ulcers, and erosions. In: Proceedings 17th Annual Waltham/OSU Symposium. Columbus, OH: 1993;108-116.
Johnson SE. Fluid therapy for gastrointestinal, pancreatic, and hepatic disease. In: DiBartola SP, ed. Fluid therapy in small animal practice. Philadelphia: WB Saunders, 1992;507-528.
Strombeck DR, Guilford WG. Chronic gastritis, gastric retention, gastric neoplasms, and gastric surgery. In: Small animal gastroenterology. Strombeck DR, Guilford WG, eds. Davis, CA: Stonegate Publishing Co., 1992.

Author Linda J. DeBowes
Consulting Editor Brent D. Jones

GASTRITIS, EOSINOPHILIC

BASICS

DEFINITION
An inflammatory disease of the stomach characterized by an infiltration of eosinophils, usually into the lamina propria.

Pathophysiology
Antigens bind to IgE on the surface of mast cells resulting in mast cell degranulation. Some of the products released are potent eosinophil chemotactants. Eosinophils likewise contain granules which contain substances which are directly damaging to the surrounding tissues. Eosinophils also can activate mast cells directly, setting up a vicious cycle of degranulation and tissue destruction.

Systems Affected
• Gastrointestinal - the stomach is seldom the only portion of the gastrointestinal tract affected • In the cat, hypereosinophilic syndrome can involve gastrointestinal tract, liver, spleen, kidney, adrenal glands and the heart

Genetics N/A

Incidence/Prevalence
Eosinophilic gastritis is reported to be more common in dogs than cats. It is less common than lymphocytic-plasmacytic gastritis.

Geographic Distribution N/A

SIGNALMENT

Species Dog and cat

Breed Predilections
German shepherd, Rottweiller, and Shar Pei may be predisposed

Mean Age and Range
• In dogs, most common in young animals less than five years of age, although any age may be affected. • In cats, a median age of 8 years with a range of 1.5–11 years has been reported.

Predominant Sex None reported

SIGNS

Historical Findings
• Intermittent vomiting, small bowel diarrhea, anorexia and weight loss are the most common owner complaints. • One report states that 50% of cats with eosinophilic gastritis/enteritis had hematochezia or melena.

Physical Examination Findings
• In cats, thickened bowel loops may be palpated.
• Evidence of weight loss may be noted.
• If hypereosinophilic syndrome is the cause of the gastrointestinal disease, enlarged peripheral lymph nodes, mesenteric lymphadenopathy, hepatomegaly and splenomegaly may be noted.

CAUSES
• Idiopathic eosinophilic gastritis • Parasitic: trichuris, visceral larval migrans, giardia
• Immune-mediated: food allergy, adverse drug reaction, associated with other forms of inflammatory bowel disease • Systemic mas-

tocytosis • Hypereosinophilic syndrome
• Eosinophilic granuloma

RISK FACTORS N/A

DIAGNOSIS

DIFFERENTIAL DIAGNOSIS
• All of the above listed causes are included in the differential diagnosis of eosinophilic gastric infiltrates. • Idiopathic eosinophilic gastritis is a diagnosis of exclusion. • Multiple fecal flotations and direct smears are imperative to rule in or out intestinal parasitism. • Intestinal biopsy will differentiate among the other causes of inflammatory bowel disease and eosinophilic gastritis. • A dietary trial will rule in or out food allergy or hypersensitivity.

CBC/BIOCHEMISTRY/URINALYSIS
• Hemogram may reveal a peripheral eosinophilia (a more common finding in cats than dogs). • Panhypoproteinemia, or hypoalbuminemia may be present if a protein losing enteropathy is also present. • Urinalysis is usually normal.

OTHER LABORATORY TESTS
A buffy coat smear is indicated to rule out systemic mastocytosis.

IMAGING
• Plain abdominal radiographs provide little information. • Barium contrast radiography may demonstrate thick intestinal walls and mucosal irregularities but do not provide any information regarding etiology or specifics regarding the nature of the thickening.
• Ultrasonography may be used to examine the liver, spleen and mesenteric lymph nodes in cats with hypereosinophilic syndrome.

OTHER DIAGNOSTIC PROCEDURES
• Definitive diagnosis requires endoscopic examination and biopsy. • Bone marrow aspirates are recommended if systemic mastocytosis is suspected. • Exploratory laparotomy may be indicated in cases where other portions of the gastrointestinal tract, unapproachable by endoscopy, are involved, and if abdominal organomegaly is present.

GROSS AND HISTOPATHOLOGIC FINDINGS
• Thickened rugal folds, erosions, ulcers and increased mucosal friability may be present in the stomach, although grossly the stomach can appear normal. • Histopathology reveals a diffuse infiltrate of eosinophils into the lamina propria, although the submucosa and muscularis can also be involved (reportedly more common in cats with this disease).

TREATMENT

INPATIENT VERSUS OUTPATIENT
Most can be successfully treated on an outpatient basis. Patients with systemic mastocyto-

sis, protein-losing enteropathies or other concurrent illnesses, may require hospitalization until they are stabilized.

ACTIVITY
No need to restrict activity unless severely debilitated

DIET
• Dietary manipulation is usually a critical component of therapy and may take several forms. In patients with severe intestinal involvement and protein losing enteropathy, total parenteral nutrition may be indicated until remission is obtained.
• Monomeric diets such as elemental diets, which have non-allergenic components can be used in patients who are not vomiting but have moderate to severe gastrointestinal inflammation, and are useful if a food allergy is suspected.
• Dietary therapy of highly digestible diets with limited nutrient sources (In the dog. Hill's prescription diets d/d and i/d, IAMS chunks and eukanuba, ANF, Hill's Science diets Maximum Stress and Canine Growth or homemade diets; in the cat, IAMS feline, Tender Vittles, Hill's prescription diet d/d) are extremely useful in getting the patients in remission and can be used once the patient is stabilized as maintenance diets.
• Once the patient is stabilized, an elimination diet trial may be instituted if food allergy or interolance in the suspected cause of the eosinophilic gastritis.

CLIENT EDUCATION
Owners need to be educated regarding the waxing/waning nature of the disease, and the necessity of life-long vigilance regarding inciting factors and the potential for long-term therapy.

SURGICAL CONSIDERATIONS N/A

MEDICATIONS

DRUGS AND FLUIDS
• Any balanced fluid such as Lactated Ringer's or Normosol-R is adequate for a patient with no other concurrent disease. Otherwise, fluids should be selected based on secondary diseases.
• Corticosteroids are the mainstay of treatment, with prednisone used most frequently (1-2 mg/kg PO q12h in dogs and 2-3mg/kg PO q12h in cats). Corticosteroids should be gradually tapered; relapses are more common in individuals who are taken off corticosteroids too quickly.
• Occasionally other immunosuppressive drugs can be used to allow a reduction in corticosteroid dose and avoid some of the adverse effects of steroid therapy. Azathioprine (1-1.5 mg/kg q24h PO in dogs and 0.3 mg/kg q48h in cats) is the most common adjunctive immunosuppressive therapy utilized.

CONTRAINDICATIONS NONE

PRECAUTIONS

Azathioprine rarely causes bone marrow suppression, usually more of a problem in cats than dogs. All individuals placed on azathioprine should have a complete blood count performed 10-14 days after the start of treatment, with rechecks monthly and then bimonthly thereafter. Usually the condition is reversible when the drug is discontinued. Pancreatitis, hepatic damage and anorexia are other potential side effects of this drug.

POSSIBLE INTERACTIONS N/A

ALTERNATE DRUGS N/A

 FOLLOW-UP

PATIENT MONITORING

• Initially, some more severely affected patients may require frequent monitoring; peripheral eosinophil counts can be helpful in monitoring therapy. The dose of corticosteroid therapy is usually adjusted during these visits. • Patients with less severe disease may be checked 2-5 weeks after their initial evaluation; and then monthly to bimonthly thereafter until prednisone therapy is completed. • Patients receiving azathioprine should be monitored as mentioned above. Patients usually do not require long term follow-up unless the problem recurs.

PREVENTION/AVOIDANCE

In cases where a food intolerance or allergy is suspected or documented, avoidance of that particular item, with strict adherence to dietary changes is required.

POSSIBLE COMPLICATIONS

• Weight loss, debilitation in refractory cases. • Unacceptable side effects of prednisone therapy. • Bone marrow suppression, pancreatitis, hepatitis or anorexia caused by azathioprine.

EXPECTED COURSE AND PROGNOSIS

• The vast majority of dogs with eosinophilic gastritis will respond to a combination of dietary manipulation and prednisone therapy. • Cats often have a more severe form of the disease, carrying a poorer prognosis than in dogs. Cats often require higher doses of prednisone for longer periods of time to bring them into remission.

 MISCELLANEOUS

ASSOCIATED CONDITIONS N/A

AGE RELATED FACTORS N/A

ZOONOTIC POTENTIAL

Only a consideration in cases of eosinophilic infiltrates secondary to parasites such an Ancylostoma, Giardia and Ascarids.

PREGNANCY

• Prednisone has been used safely in pregnant women, but corticosteroids have been associated with increased incidence of congenital defects, abortion and fetal death. • Azathioprine has been used safely in pregnant women, and may be a good substitute for corticosteroids in pregnant animals.

SYNONYMS N/A

SEE ALSO

• Enteritis, Eosinophilic • Gastritis, Lymphocytic-Plasmacytic • Enteritis, Lymphocytic-Plasmacytic • Inflammatory Bowel Disease • Mast Cell Tumors • Gastrointestinal Parasites

References

Strombeck DR, Guilford WG. Idiopathic inflammatory bowel diseases. In: Strombeck, DR, Guilford WG, eds. Small animal gastroenterology. 2nd Ed. Davis, CA: Stonegate, 1990.1

Tarris TR. Feline Inflammatory bowel disease. Vet Clin North Am, 1993;23:569-586.

Author Kelly J. Diehl

Consulting Editor Brent D. Jones

GASTRITIS, LYMPHOCYTIC-PLASMACYTIC

BASICS

DEFINITION
A form of inflammatory bowel disease characterized by a lymphocyte and/or plasma cell infiltration into the lamina propria of the stomach. Less commonly the infiltrates may extend into the submucosa and muscularis.

Pathophysiology
An abnormal immune response to environmental stimuli is most likely responsible for the initiation of gastrointestinal inflammation. Continued exposure to antigen, coupled with self-perpetuating inflammation result in disease. The exact mechanisms, antigens and patient factors involved in initiation and progression remain unknown.

Systems Affected
• Gastrointestinal - seldom is the stomach affected alone • Hemic/Lymphatic/Immune, Opthalmic, Skin/Exocrine - Other immune mediated diseases affecting the hematopoietic system (AIHA, coagulopathies), ocular (uvertia) and integument are frequently affected in humans with inflammatory bowel diseases. Animals may also develop these complications although to date they are not as well characterized.

Genetics
Basenjis and Ludenhunds have particular familial forms of inflammatory bowel disease (IBD).

Incidence/Prevalence
A common problem in both cats and dogs, representing most of the cases of inflammatory bowel disease.

Geographic Distribution N/A

SIGNALMENT

Species
Dogs and cats

Breed Predilections
Ludenhunds and basenjis have particular forms of IBD and wheat sensitive enteropathy affects Irish setters, German shepherds and shar peis have been reported to be predisposed to lymphocytic-plasmacytic gastroenteritis. There is no reported breed predilection in cats.

Mean Age And Range
Most common in middle-aged to older animals. Dogs as young as eight months and cats as young as five months of age with IBD have been reported.

Predominant Sex None reported

SIGNS

Historical Findings
• Signs associated with lymphocytic plasmacytic gastritis with or without enteritis can vary greatly between individuals in type, severity and frequency. Generally, the signs have an intermittent, chronic course but eventually increase in frequency over time. • Cats: Intermittent, chronic vomiting is the most common sign. Chronic small bowel diarrhea is the second most common sign of lymphocytic-plasmacytic gastroenteritis. • Dogs: Chronic small bowel diarrhea is the most common sign of lymphocytic-plasmacytic gastroenteritis. If only the stomach is involved, vomiting might be the most common sign. • Dogs and cats: Anorexia, sometimes alternating with periods of ravenous appetite, coupled with chronic weight loss is common. Hematochazia, hematemesis and melena are occasionally noted.

Physical Examination Findings
• Vary from a perfectly normal animal to a dehydrated, cachectic and depressed patient. • If only the stomach is involved, there may be no discernible abnormalities on physical examination.

CAUSES
Pathogenesis is most likely multi-factorial. Several causative factors have been identified.

Infectious Agents
Giardia, Salmonella, Camphylobacter, and normal resident gastrointestinal flora have been implicated but are not documented causes

Dietary Agents
Meat proteins, food additives, artificial coloring, preservatives, milk proteins, and gluten (wheat) have all been proposed as causative agents.

Genetic Factors
• Certain forms of IBD are more common in some breeds of dogs (see above). • Certain major histocompatibility genes, which are important components of normal immune responses, may render an individual susceptible to the development of IBD

RISK FACTORS See Causes

DIAGNOSIS

DIFFERENTIAL DIAGNOSIS
• Other infiltrative inflammatory bowel conditions (e.g. eosinophilic enteritis, granulomatous IBD) • Neoplastic conditions. • Infectious diseases like histoplasmosis, giardiasis, salmonellosis, Camphylobacter sp., and bacterial overgrowth. • Miscellaneous diseases like lymphagiectasia, gastrointestinal motility disorders, and exocrine pancreatic insufficiency. • In the cat, hyperthyroidism, FIP and FIV infection should be considered as well.

CBC/BIOCHEMISTRY/URINALYSIS
• Test results are often normal. • A mild non-regenerative anemia and mild leukocytosis without a left shift is sometimes seen in cats. • Neutrophilic leukocytosis with a left shift frequently seen in dogs. • Hypoproteinemia is more common in dogs than cats with IBD

OTHER LABORATORY TESTS
• Tests to eliminate other differentials (e.g. T_4 in cats, FIV/FeLV serology, fecal examinations) are recommended. • In dogs, tests to evaluate other differentials include serum trypsin-like immunoreactivity, fecal proteolytic activity using an azocasein substrate, microscopic examination of the feces and serum cobalamin and folate assays • Breath hydrogen test is useful in the diagnosis of bacterial overgrowth and malassimilation in dogs. • In cats, microscopic examination of the stool may be helpful. Most of the tests listed above have not been validated in the cat.

IMAGING
• Survey abdominal radiographs are usually normal. • Barium contrast studies occasionally reveal mucosal abnormalities and thickened bowel loops, but are generally not helpful in establishing a definitive diagnosis. They can be normal in individuals with even severe disease.

OTHER DIAGNOSTIC PROCEDURES
• A hypoallergenic diet trial may be initiated first in order to rule in/out dietary allergy or intolerance. Occasionally, certain forms of IBD will respond to dietary manipulations. However, if signs completely resolve, a diagnosis of dietary allergy or intolerance is likely, and no further work-up is necessary. • Gastric biopsy is the only way to confirm lymphocytic-plasmacytic gastritis and eliminate other infiltrative diseases. • Duodenal aspirates for Giardia sp., should be collected during endoscopy. • Intestinal fluid can be submitted for quantitative culture if bacterial overgrowth is suspected.

GROSS AND HISTOPATHOLOGIC FINDINGS
Grossly, stomach appearance can range from normal to adematous, thickened and ulcerated. The hallmark histopathologic finding is an infiltrate of lymphocytes and plasma cells in the lamina propria. The distribution may be patchy, so several biopsy specimens should be taken.

TREATMENT

INPATIENT VERSUS OUTPATIENT
Outpatient, unless the patient is debilitated from dehydration, hypoproteinemia, or cachexia.

ACTIVITY No restrictions

DIET
• Dietary therapy is an essential component of patient management.
• Patients with severe intestinal involvement and protein losing enteropathy may require total parenteral nutrition until in remission.
• Monomeric diets such as elemental diets, which have non-allergenic components, can be used in patients who are not vomiting but

have moderate to severe gastrointestinal inflammation and are useful if a food allergy is suspected.
• A highly digestible diet with limited nutrient sources (For dogs: Hill's prescription diets d/d and i/d, IAMS chunks and eukanuba, AMF, Hill's Science diets Maximum Stress and Canine Growth or homemade diets; For cats: IAMS feline, Tender Vittles, Hill's prescription diet c/d) is extremely useful in getting patients into remission and can be used once the patient is stabilized as a maintenance diet.
• Once the patient is stabilized, an elimination diet or food trial may be instituted if food allergy or intolerance is the suspected cause.

CLIENT EDUCATION
Inflammatory bowel disease is not necessarily cured as much as controlled. Relapses are common. Patience is required during the various food and medication trials that are often necessary.

SURGICAL CONSIDERATIONS
There are no surgical procedures available in veterinary patients for relief of IBD.

MEDICATIONS
DRUGS AND FLUIDS
• Any balanced fluid such as Lactated Ringer's or Normosol-R is adequate for a patient with no other concurrent disease. Otherwise, fluids should be selected based on secondary diseases.
• Corticosteroids are the mainstay of treatment for idiopathic lymphocytic-plasmacytic enteritis, with prednisone used most frequently (1–2mg/kg PO q12h in dogs and 2–3mg/kg PO q12h in cats). Cats may require a higher dose in order to control their disease. When signs resolve, gradually taper the corticosteroid dose. Relapses are more common in individuals who are taken off corticosteroids too quickly.
• Azathioprine (1–1.5 mg/kg q 24h PO in dogs and 0.3 mg/kg q 48h PO in cats) is an immunosuppressive drug that can be used to allow a reduction in corticosteroid dose and avoid some of the adverse effects of chronic steroid therapy.
• Metronidazole has antibacterial and antiprotozoal properties, and there is some evidence that it also has immune-modulating effects. The dose used for IBD in dogs and cats is 10 mg/kg PO q8h.

CONTRAINDICATIONS None

PRECAUTIONS
• Azathioprine rarely causes bone marrow suppression, usually more of a problem in cats than dogs. All individuals placed on aza-

thioprine should have a CBC performed 10–14 days after the start of treatment, with rechecks monthly and then bimonthly thereafter. Usually the condition is reversible when the drug is discontinued. Pancreatitis, hepatic damage and anorexia are other potential side effects of this drug.
• Metronidazole can cause reversible neurotoxicity and the drug is carcinogenic and mutagenic in laboratory animals. Discontinuing the drug usually reverses the neurologic signs.
• Cyclophosphamide side effects include bone marrow suppression in dogs and cats and hemorrhagic cystitis (especially in dogs). A CBC every two weeks is recommended, as side effects can occur months after initiating therapy. Cyclophosphamide is metabolized by the liver, so normal hepatic function should be established prior to use.
• Cyclosporin can cause gastrointestinal irritation, gingival hyperplasia and papillomatosis.

POSSIBLE INTERACTIONS
Cyclosporine can interfere with the metabolism of phenobarbital and phenytoin, and ketaconazole, erythromycin and cimetidine can decrease hepatic metabolism of cyclosporine. Any drugs which are potentially nephrotoxic should be used with caution in conjunction with cyclosporine.

ALTERNATE DRUGS
• Cyclophosphamide and cyclosporine can be used in place of azathioprine.
• Cyclophosphamide dose for cats and dogs is 50 mg/m^2 PO four times a week.
• Cyclosporine is currently undergoing evaluation for the treatment of inflammatory bowel disease in humans. It may be useful in the therapy of refractory cases of lymphocytic- plasmacytic gastroenteritis. A wide dose range, from 0.5 - 8.5 mg/kg PO q12h has been reported. Initiate therapy at a high dose and taper the dose as signs resolve. Cost prohibits routine use of this drug.

FOLLOW-UP
PATIENT MONITORING
• Monitor for resolution of clinical signs. Severely affected patients require frequent monitoring, with medications being adjusted during these visits. Patients with less severe disease may be checked 2–3 weeks after their initial evaluation; and then monthly to bimonthly until immunosuppressive therapy is discontinued. • Patients receiving azathioprine or cyclophosphamide should be monitored as mentioned above.

PREVENTION/AVOIDANCE
In cases where a food intolerance or allergy is suspected or documented, avoidance of that

particular item, with strict adherence to dietary changes is required.

POSSIBLE COMPLICATIONS
• Weight loss, debilitation in refractory cases.
• Unacceptable side effects of prednisone therapy. • Bone marrow suppression, pancreatitis, hepatitis or anorexia caused by azathioprine. • One author reports 4 cases of cats that developed gastrointestinal lymphosarcoma subsequent to their inflammatory bowel disease.

EXPECTED COURSE AND PROGNOSIS
Dogs and cats with mild inflammation have a good to excellent prognosis for full recovery. Patients with severe infiltrates, particularly if other portions of the GI tract are involved, carry a more guarded prognosis. Often the initial response to therapy sets the tone for a given individual's ability to recover.

MISCELLANEOUS
ASSOCIATED CONDITIONS N/A
AGE RELATED FACTORS N/A
ZOONOTIC POTENTIAL N/A
PREGNANCY
• Corticosteroids have been associated with increased incidence of congenital defects, abortion and fetal death. • Azathioprine has been used safely in pregnant women, and may be a good substitute for corticosteroids in pregnant animals. • Metronidazole is mutagenic in laboratory animals. Avoid during pregnancy.

SYNONYMS N/A

SEE ALSO
• Gastritis, Eosinophilic • Enteritis, Eosinophilic • Enteritis, Lymphocytic-Plasmacytic • Inflammatory Bowel Disease

References
Strombeck DR, Gullford WG. Idiopathic inflammatory bowel diseases. In: Strombeck DR, Gullford WG eds. Small animal gastroenterology, 2nd ed. Davis, CA: Stonegate, 1990.
Author Kelly J. Diehl
Section Editor Brent D. Jones

GASTROENTERITIS, HEMORRHAGIC—DOGS

BASICS

DEFINITION

A peracute hemorrhagic enteritis of dogs which is characterized by a sudden onset of severe bloody diarrhea which is often explosive, vomiting and hypovolemia with dramatic losses of water and electrolytes into the intestinal lumen.

Pathophysiology

Many conditions result in hemorrhagic diarrhea but the hemorrhagic gastroenteritis (HGE) syndrome of dogs appears to have unique clinical features that distinguish it as an entity separate from other causes. HGE is characterized as a peracute loss of intestinal mucosal integrity with the rapid movement of blood, fluid and electrolytes into the gut lumen. Dehydration and hypovolemic shock occur quickly. Translocation of bacteria or toxins through the damaged intestinal mucosa may result in septic or endotoxic shock.

Systems Affected

• Gastrointestinal • Cardiovascular

Genetics

Unknown, however there appears to be specific breeds represented.

Incidence and Prevalence

Common clinical condition.

Geographical Distribution   N/A

SIGNALMENT

Species   Dogs

Breed Predilections

• All breeds can be affected but the incidence is greater in small breed dogs. • Breeds most represented include miniature Schnauzers, Dachshund, Yorkshire terriers and miniature poodles.

Mean Age and Range

• Usually occurs in adult dogs with a mean age of 5 years.

Predominant Sex   N/A

SIGNS

General Comments

• Clinical findings are variable in both the course and severity of the disease. • The disease is usually peracute and associated with concurrent hypovolemic shock. • Most animals affected have been healthy with no historical environmental changes.

Historical Findings

• The signs usually begin with acute vomiting, anorexia and depression which is then followed with a bloody diarrhea. • Signs progress rapidly and become severe within a period of hours (usually 8-12 hrs.) and are the result of hypovolemic shock and hemoconcentration.

Physical Examination Findings

• The patient is generally depressed and weak and has prolonged capillary refill time and weak pulse pressure. • Skin turgor as a reflection of dehydration is normal due to the peracute nature of the disease and lag time in fluid compartmental shifts. • Abdominal palpation may be painful and fluid filled bowel detected. • Rectal examination will identify bloody diarrhea and later in the course of disease a "raspberry jam" characteristic stool develops. • Occasionally fever, but often the temperature is normal or even subnormal.

CAUSES

• The etiology is unknown. • Endotoxic or anaphylactic shock, immune mediated mechanisms directed against host enteric mucosa, or possibly infectious etiologies have been proposed. • Cultures of some dogs with HGE yield mostly pure cultures of Clostridium perfringens but the significance is unknown. • Searches for toxigenic E. coli strains have been unrewarding.

RISK FACTORS

• Unknown • Most dogs are previously healthy with no major concurrent illness.

DIAGNOSIS

DIFFERENTIAL DIAGNOSIS

• Parvovirus • Bacterial enteritis such as salmonellosis • Conditions resulting in endotoxic or hypovolemic shock • Intestinal obstruction or intussusception • Hypoadrenocorticism • Pancreatitis • Coagulopathy

CBC/BIOCHEMISTRY/URINALYSIS

• Hemoconcentration with PCV generally greater than 60% going sometimes as high as 75%. • Usually a stress leukogram. • Biochemistry profile may reveal secondary hepatic enzyme elevations and high BUN due to prerenal causes.

OTHER LABORATORY TESTS

Fecal Tests

•The stool is negative for parasites • ELISA for parvovirus is negative. • Fecal cytology will show many RBCs, occasional WBCs and possibly Clostridium perfringens spores.
• Clostridium may be cultured in high concentration but cultures are negative for other enteric pathogens.

Coagulogram

Usually normal but occasionally secondary DIC is a complication.

IMAGING

• Abdominal radiographs show fluid and gas filled small and large intestine.

OTHER DIAGNOSTIC PROCEDURES

Electrocardiogram

Cardiac arrhythmias such as ventricular premature contractions and ventricular tachycardia may be noted.

Endoscopy

• Colonoscopic examination is not indicated or helpful in the diagnosis. • May show diffuse mucosal hemorrhage, ulceration and hyperemia.

GROSS AND HISTOPATHOLOGIC FINDINGS

Changes in the intestine include gross congestion and microscopic evidence of autolysis which is devoid of marked inflammation.

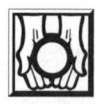

TREATMENT

INPATIENT VERSUS OUTPATIENT

Patients suspected of having HGE should be hospitalized and treated aggressively because clinical deterioration is often rapid and can be fatal.

ACTIVITY   Restricted

DIET

• NPO during acute disease.
• During recovery period a bland, low fat, low fiber diet should be fed for several days before returning to the normal diet.

CLIENT EDUCATION

• Discuss the need for immediate and aggressive medical management. With appropriate therapy mortality is usually low.
• Reoccurrence in about 10% of the cases.

SURGICAL CONSIDERATIONS   N/A

MEDICATIONS

DRUGS AND FLUIDS

• Rapid volume replacement is required in all cases.
• Balanced electrolyte solutions are given up to the rate of 40-60 ml/kg/hour IV until the PCV is less than 50%. A moderate rate of maintenance fluids are given to maintain circulatory function and to correct any potassium or other electrolyte deficits during the recovery period.
• Parenteral antibiotics are given because of the potential for septicemia and possible implications of Clostridium perfringens. Ampicillin is recommended. Alternate choices include trimethoprim-sulfa or cephalosporins. Ampicillin in combination with gentamicin or a fluroroquinolone is suggested in cases with septicemia.
• Short-acting glucocorticoids are given to dogs in shock using dexamethasone sodium phosphate 0.5-1.0 mg/kg IV.
• Excessive blood loss may require a blood transfusion.

CONTRAINDICATIONS   N/A

PRECAUTIONS

Gentamicin should be used with great care and not given to patients with dehydration or renal compromise due to potential for nephrotoxicity.

POSSIBLE INTERACTIONS N/A

ALTERNATE DRUGS

• Oral antibiotics and intestinal protectants are of little benefit and generally not administered.

• Rectal administration of mucosal protectants are of questionable value.

• Antiemetics may be given to control severe vomiting. • Intestinal motility modifiers are not considered necessary or are not recommended.

FOLLOW-UP

PATIENT MONITORING

• Monitor the PCV and total solids frequently (at least every 4-6 hours). • Modify the fluid replacement based PCV, continued GI fluid losses and circulatory function. • With a failure of clinical improvement in 24-48 hours re-evaluate the patient as other causes of hemorrhagic diarrhea are probable.

PREVENTION/AVOIDANCE N/A

POSSIBLE COMPLICATIONS

• Occasionally DIC may develop. • Neurologic signs or even seizures secondary to the hemoconcentration may occur. • Cardiac arrhythmias occur from suspected myocardial reperfusion injury.

EXPECTED COURSE AND PROGNOSIS

• The course if the disease is generally short lasting from 24-72 hours. • The prognosis is good and most patients recover with no complications. • Sudden death is uncommon but reported.

MISCELLANEOUS

ASSOCIATED CONDITIONS N/A

AGE RELATED FACTORS N/A

ZOONOTIC POTENTIAL Unknown.

PREGNANCY N/A

SYNONYMS

Acute hemorrhagic enterocolitis

SEE ALSO

• Diarrhea, Acute • Vomiting, Acute

ABBREVIATIONS

ELISA = enzyme-linked immunosorbent assay

HGE = hemorrhagic gastroenteritis

NPO = nothing per os

PCV = packed cell volume

DIC = Disseminated intravascular coagulation

RBC = red blood cells

WBC = white blood cells

References

Burrows CF. Canine hemorrhagic gastroenteritis. JAAHA. 1977 13:451-458.

Spielman BL, Garvey MS. Hemorrhagic gastroenteritis in dogs. JAAHA. 1993;29:341-344.

Strombeck DR, Guilford WG. Small animal gastroenterology. 2nd ed. Davis CA: Stonegate, 1990:338-343.

Author David C. Twedt

Consulting Editor Brent Jones

GASTROESOPHAGEAL REFLUX

BASICS

OVERVIEW
Defined as reflux of gastric or intestinal juice into the esophageal lumen. The incidence is unknown but it is probably more common than clinically recognized. Transient relaxation of the gastroesophageal sphincter or chronic vomiting may permit reflux of gastrointestinal juices into the esophageal lumen. Gastric acid, pepsin, trypsin, bile salts, and bicarbonate are all injurious to the esophageal mucosa. Esophagitis resulting from reflux may vary from mild inflammation of the superficial mucosa to severe ulceration involving the submucosa and muscularis.

SIGNALMENT
• Dogs and cats, male or female. • No breed predilections have been reported. • Reflux occurs at any age, however younger animals may be at increased risk because of developmental immaturity of the gastroesophageal sphincter. • Young animals with congenital hiatal hernia may also be at increased risk.

SIGNS

Historical Findings
• Regurgitation • Salivation • Dysphagia • Howling/crying during swallowing (odynophagia) • Anorexia

Physical Examination Findings
• Often non-remarkable • Fever and ptyalism if severe ulcerative esophagitis is present.

CAUSES AND RISK FACTORS
• Anesthesia • Failure to fast an animal prior to anesthesia • Poor patient positioning during anesthesia • Hiatal hernia • Chronic vomiting • Young age

DIAGNOSIS

DIFFERENTIAL DIAGNOSIS
Esophageal foreign body

CBC/BIOCHEMISTRY/URINALYSIS
Usually normal

OTHER LABORATORY TESTS N/A

IMAGING
Survey thoracic radiographs are usually non-remarkable. Barium contrast radiography reveals gastroesophageal reflux in some, but not all, animals.

OTHER DIAGNOSTIC PROCEDURES
Endoscopy and biopsy are probably the best means of documenting mucosal changes consistent with reflux esophagitis. Affected animals may have an irregular mucosal surface with hyperemia or active bleeding in the distal esophagus. Esophageal manometry and pHmetry may prove useful in documenting this disorder in veterinary referral centers.

TREATMENT
• Animals with reflux esophagitis are generally managed on an outpatient basis. It is not necessary to restrict activity. Food may be withheld for 1–2 days in cases of moderate to severe gastroesophageal reflux.
• Thereafter, low-fat, low-protein meals should be fed in small, frequent feedings. Fat in the diet will decrease gastroesophageal sphincter pressure and delay gastric emptying, while protein will stimulate gastric acid secretion.

MEDICATIONS

DRUGS AND FLUIDS
Specific therapy for gastroesophageal reflux may include:
Oral sucralfate suspensions (0.5–1.0 grams PO q8h)
Gastric acid anti-secretory agents (cimetidine 5–10 mg/kg PO q8h; ranitidine 0.5–1.0 mg/kg PO q12h; omeprazole 0.7 mg/kg PO q24h)
Pro-kinetic agents (cisapride 0.1–0.5 mg/kg q12h; metoclopramide 0.25–0.5 mg/kg PO q8h).

CONTRAINDICATIONS/POSSIBLE INTERACTIONS
Sucralfate suspensions may interfere with the absorption of other drugs, e.g. cimetidine, ranitidine, omeprazole, cisapride, metoclopramide.

FOLLOW-UP
• Animals affected with gastroesophageal reflux do not necessarily require follow-up endoscopy. It may be appropriate in many animal patients to simply follow clinical signs. However, endoscopy should be considered in animals that do not respond to medical therapies. • Owners should avoid feeding high fat foods as this might exacerbate gastroesophageal reflux. • The most important complications of gastroesophageal reflux are esophagitis and stricture formation.

MISCELLANEOUS

ASSOCIATED CONDITIONS
Hiatal hernia.

Reference
Evander A, et al. Composition of the reflux material determines the degree of reflux esophagitis in the dog. Gastroenterol 1987;93:280–286.
Author Robert J. Washabau
Consulting Editor Brent D. Jones

BASICS

OVERVIEW

Enteric infection of dogs with Giardia canis, a protozoan parasite; occasionally cats. Waterborne transmission of cysts. Motile (flagellated) organisms attach to surface of enterocytes in small intestine, especially duodenum through jejunum. Malabsorption syndrome with soft voluminous stools. Importance as a reservoir for human infections not known.

SIGNALMENT

Dogs (10% well-treated dogs, up to 50% pups, up to 100% kennels) and occasionally cats (up to 11%).

SIGNS

• Signs may be acute, intermittent or chronic • Soft, sometimes frothy diarrhea; rancid smell • Persistence may lead to chronic debilitation • Debilitated patient

CAUSES AND RISK FACTORS

Giardia canis transmitted by cyst usually in water supplies

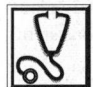

DIAGNOSIS

DIFFERENTIAL DIAGNOSIS

Other causes of maldigestion and malabsorption (e.g., pancreatic exocrine insufficiency, inflammatory bowel disease)

CBC/BIOCHEMISTRY/URINALYSIS

Usually normal

OTHER LABORATORY TESTS

• Motile organisms, tear-drop shaped, 15 x 8 µm; "falling leaf" appearance in fresh fecal drop • Cysts seen as crescent shapes with fecal flotation; 12 x 7 µm • Zinc sulfate flotation best • Fecal ELISA not superior to zinc sulfate flotation

IMAGING N/A

OTHER DIAGNOSTIC PROCEDURES

Duodenal aspirates obtained via endoscopy

TREATMENT

Treat as outpatients unless debilitated

MEDICATIONS

DRUGS AND FLUIDS

Albendazole (Valbazen) 25 mg/kg PO q12h for 2 days 90% effective; 50 times more effective than metronidazole; second 5 day course may be necessary
• Fenbendazole (Panacur) 50 mg/kg PO q24h for 3 days is effective; second 5 day course may be necessary
• Metronidazole (Flagyl) 25 mg/kg PO q12h for 5 days in dogs; 12–25 mg/kg PO q12h for 5 days in cats
• Quinacrine hydrochloride 6.6 mg/kg PO q12h for 5 days
• Fluid therapy if dehydrated

CONTRAINDICATIONS/POSSIBLE INTERACTIONS

• Metronidazole only 67% effective in dogs; bitter taste; anorexia; vomiting • Quinacrine HCl may cause lethargy, fever; not to be used in pregnant dogs, cats

FOLLOW-UP

• Serial fecal examinations to confirm efficacy of treatment. • May lead to chronic debilitation

MISCELLANEOUS

ZOONOTIC POTENTIAL

Giardiasis is the most common intestinal parasite in humans residing in North America. Giardia spp. may not be highly host specific, but there is no conclusive evidence that cysts shed by dogs and cats are infective for humans

PREGNANCY

Don't use quinicrine in pregnant animals

Reference

Barr SC, Bowman DD. Giardiasis in dogs and cats. Compend Contin Educ Pract Vet 16(5):603–614

Author Robert M. Corwin
Consulting Editor Brent D. Jones

GLAUCOMA

BASICS

DEFINITION
High intraocular pressure (IOP) that causes characteristic degenerative changes in the optic nerve and retina with subsequent loss of vision. IOP > 25-30 mm Hg (dogs) or > 31 mm Hg (cats) as determined by applanation tonometry or Schiotz tonometry (using the 1955 Friedenwald human conversion chart that accompanies the instrument) supports glaucoma.

Pathophysiology
Glaucoma develops when the normal outflow of aqueous humor is impaired. Impairment may be caused by primary eye disease (i.e., narrow or closed filtration angles and goniodysgenesis that have a genetic predisposition) or it may be secondary to other eye disease (e.g., primary lens luxation, anterior uveitis, and hyphema).

Systems Affected   Ophthalmic

Genetics
In dogs, the anomalous configuration of the filtration angles that predispose the animal to developing glaucoma is thought to be inherited, but mode of inheritance is uncertain.

Incidence/Prevalence
Although more common in certain breeds of dog, the overall prevalence of glaucoma is approximately 0.5% of all canine hospital admissions to the veterinary teaching hospitals of the colleges of veterinary medicine of North America.

Geographic Distribution   N/A

SIGNALMENT

Species
• Dogs—primary and secondary glaucoma.
• Cats—primary glaucoma is rare in cats. Secondary glaucoma is seen in cats with long-standing uveitis or lens luxation.

Breed Predilections
• Breeds predisposed to goniodysgenesis include Arctic circle breeds (i.e., Norwegian elkhound, Siberian husky, malamute, akita, samoyed), Bouvier des Flanders, basset hound, chow chow, shar pei, and spaniel breeds (i.e., American and English cocker and English and Welsh springer). • Breeds predisposed to narrow filration angels include spaniel breeds, chow, shar pei, and toy breeds (e.g., poodle, maltese, and shi tzu). • Breeds predisposed to primary lens luxations with secondary glaucoma include terriers (i.e., Boston, cairn, manchester, dandie dinmont, Norfolk, Norwich, Scottish, sealyham, West Highland white, and fox).

Mean Age and Range
• Primary glaucoma in dogs can be seen at any age, but middle-aged dogs, 4-9 years old, are predominantly affected. • Glaucoma secondary to lens luxation usually occurs in younger dogs, 2-6 years old. • Cats with chronic uveitis and secondary glaucoma tend to be older (≥ 6 years).

Predominant Sex   N/A

SIGNS

Historical Findings
• In animals with acute angle closure glaucoma, most owners report signs of apparent pain (e.g., blepharospasm, tenderness about the head, and serous to seromucoid discharge). A cloudy or red eye may also be noticed. Unless glaucoma is bilateral, most owners do not notice vision loss. • Depending on the primary disease, animals with secondary glaucoma have differing histories. Animals with uveitis-induced glaucoma may have signs of pain (for many days), scleral injection, and corneal edema. Animals with anterior lens luxation with secondary glaucoma may have signs of acute pain, shleral injection, and corneal edema and, possibly, the lens may be visible in the anterior chamber (if the corneal edema is not severe). Animals with uveitis-induced glaucoma may have seemed in pain for many days, and eyes may be reddened or cloudy. Animals with anterior lens luxation and secondary glaucoma may have historical signs of pain and a cloudy, edematous cornea. • Cats with chronic uveitis and secondary glaucoma may show no signs of pain and, owner complaint of an enlarged, seemingly painless eye or a dilated pupil is common. • Unobservant owners may note globe enlargement as the first sign in dogs or cats.

Physical Examination Findings
Acute primary glaucoma
• High IOP • Blepharospasm • Enophthalmos • Episcleral injection • Grey cloudy discoloration of the cornea • Dilated pupil • Vision loss, detected by lack of menace or dazzle response and lack of a direct or consensual pupillary light reflex in the affected eye in some animals • If the optic nerve is seen, it may appear depressed or cupped
Chronic (end-stage) glaucoma
Affected animal may have the following signs:
• Globe enlargement (buphthalmos)
• Descemet's streaks • Subluxated lens with an aphakic crescent • Optic nerve head atrophy • Retinal necrosis detected by peripapillary tapetal hyperreflectivity
Uveitis-induced glaucoma
High IOP
Affected may have following clinical signs:
• Episcleral injection • Corneal edema
• Inflammatory debris in the anterior chamber • Miotic pupil • Posterior synechia
• Iris bombé

CAUSES
• Primary glaucoma: filtration angle anomalies • Secondary glaucoma: impediments to aqueus outflow (e.g., inflammatory cells or debris in animals with uveitis; the lens or attached vitreous in animals with lens luxation; RBC in animals with hyphema; neoplastic cells in animals with ocular tumors)

RISK FACTORS
• Anterior uveitis, lens luxation, hyphema, and intraocular neoplasia. • Topically applied mydriatics may precipitate acute glaucoma in predisposed animals.

DIAGNOSIS

DIFFERENTIAL DIAGNOSIS
• See red eye chapter. • Conjunctivitis may be painful and may be a cause of a reddened eye, but IOP is not high, the pupil is not dilated, and conjunctival hyperemia is a more diffuse, red discoloration versus the episcleral vessel engorgement of glaucoma. • Uveitis may be painful and cause a reddened eye, but, at least initially, IOP is subnormal or hypotensive, and uveitis is usually associated with a miotic pupil. • Tonometry usually permits other causes of a red eye to be differentiated from glaucoma.

CBC/BIOCHEMISTRY/URINALYSIS
• Typically normal in animals with primary glaucoma. • In animals with secondary glaucoma, laboratory abnormalities are consistent with the primary systemic disease (e.g., thrombocytopenia in animals with hyphema).

OTHER LABORATORY TESTS
Serologic testing for infectious disease may be useful in diagnosing the cause of uveitis in animals with glaucoma secondary to anterior uveitis.

IMAGING
• Radiography or ultrasonography may demonstrate lesions consistent with fungal or neoplastic dissemination to the eye. • In animals with secondary glaucoma, ocular ultrasound may facilitate evaluation of the eye if the ocular media are opaque.

OTHER DIAGNOSTIC PROCEDURES
• Tonometry is essential to the diagnosis of glaucoma. • An animal with acute glaucoma should be referred to a veterinary ophthalmologist for a detailed ocular examination of both eyes, inlcuding evaluation of the drainage angles (gonioscopy).

GROSS AND HISTOPATHOLOGIC
FINDINGS   N/A

TREATMENT

INPATIENT VERSUS OUTPATIENT
Dogs with acute glaucoma should be hospitalized.

ACTIVITY   N/A

DIET   N/A

CLIENT EDUCATION
• Primary glaucoma is a bilateral disease.

• 40% or more of the canine patients will be blind in the affected eye within the first year no matter what is done medically or surgically.

SURGICAL CONSIDERATION

• Most forms of glaucoma are best treated surgically.
• Less than 10% of the dogs with primary glaucoma that have medical treatment alone will have vision at the end of the first year.
• Surgery to enhance aqueous humor outflow (filtration devices) and surgery to reduce production of aqueous humor (i.e., Nd:YAG or diode laser surgery or cyclocryosurgery to cause ciliary body ablation) are equally effective in maintaining normal IOP and vision.
• Blind painful eyes should be enucleated, and evisceration and prosthesis or one of the cycloablative procedures should be performed.

MEDICATIONS

DRUGS AND FLUIDS

Multiple drugs should be used to lower IOP into the normal range as quickly as possible in an attempt to salvage vision.

Emergency medical treatment of acute primary glaucoma in dogs should include the following:

• A topically applied miotic (either 2% pilocarpine solution q6h-q12h or demecarium bromide 0.125% [Humorsol - Merck Sharp & Dohme, West Point, PA] q12h) to constrict the pupil and enhance aqueous outflow.
• A topically applied β-adrenergic antagonist to reduce production of aqueous humor (0.5% timolol maleate [Timoptic], q8h-q12h).
• An orally administered carbonic anhydrase inhibitor diuretic (either dichlorphenamide [Daranide], 2-4 mg/kg q12h or methazolamide [Neptazane], 2-3 mg/kg q12h) to reduce production of aqueous humor.
• A hyperosmotic agent to dehydrate the vitreous humor (mannitol, 1-2 g/kg IV over 20 minutes or glycerin 1-2 ml/kg PO).

Uveitis-Induced Glaucoma in Dogs

Treated like primary glaucoma, but miotic agents should not be used and topically applied corticosteroids should be used to reduce anterior uveitis.

Cats with Chronic Smouldering Uveitis

Topically applied corticosteroids, topical β-

blockers, and carbonic anhydrase inhibitor diuretics can be used to treat glaucoma.

CONTRAINDICATIONS

• Topically applied atropine should not be used to treat glaucoma.
• Miotic agents should not be used in animals with glaucoma secondary to anterior lens luxation or uveitis.
• Intravenous administration of mannitol crystals may have fatal consequences.

PRECAUTIONS

• Topically applied pilocarpine is irritating, may cause conjunctivitis and painful brow ache, and can worsen uveitis.
• Systemic absorption of topically applied β-adrenergic antagonists can cause bronchoconstriction and bradycardia in small dogs, cats, and animals with compromised cardiovascular-pulmonary function.
• Carbonic anhydrase inhibitor diuretics cause metabolic acidosis and electrolyte imbalances that may be seen clinically as panting or heavy breathing, weakness, disorientation, and behavioral change.
• Osmotic diuretics in animals with compromised cardiovascular or pulmonary disease may initiate acute pulmonary edema.
• Diabetic animals should not be given glycerin; it will cause hyperglycemia.

POSSIBLE INTERACTIONS

Demecarium bromide is a cholinesterase inhibitor, and its use in conjunction with organophosphate flea repellant products can cause organophosphate poisoning.

ALTERNATE DRUGS

Other diuretics (e.g., furosemide and thiazides) will not reduce IOP as do the carbonic anhydrase inhibitor diuretics and are worthless in the treatment of glaucoma.

FOLLOW-UP

PATIENT MONITORING

• After discharge to the owner's care, reevaluate daily to every other day for the first week to guard against return of the ocular hypertension. Only if IOP is maintained at a hypotensive level for many weeks should drug therapy *slowly* be backed off in its intensity.
• Monitor for aforementioned drug reactions.

PREVENTION/AVOIDANCE

• Primary glaucoma is a bilateral disease. The unaffected eye should be evaluated by a veterinary ophthalmologist to determine the risk of the eye that is developing glaucoma. Prophylactic treatment in the predisposed unaffected eye (e.g., demecarium bromide, 0.125% [Humorsol], 1 drop q24h at bedtime) may delay the onset of acute angle closure glaucoma.

POSSIBLE COMPLICATIONS

• Blindness, chronic ocular pain.

EXPECTED COURSE AND PROGNOSIS

• Glaucoma is a chronic disease requiring constant medical treatment, and it causes blindness in most animals treated medically alone. • Surgically treated animals have a better chance of remaining visual longer, but most surgically managed eyes will not be visual for more than 2 years after initial diagnosis (an exception is glaucoma secondary to lens luxation, which may carry a fair prognosis with successful removal of the luxated lens).

MISCELLANEOUS

ASSOCIATED CONDITIONS N/A

AGE RELATED FACTORS N/A

ZOONOTIC POTENTIAL N/A

PREGNANCY

All of the drugs used in the medical management of glaucoma could cause problems during pregnancy. Because primary glaucoma is inherited, affected animals should not be used for reproductive purposes.

SYNONYMS N/A

SEE ALSO

• Red eye • Anterior uveitis, dogs and cats

ABBREVIATIONS

IOP = intraocular pressure

Reference

Brooks DE. Glaucoma in the dog and cat. Vet Clin North Am Small Anim Pract 1990;20:775–798.

Author J. Phillip Pickett
Consulting Editor Paul E. Miller

GLOMERULONEPHRITIS

 BASICS

DEFINITION
Glomerulonephritis is associated with intra-glomerular immune complexes, even though inflammatory cells are not always present.

Pathophysiology
Soluble circulating antigen-antibody complexes may be deposited or trapped in the glomerulus. Alternatively, in situ formation of immune complexes can occur when circulating antibodies react with "planted" antigens in the glomerular capillary wall. Subsequently, several factors, including activation of the complement system, infiltration of neutrophils and macrophages, platelet aggregation, activation of the coagulation system, and fibrin deposition, contribute to glomerular damage. The glomerulus responds to these insults by cellular proliferation and thickening of the glomerular basement membrane. If the injury persists, hyalinization and sclerosis occur, which can lead to renal failure.

Systems Affected
• Renal/Urologic—initial proteinuria can progress to chronic renal failure.
• Cardiovascular—hypoalbuminemia and sodium retention (edema and ascites), hypercholesterolemia, hypertension, hypercoagulability, and thromboembolic disease.

Genetics
Familial glomerular disease has been reported in Bernese mountain dog, samoyed, doberman pinscher, cocker spaniel, rottweiler, greyhound, soft-coated wheaten terrier, and cats.

Incidence/Prevalence
In some studies, 90% of random-source dogs have histologic evidence of glomerulonephritis. Glomerulonephritis is thought to be a leading cause of chronic renal failure in dogs.

Geographic Distribution N/A

SIGNALMENT

Species
More common in dogs than cats

Breed Predilections
In addition to the breeds listed (see Genetics), golden retriever, miniature schnauzer, and long-haired dachshund appear to be over-represented.

Mean Age and Range
• Dog—6.5 to 7.0 years; range, 0.8 to 17 years
• Cats—mean age 4.0 years

Predominate Sex
• Dogs—none

SIGNS

General Comments
• Owner complaints vary and depend on the severity and duration of proteinuria. In many animals, abnormal proteinuria is discovered on routine urinalysis in an asymptomatic animal.
• Occasionally, signs associated with an underlying infectious, inflammatory, or neoplastic disease may be the reason owners seek veterinary care.

Historical and Physical Examination Findings
• Clinical signs associated with mild to moderate urinary protein loss are usually nonspecific and include weight loss and lethargy. If protein loss is severe (i.e., serum albumin concentration < 1.5 to 1.0 g/dl), edema or ascites often develop.
• If the glomerular disease causes loss of at least three-quarters of the nephrons, renal failure and resultant azotemia, polyuria-polydipsia, anorexia, nausea, and vomiting may develop.
• Acute dyspnea or severe panting in dogs with pulmonary thromboembolism (rare)
• Acute blindness in dogs with retinal hemorrhage or detachment (rare)

CAUSES
• True autoimmune or primary glomerulonephritis has not been documented in dogs or cats. Several infectious and inflammatory diseases have been associated with secondary glomerulonephritis (see following discussion). Many cases are idiopathic. The following diseases have been associated with glomerulonephritis.
• In dogs—infectious (e.g., infectious canine hepatitis, bacterial endocarditis, brucellosis, dirofilariasis, ehrlichiosis, leishmaniasis, pyometra, borelliosis, chronic bacterial infection, Rocky Mountain spotted fever, trypanosomiasis, and septicemia), neoplastic, inflammatory (e.g., pancreatitis, systemic lupus erythematosus, polyarthritis, and prostatitis), idiopathic, familial, endocrine (e.g., hyperadrenocorticism and diabetes mellitus, and long-term administration of high-dose corticosteroids).
• In cats—infectious (e.g., FeLV, FIP, and mycoplasmal polyarthritis), neoplastic, inflammatory (e.g., pancreatitis, systemic lupus erythematosus, other immune-mediated diseases, and chronic skin disease), idiopathic, familial, and possibly endocrine (i.e., diabetes mellitus)

RISK FACTORS
See diseases and conditions listed.

 DIAGNOSIS

DIFFERENTIAL DIAGNOSIS

Other Causes of Proteinuria
• Inflammation of the urinary tract (e.g., bacterial UTI, urolithiasis, and neoplasia) is the most common cause of proteinuria. Inflammation of the urinary tract is usually associated with an active urine sediment (i.e., increased numbers of RBC, WBC, epithelial cells, and bacteria/hpf). • Amyloidosis. Similar to GN, renal amyloidosis often causes severe proteinuria with an inactive urine sediment (hyaline casts may be present). Renal biopsy is the only accurate way to distinguish amyloidosis from GN.

Other Causes of Hypoalbuminemia
• Severe liver disease (e.g., hepatic cirrhosis)
• Protein-losing enteropathies (e.g., inflammatory bowel disease, lymphangiectasia)
• Protein-losing nephropathies (e.g., amyloidosis)

CBC/BIOCHEMISTRY/URINALYSIS
• Persistent, significant proteinuria with an inactive urine sediment (hyaline casts may be observed) is the hallmark laboratory abnormality associated with GN. • Hypoalbuminemia and hypercholesterolemia are common.

OTHER LABORATORY TESTS

Urine Protein/Creatinine Ration (UP/C)
• The UP/C is used to confirm and quantify abnormal proteinuria. • The magnitude of proteinuria roughly correlates with the severity of glomerular lesions, making the UP/C a useful parameter to assess response to therapy or progression of disease. • If the glomerular disease progresses and causes loss of three-quarters of the nephrons, the resultant decreased glomerular filtration usually results in decreased proteinuria.

Protein Electrophoresis
• Urine and serum protein electrophoresis may help identify the source of the proteinuria and establish a prognosis. • Proteinuria secondary to hematuria may have an electrophoretic pattern similar to that of the serum. • Early glomerular damage usually results principally in albuminuria; however, with progression of the glomerular disease, an increasing amount of globulin may be lost as well. • Marked decreases in serum albumin and increased concentrations of larger molecular weight proteins, such as IgM, in the serum are suggestive of severe glomerular proteinuria and the nephrotic syndrome.

IMAGING
• Glomerulonephritis does not cause specific changes detected by abdominal radiography or ultrasonography; however, these tests are useful in ruling out other concurrent conditions. • Ultrasonography can be used to guide percutaneous renal biopsies.

OTHER DIAGNOSTIC PROCEDURES

Renal Biopsy
• Indicated if clinically important and persistent proteinuria with an inactive urine sediment is identified. Establishes a diagnosis (e.g., glomerulonephritis versus amyloidosis) and aids in establishing prognosis. Consider only after less invasive tests (e.g., complete blood count, serum biochemistry profile, urinalysis, and quantitation of proteinuria) and assessment of blood clotting ability have been done.

• Contraindications include a solitary kidney, thrombocytopenia or other coagulopathy, and renal lesions associated with fluid accumulation (e.g., hydronephrosis and renal cyst and abscess). Should not be attempted by inexperienced clinician or in animals that are not adequately restrained.

GROSS AND HISTOPATHOLOGIC FINDINGS

• Glomerulonephritis is usually classified according to histologic findings. Glomerular basement membrane thickening is referred to as membranous glomerulonephritis, whereas increased cellularity is referred to as proliferative glomerulonephritis. A combination of membrane thickening and increased cellularity is referred to as membranoproliferative glomerulonephritis. Glomerular scarring associated with increases in mesangial matrix is referred to as glomerulosclerosis.
• Whenever possible, immunofluorescent or immunoperoxidase staining and electron microscopy should be employed to maximize the information gained from biopsy.
• Congo red stain should also be requested to detect small amyloid deposits, which appear green and birefringent when stained with Congo red and viewed under a polarized light source.

TREATMENT

INPATIENT VERSUS OUTPATIENT

Most can be treated as outpatients. Exceptions include severely azotemic or hypertensive patients and those with thromboembolic disease.

ACTIVITY

Restricted (possible thromboembolic disease)

DIET

Sodium reduced, high quality-low quantity protein diet indicated.

CLIENT EDUCATION

If the underlying cause can not be identified and corrected, glomerulonephritis often progresses to chronic renal failure.

SURGICAL CONSIDERATIONS N/A

MEDICATIONS

DRUGS AND FLUIDS

• The most specific and effective treatment is elimination of the source of antigenic stimulation. Often difficult to accomplish because the antigen source may not be identified or be impossible to eliminate (e.g., neoplasia).
• Immunosuppressive drugs are often used in dogs and cats with glomerulonephritis as a

second course of treatment. Corticosteroids, azathioprine, chlorambucil, cyclophosphamide, and cyclosporine have been used clinically or experimentally to prevent immunoglobulin production by B cells or to alter the function of T- helper or T- suppressor cells. No controlled clinical trials in veterinary medicine have demonstrated efficacy of these drugs in treating glomerulonephritis.
• Aspirin may reduce glomerular inflammation and the risk of thromboembolism. Low-dose aspirin (0.5 mg/kg q12h) has been reported to reduce platelet aggregation in dogs more effectively than 10 mg/kg once daily and may have less of an inhibitory effect on the production of beneficial prostaglandins.
• Enalapril (0.5 mg/kg q24h), an angiotensin converting enzyme inhibitor, has been recommended for its antihypertensive and antiproteinuric effects in dogs with glomerulonephritis. However, no controlled clinical trials have demonstrated efficacy.

CONTRAINDICATIONS

Corticosteroids should not be used in azotemic patients.

PRECAUTIONS

• Caution should be exercised with use of immunosuppressive drugs.
• Dosages of highly protein bound drugs (e.g., aspirin) may need to be adjusted as serum albumin concentrations change with treatment or progression of disease.
• Enalapril should be used with caution in azotemic patients.

POSSIBLE INTERACTIONS N/A

ALTERNATE DRUGS N/A

FOLLOW-UP

PATIENT MONITORING

Urine protein:creatinine ratio most important. Immunosuppressive therapy (by altering the ratio of antigen to antibody) may worsen proteinuria. If this happens, immunosuppressive therapy should by discontinued. Also, blood pressure, body weight, serum urea nitrogen, creatinine, albumin, and electrolyte concentrations. Ideally, recheck examinations should occur at 1, 3, 6, 9, and 12 months after initiation of treatment.

PREVENTION/AVOIDANCE

Affected animals of breeds with suspected familial glomerulonephritis should not be used for breeding.

POSSIBLE COMPLICATIONS

• Nephrotic syndrome
• Hypoalbuminemia and sodium retention leading to edema/ascites
• Hypercholesterolemia/hyperlipidemia

• Hypertension
• Hypercoagulability and thromboembolic disease
• Chronic renal insufficiency or failure

EXPECTED COURSE AND PROGNOSIS

• Long-term prognosis guarded
• Glomerulonephritis often progresses to chronic renal failure despite treatment.

MISCELLANEOUS

ASSOCIATED CONDITIONS

• Nephrotic syndrome
• Pulmonary thromboembolism
• Blindness secondary to retinal hemorrhage or retinal detachment (rare)

AGE- RELATED FACTORS N/A

ZOONOTIC POTENTIAL N/A

PREGNANCY

High risk in patients with severe hypoalbuminemia or hypertension

SYNONYMS

• Glomerular disease
• Glomerulopathy
• Protein-losing nephropathy

SEE ALSO

• Nephrotic Syndrome
• Amyloidosis
• Proteinuria

ABBREVIATIONS

FIP = feline infectious peritonitis
FeLV = feline leukemia virus
GN = glomerulonephritis
RBC = red blood cells
WBC = white blood cells

References

Biewnga WJ: Proteinuria in the dog: A clinicopathological study in 51 proteinuric dogs. Res Vet Sci 41:257-264, 1986.

Center SA, Smith CA, Wilkinson E, et al. Clinicopathologic, renal immunofluorescent, and light microscopic features of glomerulonephritis in the dog: 41 cases (1975-1985). J Am Vet Med Assoc 1987; 190:81-90.

Cook AK, Cowgill LD: Clinical and pathologic features of dogs with protein-losing glomerular disease (abstr). J Vet Int Med 7:126, 1993.

Grauer GF. Glomerulonephritis. Sem Vet Med Surg Small Anim 7:187-197, 1992.

Jaenke RS, Allen TA: Membranous nephropathy in the dog. Vet Pathol 23:718-733, 1986.

Author Gregory F. Grauer
Consulting Editors Larry G. Adams and Carl A. Osborne

GLUCAGONOMA

BASICS

OVERVIEW
• A rare neoplasia of neuroendocrine tissue that secretes an excess of glucagon • Develops in areas of pancreatic islet alpha cells but could potentially develop in other areas of neuroendocrine tissue (e.g., gastrointestinal tract) • Organ systems affected include skin/exocrine, gastrointestinal, and endocrine/metabolic (i.e., hyperglycemia)

SIGNALMENT
• Dogs • On the basis of 2 presumptive reports, no breed or sex predilections • Dogs affected were 9 and 11 years old.

SIGNS
• Erythematous, crusting, and ulcerative dermatitis that begins on the feet (i.e., pads, nails, and interdigital areas) and may involve perioral, genital, perianal, and periocular areas as well (i.e., pressure points). Lesions may become pruritic and painful. • Patients often have associated staphylococcal pyodermas. • Focal truncal areas of alopecia may develop. • Vomiting • Diarrhea • Anorexia • Weight loss • Depression

CAUSES AND RISK FACTORS
See Overview

DIAGNOSIS

DIFFERENTIAL DIAGNOSIS
• Hepatocutaneous syndrome—chronic liver disease causing erythematous, crusting, and ulcerative dermatitis. Rare but more common than glucagonoma. Differentiated from glucagonoma by evidence of liver disease on laboratory tests • Drug eruptions • Zinc-re-

sponsive dermatoses • Immune-mediated skin disease • Other differential diagnoses include metabolic, gastrointestinal, inflammatory, and neoplastic causes of generalized illness.

CBC/BIOCHEMISTRY/URINALYSIS
• Mild to moderate normocytic, normochromic, nonregenerative anemia • Biohemistry analysis normal or reveals hyperglycemia • Urinalysis normal

OTHER LABORATORY TESTS
• Plasma glucagon levels are high with glucagonomas but also increased in many cases of hepatocutaneous syndrome. • Bile acids probably normal in patients with glucagonoma (not assessed in the two reported cases) but abnormal in those with hepatocutaneous syndrome

IMAGING
Ultrasonography—normal or abdominal mass. Dogs with hepatocutaneous syndrome may have microhepatica, irregular liver margins, and hepatic hyperechogenicity.

OTHER DIAGNOSTIC PROCEDURES
Skin biopsy—histopathologic findings suggest either glucagonoma or hepatocutaneous syndrome.

TREATMENT
• Diet high in fiber and carbohydrates and low in simple sugars
• Exploratory laporotomy to identify and resect pancreatic or gastrointestinal tumor

MEDICATIONS

DRUGS AND FLUIDS
• Insulin to treat diabetes mellitus
• Somatostatin analogues—(Ocreotide®; 10-

20 mg q8h-q12h may prove useful
• Glucocorticoids may help control dermatitis (prednisone, 0.5 mg/kg)

CONTRAINDICATIONS/POSSIBLE INTERACTIONS
Glucocorticoids can cause insulin resistance and create a diabetic state or make control of preexisting diabetes difficult.

FOLLOW-UP
• Monitor clinical signs and blood glucose concentration (if the patient has diabetes mellitus)
• Prognosis is poor
• Patients with hepatocutaneous syndrome—mean survival time is 5.3 months from onset of skin disease and 1.6 months from the time of diagnosis

MISCELLANEOUS

SYNONYMS
• Superficial necrolytic erythema • Necrolytic migratory erythema • Diabetic dermatopathy

Reference
Miller WH. Necrolytic migratory erythema in dogs: a cutaneous marker for gastrointestinal disease. In: Kirk RW, Bonagura JD, eds. Current veterinary therapy XI. Philadelphia: WB Saunders, 1992;561-562.
Author Mitchell A. Crystal
Consulting Editor Rhett Nichols

GLUTEN ENTEROPATHY IN IRISH SETTERS

BASICS

OVERVIEW
A rare inherited disease in which there is a predisposition to develop a sensitivity to dietary gluten present in wheat and other grains.

SIGNALMENT
• Only reported in the Irish Setter breed in the United Kingdom. • Mode of inheritance not known. • Signs develop in young to middle-aged dogs.

SIGNS
• Poor weight gain or weight loss • Mild diarrhea

CAUSES AND RISK FACTORS
The enteropathy and clinical signs are exacerbated when gluten-containing diets are fed.

DIAGNOSIS

DIFFERENTIAL DIAGNOSIS
Other chronic small intestinal diseases

CBC/BIOCHEMISTRY/URINALYSIS
Generally unremarkable

OTHER LABORATORY TESTS
• Serum folate concentrations may be subnormal, reflecting malabsorption. • Serum trypsin-like immunoreactivity and cobalamin concentrations are usually normal.

IMAGING N/A

OTHER DIAGNOSTIC PROCEDURES
Histologic examination of jejunal biopsies from affected dogs reared on a wheat-containing diet reveals partial villus atrophy and accumulation of intraepithelial lymphocytes. Jejunal abnormalities improve following gluten withdrawal but recur with gluten challenge.

TREATMENT
Avoid diets containing gluten.

MEDICATIONS

DRUGS AND FLUIDS
Folate (1.0-5.0 mg PO q24h for 2–4 weeks if serum folate is markedly subnormal (<4 µg/L)

CONTRAINDICATIONS/POSSIBLE INTERACTIONS N/A

FOLLOW-UP

PATIENT MONITORING
Monitor clinical signs

POSSIBLE COMPLICATIONS None

MISCELLANEOUS

Reference

Hall EJ, Batt RM. Dietary modulation of gluten sensitivity in a naturally occurring enteropathy of Irish setter dogs. Gut 1992;33:198–205.

Author David A. Williams
Consulting Editor Brent D. Jones

HAIR FOLLICLE TUMORS

BASICS

OVERVIEW
Hair follicle tumors are differentiated into two main groups: trichoepitheliomas, which arise from keratinocytes in the outer root sheath of the hair follicle or from both the sheath and the hair matrix; and pilomatricomas, which arise from the hair matrix. Both types are generally benign; however, a few reports of malignant pilomatricomas have been published.

SIGNALMENT
• Age, usually > 5 years • No sex predisposition • Trichoepitheliomas are common in dogs, but rare in cats. Cocker spaniels and basset hounds may be predisposed. No breed predisposition in cats. • Pilomatricomas are uncommon in both dogs and cats. Kerry blue terriers and poodles may be predisposed. No breed predisposition known for cats.

SIGNS
• Usually a solitary mass • Trichoepitheliomas are common on the back and head (cats). • Pilomatricomas are common on the back, shoulders, flanks, and limbs. • Firm, round, elevated, well-circumscribed, hairless, or ulcerated dermoepithelial masses. Cut surface is gray (trichoepithelioma) or lobulated with white chalky areas (pilomatricoma).

CAUSES AND RISK FACTORS
Unknown

DIAGNOSIS

DIFFERENTIAL DIAGNOSIS
Histopathologic examination distinguishes from basal cell tumor and squamous cell carcinoma.

CBC/BIOCHEMISTRY/URINALYSIS
Results usually normal

OTHER LABORATORY TESTS N/A
IMAGING N/A
OTHER DIAGNOSTIC PROCEDURES
Tissue biopsy

GROSS AND HISTOPATHOLOGIC FINDINGS
• Trichoepitheliomas vary in degree of differentiation and site of origin (root sheath or hair matrix). Frequent characterizations include horn cysts, lack of desmosomes, and differentiation toward hair follicle-like structures and formation of hair. • Pilomatricomas are characterized by a variable proliferation of basophilic cells resembling hair matrix cells and fully keratinized, faintly eosinophilic cells with a central unstained nucleus (shadow cells). Calcification is common.

TREATMENT
Complete excision is curative.

MEDICATIONS

DRUGS AND FLUIDS N\A
CONTRAINDICATIONS/POSSIBLE INTERACTIONS N/A

FOLLOW-UP

PATIENT MONITORING
For local recurrence

EXPECTED COURSE AND PROGNOSIS
Usually excellent

MISCELLANEOUS

Reference
Muller GH, Kirk RW, Scott DW. Neoplastic diseases. In: Muller GH, Kirk RW, Scott DW, eds. Small animal dermatology. 4th ed. Philadelphia: WB Saunders, 1989:858-866.

Author Joanne C. Graham
Consulting Editor Wallace B. Morrison

BASICS

OVERVIEW
• Microfilaremia uncommon (< 20%) • Prevalence 10% of that in unprotected dogs
• Low-average worm burden

SIGNALMENT
• Males more susceptible • No age or breed predisposition

SIGNS

Historical Findings
• Coughing • Dyspnea • Vomiting • Pulmonary thromboembolism frequently results in acute respiratory failure and death. •
Vomiting and respiratory signs predominant in cats with chronic disease

Physical Examination Findings
• Usually normal • Louder than normal bronchovesicular sounds • Murmur or gallop rhythm should increase suspicion of primary cardiac disease

CAUSES AND RISK FACTORS
• Outdoor cats have higher risk • Feline leukemia virus infection not a predisposing factor

DIAGNOSIS

DIFFERENTIAL DIAGNOSIS
• Asthma • Cardiomyopathy • Chylothorax
• Aleurostrongylus abstrusus infection • Paragonimus kellicotti infection

CBC/BIOCHEMISTRY/URINALYSIS
• Mild nonregenerative anemia • Eosinophilia inconsistent • Basophilia should increase suspicion of heartworm • Hyperglobulinemia

OTHER LABORATORY TESTS
• Microfilaria concentration tests (Knott's test): low sensitivity, high specificity • ELISA tests that detect circulating adult heartworm antigen (HWAg) are the most specific. • Low worm burdens (< 5 worms) commonly result in false-negative tests. • Negative HWAg test does not rule out heartworm disease.
• Positive HWAg provides strong evidence of heartworm disease. • ELISA tests that detect antibodies (HWAb) to circulating adult heartworm antigen are more sensitive but less specific than the HWAg test.

IMAGING

Radiographic/Angiographic Findings
• Enlarged, blunted pulmonary arteries
• Patchy, perivascular pulmonary infiltrates
• Pleural effusion • Pulmonary arterial obstruction and linear filling defects

Echocardiographic Findings
• Dilated main pulmonary artery • Worms in heart or main pulmonary artery • Exclude primary cardiac disease

OTHER DIAGNOSTIC PROCEDURES
N/A

TREATMENT
• Asymptomatic cats should not receive adulticide because of the morbidity and mortality associated with the treatment.
• Symptomatic cats should be stabilized.
• Spontaneous "cure" are probably common.

MEDICATIONS

DRUGS AND FLUIDS

Initial Stabilization
• Supplemental oxygen
• Theophylline (sustained release; 25 mg/kg PO q24h in the evening)
• Prednisolone (1-2 mg/kg PO q24h 10-14 days, then gradual reduction)
• Cautious balanced fluid therapy if indicated

Adulticide/Thromboembolism
• Thiacetarsamide (2.2 mg/kg IV q12h for 2 days)

• 20-30% mortality should be expected from adulticide therapy and pulmonary thromboembolism.
• Supportive care for pulmonary thromboembolism the same as initial stabilization
• Pulmonary thromboembolism complications most severe 5-10 days after adulticide administration

Preventatives
• Ivermectin (24 mcg/kg PO every 30 days)
• Milbemycin oxime (0.5-0.1 mg/kg PO every 30 days)

CONTRAINDICATIONS/POSSIBLE INTERACTIONS
No documented benefit from aspirin administration

FOLLOW-UP
• Serial evaluation of clinical response, thoracic radiographs, and heartworm antigen tests most informative

MISCELLANEOUS

SEE ALSO
Pulmonary thromboembolism

ABBREVIATIONS
HWAg = circulating adult heartworm antigen
HWAb = circulating adult heartworm antibody

Reference
McCall, JW, Calvert, CA, Rawlings, CA. Heartworm infection in cats: a life-threatening disease. Vet Med 1994;639-647.
Author Matthew W. Miller
Consulting Editors Larry P. Tilley and Francis W. K. Smith, Jr.

HEARTWORM DISEASE—DOGS

BASICS

DEFINITION
Disease caused by infection with Dirofilaria immitis.

Pathophysiology
• Disease is directly related to the number of worms, duration of infection, and host response. Endothelial damage leads to myointimal proliferation. Lobar arterial enlargement, tortuosity, and obstruction cause impaired compliance, loss of collateral recruitment, pulmonary hypertension, and thrombosis. Pulmonary damage is exacerbated after the death of adult worms.

Systems Affected
• Cardiavascular because of high right ventricular afterload causing hypertrophy and, in some animals, congestive heart failure (CHF)
• Renal/urologic because of immune complex glomerulopathy • Pulmonary because of embolization, allergic pneumonitis, and lymphoid granulomatosis

Genetics None

Incidence/Prevalence
• Highly variable according to climate
• Virtually 100% in unprotected dogs living in highly endemic regions.

Geographic Distribution
• Most common in tropical and semitropical zones • Common along the Atlantic and Gulf coasts and Ohio and Mississippi River basins
• Gradually extending across the US • Numerous pockets of infection in otherwise low prevalence regions • Prevalence on the rise in parts of southern Canada.

SIGNALMENT

Species Dogs and cats

Breed Predilection
• Medium- to large-breed dogs that spend a lot of time outdoors • All unprotected dogs at risk in endemic regions.

Mean Age and Range
Infection can occur at any age, but most affected animals are 3-8 years old.

Predominant Sex None

SIGNS

Historial Findings
• Animals often asymptomatic or exhibit minimal signs such as coughing • Coughing and exercise intolerance associated with moderate pulmonary damage • Cachexia, excercise intolerance, syncope, and ascites (right-sided [R-] CHF) in severely affected dogs

Physical Examination Findings
• No abnormalities in animals with mild infection and some with moderately severe infection
• Labored breathing or crackles in dogs with severe pulmonary hypertension or pulmonary

thromboembolic complications • Tachycardia, ascites, and hepatomegaly indicate R-CHF. • Hemoptysis occasionally occurs and indicates severe pulmonary thromboembolic complications.

CAUSES Infection with D. immitis

RISK FACTORS
• Residence in endemic regions • Outside habitus • Lack of prophylaxis

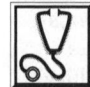

DIAGNOSIS

DIFFERENTIAL DIAGNOSIS
• Other causes of pulmonary hypertension and thrombosis such as hyperadrenocorticism
• Allergic lung disease • Other causes of ascites such as dilated cardiomyopathy • D. immitus microfilaria must be differentiated from D. reconditum.

CBC/BIOCHEMISTRY/URINALYSIS
• Anemia may be absent, mild, or moderate depending on chronicity and severity of disease and thromboembolic complications.
• Eosinophilia and basophilia vary • Hyperglobulinemia an inconsistent finding • Proteinuria common in animal with severe and chronic infection; may be caused by immune-complex glomerulonephitis or amyloidosis

OTHER LABORATORY TESTS
• Highly specific and sensitive serologic tests which identify adult D. immitis antigen are widely available. • Microfilaria identification tests include the modified Knott's test, filter tests, and direct smear.

IMAGING

Radiographic Findings
• Main pulmonary artery segment enlargement and lobar arterial enlargement and tortuosity vary from absent to severe. • Parenchymal lung infiltrates of variable severity surround lobar arteries and may extend into most or all of one or multiple lung lobes when thromboembolism occurs. • Diffuse, symmetrical, alveolar, and interstitial infiltrates occasionally occur as a manifestation of an allergic reaction to microfilaria.

Echocardiographic Findings
• Often unremarkable but may reflect right ventricular dilation and wall hypertrophy
• Parallel, linear echodensities produced by heartworms may be detected in the right ventricle, right atrium, and pulmonary arteries in dogs with high worm burdens or those with severe pulmonary hypertension.

Angiography
• Of little practical clinical importance.

OTHER DIAGNOSTIC PROCEDURES

Electrocardiographic Findings
• Usually normal • May reflect right ventricular hypertrophy in dogs with severe infection
• Heart rhythm disturbances occasionally seen (atrial fibrillation most common) in dogs with severe infection

GROSS AND HISTOPATHOLOGIC FINDINGS
• Large right heart • Pulmonary arterial myointimal proliferation • Pulmonary thromboembolism • Pulmonary hemorrhage
• Hepatomegaly and congestion in animals with severe disease

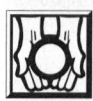

TREATMENT

INPATIENT VERSUS OUTPATIENT
• Most patients are hospitalized during adulticide administration.
• Dogs should be given microfilaricide in the morning and discharged in the evening.
• Hospitalization is recommended for dogs experiencing thromboembolic complications.

ACTIVITY
• Severe restriction of activity is required for 4 to 6 weeks after adulticide administration.
• Cage confinement is recommended for 1 to 3 weeks after adulticide administration of severe heartworm disease.
• Cage confinement for 3 to 7 days is recommended for dogs experiencing pulmonary thromboembolic complications.

DIET
Restricted sodium diet recommended for dogs with CHF

CLIENT EDUCATION
• Good prognosis for animals with mild to moderate infection
• Postadulticide pulmonary complications likely in animals with moderate to severe infection
•Reinfection can occur unless appropriate prophylaxis administered

SURGICAL CONSIDERATIONS
• Treatment of choice for animal with vena cava sydrome
• Worm removal from right heart and pulmonary artery via jugular vein by use of fluoroscopy and a long, flexible, alligator forceps is highly effective for treating high worm burden when employed by an experienced operator.

MEDICATIONS

DRUGS AND FLUIDS
• Stabilize animal with R-CHF by administration of diuretics, cage rest, and sodium restriction before adulticide treatment
• Stabilize pulmonary failure with antithrombotic agents (e.g., aspirin/heparin), anti-inflammatory dosage of corticosteroid, or bronchodilator, depending on the cause. Discontinue steroids 24 hours before adulticide administration.
• Melarsomine dihydrochloride is an adulticide drug that has the advantage of IM administration, less hepatotoxicity, and improved efficacy against both sexes of adult worms of all ages.

• Thiacetarsamide sodium, an adulticide; appropriate dosage—2 mg/kg (0.2 ml/kg) administered IV at intervals of 8-15 hours for a total of 4 doses. Feed before drug administration.
• Microfilaricide administration indicated for most dogs with circulating microfilariae, 4 to 6 weeks after adulticide. Ivermectin is administered in the morning at a dosage of 50 mcg/kg; the patient is observed for the day and discharged in the evening. Microfilaracidal dose of ivermectin not recommended in collies or shelties.

CONTRAINDICATIONS
• Icterus or hepatic failure
• Diethylcarbamazine in microfilaremic dogs

PRECAUTIONS
• Adulticide treatment is not indicated in patients with renal failure, hepatic failure, or nephrotic syndrome.
• Standard adulticide therapy in dogs with severe infection is associated with high mortality due to subsequent pulmonary thromboembolism.

POSSIBLE INTERACTIONS None

ALTERNATE DRUGS
• Heparin (75 units/kg SQ q8h) or aspirin (5-7 mg/kg PO q24h) is recommended for 1- to 3 weeks before, during, and for 3 weeks after adulticide administration in dogs with severe pulmonary arterial disease.
• Heparin (75 units/kg SQ q8h) is recommended in dogs with pulmonary thrombosis, thrombocytopenia, or hemoglobinuria.

FOLLOW-UP

PATIENT MONITORING
• A microfilaria concentration test should be performed, in appropriate patients, 3- to 4 weeks after ivermection administration. If positive, the ivermectin protocol is repeated immediately. Another microfilaria test is indicated 3 to 4 weeks later. If positive, adulticide failure should be suspected. • Heartworm prophylaxis is instituted when microfilaremia has been erradicated immediately in animal with occult infection.
• An antigen test is indicated 12 weeks after adulticide treatment. If positive, a decision must be made to either repeat the adulticide treatment or to delay for 6 to 12 months on the assumption that drug resistent, young fe-

male worms are present. • A weakly positive test result should be repeated in 1 to 3 months. • Some dogs with persistent adult infection may not require retreatment. This is determined by age, severity of infection, improvement since the first treatment, strength of the positive test result, and concomitant disease.

PREVENTION/AVOIDANCE
Heartworm prophylaxis should be provided for all dogs at risk:
• Ivermectin (Heartgard®) is a highly effective, monthly preventative that, when combined with pyrantel pamoate (Heartgard Plus®), also controls hookworm and roundworm infection. Can be given safely to microfilaremic dogs. • Milbemycine oxime (Interceptor®) is a highly effective, monthly prophylaxis that also controls hookworms, roundworms, and whipworms. The preventative dosage is microfilaricidal and acute reactions may occur when given to microfilaremic dogs. • Moxidectin is a comparatively new, monthly prophylactic drug that can be given to microfilaremic dogs. • All of the monthly prophylactic drugs can be administered safely to collies at the appropriate dosages. • Diethylcarbamazine is a safe and effective prophylactic drug which should be adminstered daily. It is marketed as tablets and chewable tablets, and, in combination with pyrantel pamoate (Filaribiti Plus®), it also controls roundworms and hookworms. Do not use in microfilaremic dogs.

POSSIBLE COMPLICATIONS
• Acute thiacetarsamide toxicity occurs in 10- to 20% of patients. • Acute, potentially lethal hepatotoxicity is uncommon. If persistent vomiting, anorexia, or icterus develops, stop the adulticide protocol, provide supportive care, and attempt adulticide treatment again 4 to 6 weeks later. • Postadulticide pulmonary thromboembolic complications may occur up to 4 to 6 weeks after treatment, and are usually most severe in dogs with severe heartworm infection and those not properly confined. • Thrombocytopenia, DIC • Skin slough with perivascular injections of thiacetarsamide. Immediately inject saline subcutaneously and apply DMSO topically at the site of perivascular injection. Melarsomine adverse effects: pulmonary thromboembolism (7-20 days after therapy). Anorexia (13% incidence), injection site reaction (myositis) 32% incidence, lethargy or depression (15%

incidence). Causes elevations of hepatic enzymes.

EXPECTED COURSE AND PROGNOSIS
• Usually uneventful with excellent prognosis in asymptomatic and mildly symptomatic animals • Guarded prognosis with higher risk of complications in dogs with severe infection

MISCELLANEOUS

ASSOCIATED CONDITIONS N/A

AGE RELATED FACTORS
"Older" dogs may not require treatment since heartworm infection may not be the life-limiting factor.

ZOONOTIC POTENTIAL N/A

PREGNANCY
• Adulticide treatment should be delayed in pregnant dogs. • Transplacental infection by microfilaria can occur.

SYNONYMS N/A

SEE ALSO
• CHF, right-sided • Disseminated intravascular coagulation • Hepatotoxins • Nephrotic syndrome • Pulmonary hypertension
• Pulmonary thromboembolism

ABBREVIATION
CHF = congestive heart failure

References
Rawlings CA, Calvert CA. Canine heartworm disease. In: Ettinger SJ, (ed). Textbook of canine and feline veterinary internal medicine. Philadelphia: WB Saunders, 1989.
Atkins CE. Heartworm disease. In: Allen DG, (ed). Small animal medicine. Philadelphia: WB Saunders, 1991.
Calvert CA. Heartworm disease. In: Birchard SJ, Sherding RG, eds. Manual of small animal practice. Philadelphia: WB Saunders, 1994.
Hribernik TN. Canine and feline heartworm disease. In: Kirk RW, ed. Current veterinary therapy X. Philadelphia: WB Saunders, 1989.

Authors Clarence A. Rawlings and Clay A. Calvert

Consulting Editors Larry P. Tilley and Francis W. K. Smith, Jr.

HEATSTROKE AND HYPERTHERMIA

BASICS

DEFINITION
• An excessively high body temperature (105-110° F, 41-43° C) that can be differentiated into fever and primary hyperthermia • Pyrogenic hyperthermia or fever—fully functional thermoregulatory mechanisms are present. Pyrogens act on hypothalamus via interleukin-1 and prostaglandins to raise the temperature set point to a higher level (e.g., septicemia). • Nonpyrogenic hyperthermia—normal heat dissipating mechanisms cannot compensate for excessive heat producing mechanisms or heat load, and the temperature rises above the hypothalamic temperature set point (e.g., animals with heatstroke, excessive exercise, seizures, tetanus, thyrotoxicosis, and malignant hyperthermia during anesthesia).

Pathophysiology
Severe hyperthermia may cause generalized cellular necrosis associated with heat denaturization of cellular proteins, enzymes, and cell membranes. The critical temperature for organ failure is 109° F.

Systems Affected
• Nervous—neuronal injury and cerebral edema • Cardiovascular—hemoconcentration, hypovolemia, and myocardial necrosis • Gastrointestinal—mucosal necrosis, bacterial translocation, and endotoxemia • Hepatobiliary—toxic thermal damage • Renal/urologic—tubular damage and acute renal failure • Hemic/lymph/immune—disseminated intravascular coagulation • Musculoskeletal—rhabdomyolysis

Genetics N/A

Incidence/Prevalence N/A

Geographic Distribution
More commonly observed in warmer climates

SIGNALMENT

Species Dogs and cats

Breed Predilection
• Breeds with a thick hair coat possibly more commonly affected • Brachycephalic breeds

Mean Age and Range
All ages can be affected

Predominant Sex None

SIGNS

Historical Findings
• Underlying cause for failure to dissipate heat (e.g., locked in a car, hot afternoon, and grooming accident) • History of laryngeal paralysis, upper respiratory disease, neurologic disease, or cardiovascular disease

Physical Examination Findings
• Panting • Hypersalivation • Hyperthermia • Dehydration • Congested mucous membranes • Tachycardia • Additional signs depend on the severity and duration of hyperthermia: • Tachyarrhythmias • Shock • Respiratory distress • Hemorrhagic vomiting and diarrhea • Petechiation • Melena • Oliguria or anuria • Seizures, stupor, and coma • Respiratory arrest

CAUSES
• Excessive environmental heat and humidity (e.g., dogs confined in cars and grooming accidents) • Exercise • Toxicosis (e.g., strychnine, organophosphates, chlorinated hydrocarbons, metaldehyde, and salicylates) • Anesthesia (i.e., malignant hyperthermia, an inherited muscle abnormality causing a rapid rise in intracellular calcium concentration with subsequent hyperthermia in response to certain inhalation anesthetics)

RISK FACTORS
• Previous episodes of heatstroke • Age extremes • Poor acclimatization to heat • Hyperthyroidism • Poor physical conditioning • Administration of drugs that compromise the patient's ability to dissipate heat (e.g., respiratory depressants) or raise the metabolic rate • Underlying cardiovascular, neurologic, or upper respiratory disease (e.g., laryngeal paralysis) • Brachycephalic breeds because of upper airway obstruction associated with confirmation • Salt or water depletion • Obesity • High heat and humidity; poor air circulation in environment • Thick hair coat

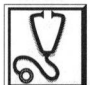

DIAGNOSIS

DIFFERENTIAL DIAGNOSIS
• Nonpyrogenic hyperthermia should be suspected when a dog is examined with a temperature exceeding 106° F and no obvious evidence of infection or neoplasia. • Panting and hypersalivation are usually not associated with fever and point to hyperthermia.

CBC/BIOCHEMISTRY/URINALYSIS
• CBC abnormalities may include a stress leukogram, thrombocytopenia, and hemoconcentration. • Biochemistry profile may reveal azotemia, high lactic dehydrogenase, high serum alkaline phosphatase, high activities of alanine and aspartate transaminate, hypernatremia, hyperchloremia, hyperglycemia, hypercalcemia, hypophosphatemia, and hypokalemia. • Urinalysis may show concentrated urine, proteinuria, cylindruria, and, occasionally, myoglobinuria.

OTHER LABORATORY TESTS
• Blood gas analysis may show a mixed acid/base disorder—respiratory alkalosis due to excessive panting and metabolic acidosis due to shock and excessive muscular activity. • Coagulation profile may show abnormalities pointing to the development of disseminated intravascular coagulation (i.e., prolonged prothrombin time [PT] and partial thromboplastin time [PTT], low fibrinogen, high fibrin degradation products [FDP], and thrombocytopenia).

IMAGING
Thoracic radiographs may identify underlying cardiovascular or respiratory disease.

OTHER DIAGNOSTIC PROCEDURES
Rectal temperature monitoring

GROSS AND HISTOPATHOLOGIC FINDINGS
Findings associated with major organ system failure

TREATMENT
• Immediate reversal of hyperthermia! The key to recovery is early recognition and treatment.
• Have the owner spray the dog with water and cool with electric fan before and during the transport to the clinic. In emergency room, continue cold water treatment, and apply alcohol on foot pads, axilla, and groin. Stop cooling when temperature has reached 103° F to avoid a precipitous drop in temperature. Ice baths are not recommended (shivering and vasoconstriction lessen heat loss).
• Stabilize vital signs—intubate comatose animals, give oxygen to cyanotic dogs, correct hypovolemia and acid/base imbalances, treat cerebral edema.
• Detect and treat possible complications (e.g., acute renal failure and disseminated intravascular coagulation).
• Remove predisposing factors.

INPATIENT VERSUS OUTPATIENT
Severe hyperthermia/heatstroke often poses an acute, life-threatening emergency situation. Most patients require intensive care for several days to weeks depending on how quickly the animal recovers.

ACTIVITY Restrict

DIET N/A

CLIENT EDUCATION
An episode of heatstroke will make the pet more susceptible to recurrence.

SURGICAL CONSIDERATIONS
Dogs with upper respiratory obstruction may require tracheostomy to facilitate breathing and heat loss.

MEDICATIONS

DRUGS AND FLUIDS
• Fluid and electrolyte replacement/shock therapy—0.45% saline with 2.5% dextrose at 50-80 ml/kg in the first hour, with additional fluids administered according to the animal's thermodynamic, metabolic, and circulatory status to maintain renal output
• Acute renal failure—dopamine infusion (2-4 mcg/kg/min IV) to increase renal blood

flow, furosemide (2 mg/kg q8h), closed urine collection system, and central venous pressure monitoring
• Cerebral edema (stupor/coma)— mannitol (0.5 g/kg over 20 min IV; do not use during initial resuscitation efforts!) and dexamethasone sodium phosphate (1-2 mg/kg IV) or prednisolone sodium succinate (10-20 mg/kg IV)
• Ventricular arrhythmias—lidocaine bolus (2 mg/kg IV) followed by infusion (25-75 mcg/kg/min IV) • Metabolic acidosis—bicarbonate (0.3 × BW{kg} × base deficit, give half as a bolus; alternatively, add 2-3 meq/kg to saline infusion)
• Disseminated intravascular coagulation—fresh frozen plasma (20 ml/kg) and heparin (50-75 U/kg SC q6h)
• Hemorrhagic diarrhea/bacterial translocation—broadspectrum antibiotics
• Seizures—diazepam (0.5 mg/kg IV) and/or phenobarbital (2 mg/kg) • Shivering or muscle rigidity—diazepam
• Anxiety, stress—oxymorphone(0.02-0.1 mg/kg IV)

CONTRAINDICATIONS

Antipyretic drugs (e.g., salicylates and flunixin meglumine) are contraindicated in animals with nonpyrogenous hyperthermia, because the temperature set point is normal and lowering it with antipyretics will not lessen hyperthermia.

PRECAUTIONS N/A

POSSIBLE INTERACTIONS

Refer to manufacturer's literature

ALTERNATE DRUGS N/A

FOLLOW-UP

PATIENT MONITORING

• Monitor temperature during cooling down, since hypothermia can develop rapidly.
• Blood pressure, central venous pressure, capillary refill time, and chest auscultation are valuable aids in detecting overhydration.
• Use a closed urine collection system to monitor urine output if renal failure is suspected. • Monitor ECG for cardiac arrhythmias. • Following the initial cool down, keep patient in a cool and well-ventilated room.
• Monitor PCV and total solids, and recheck serial blood gases, CBC, coagulation profile, serum biochemistry, and urinalysis daily to detect possible complications.

PREVENTION/AVOIDANCE

Avoid precipitating causes

POSSIBLE COMPLICATIONS

• Failure of any major organ system • Coma, seizures, and respiratory arrest secondary to cerebral edema • Acute renal failure • Disseminated intravascular coagulation • Pulmonary edema and acute respiratory distress syndrome • Cardiac arrhythmias • Rhabdomyolysis • Hepatocellular necrosis

EXPECTED COURSE AND PROGNOSIS

• The prognosis is guarded to grave, depending on the presence or absence of an underlying disease condition and the development of complications. Mortality seems to be proportional to the duration and intensity of hyperthermia and the time required to achieve a normal body temperature. • Recovering dogs may have residual neurologic deficits and nephrogenic diabetes insipidus. • Permanent damage to thermoregulatory centers is possible, predisposing to future hyperthermic episodes.

MISCELLANEOUS

ASSOCIATED CONDITIONS N/A

AGE RELATED FACTORS N/A

ZOONOTIC POTENTIAL N/A

PREGNANCY N/A

SYNONYMS
• Heatstroke • Heat prostration • Heat injury

SEE ALSO Fever

ABBREVIATION
PCV = packed cell volume

Reference

Ruslander D. Heat stroke. In: Kirk RW, Bonagura JD, eds. Current veterinary therapy. 11th ed. Philadelphia: WB Saunders, 1992:143-146.
Author Jörg Bücheler
Consulting Editors Larry P. Tilley and Francis W. K. Smith, Jr.

HELICOBACTER INFECTION

BASICS

OVERVIEW
• Helicobacteriosis is an infection of the stomach of dogs and cats. • The organism may be found in the gastric mucus, the antral mucus glands, or parietal cells.

SIGNALMENT
Dogs or cats of any breed. They are usually more than 1 year of age.

SIGNS
The predominant clinical sign is chronic vomiting.

CAUSES AND RISK FACTORS
• Helicobacter felis • Helicobacter heilmanni (formerly called Gastrospirillum spp.) • Helicobacter pylori

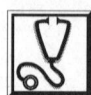

DIAGNOSIS

DIFFERENTIAL DIAGNOSIS
• Inflammatory bowel disease (IBD) • Gastric neoplasia • Obstructive pyloric disease

CBC/BIOCHEMISTRY/URINALYSIS
Usually normal

OTHER LABORATORY TESTS N/A

IMAGING N/A

OTHER DIAGNOSTIC PROCEDURES
• Gastric mucosal biopsy, generally performed via endoscopy, is the most practical diagnostic test. • Culturing or cytologic testing of gastric contents or vomitus may reveal organisms, but the diagnostic yield is much lower than by mucosal biopsies.

GROSS AND HISTOPATHOLOGIC FINDINGS
• H. heilmanni may be seen in large numbers in the gastric mucus or within the mucosal cells with H & E stain. • H. felis and H. pylori are best identified with a silver stain such as Warthan Starry. • Most cases are accompanied by an inflammatory gastritis. The most commonly found cells are lymphocytes and plasmacytes. Because this is a common finding in biopsies of cats with IBD, the two diseases can be confused.

TREATMENT N/A

MEDICATIONS

DRUGS AND FLUIDS
• Recommendations are based on treatments of similar organisms in humans. Because no drug regimen has shown 100% success in humans, a uniform approach has not been developed for veterinary patients at this time.
• Combinations of drugs are used that work in the gastric mucus and within the mucosal cells. If one is not successful, another should be tried.
• Metronidazole plus amoxicillin plus famotidine.
• Tetracycline plus metronidazole plus bismuth.
• Omeprazole plus metronidazole plus tetracycline or amoxicillin.
• Treatment should be for 14-21 days.

CONTRAINDICATIONS/POSSIBLE INTERACTIONS
Bismuth compounds contain salicylates. They can be toxic to cats if the dosage is excessive. The typical dosage is no more than 15 ml of the regular strength product per 10 pounds of body weight per day or 1 tablet per day.

FOLLOW-UP
• If clinical signs persist after treatment, consider the possibility that IBD may be concurrent. • Rebiopsy is recommended, but if that is not feasible, consider treating with corticosteroids.

MISCELLANEOUS

ABBREVIATIONS
IBD = inflammatory bowel disease

Reference

DeNovo RC, Magne ML. Current concepts in the management of helicobacter-associated gastritis. Proceedings, 13th Annu Meet Am Col Vet Int Med, Lake Buena Vista, FL, 1995:57-61.

Author Gary D. Norsworthy
Consulting Editor Fred W. Scott

HEMANGIOPERICYTOMA

BASICS

OVERVIEW
Hemangiopericytoma is a soft tissue sarcoma arising from pericytes, which are cells surrounding capillaries in subcutaneous tissue. Characteristics include:
• Locally invasive often extending far beyond visible margins • Metastasizes infrequently and does so late in the course of disease
• Local growth can interfere with limb function.

SIGNALMENT
• More common in large-breed than small-breed dogs • Rare in cats

SIGNS

Historical Findings
• Typically, slow-growing mass (weeks to months) • Rapid growth uncommon

Physical Examination Findings
• Soft tissue mass usually located on extremity • Less commonly found on trunk • Soft, fluctuant, or firm • Generally adhered to underlying tissue • Regional lymph node metastasis uncommon

CAUSES AND RISK FACTORS
Unknown

DIAGNOSIS

DIFFERENTIAL DIAGNOSIS
• Other soft tissue sarcomas (e.g., nerve sheath tumor and fibrosarcoma), lipoma, and other tumors, benign and malignant.

• Biopsy essential to confirm the diagnosis

CBC/BIOCHEMISTRY/URINALYSIS
N/A

OTHER LABORATORY TESTS N/A

IMAGING
Although metastasis is uncommon, thoracic radiographs appropriate before initiating treatment

OTHER DIAGNOSTIC PROCEDURES
Regional lymph node biopsy before treatment

TREATMENT
• Early, aggressive surgical excision is the treatment of choice.
• Microscopically, cancer cells extend far beyond gross tumor borders. Also, this tumor often has a pseudocapsule composed of cancer cells. If the tumor is "peeled out," a healthy bed of cancer cells is left behind. The tumor should be excised "en bloc." The entire sample should be submitted to a pathologist for surgical margin evaluation. Two edges of the tumor tissue should be marked with suture material to orient the pathologist if the tumor has not been clearly excised.
• In some patients, aggressive surgery means toe or limb amputation.
• Radiotherapy a good treatment option when complete surgical excision is not possible
• 1-5 year tumor control rates of 60-85% are reported with radiotherapy after surgical "debulking."

MEDICATIONS

DRUGS AND FLUIDS N/A

CONTRAINDICATIONS/POSSIBLE INTERACTIONS N/A

FOLLOW-UP
• If surgical excision is incomplete, a second surgery should be performed or radiotherapy should be started as soon as possible.
• Chemotherapy has not been consistently reported as beneficial.

EXPECTED COURSE AND PROGNOSIS
• Cure is possible when surgery is aggressive and surgical margins are tumor free. • Long-term tumor control can be achieved by radiotherapy after surgically "debulking" the tumor. Recurrence is inevitable if treatment is not aggressive.

MISCELLANEOUS

Reference
Postorino NC, et al. Prognostic variables for canine hemangiopericytoma: 50 cases (1979-1984). J Am Anim Hosp Assoc 1988;24:501-509.

Author Robyn Elmslie
Consulting Editor Wallace B. Morrison

HEMANGIOSARCOMA, BONE

BASICS

OVERVIEW
• Highly metastatic cancer • Most patients develop metastatic disease within 1 year of diagnosis and treatment. • Represents 2-3% of primary bone tumors • Axial skeleton affected slightly more than appendicular skeleton • Most common sites include the ribs and proximal humerus • When found in bone, it can be difficult to determine the primary site

SIGNALMENT
• Middle-aged dogs (mean age, 6.2 years) most common • Male to female ratio 1.6:1 • No size predilection as with other primary bone tumors • Great Dane, boxer, and German shepherd dog over-represented.

SIGNS

Historical Findings
• Long bone tumor—pain and swelling at tumor site and associated lameness (as with other primary bone tumors) • Acute fracture with little or no associated trauma • Axial skeletal tumor (e.g., rib)—signs associated with location of tumor. For example, patient with extrapleural rib mass may be asymptomatic, whereas patient with intrapleural tumor extension may have respiratory signs due to pleural fluid.

Physical Examination Findings
• Other primary bone tumors—pain on palpation, lameness, swelling • Pathologic fracture more common with hemangiosarcoma than with other primary bone tumors • Pleural effusion secondary to intrapleural extension of rib tumor

CAUSES AND RISK FACTORS
Unknown

DIAGNOSIS

DIFFERENTIAL DIAGNOSIS
• Other primary bone neoplasms • Metastatic neoplasia from another primary site • Osteomyelitis (i.e., bacterial or fungal)

CBC/BIOCHEMISTRY/URINALYSIS
Possible abnormalities include anemia, thrombocytopenia, nucleated RBC, schistocytes, and acanthocytes; also, leukocytosis with neutrophilia, a left shift, and monocytosis.

OTHER LABORATORY TESTS
Coagulation abnormalities include prolonged PT and PTT, low plasma fibrinogen, and high FDP.

IMAGING
• Radiography often shows osteolysis as the predominant change. • Thoracic radiographs to detect metastasis • Abdominal and cardiac ultrasonography to detect hemangiosarcoma at other sites • CT helpful for determining extent of disease in patients with axial tumor.

OTHER DIAGNOSTIC PROCEDURES
Biopsy and histopathologic examination of suspected tumor. Hemorrhage and large vascular spaces within the tumor often make histologic diagnosis difficult when a small specimen is examined. A biopsy specimen taken near the periphery of the tumor may be best for obtaining a distinct core of tissue, unlike other primary bone tumors for which the center of the lesion is the most diagnostic.

TREATMENT
• Amputation of affected limb followed by chemotherapy in patient with appendicular skeletal tumor • Radical surgical resection when feasible followed by chemotherapy in patient with axial skeletal tumor. Axial sites more difficult to control by surgery.

MEDICATIONS

DRUGS AND FLUIDS
• Multiple chemotherapy protocols for hemangiosarcoma have been reported. Survival data similar for single agent doxorubicin, doxorubicin + cyclophosphamide, and doxorubicin + cyclophosphamide + vincristine • Chemotherapy prolongs survival in patients whose primary tumors are removed surgically.

CONTRAINDICATIONS/POSSIBLE INTERACTIONS
Patients with pre-existing heart disease may not be able to tolerate doxorubicin because of cardiotoxicity.

FOLLOW-UP
• Thoracic radiographs monthly for 3 months followed by every third month thereafter • Abdominal and cardiac ultrasound recommended at same interval as thoracic radiographs • Survival data not reported exclusively for hemangiosarcoma of bone, but median survival for all sites of hemangiosarcoma including bone treated with surgery and chemotherapy is 180 days.

MISCELLANEOUS

ABBREVIATIONS
CT = computed tomography
FDP = fibrin degradation products
PTT = partial thromboplastin time
PT = prothrombin time

Reference
Withrow SJ, MacEwen EG. Clinical veterinary oncology. Philadelphia: JB Lippincott, 1989.

Author Joyce E. Obradovich
Consulting Editor Wallace B. Morrison

BASICS

OVERVIEW

Skin hemangiosarcoma is a malignant tumor arising from endothelial cells. It is referred to as angiosarcoma or malignant hemangioendothelioma. Primary cutaneous hemangiosarcoma develops within dermal or subcutaneous tissues.

SIGNALMENT

• Prevalence in dogs is 0.3-2.0% • Median age 9 years (range, 4.5-15 years) • Cutaneous hemangiosarcoma accounts for 14% of all hemangiosarcoma in dogs. • Pit bull, boxer, and German shepherd dog affected more commonly than other breeds • Rare in cats

SIGNS

• A solitary tumor is commonly noticed, although patient with cutaneous hemangiosarcoma can have multiple nodules clustered in one area. • Dermal hemangiosarcoma appears as small, firm, raised, dark nodules located primarily on the prepuce and ventral abdomen. • Subcutaneous hemangiosarcoma appears as firm or soft, fluctuant masses with associated bruising. These tumors are typically larger than dermal hemangiosarcoma and, although commonly located on the pelvic limbs, can arise in any location. • Ulceration is frequent.

CAUSES AND RISK FACTORS

• Vascular stasis, radio therapy, trauma and sun exposure are predisposing factors in people and may be risk factors in dogs. • Genetic predisposition in pit bull, boxer, and German shepherd dog

 DIAGNOSIS

DIFFERENTIAL DIAGNOSIS

• Trauma (i.e., subcutaneous hemangiosarcoma) • Other tumors (i.e., mast cell tumor, melanoma, basal cell carcinoma and hemangioma)

CBC/BIOCHEMISTRY/URINALYSIS

• Results normal • CBC abnormalities compatible with disseminated intravascular coagulation possible in patients with advanced or metastatic subcutaneous hemangiosarcoma

OTHER LABORATORY TESTS N/A

IMAGING

• Thoracic radiograph to detect pulmonary metastasis • Results typically normal at the time of diagnosis

OTHER DIAGNOSTIC PROCEDURES

• Histopathologic examination is required to confirm the diagnosis and differentiate between dermal and subcutaneous hemangiosarcoma. • Dermal hemangiosarcoma is well circumscribed and confined to the dermis. • Subcutaneous hemangiosarcoma is poorly circumscribed and very invasive.

 TREATMENT

• Surgical excision is the treatment of choice. • Because of size and invasive behavior, complete surgical excision of subcutaneous hemangiosarcoma is often difficult to achieve and requires aggressive surgical intervention.

 MEDICATIONS

DRUGS AND FLUIDS

• Chemotherapy is recommended after surgical excision of subcutaneous hemangiosarcoma. • Treatment with adriamycin, cyclophosphamide, and vincristine has been shown to improve survival times in dogs with aggressive hemangiosarcoma.

 FOLLOW-UP

• Median survival time in dogs with dermal hemangiosarcoma is 780 days. • Metastasis to distant dermal sites occurs in 30% of patients. • Median survival in dogs with subcutaneous hemangiosarcoma > 6 months but the behavior varies depending on the degree of invasion of the cancer. • Metastasis to lungs, other cutaneous sites, and lymph nodes can occur.

 MISCELLANEOUS N/A

ABBREVIATIONS None

Reference

Ward H, Fox LE, Calderwood-Mays MB, et al. Cutaneous hemangiosarcoma in 25 dogs: a retrospective study. J Vet Intern Med 1994;8:345-348.
Author Robyn Elmslie
Consulting Editor Wallace B. Morrison

HEMANGIOSARCOMA, SPLEEN AND LIVER

BASICS

DEFINITION
Hemangiosarcoma of the spleen and liver is a highly metastatic malignant vascular neoplasm arising from endothelial cells.

Pathophysiology
A large mass develops in the liver or spleen. These tumors metastasize rapidly via hematogenous routes most frequently to the liver (from the spleen) and lungs (from the spleen and liver). These tumors can rupture leading to acute hemorrhage, collapse, and sudden death.

Systems Affected
• Hepatobiliary • Hemic/Lymphatic/Immune-spleen • Possible metastasis to the lungs, kidneys, muscle, peritoneum, omentum, lymph nodes, mesentery, adrenal glands, spinal cord, brain, subcutaneous tissue, and diaphragm

Genetics N/A

Incidence/Prevalence
• Dogs—0.3-2.0% of recorded necropsies and 7% of all malignancies. About 50% of hemangiosarcomas are splenic and 5% are hepatic. • Cats—18 affected cats out of 3145 necropsies. The liver is the most common site.

Geographic Distribution N/A

SIGNALMENT

Species Dogs and cats

Breed Predilections
• German shepherd, boxer, great Dane, English setter, golden retriever, and pointer • Domestic shorthair cat

Mean Age and Range
• Dogs—8-10 years old • Cats—10 years old

Predominant Sex
Possible male sex predilection in dogs but none in cats

SIGNS

General Comments
• Clinical signs related to the organs involved • Signs also caused by bleeding secondary to rupture of the mass or disseminated intravascular coagulation (DIC)

Historical Findings
Sudden death because of acute blood loss, weight loss, weakness, intermittent collapse, ataxia, lameness, seizures, dementia, or paresis

Physical Examination Findings
• Pale mucous membranes • High pulse rate • Peritoneal fluid • Palpable cranial abdominal mass • Hemoabdomen

CAUSES
Unknown in dogs and cats, but includes arsenicals, vinyl chloride, and thorium dioxide in humans and methyl nitrosamine in minks.

RISK FACTORS N/A

DIAGNOSIS

DIFFERENTIAL DIAGNOSIS
• Other causes of splenic and hepatic masses including lymphosarcoma, leiomyosarcoma, liposarcoma, hematoma, hemangioma, splenic cyst, hepatoma, hepatocellular carcinoma, and hepatic cyst • 43 of 100 of splenic masses in one study were hemangiosarcoma

CBC/BIOCHEMISTRY/URINALYSIS
• Regenerative anemia with polychromasia, reticulocytosis, anisocytosis, and nucleated RBC • Leukocytosis caused by mature neutrophilia • Thrombocytopenia • High liver enzyme activity if the liver is involved

OTHER LABORATORY TESTS
• High PT, PTT, and FDP • Low FDP in patients with DIC • Evaluate clotting cascade if evidence of spontaneous hemorrhage is observed or if surgery is contemplated.

IMAGING
• Abdominal radiography of the abdomen reveals a cranial abdominal mass and possible evidence of abdominal fluid. • Thoracic radiography to detect metastasis • Area radiographs of any lameness. Pain from metastasis to bone is possible. Bone lysis with little to no proliferation is common. • Ultrasonography reveals splenic masses with multiple cavitations. Hepatic involvement is seen in most patients as multiple hypoechoic nodules. • Ultrasonography of the heart should be done in patients with evidence of pericardial effusion. Reveals a cardiac mass if the patient has primary cardiac or metastatic disease.

OTHER DIAGNOSTIC PROCEDURES
Peritoneocentesis if patient has evidence of abdominal effusion. Serosanguinous fluid or frank blood that does not clot is usually obtained. Spindle-shaped neoplastic cells are seen in a few patients.

GROSS AND HISTOPATHOLOGIC FINDINGS
• Spleen—a large, hemorrhagic, friable mass and some degree of abdominal hemorrhage in most patients • Liver—multiple, variable-sized, hemorrhagic nodules in many patients • Spleen and Liver—widespread abdominal metastasis in many patients • Histopathologic examination necessary for definitive diagnosis. Three histologic patterns predominate: (1) large blood spaces lined by endothelial cells; (2) numerous small capillary structures; and (3) solid areas of endothelial cells without apparent vascular structure.

TREATMENT

INPATIENT VERSUS OUTPATIENT
Patient should be hospitalized for initial medical and surgical management.

ACTIVITY
Restricted until after initial surgical management. Spontaneous hemorrhage can occur.

DIET No change

CLIENT EDUCATION
• Emergency surgery indicated in some patients • Sudden death possible • Follow-up chemotherapy an important part of treatment

SURGICAL CONSIDERATIONS
Surgery the initial treatment of choice

MEDICATIONS

DRUGS AND FLUIDS
• Balanced, isotonic, electrolyte solutions to correct dehydration • Fresh whole blood transfusion in animals with severe anemia • Chemotherapy with doxorubicin (30 mg/m^2 IV) and cyclophosphamide (100-150 mg/ m^2 IV) on day 1. Give diphenhydramine (2.2 mg/kg IM) 20 minutes before the doxorubicin injection to prevent anaphylactoid reaction. Give vincristine (0.75 mg/m^2 IV) on days 8 and 15. This cycle is repeated every 21 days. Generally, four cycles are given after surgery.

CONTRAINDICATIONS
• Doxorubicin should not be used in a patient with arrhythmias or reduced fractional shortening of the heart. • Chemotherapy can cause gastrointestinal, bone marrow, and cardiac toxicity. Seek advice before treatment if unfamiliar with cytotoxic drugs.

PRECAUTIONS
Monitor the WBC count and delay chemotherapy if the neutrophil count drops below 2000.

POSSIBLE INTERACTIONS None

ALTERNATE DRUGS N/A

FOLLOW-UP

PATIENT MONITORING
Thoracic and abdominal radiography and abdominal ultrasound every 3 months after treatment to monitor for evidence of recurrence or metastasis.

PREVENTION/AVOIDANCE N/A

POSSIBLE COMPLICATIONS

• Sepsis because of neutropenia • Doxorubicin-induced cardiomyopathy • Skin sloughs caused by extravasation of doxorubicin or vincristine • Vomiting and diarrhea

EXPECTED COURSE AND PROGNOSIS

• Mean time to recurrence in cats—4-5 months • Median survival time in dogs treated by surgery alone— 19-65 days • Median survival time in dogs treated by surgery plus chemotherapy—145 days (mean survival, 271 days)

 MISCELLANEOUS

ASSOCIATED CONDITIONS

DIC

AGE-RELATED FACTORS

Generally occurs in old animals, although can be seen in animals < 1 year old.

ZOONOTIC POTENTIAL None

PREGNANCY

Chemotherapy should not be used in pregnant animals.

SYNONYMS

• Malignant hemangioendothelioma
• Angiosarcoma

SEE ALSO

• Myocardial Tumors
• Hemangiosarcoma, Skin

ABBREVIATIONS

DIC= disseminated intravascular coagulation

References

Scavelli TD, Patnaik AK, Melhaff CJ, et al. Hemangiosarcoma in the cat: retrospective evaluation of 31 surgical cases. J Am Vet Med Assoc 1985;187:817-819.

Hammer AS, Couto G. Filppi J. et al. Efficacy and toxicity of VAC chemotherapy (Vincristine, Doxorubicin, and Cyclophosphamide) in dogs with hemangiosarcoma. J Vet Int Med 1991;5:160-166.

Prymals C, McKee LJ, Goldschmidt MH, et al. Epidemiologic, clinical, pathologic, and prognostic characteristics of splenic hemangiosarcoma and splenic hematoma in dogs: 217 cases (1985). J Am Vet Med Assoc 1988;193:706-712.

Brown NO, Patnaik AK, MacEwen EG. Canine hemangiosarcoma: retrospective analysis of 104 cases. J Am Vet Med Assoc 1985;186:56-58.

Johnson KA, Powers BE, Withrow SJ, et al. Splenomegaly in dogs: Predictors of neoplasia and survival after splenectomy. J Vet Intern Med 1989;3:160-166.

Author Terrance A. Hamilton

Consulting Editor Wallace B. Morrison

HEMOBARTONELLOSIS

BASICS

OVERVIEW
• Caused by rickettsial parasites that attach to the external surface of RBCs • RBC destruction and anemia caused by parasite attachment and immune response by the host

SIGNALMENT
• Occurs mostly in adult animals • In cats, more common in males • No sex prevalence in dogs

SIGNS

Cats
• Variable disease severity ranging from inapparent infection to marked depression and death • Signs include intermittent fever (only 50% of the time) during acute phase, depression, weakness, anorexia, weight loss, pale mucous membranes, splenomegaly, and icterus.

Dogs
• Mild or inapparent signs (e.g., pale mucous membranes and listlessness)——except when dogs have been splenectomized

CAUSES AND RISK FACTORS
• Haemobartonella felis (cats) and Haemobartonella canis (dogs) • Greater severity of anemia in FeLV-infected cats • Likelihood of severe anemia greatly increased in dogs with splenectomy or splenic pathologic condition

DIAGNOSIS

DIFFERENTIAL DIAGNOSIS
• Other causes of hemolytic anemia, including autoimmune hemolytic anemia, babesiosis (only in dogs in the U.S.), cytauxzoonosis (cats only), Heinz body hemolytic anemia, microangiopathic hemolytic anemia, pyruvate kinase deficiency, and phosphofructokinase deficiency (dogs only) • Differentiated from autoimmune hemolytic anemia only by recognition of parasites in blood—both disorders may be Coombs' test positive • Babesia and Cytauxzoon species are protozoal organisms that differ in morphology from Haemobartonella. • New methylene blue stains used to identify Heinz bodies • Enzyme assays or specialized DNA tests used to diagnose pyruvate kinase and phosphofructokinase deficiencies

CBC/BIOCHEMISTRY/URINALYSIS
• Anemia, most often presenting with reticulocytosis in animals with clinically important hemobartonellosis • Anemia may appear poorly regenerative if a precipitous decrease in PCV has occurred early in the disease, or if there are other concurrent disorders (e.g., FeLV or FIV infection in cats). • Auto-agglutination may be seen in feline blood samples after they cool to below body temperature. • Variable total and differential leukocyte counts are of little diagnostic assistance. • Slight hemoglobinemia rarely observed; no hemoglobinuria reported • Hyperbilirubinemia may be measured at times but is seldom severe. Substantial bilirubinuria has been recognized in some dogs. • Abnormalities related to anemic hypoxia may be demonstrated on clinical chemistry profiles, but profiles can be normal. Hypoglycemia may occur in moribund cats. • Plasma protein concentrations usually normal, but may be increased

OTHER LABORATORY TESTS
Routine blood stains (e.g., Wright-Giemsa)—to identify organism in blood films to facilitate diagnosis • Reticulocyte stains can not be used—punctate reticulocytes in cats appear similar to the parasites • H. felis organisms—small, blue-staining cocci, rings, or rods on RBC • H. canis—commonly forms chains of organisms that appear as filamentous structures on the surface of RBC • Organisms must be differentiated from precipitated stain, refractile drying or fixation artifacts, poorly staining Howell-Jolly bodies, and basophilic stippling. • Blood films must be examined for organisms before therapy is begun. • Organisms occur in cyclic parasitemias (especially in cats) and are not always identifiable in blood. • Direct Coombs' test may be positive.

IMAGING N/A

OTHER DIAGNOSTIC PROCEDURES
In nonregenerative anemia, bone marrow biopsy should be performed to assess for other disorders (e.g., myeloproliferative disease).

TREATMENT
• Without therapy, mortality may reach 30% in cats.
• Treat as outpatients, unless severely anemic or moribund.
• Alert owners that cats remain carriers even after completion of treatment, but relapse is uncommon.

MEDICATIONS

DRUGS AND FLUIDS
• Tetracycline antibiotics (20 mg/kg PO q8h) should be given for 3 weeks in cats and 2 weeks in dogs.
• Glucocorticoids such as prednisolone (1-2 mg/kg PO q12h) may be given to severely anemic animals. Gradually decrease dosage as PCV increases.
• Blood transfusions are required when anemia is considered life-threatening.
• IV fluid containing glucose is recommended in moribund animals.

CONTRAINDICATIONS/POSSIBLE INTERACTIONS
• Tetracycline antibiotics may produce fever and/or evidence of gastrointestinal disease in cats. Use a lower dosage or a different tetracycline product, or discontinue drug altogether.
• Chloramphenicol should not be used to treat cats because it causes dose-dependent erythroid hypoplasia.

FOLLOW-UP
• Examine animal after one week of therapy to assess for appropriate increase in PCV.
• Cats that recover from hemobartonellosis remain carriers, but seldom relapse with clinical disease once PCV returns to normal.

MISCELLANEOUS

ASSOCIATED CONDITIONS
• Perform FeLV test in cats with hemobartonellosis——a significant number are also FeLV-positive.

ABBREVIATIONS
FeLV = feline leukemia virus
FIV = feline immunodeficiency virus
PCV = packed cell volume
RBC = red blood cells

Reference
Harvey JW. Haemobartonellosis. In: Greene CE, ed. Infectious diseases of the dog and cat. Philadelphia: WB Saunders, 1990:434-442.,

Author John W. Harvey
Consulting Editor Alan H. Rebar

BASICS

OVERVIEW
• Amyloidosis involves the extracellular deposition of insoluble fibrillar proteins. • Dogs and cats have reactive amyloidosis. Multiple organs are often involved, but clinical signs are usually caused by renal failure. • Evidence of liver involvement includes liver failure, liver rupture, and hemoabdomen caused by hepatic vascular fragility or coagulopathy.

SIGNALMENT
• Oriental and Siamese cat; age, < 5 years (hepatic signs predominate) • Abyssinian cat (renal signs predominate) • Young adult Chinese shar pei dog. Renal signs usually predominate; rarely present for signs of liver failure or rupture.

SIGNS

Historical Findings
• History of episodic fever and swollen hocks in affected Chinese shar pei dog • Acute lethargy • Anorexia • PU/PD • Vomiting • Dehydration in patient with renal failure

Physical Examination Findings
• Icterus • Pale mucous membranes • Abdominal effusion (hemorrhage) • Hepatomegaly

CAUSES AND RISK FACTORS
• Chronic infection (coccidiodomycosis), inflammation, neoplasia, and immune disorder • Familial in Chinese shar pei dog and Abyssinian, Oriental, and Siamese cats. • Episodic fever and swollen hocks in Chinese shar pei dog ("shar -pei fever").

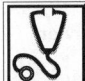

DIAGNOSIS

DIFFERENTIAL DIAGNOSIS
• Hepatic neoplasia or hepatitis • Primary coagulopathy • Abdominal trauma

CBC/BIOCHEMISTRY/URINALYSIS
• Anemia secondary to hepatic hemorrhage and rupture • Leukocytosis with left shift during febrile episodes (Chinese shar pei) • Normal to high ALP, ALT, serum bilirubin, and serum bile acid • Azotemia and dilute urine (with concurrent renal involvement and failure) • Proteinuria with concurrent renal involvement (dogs).

OTHER LABORATORY TESTS
Normal coagulation tests

IMAGING
• Radiography-hepatomegaly and possible abdominal effusion • Ultrasonography-ultrasonographic appearance has not been characterized

OTHER DIAGNOSTIC PROCEDURES
• Abdominocentesis may reveal hemorrhagic abdominal effusion. • Liver biopsy

GROSS AND HISTOPATHOLOGIC FINDINGS
• Pale, large, and friable liver with hemorrhages, hematomas, and capsular tears • Liver biopsy-acellular amorphous material in space of Disse; positive Congo red stain with polarized light. Hepatocyte atrophy and hemorrhage.

TREATMENT
• No curative treatment • Manage underlying disease when identified.

MEDICATIONS

DRUGS AND FLUIDS
• Administer fluids and blood transfusion to treat acute blood loss. • Colchicine may block formation of amyloid in the early phases (dogs, 0.03 mg/kg PO q24 h). • Dimethyl sulfoxide may promote resorption of amyloid (80 mg/kg as 18% solution in sterile water SC 3 times/week). • Vitamin C

CONTRAINDICATIONS/POSSIBLE INTERACTIONS
• Unpleasant odor of dimethyl sulfoxide limits owner compliance. • Side-effects of colchicine-vomiting, diarrhea, and bone marrow suppression

FOLLOW-UP
• Chinese shar pei may live 2 years with treatment, but will have episodes of fever and cholestasis. • Cats that survive liver hemorrhage eventually develop renal failure.

MISCELLANEOUS

SEE ALSO   Amyloidosis

ABBREVIATIONS
ALP = alkaline phosphatase
ALT = alanine aminotransferase
PU/PD = polyuria and polydipsia

References
Loeven KO. Hepatic amyloidosis in two Chinese shar-pei dogs. J Am Vet Med Assoc 1994;204:1212-1216.
Author Susan E. Johnson
Consulting Editor Albert E. Jergens

HEPATIC ENCEPHALOPATHY

BASICS

DEFINITION
A metabolic disorder affecting the CNS that develops as a result of hepatic disease

Pathophysiology
• Hepatic encephalopathy is associated with the accumulation in serum of substances that are the result of severe hepatic disorders or portal systemic shunting of blood. Slowed metabolism results in prolonged circulation of these substances. Altered membranes and functions of neurons, glial cells, and the blood brain barrier result in signs of neurologic disease. • Broad and overlapping hypotheses for the pathogenesis of hepatic encephalopathy include the following: • The ammonia hypothesis suggests that a high concentration of ammonia causes neurotoxicity. • The synergistic neurotoxin hypothesis suggests that there is a combined effect of multiple substances such as mercaptans, ammonia, indoles, scatoles, short-chain fatty acids, and other substances. Many of these are produced by intestinal bacteria. • The false neurotransmitter hypothesis suggests high concentration in the brain of depressants such as gamma–aminobutyric acid and, recently, endogenous benzodiazepam-like substances. Current evidence supports the concept of endogenous benzodiazepine-like substances as a major cause of hepatic encephaolpathy. • The amino acid hypothesis suggests that enhanced catabolism or low intake of branch chain amino acids results in a compensatory rise in aromatic amino acids, which leads to synthesis of inhibitory neurotransmitters (eg, tryptophan and serotonin).

Systems Affected
Nervous—the proposed affects on neural cells include cytotoxic edema, low excitatory receptor activity, high inhibitory receptor function, weakened blood brain barrier, and gradual degenerative changes.

Genetics N/A

Incidence/Prevalence
Uncommon in small animal practice.

Geographic Distribution N/A

SIGNALMENT
Young animals are more commonly affected by congenital portal systemic shunt, but any age animal can have severe hepatic dysfunction.

SIGNS

General Comments
• If animal has mild signs on examination, hepatic encephalopathy can be overlooked until the primary diagnosis of liver disease or portal systemic shunt is made. • Owners often comment on the intermittent and sporadic nature of the signs and its progressive course. • Owners may also have observed that signs worsen after feeding.

Historical Findings
• Ptyalism (common in cats) • Behavior changes • Visual deficits (blindness) • Circling • Pacing • Anxiety • Head pressing • Stupor • Coma • Seizures (inconsistent finding)

Physical Examination Findings
• Stunted growth • Depressed menace reflex • Visual deficits • Mentation changes and aberrant behavior as listed • Signs of liver disease (eg, icterus and ascites) in some animals • Ptyalism common in cats

CAUSES
• Abnormal portal blood flow (portosystemic shunt or acquired portal shunt) and disorders such as microvascular dysplasia, infectious or immunologic hepatitis, toxic hepatopathy, hepatic fibrosis or cirrhosis, and neoplasia • Rare, congenital, urea cycle enzyme deficiency has been reported in two dogs. • Dietary restriction of arginine can cause hyperammonemia and severe hepatic encephalopathy in cats and ferrets. Since most dietary protein contains adequate arginine, this is not currently thought to play a role in most clinical cases.

RISK FACTORS
• High-protein diet, stress, exertion, and concurrent disease can bring on signs of hepatic encephalopathy in predisposed animals. • Gastrointestinal hemorrhage causes high plasma ammonia, since digested blood provides a high protein meal. • Constipation raises ammonia, gamma aminobutyric acid, indole, and scatole concentrations by increasing time for production by bacteria and for absorption from the colon. • Hyperammonemia is worsened by the use of improperly stored RBC products.

DIAGNOSIS

DIFFERENTIAL DIAGNOSIS
• CNS trauma • Hydrocephalus • Hereditary storage disorder • Thiamine deficiency • Cerebral hypoxia • Uremic encephalopathy • Hypoglycemia • Drug intoxication • Acute ethylene glycol toxicosis • CNS tumor • Rabies • Canine distemper virus • Toxoplasmosis • Other infectious encephalopathy

CBC/BIOCHEMISTRY/URINALYSIS
• Mild to moderate nonregenerative anemia in many animals, but some with acute, fulminant hepatic failure may have normal red cell indices and abnormal leukograms. • High bilirubin, ALP, and ALT activities in many animals. The quantity of remaining "functional" hepatic mass influences serum liver enzyme activity. Cirrhotic animals may have low enzyme activity. Low serum urea nitrogen and albumin are also seen in animals with severe loss of liver function. • Ammonium biurate crystals or uroliths are helpful in confirming hepatic dysfunction.

OTHER LABORATORY TESTS
• The laboratory test of prime importance is paired serum bile acids concentration, which is high in animals with hepatic encephalopathy. Hyperbilirubinemia can interfere with the test. However, hemolytic disease can usually be ruled out by results of a hemogram. • Plasma ammonia or ammonia tolerance tests can be performed if serum bile acid test is unavailable.

IMAGING
• Abdominal radiographs and ultrasonography are advised to assess the liver size and texture and portal vessels. • CT or MRI of the CNS can be helpful in working through the differential diagnosis. • Contrast portography is frequently used.

OTHER DIAGNOSTIC PROCEDURES
• Hepatic biopsy is often needed if initial tests are not conclusive. • Electroencephalography and visual evoked potentials, if available, may be helpful in monitoring depressed or comatose patients.

GROSS AND HISTOPATHOLOGIC FINDINGS
• No specific gross pathologic findings are characteristic of hepatic encephalopathy. • Microscopic findings may include mild vacuolation of glial cells and degeneration of neurons. Cerebral edema may also be seen in severely affected animals. Hepatic findings depend on the primary hepatic condition.

TREATMENT

INPATIENT VS OUTPATIENT
Treat as inpatients until improvement is seen.

ACTIVITY
Patients should be kept quiet and warm to minimize catabolism of branched chain amino acids and proteins.

DIET
• A very low-protein diet is advised. • Oral fasting and partial parenteral nutrition with dextrose, B vitamins and vitamin K, and branched chain amino acid solutions may be helpful.

CLIENT EDUCATION
Many patients recover from hepatic encephalopathy. However, animals with chronic disease may have permanent neurologic damage. Resolution of the hepatic or portosystemic shunt is imperative.

SURGICAL CONSIDERATIONS
Surgery can correct single portosystemic shunts.

MEDICATIONS

DRUGS AND FLUIDS
• Administer antibiotics with a spectrum

against intestinal flora (aerobic and anaerobic). Neomycin (10-20 mg/kg PO q8h) and metronidazole (7.5 mg/kg PO q8h-q12h) are a good combination. In less severely affected animals, amoxicillin with clavulanic acid can be used.
• Lactulose (0.25 -0.5 mg/kg PO q6h-q8h) decreases production and absorption of ammonia. Adjust dosage to maintain soft stool.
• To treat hepatic coma, discontinue oral medications and food and give a retention enema q6h of neomycin (15 mg/kg) plus lactulose (diluted 1:2 with water; 50-200 ml total).
• Fluids: 0.9% saline or Ringer's solution supplemented with 2.5-5% dextrose and 20-30 mEq of KCl /L of maintenance fluid.
• Enemas are advocated in animals with clinical signs or constipation.

CONTRAINDICATIONS
Avoid drugs metabolized by the liver.

PRECAUTIONS
Anesthetics, sedative, tranquilizers, and analgesics should be used cautiously.

POSSIBLE INTERACTIONS
Any drug that affects or depends on hepatic metabolism must be considered carefully (e.g., cimetidine, diazepam, and barbiturates).

ALTERNATE DRUGS N/A

FOLLOW-UP

PATIENT MONITORING
• Repeated neurologic evaluations are necessary. • Monitoring of serum potassium and glucose is advised in critical animals.

PREVENTION/AVOIDANCE
Avoid stored blood in patients with liver failure.

POSSIBLE COMPLICATIONS
Chronically affected animals may have permanent neurologic damage.

EXPECTED COURSE AND PROGNOSIS
Varies with the nature of the liver disease

MISCELLANEOUS

ASSOCIATED CONDITIONS
Hepatopathy and portosystemic shunt

AGE RELATED FACTORS
Disorder specific

ZOONOTIC POTENTIAL N/A

PREGNANCY N/A

SYNONYMS N/A

SEE ALSO
• Ammonia • Portosystemic shunt

ABBREVIATIONS
ALP = alkaline phosphatase
ALT = alanine aminotransferase
CNS = central nervous system
CT = computed tomography
MRI = magnetic resonance imaging
RBC = red blood cells

References
Maddison JE. Current concepts of hepatic encephalopathy. J Vet Int Med 1992;6: 341– 353.
Strombeck DR, Guilford WG. Small animal gastroenterology. 2nd ed. Davis, Calif: Stonegate Publishing, 1990.
Author Mark E. Hitt
Consulting Editor Albert E. Jergens

HEPATIC FAILURE, ACUTE

BASICS

DEFINITION
Rapid loss of hepatic function occurring primarily because of acute hepatic necrosis. Causes vary and include drugs, toxins, infectious diseases, and hypoxia.

Pathophysiology
Hepatic necrosis occurs when the liver undergoes an insult secondary to poor perfusion, hypoxia, hepatotoxic drugs or chemicals, or infectious agents. The effect on the hepatic lobule depends on the type of insult. Most commonly, events that decrease perfusion or cause hypoxia affect zone 3 of the hepatic acinus, corresponding to the pericentral region. Many toxins affect the more metabolically-active zone 1 of the acinus, located periportally. This cellular necrosis is accompanied by enzyme leakage and, with worsening damage, impaired hepatic function and failure. Hepatic failure then causes a myriad of metabolic derangements in glucose homeostasis, protein synthesis (including coagulation factors), and detoxification, which may result in the patient's death.

Systems Affected
• Hepatobiliary—necrosis and hepatic failure • Nervous—hepatoencephalopathy • Gastrointestinal—vomiting, diarrhea, and gastrointestinal hemorrhage • Hemic/lymphatic/immune—coagulation factor deficiences and disseminated intravascular coagulation (DIC)

Genetics N/A

Incidence / Prevalence
Mild to moderate hepatic necrosis is common. Severe hepatic necrosis is less common, but its prevalence is difficult to assess since it may be caused by many disorders.

Geographic Distribution N/A

SIGNALMENT

Species
Dogs more common than cats

Breed Predilections N/A

Mean Age and Range
Varies according to cause

Predominant Sex N/A

SIGNS
• Acute onset of depression and illness • Vomiting • Icterus • Diarrhea • Encephalopathy • Seizures • Hemorrhage

CAUSES

Hepatic Hypoxia
• DIC • Thromboembolic disease • Shock • Trauma • Heatstroke • Septicemia • Acute circulatory failure from any cause

Hepatic Toxicity
Infectious agents
• Canine infectious hepatitis virus • Canine acidophil cell hepatitis virus

Drugs (see hepatotoxins for more detail)
• Anticonvulsants • Antimicrobials • Analgesics • Other drugs
Toxins (see hepatotoxins for more detail)

RISK FACTORS
Administration of any potentially hepatotoxic drug

DIAGNOSIS

DIFFERENTIAL DIAGNOSIS
• Acute gastroenteritis—laboratory data will differentiate • Acute renal failure—laboratory data will differentiate

CBC/BIOCHEMISTRY/URINALYSIS
• High ALT and AST activity • High ALP activity • High serum bilirubin concentration • Hypoglycemia • Low BUN concentration • Hypoalbuminemia • Hypercholesterolemia • Bilirubinuria

OTHER LABORATORY TESTS
• Serum bile acids—identify hepatic dysfunction • Plasma ammonia concentration—identify hepatic dysfunction • Coagulation tests—identify coagulation factor deficiencies and DIC

IMAGING
• Abdominal radiographs may identify hepatomegaly • Abdominal ultrasonography rules out biliary obstruction

OTHER DIAGNOSTIC PROCEDURES
Liver biopsy required to confirm the diagnosis of hepatic necrosis

GROSS AND HISTOPATHOLOGIC FINDINGS
• Grossly, the liver may be slightly large and discolored. • Histopathologic examination reveals hepatic necrosis. Identifying the zone affected most by necrosis helps identify the insult. Hypoxic changes are more commonly pericentral, while toxic changes are more often periportal.

TREATMENT

INPATIENT VS. OUTPATIENT
Inpatient, critical care

ACTIVITY
Restricted to promote healing and regeneration of the liver

DIET
Withold food as long as vomiting continues. After that, feed an easily digestible diet low in protein. The amount of food should be increased over several days until caloric requirements are being met.

CLIENT EDUCATION
Acute hepatic failure is a severe disease, and some patients die even with optimal treatment. The owner should attempt to identify

any predisposing cause for the hepatic necrosis, such as exposure to a drug or toxin.

SURGICAL CONSIDERATIONS N/A

MEDICATIONS

DRUGS AND FLUIDS
• Fluid administration with non-actate-containing fluid should be instituted. Additional potassium and glucose should be added if needed.
• Metoclopramide (0.2-0.4 mg/kg IV q8h) for vomiting
• Ranitidine (2 mg/kg IV q12h) for gastrointestinal hemorrhage
• Lactulose (0.2-0.4 ml/kg PO q6h-q8h) and neomycin (5 mg/kg PO q12h) or metronidazole (5 mg/kg PO q12h) for hepatoencephalopathy These drugs may be given per rectum if mentation is abnormal and swallowing impaired.
• Fresh whole blood or fresh frozen plasma may be given if coagulation tests are abnormal because of impaired hepatic synthesis.

CONTRAINDICATIONS
Drugs that use the liver for metabolism or those that alter liver blood flow or metabolic enzymes should be avoided.

PRECAUTIONS
Administration of stored blood may precipitate hepatic encephalopathy.

POSSIBLE INTERACTIONS N/A

ALTERNATE DRUGS N/A

FOLLOW-UP

PATIENT MONITORING
• Temperature, pulse, respiration, and mental status hourly for the first 24 hours • Acid-base and electrolyte balances every 12 hours for the first 48 hours • Liver enzymes and serum bilirubin every 2-3 days until marked improvement is observed

PREVENTION / AVOIDANCE
• Vaccinate dogs against infectious canine hepatitis virus. • Avoid drugs and toxins associated with hepatotoxicity.

POSSIBLE COMPLICATIONS
• Hypoglycemia • DIC • Hepatoencephalopathy • Chronic hepatitis • Cirrhosis/fibrosis of the liver • Death

EXPECTED COURSE AND PROGNOSIS
• Prognosis varies with the severity of necrosis. • Adequate support may induce hepatic regeneration.

MISCELLANEOUS

ASSOCIATED CONDITIONS
• Pancreatitis • Septicemia • Shock • DIC

AGE RELATED FACTORS N/A

ZOONOTIC POTENTIAL N/A

PREGNANCY N/A

SYNONYMS
• Acute hepatic necrosis • Acute hepatitis

SEE ALSO
• ALP/ GGT • Ammonia • AST/ ALT • Bile Acids • Bilirubin • Hepatic Encephalopathy • Hepatotoxins • Hepatitis Infectious—Dogs

ABBREVIATIONS
ALP = alkaline phosphatase
ALT = alanine aminotransferase
AST = aspartate aminotransferase
BUN = blood urea nitrogen
DIC = disseminated intravascular coagulation

References
Hughes D, King LG. The diagnosis and management of acute liver failure in dogs and cats. Vet Clin North Am Small Anim Pract 1995 (In Press.)

Maddison JE. Hepatic encephalopathy- current concepts of the pathogenesis. J Vet Int Med 1992; 6:341-353.

Author Donna S. Dimski
Consulting Editor Alfred E. Jergens

HEPATIC LIPIDOSIS

BASICS

DEFINITION
Hepatic lipidosis is the accumulation of neutral lipid within the liver associated with cholestasis and hepatic dysfunction in cats. The disease may be secondary or idiopathic hepatic lipidosis. Other species can develop hepatic lipidosis without concomitant severe liver dysfunction.

Pathophysiology
Affected cats are often obese at the onset of disease. The hallmark of hepatic lipidosis is anorexia, which promotes lipid mobilization to the liver. The liver is unable to use this lipid, and liver dysfunction ensues as lipid accumulates. The mechanism for the inability to use lipid is not fully understood, but it may be caused by protein deficiency, which leads to reduction in the synthesis of apoproteins needed to mobilize lipid from the liver.

Systems Affected
• Hepatobiliary—intrahepatic cholestasis, hepatic dysfunction, and failure • Gastrointestinal—anorexia and vomiting • Nervous—hepatoencephalopathy • Musculoskeletal—muscle wasting and weight loss

Genetics N/A

Incidence/Prevalence
The most commonly reported hepatopathy in cats

Geographic Distribution
Common in North America, but is much less commonly reported throughout the rest of the world

SIGNALMENT

Species
Cats. Hepatic lipid accumulation in dogs is usually asymptomatic.

Breed Predilections N/A

Mean Age and Range
• Mean age, 8 years; range, 1-16 years
• Primarily middle-aged adults

Predominant Sex
Possibly a slight female predilection

SIGNS
• Anorexia • Weight loss • Loss of muscle mass • Icterus • Vomiting • Encephalopathy • Hepatomegaly

CAUSES

Idiopathic Hepatic Lipidosis (common)

Secondary Hepatic Lipidosis
• Liver disease • Cholangiohepatitis
• Biliary inflammation and obstruction
• Suppurative hepatitis • Portosystemic shunt • Diabetes mellitus • Small intestinal disease • Pancreatitis • Neoplasia • Renal disease • Other systemic illness

RISK FACTORS
• Obesity • Anorexia, any cause • Illness resulting in chronic anorexia

DIAGNOSIS

DIFFERENTIAL DIAGNOSIS
• Cholangiohepatitis—differentiate by liver biopsy • Feline infectious peritonitis—differentiate by liver biopsy • Hepatic neoplasia—differentiate by liver biopsy • Pancreatitis—ascites is common; lipase concentration may not be helpful

CBC/BIOCHEMISTRY/URINALYSIS
• Nonregenerative anemia (mild) • High ALP activity • High serum bilirubin concentration • High ALT and AST activity
• Bilirubinuria

OTHER LABORATORY TESTS
• High fasting or postprandial serum bile acid concentration • High plasma ammonia concentration • Prolonged coagulation times (PT, PTT, ACT) • High FDP

IMAGING

Abdominal Radiographic Findings
Hepatomegaly

Abdominal Ultrasonography
• Hyperechogenicity characteristic of lipid accumulation in liver • Rule out biliary occlusion and pancreatitis.

OTHER DIAGNOSTIC PROCEDURES
• Examination of fine needle liver aspirate identifies vacuolar change in hepatocytes characteristic of lipidosis, but cannot rule out secondary lipidosis. • Liver biopsy definitively diagnoses hepatic lipidosis and should identify any concomitant liver disease associated with secondary lipidosis.

GROSS AND HISTOPATHOLOGIC FINDINGS
• Gross findings include diffuse and smooth hepatomegaly. The liver is yellow and appears infiltrated and may be "greasy" to the touch.
• Histopathologic examination of liver tissue reveals severe vacuolization of most hepatocytes. The vacuolization may be either macrovesicular (ie, one large vacuole taking up most of the cytoplasm) or microvesicular (ie, multiple small vacuoles). Staining of the specimen with Oil Red-O confirms the presence of lipid.

TREATMENT

INPATIENT VS. OUTPATIENT
Severely ill cats need to be managed as critical care patients. After initiation of treatment, at-home feeding and care can be continued with frequent rechecks. Outpatient care minimizes stresses that promote anorexia and compound the disease.

ACTIVITY
Most cats voluntarily restrict activity. Encourage increased activity as the disease remits.

DIET
• Dietary therapy is the cornerstone of treatment for idiopathic hepatic lipidosis.
• A high-protein, high-calorie diet should be fed in amounts designed to meet the cat's energy needs.
• For nearly all cats, this means tube feeding by nasoesophageal, esophagostomy, or gastrostomy tube. Force feeding is seldom sufficient to reverse the disease. The diet should be fed initially in small quantities, gradually increasing over a period of 3 days to amounts that meet the cat's energy needs.

CLIENT EDUCATION
• The client is responsible for continuing the tube feeding for up to 6 weeks until the cat is eating voluntarily.
• Client commitment and training in how to administer the tube feeding is essential for success.

SURGICAL CONSIDERATIONS
If an exploratory laparotomy is performed to obtain a specimen for liver biopsy, a surgical gastrostomy tube can be placed during surgery.

MEDICATIONS

DRUGS AND FLUIDS
• Lactated Ringer's solution or another balanced electrolyte solution without lactate should be used for initial management. Potassium or dextrose supplementation may be needed.
• Vomiting and gastroparesis can be managed with metoclopramide (0.2-0.4 mg/kg q8h).
• Hepatoencephalopathy can be treated with lactulose (0.2-0.4 ml/kg PO q6h-q8h) and either neomycin (5 mg/kg PO q8h) or metronidazole (10 mg/kg PO q8h).

CONTRAINDICATIONS
Do not use drugs that are primarily metabolized by the liver, or drugs that alter liver blood flow or metabolism (eg, cimetidine).

PRECAUTIONS N/A

POSSIBLE INTERACTIONS N/A

ALTERNATE DRUGS
• Antibiotics may be needed to treat concurrent infection. Antibiotics metabolized by the liver should be avoided.
• Ursodeoxycholic acid, carnitine, antioxidants (fish oil), and supplemental taurine have been advocated in the management of hepatic lipidosis. No studies have confirmed that these drugs are beneficial.
• Appetite stimulants such as diazepam, oxazepam, and cyproheptadine are seldom useful in promoting appetite in cats with hepatic lipidosis. These drugs may cause sedation.

FOLLOW-UP

PATIENT MONITORING

• Affected cats should be monitored for weight gain or loss and hydration status. Dietary and fluid therapy should be altered if needed. • Serum biochemistries should be monitored every 3-7 days. Improvement in abnormalities should be observed within 2-3 weeks after initiation of treatment. • Tube feeding should be continued until the cat eats voluntarily. The feeding tube can be removed 5-7 days after the cat eats normally.

PREVENTION/ AVOIDANCE

• Prevention of obesity decreases the risk of hepatic lipidosis. • Weight reduction in obese cats should be undertaken slowly and carefully. • Cats switched to weight reduction diets should be monitored to ensure adequate food intake. • Owners should carefully assess food intake during periods of family stress, such as the addition of a new family member or pet or moving.

POSSIBLE COMPLICATIONS

• Tube clogging or infection at gastrostomy tube entry site • Worsening hepatoencephalopathy • Disseminated intravascular coagulation • Hepatic failure and death

EXPECTED COURSE AND PROGNOSIS

• With aggressive tube feeding, 60% of cats with IHL survive. • Without aggressive dietary therapy, 10% of cats with IHL survive. • Cats with IHL have a better prognosis than cats with secondary hepatic lipidosis. • IHl seldom recurs in cats that survive the disease.

MISCELLANEOUS

ASSOCIATED CONDITIONS

• Pancreatitis • Diabetes mellitus • Other primary liver diseases

AGE RELATED FACTORS N/A

ZOONOTIC POTENTIAL N/A

PREGNANCY N/A

SYNONYMS

• Fatty liver syndrome • Hepatic steatosis

SEE ALSO N/A

ABBREVIATIONS

ACT = activated clotting time
ALP = alkaline phosphatase
ALT = alanine aminotransferase
AST = aspartate aminotransferase
FDP = fibrin degradation products
IHL = idiopathic hepatic lipidosis
PT = prothrombin time
PTT = partial thromboplastin time

References

Center SA, Crawford MA, Guida L, et al. A retrospective study of 77 cats with severe hepatic lipidosis: 1975-1990. J Vet Int Med 1993;7:349-359.

Dimski DS. Diagnosis, treatment, and pathophysiology of feline idiopathic hepatic lipidosis. Proceedings,17th Annual Waltham/Ohio State Univ Forum, Columbus, Ohio, 1993, pp. 56-62.

Akol KG, Washabau RJ, Saunders HM, Hendrick MJ. Acute pancreatitis in cats with hepatic lipidosis. J Vet Int Med 1993; 7:205-209.

Author Donna S. Dimski
Consulting Editor Albert E. Jergens

HEPATITIS, CHRONIC ACTIVE

BASICS

DEFINITION

Inflammation within the liver that is chronic and ongoing and results in accumulation of inflammatory cells and fibrosis within the hepatic parenchyma. Chronic active hepatitis is a syndrome in dogs with many causes; it is not a specific disease entity.

Pathophysiology

Initiated by any event that disrupts the normal hepatic architecture or activates cell-mediated immunity within the liver. Infectious agents and toxins are examples of inciting agents. Inflammatory cells, predominantly lymphocytes and plasma cells, accumulate initially in the periportal area, and released cytokines cause areas of hepatocyte necrosis. As the disease progresses, inflammatory cell infiltrates and hepatocyte necrosis bridge across hepatic lobules and fibrosis ensues. Cirrhosis and hepatic failure occur in the later stages of the disease.

Systems Affected

• Hepatobiliary—inflammation, necrosis, and fibrosis • Nervous—hepatoencephalopathy • Gastrointestinal—vomiting, anorexia, and ascites

Genetics

• Hepatitis caused by copper toxicity is associated with a genetic predisposition to copper accumulation in Bedlington terriers, West Highland white terriers, and perhaps other breeds (see copper hepatopathy). • Heredity may play a role in the development of chronic active hepatitis in doberman pinschers and cocker spaniels.

Incidence/Prevalence

Relatively common disease in dogs

Geographic distribution N/A

SIGNALMENT

Species

Dogs

Breed Predilections

• Bedlington terrier • West Highland white terrier • Doberman pinscher • Cocker spaniel • Labrador retriever • Skye terrier

Mean Age and Range

6 years (2-10 years)

Predominant Sex

Females overrepresented in many breeds

SIGNS

• Weight loss • Anorexia • Icterus • Ascites • Vomiting • Encephalopathy

CAUSES

Infectious

• Infectious canine hepatitis virus • Leptospirosis • Canine acidophil cell hepatitis

Immune-mediated

Toxins

• Copper hepatopathy • Drugs—anticonvulsants, diethylcarbamazine / oxibendazole

RISK FACTORS

• Breed • Sex • Age • Anticonvulsant administration • Drug administration

DIAGNOSIS

DIFFERENTIAL DIAGNOSIS:

• Acquired portosystemic shunt—differentiate by contrast radiography and liver biopsy • Hepatic neoplasia—differentiate by diagnostic imaging and liver biopsy • Other causes of ascites—right heart failure and renal or gastrointestinal loss of albumin • Other causes of icterus—biliary obstruction and hemolysis

CBC/BIOCHEMISTRY/URINALYSIS

• Nonregenerative anemia • Thrombocytopenia •High ALT and AST activities • High ALP activity • High serum bilirubin concentration • Hypoalbuminemia • Low BUN • Hypoglycemia • Bilirubinuria

OTHER LABORATORY TESTS

• High fasting or postprandial serum bile acid concentration • High plasma ammonia concentration • Prolonged coagulation times (ie, PT, PTT, ACT) • High FDP

IMAGING:

Abdominal Radiographic Findings

• Microhepatica • Ascites

Abdominal Ultrasonography

• Rules out biliary occlusion • Identifies increased echogenicity associated with hepatic fibrosis

OTHER DIAGNOSTIC PROCEDURES

Liver biopsy needed for diagnosis. Specimen can be obtained at surgery or by laparoscopy or ultrasound guidance.

GROSS AND HISTOPATHOLOGIC FINDINGS

• Gross findings may include microhepatica with cirrhosis and regenerative nodules. Acquired portosystemic shunts may be seen. • Histopathologic examination of the liver reveals accumulation of lymphocytes and plasma cells in the periportal regions. Characteristic lesions include piecemeal and/or bridging necrosis with erosion of the lobular limiting plate. Fibrosis and duplication of biliary structures may also be seen. Stains for copper should be performed to identify primary or secondary defects in copper metabolism.

TREATMENT

INPATIENT VS OUTPATIENT

Patients with severe disease require hospitalization. After stabilization, they may be managed on an outpatient basis.

ACTIVITY

Moderate restriction of activity is warranted in the initial treatment of chronic active hepatitis to promote hepatic regeneration.

DIET

Affected dogs should be fed adequate calories to promote hepatic regeneration. A diet containing small amounts of a high-quality protein source has been classically recommended. More normal protein diets are currently advocated.

CLIENT EDUCATION

• Affected dogs will probably be on medications for life.
• Many dogs with chronic active hepatitis can be managed for varying periods of time, but few dogs are cured of the disease or underlying process.

SURGICAL CONSIDERATIONS N/A

MEDICATIONS

DRUGS AND FLUIDS

• Ringer's solution supplemented with potassium and dextrose (if needed) is ideal for initial management of the nonascitic patient.
• 0.45% NaCl with 2.5% dextrose is used in patients with ascites.
• Hepatoencephalopathy must be treated appropriately (see Hepatic Encephalopathy).
• Copper hepatopathy must be appropriately managed if necessary (see Copper Hepatopathy).
• Furosemide (0.25-0.5 mg/kg IV or PO q8h-q12h) may be used to control ascites.
• Immune-mediated chronic active hepatitis is treated by immunosuppressive dosage of prednisone (1-2 mg/kg PO q12h). Azathioprine may also be used (0.5 mg/kg PO q48h).

CONTRAINDICATIONS

• Do not use drugs that are primarily metabolized by the liver, or drugs that alter liver blood flow or metabolism.
• Choleretic agents (eg, ursodeoxycholic acid) should not be used in patients with biliary obstruction.

PRECAUTIONS

• Corticosteroids may precipitate hepatic encephalopathy.
• Azathioprine depresses bone marrow function and may cause gastrointestinal toxicity and pancreatitis.

POSSIBLE INTERACTIONS

• Colchicine is available in a pure form and in combination with probenecid. Use only the pure form, because probenecid can cause vomiting and lethargy in some dogs.

ALTERNATE DRUGS

• Ursodeoxycholic acid is a choleretic that

has been used in humans with chronic active hepatitis, resulting in clinical improvement. It has been used in a few dogs with chronic active hepatitis (10-15 mg/kg/day), with reports of subjective improvement in clinical signs but minimal improvement in laboratory data or findings on histopathologic examination of the liver.
• Colchicine (0.03 mg/kg/day PO) has been used occasionally to manage cirrhosis in dogs. Studies of its efficacy are limited to anecdotal case reports.
• Chronic active hepatitis in humans is associated with low serum and liver zinc concentrations. Zinc acetate can be administered to dogs (200 mg elemental zinc/day). The dosage is adjusted to maintain a plasma zinc concentration of 200-300 mg/dl. Studies of efficacy in dogs have not been published.

FOLLOW-UP

PATIENT MONITORING
• Serum biochemical analysis should be done weekly in critically ill dogs to assess for improvement in liver enzyme activities and serum bilirubin concentration. • Monitor serum electrolytes every 2-4 weeks in dogs receiving furosemide. • Monitor CBC weekly for the first 2-4 weeks and periodically thereafter in patients receiving azathioprine.
• Monitor serum zinc concentration carefully to avoid a hemolytic crisis in patients receiving zinc acetate. • In dogs with stable disease, serum biochemicals and bile acids

should be monitored every 6-8 weeks.
• Ideally, dogs with chronic active hepatitis would have a second liver biopsy done 6 months to 1 year after initiation of treatment.

PREVENTION / AVOIDANCE
• Breeds with susceptibility to chronic active hepatitis should have serum biochemical analysis every 6 months.

POSSIBLE COMPLICATIONS
• Overwhelming infection secondary to immunosuppression • Worsening hepatoencephalopathy • Disseminated intravascular coagulation • Hepatic failure and death

EXPECTED COURSE AND PROGNOSIS
• If underlying cause can be corrected (e.g., drug administration stopped), prognosis is fair. • If immune-mediated disease is the cause, then most dogs live several months, with a maximum of 3 years.

MISCELLANEOUS

ASSOCIATED CONDITIONS N/A

AGE-RELATED FACTORS N/A

ZOONOTIC POTENTIAL N/A

PREGNANCY N/A

SYNONYMS:
• Chronic hepatitis • Doberman hepatitis

SEE ALSO
• Cirrhosis/Fibrosis of the Liver • Copper

Hepatopathy • Hepatic Encephalopathy • Hypertension, Portal

ABBREVIATIONS
ACT = activated clotting time
ALP = alkaline phosphatase
ALT = alanine aminotransferase
AST = aspartate aminotransferase
BUN = blood urea nitrogen
FDP = fibrin degradation products
PT = prothrombin time
PTT = partial thromboplastin time

References
Dill-Macky E. Chronic hepatitis in dogs. Vet Clin North Am Small Anim Pract 1995 (In Press).
Franklin JE, Saunders GK. Chronic active hepatitis in Doberman pinschers. Comp Cont Ed Pract Vet 1988; 10:1247-1254.
Leveille-Webster CR, Center SA. Chronic hepatitis: therapeutic considerations. In: Bonagura JD, ed. Kirk's current veterinary therapy XII. Philadelphia: WB Saunders, 1995;749-756.
Magne ML, Chiapella AM. Medical management of canine chronic hepatitis. Comp Cont Ed Pract Vet 1986; 8:915-921.
Strombeck DR, Miller LM, Harrold D. Effects of corticosteroid treatment on survival time in dogs with chronic hepatitis: 151 cases (1977-1985). J Am Vet Med Assoc 1988;193:1109-1113.

Author Donna S. Dimski
Consulting Editor Albert E. Jergens

HEPATITIS, GRANULOMATOUS

 BASICS

OVERVIEW

Hepatitis secondary to infection by specific bacterial, viral, parasitic, protozoal, or fungal organism resulting in granuloma formation or mononuclear phagocyte infiltration and inflammation of the liver. This process can be focal (localized) or part of a multisystemic disease, which may mask the underlying hepatic disease.

SIGNALMENT

• Dogs and cats • No breed, sex, or age predilection or known genetic basis

SIGNS

General Comments

The clinical signs range from none to signs of systemic disease.

Historical Findings

• Anorexia • Lethargy • Weight loss
• Vomiting • Diarrhea • Polyuria • Polydipsia

Physical Examination Findings

• Hepatomegaly • Abdominal pain
• Icterus • Ascites • Tachypnea • Fever

CAUSES AND RISK FACTORS

• Systemic fungal infection the most common cause (eg, blastomycosis, histoplasmosis, and coccidioidomycosis) • Bacterial infection (eg, brucellosis and mycobacterial disease)
• Neoplasia (eg, lymphosarcoma) • Parasitism (eg, visceral larval migrans, liver flukes, and dirofilariasis) • Viral (eg, feline infectious peritonitis) • Miscellaneous (eg, intestinal lymphangiectasia and idiopathic disease)

 DIAGNOSIS

DIFFERENTIAL DIAGNOSIS

Because of the multisystemic nature of this disease process, a degree of suspicion is necessary in order to make the diagnosis.

CBC/BIOCHEMISTRY/URINALYSIS

• Inflammatory or stress leukogram, nonregenerative anemia of chronic inflammation, and in some animals with parasitism. • High ALP, ALT, AST, and GGT, +/- high bilirubin; low glucose, albumin, and BUN; high or low total serum proteins, hypergammaglobulinemia, and electrolyte abnormalities in some animals with fluid and acid/base disturbances • Results of urinalysis may be normal or nonspecific, or may show proteinuria, RBC/WBC or cellular casts, other casts, and bilirubinuria.

OTHER LABORATORY TESTS

• High serum bile acid concentration • High sulfobromophthalein retention • Coagulation assays normal except in animals with end-stage liver failure • Serologic tests may reveal high fungal titer in animals with fungal disease, but these must be evaluated with caution.

IMAGING

• Radiographs may reveal hepatomegaly, abdominal mass, or loss of abdominal detail due to ascites. • Ultrasonography is useful in assessing liver size and architecture, and may assist in the diagnosis of localized lesions.

OTHER DIAGNOSTIC PROCEDURES

• Abdominocentesis with bacterial culture, sensitivity test, and cytologic examination may be useful if animal has ascites. • Laparoscopy or ultrasound guided liver biopsy are two possible means of obtaining liver tissue for definitive diagnosis. • Fungal stain, gram stain, and culture and sensitivity should be performed on blood, biopsy, or aspirated specimen.

 TREATMENT

• Must be tailored to the individual patient, depending on the underlying cause, severity of disease, and response to treatment. This is especially true in patients with multisystemic disease, which often causes granulomatous hepatitis.
• Causes of this syndrome are often difficult to treat (e.g., systemic blastomycosis and FIP), and the owners should be made aware of the guarded to poor prognosis.
• Nutritional support (enteral or parenteral nutrition) may be required if the patient is unwilling or unable to eat.

MEDICATIONS

DRUGS AND FLUIDS

• Appropriate drugs depend on the initiating cause of the granulomatous hepatic lesion. For each primary disease, consult the section that describes the treatment for that disease.
• Fluid administration should include a balanced polyionic solution such as lactated Ringer's solution and may require added dextrose (5%) and potassium. In almost all patients, potassium (10-20 mEq/L) should be added to the solution if the animal is not eating or if aggressive fluid therapy is necessary.
• Antiemetics or H2 receptor blocking drugs should be used if indicated to control vomiting or prevent gastrointestinal ulceration.

CONTRAINDICATIONS/ POSSIBLE INTERACTIONS

Because of the broad spectrum of possible causes of granulomatous hepatitis, the clinician must consider possible drug interactions once a definitive diagnosis is made.

 FOLLOW-UP

PATIENT MONITORING

Routine patient monitoring of fluid and acid/base balance and the general response to treatment. Repeat hematologic testing and ultrasound examination may be useful.

POSSIBLE COMPLICATIONS

Chronic hepatitis, cirrhosis, or hepatic failure may develop in patients with generalized granulomatous hepatitis.

EXPECTED COURSE/PROGNOSIS

This depends on the primary cause of the disease; however, in most patients, the prognosis is guarded at best due to the multisystemic nature of the problem.

 MISCELLANEOUS

ZOONOTIC POTENTIAL

Brucellosis is the main etiologic agent of concern.

PREGNANCY

No special considerations; the fetuses are likely to be affected, aborted, or stillborn.

ABBREVIATIONS

ALP = alkaline phosphatase
ALT = alanine aminotransferase
AST = aspartate aminotransferase
BUN = blood urea nitrogen
GGT = gamma glutamyl transferase
FIP = feline infectious peritonitis
RBC = red blood cell
WBC = white blood cell

Reference

Strombeck DR, Guilford WG. Diseases of the liver and biliary system. In: Strombeck DR, Guilford WG, eds. Small animal gastroenterology. 2nd ed. Davis, CA: Stonegate Publishing Co., 1990.

Author Debra L. Zoran
Consulting Editor Albert E. Jergens

HEPATITIS, INFECTIOUS—DOGS

BASICS

OVERVIEW
• Viral disease of dogs and other canidae caused by adenovirus I (CAV-1), which targets the liver, kidneys, eyes, and vascular endothelium. CAV-1 is serologically homogeneous, and antigenically distinct from CAV-2, the respiratory virus. • 4-8 days after oronasal exposure and localization in the tonsils, widespread viremia develops, resulting in virus localization in Kupffer cells and vascular endothelium. • During the initial viremic stages, saliva and feces are infectious. • The virus replicates in Kupffer cells and is eventually released, destroying nearby hepatocytes and resulting in massive viremia. • Within 10-14 days after infection, the virus is cleared from other tissues and localizes in the kidneys where it will be excreted in urine for 6-9 months. • The injury caused by the virus is also cytotoxic to the anterior uvea, which explains the appearance of severe anterior uveitis (hepatitis "blue eye") in some patients.

SIGNALMENT
• Disease of canidae, with no breed or sex predilections. • Unvaccinated dogs of any age can be affected, but primarily seen in dogs < 1 year old. • No genetic basis has been established for this disease.

SIGNS
• Determined by the immunologic status of the host. • Peracute—fever (103-106), CNS signs, vascular collapse, disseminated intravascular coagulopathy (DIC), and death within hours of onset • Acute—fever, anorexia, depression, vomiting and diarrhea, hepatomegaly, abdominal pain, ascites, vasculitis, lymphadenopathy, pyelonephritis, DIC, and hepatoencephalopathy. • Uncomplicated—depression, anorexia, transient fever, tonsillitis, vomiting and diarrhea, lymphadenopathy, hepatomegaly, and abdominal pain • Late—20% develop anterior uveitis and corneal edema 7 days after infection, and usually recover in 21 days.

CAUSES AND RISK FACTORS
• Canine adenovirus-1 • Unvaccinated status, immunosuppression, and or immunocompromise

DIAGNOSIS

DIFFERENTIAL DIAGNOSIS
Leptospirosis, suppurative hepatitis, granulomatous hepatitis, toxic hepatopathy, and any fulminant infectious disease (e.g., parvovirus and distemper).

CBC/BIOCHEMISTRY/URINALYSIS
• Initially, leukopenia caused by neutropenia and lymphopenia, but neutrophilia and lymphocytosis follow the acute, viremic stage. Also, low platelet count (animal with DIC), high nRBC count (patient with bone marrow damage caused by vasculitis or viremia), and low fibrinogen (animal with DIC) • High ALT, AST, SAP, and GGT (start to decrease in 14 days); low glucose and albumin (in animals with peracute or severe acute disease); electrolyte abnormalities because of vomiting and diarrhea (low sodium and potassium); high or low total protein • Proteinuria, WBC casts, and bilirubinuria

OTHER LABORATORY TESTS
• Bile acid assay—mild to moderately high concentration in both pre- and postprandial assays • Coagulation profile—abnormal in animals with DIC (e.g., high FDP and ACT; PT and PTT normal) • Serologic testing—IgM and IgG 4-fold increase (not routinely performed). ELISA for CAV-1 antibodies also available. • Viral isolation—anterior chamber and urine best specimens.

IMAGING
• Radiography may detect hepatomegaly or reduced abdominal detail associated with ascites. • Ultrasonography detects hepatomegaly; also may reveal hypoechoeic regions associated with hepatic necrosis, or anechoic regions will be seen if patient has ascites.

OTHER DIAGNOSTIC PROCEDURES
Liver biopsy: intranuclear inclusions in Kupffer cells and hepatocytes.

GROSS AND HISTOPATHOLOGIC FINDINGS
Hepatic necrosis, renal cortical necrosis, vasculitis, and anterior uveitis; virus can be isolated from kidneys, eyes, and tonsils, but rarely from the liver.

TREATMENT
• Provide supportive and symptomatic care depending on the severity of the clinical findings on examination. In uncomplicated cases, the patient may be treated as an outpatient. • Give the patient highly digestible diet to reduce gastrointestinal disturbances, and use antibiotics or antiemetics as indicated. • Restrict the animal's activity and access to other pets. • In complicated cases, hospitalization and aggressive supportive and symptomatic care may be required, including nutritional support if the dog is unable to eat for more than 48 hours.

MEDICATIONS

DRUGS AND FLUIDS
• Use balanced, isotonic fluids (lactated Ringer's solution) with added potassium (10-20 mEq/L) and dextrose (5%) if indicated. In dogs with fulminant hepatic failure, avoid lactate-containing fluids (Ringer's or physiologic saline are good alternatives). • Broad spectrum, bacteriocidal antibiotics (especially those effective versus gram negative and anaerobic bacteria from the gastrointestinal tract) e.g., ampicillin/amoxicillin, cephalexin/cephadroxil, amikacin/gentamycin, clindamycin/metronidazole combination therapy • Antiemetics if needed (e.g., chlorpromazine or metoclopramide). • If patient has DIC give plasma or component therapy, +/- heparin • If patient has signs of hepatoencephalopathy, consider lactulose, colonic lavage, and metronidazole antibiotic therapy.

CONTRAINDICATIONS/POSSIBLE INTERACTIONS
• Drugs requiring hepatic metabolism for activity or detoxification (eg, chloramphenicol, tetracycline, and phenobarbital) should be used with caution in patients with hepatic failure. • Avoid high protein diets in animals with hepatoencephalopathy or fulminant hepatic failure.

FOLLOW-UP

PATIENT MONITORING
Routine monitoring of fluid and acid/base balance, nutritional status, and response to treatment

PREVENTION/AVOIDANCE
• Vaccination at 6-8 weeks of age with 2 boosters 3-4 weeks apart and an annual revaccination • CAV-1 vaccines provide long-lasting immunity with a single dose, but viral shedding occurs and < 1% will develop "blue eye." • CAV-2 vaccines are effective against infectious canine hepatitis and will not cause urine shedding or anterior uveitis; however, annual revaccination is recommended.

POSSIBLE COMPLICATIONS
Pyelonephritis, DIC, glaucoma, chronic active hepatitis, septicemia due to hepatic failure, and hepatoencephalopathy

EXPECTED COURSE AND PROGNOSIS:
• Peracute—poor prognosis, death within hours of onset.

• Acute—guarded to good prognosis; in patient with a poor antibody response (titer 1:16 to 1:50) chronic hepatitis will develop; in patient with a good antibody response (> 1:500 IgG titer), complete recovery can be expected over a 5- to 7-day period.

MISCELLANEOUS

AGE RELATED FACTORS

None other than immune status and maternal immunity

ABBREVIATIONS

ACT = activated clotting time
ALP = alkaline phosphatase
ALT = alanine aminotransferase
AST = aspartate aminotransferase
CNS = central nervous system
DIC = disseminated intravascular coagulation
FDP = fibrin degradation products
GGT = gamma glutamyl transferase
PT = prothrombin time
PTT = partial thromboplastin time
nRBC = nucleated red blood cell
WBC = white blood cells

References

Greene C. Infectious canine hepatitis. In: Greene C, ed. Greene's infectious disease. 3rd ed. Philadelphia: WB Saunders, 1990.

Author Debra L. Zoran
Consulting Editor Albert E. Jergens

HEPATITIS, LEPTOSPIROSIS

BASICS

OVERVIEW

• Bacterial disease caused by the pathogenic leptospires—Leptospira interrogans.
• Serovars that have been identified in dogs include icterohemorrhagiae, canicola, pomona, grippotyphosa, ballum, bratislava, australis, tarassovi, and autumnalis. • Dogs are the maintenance hosts (carriers) for L. canicola. • The most common serovars isolated in dogs are L. icterohemorrhagiae, grippotyphosa, pomona, and canicola. • Cats are infrequently infected with leptospires, but L. bataviae, L. canicola, L. grippotyphosa, and L. pomona have been identified. • Infection occurs via oronasal exposure, primarily from contaminated water from urine of infected animals; however, transmission can occur via direct, venereal, placental, or indirect (fomites) routes including infected meat.
• The bacteria can survive for weeks in a warm, moist environment but do not survive freezing. • Leptospires can easily invade abraded skin and mucous membranes. • After infection, leptospiremia peaks in 4-12 days and is associated with a fever. • The site of primary localization and clinical signs depends on the infecting serovar, but in an animal with peracute infection death may be so rapid that it precludes development of signs of renal or liver disease.

SIGNALMENT

• Dogs and cats, but more common in dogs.
• No breed or genetic predilection • Males two times more commonly affected than females. • Severe disease occurs most commonly in young (< 1 year), unvaccinated dogs, immunocompromised dogs, and cats in a high risk environment. • Seasonal factor—prevalence higher in late summer and fall.

SIGNS

General Comments

• Clinical signs depend on which serovar is the cause of the disease, and may be acute, subacute, or chronic. • Infection with L. icterohemorrhagiae and L. canicola produces the most severe signs in dogs—hepatic necrosis and icterus and renal damage, respectively.
• L. pomona tends to cause subclinical infections and a chronic carrier state • L. grippotyphosa is often associated with development of chronic active hepatitis.

Historical Findings

• Depression • Lethargy • Anorexia
• Vomiting • Fever • Muscle stiffness
• Weight loss • Polyuria/polydipsia
• Diarrhea • Cough • Labored breathing
• Hematuria

Physical Examination Findings

• Painful abdomen • Depression • Lethargy
• Renomegaly • Hepatomegaly • Ocular/nasal discharge • Muscle stiffness • High or low body temperature • Cough • Tachypnea

CAUSES AND RISK FACTORS

Leptospira interrogans serovars icterohemorrhagiae, canicola, pomona, and grippotyphosa are the main serovars causing leptospirosis in dogs and cats; however, any of the serovars may cause disease in dogs or cats as incidental hosts. Exposure to wildlife, rodents, livestock, and the subclinical carrier are important risk factors.

DIAGNOSIS

DIFFERENTIAL DIAGNOSIS

Infectious canine hepatitis or any acute infectious disease or toxicity causing anorexia, fever, and vomiting and diarrhea, acute renal failure, and hepatopathy.

CBC/BIOCHEMISTRY/URINALYSIS

Abnormalities depend on serovar and severity of disease.
• Leukocytosis with or without a left shift, stress leukogram (ie, lymphopenia, eosinopenia, and monocytosis), leukopenia may occur in animal with peracute disease, low platelet count (animal with disseminated intravascular coagulation [DIC]); nonregenerative anemia in animals with chronic disease. • High BUN, creatinine, ALP ALT, AST, and bilirubin. Electrolyte and acid/base abnormalities may occur in association with metabolic acidosis if vomiting and diarrhea or renal failure is severe. • Isosthenuria or reduced concentrating ability, pyuria, glucosuria, hematuria, proteinuria, WBC and RBC or cellular casts, and bilirubinuria.

OTHER LABORATORY TESTS

Serologic Testing

• Paired IgM/IgG titers—peak titer at 3-4 weeks post infection; may remain positive for months or years; 4-fold increase in titer is diagnostic. • Microscopic agglutination test—most common and most definitive test if 2 titers taken over 3-4 weeks; uses specific serovars as antigens, but cross-reactions between serovars do occur; magnitude of titer does not correlate with prognosis or development of carrier state.
Titers:
1:100 = residual infection, response to infection, or vaccination.
1:100 - 1:300 = significant in unvaccinated patient.
> 1:300 = suggests active infection
> 1:1000 = diagnostic unless titer taken within 2-3 months of vaccination
• ELISA—greater sensitivity than microscopic agglutination test; paired IgM/IgG ELISA titers best. • Macroscopic plate agglutination test (rapid)—less sensitive test; > 1:40 = positive • Complement fixation test—detects recent or chronic infections

Bacterial Culture

• Leptospires are aerobic, fastidious, slow-growing, and very susceptible to environmental conditions. • The best samples are blood (acute stages only), urine (after acute stage), kidney, liver, and aqueous humor.

Darkfield Microscopy

Impractical technique because of low concentration of leptospires in urine and short survival of the bacterium in voided urine.

Coagulation Studies

High FDP, low fibrinogen, high ACT, +/- high PT and PTT if patient has DIC.

IMAGING

Radiographic Findings

Hepatomegaly and renomegaly and reduced abdominal contrast (ie, ascites) in some animals

Ultrasonographic Findings

Hepatomegaly and renomegaly, hypoechoeic regions because of hepatic necrosis, and renal cortical mineralization

OTHER DIAGNOSTIC PROCEDURES

Liver biopsy, obtaining specimen by aspiration, laparoscopy, or surgery

GROSS AND HISTOPATHOLOGIC FINDINGS

• Serovar specific • Lymphoplasmacytic and neutrophilic interstitial nephritis • Hepatic necrosis ranging from mild to severe and leading to hepatic fibrosis • In some animals, leptospires in renal or liver tissue shown by Warthin-Starry stain procedure

TREATMENT

• Supportive and symptomatic depending on the severity of disease
• Peritoneal dialysis if patient is anuric due to renal disease
• Nutritional support if vomiting and diarrhea precludes adequate nutrient intake

MEDICATIONS

DRUGS AND FLUIDS

Fluids

Balanced polyelectrolyte solutions (e.g., lactated Ringer's solution) with added potassium (10-20 mEq/L) administered IV

Antibiotics

• Procaine Pen G (40-80,000 IU/kg q12h for 14 days (for leptospiremia); adjust dosage if patient has renal failure.
• Alternatives to penicillin for treatment of leptospiremia—ampicillin, amoxicillin, cefotaxine, and ciprofloxin.
• Doxycycline (10-15 mg/kg IM q12h to eliminate renal carrrier)
• Alternative to doxycycline—minocycline and dihydrostreptomycin

Diuretics
Osmotic diuretic, loop diuretic or low-dose dopamine if patient is oliguric or anuric due to renal disease

CONTRAINDICATIONS/POSSIBLE INTERACTIONS
Use all drugs with caution because of reduced renal and hepatic elimination.

FOLLOW-UP

PATIENT MONITORING
• Monitor Leptospira titers to assess diagnostic accuracy. • Routine monitoring of renal and hepatic biochemistries to assess progress and treatment

PREVENTION/AVOIDANCE
• Vaccination is effective only for the serovars that the vaccine contains (eg, L. canicola and L. icterohemorrhagiae), and the duration of immunity is not long (6-12 months). Revaccinate show animals and hunting dogs and animals in high-risk areas more than

once yearly. Immunity to one serovar does not convey immunity to others. • Environmental control is important for prevention—control of rodents, elimination of standing water and isolation of all infected animals to reduce exposure; but elimination of the carrier state is unrealistic due to wild animal reservoirs and subclinical infections (e.g., L. canicola and L. pomona), which are widespread.

POSSIBLE COMPLICATIONS
Chronic active hepatitis and chronic renal dysfunction or shedding

EXPECTED COURSE/PROGNOSIS
• Depends on serovar, severity of disease, and host immunity. • The prognosis for recovery is good in patients with subacute infection and guarded in patients with acute infection.

MISCELLANEOUS

ZOONOTIC POTENTIAL
Contaminated urine is highly infectious to humans and animals.

ABBREVIATIONS
ACT = activated clotting time
ALP = alkaline phosphatase
ALT = alanine aminotransferase
AST = aspartate aminotransferase
BUN = blood urea nitrogen
DIC = disseminated intravascular coagulation
FDP = fibrin degradation products
PTT = partial thromboplastin time
PT = prothrombin time
RBC = red blood cells
WBC = white blood cells

References

Greene C. Leptospirosis. In: Greene C, ed. Greene's infectious diseases. 3rd ed. Philadelphia: WB Saunders, 1990.

Rentko VT, Clark N, et al. Canine leptospirosis. J Vet Int Med, 1992;6:235-44.

Author Debra L. Zoran

Consulting Editor Albert E. Jergens

HEPATITIS, SUPPURATIVE AND HEPATIC ABSCESS

BASICS

OVERVIEW
Generalized or localized infection of the liver involving pyogenic bacteria, usually bacteria from the gastrointestinal tract, and often associated with infection of other organs. Because of the liver's unique and important position as the primary interface between the gut and the rest of the body, any reduction in or inhibition of the function of the hepatic monocyte/macrophage system can result in development of hepatitis or an hepatic abscess.

SIGNALMENT
• Both dogs and cats but rare in both. • No breed or sex predilections • All ages can be affected. • No known genetic basis, but animals with genetically based immunodeficiency predisposed to infection

SIGNS
Nonspecific and may be related to other organ systems

Historical Findings
• Anorexia • Lethargy • Weight loss • Intermittent abdominal pain • Polyuria • Polydipsia

Physical Examination Findings
• Persistent fever • Hepatomegaly • Abdominal enlargement • Tachypnea • Dehydration • Lymphadenopathy • Vomiting • Diarrhea • Ascites

CAUSES/RISK FACTORS
• Hematogenous—septicemia/bacterial endocarditis, portal vein extension of gastrointestinal bacteria • Neonates—extension from umbilical vein (omphlebitis) • Direct extension—acute pancreatic abscess, peritonitis (e.g., gastrointestinal perforation and contamination from gastrointestinal surgery), and biliary tract infection • Hepatic parenchymal damage—trauma, neoplasia • Immunosuppressive disease—diabetes, Cushing's disease

DIAGNOSIS

DIFFERENTIAL DIAGNOSIS
Because of the wide range of associated conditions that often occur in animals with suppurative hepatitis, a degree of clinical suspicion is required to make the diagnosis.

CBC/BIOCHEMISTRY/URINALYSIS
• Inflammatory leukogram (leukocytosis with a left shift +/-lymphopenia and monocytosis with chronicity), nonregenerative anemia, and hypergammaglobulinemia • High ALT, AST, SAP, GGT, bilirubin (these elevations can vary and may be minor); low albumin and glucose in animals with severe hepatic compromise; electrolyte abnormalities vary, and depend on the presence of vomiting and diarrhea and other conditions that alter acid/base status. • Results of urinalysis may be normal, nonspecific, or may show proteinuria, WBC/RBC casts, and glucosuria.

OTHER LABORATORY TESTS
• Bile acid concentration may be high, the degree depending on the severity and extent of the hepatic insult. • Coagulation assays are important to evaluate whether liver compromise is severe, or whether biopsy or laparotomy is indicated. • Blood culture or culture and sensitivity and cytologic (including gram stain) examination of an abdominocentesis specimen may be indicated if a murmur is ausculted or if abdominal fluid is detected. • Screening for hyperadrenocorticism or diabetes mellitus may be indicated.

IMAGING
• Radiographic findings are nonspecific, but hepatomegaly, hepatic mass, or reduced abdominal detail due to ascites may be detected. • Ultrasonography is often useful in localizing hepatic parenchymal abnormality (e.g., mass, abscess, or infiltrative disease) and can also be used in conjunction with percutaneous biopsy to obtain tissue for histopathologic examination and bacterial culture and sensitivity test.

OTHER DIAGNOSTIC PROCEDURES
Laparoscopy could be used to visualize the liver and abdominal tissues and obtain specimens for biopsy or bacterial culture.

GROSS AND HISTOPATHOLOGIC FINDINGS
• Suppurative hepatitis or hepatic abscess may involve one or multiple lobes of the liver. If blind percutaneous biopsy is done, finding normal tissue does not rule out suppurative hepatitis. • Suppurative hepatitis is characterized by polymorphonuclear cell infiltration of hepatocytes, either in the form of a localized abscess, or as a more generalized infiltration of the hepatic parenchyma with or without maintenance of hepatic architecture.

TREATMENT
• Successful treatment is based on identifying and correcting the underlying cause of the hepatic disease. Because suppurative hepatitis is usually secondary to an infection elsewhere in the body, or caused by a disruption of the immunologic competence of the host, aggressive treatment is required to achieve a successful outcome.
• In animals with hepatic abscess, surgical removal and drainage is essential to complete recovery. This fact is complicated by the problem that the patient may already be compromised by the primary disease process that initiated the liver disease.
• The prognosis for these animals is guarded at best, and the owners should be made aware of this at the outset.

• Nutritional support may be required in patients with severe hepatic disease and debilitation.

MEDICATIONS

DRUGS AND FLUIDS
• Balanced isotonic fluids (lactated Ringer's solution +/- 5% dextrose with added potassium, 10-20 mEq/L) should be given to correct any acid/base or fluid imbalance before surgery. Note: use nonlactated Ringer's or 0.9% saline if fulminant hepatic failure is suspected or imminent.
• Antibiotics should be chosen on the basis of results of culture and sensitivity testing, but broad-spectrum (bacteriocidal against gram +/- aerobes and anaerobes) combination therapy should be instituted as soon as possible in septic patients. Intravenous administration of antibiotics is indicated if septicemia, bacterial endocarditis, or endotoxemia is suspected or imminent. Good antibiotic combinations include penicillin-derivative/aminoglycoside, cephalosporin/aminoglycoside, trimethoprim/sulfadiazine, and metronidazole/enrofloxacin.
• Antiemetics and or H2 blocking drugs may be indicated to control vomiting or prevent gastric ulceration in dogs or cats with severe hepatitis.

CONTRAINDICATIONS/POSSIBLE INTERACTIONS
Use drugs that are metabolized or excreted by hepatic mechanisms with caution.

FOLLOW-UP

PATIENT MONITORING
• Routine monitoring of fluid and acid/base balance to assure adequacy of the treatment
• Any other specific tests or management practices depend on the underlying cause of the condition.

POSSIBLE COMPLICATIONS
Fulminant hepatic failure, septicemia (if not already the underlying cause), endotoxemia, pyelonephritis or interstitial nephritis, and disseminated intravascular coagulation.

EXPECTED COURSE AND PROGNOSIS
This depends on the initial cause, the extent of the hepatic lesions, and the response to treatment.

MISCELLANEOUS

ASSOCIATED CONDITIONS
• Diabetes mellitus • Hyperadrenocorticism • Chemotherapy

ABBREVIATIONS

ALP = alkaline phosphatase
ALT = alanine aminotransferase
AST = aspartate aminotransferase
GGT = gamma glutamyl transferase
RBC = red blood cells
WBC = white blood cells

References

Strombeck DR, Guilford WG. Diseases of the liver and biliary tract. In: Strombeck DR, Guilford WG, eds. Small animal gastroenterology. 2nd ed. Davis, CA: Stonegate Publishing, 1990.

Grooters AM, Sherding RG, Biller DS, et al. Hepatic abscesses associated with diabetes mellitus in two dogs. J Vet Intern Med 1994; 8:203-206.

Author Debra L. Zoran

Consulting Editor Albert E. Jergens

HEPATOCELLULAR ADENOMA (HEPATOMA)

BASICS

OVERVIEW
Hepatocellular adenoma is a benign tumor of epithelial origin. It is more common than malignant liver tumors.

SIGNALMENT
• Rare in dogs and very rare in cats • Age and breed predispositions unknown

SIGNS
• Usually clinically silent but rupture may lead to hemoperitoneium • Single or multiple, well-circumscribed liver masses that may be pedunculated • Often highly vascular and friable

CAUSES AND RISK FACTORS
Unknown

DIAGNOSIS

DIFFERENTIAL DIAGNOSIS
• Hepatic adenocarcinoma • Hepatic abscess • Abdominal mass • Splenomegaly

CBC/BIOCHEMISTRY/URINALYSIS
• Results usually normal • Liver enzymes usually normal

OTHER LABORATORY TESTS N/A

IMAGING
• Plain radiography confirms large, asymmetrical liver. • Ultrasonography reveals mixed echopattern in the liver mass.

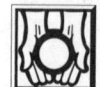

TREATMENT
Surgical excision is best.

MEDICATIONS

DRUGS AND FLUIDS N/A

CONTRAINDICATIONS/POSSIBLE INTERACTIONS N/A

FOLLOW-UP

PATIENT MONITORING
• Abdominal palpation to evaluate for recurrence every 3 months for the first year
• Abdominal imaging (i.e., radiography and ultrasonography) to evaluate for recurrence every 3 months for the first year

PREVENTION/AVOIDANCE N/A

POSSIBLE COMPLICATIONS
None unless associated with surgery

EXPECTED COURSE AND PROGNOSIS
Usually good

MISCELLANEOUS

ASSOCIATED CONDITIONS
• Histologically can be difficult to distinguish from nodular hyperplasia or normal liver tissue • Hepatoma is a confusing term and should be avoided since it refers to hepatocellular carcinoma in human medicine, although it is synonymous with hepatocellular adenoma in veterinary medicine

Reference
Klasuner JS, Hardy RM. Alimentary tract, liver, and pancreas. In: Slatter D, ed.Textbook of small animal surgery. Philadelphia: WB Saunders, 1993:2088-2105.

Author Wallace B. Morrison
Consulting Editor Wallace B. Morrison

BASICS

OVERVIEW
• Primary hepatic neoplasms are rare in dogs and cats, representing approximately 1.2% and 1.7% of all tumors in these species, respectively. • Hepatocellular carcinoma is the most common hepatic malignancy in dogs, although bile duct carcinoma is more common in cats.

SIGNALMENT
• Dogs—mean age 10-11 years • Cats—usually older than 10 years • A male predisposition reported in dogs • No breed predilection in dogs or cats

SIGNS

Historical Findings
• Highly variable; patients may have nonspecific signs for several months before diagnosis • Anorexia • Weight loss • Vomiting and/or diarrhea • Lethargy • Abdominal swelling • Signs associated with advanced disease—icterus, ascites, and CNS abnormalities (e.g., seizures and behavioral changes)

Physical Examination Findings
• Hepatomegaly • Ascites • Abdominal pain • Abdominal distension • Icterus • Palpable abdominal mass more readily detected in patients with hepatocellular carcinoma than with bile duct carcinoma.

CAUSES AND RISK FACTORS
Cause remains obscure

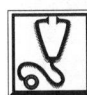

DIAGNOSIS

DIFFERENTIAL DIAGNOSIS

Gross Differentials
• Hepatocellular adenoma • Bile duct carcinoma • Nodular hyperplasia • Cirrhosis • Chronic active hepatitis • Use histologic features to differentiate. The histologic distinction between well-differentiated hepatocellular carcinoma and hepatocellular adenoma can be difficult.

CBC/BIOCHEMISTRY/URINALYSIS
• Changes in hematologic and biochemical values are common but are nonspecific for liver cancer. High serum enzyme (i.e., ALP, ALT, and AST) activities, hypoalbuminemia, hypergammaglobulinemia, hypoglycemia,

and high direct and indirect bilirubin support a diagnosis of liver disease. • Hematologically, nonregenerative anemia and leukocytosis are common.

OTHER LABORATORY TESTS
A coagulogram should be performed before biopsy or surgical procedure.

IMAGING
• Abdominocentesis and cytologic examination • Abdominal radiography to help localize the abdominal mass to the liver • Thoracic radiography to identify pulmonary metastases • Abdominal ultrasonography to assess parenchymal integrity, confirm the organ of origin, and guide fine-needle aspiration or biopsy of the tumor

OTHER DIAGNOSTIC PROCEDURES
Abdominocentesis and cytologic examination

GROSS AND HISTOPATHOLOGIC FINDINGS
• Vary from small, round, discrete lesions to large, diffuse masses > 10 cm in diameter • Hepatocellular carcinoma is usually soft and friable, unlike bile duct carcinoma which has a firm consistency. • Found in any lobe of the dog's liver, although the left lateral lobe most commonly affected • Neoplasms found in more than one liver lobe because of multiple primary lesions or intrahepatic metastases of a single neoplasm • Histologically, well-differentiated carcinoma may closely resemble normal hepatocytes or hepatocellular adenoma; the undifferentiated neoplasm has highly pleomorphic cells that are not readily recognized as hepatocyte in origin.

TREATMENT
• Surgical excision the treatment of choice for hepatic tumors • Up to 75% of the liver can be resected without marked hepatic dysfunction.

MEDICATIONS

DRUGS AND FLUIDS
No successful chemotherapy has been reported in dogs or cats.

CONTRAINDICATIONS/POSSIBLE INTERACTIONS
• Medications requiring metabolism by the liver should be used with caution in dogs and cats with hepatopathies.

• Hepatotoxicity from anticancer drugs appears to be of little or no clinical importance in small animals.

FOLLOW-UP
• Prognosis poor • Survival times of < 80 days after surgery reported in animals despite lack of evidence of metastases • The degree of invasiveness, presence of metastases, and tumor resectability are the most reliable indicators of survival. • The metastatic rate for hepatocellular carcinoma is 61%. Metastases occurs most commonly to the lungs and hepatic lymph nodes, although metastases to the heart, spleen, kidneys, intestines, brain, and ovary via the vascular system occasionally occurs. The neoplasm also spreads by direct extension to the omentum and peritoneum.

MISCELLANEOUS

ASSOCIATED CONDITIONS
• The nonneoplastic liver tissue is usually histologically normal in animals with hepatocellular carcinoma. • In contrast to humans, cirrhosis is rarely found in the liver of dogs with this carcinoma. • Hepatic neoplasms are commonly diagnosed in geriatric, debilitated animals that require concurrent management of cardiac, renal, metabolic, and electrolyte abnormalities.

PREGNANCY
Chemotherapy drugs may be carcinogenic and mutagenic.

Reference
Popp JA. Tumors of the liver, gall bladder, and pancreas. In: Moulton JE, ed. Tumors in domestic animals. 3rd ed. Berkeley, CA: University of California Press, 1990;436-449.
Author Stanley L. Marks
Consulting Editor Wallace B. Morrison

HEPATORENAL SYNDROME

 BASICS

OVERVIEW
• Failure of renal function that develops in some dogs and cats because of severe liver dysfunction • No overt pathologic changes found in the kidneys • Renal function improves if the liver disease improves. • The cause of renal dysfunction is believed to be intrarenal vasoconstriction and reduced "effective" plasma volume. • The tubules may not respond to increasing concentration of atrial natriuretic hormone. • Increase in concentrations of catecholamines and angiotensin, and decrease in glomerulopressin may precipitate further tubular dysfunction in the face of concurrent depletion of plasma volume and cardiac output reserves. • Opinions vary regarding prevalence.

SIGNALMENT
Cats or dogs may be affected at any age.

SIGNS
Urine output is initially high and then oliguric renal failure may follow.

CAUSES AND RISK FACTORS
• Liver failure caused by any common pathogenic mechanism (e.g., toxic, infectious, neoplastic, and inflammatory) is the primary risk factor. • Concurrent dehydration and ascites are hypothesized to increase the risk.

 DIAGNOSIS

DIFFERENTIAL DIAGNOSIS
• The nouveau development of acute nephrosis or prerenal azotemia or concurrent presence of chronic renal failure may be difficult to differentiate from hepatorenal syndrome if preexisting laboratory values are not available to the clinician. • Hepatorenal syndrome may be associated with the polyuria seen occasionally in dogs with liver disease. However, hepatorenal syndrome also is characterized by renal azotemia.

CBC/BIOCHEMISTRY/URINALYSIS
• Hypoalbuminemia • Hyperbilirubinemia • Creatinine is high and values may rapidly rise or gradually increase over several weeks. • Hyposthenuria

OTHER LABORATORY TESTS
Vary with the nature of the liver disease

IMAGING N/A

OTHER DIAGNOSTIC PROCEDURES
Ultrasound guided, percutaneous, or renal biopsy (after assessment of anesthetic concerns and coagulation function) can be performed at the same time as hepatic biopsy.

 TREATMENT

Treatment constitutes correction of fluid imbalances and underlying causes of hepatic disease. Particular attention to hypokalemia and metabolic alkalosis is needed.

MEDICATIONS

DRUGS AND FLUIDS
• Appropriate replacement fluids • Volume expanders (e.g., dextrans, hetastarch, and plasma proteins) • Other medication as dictated by the underlying liver disease

CONTRAINDICATIONS/ POSSIBLE INTERACTIONS
Pharmacologic selections for an animal with hepatorenal syndrome require the same concern as would any renal disorder. Aminoglycosides (nephrotoxic), furosemide (promotes dehydration), hypotensive agents (e.g., acetylpromazine), and nonsteroidal antiinflammatory drugs (cause papillary tubular necrosis) should be administered with caution.

FOLLOW-UP
• Monitoring of urine output, serum total solids, body weight, plasma osmolality, and central venous pressure may be helpful. • The prognosis is poor. In human medicine, 90% of patients do not survive.

MISCELLANEOUS

References
Strombeck DR, Guilford WG. Small animal gastroenterology. 2nd ed. Davis, CA: Stonegate Publishing, 1990:511.
Author Mark E. Hitt
Consulting Editor Albert E. Jergens

HEPATOTOXINS

BASICS

DEFINITION
Substances that induce dysfunction and clinical or overt pathologic changes in the liver. These substances can be endogenous or exogenous. If the hepatotoxin or its active metabolite causes injury that is predictable, it is called a direct or an intrinsic hepatotoxin. If it is not predictable, it is referred to as an idiosyncratic hepatotoxin.

Pathophysiology
Hepatotoxins cause cytopathic (necrosis or marked hepatocellular injury), cholestatic, or mixed patterns of histopathologic lesions. The liver can be the target of a wide array of substances because of its central role in the body's metabolic and detoxifying functions. Factors that affect susceptibility of the animal and severity of disease include, species, nutrition, drugs, concurrent disease, heredity, and prior "exposures" of the liver to the same or similar compounds.

Systems Affected
• Hepatobiliary—liver injury varies, depending on the factors listed, the concentration of the toxic substance, and the duration of exposure. The effect of hepatic toxicity ranges in clinical importance from high enzyme activity and no signs to fulminant hepatic failure. • Nervous—hepatic encephalopathy • Renal/urologic—hepatorenal syndrome (rare)

Genetics N/A

Incidence/Prevalence
Hepatotoxicity is not uncommon in most clinical practices.

Geographic Distribution N/A

SIGNALMENT

Species
Cats are generally more susceptible than dogs to hepatotoxicosis because they have lower endogenous hepatic concentrations of glucuronides and less acetylation capabilities.

Breed Predilections
Some familial lines of Siamese cats are reported to be at higher risk than other breeds because they have lower concentrations of glucuronides.

Mean Age and Range
Animals < 16 weeks old may have immature hepatic enzyme function for metabolism and excretion of drugs.

Predominant Sex N/A

SIGNS

General Comments
A detailed history of environment, medications (prescribed and over the counter), and past medical history is important.

Historical Findings
Profound malaise and anorexia in many animals

Physical Examination Findings
• Fever varies. • Icterus in some animals, but may develop later in the course of disease (e.g., 48–96 hours). • Ascites is a grave sign when induced by toxicosis. • In animals with severe hepatic failure, hepatic encephalopathy causes coma.

CAUSES

Drugs
• Acetaminophen (dogs, cats) • Diethylcarbamazine (Dirofilaria immitus microfilaria positive dogs) • Diethylcarbamazine-oxibendazole (dogs) • Glucocorticoids (dogs) • Griseofulvin (cats) • Halothane (dogs) • Mebendazole (dogs) • Megesterol acetate (cats) • Methoxyflurane (dogs) • Phenytoin (dogs) • Primidone (dogs) • Thiacetarsemide (dogs) • Trimethoprim-sulfadiazine (dogs)

Chemicals (eg)
• Aflatoxins • Chlorinated chemical compounds • Dimethylnitrosamine • Dinitrophenol • Heavy metals • Phenols

Endotoxins
• Enteric organisms (e.g., Clostridium perfringens and difficile) • Food poisoning

RISK FACTORS
• The use of medications that influence hepatic metabolism (e.g., phenobarbital, diazepam, chloramphenicol, halothane, and cimetidine) • Primary liver disease

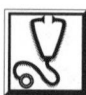

DIAGNOSIS

DIFFERENTIAL DIAGNOSIS
Any disorder that affects the liver needs to be distinguished from hepatotoxicosis. Attention to infectious canine hepatitis, feline infectious peritonitis, toxoplasmosis, suppurative cholangitis, and leptospirosis is warranted.

CBC/BIOCHEMISTRY/URINALYSIS
• The PCV and total solids are often normal or high in animals with acute hepatotoxicoses. • Extremely high serum ALT activity (proportionately greater than serum ALP activity) in animals that have not been subjected to known trauma suggests toxicosis. Because many hepatotoxins are associated with acute exposure, monitoring of serum may identify an initial peak ALT (often in the thousands) that declines quickly in 2–3 days. The concentration of ALT has no prognostic importance since hepatocytes can be irreversibly or reversibly injured. Serum ALT activity and total bilirubin concentration may be high. Loss of hepatic function varies. The albumin, urea nitrogen, and glucose concentrations may be normal, high, or low.

OTHER LABORATORY TESTS
• Monitoring of PT and PTT is important, because production of coagulation factors may be quickly reduced. Platelets and FDP should be evaluated to detect disseminated intravascular coagulopathy (DIC). • If serum bilirubin concentration is not high, then serum bile acid concentration can be used to assess hepatic function. • Drug assays are costly and results are often delayed.

IMAGING
• Radiography—liver size is normal to large in animals with acute toxicity and small, normal, or large in animals with chronic disease. • Ultrasonography—hepatic margins and parenchymal changes vary sonographically. .

OTHER DIAGNOSTIC PROCEDURES
Needle biopsy of the liver is useful to confirm diagnosis and assess severity.

GROSS AND HISTOPATHOLOGIC FINDINGS
• Findings vary. • Periportal changes suggest portal delivery of direct hepatotoxins.

TREATMENT
Principles of nursing care are critical.

INPATIENT VS OUTPATIENT
Patients should be in a critical care setting.

ACTIVITY Quiet and rest

DIET
A protein restricted diet is advised. Calories should be accurately calculated.

CLIENT EDUCATION
• The potential for 3–10 days of critical care and intensive efforts should be discussed. • The potential for future fibrosis or cirrhosis should be mentioned.

SURGICAL CONSIDERATIONS N/A

MEDICATIONS

DRUGS AND FLUIDS

Prevention or Correction of Shock
• Adequate fluids are essential in order to maintain microvascular perfusion.
• To improve delivery of oxygen and removal of waste substances, administer 1.5 times maintenance fluid rates. Initial administration is for replacement of fluid deficit, followed by maintenance dosage. Careful attention must be given to possible overhydration and monitoring of urine output. The use of 5% dextrose containing solutions is helpful in maintaining euglycemia.
• If necessary, a short acting glucocorticoid can be administered (e.g., prednisolone sodium succinate).
• Intravenous use of penicillin or ampicillin is advised for infection by normal enteric flora of aerobic and anaerobic bacteria. Concurrent parenteral use of an aminoglycoside or enrofloxacin is advised.

Nutritional support
• Branched chain amino acid solutions, supplementation of water soluble vitamins (e.g.,

B-complex), and supplementation with Vitamin K_1 in severely affected patients
• Parenteral nutritional support may be indicated.

Choleretic Agents
As oral medications become tolerated, consideration can be given to ursodeoxycholic acid (10-15 mg/kg q24h PO).

CONTRAINDICATIONS
Avoid drugs that require hepatic metabolism.

PRECAUTIONS
Drugs listed in the medications section should be used with caution.

POSSIBLE INTERACTIONS N/A

ALTERNATE DRUGS N/A

FOLLOW-UP

PATIENT MONITORING
• Prevent hypothermia • Daily assessment of blood glucose, electrolytes, and PCV is important since fluctuations can occur rapidly.
• Repeat serum biochemical analysis every 48 hours helps assess the patient's status and response to treatment.

PREVENTION/AVOIDANCE
Close scrutiny of the pet's environment is advised. Concern for future medication selection is emphasized.

POSSIBLE COMPLICATIONS
DIC, hepatic encephopathy, and progressive hepatic failure

EXPECTED COURSE AND PROGNOSIS
• In many patients, 3–5 days are needed to assess the prognosis. • The worsening of patient status, intractable emesis and hematemesis, intolerance to supportive treatment, oliguria, DIC, and hepatic encephalopathy are all poor indicators.
•The possibility of postnecrotic cirrhosis should be discussed with the client.

MISCELLANEOUS

ASSOCIATED CONDITIONS
• Hepatitis and fibrosis • Hepatic encephalopathy • Icterus

AGE RELATED FACTORS
• Young animals may have greater exposure to and ingestion of toxic substances. • Older animals may have diseases necessitating drug use that increases risk.

ZOONOTIC POTENTIAL N/A

PREGNANCY
Tetracycline can cause cholestatic liver disease in pregnant animals.

SYNONYMS N/A

SEE ALSO
• Cirrhosis/Fibrosis of the Liver • Hepatic Encephalopathy • Hepatic Failure, Acute
• Hepatorenal Syndrome • Poisoning (Intoxication)

ABBREVIATIONS
ALP = alkaline phosphatase
ALT = alanine aminotransferase
DIC = disseminated intravascular coagulation
FDP = fibrin degradation products
PCV = packed cell volume
PTT = partial thromboplastin time
PT = prothrombin time

References
Strombeck DR, Guilford WG. Small animal gastroenterology. 2nd ed. Davis, CA: Stonegate Publishing Company, 1990:511.
George CF, George RH. The liver and response to drugs. In: Wright R, et al, eds. Liver and biliary disease. Philadelphia: WB Saunders, 1985:415–452.
Author Mark E. Hitt
Consulting Editor Albert E. Jergens

HEPTAZOONOSIS

BASICS

OVERVIEW
• Infection with a protozoan of the genus Hepatozoon • Areas of involvement can include bone, liver, spleen, muscles, capillaries of the myocardium, and small intestinal epithelium.

Incidence/Prevalence
• Rare in cats in the United States (one report in a cat from Hawaii) • Uncommon in dogs, more common in southern and southwestern United States

SIGNALMENT
Breed Predilections N/A
Mean Age and Range All ages
Predominant Sex N/A

SIGNS
• Typically none • May produce severe clinical disease, including fever, inappetence, bloody diarrhea, and neurologic manifestations

CAUSES AND RISK FACTORS
• Ingestion of an infected tick of the genus Rhipicephalus • Presence of ticks of the genus Rhipicephalus

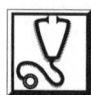

DIAGNOSIS

DIFFERENTIAL DIAGNOSIS
• Purulent inflammation • Endocarditis • Hypertrophic ostearthropy • Chagas' disease • Leishmaniasis • Babesiosis • Ehrlichiosis

CBC/BIOCHEMISTRY/URINALYSIS
Dogs—neutrophilia and associated elevated leukocyte count. Low serum glucose and high ALP activity.

OTHER LABORATORY TESTS N/A

IMAGING
Images of pelvis and lumbar vertebrae may reveal periosteal proliferation, especially in dogs under 1 year of age.

DIAGNOSTIC PROCEDURES
• Blood films to identify parasites in circulating neutrophils and monocytes • Muscle biopsy

GROSS AND HISTOPATHOLOGIC FINDINGS
• Cachexia • Muscle atrophy • Enlarged liver and spleen that may contain schizont stages on histopathology • Periosteal proliferation of bone

TREATMENT
• Hospitalization of animals in severe pain with symptomatic relief provided
• Inform the owner of the potential need to control ticks (i.e., the one-host Rhipicephalus) within their household or kennel.
• There is no reported risk to humans.

MEDICATIONS

DRUGS AND FLUIDS
• Mostly palliative; glucocorticoids may give temporary relief but should only be used for short-term to avoid immunosuppression

• Nonsteroidal antinflammatories are helpful.
• Treatment with primaquine and tetracycline reportedly offers clearance of parasitemias on rare occasions.

CONTRAINDICATIONS/POSSIBLE INTERACTIONS N/A

FOLLOW-UP
Parasitemia hard to diagnose in chronically infected animals; best to monitor signs for improvement

EXPECTED COURSE AND PROGNOSIS
Infection is often asymptomatic.

MISCELLANEOUS

Reference
Craig TM. Hepatozoonosis. In: Infectious disease of the dog and cat. Greene CE, ed. Philadelphia: WB Saunders, 1990:786-791.
Authors Dwight Bowman and Edward Pearce
Consulting Editor Fred W. Scott

BASICS

OVERVIEW

• Canine herpesvirus (CHV) is the cause of a systemic, usually fatal disease in young pups. Litter mortality is high. All organ systems are affected. Clinical disease is rare in dogs older than 3-4 weeks of age. • Mature, nonpregnant animals usually have inapparent, localized infections in the nasopharynx or external genitalia. CHV has been isolated from dogs with respiratory disease, but no causal link has been demonstrated. Transplacental infections during the last 3 weeks of gestation may result in fetal deaths, often with mummification, abortions, or the birth of dead or dying pups. Localized genital infections have been reported in both sexes. • Virus remains latent in the trigeminal nerve ganglia after primary infection, and may be excreted in nasal secretions at unpredictable intervals. Recrudescence can be provoked by stress or corticosteroid treatment. • The virus is common in the worldwide dog population, but disease is infrequent. Poor regulation of body temperature and immature immune response mechanisms are believed responsible for the exceptional susceptibility of pups less than 2-3 weeks of age.

SIGNALMENT

• Members of the dog family (dogs, coyotes, and wolves) are susceptible. • Most infected pups die between 9 and 14 days after birth; the range varies from 1 day (prenatal infection) to 1 month (neonatal infection). • The disease is most commonly reported in pure-bred dogs, although there is no breed predilection.

SIGNS

• The incubation period in neonatal pups is 4-6 days. Onset of disease is sudden, with deaths occurring 12-36 hours later. Some pups are found dead without premonitory signs. • The course is rapid. Signs in affected pups include dyspnea; serous to mucopurulent nasal discharge; anorexia; grayish-yellow or green, soft, odorless stool; persistent, agonizing crying; encephalitic signs; severe gasping before death. Occasionally, pups may present with petechial hemorrhages on the mucous membranes. • Occasionally, pups may have mild signs and survive. Pups that survive often develop ataxia, persistent vestibular signs, ataxia, or blindness. • Mature females may have lymphofollicular or hemorrhagic lesions in the vagina.

CAUSES AND RISK FACTORS

CHV is a typical herpesvirus. Only one serotype has been described, although an atypical CHV was isolated in Great Britain from "dog poxlike" lesions on the canine genital tract that was associated with male genital lesions, abortions, and stillbirths. • Young, susceptible females and their newborn pups are at greatest risk. • Paradoxically, disease is less common in closed breeding kennels where the virus is endemic and most dogs are immune. Susceptible breeding bitches that have been recently introduced into such kennels are at high risk. "Abortion storms" with massive pup losses have occurred when pregnant bitches maintained in private homes were assembled for whelping.

DIAGNOSIS

DIFFERENTIAL DIAGNOSIS

• In the absence of typical gross lesions of CHV, other causes must be sought (e.g., bacteria—brucellosis, coliform bacteria, or streptococci; toxoplasmosis; toxic substances). • Minute virus of canines (MVC, canine parvovirus type-1). MVC causes enteric or respiratory disease. Lesions characteristic of CHV are absent. • Distemper and canine adenovirus type 1 (canine hepatitis) are uncommon and there is absence of the characteristic renal lesions.

CBC/BIOCHEMISTRY/URINALYSIS

Thrombocytopenia may be observed.

OTHER LABORATORY TESTS

Serology testing is of little value.

IMAGING N/A

OTHER DIAGNOSTIC PROCEDURES

• Examination of frozen tissue sections by immunofluorescence or immunoperoxidase staining will reveal viral antigen in most organs, especially in the lesion areas. • Viral isolation in cultures of cells is readily accomplished from several tissues, especially the lung and kidney. Tissues for submission should be refrigerated but not frozen.

GROSS AND HISTOPATHOLOGIC FINDINGS

• Necropsy reveals distinctive gross changes. Characteristic lesions consist of disseminated focal necrosis and hemorrhages in several organs. Diffuse, hemorrhagic areas of necrotic foci and hemorrhagic infarcts in the kidneys of affected pups are pathognomonic. Diffuse areas of hemorrhage and necrosis also are present in the lungs, liver, adrenal glands, and, variably, in the small intestine. Generalized enlargement of lymph nodes and the spleen are consistent findings. • Typical microscopic changes include foci of perivascular necrosis with or without mild cellular infiltration in the kidney, lung, liver, spleen, small intestine, and brain. Lesions in the CNS of recovered pups may include nonsuppurative ganglioneuritis, meningoencephalitis, and necrotic changes in the cerebellum and retina. Acidophilic, intranuclear inclusions may be observed, but they are not abundant. • Necrotizing lesions may be found in fetal placentas.

TREATMENT

• Treatment is not recommended. • Antiviral drug therapy generally has been unsuccessful. • Immune sera from recovered bitches has been beneficial in reducing pup deaths, if antiserum is given before onset of illness.

MEDICATIONS

DRUGS AND FLUIDS N/A

CONTRAINDICATIONS/POSSIBLE INTERACTIONS N/A

FOLLOW-UP

• Pups that recover from the acute disease may suffer deafness, blindness, encephalopathy, or renal damage. • Normal litters can be expected from bitches that have suffered pup losses or abortions.

PATIENT MONITORING N/A

EXPECTED COURSE AND PROGNOSIS N/A

MISCELLANEOUS

• Humans and other animal species are not susceptible. • Pregnant animals, especially young bitches, should be isolated when introduced into a kennel. • There is no vaccine.

ABBREVIATION

CHV = canine herpesvirus

Reference

Carmichael LE, Greene CE. Canine herpesvirus infection. In: Greene CE, ed. Infectious diseases of the dog and cat. Philadelphia: WB Saunders, 1990:252-258.
Author Leland Carmichael
Consulting Editor Fred W. Scott

HIATAL HERNIA

 BASICS

OVERVIEW
• Protrusion of abdominal contents into the thoracic cavity through the esophageal hiatus of the diaphragm; intermittent or persistent
• Three basic types: Sliding (axial or bell)—most common, gastroesophageal junction moves cranial to the diaphragm; Paraesophageal—rare, gastroesophageal junction remains in the normal position but the gastric fundus moves cranial to the diaphragm; Combination of sliding and paraesophageal

SIGNALMENT
• Dogs and cats • Congenital in most patients (< 1 year old) but can be acquired (traumatic cause) • Possible predilection in males • No important breed predisposition although the Chinese shar-pei may be over-represented

SIGNS
• Vomiting • Regurgitation • Hypersalivation • Dyspnea • Hematemesis

CAUSES AND RISK FACTORS
• Congenital in most patients • Patient can have concurrent gastroesophageal reflux and subsequent esophagitis (depends on the amount of functional intrabdominal esophagus remaining)

 DIAGNOSIS

DIFFERENTIAL DIAGNOSIS
• Megaesophagus • Esophageal obstruction
• Gastroesophageal intussusception. This syndrome, although rare, is characterized by a highly fatal acute onset of severe vomiting, hematemesis, and abdominal pain in young, large-breed dogs with concurrent esophageal disease (usually megaesophagus).

CBC/BIOCHEMISTRY/URINALYSIS
Results normal

OTHER LABORATORY TESTS   N/A

IMAGING
• Thoracic radiography may show a dilated esophagus, soft tissue density in the caudal thorax dorsal to the vena cava, absence of the right crus of the diaphragm, or an alveolar pattern indicating aspiration pneumonia.
• Contrast esophagram evaluates esophageal size and gastric fundus location. • Fluoroscopic assistance is useful.

OTHER DIAGNOSTIC PROCEDURES
N/A

 TREATMENT

• Approach with medical treatment to control esophagitis and clinical signs. Include a low-fat diet and elevated feedings in some patients. If no response, surgical intervention is warranted.
• Untreated animals predisposed to developing chronic esophagitis with mucosal ulceration, aspiration pneumonia, strictures, and strangulation of abdominal organs
• Surgical intervention consists of anatomic replacement of herniated organs, reduction in size of the esophageal hiatus, phrenicoesophageal pexy, and a left-sided fundic gastropexy.
• The use of an antireflux surgical procedure (fundoplication) is controversial and should be reserved for patients with documented, primary incompetence of the lower esophageal sphincter.

MEDICATIONS

DRUGS AND FLUIDS
• Histamine H_2 antagonist (e.g., cimetidine and ranitidine) to reduce gastric acid production • Prokinetic agent (e.g., metoclopromide [0.2 mg/kg PO q8h]) to increase lower esophageal sphincter pressure
• Parenteral fluids and antibiotics as needed to treat concurrent aspiration pneumonia

CONTRAINDICATIONS/POSSIBLE INTERACTIONS
Avoid anticholinergic agents because of their negative effects on gastric motility.

 FOLLOW-UP
• Megaesophagus has been reported as a postoperative finding. • Aspiration pneumonia is a common secondary complication.
• Prognosis is guarded and postsurgical complications include reherniation, gastric dilatation without volvulus, and gastroesophageal reflux.

 MISCELLANEOUS

SEE ALSO Megaesophagus

References

Waldron D, Leib M. Hiatal hernia. In: Bojrab MJ, ed. Disease mechanisms in small animal surgery. 2nd ed. Philadelphia: Lea and Febiger, 1993.

Prymak C, Saunders M, Washabau R. Hiatal hernia repair by restoration and stabilization of normal anatomy. Vet Surg 1989; 18(5):386-391.

Ellison G, Lewis D, Phillips L, et al. Esophageal hiatal hernia in small animals: literature review and a modified surgical technique. J Am Anim Hosp Assoc 1987;23:391-399.

Author James E. Williams
Consulting Editor Brent D. Jones

HIP DYSPLASIA—DOGS

BASICS

DEFINITION
Hip dysplasia is the malformation and degeneration of the coxofemoral joints.

Pathophysiology
Hip dysplasia is a developmental defect initiated by a genetic predisposition to subluxation of the immature hip joint. Poor congruence between the femoral head and acetabulum creates abnormal forces across the joint, interferes with normal development (leading to irregularly shaped acetabula and femoral heads), and overloads the articular cartilage (causing microfractures and degenerative joint disease).

Systems Affected Musculoskeletal

Genetics
• Complicated, polygenetic transmission.
• Expression is determined by an interaction of genetic and environmental factors. Heritability index varies with breed (0.25-0.40).

Incidence/Prevalence
• Hip dysplasia is one of the most common skeletal diseases encountered clinically in dogs. • The actual incidence is unknown and varies with breed.

Geographic Distribution N/A

SIGNALMENT

Species Dogs

Breed Predilection
• Large breed dogs, including Saint Bernards, German shepherds, Labrador retrievers, golden retrievers, and rottweilers. • Smaller breed dogs may be affected but are less likely to demonstrate clinical signs.

Mean Age and Range
• Hip dysplasia begins in the immature dog.
• Clinical signs may develop after 4 months of age in some dogs, whereas other dogs present with clinical signs at an older age when degenerative joint disease develops.

Predominant Sex None

SIGNS

General Comments
• Clinical signs are dependent on the degree of joint laxity, amount of degenerative joint disease present, and chronicity of the disease.
• Early clinical signs are related to joint laxity; later signs are related to joint degeneration.

Historical Findings
Reported signs include reduced activity, difficulty rising, reluctance to run or jump or climb stairs, intermittent or persistent hind limb lameness (often worse after exercise), "bunny hopping" or swaying gait, and narrow stance in the hind limbs.

Physical Examination Findings
• Physical exam findings include pain, laxity, crepitus, and diminished range of motion in the hip joints. • Other findings are atrophy of thigh muscles and hypertrophy of shoulder muscles. • Joint laxity (+ Ortolani sign) is characteristic of early hip dysplasia; however, joint laxity may no longer be present in chronic cases due to periarticular fibrosis.

CAUSES
• Hip dysplasia is caused by a genetic predisposition for hip laxity. • Rapid weight gain, nutrition, and pelvic muscle mass influence the expression and progression of the disease.

RISK FACTORS N/A

DIAGNOSIS

DIFFERENTIAL DIAGNOSIS
• Degenerative myelopathy • Lumbosacral instability • Bilateral stifle disease • Panosteitis • Polyarthropathies

CBC/BIOCHEMISTRY/URINALYSIS
N/A

OTHER LABORATORY TESTS N/A

IMAGING
• Radiography—ventrodorsal, hip extended radiographs are commonly used for diagnosis of hip dysplasia. Sedation or general anesthesia may be required for accurate positioning. Radiographic signs in early disease include subluxation of the hip joint with poor congruence between the femoral head and acetabulum. The shape of the acetabulum and femoral head are normal initially, however; the acetabulum becomes shallow and the femoral head begins to flatten and the disease progresses. Radiographic evidence of degenerative joint disease eventually develops, including flattening of the femoral head, shallow acetabulum, periarticular osteophyte production, thickening of the femoral neck, sclerosis of the subchondral bone, and periarticular soft-tissue fibrosis. • Distraction radiographs can be used to quantify joint laxity and may accentuate the laxity for more accurate diagnosis of hip dysplasia. • Dorsal acetabular rim radiographs allow evaluation of the acetabular rim and assessment of dorsal coverage of the femoral head.

OTHER DIAGNOSTIC PROCEDURES
N/A

GROSS AND HISTOPATHOLOGIC FINDINGS
The femoral head and acetabulum appear normal early in the disease. Joint laxity and excess synovial fluid may be appreciated grossly. As the disease progresses, the acetabulum and femoral head are malformed and gross and histopathologic signs of synovitis and articular cartilage degeneration develop. Full thickness cartilage erosion may be present in chronically affected dogs.

TREATMENT

INPATIENT VERSUS OUTPATIENT
• Treatment options for dogs with hip dysplasia are conservative medical therapy and surgery.
• Preferred treatment depends on the dog's size, age, intended function, severity of joint laxity, the presence or absence of degenerative joint disease, clinician's preference, and the financial considerations of the owner.
• Patients are treated as outpatients unless surgery is performed.

ACTIVITY
• Exercise should be limited to the individual tolerance of the patient.
• Swimming is recommended to maintain joint mobility while minimizing weight bearing.
• Physiotherapy (passive joint motion) will reduce joint stiffness and help maintain muscle integrity.

DIET
Weight control is important to reduce the load applied to the painful joint and minimize weight gain associated with reduced exercise.

CLIENT EDUCATION
• Discuss the heritability of the disease.
• Medical therapy is palliative because the joint instability is not corrected. Joint degeneration often progresses unless corrective osteotomy procedure performed early in the disease.
• Surgical procedures can salvage joint function once severe joint degeneration is present.

SURGICAL CONSIDERATIONS
• Triple pelvic osteotomy is a corrective osteotomy procedure designed to re-establish congruity between the femoral head and acetabulum. The acetabulum is rotated in the immature patient (6-12 months) to improve the dorsal coverage of the femoral head and correct the forces acting on the joint. This will minimize the progression of degenerative joint disease and may allow development of a more normal joint if performed early (before severe degeneration develops).
• Total hip replacement is indicated to salvage function in mature dogs with severe degenerative disease unresponsive to medical therapy. Studies have indicated that pain-free joint function returns after total hip replacement in >90% of cases. Approximately 80% of cases require only unilateral joint replacement for acceptable function. Complications reported after hip replacement include luxation, sciatic neuropraxia, and infection.
• Excision arthroplasty is the surgical removal of the femoral head and neck and is used to eliminate joint pain. Results are consistently better in smaller, lighter dogs (<20 kg), and those with good hip musculature. After joint pain is eliminated, however, a slightly abnor-

mal gait often persists. Postoperative muscle atrophy is common, particularly in large dogs. Excision arthroplasty is primarily used as a salvage procedure when severe degenerative joint disease is present and pain cannot be controlled medically, or when total hip replacement is cost prohibitive.

MEDICATIONS

DRUGS AND FLUIDS

Medical therapy for hip dysplasia includes analgesics and anti-inflammatory medications to minimize joint pain (and stiffness and muscle atrophy caused by limited usage) and reduce synovitis. The biomechanical abnormality within the hip joint is not corrected, however, and the degenerative process will likely progress. Frequently, medical therapy provides only temporary relief of signs. Aspirin (10-25 mg/kg, q8h-q12h), meclofenemic acid (1.1 mg/kg divided q12h for 1 week, then maintenance) and Piroxicam (10-20 mg daily, taper down to maintenance) have been advocated.

CONTRAINDICATIONS

Corticosteroids should be avoided because of the potential side effects and the articular cartilage damage associated with long term use.

PRECAUTIONS

Gastrointestinal upset may occur with the use of nonsteroidal anti-inflammatory drugs and may preclude their use in individual cases.

POSSIBLE INTERACTIONS N/A
ALTERNATE DRUGS

Polysulfated glycosaminoglycans has been shown to have a chondro-protective effect in dogs with degenerative joint disease but has not been fully evaluated for treatment of hip dysplasia.

FOLLOW-UP

PATIENT MONITORING

Clinical and radiographic monitoring to assess progression of hip dysplasia is recommended. Clinical deterioration suggests an alternate dosage, alternate medication, or surgical intervention is indicated. Patients treated by triple pelvic osteotomy are monitored radiographically to assess osteotomy healing, implant stability, joint congruence, and progression of degenerative joint disease. Patients treated with hip replacement are monitored radiographically to assess implant stability.

PREVENTION/AVOIDANCE

Hip dysplasia is best prevented by not breeding affected dogs. Pelvic radiographs can help identify phenotypically abnormal dogs but may not identify all dogs carrying the disease. Dam/sire breedings that result in dysplastic offspring should not be repeated.

POSSIBLE COMPLICATIONS N/A
EXPECTED COURSE AND PROGNOSIS

Joint degeneration usually progresses, though most dogs can lead normal lives with proper medical or surgical management.

MISCELLANEOUS
ASSOCIATED CONDITIONS N/A
AGE RELATED FACTORS N/A
ZOONOTIC POTENTIAL N/A
PREGNANCY

Dogs with hip dysplasia should not be bred. If a dysplastic bitch becomes pregnant, the added weight may exacerbate clinical signs.

SYNONYMS N/A
ABBREVIATIONS N/A

References

Riser WH. Canine hip dysplasia: cause and control. J Am Vet Med Assoc 1974;165:360-362.

Wallace LJ. Canine hip dysplasia: past and present. Sem Vet Med Surg 1987;2:92-106.

Rettenmaier JL, Constantinescu GM. Canine hip dysplasia. Comp Cont Educ 1991;13:643-653.

Manley PA. The hip joint. In: Slatter D. ed. Textbook of small animal surgery. 2nd ed. Philadelphia; WB Saunders, 1993;1786-1804.

Author Ron M. McLaughlin
Consulting Editor Peter D. Schwarz

HISTIOCYTOMA

 BASICS

OVERVIEW
Histiocytoma is a benign skin tumor arising from Langerhans cells (i.e., histiocytes) of the skin.

SIGNALMENT
• Common in dogs but extremely rare in cats
• Over 50% of patients are dogs < 2 years old
• Boxer, dachshund, cocker spaniel, great Dane, and Shetland sheepdog breeds may be predisposed • No breed predilection in cats
• No sex predilection in cats or dogs

SIGNS
• Small, firm, dome, or button-shaped, dermoepithelial mass that may be ulcerated.
• Fast growing, nonpainful, usually solitary
• Common sites include head, ear pinna, and limbs

CAUSES AND RISK FACTORS
Unknown

 DIAGNOSIS

DIFFERENTIAL DIAGNOSIS
Histopatholigc examination and immunohistochemical stains distinguish histiocytoma from focal granulomatous inflammation, transmissible venereal tumor, lymphosarcoma, and mast cell tumor (latter stains positive with toluidine blue; histiocytoma does not).

CBC/BIOCHEMISTRY/URINALYSIS
Results usually normal

OTHER LABORATORY TESTS N/A

IMAGING N/A

OTHER DIAGNOSTIC PROCEDURES
Cytologic examination of a fine-needle aspirate characterized by plemorphic round cells, 12-24 mm in diameter, with variable-sized and shaped nuclei and variable amounts of pale blue cytoplasma that resemble monocytes. Mitotic index is usually high. Substantial lymphocyte, plasma cell, and neutrophil infiltration may be observed.

GROSS AND HISTOPATHOLOGIC FINDINGS
Histopathologic findings are characterized by uniform sheets of histiocytes that penetrate the dermis and subcutis. Cells may be densely packed in deeper layers of the dermis. Collagen fibers and skin adnexae may be displaced.

 TREATMENT

• Tumor may spontaneously regress within 3 months
• Surgical excision or cryosurgery generally curative
• Important to differentiate histiocytoma from malignant tumors of owners elect the "wait and see" approach

 **MEDICATIONS**

DRUGS AND FLUIDS N/A

CONTRAINDICATIONS/POSSIBLE INTERACTIONS N/A

 FOLLOW-UP

PATIENT MONITORING

Surgical excision is recommended of mass has not spontaneously regressed within 3 months.

EXPECTED COURSE AND PROGNOSIS

• Prognosis excelelent with surgical removal
• Spontaneous regression possible within 3 months

 MISCELLANEOUS

Reference

Madewell BR, Theilen GH. Skin tumors of mesenchymal origin. In: Theilen, GH, Madewell BR, eds. Veterinary Cancer Medicine. 2nd ed. Philadelphia: Lea & Febiger, 1987;297-299.

Author Joanne C. Graham

Consulting Editor Wallace B. Morrison

HISTOPLASMOSIS

 **BASICS**

DEFINITION
A systemic mycosis caused by the dimorphic fungus Histoplasma capsulatum.

Pathophysiology
• After inhalation of infective spores of the filamentous mold form of the organism, mild signs of respiratory disease (low-grade fever, lethargy, cough) may be observed. This initial disease often lasts for 1-2 weeks. In a high percentage of infected animals, the organism may persist in walled-off lesions in the lungs and regional lymph nodes for months to years. In a small percentage of patients (usually younger animals), extrapulmonary dissemination occurs, producing widespread clinical signs. • In some patients, there is evidence that the organism may invade by way of the gastrointestinal tract rather than the lungs.

Systems Affected
• Respiratory • Gastrointestinal • Lymph nodes, skin, eyes, bone, and CNS (rarely) may be involved in disseminated histoplasmosis.

Genetics
Unknown, but possibly there are inherited or acquired defects in host immune defenses that favor growth of the parasitic yeast form of Histoplasma in macrophages/histiocytes.

Incidence/Prevalence
Histoplasmosis is considered an uncommon disease, even in endemic areas. Dogs and cats appear to be equally susceptible.

Geographic Distribution
Found in the midwestern and eastern United States. Areas of highest incidence include the Mississippi, Missouri, and Ohio river valleys.

SIGNALMENT

Species
Occurs in both dogs and cats

Breed Predilections
• Dogs—appears to be more common in the sporting and hunting breeds • Cats—none recognized

Mean Age and Range
Most are dogs < 5 years of age and cats < 7 years of age.

Predominant Sex None recognized

SIGNS

Historical Findings
Anorexia, weight loss, weakness, dyspnea, and functional abnormalities of the gastrointestinal tract are commonly reported signs.

Physical Examination Findings
Dogs
• Affected dogs may exhibit signs of fever, wasting, lethargy, a chronic productive cough, hemoptysis, and anemia. • In many dogs, signs of gastrointestinal disease predominate. Watery to bloody diarrhea, tenesmus, and blood or mucus in the stool often are observed. Extensive blood loss through the gastrointestinal tract or protein-losing enteropathy may occur. • Disseminated histoplasmosis may progress to involve the liver, spleen, lymph nodes, bone marrow, eyes, skin, or (rarely) the CNS. Visceral lymphadenopathy, hepatosplenomegaly, jaundice, and ascites may be seen. • In some dogs, clinical signs may be restricted to the lungs and include coughing and dyspnea.
Cats
• Wasting, fever, and dyspnea may be observed. • Lymphadenopathy, hepatomegaly, lameness, ulcerative skin lesions, and ocular abnormalities (granulomatous chorioretinitis) also have been reported.

CAUSE
• Histoplasma capsulatum is a dimorphic soil fungus with a geographically restricted distribution. The organism prefers moist, humid climates and has a predilection for chicken, bat, and wild bird droppings, in which the filamentous mold form grows profusely. • Contaminated sites will continue to yield viable organisms in the soil for as long as 3-6 years after they have been abandoned.

RISK FACTORS
Aggressive nosing about in soil and underbrush, as in the sporting breeds of dogs, may expose susceptible animals to large doses of the fungus in contaminated soil. Inhalation or ingestion of the infective spores may result.

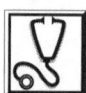 **DIAGNOSIS**

DIFFERENTIAL DIAGNOSIS
• Pulmonary lesions may resemble those of other systemic mycoses. Such lesions should be differentiated from metastatic tumors and canine distemper. • Lymphadenopathy may be seen in lymphosarcoma, other systemic mycoses, and localized bacterial infections. • Skin lesions should be differentiated from routine abscesses or other bacterial disease processes. • Bone lesions may resemble those caused by primary or metastatic bone tumors or bacterial osteomyelitis.

CBC/BIOCHEMISTRY/URINALYSIS
• Hemogram—nonregenerative anemia, neutrophilic leukocytosis, and eosinopenia (all nonspecific). Histoplasma yeast forms occasionally may be observed in circulating leukocytes. Thrombocytopenia may be present in some patients. • Serum chemistry profile—hyperglobulinemia, hypoalbuminemia, and, in some patients, bilirubinemia with abnormal liver function tests and enzyme levels • Urinalysis—few abnormalities recognized

OTHER LABORATORY TESTS
• Immunologic tests for antibodies to Histoplasma are considered unreliable (or, at best, marginally presumptive) for diagnosis. • Most cats with histoplasmosis are negative for feline leukemia virus and feline immunodeficiency virus.

IMAGING
Radiography of lung (interstitial infiltrates) and bone (osteolysis) lesions may aid in diagnosis.

OTHER DIAGNOSTIC PROCEDURES
• Microscopic identification of the small intracellular (within macrophages) Histoplasma yeast forms in biopsy/cytologic or other lesion material is the recommended method of diagnosis. In some cases of histoplasmosis the intracellular yeast forms may be present only in low numbers, necessitating a diligent search of available material. • Biopsy or cytology may reveal Histoplasma organisms within macrophages/histiocytes.

GROSS AND HISTOPATHOLOGIC FINDINGS
• Granulomatous inflammation present in many tissues • Lymph node hyperplasia • Presence of the characteristic yeast form in macrophages/histiocytes in affected tissues. In some cases the numbers of infected cells may be small.

 TREATMENT

INPATIENT VERSUS OUTPATIENT
Because treatment of histoplasmosis requires long-term therapy, the patient should be treated as an outpatient. Patients treated with amphotericin B (AMB), however, will need to be hospitalized several times a week during their initial treatment period.

ACTIVITY
Activity levels should be restricted during the period of antifungal therapy.

DIET
Because affected animals often have experienced weight loss, provision should be made for feeding a high-quality diet. Protein levels may need to be restricted, however, owing to the nephrotoxic effects of amphotericin B.

CLIENT EDUCATION
The necessity and expense of long-term therapy of a potentially fatal illness, in addition to the possible side effects of such therapy, need to be thoroughly discussed with the client. Attention should be paid to the particularly grave prognosis for cats with histoplasmosis.

SURGICAL CONSIDERATIONS N/A

 MEDICATIONS

DRUGS AND FLUIDS
Dogs
• AMB can be administered either alone or in

combination. When used alone it can be given at a dosage of 0.5 mg/kg, 3 times a week, for a total cumulative dosage of 8-10 mg/kg. It is given IV either as a slow infusion (in dogs that are gravely ill) or as a rapid bolus (in fairly healthy dogs). For slow infusion, add AMB to 250-500 ml of 5% dextrose solution and administer as a drip over a period of 4-6 hours. For a rapid bolus, add AMB to 30 ml of 5% dextrose solution and administer over a period of 5 minutes through a butterfly catheter.

• To lessen the adverse renal effects of AMB, give 0.9% NaCl (2 ml/kg/hr) for several hours before initiating AMB therapy.

• Ketoconazole (KTZ) represents an alternative to AMB in dogs that are not gravely ill. It may also be given in sequential fashion after AMB therapy has been completed, depending on the clinical response. In general, KTZ is not as effective as AMB when given alone and the response to therapy is slower. KTZ can be administered at 10-30 mg/kg PO, divided 2 or 3 times daily for 2-3 months. It should be given in the food.

• A combination of AMB and KTZ may be used in dogs that have not responded to either drug alone or that have exhibited significant toxicity. It may also be a useful alternative to therapy with AMB alone. For combination chemotherapy, administer AMB as described to a total cumulative dosage of 4-6 mg/kg, together with KTZ at 10 mg/kg PO divided daily for at least 2-3 months.

• A newer azole derivative, itraconazole (ITZ), is reportedly more effective and less toxic than KTZ, and may be curative at a dosage of 5 mg/kg PO q12h given over a period of 2-3 months. It should be given in the food.

CATS

• AMB can be administered by rapid IV bolus at a dosage of 0.25 mg/kg, 3 times a week, for a total cumulative dosage of 4 mg/kg. This can be followed by KTZ therapy, depending on the clinical response.

• KTZ can be administered at 10-20 mg/kg PO, divided 2 or 3 times daily, to cats that are not gravely ill. The medication should be given in the food. If side effects (see Precautions) occur, reduce to alternate-day therapy.

• Itraconazole has been reported to be curative with fewer side effects, at a dosage of 5 mg/kg PO q12h given over a period of 2-3 months. It should be given in the food.

CONTRAINDICATIONS

• Drugs metabolized primarily by the kidneys should not be administered along with AMB.

• Drugs metabolized primarily by the liver should not be administered along with KTZ or ITZ.

PRECAUTIONS

• Side effects of AMB therapy can be severe and include renal dysfunction, fever, inappetence, vomiting, and phlebitis.

• Side effects of KTZ or ITZ therapy include inappetence, vomiting, and hepatotoxicity. Side effects are much less common with ITZ.

POSSIBLE INTERACTIONS N/A

ALTERNATE DRUGS N/A

FOLLOW-UP

PATIENT MONITORING

• BUN should be monitored in all animals treated with AMB. Treatment should be temporarily discontinued if the BUN rises above 50 mg/dl. • Liver enzymes should be monitored in animals receiving KTZ or ITZ.

PREVENTION/AVOIDANCE

• There is no available vaccine. • Exposure to Histoplasma-contaminated soil in endemic areas should be avoided.

POSSIBLE COMPLICATIONS

• Pulmonary disease may worsen temporarily soon after therapy is begun, owing to inflammation resulting from the death of fungal cells in the lungs. • Nephrotoxicity may result from AMB therapy. • Hepatotoxicity may result from KTZ or ITZ therapy.

EXPECTED COURSE AND PROGNOSIS

• The prognosis in dogs is guarded in most patients. Those with histoplasmosis confined to the lungs have a better prognosis than those with disseminated disease. • The prognosis for cats in general is extremely poor;

most patients cannot be cured. • A relapse after treatment may occur, sometimes as long as a year after apparently successful therapy.

MISCELLANEOUS

ASSOCIATED CONDITIONS N/A

AGE RELATED FACTORS N/A

ZOONOTIC POTENTIAL

The parasitic yeast form of the fungus that is found in animal tissues is not directly transmissible to people or other animals. Under certain rare circumstances, however, there could be reversion to growth of the infective mold form of the fungus on or within bandages placed over a draining lesion or in contaminated bedding. This author recommends that prudent care be exercised whenever handling an infected dog or cat.

PREGNANCY

• AMB—no teratogenic effects have been identified • KTZ and ITZ should be used in pregnant animals only if the potential benefit justifies the potential risk to offspring.

SYNONYMS N/A

SEE ALSO N/A

ABBREVIATIONS

AMB = amphotericin B
KTZ = ketoconazole
ITZ = itraconazole

References

Legendre AM. Histoplasmosis. In: Sherding RG, ed. The cat: diseases and clinical management. 2nd ed. New York: Churchill Livingstone, 1994:557-559.

Wolf AM. Histoplasmosis. In: Greene CE, ed. Infectious diseases of the dog and cat. Philadelphia: WB Saunders, 1990:679-686.

Author Jeffrey E. Barlough
Consulting Editor Fred W. Scott

HOOKWORMS (ANCYCLOSTOMIASIS)

 BASICS

OVERVIEW
• Nematode parasites of the species Ancylostoma caninum in the small intestine of dogs, Ancylostoma tubaeforme of cats, and Ancylostoma braziliense and Uncinaria stenocephala in both dogs and cats. A. braziliense is found in Southern states, the others are also in the temperate zone. • Voracious blood-sucking adults and fourth stage larvae of A. caninum and A. tubaeforme cause blood loss anemia and enteritis. Active worms leave bite sites with continuing seepage of blood. Of special concern is infection in neonates causing acute to peracute disease. Infections may be acute to chronic-compensatory at weaning, or chronic-noncompensatory in the immunosuppressed or debilitated. Uncinaria of little clinical concern. A. braziliense is the major cause of cutaneous larva migrans. Coughing may result from larval migration to the lungs following skin penetration. • A. caninum is transmitted transcolostrally to pups. All species are transmitted by ingestion of infective larvae or by skin penetration.

SIGNALMENT
Acute disease in young, to chronic in mature dogs and cats.

SIGNS

Historical Findings
• Pale mucous membranes • Dark tarry stools • Constipation • Loss of condition • Poor appetite • Dry cough • Sudden death

Physical Examination Findings
• Poor condition • Pale mucous membranes • Dry thoracic auscultation

CAUSES AND RISK FACTORS
• Ancylostoma spp • Infected bitch or queen • Contaminated environment • Concurrent enteric infections • Other compromising conditions, e.g., pregnancy

 DIAGNOSIS

DIFFERENTIAL DIAGNOSIS
• Toxocariasis (large roundworm infection) • Coccidiosis • Strongyloidiasis • Differentiate Uncinaria eggs at 70 μm from A. caninum at 60 μm

CBC/BIOCHEMISTRY/URINALYSIS
• Eosinophilia • Anemia. May be microcytic, hypochromic due to iron deficiency.

OTHER LABORATORY TESTS
Fecal flotation; fecal egg examination: A. caninum, A. tubaeforme at 60×40 μm

IMAGING N/A

OTHER DIAGNOSTIC PROCEDURES
Necropsy of sibling pups, kittens that have died following appearance of similar clinical signs

 TREATMENT

• Pups in an environment with a history of hookworm infections should be routinely treated at 2-week intervals to weaning
• Treat acute case as inpatient to deworm and for fluid therapy including possible blood transfusion
• Alert owner to potential for sudden death
• Treat chronic compensatory including breeding female with deworming program to eliminate intestinal and somatic infections

MEDICATIONS

DRUGS AND FLUIDS

Adulticide/Larvicide Anthelmintic Activity
• Fenbendazole (Panacur) 50mg/kg bwt q24h for 3 days • Milbemycin oxime (Interceptor) 0.5mg/kg q30d

Adulticide Activity
• Butamisole (Styquin) 2.4 mg/kg bwt SQ
• Dichlorvos (Task) packets/tabs by wt bi-weekly • Febantel + praziquantel (Vercom) 10mg febantel q24h for 3 days (dogs/cats)
• Pyrantel pamoate 15 mg/kg dogs (Nemex), 20–30 mg/kg cats • Ivermectin 6 µg/kg + pyrantel pamoate (Heartgard-30 Plus)
• Supplementary intravenous fluids, vitamins

Dogs
• Adulticide/larvicide dewormer (fenbendazole) during third trimester to kill migrating larvae in somatic tissue and adults
• A/L dewormer on daily or monthly basis for pups and mature dogs
• Treat pup biweekly to weaning, if at risk
• Fluids, blood transfusion as necessary

Cats
• Adulticide/larvicide dewormer for queen prior to breeding and after littering
• Adulticide dewormer by 4 weeks for kitten

CONTRAINDICATIONS/POSSIBLE INTERACTIONS
Organophosphates: heartworm infection

 FOLLOW-UP
• Monitor fecal egg counts post-treatment
• Hematocrit if infection resulted in blood loss

 MISCELLANEOUS

AGE RELATED FACTORS
Disease more acute in young animals and chronic in adults.

ZOONOTIC POTENTIAL
Cutaneous larval migrans, especially with A. braziliense. Infective larvae penetrate skin.

SYNONYMS
Ancylostomiasis

Reference
Bowman DD. Hookworm parasites of dogs and cats. Compendium Contin Educ Pract Vet 1992;14(5):585–595.
Author Robert M. Corwin
Consulting Editor Brent D. Jones

HORNER'S SYNDROME

BASICS

OVERVIEW
Sympathetic denervation of the eye.
Anatomic pathway is very important:

Hypothalamus
↓
brainstem/cervical cord
T$_1$-T$_3$ spinal cord segments
and nerve roots
↓
vagosympathetic trunk
↓
cranial cervical ganglion
↓
middle ear
↓
ophthalmic branch CN V
↓
long ciliary nerve
↓
iris dilator muscle
↓
other fibers—smooth muscle in periorbita
upper and third eyelid

SIGNALMENT
• Idiopathic—one study suggests male golden retrievers 4-13 years old. • N/A for other causes.

SIGNS

Historical Findings N/A

Physical Examination Findings
• Miosis • Protruding third eyelid • Ptosis (drooping) of upper eyelid • Enophthalmia • Mild conjunctival hyperemia in some animals • See Table 1 for other neurologic signs.

CAUSES AND RISK FACTORS
See Table 1

DIAGNOSIS

DIFFERENTIAL DIAGNOSIS
In animals with anterior uveitis, intraocular pressure is abnormal and aqueous flare is present.

CBC/BIOCHEMISTRY/URINALYSIS
N/A

OTHER LABORATORY TESTS N/A

IMAGING See Table 1
RADIOGRAPHY
• Spinal radiographs and myelogram may reveal a spinal cord lesion. • Thoracic radiographs may reveal cause (e.g., trauma and mediastinal tumor) of injury to cranial cervical ganglion sympathetic trunk. • Skull radiographs may reveal middle ear problem. • CT and MRI may be useful in identifying a brain stem lesion, retrobulbar mass, or middle ear problem.

ULTRASONOGRAPHY
Ultrasound orbit to look for retrobulbar mass

OTHER DIAGNOSTIC PROCEDURES
• See Table 1 • CSF tap to investigate brain and spinal cord disease • Electromyography to look for brachial plexus evulsion • Pharmacologic testing: see anisocoria chapter for algorithm.

TREATMENT
• Treat underlying disease
• Idiopathic—dogs, 50-93%; cats, 45%

MEDICATIONS

DRUGS
• Treat underlying disease
• Idiopathic—none

CONTRAINDICATIONS/POSSIBLE INTERACTIONS N/A

FOLLOW-UP
• Depends on severity of underlying disease
• Idiopathic—partial or complete recovery, which can take up to 4 months

MISCELLANEOUS

SEE ALSO Anisocoria

ABBREVIATIONS
• CT = computerized tomography
• MRI = magnetic resonance imaging

Reference
De Lahunta A. Veterinary neuroanatomy and clinical neurology. 2nd ed. Philadelphia: WB Saunders, 1983:115–120.

Author David Lipsitz
Consulting Editor Paul E. Miller

Table 1.

Summary of Lesions Resulting in Horner's Syndrome

Location	Etiologies	Associated Neurologic Signs	Diagnostic Plan
brain stem	trauma, neoplasm, infectious, inflammatory	altered mental status, ipsilateral motor deficits, ipsilateral cranial nerve deficits	CT/MRI CSF
cervical spinal cord	trauma, disc, neoplasm, fibrocartilaginous embolism (FCE)	ipsilateral hemiparesis/paralysis, tetraparesis/paralysis UMN thoracic/pelvic limbs	spine films, CSF, myelogram
T1 -T3 spinal cord	trauma, disc, neoplasm, FCE	LMN thoracic limb(s) UMN pelvic limb(s)	spine films, CSF, myelogram
T1 -T3 ventral roots	brachial plexus avulsion	ipsilateral brachial plexus injury ipsilateral loss of panniculus reflex	Neurologic examination electromyography(EMG)
sympathetic trunk cranial cervical ganglion	trauma, mediastinal neoplasm, iatrogenic-surgical trauma	unilateral-none bilateral-laryngeal/pharyngeal dysfunction	chest radiographs
middle ear	trauma, neoplasm, otitis media/interna nasopharyngeal polyp(cat)	ipsilateral peripheral vestibular disease, ipsilateral facial nerve paralysis	otic examination, bullae radiographs/ CT myringotomy
retrobulbar	trauma, neoplasm, abscess	variable-none or involvement of cranial nerves II, III, IV, VI	CT/MRI ultrasound orbit

HYDROCEPHALUS

 BASICS

DEFINITION

Dilation of the ventricular system because of excessive accumulation of CSF

Pathophysiology

• Hydrocephalus is caused by obstruction of the CSF flow within the ventricular system (noncommunicating) or lack of reabsorption into the subarachnoid space (communicating). Congenital hydrocephalus is usually obstructive and can be caused by a congenitally narrow mesencephalic aqueduct or develop secondarily to prenatal infection, especially in animals with parainfluenza virus. Intracranial pressure is high or normal, and the patient may have clinical signs despite normal intracranial pressure. • Hydrocephalus ex vacuo is an incidental ventricular dilation that develops secondarily to cerebrocortical atrophy.

Systems Affected Nervous

Genetics

Autosomal recessive in Siamese cats

Incidence/Prevalence Unknown

Geographic Distribution N/A

SIGNALMENT

Species Dogs and cats

Breed Predilections

• Congenital form in small and brachycephalic dogs—bulldog, chihuahua, Maltese, Pomeranian, toy poodle, Yorkshire terrier, lhasa apso, cairn terrier, Boston terrier, pug, and Pekingese • Inherited in Siamese cats • Acquired hydrocephalus—any breed of cat or dog

Mean Age and Range

• Congenital hydrocephalus—signs usually appear a few weeks after birth up to 1 year • Acquired hydrocephalus—any age

Predominant Sex N/A

SIGNS

General Comments

Hydrocephalus may occur without clinical signs, especially in toy breeds of dog.

Historical Findings

• Behavioral abnormalities—reduced consciousness, lack of or loss of training ability (including house-training), excessive sleepiness, vocalization, sometimes hyperexcitability • Blindness • Seizures in some animals

Physical Examination Findings

• The head may appear large and dome-shaped with open fontanelles (sutures). • Signs of cerebral disease—abnormal behavior, especially dullness and sleepiness, and blindness with normal pupillary light reflexes • Gait abnormalities—incoordination, ataxia, and reduced postural reactions in some patients • In animals with the congenital form, malformation of the orbits during growth may cause ventro-lateral strabismus with normal eye movements. • High intracranial pressure may lead to fatal tentorial herniation. Clinical signs include stupor or coma, anisocoria, pinpoint or dilated fixed pupils, abnormal respiratory patterns, and decerebrate posture.

CAUSES

Communicating Hydrocephalus

Piarachnoid adhesions subsequent to meningitis (as in cats with FIP) or subarachnoid hemorrhage, and obstruction of CSF outflow at the arachnoid villi

Noncommunicating Hydrocephalus

• The precise cause of congenital hydrocephalus is unclear. • Mass lesions (e.g., tumor and abscess) and inflammatory disease are the most common causes of acquired hydrocephalus.

RISK FACTORS

Animals with compensated hydrocephalus may decompensate in the face of an insult such as infection or trauma.

 DIAGNOSIS

DIFFERENTIAL DIAGNOSIS

• Other congenital brain anomalies are usually present at birth and are nonprogressive. • Brain mass lesions or inflammatory disease that causes high intracranial pressure (hydrocephalus may coexist) might not be differentiated by historical and clinical signs alone. CSF analysis and brain imaging often are required for diagnosis. • Metabolic or toxic diseases causing cerebral dysfunction are differentiated by the symmetry of the neurologic signs and results of laboratory testing.

CBC/BIOCHEMISTRY/URINALYSIS

Results usually normal

OTHER LABORATORY TESTS

Bile acids may be necessary for a diagnosis of hepatic encephalopathy.

IMAGING

• Survey radiography may confirm a large, domed cranium with open fontanelles. The cranial vault may have a "ground glass" appearance. • CT and MRI are the most accurate and the least invasive methods of determining the diagnosis. • Ventriculography was used before the advent of CT and MRI—the ventricles are dilated with air or positive contrast by an open fontanelle or craniotomy. Radiographs then are taken to demonstrate the dilated ventricles. • Ultrasonography of the brain through an open fontanelle may reveal large ventricles.

OTHER DIAGNOSTIC PROCEDURES

• CSF can be collected and intracranial pressure measured by puncture of the cerebellomedullary cistern or lateral ventricles. Composition of the CSF is normal in the absence of other intracranial disease. • Intra-cranial pressure is normal or high. • Caution should be exercised because CSF collection in the face of high intracranial pressure may lead to fatal brain herniation through the foramen magnum or beneath the tentorium cerebelli. • CSF protein may be high and cellularity abnormal if the patient has other intracranial disease (e.g., neoplasia and inflammation). • The electroencephalographic pattern in patients with the congenital form is usually characterized by a hypersynchronous, high amplitude (25-300 microV), low frequency (1-7 Hz) pattern.

GROSS AND HISTOPATHOLOGIC FINDINGS

• The brain may be large with loss of the normal pattern of sulci and gyri. • The entire ventricular system or only that part of it rostral to an obstructive lesion may be mildly to severely distended. • Distortion of surrounding brain parenchyma may be seen, including thinning of the cerebral cortex, rupture of the septum pellucidum, and atrophy of other adjacent structures. • In animals with noncommunicating hydrocephalus, narrowing or blockage of the ventricular system due to inflammation or mass lesions may be apparent. • Brain herniation may be apparent, either of the cerebrum and midbrain under the tentorium cerebelli or of the cerebellum and caudal medulla oblongata through the foramen magnum.

 TREATMENT

INPATIENT VERSUS OUTPATIENT

• Animals with severe clinical signs or those undergoing surgery for hydrocephalus should be managed as inpatients. • Animals with mild to moderate clinical signs treated medically can be managed as outpatients.

ACTIVITY N/A

DIET N/A

CLIENT EDUCATION

Clients should observe for deterioration in mental alertness, vision, and behavior as these signal worsening of the problem.

SURGICAL CONSIDERATIONS

• Definitive treatment is by surgical shunting of CSF from the ventricles to the peritoneal cavity. • Complications are common, including infection and shunt blockage. Shunt revision is commonly needed. • Clinical signs may not resolve completely after shunting. Residual signs usually indicate irreversible brain damage. • Surgery for a brain tumor or other mass lesion should be considered if this is the underlying cause of the hydrocephalus.

MEDICATIONS

DRUGS AND FLUIDS

• Drug therapy is directed toward reducing CSF production with corticosteroids (prednisone 0.25-0.5 mg/kg PO q12h or dexamethasone 0.25 mg/kg PO q12h tapered to an alternate day regimen) or carbonic anhydrase inhibitors (e.g., acetazolamide 10 mg/kg PO q6h).
• Reduction of intracranial pressure by osmotic (slow IV infusion of mannitol 1 g/kg over 20 minutes that may be repeated twice at 6-hour intervals) and/or loop diuretics (furosemide —dogs, 2-8 mg/kg IV IM SC q12h; cats, 1-2 mg/kg IV IM SC q12h) are indicated in animals with signs of severely high intracranial pressure.
• Specific treatment for any underlying cause should be instituted when possible (e.g., antibiotics for bacterial infection).

CONTRAINDICATIONS

Fluid therapy should be used with caution in animals with severe hydrocephalus—do not overhydrate.

PRECAUTIONS

• Long-term treatment with corticosteroids may cause iatrogenic hyperadrenocorticism or hypoadrenocorticism if corticosteroids are suddenly withdrawn.
• Diuretics can cause shock or electrolyte imbalances, especially hypokalemia with furosemide administration.

POSSIBLE INTERACTIONS N/A

ALTERNATE DRUGS N/A

FOLLOW-UP

PATIENT MONITORING

Animals should be monitored for exacerbation of the hydrocephalus and for signs attributable to an underlying cause (e.g., intracranial neoplasia).

PREVENTION/AVOIDANCE N/A

POSSIBLE COMPLICATIONS

• High intracranial pressure leading to brain herniation and death • Infection and blockage when ventriculoperitoneal shunting is carried out; shunt revision and specific treatment for bacterial infection are then indicated

EXPECTED COURSE AND PROGNOSIS

• Varies depending on cause and severity of disease • Guarded to poor prognosis in animals with severe or progressive disease
• Good prognosis in animals with mild congenital form of disease; may need only occasional medical treatment

MISCELLANEOUS

ASSOCIATED CONDITIONS

Cerebellar hypoplasia in kittens congenitally infected with feline panleukopenia virus

---

AGE RELATED FACTORS

Congenital hydrocephalus most commonly seen in animals < 1 year old

ZOONOTIC POTENTIAL N/A

PREGNANCY N/A

SYNONYMS N/A

SEE ALSO N/A

ABBREVIATIONS

CSF = cerebrospinal fluid
CT = computed tomography
MRI = magnetic resonance imaging

References

Fenner WR. Diseases of the brain. In: Birchard SJ, Sherding RC, eds. Saunders manual of small animal practice. Philadelphia: WB Saunders, 1135-1136.

Kornegay JN. Congenital and degenerative diseases of the central nervous system. In: Kornegay JN, ed. Contemporary issues in small animal practice: neurologic disorders. New York: Churchill Livingstone, 1986;5:109-130.

Levesque DC, Plummer SB. Ventriculoperitoneal shunting as a treatment for hydrocephalus. Proceedings, Annu Forum Am Col Vet Int Med ACVIM, 1994:891-893.

Oliver JE, Lorenz MD. Handbook of veterinary neurology. 2nd. ed. Philadelphia: WB Saunders, 1993:285-291.

Author Mary O. Smith
Consulting Editor Joane M. Parent

HYDRONEPHROSIS

 BASICS

DEFINITION

Hydronephrosis causes progressive distention of the renal pelvis and diverticulae with atrophy of the renal parenchyma secondary to obstruction in most animals. The disease is usually unilateral and occurs secondary to complete or partial obstruction of the kidney or ureter by uroliths or because of neoplasia, retroperitoneal disease, trauma, radiotherapy, accidental ligation of the ureter during ovariohysterectomy, and after ectopic ureter surgery. Bilateral hydronephrosis is rare and usually occurs secondary to trigonal, prostatic, or urethral disease.

SIGNALMENT

Dogs are affected more often than cats.

SIGNS

Historical Findings
• None in some animals
• Anorexia
• Restlessness
• Polydipsia and polyuria
• Hematuria
• Signs of uremia in animals with bilateral hydronephrosis or if the contralateral kidney has compromised function
• Signs may be referable to the cause of obstruction

Physical Examination Findings
• Normal in some animals
• Renomegaly
• Renal, abdominal, or lumbar pain
• Abdominal mass (i.e., bladder or prostate)
• Trigonal, prostatic, or urethral mass palpated on rectal examination

CAUSES AND RISK FACTORS

Any cause of ureteral obstruction including ureteral stenosis, atresia, fibrosis (cats), or neoplasia; uroliths; trigonal mass; prostatic disease; retroperitoneal abscess, cysts, hematoma, or other mass; inadvertent ureteral ligation during ovariohysterectomy postoperative complication from ectopic ureter surgery; perineal hernia

 DIAGNOSIS

DIFFERENTIAL DIAGNOSIS
• Other causes of renomegaly (e.g., amyloidosis, neoplasia, granuloma, cysts, and perinephric pseudocysts [cats])
• Other causes of abdominal pain (e.g., pancreatitis and peritonitis)
• Intervertebral disc disease leading to lumbar pain
• Pyelonephritis without obstruction

CBC/BIOCHEMISTRY/URINALYSIS
• Results normal in some animals
• Loss of urine concentrating ability (first abnormality detected), hematuria, and pyuria
• Azotemia, hyperphosphatemia, hyperkalemia, and acidosis in animals with severe, bilateral hydronephrosis resulting in renal failure

OTHER LABORATORY TESTS N/A

IMAGING
• Abdominal radiographs may be normal or show renomegaly, prostatomegaly, uroliths, reduced retroperitoneal contrast, or urinary bladder distension.
• Excretory urography or cystography may be required to determine the location and cause of obstruction.
• Ultrasonography reveals dilation of the renal pelvis and diverticulae with thinning of the renal parenchyma. Dilation of one or both ureters are detected in some animals.

OTHER DIAGNOSTIC PROCEDURES
N/A

 TREATMENT

• Treat as an inpatient and start supportive care (fluids ± antibiotics) while pursuing diagnostics.
• Discuss renal disease versus failure and possible need for surgery with the owner.
• Specific treatment (usually surgical) depends on the cause of the hydronephrosis and presence or absence of concurrent renal failure. Hydronephrosis rarely requires emergency surgery. Metabolic and electrolyte abnormalities should be treated before surgery. Lower urinary tract obstruction should be relieved as soon as possible by catheterization, serial cystocentesis, or tube cystostomy pending surgical correction.
• A hydronephrotic kidney may not need to be removed unless severely infected or neoplastic.
• If hydronephrosis is secondary to nephroliths or ureteroliths, extracorporeal shock wave lithotripsy may be used as an alternative to surgery.

MEDICATIONS

DRUGS AND FLUIDS

• Correct fluid and electrolyte deficits with intravenous fluid therapy (0.9% NaCl or LRS) over 4-6 hours followed by maintenance fluids as needed. Some animals may be extremely polyuric necessitating higher maintenance fluid rates.

• Sodium bicarbonate should be administered to treat severe metabolic acidosis. If a measured base deficit is known, then one-quarter of the calculated dose (weight in kg $\times$ 0.3 $\times$ base deficit) of bicarbonate can be given as a slow intravenous bolus and the remainder administered with intravenous fluids. If the base deficit is not known, then bicarbonate can be given at a dosage of 3 - 9 mEq/kg depending of the estimated deficit based on the severity of the signs.

• Hyperkalemia (mild to moderate) often resolves with fluid replacement ± bicarbonate supplementation. Severe, symptomatic hyperkalemia requires more aggressive medical management such as regular insulin (0.5 u/kg IV) and 50% dextrose (2.0 g/kg IV). Some veterinary literature implies that potassium-containing solutions (e.g., lactated Ringer's solution) should be avoided in hyperkalemic patients, but current data does not support this.

• See chapters on Chronic renal failure and Acute renal failure for general treatment principles for patients with bilateral hydronephrosis.

CONTRAINDICATIONS/POSSIBLE INTERACTIONS

• Do not add or mix sodium bicarbonate with calcium-containing fluids.

• Many contraindications and potential complications are associated with the use of sodium bicarbonate and should be considered before bicarbonate administration.

• Do not give radiographic contrast material intravenously until the patient is rehydrated.

FOLLOW-UP

PATIENT MONITORING

• Ultrasonography can be repeated at 2-4 week intervals after relief of obstruction to monitor for improvement of hydronephrosis. Hydronephrosis often shows some signs of resolution by 3 months after relief of obstruction.

• Monitor BUN, creatinine, and electrolytes.

• Monitor for polyuria and postobstructive diuresis leading to hypokalemia, weight loss, and dehydration.

POSSIBLE COMPLICATIONS

Rupture of the excretory system and irreversible renal damage

EXPECTED COURSE AND PROGNOSIS

The prognosis depends on the cause of hydronephrosis, duration of obstruction, and presence or absence of concurrent infection. Irreversible damage to the kidneys usually begins 15-45 days after obstruction. If the obstruction is relieved within 1 week, renal damage is reversible. Some function may be regained with relief of obstructions present for as long as 4 weeks. Concurrent infection accelerates the severity of renal damage.

MISCELLANEOUS

Reference

Christie BA, Bjorling DE. Kidneys. In: Slatter D, ed. Textbook of small animal surgery. 2nd ed. Philadelphia, WB Saunders, 1993:1428-1442.

AUTHOR Marc G. Bercovitch

CONSULTING EDITORS Larry G. Adams and Carl A. Osborne

HYPERADRENOCORTICISM (CUSHING'S DISEASE)

BASICS

DEFINITION
A disorder caused by the deleterious effects of high circulating cortisol concentrations on multiple organ systems

Pathophysiology
Spontaneous hyperadrenocorticism is caused by excessive production of cortisol by the adrenal cortex. In 85-90% of patients, the cortisol excess is caused by bilateral adrenocortical hyperplasia resulting from pituitary corticotroph tumor or hyperplasia producing excessive amounts of adrenocorticotropic hormone (ACTH). The remaining 10-15% of patients have cortisol-secreting adrenocortical neoplasia, approximately one half of which is malignant. Iatrogenic hyperadrenocorticism is caused by excessive exogenous administration of glucocorticoids.

Systems Affected
• Renal/urologic • Skin/exocrine • Cardiovasular • Respiratory • Endocrine/metabolic • Musculoskeletal • Nervous • Reproductive • Varies between patients; in some patients, signs referable to one system may predominate, while in others, several systems are involved to a comparable degree. Signs referable to the urinary tract or skin predominate.

Genetics N/A

Incidence/Prevalence
• One of the most common endocrine disorders in dogs • Rare in cats

Geographic Distribution N/A

SIGNALMENT

Species Dogs and cats

Breed Predilections
• Poodle, dachshund, Boston terrier, boxer, and beagle have been reported to be at higher risk than other breeds. • None in cats

Predominant Sex
• No predilection in dogs with pituitary dependent hyperadrenocorticism (PDH); two thirds to three quarters of dogs with adrenal tumor are female. • None in cats

Mean Age and Range
In general, hyperadrenocorticism is a disorder of middle-aged to old animals; however, PDH can be seen in dogs as young as one year.

SIGNS
• Severity of signs varies depending on the duration and degree of cortisol excess. In some patients, the physical presence of the neoplastic process (pituitary or adrenal) contributes to clinical signs. • Polyuria and polydipsia • Pendulous abdomen • Hepatomegaly • Hair loss • Lethargy • Muscle weakness • Anestrus • Obesity • Muscle atrophy • Comedomes • Panting • Testicular atrophy • Hyperpigmentation • Calcinosis cutis • Facial nerve palsy

CAUSES
• Pituitary dependent—adenoma or hyperplasia of the corticotrophs • Adrenal tumor—adenoma or carcinoma • Iatrogenic—glucocorticoid administration

RISK FACTORS N/A

DIAGNOSIS

DIFFERENTIAL DIAGNOSIS
Depending on the exact clinical and laboratory abnormalities, differential diagnoses include hypothyroidism, sex hormone dermatosis, acromegaly, diabetes mellitus, hepatopathy, and renal disease and other causes of PU/PD.

CBC/BIOCHEMISTRY/URINALYSIS
• Eosinopenia, lymphopenia, leukocytosis, and erythrocytosis (females) in some patients • High ALP, liver enzyme activity, cholesterol, blood glucose, and total CO_2 in some patients • Low urine specific gravity (generally < 1.015, often hyposthenuric), proteinuria, hematuria, pyuria, and bactiuria in some patients

OTHER LABORATORY TESTS
Low thyroxine (T_4) and triiodithyronine (T_3)

Screening Tests for Diagnosing Hyperadrenocorticism
• See Appendix for protocols. • ACTH response test—exaggerated plasma cortisol response in patients with hyperadrenocorticism • Low-dose dexamethasone suppression test (dexamethasone [Azium]; dogs, 0.015 mg/kg; cats, 0.1 mg/kg)—failure to suppress (cortisol < 1.4 mg/dl) at 8 hours in patients with hyperadrenocorticism • Urinary cortisol-creatinine ratio (positive result must be confirmed by blood test)—high ratio in patients with hyperadrenocorticism • Note: Nonadrenal illness may cause false-positive screening test results.

Differentiating PDH from Adrenal Tumor
High-dose dexamethasone suppression test (1 mg/kg dexamethasone [Azium])—no suppression (cortisol < 50% of baseline or < 1.4 mg/dl at 4 or 8 hours) in patients with adrenal tumor. Suppression in 75% of dogs with PDH. • Plasma ACTH concentration—normal to high in patients with PDH and low in those with adrenal tumor • CRH response test—exaggerated plasma cortisol response in patients with PDH. No important change in plasma cortisol in patients with adrenal tumor

IMAGING
• Abdominal radiography may differentiate PDH from adrenal tumor (one third of adrenal tumors mineralize). Thoracic radiography to detect metastasis in patients with adrenal tumor. Other radiographic findings include hepatomegaly, osteoporosis, dystrophic calcification, congestive heart failure (rare), and pulmonary embolism (rare). • Ultrasonography, CT, and MRI often are useful for differentiating PDH from adrenal tumor as well as staging adrenal tumor. CT and MRI often are useful for revealing pituitary macroadenoma.

OTHER DIAGNOSTIC PROCEDURES
Blood pressure determination frequently documents systemic hypertension.

GROSS AND HISTOPATHOLOGIC FINDINGS
• PDH—normal-sized pituitary to pituitary macroadenoma and bilateral adrenocortical enlargement. Microscopically, pituitary adenoma or corticotroph hyperplasia of pars distalis or pars intermedia and adrenocortical hyperplasia • Adrenal tumor—variable-sized adrenal mass, atrophy of contralateral gland (bilateral tumors rare), and metastasis in some animals with adrenal carcinoma. Microscopically, adrenocortical adenoma or carcinoma.

TREATMENT

INPATIENT VERSUS OUTPATIENT
Dictated by the severity of clinical signs, the animal's overall condition, and any complicating factors (e.g., diabetes mellitus and pulmonary embolism)

ACTIVITY N/A

DIET
High-fiber diet if patient has diabetes mellitus

CLIENT EDUCATION
Lifelong therapy is required. If the patient has an adverse reaction to mitotane, discontinue the drug, give prednisone, and reevaluate in the next few days. If there is no response to prednisone in a few hours, evaluate immediately.

SURGICAL CONSIDERATIONS
• Hypophysectomy, while described, generally is not recommended for the treatment of PDH in dogs or cats because of the difficulty of the procedure and the need for intensive monitoring and lifelong hormonal supplementation.
• Bilateral adrenalectomy generally is not done to treat PDH in dogs. Cats, however, seem to tolerate the surgery better than dogs and with the appropriate personnel and facilities it is one treatment of choice for PDH in cats.
• Surgery should be considered the treatment of choice for adrenocortical adenoma and small carcinoma unless the animal is a poor surgical risk or the client refuses surgery. Medical control of hyperadrenocorticism with ketoconazole is recommended before surgery.

MEDICATIONS

DRUGS AND FLUIDS
• Mitotane (o, p'-DDD) is the drug of choice for the medical management of both PDH and adrenal tumor in dogs.

• Treatment of PDH—initial loading dosage of mitotane, 40-50 mg/kg/day until both basal and post-ACTH cortisol concentrations are in the normal resting range (1-5 mg/dl); then, 50 mg/kg/week divided into 2-3 doses; adjust dosage according to ACTH response testing. Give prednisone (0.2 mg/kg/day) during initial and subsequent loading periods. See follow-up for patient monitoring.

• Treatment for adrenal tumor—mitotane is used as chemotherapy. Goal is to obtain low to undetectable basal and post-ACTH cortisol concentrations or administer mitotane at the highest tolerated dosage. Give prednisone at 0.2 mg/kg/day.

• Drug of choice for medical management of hyperadrenocorticism in cats is controversial and further studies are indicated—mitotane (50 mg/kg/day then 50 mg/kg/week divided into 2-3 doses; adjust dosage according to ACTH response testing) or metyrapone (65 mg/kg q8-12h; adjust dosage according ACTH response testing)

CONTRAINDICATIONS N/A

PRECAUTIONS

• Side effects of mitotane are not uncommon but are mild in most dogs and include lethargy, weakness, anorexia, vomiting, diarrhea, ataxia, and iatrogenic hypoadrenocorticism. Side effects are more common in dogs with adrenal tumor that are given high doses of mitotane.

• Side effects of ketoconazole seem to be less common and include anorexia, vomiting, diarrhea, and transiently high liver enzyme activity.

POSSIBLE INTERACTIONS N/A

ALTERNATE DRUGS

• Ketoconazole (10 mg/kg q12h initially; up 20 mg/kg q12h in some dogs) is indicated in dogs unable to tolerate mitotane at a dosage necessary to control hyperadrenocorticism, for preoperative control of hyperadrenocorticism in dogs with adrenal tumor scheduled for adrenalectomy, and may be useful for palliation of clinical signs of hyperadrenocorticism in dogs with adrenal tumor. Over 25% of dogs fail to respond adequately to the drug.

• L-deprenyl is a newly-described alternative for treatment of PDH in dogs, but has not been used in cats. Further reports of long-term safety and efficacy are needed.

• For animals with pituitary macroadenomas, radiotherapy should be considered. ACTH concentration may take several months to di-minish; medical control of hyperadrenocorticism with drugs is necessary in the interim.

FOLLOW-UP

PATIENT MONITORING

Response to treatment by ACTH response testing (see references). Test after the initial 7-10 days of mitotane or ketoconazole administration to assure adequate response, then at 1, 3, and 6 months and every 6-12 months thereafter. Adequacy of any necessary mitotane reloading period is also checked by ACTH response test before a higher maintenance dosage of mitotane is initiated.

PREVENTION/AVOIDANCE N/A

POSSIBLE COMPLICATIONS

Iatrogenic hypoadrenocorticism with mitotane administration

EXPECTED COURSE AND PROGNOSIS

• Depending on the problem, clinical signs resolve within several days to months of appropriate treatment. • Untreated hyperadrenocorticism is generally a progressive disorder with a poor prognosis. • Treated PDH has a good prognosis in most patients. The average survival time for a dog with PDH treated by mitotane is 2 years with at least 10% surviving 4 years. Dogs living > 6 months tend to die of causes unrelated to their hyperadrenocorticism. • Patients with macroadenoma and neurologic signs have a poor to grave prognosis. • Adrenal adenoma carries a good to excellent prognosis in most patients and small carcinoma (not metastasized) a fair to good prognosis. • Patients with a large carcinoma or adrenal tumor with widespread metastasis generally have a poor to fair prognosis, but impressive responses to high doses of mitotane occasionally are seen.

MISCELLANEOUS

ASSOCIATED CONDITIONS

• Neurologic signs in dogs with large pituitary tumors • Glucose intolerance or concurrent diabetes mellitus • Pulmonary thromboembolism • Increased incidence of urinary tract and skin infections • Systemic hyperten-sion • Proteinuria and glomerulopathy
• Congestive heart failure (rare)

AGE RELATED FACTORS N/A

ZOONOTIC POTENTIAL N/A

PREGNANCY N/A

SYNONYMS Cushing's disease

SEE ALSO N/A

ABBREVIATIONS

ACTH = adrenocorticotropic hormone
ALP = alkaline phosphatase
CRH = corticotropin releasing hormone
CT = computed tomography
MRI = magnetic resonsance imaging
PDH = pituitary dependent hyperadrenocorticism
T$_4$ = thyroxine
T$_3$ = triiodithyronine

References

Kintzer PP, Peterson ME. Mitotane therapy of canine hyperadrenocorticism. In: Kirk RW, Bonagura JD, eds. Current veterinary therapy XII. Philadelphia: WB Saunders, 1995.

Myers NC, Bruyette DS. Feline adrenocortical diseases I: hyperadrenocorticism. Sem Vet Med Surg, August 1994.

Peterson ME. Hyperadrenocorticism. In: Kirk RW, ed. Current veterinary therapy IX. Philadelphia: WB Saunders, 1986.

Peterson ME, Kintzer PP. Medical treatment of pituitary-dependent hyperadrenocorticism in dogs. Sem Vet Med Surg 1994;9:127-131.

Author Peter P. Kintzer
Consulting Editor Rhett Nichols

HYPERANDROGENISM

BASICS

OVERVIEW
High absolute or relative concentrations of masculinizing sex hormones such as testosterone and its derivatives. Androgens are produced by testicular interstitial (i.e., Leydig) cells, ovaries, the adrenal cortex, and peripheral conversion of weak androgens to more potent androgens. Hyperandrogenism can cause behavioral changes, abnormalities of the reproductive tract, and dermatologic problems.

SIGNALMENT
• Dogs and cats • Pomeranians at higher risk than other breeds

SIGNS

Historical Findings
• Aggression • High libido • Virilization in females—lifting the leg to urinate, excessive mounting behavior, and irregular estrous cycles • Stunted growth may be caused by early closure of epiphyseal growth plates.

Physical Examination Findings
• Clitoral hypertrophy • Gynecomastia can be caused by aromatization of excess androgens to estrogens. • Priaprism • Alopecia or hirsutism • Hyperpigmentation of the skin • Seborrhea oleosa • Perianal adenoma • Prostatomegaly • Tail gland hyperplasia

CAUSES AND RISK FACTORS
• Exogenous administration of androgens and anabolic steroids • High endogenous secretion of testosterone by gonadal tissue • Testicular tumor • Exposure of female fetuses to androgens • High concentrations of gonadotrophin-releasing hormone and luteinizing hormone

DIAGNOSIS

DIFFERENTIAL DIAGNOSIS
• Hyperadrenocorticism and hypothyroidism are ruled out by endocrine testing. • Consider behavioral problems and CNS disease in overly aggressive animals • Immune-mediated skin disease can be differentiated by skin biopsy and direct immunofluorescent studies. • Rule out parasitic skin disease (e.g., mange) by examination of multiple skin scrapings. • Rule out intersex abnormality (e.g., hemaphrodites and pseudohemaphrodites) by physical examination or karyotyping.

CBC/BIOCHEMISTRY/URINALYSIS
Results usually normal

OTHER LABORATORY TESTS
Repeated serum testing, gonadotropin-releasing hormone response test, and luteinizing hormone response test superior to single serum testing to detect high concentration of testosterone. (See appendix for test protocols.)

IMAGING
Abdominal radiography, abdominal ultrasonography, and exploratory laparotomy may be useful to detect intrabdominal gonadal tissue or testosterone secreting neoplasms.

OTHER DIAGNOSTIC PROCEDURES
Skin biopsies are consistent with other endocrinopathies.

TREATMENT
• Neutering of intact animals
• Surgical excision of testosterone-secreting tumor

MEDICATIONS

DRUGS AND FLUIDS
• Megestrol acetate (Ovaban®) inhibits 5 alpha reductase in the prostate gland.
• Mitotane (Lysodren) in dogs with high adrenal androgens. (see Hyperadrenocorticism for dosaging)

CONTRAINDICATIONS/POSSIBLE
INTERACTIONS N/A

FOLLOW-UP
• Repeat serum testosterone concentration after neutering • Aggressive behavior, dermatologic abnormalities, and gynecomastia resolve after castration in some animals. • Virilization of females may be prevented by avoiding in utero exposure to androgens and exogenous administration of androgens and anabolic steroids postnatally.

MISCELLANEOUS

ASSOCIATED CONDITIONS
• High concentration of adrenal androgens associated with growth hormone-responsive dermatosis in the Pomeranian • Hyperandrogenism in male dogs enhances perianal gland adenoma and benign prostatic hyperplasia

SEE ALSO
• Dermatoses, Growth Hormone Responsive
• Dermatoses, Sex Hormone Responsive

ABBREVIATION
CNS = central nervous system

Reference

Schmeitzel LP. Growth hormone-responsive alopecia and sex hormone-associated dermatoses. In: Birchard SJ, Sherding RG, eds. Saunders manual of small animal practice. Philadelphia: WB Saunders, 1994:326-329.

Author Margaret R. Kern
Consulting Editor Rhett Nichols

BASICS

OVERVIEW
• An imbalance between coagulation factors and inhibitors that shifts the balance toward clot formation and results in an increased risk of thrombosis • Mechanisms include congenital or acquired deficiency of coagulation inhibitors or dysfibrinogenemia. • Most common mechanism is loss of antithrombin III and perhaps other factors because of protein-losing nephropathy. • Effects of thrombosis vary according to thrombus location. Pulmonary arteries are a common site of thrombosis.

SIGNALMENT
• No breed or sex predilection • Uncommon in cats

SIGNS
• None, before onset of thrombosis • Pulmonary embolism presents with respiratory distress, hepatomegaly, ventral edema, and jugular distention.

CAUSES AND RISK FACTORS
• Protein-losing nephropathy • Disseminated intravascular coagulation • Congenital deficiencies in factors related to clotting

DIAGNOSIS

DIFFERENTIAL DIAGNOSIS
• Vascular damage secondary to septicemia or trauma. Use CBC, history, and physical examination to differentiate. • Stasis of blood flow as in cardiomyopathy of cats and polycythemia (rare in dogs and cats)

CBC/BIOCHEMISTRY/URINALYSIS
• Hypoproteinemia, hypoalbuminemia, and proteinuria, if antithrombin III deficiency is secondary to protein-losing nephropathy

• Thrombocytopenia and schistocytosis in some animals with disseminated intravascular coagulation

OTHER LABORATORY TESTS
• Partial thromboplastin time, prothrombin time, fibrinogen, and fibrin degradation products—abnormal in some animals with disseminated intravascular coagulation • Thrombin time—rules out dysfibrinogenemia • Specific assays of coagulation factors and inhibitors—necessary to identify deficiencies • Urine protein/creatinine ratio, if protein-losing nephropathy is suspected

IMAGING
Angiography may be necessary to localize thrombus

OTHER DIAGNOSTIC PROCEDURES
N/A

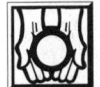

TREATMENT
• Treat animals with protein-losing nephropathy as inpatients only if thrombosis has resulted in dysfunction of important organs. Restrict activity that may lead to trauma, and warn owner of dangers of thrombosis.
• Treat animals with disseminated intravascular coagulation as inpatients by severely restricting activity.

MEDICATIONS

DRUGS AND FLUIDS

Protein-Losing Nephropathy
• Give maintenance fluids if necessary to avoid dehydration.
• Administer heparin, then warfarin, to decrease coagulation. Use aspirin as a warfarin alternative.
• Provide fresh frozen plasma or whole plasma to replace inhibitors, especially antithrombin III.

• Consider thrombolytic therapy with streptokinase or urokinase, if thrombosis has occurred.

Disseminated Intravascular Coagulation
See chapter on disseminated intravascular coagulation

CONTRAINDICATIONS/POSSIBLE INTERACTIONS
Do not treat with warfarin initially or exclusively; effect on anticoagulant proteins C and S and on vitamin K dependent factors leads to initial hypercoagulability

FOLLOW-UP
Initially, monitor prothrombin time every 3 days to titrate the dose of warfarin to 1.5-2 times the baseline prothrombin value. Use international normalization ratios to minimize the effects of test kit variability on prothrombin results. Monitor prothrombin times on a weekly basis after a stable dose has been achieved (typically no sooner than 2 weeks).

MISCELLANEOUS

SEE ALSO
• Amyloidosis • Aortic Thromboembolism
• Disseminated Intravascular Coagulation
• Disseminated Intravascular Hemolysis
• Glomerulonephritis • Pulmonary Thromboembolism

ABBREVIATION
CBC = complete blood count

Reference
Bick RL, Pegram M. Syndromes of hypercoagulability and thrombosis: a review. Sem Thromb Hemost 1994;20:109-132.
Author G. Daniel Boon
Consulting Editor Alan H. Rebar

HYPEREOSINOPHILIC SYNDROME

BASICS

OVERVIEW
• Idiopathic persistent eosinophilia—caused by sustained overproduction of eosinophils in bone marrow, which is hypothesized to result from severe reaction to an undefined antigen
• Probably includes a heterogeneous group of disorders • Multisystemic syndrome with invasion of tissues by eosinophils and subsequent organ damage and dysfunction, leading to death • Frequent tissue sites of infiltration include the gastrointestinal tract (especially intestine and liver), spleen, and lymph nodes, especially mesenteric nodes. • Less common sites are skin, kidney, heart, thyroid, lung, adrenal glands, and pancreas. Organ damage results from effects of eosinophil granule products and eosinophil-derived cytokines that are released in the tissues from activated or necrotic cells.

SIGNALMENT
• In cats, may occur more frequently in female, middle-aged domestic shorthair cats
• In dogs, occurs rarely and has been incompletely described

SIGNS
In many animals, signs occur for several weeks before presentation.

Historical Findings
• Lethargy • Anorexia • Intermittent vomiting and diarrhea • Weight loss • Less frequently, fever, pruritus, and seizures

Physical Examination Findings
• Fever • Emaciation • Hepatosplenomegaly
• Thickened (diffuse or segmental) intestine that is nonpainful • Mesenteric, and possible peripheral, lymphadenopathy • Mass lesions resulting from eosinophilic granulomatous inflammation that involves lymph nodes or organs • Pruritic erythroderma

CAUSES AND RISK FACTORS
• Unknown, but condition is believed to be a severe reaction to an underlying, but unidentifiable, antigenic stimulus • In cats, eosinophilic enteritis may be an early form.

DIAGNOSIS

DIFFERENTIAL DIAGNOSIS
Eosinophilic leukemia—distinction from hypereosinophilic syndrome is controversial, but the following differentiating criteria characterize eosinophilic leukemia:
• Immature eosinophils occur more frequently in the circulation and constitute a higher percentage of the leukocyte differential.

• Anemia occurs more often than in hypereosinophilic syndrome. Myeloid:erythroid ratio in bone marrow is higher (> 10:1) in affected cats, and blast forms are more numerous. • Tissue infiltrates consist of immature eosinophils and may show a sinusoidal pattern in the liver without fibrosis.
• In cats, chloroma-like masses in the kidneys have been reported. • Identifiable causes of eosinophilia, including parasitism, hypersensitivity disorders, infectious diseases, immune-mediated diseases, and neoplasia. In these conditions, eosinophilia is usually limited in degree and remains confined to a specific organ, such as the lung in feline asthma.

CBC/BIOCHEMISTRY/URINALYSIS
• Leukocytosis with eosinophilia (usually marked), possibly with a left shift in eosinophil series; eosinophil count range: 3200-130,000/ul • Basophilia • Anemia in some animals • In animals with organ dysfunction, biochemical abnormalities may be seen.

OTHER LABORATORY TESTS N/A

IMAGING
Intestinal mucosal irregularities and thickened intestine noted on radiographic contrast studies

OTHER DIAGNOSTIC PROCEDURES
• Bone marrow aspiration findings—hypercellular marrow, eosinophilic hyperplasia (up to 40% of nucleated cells consist of eosinophils), lack of morphologic abnormalities, and high myeloid:erythroid ratio (mean 7.27:1) • Biopsy of affected organ or mass

GROSS AND HISTOPATHOLOGIC FINDINGS
• Spleen—eosinophilic infiltrate found in red pulp, sometimes in white pulp • Gastrointestinal tract—mucosal and submucosal eosinophilic infiltrates noted in the small intestine, sometimes in the colon and stomach
• Lymph nodes—reactive hyperplasia, infiltration of cords and sinuses with eosinophils
• Heart—eosinophilic infiltrates found in myocardium and endocardium, with fibrosis and thrombus formation

TREATMENT
• Use long-term maintenance therapy to control or reduce the eosinophilia and organ damage.
• Usually, massive tissue infiltration impedes treatment attempts and results in poor prognosis.
• Occurrence of high serum IgE levels portends good response to treatment with prednisone and a better prognosis.

MEDICATIONS

DRUGS AND FLUIDS
• Corticosteroids—administer prednisolone, 1-3 mg/kg/day initially; then taper to alternate-day administration, if eosinophilia is suppressed. If eosinophilia returns, resume higher daily dose.
• Chemotherapeutic agents—try these agents if eosinophilia is steroid-resistant, but the paucity of case reports describing these therapies precludes recommending their use
• Hydroxyurea (inhibits DNA synthesis)—provide to reduce the eosinophil count after 7-14 days
• Cyclosporine—use to suppress production of eosinophilopoietic factors by T cells
• Vincristine and alkylating agents like chlorambucil are effective in humans.
• Reduce dosage or discontinue drug if toxicities such as bone marrow suppression or development of thrombocytopenia occur.

CONTRAINDICATIONS/POSSIBLE INTERACTIONS
Aggressive cytotoxic therapy has been deleterious in some human hypereosinophilic patients.

FOLLOW-UP
• Monitor CBC for eosinophil count (not always indicative of tissue infiltrates).
• Monitor clinical signs (anorexia, lethargy, vomiting, diarrhea) and any physical abnormalities.

MISCELLANEOUS

ABBREVIATIONS
CBC = complete blood count

References
Hendrick M. A spectrum of hypereosinophilic syndromes exemplified by six cats with eosinophilic enteritis. Vet Pathol 1981;18:188-200.
Huibregtse BA, Turner JL. Hypereosinophilic syndrome and eosinophilic leukemia: a comparison of 22 hypereosinophilic cats. J Anim Hosp Assoc 1994;30:591-599.

Author Karen M. Young
Consulting Editor Alan H. Rebar

BASICS

OVERVIEW

High absolute or relative concentrations of feminizing sex hormones such as estradiol, estriol, and estrone. Estrogens are produced by the ovary, testes, adrenal cortex, and by peripheral conversion of precursor hormones. The main organs affected are skin, urogenital tract, and hematopoeitic system.

SIGNALMENT

• Dogs and cats • Endogenous hyperestrogenism more common in middle-aged to old dogs

SIGNS

Historical Findings

• Low libido in males • Infertility • Males attracting other males • Failure of male dogs to lift their leg to urinate • Hematuria • Abnormal estrous cycles; prolonged proestrus or estrus • Nymphomania; excessive mounting of other females • Failure of hair to grow after clipping

Physical Examination Findings

• Testicular mass or large testicles in animals with endogenous hyperestrogenism • Bilateral testicular atrophy in animals with exogenous hyperestrogenism • Cryptorchidism • Pale mucous membranes are manifestations of anemia and bone marrow suppression in dogs. • Petechiation or other signs of hemorrhage • Large clitoris and vulva • Vaginal hyperplasia and prolapse • Pendulous prepuce • Gynecomastia • Galactorrhea • Bilateral, symmetrical alopecia beginning at the flank and perineum • Cutaneous hyperpigmentation • Prostatomegaly • Prostatic cyst or abscess • Fever, depression, and pyometra may be caused by neutropenia associated with bone marrow suppression.

CAUSES AND RISK FACTORS

• Cystic ovaries • Functional ovarian tumors (e.g., granulosa-theca cell) • A functional testicular tumor is usually a Sertoli cell tumor, but it can be a seminoma or interstitial cell tumor. • Exogenous estrogen administration

DIAGNOSIS

DIFFERENTIAL DIAGNOSIS

• Hyperadrenocorticism and hypothyroidism—rule out initially • Intersex abnormalities (e.g., hemaproditism and pseudohemaphroditism) • Allergic skin disease

• Autoimmune skin disease • Demodicosis and dermatophytosis

CBC/BIOCHEMISTRY/URINALYSIS

• Nonregenerative anemia, thrombocytopenia, and leukocytosis initially followed by leukopenia • Hematuria

OTHER LABORATORY TESTS

• High serum estrogen (estradiol) concentration to help confirm a suspected diagnosis • Serum should be separated from RBC, refrigerated, and shipped on ice. Lipemia may interfere with the radioimmunoassay. • Examination of prepucial or vaginal specimen may reveal numerous cornified cells with pyknotic nuclei or anuclear cells. • Gonadotropin-releasing hormone (GnRH) response test to detect suspected ovarian tissue after ovariohysterectomy

IMAGING

Radiography and ultrasonography to detect cryptorchid testicles or intrabdominal mass

OTHER DIAGNOSTIC PROCEDURES

• Examination of bone marrow aspirate or biopsy may reveal hypoplasia, aplasia, or fatty infiltration. • Laparoscopy or laparotomy to detect cryptorchid testicles or intraabdominal mass • Skin biopsy—findings may be consistent with those of other endocrinopathies (i.e., orthokeratotic hyperkeratosis, epidermal thinning, follicular keratosis, dilation and atrophy, increased telogen hair follicles, and sebaceous gland atrophy)

TREATMENT

• Neutering is the treatment of choice for endogenous hyperestrogenism.
• Castration of dogs with testicular neoplasia may result in permanent resolution of clinical signs.
• Ovarihysterectomy for functional ovarian tumor and cystic ovaries
• Discontinue exogenous drug administration.

MEDICATIONS

DRUGS AND FLUIDS

• Supportive and symptomatic therapy as indicated
• Whole blood transfusion or blood component therapy may be needed in patients with severe bone marrow suppression.
• Antibiotics are administered to treat secondary infection.
• Androgens and lithium may be tried to stimulate hypoplastic marrow.

• GnRH may be used to treat persistent estrus and vaginal hyperplasia caused by follicular cysts.

CONTRAINDICATIONS/POSSIBLE INTERACTIONS

• Myelosuppressive chemotherapeutic agents should not be used in patients with bone marrow suppression.
• Estrogens may increase serum concentrations of thyroxine (T_4) and triiodithyronine (T_3).

FOLLOW-UP

• Repeat CBC to monitor effectiveness of therapy or disease progression. • Male feminization signs usually have resolved by 2-6 weeks after castration without metastatic disease. • Serum estrogen concentrations should return to normal after surgical removal of functional tumors. • Bone marrow aplasia usually does not respond to castration. • Bone marrow suppression may be a permanent sequela. • Measure serum progesterone after Gn-RH administration for cystic ovaries. If ovulation occurred, serum progesterone should be > 1 ng/ml, and the bitch should be bred at the next estrus.

MISCELLANEOUS

ASSOCIATED CONDITIONS

• Canine male feminizing syndrome has been associated with hyperestrogenism and usually is caused by Sertoli cell tumor. • Hyperestrogenism also may be associated with prostatic neoplasia. • Hyperestrogenism is thought to be associated with ovarian imbalance type I dermatosis. • Exogenous estrogens should be discontinued in dogs with acute pancreatitis. • Exogenous estrogen administration is potentially hepatotoxic.

ABBREVIATION

GnRH = gonadotropin-releasing hormone

Reference

Schmeitzel LP. Growth hormone-responsive alopecia and sex hormone-associated dermatoses. In: Birchard SJ, Sherding RG, eds. Saunders manual of small animal practice. Philadelphia: WB Saunders, 1994:326-329.
Author Margaret R. Kern
Consulting Editor Rhett Nichols

HYPERPARATHYROIDISM

BASICS

DEFINITION
A pathologic, sustained high circulating concentration of parathyroid hormone (PTH)

Pathophysiology
• PTH is secreted by the parathyroid gland in response to changes in the concentration of ionized calcium in the serum. The effect of PTH is to raise the serum calcium concentration through its effects on bone and renal tubular calcium resorption and vitamin D-dependent intestinal calcium absorption.
• Hyperparathyroidism can develop as a primary condition or secondarily to a disorder of calcium homeostasis. Primary hyperparathyroidism is associated with benign (usually) adenoma of the parathyroid gland(s). Secondary hyperparathyroidism can be caused by a deficiency of calcium and vitamin D associated with malnutrition or chronic renal disease.

Systems Affected
• Renal/Urologic • Gastrointestinal
• Neuromuscular • Cardiovascular

Genetics N/A

Incidence/Prevalence
• The prevalence of primary hyperparathyroidism is unknown. • It is more commonly diagnosed in dogs than in cats. • Among causes of hypercalcemia, hyperparathyroidism is fairly common although much less so than hypercalcemia of malignancy. • Nutritional secondary hyperparathyroidism is decreasing in prevalence as the public becomes more educated in pet nutrition. • Chronic renal failure and secondary hyperparathyroidism, is extremely common, more so in cats than in dogs.

Geographic Distribution N/A

SIGNALMENT

Species Dogs and cats

Breed Predilections
• Keeshond • Siamese cat

Mean Age and Range
• Dogs—mean age, 10 years; range 5-15 years • Cats—mean age,13 years; range 8-15 years

Predominant Sex None

SIGNS

General Comments
Most dogs and cats with primary hyperparathyroidism do not appear ill Signs are usually mild and are due solely to the effects of hypercalcemia. Signs become apparent when hypercalcemia is severe and chronic.

History and Physical Examination Findings
• Polyuria • Polydipsia • Anorexia • Lethargy • Vomiting • Weakness • Urolithiasis • Stupor and coma • Note: Parathyroid ade-

noma is not palpable in dogs but sometimes can be palpated in cats. Nutritional secondary disease is sometimes associated with pathologic bone fractures and general poor body condition.

CAUSES
• Primary hyperparathyroidism is caused by PTH-secreting adenoma of the parathyroid gland. • Renal secondary hyperparathyroidism is caused by renal calcium loss and reduced gut absorption of calcium due to deficiency in calcitriol production by the renal tubular cells (renal secondary hyperparathyroidism). • Nutritional secondary hyperparathyroidism is caused by a nutritional deficiency of calcium and vitamin D.

RISK FACTORS None

DIAGNOSIS

DIFFERENTIAL DIAGNOSIS
The differential list includes causes for hypercalcemia:
• Lymphosarcoma • Anal sac apocrine gland adenocarcinoma • Other miscellaneous carcinomas • Chronic renal failure • Hypoadrenocorticism • Vitamin D rodenticide intoxication

CBC/BIOCHEMISTRY/URINALYSIS
• High serum calcium concentration • Low or low-normal serum phosphorus concentration • BUN and creatinine concentrations usually normal in patients with primary hyperparathyroidism except in those with hypercalcemia-induced renal failure

OTHER LABORATORY TESTS
• Serum ionized calcium determination—often normal in patients with chronic renal failure; high in patients with primary hyperparathyroidism and hypercalcemia associated with malignancy • Serum PTH concentration—high serum PTH is diagnostic for primary hyperparathyroidism in the absence of azotemia. Assays that measure the intact PTH molecule are most useful.

IMAGING
• Radiography can be useful to assess urolithiasis, renal morphology, and bone density and for the identification of occult neoplasia.
• Ultrasonography of the ventral cervical area sometimes reveals a parathyroid gland adenoma.

OTHER DIAGNOSTIC PROCEDURES
Surgical exploration of the ventral cervical area.

GROSS AND HISTOPATHOLOGIC FINDINGS
Parathyroid adenoma is usually a solitary, small (1 cm or less), round, light brown or reddish mass located in proximity to the thyroid gland. Occasionally multiple adenomas are found. The histologic distinctions between adenomas, hyperplasia, and carcinomas of the parathyroid gland are often unclear.

TREATMENT

INPATIENT VERSUS OUTPATIENT
• Primary hyperparathyroidism generally requires inpatient care and surgery.
• Nutritional or renal secondary hyperparathyroidism in noncritical patients can be managed on an outpatient basis.

ACTIVITY N/A

DIET
Secondary forms of hyperparathyroidism necessitate dietary calcium supplementation.

CLIENT EDUCATION
Explain signs referable to changes in calcium status, since hypocalcemia is a potential complication of parathyroidectomy.

SURGICAL CONSIDERATIONS
Surgery is the treatment of choice for primary hyperparathyroidism and is often important in establishing the diagnosis.

MEDICATIONS

DRUGS AND FLUIDS
• Normal saline is the fluid of choice for treatment of hypercalcemia.
• Diuretics (furosemide) and corticosteroids can be useful in the treatment of hypercalcemia.
• There is no medical treatment for primary hyperparathyroidism per se.

CONTRAINDICATIONS
• Until the diagnosis of lymphoma has been excluded, glucocorticoids should not be used since they can obfuscate the diagnosis.
• Calcium-containing fluids should be avoided.

PRECAUTIONS
Mithramycin has been used in patients with severe hypercalcemic crises. Its use should be avoided if possible because of associated nephrotoxicity and hepatotoxicity.

POSSIBLE INTERACTIONS N/A

ALTERNATIVE DRUGS None

FOLLOW-UP

PATIENT MONITORING
• Postoperative hypocalcemia relatively common after treatment of primary hyperparathyroidism in patients with a presurgery serum calcium concentration > 14 mg/dl. Monitor serum calcium 1-2 times daily for a period of one week after surgery. • In patients with renal impairment, monitor serum concentrations of urea nitrogen and creatinine.

PREVENTION/AVOIDANCE
• No strategies exist for prevention of primary hyperparathyroidism. • Nutritional secondary hyperparathyroidism is prevented by proper nutrition.

POSSIBLE COMPLICATIONS
Irreversible renal failure secondary to hypercalcemia

EXPECTED COURSE AND PROGNOSIS
• Untreated disease usually progresses to end-stage kidney or neurologic disease. Prognosis for treatment of parathyroid adenoma is excellent. • Recurrence is seen in a small percentage of cases.

MISCELLANEOUS

ASSOCIATED CONDITIONS
Calcium-containing urolithiasis

AGE RELATED FACTORS N/A

ZOONOTIC POTENTIAL None

PREGNANCY N/A

SYNONYMS None

SEE ALSO
• Calcium, Hypercalcemia • Renal Failure, Chronic • Hyperparathyroidism, Renal Secondary

ABBREVIATIONS
PTH = parathyroid hormone

References

Feldman EC. Disorders of the parathyroid glands. In: Ettinger SJ, Feldman EC, eds. Textbook of veterinary internal medicine. 4th ed. Philadelphia: WB Saunders, 1994;1437-1464.

Chew DJ, Nagode LA, Carothers M. Disorders of calcium: hypercalcemia and hypocalcemia. In: DiBartola SP. Fluid therapy in small animal practice. Philadelphia: WB Saunders, 1992;116-176.

Author Thomas K. Graves

Consulting Editor Rhett Nichols

HYPERPARATHYROIDISM, RENAL SECONDARY

BASICS

OVERVIEW
• Renal secondary hyperparathyroidism is a clinical syndrome characterized by a high concentration of biologically active parathyroid hormone (PTH) secondary to chronic renal failure.
• Hyperphosphatemia secondary to declining renal function reduces the activity of the 1,alpha-hydroxylase enzyme in the kidney, which in turn reduces production of calcitriol (1,25-dihydroxycholecalciferol). Low calcitriol concentration results in a low serum ionized calcium concentration, which increases PTH production and causes parathyroid gland hyperplasia. High PTH production reduces serum calcitriol and calcium concentrations at the expense of a chronically high PTH concentration.
• Calcitriol synthesis is impaired in animals with severe chronic renal failure and low numbers of renal tubules. PTH may act as a uremic toxin and may promote nephrocalcinosis and progression of chronic renal failure.

SIGNALMENT
Dogs and cats

SIGNS
• Those associated with underlying chronic renal failure are the usual reason for examination.
• Severe renal osteodystrophy or "rubber jaw" is detected in some animals, most commonly in young dogs.

CAUSES AND RISK FACTORS
Any disease that causes chronic renal failure.

DIAGNOSIS

DIFFERENTIAL DIAGNOSIS
• Hypercalcemic nephropathy is renal disease (or failure) caused by hypercalcemia and can be difficult to differentiate from renal secondary hyperparathyroidism.
• The total serum calcium concentration is usually higher in animals with hypercalcemic nephropathy than in those with renal secondary hyperparathyroidism. The ionized serum calcium concentration is usually low or normal in animals with renal secondary hyperparathyroidism and high in those with hypercalcemic nephropathy.
• Serum PTH concentration is low in animals with hypercalcemia of malignancy. Underlying causes of hypercalcemia such as lymphoma or adenocarcinoma of the anal sac may be detected.

• Primary hyperparathyroidism is initially characterized by hypercalcemia (ionized and total), normal or low serum phosphorus concentration, and high PTH concentration. Renal function is initially normal in primary hyperparathyroidism but may become compromised later in the course of disease.

CBC/BIOCHEMISTRY/URINALYSIS
• Azotemia
• Hyperphosphatemia
• Urine specific gravity < 1.030 in dogs and < 1.035 in cats
• Possible hypocalcemia (ionized calcium). The total serum calcium concentration may be low, normal, or slightly high. See Chronic Renal Failure.

OTHER LABORATORY TESTS
• Measurement of a high serum PTH concentration is necessary for definitive diagnosis and therapeutic monitoring of renal secondary hyperparathyroidism. An immunoassay for PTH directed against the amino-terminal or intact PTH molecule and validated for dogs or cats is preferred.
• A low ionized serum calcium concentration is useful for differentiating renal secondary hyperparathyroidism from other causes of hypercalcemia.

IMAGING
Radiographs may reveal low bone density, loss of the lamina dura around the teeth, and soft-tissue mineralization of the gastric mucosa or other tissues.

OTHER DIAGNOSTIC PROCEDURES
N/A

TREATMENT
• See Chronic Renal Failure for general treatment principles.
• Patients with renal secondary hyperparathyroidism should be fed a diet low in phosphorus and have free access to fresh water.

MEDICATIONS

DRUGS AND FLUIDS
Intestinal Phosphate Binders
• Prescribe if dietary management does not return phosphorus concentration to normal
• Aluminum carbonate (30-100 mg/kg/day PO with meals)
• Calcium carbonate (90-150 mg/kg/day PO with meals)
• Calcium acetate (60-90 mg/kg/day PO with meals)
• Hypercalcemia may develop when a calci-

um-containing phosphate binder is combined with calcitriol.
• Aluminum- and calcium-containing phosphate binder can be used in combination to reduce the dosage of each and minimize the risk of hypercalcemia.

Calcitriol
• Low-dose calcitriol (1.5-3.5 mg/kg PO q24h) may be used after initiation of dietary phosphorus restriction and oral phosphate binder.
• Maintain the serum phosphorus concentration within the normal range before and during calcitriol administration.

CONTRAINDICATIONS / POSSIBLE INTERACTIONS
• Calcitriol administration can result in hypercalcemia, especially if combined with a calcium-containing, intestinal phosphate binder.
• Calcium-containing intestinal phosphate binder should not be used in patients with hyperphosphatemia or with a calcium x phosphorus product > 70. Aluminum-containing intestinal phosphate binder should be used initially to correct hyperphosphatemia, followed by calcium-containing intestinal phosphate binder once the serum phosphorus concentration is normal.

FOLLOW-UP

PATIENT MONITORING
• Serum concentrations of calcium, phosphorus, creatinine, and urea nitrogen should be monitored weekly to monthly depending on treatment and the severity of chronic renal failure.
• Patients receiving calcitriol should be monitored weekly for 4 weeks then monthly for hypercalcemia and hyperphosphatemia.
• Serial evaluations of PTH concentration should document normalization of serum PTH concentration and allow for adjustments of calcitriol dosage.

PREVENTION / AVOIDANCE
Dietary phosphorus restriction in patients with chronic renal failure may delay the onset of renal secondary hyperparathyroidism.

POSSIBLE COMPLICATIONS
Renal osteodystrophy and pathologic fractures (rare)

EXPECTED COURSE AND PROGNOSIS
• Progression of the underlying chronic renal failure may be slowed by treatment of renal secondary hyperparathyroidism.
• Long-term prognosis is guarded to poor for patients with chronic renal failure and renal secondary hyperparathyroidism.

• Short-term prognosis depends on severity of chronic renal failure.

MISCELLANEOUS

AGE-RELATED FACTORS
Young animals can develop severe renal osteodystrophy and may benefit from treatment with calcitriol and calcium carbonate.

Reference

Chew DJ, Nagode LA. Calcitriol in the treatment of chronic renal failure. In: Kirk RW, Bonagura JD, ed. Current veterinary therapy XI. Philadelphia, WB Saunders, 1992:857-860.

Author Larry G. Adams
Consulting Editors Larry G. Adams and Carl A. Osborne

HYPERSENSITIVITY REACTION (ANAPHYLAXIS)

BASICS

DEFINITION
Acute manifestation of a type I hypersensitivity reaction mediated through the rapid introduction of an antigen into a host having antigen-specific antibodies of the IgE subclass. The binding of antigen to mast cells sensitized with IgE results in the release of preformed and newly synthesized chemical mediators. Anaphylactic reactions may be localized (atopy) or systemic (anaphylactic shock). Anaphylaxis not mediated by IgE is designated an anaphylactoid reaction and will not be discussed.

Pathophysiology
• First exposure of the patient to a particular antigen (allergen) causes a humoral response and results in production of IgE, which binds to the surface of mediator cells (mast cells). Patient is then considered to be sensitized to that antigen. • Second exposure to the antigen results in cross-linking of two or more IgE molecules on the cell surface, resulting in mast cell degranulation and activation. Release of mast cell granules initiates an anaphylactic reaction. • Major mast cell-derived mediators include histamine, eosinophilic chemotactic factor, arachadonic acid, metabolites (e.g., prostaglandins, leukotrienes, and thromboxanes), platelet-activating factor, and proteases. These chemical mediators cause an inflammatory response of increased vascular permeability, smooth muscle contraction, inflammatory cell influx, and tissue damage. • Clinical manifestations of the disease depend on the route of antigen exposure, the dose of antigen, and the level of the IgE response.

Systems Affected
• Skin/exocrine—pruritus, urticaria, and edema • Respiratory (cats)—dyspnea and cyanosis • Gastrointestinal—salivation, vomiting, and diarrhea • Hepatobiliary (dogs)—because of portal hypertension and vasoconstriction

Genetics
Familial basis reported for type I hypersensitivity reaction in dogs.

Incidence/Prevalence
• Localized type I hypersensitivity reactions not uncommon • Systemic type I hypersensitivity reactions rare

Geographic Distribution N/A

SIGNALMENT

Species Dogs and cats

Breed Predilections
• Numerous dog breeds documented as having a predilection for developing atopy • No cat breeds documented as having predilection for atopy

Mean Age and Range
• In dogs, age of clinical onset ranges from 3 months to several years of age. Most affected animals are 1-3 years old. • In cats, age of clinical onset ranges from 6 months to 2 years.

Predominant Sex
• In dogs, atopy affects females more than males. • In cats, there is no reported sex predilection.

SIGNS

General Comments
• Initial clinical signs vary depending on the route of exposure to the inciting antigen (allergen). • Shock is the end result of a severe anaphylactic reaction. In dogs, the shock organ is the liver. In cats, the shock organs are those of the respiratory and gastrointestinal systems.

Historical Findings
• Onset of signs is immediate (within minutes). Signs localized to the site of exposure may be seen, but these may progress to a systemic reaction. • In dogs, signs may range from localized signs such as pruritus and urticaria to more systemic signs such as vomiting, defecation, and urination. • In cats, signs may range from intense pruritus about the head to dyspnea, salivation, and vomiting.

Physical Examination Findings
• Localized cutaneous edema at the site of exposure • In some dogs, hepatomegaly • In early stages, hyperexcitability may be seen. Terminally, depression and collapse.

CAUSES
• An anaphylactic reaction can be caused by virtually any agent. • Commonly reported causes include venoms, blood-based products, vaccines, foods, and drugs.

RISK FACTORS
Previous exposure (sensitization) increases the chance of the animal developing a reaction.

DIAGNOSIS

DIFFERENTIAL DIAGNOSIS
• Other types of shock • Trauma • Varies, depending on the major organ system involved, if reaction is localized • Diagnosis can be made largely on the basis of history and clinical signs.

CBC/BIOCHEMISTRY/URINALYSIS
Because of the acute onset of disease, no tests available that reliably predict individual susceptibility

OTHER LABORATORY TESTS
• Intradermal skin testing to identify allergens
• Radioallergosorbent test to quantify the concentration of serum IgE specific for a particular antigen

IMAGING N/A

OTHER DIAGNOSTIC PROCEDURES
Limited because a severely allergic animal can develop an anaphylactic reaction when exposed to even small quantities of antigen

GROSS AND HISTOPATHOLOGIC FINDINGS
• Lesions vary, depending on severity of reaction, from localized cutaneous edema to severe pulmonary edema (in cats) and visceral pooling of blood (in dogs). • Other nonspecific findings vary and are characteristic of shock. • Nonspecific characteristics of localized reactions include edema, vasculitis, and thromboembolism.

TREATMENT

INPATIENT VERSUS OUTPATIENT
In an acutely affected animal, the reaction is considered a medical emergency requiring hospitalization of the animal.

ACTIVITY N/A

DIET
If a food-based allergen is suspected (uncommon in veterinary medicine), avoid foods associated with hypersensitivity reaction.

CLIENT EDUCATION
• Discuss the unpredictable nature of the disease.
• Discuss the need to recognize that the animal has an allergic condition that may require immediate medical care.

SURGICAL CONSIDERATIONS N/A

MEDICATIONS

DRUGS AND FLUIDS
For systemic anaphylaxis, the goal of treatment is emergency life support through the maintenance of an open airway, preventing circulatory collapse, and reestablishing physiologic parameters:
• Eliminate inciting antigen, if possible.
• Administer epinephrine hydrochloride parenterally (1:1000; 0.01 ml/kg).
• Administer fluids intravenously at shock dosages to counteract hypotension.
• Administer aminophylline in severely dyspneic patients.
• Administer catecholamines to counteract hypotension.
• Administer corticosteroids.
• Administer atropine sulfate to counteract bradycardia and hypotension.
For localized anaphylaxis, the goal is to limit the reaction, thereby preventing progression to a systemic reaction:
• Administer diphenhydramine hydrochloride (1-2 mg/kg IV or IM).
• Administer prednisolone (2 mg/kg PO).
• Administer epinephrine hydrochloride (0.15 ml SQ at site of initiation).

• If shock develops, initiate treatment for a systemic reaction.

CONTRAINDICATIONS N/A

PRECAUTIONS
Localized reaction can develop into systemic reaction.

POSSIBLE INTERACTIONS N/A

ALTERNATE DRUGS N/A

 FOLLOW-UP

PATIENT MONITORING
Closely monitor hospitalized patients for 24-48 hours.

PREVENTION/AVOIDANCE
If inciting antigen (allergen) can be identified, eliminate or reduce exposure.

POSSIBLE COMPLICATIONS N/A

EXPECTED COURSE AND PROGNOSIS
• If localized reaction is treated early, prognosis is good. • If the animal is in shock on examination, prognosis is guarded to poor.

✓ MISCELLANEOUS

ASSOCIATED CONDITIONS N/A

AGE RELATED FACTORS N/A

ZOONOTIC POTENTIAL N/A

PREGNANCY N/A

SYNONYMS N/A

SEE ALSO
• Atopy • Shock

ABBREVIATIONS
None

Reference

Mueller DL, Noxon JO. Anaphylaxis: pathophysiology and treatment. Compendium on Continuing Education for the Practicing Veterinarian 1990;12:157-170.

Author Paul W. Snyder

Consulting Editor Alan H. Rebar

HYPERTENSION, PORTAL

BASICS

DEFINITION

Portal pressure > 13 cm of H_2O

Pathophysiology

• Portal hypertension is caused by an increase in portal blood flow, an increase in resistance to portal blood flow, or a combination of these events. Portal hypertension is most frequently caused by diseases that increase resistance to portal blood flow. Obstruction to blood flow may occur in the portal system, liver, hepatic veins, caudal vena cava, or heart. The anatomic site of increased resistance is used to classify the mechanism for portal hypertension as prehepatic (portal vein), intrahepatic (liver), or posthepatic (hepatic veins, caudal vena cava, and heart). • Consequences of portal hypertension include development of multiple portosystemic shunts with subsequent hepatic encephalopathy, and alterations in abdominal lymph production and fluid homeostasis, which cause ascites. • Multiple portosystemic shunts usually connect the portal system and the caudal vena cava. They develop as a consequence of prehepatic, intrahepatic, and noncardiac posthepatic causes of portal hypertension of > 1-2 months' duration. • The ascitic fluid that forms secondary to posthepatic disorders is a modified transudate with > 2.5 gm/dl of protein. The increase in protein occurs because hepatic sinusoidal hypertension causes production of protein-rich lymph, which contributes to ascites formation. Ascites is more likely to occur when portal hypertension is accompanied by concurrent hypoalbuminemia.

Systems Affected

• Hepatobiliary—obstruction of blood flow causes distention of the venous bed behind the obstruction. Passive congestion of the spleen causes splenomegaly, and passive congestion of the liver caused by posthepatic disorders only, results in hepatomegaly. • Nervous—hepatic encephalopathy • Cardiovascular—multiple portosystemic shunts and ascites • Gastrointestinal—animals with acute portal hypertension edema of splanchnic tissues develop excessive permeability of the gut wall and endotoxemia

Genetics N/A

Incidence N/A

Geographic Distribution N/A

SIGNALMENT

Species Dogs and cats

Breed Predilections N/A

Mean Age and Range N/A

Prdominant Sex N/A

SIGNS

General Comments

Clinical signs depend on the site, degree, and rate of development of obstruction and on the underlying cause. Most disorders that cause portal hypertension are chronic.

Historical Findings

• Abdominal distention • Signs of hepatic encephalopathy may be secondary to multiple portosystemic shunts. • Additional signs reflect the underlying cause of portal hypertension. For example, cough, exercise intolerance, and dyspnea develop in animals with cardiac disorders.

Physical Examination Findings

• Abdominal effusion • Splenomegaly • Hepatomegaly (posthepatic causes only) • Jugular venous distention, positive hepatojugular reflex, muffled heart sounds, cardiac arrhythmia or murmur, and pulmonary crackles in animals with underlying cardiac causes. • Combination of ascites, hepatic encephalopathy, and icterus suggests underlying cirrhosis. • A bruit may be ausculted over the area of the liver in an animal with an hepatic arteriovenous fistula. • When acute portal hypertension occurs as a complication of surgical ligation of a congenital portosystemic shunt, signs of portal hypertension develop 24-48 hours after surgery and include abdominal distention and pain, bloody diarrhea, endotoxic shock, and death.

CAUSES

Prehepatic Disorders

• Portal vein thrombosis, stenosis, or neoplasia • Congenital portal vein atresia • Portal vein compression by a large lymph node, neoplasm, granuloma, or abscess • Postoperative complication of congenital portosystemic shunt ligation

Intrahepatic Disorders

• Cirrhosis or fibrosis of the liver • Hepatic neoplasia • Chronic hepatitis or cholangiohepatitis • Chronic biliary obstruction • Veno-occlusive disease in cocker spaniels • Liver entrapment in a diaphragmatic hernia • Atresia of intrahepatic portal vessels • Hepatic arteriovenous fistula

Posthepatic Disorders

• Right-sided congestive heart failure; heartworm disease; pericardial tamponade; constrictive pericarditis; cardiac neoplasia; cor triatriatum • Thrombosis or neoplasia of the hepatic veins or caudal vena cava • Kinked caudal vena cava • Diaphragmatic hernia with vascular entrapment

RISK FACTORS N/A

DIAGNOSIS

DIFFERENTIAL DIAGNOSIS

• Consider hypoalbuminemia (e.g., protein-losing nephropathy, protein-losing enteropathy, and liver failure), abdominal neoplasia, and diaphragmatic hernia in animals with abdominal transudate or modified transudate.

• Congenital portosystemic shunt and primary liver disorders are important causes of hepatic encephalopathy. Differentiate by liver biopsy and portogram. • Congenital portosystemic shunt is a single extrahepatic or intrahepatic shunt; it is not usually associated with portal hypertension or ascites.

CBC/BIOCHEMISTRY/URINALYSIS

• Laboratory abnormalities vary with the underlying cause of portal hypertension. In animals with chronic end-stage liver disease, findings may include high liver enzyme activity, hyperbilirubinemia, hypoalbuminemia, and coagulopathy. • Microcytosis is seen in animals with congenital or acquired portosystemic shunt.

OTHER LABORATORY TESTS

• In animals with multiple portosystemic shunts secondary to portal hypertension, serum bile acid concentration may reflect a typical "shunting pattern," with normal to moderately high fasting values and markedly high postprandial values. • Hyperammonemia and abnormal result of ammonia tolerance test are also consistent findings in animals with portosystemic shunt. • Prehepatic and intrahepatic causes of portal hypertension result in ascitic fluid that is a transudate; posthepatic disorders result in a modified transudate.

IMAGING

Radiography

• Abdominal radiographs are useful for evaluating diseases associated with portal hypertension. Findings suggesting portal hypertension include ascites and splenomegaly. Additional findings are related to the underlying cause (e.g., small liver in animals with cirrhosis). • Thoracic radiographs should be performed to detect posthepatic causes of portal hypertension and ascites.

Ultrasonography

• Findings indicating portal hypertension include dilated portal vein, splenomegaly, and multiple tortuous vessels (portosystemic shunt). • The liver should be scanned to evaluate for primary liver disease. • A dilated caudal vena cava and hepatic veins suggest a posthepatic mechanism. • Underlying cardiac disorders can be further evaluated by an echocardiogram.

OTHER DIAGNOSTIC PROCEDURES

• Cardiac causes of portal hypertension are evaluated by thoracic radiographs, ECG, central venous pressure, and echocardiography. • Primary hepatic disorders are diagnosed by liver biopsy. • Angiography is performed only after complete evaluation and exclusion of obvious cardiac and hepatic causes of portal hypertension. Portosystemic shunt can be confirmed by mesenteric portography. Hepatic arteriovenous shunts and obstruction of the portal vein or caudal vena cava are diagnosed by angiography or surgery.

• Measurement of portal pressure can be performed during laparotomy.

GROSS AND HISTOPATHOLOGIC FINDINGS

• Acquired portosystemic shunt appears as multiple tortuous vessels. • In animals with chronic end-stage liver disease, the liver is small and smooth to nodular. • Fibrosis and cirrhosis are detected histologically. • Posthepatic causes of portal hypertension lead to hepatic congestion.

TREATMENT

INPATIENT VS OUTPATIENT
Patients with hepatic encephalopathy should be hospitalized.

ACTIVITY
Depends on the underlying cause.

DIET
• Sodium restriction for ascites
• Protein restriction for hepatic encephalopathy

CLIENT EDUCATION
When portal hypertension is suspected, further testing is necessary to identify the underlying cause.

SURGICAL CONSIDERATIONS
Surgical ligation of multiple portosystemic shunt is contraindicated. Ligation may result in fatal portal hypertension. When acute portal hypertension occurs secondary to ligation of a congenital portosystemic shunt, emergency surgery to remove the ligature is indicated.

MEDICATIONS

DRUGS AND FLUIDS
• Manage hepatic encephalopathy with lactulose and antibiotics given orally (neomycin and/or metronidazole)
• Manage ascites with sodium-restriction and furosemide. Paracentesis is indicated in animals with respiratory distress or abdominal discomfort.
• Avoid high sodium fluids.
• Propranolol may lower portal pressure, but clinical efficacy is unproved.

CONTRAINDICATIONS N/A

PRECAUTIONS
• Repeated abdominocentesis with removal of large volumes of fluid may cause dehydration and hypoproteinemia.
• Overzealous use of diuretics can cause hypokalemia, metabolic alkalosis, and dehydration.

POSSIBLE INTERACTIONS N/A

ALTERNATE DRUGS N/A

FOLLOW-UP

PATIENT MONITORING
Monitor hydration status, electrolytes, and acid-base status when administering diuretics.

PREVENTION/AVOIDANCE N/A

POSSIBLE COMPLICATIONS
Animals with acute portal hypertension—portal vein thrombosis, endotoxemia, and cardiovascular collapse

EXPECTED COURSE AND PROGNOSIS
Depends on the underlying cause

MISCELLANEOUS

ASSOCIATED CONDITIONS N/A

AGE-RELATED FACTORS N/A

ZOONOTIC POTENTIAL N/A

PREGNANCY N/A

SYNONYMS N/A

SEE ALSO
• Ascites (Abdominal Effusion)
• Hepatic Encephalopathy
• Portosystemic Shunt

ABBREVIATIONS
ECG = electrocardiogram

References

Johnson S. Portal hypertension. Part I. Pathophysiology and clinical consequences. Compen Contin Educ 1987;9:741-750.

Johnson S. Portal hypertension. Part II. Clinical assessment and treatment. Compen Contin Educ 1987;9:917-930.

Author Susan E. Johnson
Consulting Editor Albert E. Jergens

HYPERTENSION, PULMONARY

BASICS

DEFINITION
A mean arterial pulmonary pressure > 25 mm Hg indicating a high pulmonary circulation pressure

Pathophysiology
• Several events lead to high pulmonary artery pressure. These include high pulmonary blood flow, left atrial hypertension, pulmonary vasoconstriction, pulmonary vessel obstructive disease, and idiopathic pulmonary hypertension. Hypoxia is a potent mediator of pulmonary vasoconstriction. • A major pathologic consequence of pulmonary hypertension is a heavy workload on the right heart leading to myocardial hypertrophy and possible right-sided congestive heart failure.
• In veterinary patients, pulmonary hypertension generally develops secondarily to an underlying disease. In human medicine, a primary idiopathic form is rarely described.

Systems Affected
Cardiovascular—cor pulmonale, pulmonary artery hypertrophy and dilation, and right-sided congestive heart failure

Genetics
No genetic basis for this disease has been found. However, pulmonary hypertension can occur secondarily to several congenital heart defects that may have a genetic basis.

Incidence/Prevalence
• The incidence and prevalence of secondary pulmonary hypertension is unknown. • No cases of idiopathic primary pulmonary hypertension have been documented in the veterinary literature.

Geographic Distribution
Geographic distribution is unknown, but there may be a relatively higher prevalence in heartworm endemic areas and at high altitudes.

SIGNALMENT
Species Dogs and cats

Breed Predilections
Breeds that are susceptible to mitral valve disease and congenital heart defects that lead to left-to-right shunting

Mean Age and Range N/A

Predominant Sex N/A

SIGNS

General Comments
Clinical signs associated with pulmonary hypertension may be superimposed on the clinical signs of the underlying primary disease.

Historical Findings
• Exercise intolerance • Dyspnea • Coughing/ hemoptysis • Syncope

Physical Examination Findings
• Dyspnea • Coughing • Hemoptysis • Loud or split second heart sound • Abnormal lung sounds • Cyanosis • Heart murmur

CAUSES

High Pulmonary Blood Flow
• Atrial septal defect • Ventricular septal defect • Left-to-right shunting patent ductus arteriosus

Left Atrial Hypertension
• Mitral valve insufficiency • Mitral valve stenosis • Left ventricular failure (i.e., cardiomyopathy)

Pulmonary Vascular Obstruction
• Pulmonary fibrosis • Pulmonary parenchymal disease
Pulmonary thromboembolism:
• Hyperadrenocorticism • Nephrotic syndrome • Sepsis • Heartworm disease • Immune-mediated hemolytic anemia • Neoplasia
• Bacterial endocarditis • Dilated cardiomyopathy • Disseminated intravascular coagulopathy • Pancreatitis

Pulmonary Vasoconstriction (Hypoxia)
• Chronic obstructive pulmonary disease
• Interstitial lung diseases • High altitude disease • Collapsing trachea • Neuromuscular disease • Pickwickian syndrome

Idiopathic Primary Pulmonary Hypertension
Not documented in dogs or cats

RISK FACTORS
• Cardiac and pulmonary disease • Failure to administer heartworm preventative • Living at high altitudes • Diseases associated with pulmonary thromboembolism (see causes)

DIAGNOSIS

DIFFERENTIAL DIAGNOSIS
• Left-sided congestive heart failure • Collapsing trachea • Right-sided congestive heart failure • Chronic obstructive pulmonary disease • Heartworm disease • Chronic bronchitis • Bronchial asthma • Pneumothorax • Pyothorax • Hemothorax

CBC/BIOCHEMISTRY/URINALYSIS
• Findings vary with underlying cause • No consistent findings associated with pulmonary hypertension • Polycythemia if pulmonary hypertension is secondary to hypoxia

OTHER LABORATORY TESTS
• Arterial blood gases (hypoxemia) • Heartworm test may be positive

IMAGING

Radiography
• Large pulmonary artery • Large right ventricle • Other findings vary with cause, but might include evidence of primary pulmonary disease, pulmonary embolism, and tracheal collapse

Echocardiography
• Right ventricular hypertrophy • Right ventricular dilatation • Pulmonary artery dilatation • If animal has tricuspid or pulmonic

valve insufficiency, pressure gradients can be estimated with Doppler and are > 25 mm Hg

OTHER DIAGNOSTIC PROCEDURES

Electrocardiography
• Right-sided mean electrical axis deviation
• Deep S waves in leads I, II, III, and aVF
• Tall T waves • Tall P waves (i.e., P pulmonale)

Cardiac Catheterization and Pulmonary Angiography
• Generally required to confirm pulmonary hypertension • Angiography may demonstrate vascular changes

GROSS AND HISTOPATHOLOGIC FINDINGS
• Consistent with underlying disease • Pulmonary artery thrombus • Dilated pulmonary artery • Right ventricular enlargement
• Medial hypertrophy of pulmonary vasculature • Intimal proliferation and sclerosis of pulmonary vasculature • Necrotizing arteritis

TREATMENT

INPATIENT VERSUS OUTPATIENT
Animals in severe respiratory distress should be hospitalized until stable.

ACTIVITY Restricted

DIET
Specific guidelines based on underlying disease. If animal has heart failure, restricted sodium diet may be beneficial.

CLIENT EDUCATION
• Diagnosis is often presumptive without catheterization or Doppler echocardiography.
• Prognosis varies with reversibility of the underlying disease.

SURGICAL CONSIDERATIONS N/A

MEDICATIONS

DRUGS AND FLUIDS
• Medical management of pulmonary hypertension is controversial. Treatment should be directed at the primary underlying disease process.
• The ideal therapeutic agent should reduce pulmonary vascular resistance and hypertension without affecting the systemic circulation. Oxygen is a compound that can accomplish this, but long-term oxygen administration is not feasible in the small animal patient. Short-term use of oxygen is beneficial.

Vasodilators
• Ideally, selection should be based on blood pressure response during cardiac catheterization.
• Choices include ACE inhibitors (e.g., enalapril), hydralazine, and nifedipine

Bronchodilators
• May be beneficial in treatment of hypoxic-mediated pulmonary hypertension in animals with bronchoconstriction
• Choices include sympathomimetics (e.g., terbutaline) and methylxanthines (e.g., theophylline, aminophylline)

Digoxin
• Not a primary treatment of pulmonary hypertension
• May be beneficial in patients with congestive heart failure

Anticoagulant Therapy
• Indicated if thromboembolic disease is diagnosed
• Choices include heparin, coumadin, and aspirin

CONTRAINDICATIONS
• Drugs or situations that worsen pulmonary hypoxia (e.g., respiratory depressants and beta blockers)
• Drugs that would cause vasoconstriction (beta blockers)

PRECAUTIONS
• Vasodilators can cause systemic hypotension.
• Vasodilators may worsen hypoxemia if pulmonary hypertension is secondary to hypoxia caused by pulmonary disease.

POSSIBLE INTERACTIONS N/A

ALTERNATE DRUGS N/A

FOLLOW-UP

PATIENT MONITORING
• Repeated physical examination with careful cardiac and pulmonary auscultation • Thoracic radiography • Measurement of arterial blood gases • Echocardiography • Electrocardiography

PREVENTION/AVOIDANCE
Client education directed at complete understanding of conditions that predispose to pulmonary hypertension

POSSIBLE COMPLICATIONS
• Right-sided heart failure • Syncope • Cardiac arrhythmias • Sudden death

EXPECTED COURSE AND PROGNOSIS
• Based on ability to reverse underlying disease • When changes are irreversible, treatment is palliative.

MISCELLANEOUS

ASSOCIATED CONDITIONS
See causes

AGE RELATED FACTORS N/A

ZOONOTIC POTENTIAL None

PREGNANCY High risk

SYNONYMS N/A

SEE ALSO
Diseases causing pulmonary hypertension

ABBREVIATION
ACE = angiotensin converting enzyme

References
Johnson LR, Hamlin RL. Recognition and treatment of pulmonary hypertension. In: Bonagura, JD, ed. Current veterinary therapy XII. Philadelphia: WB Saunders, 1995.
Hawkins EC. Disease of the lower respiratory tract. In: Ettinger SJ, Feldman EC, eds. Textbook of veterinary internal medicine. 4th ed. Philadelphia: WB Saunders, 1995.
Perry LA, Dillon AR, Bowers TL. Pulmonary hypertension. Compend Cont Ed Pract Vet 1991;13:226.
Grossman W, Braunwald E. Pulmonary hypertension. In: Braunwald E, ed. Heart disease. Volume 1. Philadelphia: WB Saunders, 1991.
Author Steven L. Marks
Consulting Editors Larry P. Tilley and Francis W. K. Smith, Jr.

HYPERTENSION, SYSTEMIC

BASICS

DEFINITION

A sustained elevation in either systolic or diastolic arterial blood pressure above the normal range

Pathophysiology

• Regulation of systemic arterial blood pressure is dependent upon the integration of complex mechanisms between the central nervous system and peripheral nerves, renal and cardiac tissues, and humoral factors, all of which synergistically affect cardiac output and peripheral vascular resistance. Systemic blood pressure equals cardiac output times peripheral vascular resistance. Cardiac output is determined by heart rate and stroke volume with the latter related to extracellular fluid volume. Extracellular fluid volume is primarily controlled by renal fluid volume mechanisms that lead to activation of the renin-angiotensin-aldosterone system. Renin is secreted within the kidney in response to reduced renal blood flow, high renal sympathetic tone, catecholamines, low distal tubular chloride concentration, and angiotensin II. Renin augments the conversion of angiotensinogen to angiotensin I, which is subsequently cleaved by angiotensin converting enzyme to angiotensin II. Angiotensin II is a potent vasoconstricter and stimulator of aldosterone secretion. Aldosterone promotes sodium and subsequent water retention leading to plasma volume expansion. • Complications of hypertension are seen in the target organs most affected by sustained, arterial blood pressure (i.e., eye, kidney, cardiovascular, and cerebrovascular systems). Vascular damage in these tissues leads to hemorrhage, thrombosis, edema, and necrosis. Hypertension causes arteriolar hypertrophy, tunica media vasorum hyperplasia, and destruction of the internal elastic lamina layer.

Systems Affected

• Cardiovascular • Renal/urologic • Ophthalmic

Genetics

Unknown

Incidence/Prevalence

Unknown, but diagnosed more frequently now that more veterinarians are monitoring blood pressure. Up to 65% of cats with chronic renal failure and up to 87% of cats with hyperthyroidism have hypertension.

Geographic Distribution N/A

SIGNALMENT

Species

Dogs and cats

Breed Predilection

None

Mean Age and Range

• Dogs—mean age 8.9 +/– 3.6 years with range of 2-14 years • Cats—mean age 15.1 +/– 3.8 years with range of 7-20 years

Predominant Sex

Male

SIGNS

• Acute blindness • Ocular hemorrhage • Dilated pupils • Retinal detachment • Swollen kidneys • Hematuria • Epistaxis • Seizures • Congestive heart failure with or without cardiac murmur • Hyperdynamic arterial pulse quality • Palpable thyroid gland

CAUSES

Primary or Essential

No known cause

Secondary

• Renal disease—end stage renal disease, glomerulonephritis, amyloidosis, renal artery stenosis • Hyperadrenocorticism • Hyperthyroidism • Diabetes mellitus • Pheochromocytoma (rare) • Hyperaldosteronism (rare) • Central nervous system disease

RISK FACTORS

See causes.

DIAGNOSIS

DIFFERENTIAL DIAGNOSIS

Differential causes of hypertension are based on physical findings and largely on the results of blood tests.

CBC/BIOCHEMISTRY/URINALYSIS

• CBC usually is normal. • Biochemistry may reveal azotemia and hyperphosphatemia (renal insufficiency), hyperglycemia (diabetes mellitus), high serum alkaline phosphatase (hyperadrenocorticism), or electrolyte imbalances. • Urinalysis may reveal proteinuria and hematuria (glomerulonephritis), poor concentration ability (renal insufficiency, hyperadrenocorticism), or glucosuria (diabetes mellitus).

OTHER LABORATORY TESTS

• Glomerulonephritis—high urine protein to urine creatinine ratio, low creatinine clearance • Renal dysfunction—low creatinine clearance • Hyperadrenocorticism—exaggerated ACTH response test, failure to suppress with dexamethasone suppression test, with high urine cortisol to creatinine ratio • Hyperthyroidism (cats)—high T4, inadequate suppression with a T3 suppression test • Hypothyroidism (dogs)—low T3, T4, free T3, free T4; possibly high T3 and T4 autoantibodies, high endogenous TSH, and depressed TSH stimulation test result • Pheochromocytoma—high urinary vanillylmandelic acid • Hyperaldosteronism—24-hour urine aldosterone and plasma aldosterone concentrations high.

IMAGING

• Thoracic radiograph to evaluate secondary cardiac changes • Abdominal radiographs to evaluate liver, adrenals, and kidneys • Echocardiogram to evaluate hypertensive heart disease • Abdominal ultrasound to evaluate kidneys and adrenal glands • CT scan if brain tumor is suspected • Thyroid scan to evaluate hyperthyroidism

OTHER DIAGNOSTIC PROCEDURES

Definitive diagnosis of hypertension requires documentation of high arterial blood pressure via direct or indirect measurement.

Direct (Invasive)

Direct intraarterial blood pressure measurement using the PDS Monitor (Baxter Company) is considered the gold standard for blood pressure accuracy, but the equipment is expensive and the technique can cause animal discomfort and is seldom performed in clinical practice.

Indirect (Noninvasive)

Indirect blood pressure measurements can be obtained using oscillometric or Doppler techniques. Requires an inflatable cuff (approximately 40% in width of the circumference of the limb at the site of placement) wrapped around a distal limb or tail. Technique using radial artery is described below. In using the tarsal artery (hindlimb), the cuff is placed at the hock for the oscillometric technique; the Doppler transducer is placed over the digital tarsal artery just proximal to the tarsal pad for the Doppler technique. Average 3-5 measurements.

Oscillometric Technique

• Dinamap (Criticon Company) • The oscillometric technique detects pulse pressure oscillations beneath the cuff bladder resulting from changes in arterial diameter. Proper cuff size is critical for accurate measurement • Animal is placed in lateral recumbency in a calm environment. Hair coat at the carpus (radial artery) is matted with alcohol and pneumatic cuff applied in snug position. Cuff is inflated and deflated automatically with blood pressure (systolic, diastolic, and mean) and heart rate automatically calculated and digitally displayed.

Doppler Technique

• Ultrasonic Doppler flow detector (Parks Medical Electronics, Oregon; Silogic, England; SDI, Wisconsin) • The Doppler technique uses ultrasound waves to detect and make audible blood flow in an artery distal to the blood pressure cuff. • Animal is placed in lateral recumbency in a calm environment. Hair coat between the carpus and elbow is matted with alcohol and pneumatic cuff applied in snug position. Distal to cuff position, transducer probe crystal is placed over the skin, just proximal to the carpal pad (digital branch of the radial artery) in a bed of ultrasound gel and taped or held in place. Cuff bladder is inflated to suprasystemic pressure with cut-off of Doppler signal. Cuff is deflated (at approximately 3 mm Hg/sec) with systolic pressure determined with return of Doppler signal. Diastolic pressure is measured when Doppler signal pitch changes abruptly or disappears.

Blood Pressure Guidelines for Dogs and Cats

Hypertension is currently defined as the following:
• Dog: Systolic > 180 mm Hg; diastolic > 100 mm HG
• Cat: Systolic > 170-180 mm Hg; diastolic > 120 mm Hg

TREATMENT

INPATIENT VERSUS OUTPATIENT

Usually outpatient unless the underlying condition requires inpatient management (e.g., fluid therapy in a cat with renal failure) or there are serious complications related to hypertension (e.g., retinal detachment)

ACTIVITY

Restrict activity until hypertension is controlled.

DIET

Choice influenced by underlying cause. Sodium restriction generally advised.

CLIENT EDUCATION

Unless underlying cause is curable (e.g., hyperthyroidism) or controllable (e.g., hyperadrenocorticism) the animal is likely to be on medication indefinitely. Alert owners to end-organ effects of hypertension (e.g., retinal hemorrhage, retinal detachment).

SURGICAL CONSIDERATIONS

Dictated by underlying cause. May be indicated for hyperthyroidism, pheochromocytoma, some forms of hyperadrenocorticism.

MEDICATIONS

DRUGS AND FLUIDS

• Treat underlying cause.
Treat hypertension with sodium restriction and medications. Single agents often are ineffective. The following stepwise approach is suggested:
• Low-sodium diet, add angiotensin-converting enzyme inhibitor (ACEI) or calcium channel blocker
• Low-sodium diet, add beta blocker or diuretic to ACEI or calcium channel blocker
• Low-sodium diet, add vasodilator with beta blocker to ACEI or calcium channel blocker

Diuretics

• Lower blood volume and cardiac output and lower peripheral vascular resistance by lowering body salt and water
• Hydrochlorothiazide (HydroDiuril)—dogs, 2-4 mg/kg PO q12h; cats, 1-2 mg/kg PO q12h
• Furosemide (Lasix)—dogs, 2-4 mg/kg PO q8-12h; cats, 1-2 mg/kg PO q12h. More likely to cause hypokalemia than a thiazide

diuretic.
• Spironolactone (Aldactone)—dogs and cats, 1-2 mg/kg PO q12h. Potassium sparing diuretic that can be used with hydrochlorothiazide or furosemide.

Beta-Adrenergic Blockers

• Lower heart rate and cardiac output and suppress renin secretion
• Propranolol (Inderal)—dogs, 0.2-1.0 mg/kg PO q8h; cats, 2.5-10 mg/cat PO q12h
• Atenolol (Tenormin)—dogs, 0.25-1 mg/kg PO q12-24h PO; cats, 6.25-12.5 mg/cat PO q24h

Angiotensin-Converting Enzyme (ACE) Inhibitors

• Lower peripheral vascular resistance and stroke volume by blocking the conversion of angiotensin I to angiotensin II
• Enalapril (Vasotec, Enacard)—dogs, 0.5 mg/kg PO q12-24h; cats, 0.25-0.5 mg/kg PO q24-48h
• Benazepril (Lotensin)—dogs and cats, 0.25-0.5 mg/kg PO q24h

Calcium Channel Blockers

• Lower peripheral vascular resistance by vasodilation. Some lower cardiac output through negative chronotropic and inotropic effects.
• Diltiazem (Cardizem)—dogs, 0.5-1.5 mg/kg PO q8h; cats, 1.5-2.5 mg/kg PO q8h
• Verapamil (Calan, Isoptin)—dogs, 1.0-3.0 mg/kg PO q8h; cats, 0.5-1.5 mg/kg PO q8h
• Amlodipine (Norvasc)—cats, 0.625 mg/cat PO q24h

Vasodilators

• Lower peripheral vascular resistance by direct action on arteriole smooth muscle
• Hydralazine HCl (Apresoline)—dogs, 0.5-3 mg/kg PO q12h; cats, 0.5-0.8 mg/kg PO q12h

CONTRAINDICATIONS

• Beta blockers might worsen bronchiolar disease, congestive heart failure, and second- and third-degree heart blocks.
• Diltiazem and verapamil should be used with caution in patients with congestive heart failure or second- or third-degree heart blocks.

PRECAUTIONS

Diuretics might induce hypokalemia and metabolic alkalosis.

POSSIBLE INTERACTIONS

See manufacturer's insert on each drug.

ALTERNATE DRUGS

Combined therapy of hydralazine (dogs, 0.5-3 mg/kg PO q12h; cats, 0.5-0.8 mg/kg PO q12h) and propranolol (dogs, 0.2-1.0 mg/kg PO q8h; cats, 2.5-10 mg/cat PO q12h). Use this combination in place of ACE inhibitor or calcium blocker.

FOLLOW-UP

PATIENT MONITORING

• Monitor blood pressure and possible complications (especially retinopathy and glomerulonephropathy). • Laboratory tests to measure clinical disease response and side effects of medications (e.g., proteinuria, hematuria, anemia, thrombocytopenia, potassium balance, sodium balance, azotemia, albumin)

PREVENTION/AVOIDANCE N/A

POSSIBLE COMPLICATIONS

• Congestive heart failure • Glomerulonephropathy (proteinuria, hematuria) • Renal failure • Retinopathy (hemorrhage, detached retina) • Stroke

EXPECTED COURSE AND PROGNOSIS

Dictated by underlying cause. In most patients, hypertension can be controlled with appropriate therapy.

MISCELLANEOUS

ASSOCIATED CONDITIONS N/A

AGE RELATED FACTORS

Renal failure and hyperthyroidism are more common in older animals

ZOONOTIC POTENTIAL N/A

PREGNANCY

Preeclampsia-associated hypertension has not been clearly identified in dogs and cats.

SYNONYM

High blood pressure

SEE ALSO

• Pheochromocytoma • Hyperthyroidism • Hyperadrenocorticism • Renal Failure, Acute • Renal Failure, Chronic • Glomerulonephritis

ABBREVIATION

ACEI = angiotensin converting enzyme inhibitor

References

Snyder PS. Canine hypertensive disease. Compend Cont Ed Pract Vet 1991;13:1785–1793.

Stiles J, et al. The prevalence of retinopathy in cats with systemic hypertension and chronic renal failure or hyperthyroidism. J Am An Hosp Assoc 1994;30:564.

Sisson D, O'Keefe D, Binns S. Blood pressure measurement in cats: comparison of three noninvasive techniques with direct measurement.Proceedings, 11th Annu Meet Am Col Vet Int Med, 1993:516–518

Author Jerry A. Thornhill
Consulting Editors Larry P. Tilley and Francis W. K. Smith, Jr.

HYPERTHYROIDISM

BASICS

DEFINITION
A pathologic, sustained, high overall metabolism caused by high circulating concentrations of thyroid hormones

Pathophysiology
Hyperthyroidism in cats most often is caused by autonomously hyperfunctioning nodules of the thyroid gland. These nodules secrete thyroxine (T_4) and triiodithyronine (T_3), uncontrolled by normal physiologic influences (e.g., pituitary thyrotropin [TSH] secretion). One or both lobes of the thyroid gland can be affected. Rare cases of feline hyperthyroidism (1-2%) are caused by hyperfunctioning thyroid carcinoma. Hyperthyroidism is extremely uncommon in dogs, but it has been seen in some dogs with thyroid carcinoma (most dogs with thyroid gland neoplasia are euthyroid) and in dogs with oversupplementation of exogenous thyroid hormone.

Systems Affected
• Musculoskeletal • Cardiovascular—myocardial hypertrophy and hypertension • Gastrointestinal—chronic cellular malnutrition, increased gastrointestinal transit time and malabsorption, and hepatocellular damage • Renal/urologic—high glomerular filtration may mask underlying chronic renal failure • Nervous • Behavioral

Genetics
No known genetic predisposition

Incidence/Prevalence
• Most common endocrine disease in cats and one of the most common diseases of late middle-aged and older cats. Its true incidence is unknown, but diagnosis of the disease is increasing. • Rare in dogs

Geographic Distribution N/A

SIGNALMENT

Species Cats and (rarely) dogs

Breed Predilections None

Mean Age and Range
Mean age in cats, approximately 13 years; range, 4-22 years

Predominant Sex None

SIGNS

General Comments
• The signs are multisystemic and reflect the overall increase in metabolism.
• Less than 10% of patients are referred to as "apathetic." These patients exhibit atypical signs (e.g., poor appetite, anorexia, depression, and weakness).

Historical Findings
• Weight loss • Polyphagia • Vomiting • Diarrhea • Polydipsia • Tachypnea • Hyperactivity • Dyspnea • Aggression

Physical Examination Findings
• Large thyroid gland (70% of patients are affected bilaterally) • Poor body condition • Heart murmur • Tachycardia • Gallop rhythm • Unkempt appearance • Thickened nails

CAUSES
• Autonomously hyperfunctioning nodules in cats. Rarely, thyroid carcinoma. • In dogs, hyperthyroidism caused by T_4 or T_3 secretion by a thyroid carcinoma.

RISK FACTORS Unknown

DIAGNOSIS

DIFFERENTIAL DIAGNOSIS
The clinical signs of feline hyperthyroidism can overlap with those of chronic renal failure, chronic hepatic disease, and neoplasia (especially intestinal lymphoma). These differentials can be excluded on the basis of routine laboratory findings and thyroid function tests.

CBC/BIOCHEMISTRY/URINALYSIS
• Erythrocytosis (mild) and, less commonly, leukocytosis, lymphopenia, and eosinopenia (stress response associated with high T_3 and T_4) • High ALT activity (common). High ALP, LDH, AST, BUN, creatinine, glucose, phosphorus, and bilirubin are less common and are caused by more severe complications of hyperthyroidism.

OTHER LABORATORY TESTS
• Serum T_4 concentration—high resting concentration confirms the diagnosis of hyperthyroidism • Serum T_3 concentration—high concentration less reliable than serum T_4
• Free T_4 (FT_4) by equilibrium dialysis—useful to diagnose mild or early hyperthyroidism in cats (these cats have normal resting serum T_4 concentrations). FT_4 more accurately reflects true thyroid gland secretory status.
• T_3 suppression test—useful to diagnose mild hyperthyroidism (see Appendix for protocol and interpretation) • Thyrotropin-releasing hormone (TRH) stimulation test—useful to diagnose mild hyperthyroidism (see Appendix for protocol and interpretation)

IMAGING
• Thoracic radiography and echocardiography may be useful in assessing the severity of myocardial disease. • In dogs, thoracic radiography should be done to detect pulmonary metastasis.

DIAGNOSTIC PROCEDURES
Treatment of hyperthyroidism can cause a significant decline in renal function. Any abnormal renal value revealed by CBC, serum biochemical testing, or urinalysis should be pursued by bacterial culture of the urine, abdominal radiography, and ultrasonography of the urinary tract.

GROSS AND HISTOPATHOLOGIC FINDINGS
Adenomatous hyperplasia of one or both lobes of the thyroid gland. Carcinoma in dogs and in 1-2% of cats.

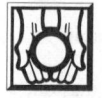

TREATMENT

INPATIENT VERSUS OUTPATIENT
Outpatient

ACTIVITY
No alterations are recommended.

DIET
Resolution of thyrotoxicosis obviates the need for dietary modifications. Poor absorption of many nutrients and high metabolism suggest the need for a highly digestible diet with high bioavailability of protein in untreated hyperthyroidism.

CLIENT EDUCATION
Inform client of side effects of antithyroid drugs (see below) and surgical complications (i.e., hypocalcemia).

SURGICAL CONSIDERATIONS
Surgical thyroidectomy is one of the recommended treatments for hyperthyroidism in cats. Surgical treatment of thyroid carcinoma (dogs and cats) usually is not curative but can be palliative.

MEDICATIONS

DRUGS AND FLUIDS
• Methimazole (Tapazole) is the antithyroid drug most often recommended (15 mg/day divided q8-12h)
• Beta-adrenergic blocking drugs are sometimes used to treat some of the cardiovascular and neurologic effects of excess thyroid hormone. These drugs can be used in combination with methimazole and mainly are used to prepare the patient for surgical thyroidectomy or radioiodine therapy.
• Fluid therapy is not used routinely in the medical management of hyperthyroidism but in conjunction with surgery. Since cardiac complications often develop, care must be taken to avoid overhydration and sodium loading.
• Radioiodine is a safe and effective treatment. Unfortunately, its use is limited because of the small number of veterinary facilities offering this treatment. High doses of radioiodine can be palliative in the treatment of carcinoma but are rarely curative.

CONTRAINDICATIONS N/A

PRECAUTIONS
• Antithyroid drugs have several side effects. Anorexia and vomiting are common side effects of methimazole. Rare side effects include self-induced excoriation of the face,

thrombocytopenia, bleeding diathesis, agranulocytosis, serum antinuclear antibodies, and hepatopathy. These effects usually develop within the first 3 months of treatment and may or may not necessitate drug cessation and alternative treatment (depending on severity).

• Bleeding, jaundice, and agranulocytosis necessitate immediate withdrawal of the drug.

POSSIBLE INTERACTIONS N/A

ALTERNATE DRUGS

• Carbimazole, another useful antithyroid drug, is not available in the United States.
• Propylthiouracil can be used if methimazole is unavailable. Side effects are more common and more severe than with methimazole.

 FOLLOW-UP

PATIENT MONITORING

Physical examination, CBC (with platelet count), serum biochemical analysis, and serum T_4 determination every 2-3 weeks for the initial 3 months of treatment. Adjust the dosage of methimazole to maintain the serum T_4 concentration in the low-normal range.

PREVENTION/AVOIDANCE N/A

POSSIBLE COMPLICATIONS

Untreated disease can lead to congestive heart failure, intractable diarrhea, renal damage, retinal detachment (as a result of hypertension), and death. Complications of surgical treatment include hypoparathyroidism, hypothyroidism, and laryngeal paralysis.

EXPECTED COURSE AND PROGNOSIS

• The prognosis for uncomplicated disease is excellent. Recurrence is possible and is most commonly associated with poor owner compliance with medical management. Regrowth of hyperthyroid tissue is possible but uncommon after surgical thyroidectomy and radioiodine treatment.
• In dogs or cats with thyroid carcinoma, the prognosis is poor. Treatment with radioiodine, surgery, or both usually is followed by recurrence of disease. Adjuvant chemotherapy is of questionable benefit.

 MISCELLANEOUS

ASSOCIATED CONDITIONS

In cats with underlying renal disease (either secondary to chronic hypertension or unrelated to thyroid disease), the prognosis is less favorable. Renal insufficiency may not become apparent until euthyroidism has been established. For this reason, a reversible form of treatment (i.e., antithyroid drugs) is recommended if renal disease is suspected in a cat with hyperthyroidism. In some patients, hyperthyroidism might best be left untreated.

AGE RELATED FACTORS N/A

ZOONOTIC POTENTIAL N/A

PREGNANCY N/A

SYNONYMS

• Thyrotoxicosis • Multinodular toxic goiter

SEE ALSO

• Hypoparathyroidism • Cardiomyopathy, Hypertrophic—Cats • Congestive Heart Failure, Left-Sided • Hypertension, Systemic

ABBREVIATIONS

ALP = alkaline phosphatase
ALT = alanine aminotransferase
AST = aspartate aminotransferase
BUN = blood urea nitrogen
LDH = lactic dehydrogenase
T_4 = thyroxine
T_3 = triiodithyronine
TSH = thyrotropin
TRH = thyrotropin-releasing hormone

References

Peterson ME. Hyperthyroid diseases. In: Ettinger SJ, Feldman EC, eds. Textbook of veterinary internal medicine. 4th ed. Philadelphia: WB Saunders, 1994.

Graves TK, Peterson ME. Occult hyperthyroidism in cats. In: Kirk RW, Bonagura, JD, eds. Current veterinary therapy XI. Philadelphia: WB Saunders, 1992.

Graves TK. Complications of treatment and concurrent illness associated with feline hyperthyroidism. In: Kirk RW, Bonagura JD. Current veterinary therapy XII. Philadelphia: WB Saunders, 1995.

Author Thomas K. Graves
Consulting Editor Rhett Nichols

HYPERTROPHIC OSTEODYSTROPHY

BASICS

DEFINITION
An inflammatory disease of bone affecting rapidly growing puppies.

Pathophysiology
Hypertrophic osteodystrophy (HOD) is characterized by nonseptic suppurative inflammation within metaphyseal trabeculae of long bones. Bones growing rapidly are affected more severely. Metaphyses are widened due to perimetaphyseal swelling and bone deposition. Trabecular microfracture and metaphyseal separation occur adjacent and parallel to the physis. Bone formation is defective. Ossifying periostitis may be extensive.

Systems Affected
• Musculoskeletal system—symmetrical distribution. Distal forelimbs are most severely affected. Costochondral junctions widened.
• Respiratory—interstitial pneumonia • Gastrointestinal—diarrhea • Soft tissue mineralization may occur in other organs

Genetics No genetic basis

Incidence/Prevalence Low

Geographic Distribution N/A

SIGNALMENT

Species Immature dogs

Breed Predilections
• Large, rapidly growing breeds • Great Danes most common • HOD has been reported in Irish wolfhound, Saint Bernard, Kuvasz, Irish setter, Weimaraner, Doberman pinscher, German shepherd, Labrador retriever, and many other breeds.

Mean Age and Range
• HOD only affects growing puppies • Average age is 3-4 months • Range of onset is 2-8 months

Predominant Sex
Males more than females

SIGNS

General Comments
• Lameness can be episodic • Degree of lameness varies; mild to non-weightbearing
• Initial episode may resolve without relapse

Historical Findings
• Based on severity of the episode • Owners often describe a depressed puppy that is reluctant to move • Inappetence is common

Physical Examination Findings
• Lameness, symmetrical, but forelimbs more severely affected • Painful, warm, swollen metaphyses • Pyrexia (can be high—106° F)
• Inappetence • Depression • Weight loss
• Dehydration • Diarrhea • Cachexia • Debilitation

CAUSES
The cause of HOD is unknown. Hypotheses proposed to explain the pathogenesis of HOD are listed below:

Metabolic
Hypovitaminosis C—eliminated because many dogs with HOD have normal ascorbic acid values; supplementation of vitamin C does not resolve HOD or prevent relapses; dogs synthesize their own vitamin C; and histologic changes differ from HOD. Hypocuprosis—copper deficiency produces histologic changes in rats similar to those seen in puppies with HOD. Copper deficiency does not cause similar changes in puppies.

Nutritional
HOD tends to occur as one or two affected puppies within a litter, yet often all puppies are receiving the same diet and supplementation. Puppies have developed HOD without overfeeding or oversupplementation. Correcting the diet does not alter the course of HOD or eliminate relapses.

Infectious
• Bacterial or fungal organisms have not been identified histopathologically in tissues from affected puppies. Attempts to transmit HOD hematogenously from affected to nonaffected puppies has failed. • Canine distemper virus RNA has been detected in bone cells of dogs with HOD. Blood taken from dogs with HOD injected into noninfected dogs resulted in development of canine distemper in 3 of 7 dogs, but HOD was not reproduced.
• The development of HOD secondary to an infectious agent may depend on the timing of exposure to the neonate.

RISK FACTORS
None proven to increase risk.

DIAGNOSIS

DIFFERENTIAL DIAGNOSIS
• Panosteitis—no metaphyseal swelling; radiographs reveal cottony intramedullary densities in long bones. • Elbow Dysplasia—no metaphyseal swelling; no fever; pain is localized to the elbow(s); radiographs reveal typical radiographic signs. • Osteochondritis Dissecans—no metaphyseal swelling or fever; pain localized to shoulder, elbow; hock or stifle; radiographs reveal subchondral defects.
• Septic polyarthritis—swelling more localized to joint capsule; radiographs localize soft tissue swelling to the joint; arthrocentesis shows septic suppurative inflammation; culture • Nonseptic polyarthritis—arthrocentesis reveals nonseptic suppurative inflammation.
• Septic metaphysitis—radiographs of the extremities not typical of HOD; asymmetrical; needle aspiration of metaphyseal lesions may reveal septic suppurative inflammation. Hematologic findings implicate bacterial infection (neutrophilia with accompanying left shift). • Retained cartilage cores—young large and giant breeds. Valgus deformity of the distal forelimbs caused by retained cartilage core in the distal ulnar physes; radiographs reveal

retained cartilage; afebrile; less perimetaphyseal swelling and less or no pain with manipulation • Canine osteochondrodysplasias—developmental disorders; various breeds. Cartilage abnormalities and abnormal bone growth result in limb shortening and bowing deformities of the distal limbs; afebrile, non-painful, heritable.

CBC/BIOCHEMISTRY/URINALYSIS
• Do not contribute to diagnosis • Stress leukogram • Normal serum parameters
• Hypocalcemia is uncommon.

OTHER LABORATORY TESTS N/A

IMAGING
• Radiography of distal extremities—irregular radiolucent zones within metaphyses, parallel and adjacent to physes; flared metaphyses. Extraperiosteal new bone may be seen extending up the diaphyses. Mineralization of perimetaphyseal soft tissues. Vertebrae and the mandible are rarely affected. • Thoracic radiography—reveals interstitial infiltrates in some dogs.

OTHER DIAGNOSTIC PROCEDURES N/A

GROSS AND HISTOPATHOLOGIC FINDINGS
• The most severe pathologic changes are found in the distal metaphyses of the radius and ulna, but all long bones will have similar abnormalities. • Gross—wide metaphyses with peripheral mineralization and soft tissue swelling. • Histological—nonseptic suppurative inflammation of the metaphysis (osteochondritis), especially adjacent to growth plates. Necrosis and probable secondary failure of osseous tissue deposition onto the calcified cartilage lattice of the primary spongiosa. Trabecular microfractures and impaction. Metaphyseal in fraction. Defective bone formation is thought to be secondary to osteochondral complex inflammation. Mineralization of perimetaphyseal soft tissues and soft tissues in other regions of the body. Interstitial pneumonia.

TREATMENT

INPATIENT VERSUS OUTPATIENT
• There is no treatment specific for HOD.
• Depends on the severity of the HOD episode, pyrexia, and the puppy's ability to maintain normal hydration and its willingness to eat.
• Some puppies will not stand or move and are prone to develop pressure sores

ACTIVITY
• Restricted; running and jumping may exacerbate metaphyseal injury and result in further inflammation.
• Confinement to a small well-padded area is recommended.
• Leash walking only.

• If the puppy is recumbent, turn every 2-4 hours to aid prevention of pressure sores and hypostatic congestion of the dependent lung.

DIET
• Normal commercial puppy ration
• Avoid supplements

CLIENT EDUCATION
• Warn the owner of the relapsing nature of HOD; boney deformities will remodel to some degree with time; bowing and valgus deformations will be permanent.
• Severe HOD will result in more severe bowing deformity.

SURGICAL CONSIDERATIONS
• In general, none
• Consider surgical methods of alimentation (pharyngostomy tube, tube gastrostomy) for debilitated puppies that will not eat or drink and have frequently relapsing episodes of acute clinical signs.

MEDICATIONS

DRUGS AND FLUIDS
• Intravenous fluid therapy—replacement fluid for dehydration; maintenance fluid thereafter.
• Nonsteroidal anti-inflammatory drugs (NSAIDs) for pain and antipyretic effects. Aspirin (10 mg/kg PO q12h) and dipyrone (25 mg/kg, injectable only) may be used. Dipyrone is an excellent antipyretic (do not overdose) and can control mild somatic and visceral pain. Prednisone (0.5 to 1.0 mg/kg PO q24h) is used only when there is no response to aspirin or dipyrone.

CONTRAINDICATIONS None

PRECAUTIONS
• If an infectious cause is proven, or if secondary infection is present, avoid immunosuppressive drugs.
• NSAIDs may cause gastric ulceration; watch for hematemesis or melena.

POSSIBLE INTERACTIONS None

ALTERNATE DRUGS None

FOLLOW-UP

PATIENT MONITORING
Puppies that improve have less metaphyseal sensitivity; they begin to get up, their appetite improves, and pyrexia resolves.

PREVENTION/AVOIDANCE N/A

POSSIBLE COMPLICATIONS
• Cachexia • Permanent bowing deformities • Secondary bacterial infection • Pressure sores • Muscle fasciculations, seizure (if hypocalcemia occurs)

EXPECTED COURSE AND PROGNOSIS
• Course: days to weeks • Most puppies have one or two episodes and recover. • Some puppies seem to have intractable relapsing episodes of pain and pyrexia and rarely die or are euthanatized as a result. • Prognosis: good for most puppies • Persistent bowing deformity after HOD will eliminate many purebred puppies from the show ring.

MISCELLANEOUS

ASSOCIATED CONDITIONS
Craniomandibular osteopathy is occasionally associated with mineralization of soft tissues (ossifying periostitis) around long bones similar to that with HOD. Lameness may result.

AGE RELATED FACTORS
HOD only occurs in immature dogs.

ZOONOTIC POTENTIAL N/A

PREGNANCY N/A

SYNONYMS
Metaphyseal osteopathy

SEE ALSO N/A

ABBREVIATIONS
HOD = hypertrophic osteodystrophy
NSAID = nonsteroidal anti-inflammatory drug

References

Bellah JR. Hypertrophic osteodystrophy. In: Bojrab MJ, ed. Disease mechanisms in small animal surgery. 2nd ed. Philadelphia: Lea & Febiger, 1993;858-864.

Lenehan TM, Fetter AW. Hypertrophic osteodystrophy. In: Newton CD, Nunamker DM. eds. Textbook of small animal orthopedics. Philadelphia: Lippincott, 1985;597-601.

Mee AP, et al. Canine virus transcripts detected in the bone cells of dogs with metaphyseal osteopathy. Bone 1993;14:59-67.

Author Jamie R. Bellah
Consulting Editor Peter D. Schwarz

HYPERTROPHIC OSTEOPATHY

BASICS

OVERVIEW
• A disease that causes high peripheral blood flow and periosteal new bone proliferation along the diaphyseal region of long bones, often beginning in the distal phalanges, metacarpal bones, and metatarsal bones
• Pathogenesis is speculative. Theories include chronic anoxia, obscure toxins, hyperestrogenism, and autonomic neurovascular reflex mechanisms mediated by afferent branches of the vagus or intercostal nerves.
• Hypertrophic osteopathy (HO) is considered a manifestation of a primary disease process.

SIGNALMENT
• More common in dogs than cats • Age of highest frequency is 8 years, which coincides with the peak incidence of pulmonary neoplasms. • Mean age is 5.6 years for dogs with nonneoplastic lung lesions. • Large-breed dogs between 1-2 years of age with embryonal rhabdomyosarcoma

SIGNS

Historical Findings
• Listlessness • Reluctance to move • Enlargement of the distal portion of the extremities

Physical Examination Findings
• Lame, sore, and painful limbs • Extremities are enlarged and firm to the touch but not edematous. • Swelling predominantly below level of elbow and stifle joints extending distally to toes

CAUSES AND RISK FACTORS
• Primary and metastatic lung tumors • Nonneoplastic thoracic conditions—pneumonia, heartworm disease, congenital/acquired heart disease, bronchial foreign bodies, Spirocerca lupi infestation of esophagus, and focal lung atelectasis • Esophageal sarcoma • Embryonal rhabdomyosarcoma of the urinary bladder

• Adenocarcinoma of the liver or prostate gland • Thoracic and abdominal mesotheliomas

DIAGNOSIS

DIFFERENTIAL DIAGNOSIS
• Osteomyelitis—bones not symmetrically affected and generally edematous; presence of lysis; history of penetrating trauma or systemic infection • Metastatic neoplasia—bones not symmetrically affected

CBC/BIOCHEMISTRY/URINALYSIS
• Dependent on the underlying cause • Serum alkaline phosphatase may be high

OTHER LABORATORY TESTS N/A

IMAGING
• Radiographs of the extremities—bilaterally symmetric extensive, rough, periosteal new bone (PNB) formation on diaphyseal region of long bones; buds of PNB project outward from the cortex and perpendicular to its long axis; PNB forms around the entire circumference of the bone; joints are not affected
• Radiographs of the thoracic and abdominal cavities to rule out various systemic disorders
• Ultrasound can be used to help identify and differentiate primary lesions.

OTHER DIAGNOSTIC PROCEDURES
N/A

TREATMENT
• Must treat underlying primary cause
• Unilateral vagotomy on the side of a lung lesion, incising through the parietal pleura, subperiosteal rib resection, or bilateral cervical vagotomy have all been suggested as methods of treatment.

MEDICATIONS

DRUGS AND FLUIDS
• Glucocorticoids (i.e., prednisone) may be used to improve clinical signs and reduce the extent of swelling.
• Dependent on the underlying cause
• Analgesics as needed

CONTRAINDICATIONS/POSSIBLE INTERACTIONS N/A

FOLLOW-UP
• Removal of the inciting cause may or may not bring about regression of clinical signs.
• Bony changes may take several months to regress. • Prognosis is guarded to poor due to the common occurrence of neoplastic causes.
• HO is an indicator of other disease processes; therefore, its diagnosis is important in recognizing the need for further diagnostic tests to identify the primary cause.

MISCELLANEOUS

SYNONYMS
• Hypertrophic pulmonary osteopathy (HPO) • Hypertrophic pulmonary osteoarthropathy (HPOA) • Hypertrophic osteoarthropathy (HOA)

ABBREVIATIONS
PNB = periosteal new bone
HO = hypertrophic osteopathy

Reference
Halliwell WH. Tumorlike lesions of bone. In: Bojrab MJ, ed. Disease mechanisms in small animal surgery. Philadelphia: Lea & Febiger, 1993.

Author Peter D. Schwarz
Consulting Editor Peter D. Schwarz

BASICS

OVERVIEW
• A collection of clinical signs that results from high viscosity of the blood • Has been associated with several primary conditions, usually neoplastic, that are characterized by marked elevations in plasma protein concentration • Rarely results from an extremely high erythrocyte count that is concurrent with normal levels of plasma proteins • Most frequent precipitating diseases include plasma cell tumor (multiple myeloma) and other lymphoid tumors or leukemias • Secretion of paraprotein (abnormal immunoglobulin) often results in total plasma protein levels > 10 g/dL; a monoclonal gammopathy is seen with serum protein electrophoresis. • Signs are related to reduced blood flow through small vessels, which results in decreased tissue oxygenation and, in some animals, hemorrhage. • Characterized by frequent occurrence of visual and neurologic deficits

SIGNALMENT
• More frequent in dogs than cats • No sex or breed predilections • More likely to occur in middle-aged and older animals

SIGNS

Historical Findings
• No consistent findings • Listlessness, weight loss, anorexia • Polyuria, polydypsia • Blindness, ataxia, seizures • Lameness, bone or joint pain • Vomiting, diarrhea

Physical Examination Findings
• Visual deficits with engorged retinal vessels, retinal hemorrhages, retinal detachment, or papilledema • Nystagmus, head tilt, ataxia, disorientation, or proprioceptive deficits • Hepatomegaly, splenomegaly, or enlarged lymph nodes • Epistaxis, bleeding gums, bleeding after venipuncture • Pallor of mucous membranes (unless polycythemic) • Tachycardia and signs of congestive heart failure

CAUSES AND RISK FACTORS
• Plasma cell tumors, multiple myeloma (IgM > IgA > IgG) • Lymphocytic leukemia or lymphoma • Chronic atypical inflammation with monoclonal gammopathy (e.g., canine ehrlichiosis, feline infectious peritonitis) • Chronic autoimmune disease (e.g., systemic lupus erythematosus, rheumatoid arthritis) • Marked polycythemia (PCV > 65%)

DIAGNOSIS

DIFFERENTIAL DIAGNOSIS
• Unexplained neurologic disease, visual deficit, or hemorrhagic diathesis • Hyperproteinemia with monoclonal gammopathy increases the likelihood of hyperviscosity syndrome.

CBC/BIOCHEMISTRY/URINALYSIS
• Nonregenerative anemia, thrombocytopenia, or leukopenia • Hyperproteinemia (total plasma protein > 9.0 g/dL) and hyperglobulinemia (> 5.0 g/dL) with monoclonal gammopathy, azotemia, hypercalcemia • Isosthenuria, proteinuria

OTHER LABORATORY TESTS
• High concentrations of IgG, IgA, or IgM detected by radial immunodiffusion • High plasma or serum viscosity (> 3.0 relative to water) • Possible increase in PT or PTT

IMAGING
Radiographic findings of focal osteolytic lesions or cardiomegaly

OTHER DIAGNOSTIC PROCEDURES
Plasma cell or lymphoid infiltrate in bone marrow biopsy

TREATMENT
• Treat as an inpatient
• Use plasmapheresis (10-15 mL/kg) to remove blood and replace isotonic fluid volume—may reduce blood viscosity to below the individual symptomatic threshold.

MEDICATIONS

DRUGS AND FLUIDS
• Provide treatment of primary neoplastic or inflammatory condition.

• See other sections for drug therapy of plasma cell tumor, lymphocytic leukemia, lymphoma, ehrlichiosis, autoimmune disease, and polycythemia.

CONTRAINDICATIONS/POSSIBLE INTERACTIONS
• Avoid use of medications that increase vascular volume.
• Do not treat with medications that impair platelet function (e.g., nonsteroidal anti-inflammatory drugs).

FOLLOW-UP
• Monitor serum or plasma total protein—return of proteins toward normal range and resolution of monoclonal gammopathy reverse signs of hyperviscosity syndrome
• Perform funduscopic examination to monitor resolution of vascular engorgement and hemorrhage. • Obtain CBC, chemistry panel, and urinalysis to monitor other lab abnormalities.

MISCELLANEOUS

SEE ALSO
• Plasmacytoma • Multiple Myeloma • Leukemia • Lymphosarcoma • Ehrlichiosis • Lupus Erythematosus • Polycythemia

ABBREVIATIONS
PCV = packed cell volume
PT = prothrombin time
PTT = partial thromboplastin time

Reference

Forrester SD, Relford RL. Serum hyperviscosity syndrome: its diagnosis and treatment. Vet Med 1992;85:48-54.

Author Robert M. Shull
Consulting Editor Alan H. Rebar

HYPHEMA

BASICS

DEFINITION
Blood in the anterior chamber

Pathophysiology
Hyphema results from any condition that causes intraocular vessel damage sufficient to allow egress of erythrocytes. The bleeding vessels are resident or acquired vessels (neovascularization). The responsible vessels are in the retina, vitreous (hyaloid artery or primary vitreous), choroid, ciliary body, or iris. Resident vessels bleed as a result of trauma, inflammation, defects in hemostasis, or neoplastic infiltration. New vessels are inherently leaky and are prone to bleed spontaneously. The most common causes of iris neovascularization are chronic retinal detachment, chronic uveitis, and intraocular neoplasia, especially lymphosarcoma. Hyphema is the presenting sign of systemic hypertension, especially in elderly cats. In most animals, hyphema does not in itself cause any adverse secondary effects. If bleeding is persistent, hyphema can result in secondary glaucoma.

Systems Affected
Ophthalmic

Genetics N/A

Incidence/Prevalence
Hyphema is a common sign on physical examination in many animals with ocular or systemic disease.

Geographic Distribution N/A

SIGNALMENT

Species Dogs and cats

Breed Predilections N/A

Mean Age and Range Birth to late in life.

Predominant Sex N/A

SIGNS

General Comments
A function of how much bleeding has occurred into the eye, whether vision is impaired, and whether hyphema is associated with systemic disease

Historical Findings
Extremely diverse, reflecting the multitude of causes. A history of vision loss is uncommon because hyphema is rarely bilateral and complete.

Physical Examination Findings
• Blood seen within the anterior chamber of the eye. • If severe, other intraocular structures cannot be seen. • Corneal edema is often present. • Blood is often seen mixed with WBC when the cause is lymphosarcoma. • Eyelid, conjunctival, or corneal lesions are often noticed if hyphema is secondary to trauma. • Intraocular pressure may be high in eyes with hyphema of long-standing duration.

CAUSES
• Trauma • Chronic retinal detachment • Uveal neoplasia, especially lymphosarcoma, hemangiosarcoma and primary uveal melanoma • Uveitis, especially if caused by feline infectious peritonitis in cats, and rickettsial disease in dogs • Coagulopathies • Vasculitis, either immune-mediated or secondary to rickettsial diseases (e.g., Rocky mountain spotted fever and ehrlichiosis) • Systemic hypertension (e.g., primary or secondary to renal disease, hyperthyroidism) • Parasite migration (e.g., ophthalmomyiasis interna) • Secondary to congenital ocular defects (e.g., collie eye anomaly, persistent primary vitreous, and severe retinal dysplasia)

RISK FACTORS
• Uveitis • Metastatic neoplasia • Chronic retinal detachment • Any disease causing vasculitis or vascular fragility • Chronic renal disease • Coagulopathies • Congenital ocular defects

DIAGNOSIS

DIFFERENTIAL DIAGNOSIS
• Bilateral hyphema usually represents a systemic disease. • Retinal detachment should be suspected in older dogs with unilateral hyphema. • A coagulopathy should be suspected in eyes with hyphema which lack conjunctival or episclera vascular injection.
• Systemic hypertension should be strongly suspected in elderly cats with hyphema and retinal hemorrhage or detachment. • Intraocular neoplasia should be suspected in animals with chronic or recurrent hyphema.

CBC/BIOCHEMISTRY/URINALYSIS
• Results of a laboratory work-up are usually normal in patients with hyphema resulting from localized ocular disease. Laboratory abnormalities are commonly found in animals with hyphema resulting from a systemic disease. • Anemia or thrombocytopenia may present if hyphema is associated with a systemic bleeding disorder. • A work-up for uveitis is indicated in animals with hyphema secondary to chronic uveitis (see dog and cat uveitis topics).

OTHER LABORATORY TESTS
When hyphema is suspected to be caused by a coagulopathy, special laboratory tests are indicated to assess hemostasis. Intrinsic coagulation is assessed by activated coagulation time and partial thromboplastin time. Extrinsic coagulation is assessed by the one-stage prothrombin time. Other tests that may be indicated are thrombocyte and reticulocyte counts, thrombin time, fibrinogen levels, and fibrin degradation products.

IMAGING
• Ocular ultrasonography is indicated whenever hyphema is severe enough to obstruct view of the intraocular structures. Retinal detachment and intraocular tumors are usually easily identified. • Thoracic radiographs and possibly abdominal ultrasound may be useful in ruling out disseminated neoplasia.

OTHER DIAGNOSTIC PROCEDURES
• Other tests that may be indicated in patients with suspected bleeding disorders are bone marrow examination and buccal bleeding time. • Measuring of blood pressure is indicated when hyphema cannot be attributed to ocular disease. • Lymph node aspiration and biopsy is indicated if lymphosarcoma is suspected.

GROSS AND HISTOPATHOLOGIC FINDINGS
• Grossly, the anterior chamber is partially or completely filled with blood. • Histologically, erythrocytes are seen in a matrix of proteinaceous fluid. Common associated findings are the presence of RBC in the iridocorneal angle and trabecular spaces and vitreal hemorrhage. Posterior synechia and inflammatory cells within the anterior uvea are common findings when hyphema is secondary to uveitis. Preiridal fibrovascular membranes are common if hyphema is secondary to retinal detachment or chronic uveitis.

TREATMENT

INPATIENT VERSUS OUTPATIENT
Usually an outpatient problem

ACTIVITY
Restricted only if hyphema is caused by a clotting disorder

DIET N/A

CLIENT EDUCATION
The client must understand that hyphema is a clinical sign and not a specific disease. No specific treatments for hyphema exist. Treatment is directed at eliminating the underlying cause.

SURGICAL CONSIDERATIONS
In animals with hyphema caused by trauma, surgical intervention is indicated to repair accompanying adnexal or corneal defects. In animals in which chronic hyphema has caused secondary glaucoma, a surgical procedure to remove (i.e., enucleation) or possibly salvage the globe (i.e., evisceration and intrascleral prosthesis) is indicated. Surgical evacuation of the blood from the anterior chamber is rarely indicated.

MEDICATIONS

DRUGS AND FLUIDS OF CHOICE

• There is no specific treatment for hyphema. Corticosteroids (1% prednisolone acetate, 0.1% dexamethasone) applied topicdally q6h are often empirically used to control uveal inflammation. Topically applied antibiotics are not indicated unless ephema is associated with conjunctival or corneal epithelial defects (trauma). Systemically administered corticosteroids are usually indicated only when the hyphema is caused by corticosteroid-responsive systemic disease (e.g., lymphosarcoma) or posterior segment inflammation. Systemic hypotensive therapy is indicated if the hyphema is caused by hypertension.
• Topically applied 1% atropine solution given to effect is indicated to prevent synechia formation unless secondary glaucoma has occurred.
• If secondary glaucoma has occurred, dichlorphenamide (2-4 mg/kg, q8h-q12h, PO) and epinephrine (1% q8h-q12h topically applied) may help lower intraocular pressure. Topically applied timolol (0.5% q12h topically applied) or dipivefrin HCl (q8h-q12h) can be used in place of epinephrine. If vision is irreversibly lost, enucleation or possibly a globe salvage procedure should be considered.
• Formed clots can be resolved if tissue plasminogen activator (0.1-0.2 mL, 250 mcg/mL) is injected into the anterior chamber within 5-7 days after the hemorrhage.

CONTRAINDICATIONS

Hyphema should not be treated with tissue plasminogen activator if a clot has not formed and if the cause of the bleeding has not been eliminated, because rebleeding is likely.

PRECAUTIONS

Pilocarpine may exacerbate breakdown of the blood aqueous barrier and may cause further bleeding.

POSSIBLE INTERACTIONS N/A

ALTERNATE DRUGS N/A

FOLLOW-UP

PATIENT MONITORING

• In animals with severe hyphema, monitor intraocular pressure daily. • Animals with less severe disease should be reexamined every 2-3 days until the hyphema resolves.

PREVENTION/AVOIDANCE

Restricted activity if hyphema is caused by a clotting disorder.

POSSIBLE COMPLICATIONS

• Glaucoma • Vision loss

EXPECTED COURSE AND PROGNOSIS

• The prognosis varies with the cause.
• The prognosis for hyphema caused by acute trauma is generally good unless the irrevocable damage has occurred to the lens, ciliary body, or retina. • Hyphema secondary to retinal detachment and anterior segment neovascularization typically will not resolve. In these animals, secondary glaucoma eventually results, necessitating some type of surgical intervention to relieve pain (e.g., enucleation and evisceration with prosthesis).

MISCELLANEOUS

ASSOCIATED CONDITIONS

• Clotting disorders • Systemic hypertension • Uveitis • Metastatic neoplasia (lymphosarcoma, hemangiosarcoma) • Retinal detachment • Von Willebrand's disease

AGE RELATED FACTORS

Systemic hypertension more common in elderly patients

ZOONOTIC POTENTIAL N/A

PREGNANCY N/A

SYNONYMS None

SEE ALSO

• Anterior Uveitis—(Dogs and Cats)
• Coagulation Factor Deficiencies
• Hypertension, Systemic • Red Eye

ABBREVIATIONS N/A

References

Nelms S, Nasisse MP, Davidson MG, Kirschner S. Hyphema associated with retinal disease in dogs: 17 cases. J Am Vet Med Assoc 1993;202:1289–1292.

Collins BK, Moore CP. Canine anterior uvea. In: Gelatt KN, ed. Veterinary ophthalmology. 2nd Ed. Philadelphia: Lea & Febiger, 1992:357–395.

Littman MP. Spontaneous systemic hypertension in 24 cats. J Vet Int Med 1994;8:79–86.

Author Mark P. Nasisse
Consulting Editor Paul E. Miller

HYPOADRENOCORTICISM (ADDISON'S DISEASE)

BASICS

DEFINITION
Endocrine disorder caused by deficient production of glucocorticoids (cortisol) or mineralocorticoids (aldosterone) or both. Primary hypoadrenocorticism is caused by disease or injury to the adrenal glands that leads to deficiencies in cortisol and aldosterone. Secondary hypoadrenocorticism is caused by exogenous administration of glucocorticosteroids or pituitary gland disease that causes reduced production of ACTH. Secondary hypoadrenocorticism causes glucocorticoid deficiency with preservation of mineralocorticoid function.

Pathophysiology
Aldosterone deficiency causes inability to excrete potassium and retain sodium. Sodium deficiency leads to diminished effective circulating volume, which in turn contributes to prerenal azotemia, hypotension, dehydration, weakness, and depression. Hyperkalemia (along with other metabolic derangements) may cause myocardial toxicity. Glucocorticoid (cortisol) deficiency contributes to anorexia, vomiting, melena, lethargy, and weight loss, predisposes to hypoglycemia, and results in impaired excretion of water free of sodium.

Systems Affected
• Multiple organ systems involved; extent of involvement varies from patient to patient • Cardiovascular • Renal/urologic • Nervous • Gastrointestinal

Genetics N/A

Incidence/Prevalence
Uncommon to rare in dogs and extremely rare in cats

Geographic Distribution N/A

SIGNALMENT
Species Dogs and cats

Breed Predilections
Great Dane, rottweiler, Portuguese water dog, standard poodle, West Highland white terrier, and wheaten terrier are at relatively increased risk. No predilection in cats.

Predominant Sex
Female dogs are at higher risk than males. No predilection in cats.

Mean Age and Range
• Dogs—median, 4 years; range, < 1-12 years • Cats—most are middle-aged; range, 1-9 years

SIGNS
General Comments
Signs vary from mild and few in number in some patients with chronic hypoadrenocorticism to severe and life-threatening in patients with acute addisonian crisis.

Historical Findings
• Dogs—lethargy, anorexia, vomiting, weight loss, waxing-waning course, diarrhea, previous response to treatment, shaking, and polyuria/polydipsia • Cats—lethargy, anorexia, vomiting, polyuria/polydipsia, and weight loss

Physical Examination Findings
• Dogs—depression, weakness, dehydration, collapse, hypothermia, slow capillary refill time, melena, weak pulse, bradycardia, painful abdomen, and hair loss • Cats—dehydration, weakness, slow capillary refill time, weak pulse, and bradycardia

CAUSES
• Primary hypoadrenocorticism—idiopathic (immune-mediated), mitotane overdose, granulomatous disease, and metastatic tumors • Secondary hypoadrenocorticism—iatrogenic after withdrawal of long-term glucocorticoid administration, isolated ACTH deficiency, panhypopituitarism, and nonfunctional pituitary tumor

RISK FACTORS N/A

DIAGNOSIS

DIFFERENTIAL DIAGNOSIS
The signs of hypoadrenocorticism are nonspecific and are seen in patients with other more common medical disorders, particularly gastrointestinal and renal diseases. Although no signs are pathognomonic, a waxing and waning course and previous response to nonspecific medical intervention (e.g., fluids and steroids) should alert the clinician to consider the diagnosis.

CBC/BIOCHEMISTRY/URINALYSIS
• Anemia, eosinophilia, and lymphocytosis in some patients • Hyperkalemia, azotemia, hyponatremia, hypochloremia, low total CO_2, hypercalcemia, high liver enzyme activity, high serum alkaline phosphatase, and hypoglycemia in some patients Some animals with hypoadrenocorticism have normal electrolytes. • Impaired urine concentrating ability is common.

OTHER LABORATORY TESTS
• Definitive diagnosis is by demonstration of an undetectable to low serum cortisol concentration that fails to increase after administration of either ACTH gel IM (dogs, 20 U; cats, 10 U) or IV administration of synthetic ACTH (dogs, 0.25 mg; cats, 0.125 mg). In hypovolemic, dehydrated animals, use IV administration of synthetic ACTH or delay testing until after initial fluid administration is completed. • Determination of the plasma ACTH concentration is indicated in animals with normal electrolytes to differentiate primary from secondary hypoadrenocorticism (sample must be collected before administration of glucocorticoids).

IMAGING
Radiography may reveal microcardia, narrow vena cava or descending aorta, hypoperfused lung fields, or megaesophagus (rare).

OTHER DIAGNOSTIC PROCEDURES
N/A

GROSS AND HISTOPATHOLOGIC FINDINGS
• Gross findings—atrophy of the adrenal glands • Microscopic findings—lymphocytic-plasmacytic adrenalitis or adrenocortical atrophy

TREATMENT

INPATIENT VERSUS OUTPATIENT
• An acute addisonian crisis is a medical emergency requiring intensive treatment. • Treatment for patients with chronic hypoadrenocorticism depends on the severity of clinical signs, although initial stabilization is conducted on an inpatient basis in most.

ACTIVITY
No alteration of activity necessary

DIET
No need to alter

CLIENT EDUCATION
• Lifelong glucocorticoid or mineralocorticoid replacement or both required • Increase in dosage of replacement glucocorticoid required during periods of stress such as travel, hospitalization, and surgery

SURGICAL CONSIDERATIONS N/A

MEDICATIONS

DRUGS AND FLUIDS
Acute Addisonian Crisis
• Treat with rapid correction of hypovolemia by use of isotonic fluids (preferably 0.9% NaCl) and parenteral administration of a rapidly acting glucocorticoid such as dexamethasone sodium phosphate or prednisolone sodium succinate; dexamethasone sodium phosphate is preferred because prednisolone cross-reacts with cortisol assays. • See Potassium, Hyperkalemia for management of severe hyperkalemia.

Chronic Primary Hypoadrenocorticism
Treat with glucocorticoid replacement (prednisone, 0.2 mg/kg/day) and mineralocorticoid replacement fludrocortisone acetate (10-20 µg/kg/day divided and adjusted by 0.05-0.1 mg increments on the basis of serial serum electrolyte determinations) or DOCP (2 mg/kg IM or SQ q21-30 days, adjusted if needed on the basis of serum electrolyte determinations).

Secondary Hypoadrenocorticism
Requires only glucocorticoid supplementation (prednisone, 0.2 mg/kg/day)

CONTRAINDICATIONS N/A
PRECAUTIONS N/A
POSSIBLE INTERACTIONS N/A
ALTERNATE DRUGS N/A

 FOLLOW-UP

PATIENT MONITORING
• The daily dosage of fludrocortisone is adjusted by 0.05-0.1 mg increments as needed on the basis of serial serum electrolyte determinations. After initiation of treatment, serum electrolyte concentrations should be monitored weekly until stabilized within the normal range. Thereafter, serum electrolyte concentrations and BUN or creatinine are checked monthly for the first 3-6 months and then every 3-12 months. In many dogs that are given fludrocortisone, the daily dose required to control the disorder increases gradually, usually during the first 6-24 months of treatment. In most dogs, the final fludrocortisone dosage needed is 20-30 µg/kg/day; very few can be controlled on 10 µg/kg/day or less. • After each of the first 2 injections of DOCP, serum electrolyte concentrations are determined, ideally at 2, 3, and 4 weeks to determine the duration of effect. Thereafter, electrolyte concentrations should be determined at the time of injection for the next 6 months (and the dosage of DOCP adjusted if necessary), and then every 6-12 months. DOCP is usually required at 3 to 4-week intervals, but a few animals need injections every 2 weeks. Alternatively, to maintain monthly injections, the dosage of DOCP can be gradually increased. Almost all patients with hypoadrenocorticism are well controlled on a maintenance DOCP dosage of 2 mg/kg/injection.

PREVENTION/AVOIDANCE
Hormonal replacement therapy must be continued for the life of the patient. The dosage of replacement glucocorticoid must be increased during periods of stress such as travel, hospitalization, and surgery.

POSSIBLE COMPLICATIONS
• PU/PD develops in some animals from prednisone administration, necessitating decreasing or discontinuing the drug. • PU/PD develops in some animals from fludrocortisone administration, necessitating a change to DOCP.

EXPECTED COURSE AND PROGNOSIS
Except for animals with primary hypoadrenocorticism caused by granulomatous or metastatic disease and secondary hypoadrenocorticism caused by a pituitary mass, the vast majority of patients with hypoadrenocorticism have a good to excellent prognosis after proper stabilization and treatment.

 MISCELLANEOUS

ASSOCIATED CONDITIONS
Concurrent endocrine gland failure occurs in up to 5% of dogs (i.e., hypothyroidism, diabetes mellitus, and/or hypoparathyroidism).

AGE RELATED FACTORS N/A

ZOONOTIC POTENTIAL N/A

PREGNANCY N/A

SYNONYM
Addison's disease (primary hypoadrenocorticism)

SEE ALSO
• Potassium, Hyperkalemia • Sodium, Hyponatremia

ABBREVIATIONS
ACTH = adrenocorticotropic hormone
DOCP = desoxycorticosterone pivilate

References
Feldman EC, Peterson ME. Hypoadrenocorticism. Vet Clin N Am Small Anim Pract 1984;14:751-766.
Kintzer PP, Peterson ME. Canine hypoadrenocorticism. In: Kirk RW, Bonagura JD, eds. Current veterinary therapy XII. Philadelphia: WB Saunders, 1995.
Peterson ME, Kintzer PP, Kass PH. Pretreatment clinical and laboratory findings in 225 dogs with hypoadrenocorticism. J Amer Vet Med Assoc 1996;208:85-91.
Greco DS, Peterson ME. Feline hypoadrenocorticism. In: Kirk RW, ed. Current veterinary therapy X. Philadelphia: WB Saunders, 1989.
Author Peter P. Kintzer
Consulting Editor Rhett Nichols

HYPOANDROGENISM

BASICS

DEFINITION
Relative or absolute deficiency of masculinizing sex hormones such as testosterone and its derivatives

Pathophysiology
• Androgens have both masculinizing and anabolic effects and are produced by the adrenal cortex, ovaries, and testes. Interstitial (Leydig's) cells of the testes primarily produce testosterone along with small amounts of dihydrotestosterone (DHT), dihydroepiandrosterone, and androstenedione. Weak androgens may be converted peripherally to more powerful androgens. • Hypoandrogenism develops because of an inadequate production of androgens, androgen receptor defect, or enzymatic defect. Androgen-responsive tissues (e.g., testes, penis, prepuce, prostate gland, and perineum) become less sensitive to the effects of androgens as a result of receptor-mediated problems. Enzymatic defects include deficiency of 5 alpha-reductase, which results in conversion failure of testosterone to DHT. Castration, testicular agenesis, and testicular hypoplasia, as well as inadequate synthesis of adrenocortical androgens, results in low androgen production.
• Affected animals usually are male phenotypes with XY chromosomes.

Systems Affected
• Renal/urologic—anatomic and functional abnormalities • Reproductive—anatomic and functional abnormalities • Skin/exocrine—alopecia and seborrheic dermatosis

Genetics
• Androgen resistance associated with testicular feminization is thought to be X-linked recessive. • Hypospadias in the Boston terrier breed are considered familial. The mode of inheritance is unknown.

Incidence/Prevalence
Uncommon

Geographic Distribution   N/A

SIGNALMENT

Species Dogs and cats

Breed Predilections
• Boston terriers—hypospadias • Calico and tortoiseshell cats—Klienfelter's syndrome (39 XXY)

Mean Age and Range
• Congenital—behavioral problems usually are recognized around puberty. • Anatomic abnormalities may be detected sooner.

Predominant Sex Male

SIGNS

Historical Findings
• Postpuberty—infertility and low libido
• Prepuberty—failure of male dogs to lift their legs to urinate; absence of urine spraying in tom cats

Physical Examination Findings
• Clinical signs vary. • Subnormal development of male secondary sex characteristcs • Smaller than expected stature for breed and age • Small, underdeveloped, or hypoplastic testes, penis, prepuce, and scrotum; soft consistency to the testes • Poor semen quality • Hypospadia • Absence of penile spines in male cats • Gynecomastia possible in male dogs • Bilaterally symmetrical alopecia and seborrhea sicca that usually begins in the perineum. • Hyperpigmentation and pruritus usually not seen • Urinary incontinence

CAUSES
• Castration • Gonadotropin deficiencies caused by hypothalamic and pituitary problems result in low GnRH, LH, and FSH concentrations, which cause low testosterone secretion and secondary hypogonadism. • Pituitary tumor may cause low LH and FSH. • Hypothalamic tumor may cause low GnRH. • Primary hypogonadism and reduced testicular size and function cause gonadotropin hyperactivity with high GnRH, LH, and FSH concentrations. • Cryptorchidism • Hyperprolactinemia inhibits LH and testosterone secretion. • Reduced sensitivity of androgen-responsive tissues

RISK FACTORS
• Drugs—ketoconazole, megesterole acetate, cimetidine, spironolactone, and some antineoplastic agents (e.g., busulfan, chlorambucil, cisplatin, cyclophosphamide, methotrexate, and vincristine) are known to decrease testosterone in humans. • Exogenous administration of steroid compounds that act by negative feeback on the pituitary gland. Anabolic steroids, estrogens, progestagens, and glucocorticoids inhibit LH and, thus, testosterone secretion.

DIAGNOSIS

DIFFERENTIAL DIAGNOSIS
• Hypothyroidism can be confirmed by a TSH stimulation test, determination of TSH concentration, or equilibrium dialysis assay for free T_4. • Intersex abnormalities (e.g., male pseudohemaphrodite and XX male syndrome) have distinct anatomic or histologic abnormalities and karyotype.

CBC/BIOCHEMISTRY/URINALYSIS
Results usually normal

OTHER LABORATORY TESTS
• Serum testosterone concentration—testosterone secretion is episodic, so repetitive testing or stimulation test is more diagnostic than a single serum test for testosterone
• GnRH stimulation test or HCG stimulation test (see Appendix for protocol)—serum testosterone concentration should not increase in response to GnRH or HCG in animals with primary gonadal problems and hypoplastic testes • Karyotyping • Neutrophils

in buccal smears may contain sex chromatin (Barr bodies) in phenotypic males. • Gonadotropin assay • Prolactin assay • Low sperm count or high numbers of abnormal sperm

IMAGING
CT and MRI to detect brain tumor

OTHER DIAGNOSTIC PROCEDURES
• Testicular biopsy may be indicated in patients with small testicles, abnormally shaped testicles, or testicles of abnormal consistency.
• Skin biopsy in patient with alopecia and seborrhea sicca

GROSS AND HISTOPATHOLOGIC FINDINGS
• Hypospadia • Testicular hypoplasia or atrophy • Persistent mullerian duct in male pseudohemaphrodites

TREATMENT

INPATIENT VERSUS OUTPATIENT
• Hormone replacement may be attempted on an outpatient basis. • Hospitalization is required for surgical procedures.

ACTIVITY N/A

DIET N/A

CLIENT EDUCATION
Affected animals should not be bred.

SURGICAL CONSIDERATIONS
Neuter animals with abnormal karyotypes and anatomic defects such as hypospadias and cryptorchidism.

MEDICATIONS

DRUGS AND FLUIDS
• Discontinue drugs that may be contributing to hypogonadism (see causes). • Replacement therapy with GnRH (Cystorelin) and gonadotropins (e.g., LH and FSH) may be attempted to increase libido in male dogs.
• Testosterone (oral methyltestosterone or injectable repositol testosterone) can be administered to castrated male dogs with testosterone responsive alopecia and urinary incontinence.

CONTRAINDICATIONS
Drugs that predispose to hypoandrogenism

PRECAUTIONS
• Testosterone can cause aggression and cholestatic liver disease. It can also aggravate chronic prostatitis and perianal adenoma.
• Chronic administration of GnRH can cause infertility by negative inhibition of the hypothalamic-pituitary-testis axis.
• Exogenous testosterone decreases testicular size and sperm counts.

POSSIBLE INTERACTIONS N/A

ALTERNATE DRUGS N/A

FOLLOW-UP

PATIENT MONITORING

Libido, sperm count, and serum testosterone concentration after initiating replacement therapy

PREVENTION/AVOIDANCE

Avoid drugs known to cause hypoandrogenism in breeding animals.

POSSIBLE COMPLICATIONS

Permanent infertility and hypogonadism

EXPECTED COURSE AND PROGNOSIS

Hypoandrogenism can be intermittent, transient, or permanent, depending on the cause.

MISCELLANEOUS

ASSOCIATED CONDITIONS

• Cryptorchidism commonly is associated with hypospadias. • Hypoandrogenism is associated with benign prostatic hyperplasia

and squamous metaplasia because of low androgen secretion and high estrogen associated with advanced age. • Hypoandrogenism is theorized to be the cause of testosterone responsive dermatosis and testosterone responsive urinary incontinence. • Idiopathic male feminizing syndrome • Intersex abnormalities—XX male syndrome

AGE RELATED FACTORS

Testosterone secretion normally diminishes with increasing age.

ZOONOTIC POTENTIAL N/A

PREGNANCY

Low adrenal androgen production by the fetus is thought to cause hypospadias.

SYNONYMS N/A

SEE ALSO

• Infertility, Male Dogs • Sexual Development Disorders • Dermatoses, Sex Hormone Responsive • Incontinence, Urinary

ABBREVIATIONS

GnRH = gonadotropin-releasing hormone
FSH = follicle-stimulating hormone
HCG = human chorionic gonadotropin
DHT = dihydrotestosterone
LH = luteinizing hormone

References

Feldman EC, Nelson RW. Canine male reproduction. In: Canine and feline endocrinology and reproduction. 2nd ed. Philadelphia: WB Saunders, 1996:672-739.

Shille VM, Olson PN. Dynamic testing in reproductive endocrinology. In: Kirk RW, ed. Current veterinary therapy X. Philadelphia: WB Saunders, 1989:1282-1288.

Meyers-Wallen VN, Patterson DF. Disorders of sexual development in dogs and cats. In: Kirk RW, ed. Current veterinary therapy X. Philadelphia: WB Saunders, 1989:1261-1269.

Purswell BJ. Pharmaceuticals used in canine reproduction. Sem Vet Med Surg (Small Anim) 1994;9:54-60.

Schmeitzel LP. Sex hormone-related and growth hormone-related alopecias. Vet Clin North Am Small Anim Pract 1990;20:1579-1601.

Author Margaret R. Kern
Consulting Editor Rhett Nichols

HYPOMYELINATION OF CENTRAL NERVOUS SYSTEM

 BASICS

DEFINITION
• All axons over 1-2 mm in diameter are invested with a covering of myelin that arises from oligodendrocytes in the CNS and Schwann's cells in the peripheral nervous system. In both forms of disease, myelin serves to insulate axons and facilitate propagation of action potentials. • Hypomyelination is a congenital condition caused by insufficient myelin production.

SIGNALMENT
• CNS hypomyelination is reported in the Welsh springer spaniel, Samoyed, chow chow, weimaraner, Bernese mountain dog, dalmatian, and an English crossbreed referred to as lurcher. In springers and Samoyeds, only male puppies are clinically affected, whereas females remain largely asymptotic carriers. No sex predisposition is reported in the other breeds. Clinical signs appear within days of birth.
• Peripheral nervous system hypomyelination is reported in golden retrievers of both sexes. Clinical signs appear at 5-7 weeks of age.

SIGNS
• CNS hypomyelination—generalized body tremors that worsen with exercise and subside during rest. Springer spaniels and Samoyeds remain affected for the remainder of their life. Clinical signs improve by 1 year of age in the other breeds. • Peripheral hypomyelination—generalized weakness, pelvic limb ataxia, muscle wasting, and hyporeflexia. These signs do not resolve with age.

CAUSES AND RISK FACTORS
• Sex-linked recessive condition proven for central hypomyelination in the springer spaniel. Genetic factors in the remaining breeds are speculative. Because clinical signs improve or resolve in the chow chow, weimaraner, Bernese mountain dog, dalmatian, and lurcher, a viral or toxic cause is possible. • The cause of peripheral hypomyelination in the golden retriever is not determined; possibly genetic

 DIAGNOSIS

DIFFERENTIAL DIAGNOSIS
CNS Hypomyelination
• Cerebellar hypoplasia or abiotrophy can cause tremors in neonatal animals; ataxia and intention tremors are less prominent in animals with CNS hypomyelination. • Storage diseases often are associated with tremors, but animals are normal at birth. • Idiopathic tremors seen in white dogs do not usually develop by 8 months of age.

Peripheral Hypomyelination
• Muscular dystrophy in the golden retriever
• Congenital myasthenia gravis • Other polyneuropathies and myopathies

CBC/BIOCHEMISTRY/URINALYSIS
Results usually normal

OTHER LABORATORY TESTS N/A

IMAGING N/A

OTHER DIAGNOSTIC PROCEDURES
Central Hypomyelination
• Diagnosis is based on clinical signs. • MRI for antemortem diagnosis • Biopsy • Necropsy

Peripheral Hypomyelination
• Electromyography—diffuse spontaneous activity • Motor nerve conduction velocity—small or no evoked potentials and slowed conduction • Nerve biopsy—insufficient myelin surrounding peripheral axons

 TREATMENT

No treatment is effective for either central or peripheral hypomyelination.

HYPOMYELINATION OF CENTRAL NERVOUS SYSTEM

 **MEDICATIONS**

DRUGS AND FLUIDS N/A

CONTRAINDICATIONS/POSSIBLE INTERACTIONS N/A

 FOLLOW-UP

Avoid breeding animals in which a genetic cause is suspected.

 MISCELLANEOUS

ABBREVIATIONS

CNS = central nervous system
MRI = magnetic resonance imaging

References

Duncan ID. Abnormalities of myelination of the central nervous system associated with congenital tremor. J Vet Inter Med 1987;1:10-23.

Matz ME, Shell L, Braund K. Peripheral hypomyelinization in two golden retriever litter mates. J Am Vet Med Assoc 1990;197:228-230.

Author Karen R. Dyer
Consulting Editor Joane M. Parent

HYPOPARATHYROIDISM

 BASICS

DEFINITION
Absolute or relative deficiency of parathyroid hormone secretion leading to hypocalcemia

Pathophysiology
• Dogs—most commonly idiopathic immune-mediated parathyroiditis • Cats—most commonly iatrogenic secondary to damaged or removed parathyroid glands during thyroidectomy for hyperthyroidism; idiopathic atrophy and immune-mediated parathyroiditis also seen (uncommon)

Systems Affected
• Nervous/neuromuscular—seizures, tetany, ataxia, and weakness caused by increased neuromuscular activity as a result of diminished neuronal membrane stability • Cardiovascular—ECG changes and bradycardia caused by altered neuromuscular activity • Gastrointestinal—anorexia and vomiting (especially cats) of unknown cause, possibly changes in gastrointestinal muscular activity • Ophthalmic—posterior lenticular cataracts of unknown cause • Respiratory—panting caused by neuromuscular weakness and anxiety associated with neurologic and neuromuscular changes • Renal/urologic—polyuria and polydipsia (PU/PD) of unknown cause

Genetics N/A

Incidence/Prevalence
• Dogs—uncommon; exact prevalence not reported • Cats—common in thyroidectomized cats (10-82% of patients, depending on surgical technique and surgical skill); spontaneous occurrence rare (only 6 cases reported)

Geographic Distribution N/A

SIGNALMENT

Species Dogs and cats

Breed Predilections
Toy poodle, miniature schnauzer, German shepherd, Labrador retriever, and Scottish terrier; mixed-breed cats

Mean Age and Range
• Dogs—mean age, 6 years; range, 6 weeks to 12 years • Cats—secondary to thyroidectomy, mean age, 12-13 years; range, 4-22 years; spontaneous, mean, 2.25 years; range, 6 months to 6.7 years

Predominant Sex
• Dogs—female • Cats—none

SIGNS

Dogs
• Seizures (54-73%) • Muscle trembling, twitching, and fasciculations (54%) • Tense, splinted abdomen (50%) • Ataxia/stiff gait (43%) • Fever (30-40%) • Panting (35%) • Posterior lenticular cataracts (15-20%) • Weakness • PU/PD • Facial rubbing • Vomiting • Anorexia • Up to 20% may have a normal physical examination

Cats (based on 6 reported cases)
• Lethargy, anorexia, and depression (100%) • Seizures (50%) • Muscle trembling, twitching, and fasciculations (83%) • Panting (33%) • Posterior lenticular cataracts (33%) • Bradycardia (17%) • Fever (17%) • Hypothermia (17%)

CAUSES
See pathophysiology.

RISK FACTORS
• Dogs—N/A • Cats—thyroidectomy for hyperthyroidism

 DIAGNOSIS

DIFFERENTIAL DIAGNOSIS
The main problems associated with hypoparathyroidism, which must be differentiated from other disease processes, are seizures, weakness, and muscle trembling, twitching, and fasciculations.

Seizures
• Cardiovascular—syncope • Metabolic—hepatoencephalopathy and hypoglycemia • Neurologic—epilepsy, neoplasia, toxin, and inflammatory disease

Weakness
• Cardiovascular—congenital anatomic defects, arrhythmias, heart failure, and pericardial effusion • Metabolic—hypoadrenocorticsm, hypoglycemia, anemia, hypokalemia (especially cats), and hypothyroidism • Neurologic/neuromuscular—myasthenia gravis, polymyositis, polyradiculoneuropathy, and spinal cord disease • Toxic—tick paralysis, botulism, chronic organophosphate exposure, and lead poisoning

Muscle Trembling, Twitching, and Fasciculations
• Metabolic—hypercalcemia, hyperadrenocorticism, and puerperal tetany (i.e., eclampsia) • Toxic—tetanus and strychnine poisoning

CBC/BIOCHEMISTRY/URINALYSIS
• Results of hemogram and urinalysis usually are normal. The importance of performing these tests is to rule out the other differential diagnoses. • Hypocalcemia (usually < 6.5 mg/dl) and normal or mild to moderate hyperphosphotemia
• Serum albumin must be evaluated carefully in all patients with hypocalcemia because hypoalbuminemia is the most common cause of hypocalcemia. In dogs with hypoalbuminemia, one of the following formulas should be used to correct the serum calcium:

$$\text{Corrected Ca} = \text{Ca (mg/dl)} - \text{albumin (g/dl)} + 3.5$$
or
$$\text{Corrected Ca} = \text{Ca (mg/dl)} - [0.4 \times \text{total protein (g/dl)}] + 3.3$$

• Hypocalcemia caused by hypoalbuminemia in cats cannot be corrected by these formulas, although it should be noted that hypoalbuminemia causes reduced serum calcium in cats. • The only other disease process that reduces serum calcium and raises serum phosphorus is renal failure, which is easily distinguished from hypoparathyroidism by the presence of azotemia.

OTHER LABORATORY TESTS
Serum PTH determination—demonstrates undetectable or very low concentration of PTH. Patients with other processes causing hypocalcemia (e.g., renal failure) have normal to high concentration of PTH.

IMAGING
Radiography and ultrasonography normal

OTHER DIAGNOSTIC PROCEDURES
• ECG changes seen in patients with hypocalcemia include prolongation of the ST and Q-T segments. Sinus bradycardia and wide T waves or T wave alternans occasionally seen. • Cervical exploration reveals absence or atrophy of the parathyroid glands.

GROSS AND HISTOPATHOLOGIC FINDINGS
• Dogs—normal tissue with mature lymphocytes, plasma cells, and fibrous connective tissue along with chief cell degeneration • Cats—parathyroid gland atrophy is more common, although histopathologic findings similar to those in dogs have been found in one cat.

 TREATMENT

INPATIENT VERSUS OUTPATIENT
Hospitalize for medical management of hypocalcemia until clinical signs of hypocalcemia are controlled and serum calcium concentration is > 7.0 mg/dl.

ACTIVITY N/A

DIET N/A

CLIENT EDUCATION N/A

SURGICAL CONSIDERATIONS N/A

 MEDICATIONS

DRUGS AND FLUIDS

Emergency/Acute Therapy
See Calcium, Hypocalcemia.

Short-Term Post-tetany Therapy
See Calcium, Hypocalcemia.

Long-Term Therapy
• Vitamin D administration is needed indefinitely. The dosage should be increased or tapered on the basis of serum calcium concentration (see table). • Shorter acting preparations of vitamin D are preferred so that overdosage (hypercalcemia) can be quickly corrected (see table). • A more economical approach to treatment is to maxi-

mize oral administration of calcium and reduce oral administration of vitamin D. Calcium is usually less expensive than vitamin D.

CONTRAINDICATIONS N/A

PRECAUTIONS

All calcium preparations given orally can cause gastrointestinal disturbances. Calcium carbonate may be less irritating because of its high calcium availability and lower dosage requirement.

POSSIBLE INTERACTIONS

• Injectable calcium solutions have been reported to be incompatible with tetracycline drugs, cephalothin, methylprednisolone sodium succinate, dobutamine, metoclopramide, and amphoteracin B.
• Thiazide diuretics used in conjunction with large doses of calcium may cause hypercalcemia.
• Patients on digitalis are more likely to develop arrhythmias if calcium is administered intravenously.
• Calcium administration may antagonize effects of calcium channel blocking agents (e.g., diltiazem, verapamil, nifedipine, and amlodipine).

ALTERNATE DRUGS N/A

FOLLOW-UP

PATIENT MONITORING

• Hypocalcemia and hypercalcemia are both concerns with long-term management.

• Serum calcium concentration monthly for the first 6 months then every 2-4 months. Goal is to maintain serum calcium between 8 and 10 mg/dl.

PREVENTION/AVOIDANCE N/A

POSSIBLE COMPLICATIONS

• Hypocalcemia • Hypercalcemia, which can lead to renal failure (see Hypercalcemia)

EXPECTED COURSE AND PROGNOSIS

• With close monitoring of serum calcium and client dedication, the prognosis for long-term survival is excellent. • Adjustments in vitamin D and oral calcium administration can be expected during the course of management, especially during the initial 2-6 months. • Cats with hypoparathyroidism secondary to thyroidectomy usually require only transient treatment because they typically regain normal parathyroid function within 4-6 months, often within 2-3 weeks.

MISCELLANEOUS

ASSOCIATED CONDITIONS

Excess muscular activity can lead to hyperthermia, which may necessitate treatment.

AGE RELATED FACTORS N/A

ZOONOTIC POTENTIAL N/A

PREGNANCY

Hypocalcemia can lead to weakness and dystocia.

SYNONYMS None

SEE ALSO

• Calcium, Hypocalcemia • Hyperthyroidism

ABBREVIATIONS

Ca = calcium • ECG = electrocardiography
PTH = parathyroid hormone
PU/PD = polyuria and polydipsia

References

Feldman EC, Nelson RW. Hypocalcemia and primary hypoparathyroidism. In: Feldman EC, Nelson RW, eds. Canine and feline endocrinology and reproduction. Philadelphia: WB Saunders, 1996:497-516.

Bruyette DS, Feldman EC. Primary hypoparathyroidism in the dog. Report of 15 cases and review of 13 previously reported cases. J Vet Int Med 1988;2:7-14.

Waters CB, Scott-Moncrieff JCR. Hypocalcemia in cats. Compend Contin Educ Pract Vet 1992;14:497-507.

Peterson ME, James KM, Wallace M, Timothy SD, Joseph RJ. Idiopathic hypoparathyroidism in five cats. J Vet Int Med 1991;5:47-51.

Author Mitchell A. Crystal
Consulting Editor Rhett Nichols

Table 1.

Vitamin D and Calcium Preparations			
Preparation	*Dose*	*Maximal Effect*	*Size*
1,25 dihydroxycholecalciferol (active vitamin D₃, calcitriol)	0.03-0.06 mg/kg/day	1-4 days	0.25 and 0.5 mg capsules
Dihydrotachysterol	Initial: 0.02-0.03 mg/kg/day Maint: 0.01-0.02 mg/kg/24-48 hrs.	1-7 days	0.125, 0.2, 0.4, and 0.125 mg capsules, 0.25 mg/ml syrup
Ergocalciferol (vitamin D₂)	Initial: 4000-6000 U/kg/day Maint: 1000-2000 U/kg/day-week	5-21 days	25,000 and 50,000 U capsules and 8,000 U/ml syrup
Preparation	*Dose*	*Maximal Effect*	*Size*
Calcium carbonate	Dogs: 1-4 g/day Cats: 0.5-1 g/day	40%	350-1500 mg tablets
Calcium gluconate	Dogs: 1-4 g/day Cats: 0.5-1 g/day	10%	325, 500, 650 and 1000 mg tablets
Calcium lactate	Dogs: 1-4 g/day Cats: 0.5-1 g/day	13%	325 and 650 mg tablets

HYPOPITUITARISM

BASICS

OVERVIEW
A condition resulting from destruction of the pituitary gland by a neoplastic, degenerative, or anomalous process. Associated with low production of pituitary hormones including thyroid stimulating hormone (TSH), adrenocorticotropin hormone (ACTH), leutinizing hormone, follicle stimulating hormone, and growth hormone (GH)

SIGNALMENT
• Age—2-6 months • Breeds—German shepherd dog, Carnelian bear dog, spitz, toy pinscher, and weimaraner

Genetics
Simple autosomal recessive in German shepherd dog and Carnelian bear dog

SIGNS

Historical Findings
• Mental retardation manifested as difficulty in house-breaking • Slow growth noticed in first 2-3 months of life • Proportionate dwarfism

Physical Examination Findings
• Retained puppy haircoat • Thin, hypotonic skin • Shrill bark • Trunkal alopecia • Cutaneous hyperpigmentation • Infantile genitalia • Delayed dental eruption

CAUSES AND RISK FACTORS

Congenital
• Cystic Rathke's pouch • Isolated GH deficiency

Acquired
• Pituitary tumor • Trauma • Radiotherapy

DIAGNOSIS

DIFFERENTIAL DIAGNOSIS
• Hypothyroid dwarfism. Breed predilection and disproportionate dwarfism observed in patients with hypothyroidism. • Other causes of stunted growth: portosystemic shunt, diabetes mellitus, hyperadrenocorticism, malnutrition, parasitism

CBC/BIOCHEMISTRY/URINALYSIS
• Eosinophilia • Lymphocytosis • Hypophosphatemia • Hypoglycemia

OTHER LABORATORY TESTS

Corticotropin and TSH Response Tests
Subnormal response to TSH and ACTH

Growth Hormone and Insulin-like Growth Factor Assays
Growth hormone assay not currently available in the United States; recommend measurement of IGF-1, which is low.

IMAGING
Radiography may reveal epiphyseal dysgenesis and abnormal retention of physeal growth plates.

OTHER DIAGNOSTIC PROCEDURES
N/A

TREATMENT
Treatment consists of replacing deficient hormones.

MEDICATIONS

DRUGS AND FLUIDS
• Growth hormone, human, porcine, or bovine, if available (0.1 IU/kg SQ 3 times weekly for 4-6 weeks; repeat if necessary) • Treat hypothyroidism with levothyroxine (22 mcg/kg PO q24h) • Glucocorticoid (e.g., prednisone, 0.2 mg/kg PO q24h) if ACTH response test results are subnormal. Higher dosage of steroids needed during periods of stress.

CONTRAINDICATIONS/POSSIBLE INTERACTIONS
Hypersensitivity reactions and carbohydrate intolerance may develop with growth hormone supplemention.

FOLLOW-UP

PATIENT MONITORING
Blood and urine glucose concentration. Stop growth hormone supplementation if glucosuria develops or blood glucose is > 150 mg/dl

POSSIBLE COMPLICATIONS
Neurologic complications of expansion of Rathke's pouch are possible.

EXPECTED COURSE AND PROGNOSIS
• Skin and hair coat improve within 6-8 weeks of initiating growth hormone and thyroid supplementation • Generally no increase in stature because growth plates usually closed at the time of diagnosis • Dogs often die at a young age (3-4 years) because of neurologic complications. • Poor long-term prognosis

MISCELLANEOUS

SEE ALSO
• Hypothyroidism • Hypoadrenocorticism (Addison's Disease)

ABBREVIATIONS
TSH = thyroid stimulating hormone
ACTH = Adrenocorticotropin
GH = growth hormone

References
Campbell KL. Growth hormone-related disorders in dogs. Compend Cont Educ Pract Vet 1988;10:477-482.
Author Deborah S. Greco
Consulting Editor Rhett Nichols

BASICS

OVERVIEW

Both appear as white anterior chamber opacities. Hypopyon, the more common of the two conditions, is an accumulation of WBC in the anterior chamber which develops in animals with extreme breakdown of the blood aqueous barrier. The cellular components typically settle homogeneously in the ventral anterior chamber, forming a horizontal line. Lipid flare refers to the presence of lipid-laden aqueous humor in the anterior chamber, giving the entire aqueous humor a milky-white color. The aqueous becomes laden with lipids when breakdown of the blood aqueous barrier and concurrent hyperlipidemia occurs.

SIGNALMENT

• Hypopyon is seen in dogs and cats of any age, breed, or sex that have severe anterior uveitis from any cause. • Hyperlipidemic miniature schnauzers are prone to lipid flare. • Lipid flare is rare in cats.

SIGNS

• Turbidity of aqueous humor, diffuse in animals with lipid flare and ventral in animals with hypopyon • Signs of anterior uveitis, the degree depending on the severity of disease

CAUSES AND RISK FACTORS

• Hypopyon may be composed of inflammatory cells in animals with severe keratitis and anterior uveitis or neoplastic cells in animals with intraocular neoplasia (e.g., lymphosarcoma). • Any cause of anterior uveitis can lead to hypopyon or lipid flare (see anterior uveitis). • In addition to anterior uveitis, factors involved in the genesis of lipid flare include the following:

Primary Hyperlipidemia
• Idiopathic hyperlipidemia in miniature schnauzers • Lipoprotein lipase deficiency in cats

Secondary Hyperlipidemia
• Diabetes mellitus • Pancreatitis • Hypothyroidism • Cholestatic liver disease • Hyperadrenocorticism • Nephrotic syndrome

DIAGNOSIS

DIFFERENTIAL DIAGNOSIS

Aqueous flare due solely to a high anterior chamber protein concentration will not be milky-white like lipid flare and will not obscure one's ability to see the iris as in animals with hypopyon.

CBC/BIOCHEMISTRY/URINALYSIS

• Results are typically normal in dogs with hypopyon unless it is secondary to a systemic disease. • In animals with lipid flare, high serum cholesterol or triglyceride concentration is common. A cholesterol concentration of up to 500 mg/dL is mild, from 500 to 750 mg/dL is moderate, and > 750 mg/dL is marked. A high serum triglyceride concentration up to 400 mg/dL is mild, 400 to 1000 mg/dL is moderate, and > 1000 mg/dL is marked. Lower cutoff points are appropriate for cats.

OTHER LABORATORY TESTS

• Standing plasma test to determine if lipemia is caused by chylomicrons, very low-density lipoproteins, or both. Chylomicrons form a cream layer on top of the sample and very low-density lipoprotein particles remain suspended. • Lipoprotein electrophoresis • Measurement of lipoprotein lipase activity to detect low activity of this enzyme

IMAGING N/A

OTHER DIAGNOSTIC PROCEDURES

• Work-ups for ulcerative keratitis or anterior uveitis may be indicated. • Anterior chamber paracentesis is seldom worthwhile unless globe perforation has occurred and bacterial endophthalmitis is suspected or if lymphosarcoma is suspected.

TREATMENT

• Patients with hypopyon should be hospitalized for aggressive medical therapy and owners should be warned of the potential for blindness.
• Patients with primary hyperlipidemia or secondary hyperlipidemia not responding to treatment of primary disease should be fed a diet low in fat and calories. They may be treated as outpatients.

MEDICATIONS

DRUGS AND FLUIDS

• Unless globe perforation has occurred, hypopyon is usually sterile. If hypopyon is secondary to corneal ulceration, however, the cornea may be infected and aggressive antibiotic therapy is indicated (see ulcerative keratitis).
• If the cornea is not ulcerated, topically applied 1% prednisolone acetate or 0.1% dexamethasone q 1-2h initially, then q4h-q8h in animals with severe hypopyon and q6h-q8h in animals with lipid flare.
• Subconjunctivally applied steroids (e.g., triamcinolone acetonide , 4-8 mg/eye) as an adjunct to topical treatment.

• Systemically administered corticosteroids (1.0-2.0 mg/kg/day for 7 days, then gradually decrease dosage).
• Atropine applied topically 1% q4h-q6h initially in animals with severe disease, then q6h-q12h.
• Alternatively, topically applied nonsteroidal antiinflammatory drugs (e.g., flurbiprofen or suprofen) may be used q6h in animals with severe hypopyon when topically applied corticosteroids are contraindicated.

CONTRAINDICATIONS/POSSIBLE INTERACTIONS

• Avoid topically or subconjunctivally applied corticosteroids if the cornea is ulcerated.
• The safety of topically applied NSAIDS in cats is undetermined.
• Atropine should be used with caution or not at all if intraocular pressure is high.

FOLLOW-UP

• Monitor with frequent (initially daily) ocular examinations, including tonometry to rule out secondary glaucoma. • The prognosis for hypopyon is guarded and depends on the response to treatment. • Lipid flare usually resolves quickly with topical treatment and treatment of the primary disease.

MISCELLANEOUS

PREGNANCY

Avoid systemically administered steroids in pregnant animals.

SEE ALSO
• Anterior Uveitis (Dogs and Cats)
• Keratitis, Ulcerative

Reference

Collins BK, Moore CP. Canine anterior uvea. In: Gelatt KN, ed. Veterinary ophthalmology. 2nd ed. Philadelphia: Lea & Febiger, 1991:357–395.

Author Michael J. Ringle
Consulting Editor Paul E. Miller

HYPOTHYROIDISM

 BASICS

DEFINITION

The clinical state associated with deficiency of thyroxine (tetraiodothyronine [T_4] and tri-iodothyronine [T_3]), which causes low cell metabolism in most tissues of the body

Pathophysiology

• Primary acquired hypothyroidism (90% of dog patients) is caused by lymphocytic thyroiditis or idiopathic follicular atrophy, resulting in thyroid dysfunction. Less common causes include dietary iodine deficiency and thyroid destruction by neoplasia or infection. Hypothyroidism in cats is uncommon and is usually iatrogenic, caused by bilateral thyroidectomy or radiotherapy for hyperthyroidism. • Secondary hypothyroidism is caused by impaired thyroid-stimulating hormone (TSH) secretion as a result of congenital malformation of the pituitary or destruction of the pituitary by neoplasia or infection. Congenital hypothyroidism causes cretinism (dwarfism) because thyroid hormone is necessary for normal development of the skeletal and central nervous systems. Glucocorticoids, concurrent illness, and malnutrition can also impair TSH secretion.

Systems Affected

• Skin/exocrine • Cardiovascular • Nervous • Neuromuscular • Reproductive • Gastrointestinal • Ophthalmic • Endocrine/metabolic

Genetics

Unproven, although genetic factors are suggested by breed predilections

Incidence/Prevalence

• Most common endocrinopathy in dogs. Prevalence, 1:156-1:500. • Prevalence in cats extremely low

Geographic Distribution N/A

SIGNALMENT

Species

Dogs and (rarely) cats

Breed Predilections

Airedale terrier, boxer, cocker spaniel, dachshund, Doberman pinscher, golden retriever, Great Dane, Irish setter, miniature schnauzer, Old English sheepdog, Pomeranian, poodle, and Shetland sheepdog

Mean Age and Range

4-10 years

Predominant Sex

Female (2.5:1); spayed females have a higher relative risk than intact females

SIGNS

General Comments

Signs develop gradually and vary widely.

Historical Findings

Include lethargy, mental depression, exercise intolerance, increased sleeping, personality change, unexplained weight gain, heat seeking, infertility or low libido in breeding animals, and gradual hair loss

Physical Examination Findings
Dermatologic Abnormalities
• Most common • Bilaterally symmetric alopecia beginning on the tail ("rat tail") and becoming generalized • Hyperpigmentation and hyperkeratosis • Dry or oily seborrhea • Dry, dull, brittle, and easily epilated hair coat; change in coat color possible • Poor wound healing and easy bruising • Increased prevalence of pyoderma and otitis externa • Thick, cool, puffy skin; myxedema with "tragic expression"
Cardiovascular
• Bradycardia • Weak apex beat and peripheral pulses
Neuromuscular
• Localized peripheral neuropathies, including facial and vestibular nerve neuropathies, laryngeal paralysis, and Horner's syndrome • Generalized peripheral neuropathies (uncommon) characterized by weakness and hyporeflexic spinal reflexes • Generalized myopathies characterized by stiff gait and weakness
Gastrointestinal
• Constipation • Regurgitation caused by diffuse megaesophagus
Reproductive
• Infertility in intact animals common • In females, duration of estrus shortened and anestrus prolonged • Low libido and testicular atrophy in males
Ophthalmic
Hyperlipidemia may cause corneal lipidosis and anterior uveitis.

CAUSES

• See pathophysiology. • Lymphocytic thyroiditis • Idiopathic follicular atrophy • Iatrogenic • Iodine deficiency • Congenital • Neoplasia • Infection

RISK FACTORS

Though unproven, neutering may be associated with a relatively higher risk of hypothyroidism.

 DIAGNOSIS

DIFFERENTIAL DIAGNOSIS

The differential diagnosis is extensive. Other causes of endocrine alopecia should be considered, including hyperadrenocorticism and sex hormone responsive dermatoses.

CBC/BIOCHEMISTRY/URINALYSIS

• Mild normocytic, normochromic nonregenerative anemia • Hypercholesterolemia, hypertriglyceridemia, and high creatine kinase activity • Results of urinalysis usually normal

OTHER LABORATORY TESTS

Note: See appendix for table of endocrine test protocols.

Hormone Radioimmunoassay (RIA)

• Serum T_4 and T_3—low values are consistent with hypothyroidism; however, many factors can lower T_3 and T_4 concentrations, including nonthyroidal disease and medications (e.g., glucocorticoids and anticonvulsants) • Free T_4 (FT_4)—in theory, the serum concentration of FT_4 is not significantly affected by changes in serum binding associated with no thyroidal disease or drug therapy. Therefore, measurement of FT_4 may be more accurate than T_4 in diagnosing hypothyroidism. Selection of assay type and laboratory quality assurance is extremely important because some methods of analysis have low diagnostic accuracy.

Thyrotropin (TSH) Stimulating Test

• In the past, considered the most definitive test for the diagnosis of hypothyroidism; measures serum T_4 concentration before and after administration of bovine TSH • Post-TSH T_4 concentration below the normal range confirms a diagnosis of hypothyroidism. • Variable availability and high cost of TSH has limited the usefulness of this test.

Thyrotropin-Releasing Hormone (TRH) Stimulation Test

• Measures the pituitary release of TSH in response to exogenous TRH by measuring serum T_4 concentration • TRH more readily available and less expensive than TSH • In theory, dogs with hypothyroidism would not respond to TRH; however, interpretation of test results can be difficult because of relatively small increases in serum T_4 after TRH administration.

TSH Assay

A validated TSH assay for dogs is now available. A high concentration is consistent with primary hypothyroidism; however, nonthyroidal illness may also cause a high TSH concentration.

IMAGING

Echocardiography may indicate diminished myocardial contractility.

OTHER DIAGNOSTIC PROCEDURES

Electrocardiography may reveal low voltage R waves (< 1.0 mV) and sinus bradycardia.

GROSS AND HISTOPATHOLOGIC FINDINGS

• Primary hypothyroidism—significant loss of follicular epithelium, usually with associated lymphocytic thyroiditis • Secondary hypothyroidism—follicles distended with colloid

 TREATMENT

INPATIENT VERSUS OUTPATIENT

Outpatient, except in patients with myxedema coma

ACTIVITY N/A

DIET

Avoid high-fat diets. Most obese patients lose weight with proper medical management.

CLIENT EDUCATION

• Successful management is possible and prognosis is good.

• Hormone supplementation is required for the remainder of the patient's life.

• Dosages of thyroid hormone vary and must be individualized to the patient. Frequent rechecks to evaluate thyroid hormone concentrations may be necessary. Improper dosaging or frequency of administration (failure of compliance) of thyroid supplement may significantly affect response.

• Response to thyroid supplement is gradual and a minimum 3 months of treatment is recommended before effectiveness is judged.

• The recommended dosage of thyroid supplement greatly exceeds human dosages because of differences in metabolism.

SURGICAL CONSIDERATIONS N/A

MEDICATIONS

DRUGS AND FLUIDS

Treatment of choice is synthetic sodium levothyroxine (L-thyroxine). Dosage of 0.02 mg/kg/day is recommended initially. Extremely large or small dogs are more accurately dosaged on the basis of body surface area (0.5 mg/m^2/day, divided q12h if needed). Approximately 4 weeks of treatment is necessary to reach steady state.

CONTRAINDICATIONS None

PRECAUTIONS

• In patients with diabetes mellitus or heart disease, a lower starting dosage of L-thyroxine is advised to allow adaptation to high metabolic rate. • Patients with concurrent hypoadrenocorticism should be controlled with adrenocortical supplementation before initiating thyroid replacement.

POSSIBLE INTERACTIONS

Concurrent administration of drugs that inhibit serum protein binding (e.g., glucocorticoids, salicylates, and phenytoin) may necessitate higher dosage or q12h treatment with L-thyroxine.

ALTERNATE DRUGS

Triiodothyronine is rarely indicated, because it has an extremely short half-life and is more likely to cause iatrogenic hyperthyroidism.

FOLLOW-UP

PATIENT MONITORING

• Improvement in patient activity and attitude is often observed within 7-10 days of initiating treatment. Visible improvement in skin and hair coat may take 6-8 weeks. Treatment failure usually indicates erroneous diagnosis. • Assess postpill serum T$_4$ concentration after about 8 weeks of treatment. Peak serum T$_4$ concentration 4-8 hours after administration of L-thyroxine should be near or slightly above normal range. Prepill (or trough) concentration just before next dosing should be in the low-normal range. If postpill concentration is adequate but prepill concentration is low, dosage frequency should be increased (i.e., from q24h to q12h). If both are low, inadequate dosage, intestinal malabsorption, use of an out-of-date or ineffective product, or failure of owner compliance should be considered. Less commonly, circulating antibodies to T$_3$ or T$_4$ may interfere with measurement of thyroid hormone (in which case only clinical response can be used to assess treatment protocol).

PREVENTION/AVOIDANCE

Lifelong administration of proper replacement therapy and periodic postpill T$_4$ assessments to assure adequate control prevents recurrence of clinical disease.

POSSIBLE COMPLICATIONS

Overdosage of L-thyroxine can cause anxiety, polyuria, polydipsia, weight loss, diarrhea, and tachyarrhythmias.

EXPECTED COURSE AND PROGNOSIS

• Prognosis for adult dogs with primary hypothyroidism given proper thyroid replacement therapy is good and life expectancy is expected to be normal. • Prognosis for patients with acquired secondary or tertiary hypothyroidism is guarded to poor because of the potential for destructive, space-occupying lesions expanding into the brain stem.

• Prognosis for congenital hypothyroid or cretin puppies is guarded because of the potential for irreversible musculoskeletal abnormalities.

MISCELLANEOUS

ASSOCIATED CONDITIONS N/A

AGE RELATED FACTORS N/A

ZOONOTIC POTENTIAL N/A

PREGNANCY N/A

SYNONYMS N/A

SEE ALSO

Myxedema and Myxedema Coma

ABBREVIATIONS

T$_3$ = triiodothyronine

T$_4$ = tetraiodothyronine

TSH = thyroid-stimulating hormone or thyrotropin

TRH = thyroid-releasing hormone

FT$_4$ = free tetraiodothyronine

References

Chastain CB, Panciera DL. Hypothyroid diseases. In: Ettinger SJ, Feldman EC, eds. Textbook of veterinary internal medicine. 4th ed. Philadelphia: WB Saunders, 1995:1487-1501.

Ferguson DC. Update on diagnosis of canine hypothyroidism. Vet Clin North Am Small Anim 1994;24:515-539.

Panciera DL. Hypothyroidism in dogs: 66 cases (1987-1992). J Am Vet Med Assoc 1994;204:761-767.

Author Leland Thompson

Consulting Editor Rhett Nichols

IMMUNODEFICIENCY DISORDERS, PRIMARY

BASICS

DEFINITION
Diminished ability to mount an effective immune response. Primary immunodeficiency disease is caused by heritable defects in the immune system. Secondary immunodeficiency disease is a diminished immune response acquired as a consequence of some other primary disease. This topic covers primary immunodeficiency disorders.

Pathophysiology
The types and causes of primary immunodeficiency diseases are diverse. The identification of a specific defect in the immune response requires an adequate understanding of the cellular and genetic basis of the immune system. Primary immunodeficiencies involving the cell-mediated, humoral, complement, and phagocytic systems have all been described in the veterinary literature. Defects involving the humoral immune response are associated with a high susceptibility to bacterial infection. Defects involving the cell-mediated immune response are associated with a high susceptibility to viral, fungal, and protozoal infections. Defects in the phagocytic or complement system are associated with disseminated infection.

Systems Affected
• Hemic/lymph/immune—defect in a specific cell population in lymphoid tissue
• Skin/exocrine, respiratory, gastrointestinal—chronic or recurrent infections
• Musculoskeletal—failure to thrive • Other organ systems—dissemination of infection

Genetics
Primary immunodeficiencies are typically breed-specific with variable modes of inheritance.

Incidence/Prevalence
Rare

Geographic Distribution N/A

SIGNALMENT

Species
Dogs and cats

Breed Predilections
• X-linked severe combined immunodeficiency—bassett hound • IgA deficiency—beagle, German shepherd, and shar-pei • IgM deficiency—Doberman pinscher • Thymic hypoplasia—dwarfed weimaraners • Cyclic hematopoiesis—gray collie • Chédiak-Higashi syndrome—Persian cat • Leukocyte adhesion deficiency—Irish setter • Complement deficiency—Brittany spaniel • Bactericidal defect—Doberman pinscher • Transient hypogammaglobulinemia—Samoyed

Mean Age and Range
Primary immunodeficiency diseases typically are expressed in the first year of life.

Predominant Sex
X-linked recessive severe combined immunodeficiency disease of the bassett hound—males are affected and females are carriers for the defect.

SIGNS

General Comments
Clinical signs depend on the level at which the immune response is defective, and range from chronic respiratory and gastrointestinal signs and skin infections to life-threatening conditions.

Historical Findings
• High susceptibility to infection and failure to respond to appropriate, conventional antibiotic therapy • Signs include lethargy, anorexia, skin infection, and failure to thrive. • Clinical signs often appear when maternal antibody concentrations decline. • Vaccine-induced disease by modified live virus preparations

Physical Examination Findings
• Failure to thrive is the hallmark of primary immunodeficiency disease. • Clinical signs are attributable to infections.

CAUSES
Congenital

RISK FACTORS
N/A

DIAGNOSIS

DIFFERENTIAL DIAGNOSIS
•Patient must be rigorously evaluated for underlying disease processes that may cause secondary (acquired) immunodeficient state.
• Patients with primary (heritable) immunodeficiencies typically are young animals examined because of recurrent infection that fails to respond to conventional treatment.

CBC/BIOCHEMISTRY/URINALYSIS
CBC results may indicate deficiencies in specifically affected cell lines or a chronic inflammatory process.

OTHER LABORATORY TESTS
• Serum protein electrophoresis can be used to demonstrate gross deficiencies in immunoglobulin concentrations. • Serum immunoglobulin quantitation can be used to evaluate the humoral immune system and identify selective immunoglobulin deficiencies or support a diagnosis of agammaglobulinemia. • The lymphocyte transformation test can be used to evaluate the cell-mediated immune system and identify animals with T lymphocyte deficiencies. • Bactericidal assays can be used to evaluate neutrophil function. • Serum concentrations of complement components can diagnose complement deficiencies. • Enumeration of lymphocyte subsets by immunofluorescence with monoclonal antibodies can be used to identify deficiencies of specific cell lines. • Other more specific tests

to evaluate immune function in veterinary species are available but generally require access to research laboratories that perform the tests to get reliable results.

IMAGING N/A

OTHER DIAGNOSTIC PROCEDURES
In some patients, bone marrow and lymph node biopsies can aid in classifying the type of immune deficiency.

GROSS AND HISTOPATHOLOGIC FINDINGS
• Lesions vary; most are the result of recurrent or opportunistic infection involving the skin, ear canal, respiratory, and gastointestinal systems. • Lesions of septicemia are common in animals with severe defects. • Lesions related to the primary immunodeficiency vary depending on the specific defect. • T lymphocyte defects can cause hypoplastic or dysplastic lesions of the thymus and T lmyphocyte-dependent areas of secondary lymphoid tissues. • B lymphocyte defects can cause hypoplastic or dysplastic lesions of the bone marrow or B lymphocyte-dependent areas of secondary lymphoid tissues. • Lymphoid hypoplasia or hyperplasia may be seen, depending on the overall defect and the presence or absence of infection.

TREATMENT

INPATIENT VERSUS OUTPATIENT
• Hospitalization may be necessary to control life-threatening infection. • Outpatient management is possible for some patients' primary immunodeficiencies.

ACTIVITY
The patient's activity is determined largely by the severity of the defect and the presence or absence of infection.

DIET
• Dietary management may be required to ensure that the patient is maintained at an adequate level of nutrition.
• Potential sources of infectious agents such as raw meat must be avoided.

CLIENT EDUCATION
• Discuss the fact that with a primary immunodeficiency the animal cannot be cured.
• Discuss why the patient has increased susceptibility to infection.
• Discuss and advise as to the heritability of the disease.
• Discuss the possibility of other littermates being affected.

SURGICAL CONSIDERATIONS N/A

MEDICATIONS

DRUGS AND FLUIDS
• Antibiotics to control infections
• Gamma globulin or plasma preparations can be used in conjunction with antibiotics to control infection in patients with humoral defects.
• Symptomatic treatment for secondary disease states

CONTRAINDICATIONS
Gamma globulin or plasma preparations should not be administered to patients with selective IgA deficiency because many affected patients have high concentrations of anti-IgA antibodies and may develop an anaphylactic reaction.

PRECAUTIONS
Modified live virus vaccines should not be administered to patients with suspected T lymphocyte deficiencies because it may induce disease in these patients.

POSSIBLE INTERACTIONS N/A

ALTERNATE DRUGS N/A

FOLLOW-UP

PATIENT MONITORING
• Patient should be monitored for clinical signs of secondary infection. • Routine physical examination to assess efficacy of antibiotic therapy for control of secondary infection

PREVENTION/AVOIDANCE
• Affected animals should not be used in a breeding program. • Pedigree analysis to determine the mode of inheritance and to prevent propagating the defect

POSSIBLE COMPLICATIONS N/A

EXPECTED COURSE AND PROGNOSIS
• The severity of the defect determines the course of disease and prognosis. • Patients with minor defects can be successfully managed.

MISCELLANEOUS

ASSOCIATED CONDITIONS
Opportunistic infection

AGE RELATED FACTORS
Primary immunodeficiencies usually are expressed early in life.

ZOONOTIC POTENTIAL N/A

PREGNANCY N/A

SYNONYMS N/A

SEE ALSO
Leukopenia

ABBREVIATIONS N/A

References

Guliford WG. Primary immunodeficiency diseases of dogs and cats. Compend Cont Ed Small Anim 1987;9:641-648.

Lewis RM, Picut CA. Veterinary clinical immunology. Philadelphia: Lea & Febiger, 1989.

Morgan RV. Handbook of small animal practice. New York: Churchill Livingstone, 1992.

Author Paul W. Snyder
Consulting Editor Alan H. Rebar

IMMUNOPROLIFERATIVE ENTEROPATHY IN BASENJIS

BASICS

OVERVIEW
• An immunologically-mediated disease characterized by chronic intermittent diarrhea, anorexia, and weight loss associated with lymphoplasmacytic enteritis, protein-losing enteropathy, malabsorption, maldigestion, and hypergammaglobulinemia due to increased concentrations of serum IgA.
• Pathogenesis unclear but related to abnormal immune responses. • Systems affected include gastrointestinal, immune, skin, kidney, endocrine, and liver.

SIGNALMENT
• Young to middle aged Basenjis • Related dogs often affected

SIGNS
• Chronic intermittent diarrhea • Severe progressive weight loss • Anorexia often precedes diarrhea • Bilaterally symmetric alopecia • Scaling and ulceration of ear margins • Attitude is usually bright and alert

CAUSES AND RISK FACTORS
Episodes of diarrhea are associated with stressful events (boarding, estrus, transport, vaccination).

DIAGNOSIS

DIFFERENTIAL DIAGNOSIS
• Lymphangiectasia, lymphoplasmacytic enteritis, eosinophilic enteritis, histoplasmosis, EPI, intestinal lymphosarcoma, metabolic disorders. • Signalment, age of onset, serum IgA levels, and gastrointestinal histology are used to differentiate.

CBC/BIOCHEMISTRY/URINALYSIS
• Poorly regenerative anemia and moderately increased hepatic enzymes in severely affected dogs. • Severe hypoalbuminemia.

OTHER LABORATORY TESTS
• Hypergammaglobulinemia due to increased serum IgA. • Depression of BT-PABA and xylose curves that correlates with severity of clinical disease. • Hypergastrinemia and hyperchlorhydria may be present. • SIBO may cause functional EPI.

IMAGING N/A

OTHER DIAGNOSTIC PROCEDURES
• Endoscopic appearance of the small bowel is typically abnormal.

GROSS AND HISTOPATHOLOGIC FINDINGS
• Consistent pathologic lesions include uniform thickening of the small bowel, generalized infiltration of the intestinal lamina propria with lymphocytes and plasma cells, and blunting and fusion of villous tips. • Gastric mucosal hypertrophy, lymphocytic gastritis, parietal and chief cell hyperplasia, and gastric ulceration may be present. • Presence and severity of gastric lesions do not correlate with severity of intestinal lesions. • Other associated lesions include thyroid parafollicular cell atrophy, acinar atrophy, and glomerulonephritis.

TREATMENT
• Advise owners not to breed affected dogs or their littermates.
• Minimize stressful episodes
• Dietary trials should be used to determine which diet is best tolerated.

MEDICATIONS

DRUGS AND FLUIDS
• Use antibiotics to treat SIBO.
• Use corticosteroids for immunosuppression.
• Antibiotics: Metronidazole (10-20 mg/kg q12h-q24h), Tylosin (10 mg/kg PO q12h), Oxytetracycline (10-20 mg/kg q8h)
• Corticosteroids: Prednisone (1 mg/kg PO q12h tapered to 0.5-1 mg/kg q48h)

CONTRAINDICATIONS/POSSIBLE INTERACTIONS
Avoid anticholinergics

FOLLOW-UP
• Initial improvement in diarrhea and weight loss usually occurs with antibiotic or corticosteroid therapy. • Recurrence of signs is common • Long term prognosis is poor.

MISCELLANEOUS

ABBREVIATIONS
EPI = exocrine pancreatic insufficiency
SIBO = small intestinal bacterial overgrowth

Reference

Breitschwerdt EB. Immuno-proliferative enteropathy of Basenjis. Semin Vet Med Surg (Sm Anim) 1992;7:153-161.
Author Amy M. Grooters
Consulting Editor Brent D. Jones

INFLAMMATORY BOWEL DISEASE (IBD)

BASICS

DEFINITION
A group of gastrointestinal diseases characterized by inflammatory cellular infiltrates in the lamina propria of the small or large intestine with associated clinical signs.

Pathophysiology
An abnormal mucosal immune response to certain causative factors which results in the recruitment of inflammatory cells to the intestine. Damage results from the elaboration of cytokines, release of proteolytic and lysosomal enzymes, complement activation secondary to immune complex deposition and generation of oxygen free radicals. Certain environmental agents and hereditary factors may also influence the development of inflammatory bowel disease.

Systems Affected
Gastrointestinal, hepatobiliary and rarely musculoskeletal, ophthalmic, hemic/lymphatic/immune, skin/exocrine and respiratory.

Genetics N/A

Incidence/Prevalence
Not uncommon

Geographic Distribution N/A

SIGNALMENT

Species Dogs and cats

Breed Predilections
Breed predisposition with some forms of the disease, e.g., immunoproliferative disease of Basenjis and Lunderhunds, histiocytic colitis of French Bulldogs and Boxers, and wheat sensitive enteropathy in Irish Setters.

Mean Age and Range
More common in animals greater than two years of age although even young animals can be affected.

Predominant Sex N/A

SIGNS

Historical Findings
• Dogs: Intermittent, chronic vomiting, diarrhea and weight loss are common • Cats: The most common sign is vomiting, followed by diarrhea. • Borborygmus, flatulence, anorexia/ravenous appetite, hematochezia, abdominal pain and mucoid stools are less commonly reported.

Physical Examination Findings
Vary from an apparently healthy animal to a thin, depressed one. Poor haircoat is frequently noted. Abdominal palpation may reveal pain, thickened bowel loops and mesenteric lymphadenopathy.

CAUSES
The pathogenesis of this disease is most likely multi-factorial. Several causative factors have been identified:

Infectious Agents
No convincing link between one microbial agent and IBD has been definitively established. Giardia, Salmonella, Camphylobacter, and normal resident gastrointestinal flora have been implicated.

Dietary Agents
Meat proteins, food additives, artificial coloring, preservatives, milk proteins, gluten (wheat) have all been proposed as dietary causative agents.

Genetic Factors
• Certain forms of IBD are more common in some breeds of dogs (see above). • Inherited chromosome fragility has been suggested to be associated with IBD in humans. • Certain major histocompatibility genes, which are important components of normal immune responses, may render an individual susceptible to the development of IBD.

RISK FACTORS
See Causes

DIAGNOSIS

DIFFERENTIAL DIAGNOSIS
• Cats: hyperthyroidism, intestinal neoplasia, dietary intolerance/hypersensitivity, granulomatous FIP, exocrine pancreatic insufficiency, intestinal parasitism and bacterial overgrowth are primary differentials • Dogs: intestinal neoplasia, motility disorders, dietary intolerance/hypersensitivity, lymphangiectasia, exocrine pancreatic insufficiency, intestinal parasitism and bacterial overgrowth are primary differentials

CBC/BIOCHEMISTRY/URINALYSIS
• Test results often normal. These tests assist in ruling in or out some of the other differential diagnoses. • Occasionally a mild nonregenerative anemia and mild leukocytosis without a left shift is present in cats. • Dogs with IBD frequently have a mature neutrophilic leukocytosis with a left shift. •Hypoproteinemia tends to be a more common finding in dogs with IBD than cats.

OTHER LABORATORY TESTS
• Tests to eliminate other differentials (i.e., T4 in cats, FIV/FeLV serology), • Fecal examinations • Dogs: other supportive laboratory tests include serum trypsin like immunoreactivity (to rule in or out exocrine pancreatic insufficiency), fecal proteolytic activity using an azocasein substrate, microscopic examination of the feces and serum cobalamin and folate assays. Breath hydrogen test is useful in the diagnosis of bacterial overgrowth and malassimilation. • Cats: microscopic examination of the stool may be helpful. Most of the tests listed above have not been validated in the cat.

IMAGING
• Survey abdominal radiographs are usually normal. • Barium contrast studies occasionally reveal mucosal abnormalities, and thickened bowel loops, but are generally not helpful in establishing a definitive diagnosis. They can be normal in individuals with severe disease.

OTHER DIAGNOSTIC PROCEDURES
• A hypoallergenic diet trial may be initiated first in order to rule in or out dietary allergy or intolerance. Occasionally, certain forms of IBD will respond to dietary manipulations. However, if signs completely resolve, a diagnosis of dietary allergy/intolerance is likely and no further work-up is necessary. • Intestinal biopsy is the only way to definitively diagnose IBD and eliminate other differentials. • Duodenal aspirates for Giardia spp. should be collected during endoscopy. • Intestinal fluid can be submitted for quantitative culture if bacterial overgrowth is suspected.

GROSS AND HISTOPATHOLOGIC FINDINGS
Infiltration of intestines with inflammatory cells. See specific disease chapters

TREATMENT

INPATIENT VERSUS OUTPATIENT
Most of these patients can be treated on an outpatient basis, unless the patient is debilitated from dehydration, hypoproteinemia, or cachaxia.

ACTIVITY
In general, these patients don't require exercise restriction.

DIET
Dietary manipulation is important. A more detailed description of possible dietary regimes is discussed under each disease in the disease section.

CLIENT EDUCATION
It must be emphasized to the owner that inflammatory bowel disease is not necessarily cured as much as controlled. Relapses are common, and the client must be prepared to be patient during the various food and medication trials that are often necessary to get the disease under control. In a severely debilitated animal, hospitalization and, potentially, parenteral nutrition may be needed.

SURGICAL CONSIDERATIONS
Unlike the situation in human beings, there are no surgical procedures available in veterinary patients for relief of IBD.

MEDICATIONS

DRUGS AND FLUIDS
• See also discussion of specific diseases.
• If the patient is dehydrated or must be NPO because of vomiting, balanced fluids

such as Normosol-R or lactated Ringer's are indicated. If the patient has concurrent diseases (i.e., renal disease, cardiac diseases) fluids should be selected that are best suited for those problems.

CONTRAINDICATIONS

If secondary problems are present, therapeutic agents which might be contrindicated for those conditions should be avoided.

PRECAUTIONS

As mentioned above

POSSIBLE INTERACTIONS

See discussion of individual diseases

ALTERNATE DRUGS

See discussion under specific diseases

FOLLOW-UP

PATIENT MONITORING

Periodic re-evaluation may be necessary until the patient's condition stabilizes. No other follow-up may be required except for yearly physical examinations, and assessment during times of relapse.

PREVENTION AVOIDANCE N/A

POSSIBLE COMPLICATIONS

Dehydration, malnutrition, adverse drug reactions, hypoproteinemia, anemia, and diseases secondary to therapy or as a result of the above mentioned problems can occur.

EXPECTED COURSE AND PROGNOSIS

Varies with specific type of IBD. See specific diseases.

MISCELLANEOUS

ASSOCIATED CONDITIONS

See Possible Complications and refer to specific diseases

AGE RELATED FACTORS

• See discussion of specific diseases • The work-up and differentials are essentially the same, regardless of age. Some differentials are more likely in younger individuals (i.e., intestinal parasitism versus neoplasia).
• Younger individuals with confirmed inflammatory bowel disease may have other immune system defects, and owners should be counseled regarding breeding, and monitoring for the appearance of other diseases.

ZOONOTIC POTENTIAL N/A

PREGNANCY

(see discussion of individual problems)

SYNONYMS N/A

SEE ALSO

• Gastritis, Lymphocytic-Plasmacytic
• Enteritis, Lymphocytic-Plasmacytic
• Gastritis, Eosinophilic • Enteritis, Eosinophilic • Colitis and Proctitis

References

Strombeck DR, Guilford WG. Idiopathic inflammatory bowel diseases. In: Strombeck, DR, Guilford WG, eds. Small animal gastroenterology. 2nd ed. Stonegate, Davis, CA: 1990.

Tams TR. Feline inflammatory bowel disease. Vet Clin North Am, 1993;23.

Author Kelly J. Diehl
Consulting Editor Brent D. Jones

INSULINOMA

BASICS

DEFINITION
Pancreatic islet beta-cell neoplasm, which secretes an excess quantity of insulin

Pathophysiology
Excessive insulin secretion leads to excerssive glucose uptake and utilization by insulin-sensitive tissues and reduced hepatic production of glucose. This causes hypoglycemia and its associated clinical signs.

Systems Affected
• Nervous—seizures, disorientation, abnormal behavior, collapse, posterior paresis, and ataxia • Musculoskeletal—weakness and muscle fasciculations • Gastrointestinal—polyphagia and weight gain

Genetics N/A

Incidence/Prevalence
• Dogs—uncommon • Cats—rare (4 reports)

Geographic Distribution N/A

SIGNALMENT

Species
Dogs and cats

Breed Predilections
• Dogs—standard poodle, boxer, fox terrier, Irish setter, German shepherd, golden retriever, and collie • Cats—none; possibly Siamese

Mean Age and Range
• Dogs—middle-aged to old; mean, 10.5 years; range, 3-14 years (rare in dogs < 6 years old) • Cats—(4 cases) mean, 14.75 years; range, 12-17

Predominant Sex None

SIGNS

General Comments
• Clinical signs are episodic. • Signs may or may not be related to fasting, excitement, exercise, and eating. • Dogs usually demonstrate more than one clinical sign and signs progress with time.

Historical Findings
• Dogs—seizures (generalized and focal) most common. Also, posterior paresis, weakness, collapse, muscle fasciculations, abnormal behavior, lethargy and depression, ataxia, polyphagia, weight gain, polyuria and polydipsia, and exercise intolerance • Cats—seizures, ataxia, muscle fasciculations, weakness, lethargy and depression, anorexia, weight loss, and polydipsia

Physical Examination Findings
• Usually within normal limits • Obesity in some dogs • Rarely, polyneuropathy in dogs

CAUSES
Most patients have malignant, insulin-producing carcinoma or adenocarcinoma of the pancreas. Tumors believed to be benign according to histopathologic findings usually metastasize later.

RISK FACTORS
Fasting, excitement, exercise, and eating may increase the risk of hypoglycemic episodes.

DIAGNOSIS

DIFFERENTIAL DIAGNOSIS
• Extrapancreatic tumor hypoglycemia—paraneoplastic hypoglycemia has been documented in dogs with hepatocellular carcinoma, metastatic mammary carcinoma, primary pulmonary carcinoma, and others. These tumors secrete insulin or insulin-like factors. Differentiation from beta-cell pancreatic tumor is by a complete hypoglycemic workup, including imaging. • Seizures and collapse—must consider cardiovascular (e.g., syncope), metabolic (e.g., hepatoencephalopathy, hypocalcemia, and hypoadrenocorticism) and neurologic (e.g., epilepsy, neoplasia, toxin, and inflammatory disease) causes • Posterior paresis and weakness—consider cardiovascular (e.g., congenital anatomic defect, arrhythmias, heart failure, and pericardial effusion), metabolic (e.g., hypoadrenocorticsm, hypocalcemia, anemia, hypokalemia, and hypothyroidism), neurologic and neuromuscular (e.g., spinal cord disease, myasthenia gravis, polymyositis, and polyradiculoneuropathy) and toxic (e.g., tick paralysis, botulism, chronic organophosphate exposure, and lead poisoning) causes • Muscle fasciculations—consider metabolic (e.g., hypercalcemia, hypocalcemia, and hyperadrenocorticism) and toxic (e.g., tetanus and strychnine poisoning) causes

CBC/BIOCHEMISTRY/URINALYSIS
Results usually normal, except hypoglycemia (< 70 mg/dl in more than 90% of patients)

OTHER LABORATORY TESTS
• Simultaneous fasting glucose and insulin determination—on initiating fasting, collect blood samples hourly or bihourly for serum glucose determination and serum storage. When the serum glucose drops below 60 mg/dl (usually within 8-10 hours in dogs), that serum sample is submitted for serum insulin determination. Interpretation: high insulin, insulinoma likely; normal insulin, insulinoma possible; low insulin, insulinoma unlikely. • Amended insulin-glucose ratio (AIGR)—this test is intended to diagnose insulinoma when the insulin concentration is within the normal range but inappropriately high for the degree of hypoglycemia. • AIGR = (plasma insulin [mcU/ml] x 100)/(plasma glucose [mg/dl] - 30); use 1 as denominator if glucose is < 30 • AIGR > 30 suggests insulinoma • AIGR = 19-30 gray zone, repeat test • AIGR < 19 insulinoma unlikely • Note: False-positive results are possible, especially when serum glucose is < 40 mg/dl.

IMAGING
Thoracic and abdominal radiography and abdominal ultrasonography are usually normal, but help evaluate for extrapancreatic tumor hypoglycemia as well as some other differential diagnoses.

OTHER DIAGNOSTIC PROCEDURES
N/A

GROSS AND HISTOPATHOLOGIC FINDINGS
• Insulinoma is usually a small, solitary nodule, although multiple nodules or diffuse infiltration are seen. Most insulinomas can be identified grossly at surgery. Metastasis is seen in 40% of patients at surgery. Common areas include the regional lymph nodes and liver; other areas include the duodenum, mesentery, omentum, and spleen. • Histopathologically appear as either carcinoma or adenoma, but both behave malignantly.

TREATMENT

INPATIENT VERSUS OUTPATIENT
• Hospitalize for workup, surgery, and, if clinically hypoglycemic, treatment.
• Treat as outpatient if the owner declines surgery and the animal is not clinically hypoglycemic.

ACTIVITY Restricted

DIET
The first and most important aspect of management (with or without surgery). Feed 4-6 small meals a day. Diet should be high in protein, fat, and complex carbohydrates and low in simple sugars (avoid semimoist food).

CLIENT EDUCATION
Owner should be aware of signs of hypoglycemia and seek immediate attention if they occur.

SURGICAL CONSIDERATIONS
Confirms diagnosis, improves survival time, has potential to provide prolonged remission, and improves response to medical treatment.

MEDICATIONS

DRUGS AND FLUIDS

Emergency/Acute Therapy
See Hypoglycemia.

Long-Term Therapy
• Glucocorticoids (prednisone at an initial dosage of 0.25 mg/kg PO q12h; can increase to 2-3 mg/kg PO q12h if needed) constitute initial medical treatment once diet alone has proven ineffective. Begin with the low dosage and gradually increase as signs of hypoglycemia recur.
• Diazoxide (Proglycem, 5 mg/kg PO q12h; can gradually increase to 30 mg/kg PO q12h if needed) is added after diet and glucocorticoids have proven ineffective.

• A synthetic somatostatin analogue (Octreotide, 10-20 mg q8-12h) prevents hypoglycemia in some dogs refractory to conventional treatment. Can be used with diet, steroids, and diazoxide. This drug is expensive.

CONTRAINDICATIONS Insulin

PRECAUTIONS

• Dextrose bolus—suitable for acute hypoglycemic crisis followed by continuous fluids with dextrose • Glucocorticoids used at high dosages and for prolonged periods can cause iatrogenic hyperadrenocorticism. • Diazoxide can cause gastrointestinal irritation and has been found in humans to cause bone marrow suppression, cataract formation, aplastic anemia, tachycardia, and thrombocytopenia.

POSSIBLE INTERACTIONS N/A

ALTERNATE DRUGS N/A

FOLLOW-UP

PATIENT MONITORING

• For return or progression of clinical signs of hypoglycemia
• Serum glucose concentration; adjust medication as needed

PREVENTION/AVOIDANCE N/A

POSSIBLE COMPLICATIONS

Recurrent or progressive episodes of hypoglycemia

EXPECTED COURSE AND PROGNOSIS

• Dogs and cats—likelihood of malignancy is high. Metastasis is seen in 40% of patients at the time of surgery. • Dogs—mean survival time, about 16-19 months; range, 2-60 months. Surgery improves survival time. • Cats—mean survival time, about 6.5 months; range, 0-18 months

MISCELLANEOUS

ASSOCIATED CONDITIONS

Obesity

AGE RELATED FACTORS

Younger dogs have shorter survival times.

ZOONOTIC POTENTIAL N/A

PREGNANCY N/A

SYNONYMS

• Insulin-secreting tumor • B-cell tumor • Hyperinsulinism • Islet cell tumor • Islet cell adenocarcinoma • Insulin-producing pancreatic tumor

SEE ALSO

Glucose, Hypoglycemia

ABBREVIATIONS

AIGR = amended insulin-glucose ratio

References

Feldman EC, Nelson RW. Feldman beta-cell neoplasia: insulinoma. In: Feldman EC, Nelson RW, eds. Canine and feline endocrinology and reproduction. 2nd ed. Philadelphia: WB Saunders, 1996:422-441.

Hawks D, Peterson ME, Hawkins KL, Rosebury WS. Insulin-secreting pancreatic (islet cell) carcinoma in a cat. J Vet Int Med 1992;6:193-196.

Peterson ME. Islet cell tumors secreting insulin, pancreatic polypeptide, gastrin, or glucagon. In: Kirk RW, Bonagura JD, eds. Current veterinary therapy XI. Philadelphia: WB Saunders, 1992:368-375.

Author Mitchell A. Crystal
Consulting Editor Rhett Nichols

INTERSTITIAL CELL TUMOR, TESTICLE

 BASICS

OVERVIEW
Interstitial cell tumor is a benign tumor of testicle that arises from interstitial (i.e., Leydig) cells. It is common in dogs and rare in cats.

SIGNALMENT
Usually, older male dogs

SIGNS
• Usually none unless associated with estrogen secretion causing feminization and bone marrow hypoplasia (see sertoli cell tumor)
• Single or multiple discrete tumor masses (usually 1 to 2 cm) may be present within a single testis

CAUSES AND RISK FACTORS
Cryptorchidism may predispose but generally unknown

 DIAGNOSIS

DIFFERENTIAL DIAGNOSIS
• Sertoli cell tumor • Seminoma • Hyper-adrenocorticism if feminization is observed
• Hypothyroidism if feminization is observed

CBC/BIOCHEMISTRY/URINALYSIS
• Results usually normal unless estrogen excess causes bone marrow hypoplasia • Patient with estrogen excess may have various cytopenias

OTHER LABORATORY TESTS N/A

IMAGING
Ultrasonography—tumors < 3 cm diameter tend to be hypoechoic and tumors > 5 cm tend to have mixed echogenic patterns

OTHER DIAGNOSTIC PROCEDURES
N/A

 TREATMENT

Castration and histopathologic examination

MEDICATIONS

DRUGS AND FLUIDS
• None unless patient has bone marrow hypoplasia
• Recombinant hematopoietic colony-stimulating factors may be useful in treating bone marrow hypoplasia

CONTRAINDICATIONS/POSSIBLE INTERACTIONS N/A

FOLLOW-UP

POSSIBLE COMPLICATIONS
Cytopenias from extrogen excess

EXPECTED COURSE AND PROGNOSIS
Usually excellent

MISCELLANEOUS

ASSOCIATED CONDITIONS
• Prostate disease is common in patient with testicular tumor • Reported as a functional ectopic tumor in one cat

Reference
Suess RP, Barr SC, Sacre BJ, et al. Bone marrow hypoplasia in a feminized dog with and interstitial cell tumor. J Am Vet Med Assoc 1992;200:1346-1348.
Author Wallace B. Morrison
Consulting Editor Wallace B. Morrison

INTERVERTEBRAL DISK DISEASE, CERVICAL

BASICS

DEFINITION
Cervical, intervertebral disk disease is an age-related change within the intervertebral disk which can result in disk protrusion or extrusion.

Pathophysiology
• Intervertebral disk disease is classified as either Hansen type I or Hansen type II • Hansen type I disease involves chondroid degeneration of the disk, disk mineralization, and acute extrusion • Hansen type II disease involves gradual fibroid metaplasia of the disk, with an insidious bulging or protrusion of the dorsal annulus.

Systems Affected
Nervous—due to focal compressive myelopathy

Genetics
No known genetic basis. Chondrodystrophoid breeds such as dachshund, beagle and Pekingese are predisposed to Hansen type I disease; large breeds, especially Doberman pinscher, are predisposed to Hansen type II disease.

Incidence and Prevalence
Unknown. Cervical lesions account for 14 to 16% of intervertebral disk disease in dogs.

Geographic Distribution N/A

SIGNALMENT

Species Dogs

Breed Predilections
• Type I disease—beagle, toy poodle, dachshund, and all chondrodystrophoid breeds
• Type II disease—Doberman pinscher

Mean Age and Range
• Hansen type I disease—3-6 years • Hansen type II disease: 8-10 years

Predominant Sex None

SIGNS
Clinical signs of cervical disk disease are variable depending on the type of disk disease and the severity of disk extrusion.

Historical Findings
• Based on the degree of disk extrusion, reported signs include pain when the dog is picked up or its neck is manipulated, failure to flex the neck to eat or drink, and failure to turn the head and neck to the right and left.
• Spasms of the cervical and shoulder muscles may occur. • If the disk extrusion impinges on a lower cervical nerve root, the dog may hold one front limb off the ground (root signature sign). • Paresis or paralysis of all four limbs may occur but is less common than neck pain only.

Physical Examination Findings
• Neck pain is the most common finding upon physical examination. Pain is elicited by flexing and extending the neck or turning the neck side to side. Pain is also elicited on deep palpation of the cervical muscles. • Approxi-

mately 50% of dogs with cervical disk disease have root signature sign. • Less frequently, dogs will have paresis or paralysis involving all four limbs. In nonchondrodystrophoid breeds with Hansen type II disease, hind limb paresis may be more pronounced than fore-limb paresis. • Depending on the severity and location of the disk extrusion, dogs may or may not have decreased spinal reflexes in the fore-limbs. Hind limb reflexes are normal to exaggerated.

CAUSES
• Age related, chondroid degeneration with Hansen type I disease. • Age related, fibroid metaplasia with Hansen type II disease

RISK FACTORS Obesity

DIAGNOSIS

DIFFERENTIAL DIAGNOSIS
• Hansen type I disease—diskospondylitis, meningitis, trauma, and neoplasia. • Hansen type II disease—lower cervical vertebral instability (Wobbler's syndrome), neoplasia, diskospondylitis, and meningitis

CBC/BIOCHEMISTRY/URINALYSIS
N/A

OTHER LABORATORY TESTS

IMAGING
• Cervical spinal radiographs—spinal radiographs often reveal narrowed, wedged-shaped disk space, small intervertebral foramen, and collapsed articular facets. With Hansen type I disease, mineralized disk material may be seen within the spinal canal or intervertebral foramen. The dorsolateral view is extremely valuable in cervical disk herniation. This view may reveal a round, button shaped density seen overlying the disk space. When this round density is seen extending beyond the vertebral endplates, disk extrusion into the spinal canal is likely. • Myelography is indicated when the exact location of the lesion is uncertain following plain radiographs, when the neurologic exam is in conflict with the radiographic findings, and when multiple lesions are evident on plain radiographs. Cisternal injections are usually used for cervical lesions. Following injection, the lateral view often reveals dorsal deviation of the ventral contrast column at the location of disk extrusion. On the dorsoventral view, the contrast column may deviate to one side or the other, or the right to left columns may widen at the site of disk extrusion.

OTHER DIAGNOSTIC PROCEDURES
In most patients, none are needed except those discussed under imaging. If signalment, history, or neurologic examination findings are inconsistent with disk disease, cerebrospinal fluid should be collected and analyzed at the time of myelography.

GROSS AND HISTOPATHOLOGIC FINDINGS
• Grossly, the extruded disk material is white to yellow and granular in consistency. The disk material may be clumped together, especially in chronic cases. • Histologically, water and proteoglycans are low, collagen is high, the disk becomes more cartilaginous, and the nucleus becomes granular and calcified.

TREATMENT

INPATIENT VERSUS OUTPATIENT
• Dogs with cervical disk disease can be broken down into three categories: 1) those with a first time episode of neck pain; 2) those with repeated episodes of neck pain, and 3) those with neck pain plus neurologic deficits.
• Dogs in the first category are usually treated as outpatients.

ACTIVITY
• All dogs with disk disease should have reduced activity levels. Harnesses rather than collars should be used for leash walking and animals should be discouraged from any form of jumping.
• In cases with an initial episode of neck pain only, cage confinement for 2-4 weeks may alleviate signs and should be tried prior to surgical treatment.

DIET
All obese dogs should be placed on a reducing diet.

CLIENT EDUCATION
Signs of spinal cord compression should be discussed with the client. In animals treated conservatively, the importance of cage rest must be emphasized.

SURGICAL CONSIDERATIONS
• Surgery is indicated for most animals with repeated episodes of neck pain and all animals with neurologic deficits. The specific surgical procedure for animals with neck pain only is controversial. Some surgeons prefer ventral disk fenestration as the treatment of choice, while others prefer the ventral slot procedure. If imaging reveals disk material within the spinal canal, the ventral slot procedure is the surgical treatment of choice.
• In animals with neurologic deficits, the ventral slot procedure is the surgical treatment of choice.

MEDICATIONS

DRUGS AND FLUIDS
Although the key to successful conservative management of cervical disk disease is cage rest, low doses of glucocorticoids such as prednisone can be used to decrease pain.

CONTRAINDICATIONS N/A

INTERVERTEBRAL DISK DISEASE, CERVICAL

PRECAUTIONS
• The use of glucocorticoids without concurrent cage confinement can decrease the dog's pain, encourage excessive activity, and result in further disk extrusion. The dog must be cage rested if conservative treatment is attempted.
• The use of nonsteroidal anti-inflammatory drugs (NSAIDs) may result in life-threatening gastrointestinal hemorrhage. NSAIDs should be avoided in all patients.

POSSIBLE INTERACTIONS
The use of NSAIDs in combination with glucocorticoid increases the risk of life-threatening gastrointestinal hemorrhage. This combination of drugs should be avoided in all patients.

ALTERNATIVE DRUGS None

FOLLOW-UP

PATIENT MONITORING
Dogs with cervical disk disease should be reevaluated for worsening neurologic signs weekly until clinical signs have resolved.

PREVENTION/AVOIDANCE
• Disk disease is unavoidable in certain breeds. • The exacerbation of clinical signs might be slowed or avoided by keeping the dog's body weight lean, and avoiding strenuous exercise and jumping.

POSSIBLE COMPLICATIONS
• Recurrence of neck pain with or without neurologic deficits is possible. • Animals treated surgically may be less likely to have recurrences. • Catastrophic spinal cord compression almost never occurs with cervical disk disease.

EXPECTED COURSE AND PROGNOSIS
• Many animals treated conservatively have recurrence and ultimately require surgery.
• Most animals treated surgically do not have recurrent episodes.

MISCELLANEOUS

ASSOCIATED CONDITIONS
The same breeds predisposed to cervical disk disease are predisposed to thoracolumbar disk disease.

AGE-RELATED FACTORS N/A
ZOONOTIC POTENTIAL N/A

SYNONYMS N/A
SEE ALSO
Intervertebral Disk Disease, Thoracolumbar

ABBREVIATIONS
NSAID = nonsteroidal anti-inflammatory drug

References
Toombs JT, Bauer MB. Intervertebral disk disease. In: Slatter DH, ed. Textbook of small animal surgery. 2nd ed. Philadelphia: WB Saunders, 1993;1070.

Braund KG. Canine intervertebral disk disease. In: Bojrab MJ, ed. Disease mechanisms in small animal surgery. Philadelphia: WB Saunders, 1993:960-969.

Oliver JE, Lorenz MD. Handbook of veterinary neurology. 2nd ed. Philadelphia: WB Saunders, 1993;170.

Waters DJ. Nonambulatory tetraparesis secondary to cervical disk disease in the dog. J Am Anim Hosp Assoc 1989;25:647-653.

Seim HB. Prata RG. Ventral decompression for the treatment of cervical disk disease in the dog: A review of 54 cases. J Am Anim Hosp Assoc 1982;18:233-240.

Author Michael S. Bauer
Consulting Editor Peter D. Schwarz

INTERVERTEBRAL DISK DISEASE, THORACOLUMBAR

BASICS

DEFINITION
Thoracolumbar, intervertebral disk disease is an age-related change within the intervertebral disk that can result in disk protrusion or extrusion.

Pathophysiology
Intervertebral disk disease is classified as either Hansen type I or Hansen type II. Hansen type I disease involves chondroid degneration of the disk, disk mineralization, and acute extrusion. Hansen type II disease involves gradual fibroid metaplasia of the disk, with an insidious bulging or protrusion of the dorsal annulus. Disk extrusion results in focal myelopathy. Varying degrees of spinal cord compression lead to ischemia and emyelination.

Systems Affected
Nervous—due to focal compressive myelopathy

Genetics
• No known genetic basis • Chondrodystrophoid breeds such as dachshund, beagle, and Pekingese are predisposed to Hansen type I disease, and large breeds are predisposed to Hansen type II disease.

Incidence/Prevalence
Unknown, although thoracolumbar disk disease accounts for approximately 85% of disk disease in dogs

Geographic Distribution N/A

SIGNALMENT

Species Dogs

Breed Predilections
• Hansen type I disease—dachshund, shih tzu, Pekingese, Welsh corgi, beagle, and all chondrodystrophoid breeds • Hansen type II disease—large breeds

Mean Age and Range
• Hansen type I disease—3-6 years • Hansen type II disease—8-10 years

Predominant Sex None recognized

SIGNS

General Comments
Clinical signs of thoracolumbar disk disease are variable depending on the type of disk disease and the severity of disk extrusion.

Historical Findings
• Based on the degree of disk extrusion, reported signs include back pain only and back pain with hindlimb ataxia to complete paraparesis. • Onset of signs may follow jumping. • There is usually no history of trauma. • Small-breed dogs with Hansen type I disease usually have acute onset of clinical signs. • Large-breed dogs with Hansen type II disease usually have insidious onset of clinical signs.

Physical Examination Findings
• Thoracolumbar pain is a common finding on physical examination. Pain is elicited on deep palpation of the epaxial muscles. • Varying degress of paraparesis may be present. • Hindlimb proprioception is usually diminished or absent. • Spinal reflexes are usually normal to exaggerated. • Lack of deep pain perception in the hindlimbs may be diminished or absent. Absence of deep pain sensation is indicative of a worse prognosis.

CAUSES
• Age related, chondroid degeneration with Hansen type I disease • Age related, fibroid metaplasia with Hansen type II disease

RISK FACTORS Obesity

DIAGNOSIS

DIFFERENTIAL DIAGNOSIS
• Hansen type I disease—trauma, neoplasia, and fibrocartilaginous embolism can be differentiated by history and radiography (myelography) • Hansen type II disease—degenerative myelopathy, neoplasia, and diskospondylitis can be differentiated by history and radiography (myelography)

CBC/BIOCHEMISTRY/URINALYSIS
N/A

OTHER LABORATORY TESTS N/A

IMAGING
• Thoracolumbar spinal radiography—spinal radiographs often reveal narrowed, wedge-shaped disk space, small intervertebral foramen, and collapsed articular facets. With Hansen type I disease, mineralized disk material may be seen within the spinal canal or intervertebral foramen. • Myelography is indicated when the exact location of the lesion is uncertain following plain radiography, when the neurologic exam is in conflict with the radiographic findings, and when multiple lesions are evident on plain radiographs. Injections for thoracolumbar disk disease are usually made at the T5-6 intervertebral space. Following injection, the lateral view often reveals obliteration of contrast columns or dorsal deviation of the ventral contrast column at the location of disk extrusion. On the dorsoventral view, the contrast column may be obliterated, may be deviated to one side or the other, or the right to left columns may widen at the site of disk extrusion.

OTHER DIAGNOSTIC PROCEDURES
In most patients, none are needed except those discussed under imaging. If signalment, history, or neurologic exam findings are inconsistent with disk disease, cerebrospinal fluid should be collected and analyzed at the time of myelography.

GROSS AND HISTOPATHOLOGIC FINDINGS

Gross Findings
The extruded disk material is white to yellow and granular in consistency. The disk material may be clumpted together, especially in chronically affected patients.

Histopathologic Findings
Water and proteoglycans are decreased, collagen is increased, the disk becomes more cartilaginous, and the nucleus becomes granular and calcified.

TREATMENT
Dogs with thoracolumbar disk disease can be broken down into four categories: 1) those with a first-time epidose of back pain only, 2) those with repeated episodes of back pain, 3) those with varying degrees of paraparesis with the presence of deep pain perception, and 4) those with complete paraparesis and loss of deep pain perception.

INPATIENT VERSUS OUTPATIENT
• Dogs in the first category may be treated as outpatients.
• Animals with mild neurologic deficits should be monitored closely for worsening signs.

ACTIVITY
• All dogs with disk disease should have restricted activity levels.
• In dogs with an initial episode of back pain only, cage confinement for 2-4 weeks may alleviate signs and should be tried before surgical treatment.

DIET
All obese dogs should be placed on a reducing diet.

CLIENT EDUCATION
• Signs of spinal cord compression should be discussed with the client. Animals with deterioration of clinical signs should be immediately reevaluated.
• The importance of cage rest must be emphasized when conservatively treating an animal.

SURGICAL CONSIDERATIONS
• Surgery is indicated for animals with repeated episodes of back pain and most animals with neurologic deficits. The specific surgical procedure is controversial. Some surgeons prefer ventral or lateral disk fenestration as the treatment of choice for dogs with back pain only, while others prefer decompression. Decompression is usually performed via hemilaminectomy. If neurologic deficits are present, decompression is the treatment of choice. The use of concurrent prophylactic fenestration may be used but is controversial.
• In animals with loss of deep pain perception, the prognosis is unknown but generally considered guarded to poor. Animals with acute loss of deep pain perception may benefit from emergency decompressive surgery.

INTERVERTEBRAL DISK DISEASE, THORACOLUMBAR

MEDICATIONS

DRUGS AND FLUIDS

Animals with acute spinal cord compression are treated with methylprednisolone (30 mg/kg, IV) as soon as possible.

PRECAUTIONS

• The use of glucocorticoids without concurrent cage confinement can lessen the dog's pain, encourage excessive activtiy, and result in further disk extrusion. The dog must be cage-rested if conservative treatment is attempted.
• Prolonged use of glucocorticoids may predispose the animal to gastrointestinal hemorrhage or even colonic perforation.
• The use of nonsteroidal antiinflammatory drugs may result in life-threatening gastrointestinal hemorrhage and should be avoided in all cases.

POSSIBLE INTERACTIONS

The use of nonsteroidal antiinflammatory drugs in combination with glucocorticoids increases the risk of life-threatening gastrointestinal hemorrhage. This combination of drugs should be avoided in all patients.

ALTERNATE DRUGS None

FOLLOW-UP

PATIENT MONITORING

• Dogs with thoracolumbar disk disease treated conservatively should be reevaluated for worsening neurologic signs twice daily for the first few days after onset. • Dogs treated conservatively, with stable neurologic signs, should be reevaluated weekly until clinical signs have resolved. • After surgery, dogs should be evaluated twice daily until improvement is evident. • Urinary bladder function should be closely monitored. Manual expression (tid to qid) often is necessary in dogs unable to ambulate.

PREVENTION/AVOIDANCE

• Disk disease is unavoidable in certain breeds. • The exacerbation of clinical signs might be slowed or avoided by keeping the dog's body weight lean and avoiding strenuous exercise and jumping.

POSSIBLE COMPLICATIONS

• Recurrence of signs is possible. • Animals treated surgically may be less likely to have recurrences. • Catastrophic spinal cord compression may occur with thoracolumbar disk disease.

EXPECTED COURSE AND PROGNOSIS

• Many animals treated conservatively may have recurrence and ultimately require surgery. • Most animals treated surgically do not have recurrent episodes.

MISCELLANEOUS

ASSOCIATED CONDITIONS

The same breeds predisposed to thoracolumbar disk disease are predisposed to cervical disk disease.

AGE RELATED FACTORS N/A

ZOONOTIC POTENTIAL N/A

SYNONYMS N/A

SEE ALSO

Intervertebral Disk Disease, cervical

ABBREVIATIONS N/A

References

Toombs JT, Bauer MB. Intervertebral disk disease. In: Slatter DH, ed. Textbook of small animal surgery. 2nd ed. Philadelphia: WB Saunders, 1993:1070-1086.

Braund K.G. Canine intervertebral disk disease. In: Bojrab MJ, ed. Disease mechanisms in small animal surgery. Philadelphia: Lea & Febiger, 1993:960-969.

Oliver JE, Lorenz MD. Handbook of veterinary neurology. 2nd ed. Philadelphia: WB Saunders, 1993.

Levine SH, Caywood DD. Recurrence of neurological deficits in dogs treated for thoracolumbar disk disease. J Am Anim Hosp Assoc 1984;20:889-894.

Prata RG. Neurosurgical treatment of thoracolumbar disks: the rationale and value of laminectomy with concomitant disk removal. J Am Anim Hosp Assoc 1981;17:17-26.

Author Michael S. Bauer
Consulting Editor Peter D. Schwarz

INTUSSUSCEPTION

BASICS

DEFINITION
A prolapse or invagination of one portion of the gastrointestinal tract into the lumen of an adjoining segment. The invaginated segment is the intussusceptum and the ensheathing segment is the intussuscipiens. Intussusceptions are classified according to location within the alimentary tract: enterocolic (ileocolic; most common location), cecocolic, enteroenteric, duodenogastric, gastroesophageal. High intussusceptions may be defined as those proximal to the jejunum whereas low intussusceptions are those distal to the duodenum.

Pathophysiology
• Although the exact physical and mechanical events that lead to intussusception are unknown, uncoordinated peristalsis is probably involved. Vigorous contraction of a bowel segment causes invagination of that segment into an adjacent flaccid segment. Regions of the GI tract that undergo abrupt change in anatomic diameter (e.g., ileocolic or gastroesophageal junctions) seem to be at high risk. • Intussusception results in partial or complete GI obstruction leading to hypovolemia and dehydration. Vascular compromise is common, especially to the intussusceptum. Compromise can range from venous and lymphatic obstruction to arterial obstruction with full-thickness necrosis. There may be disruption of the mucosal barrier allowing absorption of bacteria and/or endotoxin and exacerbation of shock.

Systems Affected
• Gastrointestinal • Cardiovascular—hypovolemic or septic shock • Multiple organ failure may ensue in severe untreated cases.

Genetics
Heritability is unproven although gastroesophageal intussusception (GEI) has been reported in multiple littermates.

Incidence/Prevalence Unknown.

Geographic Distribution N/A

SIGNALMENT

Species
• Dogs and cats • GEI-Only reported in dogs.

Breed Predilections
German shepherd dogs and Siamese cats. German shepherd dogs have an especially high prevalence of GEI (64%)

Mean Age and Range
• There is a higher incidence of intussusception in puppies and kittens with approximately 80% of affected animals being less than one year of age. Age predilection is even more pronounced for GEI with 80% of dogs being less than 3 months of age. • Reported age range: 5 days-9 years.

Predominant Sex
No sex predilection for intussusception in general. Male:Female ratio approximately 2:1 for GEI.

SIGNS

General Comments
Clinical signs and disease progression vary markedly depending upon location of the intussusception, degree of vascular compromise, and completeness of obstruction. In general, high intussusceptions have a more acute onset of signs and a more rapid clinical deterioration with higher mortality when compared to low intussusceptions.

Historical Findings
• High intussusceptions—frequent vomiting, regurgitation, hematemesis, dyspnea, abdominal discomfort, and collapse • Low intussusceptions—may include bloody mucoid diarrhea, tenesmus, intermittent vomiting, and weight loss.

Physical Examination Findings
• Cardinal signs are intermittent vomiting, bloody mucoid stools and palpation of a sausage-shaped abdominal mass. Since ileocolic intussusception is most common, the palpable mass is typically located in the cranial abdomen. • Most animals will be mildly to severely dehydrated. • Signs of shock may be present. • Abdominal pain is variable. • Ileocolic intussusception may present with the intussusceptum protruding through the anus.

CAUSES
• Most are idiopathic • Enteritis (viral, bacterial) • Foreign bodies • Intestinal parasites • Previous abdominal surgery • Intestinal mass • Megaesophagus associated with GEI

RISK FACTORS
Any condition leading to altered GI motility will predispose a patient to intussusception.

DIAGNOSIS

DIFFERENTIAL DIAGNOSIS
• As many of the disease conditions that may mimic intussusception are also predisposing factors for development of intussusception, thorough examination and close patient monitoring are of utmost importance. • Viral enteritis can usually be diagnosed on the basis of typical changes in CBC (leukopenia) and commercial antigen test kits. • Foreign bodies may be radiopaque or may cause plication of intestinal loops (linear foreign bodies). Contrast studies can usually differentiate a foreign body from an intussusception, although the distinction is often made at the time of exploratory celiotomy. • Mesenteric volvulus can present with similar signs as intussusception and plain radiographic distinction may be difficult. Mesenteric volvulus tends to have a more rapidly fatal course than intussusception and emergency celiotomy is indicated to differentiate the two conditions. • Intestinal parasites are diagnosed by fecal examination and response to appropriate anthelminthic. • Hemorrhagic gastroenteritis (HGE) can be differentiated on the basis of a lack of radiographic signs of obstruction. • An ileocolic intussusception with the intussusceptum protruding through the anus is differentiated from rectal prolapse by passage of a blunt probe between the prolapsed segment and the anus. If the probe passes into the pelvic canal then the protrusion is due to an intussusception. • Gastroesophageal intussusception has inappropriately been confused with hiatal hernia

CBC/BIOCHEMISTRY/URINALYSIS
• Leukogram is variable ranging from leukopenia in cases with underlying viral enteritis to leukocytosis with massive bowel necrosis or peritonitis. Hematocrit may be low if significant GI hemorrhage has occurred or high with dehydration. • Electrolyte abnormalities. Hyponatremia, hypochloremia, and hypokalemia tend to be more profound with high intussusceptions. • Urinalysis is usually normal

OTHER LABORATORY TESTS
Blood gas evaluation usually reveals a metabolic acidosis. Early in the course of a high intussusception, metabolic alkalosis may prevail due to loss of gastric acid in the vomitus

IMAGING
• Although definitive diagnosis of intussusception with plain films may be difficult, radiographic signs of obstruction (bowel loops distended with gas and fluid) are usually present and are more pronounced with complete obstruction. A tissue-dense tubular mass lends strong support to a diagnosis of intussusception. • In cases of GEI, thoracic radiographs show dilation of the thoracic esophagus with a tissue-dense mass in the caudal esophagus. The normal gastric air bubble may be absent in the cranial abdomen. • Abdominal ultrasound can be used to identify the intussusception. A cylindrical intestinal mass with a characteristic "double ring" is highly specific for intussusception. • Contrast studies (upper GI, barium enema) can be used to outline an intussusception, however often at the expense of unnecessary delays in definitive treatment.

OTHER DIAGNOSTIC PROCEDURES
• Esophagoscopy can identify a soft tissue mass (stomach) within the lumen of the esophagus in patients with GEI • Colonoscopy may be helpful in identifying enterocolic or cecocolic intussusceptions.

GROSS AND HISTOPATHOLOGIC FINDINGS
• The basic lesion is grossly obvious. • Histopathologic changes in the affected bowel range from areas of mucosal erosion

and hemorrhages to full-thickness mural necrosis.

TREATMENT

INPATIENT VERSUS OUTPATIENT
Admit the patient for immediate treatment. Intussusception should be considered a life-threatening condition.

ACTIVITY
Restrict activity during the treatment and postoperative periods (approximately 7-10 days).

DIET
• Vomiting patients should be maintained NPO.
• Following surgical correction, oral intake of fluid and food can usually be initiated in the first 24 hours. Early oral alimentation, in the form of small frequent meals, promotes normal peristalsis and avoids ileus.

CLIENT EDUCATION
• A poor to grave prognosis is associated with nonoperative treatment of intussusception. Early surgery affords the best prognosis.
• Gastroesophageal intussusception is associated with a high mortality in all cases.
• Correction of intussusception may not correct the underlying GI disorder.

SURGICAL CONSIDERATIONS
• A surgical emergency. Celiotomy and correction should follow initial patient stabilization. • Manual reduction of the intussusception should be attempted by gently "milking" the invaginated segment.
• Bowel viability is assessed using criteria of color, pulsation, intestinal contraction, and Wood's lamp fluorescence following IV fluorescein injection.
• If the intussusception is non-reducible or non-viable then resection and anastomosis are indicated.
• Risk of postoperative recurrence can be minimized by enteroplication of the small intestines.

MEDICATIONS

DRUGS AND FLUIDS
• Aggressive intravenous fluid support is required to correct hydration deficits and replace ongoing GI losses. Generally a balanced electrolyte solution (e.g., lactated Ringer's solution) is appropriate. With profound hyponatremia and hypochloremia, 0.9% NaCl is the fluid of choice. Potassium supplementation should be based on measured serum levels.

• Broad spectrum antibiotics or combinations with efficacy against coliforms and anaerobes should be administered prior to surgery and preferentially given by the intravenous route.
• Histamine blockers (e.g., cimetidine) and/or protectants (e.g., sucralfate) may be indicated if GI ulceration is suspected.

CONTRAINDICATIONS
Motility enhancing antiemetics (e.g., metoclopromide) should not be used in patients with GI obstruction. Antiemetics in general will only mask the signs of obstruction.

PRECAUTIONS
Anticholinergics exacerbate postoperative ileus and are not recommended.

POSSIBLE INTERACTIONS N/A

ALTERNATE DRUGS N/A

FOLLOW-UP

PATIENT MONITORING
• Monitor closely for recurrence or worsening of signs for the first 3-5 days following surgery, as this is when serious complications are likely to occur. • Recurrence of intussusception is common (20-30%) in patients that do not receive enteroplication and usually occurs within three days. • Anastomotic dehiscence or leakage should be suspected with a deterioration of clinical signs. Diagnostic peritoneal lavage is the most sensitive method to detect dehiscence.

PREVENTION/AVOIDANCE
Routine veterinary care of puppies and kittens (e.g., vaccinations and treatment of intestinal parasites) will eliminate many of the predisposing factors for intussusception.

POSSIBLE COMPLICATIONS
• Recurrence of intussusception • Persistence of underlying GI problem if undiagnosed • Peritonitis • Complications associated with short bowel syndrome if large segment of intestine was resected

EXPECTED COURSE AND PROGNOSIS
• Presence and severity of underlying conditions will affect prognosis. • Expect <20% overall mortality with proper treatment.
• Mortality with GEI is high (approximately 95%).

MISCELLANEOUS

ASSOCIATED CONDITIONS
May accompany other GI abnormalities.

AGE RELATED FACTORS
Intussusception in older animals may be more commonly associated with mural mass lesions. Resected segments in older patients should routinely be submitted for histopathology.

ZOONOTIC POTENTIAL N/A

PREGNANCY
The stress of the metabolic and hemodynamic derangements coupled with anesthesia and surgery may result in pregnancy termination.

SYNONYMS
Cecocolic intussusception is commonly termed cecal inversion.

SEE ALSO
• Shock • Peritonitis

ABBREVIATIONS
GEI = gastroesophageal intussusception
GI = gastrointestinal

References
Leib MS, Blass CE. Gastroesophageal intussusception in the dog: a review of the literature and a case report. JAAHA. 1984;20:783-790.
Lewis DD. Intussusception in dogs and cats. Compend Contin Educ Pract Vet. 1987;9:523–533.
Orsher RJ, Rosin E. Small intestine. In: Slatter D, ed. Textbook of small animal surgery. 2nd ed. Philadelphia: WB Saunders, 1993;593–612.
Oakes MG, Lewis DD, Hosgood G, et al. Enteroplication for the prevention of intussusception recurrence in dogs: 31 cases. JAVMA. 1994;205:72–75.
Author Bradford C. Dixon
Consulting Editor Brent D. Jones

IRIS ATROPHY

 BASICS

OVERVIEW
Degeneration of the pupillary margin or stroma (or both portions) of the iris, resulting in an iris that is thin or that has areas of full-thickness tissue loss. Can be a senile or secondary change. Secondary iris atrophy can be a sequelae to chronic inflammation (uveitis) or high intraocular pressure (glaucoma). Frequently, the iris sphincter muscle is affected, resulting in incomplete pupillary constriction. In some animals, the margin remains unaffected, with loss of stroma and iris dilator muscle causing large holes in the iris that resemble multiple pupillary openings. Vision is unaffected.

SIGNALMENT
• A common aging change seen in all breeds of dog, with small breeds (e.g., miniature and toy poodle, miniature schnauzer, and chihuahua) affected more commonly. • Uncommon in cats but appears to be most common in cats with blue irides. • Secondary iris atrophy can occur in any breed of dog or cat.

SIGNS
Historical Findings
• Photophobia • Previous episodes of uveitis or glaucoma

Physical Examination Findings
• Incomplete pupillary light reflex, accompanied by a normal menace response • Irregular, scalloped edge to the pupillary margin • Transillumination reveals thin or absent areas of iris • Strands of iris occasionally remain, spanning across portions of the pupil • Holes within the iris stroma may resemble additional pupils • Secondary iris atrophy can be accompanied by any of the signs associated with chronic glaucoma or uveitis, including, but not limited to, conjunctival or episcleral injection, corneal edema, posterior synechiae, high intraocular pressure, and buphthalmia.

Causes and Risk Factors
• Normal aging • Uveitis • Glaucoma

 DIAGNOSIS

DIFFERENTIAL DIAGNOSIS
Must differentiate from congenital iris anomalies:
• Iris aplasia (rare in dogs and cats) • Iris hypoplasia • Iris coloboma (i.e., a complete, full-thickness area of lack of development of all layers of the iris) is frequently associated with the merle condition. Absence of the lens zonules and indentation of the lens deep to the colobomatous area may also be associated. • Polycoria—more than one pupil, each with the ability to constrict • Persistent pupillary membranes, which arise from the collarette (midportion) of the iris, not from the free pupillary margin

CBC/BIOCHEMISTRY/URINALYSIS
N/A

OTHER LABORATORY TESTS N/A

IMAGING N/A

OTHER DIAGNOSTIC PROCEDURES
Tonometry:
• High intraocular pressure if secondary to glaucoma • Possibly low intraocular pressure if atrophy is secondary to uveitis

 TREATMENT

• Iris atrophy is nonreversible.
• When secondary to uveitis or glaucoma, treatment should be aimed at controlling the underlying disease. Effective treatment may halt the progression of the condition.
• Provide the animal with adequate shade because it may exhibit photophobia due to inability to constrict its pupil.

MEDICATIONS

DRUGS AND FLUIDS
• None for senile iris atrophy.
• Treat the underlying disease if iris atrophy is secondary (see chapters on glaucoma and uveitis).

CONTRAINDICATIONS/POSSIBLE INTERACTIONS
Atropine topically applied exacerbates signs of photophobia and pupillary dilation.

 FOLLOW-UP

Senile iris atrophy may continue to progress with age. Secondary iris atrophy does not usually progress once the primary disease is controlled.

 MISCELLANEOUS

SEE ALSO
• Anterior Uveitis (Dogs and Cats)
• Glaucoma

Reference

Collins BK, Moore CP. Canine anterior uvea. In: Gelatt KN, ed. Veterinary ophthalmology. Philadelphia: Lea & Febiger, 1991:357–395.

Author Stephanie L. Smedes
Consulting Editor Paul E. Miller

IRRITABLE BOWEL SYNDROME

BASICS

DEFINITION
A functional disorder that causes chronic intermittent signs of colonic dysfunction in the absence of structural gastrointestinal pathology.

Pathophysiology
The pathophysiology of irritable bowel syndrome (IBS) is unclear. Potential causes include abnormal colonic myoelectrical activity and motility, dietary fiber deficiency, dietary intolerances, stress, and changes in neural or neurochemical regulation of colonic function.

Systems Affected
Gastrointestinal

Genetics N/A

Incidence/Prevalence
It has been estimated that 10-15% of dogs with chronic large bowel diarrhea have IBS. However, because this disorder is poorly characterized and the diagnosis is based on exclusion of other causes, it is difficult to accurately assess its prevalence.

Geographical Distribution N/A

SIGNALMENT

Species Dogs

Breed Predilections
Any breed; especially working dogs

Mean Age and Range
Any age can be affected.

Predominant Sex No sex predilection.

SIGNS

Historical Findings
• Chronic, intermittent signs of large bowel diarrhea, including frequent passage of small amounts of feces and mucus, and dyschezia.
• Hematochezia is uncommon.
• Abdominal pain, bloating, vomiting, and nausea may also occur.

Physical Examination Findings
Physical examination is often unremarkable. Abdominal pain may be evident.

CAUSES
Unknown

RISK FACTORS
Stress, such as changes in the household or being left alone for extended periods, may be associated with episodes of diarrhea. However, in many dogs with IBS, stress does not appear to play a role.

DIAGNOSIS

The diagnosis of IBS is based on the exclusion of all other potential causes of large bowel diarrhea, and should be reserved for patients that have undergone a thorough diagnostic evaluation, therapeutic deworming, and bland diet trials without resolution of signs.

DIFFERENTIAL DIAGNOSIS
• Whipworms • Inflammatory colitis
• Clostridium perfringens • Fiber-responsive large bowel diarrhea • Dietary indiscretion
• Giardia • Histoplasmosis • Colonic neoplasia • Cecal inversion

CBC/BIOCHEMISTRY/URINALYSIS
Normal

OTHER LABORATORY TESTS
Direct fecal examination, fecal flotation, fecal cytology are normal.

IMAGING
Survey and contrast radiographic studies of the abdomen are normal.

OTHER DIAGNOSTIC PROCEDURES
• Colonoscopy is generally normal. Colonic spasm, excessive intraluminal mucus, and hypermotility are occasionally present. • Mucosal biopsy specimens from multiple areas in the colon are histologically normal.

GROSS AND HISTOPATHOLOGIC FINDINGS
Normal

TREATMENT

INPATIENT VERSUS OUTPATIENT
Usually treat as outpatient.

ACTIVITY N/A

DIET
Feeding a highly digestible diet with added soluble fiber (Metamucil®, 1-3 tablespoons per day) will often improve the diarrhea, but rarely results in complete resolution of clinical signs.

CLIENT EDUCATION
• Clients should be informed that response to treatment is variable, and affected dogs may have long term intermittent clinical signs.
• Any stressful factors in the dog's environment should be eliminated if possible.

SURGICAL CONSIDERATIONS
N/A

MEDICATIONS

DRUGS AND FLUIDS
• Drug therapy is instituted for several days up to 1-2 weeks during episodes in which signs occur.
• Motility modifiers (opiate anti-diarrheals) improve signs of diarrhea by increasing rhythmic segmentation.
• Combination antispasmodic-tranquilizer preparations are used to relieve abdominal cramping, bloating, and distress.
• If nausea and vomiting preclude the use of oral medication, parenteral antiemetics should be administered for 1-2 days.

Motility Modifiers
• Loperamide (Imodium®), 0.1-0.2 mg/kg PO q8h • Diphenoxylate (Lomotil®), 0.05-0.1 mg/kg PO q8h-q12h

Antispasmodic-Tranquilizer Combinations
• Chlordiazepoxide and clidinium bromide (Librax®), 0.1-0.25 mg of clidinium/kg PO q8h-q12h • Isopropamide and prochlorperazine (Darbazine®), 0.14-0.22 mg/kg SQ q12h; oral: see package insert

Parenteral Antiemetics
Chlorpromazine (Thorazine®), 0.2-0.5 mg/kg q6h-q24h SQ or IM

CONTRAINDICATIONS
• Opiates are contraindicated with respiratory dysfunction, hepatic encephalopathy, severe debilitation • Anticholinergics are contraindicated with cardiac disease, hepatic disease, renal disease, hypertension, hyperthyroidism.

PRECAUTIONS N/A

POSSIBLE INTERACTIONS N/A

ALTERNATE DRUGS
• Sulfasalazine (Azulfidine®), 22-30 mg/kg PO q8h has been reported to improve signs in some dogs with significant dyschezia.

FOLLOW-UP

PATIENT MONITORING
Have owner monitor fecal consistency and watch for signs of dyschezia and abdominal discomfort.

PREVENTION/AVOIDANCE
Minimize any stressful factors in the animal's environment that might have precipitated an episode.

POSSIBLE COMPLICATIONS N/A

EXPECTED COURSE AND PROGNOSIS
• Improved stools, decreased mucus, and relief of dyschezia and abdominal distress should be apparent with 1-2 days of starting medication.
• In some dogs with IBS, signs will completely resolve following treatment and dietary alterations, while others will have long term episodic signs.

MISCELLANEOUS

ASSOCIATED CONDITIONS N/A

AGE RELATED FACTORS N/A

ZOONOTIC POTENTIAL N/A

PREGNANCY N/A

IRRITABLE BOWEL SYNDROME

SYNONYMS
• Spastic colon, nervous colon, spastic colitis, mucous colitis

SEE ALSO
• Diarrhea, Chronic—Dogs • Colitis and Proctitis

ABBREVIATIONS
IBS = Irritable bowel syndrome

References

Tams TR. Irritable bowel syndrome. In: Kirk RW, Bonagura JD, eds. Current veterinary therapy XI. Philadelphia: WB Saunders, 1992;604-608.

Leib MS, Monroe WE, Codner EC. Management of chronic large bowel diarrhea in dogs. Vet Med 1991;86:922-929.

Strombeck DR, Guilford WG. Small animal gastroenterology. Davis, CA: Stonegate, 1990.

Author Amy M. Grooters
Consulting Editor Brent D. Jones

IVERMECTIN TOXICITY

BASICS

OVERVIEW
• Some dogs are unusually sensitive to the toxic effects of ivermectin. • Toxicity occurs in dogs given large extra-label dosages (10-15x or greater than recommended dosage). • Ivermectin potentiates the release and binding of a neuroinhibitory substance, gamma-aminobutyric acid (GABA), at certain synapses in the CNS. • Differing sensitivities to ivermectin toxicity may relate to a defect in the blood-brain barrier, presence of higher than normal amount of unbound ivermectin in the plasma, or an ivermectin-specific blood brain transport mechanism in sensitive dogs. • Ivermectin is metabolized and excreted by the liver.

SIGNALMENT
• Most commonly seen in collies, followed by Australian shepherds. Not all collies are sensitive. • May be a genetic component in sensitive animals • No age or sex predilection.

SIGNS
• Mydriasis • Depression • Drooling • Vomiting • Ataxia • Tremors • Disorientation • Weakness, recumbency • Nonresponsiveness • Blindness • Bradycardia • Hypoventilation • Coma • Death

CAUSES AND RISK FACTORS
• Extra label use at high dosage • Breed sensitivity (eg, collie and Australian shepherd)

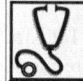

DIAGNOSIS

DIFFERENTIAL DIAGNOSIS
• Overdoses of other avermectin compounds such as milbemycin oxime • Other toxicants or diseases affecting CNS • No specific tests are useful in confirming a diagnosis of ivermectin toxicity. The diagnosis is based on history and clinical signs.

CBC/BIOCHEMISTRY/URINALYSIS
N/A

OTHER LABORATORY TESTS
Arterial blood gases may reveal a high Pa_{CO2} and a low Pa_{O2} caused by respiratory depression and hypoventilation.

IMAGING N/A

OTHER DIAGNOSTIC PROCEDURES
A temporary (30-40 minute) return to consciousness or resumed alertness and muscle activity after the administration of physostigmine (1 mg IV) supports, but does not confirm, a diagnosis of ivermectin toxicity. Treatment with glycopyrrolate before pysostigmine administration may prevent severe bradycardia. The use of physostigmine does not speed recovery and therefore has no indication for treating ivermectin toxicity.

TREATMENT
• Mainstay of management is supportive and symptomatic care. • Proper fluid therapy and maintenance of electrolyte balance, nutritional support, and prevention of secondary complications are important therapeutic goals. • Since severe CNS depression or coma may last for weeks, institute nutritional support early in the course of treatment (preferably within the first 2-3 days). • Affected animals may remain recumbent for long periods, and thus frequent turning of the dog, appropriate bedding, physical therapy, attentive nursing care, and other standard treatment measures for a recumbent animal are important. • Apply ocular lubricants. • Mechanical ventilation may be required in patients with respiratory depression.

MEDICATIONS

DRUGS AND FLUIDS
• Administer balanced electrolyte solutions intravenously. • There is no known reversal agent. • Atropine or glycopyrrolate can be administered as needed to treat bradycardia.

CONTRAINDICATIONS/POSSIBLE INTERACTIONS
Avoid other drugs that stimulate the GABA receptor (eg, benzodiazepine tranquilizers).

FOLLOW-UP
• The prognosis and eventual outcome are dependent on a number of factors including individual and breed sensitivity, the amount of drug ingested or injected, how rapidly clinical signs develop, response to supportive treatment, and the overall health of the animal. • While convalescence may be prolonged (several weeks), good supportive care in many seemingly hopeless cases has resulted in complete recovery.

MISCELLANEOUS

SEE ALSO
• Heartworm Disease—Dogs • Poisoning (Intoxication)

ABBREVIATIONS
• CNS = central nervous system
• GABA = gamma-aminobutyric acid

Reference

Paul AJ, Tranquilli WJ. Ivermectin. In: Kirk RW, ed. Current veterinary therapy X. Philadelphia: WB Saunders, 1989:140-142.

Author Allan J. Paul
Consulting Editor Gary Osweiler

KERATITIS, NONULCERATIVE

BASICS

DEFINITION
Any inflammation of the cornea that does not retain fluorescein stain. In some animals, it may progress to corneal ulceration. Keratitis can be classified further by cause, predominant inflammatory cell type, microbial agent, or location in the cornea. Examples include eosinophilic keratitis, neurotrophic keratitis, bacterial keratitis, and interstitial keratitis.

Pathophysiology
Alteration of corneal clarity indicates a pathologic response (e.g., keratitis). Pathologic responses include edema, neovascularization, inflammatory cell infiltration, pigmentation, lipid or calcium deposition, enzymatic destruction, and scarring. Neovascularization can be superficial or deep. Superficial vessels are dendritic or tree-branching in appearance and usually indicate superficial or external eye disease. Deep vessels are shorter and straighter, resulting in a paintbrush appearance around the perilimbal cornea. Deep vessels indicate deep corneal or intraocular disease (e.g., uveitis).

Systems Affected Ophthalmic

Genetics
• There is no proven genetic basis for nonulcerative keratitis in dogs or cats. • Breed predilections suggest there may be genetic influences in some animals. • Chronic superficial keratitis (pannus) in the German shepherd may be inherited recessively with variable expression. Environmental factors (e.g., altitude and solar radiation) modify the occurrence of this disease.

Incidence/Prevalence
Common cause of eye disease in dogs and, to a lesser extent, in cats.

Geographic Distribution
Altitude but not latitude or longitude is an important risk factor. The greatest number of cases in the USA occur in Colorado.

Signalment

Species
Dogs
• Chronic superficial keratitis (pannus)
• Nodular granulomatous episclerokeratitis
• Pigmentary keratitis (or corneal pigmentation) • Keratoconjunctivitis sicca (KCS)
Cats
• Herpetic keratitis (stromal form)
• Eosinophilic keratitis • Corneal sequestration • KCS is uncommon and is usually secondary to chronic herpesvirus infection.

Breed Predilections
Dogs
• Chronic superficial keratitis can occur in any breed, but prevalence is higher in the German shepherd and Belgian tervuren.

• Nodular granulomatous episclerokeratitis occurs primarily in the collie. Other breeds include the shetland sheepdog and border collie. • Brachycephalic breeds with prominent nasal folds, nasal trichiasis, and exposure keratopathy are predisposed to corneal pigmentation, notably the pug, Pekingese, lhasa apso, and shih tzu. • Brachycephalic breeds are predisposed to KCS. Notable breeds include the English bulldog, cocker spaniel, cavalier King Charles spaniel, lhasa apso, shih tzu, pug, Pekingese, and the West Highland white terrier.
Cats
• No known breed predilection for eosinophilic or herpetic keratitis. • Corneal sequestration is most prevalent in the Persian, Siamese, Burmese, and Himalayan breeds.

Mean Age and Range
Dogs
• Chronic superficial keratitis can occur at any age, but dogs between 4-7 years are at comparatively higher risk. • Nodular granulomatous episclerokeratitis is a disease of young to middle-aged collies with a mean age of 3.8 years. • KCS is usually a disease of middle-aged or older dogs.
Cats
• Herpetic keratitis affects cats of all ages.
• Eosinophilic keratitis and corneal sequestration affect cats of all ages except neonates.

Predominant Sex
In dogs, a female predisposition for KCS has been suggested.

SIGNS

Historical Findings
• Keratitis may cause variable corneal discoloration. • Depending on the specific keratitis, a history of ocular discomfort (i.e., squinting, tearing, blepharospasm, rubbing at eye) may be reported.

Physical Examination Findings
Keratitis associated with or secondary to chronic uveitis or glaucoma can be unilateral or bilateral and is often characterized by diffuse and marked corneal edema (bluish-white), circumcorneal and deep vascularization, and evidence of ocular discomfort.
Dogs
• Chronic superficial keratitis usually appears as bilateral and often symmetrical pinkish-white lesions with variable pigmentation (i.e., granulation tissue) that begin at the lateral or ventrolateral cornea. The lateral, medial, ventral, and dorsal corneal quadrants are usually affected in that order. White lipid deposits may occur in adjacent corneal stroma. In animals with advanced chronic superficial keratitis, blindness can occur. The third eyelids can also be affected and may appear thickened or depigmented. • Nodular granulomatous episclerokeratitis usually appears as bilateral, raised, pink, vascular, and often symmetrical lesions of the lateral cornea. Lesions may be slowly or rapidly progressive. White lipid de-

posits may occur in adjacent corneal stroma. The third eyelids can also be affected and may appear thickened. • Pigmentary keratitis appears as focal to diffuse brown or black discoloration of the cornea, often in association with corneal neovascularization or scarring. It can be unilateral or bilateral.
• Findings with KCS are variable, and the condition can be unilateral or bilateral. Early signs include mucoid or mucopurulent ocular discharge and conjunctival hyperemia. With chronicity or greater severity, corneal neovascularization, pigmentation (brown), and variable scarring occur.
Cats
• Herpetic nonulcerative (stromal) keratitis can be unilateral or bilateral and often occurs with ulceration. It causes stromal edema (bluish-white), scarring, and vascularization. Stromal scarring can be severe enough to threaten vision. • Eosinophilic keratitis is most often unilateral and affects the lateral or medial cornea, but any quadrant can be affected. It appears as a white, pinkish-white, or grey corneal plaque usually with a roughened or cobblestone surface. The corneal epithelium is usually intact, but some fluorescein stain retention is possible. vascularization is variable. • Corneal sequestration is usually unilateral but can be bilateral and appears as an amber, brown, or black, oval to circular plaque of the central or paracentral cornea. Affected cornea is usually ulcerated but retains fluorescein stain only at the periphery of the lesion. Corneal vascularization is variable. The edges of the plaque are usually slightly elevated because of edema, thickened epithelium, or granulation tissue.

CAUSES
Dogs
• Chronic superficial keratitis is presumed to be an immune-mediated disease that is influenced by environmental factors, notably altitude and solar radiation; the disease has a breed predilection. • Nodular granulomatous episclerokeratitis is presumed to be an immune-mediated disease; the disease has a breed predilection. • Pigmentary keratitis is a secondary condition, and the primary cause should be sought. It is most often associated with exposure keratopathy, nasal trichiasis, nasal folds, KCS, or chronic superficial keratitis. Some breeds, notably the Pekingese and pug, appear to have a congenital predisposition to this condition. • Most cases of keratoconjunctivitis sicca are caused by immune-mediated dacryoadenitis. (See KCS chapter.)
Cats
• Herpetic stromal keratitis is believed to be an immune-mediated, T-cell lymphocyte reaction to herpesvirus antigen rather than a cytopathic effect of the virus. • The cause of eosinophilic keratitis is unknown. Some cats are concurrently infected with feline herpesvirus. • The cause of corneal sequestra-

tion is unknown. Most but not all cats have some evidence of previous corneal trauma or irritation. A relationship between herpesvirus keratitis and subsequent corneal sequestration has been suggested.

RISK FACTORS

Dogs
• Chronic superficial keratitis is more likely to occur in dogs living at high altitudes with more intense exposure to solar radiation.
• See breed predilections for nodular granulomatous episclerokeratitis, pigmentary keratitis, and KCS.

Cats
• Herpesvirus infection may be a risk factor for corneal sequestration. • See breed predilections for corneal sequestration.

DIAGNOSIS

DIFFERENTIAL DIAGNOSIS

Dogs
• Infectious keratitis is usually ulcerative and painful. • The causes of noninfectious and nonulcerative keratitis can be differentiated from one another by breed predilections or ocular findings as described. • Nodular granulomatous episclerokeratitis is distinguished from neoplasia by age of onset, breed predilection, bilateral nature, and therapeutic response to antiinflammatory therapy.

Cats
• Herpetic stromal keratitis may or may not be associated with corneal ulceration or respiratory disease. • Eosinophilic keratitis is relatively unique in appearance but should be distinguished from fungal keratitis, acid-fast granuloma, neoplasia, and granulation tissue of other causes, including herpetic keratitis, foreign body granuloma, and healing corneal ulcers. Microbial culture and cytologic and histopathologic examinations of appropriate specimens aid the differential diagnosis.
• Corneal sequestration is unique in appearance but should be distinguished from melanoma. Sequestration usually affects the central or paracentral cornea, whereas melanoma affects the limbal cornea and sclera.

CBC/BIOCHEMISTRY/URINALYSIS

Results are usually normal.

OTHER LABORATORY TESTS
• Cats with herpetic keratitis, corneal sequestration, or KCS may have a positive serologic test for herpesvirus, with titers > 1:100 considered significant (Nasisse MP, personal communication, 1994). • Viral culture or immunofluorescent antibody test (IFA) for herpesvirus from conjunctival scrapings may be positive in cats with herpesvirus keratitis, eosinophilic keratitis, corneal sequestration, or KCS (see diagnostic procedures).

IMAGING N/A

OTHER DIAGNOSTIC PROCEDURES

Dogs
• For dogs with chronic superficial keratitis, cytologic evaluation of corneal or conjunctival scrapings reveals a preponderance of lymphocytes and plasma cells. • For dogs with pigmentary keratitis, suspected KCS, or any corneal disease of undetermined cause, a Schirmer tear test should be performed—values > 15 mm/minute are normal; values <10 mm/minute are consistent with KCS; values between 10-15 suggest KCS but should be interpreted with consideration of the breed and concurrent ocular findings.

Cats
• For cats with herpetic keratitis, cellular material obtained by conjunctival or corneal scraping can be placed on a glass slide, air-dried, and submitted for IFA testing (Virology Laboratory, College of Veterinary Medicine, University of Tennessee, Knoxville, TN 37996, phone: 615-974-5643). • For cats with eosinophilic keratitis or corneal sequestration, histopathologic examination of affected cornea obtained by superficial keratectomy is diagnostic, but diagnosis is usually possible by clinical signs alone.

GROSS AND HISTOPATHOLOGIC FINDINGS

Dogs
• For dogs with chronic superficial keratitis, histopathologic examination of affected cornea reveals fibrovascular infiltrate of the superficial stroma accompanied by lymphocytes, plasma cells, and variable pigmentation. • For dogs with ocular granulomatous episclerokeratitis, histopathologic testing reveals increased vascularization of the limbal cornea with variable numbers of lymphocytes, plasma cells, and histiocytes. Reticulin fibers may be present, but fibrosis is not a prominent feature. Corneal and conjunctival epithelium are intact.

Cats
• For cats with eosinophilic keratitis, histopathologic examination of affected cornea usually reveals granulomatous inflammation of the superficial stroma with eosinophils, lymphocytes, plasma cells, and histiocytes. Mast cells may also be seen. Epithelium may be intact, thin, or ulcerated.
• For cats with corneal sequestration, coagulation necrosis of the corneal stroma with ulceration or necrosis of the epithelium is seen. Vascularization and variable numbers of polymorphonuclear and mononuclear inflammatory cells are present.

TREATMENT

INPATIENT VERSUS OUTPATIENT
• Treat initially on an outpatient basis.
• Lack of adequate therapeutic response or

continued ocular discomfort may warrant hospitalization and surgery (see surgical considerations).

ACTIVITY
Normal activity unless surgery is performed. Restricted activity in the immediate postoperative period.

DIET N/A

CLIENT EDUCATION

Dogs
• Chronic superficial keratitis is controlled rather than cured. Clinical exacerbations may occur during the warmer times of the year.
• Nodular granulomatous episclerokeratitis is controlled rather than cured. • For dogs with pigmentary keratitis, the primary cause must be sought and corrected to prevent progression. • Keratoconjunctivitis sicca requires lifelong treatment and sometimes surgery.

Cats
• For cats with herpetic keratitis, ocular discomfort and corneal opacity are often recurrent. • Eosinophilic keratitis is controlled rather than cured. • A corneal sequestrum may slough spontaneously, but this requires months or even years. The clinical course is prolonged without surgery. If keratectomy is performed, removal of the sequestrum may be incomplete, or sequestration may recur postoperatively.

SURGICAL CONSIDERATIONS

Dogs
• For dogs with chronic superficial keratitis: superficial keratectomy can be performed in animals with severe disease, but this is usually unnecessary, and indefinite medical treatment is still required to prevent recurrence. Beta-irradiation with a Strontium-90 probe is noninvasive and may be preferred because lymphocytes, plasma cells, and melanocytes are sensitive to effects of irradiation. • For dogs with nodular granulomatous episclerokeratitis, superficial keratectomy is diagnostic but usually unnecessary and only temporarily resolves clinical signs. Medical treatment is preferred. • For dogs with pigmentary keratitis, superficial keratectomy can be performed but should be done only after the initial problem is corrected. It is indicated only if severe enough to be visually threatening. Beta-irradiation and cryotherapy have been used to resolve pigmentary keratitis.
• Parotid duct transposition surgery or partial permanent tarsorrhaphy may be indicated in some dogs with KCS.

Cats
• For cats with eosinophilic keratitis, superficial keratectomy is diagnostic but usually unnecessary and only temporarily resolves clinical signs. Medical treatment is preferred.
• For cats with corneal sequestration, keratectomy is curative in some cats but recurrence is possible. The primary indication for surgery is ocular discomfort.

KERATITIS, NONULCERATIVE

MEDICATIONS

DRUGS AND FLUIDS

Dogs
• For animals with chronic superficial keratitis, topically applied corticosteroids are used q6h-q12h to cause regression of corneal blood vessels. Prednisolone, dexamethasone, flumethasone, and betamethasone are acceptable. In animals with severe disease, corticosteroids can be administered by subconjunctival injection as an adjunct to topical therapy. Acceptable dosages are triamcinolone acetonide (Vetalog®), 4-8 mg; methylprednisolone acetate (Depo-Medrol¨), 4-8 mg; and betamethasone phosphate/acetate (Betasone®), 0.75-1.5 mg. Topically applied, 1% or 2% cyclosporine solution can be used q8h-q12h alone or in combination with topically applied corticosteroids. The two together may be synergistic. • For animals with nodular granulomatous episclerokeratitis , topically or subconjunctivally applied corticosteroids are used in a manner similar to that for animals with chronic superficial keratitis. Systemically administered azathioprine initiated at 2 mg/kg/day followed by gradual reduction is effective when used alone or in combination with topically applied corticosteroids and may be the treatment of choice. • For animals with pigmentary keratitis, topical treatment is directed at the primary cause (e.g., chronic superficial keratitis or KCS). This may include topically applied corticosteroids if the primary condition is inflammatory, or lubricants or cyclosporine if the primary condition is exposure keratopathy or KCS. • For keratoconjunctivitis sicca, topically applied 1% or 2% cyclosporine is the treatment of choice (see KCS).

Cats
• Topically applied antiviral agents such as trifluridine (Viroptic®) or idoxuridine (Herplex®) should be used q4h-q6h. Nonulcerative (stromal) keratitis may benefit from concurrent topical application of corticosteroids, but these should be used judiciously because viral recrudescence is possible. • Eosinophilic keratitis usually responds well to topically applied corticosteroids q6h-q12h to cause remission, as in dogs. In difficult to manage cases, megestrol acetate (Ovaban¨) can be administered (5 mg q24h PO for 5 days, then 5 mg q48h for 1 week, then 5 mg weekly for maintenance). • For corneal sequestration, the initial problem should be treated when possible. Topically applied antibiotics q6h-q12h (e.g., triple antibiotic) are usually indicated. If herpesvirus is suspected, antiviral drugs can also be used. Topically applied 1% atropine ointment is started q12h and then reduced to q24h or q48h to relieve discomfort associated with concurrent uveitis.

CONTRAINDICATIONS
• Topically applied corticosteroids are contraindicated in the presence of a corneal ulcer. • Megestrol acetate is contraindicated in sexually intact female cats or cats with marginal liver function. • Topically applied atropine is contraindicated in animals with glaucoma and lens luxation and is a relative contraindication for animals with KCS.

PRECAUTIONS
• Azathioprine can cause gastrointestinal signs, hepatotoxicity, and myelosuppression. • Megestrol acetate is not FDA approved for use in cats. Possible side-effects include polyphagia, transient diabetes mellitus, mammary hyperplasia, mammary neoplasia, and pyometra.

POSSIBLE INTERACTIONS N/A

ALTERNATE DRUGS N/A

FOLLOW-UP

PATIENT MONITORING
• Periodic ocular examination is recommended to evaluate efficacy of topically and systemically administered medications. Recheck examinations should be at 1 to 2-week intervals followed by gradual reduction with remission or resolution of signs.

PREVENTION/AVOIDANCE
For animals with chronic superficial keratitis, minimizing exposure to solar radiation may reduce severity of clinical signs.

POSSIBLE COMPLICATIONS
• Visual deficit or blindness is possible in animals with advanced chronic superficial keratitis, nodular granulomatous episclerokeratitis, pigmentary keratitis, KCS, eosinophilic keratitis, or herpetic keratitis. • Continued ocular discomfort is possible with herpetic keratitis or corneal sequestration. Ocular discomfort is minimal or variable with other conditions given in this chapter.

EXPECTED COURSE AND PROGNOSIS See client education

MISCELLANEOUS

ASSOCIATED CONDITIONS N/A

AGE RELATED FACTORS N/A

ZOONOTIC POTENTIAL N/A

PREGNANCY
Corticosteroids and azathioprine should be avoided or used cautiously in pregnant animals.

SYNONYMS

Dogs
• Chronic superficial keratitis is also called pannus, degenerative pannus, German shepherd pannus, chronic immune-mediated keratoconjunctivitis syndrome, and überreiter's syndrome. • Nodular granulomatous episclerokeratitis has also been called fibrous histiocytoma, nodular fasciitis, proliferative keratoconjunctivitis, collie granuloma, and pseudotumor. • Pigmentary keratitis is also called corneal pigmentation.

Cats
Corneal sequestration has been called corneal nigrum and corneal mummification.

SEE ALSO
• Corneal Degenerations and Infiltrations • Corneal Dystrophies • Episcleritis • Keratitis, Ulcerative • Keratoconjunctivitis sicca

ABBREVIATIONS
• IFA = immunofluorescent antibody • KCS = keratoconjunctivitis sicca

References

Chavkin MJ, Roberts SM, Salman MD, Severin GA, Scholten NJ. Risk factors for development of chronic superficial keratitis in dogs. J Am Vet Med Assoc 1994;204:1630–1634.

Paulsen ME, Lavach JD, Snyder SP, Severin GA, Eichenbaum JD. Nodular granulomatous episclerokeratitis in dogs: 19 cases (1973-1985). J Am Vet Med Assoc 1987;190:1581–1587.

Nasisse MP. Feline herpesvirus ocular disease. Vet Clin North Am Small Anim Pract 1990;20:667–680.

Paulsen ME, Lavach JD, Severin GA, Eichenbaum JD. Feline eosinophilic keratitis. A review of 15 clinical cases. J Am Anim Hosp Assoc 1987;23:63–69.

Pentlarge VW. Corneal sequestration in cats. Comp Cont Educ Pract Vet 1989;11:24–32.

Author B. Keith Collins
Consulting Editor Paul E. Miller

BASICS

DEFINITION
Inflammation of the cornea associated with loss of the corneal epithelium (corneal erosion) and, possibly, variable amounts of underlying corneal stroma (corneal ulcer). Because clinical distinction between an ulcer and the less severe corneal erosion is sometimes difficult, this chapter will refer to both disorders as ulcerative keratitis.

Pathophysiology
Any condition that disrupts the corneal epithelium or stroma may result in ulcerative keratitis. In dogs and cats, causes are both traumatic and nontraumatic. Ulcers can be classified as superficial or deep, uncomplicated or complicated. A superficial ulcer involves only the epithelium and possibly the superficial stroma. Deep ulcers involve a greater thickness of stroma and may extend to Descemet's membrane, which may cause the globe to rupture. Complicated ulcers occur with persistence of the inciting cause, microbial infection, or production of degradative enzymes.

After the occurrence of an epithelial wound, adjacent epithelial cells loosen and begin to migrate over the defect within a few hours. Mitosis occurs within a few days, normal epithelial thickness is restored, and the healing process is complete in 5-7 days.

Stromal wound healing is slower, more complex, and can occur in an avascular or vascular manner. If the stromal wound is relatively shallow, epithelial migration and mitosis may be sufficient to fill the defect. The epithelium can occasionally cover some stromal ulcers, even when epithelial and stromal regeneration are insufficient to restore normal corneal thickness. Such a nonulcerated, crater-like defect is called a facet. Most stromal ulcers heal by fibrovascular infiltration that may require several weeks. It is common for stromal ulcers to be complicated by microbial infection or enzymatic destruction initiated by corneal epithelial or stromal cells, host inflammatory cells, or microbial organisms.

Epithelial basement membrane disease (EBMD) delays healing of some superficial ulcers because it interferes with attachment of the regenerating epithelium to the underlying stroma. This results in a protracted clinical course and is referred to as a refractory ulcer (see synonyms).

Excessive enzymatic destruction may result in a tenacious or gelatinous appearance of the corneal stroma. This is termed a melting or collagenase ulcer.

Systems Affected Ophthalmic

Genetics
• No proven genetic basis, but breed predilections suggest that there may be genetic influences. • Ulcers may occur secondary to other corneal diseases that have breed predispositions and, presumably, a genetic basis. Examples include corneal epithelial dystrophy in the shetland sheepdog and corneal endothelial dystrophy in the Boston terrier.

Incidence/Prevalence
Common cause of eye disease in both dogs and cats

Geographic Distribution N/A

SIGNALMENT

Species Dogs and cats

Breed Predilections
• Brachycephalic breeds of dog • Refractory ulcers occur most often in the boxer but may occur in any breed. • Persian, Himalayan, Siamese, and Burmese cats are predisposed to feline corneal sequestration (see nonulcerative keratitis)

Mean Age and Range
• Age of onset is highly variable and is determined by the cause of the ulcer. • Refractory ulcers tend to affect middle-aged and older dogs.

Predominant Sex
No proven sex predilection

SIGNS

Historical Findings
• The condition may be acute or chronic.
• Client complaints range from tearing, squinting, and rubbing at the eyes to the appearance of a film over the eye (e.g., corneal edema and prolapsed third eyelid). • A history of trauma exists in some animals.
• Cats with herpetic ulcers may have a history of respiratory disease

Physical Examination Findings
• Nonspecific ocular findings may include serous to mucopurulent ocular discharge, blepharospasm, photophobia, nictitans prolapse, and conjunctival hyperemia (i.e., a red eye).
• Closer inspection of the cornea may reveal one or more circumscribed, linear, or geographic (map-like) defects in the cornea. Deep stromal ulcers or descemetoceles may appear as a crater-like defect. • Depending on the size, cause, and duration of the ulcer, additional pathologic findings may include neovascularization, pigmentation, edema, scarring, mineral or lipid deposition, inflammatory cell infiltrate, and collagenolytic activity (or melting) of the corneal stroma. This may cause focal to diffuse areas of corneal opacity. • Refractory ulcers have loose or redundant epithelial edges, and they may demonstrate undermining of fluorescein stain in areas with seemingly intact epithelium.
• In an otherwise normal eye, a corneal ulcer usually stimulates tear production, possibly resulting in overflow of tears onto the face (i.e., epiphora). The absence of obvious lacrimation suggest concurrent dry eye component or keratoconjunctivitis sicca (KCS).

• "Reflex anterior uveitis" that may be mild or severe occurs secondarily to corneal ulceration. Signs of concurrent uveitis may include variable pupil constriction (miosis) or reduced intraocular pressure when compared with the normal eye and possibly visible exudates in the anterior chamber (e.g., fibrin, hypopyon, and hyphema). Visible anterior chamber exudates are most common in animals with ulcers caused by penetrating corneal wounds or with concurrent bacterial infection. In the latter instance, the exudate is usually sterile and is a response to toxins elaborated by the microbial agent(s).

CAUSES
• Trauma—blunt, penetrating, or perforating • Adnexal disease—distichiasis, ectopic cilia, entropion, ectropion, trichiasis, eyelid mass. • Tear film abnormality—quantitative tear deficiency such as KCS, or qualitative tear deficiency caused by conjunctival goblet cell (or mucin) deficiency or some other unidentified tear abnormality. • Infection—primary corneal infection is most common in cats and is caused by herpesvirus. • Lagophthalmos (or inability to close the eyelids completely)—this results in exposure keratitis and drying. It may be breed-related in brachycephalic dogs and, to a lesser extent, in some cat breeds, or it may be caused by exophthalmos, buphthalmos, or neuroparalytic from idiopathic facial nerve paralysis (especially in cocker spaniels). • Innate corneal disease—EBMD, endothelial dystrophy, or other endothelial disease. • Miscellaneous—foreign body, chemical burns, neurotrophic keratitis (loss of trigeminal sensation), immune-mediated disease.

RISK FACTORS
• Trauma • KCS from any cause • Feline herpesvirus infection

DIAGNOSIS

DIFFERENTIAL DIAGNOSIS
• Fluorescein dye retention is diagnostic for ulcerative keratitis. • Other causes of a red and painful eye, notably conjunctivitis, KCS, uveitis, and glaucoma (see red eye chapter).
• Ulcerative keratitis may develop concurrently with other causes of a red eye (e.g., secondary to KCS).

CBC/BIOCHEMISTRY/URINALYSIS
Results usually normal

OTHER LABORATORY TESTS
Positive serologic test for feline herpesvirus may confirm the cause of a corneal ulcer in a cat, although a negative test result does not rule out herpesvirus infection. A titer > 1:100 is considered consistent with infection (Nasisse MP, personal communication, 1994).

IMAGING N/A

KERATITIS, ULCERATIVE

OTHER DIAGNOSTIC PROCEDURES

• Three fluorescein staining patterns are recognized: 1) superficial or stromal ulcers stain a homogenous green. Ulcers may be circular, irregular, linear, or any combination thereof. Interpretation of depth is subjective; 2) a "crater-like" defect that retains stain at the periphery and is clear at the center is a descemetocele. Descemet's membrane may be seen bulging anteriorly; 3) a "crater-like" defect that pools stain transiently but from which stain is rinsed easily indicates a previous stromal ulcer that has reepithelialized (facet). Such a defect must be distinguished from a descemetocele. • Application of rose bengal stain to the eye may facilitate diagnosis of superficial linear ulcers (dendritic ulcers) caused by herpesvirus. Dendritic ulcers are considered pathognomonic for herpesvirus infection in cats. • Microbial culture and susceptibility testing for aerobic bacteria and fungi is indicated in animals with rapidly progressive or deep corneal ulcers. • A Schirmer tear test identifies KCS-associated ulceration. • Cytologic evaluation of cells obtained by corneal scraping followed by Gram, Giemsa or Wright's staining may reveal microbial organisms. These results may direct initial antimicrobial therapy.

GROSS AND HISTOPATHOLOGIC FINDINGS N/A

TREATMENT

INPATIENT VERSUS OUTPATIENT
Animals with deep or rapidly progressive ulcers may require hospitalization for surgery and/or frequent medical treatments.

ACTIVITY
• Restrict if the animal has a deep stromal ulcer or descemetocele because a deep ulcer could rupture. • Self-trauma to the eye should be prevented. An Elizabethan collar should be applied if this is a problem.

DIET N/A

CLIENT EDUCATION
• If more than one ophthalmic solution is applied to the eye(s) for treatment, the client should allow at least 5 minutes between application of different drugs to prevent chemical incompatibility or dilutional factors from reducing treatment efficacy. • The client should be instructed to contact the veterinarian if the animal appears more painful or if the ulcer appears to be deteriorating.

SURGICAL CONSIDERATIONS
• Superficial ulcers do not usually require surgery if the inciting cause has been eliminated (e.g., the entropion repaired, the foreign body removed). Refractory ulcers are an exception. • Refractory ulcers should be debrided with a dry, sterile, cotton-tipped swab to remove loose epithelial edges after topical

anesthesia is applied. Additional procedures that may be beneficial include creating a nictitans flap, keratotomy, superficial keratectomy, and conjunctival flap surgery. The techniques of punctate or grid keratotomy are performed easily and are recommended as the first surgical procedure after corneal debridement. • An ulcer that extends to one-half or greater corneal thickness, and particularly to Descemet's membrane, may benefit from surgery. A descemetocele should be considered a surgical emergency. A variety of surgical procedures are described, but the author finds the rotational pedicle conjunctival flap to be the most versatile and amenable to use by the clinical practitioner. • Full-thickness corneal lacerations should be repaired immediately (refer to surgical text).

MEDICATIONS

DRUGS AND FLUIDS

Antibiotics
Topically applied antibiotics are indicated in the treatment of all corneal ulcers. The frequency of antibiotic application is determined both by the severity of the ulcer and by the preparation used. Ointments have a longer contact time and should be applied q6h-q12h, whereas solutions require more frequent application (e.g., 4, 6, or even 8 times daily), particularly in the initial treatment of complicated ulcers. Antibiotics commonly used include chloramphenicol, oxytetracycline/polymyxin B (Terramycin®), erythromycin, triple antibiotic, gentamicin, and tobramycin (Tobrex®). The combination of neomycin, polymyxin B, and bacitracin (i.e., triple antibiotic) is an excellent first choice for treatment because of its broad-spectrum of antimicrobial activity. Gentamicin and tobramycin are good choices for rapidly progressive ulcers in which Pseudomonas sp. or another gram-negative organism is suspected. For aminoglycoside-resistant Pseudomonas sp., a topically applied fluoroquinolone solution (Ciloxan®) is available.

Atropine
Atropine 1% ointment or solution is used to treat the "reflex anterior uveitis" that occurs with corneal ulcers. It should be used with enough frequency to cause mydriasis (usually q8h-q24h) followed by gradual reduction.

Antiviral Agents
Antiviral agents are indicated for treatment of herpetic ulcers in cats. Trifluridine (Viroptic®) or idoxuridine (Herplex®) solutions should be applied q4h-q6h until clinical response is observed and then at reduced frequency for 1-2 weeks after clinical signs have subsided.

Anticollagenolytic Agents
Acetylcysteine (Mucomyst®) has been used

most commonly for the treatment of melting ulcers, but its efficacy is controversial. The 20% stock solution can be diluted to 5-10% with artificial tears and applied every 2-4 hours. Alternatively, it can be mixed with antibiotics in the following manner: 5 mL 20% acetylcysteine, 2 mL gentamicin injection (50 mg/mL), and 8 mL artificial tear solution for a concentration of 0.6% gentamicin and 6.6% acetylcysteine.

Analgesic/Antiinflammatory Agents
Nonsteroidal antiinflammatory drugs (NSAID) may be indicated both for their anti-inflammatory and analgesic properties. Aspirin can be used in dogs (10-15 mg/kg q12h PO) and in cats judiciously (10 mg/kg PO q48h).

Contact Lenses
Therapeutic contact lenses act as a bandage to reduce both frictional irritation from the eyelids and pain sensation (available from The Cutting Edge, Ltd, Diamond Springs, CA 95619-9969, 1-800-468-2275.) They may also provide sustained drug release. Additional advantages include easy application with only topical anesthesia and continued visualization of the eye. They are of greatest benefit in treating refractory ulcers and can be used as an alternative to or in conjunction with surgery. Disadvantages include relatively high cost (about $13-$15/lens) and the fact that the contact lens can be displaced by the third eyelid. Contact lenses with different diameters (13.5-17.0 mm) and base curvature (8.5-9.0 mm) are available for use in different breeds. Contact lenses with a shorter radius of curvature (i.e., more curved) may provide a better fit for small-breed dogs.

CONTRAINDICATIONS
• Topically applied corticosteroids are contraindicated in a patient with a corneal erosion or ulcer. • Topically applied NSAID are contraindicated in the treatment of herpetic ulcers. • Topically applied atropine is contraindicated in animals with glaucoma and lens luxation and is a relative contraindication in those with KCS. • Topically applied cyclosporine is contraindicated in animals with distemper or herpesvirus-associated ulcers.

PRECAUTIONS
• Atropine should be used judiciously (if at all) in treating ulcers associated with KCS because atropine further compromises tear production. Schirmer tear tests should be performed if KCS is suspected as the cause of the ulcer, or periodic tear tests may be indicated if atropine is to be used for an extended period of time. • Topically applied NSAID such as flurbiprofen (Ocufen®) and diclofenac (Voltaren®) may delay corneal healing, but they do not potentiate enzymatic corneal destruction in the manner that corticosteroids will. • Topically applied cyclosporine (primarily used to treat KCS) can be used safely

in the presence of a corneal ulcer unless it is related to canine distemper or feline herpesvirus infection.

POSSIBLE INTERACTIONS N/A

ALTERNATE DRUGS
Some ophthalmologists use autologous plasma (collected in EDTA) in place of acetylcysteine as an anticollagenolytic agent. Keep refrigerated, avoid contamination, and discard after 48 hours.

FOLLOW-UP

PATIENT MONITORING
• The ulcerated eye(s) should be stained periodically with fluorescein solution to assess healing. Superficial ulcers should be restained in 3-5 days. • A superficial ulcer that persists for 7 days or longer suggests that either the inciting cause has not been eliminated or the patient has EBMD. In the latter instance, the eye should be treated as a refractory ulcer (see surgical considerations). • Deep stromal or rapidly progressive ulcers should be assessed every 1-2 days initially (if the patient is not hospitalized) until improvement is seen or the ulcer has stabilized. Many of these patients are hospitalized or go immediately to surgery.

PREVENTION/AVOIDANCE
• Lubricant ointment administration (e.g., Lacrilube®), permanent partial tarsorrhaphy surgery, or both may be helpful in preventing recurrent ulceration in brachycephalic dogs.
• Dogs with KCS-related ulcers require continued medical treatment of KCS or parotid duct transposition surgery to prevent continued ulceration. • Chronic or intermittent antiviral therapy may be necessary to prevent recurrent ulceration in cats with herpesvirus.

POSSIBLE COMPLICATIONS
Progressive corneal ulceration may result in rupture of the globe, endophthalmitis, secondary glaucoma, phthisis bulbi, and blindness. A blind and painful eye may require enucleation.

EXPECTED COURSE AND PROGNOSIS
• An uncomplicated superficial ulcer should usually heal in 5-7 days or about 1 mm/day.
• A refractory ulcer may persist for weeks or even months in spite of medical therapy. It will often heal within 2 weeks after punctate or grid keratotomy (see surgical considerations). • If the client elects medical therapy as the sole treatment for a deep corneal ulcer, several weeks may be required for fibrovascular infiltrate to reach the defect, and even then the ulcer does not always granulate satisfactorily. Continued deterioration of the ulcer and globe rupture are possible. • Surgical repair of a deep ulcer with a conjunctival flap frequently results in more comfort for the patient within a few days after surgery. If healing is uneventful, the conjunctival flap can often be removed in 4-6 weeks.

MISCELLANEOUS

ASSOCIATED CONDITIONS N/A

AGE-RELATED FACTORS N/A

ZOONOTIC POTENTIAL N/A

PREGNANCY N/A

SYNONYMS
Refractory ulcers are also called persistent corneal erosions, indolent ulcers, boxer ulcers, and recurrent erosions.

SEE ALSO
• Corneal Degenerations and Infiltrations
• Corneal Dystrophies
• Keratitis, Nonulcerative
• Keratoconjunctivitis Sicca
• Red Eye

ABBREVIATIONS
• EBMD = epithelial/basement membrane disease
• KCS = keratoconjunctivitis sicca
• NSAID = nonsteroidal antiinflammatory drugs

References

Nasisse MP. Canine ulcerative keratitis. Comp Cont Educ Pract Vet 1985;7:686–701.

Kirschner SE. Persistent corneal ulcers: What to do when ulcers won't heal. Vet Clin North Am Small Anim Pract 1990;20:627–642.

Collins BK. Diseases of the globe: cornea and sclera. In: Bojrab MJ, ed. Disease mechanisms in small animal surgery. 2nd ed. Philadelphia: Lea & Febiger, 1993;130–138.

Hakanson NE, Merideth RE. Conjunctival pedicle grafting in the treatment of corneal ulcers in the dog and cat. J Am Anim Hosp Assoc 1987;23:641–648.

Author B. Keith Collins
Consulting Editor Paul E. Miller

KERATOCONJUNCTIVITIS SICCA (KCS)

BASICS

OVERVIEW
A deficiency of aqueous tear film resulting in drying and inflammation of the cornea and conjunctiva.

SIGNALMENT
• Very common in dogs; much rarer in cats.
• Many breeds of dogs are predisposed, including the cocker spaniel, bulldog, West Highland white terrier, lhaso apso, and shih tzu. • Inheritance is not defined. • Age of onset depends on the inciting cause. • Some studies report females are predisposed.

SIGNS
Cats tend to be less symptomatic than dogs:
• Blepharospasm • Conjunctival hyperemia
• Chemosis • Prominent nictitans
• Mucoid to mucopurulent ocular discharge
• Corneal changes, including superficial vascularization, pigmentation, and ulceration, in animals with chronic disease • Impaired or loss of vision if superficial keratitis becomes severe

CAUSES AND RISK FACTORS
• Immunologic—most common cause is immune-mediated adenitis, which is often associated with other immune-mediated diseases, such as atopy • Congenital—pug and Yorkshire terrier • Neurogenic—occasionally seen after traumatic proptosis or neurologic disease that interrupts innervation of the lacrimal gland • Drug-induced—general anesthesia and atropine cause transient reduction in tear production • Drug toxicity— some sulfa-containing drugs such as trimethoprim and sulfamethoxazole can cause transient or permanent KCS in some animals; also associated with 5-aminosalicylic acid and phenazopyridine • Iatrogenic—removal of the nictitans gland may predispose animal to KCS; especially true of at-risk breeds
• Radiotherapy— when the periocular area is in or near the primary beam • Systemic disease—canine distemper virus or any debilitating disease • Chronic conjunctivitis—occasionally seen in cats with chronic herpes or chlamydia conjunctivitis • Chronic blepharoconjunctivitis in dogs • Breed-related predisposition

DIAGNOSIS

DIFFERENTIAL DIAGNOSIS
KCS is often confused with bacterial conjunctivitis. Most dogs with chronic KCS have secondary bacterial overgrowth. Differentiate by use of the Schirmer tear test.

CBC/BIOCHEMISTRY/URINALYSIS
N/A

OTHER BLOOD TESTS N/A

IMAGING N/A

OTHER DIAGNOSTIC PROCEDURES
• Decreased Schirmer Tear test is diagnostic. Normal value in dogs is at least 15 mm/minute of wetting. Most animals that are symptomatic have Schirmer tear test values below 10 mm/min of wetting.
• Fluorescein staining should be performed to evaluate for corneal ulceration. • Bacterial culture and sensitivity testing may be indicated if initial treatment is unsuccessful; however, since most animals with chronic KCS have bacterial overgrowth, cultures are not routinely recommended. • Cytologic examination of conjunctiva may indicate the nature and degree of bacterial overgrowth.

TREATMENT

• Treat on an out-patient basis, unless secondary disease such as ulcerative keratitis is identified.
• Clean eyes before instilling medication.
• Instruct owners to keep the animal's eyes and periocular area clean and free of dried discharge.
• Advise owners that if the animal experiences an increase in ocular pain, they should call at once, because animals with KCS are predisposed to severe corneal ulceration.
• Parotid duct transposition is a surgical procedure whereby the parotid duct is rerouted to deliver saliva to the inferior cul-de-sac. This procedure is performed much less frequently since cyclosporine was introduced. Saliva is often irritating to the cornea, and some animals are uncomfortable after this surgery.

MEDICATIONS

DRUGS AND FLUIDS

• Cyclosporine A is the drug of choice for treating KCS in dogs. It is most effective in the immune-mediated type of KCS, and one study showed it to be effective in promoting lacrimation in 80% of animals. It can be used as a 2% or 1% solution, q12h initially, and then q12h or q24h thereafter depending on response.

• Topically or orally administered pilocarpine is occasionally effective in improving lacrimation via direct stimulation of the gland. It is given as 1-2 drops on food q12h, or in the affected eye q12h. Generally, a 1% or 2% solution is used.

• Artificial tears and lubricant ointments help moisten the cornea but must be used frequently, and they only transiently relieve drying.

• Topically applied, broad-spectrum antibiotics, either in the form of solutions or ointments, are indicated frequently in the initial treatment of a dog with chronic KCS and secondary bacterial overgrowth. Once the bacterial overgrowth is controlled and tear production improved, antibiotics are not indicated.

• Topically applied corticosteroids were frequently used in animals with KCS before cyclosporine use. They minimize inflammation and are effective in reducing corneal vascularization and pigmentation. Because cyclosporine serves these functions without the risk of exacerbating a corneal ulcer, corticosteroids are used less frequently to treat KCS.

• Mucolytic agents such as acetylcysteine are occasionally used to help break up tenacious mucous discharge. Mucolytics add significantly to the cost of treatment and are rarely indicated once tear production has improved.

CONTRAINDICATIONS/POSSIBLE INTERACTIONS

• Topically applied cyclosporine is irritating in some animals.

• Topically applied pilocarpine is initially irritating; however, animals seem to develop a tolerance.

• Orally administered pilocarpine causes vomiting and diarrhea in some animals.

• Topically applied corticosteroids should be avoided in animals with ulcerative keratitis.

FOLLOW-UP

• Patients should be rechecked at regular intervals to monitor response and progress. Schirmer tear test should be performed 4-6 weeks after initiating cyclosporine to evaluate response (the animal should have received the drug the day of the visit). • Most animals with immune-mediated KCS will need lifelong treatment. Other types of KCS may be transient (e.g., post-anesthesia), and treatment need only continue until tear production returns.

MISCELLANEOUS

ABBREVIATIONS

• KCS = keratoconjunctivitis sicca
• PDT = parotid duct transposition
• STT = Schirmer tear test

Reference

Gelatt KN. Veterinary ophthalmology. 2nd ed. Philadelphia: Lea & Febiger, 1991.
Author Erin S. Champagne
Consulting Editor Paul E. Miller

LARYNGEAL DISEASE

BASICS

DEFINITION
The term laryngeal disease suggests the presence of a disease process that alters normal structure and, usually, function of the larynx.

Pathophysiology
A variety of signs are seen depending upon the cause and severity of the resulting laryngeal dysfunction. With severe obstruction to laryngeal airflow, hyperpyrexia and heat prostration become potential complications; the syndrome of air hunger (i.e., hypoventilation, hypoxemia) may result in retching, vomiting, aspiration pneumonia, and even respiratory or cardiac arrest.

Systems Affected
• Respiratory—as a result of interference with air/oxygen delivery to the alveoli (i.e., hypoventilation). Other respiratory complications include aspiration pneumonia and even pulmonary edema in some dogs. • Gastrointestinal—as a result of retching and vomiting secondary to severe hypoxemia
• Cardiovascular and nervous—as a result of hyperpyrexia and heat prostration

Genetics
Laryngeal Paralysis
• Hereditary laryngeal paralysis has been reported in the Bouvier des Flandres (autosomal dominant trait) and in the Siberian husky and husky mixed breeds (mode of inheritance under study). Dalmations may show laryngeal paralysis as part of generalized polyneuropathy syndrome. • The acquired form is overrepresented by certain giant (i.e., Saint Bernard, Newfoundland) and large (Irish setters, Labrador and golden retriever) breeds of dogs; however, no genetic studies have been reported. • No genetic studies have been reported in cats.

Incidence/Prevalence
Laryngeal Paralysis
• High incidence of hereditary forms • Fairly high prevalence, undefined incidence of acquired (i.e., idiopathic) form • Extremely rare in the cat
Laryngeal Trauma
Rare in both the dog and cat
Laryngeal Tumors
• Both primary and as part of a generalized neoplastic process are rare in dogs • More common in domestic cats, but incidence is poorly defined

Geographic Distribution N/A

SIGNALMENT

Species Dogs and cats

Breed Predilections See genetics.

Mean Age and Range
Laryngeal Paralysis
• In the hereditary form, variant signs first appear at 4-8 months of age. • In the idio-

pathic form, clinical signs develop between 2 and 12 years of age (mean ranges from 9-12 years in various reports). • Too few cases have been reported in cats to provide meaningful statistics, although it usually occurs in old cats.
Laryngeal Neoplasia
Middle-aged to old dogs and cats are affected.

Predominant Sex
Laryngeal Paralysis
• In the hereditary form, a 3:1 male predominance is reported. • In the idiopathic form, a small to moderate male predominance is reported.

SIGNS

General Comments
Clinical signs appear to be directly related to the degree of impairment on laryngeal airflow imposed by the laryngeal disease process.

Historical Findings
• The most common signs reported include change in character of bark or meow, occasional coughing, reduced activity, exercise intolerance, and abnormal breathing sounds with exertion and/or stress. • Other signs occurring under exertion and/or stress or heat may include severely difficult breathing, gagging/retching, vomiting, weakness/lethargy, collapse, and even sudden death.

Physical Examination Findings
• Noisy respiration and a high pitched inspiratory sound, (i.e., stridor) are the most common abnormalities on patient presentation. In cats, the inspiratory stridor is less characteristic than in dogs. • Upper airway sounds are referred over the trachea and to hilar lung fields, bilaterally. • If aspiration has occurred, focal or bilateral rales may be auscultated.
• In most affected animals, the rectal temperature is elevated.

CAUSES
Laryngeal Paralysis
• Congenital • The idiopathic form has been ascribed variously to hormonal deficiencies (i.e., hypothyroidism), central or peripheral vagal nerve abnormalities, cervical trauma, abnormalities involving the recurrent laryngeal nerves, generalized peripheral neuropathies, myopathies, and other immune-mediated disorders. • Thyroid adenocarcinoma can cause impingement on or invasion of recurrent laryngeal nerves.
Laryngeal Trauma
• Penetrating (i.e., bite wounds) or blunt neck trauma • Injury secondary to ingested foreign materials (i.e., bones, sticks, needles, pins, etc.)
Laryngeal Neoplasia
• Squamous cell adenocarcinoma is the most common laryngeal tumor in dogs. Other reported tumors include leiomyoma, rhabdomyosarcoma, osteosarcoma, hemangiosarcoma, mast-cell tumors, and lymphosarcoma.
• In cats, squamous cell adenocarcinoma and lymphosarcoma occur with nearly equal frequency, but both are quite rare.

RISK FACTORS
• See causes above for various systemic disorders that may play a role in predisposition to idiopathic laryngeal paralysis. • Concomitant pulmonary abnormalities

DIAGNOSIS

DIFFERENTIAL DIAGNOSIS
• Laryngeal collapse is a potential complication of long-standing brachycephalic syndrome and, rarely, laryngeal paralysis. There is a noisy, obstructed breathing pattern but absence of inspiratory stridor resulting from the presence of other obstructing structures. Clinical signs in a brachycephalic breed make laryngeal collapse a more likely possibility, but a complete laryngeal examination under heavy sedation must be carried out to confirm the diagnosis. • Chronic proliferative, pyogranulomatoius laryngitis can cause a mass lesion requiring surgical removal, histopathologic examination, and tapered administration of corticosteroids. • Obstructing processes involving the trachea and the tracheobronchial junction frequently mimic laryngeal diseases on physical examination. Potential causes include tracheal collapse (i.e., tracheomalacia), as well as intraluminal and peritracheal masses.

CBC/BIOCHEMISTRY/URINALYSIS
There may be a high white blood cell count with a left shift when aspiration pneumonia has complicated the laryngeal disorders. Otherwise, the hemogram, serum chemistry profile, and urinalysis usually are normal.

OTHER LABORATORY TESTS
• Arterial blood gas analysis defines the presence of hypoxemia and respiratory acidosis. • Whereas hypothyroidism has been suggested as a cause for idiopathic laryngeal paralysis, and thyroid testing is routinely performed, less than 10% of dogs we have seen with this condition are hypothyroid. The few dogs in which we have attempted thyroid replacement have not shown improvement in laryngeal function.

IMAGING
• Routine imaging procedures are of little benefit in primary diagnostics, but radiography, fluoroscopy, and bronchoscopy are useful in ruling out the differential diagnoses and evaluating patients for the presence of aspiration pneumonia. • Barium swallow with or without fluoroscopy should be performed in each dog with laryngeal dysfunction in which occasional vomiting is reported in the history. A low incidence (i.e., < 10 %) of esophageal motor dysfunction is present in dogs with idiopathic laryngeal paralysis.

OTHER DIAGNOSTIC PROCEDURES
• Visual inspection of the larynx with a laryngoscope under heavy sedation or anesthesia is required for proper evaluation of a patient

with laryngeal disease. The use of even light barbiturate anesthesia makes evaluation of laryngeal function difficult in the dog with laryngeal paralysis; therefore, the use of acepromazine (0.033 mg/kg IM or SQ) is recommended. In cats, the use of ketamine HCl (6-10 mg/kg IV) alone, ketamine HCl (3-5 mg/kg) in combination with diazepam (0.1-0.2 mg/kg) or Telazol (9-12 mg/kg IM or SC) provides sedation without interfering with laryngeal function. • Electromyography (EMG) studies define the presence of partial or complete denervation—denervation potentials (fibrillation and/or positive waves) with or without pseudomyotonia.

GROSS AND HISTOPATHOLOGIC FINDINGS

• Gross abnormalities include redness and swelling of the mucosa over the arytenoid cartilages and the vocal folds. • Histopathologic findings encompass inflammation and edema of the perilaryngeal mucous membranes and denervation atrophy of the laryngeal muscles that were examined.

TREATMENT

INPATIENT VERSUS OUTPATIENT

• Stable patients can be managed as outpatients while awaiting surgery.
• Patients with significant respiratory distress should be managed as an emergency with either emergency tracheotomy and/or oxygen therapy combined with sedation and corticosteroids (dexamethasone sodium phosphate, 1-2 mg/kg, IV, then 0.5-1.0 mg/kg SQ, q12h for 24 hours then 0.2 mg/kg SQ q12h in tapering doses).

ACTIVITY

Severe restriction in patients pending surgery or in those in which the owner refuses surgery

DIET N/A

CLIENT EDUCATION

• Discuss potential complications of heat prostration, aspiration pneumonia, and asphyxia if surgery is not pursued. Also discuss the improved quality of life and normal life expectancy with successful surgery.
• Discuss the hereditability of the congenital forms of laryngeal paralysis.
• Increased risk for aspiration pneumonia after surgery

SURGICAL CONSIDERATIONS

Laryngeal Paralysis

• Surgical management is the treatment of choice.
• Variety of procedures reported; efficacy of any one procedure depends on the surgeon's experience and expertise, and perhaps other minor factors

Laryngeal Trauma

Temporary tracheotomy may be life saving and curative

Laryngeal Neoplasia

• Tumor excision with or without modified surgery to enlarge the laryngeal airway may be curative in dogs with certain neoplasms.
• For squamous cell adenocarcinoma, surgical excision coupled with radiation therapy is the management of choice.
• Tonsillar lymphosarcoma responds to chemotherapy.
• Permanent tracheostomy may improve quality of life.

MEDICATIONS

DRUGS AND FLUIDS

Dogs with idiopathic laryngeal paralysis in which surgery is declined by the owner may benefit from the use of mild sedatives (i.e., acepromazine, promazine, or diazepam) and corticosteroids (prednisone 2.2 mg/kg divided q12h initially, then gradually reduce to alternate-day therapy).

CONTRAINDICATIONS N/A

PRECAUTIONS

• Heavy sedation without a tracheotomy in a hot environment may predispose to heat prostration.
• Chronic use of corticosteroids may predispose patients to gastric ulcerations and susceptible dogs and cats to diabetes mellitus and systemic and/or focal infections.

POSSIBLE INTERACTIONS N/A

ALTERNATE DRUGS N/A

FOLLOW-UP

PATIENT MONITORING

• Reexamination of larynx is recommended 3-4 weeks postoperatively. • Arterial blood gases should show normalization postoperatively. • Improvement in activity and exercise tolerance is reported by owner after surgery.

PREVENTION/AVOIDANCE

Dogs with inheritable laryngeal paralysis should not be used for breeding

POSSIBLE COMPLICATIONS

• Recurrence of clinical signs with tumor regrowth or with inadequate surgery for laryngeal paralysis • Laryngeal web formation in dogs that had bilateral vocal cord resection as a surgical procedure (transect and treat with tapered corticosterioids) • Increased risk of aspiration pneumonia after any of the laryngeal surgical protocols

EXPECTED COURSE AND PROGNOSIS

Laryngeal Paralysis

• Long-term prognosis good to excellent with

successful surgery. • Additional surgery may improve prognosis if initial surgery was unsatisfactory.

Laryngeal Trauma

Most patients progress satisfactorily with conservative management, even after emergency tracheotomy

Laryngeal Neoplasia

• Prognosis is poor in both dogs and cats with squamous cell adenocarcinoma, even with radiation therapy. • Prognosis in cats with lymphosarcoma is variable, depending upon the chemotherapy used and patient responsiveness.

MISCELLANEOUS

ASSOCIATED CONDITIONS

• Cervical masses, notably thyroid adenocarcinoma, may be present (see causes). • A low incidence of generalized esophageal motor dysfunction is present in dogs with idiopathic laryngeal paralysis, suggesting a polyneuropathy.

AGE RELATED FACTORS

Onset of clinical signs within the first year of life with the hereditary form of laryngeal paralysis

ZOONOTIC POTENTIAL N/A

PREGNANCY

Increased risk in those animals experiencing clinical signs of laryngeal dysfunction

SYNONYMS N/A

SEE ALSO

• Brachycephalic Airway Syndrome
• Tracheal Collapse • Stertor and Stridor

ABBREVIATIONS N/A

References

Venker-van Haagen AJ. Laryngeal disease of dogs and cats. In: Kirk RW, ed. Current veterinary therapy IX. Philadelphia: WB Saunders, 1986.

Venker-van Haagen AJ. Diseases of the larynx. Vet Clin North Am. Vol. 22. Philadelphia: WB Saunders, 1992.

Harvey CE. The larynx. In: Bojrab MJ, ed. Pathophysiology In small animal surgery. Philadelphia: Lea & Febiger, 1981.

Ford RB. Noninfectious diseases of the upper respiratory tract. In: Sherding RG, ed. The cat. Diseases and clinical management. New York: Churchill Livingstone, 1989.

Author Neil K. Harpster

Consulting Editors Lynelle Johnson and Bradley L. Moses

LEAD POISONING

BASICS

DEFINITION
Intoxication (blood lead > 0.4 ppm) due to either acute or chronic ingestion of some form of lead.

Pathophysiology
• Lead interacts with sulfhydryl groups and interferes with numerous enzymes, including those involved in heme synthesis. This causes fragility and reduced survival of RBC. Reticulocytes and nucleated RBC are released from the bone marrow. Inhibition of 5-pyrimidine nucleotidase causes retention of RNA degradation products and aggregation of ribosomes (ie, basophilic stippling).
• Damage to CNS capillaries may account for brain lesions. A weaker blood-brain barrier in young animals may permit more lead to reach the brain.

Systems Affected
• Hemic/Lymph/Immune—interference with hemoglobin synthesis • Gastrointestinal—unknown mechanism • Nervous—capillary damage and possible direct toxic effect • Renal/Urologic—damage to proximal renal tubule cells

Genetics N/A

Incidence/Prevalence
• Incidence in pets is unknown. • Less prevalent in dogs due to elimination of sources. • More prevalent in cats because of increased awareness and better diagnosis. • Higher number of cases during warm months of the year.

Geographic Distribution
Low socioeconomic status of the pet-owning family is associated with high blood lead concentration in pets.

SIGNALMENT

Species
Dogs commonly affected, followed by cats.

Breed Predilections N/A

Mean Age and Range
Mainly dogs <1 year old

Predominant Sex N/A

SIGNS

General Comments
• Primarily gastrointestinal and neurologic. Gastrointestinal signs often precede CNS signs. • CNS signs occur more often with acute exposure to lead. • Gastrointestinal signs predominate in animals with chronic, low-level exposure. • History of renovation of older home or ingestion of lead objects

Gastrointestinal Signs
• Vomiting • Diarrhea • Anorexia
• Abdominal pain

CNS Signs
• Lethargy • Hysteria • Seizures • Blindness

CAUSES
Ingestion of some form of lead:
• Paint and paint residue or dust from sanding • Car battery • Linoleum • Solder
• Plumbing materials and supplies • Lubricating compound • Putty • Tar paper
• Lead foil • Golf ball • Improperly glazed ceramic food or water bowl • Lead object (eg, shot, fishing sinkers, and drapery weight)

RISK FACTORS
• Age <1 year • Living in economically depressed areas • Living in old home or building that is being renovated

DIAGNOSIS

DIFFERENTIAL DIAGNOSIS

Dogs
• Canine distemper • Infectious encephalitides • Bromethalin or methylxanthine toxicosis • Nonsteroidal anti-inflammatory toxicity • Heat stroke • Intestinal parasitism • Intussusception • Pancreatitis • Infectious canine hepatitis

Cats
• Degenerative or storage disease • Hepatic encephalopathy • Infectious encephalitides • Organophosphate poisoning

CBC/BIOCHEMISTRY/URINALYSIS
• 5-40 nucleated RBC/100 WBC without anemia • Anisocytosis, polychromasia, poikilocytosis, target cells, hypochromasia. • Basophilic stippling of RBC • Absence of RBC changes does not rule out lead poisoning. • Neutrophilic leukocytosis • Results of urinalysis indicative of mild, non-specific renal damage

OTHER LABORATORY TESTS
• Antemortem whole blood lead and postmortem liver or kidney lead concentration. Blood lead concentration ≥ 0.4 ppm (40 mcg/dl) or liver/ kidney concentration > 5 ppm (wet weight) indicates lead poisoning. Lower concentration must be interpreted in conjunction with history and clinical signs. Blood lead concentration does not correlate with occurrence or severity of clinical signs.
• CaNa₂EDTA mobilization test requires two 24-hour urine samples. A 24-hour urine sample is collected, CaNa₂EDTA is administered (75 mg/kg IM), and a second 24-hr urine sample is collected. Post-EDTA urine lead increases 10- to 60-fold in animals with lead toxicity.

IMAGING
Radiopaque material in gastrointestinal tract, but presence or absence does not rule in or rule out lead poisoning

OTHER DIAGNOSTIC PROCEDURES
N/A

GROSS AND HISTOPATHOLOGIC FINDINGS
• Generally, no gross findings. Paint chips or lead object in the gastrointestinal tract in some animals. • Intranuclear inclusion bodies in hepatocytes or renal tubule epithelial cells in some animals. Inclusion bodies are an intracellular storage form of lead considered pathognomonic for lead poisoning.

TREATMENT

INPATIENT VS OUTPATIENT
Inpatient for first course of chelation, depending on the severity of clinical signs. Orally administered chelators for outpatient treatment .

ACTIVITY N/A

DIET N/A

CLIENT EDUCATION
Inform the client of potential adverse human health effects of lead. Public health officials should be notified and the source of lead determined.

SURGICAL PROCEDURES
Remove lead objects from the gastrointestinal tract.

MEDICATIONS

DRUGS AND FLUIDS
• Evacuate the gastrointestinal tract with saline cathartics such as sodium sulfate (2 to 25 gm in dogs and 2 to 5 gm in cats PO as 20% solution or less). Gastric or enterogastric lavage may be indicated. • Seizures controlled with diazepam (0.25 to 0.5 mg/kg IV; repeat if necessary) or phenobarbital (dosage IV to effect). In addition, mannitol (1 to 2 gm/kg IV slow infusion over 30 min) and dexamethasone (5 to 8 mg/kg IV) may alleviate CNS signs. • Lead body burden is reduced with CaNa₂EDTA (dogs and cats, 25 mg/kg SQ q6h for 5 days). CaNa₂EDTA should be diluted to a 1% solution with 5% dextrose in water before administration. Animals with blood lead concentrations of 1 ppm or greater will most likely need multiple treatments. Five-day rest periods should separate treatments.

CONTRAINDICATIONS
• EDTA should not be administered to animals with renal impairment or anuria. Urine flow should be established before administration. • D-penicillamine should not be given if there is lead in the gastrointestinal tract

(increases absorption). Succimer does not increase gastrointestinal absorption of lead.

PRECAUTIONS N/A

POSSIBLE INTERACTIONS N/A

ALTERNATE DRUGS

Alternatives to CaNa$_2$EDTA include:
• D-penicillamine (8 mg/kg, PO, q6h for 7 to 14 days). Multiple treatments should be separated by 7-day rest periods. • Succimer, a new orally administered chelating agent, may become the future drug of choice (10 mg/kg PO, q8h for 5 days followed by 10 mg/kg PO, q12h for 2 weeks). Extended treatment should be separated by a 2-week rest period.

 FOLLOW-UP

PATIENT MONITORING

Blood lead should be < 0.4 ppm. Assay blood lead 10 to 14 days after chelation.

PREVENTION/AVOIDANCE

Determine source of lead and remove it from the pet's environment.

POSSIBLE COMPLICATIONS

Permanent neurologic signs (eg, blindness) occasionally

EXPECTED COURSE AND PROGNOSIS

• Signs should dramatically improve within 24 to 48 hours of initiating chelation.
• Prognosis is favorable in treated animals.
• Uncontrolled seizures warrant a guarded prognosis.

 MISCELLANEOUS

ASSOCIATED CONDITIONS N/A

AGE RELATED FACTORS

Dogs <1 year of age more likely to be poisoned

ZOONOTIC POTENTIAL

None. However, humans in the same environment may be at risk for exposure.

PREGNANCY

Transplacental passage may cause neonatal poisoning. Lead mobilized from bone during lactation is unlikely to poison nursing animals.

SYNONYMS

Plumbism

SEE ALSO

Poisoning (Intoxication)

ABBREVIATIONS

CNS = central nervous system
RBC = red blood cells
RNA = ribonucleic acid
WBC = white blood cells

References

Braton R, Kowalczyk D. Lead poisoning. In: Kirk R, ed. Current veterinary therapy X. Philadephia: WB Saunders, 1989.

Morgan RV. Lead poisoning in small companion animals: An update: (1987-1992). Vet Hum Toxicol 1994;36:18.

Morgan RV, et al. Demographic data and treatment of small companion animals with lead poisoning: 347 cases (1977-1986). J Am Vet Med Assoc 1991;199:98.

Morgan RV, et al. Clinical and laboratory findings in small companion animals with lead poisoning: 347 cases (1977-1986) J Am Vet Med Assoc 1991;199:93.

VanAlstine WG, et al. Acute lead toxicosis in a household of cats. J Vet Diagn Invest 1993;5:496.

Author Robert H. Poppenga
Consulting Editor G. Osweiler

LEGG-CALVÉ-PERTHES DISEASE

BASICS

DEFINITION
Legg-Calvé-Perthes Disease (LCPD) is a spontaneous degeneration of the femoral head and neck leading to collapse of the coxofemoral joint and osteoarthritis

Pathophysiology
The precise cause of LCPD is unknown. Histologic evidence points to infarction of vessels serving the proximal femur. Necrosis of subchondral bone leads to collapse and deformation of the femoral head during normal loading. The articular cartilage becomes thickened with cleft development and fraying of superficial layers. Although a specific vascular lesion has not been identified, the simultaneous processes of osseous degeneration and repair seen in LCPD are characteristic of ischemia and revascularization of bone.

Systems Affected
Musculoskeletal—Legg-Calvé-Perthes disease causes hind limb lameness that is insidious in onset

Genetics
• The Manchester terrier exhibits a multifactorial inheritance pattern with a high degree of heritability of LCPD. • A hereditary predispostion is considered likely in dogs with this disease.

Incidence and Prevalence
Although LCPD is a common orthopedic disease among small dogs, no accurate estimates of incidence/prevalence are available.

Geographic Distribution N/A

SIGNALMENT

Species Dogs

Breed Predilections
Toy breeds and terriers are most susceptible. Manchester terriers, miniature pinschers, toy poodles, Lakeland terriers, West Highland white terriers, and cairn terriers have a higher than expected incidence of LCPD.

Mean Age and Range
Most affected dogs are 5-8 months of age with a range of 3-13 months.

Predominant Sex
Both sexes appear to be equally susceptible.

SIGNS

GENERAL COMMENTS
Legg-Calvé-Perthes disease is usually a unilateral problem with only 12-16% biltateral.

Historical Findings
Lameness usually has a gradual onset over a 2-3 month period. It is a weight-bearing lameness with occasional periods when the leg is carried. There is no history of significant trauma.

Physical Examination Findings
Pain on manipulation of the hip is the prima-ry physical finding. Crepitation of the joint is inconsistent, but atrophy of the thigh muscles is nearly always present. The physical examination is otherwise normal.

CAUSES
The cause of LCPD is not known, but tamponade of the intracapsular, subsynovial vessels serving the femoral head is a suggested cause of ischemia leading to the pathologic changes.

RISK FACTORS
• Toy and miniature breeds are at increased risk. • Trauma to the hip region

DIAGNOSIS

DIFFERENTIAL DIAGNOSIS
Medial patellar luxation (which can occur independently) is the primary differential diagnosis of LCPD in the young dog. In older dogs with chronic LCPD, rupture of the cranial cruciate ligament is the primary rule out.

CBC/BIOCHEMISTRY/URINALYSIS
• Hematology—normal • Clinical chemistries—normal • Urinalysis—normal

OTHER LABORATORY TESTS N/A

IMAGING
Early radiographic changes include widening of the joint space, decreased bone density of the epiphysis, and sclerosis and thickening of the femoral neck. Later, there are lucent areas within the femoral head. Flattening and extreme deformation of the femoral head and severe osteoarthritis are endstage changes of LCPD.

OTHER DIAGNOSTIC PROCEDURES
Orthopedic examination and radiography are used to confirm the diagnosis.

GROSS AND HISTOPATHOLOGIC FINDINGS
The femoral head removed during femoral head and neck excision is usually deformed with a thickened irregular articular surface. Early LPD is characterized histologically by loss of lacunar osteocytes and necrosis of marrow elements. At the same time, granulation tissue surrounds trabeculae. Later, metaphyseal trabeculare thicken and there is a mixture of necrosis and repair tissue typical of revascularization of bone. Advanced changes include osteoclastic activity and new bone formation.

TREATMENT

One patient was successfully managed with an Ehmer sling, which was maintained for 10 weeks. Unfortunately, the insidious onset of LCPD will frequently prevent early recognition and conservative treatment. Femoral head and neck excision with early and vigor-ous exercise after surgery is the treatment of choice for LCPD. Conservative treatment consisting of rest and analgesics reportedly is successful in alleviating signs of lameness in a minority of patients.

INPATIENT VERSUS OUTPATIENT
Surgical patients are hospitalized for 1-3 days after surgery.

ACTIVITY
Early activity after surgery is encouraged to improve limb use. When conservative therapy is chosen, restricted activity is recommended.

DIET
There are no special dietary requirements for treating LCPD, but avoidance of obesity is beneficial.

CLIENT EDUCATION
Owners of Manchester terriers should be aware of the genetic basis of LCPD in that breed and the inadvisability of breeding affected dogs.

SURGICAL CONSIDERATIONS
Femoral head and neck excision is the treatment of choice for LCPD.

MEDICATIONS

DRUGS AND FLUIDS
Nonsteroidal antiinflammatory drugs (NSAIDs) can be used pre- or postoperatively to minimize joint pain and reduce synovitis. Aspirin, buffered or enteric coated (10-25 mg/kg PO q8h or q12h); phenylbutazone (3-7 mg/kg PO q8h, total dose < 800 mg/day); meclofenemic acid (0.5 mg/kg PO q12h; and piroxicam (0.3 mg/kg PO q24h for 3 days then every other day) are commonly used.

CONTRAINDICATIONS
Intolerance to NSAIDs is indicated by gastrointestinal upset and may preclude their use in individual patients.

PRECAUTIONS
• Inhibition of platelet activity by NSAIDs may increase hemorrhage at surgery. Aspirin should be discontinued at least 1 week before surgery if possible.
• Most NSAIDs cause some degree of gastric ulceration.
• Acetaminophen is unsuitable as an analgesic because of its potential for toxicity.

POSSIBLE INTERACTIONS
NSAIDs should not be used in conjunction with glucocorticoids because of risk of gastrointestinal tract ulceration.

ALTERNATE DRUGS
Chondroprotective drugs such as polysulfated glycosaminoglycans have little use once advance disease is present. There is no evidence to suggest that these drugs will prevent the disease.

FOLLOW-UP

PATIENT MONITORING

• Postsurgical progress checks (at 2-week intervals) are necessary to ensure patient compliance with exercise recommendations.
• Patients selected for conservative therapy should be reevaluated (physical exam, radiographs) to determine if surgery is needed.

PREVENTION/AVOIDANCE

• Breeding of affected animals is to be discouraged. • Dam/sire breedings that result in LCPD should not be repeated.

POSSIBLE COMPLICATIONS

Limiting postoperative exercise after femoral head and neck excision may result in less than optimal limb use.

EXPECTED COURSE AND PROGNOSIS

With surgery (FHNE), the prognosis for full recovery is good to excellent (84-100% success rate). Conservative therapy is reported to alleviate lameness after 2-3 months in about 25% of affected dogs.

MISCELLANEOUS

ASSOCIATED CONDITIONS N/A

AGE RELATED FACTORS

Although LCPD affects juvenile, small-breed dogs, older dogs may be affected by chronic LCPD.

ZOONOTIC POTENTIAL N/A

PREGNANCY N/A

SYNONYMS

• Perthes disease • Coxa plana • Coxa magna
• Avascular necrosis of the femoral head
• Aseptic necrosis of the femoral head
• Osteochondritis juvenilis

SEE ALSO N/A

ABBREVIATIONS

LCPD = Legg-Calvé-Perthes disease
NSAID = nonsteroidal antiinflammatory drug

References

Smith MM. Perthes disease. In: Slatter DH, ed. Textbook of small animal surgery. 2nd ed. Philadelphia: WB Saunders, 1993:1981-1984.

Gambardella PC. Legg-Calvé-Perthes disease in dogs. In: Bojrab MJ, ed. Disease mechanisms in small animal surgery. 2nd ed. Philadelphia: WB Saunders, 1993:804-807.

Brinker WO, Piermattei DL, Flo GL. Diagnosis and treatment of orthopedic conditions of the hind limb. In: Handbook of small animal orthopedics and fracture treatment. 2nd ed. Philadelphia: WB Saunders, 1990:376-377.

Gibson KL, Lewis DD, Perchman RD. Use of external coaptation for the treatment of avascular necrosis of the femoral head in a dog. J Am Vet Med Assoc 1990;197:868.

Author Larry Carpenter
Consulting Editor Peter D. Schwarz

LEIOMYOMA, STOMACH, SMALL AND LARGE INTESTINE

BASICS

OVERVIEW
Leiomyoma is an uncommon benign tumor arising from the smooth muscle of the stomach and intestinal tract.

SIGNALMENT
• Middle-aged to older (> 6 years) dogs and cats • Dogs more commonly affected than cats • No breed predisposition

SIGNS

Historical Findings
• Usually nonspecific • Stomach—vomiting • Small intestine—vomiting, weight loss, borborygmus, and flatulence • Large intestine and rectum—tenesmus, sometimes leading to rectal prolapse

Physical Examination Findings
• Stomach—no specific abnormalities • Small intestine—midabdominal mass and occasionally distended, painful loops of small bowel • Large intestine and rectum—palpable mass per rectum

CAUSES AND RISK FACTORS
Unknown

DIAGNOSIS

DIFFERENTIAL DIAGNOSIS
• Gastric foreign body • Gastrointestinal adenocarcinoma • Leiomyosarcoma or malignant lymphoma • Pancreatitis

CBC/BIOCHEMISTRY/URINALYSIS
• Results usually normal • Hypoglycemia in a few patients

OTHER LABORATORY TESTS N/A

IMAGING
• Abdominal ultrasound may reveal a thickened wall of stomach or bowel. • Stomach and small intestine—positive contrast radiography may reveal a space-occupying mass. Upper gastrointestinal-tract endoscopy and mucosal biopsy should be done but is frequently nondiagnostic because the tumors are deep to the mucosal surface. Surgical biopsy often is required to confirm the diagnosis. • Large intestine and rectum—double-contrast radiography reveals a space-occupying mass; colonoscopy may reveal a mass, but mucosal biopsy is sometimes nondiagnostic because of normal mucosal covering of the tumor; deep surgical biopsy should be done if possible.

OTHER DIAGNOSTIC PROCEDURES
N/A

TREATMENT
• Surgical resection the treatment of choice • If the tumor is resectable, surgery is curative.

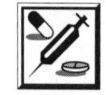

MEDICATIONS

DRUGS AND FLUIDS N/A

CONTRAINDICATIONS/POSSIBLE INTERACTIONS N/A

FOLLOW-UP
• If complete resection has been done, normal postoperative care should be given after surgery. • No additional follow-up is necessary.
• Some dogs have clinical signs of hypoglycemia (e.g., weakness and seizures).
• Hypoglycemia has recently been recognized as an associated paraneoplastic syndrome.

MISCELLANEOUS

Reference
Theilen GH, Madewell BR. Tumors of the digestive tract. In: Theilen GH, Madewell BR, eds. Veterinary cancer medicine. 2nd ed. Philadelphia: Lea & Febiger, 1987.
Author Ralph C. Richardson
Consulting Editor Wallace B. Morrison

LEIOMYOSARCOMA, STOMACH, SMALL, AND LARGE INTESTINE

BASICS

OVERVIEW
• Uncommon malignant tumor arising from the smooth muscle of the stomach and intestinal tract • Tends to be locally invasive and slow to metastasize • Early diagnosis and complete resection may be curative

SIGNALMENT
• Mostly middle-aged to older (> 6 years) dogs and cats • Dogs more commonly affected than cats • No breed predisposition

SIGNS

Historical Findings
• Stomach—abdominal discomfort, weight loss, and vomiting • Small intestine—vomiting, weight loss, borborygmus, and flatulence • Large intestine and rectum—tenesmus leading to rectal prolapse in some animals

Physical Examination Findings
• Stomach—nonspecific • Small intestine—midabdominal mass and, in some animals, distended, painful loops of small bowel on abdominal palpation • Large intestine and rectum—palpable mass per rectum

CAUSES AND RISK FACTORS
Unknown

DIAGNOSIS

DIFFERENTIAL DIAGNOSIS
• Gastric foreign body • Gastrointestinal adenocarcinoma • Leiomyoma • Malignant lymphoma • Pancreatitis

CBC/BIOCHEMISTRY/URINALYSIS
• Results usually normal • Hypoglycemia has been reported as a paraneoplastic syndrome.

OTHER LABORATORY TESTS N/A

IMAGING
• Abdominal ultrasonography reveals a thickened wall of the stomach or bowel in some animals. • Stomach and small intestine—positive contrast radiography reveals a space-occupying mass in some animals; upper gastrointestinal tract endoscopy and mucosal biopsy should be done but results frequently nondiagnostic because the tumor is deep to the mucosal surface; surgical biopsy often required to confirm the diagnosis • Large intestine and rectum—double contrast radiography reveals a space-occupying mass; colonoscopy may reveal a mass, but mucosal biopsy is sometimes nondiagnostic if the tumor is intramural; collect deep biopsy specimen if possible

OTHER DIAGNOSTIC PROCEDURES N/A

TREATMENT
• Surgery can be curative since this tumor is usually confined to the gastrointestinal tract and is slow to metastasize.
• Careful evaluation for metastasis should be conducted before extensive surgery. Sites examined should include the mesenteric lymph nodes, liver, and lungs.

MEDICATIONS

DRUGS AND FLUIDS None reported

CONTRAINDICATIONS/POSSIBLE INTERACTIONS N/A

FOLLOW-UP
• If resection is complete, routine physical examination and abdominal and thoracic radiography at 1, 3, 6, 9, and 12 months after surgery. • If resection is incomplete, symptomatic support to relieve clinical signs.

MISCELLANEOUS

Reference
Theilen GH, Madewell BR. Tumors of the digestive tract. In: Theilen GH, Madewell BR, eds. Veterinary cancer medicine. 2nd ed. Philadelphia: Lea & Febiger, 1987.

Author Ralph C. Richardson
Consulting Editor Wallace B. Morrison

LEISHMANIASIS

BASICS

OVERVIEW
• Infection with a protozoan of the genus Leishmania • Two types—cutaneous and visceral • Liver, spleen, skin, kidneys, and eyes can be involved.

Incidence/Prevalence
Not endemic in the United States. Most cases are imported. Rare and isolated foci of autochthonous transmission of both forms.

SIGNALMENT
Visceral in dogs—no breed predilection
Cutaneous in cats (rare)—no breed predilection

Mean Age and Range
All ages

Predominant sex
Male (visceral)

SIGNS

Visceral
• Weight loss, exercise intolerance, and anorexia • Nonpruritic skin lesions, symmetric alopecia, and scaling • Onychogryposis • Enlargement of spleen, lymph nodes, and liver • Glomerulonephritis • Polyarthritis • Ocular lesions

Cutaneous
Suppurating skin lesions, typically on extremities, ear, nose, etc.

CAUSES AND RISK FACTORS
• Bites from infected flies or possibly by transfusion • Travel to endemic areas

DIAGNOSIS

DIFFERENTIAL DIAGNOSIS
Chronic visceral infection may present with signs suggestive of systemic mycoses (e.g., histoplasmosis). • Cutaneous leishmaniasis may be similar to lesions of cryptococcosis or mosquito allergy.

CBC/BIOCHEMISTRY/URINALYSIS
Anemia, leukopenia, thrombocytopenia, azotemia, hypergammaglobulinemia, hypoalbuminemia, and proteinuria

OTHER LABORATORY TESTS
The Coomb's antinuclear antibody test and antiplatelet antibody tests may be positive.

IMAGING N/A

OTHER DIAGNOSTIC PROCEDURES
• Culture of biopsy specimens by Communicable Disease Center (CDC) • Cytologic or histopathologic identification of organisms in macrophages in dermal lesion scrapes or biopsies or fine needle aspirates of lymph nodes, bone marrow, or spleen • Serologic testing is available.

GROSS AND HISTOPATHOLOGIC FINDINGS
Biopsy may reveal causative organisms.

TREATMENT
• Outpatient therapy with concern for the potential of local transmission by competent United States vector flies.
• Owner should be advised of potential zoonotic transmission of organisms in lesions to humans.
• Cutaneous lesions on cats' ears have been treated by the surgical removal of the pinna.

MEDICATIONS

DRUGS AND FLUIDS

Dogs
• Sodium stibogluconate (an antimonial compound available through CDC)—10-50 mg/kg daily for 10-30 days.
• Alternative treatments include antifungal agents and allopurinol (used in human infections).
• Experimental treatment of people with gamma-interferon and antimonials has shown success.

CONTRAINDICATIONS/POSSIBLE INTERACTIONS N/A

FOLLOW-UP
Repeat biopsies after treatment.

EXPECTED COURSE AND PROGNOSIS
• Dogs usually are not cured by antimonial therapy. • Relapses may occur often. • Consider euthanasia.

MISCELLANEOUS

Reference
Bravo L, Frank LA, Brenneman KA. Canine leishmaniasis in the United States. Comp Cont Ed Pract Vet 1993;15:699-708.

Authors Dwight Bowman and Edward Pearce

Consulting Editor Fred W. Scott

BASICS

OVERVIEW

Lens luxation into the anterior chamber or posterior segment occurs when the lens capsule separates for 360° from the zonules which hold the lens in place. Subluxation is a partial separation of the lens from its zonular attachments. The subluxated lens remains in its normal or near-normal position in the pupil. Primary lens luxation is the result of an inherited tendency for the zonules to weaken and break, or rarely, a congenital malformation of the zonular attachments. Congenital luxations are often associated with microphakia. Secondary lens luxation (the most common form in cats) results from zonular rupture caused by globe stretching, chronic intraocular inflammation, or intraocular neoplasia.

SIGNALMENT

• Primary lens luxation is usually seen in adult dogs. The poodle, shar pei, whippet, Norwegian elkhound, and terrier breeds are most commonly affected. • Secondary lens luxation occurs in dogs and cats.

SIGNS

• Acute or chronically painful eye with episcleral injection and diffuse corneal edema, especially if glaucoma is present • Central corneal edema—can be caused by the lens touching the endothelium, resulting in mechanical disruption of endothelial cells • Abnormally shallow or deep anterior chamber • Iridodonesis • Aphakic crescent (an area of pupil devoid of the lens) • Malpositioned clear lens sometimes observed in an otherwise asymptomatic eye

CAUSES AND RISK FACTORS

• The inheritance pattern of primary lens luxation is uncertain. • Although lens luxation may cause secondary glaucoma, longstanding glaucoma can cause buphthalmia and lens luxation. History usually differentiates these two conditions. • Primary lens luxation and primary glaucoma may occur simultaneously in some breeds, such as the Jack Russell terrier and shar pei. • Uveitis, especially chronic lens-induced uveitis. • Intraocular neoplasia may physically luxate the lens. • Trauma rarely causes a normal lens to luxate without signs of severe uveitis or hyphema.

DIAGNOSIS

DIFFERENTIAL DIAGNOSIS

• Uveitis and glaucoma also cause painful, red eyes with corneal edema. • Corneal endothelial dystrophy can also cause corneal edema and make it difficult to see the intraocular structures. • Careful ophthalmic examination usually permits differentiation of lens luxation from other ocular diseases.

CBC/BIOCHEMISTRY/URINALYSIS

• Results normal unless lens luxation is the sequela of a systemic disease that causes uveitis or dissemination of neoplasia.

OTHER LABORATORY TESTS N/A
IMAGING

• Thoracic radiographs and abdominal ultrasonography may be indicated if luxation is secondary to intraocular neoplasia. • Ocular ultrasonography is helpful in animals with corneal edema or cloudy ocular media.

OTHER DIAGNOSTIC PROCEDURES

Complete ophthalmic examination, including tonometry, is indicated.

TREATMENT

Lens luxation is treated both surgically and medically in potentially visual eyes with the goal of preventing glaucomatous damage to the retina and optic nerve. In general, lens luxation in a potentially visual eye is best treated by removing the lens. Irreversibly blind eyes or eyes with lens luxation secondary to intraocular neoplasia are often best treated by enucleation or, if appropriate, one of the globe salvage procedures (e.g., cyclocryosurgery, evisceration, and intrascleral prosthesis).

MEDICATIONS

DRUGS AND FLUIDS

• If the intraocular pressure is normal, the lens luxation is primary, and the lens is in the posterior segment, topically applied miotic (i.e., 0.125% demecarium bromide, q12h-q24h) potentially lessens the chance of anterior lens luxation and secondary glaucoma.

• High intraocular pressure (> 40mmHg) is treated with mannitol (1g/kg/IV over 20 minutes).
• Carbonic anhydrase inhibitors (e.g., dichlorphenamide, 2-4 mg/kg q12h PO) should also be initiated to reduce aqueous production.
• Topically applied antiinflammatory (e.g., 0.1% dexamethasone sodium phosphate, q6h) is also indicated.
• These medications should be initiated, and if the eye has the potential for vision, the patient should be referred to a veterinary ophthalmologist immediately for intracapsular lens extraction.

CONTRAINDICATIONS/POSSIBLE INTERACTIONS

Topically applied miotics are contraindicated if the lens is in the anterior chamber.

FOLLOW-UP

• If surgery is not performed and a primary, posterior luxation is being managed medically, intraocular pressure should be reevaluated initially 24 hours after starting medical treatments and frequently thereafter. Once intraocular pressure remains stable, patients should be examined at least quarterly.
• Secondary glaucoma and retinal detachment can occur. • If only one lens is involved at the time of examination, the other lens may become involved at a later date.

MISCELLANEOUS

Reference

Gelatt KN. The canine lens. In: Gelatt KN, ed. Veterinary ophthalmology. Philadelphia: Lea and Febiger, 1991:429–460.

Author Denise M. Lindley
Consulting Editor Paul E. Miller

LEPTOSPIROSIS

 BASICS

DEFINITION

Leptospirosis is a worldwide problem and an important cause of acute and chronic disease of dogs (septicemia, hepatitis, nephritis, abortion, and stillbirths) and other animals and is caused by pathogenic members of the genus Leptospira. The vaccine for dogs contains the serovars L. canicola and L. icterohaemorrhagiae that promote immunity to homologous serovars but may not prevent colonization of the dog's kidneys, resulting in a chronic carrier state. Vaccination is serovar-specific and does not promote protection against other serovars present in nature.

Pathophysiology

Leptospira penetrate intact or cut skin or mucus membranes, rapidly invade the bloodstream (4-7 days), and spread to all parts of the body (2-4 days), resulting in fever, leukocytosis, transitory anemia (hemolysis), hemoglobinuria, and albuminuria The fever and bacteremia soon resolve and cytotoxic capillary and endothelial cell damage occurs (petechial hemorrhages). Leptospira rapidly invade and multiply in the liver (hepatic necrosis) and kidney (leptospiruria), and early serum antibody appears. At this point, death may result from acute septicemia or hemolytic anemia, or kidney parenchyma localization may result in focal interstitial nephritis and vascular damage. Because of tubular damage, leptospira may localize in renal tubules, resulting in prolonged leptospiruria. Death may result from interstitial nephritis and renal failure.

Systems Affected

Subacute to Acute/Severe Disease
• Renal/urologic—focal interstitial nephritis, hemoglobinuric nephrosis, tubular damage/failure • Hepatobiliary—hepatitis, dysfunction, necrosis • Cardiovascular—endothelial cell damage, hemorrhage • Nervous—meningitis
Chronic Disease
• Urogenital—chronic renal failure, abortion, weak puppies • Ophthalmic—anterior uveitis

Genetics N/A

Incidence/Prevalence

• Usually one or more serovars account for endemic disease in a geographic area.
• Traditionally, serovars L. canicola and L. icterohaemorrhagiae cause clinical disease in dogs; however, L. grippotyphosa and L . pomona are becoming more prominent.
• Reported incidence is falsely low. Most infections in dogs are inapparent and remain undiagnosed. • L. canicola infections are the most common worldwide (L. icterohaemorrhagiae in Australia). • Prevalence in city dogs is higher (37.8%) than in suburban dogs (18.7%).

Geographic Distribution

Worldwide occurrence, especially in warm, wet climates or seasons; standing water and soil of neutral or slightly alkaline pH promotes presence in environment

SIGNALMENT

Species Dogs and, rarely, cats

Breed Predilections N/A

Mean Age and Range

• Young dogs without passive maternal antibody are more likely to exhibit severe disease.
• Older dogs with adequate antibody titer levels seldom exhibit clinical disease unless exposed to a serovar not in the vaccine.

Predominant Sex

Male dogs are more commonly affected.

SIGNS

General Comments

• Clinical signs vary with the age and immune status of the animal, environmental factors affecting leptospira survival, and virulence of the infecting serovar. • Disease/infection is rare in cats. • Primary reservoir host—may spread particular leptospira serovar via urine shedding without demonstrating clinical signs or with demonstration of less severe disease (acute diffuse to chronic interstitial nephritis [e.g., L. canicola in dogs with relatively weak antibody response]) • Incidental (accidental) host—acute severe form (fulminant, fever, hemorrhage, anemia, jaundice [e.g., L. icterohaemorrhagiae in dogs with severe antibody response])

Historical Findings

• Peracute to subacute disease—fever, sore muscles, stiffness, shivering, weakness, anorexia, depression, vomiting, rapid dehydration, diarrhea (with or without blood), icterus, spontaneous cough, difficulty breathing, PU/PD (later no urination), bloody vaginal discharge, and death (without clinical signs) • Chronic disease—no apparent illness, fever of unknown origin, and PU/PD (chronic renal failure)

Physical Examination Findings

Peracute to acute disease—fever, weakness, anorexia, vomiting, tachypnea, rapid irregular pulse, poor capillary perfusion, hematemesis, hematochezia, melena, epistaxis, injected mucous membranes, widespread petechial and ecchymotic hemorrhages, icterus, reluctance to move/paraspinal hyperesthesia/stiff gait, conjunctivitis, rhinitis, hematuria, and mild lymphadenopathy

CAUSES

Pathogenic serovars of the genus Leptospira capable of infecting the dog (L. canicola, icterohaemorrhagiae, pomona, grippotyphosa, bratislava, copenhagenii, australis, autumnalis, ballum, bataviae) and cat (L. canicola, grippotyphosa, pomona, bataviae)

RISK FACTORS

• Direct transmission—host-to-host contact via infected urine, postabortion discharge, infected fetus/discharge, and sexual contact (semen) • Indirect transmission—exposure to (via urine) a contaminated environment (vegetation, soil, food, water, bedding) under conditions in which leptospira can survive

Disease Agent

Leptospira serovar, its particular virulence factors, infectious dose, and route of exposure

Host Factors That Increase Susceptibility to Disease

• Vaccine status—vaccine protection is serovar-specific; will prevent clinical disease as a result of homologous serovar but not necessarily kidney colonization and urine shedding; nonvaccine serovars may infect and cause disease in the vaccinated host • Males and young dogs are at greater risk. • Outdoor animals/hunting dogs—exposure of mucous membrane to water and exposure of abraded or water-softened skin increases risk of infection

Environmental Factors

Favorable conditions for survival of leptospira outside of the host:
• Warm and moist environment (temperature ranges of 7-10° C (44.6-50° F) to 34-36° C (93-96° F) • Presence of standing water of neutral or slightly alkaline pH; survives 180 days in wet soil and longer in standing water; survives better in stagnant versus flowing water; higher incidence of disease in wet season (high rainfall areas) of temperate regions; low lying areas that are marshy/muddy/irrigated; warm humid climates of the tropical and subtropical regions • Dense animal population (kennels and urban settings versus rural settings) which increases chances of urine exposure. • Exposure to rodents and to wildlife

 DIAGNOSIS

DIFFERENTIAL DIAGNOSIS

• Subclinical infections and chronic carrier states go undetected

Subacute to Acute Disease

Dogs
Heartworm disease, immune-mediated hemolytic anemia, bacteremia/septicemia (bite wound, prostatitis, endocarditis, dental disease), infectious canine hepatitis virus, canine herpesvirus, hepatic neoplasia, trauma, lupus, RMSF, ehrlichiosis, toxoplasmosis, renal neoplasia, renal calculi
Cats
Hemobartonellosis, drugs (acetaminophen), bacteremia/septicemia, FIV and FeLV associated diseases, cholangitis, toxoplasmosis, FIP, hepatic neoplasia, autoimmune disease (e.g., SLE), trauma, renal calculi, renal neoplasia

Reproductive/Neonatal Disease

Dogs
Brucellosis, distemper, herpes
Cats
FIP, FeLV, panleukopenia, herpesvirus, toxoplasmosis, salmonellosis

CBC/BIOCHEMISTRY/URINALYSIS

CBC
PCV and total plasma solids high (dehydration) or PCV low (hemolyisis); leukocytosis with left shift (leukopenia initially during leptospiremic phase); thrombocytopenia; increased fibrin degradation products (FDP)

Serum Chemistry Profile
BUN and creatinine high (dependent on degree of renal failure); electrolyte alterations (dependent on degree of renal and GI dysfunction): hyponatremia, hypochloremia, hypokalemia (hyperkalemia with kidney failure), hyperphosphatemia; hypoalbuminemia; serum bicarbonate low; high ALT (serum alanine aminotransferase), AST (serum aspartate aminotransferase), LDH (serum lactate dehydrogenase), SAP (serum alkaline phosphatase)

Urinalysis
Proteinuria, isosthenuria, glucosuria (acute renal failure)

OTHER LABORATORY TESTS
• Serology—microscopic agglutination test (MAT) performed in acute stage and 3-4 weeks later (convalescent serum); in unvaccinated animal, titers initially may be low (1:100-1:200) but may rise in the convalescent sample to 1:800-1:1600 or higher if a homologous leptospira serovar is tested; in vaccinated animals, expect low (usually not higher than 1:400) titers for the vaccine serovars L. canicola and L. icterohaemorrhagiae, and for other serovars the above information is the same; ideally, all serum samples should be run at the same time • Dark-field microscopy and fluorescent antibody of urine—dark-field exam is inconclusive, difficult to read, and requires fresh urine; FA tests of centrifuged and uncentrifuged urine are more conclusive, and leptospiras do not need to be viable for the test (submit urine to lab on ice by overnight courier); need to correlate FA results with clinical history

IMAGING N/A

OTHER DIAGNOSTIC PROCEDURES
• Culture of body fluids antemortem (urine, blood, aqueous humor) and tissues postmortem (kidney, liver, fetus, placenta) is usually not practical because of the fastidiousness of leptospiras; contact your laboratory for the proper leptospira transport medium if culture is attempted. • FA should be done on all tissues submitted for postmortem workup, especially kidney and liver. • Special stains (Warthin-Starry silver stain)—immunohistochemistry with monoclonal antibodies should be attempted on formalin-fixed sections of kidney, liver, and fetal/placental tissues

GROSS AND HISTOPATHOLOGIC FINDINGS
Depend on the leptospira serovar involved and the host's immunity; cats in general have less severe lesions

TREATMENT

INPATIENT VERSUS OUTPATIENT
Acute severe cases must be treated as inpatients; the extent of supportive therapy depends on the severity of the disease.

ACTIVITY
Acutely ill animals and bacteremic/septicemic animals should have restricted activity with cage rest, monitoring, and warmth.

DIET
Severely ill patients often are anorexic, in shock, and lethargic.

CLIENT EDUCATION
Zoonotic potential from contaminated urine of affected dogs

SURGICAL CONSIDERATIONS N/A

MEDICATIONS

DRUGS AND FLUIDS
• Appropriate therapy depends on severity of illness. • Patients with dehydration and shock should be treated with parenteral, balanced, polyionic, isotonic IV solution (lactated Ringer's).
• If severe hemorrhage is present, a blood transfusion may be needed.
• Oliguria or anuria—initially treat with rehydration; then IV osmotic diuretics, tubular diuretics; peritoneal dialysis may be necessary
• Antimicrobial therapy—use procaine penicillin G (40,000-80,000 U/kg, IM, q24h or divided q12h) until kidney function returns; to eliminate leptospiras from the kidney interstitial tissues, use dihydrostreptomycin (10-15 mg/kg, IM, q12h for 2 weeks), streptomycin if not in renal failure, or doxycycline (unapproved; 5.0 mg/kg PO q24h)

CONTRAINDICATIONS N/A

PRECAUTIONS
Aminoglycosides cannot be used in patients until kidney function has been restored.

POSSIBLE INTERACTIONS N/A

ALTERNATE DRUGS
Ampicillin or amoxicillin in the place of penicillin; erythromycin

FOLLOW-UP

PATIENT MONITORING
Prognosis is guarded in acute severe disease. Kidney and liver function and electrolytes should be monitored. Changes in BUN, serum creatinine concentration, and urine specific gravity in dogs with renal failure are indicators of prognosis.

PREVENTION/AVOIDANCE
• Vaccinate dogs per current label recommendations; bacteria-induced immunity lasts only 6-8 months and is serovar specific (i.e., no cross-protection outside of the serogroup); revaccination at least yearly; dogs at risk (hunter, show dogs, dogs with access to water/ponds) vaccinate every 4-6 months, especially in endemic areas • Strict kennel sanitation to avoid contact of animals with infected urine • Monitor and remove carrier dogs from kennels until treated. • Isolate affected animals during treatment. • Rodent control in kennels • Limit access to marshy/muddy areas, ponds, low lying areas with stagnant surface water, and heavily irrigated pastures. • Limit access to wildlife.

POSSIBLE COMPLICATIONS
• Most infections are subclinical or chronic. • Guarded prognosis for severely ill animals; DIC reactions possible • Liver and kidney dysfunction may be permanent. • Uveitis and abortion sequelae possible

EXPECTED COURSE AND PROGNOSIS
• Most infections are subclinical or chronic.
• Prognosis is guarded in acute severe disease.

MISCELLANEOUS

ASSOCIATED CONDITIONS N/A

AGE RELATED FACTORS
Severe clinical disease in young dogs (nonvaccinated or lacking maternal antibody)

ZOONOTIC POTENTIAL
• High zoonotic potential • Leptospira organisms spread in the urine of infected animals.
• Strict kennel hygiene and disinfection of premises (iodine-based disinfectant or stabilized bleach solutions) • Acutely infected and carrier animals must be treated.

PREGNANCY
Possible abortion sequelae to leptospirosis; antimicrobial therapy must take into account the effect of drug on developing fetus

SYNONYMS
Weil's disease, swineherd's disease, rice field disease, water-fever or cane-fever disease (all synonyms for disease in humans)

SEE ALSO N/A

ABBREVIATIONS N/A

References
Baldwin CJ, Atkins CE. Leptospirosis in dogs. Compen Con Ed Pract Vet 1987;9:499-508.
Heath SE, Johnson R. Leptospirosis. JAVMA 1994;205:1518-1523.
Author Patrick L. McDonough
Consulting Editor Fred W. Scott

LEUKEMIA, ACUTE LYMPHOBLASTIC

 BASICS

OVERVIEW
• Acute lymphoblastic leukemia is defined as the presence of circulating neoplastic prolymphocytes and lymphoblasts in the blood.
• Animals with acute lymphoblastic leukemia have impaired humoral and cellular immunity. • acute lymphoblastic leukemia is characterized by bone marrow infiltration (and extramedullary sites) and displacement of normal hematopoietic stem cells. • Other organs can be infiltrated.

SIGNALMENT
• Dogs—male to female ratio is 3:2, with a mean age of 6.2 years (range 1 to 12 years).
• Rare in cats.

SIGNS
• Often nonspecific. Enlarged liver and spleen, lymphadenomegaly, and other signs reflecting specific organ infiltration. Petechial or ecchymotic hemorrhages may result from thrombocytopenia.

CAUSES AND RISK FACTORS
• Dog: Ionizing radiation, oncogenic viruses, and chemical agents, suspected but unproved
• Cat: Feline leukemia virus infection.

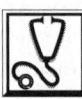 **DIAGNOSIS**

DIFFERENTIAL DIAGNOSIS
• Acute or chronic infections (toxoplasmosis, canine distemper or ehrlichiosis • Aplastic anemia • Metastatic neoplasia • Multicentric lymphosarcoma: all patients usually have only moderately enlarged peripheral lymph nodes, marked splenomegaly and have signs of systemic illness of relatively acute onset.
• Other leukemias

CBC/BIOCHEMISTRY/URINALYSIS
• CBC: normocytic, normochromic, non-regenerative anemia; thrombocytopenia; lymphoblastosis; leukocytosis or leukopenia
• Serum chemistry profile: elevations in liver enzymes

OTHER LABORATORY TESTS
• Immunohistochemistry or enzymatic biochemistry may be needed to differentiate from other leukemic cells.

IMAGING N/A

OTHER DIAGNOSTIC PROCEDURES
• Bone marrow cytology or core biopsies: lymphoblastic infiltration with decreased numbers of myeloid and erythroid precursors and low numbers of megakaryocytes.

 TREATMENT

• Usually as outpatients unless ill.
• Patients are immunocompromised and should not be exposed to infectious diseases.

 MEDICATIONS

DRUGS AND FLUIDS
• Transfusions as indicated to restore red blood cells, platelets or coagulation factors.

• Combination chemotherapy with prednisone (20 mg/M^2 PO q12h) and vincristine (0.7 mg/M^2 IV weekly) may result in partial or short-lived complete remissions in some cases.

CONTRAINDICATIONS/POSSIBLE INTERACTIONS
Chemotherapy can have toxic side effects. Seek advice prior to starting treatment if you are unfamiliar with cytotoxic drugs.

 FOLLOW-UP

• Monitor peripheral blood counts and bone marrow to judge success and toxicity of therapy.
• Hemorrhage from thrombocytopenia is major cause in dogs with acute lymphoblastic leukemia. • Prognosis is grave.

 MISCELLANEOUS

Chemotherapy is contraindicated in pregnant animals

ABBREVIATIONS N/A

Reference

Leifer CE, Matus RE. Lymphoid leukemia in the dog: acute lymphoblastic leukemia and chronic lymphocytic leukemia. Vet Clin North Am Small Anim Pract 1985;15:723-739.
Author Linda S. Fineman
Consulting Editor Wallace B. Morrison

BASICS

OVERVIEW
Chronic lymphocytic leukemia has the following characteristics:
• Circulating neoplastic lymphocytes that are mature and well-differentiated • Patients may have impaired humoral and cellular immunity • Systems affected include hematopoietic, lymphatic, and integument

SIGNALMENT
• Dogs—male to female ratio, 2:1; mean age, 9.4 years (range, 3 to 15 years) • Rare in dogs and cats

SIGNS
Nonspecific, including polydypsia and polyuria, lymphadenopathy, lameness, fever, and bruising

CAUSES AND RISK FACTORS
Ionizing radiation, oncogenic viruses, and chemical agents suspected but unproved

DIAGNOSIS

DIFFERENTIAL DIAGNOSIS
• Lymphosarcoma may have a leukemic phase • Immune-mediated hematologic diseases

CBC/BIOCHEMISTRY/URINALYSIS
• Mild to moderate normocytic, normochromic anemia • Normal to low platelet count • Lymphocytosis (ranging from 5,000 to >100,000 lymphocytes per mm^3) • Normal to mildly high serum globulins • High ALP in some animals

OTHER LABORATORY TESTS
• Serum protein electrophoresis detects monoclonal spikes (usually IgM) in about 50% of patients. • Bence Jones proteinuria in about 50% of patients. • Direct Coomb's test may be positive in patient with secondary immune-mediated hemolytic anemia.

IMAGING
Radiography and ultrasonography reveal cranial organomegaly or internal lymphadenomegaly in some animals.

OTHER DIAGNOSTIC PROCEDURES
In advanced stages of disease, cytologic examination of bone marrow and core biopsy reveal high numbers of mature lymphocytes with crowding out of normal cell lines.

TREATMENT
• Usually managed as outpatients
• Splenectomy indicated in patient with secondary, immune-mediated hemolytic anemia or thrombocytopenia, or if hypersplenism cannot be controlled medically
• Treatment advised only when patient is symptomatic

MEDICATIONS

DRUGS AND FLUIDS
• Chlorambucil (0.2 mg/kg PO q24h 7 days, then 0.1 mg/kg q24h to effect)
• Prednisone (20 mg/M^2 PO q12h) in combination with chlorambucil

CONTRAINDICATIONS/POSSIBLE INTERACTIONS
Patients receiving chemotherapy should be monitored for myelosuppression; dosage may need to be altered depending on neutrophil and platelet counts.

FOLLOW-UP
• Periodic cytologic examination of bone marrow and weekly CBC to determine response to treatment and progression of disease.
• Variable course, but progressive. Severe hemolytic anemia and pneumonia may cause death.

MISCELLANEOUS
Chemotherapy drugs contraindicated in pregnant animals

ABBREVIATIONS
ALP = alkaline phosphatase

Reference

Leifer CE, Matus RE. Lymphoid leukemia in the dog: acute lymphoblastic leukemia and chronic lymphocytic leukemia. Vet Clin North Am (Small Anim Pract) 1985;15:723-739.
Author Linda S. Fineman
Consulting Editor Wallace B. Morrison

LEUKOCYTOCLASTIC VASCULITIS

BASICS

OVERVIEW
• Inflammation of small blood vessels (arterioles, capillaries, and venules), which usually affects the skin and sometimes other organs
• Mechanism involves a type III hypersensitivity reaction with deposition of immune complexes in the vessel wall. Complement is activated and neutrophils infiltrate the vessel wall. Release of lysosomal enzymes by neutrophils causes necrosis of the vessel wall, which may result in thrombosis, hemorrhage, and infarction. • May occur as a hypersensitivity reaction to microorganisms and drugs, or as a manifestation of systemic lupus erythematosus or rheumatoid arthritis

SIGNALMENT
• Predisposition in Doberman pinschers to development of a hypersensitivity reaction to sulfadiazine and related sulfa-compounds • In Scottish terriers, manifests as an apparently hereditary leukocytoclastic vasculitis of the nasal planum, nostrils, and nasal mucosa
• Rare in cats

SIGNS
Historical Findings
• Acute or insidious onset of symptoms
• Skin lesions • Depression • Fever, if systemic • Recent initiation of drug treatment

Physical Examination Findings
• Usually one or more erythematous maculae or papules (palpable purpura), hemorrhagic bullae, necrosis or ulcers • Possible depigmentation • Frequent involvement of the nasal planum, pinnae, paws, tail, lips, and oral cavity • Possible swelling of lymph nodes
• Possible signs related to an underlying disease process

CAUSES AND RISK FACTORS
• Hereditary (Scottish terrier) or genetic predisposition (Doberman pinscher) • Concurrent systemic lupus erythematosus, rheumatoid arthritis • Vaccine-induced condition (rabies) • Staphyloccocal hypersensitivity • Drug hypersensitivity • Contact with infectious agents (eg, Ehrlichia canis, Erysipelothrix rhusiopathiae) • Idiopathic in many cases

DIAGNOSIS

DIFFERENTIAL DIAGNOSIS
• Urticaria • Systemic lupus erythematosus or rheumatoid arthritis—determined by positive antinuclear antibody or rheumatoid factor test • Cellulitis • Thrombocytopenia—flat purpura, low platelet count • Disseminated intravascular coagulation—abnormal clotting times, high fibrin split products • Sepsis—positive blood culture

CBC/BIOCHEMISTRY/URINALYSIS
• Abnormalities in routine tests • Neutrophilic leukocytosis found in many animals

OTHER LABORATORY TESTS
Additional tests (cultures, serology, immune tests, clotting tests) often necessary to determine underlying cause

IMAGING N/A

OTHER DIAGNOSTIC PROCEDURES
Skin biopsy for definitive diagnosis

GROSS AND HISTOPATHOLOGIC FINDINGS
• Necrosis of the wall of small blood vessels with deposition of fibrinoid material and neutrophils with nuclear debris • Possible edema, hemorrhage, and necrosis of surrounding tissue

TREATMENT
• Provide treatment to eliminate underlying cause and reduce inflammatory reaction.
• Treatment approach depends on the underlying cause.
• Use corticosteroids except in the case of an underlying infectious disease.

MEDICATIONS

DRUGS AND FLUIDS
• Corticosteroids—prednisone (2 mg/kg PO for 10-14 days)
• If glucocorticoid therapy is not successful, administer dapsone (1 mg/kg PO q8h) or sulfasalazine (20-40 mg/kg PO q8h).

CONTRAINDICATIONS/POSSIBLE INTERACTIONS
• Avoid the use of corticosteroids until infections have been ruled out.
• Dapsone can cause hepatotoxicity, thrombocytopenia, and mild anemia and leukopenia. Pyrimethamine increases the toxicity of dapsone.

FOLLOW-UP
• Reexamine the patient once a week until vasculitis has regressed. Additional follow-up depends on the underlying disease. • Monitor the patient every other week during dapsone therapy for side effects. • Prognosis depends on identification and nature of the underlying disease. If no underlying disease can be identified, the prognosis is guarded.

MISCELLANEOUS

SEE ALSO
• Lupus Erythematosus, Systemic • Vasculitis

Reference
Muller GW, Kirk RW, Scott DW. Small animal dermatology. 4th ed. Philadelphia: WB Saunders, 1989:533-535.
Author Harm HogenEsch
Consulting Editor Alan H. Rebar

BASICS

OVERVIEW
Progressive, degenerative, demyelinating disease primarily affecting the spinal cord in the rottweiler worldwide

SIGNALMENT
• Rottweilers of either sex, 1.5-4 years old
• Probably an autosomal recessive inherited disease

SIGNS
• No history of injury or illness preceding the clinical signs • Owners do not report discomfort. • Insidious, progressive onset
• Proprioceptive ataxia and upper motor neuron weakness involving all four limbs. Proprioceptive positioning disappears as the disease progresses. • Spinal reflexes normal to exaggerated • In later stages of the disease, crossed extensor reflexes in all four limbs

CAUSES AND RISK FACTORS
Unknown

DIAGNOSIS

DIFFERENTIAL DIAGNOSIS
• Neuroaxonal dystrophy and distal sensorimotor polyneuropathy; two other neurologic disorders in the rottweiler, are differentiated on the basis of neurologic deficits. With the former, neuroaxonal dystrophy; deficits relate to the cerebellum; with the latter, the tetra-paresis is associated with lower motor neuron signs. • Patients with diskospondylitis and fracture or luxation are in discomfort on examination. Intervertebral disc disease is painful and usually not seen in large-breed dogs of that young age. • Cervical vertebral instability (wobbler) is differentiated on the basis of spinal survey and myelographic studies, which reveal stenosis of the vertebral canal. • Myelitis caused by canine distemper virus or other inflammatory causes progresses faster. Results of CSF analysis are abnormal.
• Primary spinal cord tumor is seen in older dogs. Myelography reveals spinal cord compression.

CBC/BIOCHEMISTRY/URINALYSIS
Results normal

OTHER LABORATORY TESTS N/A

IMAGING
Spinal cervical survey radiographs normal

OTHER DIAGNOSTIC PROCEDURES
• Results of CSF analysis normal • Results of myelography normal

TREATMENT
• Treat as outpatient unless the severity of neurologic deficits precludes nursing care at home
• Activity is whatever can be tolerated by the animal.
• Insure proper intake of food. The animal may have difficulty reaching the feeding area.
• The neurologic status slowly and progressively deteriorates to the point that the animal is unable to walk or get up.

MEDICATIONS

DRUGS AND FLUIDS
No treatment available

CONTRAINDICATIONS/POSSIBLE INTERACTIONS N/A

FOLLOW-UP
• Neurologic examination monthly to monitor progression of disease • Bed sore and urine and fecal scalds can be avoided by keeping the animal on a clean, dry, and cushioned pad (e.g., synthetic sheepskin). • Severe tetraparesis occurs within 6-12 months after onset of the clinical signs. • Euthanasia is usually performed because of severe debility.

MISCELLANEOUS

ABBREVIATIONS
CSF = cerebrospinal fluid

Reference
Chrisman CL. Neurological diseases of rottweilers: neuroaxonal dystrophy and leukoencephalomalacia. J Small Anim Pract 1992;33:500-504.
Author Joane M. Parent
Consulting Editor Joane M. Parent

LIPOMA, INFILTRATIVE

BASICS

OVERVIEW
• An invasive, nonencapsulated, lipoma variant • Although a benign neoplasm, the tumor infiltrates soft tissues, particularly muscles, but also fasciae, tendons, blood vessels, lymph nodes, joint capsules, and nerves. • Muscle infiltration is typically so extensive that surgical cures are nearly impossible. • Occurs much less frequently than lipoma

SIGNALMENT
• No breed predilection, but develops more frequently in females (female to male ratio, 3:1) • Affects mostly middle-aged animals

SIGNS

Physical Examination Findings
• Large, diffuse, soft tissue mass that clinically appears as localized muscle swelling • Mostly affects muscles of the pelvis, thigh, shoulder, sternum, and lateral cervical region • The lower extremities and abdominal wall affected less frequently

CAUSES AND RISK FACTORS
Unknown

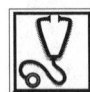

DIAGNOSIS

DIFFERENTIAL DIAGNOSIS
• Rhabdomyoma or rhabdomyosarcoma • Lipoma or liposarcoma • Mast cell neoplasia • Fibrosarcoma

CBC/BIOCHEMISTRY/URINALYSIS
Results normal

OTHER LABORATORY TESTS N/A

IMAGING
Radiography reveals fat dense tissue between soft tissue dense structures.

OTHER DIAGNOSTIC PROCEDURES
Cytologic examination of aspirate diagnostic for mature adipocytes

GROSS AND HISTOPATHOLOGIC FINDINGS
• Histologic analysis diagnostic for well-differentiated adipocytes, but they can be indistinguishable from normal adipose tissue • Distinctive feature is infiltration into and between muscle bundles.

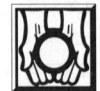

TREATMENT
• The characteristic invasiveness makes surgical excision extremely difficult.
• Clients should be informed that at least 50% of patients have recurrence after surgery, except for those that have limb amputation for appendicular tumor
• Amputation of an affected limb should be recommended only when the tumor affects the animal's quality of life; this tumor causes little problem unless it interferes with movement, causes pressure-related pain, or develops in a vitally important anatomic site.

MEDICATIONS

DRUGS AND FLUIDS N/A

CONTRAINDICATIONS/POSSIBLE INTERACTIONS N/A

FOLLOW-UP
• Responsibility focuses on deciding whether or when to recommend surgery. • Follow-up evaluations should be scheduled as dictated by tumor growth characteristics.

MISCELLANEOUS
Infiltrative lipoma has not been reported to metastasize. However, there is one report of bone and joint invasion.

Reference
Frazier KS, Herron AJ, Dee JF, et al. Infiltrative lipoma in a canine stifle joint. J Am Anim Hosp Assoc 1993;29:81.

Author James P. Thompson
Consulting Editor Wallace B. Morrison

BASICS

OVERVIEW
• The only two poisonous lizards in the world are found in the southwestern United States and Mexico. They are *Heloderma suspectum* (Gila Monster) and *Heloderma horridum* (Mexican Beaded Lizard). • They have a tenacious bite, and deliver the venom from venom glands on the lower jaw by aggressive chewing action over grooved teeth. • These lizards are nonaggressive and animal envenomations are rare. • Their venom components are less well charaterized than other venoms. • There is no evidence that the venom alters coagulation in the victim.

SIGNALMENT
Dogs and cats

SIGNS

Historical Findings
• Sudden outset of pain • Most are bitten on the face, especially the lower lip. • Victim may still have the lizard attached to it (pathoneumonic).

Physical Examination Findings
• Bleeding from bite site • Hypotension in some animals • Extremely painful bite site • Localized swelling • Ptyalism (excessive salivation) • Excessive lacrimation • Frequent urination and defecation • Aphonia (some cats) • Exophthalmus secondary to retrobulbar hemorrhage

CAUSES AND RISK FACTORS
Outdoor activities

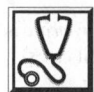

DIAGNOSIS

DIFFERENTIAL DIAGNOSIS
• Trauma • Venomous snake bite, which usually has fewer punctures; and the patient is more affected by depression and clotting abnormalities.

CBC/BIOCHEMISTRY/URINALYSIS
N/A

OTHER LABORATORY TESTS N/A

IMAGING N/A

OTHER DIAGNOSTIC PROCEDURES
Electrocardiography may detect arrhythmias.

TREATMENT
• Remove lizard if still attached to patient. This can be accomplished by placing a prying instrument between the jaws and pushing into the back of the mouth. Also, a flame underneath the lizard's jaw often causes it to release its grip. • Hospitalize patient to monitor and treat hypotension if present. • Flush bite site with lidocaine and probe bite site to identify and remove fragments of lizard teeth. If teeth are not removed, they will become sequestra and abscess. • Soak bitten area with Burow's solution or similar solution q8h.

MEDICATIONS

DRUGS AND FLUIDS
• Start crystalloid fluid therapy to prevent or correct hypotension. • Control pain with aspirin (dogs) or narcotics (if severe pain). • Broad spectrum antibiotics are indicated.

CONTRAINDICATIONS/POSSIBLE INTERACTIONS
• The author generally does not employ corticosteriods in the treatment of lizard envenomations, unless marked hypotension is manifest. • Antihistamines are not useful in animals with lizard bites.

FOLLOW-UP
• ECG monitoring for arrhythmias
• Monitor site of bite for infection.

MISCELLANEOUS

Reference
Peterson ME, Meerdink G. Bites and stings of venomous animals. In: Kirk, ed. Current veterinary therapy X. Philadelphia: WB Saunders, 1989;177-186.

Author Michael E. Peterson

Consulting Editor Gary Osweiler

LOWER URINARY TRACT INFECTION

 BASICS

DEFINITION

Lower urinary tract infection results from microbial colonization of the urinary bladder and/or proximal portion of the urethra.

Pathophysiology

Microbes, usually aerobic bacteria, ascend the urinary tract under conditions that permit the organisms to persist in the urine or adhere to the epithelium and subsequently multiply. Colonization of the urinary tract requires at least transient impairment of the mechanisms that normally defend against urinary tract infection. Inflammation of infected tissues results in the clinical signs and laboratory test abnormalities exhibited by patients with urinary tract infection.

Systems Affected

Renal/Urologic—lower urinary tract

Genetics N/A

Incidence/Prevalence

Common in female dogs, less common in male dogs, and uncommon in cats

Geographic Distribution N/A

SIGNALMENT

Species

More common in dogs than in cats

Breed Predilections None

MEAN AGE AND RANGE

All ages affected; however, occurrence increases with age because of a greater frequency of other urinary lesions (e.g., uroliths, prostate disease, and tumors) that predispose to secondary urinary tract infection.

Predominant Sex

More common in female than male dogs, but occurrence in male and female cats is similar.

SIGNS

Historical Findings

- None in some animals
- Pollakiuria (ie, frequent voiding of small volumes)
- Dysuria
- Urgency (or an apparent loss of ability to control urination during periods of confinement)
- Urinating in places that are not customary
- Hematuria and cloudy or malodorous urine in some animals

Physical Examination Findings

- Acute lower urinary tract infection—bladder or urethra may be tender on palpation. Palpation of the bladder may stimulate urination.
- Chronic lower urinary tract infection—wall of the bladder or urethra may be palpably thickened or abnormally firm
- Secondary urinary tract infection—findings referable to the underlying problem

CAUSES

- Aerobic bacteria are the most common cause.
- Most common—*Escherichia, Staphylococcus,* and *Proteus* spp (more than half of all cases)
- Common—*Streptococcus, Klebsiella, Enterobacter, Pseudomonas,* and *Corynebacterium* spp
- Rare—a few other bacterial and fungal agents

RISK FACTORS

- Conditions that cause urine stasis or incomplete emptying of the bladder
- Conditions that disrupt mucosal defense properties
- Conditions that reduce of bypass anatomic and functional barriers to microbial ascent of the urinary tract (e.g., loss of muscle tone or length of the urethra and the vesicoureteral junctions)
- Conditions that compromise the antibacterial properties of urine (e.g., changes in urine pH osmolality and high concentrations of urea and certain organic acids)

 DIAGNOSIS

DIFFERENTIAL DIAGNOSIS

Any other disease of the bladder or urethra
- Conditions that are commonly confused with or complicated by urinary tract infection included urolithiasis and neoplasia. In cats, idiopathic hemorrhagic cystitis is also a common problem that must be distinguished from urinary tract infection.
- Lower urinary tract disease can become complicated by secondary urinary tract infection. This is termed complicated urinary tract infection and requires different therapeutic strategies than those used for uncomplicated (i.e., simple) episodes of urinary tract infection.
- Frequent reinfection (more than one episode of newly aquired urinary tract infection within a year) usually indicates impaired host defense mechanisms. Search for an underlying cause. If the underlying cause can not be identified and corrected, consider prophylactic antibacterial drug therapy.

CBC/BIOCHEMISTRY/URINALYSIS

- Results of CBC and serum biochemistry normal
- Pyuria is most commonly associated with urinary tract infection, but noninfectious urinary lesions can also cause pyuria. Hematuria and proteinuria are also common. Bacteria may or may not be detected by microscopic examination of urine sediment. Furthermore, bacteriuria is sometimes reported in animals that do not have urinary tract infection.

OTHER LABORATORY TESTS

Urine Culture and Sensitivity Testing

- Urine culture is necessary for definitive diagnosis of urinary tract infection.
- Correct interpretation of urine culture results requires obtaining the specimen in a manner that minimizes contamination, handling and storing the specimen so that numbers of viable bacteria do not change in vitro, and a quantitative culture method. Keep the specimen in a sealed sterile container, and if the culture is not started right away, the urine can be refrigerated up to 8 hours without important change in the results.
- Cystocentesis is the preferred technique for obtaining urine for culture.
- Cutoff values for significant bacteriuria in urine of dogs—obtained by cystocentesis, > 1,000/ml; obtained by catheterization, > 10,000/ml; and voided urine specimen, > 100,000/ml.
- Cutoff values for significant bacteriuria in urine of cats—obtained by cystocentesis or catheterization, > 1,000/ml; and voided urine specimen, > 10,000/ml.
- Values that approach but do not exceed these cutoffs (ie, < one order of magnitude below) are suspicious, and retesting is indicated. Urine cultures that produce values > one order of magnitude below these cutoffs are negative.
- In vitro susceptibility testing that determines the MIC of each drug against the isolated organism is preferred for urinary pathogens. Drugs commonly used to treat urinary tract infection are highly concentrated in the urine, and any drug with an MIC value $\leq$ one fourth of the average urine concentration of the drug during treatment is likely to be effective.

IMAGING

Survey and contrast radiograpy as well as ultrasound of the bladder or urethra may detect underlying urinary tract lesion (i.e., complicated urinary tract infection).

OTHER DIAGNOSTIC PROCEDURES

N/A

GROSS AND HISTOPATHOLOGIC FINDINGS NA

 TREATMENT

INPATIENT VERSUS OUTPATIENT

Treat as outpatient unless animal also has other urinary abnormality (e.g., obstruction) that requires inpatient treatment.

ACTIVITY

- Unrestricted
- Regulating the animal's urination so that it coordinates with antibacterial drug treatments may improve therapeutic efficacy.

DIET

Dietary restrictions not necessary for treatment of lower urinary tract infection, but dietary modification may be indicated for other concurrent urinary diseases (e.g., urolithiasis).

CLIENT EDUCATION

Prognosis for cure of simple urinary tract infection is excellent, but prognosis for complicated urinary tract infection depends on the underlying abnormality. Compliance with recommendations for treatment and follow-up evaluations is crucial for optimum results.

SURGICAL CONSIDERATIONS

Except when a concomitant disorder requires surgical intervention, management of lower urinary tract infection does not involve surgery.

MEDICATIONS

DRUGS AND FLUIDS

Antibiotics

• An appropriate drug can be selected on the basis of the genus of the infecting bacteria—penicillin (eg, ampicillin and amoxicillin) for *staphylococci, streptococci,* and *Proteus*; trimethoprim-sulfa product for *E. coli*; cephalexin for *Klebsiella*; tetracycline for *Pseudomonas.*
• For an organism for which predictable susceptibility to a specific drug is not known or that does not respond as expected to the first drug, base choice of drug on results of sensitivity test.
• Antibacterial drugs are usually most effective when given q8h; however, fluoroquinolones and trimethoprim-sulfa products are effective when given q12h.
• For acute uncomplicated lower urinary tract infection, treat with antimicrobial drugs for 7-14 days. For chronic bacterial cystitis, treatment up to 4-6 weeks may be necessary. Appropriate duration of treatment for complicated lower urinary tract infection depends on the nature of the underlying problem.
• Low-dose, bedtime antibacterial therapy can be used to prevent urinary tract infection in animals that have frequent reinfections. Such prophylactic treatment is started immediately after cure of the most recent episode of urinary tract infection by conventional treatment. Administer an appropriate antibacterial drug, usually ampicillin or nitrofurantoin, once daily for 4-6 months or longer. Dosage should be about one third of the conventional daily dosage, and the drug should be given after the animal has urinated for the last time each evening.

CONTRAINDICATIONS

Allergic reaction to a drug is a contraindication to further use of that drug

PRECAUTIONS

• Long-term or repeated use of antimicrobial drugs is associated with adverse effects in some animals (e.g., allergic reaction).
• Keratoconjunctivitis sicca is associated with administration of trimethoprim-sulfa products.
• Because of potential nephrotoxicity with long-term administration, aminoglycosides should be used only when there are no alternatives.

POSSIBLE INTERACTIONS

In patients with impaired renal function, urinary excretion of drugs used to treat urinary tract infection may be reduced. Besides leading to unintended drug accumulation in such patients, impaired urinary excretion of the drug might reduce its effectiveness.

ALTERNATE DRUGS

• Enrofloxacin and nitrofurantoin
• Ceftiofur, gentamicin, and amikacin, which must be given by injection

FOLLOW-UP

PATIENT MONITORING

• When antibacterial drug efficacy is in doubt, begin urine culture 2-3 days after starting treatment. If the drug is effective, the culture will be negative.
• Continue treating at least 1 week after resolution of hematuria, pyuria, and proteinuria. Failure of urinalysis findings to return to normal while an episode of urinary tract infection is being treated with an effective antibiotic (ie, as indicated by negative urine culture) generally means that there is some other urinary tract abnormality (e.g., urolith, tumor). Rapid recrudescence of signs when treatment is stopped generally indicates that there is a concurrent urinary tract abnormality or that the infection extends into some deep-seated site (e.g., prostatic or renal parenchyma).
• Successful cure of an episode of urinary tract infection is best demonstrated by performing a urine culture 7-10 days after completing antimicrobial therapy.
• Animals given low-dose bedtime prophylactic antibacterial therapy for frequent reinfection should have a urine culture performed via cystocentesis every 1-2 months.

PREVENTION/AVOIDANCE

• Avoid indiscriminate use of urinary catheters
• Animals with frequent reinfection can be given bedtime therapy to augment host defenses and prevent reinfection.

POSSIBLE COMPLICATIONS

Failure to detect or effectively treat lower urinary tract infection may lead to pyelonephritis or formation of struvite uroliths.

EXPECTED COURSE AND PROGNOSIS

• If not treated, expect lower urinary tract infection to persist indefinitely. Associated health risks include development of urolithiasis and extension of infection to other portions of the urinary tract (eg, the kidneys) or beyond (e.g, septicemia, discospondylitis, and bacterial endocarditis).

• Generally, the prognosis for animals with uncomplicated lower urinary tract infection is good to excellent. Animals that have frequent reinfection are candidates for low-dose bedtime prophylactic therapy as described , but even these patients usually do well. The prognosis for animals with complicated lower urinary tract infection is determined by the prognosis for the other urinary abnormality.

MISCELLANEOUS

ASSOCIATED CONDITIONS

• Struvite uroliths
• Diabetes mellitus or hyperadrenocorticism

AGE- RELATED FACTORS

Complicated urinary tract infection is more common in middle-aged to old than young animals

ZOONOTIC POTENTIAL

None

PREGNANCY

Depending on the stage of pregnancy, intensity of signs, and presence or absence of concomitant abnormalities, consider deferring treatment. Avoid using tetracycline, nitrofurantoin, or enrofloxacin.

SYNONYMS

Bacterial cystitis, urethrocystitis, and urethritis

SEE ALSO

Pyelonephritis
Urolithiasis, Struvite—Dogs and Cats

ABBREVIATIONS

MIC = minimum inhibitory concentration

References

Grauer GF. Urinary tract infections. In: Nelson RW, Couto CG, eds. Essentials of small animal internal medicine. St Louis: Mosby-Year Book, 1992:494-500.
Lees GE, Rogers KS. Treatment of urinary tract infections in dogs and cats. J Amer Vet Med Assoc 1986;189:648-652.
Author George E. Lees
Consulting Editors Larry G. Adams and Carl A. Osborne

LUMBOSACRAL STENOSIS

BASICS

DEFINITION
Clinical syndrome caused by dorsoventral narrowing of the lumbosacral vertebral canal with compression of the L7, sacral, or caudal nerve roots

Pathophysiology
• In patients with congenital lumbosacral stenosis, abnormal development of the dorsal arch of the L7-S1 vertebrae causes congenital narrowing of the lumbosacral spinal canal. Chronic biomechanical stress may contribute to degenerative changes that reduce the canal diameter and cause compression of the spinal nerve roots. If the canal is congenitally small, less stenosis is required before clinical signs appear. • Acquired lumbosacral stenosis caused by bony and soft tissue degenerative changes, leads to gradual but progressive reduction in the lumbosacral spinal canal.

Systems Affected
Nervous—specifically nerve roots, from L7 caudally

Genetics No known genetic basis

Incidence/Prevalence Unknown

Geographic Distribution N/A

SIGNALMENT

Species Common in dogs, rare in cats

Breed Predilections
• Congenital stenosis—small to medium-sized dogs • Acquired stenosis—large-breed dogs. German shepherds may be predisposed.

Mean Age and Range
Both forms—mature to middle-aged dogs

Predominant Sex
• Congenital form—males and females
• Acquired form—males

SIGNS
• Clinical signs relate to various degrees of compression of the nerve roots L7, sacral, and caudal. Lumbosacral pain is the salient clinical feature. • Sciatic nerve dysfunction may manifest initially as lameness, but progresses to pelvic limb weakness, muscle wasting, and postural reaction deficits. • Pudendal nerve root involvement causes urinary or fecal incontinence. • Caudal nerve root involvement causes weakness to paralysis of the tail. • Compression of both meninges and nerve roots causes sensory disturbances that vary from unpleasant sensations to obvious low lumbar pain. Self mutilation is a common clinical sign in patients with congenital lumbosacral stenosis. • In patients with both forms, extension of the pelvic limbs or dorsoflexion of the tail over the back reduces the lumbosacral canal diameter and usually elicits a painful response.

CAUSES
Congenital vertebral malformation, type II disc protrusion, hypertrophy or hyperplasia of the interarcuate ligament, proliferation of the articular facets, and subluxation or instability of the lumbosacral junction

RISK FACTORS N/A

DIAGNOSIS

DIFFERENTIAL DIAGNOSIS
• A thorough orthopaedic examination is necessary, because early low lumbar pain may be difficult to distinguish from hip dysplasia or other orthopaedic injury. • Chronic diskospondylitis, osteomyelitis, and primary or metastatic vertebral tumor of the lumbosacral region cannot be differentiated by clinical signs alone. • Vertebral fracture and subluxation are acute and characterized by more bilateral signs. • Localized myelitis or radiculoneuritis usually causes more diffuse pain.

CBC/BIOCHEMISTRY/URINALYSIS
• Results usually normal • Urinalysis may indicate lower urinary tract infection secondary to urinary incontinence.

OTHER LABORATORY TESTS N/A
IMAGING
• Spondylosis at the lumbosacral junction, narrowing of the L7-S1 disc space, and ventral displacement of the sacrum relative to the lumbar vertebrae are common findings. However, these changes should be interpreted with caution since all can be seen in clinically normal animals. • Myelography is rarely of benefit because the subarachnoid space rarely extends beyond the sixth lumbar vertebrae in large-breed dogs. However, myelography is indicated to rule out lesions rostral to the lumbosacral junction. • Epidurography may outline a space-occupying mass over the lumbosacral disc space. • Discography of the L7-S1 disc space may help highlight elevation of the dorsal annulus fibrosis. • Intraosseous venography is technically difficult and is the least reliable diagnostic procedure. • CT and MRI are newer techniques that may enhance the ability to recognize this condition.

OTHER DIAGNOSTIC PROCEDURES
Electromyography is used diagnostically and prognostically. Denervation may or may not be detected in the muscles innervated by the nerve roots L7 to caudal. If found, it confirms the localization of the lesion and implies permanent deficits.

GROSS AND HISTOPATHOLOGIC FINDINGS
One or more of the following pathologic features may be seen: hypertrophy of the ligamentum flavum, type II disc disease, hypertrophy of the interarcuate ligament, spondylosis causing stenosis of the intervertebral foramen with ensuing compression of nerve roots, ventral displacement of the sacrum with regard to lumbar vertebrae, proliferation of articular facets, congenital malformation consisting of shortened pedicles, and thickened and sclerotic lamina and articular processes.

TREATMENT

INPATIENT VERSUS OUTPATIENT
• Patients that are urinary continent can be discharged pending surgery.
• Patients with urinary incontinence should be hospitalized for initial medical management.

ACTIVITY
• Confinement and restricted leash walks, alone or combined with corticosteroid administration, frequently alleviate the pain associated with this condition. However, clinical signs often return with increasing levels of exercise.
• Exercise should be restricted for 4 weeks after surgery.

DIET
Obesity should be avoided because excess weight increases biomechanical stress on the spine.

CLIENT EDUCATION
• Without treatment, the syndrome causes progressive neurologic impairment of the pelvic limbs, urinary and fecal incontinence, and paralysis of the tail. Medical management alone is usually unsatisfactory.
• Pelvic limb lameness and self-mutilation result from pain associated with nerve root irritation and compression.
• Surgical treatment stops the progression of the disease and removes the source of pain, but some of the neurologic deficits may remain.

SURGICAL CONSIDERATIONS
• Surgical decompression is the preferred treatment.
• Dorsal laminectomy of the L7-S1 vertebrae effectively relieves compression in most patients. If nerves roots are being compressed by spondylitic bone, a dorsal laminectomy can be combined with facetectomy or foraminotomy.
• If the lumbosacral junction appears unstable either radiographically or by visualization during surgery, fusion of the lumbosacral joint may be necessary. This can be accomplished by fixation of the L7-S1 articular process to the wing of the ileum through a dorsal approach, or by a ventral approach with an ileal graft placed in a ventral slot.

MEDICATIONS

DRUGS AND FLUIDS
Conservative treatment by use of nonsteroidal antiinflammatory drugs (NSAIDs) or corticosteroids is usually unsatisfactory.

CONTRAINDICATIONS N/A

PRECAUTIONS N/A

POSSIBLE INTERACTIONS N/A

ALTERNATE DRUGS N/A

 FOLLOW-UP

PATIENT MONITORING
• After surgery, catheterize the bladder manually and express it three to four times daily until adequate voluntary control returns.
• Monitor carefully for urinary tract infection and administer appropriate antibiotics if necessary.

PREVENTION/AVOIDANCE N/A

POSSIBLE COMPLICATIONS
• Seroma formation is a frequent sequel to surgery; can be effectively managed by cage rest and surgical drainage • While infrequent, recurrence of clinical signs may be caused by excessive fibrous tissue formation (laminectomy membrane) in the surgical area. Proper surgical technique should minimize this complication. Surgical removal of laminectomy membranes is difficult and has a lower success rate than the initial dorsal laminectomy.

EXPECTED COURSE AND PROGNOSIS
• Prognosis varies with the degree of neurologic injury. • Dogs that have low lumbar pain and mild neurologic deficits have a good prognosis after surgery. Most recover fully within a few months. • Dogs with fecal and urinary incontinence have a guarded prognosis.

 MISCELLANEOUS

ASSOCIATED CONDITIONS
Lower urinary tract infections frequently accompany urinary incontinence.

AGE RELATED FACTORS N/A

ZOONOTIC POTENTIAL N/A

PREGNANCY N/A

SYNONYMS
• Lumbosacral malarticulation-malformation
• Lumbosacral instability • Lumbosacral spondylopathy • Lumbosacral spondylolisthesis

SEE ALSO
• Intervertebral Disc Disease • Discospondylitis

ABBREVIATIONS
CT = computerized tomography

MRI = magnetic resonance imaging
NSAID = nonsteroidal antiinflammatory drug

References
Morgan JP, Bailey CS. Cauda equina syndrome in the dog: radiographic evaluation. J Small Anim Pract 1990;31:69-77.

Oliver JE Jr, Selcer RR, Simpson S. Cauda equina conpression from lumbosacral malarticulation and malformation in the dog. J Am Vet Med Assoc 1978;173:207-214.

Sisson AF, LeCouteur RA, Ingram JT, Park RD, Child G. Diagnosis of cauda equina abnormalities by using electromyography, discography, and epidurography in dogs. J Vet Int Med 1992;6:253-263.

Slocum B, Devine T. L7-S1 fixation-fusion for treatment of cauda equina compression in the dog. J Am Vet Med Assoc 1986;188:31-35.

Tarvin G, Prada RG. Lumbosacral stenosis in dogs. J Am Vet Med Assoc 1980;177:154-159.

Author Karen R. Dyer

Consulting Editor Joane M. Parent

LUNG LOBE TORSION

BASICS

OVERVIEW
• Twisting of lung lobe(s) at the hilus with occlusion of the bronchus, lymphatics, vein and, finally, the arteries • The right middle lobe is the most commonly affected but other lobes can twist singly or in pairs. • Initially, the lobe becomes engorged with blood, causing its enlargement. • Infarction and necrosis may occur. • Hemorrhagic pleural effusion typically occurs. • Chronic survivors may have shrinkage and fibrosis of the lobe.

SIGNALMENT
• Most common in large, deep-chested dogs
• Less common in cats

SIGNS
• Depression, fever, weakness, collapse
• Dyspnea, orthopnea, cough, hemoptysis
• Ventral thoracic dullness, tachycardia, cyanosis, shock

CAUSES AND RISK FACTORS
• Lobar torsion usually is associated with a preexisting condition that results in pleural effusion (e.g., trauma, neoplasia, chylothorax). • Thoracic or diaphragmatic surgery
• Spontaneous, idiopathic

DIAGNOSIS

DIFFERENTIAL DIAGNOSIS
• Pulmonary contusion • Diaphragmatic hernia • Pulmonary abscess or infarction
• Neoplasia, lymphomatoid granulomatosis
• Coagulopathies • Pneumonia, embolization, thrombosis • Uncomplicated pleural effusion and compression atelectasis • Fungal or foreign body granuloma • Lobar consolidation or bronchial obstruction from a foreign body

CBC/BIOCHEMISTRY/URINALYSIS
N/A

OTHER LABORATORY TESTS N/A

IMAGING
• Radiology initially may reveal air bronchograms with disorientation of the torsed bronchus. Pleural effusion is suggested by ventral leafing and interlobar fissures. Consolidation and swelling of the torsed lobe typically are seen with possible displacement of the heart and mediastinum. There may be a lack of expansion of other lobes. Thoracentesis may allow improved visualization and provide therapeutic benefits.
• Ultrasound may allow further characterization, but fine needle aspiration is contraindicated.

OTHER DIAGNOSTIC PROCEDURES
• The pleural effusion typically is hemorrhagic, with a PCV and white blood cell count similar to that of peripheral blood. Platelets are absent from the pleural fluid. • Chronicity or preexisting effusions such as chyle may alter the observed effusion. • Bronchoscopy can reveal occlusion of the associated bronchus.
• Surgical exploration leads to definitive diagnosis and therapy.

TREATMENT
• Thoracentesis or chest tube placement
• Reexpansion pulmonary edema can be a serious problem (especially in cats) if large volumes of pleural fluid are withdrawn quickly or if chronically compressed lungs are acutely inflated at surgery.
• Oxygen therapy and shock therapy when indicated • Anesthesia requires adequate ventilatory support, careful monitoring, and effective response to the patient's needs.
• Surgical removal of the involved lobe(s) is the only effective therapy.
• The torsed lung lobe(s) should not be salvaged because recurrence or necrosis may result.
• In situ ligation of the vessels or alternately clamping with noncrushing forceps has been advocated.

• The remaining thoracic structures are closely inspected for any abnormalities.
• Postoperative monitoring, supportive care, and tube drainage are indicated.

MEDICATIONS

DRUGS AND FLUIDS
• Perioperative antibiotics
• IV fluid therapy
• Shock therapy when indicated

CONTRAINDICATIONS/POSSIBLE INTERACTIONS N/A

FOLLOW-UP
• Observe for recurrence of pleural effusion.
• Radiograph chest before discharge and as needed thereafter. • If no underlying abnormality remains, the prognosis is good.

MISCELLANEOUS

Reference
Slatter DH. Textbook of small animal surgery. 2nd ed. Philadelphia: W B Saunders, 1993.
Author Bradley L. Moses
Consulting Editors Lynelle Johnson and Bradley L. Moses

LUPUS ERYTHMATOSUS, CUTANEOUS (DISCOID)

BASICS

OVERVIEW
• Considered to be a benign variant of systemic lupus erythematosus. • Second most common immune-mediated skin disease in dogs, after pemphigus foliaceus. • Predominantly involves skin and mucous membranes.

SIGNALMENT
• Seen in both dogs and cats. • Predisposed breeds: collies, German shepherd dogs, Siberian huskies, shetland sheepdogs, Alaskan malamutes, and their crosses. • May be more common in females. • No age predilection.

SIGNS
• Often starts with depigmentation of nose and/or lips. • Depigmentation progresses to erosions and ulcerations. • Eventual tissue loss and scarring. • May also involve pinnae, periocular region, feet, and genitalia.

CAUSES AND RISK FACTORS
• Some evidence suggests that the disorder may be associated with interaction of a virus with a disturbed immune system in a genetically predisposed host. • Exposure to ultraviolet light is a complicating but not causative factor.

DIAGNOSIS

DIFFERENTIAL DIAGNOSIS
• Nasal discoid lupus erythematosus (DLE) must be differentiated from other causes of nasal dermatitis, including systemic lupus erythematosus, pemphigus foliaceus, pemphigus erythematosus, uveodermatologic syndrome, nasal pyoderma, nasal solar dermatitis, demodicosis, zinc-responsive dermatosis, dermatomyositis, trauma, nasodigital hyperkeratosis, contact dermatitis, drug eruption, squamous-cell carcinoma, and several systemic fungal infections. • Non-nasal forms of DLE must be differentiated from the other immune-mediated skin disorders, demodicosis, dermatophytosis, and hypersensitivity disorders.

CBC/BIOCHEMISTRY/URINALYSIS
Routine hematology, biochemistry, and urinalysis usually normal or negative.

OTHER LABORATORY TESTS
ANA, LE preparation, and Coombs' tests usually normal or negative.

IMAGING N/A

OTHER DIAGNOSTIC PROCEDURES
• Biopsies of non-ulcerated, primary lesions, which are often characterized by interface dermatitis and excessive dermal mucin.

GROSS AND HISTOPATHOLOGIC FINDINGS
• Immunopathologic examination of non-ulcerated samples preserved in Michel's solution. • Reveals characterisitic "lupus band."

TREATMENT
• Not a life-threatening disease; therefore, important not to overtreat.
• Avoid direct solar exposure and use waterproof sunblocks with an SPF>15.
• Vitamin E, 10-20 IU/kg PO q12h may help limit scarring.

MEDICATIONS

DRUGS AND FLUIDS
• Tetracycline and niacinamide - 250 mg of each q8h for dogs < 10 kg; 500 mg q8h for larger dogs.
• Topical corticosteroids—initially a potent fluorinated product (e.g., 0.1% amcinonide) q24h for 14 days; then q48h-q72 h for 28 days; if in remission switch to less potent product such as 0.5% or 2.5% hydrocortisone.
• For severe cases, consider prednisone 2 mg/kg/day combined with azathioprine 2 mg/kg on alternate days.

CONTRAINDICATIONS/POSSIBLE INTERACTIONS N/A

FOLLOW-UP

PATIENT MONITORING
• Recheck 14 days after initiating treatment for clinical response. • Routine hematology and biochemistry every 3 months if using topical or oral corticosteroids for control.

PREVENTION/AVOIDANCE
• Avoid using affected animals for breeding.
• Solar avoidance for those prone to DLE.

POSSIBLE COMPLICATIONS
• Scarring • Secondary pyoderma

EXPECTED COURSE AND PROGNOSIS
Progressive but not usually life-threatening if left untreated.
With proper treatment, expect remission in about 75% of patients.
Need for chronic immunosuppressive therapy suggests a worse prognosis.

MISCELLANEOUS

ABBREVIATIONS
ANA = antinuclear antibody
DLE = discoid lupus erythematosus
LE = lupus erythematosus

References

Nesbitt GH; Ackerman LJ: Dermatology for the small animal practitioner. Trenton, NJ: Veterinary Learning Systems, 1991.
Author Lowell Ackerman
Consulting Editor Lowell Ackerman

LUPUS ERYTHEMATOSUS, SYSTEMIC (SLE)

 BASICS

DEFINITION
A multisystem autoimmune disease characterized by the formation of autoantibodies against a wide array of self-antigens and circulating immune complexes

Pathophysiology
The cause of SLE is unknown. An immunoregulatory defect causes the production of autoantibodies to non–organ-specific nuclear and cytoplasmic antigens and to cell and organ-specific antigens. Immune complexes are formed and deposited in the glomerular basement membrane, synovial membrane, skin, blood vessels, and other sites. Tissue injury is caused by activation of complement by immune complexes and infiltration of inflammatory cells. In addition, a direct cytotoxic effect of autoantibodies against membrane-bound antigens contributes to tissue damage. Clinical manifestations of the disease depend on the localization of the immune complexes and the specificity of the autoantibodies.

Systems Affected
• Musculoskeletal—deposition of immune complexes in the synovial membranes
• Skin/exocrine—deposition of immune complexes in skin • Renal/urologic—deposition of immune complexes in the glomeruli
• Hemic/lymph/immune—autoantibodies against RBC, leukocytes, or platelets.
• Other organ systems if there is deposition of immune complexes or autoantibodies

Genetics
Hereditary in a colony of German shepherds; linked to the major histocompatibility complex allele DLA-A7

Incidence/Prevalence
Rare, but probably underdiagnosed

Geographic Distribution N/A

SIGNALMENT

Species Dogs and cats

Breed Predilections None

Mean Age and Range
The mean age is 6 years, but SLE can occur at any age.

Predominant Sex None

SIGNS

Historical Findings
• The onset can be acute or insidious with signs varying depending on the site of immune complex deposition and specificity of the autoantibodies. • Waxing and waning course with clinical manifestations often changing over time • Signs include lethargy, anorexia, shifting leg lameness, skin lesions, and altered behavior.

Physical Examination Findings
• Joints may be swollen and painful.
• Symmetric or focal cutaneous lesions may

be characterized by erythema, scaling, ulceration, and alopecia. Mucocutaneous and oral lesions are common. • Fever • Lymphadenopathy and hepatosplenomegaly • Arrhythmias, heart murmurs, and pleural frictions rubs (i.e., associated with myocarditis, pericarditis, or pleuritis) • Muscle wasting

CAUSES
• Definitive causes of SLE have not been identified.
• Exposure to drugs and viral infections are suspected causes.

RISK FACTORS
Exposure to ultraviolet light may exacerbate the disease.

 DIAGNOSIS

• Definitive diagnosis requires a positive antinuclear antibody (ANA) or lupus erythematosus (LE) cell test or both and two major signs or one major and two minor signs. Probable diagnosis of SLE requires positive ANA or LE cell test or both and one major or two minor signs. • Major signs are polyarthritis, proteinuria, dermatitis, hemolytic anemia, leukopenia, thrombocytopenia, and polymyositis. • Minor signs are fever of unknown origin, oral ulcers, peripheral lymphadenopathy, pleuritis, pericarditis, myocarditis, depression, and seizures.

DIFFERENTIAL DIAGNOSIS
A patient with a disease such as neoplasia has similar signs on examination as those associated with SLE. It is important to rule out infectious disease because SLE is treated with immunosuppressive drugs.

CBC/BIOCHEMISTRY/URINALYSIS
• CBC may reveal anemia, leukopenia, and thrombocytopenia. Anemia can be moderate and nonregenerative (e.g., anemia of chronic disease) or severe and regenerative (e.g., hemolytic). Alternatively, the CBC may reveal leukocytosis (i.e., monocytosis and neutrophilia) resulting from chronic inflammation.
• Results of biochemical analysis vary widely depending on the organ(s) affected. • High urine protein/urine creatinine ratio (> 1) indicates true proteinuria that may be caused by glomerulonephritis. Patients with hemolytic anemia may have bilirubinuria.

OTHER LABORATORY TESTS
• Serum electrophoresis usually shows an increase of β- and γ-globulins. • ANA test—sensitive assay. Positive test result supports a diagnosis of SLE. False-positive results are associated with some infectious diseases (e.g., leishmaniasis and subacute bacterial endocarditis in dogs; FeLV, cholangiohepatitis, and treatment with propylthiouracil in cats).
• LE test—positive test result supports a diagnosis of SLE. Less sensitive than the ANA test and cumbersome to perform. • Direct

antiglobulin test (Coombs' test)—positive in patients with immune-mediated hemolytic anemia

IMAGING
Radiography of affected joints reveals nonerosive arthritis, this in contrast to the erosive lesions of rheumatoid arthritis.

OTHER DIAGNOSTIC PROCEDURES
• Arthrocentesis in patients with lameness or swollen joints. High cell count with nondegenerate neutrophils and monocytes and low viscosity are characteristic findings. • Bacterial culture of synovial fluid is negative. • Skin biopsy in patients with skin lesions. Save specimen in 10% buffered formalin (for histopathologic examination) and Michel's solution (for immunofluorescence testing).
• Bone marrow biopsy in affected patients with nonregenerative anemia reveals excess iron deposition (anemia of chronic disease).

GROSS AND HISTOPATHOLOGIC FINDINGS
• Nonerosive polyarthritis with infiltration of synovial membrane by neutrophils and lymphocytes; no pannus formation • Membranous or membranoproliferative glomerulonephritis • Mononuclear interface dermatitis with hydropic degeneration of keratinocytes and eosinophilic round bodies representing apoptotic basal keratinocytes. Vasculitis of dermal blood vessels and panniculitis in some patients. Immunofluorescence demonstrates deposition of immune complexes along the basement membrane of the dermal-epidermal junction. • Vasculitis may be seen in any organ, especially myocardium, pericardium, and meninges. • Reactive lymphoid hyperplasia in the lymph nodes and spleen

 TREATMENT

INPATIENT VERSUS OUTPATIENT
• Hospitalization may be necessary for initial management (e.g., in a patient with hemolytic crisis).
• Outpatient management usually is possible.

ACTIVITY
During episodes of acute polyarthritis, enforced rest is indicated.

DIET
Dietary protein restriction is recommended in animals with severe renal disease caused by glomerulonephritis.

CLIENT EDUCATION
• Discuss the progressive and unpredictable course of the disease.
• Discuss the need for long-term, immunosuppressive therapy and its side effects.
• Discuss hereditability of the disease.

SURGICAL CONSIDERATIONS N/A

MEDICATIONS

DRUGS AND FLUIDS
• The goal of treatment is to control the abnormal immune response and to reduce the inflammation. Corticosteroids target both objectives and are the basis of the treatment.
• Prednisone (1-2 mg/kg PO q12h)
• Add a cytotoxic immunosuppressive drug when prednisone fails to improve the condition or when the patient is steroid intolerant. Reduce prednisone to 0.5-1 mg/kg PO q12h. Use azathioprine (dogs, 2 mg/kg PO q24h), cyclophosphamide (50 mg/m^2 PO for 4 consecutive days, then 3 days off, repeat weekly) or chlorambucil (dogs, 2-3 mg/m^2 PO; cats,1.5 mg/m^2 PO).
• Reduce immunosuppressant drug dosage to lowest possible once remission is achieved.
• Aspirin (dogs, 10-25 mg/kg PO q12h; cats, 10-40 mg/kg PO q72h) may be given to animals with painful joints.

CONTRAINDICATIONS
Aspirin should not be give to patients with thrombocytopenia or gastrointestinal ulcers.

PRECAUTIONS
• Cats are susceptible to azathioprine toxicity and this drug should be used with caution, if at all (dosage, 1 mg/cat PO q48h).
• Cyclophosphamide can induce hemorrhagic cystitis and bone marrow suppression.
• Treatment with immunosuppressive drugs increases the risk of severe infection.

POSSIBLE INTERACTIONS
Concurrent use of aspirin and prednisone increases the risk of gastrointestinal ulceration.

ALTERNATE DRUGS
Cyclosporin A (5-10 mg/kg PO q12h) may be tried in refractory patients. Use with caution and withdraw if side effects occur (e.g., gastritis, lymphocytoid dermatitis, papillomatosis, and gingival hyperplasia).

FOLLOW-UP

PATIENT MONITORING
• Weekly physical examination • CBC and biochemical analsysis to monitor side effects of the immunosuppressive drugs. Initially, on a weekly basis. • ANA remains high during remission and is *not* useful to monitor the disease.

PREVENTION/AVOIDANCE
Do not breed affected animals.

POSSIBLE COMPLICATIONS N/A

EXPECTED COURSE AND PROGNOSIS
The prognosis is guarded to poor. The presence of hemolytic anemia and glomerulonephritis and the development of bacterial infection warrant a poor prognosis.

MISCELLANEOUS

ASSOCIATED CONDITIONS N/A

AGE RELATED FACTORS N/A

ZOONOTIC POTENTIAL N/A

PREGNANCY
The use of cytotoxic immunosuppressive drugs in pregnant animals is contraindicated.

SYNONYMS N/A

SEE ALSO
• Anemia, Immune-Mediated • Thrombocytopenia, Immune-Mediated • Glomerulonephritis • Arthritis

ABBREVIATIONS
ANA = antinuclear antibody
RBC = red blood cells
SLE = systemic lupus erythematosus

References

Lewis RM, Picut CA. Veterinary clinical immunology. Philadelphia: Lea & Febiger, 1989.

Halliwell REW, Gorman NT. Veterinary clinical immunology. Philadelphia: WB Saunders, 1989.

Pedersen NC, Barlough JE. Systemic lupus erythematosus in the cat. Feline Pract 1991;19:5-13.

Author Harm HogenEsch
Consulting Editor Alan H. Rebar

LYME DISEASE

BASICS

DEFINITION
Lyme disease is one of the most common tick-transmitted zoonotic diseases in the world, caused by the spirochete Borrelia burgdorferi. The dominant clinical feature in dogs is a recurrent acute arthritis with lameness, sometimes with anorexia and depression. Dogs may develop cardiac, neurologic, or renal diseases. Lyme disease has also been reported in horses, cattle, and cats.

Pathophysiology
The pathogenesis of Lyme arthritis is still unclear. Local skin infestation after a tick bite is followed by a generalized infection of predominantly connective tissues, joint capsules, muscle, and lymph nodes. It is presently not known whether arthritis is caused directly by persistent spirochetes or by immune complexes. The incubation period in experimental dogs is 2-5 months.

Systems Affected
• Persistent B. burgdorferi can be found in skin, muscle, connective tissues, joints, and lymph nodes but rarely in body fluids like blood, CSF, or synovial fluid. • Pathologic changes with few exceptions are restricted to joints, local lymph nodes, and the skin at the site of the tick bite.

Genetics
A genetic basis for Lyme disease is known in mice but has not been established for dogs.

Incidence/Prevalence
• The percentage of seropositive dogs within a dog population varies greatly with the exposure to infected ticks in endemic areas. A range of 5-80% has been reported. • Only approximately 5% of seropositive dogs in endemic areas develop Lyme disease.

Geographic Distribution
Lyme disease has a worldwide distribution. However, there is a great variation in the distribution of endemic areas. In the United States, more than 90% of all cases occur in the northeast, followed by the upper Mississippi region, California, and some southern states.

SIGNALMENT
In endemic areas, Lyme disease is fairly common in dogs but rarely seen in cats. There is no known breed or sex predilection in dogs. However, young dogs appear to be more susceptible than older dogs. Only about 5% of seropositive dogs develop disease.

SIGNS
• The dominant clinical feature in dogs is recurrent acute arthritis with lameness, sometimes with fever, anorexia, and depression. During the acute lameness, one or more joints may be swollen and warm, and a pain response is elicited by palpation. Dogs may walk stiffly with an arched back and may be sensitive to touch. Prescapular and/or popliteal lymph nodes may be swollen. Lameness usually lasts for only 3-4 days and responds well to antibiotic treatment. • Cardiac signs, including complete heart block and neurologic complications, have been reported but are rare. More recently, a fatal renal failure with protein loss in urine and immune complexes in glomeruli has been reported. • Blood and urine analysis is usually unremarkable. On rare occasions, spirochetes have been detected in Giemsa-stained blood smears.

CAUSES
• Lyme disease is caused by the spirochete Borrelia burgdorferi or related Borrelias that are transmitted by the small, hard-shell deer tick Ixodes scapularis or related Ixodes ticks. Infection only takes place after the tick (nymphal stage in spring or adult female in fall) is partially engorged, 24-48 hours after the initial infestation. • Ixodes ticks have a 2-year life cycle. Larvae hatch in spring and become infected by feeding on white-footed mice, Peromyscus leucopus, which are persistently infected. The larvae molt into nymphs in the spring of the following year and stay infected or become infected by feeding on mice. Nymphs molt into adults in late fall of the second year. Adult female ticks engorge after mating on deer or other mammals, fall off, and hide under leaves until the following spring when they each lay about 2,000 eggs. Adult male ticks tend to stay on the deer.

RISK FACTORS
Roaming in tick infested areas in Lyme-endemic areas poses the greatest risk. It has been speculated that vectors other than ticks and urine from infected dogs may be sources of infection. However, there is very little evidence for either.

DIAGNOSIS

DIFFERENTIAL DIAGNOSIS
Lyme arthritis should be differentiated from septic arthritis caused by streptococcal or strephylococcal infection by Giemsa stains and by culture of synovial fluid. Other infectious diseases such as Rocky Mountain spotted fever or canine ehrlichiosis can be ruled out by serology and platelet counts. Degenerative joint disease, osteochondritis dissecans, or panosteitis would not respond to antibiotic treatment like Lyme arthritis. Immune-mediated diseases should be ruled out by testing for antinuclear antibodies (ANA), lupus erythematosis (LE) preparations, and rheumatoid arthritis (RA) factor.

CBC/BIOCHEMISTRY/URINALYSIS
Hematological and biochemical analysis of blood and urine is unremarkable.

OTHER LABORATORY TESTS
Positive serology by ELISA and Western blots indicates previous exposure to B. burgdorferi and may be indicative of Lyme disease. While the ELISA test cannot differentiate between sera from vaccinated and from naturally infected dogs, the Western blot can. Cross-reactions with antibody responses to Leptospira species are minimal.

IMAGING
Radiographs would only be helpful for the differential diagnosis of lameness.

OTHER DIAGNOSTIC PROCEDURES
B. burgdorferi frequently can be isolated from skin biopsy specimens of infected dogs. However, the process is time-consuming and expensive and, therefore, not practical.

GROSS AND HISTOPATHOLOGIC FINDINGS
• The only gross findings would be swollen joint(s) with excess synovial fluid and sometimes enlarged lymph nodes. Histopathology of acute arthritis would show a fibrino purulent synovitis. Other joints may have a mild synovitis with infiltration of lymphocytes and plasma cells. Lymph nodes may show cortical hyperplasia with multiple enlarged follicles and expanded parafollicular areas. • In the skin near the site of the tick bite, there may be perivascular infiltrates of plasma cells, lymphocytes, and some mast cells in the superficial dermis.

TREATMENT

INPATIENT VERSUS OUTPATIENT
Dogs with Lyme disease should be treated as outpatients.

ACTIVITY
Reduced activity is advisable until clinical signs improve.

DIET
A change in diet is not needed.

CLIENT EDUCATION
The most important rule in treatment is the regular application of antibiotics as prescribed.

SURGICAL CONSIDERATIONS
Aspiration of synovial fluid for diagnostic purposes may be considered.

MEDICATIONS

DRUGS AND FLUIDS
The antibiotics most commonly used to treat Lyme disease are doxycycline (5 mg/kg q12h PO) or amoxicillin (20 mg/kg q8-12h PO). The duration of treatment is debatable and it is presently not known whether antibiotics eliminate persistent infection of B. burgdorferi. A treatment period of 2-4 weeks usually is recommended.

CONTRAINDICATIONS N/A

PRECAUTIONS

Young and growing animals should not be treated with tetracyclines (doxycycline).

POSSIBLE INTERACTIONS

The rare occurrence of Jarisch-Herxheimer reaction within the first 3 days of antibiotic treatment has been reported in humans but is not known in animals. Toxic by-products from killed spirochetes may intensify signs.

ALTERNATE DRUGS

Corticosteroids may ameliorate signs. However, they would mask the effect of antibiotics for a diagnostic purpose.

FOLLOW-UP

PATIENT MONITORING

Improvement should be seen within 3 days of antibiotic treatment. If improvement is not seen, a differential diagnosis should be considered.

PREVENTION/AVOIDANCE

• Lyme disease can be prevented by either avoiding tick infestation or by vaccination.
• Tick engorgement on dogs may be prevented by tick repellents containing DEET or permethrin, tick collars, and/or by grooming dogs daily. Controlling the tick population in the environment would be limited to small areas. Attempts to reduce the deer and/or rodent population had limited results. • For vaccination of dogs, two commercial bacterins consisting of killed B. burgdorferi in adjuvant are currently on the market. One vaccine was shown to reduce the incidence of disease from 4.7% of seropositive dogs to about 1%. However, the value of these bacterins are still debatable and it would be more desirable to have a single protein vaccine such as the OspA that protects dogs from infec-

tion. Field trials for such a vaccine are presently being conducted.

POSSIBLE COMPLICATIONS

Although arthritis with lameness is the dominant symptom, heart block, CNS disorders, and a fatal renal failure may be complications of Lyme disease in dogs.

EXPECTED COURSE AND PROGNOSIS

Recovery should be expected by 2 or 3 days after initiation of antibiotic treatment. However, the disease may be recurrent with intervals of weeks to months. Recurrent disease responds again to antibiotic treatment. The nonresponsive chronic arthritis seen in humans is not known in dogs.

MISCELLANEOUS

ASSOCIATED CONDITIONS N/A

AGE RELATED FACTORS

Young pups appear to be more susceptible to Lyme disease than older dogs. However, the disease can occur in dogs of all ages and there is no difference in treatment.

ZOONOTIC POTENTIAL

• Lyme disease occurs in humans as in dogs and the source of infection is ticks. It has been speculated that B. burgdorferi in the saliva or urine of infected dogs might be transmissible to humans. Our experiments to test this hypothesis have failed to provide any evidence of transmission. • It also has been speculated that dogs can transport ticks home and the ticks become attached to humans. Ixodid ticks are not intermittent feeders. Ixodid ticks attach quickly. Once a tick starts feeding on a dog, it will feed to repletion and not change hosts.

PREGNANCY

Although possible, there is no convincing evidence that B. burgdorferi infection is transmitted in utero in dogs. Pregnant animals tolerate antibiotic treatment, but tetracyclines should not be used.

SYNONYMS

• Lyme disease • Lyme borreliosis • Lyme arthritis

SEE ALSO N/A

ABBREVIATIONS N/A

References

Magnarelli L A, Anderson JF, Schreier AB, et al. Clinical and serologic studies of canine borreliosis. J Am Vet Med Assoc 1987;191:1089-1094.

Codner EC. Infectious polyarthritis in the dog and cat. In: Kirk R, Bonagura JD, eds. Current veterinary therapy, vol. XI. Small animal practice. Philadelphia: WB Saunders, 1992:246-252.

Appel MJG, Allan S, Jacobson RH, et al. Experimental Lyme disease in dogs produces arthritis and persistent infection. J Infec Dis 1993;167:651-664.

Levy SA, Barthold SW, Daubach DM, et al. Canine Lyme borreliosis. Compend Cont Ed Pract Vet 1993;15:833-848.

Appel MJG, Jacobson RH. Canine Lyme disease: an update. In: Kirk R, ed. Current veterinary therapy, XII. Philadelphia: WB Saunders (in press).

Author M. J. G. Appel
Consulting Editor Fred W. Scott

LYMPHADENITIS

 BASICS

DEFINITION
Inflammation of one or more lymph nodes. Lymphoid hyperplasia is not a form of lymphadenitis.

Pathophysiology
Lymphadenitis is usually the result of an infectious agent gaining access to a lymph node and establishing infection. Because of the filtration functions of lymph nodes, they are quite likely to be exposed to infectious agents. Although many organisms may produce lymphadenitis, those agents such as fungi and mycobacteria that reside within macrophages and elicit a granulomatous inflammatory response are especially prone to establish infection within lymph nodes. Noninfectious lymphadenitis is an infrequent occurrence. One example is eosinophilic lymphadenitis that occurs as an occasional component of eosinophilic inflammatory diseases.

Systems Affected
Hemic/lymphatic/immune. However, lymphadenitis frequently is a component of more widespread infectious disease.

Genetics
No known genetic basis for lymphadenitis exists except for rare cases of immunodeficiency. An example is the familial susceptibility of certain basset hounds to mycobacteriosis; lymphadenitis is a frequent manifestation of that syndrome.

Incidence/Prevalence
Because it is a frequent manifestation of a number of infectious diseases, lymphadenitis is a relatively common occurrence.

Geographic Distribution
Geographic differences in occurrence of lymphadenitis would be anticipated in the systemic fungal infections such as histoplasmosis (central United States) and blastomycosis (central and eastern United States) and in less common infections such as leishmaniasis (southern and southwestern United States).

SIGNALMENT
Species Dogs and cats

Breed Predilection None

Mean Age and Range
Because of their susceptibility to infection, neonates may have an increased occurrence of lymphadenitis.

Predominant Sex None

SIGNS
General Comments
When lymphadenitis is a complication of infection in another organ, clinical signs usually relate to that organ rather than to the inflamed lymph node. Clinical signs in animals with lymphadenitis that is a component of systemic infection are those associated with systemic inflammatory disease: fever, malaise, anorexia

Historical Findings
Lymphadenitis seldom causes lymph node enlargement that is so severe as to be observed by animal owners. They are more likely to report either the systemic signs of inflammatory disease or signs associated with specific organ dysfunction.

Physical Examination Findings
Inflamed lymph nodes are typically enlarged, firm, and may be painful. A few animals with bacterial lymphadenitis will develop abscesses within the nodes. Such abscesses may open to the exterior and present as draining tracts. Animals with lymphadenitis may also have fever and other systemic signs of infection.

CAUSES
• Bacteria: Most pathogenic aerobic and anaerobic bacteria are occasional causes of lymphadenitis. Among the more likely agents are Pasteurella, Bacteroides, and Fusobacterium species. A few bacteria such as Yersinia pestis (bubonic plague) and Francisella tularensis (tularemia) have a particular affinity for lymph nodes and are especially likely to have lymphadenitis as a manifestation of disease. • Fungi: Fungal infections commonly include lymphadenitis as one manifestation of systemic disease. Commonly implicated organisms include Blastomyces, Cryptococcus, Histoplasma, Coccidiodes, and Sporothrix. Many other mycotic agents are occasional causes of lymphadenitis. • Protozoa: Animals with toxoplasmosis and leishmaniasis frequently have lymphadenitis, although it is unlikely to be the most obvious clinical finding. • Algae: Lymphadenitis often is one manifestation of canine protothecosis. • Viruses: Although many viral infections cause lymphadenopathy due to lymphoid hyperplasia, the feline infectious peritonitis coronavirus actually causes lymphadenitis. The mesenteric lymph nodes are most commonly affected. • Noninfectious lymphadenitis such as that associated with pulmonary or systemic eosinophilic disease is usually of unknown cause.

RISK FACTORS
Any intrinsic or extrinsic factor that compromises immune function increases the susceptibility of animals to lymphadenitis. Among the more common extrinsic factors in veterinary medicine are feline leukemia virus and feline immunodeficiency virus infection.

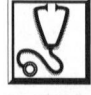 **DIAGNOSIS**

DIFFERENTIAL DIAGNOSIS
Lymphadenitis frequently cannot be distinguished on the basis of clinical findings from other causes of lymphadenopathy. The most common ones are lymphoid hyperplasia, malignant lymphoma, and metastatic neoplasia.

Fever and painful lymph nodes are more likely to be associated with lymphadenitis. Both malignant lymphoma and lymphoid hyperplasia are more common causes of generalized lymph node enlargement than is lymphadenitis.

CBC/BIOCHEMISTRY/URINALYSIS
• Although animals with lymphadenitis may have an inflammatory leukogram, the absence of such changes certainly does not exclude lymphadenitis. • Some animals with systemic causes of lymphadenitis (fungal infections, leishmaniasis) may have marked hyperglobulinemia. • Circulating eosinophilia, often severe, is a relatively consistent finding in animals with eosinophilic diseases that are sufficiently extensive and severe as to cause lymphadenitis.

OTHER LABORATORY TESTS
Serologic tests for the various systemic fungal diseases can be useful in their identification, although these tests are best utilized only when attempts to demonstrate the organisms fail.

IMAGING
Imaging techniques (radiography and ultrasonography) can be of benefit in determining the involvement of deep nodes such as those in the thoracic and abdominal cavities in systemic inflammatory diseases. They can also be valuable in assessing involvement of other organs, e.g. pneumonia in blastomycosis or histoplasmosis.

OTHER DIAGNOSTIC PROCEDURES
• Fine needle aspiration cytology can be used to identify most cases of lymphadenitis. Cytologic findings characteristic of lymphadenitis include increased proportions of neutrophils, macrophages, eosinophils, or some combination of those cell types. Occasional neutrophils, macrophages, and eosinophils are found in aspirates from normal nodes. • Bacteria, fungal agents, protozoa, and algal organisms are often present in fine needle aspirates of lymph nodes from animals with those infections. Cytologic examination frequently is the most efficient means of detecting and identifying specific infectious agents in animals with either lymphadenitis of an isolated node or systemic infection. • Eosinophilic lymphadenitis should not be diagnosed on cytologic specimens unless the proportion of eosinophils is markedly increased, because mild eosinophilic infiltrates occur commonly in peripheral nodes of animals with allergic or parasitic skin disease. In most such cases in which lymphadenopathy is present, it is due primarily to lymphoid hyperplasia rather than eosinophilic lymphadenitis. • When a diagnosis is not made by cytologic examination, a lymph node biopsy may be indicated. Such specimens can be used for both histopathologic evaluation and culture.

GROSS AND HISTOPATHOLOGIC FINDINGS

• Although lymph nodes affected with lymphadenitis may be grossly normal, they more frequently are enlarged and firm. The extent of enlargement varies widely, and it often distorts the shape of the node. Severe lymphadenitis may extend through the capsule of the node into the adjacent tissues. • On cut surface, affected nodes are often hyperemic and may have poorly defined nodules. In the extreme examples of purulent lymphadenitis, abscesses may develop. • Histologic lesions of purulent lymphadenitis include diffuse or multifocal infiltration of the affected node by neutrophils. The normal cortical-medullary architecture of the node may be disrupted. Granulomatous lymphadenitis is characterized by accumulations of activated macrophages involving the parenchyma of the node. In eosinophilic lymphadenitis, large numbers of eosinophils occur both within sinuses and in the cortical parenchyma. Necrosis is common in all forms of lymphadenitis.

TREATMENT

Because lymphadenitis is a lesion rather than a specific disease, no single set of therapeutic recommendations is appropriate. Identifying the characteristics of the inflammation and the causative agent will dictate appropriate therapy.

INPATIENT VERSUS OUTPATIENT
N/A

ACTIVITY N/A

DIET N/A

CLIENT EDUCATION N/A
SURGICAL CONSIDERATIONS N/A

MEDICATIONS

DRUGS AND FLUIDS

Effective drug therapy for lymphadenitis requires identification of the causative agent. Purulent lymphadenitis of a single lymph node is likely to be of bacterial etiology and can be treated with broad spectrum systemic antibiotics if no organism is detected on initial cytologic evaluation.

CONTRAINDICATIONS N/A

PRECAUTIONS N/A

POSSIBLE INTERACTIONS N/A

ALTERNATE DRUGS N/A

FOLLOW-UP

PATIENT MONITORING N/A
PREVENTION/AVOIDANCE N/A
POSSIBLE COMPLICATIONS N/A
EXPECTED COURSE AND PROGNOSIS N/A

MISCELLANEOUS

ASSOCIATED CONDITIONS

Lymphadenitis involving multiple lymph nodes is frequently one manifestation of systemic infection that also affects many other organs. Also, detection of fungal, protozoal, or algal organisms in any inflamed node should alert one to the possibility of systemic infection by that agent.

AGE RELATED FACTORS N/A

ZOONOTIC POTENTIAL

• Direct transmission of infection with agents responsible for lymphadenitis is unlikely with the exception of Sporothrix schenckii. Cats with sporotrichosis present some risk of human infection. • Caution should be exercised when performing fine needle aspirations if infectious lymphadenitis is suspected.

PREGNANCY N/A

SYNONYMS N/A

SEE ALSO
See Causes

ABBREVIATIONS N/A

References

Duncan JR The lymph nodes. In: Diagnostic cytology of the dog and cat. RL Cowell, RD Tyler, eds. Goleta, CA: American Veterinary Publications, 1989;93-98.
Rogers KS, Barton CL, Landis M: Canine and feline lymph nodes. II. Diagnostic evaluation of lymphadenopathy. Compend Contin Educ Pract Vet. 15(11) 1493-1503.
Author Edward A. Mahaffey
Consulting Editor Alan H. Rebar

LYMPHANGIECTASIA

BASICS

DEFINITION
An obstructive disorder involving the lymphatic system of the gastrointestinal tract, resulting in protein-losing enteropathy.

Pathophysiology
Lymphatic obstruction results in dilation and rupture of intestinal lacteals with subsequent loss of lymphatic contents (plasma proteins, lymphocytes, and chylomicrons) into the intestinal lumen. Although the proteins may be digested and reabsorbed, excessive enteric loss will result in hypoproteinemia. Hypoproteinemia will cause a decrease in plasma oncotic pressure, leading to edema formation, ascites, and pleural effusion.

Systems Affected
- Gastrointestinal - diarrhea, ascites
- Skin/Exocrine - subcutaneous edema
- Respiratory - pleural effusion

Genetics
Familial tendency for protein-losing enteropathy has been reported in soft-coated Wheaten terriers, basenjis, and Lundehunds. The mode of inheritance is unknown.

Incidence/Prevalence Uncommon

Geographic Distribution N/A

SIGNALMENT

Species Dogs

Breed Predilections
An increased incidence has been reported in soft-coated Wheaten terriers, basenjis, Lundehunds, and Yorkshire terriers.

Mean Age and Range
The mean age is 4.9 ± 1.9 years, and the age range is 2-9 years.

Predominant Sex
An increased incidence has been seen in female soft-coated Wheaten terriers.

SIGNS
Clinical signs are variable but may include:
- Diarrhea - chronic, intermittent of watery to semi-solid consistency • Ascites • Subcutaneous edema • Dyspnea from pleural effusion • Weight loss • Flatulence • Vomiting

CAUSES

Primary or Congenital Lymphangiectasia
- Focal (intestinal lymphatics only) • Diffuse lymphatic abnormalities (e.g. chylothorax, lymphedema, chylous ascites, thoracic duct obstruction)

Secondary Lymphangiectasia
- Right heart failure • Constrictive pericarditis • Budd-Chiari syndrome • Neoplasia (lymphosarcoma)

RISK FACTORS N/A

DIAGNOSIS

DIFFERENTIAL DIAGNOSIS
- Must differentiate from other causes of hypoproteinemia and dependent edema.
- Hypoalbuminemia can be caused by decreased hepatic synthesis due to severe hepatic disease. Globulins will often be normal or increased. • Hypoalbuminemia can be caused by glomerulonephritis or amyloidosis, and proteinuria should be detected on urinalysis. • Acute or chronic blood loss can cause hypoproteinemia. • A rare cause of hypoproteinemia is inadequate protein intake (i.e., starvation).

CBC/BIOCHEMISTRY/URINALYSIS
- Lymphopenia is usually present • Hypoalbuminemia and hypoglobulinemia (panhypoproteinemia) • Hypocholesterolemia • Hypocalcemia

OTHER LABORATORY TESTS
- Serum protein electrophoresis can be performed to quantitate and identify protein loss. Gastrointestinal protein loss will be characterized by loss of albumin and globulins. Liver disease will be characterized by low levels of albumin with normal or high globulins, and renal disease characteristically causes hypoalbuminemia with normal serum globulins. • Urine protein:creatinine ratio can be performed to rule out proteinuria. • Serum bile acids (pre- and post-prandial) or an ammonia tolerance test can be performed to assess hepatic function. • Fluid analysis of body cavity effusions can be performed since the effusion associated with lymphangiectasia is usually a transudate, but chylous ascites and chylothorax are occasionally present.

IMAGING
- Survey thoracic and abdominal radiographs are taken to rule out cardiac disease and neoplasia. Radiographs can also detect or confirm ascites or pleural effusion. • Cardiac ultrasound can be performed to rule out right-sided congestive heart failure.

OTHER DIAGNOSTIC PROCEDURES
- An ECG can be performed to aid in evaluating the heart and ruling out right-sided congestive heart failure. • Endoscopy allows for mucosal visualization and biopsy. • Laparotomy allows for surgical biopsies of intestines and lymph nodes to be obtained.

GROSS AND HISTOPATHOLOGIC FINDINGS
- Gross findings at laparotomy may include dilated lymphatics which are visible as a web-like network throughout the mesentery and serosal surface. Small yellow-white nodules and foamy granular deposits may be seen adjacent to lymphatics. • Histopathology findings include a ballooning distortion of villi caused by markedly dilated lacteals. The villi can be edematous, and some have a blunted appearance. Mucosal edema is usually present, and diffuse or multifocal accumulations of lymphocytes and plasma cells can be identified in the lamina propria.

TREATMENT

INPATIENT VERSUS OUTPATIENT
Most treated as outpatients. Hospitalization may be required if patient requires plasma transfusion.

ACTIVITY
Normal

DIET
Dietary long-chain triglycerides serve as the stimulus for intestinal lymph flow and subsequent protein loss. Therefore, dietary therapy involves feeding a low-fat diet with an ample supply of high quality protein such as Prescription Diet® r/d® or w/d® (Hill's Pet Products, Topeka, KS). To supplement fat and increase the calories in this diet, medium-chain triglycerides (MCTs) are fed. Commercial sources of MCTs are MCT oil® (Mead Johnson, Evansville, IN) or Portagen® (Mead Johnson, Evansville, IN). The diet should also be supplemented with fat-soluble vitamins (A, D, E, and K).

CLIENT EDUCATION
Discuss prognosis and response to therapy with owners as they can be unpredictable.

SURGICAL CONSIDERATIONS
- When intestinal lymphangiectasia occurs secondary to an identifiable lymphatic obstruction, surgery should be considered to relieve the obstruction. • Pericardiectomy is indicated in cases of constrictive pericarditis.

MEDICATIONS

DRUGS AND FLUIDS
- Corticosteroids can be used if dietary therapy is unsuccessful. Oral prednisone is administered at a dose of 1-2 mg/kg q12h. Once remission of the disease has occurred, the dosage should be adjusted to a lower maintenance level. • Antibiotics can be administered to control secondary bacterial overgrowth. Tylosin (10-20 mg/kg PO q12h) and metronidazole (10-20 mg/kg PO q12h) have been used for this purpose.

CONTRAINDICATIONS N/A

PRECAUTIONS N/A

POSSIBLE INTERACTIONS N/A

ALTERNATE DRUGS N/A

FOLLOW-UP

PATIENT MONITORING

Monitor body weight, serum protein concentration, and evidence of return of clinical signs (pleural effusion, ascites, edema) every 7-14 days.

PREVENTION/AVOIDANCE N/A

POSSIBLE COMPLICATIONS

- Respiratory difficulty from pleural effusion.
- Severe protein-calorie depletion.
- Intractable diarrhea.

EXPECTED COURSE AND PROGNOSIS

Prognosis is guarded. Some animals fail to respond to treatment. Remissions of several months to greater than 2 years can be maintained in other animals.

 MISCELLANEOUS

ASSOCIATED CONDITIONS

Soft-coated Wheaten terriers may also have protein-losing nephropathy.

AGE RELATED FACTORS N/A

ZOONOTIC POTENTIAL N/A

PREGNANCY N/A

SYNONYMS N/A

SEE ALSO

Protein-Losing Enteropathy

ABBREVIATIONS N/A

References

Fossum TW, Sherding RG, Zack PM, et al. Intestinal lymphangiectasia associated with chylothorax in two dogs. J Am Vet Med Assoc 1987;190:61-64.

Fossum TW. Protein-losing enteropathy. Semin Vet Med Surg (Sm Anim) 1989;4:219-225.

Meschter CL, Rakich PM, Tyler DE. Intestinal lymphangiectasia with lipogranulomatous lymphangitis in a dog. J Am Vet Med Assoc 1987;190:427-430.

Suter MM, Palmer DG, Schenk H. Primary intestinal lymphangiectasia in three dogs: a morphological and immunopathological investigation. Vet Pathol 1985;22:123-130.

Tams TR, Twedt DC. Canine protein-losing gastroenteropathy syndrome. Compend Contin Educ Pract Vet 1981;3:105-114.

Author Mollyann Holland
Consulting Editor Brent D. Jones

LYMPHEDEMA

BASICS

OVERVIEW
• Abnormal accumulation of protein rich lymph fluid into interstitial spaces, especially subcutaneous fat • Chronic lymphedema causes tissue fibrosis. • May be congenital or acquired

SIGNALMENT
• More common in dogs than cats • Congenital in bulldogs and hereditary/congenital in a family of poodles; possible breed predilection in Labrador retrievers and Old English sheepdogs

SIGNS

Historical Findings
• Primary/congenital—peripheral limb swelling usually present at birth or develops in first several months • Edema typically starts at distal extremity and slowly advances proximally.

Physical Examination Findings
• Edema most common in limbs, especially pelvic limbs; may be unilateral or bilateral • Edema less common in ventral thorax, abdomen, ears, and tail • Edema is pitting, nonpainful, and temperature of affected area is normal. • Pitting nature lost with chronicity as fibrosis occurs • Lameness and pain uncommon unless cellulitis develops

CAUSES AND RISK FACTORS
• Hereditary/congenital malformation of the lymphatic system (i.e., aplasia, valvular incompetence, and lymph node fibrosis) • Excessive interstitial fluid production secondary to venous hypertension (associated with congestive heart failure and obstruction of venous drainage) or increased vascular permeability (associated with infection, trauma, heat, and irradiation) • Secondary damage to lymphatic vessels or lymph nodes associated with trauma, infection and neoplasia

DIAGNOSIS

DIFFERENTIAL DIAGNOSIS
• Edema caused by venous stasis (e.g., congestive heart failure and cirrhosis). Look for varices, hyperpigmentation, and ulceration. • Arterio-venous fistulae. Listen for machinery murmur, feel for pulsatile vessels. Confirm with angiogram. • Edema caused by hypoproteinemia (protein losing nephropathy or enteropathy, hepatic failure, serum loss from burns or hemorrhage). Check serum protein concentration. • Trauma. Review history; look for bruising and lacerations. • Neoplasia. If swelling is firm, obtain aspirate and perform cytologic examination. • Cellulitis. Look for fever, pain, and warm swelling.

CBC/BIOCHEMSITRY/URINALYSIS
Results normal

OTHER LABORATORY TESTS N/A

IMAGING
Lymphography useful in documenting abnormalities within the lymphatic system. Best studies obtained with an injection of aqueous based contrast media directly into a lymphatic vessel. See references for detailed description of the technique.

OTHER DIAGNOSTIC PROCEDURES
N/A

TREATMENT

• No curative treatment, although there are a number of surgical and medical treatments that may be tried.
• Rest and massage of the affected limbs does not help.
• Conservative care consists of long-term use of pressure wraps, coupled with skin care and use of antibiotics to treat cellulitis and lymphangitis. This course may be successful in some animals.
• Surgical procedures that can be attempted when conservative care and medications fail include lymphangioplasty, bridging techniques, lymphaticovenous shunts, superficial and deep lymphatic anastomosis, and excisional procedures. None of these techniques is consistently beneficial, and only excisional procedures have been reported in dogs.

MEDICATIONS

DRUGS AND FLUIDS
• Diuretics, steroids, anticoagulants, and fibrinolytic agents have been used, but beneficial effects have not been confirmed.
• Benzopyrones reduce high protein edema by stimulating macrophages to release proteases. Oral dosages recommended in humans are 3 g/day of either rutoside, diosmin or rutin, or 440 mg/day of coumarin. Beneficial effects recorded in experimental studies in dogs.

CONTRAINDICATIONS/POSSIBLE INTERACTIONS
Diuretics—they initially reduce swelling but increase protein content of interstitial fluid, resulting in further tissue damage and fibrosis.

FOLLOW-UP

• Puppies with severe lymphedema may die.
• Resolution has been seen in some puppies with pelvic limb involvement only.

MISCELLANEOUS

References

Fossum TW, Miller MW. Lymphedema: etiopathogenesis. J Vet Int Med 1992; 6:283-293.

Fossum TW, King LA, Miller MW, et al. Lymphedema: clinical signs, diagnosis, and treatment. J Vet Int Med 1992; 6:312-319.

Author Francis W. K. Smith Jr.

Consulting Editors Larry P. Tilley and Francis W.K. Smith, Jr.

BASICS

OVERVIEW
Lymphomatoid granulomatosis is characterized by angiocentric and angiodestructive infiltration by atypical lymphoid cells. It is a rare pulmonary disease of dogs.

SIGNALMENT
• Median age, 5.75 years (range, 1.5-14 years) • No breed predilection • More common in large-breed and pure-breed than other dogs

SIGNS
• Progressive respiratory signs including cough and dyspnea • Exercise intolerance • Weight loss • Anorexia • Fever in 50% of patients • Duration of signs is days to weeks

CAUSES AND RISK FACTORS
Unknown

DIAGNOSIS

DIFFERENTIAL DIAGNOSIS
• Mycotic, bacterial, or aspiration pneumonia • Primary or metastatic pulmonary neoplasia

CBC/BIOCHEMISTRY/URINALYSIS
• Neutrophilic leukocytosis in many patients • Eosinophilia in many patients • Basophilia in many patients

OTHER LABORATORY TESTS N/A

IMAGING
• Radiographic features are lobar pulmonary consolidation (i.e., mass lesions), hilar lymphadenomegaly, and pleural effusion.

• Lesions are unilateral or bilateral.

OTHER DIAGNOSTIC PROCEDURES
Biopsy for definitive diagnosis

GROSS AND HISTOPATHOLOGIC FINDINGS
• Histologically characterized by pleomorphic, angioinvasive mononuclear cells that often cause vascular obliteration • Cytologically, may appear as sterile eosinophilic and neutrophilic inflammation with reactive macrophages

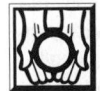

TREATMENT
Cytotoxic drugs combined with surgical excision when appropriate

MEDICATIONS

DRUGS AND FLUIDS
Combination protocol with prednisone, cyclophosphamide, and vincristine suitable for lymphosarcoma

CONTRAINDICATIONS/POSSIBLE INTERACTIONS
• Myelosuppression caused by cytotoxic drugs • Hemorrhagic cystitis caused by cyclophosphamide

FOLLOW-UP

PATIENT MONITORING
• Same as for dogs with lymphosarcoma treated by chemotherapy • Some dogs may survive longer than 2 years, but survival after

chemotherapy is usually short.

POSSIBLE COMPLICATIONS
• Dyspnea as disease progresses • Depression • Anorexia • Myelosuppression caused by chemotherapy

MISCELLANEOUS
Not a granulomatous disease as previously reported

SYNONYMS
• Eosinophilic pulmonary granulomatosis • Lymphoid granulomatosis • Lymphoproliferative angiitis • Granulomatosis

ASSOCIATED CONDITIONS
May progress to lymphosarcoma

Reference
Berry CR, Moore PF, Thomas WP, et al. Pulmonary lympomatoid granulomatosis in seven dogs (1976-1987). J Vet Int Med 1990;4:157-166.
Author Wallace B. Morrison
Consulting Editor Wallace B. Morrison

LYMPHOSARCOMA—CATS

BASICS

DEFINITION
Malignant transformation of lymphocytes that reside mainly in lymphoid tissues

Pathophysiology
Depends on the organs involved

Systems Affected
• Hemic/lymphatic/immune • Gastrointestinal • Renal/urologic • Ophthalmic • Nervous • Skin/exocrine

Genetics N/A

Incidence/Prevalence
• About 90% of hematopoietic tumors and 33% of all tumors in cats • Prevalence ranges from 41.6-200 per 100,000 cats.

Geographic Distribution
• On the East coast, mediastinal lymphosarcoma most common (40-52% of all patients)
• On the West coast, alimentary lymphosarcoma most common (36% of all patients)

SIGNALMENT

Species Cats

Breed Predilections None

Mean Age and Range
• Mean age of FeLV-positive cats, 3 years Mean age of FeLV-negative cats, 7 years
• Median age of cats with localized extranodal lymphosarcoma, 13 years

SIGNS

General Comments
History and examination findings depend on anatomic form

Historical Findings
• Mediastinal form—open-mouthed breathing, coughing, regurgitation, anorexia, and weight loss • Alimentary form—anorexia, weight loss, lethargy, vomiting, constipation, diarrhea, melena, and frank blood in the stool
• Renal form—signs consistent with renal failure such as vomiting, anorexia, polydipsia, polyuria, and lethargy • Multicentric form—possibly none in early stages, but anorexia, weight loss, depression with progression of disease • Solitary form—depends on the location. Nasal lymphosarcoma, sneezing and nasal discharge; spinal cord lymphosarcoma, posterior paresis, cutaneous lymphoma, pruritic, hemorrhagic, or alopecic dermal masses

Physical Examination Findings
• Mediastinal form—noncompressible cranial thorax • Alimentary form—thickened intestines or abdominal masses • Renal form—large, irregular kidneys • Multicentric form—generalized lymphadenomegaly • All forms—fever, dehydration, depression, cachexia in some patients

CAUSES
• FeLV is the cause of lymphosarcoma in cats. • Cats inconsistently test positive for the virus during illness (85% with mediastinal, 45% with renal, 20% of multicentric, and 15% with alimentary).

RISK FACTORS FeLV exposure

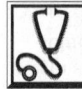

DIAGNOSIS

DIFFERENTIAL DIAGNOSIS
• Mediastinal lymphosarcoma—congestive heart failure, cardiomyopathy, chylothorax, pyothorax, hemothorax, pneumothorax, diaphragmatic hernia, allergic lung disease, thymoma, ectopic thyroid carcinoma, pleural carcinomatosis, and acetaminophen toxicity
• Alimentary lymphosarcoma—foreign body ingestion, intestinal ulceration, intestinal fungal infection, inflammatory bowel disease, intussusception, lymphangiectasia, and other gastrointestinal tumor • Renal lymphosarcoma—pyelonephritis, amyloidosis, glomerulonephritis, and chronic renal failure Multicentric lymphosarcoma—systemic mycotic infection, immune-mediated disease, toxoplasmosis, lymphoid hyperplasia, and hypersensitivity reaction

CBC/BIOCHEMISTRY/URINALYSIS
In some patients:
• Anemia, leukocytosis, and lymphoblastosis
• High creatinine, high serum urea nitrogen, high hepatic enzyme activity, hypercalcemia, and monoclonal gammopathies • Isosthenuria, bilirubinuria, and proteinuria

OTHER LABORATORY TESTS
FeLV testing

IMAGING
• Thoracic radiography to reveal a mediastinal mass, pleural effusion, abnormal pulmonary parenchymal patterns (rare), or perihilar or retrosternal lymphadenomegaly
• Abdominal radiography to detect masses, hepatomegaly, splenomegaly, mesenteric or sublumbar lymphadenomegaly, or unilateral or bilateral renomegaly • Abdominal ultrasonography to reveal diffuse echotexture changes in the liver, spleen, or kidneys, and focal thickening of the intestines

OTHER DIAGNOSTIC PROCEDURES
• Examination of bone marrow aspirate or core biopsy to evaluate bone marrow reserves
• Cytologic examination of a mass or lymph node • Biopsy of mass or lymph node

GROSS AND HISTOPATHOLOGIC FINDINGS

Gross Findings
Likely to be white to gray in color with areas of hemorrhage and necrosis

Cytologic Findings
Monomorphic population of pleomorphic lymphoid cells, sometimes with prominent, multiple nucleoli and coarse nuclear chromatin

Histopathologic Findings
• Vary • Several morphologic classification schemes in use

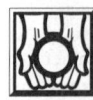

TREATMENT

INPATIENT VERSUS OUTPATIENT
Treat as an outpatient whenever possible

ACTIVITY Normal activity

DIET No change

CLIENT EDUCATION
• Cure possible but not likely
• Goal to induce remission and achieve a good quality of life for patient for as long as possible

SURGICAL CONSIDERATIONS
• Surgery used to relieve intestinal obstructions and remove solitary masses
• Surgery used to obtain specimens for histopathologic examination

MEDICATIONS

DRUGS AND FLUIDS
• Chemotherapy used in a combination or sequential protocol
• Some protocols have an induction period and maintenance period.
• Combination chemotherapy—vincristine (0.5 mg/m^2 IV once weekly), cyclophosphamide (50 mg/m^2 PO q48h), cytosine arabinoside (100 mg/m^2 SQ first 2 days), and prednisone (40 mg/m^2 q24h for 1 week then 20 mg/m^2 PO q48h). This is used for 6 weeks as the induction protocol.
• Maintenance chemotherapy—methotrexate (2.5 mg/m^2 PO 3 times a week), chlorambucil (20 mg/m^2 PO q2wk), prednisone (20 mg/m^2 PO q48h), and vincristine (0.5 mg/m^2 IV q4wk)
• Sequential chemotherapy: Week 1—vincristine (0.025 mg/kg IV), L-asparaginase (400 IU/kg IM), and prednisone (2 mg/kg PO divided twice a day). Week 2—cyclophosphamide (10 mg/kg IV). Week 3—vincristine (0.025 mg/kg IV) Week 4—methotrexate (0.8 mg/kg IV). The cycle is repeated. Maintenance is lengthening the time between each treatment.
• Drugs useful to treat relapsing lymphoma in cats include doxorubicin, vinblastine, actinomycin-D, and mitoxantrone.
• Radiotherapy can be used for localized lymphoma. Relapses outside the radiation field are not uncommon.

CONTRAINDICATIONS None

PRECAUTIONS
• Myelosuppression secondary to chemotherapy more common than average in FeLV-positive cats

• Seek advice before initiating treatment if you are unfamiliar with cytotoxic drugs.

POSSIBLE INTERACTIONS None

ALTERNATE DRUGS
Prednisone alone for temporary palliation

FOLLOW-UP

PATIENT MONITORING
• Physical examination, CBC, and platelet count before each weekly cycle • Radiography as necessary

PREVENTION/AVOIDANCE
Avoid exposure to or breeding FeLV positive cats.

POSSIBLE COMPLICATIONS
Leukopenia and sepsis

EXPECTED COURSE AND PROGNOSIS
• Depends on initial response to chemotherapy, anatomic type, FeLV status, and tumor burden • Cats that have complete remission in response to chemotherapy—median survival time, 7 months • Partial remission—median survival time, 2.5 months • No response—median survival time, 1.5 months • About 10% of cats with mediastinal lymphosarcoma live > 2 years. • Cats with alimentary lymphosarcoma—median survival time, 8 months • Cats with peripheral multicentric lymphosarcoma—median survival time, 23.5 months • FeLV-negative cats with renal lymphosarcoma—median survival time, 11.5 months • FeLV-positive cats with renal lymphosarcoma—median survival time, 6.5 months • FeLV-negative cats with lymphosarcoma—median survival time, 7 months • FeLV-positive cats with lymphosarcoma—median survival time, 3.5 months • FeLV-negative cats with a low tumor burden—median survival time, 17.5 months • FeLV-positive cats with a low tumor burden—median survival time, 4 months • Cats treated with prednisone alone live 1.5-2 months. • Cats with localized lymphosarcoma, achieving complete remission—median duration remission, 114 weeks

MISCELLANEOUS

ASSOCIATED CONDITIONS
• Hypoglycemia (rare) • Monoclonal gammopathy (rare) • Hypercalcemia (rare)

AGE RELATED FACTORS
Young cats with lymphoma are generally FeLV positive.

ZOONOTIC POTENTIAL None

PREGNANCY
Chemotherapy should not be used in pregnant animals.

SYNONYMS
• Lymphoma • Malignant lymphoma

SEE ALSO N/A

ABBREVIATION
FeLV = feline leukemia virus

References

Jeglum KA, Whereat A, Young KA. Chemotherapy of lymphoma in 75 cats. J Am Vet Med Assoc 1987;190:174-178.

Mooney SC, Hayes AA, Matus RE, et al. Renal lymphoma in cats: 28 cases (1977-1984). J Am Vet Med Assoc 1987;191:1473-1477.

Mooney SC, Hayes AA, MacEwen EG, et al. Treatment and prognostic factors in lymphoma in cats: 103 cases (1977-1981). J Am Vet Med Assoc 1989;194:696-699.

Elmslie RE, Ogilive GK, Gillette EL, et al. Radiotherapy with and without chemotherapy for localized lymphoma in 10 cats. Vet Radiol 1991;32:277-280.

Author Terrance A. Hamilton
Consulting Editor Wallace D. Morrison

LYMPHOSARCOMA—DOGS

BASICS

DEFINITION
Lymphosarcoma (malignant lymphoma) is a clonal proliferation of neoplastic lymphocytes in solid tissues, primarily in lymph nodes, bone marrow, and visceral organs.

Pathophysiology
Usually unifocal in origin with follicle-associated B lymphocytes that retain growth characteristics and ability to migrate. Ease of migration may account for spread of clinical disease. High growth fraction may account for sudden onset of clinical signs.

Systems Affected
• Hepatobiliary—generalized, often peripheral lymphadenomegaly with or without splenic or hepatic involvement • Hemic/lymphatic • Gastrointestinal—infiltration of stomach, intestines, and associated lymph nodes • Respiratory—proliferation of neoplastic lymphocytes in mediastinal lymph nodes and thymus • Miscellaneous (extranodal)—proliferation of or invasion by neoplastic lymphocytes in the bone marrow, ocular, cutaneous, mucocutaneous, neural, renal, cardiac, and other tissues

Genetics
No consistent documentation of genetic basis

Incidence/Prevalence
6-30 per 100,000 dogs per year

Geographic Distribution N/A

SIGNALMENT

Species Dogs

Breed Predilections
• Reported high risk breeds—boxer, basset hound, golden retriever, Saint Bernard, Scottish terrier, Airedale terrier, and bulldog • Reported low risk breeds—dachshund and Pomeranian

Mean Age and Range
Patients usually 5-10 years old

Predominant Sex None

SIGNS

General Comments
Clinical signs depend on anatomic form and stage of disease

Historical Findings
• For all forms of malignant lymphoma—clinical signs nonspecific: anorexia, lethargy, weight loss, etc. • Multicentric—generalized, painless lymphadenomegaly most common clinical sign; distended abdomen (i.e., hepatomegaly, splenomegaly, or ascites) in some patients • Gastrointestinal—vomiting, diarrhea, anorexia, and abdominal discomfort • Mediastinal—coughing, difficulty swallowing, anorexia, drooling, labored breathing, and exercise intolerance

Extranodal—clinical signs vary with the anatomic site:
• Ocular—photophobia and conjunctivitis • CNS— seizures • Cutaneous—plaque-like lesions • Renal—lumbar pain • Cardiac—exercise intolerance or syncope

Physical Examination Findings
• Multicentric—generalized, painless, irregular, movable, large lymph node(s) with or without hepatosplenomegaly • Gastrointestinal—marked weight loss or palpable abdominal mass • Mediastinal—dyspnea, tachypnea, or muffled heart sounds (i.e., pleural effusion) • Physical changes vary with form of extranodal malignant lymphoma: • Ocular—anterior uveitis, retinal hemorrhages, and hyphema • Cutaneous—raised plaque • Neural—dementia, seizures, and paralysis • Renal—renomegaly and renal failure • Cardiac—arrhythmias

CAUSES
No specific cause proven

RISK FACTORS N/A

DIAGNOSIS

DIFFERENTIAL DIAGNOSIS
• Infectious, neoplastic, immune-mediated, and inflammatory disease • Cytologic and histologic evaluation and complete staging will differentiate malignant lymphoma from other diseases.

CBC/BIOCHEMISTRY/URINALYSIS
• Anemia, lymphocytosis, lymphopenia, neutrophilia, monocytosis, circulating blasts, and thrombocytopenia in many patients • High ALT or ALP activity hypercalcemia in many patients • Results of urinalysis usually normal

OTHER LABORATORY TESTS N/A

IMAGING
• Thoracic radiography reveals sternal or tracheobronchial lymphadenomegaly, widened mediastinum, pulmonary densities, and pleural effusion. • Abdominal radiography reveals sublumbar or mesenteric lymphadenomegaly, intestinal mass, abdominal effusions, or hepato(spleno)megaly. • Ultrasonography reveals lymphadenomegaly (obscured by effusion) or nodules in visceral organs. • Evaluate cardiac contractility before anthracycline administration.

OTHER DIAGNOSTIC PROCEDURES
• Examination of bone marrow aspirate and core biopsy to identify the extent of disease which impacts on the chemotherapy choices • CSF tap if patient has CNS signs • ECG to identify chamber abnormalities or arrhythmias before doxorubicin administration

GROSS AND HISTOPATHOLOGIC FINDINGS
• Homogenous, white masses with areas of necrosis on cut section • Monomorphic population of discrete round neoplastic cells that efface and replace parenchyma of lymph nodes and visceral organs or bone marrow

TREATMENT

INPATIENT VERSUS OUTPATIENT
• Administer chemotherapy in-hospital. • Once remission is achieved, some protocols include drugs administered orally by the owner at home.

ACTIVITY
Restrict activity in patient with low WBC or platelet count.

DIET N/A

CLIENT EDUCATION
• Chemotherapy not curative—relapse usually occurs • Side effects of chemotherapy drugs depend on the type used. • Most dogs have leucopenia by day 7-10. • Most chemotherapies have a 70-80% response rate. • Quality of life is good while the patient is receiving chemotherapy and while in remission.

SURGICAL CONSIDERATIONS
Rarely successful unless limited to one accessible site

MEDICATIONS

DRUGS AND FLUIDS
• Many combination chemotherapy protocols exist with similar remission and survival times. • Single-agent therapy with doxorubicin is associated with similar remission and survival time as that for combination chemotherapy. • Corticosteroids alone are effective short term (i.e., 1-2 months).

Doxorubicin Protocol
30 mg/m^2 (1 mg/kg if patients weighs < 10 kg) IV q21 days for 2 treatments past complete remission (3-4 treatments)

Combination Chemotherapy Protocol
Induction
• Vincristine 0.5 mg/m^2 IV day 1 • Cyclophosphamide 50 mg/m^2 PO days 4-7 • Prednisone 20 mg/m^2 PO q12h • Repeat weekly for 6 weeks, then begin maintenance
Maintenance
• Methotrexate 5.0 mg/m^2 PO days 1 and 5 • Cyclophosphamide 100 mg/m^2 PO day 3 • Prednisone 20 mg/m^2 q48h • Maintenance continued for 6 weeks followed by 1 week of induction, then 6 weeks of maintenance. Continue for 1 year or until relapse.

CONTRAINDICATIONS N/A

PRECAUTIONS
• Use doxorubicin cautiously or not at all in patients with poor cardiac contractility or arrhythmias.
• Use anthracyclines cautiously in dogs with marked bone marrow involvement (80-90%).
• Always use a catheter when administering intravenous drugs.

POSSIBLE INTERACTIONS
All chemotherapy drugs need to be given according to published protocols, since many have overlapping side effects.

ALTERNATE DRUGS
Many alternate treatment protocols exist.

 FOLLOW-UP

PATIENT MONITORING
• Physical examination and cytologic or histologic evaluation of all nonresponsive lymph nodes. • CBC and platelet count on day 10 after first treatment. If patient has severe leucopenia or neutropenia (WBC < 2000 cells/mm^3; neutrophils < 1000 cells/mm^3), dosage can be reduced (15-25%) or colony stimulating factors added to current protocol.
• CBC and platelet count before each anthracycline chemotherapy or once weekly (day 1) with combination chemotherapy. If patient has moderate or severe leucopenia (WBC < 4000 cells/mm^3), delay treatment until cell counts are in normal range (usually 1 week).
• Repeat tests with abnormal results before

treatment after 2-3 courses of chemotherapy to confirm response to treatment. • Echocardiography and ECG periodically during and after doxorubicin administration to identify development of cardiotoxicity

PREVENTION/AVOIDANCE N/A

POSSIBLE COMPLICATIONS
• Leucopenia and neutropenia • Vomiting and diarrhea • Anorexia • Cardiotoxicity (usually after total cumulative dose of 180-240 mg/m^2) • Alopecia • Pancreatitis • Sepsis • Tissue sloughing with extravasated dose

EXPECTED COURSE AND PROGNOSIS
• Median duration of first remission in dogs treated with combination chemotherapy or doxorubicin—6 months (range, 52-486 days) with 58-89% of dogs achieving a complete remission • Median survival time in dogs treated with combination chemotherapy or doxorubicin—6-12 months (range, 112-365 days) • Dogs with mediastinal form and/or hypercalcemia have a poorer prognosis.
• Primary CNS, diffuse gastrointestinal, and multi-site cutaneous forms associated with poor response to treatment

 MISCELLANEOUS

ASSOCIATED CONDITIONS N/A
AGE RELATED FACTORS N/A

ZOONOTIC POTENTIAL N/A

PREGNANCY
Treatment of pregnant dogs contraindicated

SYNONYMS
Lymphoma or lymphosarcoma

SEE ALSO
• Leukemia • Hypercalcemia • Colony stimulating factors

ABBREVIATIONS
ALP = alkaline phosphatase
ALT = alanine transaminase
ECG = electrocardiography

References

MacEwan EG, Young KM. Hematopoietic tumors: canine lymphoma and lymphoid leukemias. In: Withrow SJ, MacEwan EG, eds. Clinical veterinary oncology. Philadelphia: JB Lippincott, 1989:380-393.

Madewell BR, Theilen GH. Hematopoietic neoplasms, sarcomas, and related conditions: part IV canine. In: Theilen GH, Madewell BR, eds. Veterinary cancer medicine. Philadelphia: Lea & Febiger, 1987.

Vonderhaar MA. Evaluation of dogs with malignant lymphoma treated with doxorubicin or epirubicin as single agent therapy [Dissertation]. West Lafayette, Indiana: Purdue University, 1994.

Couto CG. Canine lymphomas: something old, something new. Compend Cont Ed Pract Vet 1985;7:291-302.

Author Mary Ann Vonderhaar
Consulting Editor Wallace B. Morrison

MALASSEZIA DERMATITIS

BASICS

OVERVIEW

Malassezia dermatitis (MD) occurs when the organism Malassezia pachydermatis, normally a skin and ear canal commensal, causes pruritus and inflammation of the skin. The number of organisms on affected skin is usually higher than normal, but does not always correlate with the degree of pruritus. Most cases are secondary to other seborrheic skin disorders, although primary infections are sometimes seen.

SIGNALMENT

• Malassezia dermatitis is seen mainly in dogs with seborrheic skin disorders; therefore, breeds commonly affected with primary or secondary seborrhea are predisposed. • Rare cases have been reported in cats with systemic illnesses and in cases of recalcitrant chin acne. No sex predilection has been reported.
• Older dogs with chronic dermatoses may be predisposed.

SIGNS

Historical Findings
• Pruritus is poorly responsive to cortisone.
• Previously affected with a milder, chronic dermatosis. • Owners have noted a strong, rancid odor.

Physical Examination Findings
• Pruritus • Erythema • Scale • Sebaceous crusts • Malodor • Lichenification
• Face, ventral neck, axillae, groin, perineum, and paws commonly affected.

CAUSES AND RISK FACTORS
• Primary seborrhea (hereditary keratinization disorders). • Secondary seborrhea due to underlying hypersensitivity dermatoses (flea allergy dermatitis, atopy, food hypersensitivity, contact hypersensitivity), endocrinopathies (hypothyroidism, reproductive hormone imbalances, hyperadrenocorticism), and ectoparasitism (flea infestation, demodicosis, sarcoptes). • Chronic antibiotic therapy.

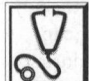

DIAGNOSIS

DIFFERENTIAL DIAGNOSIS
• The differential diagnoses include primary seborrhea and the numerous causes of secondary seborrhea. • Secondary pyoderma may result in signs similar to Malassezia infection.

CBC/BIOCHEMISTRY/URINALYSIS
N/A

OTHER LABORATORY TESTS N/A

IMAGING N/A

OTHER DIAGNOSTIC PROCEDURES
• Skin cytology (touch preparation, cotton swab preparation, or cellophane tape preparation) reveals increased numbers of budding yeast organisms. • Evidence of concurrent pyoderma may also be present.

GROSS AND HISTOPATHOLOGIC FINDINGS
• Histopathology may also be diagnostic, although organisms are less easily demonstrated than with skin cytology.
• Other histological changes will depend on the underlying dermatosis.

TREATMENT
• Underlying skin disorders should be evaluated and specifically treated when possible. MD may recur when the seborrheic skin changes are not reversed.
• Keratolytic shampoos containing sulfur, salicylic acid, tar, or benzoyl peroxide are often used in conjunction with an antifungal shampoo containing miconazole, ketoconazole, or chlorhexidine.
• Bathing every 2-3 days is often helpful in cases of MD.

MEDICATIONS

DRUGS AND FLUIDS
• Localized cases may respond to topical antifungal creams or lotions (miconazole, ketoconazole, or clotrimazole) applied once to twice daily.
• Ketoconazole (10 mg/kg q24h for 2-4 weeks) is indicated in widespread or locally severe cases.

CONTRAINDICATIONS/POSSIBLE INTERACTIONS
Imidazole antifungal drugs have been associated with life-threatening cardiac arrhythmias in man when administered concomitantly with the antihistamines astemazole and terfenidine.

FOLLOW-UP
• Monitor response with physical examinations and skin cytology findings after 2-4 weeks of therapy. • Treatment should be continued until only rare organisms can be demonstrated or 7 days after a complete response is achieved. Pruritus and odor are usually noticeably improved within 1 week.
• Recurrences are common when underlying dermatoses are not well controlled. • Regular bathing with antifungal shampoos will help decrease recurrence.

MISCELLANEOUS
Ketoconazole is contraindicated during pregnancy.

ABBREVIATIONS
MD = malassezia dermatitis

Reference
Scott DW, Miller WH, Griffin CE. Muller and Kirk's small animal dermatology. 5th ed. Philadelphia: WB Saunders, 1995:351.
Author Jon D. Plant
Consulting Editor Lowell Ackerman

MALIGNANT FIBROUS HISTIOCYTOMA (GIANT CELL TUMOR)

BASICS

OVERVIEW
Malignant fibrous histiocytoma (giant cell tumor) has the following characteristics:
• Mesenchymal neoplasm • Name based on its histologic features of fibroblast-like cells accompanied by histiocyte-like cells and pleomorphic, multinucleated giant cells • Malignant giant cell tumor of soft parts is a malignant tumor of superficial and deep connective tissue; considered a possible variant of malignant fibrous histiocytoma • These tumors believed to arise from a primitive, pleomorphic sarcoma cell, which exhibits partial fibroblastic and histiocytic differentiation • Both tumors are locally invasive, firm, subcutaneous masses • Despite previous reports to the contrary, their metastatic potential in dogs appears to be high

SIGNALMENT
• Reported more commonly in cats than dogs • No breed or sex predilection • Mean age for cats, 9 years (range, 2-12 years) • Median age for dogs, 8.4 years (range, 3-10.3 years)

SIGNS

Historical Findings
• Anorexia, weight loss, and lethargy in some patients • Other complaints depend on site of involvement

Physical Examination Findings
• Firm, invasive tumor arising in subcutaneous tissue • May exhibit deep extension into underlying skeletal muscle • May develop adjacent to bone and induce bone destruction and proliferation • The dorsal thoracic and scapular area, limbs, and pelvic region are the most common sites • Distant metastasis common

CAUSES AND RISK FACTORS Unknown

DIAGNOSIS

DIFFERENTIAL DIAGNOSIS
• Fibrosarcoma • Chondrosarcoma • Osteosarcoma • Mast cell neoplasia • Rhabdomyoma or rhabdomyosarcoma • Liposarcoma

CBC/BIOCHEMISTRY/URINALYSIS
• CBC results vary; may be normal • Regenerative or nonregenerative anemia in some patients • Biochemistry variably abnormal • Urinalysis is usually normal

OTHER LABORATORY TESTS N/A

IMAGING
• Radiography reveals soft tissue dense mass • Bone proliferation or destruction observed in some patients

OTHER DIAGNOSTIC PROCEDURES
• Cytologic examination of aspirate may reveal histiocytelike and fibroblastlike cells. • Histologic examination necessary for definitive diagnosis

TREATMENT
• The local invasive nature makes surgical excision difficult; recurrence rate high • Amputation of an affected limb may be an appropriate treatment for metastasis • Radiotherapy may be helpful • Chemotherapy may be helpful

MEDICATIONS

DRUGS AND FLUIDS N/A

CONTRAINDICATIONS/POSSIBLE INTERACTIONS N/A

FOLLOW-UP
Schedule follow-up examinations according to growth of tumor.

MISCELLANEOUS
Considerable debate exists among pathologists regarding classification of these tumors. This may account for the apparent differences in behavior reported in the literature.

Reference

Waters CB, Morrison WB, DeNicola DB, et al. Giant cell variant of malignant fibrous histiocytoma in dogs: 10 cases (1986-1993). J Am Vet Med Assoc 1994;205:1420-1424.

Author James P. Thompson
Consulting Editor Wallace B. Morrison

MAMMARY GLAND HYPERPLASIA—CATS

 BASICS

OVERVIEW
• This condition is also called benign mammary hypertrophy, mammary fibroadenomatosis, and fibroglandular mammary hypertrophy. • It is a progesterone-dependent enlargement of one or more mammary glands.

SIGNALMENT
Young, intact, cycling or pregnant queens and cats of either gender receiving an exogenous progestogen (e.g., megestrol acetate)

SIGNS
• Localized or diffuse enlargement of one or more mammary glands • The masses are firm and nonpainful. • No concurrent signs of systemic illness

CAUSES AND RISK FACTORS
• Secondary to a progesterone influence
• High progesterone a finding in queens experiencing false pregnancy (induced to ovulate but nonpregnant) for 40-50 days after ovulation induction, pregnant queens throughout gestation, and in cats receiving exogenous progestogens.

 DIAGNOSIS

DIFFERENTIAL DIAGNOSIS
• Mastitis—mastitis occurs when the queen is lactating, and the mammary glands are erythematous and painful. The queen is systemically ill with fever and immature neutrophilia. Fluid expressed from the affected gland(s) contains inflammatory cells and bacteria.
• Mammary neoplasia—neoplasia occurs in old queens (> 6 years of age). The gross appearance of neoplastic mammary masses may be indistinguishable from that of mammary hyperplasia, necessitating differentiation by biopsy of affected tissue.

CBC/BIOCHEMISTRY/URINALYSIS
Results normal

OTHER LABORATORY TESTS N/A

IMAGING N/A

OTHER DIAGNOSTIC PROCEDURES
• Cytologic examination of fluid expressed from affected glands is non-inflammatory.
• Benign fibroglandular proliferation with no inflammation or necrosis is demonstrated by excision biopsy.

 TREATMENT

• Hypertrophy due to high endogenous progesterone regresses when progesterone falls at the end of false pregnancy or gestation.
• Consider ovariohysterectomy in cats not intended for breeding.
• Hypertrophy due to administration of exogenous progestogens regresses when the medication is withdrawn.

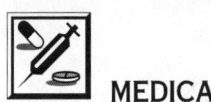 **MEDICATIONS**

DRUGS AND FLUIDS N/A

CONTRAINDICATIONS/POSSIBLE INTERACTIONS N/A

 FOLLOW-UP

• The likelihood of recurrence in cats left intact is unknown. • The correlation between appearance of this condition and other abnormal conditions of the reproductive tract is unknown.

 **MISCELLANEOUS**

Reference

Hayden DW, Johnston SD, Krang DT, et al. Feline mammary hypertrophy/fibroadenoma complex: clinical and hormonal aspects. Am J Vet Res 1981; 42:1699-1703.

Author Margaret V. Root

Consulting Editor Sara K. Lyle

MAMMARY GLAND TUMORS—CATS

BASICS

DEFINITION
Malignant and benign mammary gland tumors of cats

PATHOPHYSIOLOGY
Hormonal influences appear to be involved in the etiopathogenesis of mammary dysplasias in cats, but recent evidence suggests that an association with mammary tumor deveopment is less certain than previously believed. • Almost all are malignant.

SYSTEMS AFFECTED
• Reproductive—mammary glands and metastatic sites • At the time of euthanasia, more than 80% of cats have metastases to one or more of the following organs: lymph nodes, lungs, pleura, liver, diaphragm, adrenal gland, and kidneys.

GENETICS
• Unknown • Siamese cats have a significantly higher risk and tumor development occurs at a younger age than other breeds.

INCIDENCE/PREVALENCE
• Third most commonly reported neoplasm in female cats after hematopoietic and skin tumors • Prevalence 25.4/100,000 female cats

GEOGRAPHIC DISTRIBUTION
N/A

SIGNALMENT
Species Cats

BREED PREDILECTIONS
• Most often reported in domestic shorthair and Siamese breeds. • Siamese cats have twice the risk of developing mammary carcinoma than other breeds.

MEAN AGE AND RANGE
Mean age, 10.7 years (range, 9 months-21 years)

PREDOMINANT SEX
Almost all (99%) mammary tumors appear in intact females.

SIGNS
General Comments
• Many cats have advanced disease on examination. • Approximately 60% of cats have multiple gland involvement, and 1/3 of cats have simultaneous involvement of the left and right mammary gland chains.

Historical Findings
Mass or masses in the mammary area that may or may not be ulcerated

Physical Examination Findings
• Solitary mass in one location or multiple masses in more than one location • Usually firm and nodular • Ulceration common • Infiltrated lymphatic vessels may appear as subcutaneous, firm, thick cords. • The pelvic limbs may be edematous and swollen with discomfort because of tumor thrombi or impaired vascular return.

CAUSES
• Unknown • Hormonal influences, particularly that of progestins, associated with tumor development • Type-C and type-A viral particles have been identified in feline neoplastic mammary tissue, although the importance of these has not been determined.

RISK FACTORS
• Intact female cats have an approximately seven-fold higher risk than spayed females • Endogenous progesterone or administration of exogenous progestins such as megestrol acetate is associated with relatively higher risk for dysplasia.

DIAGNOSIS

DIFFERENTIAL DIAGNOSIS
• Lobular hyperplasia • Fibroepithelial hyperplasia • Papillary cystic hyperplasia • Mastitis • Cysts

CBC/BIOCHEMISTRY/URINALYSIS
Results usually normal

OTHER LABORATORY TESTS N/A

IMAGING
• Thoracic radiography to detect lung metastasis • Abdominal radiography or ultrasonography and cytologic examination of fine-needle aspirate of sublumbar lymph nodes or ascites if clinically warranted

OTHER DIAGNOSTIC PROCEDURES
• Because of the aggressive nature of these tumors, a preliminary biopsy is not recommended. Tissue for histopathologic examination should be obtained at the time of mastectomy. • Cytologic examination of fine-needle aspirate of lymph nodes if metastasis is suspected

GROSS AND HISTOPATHOLOGIC FINDINGS
Gross
Tumors usually develop in the subcutaneous tissue adjacent to the nipple and may adhere to the overlying skin.

Histopathology
• Tubular and papillary adenocarcinomas most common • Scirrhous carcinoma rare • A few mammary sarcomas reported • Tumors often contain extensive areas of necrosis with lymphocytic and plasma cell infiltration.

TREATMENT

INPATIENT VERSUS OUTPATIENT
Stable patients can be discharged after surgery or chemotherapy.

ACTIVITY N/A

DIET N/A

CLIENT EDUCATION
• Discuss importance of early detection and treatment.
• Discuss potential benefits of early ovariohysterectomy.

SURGICAL CONSIDERATIONS
• Cats with no radiographic evidence of metastasis should have radical mastectomy (removal of all four glands of the affected mammary chain plus the ipsilateral axillary and inguinal lymph nodes).
• If tumors are present in both mammary chains, two radical mastectomies are performed, usually 1 month apart.

MEDICATIONS

DRUGS AND FLUIDS
Combination chemotherapy with doxorubicin (25 mg/m² IV over 20 to 30 minutes) and cyclophosphamide (100 mg/m² PO) on days 3, 4, 5, and 6 after doxorubicin. Repeat every 3 to 5 weeks. This protocol has been shown to induce short-term partial and complete responses in 50% of cats with metastatic or nonresectable local disease.

CONTRAINDICATIONS
• Compromised myocardial function
• Severe myelosuppression

PRECAUTIONS
Do not exceed doxorubicin cumulative dose of 200 mg/m²
• Chemotherapy can be toxic. Seek advice before initiating treatment if you are unfamiliar with cytotoxic drugs.
• Hepatic disease
• Renal insufficiency

POSSIBLE INTERACTIONS
Verapamil can potentiate doxorubicin-induced cardiotoxicity, and concurrent use should be avoided.

ALTERNATE DRUGS
• Responses occasionally reported to a combination of vincristine (0.5 mg/m² IV once weekly), cyclophosphamide (50 mg/m² PO q48h), and methotrexate (2.5 to 5 mg/m² PO 2-3 times weekly).
• No effective biological response modifier is available that has shown to be efficacious in cats with mammary tumors.

FOLLOW-UP

PATIENT MONITORING
• Complete physical examination bimonthly with emphasis on palpation of the previous incision line(s), the remaining mammary glands, and the axillary and inguinal lymph node regions. • Thoracic radiography every 1-3 months

PREVENTION/AVOIDANCE

Ovariectomized cats have only 0.6% the risk of intact cats of developing mammary carcinoma, but the optimum age for ovariectomy to be sparing is unknown.

POSSIBLE COMPLICATIONS

From Tumor

Anemia, osteoporosis, hypercalcemia, disseminated intravascular coagulopathy

From Chemotherapy

• Dilated cardiomyopathy • Myelosuppression • Anorexia • Gastrointestinal toxicity • Renal insufficiency • Hepatopathy

EXPECTED COURSE AND PROGNOSIS

• High incidence of recurrence and metastases • The type of surgery is significantly related to the time of disease-free interval. Cats treated by radical mastectomy have a longer disease-free interval (575 days) than cats treated by conservative surgery (325 days). A similar but nonsignificant trend was observed for survival time (800 vs 500 days). • The single most important prognostic factor is tumor size. Cats with tumors > 3 cm in diameter have a median survival of 6 months after surgery. Cats with tumors < 2 cm in diameter have a significantly better prognosis, with a median survival of approximately 3 years.
• Cats with well-differentiated tumors with few mitotic figures have been shown to have comparatively higher survival times.

MISCELLANEOUS

ASSOCIATED CONDITIONS

Mastitis, uterine disease, and other unrelated tumors

AGE RELATED FACTORS

Middle-aged cats most commonly affected, with highest incidence in the 10 to 14-year-old age group.
Siamese cats develop mammary gland tumors at a younger age, but the incidence does not significantly increase after the 7-9 year risk plateau.

ZOONOTIC POTENTIAL None

PREGNANCY

Chemotherapy should not be used in pregnant animals.

SYNONYMS None

SEE ALSO N/A

ABBREVIATIONS N/A

References

Moulton JE. Mammary tumors of the cat. In: Moulton JE, ed. Tumors in domestic animals 3rd ed. University of California Press, Berkeley, 1990;547-552.

Hayes AA, Mooney S. Feline mammary tumors. Vet Clin North Am Small Anim Pract 1985;15:513-520.

Ogilvie GK. Feline mammary neoplasia. Compend Cont Ed Pract Vet 1983;5:384-393.

Jeglum KA, deGuzman E, Young KM. Chemotherapy of advanced mammary adenocarcinoma. J Am Vet Med Assoc 1985;87:157-160.

Author Stanley L. Marks
Consulting Editor Wallace B. Morrison

MAMMARY GLAND TUMORS—DOGS

BASICS

DEFINITION
Benign or malignant tumors of the mammary glands

Pathophysiology
• Dogs spayed before first estrous cycle have 0.5% risk compared with intact bitch. • Dogs spayed before second estrous cycle have 8.0% risk compared with intact bitch. • Dogs spayed after second estrus have 26% risk compared with intact bitch. • Dogs spayed after 2.5 years of age—no sparing effect on risk

Systems Affected
• Reproductive • Respiratory

Genetics N/A

Incidence/Prevalence
• 198.8/100,00 female dogs • about 50% are malignant • Almost exclusively affects females • About 50% of patients have multiple tumors.

Geographic Distribution
Similar worldwide

SIGNALMENT
• Extremely rare in males • Primarily middle-aged and old females

Species Dogs

Breed Predilections None

Mean Age and Range
• Median age about 10.5 years (range, 1-15 years) • Uncommon in dogs < 5 years

Predominant Sex Female

SIGNS

General Comments
• Lymphatic connections exist between right and left series of glands. • Generally, cranial glands drain to axillary lymph nodes and caudal glands drain to inguinal lymph nodes. Glands in-between drain variably to either or both the axillary and inguinal lymph lodes. • Plexiform connections exist that help explain the occurrence of lymphatic metastasis against predicted lymph flow.

Historical Findings
Usually slow growing single or multiple mammary gland masses

Physical Examination Findings
• Single or multiple mammary gland masses • Ulcerated in some patients • Freely movable in some patients (implies benign behavior) • Fixed to skin or body wall in some patients (implies malignant behavior)

CAUSES AND RISK FACTORS
• None known • Circumstantial evidence in some studies incriminates treatment with progestins and estrogen in combination, prolactin, and growth hormone.

DIAGNOSIS

DIFFERENTIAL DIAGNOSIS
• Lipoma • Mast cell tumor • Mammary hyperplasia • Mastitis

CBC/BIOCHEMISTRY/URINALYSIS
• Results usually normal • Hypercalcemia occasionally reported

OTHER LABORATORY TESTS N/A

IMAGING
• Thoracic radiography to detect metastasis • Abdominal radiography to detect metastasis to iliac (sublumbar) lymph nodes • Radionuclide bone scanning rarely positive in dogs

OTHER DIAGNOSTIC PROCEDURES
• Examination of cytologic preparations often misleading. Inflammation may mimic criteria of malignancy. • Excisional biopsy for definitive diagnosis.

GROSS AND HISTOPATHOLOGIC FINDINGS

Gross Findings
• Considerable inflammation associated • Ulceration in some patients

Histopathologic Findings
• 50% benign • 42% adenocarcinoma • 4% inflammatory carcinoma • 4% sarcoma

TREATMENT
• Surgery the primary mode of treatment • Chemotherapy infrequently reported

INPATIENT VERSUS OUTPATIENT
N/A

ACTIVITY N/A

DIET N/A

CLIENT EDUCATION
• Never leave a mammary lump in place and observe. • Early surgical intervention is best. • Advise spaying before first estrus.

SURGICAL CONSIDERATIONS
• Local excision (ie, simple, regional , or unilateral mastectomy) with wide and deep margins (at least 2 cm in all directions) can be as effective in terms of disease free interval as radical bilateral mastectomy. • Chemotherapy is infrequently reported, but it may be effective in some patients.

MEDICATIONS

DRUGS AND FLUIDS
Doxorubicin (30 mg/mg^2 IV q 21days) reported to have induced a partial remission for 12 and 16 months in two dogs

CONTRAINDICATIONS N/A

PRECAUTIONS
Chemotherapy can be toxic. Seek advice before treatment if you are unfamiliar with cytotoxic drugs.

POSSIBLE INTERACTIONS
Myelotoxicity, vomiting and diarrhea, pancreatitis, and cardiac damage possible side effects of doxorubicin administration

ALTERNATE DRUGS
Although tamoxifen is helpful in some women with breast cancer, do not use it in dogs.

FOLLOW-UP

PATIENT MONITORING
Physical examination and thoracic radiographs at 1, 3, 6, 9, and 12 months after treatment

PREVENTION/AVOIDANCE
Spay before first estrus.

POSSIBLE COMPLICATIONS N/A

EXPECTED COURSE AND PROGNOSIS
• Median survival of patient with tubular adenocarcinoma after mastectomy, 24.6 months • Median survival of patient with solid carcinoma after mastectomy, 6.5 months • Patient with benign tumor has excellent prognosis after mastectomy • Patient with carcinoma 5 cm in diameter usually has a good prognosis • Inflammatory carcinoma represents a very aggressive subtype of mammary gland tumor in dogs, characterized by rapid growth, firmness, diffuse involvement, erythema, limb edema, color change, and pain. Patient may be anemic, have leukocytosis, and develop DIC. The tumor can be mistaken for mastitis, abscess, or dermatitis. Prognosis is poor.

MISCELLANEOUS

ASSOCIATED CONDITIONS
• Hypertrophic osteopathy • Metastasis to lungs and CNS

AGE RELATED FACTORS N/A

ZOONOTIC POTENTIAL N/A

PREGNANCY N/A

SYNONYMS N/A

SEE ALSO N/A

ABBREVIATIONS
CNS = central nervous system
DIC = disseminated intravascular coagulation

MAMMARY GLAND TUMORS—DOGS

References

Hahn KA, Richardson RC, Knapp DW. Canine malignant mammary neoplasia: biological behavior, diagnosis, and treatment alternatives. J Amer Anim Hosp Assoc 1992;28:251-256.

Morris JS, Dobson JM, Bostock DE. Use of tamoxifen in control of canine mammary neoplasia. Vet Rec 1993;133:539-542.

Allen SW, Mahaffey EA. Canine mammary neoplasia: prognostic indicators and response to surgical therapy. J Am Anim Hosp Assoc 1989;25:540-546.

Author Wallace B. Morrison
Consulting Editor Wallace B. Morrison

MAST CELL TUMORS

BASICS

DEFINITION
Neoplasia rising from mast cells

Pathophysiology
• Histamine and other vasoactive substances within the cytoplasmic granules of mast cell tumors can cause erythema and edema.
• Heparin within the cytoplasmic granules increases the likelihood of bleeding.

Systems Affected
• Skin/exocrine—skin and subcutaneous tissue the most common location in dogs and cats • Hemic/lymphatic—the spleen is a common primary location in cats; the spleen is an uncommon primary location in dogs • Gastrointestinal—intestinal mast cell tumor uncommon in cats and rare in dogs • In dogs, mast cell tumors located in the inguinal region tend to behave more aggressively than similarly graded tumors in other locations.

Genetics N/A

Incidence/Prevalence
• Mast cell tumors represent 20-25% of all skin and subcutaneous tumors in dogs.
• Cutaneous mast cell tumor is the fourth most common skin tumor in cats after basal cell tumor, squamous cell carcinoma, and fibrosarcoma.

Geographic Distribution N/A

SIGNALMENT

Species
Dogs and cats

Breed Predilections
• Boxers and Boston terriers • Siamese are predisposed to histiocytic cutaneous mast cell tumors.

Mean Age and Range
• Dogs—mean age, 8 years • Cats—mean age, 10 years • Reported in animals < 1 year old and in cats as old as 18 years

Predominant Sex
• No sex predilection in dogs • Male cats may be more commonly affected than females.

SIGNS

General Comments
Clinical signs depend on the location and grade of the tumor.

Historical Findings
Dogs
• Patient may have had skin or subcutaneous mast cell tumor for days to months at the time of examination • Recent rapid growth after months of quiescence common • Recent onset of erythema and edema more common with high-grade skin and subcutaneous tumors
Cats
• Anorexia is the most common complaint in cats with splenic mast cell tumor. • Vomiting can occur secondary to both splenic and gastrointestinal mast cell tumor.

Physical Examination Findings
Dogs
• Extremely variable; tumors can resemble any other type of skin or subcutaneous tumor, both benign and malignant • Primarily a skin or subcutaneous mass • Most tumors are solitary, although they can be multifocal. • Approximately 50% are located on the trunk and perineum, 40% on the extremities, and 10% on the head and neck region. • Regional lymphadenopathy may develop when a high-grade tumor metastasizes to draining lymph nodes. • Hepatomegaly and splenomegaly are features of disseminated mast cell neoplasia.
Cats—Cutaneous Mast Cell Tumors
• Develop primarily in the subcutaneous tissue or dermis • Can be papular or nodular, solitary or multiple, and hairy, alopecic, or have an ulcerated surface • Slight predilection for the head and neck regions • Cats with solitary dermal masses have a 15-45% metastatic rate.
Cats—Splenic Mast Cell Tumor
• Splenomegaly the only consistent physical finding • Cats may also have gastric or duodenal ulcers, presumably because of the release of histamine by the tumor. • Mastocythemia and anemia develop in some cats, the latter caused by erythrophagocytosis by the tumor, splenic sequestration, hemorrhage at the site of gastrointestinal ulceration, or splenic rupture.
Cats—Intestinal Mast Cell Tumor
Firm, segmental thickenings of the small intestinal wall, measuring from 1-7 cm in diameter. Metastasize to mesenteric lymph nodes, spleen, liver, and, rarely, the lungs.

CAUSES N/A

RISK FACTORS
• Hereditary • Previous inflammation

DIAGNOSIS

DIFFERENTIAL DIAGNOSIS
• Clinical findings on examination of dogs with mast cell tumor are extremely variable; tumor can resemble any other skin or subcutaneous tumor. • Splenic mast cell tumor is the most common cause of splenomegaly in cats. • Intestinal mast cell tumor in cats can resemble any primary gastrointestinal disorder (i.e., inflammatory and neoplasia).

CBC/BIOCHEMISTRY/URINALYSIS
Anemia and mastocythemia in some cats with splenic mast cell tumor and some dogs with systemic mastocytosis

OTHER LABORATORY TESTS N/A

IMAGING
Abdominal radiography reveals splenomegaly in some cats with splenic mast cell tumor and some dogs with systemic mastocytosis.

OTHER DIAGNOSTIC PROCEDURES
• Cytologic examination of fine-needle aspirate is the most important preliminary diagnostic test; reveals round cells with basophilic cytoplasmic granules that do not form sheets or clumps. If the malignant mast cells are agranular, the presence of a large eosinophilic infiltrate may suggest mast cell tumor.
• Tissue biopsy is necessary for definitive diagnosis and tumor grading. • Staging the mast cell tumor allows one to determine the extent of disease and determine appropriate treatment. • Diagnostic tests, in addition to those listed above, to achieve complete staging, include cytologic examination of bone marrow aspirate, cytologic examination or biopsy of local lymph node, thoracic radiography, and abdominal ultrasonography.

GROSS AND HISTOPATHOLOGIC FINDINGS
• Histopathologic examination allows grading of the tumor to predict biologic behavior. Mast cell tumors in dogs are graded I to III, with grade III being the most aggressive type. Survival times (Bostock):
• Grade I—77% alive 6 months after surgery
• Grade II—45% alive 6 months after surgery • Grade III—13% alive 6 months after surgery
• A grading system for cats with cutaneous mast cell tumor is not available, but histopathologic examination allows differentiation between benign histiocytic cutaneous mast cell tumor and the potentially malignant types.

TREATMENT
• Aggressive surgical excision is the treatment of choice for mast cell tumor in dogs.
• When histopathologic examination reveals mast cell tumor cells extend close to surgical margins, a second aggressive surgery should be performed as soon as possible.
• It is impossible to comment on completeness of surgical excision and predict biologic behavior of mast cell tumors without histopathologic evaluation of the entire, surgically excised tissue.
• Cutaneous mast cell tumor in cats tends to be somewhat less invasive than their canine counterpart.
• At least 2 cm surgical margins should be obtained.
• Splenectomy is the treatment of choice in cats with splenic mast cell tumor.
• Biopsy of lymph nodes and other suspicious visceral organs is appropriate.
• Radiotherapy is a good treatment option for a patient with cutaneous mast cell tumor in a location that does not allow aggressive surgical excision. If possible, surgery should be performed before radiotherapy to reduce the tumor to a microscopic volume.

• Mast cell tumor located on an extremity responds better to radiotherapy than do tumors located on the trunk.

INPATIENT VERSUS OUTPATIENT
N/A

ACTIVITY N/A

DIET N/A

CLIENT EDUCATION
• A patient that has had more than one cutaneous mast cell tumor is predisposed to developing new mast cell tumors.
• Fine needle aspiration and cytologic examination should be performed as soon as possible on any new mass.
• Appropriate surgical excision should be done as soon as possible.

MEDICATIONS

DRUGS AND FLUIDS
• When cutaneous mast cell tumor cannot be controlled by surgery or radiotherapy, medical treatment is appropriate.
• Prednisone has been the mainstay of treatment, but recent evidence suggests that prednisone alone achieves very short-term remission.
• Chemotherapy drugs such as vinblastine, vincristine, and cyclophosphamide can be added to the protocol to lengthen the remission of prednisone-sensitive mast cell tumors.
• Chemotherapy does not appear to be beneficial in the treatment of prednisone-resistant mast cell tumor.
• Prednisone and chemotherapy are indicated in cats with evidence of systemic mastocytosis after splenectomy.
• All cats with intestinal mast cell tumor should be treated with prednisone and chemotherapy after surgery.
• Histamine-blocking agents (e.g., cimetidine and ranitidine) are helpful, particularly in pa-

tients with systemic mastocytosis or when massive histamine release is a concern.

CONTRAINDICATIONS N/A

PRECAUTIONS N/A

POSSIBLE INTERACTIONS N/A

ALTERNATE DRUGS N/A

FOLLOW-UP

PATIENT MONITORING
• Any new mass that develops should be evaluated either cytologically or histologically to determine whether new mast cell tumors are developing. • Regional lymph nodes should be evaluated at regular intervals to detect metastasis of grade II to III mast cell tumor.

PREVENTION/AVOIDANCE N/A

POSSIBLE COMPLICATIONS
• Bleeding • Hemorrhagic gastroenteritis

EXPECTED COURSE AND PROGNOSIS

Dogs
• See histopathologic section for prognosis in dogs. • Survival may be prolonged if prednisone and chemotherapy are used in patients in which complete surgical excision is not possible or that have evidence of metastasis to local lymph nodes.

Cats
• Survival times of > 1year reported after splenectomy for splenic mast cell tumor.
• Prognosis is poor if mastocythemia occurs concurrently, although prednisone and chemotherapy may achieve short-term remission. • The prognosis for intestinal mast cell tumor is poor with survival times rarely > 4 months after surgery.

MISCELLANEOUS

ASSOCIATED CONDITIONS N/A

AGE RELATED FACTORS N/A

ZOONOTIC POTENTIAL N/A

PREGNANCY N/A

SYNONYMS N/A

SEE ALSO N/A

ABBREVIATIONS N/A

References

Bostock DC. The prognosis following surgical removal of mastocytomas in dogs. J Small Anim Pract 1973;14:27-40.

Patniak AK, Ehler WN, MacEwen EG. Canine cutaneous mast cell tumors: morphologic grading and survival time in 83 dogs. Vet Pathol 1984;21:469-474.

Turrel JM, Kitchell BE, Miller LM, et al. Prognostic factors for radiation treatment of mast cell tumor in 85 dogs. J Am Vet Med Assoc 1988;193:936-940.

Buerger RG, Scott DW. Cutaneous mast cell neoplasia in cats: 14 cases (1975-1985). J Am Vet Med Assoc 1987;190:1440-1444.

Liska WD, MacEwen EG, Zaki FA, et al. Feline systemic mastocytosis: a review and results of splenectomy in seven cases. J Am Anim Hosp Assoc 1979;15:589-597.

Author Robyn E. Elmslie
Consulting Editor Wallace B. Morrison

MASTITIS

BASICS

OVERVIEW
• Bacterial infection of one or more lactating glands • Develops because of ascending infection, trauma to the gland, or hematogenous spread • Escherichia coli, Staphylococci, and B-hemolytic Streptococci most commonly involved • Potentially life-threatening infection that may lead to septic shock
• Direct effect on mammary glands with systemic involvement if sepsis develops

SIGNALMENT
Postpartum bitch and queen

SIGNS

Historical Findings
• Anorexia • Lethargy • Neglect of puppies or kittens • Failure of puppies or kittens to thrive

Physical Examination Findings
• Firm, swollen, warm, and painful mammary gland(s) from which purulent or hemorrhagic fluid can be expressed • Fever, dehydration, and septic shock if patient has systemic involvement • Abscessation or gangrene of gland(s)

CAUSES AND RISK FACTORS
• Trauma inflicted by puppy or kitten toenails and teeth • Poor hygiene • Systemic infection originating elsewhere (e.g., metritis)

DIAGNOSIS

DIFFERENTIAL DIAGNOSIS
• Galactostasis—no systemic illness; cytologic examination and culture of milk and culture help differentiate • Inflammatory mammary adenocarcinoma—affected gland does not produce milk; biopsy differentiates

CBC/BIOCHEMISTRY/URINALYSIS
• Leukocytosis with left shift • Leukopenia in patients with sepsis • Mildly high PCV, total protein, and BUN in dehydrated patients

IMAGING N/A

OTHER LABORATORY TESTS N/A

OTHER DIAGNOSTIC PROCEDURES
• Milk analysis—normal milk is slightly more acidic than serum but may become alkaline with infection. Neutrophils, macrophages, and other mononuclear cells are common; degenerative neutrophils with intracellular bacteria indicate septic mastitis. • Bacterial culture of the milk identifies the organism.

TREATMENT
• Treat as inpatient until stable
• Puppies and kittens usually hand raised or placed on healthy surrogate dam. In selected patients, neonates may be allowed to continue nursing, with special attention paid to antibiotics used and weight gain of neonates.
• Abscessed or gangrenous glands require surgical debridement.

MEDICATIONS

DRUGS AND FLUIDS
• Correct electrolyte imbalances and hypoglycemia.
• Treat shock if indicated.
• If milk is acidic, use weak bases (e.g., erthomycin and lincomycin;); if milk is alkaline, use weak acids (e.g., amoxicillin and cephalosporin.) Chloramphenical and enrofloxacin effective for both.
• Apply warm compress and milk out affected glands several times daily.
• Affected glands can be infused with 1% betadine solution by lacrimal cannula

CONTRAINDICATIONS/ COMPLICATIONS
• If puppies or kittens continue to nurse, avoid tetracycline, enrofloxacin, and chloramphenicol.
• Cephalosporins, amoxicillin, and amoxicillin with clavulanic acid can be used.

FOLLOW-UP

PATIENT MONITORING
• Physical examination and CBC

PREVENTION/AVOIDANCE
Keep environment clean, shave hair from around mammary glands, clip toenails of puppies and kittens

POSSIBLE COMPLICATIONS
• Abscessation or gangrene can cause loss of gland(s) • Handraising of puppies and kittens requires considerable commitment by the owner

EXPECTED COURSE AND PROGNOSIS
Prognosis is good with treatment.

MISCELLANEOUS

Reference

Olson JD, Olson PN. Disorders of the canine mammary gland. In: Morrow DA, ed. Current therapy in theriogenology 2. Philadelphia: WB Saunders, 1986:506-509.
Author Joni L. Freshman
Consulting Editor Sara K. Lyle

BASICS

OVERVIEW
• An inflammatory process involving the mediastinal space, which is usually the result of an infectious process. • In the acute disease, severe infection may be life-threatening with spread to the pleural space or the development of sepsis; in chronic disease, the development of mediastinal granuloma or abscess may result in superior vena cava syndrome.
• Primary effects on the cardiovascular system as a result of interference with venous return, or the respiratory system secondary to intrathoracic mass effect or pleural effusion. May also interfere with esophageal function.

SIGNALMENT
Rare condition in both dogs and cats

SIGNS
• Lethargy, weakness • Dysphagia, regurgitation • Edema of head, neck, forelimbs
• Polypnea, dyspnea

CAUSES AND RISK FACTORS
• Acute disease most commonly is the result of esophageal perforation or tracheal tears, but may also occur secondary to neck wounds (bites or gunshots), sepsis, pneumonia, pericarditis, or pyothorax. • Gram-negative bacteria may complicate esophageal perforation.
• Chronic disease usually is the result of a bacterial (i.e., Actinomyces spp., Nocardia spp.) or fungal (i.e., Coccidioides, Cryptococcus, Blastomyces, and Histoplasma species) infection. • Predisposing factors include esophageal foreign bodies, cervical or thoracic trauma, and the immune suppressed state.

DIAGNOSIS

DIFFERENTIAL DIAGNOSIS
• Isolated pericarditis, pyothorax, pneumonia
• Cranial mediastinal masses, including lymphosarcoma, thymoma, thyroid and parathyroid tumors, neurogenic tumors, mesenchymal tumors (i.e., usually lipoma or other fat accumulation), and mediastinal cysts
• Esophageal motor dysfunction, other esophageal abnormalities, and gastroesophageal disorders

CBC/BIOCHEMISTRY/URINALYSIS
• Elevated WBC count with left shift on hemogram • May also be elevated PCV and total protein as a result of volume depletion

OTHER LABORATORY TESTS N/A

IMAGING
• Thoracic radiographs will define the presence of mediastinal widening. Pneumothorax and/or a bilateral pleural effusion may also be seen. • Esophageal contrast study to evaluate for esophageal perforation or other abnormalities (a water-soluble contrast media should be used when perforation is suspected).
• Thoracic ultrasound is beneficial in differentiating between mediastinal fluid accumulation (i.e., cysts, abscesses), inflammatory reactions, and tumors. CT and MRI will supply the same information more definitively.

OTHER DIAGNOSTIC PROCEDURES
Thoracentesis of any pleural effusion, or when absent, transthoracic fine-needle aspirate or cutting-needle biopsy of the mediastinal "enlargement" to establish cytologic diagnosis. All samples should be submitted for culture and sensitivity.

TREATMENT
• Treat as an inpatient with restricted activity until infection is controlled and patient's condition is stable.
• Owners should be aware that this is a serious disease with a guarded prognosis.
• Pleural effusion of significant quantity or pyothorax of any degree should be managed by tube thoracostomy.
• Esophageal perforation is a surgical emergency. After surgical repair, either parenteral alimentation or gastric tube feeding should be enforced for 3-5 days.
• Chronic mediastinitis is best treated by surgical exploration whether associated with an abscess or a granuloma.
• Postoperatively, tube thoracostomy should be maintained by continuous water seal suction for 5-7 days or until negligible fluid is removed. In the absence of surgery, a similar course should be followed with or without pleural cavity lavage.

MEDICATIONS

DRUGS AND FLUIDS
• Broad-spectrum, bactericidal antibiotics based on culture and sensitivity results should be administered parenterally for at least the first week of therapy, then orally.
• Physiologically balanced electrolyte solutions should be administered parenterally until oral alimentation is acceptable or the patient's water and food intake returns to normal or near normal.

CONTRAINDICATIONS/POSSIBLE INTERACTIONS
Aminoglycoside antibiotics should be avoided or the dosage based accurately on creatinine clearance in patients with azotemia.

FOLLOW-UP
• Patient monitoring should include temperature recording daily, repeating hemograms every 2-3 days during hospitalization (usually 7-10 days), and thoracic radiographs at 7 to 10-day intervals. • Antibiotic therapy should be continued for 1 week after the hemogram and radiographs return to normal. • Potential complications include pyothorax, sepsis, and mediastinal fibrosis. • The prognosis with early diagnosis and aggressive treatment is fair to good; however, with the development of mediastinal fibrosis, the long-term prognosis is guarded to poor.

MISCELLANEOUS

ABBREVIATIONS
CT = computerized tomography
MRI = magnetic resonance imaging

Reference

Bauer T. Mediastinal, pleural and extrapleural diseases. In: Ettinger SJ, ed. Textbook of veterinary internal medicine. 3rd ed. Philadelphia: WB Saunders, 1989.
Author Neil K. Harpster
Consulting Editors Lynelle Johnson and Bradley L. Moses

MEGACOLON

BASICS

DEFINITION
A condition of persistent increased large bowel diameter associated with chronic constipation/obstipation and low to absent colonic motility.

Pathophysiology
Acquired megacolon results from chronic retention of fecal material which leads to colonic absorption of fecal water and solidified fecal concretions. Prolonged distention of the colon results in irreversible changes in colonic motility leading to colonic inertia. Congenital absence of colonic ganglionic cells (Hirschsprung's disease) has not been clearly documented in small animals.

Systems Affected Gastrointestinal

Genetics
Heritability is unproven in animals

Incidence/Prevalence Unknown

Geographic Distribution N/A

SIGNALMENT

Species
• Idiopathic megacolon primarily in cats
• Megacolon secondary to outlet obstruction can occur in both cats and dogs.

Breed Predilections
Some evidence for increased risk in Manx cats

Mean Age and Range
Idiopathic megacolon occurs most frequently in middle-aged to older cats. A mean age of 4.9 years with a range of 1-15 years has been reported.

Predominant Sex None

SIGNS

Historical Findings
• Megacolon typically has a chronic insidious onset. Signs are often present for months to years. • Chronic constipation • Tenesmus • Anorexia • Intermittent vomiting • Weight loss • Paradoxical diarrhea

Physical Examination Findings
• Abdominal palpation reveals an enlarged colon with a hard fecal mass. • Digital rectal examination may indicate an underlying (obstructive) cause and confirms a palpable fecal impaction. • Dehydration • Scruffy, unkept hair coat

CAUSES
• Idiopathic (most common) • Mechanical obstruction due to: pelvic fracture malunion, foreign body or improper diet (especially bones), stricture, tumor, anal or rectal atresia. • Trauma to colonic innervation • Congenital anomalies of the caudal spine (especially Manx cats) • Congenital or acquired abnormalities in the intrinsic nerve supply (unconfirmed)

RISK FACTORS
• Pelvic trauma in cats • Possible association with low physical activity.

DIAGNOSIS

DIFFERENTIAL DIAGNOSIS
• Other causes of palpable colonic masses (e.g., lymphoma, carcinoma, intussusception) can be distinguished on the basis of texture, rectal exam and radiographic appearance.
• Owners often report "constipation" in cats with urinary obstruction. Palpation of an enlarged urinary bladder should readily distinguish the two conditions.

CBC/BIOCHEMISTRY/URINALYSIS
• May show evidence of dehydration (elevated packed cell volume, total protein) and stress leukogram. • Electrolyte abnormalities may develop depending on duration of obstipation. • Urinalysis reveals no consistent changes

OTHER LABORATORY TESTS N/A

IMAGING
• Radiographs are indicated to try and identify an underlying cause. • The enlarged, fecal-filled colon is easily seen on plain abdominal radiographs. • Radiographic evidence of previous spinal or pelvic trauma may indicate an underlying cause.

OTHER DIAGNOSTIC PROCEDURES
Colonoscopy may be necessary to rule out mural or intramural obstructive lesions

GROSS AND HISTOPATHOLOGIC FINDINGS
• The most severe dilation typically occurs in the transverse and descending colon although the entire length of colon can be involved.
• The colon is for the most part histologically normal. Consistent changes in number or appearance of ganglion cells have not been identified.

TREATMENT

INPATIENT VERSUS OUTPATIENT
• Initial management will usually require hospitalization.
• If the patient is to be treated medically it will usually require anesthesia and manual evacuation of the colon using warm water enemas and gentle extraction of feces with sponge forceps. Care must be taken not to excessively traumatize the colonic mucosa.
• Long-term therapy is continued at home.

ACTIVITY
• Encourage activity and exercise. • Restrict activity in the postoperative period if surgery is performed.

DIET
• A high fiber is recommended (e.g. Hill's r/d or w/d). • A more palatable maintenance-type diet can be supplemented with products such as Metamucil or pumpkin pie filler.

CLIENT EDUCATION
• Medical therapy is life-long and often frustrating. Owner compliance and a semi-cooperative patient are a must.
• If medical therapy fails then surgery should be undertaken prior to severe patient debilitation.

SURGICAL CONSIDERATIONS
• If an underlying obstructive cause of megacolon is identified then it must be surgically corrected.
• Subtotal colectomy with ileorectal or colorectal anastomosis is the treatment of choice for idiopathic megacolon refractory to medical management.
• Diarrhea should be expected for several months after colectomy. The stools will become more formed as the ileum adapts by increasing reservoir capacity and water absorption.

MEDICATIONS

DRUGS AND FLUIDS
• Most cases will require parenteral fluid support to correct dehydration. Intravenous administration of balanced electrolyte solutions is the preferred route. • Recent reports have claimed dramatic results in improving colonic motility using cisapride, a GI prokinetic drug. The recommended dosage is 0.5 mg/kg PO q8h-q24h. Cats weighing up to 4.5 kg are started at 2.5 mg q8h whereas cats greater than 4.5 kg get 5.0 mg PO q8h. Cisapride is given 30 minutes prior to feeding. • Stool softeners (e.g., lactulose, 2-3 ml PO q8h) are recommended in conjunction with cisapride and diet. Dosage and frequency can be adjusted based upon response. • Broad spectrum prophylactic antibiotics are recommended prior to colon evacuation and during the perioperative period if surgery is elected.

CONTRAINDICATIONS
• Hypertonic sodium phosphate enemas (e.g., Fleet® enema) should not be used in cats or small dogs due to potentially fatal electrolyte derangements, most notably hypocalcemia.
• Mineral oil is extremely dangerous if given orally due to a high risk of fatal aspiration.

PRECAUTIONS
Common hair ball laxatives (e.g., Laxatone®, Cat-A-Lax® are not likely to be beneficial in treating constipation.

POSSIBLE INTERACTIONS N/A

ALTERNATE DRUGS
Docusate sodium (DSS®, Colace® can be used as a stool softener in place of lactulose.

FOLLOW-UP

PATIENT MONITORING

• Following colonic resection and anastomosis, patients should be closely monitored for 3-5 days for signs of dehiscence and peritonitis. Clinical deterioration warrants abdominocentesis and peritoneal lavage to detect anastomotic leakage. • Fluid support should be continued until the patient is willing to eat and drink.

PREVENTION/AVOIDANCE

• Pelvic fractures that cause a narrowing of the pelvic canal should be repaired at the time of injury. • Foreign bodies and feeding of bones should be avoided if possible.

POSSIBLE COMPLICATIONS

• Recurrence or persistence of the problem is the most common complication. • Potential surgical complications include peritonitis, persistent diarrhea, stricture formation, and recurrence of obstipation. • Traumatic perforation of the colon is a serious complication of overzealous fecal evacuation.

EXPECTED COURSE AND PROGNOSIS

• Historically, medical management has been unrewarding. Although still too early to make definitive conclusions, the use of cisapride appears to improve the prognosis with medical management. • Although subtotal colectomy is well tolerated by cats in general, constipation recurrence rates of up to 45% have recently been reported with long-term follow-up.

MISCELLANEOUS

ASSOCIATED CONDITIONS

Perineal Hernia

AGE RELATED FACTORS

Due to the advanced age of many cats with megacolon, other medical conditions associated with older cats (e.g., chronic renal insufficiency, hyperthyroidism) may be concurrently diagnosed.

ZOONOTIC POTENTIAL N/A

PREGNANCY

• The effect of cisapride on the fetus is unknown. • Animals with megacolon would be at increased risk for dystocia if they carried a pregnancy to term.

SYNONYMS N/A

SEE ALSO

• Perineal Hernia • Peritonitis

ABBREVIATIONS N/A

References

Bertoy RW. Megacolon. In: Bojrab MJ, ed. Disease mechanisms in small animal surgery. 2nd ed. Philadelphia: Lea & Febiger, 1993;262-265.

Holt D, Johnston DE. Idiopathic megacolon in cats. Compend Contin Educ Pract Vet. 1991;13:1411–1416.

Aronsohn M. Large intestine. In: Slatter D, ed. Textbook of small animal surgery. 2nd ed. Philadelphia: WB Saunders, 1993:613-627.

Burrows CF. Medical diseases of the colon. In: Jones BD, ed. Canine and feline gastroenterology. Philadelphia: WB Saunders, 1986:221-256.

Tams TR. Cisapride: clinical experience with the newest GI prokinetic drug. [Abstract] Proceedings of the 12th Annual Veterinary Medical Forum–ACVIM. 1994;100–101.

Author Bradford C. Dixon

Consulting Editor Brent D. Jones

MEGAESOPHAGUS

BASICS

DEFINITION
Rather than a single disease entity, megaesophagus refers to esophageal dilation and hypomotility which may be present as a primary disorder or secondary to esophageal obstruction or neuromuscular dysfunction.

Pathophysiology
With megaesophagus, esophageal motility is decreased or absent resulting in accumulation and retention of food and liquid within the esophagus. Reflex esophageal motility begins when food stimulates sensory afferents in the esophageal mucosa which then sends afferent messages to the brain stem swallowing center via the vagus nerve. Efferent messages from lower motor neurons in the nucleus ambiguous travel via the vagus to stimulate contraction of esophageal striated and smooth muscle. Lesions anywhere along this pathway, including the myoneural junction, may result in esophageal hypomotility and distention. Increased lower esophageal sphincter tone is not an important cause of megaesophagus in veterinary patients.

Systems Affected
Gastrointestinal • Neuromuscular • Respiratory (if aspiration pneumonia occurs)

Genetics
Congenital idiopathic megaesophagus is heritable in wirehaired fox terriers (simple autosomal recessive) and miniature Schnauzers (simple autosomal dominant or 60% penetrance autosomal recessive).

Incidence/Prevalence
Megaesophagus is the most common cause of regurgitation in dogs and cats. The incidence of megaesophagus at the University of Missouri over an eight year period was reported to be approximately one per thousand admissions (Guilford).

Geographic Distribution N/A

SIGNALMENT

Species
Dogs and cats. More common in dogs than cats.

Breed Predilections
Hereditary in wirehaired fox terriers and miniature Schnauzers. Familial predispositions have been reported in the German shepherd, Newfoundland, Great Dane, Irish setter, shar pei, pug, greyhound and cats.

Mean Age and Range
With congenital megaesophagus signs of regurgitation first appear at weaning. Acquired forms are most often reported in young adults to middle aged animals.

Predominant Sex N/A

SIGNS

Historical Findings
• History relating to megaesophagus may include regurgitation of food and water, weight loss or poor growth, salivation and a gurgling sound. With congenital megaesophagus regurgitation of liquids through the nostrils and a poor hair coat may be seen. • History relating to the underlying cause of megaesophagus may include weakness, paresis or paralysis, ataxia, gagging, dysphagia, pain or depression. • Coughing, mucopurulent nasal discharge and dyspnea with aspiration pneumonia

Physical Examination Findings
• Occasionally normal • Signs related to megaesophagus: Regurgitation, cachexia, auscultation of retained fluid and food in the esophagus, halitosis, ptyalism, bulging of the esophagus at the thoracic inlet and pain associated with palpation of the cervical esophagus • Signs related to cause or sequelae of megaesophagus: Respiratory crackles, tachypnea, pyrexia, myalgia, muscle weakness, muscle atrophy, hyporeflexia, proprioceptive and postural deficits, autonomic disorders (mydriasis with loss of pupillary light reflex, dry nasal and ocular mucous membranes, diarrhea, bradycardia), cranial nerve deficits (especially cranial nerves IX and X), paresis or paralysis and mentation changes.

CAUSES

Congenital Idiopathic Megaesophagus

Esophageal Obstruction
• Esophageal foreign body, stricture, neoplasia, granuloma • Vascular ring anomalies (e.g., persistent right aortic arch) • Periesophageal compression

Neuromuscular Diseases
• Myasthenia gravis, polymyositis, polyneuritis, dysautonomia, systemic lupus erythematosus (SLE), polyradiculoneuritis, central nervous system disorders (degenerative, infectious/inflammatory, neoplasia, traumatic disorders of the brain stem and spinal cord), botulism, bilateral vagal damage.

Miscellaneous Causes
• Esophagitis, hypothyroidism, hypoadrenocorticism, thymoma, toxicosis (lead, thallium, acetylcholinesterase).

RISK FACTORS N/A

DIAGNOSIS

DIFFERENTIAL DIAGNOSIS
• Differentiate from other disorders causing regurgitation. Obstructive pharyngeal disease (foreign bodies, inflammation, neoplasia, cricopharyngeal achalasia) and palate disorders may produce regurgitation with normal esophageal motility. Pharyngeal pain and dysphagia are often present with obstructive pharyngeal disease. • Regurgitation must be distinguished from dysphagia and vomition.

Regurgitation is a passive process with no forceful abdominal contraction, anticipatory salivation, nausea or retching. The presence of bile stained ingesta suggests vomition. The time relationship between eating and expulsion of food is not useful in distinguishing regurgitation and vomiting.

CBC/BIOCHEMISTRY/URINALYSIS
No characteristic findings, but may aid in identifying the underlying cause of megaesophagus.

OTHER LABORATORY TESTS
• Acetylcholine receptor antibody titers to screen for myasthenia gravis • Antinuclear antibody titers and LE cell prep to evaluate for immune cause • ACTH stimulation to evaluate adrenal function • Blood lead level • T_4 to evaluate thyroid function

IMAGING

Survey Thoracic Radiographs
Esophagus dilated with gas, fluid or ingesta. The trachea is often displaced ventrally by the distended esophagus.

Contrast Esophagram and Fluoroscopy
• An esophagram using either barium liquid or paste may demonstrate contrast pooling and abnormal esophageal motility. • Abnormal primary and secondary esophageal peristalsis can be visualized with fluoroscopy. • Contrast studies are not necessary for diagnosing most cases of megaesophagus and should be used with caution in animals known to have megaesophagus.

OTHER DIAGNOSTIC PROCEDURES
• Endoscopy: Can be used to visualize dilated esophagus, foreign bodies, neoplasia and esophagitis. Mucosal biopsies and cytology samples may be obtained. Esophageal foreign bodies may be removed via endoscopy. • Electromyography (EMG) and nerve conduction velocity (NCV): Fibrillation potentials, positive sharp waves and complex repetitive discharges suggest neuromuscular disease. Prolonged NCV suggests peripheral neuropathy. • Muscle and nerve biopsy: May provide diagnosis of inflammatory, degenerative and immune-mediated peripheral nerve and muscle disease. • Repetitive nerve stimulation and Tensilon testing: Resolution of muscular weakness following edrophonium chloride (0.1-0.2 mg/kg IV) and a decremental response of the compound action potential provide support the diagnosis of myasthenia gravis. • Cerebrospinal fluid analysis: Pleocytosis and/or protein elevations suggest central nervous system disease.

GROSS AND HISTOPATHOLOGIC FINDINGS
Gross and histopathologic findings vary depending on the underlying disease.

TREATMENT

INPATIENT VERSUS OUTPATIENT
Many patients treated as outpatients. Patients with aspiration pneumonia, obstruc-

tive megaesophagus, severe debilitation or advanced neurological disease should be hospitalized.

ACTIVITY

No change in activity is necessary for megaesophagus alone.

DIET

• Feed in upright position (45-90° angle to floor) and maintain position for 10-15 following feeding.
• Feeding a gruel often produces the least regurgitation, although the consistency of the diet must be individualized for each patient. The consistency of food which produces the least regurgitation may change with time.
• Parenteral feeding via gastrotomy tube may be necessary in some patients with severe regurgitation.

CLIENT EDUCATION

The danger of aspiration pneumonia and importance of the special feeding requirements must be emphasized to the client.

SURGICAL CONSIDERATIONS

Surgery may be necessary to remove esophageal foreign bodies, neoplasia or correct vascular ring anomalies. There are no surgical procedures which improve esophageal motility, however the modified Heller's cardiomyotomy reduces lower esophageal tone and may improve gravity facilitated movement of ingesta into the stomach. Surgical treatment of megaesophagus has not been critically evaluated in dogs and cats and is not currently recommended in most patients.

MEDICATIONS

DRUGS AND FLUIDS

• There are no drugs commonly used to treat megaesophagus alone. Treatment should be directed at the underlying disease or associated conditions (e.g., aspiration pneumonia).
• Metoclopramide increases gastric emptying and may increase distal esophageal motility. However, metoclopramide also increases gastroesophageal sphincter tone. Metoclopramide is more useful when feeding through a gastrotomy tube.

• Broad spectrum antibiotics are necessary for patients with aspiration pneumonia. Parenteral antibiotics or enteral administration via a gastrotomy tube may be required for patients with severe regurgitation.
• Immunosuppression (prednisone, cyclophosphamide, azothioprine) is required for immune-mediated neuromuscular disease and SLE.
• Prednisone and acetylcholinesterase inhibitors (pyridostimine) are used to treat myasthenia gravis.

CONTRAINDICATIONS N/A

PRECAUTIONS

Although corticosteroids may be necessary to treat conditions causing megaesophagus, they should be used with caution in patients with aspiration pneumonia.

POSSIBLE INTERACTIONS N/A

ALTERNATE DRUGS N/A

FOLLOW-UP

PATIENT MONITORING

• Patients should be re-examined if signs of aspiration pneumonia develop (fever, cough, mucopurulent nasal discharge). • Repeat thoracic radiographs, esophagrams, fluoroscopic and neurologic examinations as necessary to follow progression or resolution of megaesophagus.

PREVENTION/AVOIDANCE

Esophageal obstruction may be prevented if pets are not allowed access to bones, garbage or other tempting items.

POSSIBLE COMPLICATIONS

Aspiration pneumonia.

EXPECTED COURSE AND PROGNOSIS

• Prognosis is poor with or without treatment. Aspiration pneumonia, owner noncompliance and malnutrition are leading causes of death. • Additional neurologic abnormalities may develop if the megaesophagus is caused by neuromuscular disease. • Megaesophagus caused by myasthenia gravis may improve with treatment.

• Occasionally congenital idiopathic megaesophagus may resolve with time, although this probably occurs much less frequently than previously reported.

MISCELLANEOUS

ASSOCIATED CONDITIONS

Aspiration pneumonia.

AGE RELATED FACTORS

Regurgitation at weaning is suggestive of congenital or obstructive megaesophagus.

ZOONOTIC POTENTIAL

Rabies vaccination status should be obtained in all patients with megaesophagus.

PREGNANCY N/A

SYNONYMS

Achalasia, a term used to describe esophageal hypomotility and lower esophageal sphincter hypertonicity in man, should not be used because megaesophagus in animals is rarely associated with lower esophageal sphincter hypertonicity.

SEE ALSO

Dysphagia • Pneumonia, Bacterial
• Myasthenia Gravis

ABBREVIATIONS N/A

References

Boudrieau RJ. Megaesophagus in the dog: a review of 50 cases. JAAHA 1985;21:33-40.

Guilford WG. Megaesophagus in the dog and cat. Sem Vet Med Surg (Small Anim) 1990;5:37-45.

Leib MS. Megaesophagus. In: Bojrab MJ, ed. Disease mechanisms in small animal surgery. 2nd ed. Philadelphia: Lea and Febiger, 1993:205-209.

Author Randall C. Longshore
Consulting Editor Brent D. Jones

MELANOCYTIC TUMORS, ORAL

 BASICS

OVERVIEW
Oral melanocytic tumors are characterized by progressive invasion of neoplastic melanocytes within the oral cavity of dogs and cats. The most common oral malignancy in dogs and third most common in cats. Tumors arise from the gingival surface, grow rapidly, and are highly invasive to bone. Metastasis is common, with spread to lymph nodes more common than the lungs.

SIGNALMENT
No sex or breed predisposition

SIGNS
Historical Findings
• Excessive salivation • Halitosis • Dysphagia • Bloody oral discharge • Weight loss

Physical Examination Findings
• Oral mass • Loose teeth • Facial deformity • Occasional cervical lymphadenopathy

CAUSES AND RISK FACTORS N/A

 DIAGNOSIS

DIFFERENTIAL DIAGNOSIS
• Other oral malignancy • Epilus • Ameloblastoma • Benign polyp • Abscess

CBC/BIOCHEMISTRY/URINALYSIS
Results usually normal

OTHER LABORATORY TESTS N/A

IMAGING
• Skull radiography to evaluate for bone involvement deep to mass • Thoracic radiography to evaluate lungs for metastasis

OTHER DIAGNOSTIC PROCEDURES
• A deep tissue biopsy (down to the bone) required for definitive diagnosis • Carefully palpate regional lymph nodes (i.e., mandibular and retropharyngeal)

 TREATMENT

• Radical surgical excision required (e.g., hemimaxillectomy-maxillectomy) and is usually well-tolerated by the patient
• Margins of at least 2 cm necessary
• Median and mean survival after complete surgical excision in dogs—340 days and 567 days, respectively
• Median and mean survival after incomplete surgical excision in dog—is 260 days and 210 days, respectively
• Survival after any form of surgical excision in cats usually < 60 days
• Radiotherapy may be helpful in come patients
• Survival in dogs after treatment—0-19 months
• Response to radiotherapy in cats unreported
• Radiation therapy combined with low-dose cisplatin chemotherapy may improve overall survival.
• No effective chemotherapy has been reported for local or systemic control in dogs or cats. Local control with intralesionally administered cisplatin have been reported.

MEDICATIONS

DRUGS AND FLUIDS
Cisplatin or doxorubicin as single-agent chemotherapy

CONTRAINDICATIONS/POSSIBLE INTERACTIONS N/A

FOLLOW-UP
• Repeat a head and neck examination with survey thoracic radiography at 1, 2, 3, 6, 9, 12, 15, 18, and 24 months after treatment. • Factors at the time of diagnosis indicating good prognosis include location (i.e., accessible to surgery), small tumor size (< 8.0 cm³), absence of bone invasion, and low mitotic index. • Cause of death is secondary to local recurrence, metastasis, and cachexia. • The overall prognosis is poor in cats because most tumors are locally invasive and diagnosed late in the course of the disease.

MISCELLANEOUS

ASSOCIATED CONDITIONS N/A

Reference

Hahn KA, DeNicola DB, Richardson RC, et al. Canine oral malignant melanoma: prognostic utility of an alternative staging system. J Small Anim Pract 1994;35:251-256.
Author Kevin A. Hahn
Consulting Editor Wallace B. Morrison

MELANOCYTIC TUMORS, SKIN AND DIGIT

BASICS

DEFINITION
Benign or malignant neoplasm arising from melanocytes and melanoblasts (melanin-producing cells)

Pathophysiology
• Locally invasive • Malignant melanoma can invade bone or metastasize to regional lymph nodes.

Systems Affected
• Skin/exocrine • Metastatic sites (e.g., bone, lymph nodes, lung, and viscera)

Genetics Unknown

Incidence/Prevalence
• Dogs—4-20% of all skin tumors • Cats—0.8-7% of all skin tumors

Geographic Distribution N/A

SIGNALMENT

Species
Dogs and cats

Breed Predilections
• Scottish terrier, Boston terrier, Airedale terrier, cocker spaniel, boxer, springer spaniel, Irish setter, Irish terrier, chow chow, Chihuahua, and Doberman pinscher • No breed predisposition in cats

Mean Age and Range
• Dogs—9 years • Cats—8-14 years

Predominant Sex
• Males may be predisposed in dogs. • No sex predilection in cats

SIGNS

Historical Findings
• Slow or rapidly growing mass • Lameness if digit is involved

Physical Examination Findings
• Pigmented or nonpigmented (amelanotic) mass, usually solitary • Occurs anywhere but may be more common on face, trunk, feet, and scrotum in dogs, and head and pinna in cats • Regional lymph nodes may be large.
• Patients with advanced disease may have dyspnea or harsh lung sounds because of pulmonary metastasis.

CAUSES Unknown

RISK FACTORS Unknown

DIAGNOSIS

DIFFERENTIAL DIAGNOSIS
Histopathologic examination and special stains may distinguish amelanotic tumor from poorly differentiated mast cell tumors, lymphosarcoma, and carcinoma.

CBC/BIOCHEMISTRY/URINALYSIS
Results usually normal

OTHER LABORATORY TESTS
Immunohistochemical stains may be helpful for differentiating melanoma (especially amelanotic) from other tumors. Melanoma stains positive with vimentin, S-100, and neuron specific enolase.

IMAGING
• Thoracic radiography to detect metastasis
• Area radiography to determine if underlying bone involved, especially in patients with melanoma of the digit

OTHER DIAGNOSTIC PROCEDURES
Cytologic examination of fine-needle aspirate reveals brown, rod-like intracellular granules (melanin) in various-sized and shaped cells. Pigment may be absent in the case of amelanotic melanoma. Macrophages (melanophages) containing phagocytosed melanin may be seen.

GROSS AND HISTOPATHOLOGIC FINDINGS

Gross Findings
• Masses vary in color and appearance. In general, benign melanoma is slow-growing, brown to black, and vary from macules and plaques to firm, dome-shaped nodules, 0.5-2 cm in diameter. In general, malignant melanoma is rapidly growing and amelanotic to dark brown, gray, or black. Both benign and malignant masses may be ulcerated.
• Melanoma involving the digit (dog) and eyelid (cat) tend to be malignant.

Histopathologic Findings
• Often difficult to distinguish benign from malignant lesions since either may have cells that vary in shape (i.e., epithelioid, fusiform, dendritic, and mixed), degree of pigmentation, and cytoplasmic morphology. In general, malignant melanomas have a high mitotic index, nuclear and nucleolar pleomorphism, and are invasive into surrounding tissues. Amelanotic malignant melanoma poses a diagnostic challenge; special stains may be particularly useful. • The patient may have inflammation, predominantly lymphoplasmacytic, in association with benign and malignant lesions.

TREATMENT

INPATIENT VERSUS OUTPATIENT
Treat as an inpatient if undergoing surgery

ACTIVITY
Depends on location of tumor. In general, restrict activity until sutures are removed.

DIET
Normal diet

CLIENT EDUCATION
• Discuss the need for early surgical removal.
• Avoid a "wait and see" approach.
• Malignant melanoma may metastasize early in the course of the disease; prognosis is guarded.

SURGICAL CONSIDERATIONS
• Wide surgical excision the treatment of choice
• Melanoma involving the nail bed or digit requires amputation of the digit.

MEDICATIONS

DRUGS AND FLUIDS
Adjunctive chemotherapy recommended if surgical excision is incomplete or the mass is nonresectable. Dacarbazine and doxorubicin have been reported to induce partial and complete remission in a small number of animals and may be the drugs of choice.

CONTRAINDICATIONS
Doxorubicin is cardiotoxic and contraindicated in patients with preexisting heart disease.

PRECAUTIONS
Veterinarians administering chemotherapeutics should follow published guidelines on the safe use of these drugs and should be familiar with potential side effects.

POSSIBLE INTERACTIONS
None reported

ALTERNATE DRUGS
Cimetidine has been shown to be of some benefit in horses and humans with malignant melanoma. The drug is believed to act as a biologic response modifier by reversing suppressor T cell-mediated immune suppression. This drug has not been evaluated for this purpose in dogs and cats.

FOLLOW-UP

PATIENT MONITORING
• Evaluate for evidence of recurrence and metastasis at 1, 3, 6, and 12 months after surgery or if the owner feels the mass is returning or if the patient is otherwise not normal. • Thoracic radiography at the time of rechecks and periodically thereafter

PREVENTION/AVOIDANCE N/A.

POSSIBLE COMPLICATIONS N/A

EXPECTED COURSE AND PROGNOSIS
• 25-50% of melanomas in dogs are reported to be malignant. Those occurring on the digit and scrotum have a greater likelihood of being malignant. • Mean survival time for dogs with benign melanomas > 24 months (skin) and 19.3 months (digit) with 2-year survival times of 94.3% (skin) and 38% (digit) • Survival time for dogs with malignant melanoma 8-13.5 months (skin) and 16.9 months (digit) with 2-year survival times of 34.1% (skin) and 22-36% (digit) • 35-50% of melanomas in cats are reported to be malignant. • Survival times for cats with melanoma of the skin or digit have not fre-

quently been reported. One study of 8 cats with melanoma reported a mean survival time of 13.5 months for three cats with malignant palpebral melanoma, and of five cats with dermal melanoma, three were still alive after 12 months, one died of metastasis at 90 days, and one died of unrelated causes.

MISCELLANEOUS

ASSOCIATED CONDITIONS None

AGE RELATED FACTORS None

ZOONOTIC POTENTIAL None

PREGNANCY N/A

SYNONYMS
• Benign—melanocytic nevus, melanocytoma
• Malignant—melanosarcoma (rarely used)

SEE ALSO N/A

ABBREVIATIONS N/A

References

Miller WH, Scott DW, Anderson WI. Feline cutaneous melanocytic neoplasms: a retrospective analysis of 43 cases (1979-1991). Vet Dermatol 1993;4:19-26.

Patnaik AK, Mooney S. Feline melanoma: a comparative study of ocular, oral, and dermal neoplasms. Vet Pathol 1988;25:105-112.

Bostock DE. Prognosis after surgical excision of canine melanomas. Vet Pathol 1979;16:32-40.

Aronsohn MG, Carpenter JL. Distal extremity melanocytic nevi and malignant melanomas in dogs. J Am Anim Hosp Assoc 1990;26:605-612.

Pulley LT, Stannard AA. Tumors of the skin and soft tissues. In: Moulton JE, ed. Tumors in domestic animals. 3rd ed. Berkeley: University of California Press, 1990:75-82.

Author Joanne C. Graham

Consulting Editor Wallace B. Morrison

MENINGIOMA—CATS

BASICS

OVERVIEW
Tumors of the meninges most commonly found intracranially, over the cerebrum • Usually solitary masses but are occasionally multiple • Also develop along the spinal cord but less frequently and with an intradural, extramedullary predilection site • The tumor compresses the adjacent tissue causing vasogenic edema. Edema resolution accounts for improvement in neurologic signs that occurs with corticosteroid administration.

SIGNALMENT
• Most cats > 9 years old but can be 1-24 years old • Males may be predisposed.

SIGNS
• Neurologic signs vary with the tumor location. • The clinical course is typically chronic and insidiously progressive over weeks to months. • Lateralizing deficits predominate.

Intracranial Meningioma
• The most common neurologic abnormalities relate to the cerebrum—abnormal behaviour and mentation, blindness, contralateral proprioceptive deficits, and seizures. • Signs suggesting herniation (e.g., anisocoria and stupor) in some cats

Intraspinal Meningiomas
• The nature of the ataxia and motor dysfunction varies with location of the lesion along the spinal column. • Spinal hyperpathia

CAUSE AND RISK FACTORS
• Cause is uncertain • Its documentation in young cats with mucopolysaccharidosis suggests a causal relationship.

DIAGNOSIS

DIFFERENTIAL DIAGNOSIS
Other primary CNS (e.g., glioma) or secondary (e.g., extensional or metastatic) tumors differentiated on the basis of a more rapid onset and progression of signs and on brain imaging.

CBC/BIOCHEMISTRY/URINALYSIS
Results usually normal

OTHER LABORATORY TESTS
• Computed tomography (CT) and magnetic resonance imaging (MRI) of the cranial vault are the preferred diagnostic techniques. On CT scans, homogenous enhancement of well-circumscribed lesions more typical than ring enhancement in post-contrast scans.
• Skull radiography and CT may reveal hyperostosis of the calvaria adjacent to the meningioma and increased tissue density if the tumor is calcified. • CSF analysis infrequently performed because of the characteristic results of diagnostic imaging; results are normal or the protein is high with or without suppurative inflammation if the tumor is necrotic. • Electroencephalography reveals slow wave, medium-voltage activity indicative of cortical depression. In a minority of cats, paroxysmal waveforms characteristic of seizure activity are observed. • In cats with spinal meningioma, myelography typically reveals an intradural-extramedullary mass showing a "golf tee" appearance making it difficult to differentiate from a nerve sheath tumor without biopsy.

TREATMENT
• If treated medically, treat as outpatient unless the cat is dehydrated and anorexic or has frequent seizures
• Surgical excision necessary for definitive management and is successful in most cats in which the tumor is accessible
• Medical management only palliative and the cat is expected to deteriorate over time

MEDICATIONS

DRUGS AND FLUIDS
• Administer corticosteroids to improve neurologic deficits associated with vasogenic edema and anticonvulsants if seizures occur more frequently than one per 6-8 weeks.
• If the cat is stuporous, severely ataxic, or showing signs of herniation, administer dexamethasone sodium phosphate (4-6 mg/kg IV). If the cat continues to deteriorate or is not improving, administer 0.5-2.0 g/kg of 20% mannitol solution in a drip over 20 minutes.
• Once the cat is stable, administer prednisone (1 mg/kg q12h) or dexamethasone (0.25 mg/cat PO q8h). For seizure control, administer phenobarbital (2 mg/kg PO q8h-q12h) or diazepam (0.5 mg/kg PO q8h-q12h).
• Avoid overzealous fluid administration as it may exacerbate cerebral edema and neurologic deficits.

CONTRAINDICATIONS/POSSIBLE INTERACTIONS
Avoid chloramphenicol and cimetidine if phenobarbital is being administered because they delay its metabolism.

FOLLOW-UP
• Serial neurologic examinations to detect marked improvement in deficits within 24-48 hours after initiation of corticosteroids.
• Prognosis good in approximately 70% of cats that have excision. Tumor regrowth may occur and seizure activity may persist.
• In cats that have medical management, neurologic deficits become more severe, but it may take many months since meningiomas tend to be slow growing. Thoracolumbar meningioma progresses to cause paralysis and inability to control urination and causes urinary retention and, possibly, bladder atony and cystitis.

MISCELLANEOUS

ABBREVIATIONS
CNS = central nervous system
CSF = cerebrospinal fluid
CT = computed tomography
MRI = magnetic resonance imaging

Reference
Braund KG, Ribas JL. Central nervous system meningiomas. Compend Contin Educ Pract Vet 1986;8:241-248.
Author Richard J. Joseph
Consulting Editor Joane M. Parent

BASICS

OVERVIEW
Meningioma is a tumor arising from meningiocytes (e.g., arachnoid cells of the dura mater, the arachnoid, and the pa mater that surround the brain and spinal cord) and has the following characteristics:
• Second most common CNS tumor in dogs
• Location can be paranasal or retrobulbar in location
• Most grow by expansion, but some can infiltrate the surrounding brain • Slow growing
• Can be multiple

SIGNALMENT
• Dogs—no gender or breed predilection; most dogs over 7 years old (range, 16 months-14 years)

SIGNS
• Depend on location of tumor(s) and secondary effects • Common signs include circling, pacing, visual deficits, seizures, lethargy, and aggression, often combined with cranial nerve deficits

CAUSES AND RISK FACTORS N/A

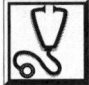

DIAGNOSIS

DIFFERENTIAL DIAGNOSIS
• Other primary or metastatic intracranial tumors • Granulomatous meningoencephalitis
• Metabolic encephalopathy • Degenerative myelopathy • Distemper • Rabies

CBC/BIOCHEMISTRY/URINALYSIS
Results usually normal

OTHER LABORATORY TESTS N/A

IMAGING
• Myelography to detect spinal signs • CT or MRI to detect intracranial signs

OTHER DIAGNOSTIC PROCEDURES
Results of CSF analysis usually normal

TREATMENT
Radiotherapy and surgical excision reported to be successful

MEDICATIONS

DRUGS AND FLUIDS N/A

CONTRAINDICATIONS/POSSIBLE INTERACTIONS N/A

FOLLOW-UP
• Repeat primary imaging studies at 3, 6, 9, 12 months after treatment or whenever clinical signs recur • Prognosis after surgery guarded and depends on surgical accessibility, skill of surgeon, and postoperative care; cure possible • Radiotherapy can be curative.

MISCELLANEOUS

ABBREVIATIONS
CSF = cerebral spinal fluid
CNS = central nervous system
CT = computed tomography
MRI = magnetic resonance imaging

Reference

Braund KG, Ribas JL. Central nervous system meningiomas. Comp Cont Ed Pract Vet 1986; 8:241-248.
Author Wallace B. Morrison
Consulting Editor Wallace B. Morrison

MENINGITIS, ASEPTIC

 BASICS

OVERVIEW
The most common form of meningitis in dogs; causes cervical and thoracolumbar spinal pain in young, large-breed dogs.

SIGNALMENT
• Most affected dogs 4-24 months old
• Large-breed dogs most common • Males and females

SIGNS
• Severe neck pain • Hunched back
• Reluctance to move • Stiff, stilted gait
• No neurologic deficits in most dogs
• Fever and depression in some dogs • Signs may be intermittent initially • If not treated, some dogs develop neurologic deficits (e.g., weakness, paralysis, and blindness)

CAUSES AND RISK FACTORS
Unknown

 DIAGNOSIS

DIFFERENTIAL DIAGNOSIS
• Infectious causes of meningitis must be differentiated on the basis of CSF analysis, bacterial culture, and serologic testing. • Cervical disk disease causes cervical pain but patients have no fever, leucocytosis, or abnormal CSF.
• Polyarthritis can cause cervical pain and lameness but results of CSF analysis are normal and cytologic examination of joint fluid shows inflammation. • Cervical diskospondylitis causes neck pain and fever but the results of CSF examination are usually normal and radiographs of the affected vertebrae should be diagnostic.

CBC/BIOCHEMISTRY/URINALYSIS
• Leucocytosis with neutrophilia in some patients • Results of biochemical analysis and urinalysis normal

OTHER LABORATORY TESTS N/A
Serologic tests for infectious agents are negative.

IMAGING N/A

OTHER DIAGNOSTIC PROCEDURES
• CSF examination—dramatic increase in mature, nontoxic neutrophils and high protein. • Bacterial culture of CSF, blood, and urine negative • Histopathologic findings not well documented because of responsiveness to treatment

 TREATMENT

• Treat as inpatient until signs resolve
• Restrict activity.

MEDICATIONS

DRUGS AND FLUIDS

• Prednisone (2-4mg/kg PO q24h). Dogs should respond within 48 hours. Gradually decrease prednisone dosage after 2 weeks and administer maintainence dosage (1 mg/kg q48h) for at least 2 months.
• Medication can be discontinued in some dogs after 2-4 months. Treatment for 4-6 months may be necessary.

CONTRAINDICATIONS/POSSIBLE INTERACTIONS N/A

FOLLOW-UP

• Monitor for presence of neck pain and leucocytosis • Continue prednisone medication for at least 2 months after the patient is free of signs to reduce the likelihood of relapse.
• The disorder may resolve spontaneously at 18-24 months of age in some dogs.

MISCELLANEOUS

SYNONYMS

Corticosteroid responsive meningitis

SEE ALSO

• Meningitis, Bacterial • Meningoencephalitis • Meningomyelitis

ABBREVIATION

CSF = cerebrospinal fluid

Reference

Meric SM. Meningitis-a changing emphasis. J Vet Int Med 1988;2:26-35.
Author Susan M. Taylor
Consulting Editor Joane M. Parent

MENINGITIS/MENINGOENCEPHALITIS/MENINGOMYELITIS, BACTERIAL

BASICS

DEFINITION
• Meningitis—inflammation of the meninges • Meningoencephalitis—inflammation of the meninges and brain • Meningomyelitis—inflammation of the meninges and spinal cord

Pathophysiology
Bacterial infection of the CNS by extension of an infected extraneural site or by hematogenous route. Inflammation of the meninges can lead to secondary inflammation of the brain or spinal cord, resulting in neurologic deficits.

Systems Affected
• Nervous—meninges, brain, or spinal cord • In addition, multisystemic signs may develop since the bacterial infection usually originates in an extraneural site.

Genetics N/A

Incidence/Prevalence Rare

Geographic Distribution N/A

SIGNALMENT

Species Dogs and cats

Breed Predilections N/A

Mean Age and Range
• Animals of any age are affected. • Neonates may have a relatively higher risk because of omphalophlebitis.

Predominant Sex N/A

SIGNS

General Comments
Patients with bacterial meningoencephalitis/ myelitis are nearly always systemically ill; they may have depression, shock, hypotension, and disseminated intravascular coagulation.

Physical Examination Findings
• A site of underlying infection may be found. • Cervical rigidity, hyperesthesia, and pyrexia are characteristic in patients with meningeal involvement. • Vomiting and bradycardia in some patients

Neurologic Examination Findings
• Because the infection can spread to any part of the CNS, the deficits reflect the location of the parenchyma that is involved. • Signs of high intracranial pressure, such as stupor, coma, anisocoria or poor physiological nystagmus, may be seen.

CAUSES
• Bacterial meningitis is usually secondary to local extension from infection of the ears, eyes, sinuses, nasal passages, or areas of diskospondylitis or osteomyelitis. • Less often, hematogenous spread of bacterial infection occurs from extracranial foci in dogs with bacterial endocarditis, prostatitis, metritis, or diskospondylitis. • A point of origin is not always found.

RISK FACTORS
• Untreated bacterial infection • Immunocompromised patient • Injury involving the CNS or adjacent structures

DIAGNOSIS

DIFFERENTIAL DIAGNOSIS
• Fungal meningitis—affected extraneural sites are common in dogs with CNS cryptococcus (e.g., nasal, skin, and bone), blastomycosis (e.g., lung, lymph nodes, eyes, skin, and bone), or coccidioidomycosis (e.g., lung, bones, and joints), and the diagnosis can often be made by biopsy or cytologic examination of these affected tissues. Serologic testing is also available for these agents. Organisms are sometimes observed in the CSF and can be cultured. • Distemper virus meningoencephalitis—usually seen in young, unvaccinated dogs. CNS signs may be preceded by mild gastrointestinal and respiratory signs. Chorioretinitis is common. Inclusion bodies may be observed on cytologic examination or the virus detected in a conjunctival scraping or tracheal wash specimen by fluorescent antibody technique. CSF analysis typically reveals a high number of small lymphocytes and high protein concentration, primarily albumin. Neutrophils are not present. • FIP virus meningoencephalitis—often accompanied by uveitis and chorioretinitis. Affected cats are generally < 3 years old and, contrary to bacterial CNS infection, may have a protracted history. • Toxoplasma meningoencephalitis—may be accompanied by pneumonia, hepatitis, myositis, and uveitis, especially in cats. Toxoplasmosis is usually seen in young dogs, frequently involving the nerve roots and muscles. The serum toxoplasma titer may rise with active infection. Serum IgM may be detected in the serum and CSF of affected dogs. Biopsy of affected tissues may reveal the organism. • Aseptic (immune-mediated) meningitis—observed mainly in young, large-breed dogs that have cervical pain alone on examination and are not systemically ill. • In patients with neoplasia of the CNS, the signs are limited to the CNS. Results of standard laboratory tests are normal. The diagnosis is made by CT and CSF analysis. • Granulomatous meningoencephalomyelitis—differentiated by clinical signs (usually not systemic), CSF analysis (i.e., lymphocytes, monocytes, occasional plasma cells and aplastic mononuclear cells, and sometimes mature nontoxic neutrophils), and negative CSF culture

CBC/BIOCHEMISTRY/URINALYSIS
• Leukocytosis common; left shift or toxicity in some patients • Evidence of other organ involvement (e.g., liver and kidney) and hyperglobulinemia in response to chronic infection • Pyuria and bacteriuria in animals with underlying urinary tract or prostatic infection

and animals with hematogenous spread of bacteria

OTHER LABORATORY TESTS
• Positive serologic tests can differentiate fungal, protozoal, rickettsial, and viral from bacterial disease. In cats, toxoplasma titer can be positive without clinical disease. • Cytologic examination of infected tissues (e.g., skin, eyes, nasal discharge, and sputum) to help identify the organism, especially in patients with fungal disease • Blood and urine culture may be positive.

IMAGING
• Spinal radiography to look for diskospondylitis as a focus of infection • Skull radiography in patients in which the sinus, nasal cavity, or ear is the suspected initiating site • Echocardiography in patients with suspected valvular endocarditis

OTHER DIAGNOSTIC PROCEDURES
• CSF collection contraindicated if the patient has signs suggesting high intracranial pressure because it can precipitate brain herniation • CSF analysis—neutrophilic pleocytosis with high protein concentration. In some patients, the neutrophils appear toxic or degenerated and bacteria are seen. It is difficult to differentiate aseptic meningitis from bacterial meningitis by CSF analysis alone. • CSF culture (aerobic or anaerobic) may be positive. • Biopsy of infected tissue may help identify the organism.

GROSS AND HISTOPATHOLOGIC FINDINGS
• Subdural empyema, herniation, or purulent material on the surface of the brain in some patients • Microscopically, diffuse suppurative leptomeningeal infiltration is common.

TREATMENT

INPATIENT VERSUS OUTPATIENT
Patients should be aggressively treated as inpatients.

ACTIVITY Restricted

DIET N/A

CLIENT EDUCATION
Rapid and aggressive treatment is important.

SURGICAL CONSIDERATIONS N/A

MEDICATIONS

DRUGS AND FLUIDS
• Antibiotics that penetrate the blood brain barrier (e.g., chloramphenicol, trimethoprim, sulfonamides, metronidazole, moxalactam, and cefotaxime). Whenever possible, the organism should be identified and isolated to determine drug sensitivity (e.g., CSF culture, blood and urine culture, and culture of primary

MENINGITIS/MENINGOENCEPHALITIS/MENINGOMYELITIS, BACTERIAL

site). If cultures cannot be obtained, the antibiotic chosen should be broad in spectrum and effective against aerobes and anaerobes.
• In patients with inflammation and suspected staphylococcal infection, use penicillin or ampicillin, which enter the CNS. This is then administered in combination with another antibiotic that enters the CNS.
• Anticonvulsants (i.e., diazepam initially and then phenobarbital) in patients with seizures.

CONTRAINDICATIONS
Aminoglycosides and first generation cephalosporins do not penetrate the blood-brain barrier even in the presence of inflamed meninges and should not be used.

PRECAUTIONS N/A

POSSIBLE INTERACTIONS
Do not administer chloramphenicol to animals also treated with phenobarbital. Chloramphenicol inhibits the hepatic metabolism of phenobarbital leading to a toxic concentration of phenobarbital.

ALTERNATE DRUGS N/A

FOLLOW-UP

PATIENT MONITORING
Nervous system signs, fever, leukocytosis, and systemic signs

PREVENTION/AVOIDANCE
Local infection adjacent to the CNS (i.e., eyes, ears, sinuses, nose, and spine) should be treated early and aggressively to prevent extension to the CNS.

POSSIBLE COMPLICATIONS
Damage caused by inflammation of the brain and spinal cord or associated thrombosis may be irreversible.

EXPECTED COURSE AND PROGNOSIS
• The response to antibiotics is variable and the prognosis guarded. • Many patients die despite treatment. • Some patients recover completely; treatment for at least 4 weeks past resolution of all signs is recommended.

MISCELLANEOUS

ASSOCIATED CONDITIONS N/A
AGE RELATED FACTORS N/A
ZOONOTIC POTENTIAL N/A
PREGNANCY N/A
SYNONYMS N/A
SEE ALSO
• Meningitis, Aseptic • Encephalitis • Meningoencephalomyelitis, Granulomatous

ABBREVIATIONS
CNS = central nervous system
CSF = cerebrospinal fluid
CT = computed tomography

References
Dow SW, LeCouteur RA, Henik RA, et al. Central nervous system infection associated with anaerobic bacteria in two dogs and two cats. J Vet Int Med 1988;2:171-176.
Fenner WR. Meningitis. In: Kirk R, ed. Current veterinary therapy IX. Philadelphia: WB Saunders, 1986:814-818.
Fenner WR. Bacterial Infections of the central nervous system. In: Greene CE, ed. Infectious diseases of the dog and cat. Philadelphia: WB Saunders, 1990:184-196.
Meric SM. Canine meningitis. J Vet Int Med 1988;2:26-35.
Thomas WB, Sorjonen DC, Steiss JE. A retrospective evaluation of 38 cases of canine distemper encephalomyelitis. J Am Anim Hosp Assoc 1993;29:129-133.

Author Susan M. Taylor
Consulting Editor Joane M. Parent

MENINGOENCEPHALOMYELITIS, EOSINOPHILIC

 BASICS

OVERVIEW
• Diffuse or multifocal meningoencephalomyelitis • CSF analysis reveals eosinophilic pleocytosis. • Eosinophils are in response to a parasite or an allergic reaction. • The underlying cause of the idiopathic syndrome is unknown. • Meningeal involvement can be marked.

SIGNALMENT
• Any dog. The golden retriever may be predisposed. • Male > females • 14 weeks–5.5 years

SIGNS
• Clinical signs vary in location and severity. • Neurologic abnormalities relate to the cerebrum in many patients—dementia, seizures, circling, and cortical blindness.

CAUSES AND RISK FACTORS
• Idiopathic/allergic—more common than other causes • Neoplasia—as a reaction to foreign material • Parasitic—cerebral cysticerci, Neospora caninum, Toxoplasma gondii, Dirofilaria immitis

 DIAGNOSIS

DIFFERENTIAL DIAGNOSIS
• This syndrome cannot be differentiated from the other encephalitides on the basis of clinical signs alone. CFS analysis must be done. • Once the presence of eosinophils in the CSF is confirmed, there are three considerations—parasite, allergic response, and tumor. • Parasitic diseases are differentiated on the basis of systemic signs, laboratory data, and serologic test results. • Patients with the allergic and idiopathic disease usually have a predominance of cerebral signs, negative serologic test results, and marked eosinophilic pleocytosis. • Patients with a brain tumor are older, have a longer history, and have clinical signs related to a focal lesion. Although eosinophils may be found, the number is usually low. The diagnosis of a brain tumor is confirmed by brain imaging and biopsy.

CBC/BIOCHEMISTRY/URINALYSIS
• Peripheral eosinophilia in some patients is not a reliable indicator of brain disease. The degree of peripheral eosinophilia does not correlate with the number of eosinophils in the CSF. • Results of biochemical analysis and urinalysis are usually normal in patients with idiopathic and allergic disease. Liver enzyme activity and creatine kinase may be high in patients with protozoal disease.

OTHER LABORATORY TESTS N/A

IMAGING N/A

OTHER DIAGNOSTIC PROCEDURES
• CSF analysis—marked eosinophilic pleocytosis in patients with idiopathic and allergic disease. In patients with parasitic disease, the pleocytosis is of a lesser degree and may be accompanied by neutrophils. In patients with neoplasia, the WBC count is low, and eosinophils are present but in small numbers. • Once CSF analysis confirms the presence of eosinophils, parasitic disease should be looked for thoroughly. • Serologic testing for heartworm, Neospora caninum, and Toxoplasma gondii should always be done.

 TREATMENT

• Most patients need to be hospitalized because of the severity of the clinical signs. • Activity according to what the patient can tolerate • Regular diet
• The idiopathic form of the disease carries a good prognosis provided treatment is early and aggressive.

MEDICATIONS

DRUGS AND FLUIDS

• Idiopathic disease is treated by steroid administration—dexamethasone (0.25 mg/kg q12h for 3 days, then q24h for 3 days). This is followed by prednisone (1 mg/kg q24h for 2 weeks then q48h 6-8 weeks). The steroids can then be slowly weaned off over 6 weeks.
• Clindamycin, sulfonamides, and pyrimethamine are used to treat protozoal disease.
• If heartworm is diagnosed, it should be treated later on. Microfilarial migration to the CNS is rare. No treatment available other than supportive.

CONTRAINDICATIONS/POSSIBLE INTERACTIONS

Steroids are contraindicated if the patient has protozoal disease.

FOLLOW-UP

• Neurologic examination should be repeated every 6 hours to monitor progress. • The idiopathic form carries a good prognosis with early and aggressive treatment. Improvement is usually seen in the first 72 hours with full recovery in 6-8 weeks. CSF analysis can then be repeated to determine if treatment can be stopped. • Patients with protozoal disease have a poor to grave prognosis. • With larval migration such as in patients with heartworm disease, prognosis varies with the location of the lesion. In time, signs may resolve, but often the larvae continue to migrate and death may ensue. Prognosis is guarded to poor.
• Regardless of the cause of the presence of eosinophils in the CNS, their degradation is toxic to nervous tissue. The patient may have permanent deficits, not only from the primary disease, but also from the effects of the eosinophils.

MISCELLANEOUS

ABBREVIATION

CSF = cerebrospinal fluid

Reference

Smith-Maxie LL, Parent JM, Rand J, et al. Cerebrospinal fluid analysis and clinical outcome of eight dogs with eosinophilic meningoencephalomyelitis. J Vet Int Med 1989;3:167-174.
Author Joane M. Parent
Consulting Editor Joane M. Parent

MENINGOENCEPHALOMYELITIS, GRANULOMATOUS

BASICS

DEFINITION
Progressive, idiopathic, inflammatory disease of the CNS in dogs

Pathophysiology
Immunohistologic studies and the histologic resemblance to experimental allergic encephalomyelitis support an immunologic basis for this disease. However, there are also similarities between this disease and viral encephalomyelitis, suggesting that an altered host response to an infectious agent is also possible. No infectious agents have been identified.

Systems Affected
• Nervous • Ophthalmic—an ocular form occasionally is seen in combination with the CNS form or alone

Genetics
No heritability demonstrated

Incidence/Prevalence
Although the literature reports it as a sporadic disorder, field evidence suggests that it may be one of the most common causes of progressive CNS dysfunction in adult dogs.

Geographic Distribution N/A

SIGNALMENT
Species Dogs

Breed Predilections
• Poodles and terriers may be predisposed. • Other small breeds are also commonly affected. • Large-breed dogs may be affected, particularly with the disseminated form of the disease.

Mean Age and Range
• Mean age 5 years, 6 months-10 years • Older dogs occasionally affected • Approximately 30% of affected dogs < 2 years old

Predominant Sex
Both sexes affected with a higher prevalence in females

SIGNS
Historical Findings
Focal form
• Acts as a slowly enlarging, space-occupying mass • Signs progress over 3-6 months. • Most often affects the brainstem, cerebral cortex, cerebellum, or cervical spinal cord
Disseminated form
• Acute onset of CNS signs with rapid progression over 1-8 weeks • 25% die within 1 week • Most often affects the caudal brainstem (vestibular system), cervical cord, and meninges • Fever in some patients

Neurologic Examination Findings
• Abnormalities reflect the location of the lesion(s). • Ataxia, seizures, circling, head pressing, and blindness indicate cerebral involve-

ment. • Head tilt, nystagmus, and trigeminal or facial paralysis indicate brainstem involvement. • Patients with the ocular form have acute blindness with bilaterally dilated nonresponsive pupils. • Cervical pain and paresis or paralysis commonly occur in patients with meningeal and spinal cord involvement.

CAUSES Unknown
RISK FACTORS N/A

DIAGNOSIS

DIFFERENTIAL DIAGNOSIS
• Granulomatous meningoencephalomyelitis cannot be differentiated from other causes of meningoencephalomyelitis by clinical signs alone. • Infectious causes of meningoencephalomyelitis such as viral, fungal, rickettsial, and protozoal disease can be differentiated by the presence of systemic signs, results of serologic testing, and results of CSF analysis and culture. • Dogs with aseptic (immune-mediated) meningitis have cervical pain without neurologic deficits, and results of CSF analysis usually reveal neutrophilic pleocytosis. • Brain tumors are differentiated from the focal form by CSF analysis combined with CT scan.

CBC/BIOCHEMISTRY/URINALYSIS
Results usually normal

OTHER LABORATORY TESTS
None required. Serum titers are helpful in ruling out infectious disease.

IMAGING
CT scan and MRI are useful to determine the form of disease and the location and the extent of the inflammatory process.

OTHER DIAGNOSTIC PROCEDURES
• CSF examination—mononuclear pleocytosis with a high number of lymphocytes and monocytes and occasional plasma cells. Large, foamy mononuclear cells frequently are seen. The neutrophil population varies from 1-20% in most patients. • CSF protein is mildly to moderately high.

GROSS AND HISTOPATHOLOGIC FINDINGS
• Grossly, the meninges may be thickened and cloudy. • Sections of the brain may have circumscribed areas that are soft and grayish in color. • The optic nerves are large in patients with the ocular form. • Dense, perivascular aggregations of mononuclear cells arranged in a whirling pattern are characteristic.

TREATMENT

INPATIENT VERSUS OUTPATIENT
• Patients with serious or progressive disease should be hospitalized for initial treatment. • Stable patients can be discharged after the diagnosis has been made.

ACTIVITY Restricted
DIET N/A
CLIENT EDUCATION
• This disorder is fatal, although some dogs respond to treatment for a short time (weeks to a few months). • The initial diagnostic evaluation is important to differentiate granulomatous meningoencephalomyelitis from more treatable disorders.

SURGICAL CONSIDERATIONS N/A

MEDICATIONS

DRUGS AND FLUIDS
Corticosteroids (prednisone 1-2 mg/kg/day PO). If at all, improvement occurs in the first 2 weeks of treatment. The dose can then be gradually decreased. Most patients require continued treatment to prevent recurrence.

CONTRAINDICATIONS
It is important to eliminate infectious differentials before treating with corticosteroids.

PRECAUTIONS N/A
POSSIBLE INTERACTIONS N/A
ALTERNATE DRUGS
• In patients in which prednisone is ineffective, cyclophosphamide may be tried. • In selected patients, azathioprine (2mg/kg/day) is added to the treatment regimen when the side effects of prednisone (eg, polyuria and polyphagia) are too pronounced or when prednisone has failed. • Radiotherapy may be beneficial.

FOLLOW-UP

PATIENT MONITORING
• Nervous system signs • CBC and biochemical analysis regularly to monitor for toxicity if azathioprine or cyclophosphamide is administered

PREVENTION/AVOIDANCE
Too rapid a decrease in corticosteroid dosage may cause rapid deterioration.

POSSIBLE COMPLICATIONS
Disease may progress despite appropriate treatment.

EXPECTED COURSE AND PROGNOSIS
• The progression of signs can sometimes be slowed or reversed by corticosteroid administration. • Corticosteroids need to be continued for life. • Disease progresses in most patients despite treatment.

MISCELLANEOUS

ASSOCIATED CONDITIONS N/A

MENINGOENCEPHALOMYELITIS, GRANULOMATOUS

AGE RELATED FACTORS N/A

ZOONOTIC POTENTIAL N/A

PREGNANCY

Prednisone administration and the short life expectancy of affected dogs make successful gestation unlikely.

SYNONYMS

Reticulosis, inflammatory and neoplastic

SEE ALSO

• Encephalitis • Meningitis

ABBREVIATIONS

CNS = central nervous system
CT = computed tomography
CSF = cerebrospinal fluid
MRI = magnetic resonance imaging

References

Braund KG. Clinical syndromes in veterinary neurology. 2nd ed. St. Louis: Mosby, 1994:135.

Meric SM. Canine meningitis. J Vet Int Med 1988;2:26-35.

Thomas JB, Eger C. Granulomatous meningoencephalomyelitis in 21 dogs. J Small Anim Pract 1989;30:287-293.

Author Susan M. Taylor

Consulting Editor Joane M. Parent

MESOTHELIOMA

BASICS

OVERVIEW
Mesothelioma is a rare tumor of the epithelial lining of body cavities and has the following characteristics:
• Primary tumors in dogs involve the thoracic cavity, pericardial sac, abdominal cavity, and vaginal tunic of the scrotum. • Primary tumors in cats involve the thoracic cavity, pericardial sac, and the abdominal cavity.

SIGNALMENT
• Sclerosing mesotheliomas seen primarily in male dogs • German shepherd dog the most commonly affected breed

SIGNS
• Effusion (hemorrhagic) and displacement of organs • Dyspnea • Exercise intolerance • Mediastinal mass • Vomiting

CAUSES AND RISK FACTORS
Exposure to asbestos

DIAGNOSIS

DIFFERENTIAL DIAGNOSIS
• Any cause of effusion such as congestive heart failure, liver disease, hypoalbuminemia, pyothorax, lymphosarcoma, and idiopathic pericardial effusion • Other causes of mediastinal masses such as Iymphosarcoma, thymoma, thyroid carcinoma, and chemodectoma

CBC/BIOCHEMISTRY/URINALYSIS
No specific abnormalities

OTHER LABORATORY TESTS N/A

IMAGING
• Radiographs show body cavity effusion.
• Ultrasound may detect pericardial sac thickening and effusion with mesothelioma of the pericardial sac.

OTHER DIAGNOSTIC PROCEDURES
• Results of cytologic examination of fluid should be interpreted cautiously because it can be difficult to distinguish mesothelioma from physiological mesothelial proliferation.
• Exploratory surgery or laparoscopy reveals nodules, plaques, or thickenings of the mesothelial lining of the body cavity. • Histologic evaluation reveals morphologic characteristics of epithelial neoplasms and mesenchymal proliferation.

TREATMENT
• Patients can be treated as outpatients, but restrict the activity of patients with dyspnea.
• Partial pericardectomy is useful to relieve pericardial effusion.
• Palliation effusion by centesis or pleurodesis.

MEDICATIONS

DRUGS AND FLUIDS
• Cisplatin chemotherapy has been used successfully.
• Cisplatin can be given intracavitary but penetrates tumor only a few cells deep and is not effective.
• Give cisplatin according to established protocols that include adequate diuresis.

CONTRAINDICATIONS/POSSIBLE INTERACTIONS
• Cisplatin can not be used in cats.
• Cisplatin should not be used in dogs with renal disease.

FOLLOW-UP
• Thoracic radiography with every treatment and every 3 months after treatment • Avoid exposure to asbestos. • Laboratory tests to assess renal status after cisplatin administration.
• Of 3 dogs treated by intracavitary cisplatin, the survivals were 410 days, >129 days, and >306 days.

MISCELLANEOUS
These are highly effusive tumors.

Reference

Moore AS, Kirk C, Cardona A. Intracavitary cisplatin chemotherapy experience with six dogs. J Vet Intern Med 1991;5: 227-231.
Author Terrance A. Hamilton
Consulting Editor Wallace B. Morrison

BASICS

DEFINITION
Metaldehyde is a polycyclic polymer of acetaldehyde that primarily affects the nervous system. It is an ingredient of slug and snail baits and is used as solid fuel for some camp stoves. Baits may be liquid or dry; however, most are dry pellets of metaldehyde mixed with feed material such as soybeans, rice, oats, sorghum, and apples. Some baits that contain metaldehyde contain other toxicants, such as arsenate and insecticides.

Pathophysiology
The exact mechanism of metaldehyde toxicosis is unknown. It may increase excitatory neurotransmitters or decrease inhibitory neurotransmitters.

Systems Affected
• Nervous • Respiratory—death usually due to respiratory failure • Hepatobiliary—if the animal survives the initial convulsive period, it may die of liver disease 2-3 days later.

Genetics N/A

Incidence/Prevalence
Varies with geography

Geographic Distribution
This toxicosis is more commonly found in coastal and low-lying areas, with a higher prevalence of snails and slugs than other areas.

SIGNALMENT

Species Dogs and cats

Breed Predilections N/A

Mean Age and Range Any

Predominant Sex N/A

SIGNS

General Comments
Clinical signs may occur immediately after ingestion, or may be delayed for up to 3 hours.

Historical Findings
Most often, owners report bizarre behavior, ataxia, and convulsions.

Physical Examination Findings
• Convulsions—may be continuous or intermittent. Between convulsions, the animal may have muscle tremors, anxiety, and be hyperesthetic. Seizures are not necessarily evoked by external stimuli. • Hyperthermia —temperature of up to 108° F is common and is probably caused by excessive muscle activity. • Tachycardia • Nystagmus • Mydriasis • Hyperpnea • Hypersalivation • Ataxia • Vomiting • Cyanosis • Diarrhea • Dehydration • Depression or narcosis may occur late in the course of toxicosis. • Death is usually due to respiratory failure and occurs 4-24 hours after exposure. • If the animal survives the initial convulsive period, it may die of liver disease in 2-3 days.

CAUSES
Ingestion of metaldehyde

RISK FACTORS N/A

DIAGNOSIS

DIFFERENTIAL DIAGNOSIS
• Strychnine toxicosis causes intermittent seizures that can be evoked by external stimuli. • Penitrem A is a mycotoxin usually found in moldy English walnuts or cream cheese, but it has been reported in other foodstuffs. This toxin causes a tremorgenic syndrome. • Roquefortine is a mycotoxin found in moldy bleu cheese and other foodstuffs and causes a tremorgenic syndrome. • Lead toxicosis can cause seizures as well as behavior changes, blindness, and gastrointestinal upset. • Organochlorine insecticides can cause seizures in most mammals. • Anticholinesterase insecticides (e.g., organophosphates and carbamates) can cause seizures, usually accompanied by excessive salivation, lacrimation, urination, and defecation. • Seizures can be caused by a host of nontoxic conditions that affect the nervous system, including neoplasia, trauma, infection, metabolic disorder, and congenital disorder.

CBC/BIOCHEMISTRY/URINALYSIS
Results usually not diagnostic

OTHER LABORATORY TESTS
Metaldehyde testing can be done on vomitus, stomach contents, or serum.

IMAGING N/A

OTHER DIAGNOSTIC PROCEDURES
Cerebrospinal fluid analysis not diagnostic

GROSS AND HISTOPATHOLOGIC FINDINGS
• Hepatic, renal, and pulmonary congestion
• Petechial and ecchymotic hemorrhages
• Subendocardial and subepicardial hemorrhages

TREATMENT

INPATIENT VS OUTPATIENT
Patients should be hospitalized until convulsions cease.

ACTIVITY
Restricted

DIET
Do not feed animals that are vomiting, convulsing, or heavily sedated.

CLIENT EDUCATION N/A

SURGICAL CONSIDERATIONS N/A

MEDICATIONS

DRUGS AND FLUIDS
• No antidote available • Prevent further absorption by use of emetics or gastric lavage followed by administration of activated charcoal. • Tranquilize convulsing animals with diazepam or barbiturates. • Fluids may be necessary to treat dehydration or acidosis.

CONTRAINDICATIONS
Never induce vomiting in a convulsing animal.

PRECAUTIONS
• Do not use depressants if animal is already depressed. • Barbiturates can lead to cardiac arrest.

POSSIBLE INTERACTIONS N/A

ALTERNATE DRUGS N/A

FOLLOW-UP

PATIENT MONITORING
Periodically allow tranquilizers to wear off and reevaluate convulsive condition.

PREVENTION/AVOIDANCE
Do not apply metaldehyde in areas accessible to pets.

POSSIBLE COMPLICATIONS
Patient may develop liver disease if it survives the initial convulsive phase.

EXPECTED COURSE AND PROGNOSIS
• Prognosis depends mostly on the amount ingested. • Death occurs in 4-24 hours after exposure if the animal is not successfully treated. • Liver disease can be a secondary problem. • Reported sequelae include diarrhea, memory loss, and temporary blindness.

MISCELLANEOUS

ASSOCIATED CONDITIONS
Some types of molluscicides contain toxicants such as arsenate and insecticides in addition to metaldehyde. These compounds can cause concurrent toxicoses.

AGE RELATED FACTORS N/A

ZOONOTIC POTENTIAL N/A

PREGNANCY
Not known to be mutagenic, genotoxic, or immunotoxic.

SYNONYMS
• Polyacetaldehyde • Limovet • Limax
• Antimilace • Snail bait

SEE ALSO Poisoning (Intoxication)

ABBREVIATIONS N/A

References
Booze TF, Oehme FW. Metaldehyde toxicity: a review. Vet Hum Toxicol 1985; 27:11-19.
Von Burg R, Stout T. Metaldehyde. J Appl Toxicol 1991;11:377-378.
Andreasen JR. Metaldehyde toxicosis in ducklings. J Vet Diagn Invest 1993;5:500-501.
Author Konstanze H. Plumlee
Consulting Editor Gary D. Osweiler

METRITIS

BASICS

OVERVIEW
• Bacterial uterine infection that develops in the immediate postpartum period (usually within the first week); occasionally develops after an abortion or breeding • Bacteria ascend through the open cervix to the uterus. • A large, flaccid, postpartum uterus provides an ideal environment for bacterial growth. • Gram negative bacteria such as Escherichia coli commonly isolated • Potentially life-threatening infection that can lead to septic shock • Directly affects uterus with systemic involvement as sepsis develops

SIGNALMENT
• Postpartum bitch and queen • No age or breed predilection

SIGNS
Historical Findings
• Malodorous, purulent, sanguinopurulent or dark green vulvar discharge • Depression • Anorexia • Neglect of puppies and kittens • Reduced milk production

Physical Examination Findings
• Fever • Large uterus on abdominal palpation • Dehydration • Injected mucous membranes • Tachycardia as sepsis develops.

CAUSES AND RISK FACTORS
• Dystocia • Obstetric manipulation • Retained fetuses or placenta • Post abortion and post natural or artificial insemination (rare)

DIAGNOSIS

DIFFERENTIAL DIAGNOSIS
• Subinvolution of placental sites—no sign of infection on cytologic examination of vagina • Eclampsia—serum calcium concentration differentiates • Mastitis—physical examination findings differentiate

CBC/BIOCHEMISTRY/URINALYSIS
• Neutrophilia with left shift; leukopenia in occasional patient with endotoxic shock • High PCV, total protein, creatinine, BUN, and urine specific gravity secondary to dehydration. • High liver enzyme activity in patients with endotoxemia • Urine specific gravity low in some patients with endotoxemia

OTHER LABORATORY TESTS N/A

IMAGING
• Radiography reveals retained fetuses and maybe a large uterus • Ultrasonography reveals intrauterine fluid accumulation and retained placenta and fetuses as well as abdominal effusion secondary to uterine rupture

OTHER DIAGNOSTIC PROCEDURES
• Vaginal cytologic examination to detect degenerative neutrophils with intracellular and extracellular bacteria. • Anterior vaginal culture for aerobes and anaerobes to identify organism

TREATMENT
• As inpatient until systemic signs resolve • Ovariohysterectomy is the treatment of choice if patient has a retained fetus or placenta, uterine rupture, severe infection, or if future breeding not desired. • In chronically affected animals that do not respond to medical treatment, hysterotomy and lavage can be performed as long as the uterus has no friable areas. • A friable uterus should be packed off and handled gently at surgery.

MEDICATIONS

DRUGS AND FLUIDS
• IV administration of balanced electrolyte solution to treat dehydration • Treat shock. • Correct electrolyte imbalances and hypoglycemia identified by serum chemistry profile. • Start broad-spectrum bactericidal antibiotics—oral administration if patient is stable, intravenous if patient is in shock • Antibiotic choice should be confirmed by bacterial culture and continued at least 14 days. • Oxytocin (0.5-1.0 U/kg IM repeated in 1-2 hours) • Prostaglandin F_{2a} (100-250 mcg/kg SQ q12h for 5-8 days to evacuate uterus)

CONTRAINDICATIONS/POSSIBLE INTERACTIONS
• Prostaglandin can induce uterine rupture if the tissue is devitalized.
• Oxytocin may not be effective beyond 48 hours postpartum.
• Flushing of uterus may cause rupture of devitalized wall.

FOLLOW-UP

PATIENT MONITORING
• CBC, temperature, vaginal cytologic examination, and clinical signs. • Ultrasonography to monitor evacuation of uterine fluid

PREVENTION/AVOIDANCE
• If medical treatment is ineffective, ovariohysterectomy is necessary. • Uterine rupture and peritonitis may occur with medical treatment.

EXPECTED COURSE AND PROGNOSIS
• Prognosis for recovery in patients that have ovariohysterectomy is good. • Prognosis for recovery in patients that have medical treatment is fair, but future reproduction may be adversely affected. • Old bitches and queens should have ovariohysterectomy.

MISCELLANEOUS

Reference
Magne ML. Acute metritis in the bitch. In: Morrow DA, ed. Current therapy in theriogenology 2. Philadelphia: WB Saunders, 1986;505-506.

Author Joni L. Freshman
Consulting Editor Sara K. Lyle

BASICS

OVERVIEW
• Form of cardiac dysfunction associated with an abnormal number of moderator bands spanning the ventricular cavity, interventricular septum, papillary muscles, or ventricular free walls • Can cause systolic and diastolic dysfunction

SIGNALMENT
• Seen primarily in cats • All ages affected

SIGNS

Historical Findings
• Lethargy • Tachypnea/dyspnea • Anorexia • Weight Loss • Hind limb paresis/paralysis due to thromboembolic disease

Physical Examination Findings
• Gallop rhythm • Systolic murmur • Arrhythmias • Hypothermia • Left or right-sided congestive heart failure (CHF)

CAUSES AND RISK FACTORS
• Congenital anomaly • Secondary to acquired myocardial disease

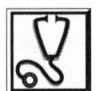

DIAGNOSIS

DIFFERENTIAL DIAGNOSIS
• Restrictive cardiomyopathy • Hypertrophic cardiomyopathy • Dilated cardiomyopathy • Hypertension • Other congenital defects

CBC/BIOCHEMISTRY/URINALYSIS
Azotemia and hypokalemia may affect treatment and prognosis.

OTHER LABORATORY TESTS
Plasma taurine concentration useful in diagnosing taurine-responsive dilated cardiomyopathy

IMAGING

Thoracic Radiography
Radiographs may reveal one or more of the following:
•Generalized cardiomegaly • Atrial enlargement • Pulmonary edema • Pleural effusion • Ascites

Echocardiography
Two-dimensional echocardiography may confirm the presence of excessive moderator bands.

OTHER DIAGNOSTIC PROCEDURES
• ECG to detect arrhythmias • Blood pressure determination

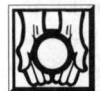

TREATMENT
• Treat as inpatient if animal has CHF.
• Minimize stress during initial treatment.
• Treatment strategy may vary and should be based on underlying pathophysiolgic process
• Alert owner to possibility of animal developing thromboembolic disease.
• Sudden death is a possibility.

MEDICATIONS

DRUGS AND FLUIDS

Congestive Heart Failure
• Furosemide—1 mg/kg IV initially, then switch to 1 mg/kg SC or PO q8h-q12h
• 2% nitroglycerin ointment—apply 1/8-1/4 inch topically to hairless area q4h-q6h until congestive signs resolve (e.g., pulmonary edema).
• Manually remove pleural fluid.
• Administer oxygen

Long-Term Management (in addition to diuretic administration)
• Digoxin to increase myocardial contractility or treat supraventricular tachyarrhythmias—1/4 of a 0.125-mg tablet per cat PO q48h-q72h

• Diltiazem to improve myocardial relaxation or treat supraventricular tachyarrhythmias—1-2.5 mg/kg PO q8h
• Enalapril for balanced vasodilation—0.5 mg/kg PO q24h-q48h
• Treat thromboembolic disease if present.

CONTRAINDICATIONS/POSSIBLE INTERACTIONS
• Concurrent azotemia warrants judicious use of diuretics; azotemia is a relative contraindication for the use of enalapril and requires careful monitoring.
• Hypokalemia may predispose animal to digoxin toxicity.

FOLLOW-UP
• Monitor radiographs for resolution of congestive state. • Monitor serial ECG for arrhythmias. • Monitor serum biochemical analysis for azotemia and electrolyte imbalances.

MISCELLANEOUS

SEE ALSO
• Dilated Cardiomyopathy, Cats • Hypertension, Systemic • Hypertrophic Cardiomyopathy, cats • Restrictive Cardiomyopathy, Cats

ABBREVIATIONS
CHF = congestive heart failure
ECG = electrocardiogram

Reference
Fox RP. Canine and feline cardiology. New York: Churchill Livingstone Inc., 1988.
Author Michael B. Lesser
Consulting Editors Larry P. Tilley and Francis W.K. Smith, Jr.

MUCOPOLYSACCHARIDOSIS

 **BASICS**

OVERVIEW
• The mucopolysaccharidoses (MPS) are a group of heritable lysosomal storage disorders caused by deficiency of lysosomal enzymes needed for the stepwise degradation of glycosaminoglycans (mucopolysaccharides). Undegraded glycosaminoglycans are stored in lysosomes, causing progressive tissue and organ dysfunction. Features of the different types of MPS depend on the specific lysosomal enzyme deficiency, type of undegraded glycosaminoglycans stored, and the tissues in which storage occurs.
• In reports in dogs and cats, the enzyme deficiencies and types of undegraded glycosaminoglycans stored are as follows: MPS I, alpha-L-iduronidase deficiency, dermatan and heparan sulfate stored; MPS VI, arylsulfatase B deficiency, dermatan sulfate stored; MPS VII, beta-glucuronidase deficiency, dermatan and chrondroitin sulfate stored.

SIGNALMENT
• MPS I and VI have been reported in cats (domestic shorthair and Siamese, respectively).
• MPS I, VI, and VII have been reported in dogs (Plott hound, miniature pinscher, and mixed breed, respectively). Both sexes are affected equally because inheritance is autosomal recessive.

SIGNS
• Common features include dwarfism (except cats with MPS I); severe bone disease (dysostosis multiplex); degenerative joint disease, including hip subluxation, facial dysmorphia, hepatomegaly (except cats with MPS VI); corneal clouding, large tongue (MPS dogs); thickening of heart valves, excess urinary excretion of undegraded glycosaminoglycans; and metachromatic granules (Alder-Reilly bodies) in blood leukocytes. • Disease is progressive, with clinical signs apparent at age 2-4 months. Affected animals may live several years, but locomotor difficulty is progressive. Corneal clouding, caused by fine granular opacities in the corneal stroma, is first apparent at approximately 8 weeks of age. • Facial dysmorphia is more evident in Siamese cats, which normally have an elongated face.
• Skeletal abnormalities are more severe in cats with MPS VI than those with MPS I, and some MPS VI cats develop posterior paresis as a result of spinal cord compression. Manipulation of the head or neck is usually painful. • CNS disease is not clinically apparent in dogs and cats with any of the types of MPS reported, although microscopic evidence of neuronal storage has been reported.

CAUSES AND RISK FACTORS
• Autosomal recessive transmission, with the exception of MPS II, which is X-linked recessive, has not been reported in dogs or cats.
• Inbreeding increases the risk if the defective gene is in the family.

 DIAGNOSIS

DIFFERENTIAL DIAGNOSIS
• Metachromatic granules within neutrophils and lymphocytes suggest MPS but can be observed in other lysosomal storage diseases in dogs and cats such as GM_2 gangliosidosis, which, unlike MPS, is characterized by progressive neurologic disease and early death. Similar granules are also observed in the neutrophils of some Birman cats. Lymphocytes are normal in Birman cats, and there are no clinical abnormalities. Very rarely, toxic granulation of neutrophils can have a similar appearance. • Corneal clouding is characteristic of numerous other lysosomal storage diseases, including acid lipase deficiency, GM and GM_2 gangliosidosis, and mannosidosis; lysosomal enzyme panels can be performed to definitely diagnose the type of storage disorder. Corneal edema and corneal dystrophy can appear similar to storage-induced corneal clouding. • Although the radiographic findings in animals with MPS are characteristic, other disorders with similar findings include congenital hypothyroidism, epiphyseal dysplasia, and hypervitaminosis A.

CBC/BIOCHEMISTRY/URINALYSIS
Wright's stained blood films reveal neutrophils and monocytes that contain numerous distinctive metachromatic granules. These granules are more distinct in animals with MPS VI and VII than in those with MPS I. Granules are usually not apparent when stained with Diff-Quik. Occasional lymphocytes have vacuoles that contain metachromatic granules, particularly in MPS VII.

OTHER LABORATORY TESTS
• Wright's stained cytologic preparations of lymph nodes, liver, bone marrow, and joint fluid reveal characteristic metachromatic granules within cells. Distended lysosomes are evident in cells of many tissues evaluated by light and electron microscopy. • Excess undegraded glycosaminoglycans in urine usually indicate MPS. • Definitive diagnosis is made by measuring lysosomal enzyme activity in serum, leukocyte pellets, or frozen liver.

IMAGING
• Radiography reveals low bone density with thin cortices. • Epiphyseal abnormalities vary from slight irregularities to large, scalloped defects in subchondral bone. • Joint changes include acetabular flattening and periarticular osteophyte formation. • Proliferative bone is present around all articular facets of vertebrae, resulting in fusion of cervical vertebrae in some cats.

OTHER DIAGNOSTIC PROCEDURES
N/A

 TREATMENT

Replacement of missing lysosomal enzymes has been attempted. Bone marrow transplantation is most successful. After engraftment, donor-derived normal leukocytes provide missing enzyme to various tissues. Although bone marrow transplant, when performed at a very early age, allows MPS-affected animals to lead near-normal lives, it is expensive, life-threatening, and a normal sibling must be the donor. It is not as helpful when performed after skeletal maturity and is somewhat impractical in animals with lysosomal storage disorders. Evaluation of bone marrow transplant in animals has been performed to determine effectiveness in children.

MEDICATIONS

DRUGS AND FLUIDS
• Animals with MPS are more susceptible to viral and bacterial respiratory infection; antibiotics may be indicated. • They are also prone to dehydration; fluids are given SQ as indicated. • With increasing age, immobility and difficulty eating progress; a diet of soft food may be helpful.

CONTRAINDICATIONS/POSSIBLE INTERACTIONS N/A

FOLLOW-UP

PREVENTION/AVOIDANCE
Avoid inbreeding if history of affected animals in family. When applicable, perform enzyme assay to diagnose heterozygotes.

EXPECTED COURSE AND PROGNOSIS
Prognosis is reasonably good in animals treated by bone marrow transplantation. Untreated animals usually die within the first 3 years of life.

MISCELLANEOUS

ABBREVIATION
MPS = mucopolysaccharidoses

Reference

Gasper PW, Thrall MA, Wenger DW, et al. Correction of feline arylsulphatase B deficiency (mucopolysaccharidosis VI) by bone marrow transplantation. Nature 1984;312:467-469.

Author Mary Anna Thrall

Consulting Editor Alan H. Rebar

MULTIPLE MYELOMA

BASICS

DEFINITION
• Rare malignant neoplasm of hematopoietic tissue derived from a monoclonal population of plasma cells in bone marrow • Two of four defining features must be present for diagnosis—monoclonal gammopathy, bone marrow invasion by plasma cells, Bence Jones proteinuria, and lytic bone lesions.

Pathophysiology
• Proliferation of a single clone of plasma cells that produces immunoglobulins (IgA or IgG) or subunits (heavy or light chains) • Polymerized IgA or IgG may increase serum viscosity. • Bleeding in some patients caused by effect of protein on platelet function and coagulation factors • Nephrotoxicity secondary to protein deposition as amyloid or to direct effect on renal tubules

Systems Affected
• Musculoskeletal—multiple areas of active bone marrow in the skelton, including vertebral column (especially lumbar), pelvis, skull, and, occasionally, appendicular bones • Neoplastic plasma cells may be present in soft tissue extraskeletal sites (e.g., liver, spleen, lymph nodes, kidney, and gastrointestinal tract). • Nervous, cardiovascular and respiratory changes secondary to hyperviscosity

Genetics N/A

Incidence/Prevelance
• Dog—reported prevalence < 1% of all malignant tumors and < 8% of hematopoietic malignant tumors • Cat—reported prevalence < 1% of hematopoietic tumors

Geographic Distribution N/A

SIGNALMENT

Species Dogs and cats

Breed Predilections N/A

Mean Age and Range
Primarily middle-aged or old dogs and cats (6-13 years)

Predominant Sex N/A

SIGNS

General Comments
Attributed to area(s) of bony infiltrate, effects of proteins produced (e.g., hyperviscosity and nephrotoxicity), or organ(s) infiltrated

Historical Findings
• Depend on location and extent of disease • Include lameness, pain, urinary incontinance, uni- or bilateral, epistaxis, blindness, dementia, malaise, dyspnea, and polyuria and polydipsia

Physical Examination Findings
Dogs
• Bleeding (nose or mucous membranes) • Blindness, retinal hemmorhage, or dialated retinal vessels • Lameness, bone pain, and

weakness in patients with lytic bone lesions • Dementia, malaise, and coma (rare) • Polyuria and polydipsia in patients with hypercalcemia or renal dysfunction • Pale mucous membranes, fever, lethargy, and hepato(spleno)megaly
Cats
Anorexia, weight loss, malaise, PU/PD, chronic infection, and fever

CAUSES Unknown
RISK FACTORS N/A

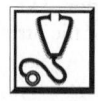

DIAGNOSIS

DIFFERENTIAL DIAGNOSIS
• Infectious disease—bacterial, fungal, or parasitic (e.g., ehrlichiosis) • Neoplastic disease—metastatic (e.g., carcinoma, sarcoma, mast cell tumor, lymphoma, and lymphoid leukemia) • Immune-mediated—benign hypergammaglobinemia, plasmacytic gastroenterocolitis

CBC/BIOCHEMISTRY/URINALYSIS
• Hemogram may indicate anemia, neutropenia (rarely leucopenia), thrombocytopenia, eosinophilia and, very rarely, plasma cell leukemia. • High RBC Rouleux formation, high serum viscosity, or high serum total protein with hypoalbuminemia and hyperglobulinemia • Hypercalcemia and high BUN, creatinine, ALP, or ALT • Proteinuria, isosthenuria, cylindruria, pyuria, hematuria, and bacteuria

OTHER LABORATORY TESTS
• Serum protein electrophoresis to identify monoclonal gammopathy (i.e., protein spike) • Serum immunoelectrophoresis • Serum immunoglobulin quantification • Urine protein electrophoresis to detect Bence Jones proteins (30-40% of dogs) • Coagulation profile • Serum viscosity

IMAGING

Radiography
• Dogs—radiographs of axial and appendicular skeleton show multifocal, lytic ("punched-out") lesions (50% of dogs) • Cats—boney changes rare • Extraskeletal sites may be identified by organomegaly.

Ultrasonography
Detects changes in echotexture of visceral organs (i.e., infiltration) in some patients

OTHER DIAGNOSTIC PROCEDURES
Cytologic examination of bone marrow and skeletal and extraskeletal lesions to detect whether > 20-25% of normal cell population are plasma cells

GROSS AND HISTOPATHOLOGIC FINDINGS

Gross Findings
Red-gray to greenish in color

Histopathologic Findings
Sheets or discrete round cells with eosinophillic cytoplasm, eccentric nuclei, perinuclear clear zone, and "cartwheel" appearance of nuclear chromatin. Neoplastic cells may grow between osseous trabeculae or cause erosion and lysis of boney trabeculae and cortex.

TREATMENT

INPATIENT VERSUS OUTPATIENT
• If patient has azotemia, hypercalcemia, or clinically important bacterial infection, treat as inpatient • Phlebotomy and replacement with an equal volume of isotonic fluids IV if patient has signs of hyperviscosity

ACTIVITY
• Treat patients with multiple myeloma as immunologic cripples.
• Care should be taken to prevent exposure to infection.

DIET N/A

CLIENT EDUCATION
• Chemotherapy is palliative, but long remissions are possible.
• Relapse will occur.
• Side effects depend on drugs used.

SURGICAL CONSIDERATIONS
Areas nonresponsive to chemotherapy or solitary lesions can be removed surgically.

MEDICATIONS

DRUGS AND FLUIDS

Dogs
• Melphalan—0.1 mg/kg PO q24h for 10 days, then 0.05 mg/kg PO q24h continuously • Prednisone—0.5 mg/kg PO q24h for 10 days, then 0.5 mg/kg on alternate days for 60 days, then stop • Cyclophosphamide can be used in addition to or in place of melphalan—200-300 mg/m^2 IV once weekly or 50 mg/m^2 PO q24h for 4 days/week

Cats
• Melphalan—0.5mg q24h for 10 days, then 0.5 mg PO q48h • Prednisone—2.5 mg PO q24h • Treat hypercalcemia and renal failure appropriately. • Treat bacterial infection aggressively with appropriate antibiotics.

CONTRAINDICATIONS N/A
PRECAUTIONS
• Melphalan is very bone marrow suppressive, especially to platelets. Patients with thrombocytopenia may benefit from a substitution of cyclophosphamide for melphalan. • Since these patients may have low numbers of neutrophils or nonfunctional lymphocytes,

care should be taken to minimize exposure to infectious agents (i.e., viral, bacterial, fungal, etc). Aseptic or very clean technique is recommended when performing any invasive techniques, even drawing blood.
• Chemotherapy can be toxic. Seek advice before initiating treatment if you are unfamiliar with cytotoxic drugs.

POSSIBLE INTERACTIONS N/A

ALTERNATE DRUGS

A more agressive combination chemotherapy protocol for dogs includes the following:
• Cyclophosphamide200 mg/m² IV q14days
• Vincristine—0.7 mg/m² IV q14 days
• Melphalan—0.10 mg/kg q24h PO for 10 days, then 0.05 mg/kg PO q24h
• Prednisone—0.5 mg/kg PO q24h

FOLLOW-UP

PATIENT MONITORING

• CBC and platelet counts weekly for at least 4 weeks to assess the bone marrow response
• Repeat tests with abnormal results.

PREVENTION/AVOIDANCE N/A

POSSIBLE COMPLICATIONS

• Bleeding, secondary infection, and pathologic fractures • Even with treatment, it may be several months until clinical signs resolve.
• Chemotherapy may cause leukopenia or thrombocytopenia, anorexia, alopecia, hemmorhagic cystitis, or pancreatitis.

EXPECTED COURSE AND PROGNOSIS

In patients that respond to treatment:
• Dogs—survival time, 6-12 months • Cats—survival time, 4-12 months • Continued care must be taken to protect the patient from secondary infections.

MISCELLANEOUS

ASSOCIATED CONDITIONS N/A

AGE RELATED FACTORS N/A

ZOONOTIC POTENTIAL N/A

PREGNANCY

Chemotherapy contraindicated in pregnant animals

SYNONYMS

Plasma cell myeloma, plasmacytoma, myelocytoma, myelosarcoma, plasma cell leukemia, erythrocytoma, and lymphocytoma

SEE ALSO

• Hypercalcemia • Renal Failure

ABBREVIATIONS

ALP = alkaline phosphatase
ALT = alanine transferase
BUN = blood urea nitrogen
PU = polyuria
PD = polydipsia

References

MacEwan EG, Young KM. Hematopoietic tumors: plasma cell neoplasms. In: Withrow SJ, MacEwan EG, eds. Clinical veterinary oncology. Philadelphia: JB Lippincott, 1989:402-411.

Theilen GH, Madewell BR. Tumors of the skeleton. In: Theilen GH, Madewell BR, eds. Veterinary cancer medicine. Philadelphia: Lea & Febiger, 1987.

Thompson JP. Immunologic diseases. In: Ettinger SJ, ed. Textbook of veterinary internal medicine. 3rd ed. Philadelphia: WB Saunders, 1989:2002-2031.

Couto CG. Oncology. In: Sherding RG, ed. The cat diseases and clinical management. New York: Churchill Livingstone, 1989:589-647.

Hammer AS, Couto GC. Complicatons of multiple myeloma. J Am Anim Hosp Assoc 1994;30:9-14.

Author Mary Ann Vonderhaar
Consulting Editor Wallace B. Morrison

MUSHROOM POISONING

 BASICS

OVERVIEW

Toxic mushrooms are classified into four categories on the basis of clinical signs and their time of onset, and into seven categories on the basis of the toxin they contain. Amanita sp. is the most important group. Systems affected include hepatobiliary (hepatic necrosis), renal/urologic (renal tubular necrosis), and nervous (autonomic and central).

• Category A mushrooms—the most toxic and the cause of cellular destruction, most often of liver and kidneys. Group I toxins (ie, cyclopeptides) are found in Amanita sp. and Galerina sp. Group II toxins (ie, monomethylhydrazine) are found in Gyromitra sp.; onset of signs is > 6 hours after ingestion.

• Category B mushrooms—affect the autonomic nervous system and includes Coprinus sp. (ie, coprine poisoning, group III toxin) and Clitocybe and Inocybe (ie, muscarinic effects, group IV toxin). • Category C mushrooms—affect the CNS causing delirium; includes group V toxins (ie, ibotenic acid-muscimol, Amanita sp.) and group VI toxins (Psilocybe and Panceobus sp.), which are hallucinogenic • Category D mushrooms—various genera containing group VII toxins which induce gastrointestinal irritation 30 minutes to 3 hours after ingestion. • Onset of signs after ingestion of category B, C, or D mushrooms is 20 minutes to 3 hours.

SIGNALMENT

Primarily in dogs; mostly puppies

SIGNS

General Comments

• The clinical course depends on the type of mushroom. • Toxicity of mushroom species varies, depending on the location of growth.

Physical Examination Findings

General signs

• Vomiting • Diarrhea • Abdominal pain
• Lethargy • Icterus • Ataxia • Seizures
• Coma

Signs caused by Group IV toxins (muscarinic effects)

• Ptyalism (excess salivation) • Lacrimation
• Diarrhea

CAUSES AND RISK FACTORS

Exposure to and ingestion of toxic mushroom

 DIAGNOSIS

DIFFERENTIAL DIAGNOSIS

• Diagnosis in most animals relies on owner observation. • Seasonal occurrence; primarily summer and fall

CBC/BIOCHEMISTRY/URINALYSIS

• High ALT, AST, and total bilirubin and high BUN and creatinine, which may be delayed for 24-48 hours after ingestion • Hypoglycemia • Hypokalemia

OTHER LABORATORY TESTS

Identification of mushrooms or spores in vomitus or stomach contents by an experienced mycologist. Refrigerate and submit mushroom.

IMAGING N/A

OTHER DIAGNOSTIC PROCEDURES
N/A

GROSS AND HISTOPATHOLOGIC FINDINGS

Hepatocellular and renal tubular necrosis

 TREATMENT

• NPO if vomiting • Caution owner that temporary improvement in gastrointestinal signs in patients with group I toxicity is often followed by delayed onset of hepatic and renal failure.

MEDICATIONS

DRUGS AND FLUIDS

• Induce emesis (Ipecac syrup 1-2 ml/kg up to 15 ml or apomorphine 0.04 mg/kg IV) • Activated charcoal (1-5 g/kg q3h-q6h for 24-36 h; mix charcoal in water as follows: 1 gram charcoal/5 - 10 ml water) • Parenteral fluids to maintain hydration and diuresis • Furosemide (5 mg/kg IV q6h-q8h) if oliguric or anuric renal failure develops in patients with normal hydration status • Atropine (0.2 - 0.4 mg/kg 1/2 dose IV, 1/2 dose IM) to block muscarinic signs (group IV toxins only) • Benzylpenicillin (penicillin G 20,000 U/kg IM q12h-q24h) • Diazepam for seizures (0.5-1.5 mg/kg IV or IM)

CONTRAINDICATIONS/POSSIBLE INTERACTIONS

Atropine contraindicated except in animals with group IV toxins

FOLLOW-UP

• Monitor hepatic and renal function for at least 48 hours. • Good prognosis except in animals that have ingested category A group 1 toxins (cyclopeptides). Temporary improvement in gastrointestinal signs in patients with group I toxicity is often followed by delayed onset of hepatic and renal failure.

MISCELLANEOUS

SEE ALSO Poisoning (Intoxication)

ABBREVIATIONS

ALP = alkaline phosphatase
ALT = alanine transaminase
AST = apartate transaminase
BUN = blood urea nitrogen
CNS = central nervous system
NPO = nothing per os

Reference

Lincoft G, Mitchel DH. Toxic and hallucinogenic mushroom poisoning. New York: Van Nostrano Reinhold, 1977.

Author Ronald B. Wilson
Consulting Editor Gary Osweiller

MYASTHENIA GRAVIS

BASICS

DEFINITION
Myasthenia gravis is a disorder of neuromuscular transmission characterized by muscular weakness and excessive fatigability.

Pathophysiology
Transmission failure at the neuromuscular junction (NMJ) results from structural or functional abnormalities of the nicotinic acetylcholine receptors (AChR) in the congenital form of myasthenia gravis and from autoantibody-mediated destruction of AChRs and postsynaptic membranes in the acquired form of myasthenia gravis.

Systems Affected
• Neuromuscular—as a result of abnormalities or destruction of AChR • Respiratory—if aspiration pneumonia occurs secondary to megaesophagus

Genetics
• Congenital familial forms of myasthenia gravis–Jack Russell terriers, springer spaniels, and smooth fox terriers with an autosomal-recessive mode of inheritance • Acquired myasthenia gravis, like other autoimmune diseases, requires the appropriate genetic background for the disease to occur. Development of the disease is multifactorial, involving environmental, infectious, and hormonal influences.

Incidence/Prevalence
• Congenital myasthenia gravis is rare.
• Acquired myasthenia gravis is not uncommon in the dog, rare in the cat

Geographic Distribution Worldwide

SIGNALMENT

Species Dogs and cats

Breed Predilections
• Congenital myasthenia gravis-Jack Russell terriers, springer spaniels, and smooth fox terriers • Acquired myasthenia gravis-several breeds, including golden retrievers, German shepherds, Labrador retrievers, dachshunds, Scottish terriers

Mean Age and Range
• Congenital myasthenia gravis—6-8 weeks of age • Acquired myasthenia gravis—bimodal age of onset with a younger group of dogs at 1-4 years of age and an older group at 9-13 years of age

Predominant Sex
• Congenital myasthenia gravis-no sex predilection • Acquired myasthenia gravis-there may be a slight predilection for females in the young age group with no difference in the older age group

SIGNS

General Comments
• Acquired myasthenia gravis may have several clinical presentations ranging from focal in-

volvement of the esophageal, pharyngeal, and extraocular muscles to acute generalized collapse. • Myasthenia should be on the differential diagnosis of any dog with acquired megaesophagus or lower motor neuron weakness.

Historical Findings
• Owners will commonly report vomiting. It is important to differentiate whether this is vomiting or regurgitation. • Voice change
• Exercise related weakness • Acute collapse

Physical Examination Findings
• The dog or cat may look normal at rest.
• Excessive drooling, regurgitation, and repeated attempts at swallowing. Muscle atrophy usually not present. • Dyspnea, if aspiration pneumonia is present. • Fatigue or "cramping" with mild exercise • Upon careful neurological examination, subtle findings including a diminished or absent palpebral reflex and a poor or absent gag reflex may be found. The palpebral reflex may be fatigable. Spinal reflexes are usually normal but fatigable. Rarely spinal reflexes are absent and the dog unable to support its weight.

CAUSES
• Congenital • Immune-mediated • Paraneoplastic

RISK FACTORS
• Appropriate genetic background • Neoplasia, in particular thymoma • Methimazole treatment in cats may result in reversible myasthenia

DIAGNOSIS

DIFFERENTIAL DIAGNOSIS
• Other disorders of neuromuscular transmission, including tick paralysis, botulism, and cholinesterase toxicity • Acute or chronic polyneuropathies • Polymyopathies, including polymyositis • Differentiation of myasthenia from other neuromuscular disorders is dependent upon a careful history, a thorough physical and neurologic examination, and specialized laboratory testing.

CBC/BIOCHEMISTRY/URINALYSIS
• No abnormalities are found on standard laboratory testing and urinalysis. • Serum CK normal with myasthenia • Serum CK may be elevated if polymyositis is present associated with concurrent thymoma

OTHER LABORATORY TESTS
• Serum acetylcholine receptor antibody titer is diagnostic for acquired myasthenia gravis.
• Evaluation of thyroid and adrenal function; abnormalities may occur in association with acquired myasthenia gravis

IMAGING
Thoracic radiographs, megaesophagus, and cranial mediastinal mass

OTHER DIAGNOSTIC PROCEDURES
• Ultrasound guided biopsy of a cranial mediastinal mass may support a diagnosis of thy-

moma. • Dramatic increase in muscle strength following the intravenous administration of edrophonium chloride (0.1 mg/kg IV) may have false negatives and false positives. If the patient has diminished or absent palpebral reflex present, administration of edrophonium chloride may result in return of the reflex. • With increased availability of acetylcholine receptor antibody testing, the necessity of performing electrophysiologic evaluation for the diagnosis of myasthenia is questionable. Many animals with acquired myasthenia are poor anesthetic risks. • An electrocardiogram should be performed if bradycardia is present. Third-degree heart block has been recently documented in some patients with acquired myasthenia.

GROSS AND HISTOPATHOLOGIC FINDINGS
Biopsy of a cranial mediastinal mass may reveal thymoma or thymic hyperplasia

TREATMENT

INPATIENT VERSUS OUTPATIENT
• Initial management as an inpatient until adequate dosages of anticholinesterase drugs are achieved
• A patient with aspiration pneumonia may require intensive care.
• A gastrostomy tube may be required if the animal is unable to eat or drink without regurgitation.

ACTIVITY
The severity of the muscle weakness and extent of aspiration pneumonia will itself limit the animal's activity.

DIET
• Elevation of food and water
• Different consistencies of food may be tried, including gruel, hard food or soft food to evaluate what is best tolerated.

CLIENT EDUCATION
• It is important to advise the owner that although myasthenia gravis is a treatable disorder, it will require, in most patients, months of special feeding and medication.
• A dedicated owner is important to a favorable outcome with acquired myasthenia.

SURGICAL CONSIDERATIONS
• Cranial mediastinal mass (thymoma)
• Before attempting surgical removal, the animal should be stabilized on anticholinesterase drugs and aspiration pneumonia treated.
• Weakness may not be present initially
• Any animal with a suspected thymoma should be tested for acquired myasthenia gravis before surgery.

MEDICATIONS

DRUGS AND FLUIDS
• Anticholinesterase drugs prolong the action of acetylcholine at the neuromuscular junc-

tion. Pyridostigmine bromide syrup (Mestinon syrup, Roche Laboratories) 1-3 mg/kg q8h-q12h PO diluted half and half in water.

• If there is a poor response to pyridostigmine or if there is no response to the edrophonium chloride challenge, corticosteroids at 0.5 mg/kg daily should be initiated.

• Prednisone at immunosuppressive dosages may initially worsen weakness.

CONTRAINDICATIONS

Avoid drugs that may reduce the safety margin of neuromuscular transmission-aminoglycoside antibiotics, antiarrhythmic agents, phenothiazines, anesthetics, narcotics, muscle relaxants, and magnesium

PRECAUTIONS

• Avoid large volumes of barium to evaluate megaesophagus.

• If a large, air filled esophagus is seen on survey radiographs, a barium study is not indicated

POSSIBLE INTERACTIONS N/A

ALTERNATE DRUGS N/A

FOLLOW-UP

PATIENT MONITORING

• Return of muscle strength should be evident. • Thoracic radiographs should be evaluated every 4-6 weeks for resolution of megaesophagus. • AChR antibody titers should be evaluated every 6-8 weeks because they return to the normal range with clinical remission of disease.

PREVENTION/AVOIDANCE N/A

POSSIBLE COMPLICATIONS

• Aspiration pneumonia • Respiratory arrest

EXPECTED COURSE AND PROGNOSIS

• In the absence of a severe aspiration pneumonia or pharyngeal weakness, the prognosis for complete recovery is good. Time frame for resolution on average is 4-6 months. • If thymoma is present, prognosis is guarded unless complete surgical removal and control of myasthenic signs are achieved.

MISCELLANEOUS

ASSOCIATED CONDITIONS

• Other autoimmune disorders including thyroiditis, skin disorders, and hypoadrenocorticism • Disorders of the thymus, including thymoma and thymic hyperplasia • Other neoplasias

AGE RELATED FACTORS

Bimodal age of onset with a younger group showing clinical signs at 1-4 years of age and an older group at 9-13 years of age

ZOONOTIC POTENTIAL N/A

PREGNANCY

• In human myasthenia gravis, there may be some resolution of weakness during pregnancy with worsening noted after delivery. Myasthenia has been documented in dogs after whelping. • In some newborn infants of myasthenia gravis mothers there is a temporary type of myasthenia gravis weakness that lasts from several days to weeks as a result of the transfer of autoantibodies from the mother to the fetus before the baby is born.

SYNONYMS N/A

SEE ALSO

• Autoimmune Diseases • Megaesophagus, Acquired

ABBREVIATIONS

Ach = acetylcholine
AChR = acetylcholine receptor

References

Shelton GD. Canine myasthenia gravis. In: Kirk RW, Bonagura JD, eds. Current veterinary therapy XI. Philadelphia: WB Saunders, 1992:1039-1040.

Shelton GD. Megaesophagus secondary to myasthenia gravis. In: Kirk RW, Bonagura JD, eds. Current veterinary therapy XI. Philadelphia: WB Saunders, 1992:580-583.

Drachman DB. Myasthenia gravis. N Engl J Med 1994;330:1797-1810.

Author G. Diane Shelton
Consulting Editor Peter D. Schwarz

MYCOBACTERIAL INFECTIONS

BASICS

OVERVIEW

• Mycobacteria are gram-positive, non-branching, acid-fast bacteria that can cause sporadic disease in humans and animals.
• Mycobacterium spp. cause three main syndromes in dogs and cats: systemic mycobacteriosis (tuberculosis [TB]) feline leprosy (FL), and atypical mycobacteriosis (AM) • Systemic mycobacteriosis is caused by M. Bovis, M. avium-intracellular complex, M. tuberculosis, and M. microti. In dogs, infections with M. tuberculosis are prevalent; M. bovis is the most common isolate in cats with systemic mycobacteriosis. Clinical signs are the result of internal tubercular granuloma formation.
• Feline leprosy is caused by M. lerpaemurium, the same organism that causes leprosy in humans. Rodent bites may play a role in disease transmission. Disease appears more commonly in seaport communities and coastal areas. Patients typically present with localized cutaneous nodules. • Atypical mycobacteriosis is caused by several species of saprophytic, nontuberculous, nonlepromatous mycobacterium. These organisms are ubiquitous in nature and infections are thought to be acquired from the environment and not from other animals. Infections present as spreading, primarily subcutaneous inflammation.

SIGNALMENT

• Basset hounds and Siamese cats appear to be overrepresented in reports of M. avium-intracellulare complex infections. Incidence of M. tuberculosis infections in animals would be expected to parallel that seen in human populations: higher incidence in densely populated or economically depressed regions, particularly on the Atlantic coast and southeastern regions of North America. Animal infections generally are rare. No sex or age predilections reported. • Feline leprosy typically is seen in young to middle-aged cats that are allowed to roam and live in a cool, moist, coastal climate. No breed predilection reported. Newborn kittens are more susceptible than older cats. Infections generally are rare except in those areas noted above. • Atypical mycobacteriosis is more prevalent in cats than dogs. No age, sex, or breed predilection noted.

SIGNS

Historical Findings

• Animals with systemic tuberculosis may have a history of living on a farm or long-term exposure to cattle or poultry. The pet owners may have history of active infection with the same causative agent or positive tuberculin tests. • Cats with feline leprosy may come from seaport/coastal regions or have lived in such an area previously. History of unknown bite trauma may be found.

• Patients with atypical mycobacteriosis may have history of cat bites/scratches, abrasions, automobile accidents, surgical incisions, or nonsterile injections before the development of lesions.

Physical Examination Findings

Systemic Mycobacteriosis
Usually a subclinical disease; however, of the three main syndromes caused by mycobacterial infection, tuberculosis is the disease most likely to present with signs of systemic illness. There is some variation in the predominant signs in dogs when compared to cats. • Dogs more commonly develop respiratory signs secondary to bronchopneumonia, pulmonary nodule formation, and hilar lymphadenopathy. Fever, weight loss, retching, ptyalism, and tonsillar enlargement all may be seen if oropharyngeal lesions develop. • Cats develop intestinal lesions with greater frequency than do dogs. Signs exhibited may include weight loss, anemia, vomiting, and diarrhea. Abdominal palpation may reveal enlarged mesenteric lymph nodes or effusion. • When disseminated disease develops, signs reflect the site of granuloma formation. These signs may include pleural effusion, pericardial effusion, generalized lymphadenopathy, weight loss, fever, sudden death, visceral masses, dermal nodules, nonhealing draining ulcers, uveitis, lameness, CNS signs, and spontaneous fractures.
Feline Leprosy
Single or multiple cutaneous nodules may be noted, most often involving the head and/or extremities. Lesions may be ulcerated or abscessed. Nodules are usually nonpainful and freely moveable. Cats seldom appear systemically ill.
Atypical Mycobacteriosis
Lesions may develop more slowly than those cats with feline leprosy. Chronic nonhealing wounds located on the thorax, abdomen, or in the lumbar or groin regions are standard. Ulcers and draining fistulae are present secondary to subcutaneous abscessation. Fever may occur but other signs of chronic infection such as anorexia or weight loss are usually absent.

CAUSES AND RISK FACTORS

• Exposure to infected carrier animals/humans or crowded conditions (TB)
• Depressed cell-mediated immunity (TB, probably FL and AM as well) • Open wounds (AM) • Rodent bites (FL, theoretical cause)
• FIV positive status (FL, theoretical risk)
• Drinking unpasteurized milk or eating raw offal

DIAGNOSIS

DIFFERENTIAL DIAGNOSIS

Systemic Mycobacteriosis

Must be differentiated from other mycobacterial infections, neoplasia, deep mycotic infections, foreign body abscesses, and other infectious or inflammatory causes of diffuse

granuloma formation. Differentiation is based on biopsy, cytology, bacterial culture, laboratory animal inoculation, and bacilli Calmette-Guerin test (BCG test; dogs only).

Feline Leprosy

Must be differentiated from other mycobacterial infections, deep mycotic infections, neoplasia, eosinophilic granuloma complex, foreign body dermatitis, mycetomas, dermatophyte pseudomycetomas, and chronic bacterial infections. Differentiate based on compatible history, biopsy, cytology, bacterial culture, and laboratory animal inoculation.

Atypical Mycobacteriosis

Must be differentiated from systemic mycobacteriosis, feline leprosy (cats only), foreign body dermatitis, deep mycotic infections, mycetomas, dermatophyte pseudomycetomas, chronic bacterial infections, generalized demodicosis (dogs mostly), sterile nodular panniculitis, pansteatitis, eosinophilic granuloma complex, and neoplasia. Differentiate based on biopsy and bacterial culture results. Lack of tissue grains helps differentiate from nocardiosis.

CBC/BIOCHEMISTRY/URINALYSIS

• Nonspecific and variable findings. Changes will reflect organ involvement in diffuse or disseminated disease. • Moderate leukocytosis, anemia, hyperglobulinemia, and normal-to-reduced albumin levels may be noted in systemic mycobacteriosis.

OTHER LABORATORY TESTS

Serologic testing, including hemagglutination and complement fixation tests, are unreliable but have been used to detect infected dogs and cats when skin testing results were considered inconclusive. (This applies to TB only.)

IMAGING

Thoracic Radiography (TB Only)

Visible masses may be apparent on chest radiographs associated with any of the organ systems present. Any of the following may be seen:
• Tracheobroncial lymphadenopathy • Interstitial lung infiltration • Diffuse radiopaque densities in lung lobes • Calcified pulmonary lesions • Diffuse miliary densities • Pleural effusion • Globoid enlargement of cardiac silhouette as a result of pericardial effusion

Abdominal Radiography (TB Only)

Enlargement of abdominal viscera may be noted as generalized organomegaly or solitary masses. Abdominal effusion or calcified mesenteric lymph nodes may be seen.

Skeletal Radiography (TB Only)

Small, circumscribed, lucent bony lesions may be noted. Vertebral osteomyelitis or changes consistent with hypertrophic osteopathy may be seen.

OTHER DIAGNOSTIC PROCEDURES

• Ocular exam may reveal changes consistent with granulomatous urveitis (TB only).

• CSF tap and neurodiagnostics may be abnormal depending on the degree of CNS involvement (TB only). • Cytology of direct smears of exudates or granuloma aspirates with acid-fast staining may provide diagnosis. Look for intracellular bacilli with characteristic clubbed shape and beaded appearance.
• Intradermal skin testing has been used to evaluate delayed-type hypersensitivity for TB in dogs but is generally considered unreliable and may produce false-positives. • Bacterial culture—pathogenic mycobacterium are slow-growing and isolation may take several weeks. Isolation should be attempted only if laboratory has proper biocontainment facilities. The causative agent of feline leprosy is much more difficult to grow than the other two main mycobacteria-related syndrome organisms. • Laboratory animal inoculation.

GROSS AND HISTOPATHOLOGIC FINDINGS

Systemic Mycobacteriosis

Gross lesions—generalized emaciation may be recognized. Multifocal granulomas typically are grayish-white to yellow circumscribed nodular lesions that may be noted in multiple organs. Primary lesion sites in dogs are lung and bronchial lymph nodes; ileocecal and mesenteric nodes are more commonly involved in cats.

Feline Leprosy

Gross lesions—solitary or multiple raised, painless plaquelike lesions, 1-3.5 cm in diameter in the skin and underlying subcutis. Lesions may be ulcerated but are not typically fistulated and exudative. Lesions tend to be concentrated on the head and limbs but may be anywhere.

Atypical Mycobacteriosis

Gross lesions—draining, fistulated wounds several centimeters in diameter predominantly in the inguinal area, lumbosacral region, ventral abdomen, flank and chest wall. Regional lymph nodes may be enlarged.

TREATMENT

• Because of public health risk involved in treating pets with systemic mycobacteriosis, treatment is not advised in many circumstances. Family physicians and public health officials should be notified and consulted with by the owners before making decisions regarding treatment versus humane euthanasia.

• Treatment may not be required in all cats of feline leprosy. Small lesions that appear to be in regression at time of diagnosis may warrant no further therapy in some animals.
• Dogs with atypical mycobacteriosis may achieve remission more readily than cats.
• Surgical debulking should be considered in combination with medical therapy in many cases of both feline leprosy or atypical mycobacteriosis. Surgical treatment may be more effective in dogs with atypical mycobacteriosis.
• Avoid concurrent immunosuppressive therapy.

MEDICATIONS

DRUGS AND FLUIDS

Systemic Mycobacteriosis

• If treated (see above), two or more of the following drugs are typically used. Isoniazid in combination with ethambutol (or pyrazinamide) and rifampin may be the most effective combination.
• Isoniazid 10-20-mg/kg PO q24h x 6-12 months (no more than 300 mg total per patient per day) • Rifampin 10-20 mg/kg PO q12-24h x 6-9 months (no more than 600 mg total per patient per day)
• Ethambutol 15 mg/kg PO q24h x 6-12 months • Dihydrostreptomycin 15 mg/kg IM q24h x 6-9 months
• Pyrazinamide 15-40 mg/kg PO q24h x 6-9 months
• The above drug dosages are for dogs only. Little is known regarding combination drug therapy for systemic mycobacteriosis in cats.

Feline Leprosy

• Dapsone 1 mg/kg up to 50 mg/cat PO q8-12h x 2-4 weeks. Start at 1 mg/kg PO q12h.
• Clofazimine 2-8mg/kg PO q24h x 6 weeks, then q3-4 days for 1-2 months
• Rifampin 10-20 mg/kg PO q12h x 3-4 weeks

Atypical Mycobacteriosis

• Typically, 2-6 weeks treatment
• Erythromycin 11 mg/kg PO q24h (dogs and cats) • Chloramphenicol 15-25 mg/kg PO q8h (dogs) or q12h (cats)
• Tetracycline 22 mg/kg PO q8h (dogs and cats)
• Enrofloxacin 2.5-15 mg/kg PO q12h (dogs and cats)
• Clofazimine 8-12 mg/kg PO q24h (dogs and cats)
• Amikacin 5-7 mg/kg IM, SC q12h x 2-4 weeks (dogs and cats)

CONTRAINDICATIONS/POSSIBLE INTERACTIONS

• Dapsone can be toxic in cats and produce hemolytic anemia and liver disease.
• Clofazimine can cause a pinkish-orange discoloration of the subcutaneous fat and possible weight loss. High serum alkaline phosphatase may also be seen. Capsules must be reformulated to achieve proper dose.
• Monitor patients on amikacin for signs of nephrotoxicity.
• Myelosuppression may occur with chloramphenicol.

FOLLOW-UP

Owners should be alerted to look for recurrence of lesions after surgical or medical therapies.

EXPECTED COURSE AND PROGNOSIS

Systemic Mycobacteriosis

Generally poor if multiple organ involvement or severe compromise

Feline Leprosy

Animals are generally in good health overall, and prognosis is determined largely by the spread of the lesions.

Atypical Mycobacteriosis

Prognosis is generally better in dogs than cats. Multiple surgeries and attempts at medical therapy may be required.

MISCELLANEOUS

ABBREVIATIONS

TB = tuberculosis
FL = feline leprosy
AM = atypical mycobacteriosis

Reference

Green CE. Mycobacterial infections. In: Green CE, ed. Infectious disease of the dog and cat. Philadelphia: WB Saunders, 1990:558-572.
Author Matthew S. Mellema
Consulting Editor Fred W. Scott

MYCOPLASMA

BASICS

DEFINITION
• Belongs to class Mollicutes; Latin—*mollis,* soft; *cutis,* skin • Over 80 genera, classified into three families: mycoplasmas, T-mycoplasmas (ureaplasmas), and acholeplasmas • Smallest (0.2-0.3 mm) and simplest procaryotic cells capable of self-replication • Fastidious, facultative anaerobic, gram-negative rods; reproduce by binary fission • Genome replication not necessarily synchronized with cell division, resulting in budding forms and chains of beads • Ubiquitous in nature as parasites, commensals, or saprophytes in animals, plants, and insects • Many are pathogens of humans, animals, plants, and insects • Lack a cell wall and consequently are plastic, highly pleomorphic, and sensitive to lysis by osmotic shock, detergents, alcohols, and specific antibody plus complement • Enclosed by a trilayered cell membrane built of amphipathic lipids (phospholipids, glycolipids, lipoglycans, sterols) and proteins • Most species require sterols for growth. • Differ from wall-defective or wall-less L-phase variants of bacteria, which can revert to the bacterial form

Pathophysiology
• Mycoplasmas are often part of the resident flora as commensals on mucous membranes of the upper respiratory, digestive, and genital tracts. • Consequently, the pathogenicity and role of mycoplasmas in disease are often controversial. • Mechanisms by which mycoplasma cause disease are poorly understood. • Mycoplasma species show considerable host specificity. • Some species attach to cells by specific receptors. • Small size and plastic nature enable them to adapt to the shape and contours of host cell surfaces. • Intimate contact with host cells is necessary for assimilation of vital nutrients and growth factors (e.g., nucleic acid precursors), which mycoplasmas cannot synthesize. • Products produced during growth include capsular carbohydrate, hemolysins, proteolytic enzymes, ammonia, and endonucleases. • Accumulation of mycoplasma metabolites (i.e., H_2O_2, NH_3) may contribute to cytopathic effects and tissue damage. • Cytotoxic glycoproteins and proteins have been isolated from the membranes of several species. • Intimate association with surface of host's cell and tendency of exogenous proteins to bind to mycoplasmal membrane may allow mycoplasma to evade the host's immune response • May incorporate host cell antigen onto mycoplasma membrane (capping) because not separated by a cell wall • Conversely, mycoplasmal protein antigen may become incorporated onto surface of host cell and thereby involve host cell in deleterious immunologic reactions intended against the mycoplasma • Immune re-

sponse predominately humoral; as with bacterial infections, first antibodies to appear are IgM and IgA, followed by IgG • Complement fixing antibodies (mostly IgM) are found early in infection, IgG antibodies are mycoplasmacidal and may persist for many months; IgA antibodies temporarily block adherence of mycoplasmas to host cells. • Secondary bacterial invaders common (e.g., attachment to cells of respiratory tract may result in destruction of cilia, predisposing to secondary bacterial infection) • Fibrinous exudate accompanying infections protects mycoplasma from antibody and antimicrobial drugs and contributes to chronicity.

Systems Affected
Dogs
• Respiratory—pneumonia and upper respiratory infections caused by M. cynos, and associated with M. canis, M. spumans, M. edwardii, M. feliminutum, M. gateae, and M. bovigenitalium • Renal/urologic—urinary and genital tract infections caused by M. canis and M. spumans (i.e., balanoposthitis, urethritis, prostatitis, cystitis, nephritis, vaginitis, endometritis) • Reproductive—mycoplasma and ureaplasma associated with infertility, early embryonic death, abortion, stillbirths or weak newborns, and neonatal mortality • Musculoskeletal—arthritis resulting from M. spumans • Gastrointestinal—associated with colitis
Cats
• Ophthalmic—feline conjunctivitis associated with M. felis (5-25%) • Respiratory—feline pneumonia associated with M. gateae, M. feliminutum, and M. felis; upper respiratory infections associated with M. felis • Musculoskeltal—chronic fibrinopurulent polyarthritis and tenosynovitis associated with M. gatea and unspecified mycoplasmal organisms • Renal/urologic—urinary tract infections • Reproductive—abortions and fetal deaths associated with M. gateae and ureaplasmas • Skin/exocrine—chronic cutaneous abscesses

Genetics N/A

Incidence/Prevalence
• Frequent inhabitants of mucosal membranes (e.g., M. gatea and/or M. felis found in oral cavity or urogenital tract of 70-80% of healthy cats) • Rate of isolation of mycoplasmas increases significantly in diseased versus normal dogs (e.g., lung, uterus, prepuce).

Geographic Distribution Ubiquitous

SIGNALMENT N/A

SIGNS

General Comments
Pathogenic role controversial

Historical Findings
• Polyarthritis—chronic intermittent lameness, reluctance to move, joint pain, fever, malaise • Conjunctivitis—uni- or bilateral

Physical Examination Findings
• Polyarthritis—diffuse limb edema, joint swelling, pain • Conjunctivitis—blepharospasm, chemosis, conjunctival hyperemia, epiphora, and serous or purulent ocular discharge • Mild rhinitis—sneezing

CAUSES
• Mycoplasma flora of the dog consists of M. canis, M. spumans, M. maculosum, M. edwardii, M. cynos, M. molare, M. opalescens, M. feliminutum, M. gateae, M. arginini, M. bovigenitalium, Acholeplasma laidlawii, and ureaplasmas • Mycoplasma flora of the cat consists of M. felis, M. gateae, M. feliminutum, M. arginini, M. pulmonis, M. arthritidis, M. gallisepticum, Acholeplasma laidlawi, and ureaplasmas

RISK FACTORS
• Commensals occasionally cause systemic infection in association with immunodeficiency, immunosuppression, or cancer. • Impaired resistance of the host may allow mycoplasmas to cross the mucosal barrier and disseminate. • Mycoplasma may be opportunistic as one factor in a multifactorial etiologic complex. • Various stresses predispose to infection (e.g., reproductive problems associated with overcrowded operations [kennel]). • Impaired pulmonary clearance resulting from viral infection may allow mycoplasmas to establish infection in lungs as secondary opportunistic pathogens. • Urinary tumors and urinary calculi may predispose to urinary mycoplasma infection.

DIAGNOSIS

DIFFERENTIAL DIAGNOSIS
• Canine and feline upper respiratory infection—viruses (parainfluenza virus, canine distemper, herpesvirus, feline calcivirus, reovirus), Chlamydia psittaci, bacteria (Bordetella bronchiseptica, staphylococci, streptococci, coliforms) • Canine and feline urinary tract infection—bacteria (staphylococci, streptococci, coliforms), fungus (Candida), parasites • Canine infertility, early embryonic death, abortion, stillbirths or weak newborns, and neonatal mortality—bacteria (Brucella, Salmonella, Campylobacter, E. coli, streptococcus), viruses (canine herpesvirus, canine distemper, canine adenovirus), Toxoplasma gondii, endocrinopathies (progesterone deficiency, hypothyroidism) • Canine prostatitis—bacteria (E. coli, Brucella canis), fungi (Blastomyces, Cryptococcus) • Canine and feline arthritis—immune-mediated, bacteria (staphylococci, streptococci, coliforms, anaerobes), bacterial L-forms, rickettsia (Ehrlichia), Borrelia burgdoferi, fungal (Coccidioides, Cryptococcus, Blastomyces), protozoa (Leishmania), viral (feline calicivirus) • Feline conjunctivitis—feline herpesvirus, feline cali-

civirus, feline reovirus, Chlamydia psittaci, bacteria

CBC/BIOCHEMISTRY/URINALYSIS

Polyarthritis
• Hemogram— mild anemia, neutrophilic leukocytosis • Biochemistry—hypoalbuminemia, hypoglobulinemia • Urinalysis—proteinuria resulting from immune-complex glomerulonephritis

OTHER LABORATORY TESTS

Serologic tests (complement fixation, agar gel immunodiffusion, enzyme-linked immunosorbent assay [ELISA]) to detect organism.

IMAGING

Polyarthritis—no radiographic changes

OTHER DIAGNOSTIC PROCEDURES

• Extremely pleomorphic; in smears (e.g., conjunctival scrapings) seen as coccobacilli, coccal forms, ring forms, spirals, and filaments • Stain poorly (gram-negative); preferred staining method is by Giemsa or other Romanowsky stains • Definitive diagnosis based on isolation and identification or detection of the mycoplasmas in tissues by a fluorescent antibody procedure. • Can submit cotton swabs placed in Hayflick's broth medium or commercially available swabs • Fragile organisms; therefore specimens should be refrigerated and delivered to the laboratory within 48 hours • Mycoplasma in tissues can be preserved for longer periods by freezing. • Because of limited biosynthetic abilities, require complex media for growth • Usually grown on solid media consisting of beef heart infusion, peptone, horse serum, yeast extract, inhibitors of bacterial growth (penicillin for gram-positives, thallium acetate for gram-negatives), some additives required for growth of some species • Optimum temperature for growth of species from animals is 36-37º C. • Facultative anaerobe, grown under anaerobic conditions (95% N_2 + 5% CO_2) • Form minute fried-egg shaped colonies (0.01-1.00 mm diameter) consisting of an opaque, granular central area embedded into the agar medium and a flat translucent peripheral ring on its surface • Dark-field and phase contrast microscopy used for studying morphology in liquid media • Differentiate mycoplasma species by cultural (i.e., sensitivity to digitonin), biochemical (i.e., fermentative behavior, urease formation), and antigenic characteristics. • Other tests helpful in identification include hemolysis and hemadsorption, reduction of tetrazolium chloride, liquefaction of heat-aggregated serum, and requirement for coenzymes. • Definitive species identification requires specific antiserums and monoclonal antibodies. • Polyarthritis—synovial fluid contains high numbers of nondegenerative neutrophils • Prostatic fluid— inflammatory cells with negative bacterial culture

TREATMENT

Result of absence of a cell wall readily killed by drying, sunshine, and chemical disinfection

MEDICATIONS

DRUGS AND FLUIDS

• Sensitive to antibiotics that specifically inhibit synthesis in procaryotes (ie, tetracyclines, doxycycline, chloramphenicol) • No standardized procedure for in vitro antimicrobial susceptibility tests • Topical antibiotic for conjunctivitis

CONTRAINDICATIONS

Improper use of topical steroid ointments in animals with with conjunctivitis may prolong infection and predispose to corneal ulceration.

PRECAUTIONS

Lack of cell walls allows mycoplasms to be resistant to sulfonamides and b-lactans that inhibit peptidogtycan synthesis.

POSSIBLE INTERACTIONS

See age related factors and pregnancy.

ALTERNATE DRUGS

Gentamicin, kanamycin, spectinomycin, spiramycin, tylosin, erythromycin, nitrofurans, and fluorquinolones

CONTRAINDICATIONS/POSSIBLE INTERACTIONS N/A

FOLLOW-UP

PATIENT MONITORING

Treat for an extended period of time

POSSIBLE COMPLICATIONS

See age related factors and pregnancy.

MISCELLANEOUS

ASSOCIATED CONDITIONS

M. pneumoniae infects respiratory tracts in humans worldwide, causing mycoplasma pneumonia, bronchitis, or upper respiratory infection, which is usually self-limited and rarely fatal.

AGE RELATED FACTORS

Avoid tetracyclines in puppies.

ZOONOTIC POTENTIAL

• Not generally considered zoonotic • Suppurative mycoplasmal tenosynovitis developed in veterinarian after scratch from cat being treated for colitis

PREGNANCY

Tetracycline and chloramphenicol should not be used in pregnant animals.

SYNONYMS

Pleuropneumonialike organisms (PPLO)

SEE ALSO N/A

ABBREVIATIONS N/A

References

Rosendal S. Mycoplasma infections. In: Greene CE, ed. Infectious diseases of the dog and cat. Philadelphia: WB Saunders, 1990:446-449.
Pedersen NC. Mycoplasmal infections. In: Holzworth J, ed. Diseases of the cat. Philadelphia: WB Saunders, 1987:308-311.
Author J. Paul Woods
Consulting Editor Fred W. Scott

MYELODYSPLASTIC SYNDROMES

BASICS

OVERVIEW
Myelodysplasia is the term for the "pre-leukemic" phase of a myeloproliferative disorder.

SIGNALMENT
More common in cats than dogs

SIGNS
• Pale mucous membranes • Lethargy
• Weight loss • Hepatosplenomegaly
• Peripheral lymphadenomegaly varies

CAUSES AND RISK FACTORS
• Associated with FeLV infection in cats
• Bone marrow dysplasia can be caused by ehrlichiosis and Rocky Mountain spotted fever. • Drugs such as trimethoprim and a sulfa combination, estrogen, butazolidin, and cytotoxic anticancer agents can cause myelodysplasia.

DIAGNOSIS

DIFFERENTIAL DIAGNOSIS
Myelodysplasia must be differentiated from infectious causes and drug toxicity (see previous section).

CBC/BIOCHEMISTRY/URINALYSIS
• Cytopenias • Megaloblastic anemia
• Circulating nucleated RBC • Large bizarre platelets • Immature granulocytes with ab-

normal morphologic characteristics
• Monocytosis

OTHER LABORATORY TESTS N/A

IMAGING N/A

OTHER DIAGNOSTIC PROCEDURES
Examination of bone marrow aspirate and core biopsy reveals ineffective erythropoiesis and granulopoiesis within a specimen with normal cellularity.

TREATMENT
Intensive nursing care often necessary

MEDICATIONS

DRUGS AND FLUIDS
Supportive care includes multiple blood transfusion, nutritional support, and antibiotics for secondary bacterial infection in some animals.

CONTRAINDICATIONS/POSSIBLE INTERACTIONS N/A

FOLLOW-UP
• Transfuse as necessary • Repeat CBC and cytologic examination of bone marrow aspirate or biopsy to monitor progression of the

disease • Prognosis guarded to poor • Possible complications include sepsis, hemorrhage, and profound anemia.

MISCELLANEOUS

ABBREVIATIONS
FeLV = feline leukemia virus
RBC = red blood cells

Reference
Harvey JW. Myeloproliferative disorders in dogs and cats. Vet Clin North Am Small Anim Pract 1981;11:349-381.

Author Linda S. Fineman
Consulting Editor Wallace B. Morrison

MYELOMALACIA (DIFFUSE, HEMORRHAGIC)

BASICS

OVERVIEW
• Acute, progressive, ischemic necrosis of the spinal cord following acute spinal cord trauma • Myelomalacia first appears at the site of injury and then progresses both cranially and caudally. • Death may be caused by respiratory paralysis because the intercostal and phrenic nerves are affected.

SIGNALMENT
Any age or breed. Because there is a close association between acute type I disc herniation and myelomalacia, breeds predisposed to the former are more commonly affected.

SIGNS
• Acute paralysis from spinal injury is the initial clinical sign. If the injury is to the thoracolumbar spine, the patient is paralyzed with exaggerated spinal reflexes in the pelvic limbs. Pain perception is usually absent caudal to the lesion. Within 72 hours, the spinal cord malacia progresses to involve the lumbosacral spinal segments, causing pelvic limb areflexia and atonia, dilated anus, and flaccid, easily expressed urinary bladder. Involvement of the thoracic and cervical spinal cord segments may develop 7-10 days after the initial insult. • Subarachnoid hemorrhage secondary to necrosis of the microvasculature in the spinal cord may cause hyperthermia and extreme meningeal pain.

CAUSES AND RISK FACTORS
• Vertebral or spinal cord trauma • Type I disc disease

DIAGNOSIS

DIFFERENTIAL DIAGNOSIS
Initially cannot be differentiated from spinal trauma. Hind limb upper motor neuron paralysis progressing to a lower motor neuron paralysis and a rostrally advancing line of analgesia are necessary for this diagnosis.

CBC/BIOCHEMISTRY/URINALYSIS
• Results usually normal, initially. If cause of injury is a road accident, nonspecific abnormalities related to other organ injury. • Once myelomalacia has developed, degenerative left shift caused by massive spinal cord necrosis in some patients

OTHER LABORATORY TESTS N/A

IMAGING
• Spinal survey radiography reveals evidence of herniated disc, vertebral fracture, or luxation. • Myelogram indicates cord compression or edema.

OTHER DIAGNOSTIC PROCEDURES
N/A

TREATMENT
• No treatment will reverse spinal cord damage. • Agents proven useful in treating the secondary effects of spinal cord trauma (i.e., methylprednisolone sodium succinate or 21-aminosteroid compounds) have not been evaluated in patients with myelomalacia; they may be useful in halting progression of the malacia.

MEDICATIONS

DRUGS AND FLUIDS
Methylprednisolone sodium succinate (30 mg/kg IV initially followed by 15 mg/kg IV 2 and 6 hours after the initial dose followed by 2.4 mg/kg/hour for 42 hours)

CONTRAINDICATIONS/POSSIBLE INTERACTIONS
Rise in incidence of infection associated with methylprednisolone administration in humans

FOLLOW-UP
• In a few patients, myelomalacia only progresses caudally. While paralysis is permanent, respiratory compromise does not occur. • Myelomalacia has been reported after decompressive laminectomy, suggesting that surgery does not prevent its occurrence.

MISCELLANEOUS

Reference

Griffiths IR. The extensive myelopathy of intervertebral disc protrusions in dogs (the ascending syndrome). J Small Anim Pract 1972;13:425-428.
Author Karen R. Dyer
Consulting Editor Joane M. Parent

MYELOPATHY, DEGENERATIVE

BASICS

DEFINITION
Syndrome characterized by slow, progressive degeneration of axons and myelin in the spinal cord

Pathophysiology
Attempts have been made to link degenerative myelopathy to vitamin B_{12} deficiency, vitamin E deficiency, progressive increase in circulating suppressor T lymphocytes, an autoimmune response to a neural antigen, and "dying back" neuropathy. None has been established as an important pathophysiologic factor.

Systems Affected
Nervous

Genetics
A hereditary basis is suspected but not proven in the German shepherd, German shepherd mixed-breed, and Siberian husky.

Incidence/Prevalence
• Data is not available, but degenerative myelopathy is the most common cause of pelvic limb paresis in middle-aged, German shepherd, and German shepherd mixed-breed dogs. • Rare in other breeds of dogs and in cats

Geographic Distribution N/A

SIGNALMENT

Species Dogs and cats

Breed Predilections
• German shepherd and German shepherd mixed-breed most commonly affected breeds • Other large and medium breeds occasionally affected—collie and collie cross, Labrador retriever, Siberian husky, Chesapeake Bay retriever, Kerry blue terrier, and Welsh corgi (observed in latter breed by author)

Mean Age and Range
• Mean age of onset, 9.6 years; range, 4-14 years • Reported in of two German shepherds, 6 and 7 months old

Predominant Sex Male > female

SIGNS

Historical Findings
• Insidious onset • Initial signs, mild ataxia and paresis of the pelvic limbs; thoracic limbs not affected • Owners often bring their dog in for examination several months after onset of clinical signs, suspecting arthritis. • Knuckling and scuffing of the toes of the pelvic limbs is the most common complaint. Crossing over and swaying of the rear quarters often occur when the animal is turning. • The signs are bilateral but not necessarily symmetrical. • Voluntary control of urination and defecation is retained until extremely late in the course of the disease. In later stages of the disease, the caudal paraspinal and pelvic limb muscles often atrophy from disuse. • Pain or discomfort not evident in affected dogs

Neurologic Examination Findings
• Deficits limited to the pelvic limbs • Ataxia and upper motor neuron paresis localized to the T3-L3 spinal cord segments • In early stages, proprioception deficits are worse than expected for the mild degree of paresis observed. Proprioceptive deficits may be considerably asymmetric • Withdrawal reflexes are normal to exaggerated; some patients have a crossed extensor reflex. • Anal sphincter tone, perineal reflex, and tail tone are normal. • Most patients have normal to exaggerated patellar reflexes, but some have impaired or absent patellar reflexes unilaterally or bilaterally because of degeneration of the dorsal root ganglia or dorsal gray matter of the spinal cord. The ventral motor roots are not affected, so this is not a true lower motor neuron sign. This sign indicates degenerative myelopathy. • Pain perception is preserved.

CAUSES Unknown

RISK FACTORS N/A

DIAGNOSIS

DIFFERENTIAL DIAGNOSIS
• Hansen's type II intervertebral disc protrusion and spinal neoplasia are the two conditions most likely to resemble degenerative myelopathy. Although back pain at the lesion site is a common finding in these conditions, it may not be observed. Survey radiography and myelography should be done to rule out these potentially treatable diseases. • Myelitis is usually more acute and progressive. It is ruled out by CSF analysis at the time of myelography. • Discospondylitis is differentiated by the presence of back pain, which is usually severe. Survey radiography is also helpful. • Lumbosacral stenosis generally causes hyperesthesia at the lumbosacral region, but electromyography and epidurography may be needed in some patients to exclude this possibility. • Vertebral spondylosis and dural ossification are common radiographic findings in old, large-breed dogs, but almost never cause clinical signs.

CBC/BIOCHEMISTRY/URINALYSIS
Results usually normal

OTHER LABORATORY TESTS
Abnormal cell-mediated immune studies—most dogs with degenerative myelopathy are reported to have depressed cell-mediated immune responses to concanavalin A, phytohemagglutinin P, and pokeweed mitogens. These tests are not readily available, and their diagnostic accuracy has not been confirmed by double-blind case studies.

IMAGING
• Thoracic and abdominal radiography to screen for metastatic disease, considering the age of the patients and the possibility of spinal neoplasia • Spinal survey radiographs generally normal or may reveal dural ossification or spondylosis; these findings generally of no clinical importance • Myelography—normal • CT—normal • MRI—lesions may be found throughout the lumbar spinal cord in patients with degenerative myelopathy. If confirmed and consistent, this may be a relatively noninvasive way of confirming the diagnosis.

OTHER DIAGNOSTIC PROCEDURES
CSF analysis—in most patients, the spinal fluid collected from the lumbar subarachnoid space contains a high protein concentration (40-100 mg/dl) with a normal WBC count. Unfortunately, these findings are the same in patients with type II disc protrusion, the main differential.

GROSS AND HISTOPATHOLOGIC FINDINGS
• Gross necropsy findings are normal. • Histologic examination reveals demyelination, axonal degeneration, and astrocytosis of the white matter. The most severe lesions are in the thoracic spinal cord in dorsolateral and ventromedial funiculi. Lesions are generally not symmetrical and not continuous throughout the spinal cord. Some patients have marked degeneration in the lumbar dorsal nerve roots but not the ventral nerve roots; these also have loss of neurons in the dorsal and intermediate gray matter of the spinal cord.

TREATMENT

INPATIENT VERSUS OUTPATIENT
Patients generally treated as outpatients. Hospitalization is only briefly needed for the diagnostic workup.

ACTIVITY
Exercise should be encouraged to prevent muscle atrophy. The stronger and more active the dog is, the longer he will stay ambulatory as the paresis progresses.

DIET Avoid excess weight.

CLIENT EDUCATION
• This is a nontreatable disease that progresses slowly and steadily. • The owner should keep the dog active as long as possible to delay onset of a nonambulatory state. • Once the dog becomes nonambulatory, careful attention is needed to prevent pressure sores. • The use of a cart may be beneficial. • Euthanasia is generally indicated once a nonambulatory state is reached.

SURGICAL CONSIDERATIONS
• No effective surgery available • It is possible for a dog to have both a type II disc protrusion and degenerative myelopathy. Unless the spinal cord compression caused by the disc protrusion is extreme, surgery should

not be done until a therapeutic trial of corticosteroids is completed. If marked improvement is seen, then decompressive surgery is warranted. Surgery to remove a type II disc protrusion in a dog whose clinical signs are actually the result of degenerative myelopathy often causes irreversible neurologic deterioration.

MEDICATIONS

DRUGS AND FLUIDS
• No proven effective treatment available
• One author has proposed a combination of exercise, vitamin supplements, and epsilon aminocaproic acid (EACA; Amicar, Lederle, NY; 500 mg PO q8h mixed with a hematinic compound). This treatment apparently slows the progression in 50% of patients, and 15-20% of dogs have no further deterioration if treatment is maintained. However, no controlled trials have been done to support this claim.

CONTRAINDICATIONS
• Since corticosteroid administration is not beneficial in the treatment of this disease, it should not be used.
• Steroid myopathy may worsen muscle atrophy and pelvic limb weakness, hastening the onset of a nonambulatory state.

POSSIBLE INTERACTIONS N/A
ALTERNATIVE DRUGS N/A

FOLLOW-UP

PATIENT MONITORING
• If EACA administration is effective, improvement should be seen within 8 weeks; a neurologic examination is done at that time to assess therapeutic response. If deterioration is observed, treatment is discontinued because it is expensive. • Dogs with degenerative myelopathy should be reevaluated on a regular basis to monitor progression and avoid complications.

PREVENTION/AVOIDANCE N/A
POSSIBLE COMPLICATIONS
Pressure sores and urine scalding once a nonambulatory state is reached

EXPECTED COURSE AND PROGNOSIS
• Most affected dogs gradually lose function in the pelvic limbs, reaching a nonambulatory state within 6 months-2 years after onset of signs. • If the dog is maintained in a nonambulatory state, thoracic limb function is eventually lost and urinary and fecal incontinence may develop.

MISCELLANEOUS

ASSOCIATED CONDITIONS
• Some dogs have enteropathy that leads to subnormal serum vitamin B_{12} and vitamin E concentrations. It is speculated that the enteropathy may be caused by degenerative myelopathy causing autonomic nerve dysfunction, which in turn leads to impaired intestinal motility and intestinal bacterial overgrowth. • Some dogs have depressed cell-mediated immunity. It is not known if this is a response to the lesion or an indication that degenerative myelopathy has an immunologic basis.

AGE RELATED FACTORS
• Clinical signs develop after age 4. • A few cases have been reported of a similar syndrome in dogs < 1 year old.

ZOONOTIC POTENTIAL N/A

PREGNANCY
Due to the slowly progressive nature of degenerative myelopathy, an affected dog that is still ambulatory should reach term normally; however, the probable heritability of degenerative myelopathy should be discussed.

SYNONYMS
Degenerative radiculomyelopathy of the aged German shepherd

SEE ALSO
Intervertebral Disc Disease

ABBREVIATIONS
CT = computed tomography
CSF = cerebrospinal fluid
EACA = epsilon aminocaproic acid
MRI = magnetic resonance imaging
WBC = white blood cells

References
Clemmons RM. Degenerative myelopathy. In: Kirk RW, ed. Current veterinary therapy X. Philadelphia: WB Saunders, 1989:830-833.
Kornegay JN. Congenital and degenerative diseases of the central nervous system: axonal and myelin lesions—degenerative myelopathy. In: Kornegay JN, ed. Neurologic disorders. New York: Churchill Livingstone, 1986:120-122.
LeCouteur RA, Child G. Diseases of the spinal cord: degenerative myelopathy of dogs. In: Ettinger SJ, ed. Textbook of veterinary internal medicine. 3rd ed. Philadelphia: WB Saunders, 1989:648-649.
Longhofer SL, Duncan ID, Messing A. A degenerative myelopathy in young German shepherd dogs. J Small Anim Pract 1990;31:199-203.
Oliver JE, Lorenz MD. Handbook of veterinary neurology. 2nd ed. Philadelphia: WB Saunders, 1993:143-145.

Author Allen Sisson
Consulting Editor Joane M. Parent

MYELOPROLIFERATIVE DISORDERS

BASICS

OVERVIEW
• Neoplastic proliferation of one or more bone marrow cell lines • Believed to represent a spectrum of disorders in which the stem cell involved is a hematopoietic precursor capable of differentiating into all blood cell types except lymphocytes

SIGNALMENT
• Dogs and cats • More common in cats

SIGNS
• Pale mucous membranes • Lethargy • Weight loss • Hepatosplenomegaly • Peripheral lymphadenomegaly in a few patients

CAUSES AND RISK FACTORS
• Cats— the syndrome most commonly associated with FeLV infection • Cats recovering from panleukopenia or haemobartonellosis may have a relatively higher risk of developing a mutant cell line induced by FeLV.
• Dogs—unknown

DIAGNOSIS

DIFFERENTIAL DIAGNOSIS
• Acute lymphocytic leukemia—usually differentiated by special staining techniques
• Eosinophilia (e.g., parasitism, allergic disease, and eosinophilic gastroenteritis) must be differeintiated from eosinophilic leukemia.

• Severe hemolytic anemia must be differentiated from acute erythroleukemia. • Severe, nonregenerative anemia • Circulating nucleated RBC • Megaloblastic erythrocytes • Leukocytosis or leukopenia • Thrombocytopenia with abnormal platelet morphology

OTHER LABORATORY TESTS N/A

IMAGING N/A

OTHER DIAGNOSTIC PROCEDURES
• Cytologic examination of bone marrow aspirate or core biopsy reveals hypercellular bone marrow with abnormal morphologic changes in all cell lines and neoplastic proliferation or absence of one cell line. • Special or immunohistochemical stains to determine cell type may be necessary.

TREATMENT
Outpatient or inpatient

MEDICATIONS

DRUGS AND FLUIDS
• Supportive care consists of blood transfusions and fluid therapy to correct dehydration; antibiotics indicated in some patients to combat secondary infection.
• Little information available in the veterinary literature regarding treatment of myeloproliferative disease
• Cytosine arabinoside can be used (100 mg/m^2 SQ divided q12h 4 days per week).

CONTRAINDICATIONS/POSSIBLE INTERACTIONS
Chemotherapy can be toxic. Seek advice before treatment if unfamiliar with cytotoxic drugs.

FOLLOW-UP
• CBC and examinaiton of bone marrow aspirate to determine response to treatment and progression of disease
• Prognosis grave, with a rapid and fatal clinical course in most patients

MISCELLANEOUS
Chemotherapy drugs are contraindicated in pregnant animals.

ABBREVIATIONS
FeLV = feline leukemia virus
RBC = red blood cells

Reference
Harvey JW. Myeloproliferative disorders in dogs and cats. Vet Clin North Am (Small Anim Pract) 1981;11(2):349-381.
Author Linda S. Fineman
Consulting Editor Wallace B. Morrison

BASICS

OVERVIEW

• The rapid development of myocardial necrosis resulting from a sustained and complete reduction of blood flow to a portion of the myocardium caused by thrombus formation • Uncommon as a naturally occurring disease in dogs • Microscopic intramural myocardial infarctions and focal areas of myocardial fibrosis are common findings in dogs with acquired cardiovascular disease. • Consistent ECG characteristics of spontaneous myocardial infarction are not well characterized in dogs and cats.

SIGNALMENT

Rare in dogs and cats

SIGNS

Historical Findings

• Lethargy • Anorexia • Weakness • Dyspnea • Collapse • Vomiting • Obesity • Unexpected death

Physical Examination Findings

• Lameness • Tachycardia • Heart murmur • Cardiac rhythm disturbances • Low-grade fever

CAUSES AND RISK FACTORS

• Atherosclerosis and coronary artery disease • Nephrotic syndrome • Vasculitis • Hypothyroidism • Bacterial endocarditis • Neoplasia • Septicemia • Intramural coronary arteriosclerosis in older dogs • Subvalvular aortic stenosis

Cats

• Cardiomyopathy • Thromboembolism

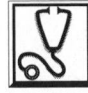

DIAGNOSIS

Generally presumptive based on acute onset of signs in a patient with predisposing factors and consistent ECG changes.

DIFFERENTIAL DIAGNOSIS

Other causes of S-T segment changes

• Normal variation • Myocardial ischemia/ hypoxia • Hyper, hypokalemia • Digitalis toxicity • Trauma to the heart • Pericarditis • Artifact—i.e., wandering baseline

Other Causes of Weakness and Collapse

• Trauma • Neurologic disease • Thromboembolism • Pericardial effusion • Arrhythmia

CBC/BIOCHEMISTRY/URINALYSIS

• Mild leukocytosis • High liver enzymes • Hyperlipidemia (if animal is hypothyroid) • High amylase • High creatinine and cardiac isoenzymes • High LDH

OTHER LABORATORY TESTS

Low T_4 and T_3

IMAGING

• Echocardiography—2D and M-mode echocardiography useful in evaluating wall motion abnormalities and overall left ventricular function. • Angiocardiography—coronary angiography is rarely, if ever, used in clinical veterinary cardiology.

OTHER DIAGNOSTIC PROCEDURES

Electrocardiographic Findings

• Sudden deviation of the ST segment • Tall peaked T waves (first few hours) • Sudden development of Q waves or a change in direction of the T wave • Axis shift of the frontal plane • Low voltage QRS complexes • Sudden development of bundle branch block or heart block • Sudden onset of ventricular arrhythmias because of myocardial ischemia • A sloppy "R" wave descent may be associated with intramural myocardial infarction

TREATMENT

• Treatment should be directed at the underlying disorder as should the symptomatic therapy (i.e., CHF)
• Imperative to identify and immediately treat life-threatening arrhythmias
• Restrict activity

MEDICATIONS

DRUGS AND FLUIDS

• Thrombolytic agents, IV—(e.g., streptokinase—however, cost prohibitive and lack of experience in veterinary medicine with dosage and use)
• Lidocaine for ventricular arrhythmias
• Beta blockers (use cautiously with dilated cardiomyopathy because of possible development of low output congestive heart failure)
• Propranolol —dogs, 0.2-1.0 mg/kg PO q8h; cats, 2.5- 5 mg/cat PO q12h-q8h
• Atenolol—dogs, 0.25-1.0 mg/kg PO q24h-q12h; cats, 6.25-12.5 mg PO q24h
• Antithrombotic agents (e.g., warfin, heparin, and aspirin)

CONTRAINDICATIONS/POSSIBLE INTERACTIONS N/A

FOLLOW-UP

• Determined by clinical status and diagnosis of underlying disorder • Monitor anticoagulated patient; perform CBC and bleeding profiles, including fibrinogen

MISCELLANEOUS

SEE ALSO

• Ventricular Tachycardia • Atherosclerosis

ABBREVIATIONS None

References

Tilley LP. Essentials of canine and feline electrocardiography. 3rd ed. Baltimore: Williams & Wilkins, 1992.

Liu SK , Tilley LP. Clinical and pathologic findings in dogs with artheriosclerosis: 21 cases (1970-1983). JAVMA 1986;189:227.

Authors Larry P. Tilley and T. Arch Robertson

Consulting Editors Larry P. Tilley and Francis W.K. Smith, Jr.

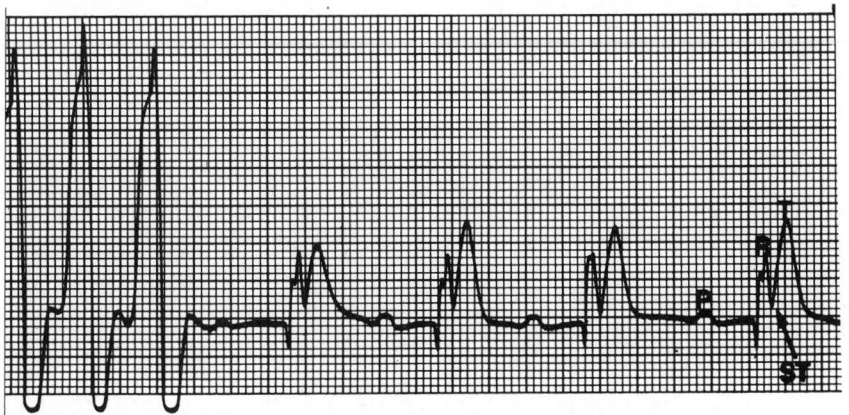

Transmural infarction of the left ventricle in a dog with arteriosclerosis and hypothroidism. The first three rapid successive complexes represent ventricular tachycardia. The sinus rhythm that follows illustrates small complexes, marked elevation of the S-T segment, and first degree AV block (prolonged P-R interval). (From: Tilley LP. Essentials of canine and feline electrocardiography. 3rd ed. Baltimore: Williams & Wilkins, 1992, with permission).

MYOCARDIAL TUMORS

 BASICS

OVERVIEW
Myocardial tumors are rare. Types reported include hemangiosarcoma, hemangioma, fibrosarcoma, fibroma, lymphosarcoma, myxosarcoma, myxoma, rhabdomyoma, and neurofibroma.

SIGNALMENT
More common in old animals

SIGNS
• Depend on tumor location and infiltration
• Include sudden collapse caused by cardiac arrhythmia or signs of heart failure because of pericardial effusion, venous obstruction, myodynamic failure, or valvular obstruction

 DIAGNOSIS

DIFFERENTIAL DIAGNOSIS
• Idiopathic pericardial effusion • Pericarditis
• Cardiomyopathy • Congestive heart failure
• Valvular insufficiency

CBC/BIOCHEMISTRY/URINALYSIS
Anemia in a few patients

OTHER LABORATORY TESTS N/A

IMAGING
• Thoracic radiography to evaluate heart size and shape • Echocardiography to assess myocardial texture

OTHER DIAGNOSTIC PROCEDURES
• Electrocardiography to determine presence of arrhythmia • Surgical biopsy

 TREATMENT

• Treat as inpatient and restrict activity until recovered from surgery
• Surgical excision can be curative for benign tumors
• Pericardiectomy can provide relief from cardiac tamponade
• Chemotherapy probably most effective after surgical excision
• Alert the owner to the potential for sudden death

MEDICATIONS

DRUGS AND FLUIDS
• Lidocaine infusion (25-75 µg/kg/min) or procainamide (8-20 mg/kg PO q8h) to treat ventricular premature contractions and ventricular tachycardia.
• Atenolol (6.25-12.5 mg/cat PO q12h), (0.25-1.0 mg/kg PO q12h-q24h) in dog or propranolol (0.2-1 mg/kg PO q8h) (dog) to treat paroxysmal atrial tachycardia.
• Combination chemotherapy with doxorubicin. (30 mg/m^2 q3wk), cyclophosphamide (100-150 mg/m^2 q3wk), and vincristine (0.7 mg/m^2 wk 2 and wk 3) has been used successfully to treat cardiac hemangiosarcoma.

CONTRAINDICATIONS/POSSIBLE INTERACTIONS
• Chemotherapy can have gastrointestinal, bone marrow, cardiac, and other toxicities. Seek advice before treatment if you are unfamiliar with cytotoxic drugs.

FOLLOW-UP
• Serial cardiac ultrasonography to monitor response to treatment and doxorubicin toxicity • Thoracic radiography to monitor effusion and metastasis • CBC and platelet count to monitor chemotherapy myelosuppression • Prognosis for myocardial tumors guarded

MISCELLANEOUS
Chemotherapy should not be used in pregnant animals.

Reference
deMadron NE, Helfand SC, Stebbins KE. Use of chemotherapy for treatment of cardiac hemangiosarcoma in a dog. J Am Vet Med Assoc 1987;190:887-891.
Author Terrance A. Hamilton
Consulting Editor Wallace B. Morrison

MYOCARDITIS

BASICS

DEFINITION

Inflammation of the heart muscle, often caused by infectious agents affecting the myocytes, interstitium, vascular elements, or pericardium. Viral, bacterial, rickettsial, fungal, and protozoal diseases are all associated with myocardial inflammation (i.e., myocarditis). Pharmacologic agents (e.g., Doxorubicin) can also be causative.

Pathophysiology

• The mechanisms involved in the inflammatory process include toxin production, direct invasion of myocardial tissue, and immune-mediated myocardial damage. Vasculitis associated with systemic disease may be involved. Allergic reactions and direct myocyte damage caused by pharmacologic agents can lead to myocardial inflammation. Protozoal agents (e.g., Trypanasoma cruzi) lead to granulomatous myocarditis, while viral myocarditis is associated with cell-mediated immunologic reactions. • Myocardial involvement may be focal or diffuse. Clinical manifestations depend on the extent of the lesions. Diffuse, severe involvement may lead to global myocardial damage and congestive heart failure, while discreet lesions involving the conduction system may cause profound arrhythmias.

Systems Affected

• Systemic organ involvement depending on the causative agent • Cardiovascular due to myocardial failure or arrhythmias. • Respiratory, if pulmonary edema develops

Genetics N/A

Incidence/Prevalence

• Viral myocarditis (e.g., caused by parvovirus, distemper virus, and herpesvirus) is rarely seen. Very young puppies in their first months of life may be profoundly affected. A second form occurs (parvoviral) in which dilated cardiomyopathy develops in dogs 5-6 months of age that were infected during their first weeks of life. • Protozoal myocarditis associated with Trypanasoma cruzi (i.e., Chagas' disease) is reported in dogs less than 2 years old from the southeastern United States. Males are more commonly affected than females. Toxoplasma gondii occasionally causes myocarditis. Animals that are immunosuppressed (e.g., cats with feline leukemia virus) are at high risk. Hepatozoon canis has been reported in dogs in the Texas Gulf. • Fungal myocarditis is primarily seen in association with systemic fungal infection. Myocardial involvement varies with regional prevalence and prevalence of the systemic manifestation. • Bacterial myocarditis can be caused by generalized sepsis and bacteremia. Doxorubicin cardiotoxicity has been reported in dogs receiving cumulative doses ranging from 240 mg/M^2 to 150 mg/M^2 or less.

• Spirochetal myocarditis associated with Borrelia burgdorferi has been documented in 10% of humans with Lyme's disease. The incidence and prevalence in dogs is not well documented.

Geographic Distribution

Myocarditis associated with infectious agents should be suspected wherever these diseases are endemic (see above).

SIGNALMENT

Species Dogs and cats

Breed Predilections N/A

Mean Age And Range
• Viral myocarditis is seen primarily in young animals, less than one year in age.

Predominate Sex N/A

SIGNS

General Comments

•Clinical signs related to the degree and location of myocardial involvement • Range from signs of arrhythmias to those of congestive heart failure • The onset of cardiac dysfunction in association with systemic illness or the use of specific pharmacologic agents is often the hallmark of myocarditis.

Historical Findings

• Coughing, exercise intolerance, dyspnea are associated with congestive heart failure. • Syncope and weakness are associated with arrhythmias. • Concurrent systemic manifestations are often seen in association with infective myocarditis. • The use of antineoplastic or other pharmacologic agents is associated with the onset of cardiac dysfunction.

Physical Examination Findings

• A gallop rhythm or murmur may be found, depending on the nature of the myocardial damage. • Arrhythmias may be ausculted.
• Fever is common in animals with active infection associated with myocarditis.

CAUSES

• Virus (e.g., parvovirus, distemper virus, herpesvirus) • Protozoa (e.g., Trypanosoma cruzi, Toxoplasma gondii, and Hepatazoon canis) • Bacteria • Fungus (e.g., Cryptococcus neoformans, Coccidioides immitis, and Aspergillus terreus) • Algae (e.g., Prototheca spp.) • Doxorubicin

RISK FACTORS

• Exposure to infectious agents • Use of myocardiotoxic compounds • Immunosuppression • Debilitating diseases

DIAGNOSIS

DIFFERENTIAL DIAGNOSIS

• Preexisting heart disease including congenital defects, cardiomyopathy, and acquired valvular disease should always be considered.
• History of a heart murmur or the presence of arrhythmias before onset of systemic illness

helps differentiate myocarditis from other diseases. • Presence of extracardiac organ involvement and identification of infectious agents may help in the diagnosis of myocarditis.

CBC/BIOCHEMISTRY/URINALYSIS

Abnormalities vary depending on organ involvement.

Other Laboratory Tests

• Serologic tests to help identify an infectious agent. • Cytologic examination of pericardial, pleural, and peritoneal effusions to identify the infectious organism. • Blood culture to diagnose bacteremia.

IMAGING

Thoracic Radiographic Findings

• The cardiac silhouette may appear large or normal depending on the extent of involvement. • Pulmonary edema, congestion, or pleural effusion in animals with congestive heart failure (CHF) • Globoid heart in some animals with pericardial effusion • Pulmonary granuloma may be found in animals with granulomatous myocardial infection.

Echocardiographic Findings

• Reflect the extent of myocardial damage; may be normal if lesions are small or primarily affect the conduction system. • Pericardial effusion in some animals. The pericardium may appear thickened and hyperechoic depending on the extent of pericardial involvement. • The myocardium may appear mottled with patchy areas of hyperechogenicity caused by myocardial inflammation, fibrosis, or granulomas. • Regional dyskenisis caused by focal involvement may be appreciated on 2-D echocardiography.

Angiography

• Because of the quality and noninvasive nature of echocardiography, cardiac catheterization is rarely indicated in the diagnosis of myocarditis. • Angiography may be used if echocardiography is not available to detect specific chamber involvement, or the presence of pericardial effusion.

OTHER DIAGNOSTIC PROCEDURES

Electrocardiographic Findings

• Left ventricle, left atrium, right ventricle, or right atrium enlargement patterns in some animals depending on the extent of chamber involvement. • Arrhythmias include both atrial and ventricular tachyarrhythmias.
• Right and left bundle branch blocks and hemiblocks should be differentiated from ventricular enlargement patterns. • Atrioventricular nodal conduction disturbances in some animals.

Endomyocardial Biopsy

Useful in the detection of infectious agents such as protozoa, fungal elements, or inflammatory cell infiltrates.

Pericardiocentesis

• Alleviates pericardial effusion • Submit fluid for cytologic examination and possible bacterial culture.

Holter Monitor Study
• For detecting arrhythmias, frequency and severity • For monitoring antiarrhythmic therapy

GROSS AND HISTOPATHOLOGIC FINDINGS
• Dilated cardiac chambers with patchy areas of hyperemia, necrosis, or fibrosis • Granulomas seen grossly in some animals • Microscopic examination of the myocardium or pericardium may reveal the presence of inflammatory cells (e.g., lymphocytes, plasma cells, and macrophages), patchy fibrosis, or the infectious agents themselves. • Myofiber dropout is seen in animals with Doxorubicin toxicity.

TREATMENT

INPATIENT VERSUS OUTPATIENT
• Patients with CHF should be hospitalized for initial medical management.
• Patients with severe ventricular arrhythmias should be hospitalized for initial anti-arrhythmic therapy.
• Patients with severe systemic manifestations should be hospitalized for aggressive medical therapy.

ACTIVITY Restricted

DIET
Sodium restriction if animal has CHF

CLIENT EDUCATION
• Cardiac manifestations may persist even with resolution of systemic illness.
• Certain arrhythmias (i.e., ventricular tachyarrhythmias) may predispose animal to sudden death.
• It may be difficult to make an antemortem diagnosis.
• Some infectious agents may pose a public health risk.

SURGICAL CONSIDERATIONS
Complete atrioventricular block may require pacemaker implantation.

MEDICATIONS

DRUGS AND FLUIDS OF CHOICE
• If a specific etiologic agent is identified, treatment should be directed against the agent itself.
• Antiarrhythmic therapy should be tailored to the predominate arrhythmia.
• CHF is treated with furosemide (1-2 mg/kg PO q6h-q12h), enalapril (0.25-0.5 mg/kg PO q12h-q24h) and digoxin (0.22 mg/M^2).

CONTRAINDICATIONS
Because of the public health significance, treatment of some infectious diseases (i.e., T. cruzi) may not be undertaken.

PRECAUTIONS
• All antiarrhythmic drugs have proarrhythmic properties and should be monitored closely.
• Systemic organ involvement (e.g., renal involvement) may necessitate the modification of drug dosages or use of various cardiac drugs. Therefore, careful monitoring of systemic function is essential.

POSSIBLE INTERACTIONS N/A

ALTERNATE DRUGS N/A

FOLLOW-UP

PATIENT MONITORING
• Monitor antiarrhythmic therapy with frequent auscultation and ECG. • Monitor serologic titers when appropriate. • Auscultation and follow-up radiographs help monitor treatment of CHF. • Hemograms and serum biochemical analysis monitor systemic effects of the disease.

PREVENTION/AVOIDANCE
• Avoid breeding animals with a poor vaccination history. • Avoid endemic areas if possible. • Monitor ECG and echocardiogram when using doxorubicin.

EXPECTED COURSE AND PROGNOSIS
• Depends on the extent and severity of myocardial involvement. • Many systemic fungal and protozoal diseases do not respond well to medical management. • Patients with extensive myocardial inflammation and degeneration and signs of CHF have a very poor prognosis. • Patients with isolated, controllable arrhythmias have a good prognosis if the underlying cause can be treated successfully.

MISCELLANEOUS

ASSOCIATED CONDITIONS
Often accompanies systemic illness

AGE RELATED FACTORS
Viral myocarditis is most often seen in young animals < 1 year old

ZOONOTIC POTENTIAL
• Varies with infectious agent involved. • Protozoal and mycotic infections may have a high zoonotic potential.

PREGNANCY
Some viral diseases such as canine herpesvirus and parvovirus have been shown to be passed to the fetus during pregnancy.

SYNONYMS N/A

SEE ALSO
• Infectious diseases listed under causes
• Ventricular Premature Complexes
• Ventricular Tachycardia

ABBREVIATIONS
CHF = congestive heart failure
LA = left atrium
RA = right atrium
LV = left ventricle
RV = right ventricle

References

Fox PR. Myocardial diseases. In: Ettinger SJ, ed. Textbook of veterinary internal medicine. 3rd ed. Philadelphia: WB Saunders, 1989.

Liu SK. Cardiovascular pathology. In: Fox PR, ed. Canine and feline cardiology. New York: Churchill Livingstone Inc., 1988.

Wynne J, Braunwald E. The cardiomyopathies and myocarditides: toxic, chemical, and physical damage to the heart. In: Braunwald E, ed. Heart disease: a textbook of cardiovascular medicine. 4th ed. Philadelphia: WB Saunders, 1992.

Author Michael B. Lesser
Consulting Editors Larry P. Tilley and Francis W. K. Smith, Jr.

MYOCLONUS

 BASICS

OVERVIEW
• Coarse, repetitive, rhythmic contractions of a portion of a muscle, entire muscle, or group of muscles • May affect one or multiple muscle groups • A CNS dysfunction involving the lower motor neurons and interneurons at the segmental level or, in rare patients, at the basal nuclei • Myoclonus is a clinical sign and although reported as secondary to canine distemper virus infection, many abnormalities at the right location can be causative.

SIGNALMENT
Acquired
• Any dog • Rarely reported in cats

CONGENITAL
• Familial reflex myoclonus an inherited disorder of the Labrador retriever with onset at 3 weeks • Neonatal myoclonus of the paravertebral muscles caused by spongy degeneration reported in the silky terrier

SIGNS
Historical Findings
• Myoclonus is observed after a bout of gastrointestinal signs, cough, or ocular or nasal purulent discharge. It persists at rest and even during sleep. The frequency remains consistent in a given patient. • A diagnosis of canine distemper may have preceeded the myoclonus by months to years; myoclonus occurs more frequently in the chronic phase of distemper. • Familial reflex myoclonus is observed when the animal starts to ambulate. Myoclonus is intermittent and induced by auditory or tactile stimulus and by exercise. Affected patients are often unable to walk.

Physical Examination Findings
• Masticatory and appendicular muscles the most frequent groups of muscles affected in dogs with distemper virus-induced myoclonus • The dog may have other signs suggesting distemper virus infection such as hard pads, ocular and nasal purulent discharge, and chorioretinitis. • Neurologic deficits suggesting multifocal lesions seen in some patients • The animal may be otherwise healthy.

CAUSES AND RISK FACTORS
Congenital
• Familial reflex myoclonus in the Labrador retriever • Spongy degeneration in the silky terrier • Other congenital anomalies of unknown cause

Acquired
• Canine distemper virus (most frequent cause)—the only CNS disease repeatedly associated with acquired myoclonus in dogs. Unvaccinated dogs are at risk. • Encephalitis of any cause • Degenerative disease, especially spongy degeneration

 DIAGNOSIS

DIFFERENTIAL DIAGNOSIS
• The presence of systemic signs such as gastroenteritis, pneumonia, and ocular purulent discharge suggest canine distemper virus infection. • Acquired myoclonus must be differentiated from other movement disorders that are limited to parts of the body. • Doberman, Labrador retriever, and English bulldog occasionally have head nods in a "yes" or "no" direction. The movement is limited to the head, appears intermittently, and lasts from few seconds to one minute. The animal continues its activity and is otherwise normal. • Dancing doberman disease differentiated on the basis of breed and the type of movements observed, e.g., the dog holds one pelvic limb flexed while standing. In most patients, both limbs become affected giving a dancing aspect to the standing position.

CBC/BIOCHEMISTRY/URINALYSIS
• Normal in patients with congenital myoclonus or myoclonus secondary to canine distemper virus infection • In patients with other forms of acquired myoclonus, results may suggest a specific cause if the patient has infectious encephalomyelitis. Otherwise, results normal

OTHER LABORATORY TESTS N/A

IMAGING N/A

OTHER DIAGNOSTIC PROCEDURES
• In patients with acute development of myoclonus, CSF analysis, serologic testing, and brain imaging (computed tomography and magnetic resonance imaging) may help determine a diagnosis. • Electrodiagnostic techniques may help to localize the lesion site responsible for the myoclonus.

 TREATMENT

• Patients with active encephalomyelitis should be hospitalized to establish a diagnosis and initiate treatment.
• Exercise according to the patient's tolerance.
• Insure proper nutrition if the animal suffers from active CNS disease. Modification of the diet may be necessary if patient has vomiting or diarrhea.
• Myoclonus usually persists for the life of the animal regardless of the cause.
• In the familial myoclonus of the Labrador, clinical signs are severe and usually not compatible with quality of life.

MEDICATIONS

DRUGS AND FLUIDS
• In most patients, myoclonus is associated with the chronic inactive phase of canine distemper. There is no treatment.
• Treat patients with active encephalomyelitis accordingly.

CONTRAINDICATIONS/POSSIBLE INTERACTIONS N/A

 FOLLOW-UP
• Monitor CNS disease. • Myoclonus usually persists indefinitely. Remission is occasionally seen. • Dogs with active distemper virus infection have a poor to grave prognosis.

 MISCELLANEOUS

ABBREVIATIONS
CNS = Central nervous system
CSF = Cerebrospinal fluid

SYNONYMS
• Flexor spasm • Canine chorea

Reference
Oliver JE, Lorenz MD. Handbook of veterinary neurology. 2nd ed. Philadelphia: WB Saunders, 1993:247-257.
Author Joane M. Parent
Consulting Editor Joane M. Parent

MYOPATHY, FOCAL INFLAMMATORY—MASTICATORY MUSCLE MYOSITIS AND EXTRAOCULAR MYOSITIS

BASICS

DEFINITION
Masticatory muscle myositis (MMM) is a focal inflammatory myopathy affecting the muscles of mastication (temporalis and masseter muscles) and sparing the limb muscles. Extraocular muscle myositis (EOM) selectively affects the extraocular muscles, sparing limb and masticatory muscles.

Pathophysiology
An immune-mediated etiology is suspected for MMM based on the presence of autoantibodies against type 2M fibers and a positive clinical response to immunosuppresive dosage of corticosteroids. An immune-mediated etiology is also suspected for EOM as a result of positive clinical response to corticosteroids.

Systems Affected
Neuromuscular—the muscles of mastication and extraocular muscles

Genetics
Unknown; however, as with autoimmune diseases in general, the appropriate genetic background must be present for the development of an autoimmune disease. • Golden retrievers may have a genetic predisposition to EOM.

Incidence/Prevalence
Unknown; however, MMM is not rare

Geographic Distribution
Probably worldwide

SIGNALMENT

Species Dogs

Breed Predilections
• Various large and small breeds of dogs
• EOM—golden retrievers

Mean Age and Range
No obvious age predisposition

Predominant Sex
No obvious sex predisposition

SIGNS

General Comments
• With MMM, clinical signs are usually related to abnormalities of jaw movement and jaw pain. • This disorder is not a "table top" diagnosis, and laboratory testing is usually required to confirm a suspected diagnosis.

Historical Findings
• MMM—acute or chronic pain on opening the jaw, inability to pick up a ball, or get food into the mouth, acutely swollen muscles, or progressive muscle atrophy • EOM—bilateral exopthalmos

Physical Examination Findings
• MMM—marked jaw pain with manipulation and/or trismus, acute muscle swelling with exopthalmos, or muscle atrophy with enophthalmos • Inability to open the jaw un-

der anesthesia. May be confused with a retroorbital abscess. • EOM—bilateral proptosis and impaired vision

CAUSES
Immune-mediated for both MMM and EOM

RISK FACTORS
• Appropriate genetic background • Possible previous bacterial or viral infection

DIAGNOSIS

DIFFERENTIAL DIAGNOSIS
• Retroorbital abscess—probe behind last upper molar • Temporomandibular joint disease—radiographically abnormal TM joints • Polymyositis—markedly high serum creatine kinase (CK), generalized EMG abnormalities, and diagnostic muscle biopsies • Neurogenic atrophy of temporalis muscles—determine by EMG and muscle biopsy • Atrophy of masticatory muscles due to cortiosteroids—previous history of corticosteroid use, and characteristic changes on muscle biopsy

CBC/BIOCHEMISTRY/URINALYSIS
Serum creatine kinase (CK) normal or mildly elevated

OTHER LABORATORY TESTS
• Muscle biopsy—diagnostic test of choice for MMM • Immunocytochemical assay for the demonstration of autoantibodies against masticatory muscle type 2M fibers—negative in patients with polymyositis and EOM

IMAGING
• Radiographic evaluation of the temporomandibular joints • Orbital sonogram in patients with EOM demonstrates swollen extraocular muscles

OTHER DIAGNOSTIC PROCEDURES
Electromyographic evaluation (EMG) to differentiate EOM from polymyositis (PM). Abnormal masticatory muscles only with MMM, generalized abnormalities with PM.

GROSS AND HISTOPATHOLOGIC FINDINGS
• MMM—swelling or atrophy of the masticatory muscles should be present • The biopsy specimen may contain myofiber necrosis, phagocytosis, and mononuclear cell infiltration with a mulitfocal and perivascular distribution. Myofiber atrophy and fibrosis with chronicity. Eosinophils rarely present. • EOM—mononuclear cell infiltration restricted to extraocular muscles

TREATMENT

INPATIENT VERSUS OUTPATIENT
Treatment may be performed on an outpatient basis.

ACTIVITY N/A

DIET
• MMM—liquid food or gruel may be required until patient regains jaw mobility
• May need a gastric feeding tube to facilitate fluid and caloric intake

CLIENT EDUCATION
• Long-term corticosteroid therapy may be required.
• Chronic MMM—residual muscle atrophy

SURGICAL CONSIDERATIONS
Surgical intervention is not indicated.

MEDICATIONS

DRUGS AND FLUIDS
MMM and EOM—immunosuppressive dosages of corticosteroids. Decrease dosage as jaw mobility, swelling, and serum CK return to normal. Maintain on lowest alternate-day dosage that prevents restricted jaw mobility. Treat for minimum of 6 months.

CONTRAINDICATIONS N/A

PRECAUTIONS
• Continual observation for infection and undesirable side effects of corticosteroids.
• Clinical signs may recur if treatment is stopped too soon.

POSSIBLE INTERACTIONS N/A

ALTERNATE DRUGS
If side effects of corticosteroids are intolerable, a lower dosage of corticosteroids combined with another drug such as azothiaprine should be instituted.

FOLLOW-UP

PATIENT MONITORING
• MMM—return of jaw mobility and low CK • EOM—reduced swelling of extraocular muscles

PREVENTION/AVOIDANCE N/A

POSSIBLE COMPLICATIONS
• Undesirable side effects of corticosteroids
• Recurrence of clinical signs if treatment is stopped too early • Poor clinical response if high enough dosages of corticosteroids are not used

EXPECTED COURSE AND PROGNOSIS
• MMM—jaw mobility should return to normal unless chronic with severe fibrosis
• Prognosis is good if treated early with adequate dosages of corticosteroids • EOM—good response to corticosteroids. Prognosis is good.

MYOPATHY, FOCAL INFLAMMATORY—MASTICATORY MUSCLE MYOSITIS AND EXTRAOCULAR MYOSITIS

MISCELLANEOUS

ASSOCIATED CONDITIONS
May have other, concurrent, autoimmune disorders

AGE RELATED FACTORS N/A

ZOONOTIC POTENTIAL N/A

PREGNANCY Not known

SYNONYMS
• Eosinophilic myositis • Atrophic myositis

SEE ALSO
• Immune-Mediated Disorders • Myopathies, Inflammatory

ABBREVIATIONS
MMM = masticatory muscle myositis
EOM = extraocular myositis
PM = polymyositis
EMG = electromyogram
CK = serum creatine kinase

References

Shelton GD. Canine masticatory muscle disorders. In: Kirk RW, ed. Current veterinary therapy X. Philadelphia: WB Saunders, 1989;816-819.

Orvis JS, Cardinet GH III. Canine muscle fiber types and susceptibility of masticatory muscles to myositis. Muscle Nerve 1981;4:354-359.

Shelton GD, Cardinet GH III, Bandman E. Canine masticatory muscle disorders: a clinicopathological and immunochemical study of 29 cases. Muscle Nerve 1987;10:753-766.

Carpenter JL, Schmidt GM, Moore FM, et al. Canine bilateral extraocular polymyositis. Vet Pathol 1989;26:510-512.

Author G. Diane Shelton

Consulting Editor Peter D. Schwarz

MYOPATHY, GENERALIZED INFLAMMATORY—POLYMYOSITIS AND DERMATOMYOSITIS

BASICS

DEFINITION
Polymyositis is a condition in which skeletal muscles are damaged by a nonsuppurative inflammatory process dominated by lymphocytic infiltration. The term dermatomyositis is used when polymyositis is associated with characteristic skin lesions.

Pathophysiology
Inflammation of skeletal muscles results in muscle weakness, myalgia, and atrophy. Muscle inflammation may be a result of immune-mediated, infectious, or paraneoplastic disorders or it may be a sequellae to certain drug therapies.

Systems Affected
• Neuromuscular—generalized muscle involvement including masticatory and limb muscles • Gastrointestinal—in particular the pharyngeal and esophageal muscles because they are composed predominantly of skeletal muscle in the dog • Skin/exocrine—in particular if related to a generalized immune-mediated connective tissue disorder

Genetics
• Unknown; however, as with autoimmune diseases in, general, the appropriate genetic background must present • Dermatomyositis in rough coated collies and Shetland sheepdogs has been reported to have an autosomal dominant inheritance pattern.

Incidence/Prevalence
Unknown; however, generalized inflammatory myopathies are not common

Geographic Distribution
Probably worldwide

SIGNALMENT
Species Dogs and rarely in cats

Breed Predilections
• Various breeds of dogs and cats may be affected with polymyositis. • Dermatomyositis has been reported in rough coated collies, Shetland sheepdogs, and Australian cattle dogs.

Mean Age and Range
• No obvious age predisposition for polymyositis • 3-5 months of age for familial dermatomyositis

Predominant Sex
No obvious sex predisposition for polymyositis or dermatomyositis

SIGNS
General Comments
• Polymyositis is usually associated with a stiff-stilted gait, muscle pain, and or muscle weakness. • It is important to remember that an elevated serum creatine kinase (CK) is supportive of but not diagnostic of myositis. • A muscle biopsy is necessary to confirm the diagnosis.

Historical Findings
• Acute or chronic history of stiff-stilted gait • Muscle swelling and/or muscle atrophy • Generalized muscle pain • Generalized muscle weakness and exercise intolerance • Regurgitation of food or difficulty swallowing

Physical Examination Findings
• Pain upon palpation of muscle groups • Generalized muscle atrophy, including the muscles of mastication • Gait abnormalities, including a stiff-stilted gait • Neurologic examination not abnormal. There may be a diminished gag reflex if the pharyngeal muscles are affected. • Typical skin lesions in dogs with dermatomyositis

CAUSES
• Immune-mediated • Infectious (Toxoplasma gondii, Neospora canis, Hepatozooan canis, Ehrlichia canis, bacterial infection uncommon) • Drug-induced • Paraneoplastic syndrome

RISK FACTORS
• Appropriate genetic background for dermatomyositis and immune-mediated causes of polymyositis • Possible previous bacterial or viral infection • Neoplasia, possibly occult

DIAGNOSIS

DIFFERENTIAL DIAGNOSIS
• Polyarthritis—physical examination, evaluation of joint fluid • Noninflammatory muscle disorders—muscle biopsy should differentiate • Polyneuropathy—neurological exam, electrophysiology, and muscle biopsy should differentiate • Chronic intervertebral disc disease—physical examination and serum CK should differentiate

CBC/BIOCHEMISTRY/URINALYSIS
Serum creatine kinase (CK) should be markedly elevated.

OTHER LABORATORY TESTS
• Serum antinuclear antibody titer may be positive with connective tissue disorders • May have concurrent hypothyroidism

IMAGING
• If regurgitation is present a thoracic radiography to evaluate for the presence of esophageal dilitation. • If pharyngeal weakness is present, a dynamic study to evaluate the swallowing process.

OTHER DIAGNOSTIC PROCEDURES
• Evaluation of a muscle biopsy sample is the single most important test in the diagnosis of polymyositis. Multiple muscles should be sampled because a patchy distribution may be present that could be missed with a single sample. • Electromyographic evaluation (EMG) should be performed to determine the distribution of muscle involvement and the muscles to be biopsied. Should also help differentiate myopathic from neuropathic causes of muscle weakness.

GROSS AND HISTOPATHOLOGIC FINDINGS
• Muscle swelling or atrophy • Biopsy specimens usually contain mononuclear cell infiltrates. • Rarely neutrophils or eosinophils may be present. • Regenerating myofibers may also be observed. • Rarely, an intramyofiber parasite cyst may be present. • With chronicity, extensive myofiber atrophy and fibrosis may occur.

TREATMENT

INPATIENT VERSUS OUTPATIENT
Treatment may be performed on an outpatient basis.

ACTIVITY
Activity and muscle strength should improve as muscle inflammation resolves.

DIET
• If megaesophagus is present, feeding from an elevation may be required. Foods of different consistencies should be tried.
• If regurgitation is severe, a gastric feeding tube may be needed to maintain hydration and nutrition.

CLIENT EDUCATION
• Long-term immunosuppressive therapy may be required in patients with immune-mediated conditions.
• Residual muscle atrophy may be present in patients with chronic conditions and extensive fibrosis.
• Genetic counseling for familial disorders

SURGICAL CONSIDERATIONS
Surgery only for concurrent neoplasia if present

MEDICATIONS

DRUGS AND FLUIDS
• In immune-mediated polymyositis, immunosuppressive dosages of corticosteroids usually result in clinical improvement.
• Corticosteroid dosages should be decreased to the lowest alternate-day dosage that maintains normal CK and improved muscle strength and mobility. Long-term therapy may be necessary.
• If an infectious agent is identified, specific therapy should be initiated (refer to sections on specific infectious agent for treatment).

CONTRAINDICATIONS N/A

PRECAUTIONS
• Continual observation for infection and undesirable side effects of corticosteroids
• It is important to remember that muscle atrophy may occur as a result of chronic corticosteroid therapy.

POSSIBLE INTERACTIONS N/A

MYOPATHY, GENERALIZED INFLAMMATORY—POLYMYOSITIS AND DERMATOMYOSITIS

ALTERNATE DRUGS

If side effects of corticosteroids are intolerable, a lower dose of corticosteroids combined with another drug such as azothiaprine should be instituted.

FOLLOW-UP

PATIENT MONITORING

• Periodic evaluation of serum CK • The serum CK, if elevated, should decrease into the normal range. • Side effects of corticosteroids

PREVENTION/AVOIDANCE N/A

POSSIBLE COMPLICATIONS

• Undesirable side effects of corticosteroids • Recurrence of clinical signs if treatment is stopped too early • Poor clinical response if inadequate dosages of corticosteroids are used

EXPECTED COURSE AND PROGNOSIS

• Prognosis is good to fair for immune-mediated polymyositis. • Prognosis is guarded if polymyositis is a paraneoplastic disorder and associated with occult neoplasia.

MISCELLANEOUS

ASSOCIATED CONDITIONS

• May have other concurrent autoimmune disorders • May have associated neoplasia

AGE RELATED FACTORS N/A

ZOONOTIC POTENTIAL N/A

PREGNANCY Not known

SYNONYMS N/A

SEE ALSO Immune-Mediated Disorders

ABBREVIATIONS

CK = creatine kinase

References

Kornegay JN, Gorgacz EJ, Dawe DL, et al. Polymyositis in dogs. J Am Vet Med Assoc 1980;176:431-438.

Hargis AM, Haupt KH, Prieur DJ, Moore MP. A skin disorder in three Shetland sheepdogs: comparison with familial canine dermatomyositis of collies. Compend Contin Educ Pract Vet 1985;7:306-318.

Shelton GD, Cardinet GH III. Pathophysiologic basis of canine muscle disorders. J Vet Int Med 1987;1:36-44.

Author G. Diane Shelton
Consulting Editor Peter D. Schwarz

MYOPATHY, NONINFLAMMATORY—ENDOCRINE

BASICS

DEFINITION
Myopathies associated with various endocrinopathies including hypo- and hyperthyroidism, and hypo- and hyperadrenocorticism and those associated with exogenous corticosteroid use (steroid myopathy)

Pathophysiology
Muscle Disorders with Adrenal Dysfunction
• Glucocorticoid excess - impaired muscle protein metabolism may accelerate the degradation of myofibrillar and soluble protein in skeletal muscle; impairment of carbohydrate metabolism due to induction of an insulin resistant state. Elevated levels of ACTH may also be myopathic. • Adrenal insufficiency, circulatory insufficiency, fluid and electrolyte imbalance and impaired carbohydrate metabolism.

Muscle Disorders with Thyroid Disease
• Hyperthyroidism - increased mitochondrial respiration, accelerated protein degradation and lipid oxidation, glycogen depletion, and impaired glucose uptake. • Hypothyroidism - impaired muscle energy metabolism by reduced glycogen breakdown, gluconeogenesis, and oxidative and glycolytic capacity. Impaired insulin stimulated carbohydrate metabolism.

Systems Affected
• Neuromuscular - impaired energy metabolism • Cardiovascular - impaired energy metabolism, circulatory disorders

Genetics N/A

Incidence/Prevalence
• Exact incidence not known • Myopathies related to exogenous corticosteroids common • Myopathies associated with Cushing's syndrome and hypothyroidism not uncommon

Geographic Distribution
Probably worldwide

SIGNALMENT

Species
• Dogs - steroid myopathy, and weakness associated with hyper- and hypoadrenocorticism and hypothyroidism • Cats - hyperthyroid associated weakness

Breed Predilections
Several breeds affected

Mean Age and Range
• Steroid myopathy may occur in dogs of any age • For other disorders, see sections related to specific disease

Predominant Sex
No sex predilection has been found for endocrine myopathies

SIGNS

General Comments
Dog muscle is very susceptible to the effects of exogenous corticosteroids. Muscle atrophy is not uncommon with prolonged corticosteroid use, particularly of the masticatory muscles.

Historical Findings
• Muscle weakness, atrophy, and stiffness that may not be associated with other clinical signs of an endocrine disorder. • Regurgitation, dysphagia, and dysphonia

Physical Examination Findings
• Muscle weakness, stiffness, cramping, and myalgia • Muscle hypertrophy or atrophy • May or may not have other clinical signs of an endocrine disorder

CAUSES
• Endocrine dysfunction • Autoimmune • Neoplastic

RISK FACTORS N/A

DIAGNOSIS

DIFFERENTIAL DIAGNOSIS
• Inflammatory myopathies; muscle biopsy should differentiate • Non-inflammatory myopathies; muscle biopsy should differentiate

CBC/BIOCHEMISTRY/URINALYSIS
• Abnormalities consistent with endocrine disorder on baseline testing • Serum creatine kinase is usually normal

OTHER LABORATORY TESTS
Evaluation of thyroid and adrenal function should be diagnostic

IMAGING
• If regurgitation and dysphagia present, dynamic studies for evaluation of pharyngeal and esophageal function • Cardiac evaluation in hyperthyroid cats

OTHER DIAGNOSTIC PROCEDURES
• Muscle biopsy, using fresh frozen muscle sections. • Electromyography

GROSS AND HISTOPATHOLOGIC FINDINGS
• Hyperadrenocorticism and steroid myopathy—selective atrophy of type 2 muscle fibers, lobulated to "ragged-red" like fibers in some cases with associated myotonia. • Hypoadrenocorticism—no abnormalities • Feline hyperthyroidism—not known if pathologic abnormalities occur within muscle • Hypothyroidism—atrophy of type 2 fibers occasionally with a shift to an increased population of type 1 fibers, may see PAS positive deposits in type 2 fibers.

TREATMENT

INPATIENT VERSUS OUTPATIENT
Refer to treatment for specific endocrine disorders

ACTIVITY
In humans, inactivity will worsen clinical corticosteroid myopathy and increased muscle activity may partially prevent atrophy. Physical therapy may be useful in preventing and treating muscle weakness and wasting in dogs receiving glucocorticoids.

DIET
• Feeding from an elevation if regurgitation and megaesophagus are present • Loose consistency of food best tolerated if dysphagia and esophageal dilation are present • Placement of gastric feeding tube if oral feeding not tolerated

CLIENT EDUCATION
• Refer to sections on specific endocrine disorders • Prognosis is poor for resolution of myotonia associated with hyperadrenocorticism

SURGICAL CONSIDERATIONS
Surgical removal of neoplasia if present

MEDICATIONS

DRUGS AND FLUIDS
• Refer to sections on treatment for specific endocrine disorders • Corticosteroid myopathy-reduces the corticosteroid dosage to the lowest possible level. Use a nonfluorinated corticosteroid, alternate-day dosage. • If intramyofiber lipid storage is present in steroid myopathy, use of L-carnitine (50 mg/kg q12h) may result in improved muscle strength.

CONTRAINDICATIONS N/A

PRECAUTIONS
Refer to sections on specific endocrine disorders

POSSIBLE INTERACTIONS N/A

ALTERNATE DRUGS
The fluorinated corticosteroids, triamcinolone, betamethasone, and dexamethasone, are most likely to produce muscle weakness. Use an equivalent dosage of another corticosteroid.

FOLLOW-UP

PATIENT MONITORING
• Refer to sections on specific endocrine disorders • Muscle strength and mass should return in patients with steroid myopathy with decreased steroid use. This recovery may take weeks.

PREVENTION/AVOIDANCE N/A

POSSIBLE COMPLICATIONS
Refer to sections on specific endocrine disorders

EXPECTED COURSE AND PROGNOSIS
• Prognosis is poor for resolution of myotonia

in patients with hyperadrenocorticism • Prognosis good for return of muscle strength and mass with steroid myopathy • Improvement in muscle pain and stiffness likely with hypothyroid myopathy • Prognosis good for return of muscle strength in feline hyperthyroidism with return to euthyroid state • Prognosis good for return of muscle strength with hypoadrenocorticism • Dysphagia and regurgitation may resolve with adequate treatment

MISCELLANEOUS

ASSOCIATED CONDITIONS
• Multiple endocrinopathies may be present

• Myasthenia gravis may occur concurrently in some hypothyroid dogs

AGE RELATED FACTORS N/A

ZOONOTIC POTENTIAL N/A

PREGNANCY Unknown

SYNONYMS N/A

SEE ALSO N/A

ABBREVIATIONS N/A

References

LeCouteur RA, Dow SW, Sisson AF. Metabolic and endocrine myopathies of dogs and cats. Sem Vet Med Surg (Small Anim) 1989;4:146-155.

Shelton GD, Cardinet III GH. Pathophysiologic basis of canine muscle disorders. J Vet Int Med 1987;1:36-44.

Jaggy A, Oliver JE, Ferguson DC, et al. Neurological manifestations of hypothyroidism: A retrospective study of 29 cases. J Vet Int Med 1994;8:328.

Author G. Diane Shelton

Consulting Editor Peter D. Schwarz

MYOPATHY, NONINFLAMMATORY—HEREDITARY LABRADOR RETRIEVER

BASICS

OVERVIEW
• An inherited progressive and degenerative generalized myopathy of Labrador retrievers • Simple autosomal recessive mode of inheritance • Pathophysiologic mechanism(s) unknown • Histologic examination of muscle is more typical of a neurogenic rather than a myopathic cause but no morphologic changes in the CNS or peripheral nerves have been identified.

SIGNALMENT
• Seen in both black and yellow Labrador retrievers. • Males and females can be affected. • Age of onset is variable (6 weeks to 7 months) but most commonly 3-4 months

SIGNS
• Severity of clinical signs varies and may include stilted gait, muscle weakness, "bunny hopping" pelvic limb gait, ventroflexion of the neck, arched back, and abnormal joint posture (cow hocked stance, hyperextended carpii). • Clinical signs worsen with exercise and dogs may collapse with forced exercise. • Rest results in some improvement. • Signs are made worse by excitement and cold weather. • Generalized muscle atrophy varies from mild to severe. • Atrophy of proximal limb and masticatory muscles is often most prominent. • Tendon reflexes may be normal, hypoactive, or absent. • Occasionally dogs become recumbent or develop megaesophagus.

CAUSE AND RISK FACTORS
Autosomal recessive mode of inheritance

DIAGNOSIS

DIFFERENTIAL DIAGNOSIS
• In dogs with little muscle atrophy, exercise intolerance may mimic signs of myasthenia gravis or cardiac or orthopaedic disease. • In dogs with marked muscle atrophy, other myopathies (infectious, immune-mediated, metabolic, congenital) and generalized lower motor neuron disorders should also be considered.

CBC/BIOCHEMISTRY/URINALYSIS
Creatine kinase may be normal or mildly or moderately elevated.

OTHER LABORATORY TESTS N/A

IMAGING N/A

OTHER DIAGNOSTIC PROCEDURES
• Spontaneous activity, including complex repetitive discharges seen on EMG especially in proximal limb and masticatory muscles. Mildly affected dogs may have no EMG abnormalities. • Muscle histology shows variation in fiber size, angular atrophy of both type l and type ll myofibers, grouped atrophy, increase in central nuclei, muscle degeneration and regeneration, and fibrosis. In some cases there is a deficiency in type ll myofibers and in others an increase in type ll myofibers.

TREATMENT
• No specific treatment
• Avoid cold because it exacerbates clinical signs.
• Breeding of affected animals is to be discouraged.

• Dam/sire breedings that result in offspring with this myopathy should not be repeated.

MEDICATIONS

DRUGS AND FLUIDS
Diazepam may be beneficial.

CONTRAINDICATIONS/POSSIBLE INTERACTIONS None known

FOLLOW-UP
• Clinical signs generally stabilize. • Mildly affected dogs can be acceptable pets and, with time, may show some improvement in exercise tolerance. • Aspiration pneumonia a risk in dogs with megaesophagus

MISCELLANEOUS

ASSOCIATED CONDITIONS N/A
AGE RELATED FACTORS N/A
ZOONOTIC POTENTIAL N/A
PREGNANCY N/A

Reference

McKerrell RE, Braud KG. Hereditary myopathy of Labrador retrievers. In: Kirk RW, Bonagura JD, eds. Current veterinary therapy X. Philadelphia: WB Saunders, 1989:820-821.

Author Georgina Child
Consulting Editor Peter D. Schwarz

MYOPATHY, NONINFLAMMATORY—HEREDITARY MYOTONIA

BASICS

OVERVIEW
• Myopathy characterized by persistent contraction of muscle fibers on initiation of movement or when stimulated to contract
• Can affect all skeletal muscles • Condition may be congenital or acquired • Congenital myotonia may be associated with abnormal chloride conductance of muscle membrane.

SIGNALMENT
Congenital myotonia is described in young chow chows and rarely other dog breeds.

SIGNS

Historical Findings
• Difficulty rising • Stiffness after rest
• Dyspnea, dysphagia, and/or regurgitation may be seen. • Clinical signs improve with exercise. • Cold exacerbates signs.

Physical Examination Findings
• Proximal limb and neck muscles; tongue hypertrophied • Abduction of thoracic limbs
• "Bunny hopping" pelvic limb gait • May fall and remain rigid in lateral recumbency for short periods

CAUSES AND RISK FACTORS
Autosomal recessive mode of inheritance suspected in chow chows

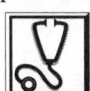

DIAGNOSIS

DIFFERENTIAL DIAGNOSIS
Other myopathies. Distinguished by characteristic signalment, clinical, and electromyographical findings.

CBC/BIOCHEMISTRY/URINALYSIS
Creatinine kinase may be slightly elevated.

OTHER LABORATORY TESTS N/A

IMAGING N/A

OTHER DIAGNOSTIC PROCEDURES
• Percussion of muscles and tongue in conscious and anesthetized dogs causes sustained dimpling. • Electromyography shows multifocal or generalized high frequency discharges that wax and wane in amplitude and frequency ("dive-bomber" sounding potentials). These are increased after muscle percussion.
• Histologic examination of muscle shows mild changes (some angular atrophy, central nuclei, variation in fiber size).

TREATMENT
• Avoid cold.
• Respiratory obstruction caused by adduction of vocal cords or regurgitation is a possible risk when inducing and postanesthesia
• Inherited condition in chow chows, so advise owner regarding breeding.
• Breeding of affected animals is to be discouraged.
• Dam/sire breedings that result in offspring with myotonia should not be repeated.

MEDICATIONS

DRUGS AND FLUIDS
Membrane stabilizing drugs procainamide and quinidine may decrease severity of clinical signs.

CONTRAINDICATIONS/POSSIBLE INTERACTIONS None

FOLLOW-UP
• Prognosis guarded • Signs may stabilize or may worsen with age. • Respiratory obstruction and/or aspiration of regurgitated food can be life-threatening.

MISCELLANEOUS

ASSOCIATED CONDITIONS N/A

AGE RELATED FACTORS N/A

ZOONOTIC POTENTIAL N/A

PREGNANCY N/A

Reference
Duncan ID, Griffiths IR. Myotonia in the dog. In: Kirk RW, ed. Current veterinary therapy VIII. Philadelphia: WB Saunders, 1983:686-689.

Author Georgina Child
Consulting Editor Peter D. Schwarz

MYOPATHY, NONINFLAMMATORY—HEREDITARY SCOTTY CRAMP

BASICS

OVERVIEW
• Inherited neurologic disorder in Scottish terriers characterized by episodic muscle hypertonicity or cramping • It is not associated with any morphologic changes in muscle, peripheral nerve, or CNS. • The abnormality is thought to be the result of disordered serotonin metabolism within the CNS.

SIGNALMENT
A similar condition reported in young dalmatians and Labrador retrievers may be result of low number of neurotransmitter glycine receptors in the CNS.

SIGNS
• Affected dogs are normal at rest and on initial exercise. • With further exercise or excitement, clinical signs become apparent, including abduction of the thoracic limbs, arching of the lumbar spine, and stiffening or overflexion of the pelvic limbs (goose stepping gait). • Dogs may fall with tail and pelvic limbs flexed tightly against the body, respiration may cease for a short time, and facial muscles may be contracted. • No loss of consciousness. Severity of signs varies. • Episodes may last up to 30 minutes.

CAUSES AND RISK FACTORS
Inherited condition with probable recessive mode of transmission

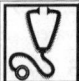

DIAGNOSIS

DIFFERENTIAL DIAGNOSIS
Seizure disorder. Scotty cramp distinguished on basis of family history, typical clinical signs with no loss of consciousness, and induction of signs with serotonin antagonists.

CBC/BIOCHEMISTRY/URINALYSIS
No abnormalities

OTHER LABORATORY TESTS N/A

IMAGING N/A

OTHER DIAGNOSTIC PROCEDURES
Clinical signs may be induced with serotonin antagonist methysergide.

TREATMENT
• Behavioral modification and/or environmental changes to eliminate situations triggering episodes of cramping (excitement, stress) may be adequate treatment.
• Breeding of affected animals is to be discouraged.
• Dam/sire breedings that result in offspring with Scotty cramp should not be repeated.

MEDICATIONS

DRUGS AND FLUIDS
Acepromazine, diazepam, or vitamin E may reduce the incidence and severity of episodes.

CONTRAINDICATIONS/POSSIBLE INTERACTIONS
• Serotonin antagonists increase severity of clinical signs.
• Aspirin, indomethacin, phenylbutazone, banamine, and penicillin may exacerbate clinical signs.

FOLLOW-UP
Disorder is nonprogressive

MISCELLANEOUS

ASSOCIATED CONDITIONS N/A

AGE RELATED FACTORS N/A

ZOONOTIC POTENTIAL N/A

PREGNANCY N/A

ABBREVIATIONS
CNS = central nervous system

Reference
Meyers KM, Clemmons RM. Scotty cramp. In: Kirk RW, ed. Current veterinary therapy Vlll. Philadelphia: WB Saunders, 1983:702-704.

Author Georgina Child
Consulting Editor Peter D. Schwarz

MYOPATHY, NONINFLAMMATORY—HEREDITARY X-LINKED MUSCULAR DYSTROPHY

BASICS

OVERVIEW
• Inherited, progressive, and degenerative generalized myopathy with X-linked mode of inheritance • Affected dogs lack muscle membrane associated protein dystrophin. • An RNA processing defect has been identified in golden retrievers, Irish terriers, Samoyeds, rottweilers, Belgian shepherds, and one miniature schnauzer.

SIGNALMENT
• The disease also has been described in cats. • Seen primarily in males • Females carry the gene defect but homozygotes also may be affected.

SIGNS
• Clinical signs described in golden retrievers include exercise intolerance, stilted gait, "bunny hopping" pelvic limb gait, plantigrade stance, partial trismus, muscle atrophy (especially the truncal and temporalis muscles), hypertrophy of some muscles (especially the tongue), kyphosis, lordosis, drooling, dysphagia, and aspiration pneumonia as a result of pharyngeal and/or esophageal involvement. • Clinical signs vary in severity, onset, and progression but may be seen as early as 6 weeks and tend to stabilize by 6 months. • Stunting and ineffective suckling may be evident in younger pups. • Cardiac failure as a result of cardiomyopathy and severe muscle contractures may occur. • Spinal reflexes are normal initially but may become hypoactive. • Clinical signs in other dog breeds are similar and include vomiting and megaesophagus. • Clinical signs in dystrophin deficient cats include muscle hypertrophy, stiff gait, cervical rigidity, exercise intolerance, and vomiting. • Clinical signs were not apparent in one cat until 21 months of age.

CAUSES AND RISK FACTORS
Inherited defect on X chromosome

DIAGNOSIS

DIFFERENTIAL DIAGNOSIS
Other inherited, infectious (protozoal), immune-mediated, or metabolic myopathies. Distinguished by histologic examination of muscle and demonstration of dystrophin deficiency.

CBC/BIOCHEMISTRY/URINALYSIS
Marked elevation in serum creatine kinase (may be > 10,000 UL); further increase after exercise

OTHER LABORATORY TESTS
Dystrophin deficiency demonstrated immunocytochemically or by Western blot analysis

IMAGING N/A

OTHER DIAGNOSTIC PROCEDURES
• Electromyography shows complex repetitive discharges. • Histologic examination of muscle shows muscle fiber necrosis and regeneration, presence of myofiber mineralization that may be dramatic, and myofiber hypertrophy that may be variation in myofiber size or fibrosis

TREATMENT
• No proven effective treatment
• Breeding of affected animals is to be discouraged.

• Dam/sire breedings that result in offspring with X-linked muscular dystrophy should not be repeated.

MEDICATIONS

DRUGS AND FLUIDS
Glucocorticosteriods may provide some improvement (reason unknown).

CONTRAINDICATIONS/POSSIBLE INTERACTIONS None

FOLLOW-UP
• Signs tend to stabilize at 6 months in golden retrievers. • Progression in other breeds and cats variable • Aspiration pneumonia or cardiomyopathy may be life-threatening.

MISCELLANEOUS

ASSOCIATED CONDITIONS N/A

AGE RELATED FACTORS N/A

ZOONOTIC POTENTIAL N/A

PREGNANCY N/A

Reference

Kornegay JN. The X-linked muscular dystrophies. In: Kirk RW, Bonagura JD, eds. Current veterinary therapy XI. Philadelphia: WB Saunders, 1992:1042-1047.

Author Georgina Child
Consulting Editor Peter D. Schwarz

MYOPATHY, NONINFLAMMATORY—METABOLIC

BASICS

DEFINITION
Metabolic myopathies are those associated with disorders of glycogen metabolism, lipid metabolism, or oxidative-phosphorylation and mitochondrial metabolism. Currently they are poorly characterized in veterinary medicine.

Pathophysiology
This group of disorders is usually associated with inherited or acquired enzyme defects involving major metabolic pathways. This may result in storage of the abnormal metabolic by-product or morphologic abnormalities of mitochondria.

Systems Affected
• Neuromuscular—dependence on oxidative metabolism for energy • Nervous system—dependence on glycolytic and oxidative metabolism for energy • Cardiovascular—dependence on oxidative metabolism for energy • Hemic/lymphatic—red blood cells dependent on glycolytic metabolism

Genetics
Not yet determined for any of the metabolic myopathies

Incidence/Prevalence
Most metabolic myopathies, with the exception of the lipid storage myopathies, are rare.

Geographic Distribution
Unknown, probably worldwide

SIGNALMENT

Species Dogs and cats

Breed Predilections
• Inherited muscle phosphofructokinase deficiency—English springer spaniels • Acid maltase deficiency—Lapland dogs • Debranching enzyme deficiency—German shepherds • Suspected mitochondrial abnormalities—clumber spaniel, Sussex spaniel, Old English sheepdog

Mean Age and Range
• Inherited metabolic defects, approximately 2-3 months • Acquired metabolic defects, adult animals

Predominant Sex
No sex predominance has been found.

SIGNS

General Comments
Very few metabolic myopathies have been adequately described. Our knowledge in this area should greatly expand in the coming years.

Historical Findings
• Muscular weakness, exercise intolerance, cramping, and collapse • Regurgitation and/or dysphagia, and esophageal and/or pharyngeal abnormalities • Dark colored urine, myoglobinuria, and hemoglobinuria • Encephalopathy • Vomiting

Physical Examination Findings
• Exercise-related weakness, stiffness, and cramping • Abnormal neurological examination, disorientation, stupor, and coma • Abdominal distension, and storage product accumulation in liver • May be normal in appearance with fluctuating clinical signs

CAUSES
• Inborn error of metabolism • Acquired metabolic defect, viral infections, drug-induced, and environmental factors

RISK FACTORS
• Inherited disorders and appropriate genetic background • Others unknown

DIAGNOSIS

DIFFERENTIAL DIAGNOSIS
• Inflammatory myopathies; muscle biopsy should differentiate • Other noninflammatory myopathies; muscle biopsy should differentiate • Other metabolic encephalopathies; laboratory evaluation should differentiate

CBC/BIOCHEMISTRY/URINALYSIS
• Elevated resting or postexcercise plasma lactate concentration in patients with disorders of fatty acid oxidation or oxidative phosphorylation • No elevation in postexercise plasma lactate with glycolytic disorders • Serum creatine kinase concentration may be elevated with exercise and normal at rest or persistently elevated. • Hypoglycemia may be present with some glycolytic and oxidative disorders. • Hyperammonemia may be present with urea cycle defects.

OTHER LABORATORY TESTS
• Quantitation of plasma and urine amino acids - abnormal accumulations • Quantitation of urine organic acids - demonstrates abnormal organic acid production • Quantitation of plasma, urine, and muscle carnitine - may be low with primary disorders of carnitine, and primary organic acidurias • Specific enzyme assays depending on suspected metabolic defect • Establish fibroblast cultures for study of metabolic defect

IMAGING
Evaluation of the central nervous system by magnetic resonance imaging; abnormalities found in humans with metabolic encephalopathies

OTHER DIAGNOSTIC PROCEDURES
• Muscle biopsy—demonstration of storage products (glycogen, lipid) or abnormal mitochondria by light microscopy using fresh frozen muscle sections • Electron microscopy of muscle—abnormal mitochondria and paracrystalline inclusions, glycogen accumulation • Cardiovascular system evaluation—may have concurrent cardiomyopathy • Other organ biopsies if organomegaly

GROSS AND HISTOPATHOLOGIC FINDINGS
• Triglyceride droplets in muscle, lipid stor-
age myopathy • Ragged red fibers in muscle, mitochondrial myopathy • Glycogen deposition in muscle, glycogen storage disorders

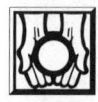

TREATMENT

INPATIENT VERSUS OUTPATIENT
• May require intensive care if patients have severe encephalopathy, seizures, lactic acidemia, hypoglycemia, or hyperammonemia • If clinical signs are only related to neuromuscular system, may treat on an outpatient basis

ACTIVITY
Exercise restriction if patient has muscle weakness, stiffness, or collapse induced by exercise

DIET
• Avoid prolonged periods of fasting. • Dietary restrictions may be made depending on underlying metabolic defect. • Vitamin and cofactor therapy as determined by underlying defect

CLIENT EDUCATION
• Most inherited metabolic defects are not curable at present time. Some are treatable. • Advise not breeding affected animals.

SURGICAL CONSIDERATIONS N/A

MEDICATIONS

DRUGS AND FLUIDS
• Specific treatments depend on the metabolic abnormality and clinical signs. • Lipid storage myopathies - L-carnitine (50 mg/kg q12h, PO), riboflavin (50-100 mg/day PO), coenzyme Q (1mg/kg daily PO) • Mitochondrial myopathies, may benefit from therapy similar to that for lipid storage myopathies

CONTRAINDICATIONS
None known at this time

PRECAUTIONS
Avoid fasting and strenuous exercise if precipitates clinical signs

POSSIBLE INTERACTIONS N/A

ALTERNATE DRUGS N/A

FOLLOW-UP

PATIENT MONITORING
• Lipid storage myopathies, return of muscle strength, and elimination of muscle pain • Serum CK should return to normal if previously elevated

PREVENTION/AVOIDANCE N/A

POSSIBLE COMPLICATIONS
Severe neurologic impairment

EXPECTED COURSE AND PROGNOSIS
• Poor if an untreatable disorder • Lipid storage myopathies may be good without underlying organic acidemia.

MISCELLANEOUS

ASSOCIATED CONDITIONS
• Iatrogenic and naturally occuring Cushing's syndrome; lipid storage myopathies have been found in some dogs • Hemolytic anemia due to underlying metabolic defect

AGE RELATED FACTORS
Inborn errors usually in young dogs.
• Acquired defects in adult dogs

ZOONOTIC POTENTIAL N/A

PREGNANCY Unknown

SYNONYMS
• Lipid storage myopathies • Mitochondrial myopathies • Glycogen storage disorders • Cori's disease (glycogenosis type III) • Phosphofructokinase deficiency (glycogenosis type VII) • Acid maltase deficiency (glycogenosis type II)

SEE ALSO N/A

ABBREVIATION
CK = serum creatine kinase

References
LeCouteur RA, Dow SW, Sisson AF. Metabolic and endocrine myopathies of dogs and cats. Sem Vet Med Surg (Small Animal) 1989;4:146-155.
Shelton GD. Canine lipid storage myopathies. In: Bonagura JD, Kirk RW, eds. Current veterinary therapy XII. Philadelphia: WB Saunders, 1995;1161-1163.
Shelton GD, Gardinet GH III. Pathophysiologic basis of canine muscle disorders. J Vet Int Med 1987;1:36-44.
Author G. Diane Shelton
Consulting Editor Peter D. Schwarz

MYXEDEMA AND MYXEDEMA COMA

BASICS

OVERVIEW

• Myxedema coma is a severe clinical syndrome of long-standing, untreated hypothyroidism characterized by hypothermia, mental dullness, bradycardia, hypoventilation, hypotension, and depression or coma. • The condition derives its name from the characteristic, nonpitting edema that develops in almost any organ as a result of severe hypothyroidism. • Pathogenesis is unclear, but clinical signs may be caused by a profound reduction of metabolic activity and oxidative processes throughout the body. • Mortality rate is high.

SIGNALMENT

Only four dogs with myxedema coma are described in the veterinary literature. Three were doberman pinschers. Two were intact males, and two intact females. Age ranged from 2.5- 5 years.

SIGNS

• Typical signs of hypothyroidism (see Hypothyroidism) • Profound hypothermia (usually without shivering) • Nonpitting edema of the skin (especially the face, resulting in "tragic facies") • Mental dullness ranging from depression to complete unresponsiveness • Bradycardia with cyanosis

CAUSES AND RISK FACTORS

• Myxedema coma develops in patients with long-standing, untreated hypothyroidism stressed by infection, trauma, or exposure to cold. • Neurologic or respiratory depressant medication may also predispose to the development of coma.

DIAGNOSIS

DIFFERENTIAL DIAGNOSIS

• Metabolic disturbances • Addisonian crisis • Ketoacidotic diabetes mellitus • Hypoglycemia

• Hepatoencephalopathy • Cardiac failure

CBC/BIOCHEMISTRY/URINALYSIS

• Mild normocytic normochromic anemia • Hypercholesterolemia • Hypoglycemia • Hyponatremia (probably dilutional)

OTHER LABORATORY TESTS

Thyroxine concentration and response to TSH stimulation are usually severely depressed (see hypothyroidism).

IMAGING N/A

OTHER DIAGNOSTIC PROCEDURES
N/A

TREATMENT

Myxedema coma is a medical emergency. Rapid replacement of thyroid hormone is important to successful treatment since most signs are caused by profound hypometabolism. Once euthyroidism is restored, normal metabolic processes contribute considerably to recovery.

MEDICATIONS

DRUGS AND FLUIDS

• Hormone replacement—administer 0.02mg/kg IV (or 0.5 mg/m² IV) levothyroxine sodium (Synthroid® powder for injection). The dosage is best titrated to response and should be followed by oral thyroid hormone replacement when possible.
• Supportive care—passive warming with blankets, cautious IV fluid therapy with glucose supplementation if necessary, and oxygen therapy (if results of blood gas analysis warrant).
• Other treatment—corticosteroids recommended because of the potential impairment of the adrenocortical response to stress. Administration of a broad-spectrum antibiotic indicated to treat infection that may predispose to myxedema coma.

CONTRAINDICATIONS/POSSIBLE INTERACTIONS

• Avoid aggressive fluid therapy until thyroid replacement is achieved to support cardiac function.
• Active warming with heating pads may reduce peripheral vascular tone and should be avoided.

FOLLOW-UP

• Successful treatment results in improvement of vital signs within 4-6 hours. However, improvement may be transient unless underlying infection or other stresses are controlled. • Prognosis is grave; all four reported canine patients died or were euthanatized despite aggressive treatment.

MISCELLANEOUS

ABBREVIATIONS

TSH=Thyroid stimulating hormone

References

Chastain CB, Graham CL, Riley MG. Myxedema coma in two dogs. Canine Pract 1982;9:20-34.

Kelly MJ, Hill JR. Canine myxedema stupor and coma. Compend Contin Ed Pract Vet 1984;6:1049-1055.

Author Leland Thompson

Consulting Editor Rhett Nichols

BASICS

OVERVIEW

Sleep Disorders
Narcolepsy
Excessive daytime sleepiness, lethargy, or brief periods of "collapse" and unconsciousness that resolve spontaneously
Cataplexy
Brief episodes of muscle paralysis with loss of tendon reflexes; the animal stays alert and will follow with its eyes. These brief episodes of motor inhibition are completely and spontaneously reversible.

SIGNALMENT
• Multiple breeds of dog. Proven hereditary in Labrador retriever, poodle, dachshund, and doberman pinscher. Genetic studies of Labrador and doberman support a recessive inheritance with complete penetrance.
• Clinical signs usually appear before 6 months of age. • Rare in cats

SIGNS
• Results of physical and neurologic examination normal except during an attack
• Onset of signs is rapid (peracute) in both conditions; attacks usually last only a few seconds to minutes, but can last up to 30 minutes. • Episodes usually characterized by collapse into lateral or sternal recumbency with no movements and atonic muscles • Eye movements, muscular twitching and whining (as in REM sleep), frequently observed during episodes • Animals usually aroused by loud noises, petting, or other external stimuli
• Affected animals can have multiple episodes in one day. • Episodes most commonly elicited during eating, excitement, playing, and sexual activity

CAUSES AND RISK FACTORS
• Unknown • Neurotransmitter disturbance
• Possible immune system involvement

DIAGNOSIS

DIFFERENTIAL DIAGNOSIS
• In contrast with seizure activity—urinary or fecal incontinence, excessive salivation, and muscle rigidity are not characteristic of sleep disorders. • Other considerations for cataplexy—myasthenia gravis, hypoglycemia, hypocalcemia, hypokalemia, adrenal insufficiency, polymyositis, syncope, and nonconvulsive seizure (drop attacks) • Other considerations for narcolepsy—hypothyroidism, chronic hypoxia, obesity (Pickwickian syndrome), and other metabolic illnesses.

CBC/BIOCHEMISTRY/URINALYSIS
Results normal; tests only performed to rule out differentials.

OTHER LABORATORY TESTS N/A

IMAGING N/A

OTHER DIAGNOSTIC PROCEDURES
• If a consistent activity that elicits attacks can be identified, attempt to simulate the activity so that an attack can be observed. This will probably only be helpful in severely affected animals. • Food elicited cataplexy test—place 10 pieces of food in a row 12-24 inches apart. Record the time required for the patient to eat all the pieces and the number, type, and duration of any cataplectic attacks that occur. Normal dogs eat all food in < 45 seconds and have no attacks; cataplectic dogs take > 2 minutes to eat the food and can have 2-20 attacks. • Yohimbine challenge—give 25-50 mcg/kg IV bolus. A positive test is a 90% reduction in the number or severity of cataplectic attacks. The response should take place within 20-30 minutes after administration and last for about 4 hours. • Physostigmine challenge—give 0.025 mg/kg IV; 5-15 minutes after the injection, repeat the food-elicited cataplexy test. May have to increase dosage (0.05 mg/kg, 0.075 mg/kg, and 0.10 mg/kg). This test produces signs in affected patients, causing up to a 300% increase in the number and duration of episodes. The effects of each dose last 15-45 minutes.

TREATMENT
• Primary goal is to reduce the severity and frequency of cataplectic attacks.
• Inform client that cataplexy is not a fatal disease, that choking on food and airway obstruction do not occur, that the pet is not suffering but that situations like hunting, swimming, and unleashed activities put the animal at risk.

MEDICATIONS

DRUGS AND FLUIDS
• Yohimbine (drug of choice)—50-100 mcg/kg SQ or PO q8h-q12h
• Imipramine (Tofranil—0.5-1.0 mg/kg PO q8h
• Methylphenidate (Ritalin—5-10 mg PO q24h
• Dextroamphetamine—5-10 mg PO q24h

CONTRAINDICATIONS/POSSIBLE INTERACTIONS
• Many patients develop drug tolerance and change of drug may become necessary
• Monamine oxidase inhibitors contraindicated in dogs because of possible toxic cardiovascular side effects

FOLLOW-UP
• Avoidance of inciting activities may reduce episodes so that medication is not needed.
• Animals with the inherited form may improve with age. • Prognosis varies since the disease is not curable, and even with treatment some patients remain symptomatic.

MISCELLANEOUS

ABBREVIATION N/A

Reference
Fenner WR. Seizures, narcolepsy, and cataplexy. In: Birchard SJ, Sherding RG, eds. Saunders manual of small animal practice. Philadelphia: WB Saunders, 1994: 1147-1156.

Author T. Mark Neer
Consulting Editor Joane M. Parent

NASAL AND NASOPHARYNGEAL POLYPS

BASICS

OVERVIEW
• Polyps are protruding, pink, polypoid growths (benign) from the mucous membranes. • Nasal polyps originate from the nasal mucosa in dogs and cats. • Nasopharyngeal polyps originate from the base of the eustachian tube in cats. • The nasopharyngeal polyps can extend into the external ear canal and the middle ear as well as the pharynx and nasal cavity.

SIGNALMENT
• Nasopharyngeal polyps in kittens and young adults • Nasal polyps can occur in dogs or cats.

SIGNS

Nasal Polyps
Signs are nonresponsive to antibiotic therapy or are recurrent. • Chronic mucopurulent nasal discharge • Noisy breathing • Nasal congestion • Sneezing or epistaxis • Unilateral decreased nasal airflow

Nasopharyngeal Polyps
• Signs as above • Inspiratory dyspnea • Dysphagia • Chronic nonresponsive otitis • Head tilt • Horner's syndrome

CAUSES AND RISK FACTORS
The origin of either polyp type is unknown.

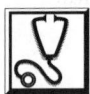

DIAGNOSIS

DIFFERENTIAL DIAGNOSIS
• Upper respiratory infection • Upper airway obstruction • Chronic otitis • Neurologic disease • Nasopharyngeal stenosis • Foreign body • Neoplasia

CBC/BIOCHEMISTRY/URINALYSIS
N/A

OTHER LABORATORY TESTS N/A

IMAGING

Nasal Polyps
Radiographs of the nasal cavity may show a soft tissue structure within the nasal passages.

Nasopharyngeal Polyps
• Radiographs show a soft tissue mass within the nasopharynx. • Radiographs should be closely evaluated for involvement of the tympanic bullae.

OTHER DIAGNOSTIC PROCEDURES
• Rhinoscopy allows visualization and biopsy of the mass. • Palpation and visual examination of the nasopharynx often reveal the presence of a polyp. • Deep otoscopic examination

TREATMENT
• Polyps should be treated surgically; surgical excision via the oral cavity or rhinotomy in the case of nasal polyps.
• Concurrent bulla osteotomy may prevent recurrence of nasopharyngeal polyps.

MEDICATIONS

DRUGS AND FLUIDS
Therapy for secondary bacterial or yeast infections in the nasal or otic cavity should be employed.

CONTRAINDICATIONS/POSSIBLE INTERACTIONS N/A

FOLLOW-UP
• Incomplete removal of the polyp and stalk may result in recurrence.
• Horner's syndrome or facial paralysis may occur after bulla osteotomy. They are generally transient.

MISCELLANEOUS N/A

Reference
Ettinger SJ, Feldman EC. Textbook of veterinary internal medicine. 4th ed. Philadelphia: WB Saunders, 1995.
Author James C. Prueter
Consulting Editors Lynelle Johnson and Bradley L. Moses

BASICS

OVERVIEW
Formation of a thin but tough membrane at the internal nasal meatus, resulting in the narrowing of this orifice from a 5-6 mm oval opening to a 1-2 mm diameter opening. The presence of chronic inflammation and fibrosis on histologic examination suggests an infectious or allergic etiology.

SIGNALMENT
• Cats of any breed or sex may be affected. Patients have ranged in age from 8 months to 10 years old. • It would seem that any age cat could present with this disease entity as long as ample time has passed since exposure to the inciting cause.

SIGNS
• Evidence of upper respiratory obstruction • Whistling or snoring noise • Minimal nasal discharge • Duration of at least several months • Aggravation of signs during eating • Failure to respond to antibiotics and corticosteroids

CAUSES AND RISK FACTORS
• Viral upper respiratory or chlamydial infections • Foreign body or irritant contacting affected area

DIAGNOSIS

DIFFERENTIAL DIAGNOSIS
• Nasopharyngeal polyps (can be visualized during oral examination or by radiographic evaluation) • Chronic rhinitis or sinusitis (moderate to severe nasal discharge and sneezing; obvious radiographic changes commonly noted) • Foreign bodies (unilateral mucopurulent nasal discharge; radiographic abnormalities) • Intranasal neoplasia (unilateral obstruction; nasal discharge often bloody; radiographic changes) • Mycotic rhinitis (moderate to severe nasal discharge, often hemorrhagic; radiographic changes) • Laryngeal diseases (no improvement with open-mouth breathing; lack of snorting and nasal discharge; abnormalities on oral examination)

CBC/BIOCHEMISTRY/URINALYSIS
N/A

OTHER LABORATORY TESTS N/A

IMAGING
Near normal radiographic findings

OTHER DIAGNOSTIC PROCEDURES
• Inability to pass a 3.5 French catheter through the ventral meatus into the pharynx • Visualization of the membrane using a retroflexed pediatric bronchoscope or a dental mirror

TREATMENT
• Hospitalization and surgery are necessary in all patients. • While under general anesthesia and in dorsal recumbency with the mouth wide open, the soft palate is incised and the membrane resected. • The soft palate is sutured.

MEDICATIONS

DRUGS AND FLUIDS
Postoperative antibiotics are recommended.

CONTRAINDICATIONS/POSSIBLE INTERACTIONS N/A

FOLLOW-UP
• The owner must be warned that recurrences are possible. • High levels of corticosteroids should be considered if a second surgery is necessary.

MISCELLANEOUS

Reference

Mitten RW. Acquired nasopharyngeal stenosis in cats. In: Kirk RW, Bonagura JD, eds. Current veterinary therapy XI. Philadelphia: WB Saunders, 1992;801-803.
Author Justin H. Straus
Consulting Editors Lynelle Johnson and Bradley L. Moses

NEOSPOROSIS

 BASICS

OVERVIEW
• Neospora caninum is a recently recognized coccidian protozoa previously confused with Toxoplasma gondii. Tachyzoites and tissue cysts resemble T. gondii under light microscopy. • Complete life cycle is unknown. • Disease is caused by necrosis associated with tissue damage from cyst rupture and tachyzoite invasion. • Only natural mode of transmission identified at this time is congenital.

SIGNALMENT
• Natural infections occur in dogs. Cats have been experimentally infected. • Puppies mainly infected • Hunting dogs are overrepresented.

SIGNS
• Signs are similar to those of toxoplasmosis except the neurologic and muscular abnormalities predominate and are often more severe.
• Young dogs (< 6 months) more commonly develop ascending paralysis distinguishable from other forms of paralysis by gradual muscle atrophy, and stiffness with pelvic limbs more affected than thoracic limbs. Progresses to rigid contracture of limbs. • Cervical weakness and dysphagia develop with time, eventually leading to death. • Virtually all organs are infected, including skin. • Older dogs usually show CNS involvement (seizures, tremors), polymyositis, myocarditis, and dermatitis.

CAUSES AND RISK FACTORS N/A

 DIAGNOSIS

DIFFERENTIAL DIAGNOSIS
• In young dogs, consider other causes of peripheral multifocal neurologic signs.
• In young dogs, consider infectious diseases (toxoplasmosis, distemper) and progressive polyradiculomyositis.
• Other causes of diffuse lower motor neuron muscular diseases in young dogs are rare.
• In older dogs with CNS disease, consider other infectious diseases (fungal, rabies, pseudorabies), toxicity (lead, organophosphorus, carbamate, chlorinated hydrocarbon, strychnine), nonsuppurative encephalitis, meningitis, granulomatous meningoencephalitis, and metabolic disease (hypoglycemia, hepatic encephalopathy).

CBC/BIOCHEMISTRY/URINALYSIS
CBC, biochemical panel, and urinalysis findings vary depending on the organ system involved. CPK and AST activities can be increased with muscle involvement.

OTHER LABORATORY TESTS
• Serologic testing (IFA) on cerebral spinal fluid (CSF) or serum • Antibodies do not cross-react with T. gondii.

IMAGING N/A

OTHER DIAGNOSTIC PROCEDURES
• Cerebral spinal fluid (CSF)—slight increase in protein and nucleated cell numbers. Cells mainly are mononuclear but neutrophils can be present. • Biopsy—may allow differentiation from T. gondii by its location in host cell cytoplasm and not within a parasitophorous vacuole such as T. gondii. Tissue cysts of N. caninum have thicker walls, and can be differentiated from T. gondii by immunohistochemical staining.

 TREATMENT

• Once muscle contracture or ascending paralysis has occurred, the prognosis for clinical improvement is poor.
• Progression of clinical disease might be arrested by treatment.

MEDICATIONS

DRUGS AND FLUIDS
• See toxoplasmosis • Clindamycin (25-50 mg/kg per day, divided into 2 doses, PO or IM) for at least 2 weeks after clinical signs cleared

CONTRAINDICATIONS/POSSIBLE INTERACTIONS N/A

 FOLLOW-UP

PATIENT MONITORING N/A
Treat for an extended period of time

EXPECTED COURSE AND PROGNOSIS N/A

 MISCELLANEOUS

ZOONOTIC POTENTIAL
Unlike T. gondii, N. caninum has not been identified to have zoonotic potential to date.

ABBREVIATIONS
AST = aspartate aminotransferase
CPK = creatine phosphokinase
CNS = central nervous system
CSF = cerebral spinal fluid

Reference

Dubey JP. Neosporosis. In: Proc. ACVIM 11th Annual Meeting, May 1993:710-712.
Author Stephen C. Barr
Consulting Editor Fred W. Scott

NEPHROLITHIASIS

BASICS

DEFINITION
Nephroliths are uroliths (i.e., polycrystalline concretions or calculi) located in the renal pelvis or collecting diverticula of the kidney. Nephroliths or nephrolith fragments may pass into the ureters (ureteroliths). Nephroliths that are not infected, not causing obstruction or clinical signs, and not progressively enlarging are termed "inactive" nephroliths.

Pathophysiology
Nephroliths can obstruct the renal pelvis or ureter, predispose to pyelonephritis, and result in compressive injury to the renal parenchyma leading to renal failure. See chapters on the different urolith types for pathophysiology of urolithiasis. In cats, nephroliths composed of blood clots mineralized with calcium phosphate can form secondarily to chronic renal hematuria.

Systems Affected
• Renal/Urologic—the urinary tract is affected, with potential for obstruction, recurrent urinary tract infection, and renal failure.
• Obstruction of the renal pelvis or ureter in an animal with pyelonephritis can cause septicemia (urosepsis), thereby affecting any body system.

Genetics N/A

Incidence/Prevalence
• Nephroliths compose approximately 1.3–4% of uroliths in dogs and cats submitted to stone centers for analysis. The true incidence of nephroliths is likely much higher because many animals with nephroliths are asymptomatic. • The most common mineral compositions of nephroliths in dogs submitted for analysis, in descending frequency, are: calcium oxalate, struvite, ammonium urate, mixed, and calcium phosphate. • The most common mineral compositions of nephroliths in cats submitted for analysis, in descending frequency, are: calcium oxalate, matrix, calcium phosphate, mixed, and struvite.

Geographic Distribution N/A

SIGNALMENT

Species Dogs and cats

Breed Predilections
Dogs
• Calcium oxalate nephroliths—miniature schnauzer, lhasa apso, Yorkshire terrier, miniature poodle, and shih tzu • Struvite nephroliths—miniature schnauzer, bichon frise, shih tzu, Yorkshire terrier, lhasa apso, cocker spaniel, and miniature poodle • Urate nephroliths—Dalmatian, Yorkshire terrier, and English bulldog
Cats
• Domestic shorthair (43%), domestic longhair (13%), Siamese (8%), and Persian (4%).

In another study, Siamese cats appeared to be predisposed compared with the overall hospital population.

Mean Age and Range
Dogs—mean age of affected animals is 9 years (range, 4 months to 14 years)
Cats—mean age of affected animals is 8 years (range, 2 months to 18 years)

Predominant Sex
• Overall, nephroliths in dogs slightly more common in females (55%) than males (41%) with 4% unspecified • Struvite nephroliths—female > males • Calcium oxalate, cystine, and urate nephroliths—males > females
• Male cats (67%) more commonly affected than female cats (33%)

SIGNS

General Comments
Many patients are asymptomatic, and the nephroliths are diagnosed during work-up of other problems.

Historical Findings
No signs or hematuria, vomiting, recurrent urinary tract infection, and dysuria or pollakiuria in animals with urinary tract infection • Signs attributable to uremia in animals with bilateral obstruction or renal failure • Signs referable to lower urinary tract urolithiasis if uroliths are present in the upper and lower urinary tract • So-called "renal colic" in animals with acute abdominal or lumbar pain and vomiting is uncommon.

Physical Examination Findings
Abdominal or lumbar pain on palpation

CAUSES
For an extensive list of causes, see chapters on each urolith type. Oversaturation of the urine with calculogenic minerals may contribute to urolithiasis. • Calcium oxalate urolithiasis—hypercalciuria, hypercalcemia, hypocitraturia, hyperoxaluria, primary hyperparathyroidism, and excessive dietary calcium intake • Calcium phosphate urolithiasis—chronic renal bleeding (cats), hypercalcemia, hyperparathyroidism, excessive dietary calcium and phosphorus, and renal tubular acidosis • Cystine urolithiasis—cystinuria
• Struvite urolithiasis—pyelonephritis, urinary tract infection with urease-producing microbes, and diets that produce alkaline urine • Urate urolithiasis—genetic defect in conversion of uric acid to allantoin (Dalmatians) and portosystemic shunt
• Xanthine urolithiasis—allopurinol administration and high dietary purine intake in dogs predisposed to urate urolithiasis

RISK FACTORS
Alkaline urine for struvite and calcium phosphate uroliths • Acid urine for calcium oxalate, cystine, urate, and xanthine uroliths • Urine retention and formation of highly concentrated urine • Lower urinary tract infection for ascending infection and pyelonephritis • Additional risk factors include conditions that predispose to urinary

tract infection (e.g., perineal urethrostomy, ectopic ureters, and hyperadrenocorticism), vesicoureteral reflux, and exogenous steroid administration or hyperadrenocorticism (calcium oxalate uroliths).

DIAGNOSIS

DIFFERENTIAL DIAGNOSIS
Nephroliths should be considered in any patient with renal failure, recurrent urinary tract infection, acute vomiting (e.g., acute pancreatitis, acute gastroenteritis, intestinal and gastric obstruction), or abdominal or lumbar pain (e.g., intervertebral disc protrusion and peritonitis). Nephroliths are usually confirmed by radiographs or ultrasonography. In cats, mineralization of the renal pelvis or collecting diverticula must be differentiated from true nephrolithiasis.

CBC/BIOCHEMISTRY/URINALYSIS
CBC results are usually normal unless the patient has pyelonephritis. Animals with pyelonephritis may have leukocytosis and neutrophilia with a left shift. • Serum biochemistry analysis is usually normal unless bilateral obstruction, pyelonephritis, or compressive renal injury leads to renal failure (azotemia with an inappropriate urine specific gravity, hyperphosphatemia). Hypercalcemia may contribute to formation of calcium oxalate or calcium phosphate nephroliths in some patients. • Urinalysis may reveal hematuria and crystalluria; crystal type may indicate mineral composition of the nephrolith(s). Pyuria, proteinuria, and bacteriuria may also be seen in animals with urinary tract infection.

OTHER LABORATORY TESTS
Submit all retrieved nephroliths or nephrolith fragments for quantitative analysis to allow implementation of appropriate preventative strategies. Although definitive identification of nephrolith type requires quantitative analysis, nephrolith composition can frequently be predicted on the basis of signalment, radiographic appearance, and urinalysis findings. • Results of bacterial culture of urine may confirm urinary tract infection in animals with concurrent pyelonephritis.

IMAGING
Radiopaque nephroliths (e.g., calcium phosphate, calcium oxalate, and struvite) can be detected by survey radiography. Cystine, urate, and xanthine are radiolucent to slightly radiopaque. • Ultrasonography or excretory urography may confirm the presence, size, and number of nephroliths or ureteroliths regardless of radiographic density.

OTHER DIAGNOSTIC PROCEDURES
After extracorporeal shock wave lithotripsy (ESWL), nephrolith fragments can be retrieved for quantitative analysis by voiding, catheter-assisted retrieval, or voiding urohydropropulsion.

GROSS AND HISTOPATHOLOGIC FINDINGS

Histopathologic examination is not required except to confirm the presence of secondary renal lesions.

TREATMENT

INPATIENT VERSUS OUTPATIENT
Animals with inactive nephroliths are managed as outpatients. Medical dissolution protocols can be administered to outpatients. Removal of nephroliths by surgery or ESWL requires hospitalization.

ACTIVITY Unlimited

DIET
Medical dissolution of nephroliths requires feeding an appropriate diet for the specific nephrolith type. See Medications section.

CLIENT EDUCATION
• Inactive nephroliths may not require removal; however, they should be monitored periodically by urinalysis, urine culture, and radiography. Inactive nephroliths have the potential to cause obstruction at any time, which can result in hydronephrosis without clinical signs. Therefore, conservative management and monitoring of inactive nephroliths is associated with a slight risk of undetected and potentially irreversible renal damage. This risk must be weighed against the potential renal damage caused by nephrotomy.
• Nephroliths (especially metabolic uroliths) tend to recur after removal; therefore, the patient should be monitored periodically.

SURGICAL CONSIDERATIONS
• Indications for removal of nephroliths include obstruction, recurrent infection, symptomatic nephroliths, progressive nephrolith enlargement, and a nonfunctional contralateral kidney.
• Treatment options for nephroliths include medical dissolution, surgery, and ESWL. Calcium oxalate nephroliths, the most common mineral compostion in dogs and cats, are not amenable to medical dissolution. Ureteroliths or obstructing nephroliths are also not amenable to medical dissolution.
• Surgical options include nephrotomy and pyelolithotomy. Because the nephroliths are surrounded by renal tissue, nephrotomy is required in most dogs and cats. Nephrolith removal by percutaneous nephrolithomy has also been reported in dogs experimentally.
• ESWL is a safe and effective method of treating nephroliths and ureteroliths in dogs. Nephrolith fragments pass down the ureter into the bladder and are voided in the urine. Cats have not been treated with ESWL.

MEDICATIONS

DRUGS AND FLUIDS
• Antibiotics on the basis of urine culture and sensitivity testing as needed. Periprocedural antibiotics are recommended when infected nephroliths are treated by ESWL or are surgically removed.
• Medical dissolution protocols are limited to struvite, urate, and cystine uroliths.
• Medical dissolution protocols for *struvite* nephroliths include a calculolytic diet (Prescription Diet s/d, Hill's Pet Products) and appropriate antibiotic administration (i.e., if patient has urinary tract infection) for the duration of treatment.
• Medical dissolution of canine *urate* nephroliths can be attempted by a protein- and purine-restricted, alkalinizing diet (Prescription Diet Canine u/d, Hill's Pet Products), allopurinol (15 mg/kg PO q12h), and supplemental potassium citrate as needed to maintain a urine pH of approximately 7.0.
• Medical dissolution of canine *cystine* nephroliths can be attempted by a protein-restricted, alkalinizing diet (Prescription Diet Canine u/d, Hill's Pet Products), 2-MPG (Thiola®, 15 mg/kg PO q12h), and supplemental potassium citrate as needed to maintain a urine pH of approximately 7.5.

CONTRAINDICATIONS
• Allopurinol should not be used without dietary purine restriction because it may cause xanthine nephrolithiasis in dogs predisposed to urate urolithiasis.
• Acidifying diets should not be fed to azotemic patients.

PRECAUTIONS N/A

POSSIBLE INTERACTIONS N/A

ALTERNATE DRUGS N/A

FOLLOW-UP

PATIENT MONITORING
Abdominal radiography (ultrasonography for radiolucent uroliths), urinalysis, and urine culture every 3 to 6 months to monitor for nephrolith recurrence. Dogs treated with ESWL should be monitored every 2 to 4 weeks by radiographs and ultrasonography until nephrolith fragments have passed out through the excretory system.

PREVENTION/AVOIDANCE
Elimination of factors predisposing to individual urolith type, augmentation of urine volume, and correction of factors contributing to urine retention

POSSIBLE COMPLICATIONS
Hydronephrosis, renal failure, recurrent urinary tract infection, and pyelonephritis

EXPECTED COURSE AND PROGNOSIS
• Course is highly variable depending on nephrolith type, location, and size, and the presence of secondary complications (e.g., obstruction, infection, and renal failure).
• Inactive nephroliths may remain inactive for years, resulting in an excellent prognosis.
• The prognosis for patients with renal failure caused by nephrolithiasis is determined by the severity and rate of progression of the renal failure. • We have had excellent results treating dogs with nephroliths with ESWL, including a return to normal health and an excellent prognosis.

MISCELLANEOUS

ASSOCIATED CONDITIONS
Hyperadrenocorticism and chronic glucocorticoid administration are associated with calcium oxalate uroliths and urinary tract infections that cause struvite urolithiasis.

AGE RELATED FACTORS
Geriatric dogs that are poor surgical candidates can be treated with ESWL.

ZOONOTIC POTENTIAL N/A

PREGNANCY
Pregnancy is a contraindication to ESWL.

SYNONYMS
• Kidney stones • Renal calculi • Renoliths • Kidney calculi

SEE ALSO
• Renal Failure, Chronic • Hydronephrosis
• Pyelonephritis • Urinary Tract Obstruction
• Urolithiasis, Calcium Oxalate • Urolithiasis, Calcium Phosphate • Urolithiasis, Cystine • Urolithiasis, Struvite—Cats
• Urolithiasis, Struvite—Dogs • Urolithiasis, Urate • Urolithiasis, Xanthine

ABBREVIATIONS
ESWL = extracorporeal shock wave lithotripsy

References

Block G, Adams LG, Widmer WR, et al. The use of extracorporeal shock wave lithotripsy for treatment of spontaneous nephrolithiasis and ureterolithiasis in dogs. J Am Vet Med Assoc 1995;208:531-536.

Osborne CA, Lulich JP, Polzin DJ, et al. Canine and feline nephrolithiasis: causes and cure. In: Proceedings, 11th Annu Forum Am Col Vet Int Med 1993;370-373.

Carter WO, Hawkins EC, Morrison WB. Feline nephrolithiasis: eight cases (1984 through 1989). J Am Anim Hosp Assoc 1993;29:247-256.

Stone EA. Canine nephrotomy. Compend Contin Ed Pract Vet 1987;9:883-888.

Author Larry G. Adams
Consulting Editors Larry G. Adams and Carl A. Osborne

NEPHROTIC SYNDROME

 BASICS

DEFINITION

Nephrotic syndrome is characterized by the combination of clinically important proteinuria, hypoalbuminemia, ascites or edema, and hypercholesterolemia. In addition, systemic hypertension and hypercoagulability are commonly associated. Nephrotic syndrome usually occurs secondary to either glomerulonephritis or amyloidosis.

Pathophysiology

• Persistent protein loss > 3.5 g/day often leads to clinical signs of nephrotic syndrome. Consequences of severe proteinuria include sodium retention and edema, hypercholesterolemia, hypertension, hypercoagulability, muscle wasting and weight loss.

• A combination of low plasma oncotic pressure and intrarenal sodium retention often causes ascites and edema. The hypercholesterolemia associated with nephrotic syndrome is probably caused by a combination of low catabolism of proteins and lipoproteins and high hepatic synthesis of proteins and lipoproteins. This results in the accumulation of large molecular weight, cholesterol-rich lipoproteins.

• Systemic hypertension probably develops because of a combination of sodium retention, glomerular capillary and arteriolar scarring, low renal production of vasodilators, high responsiveness to normal pressor mechanisms, and activation of the renin-angiotensin system.

• Hypercoagulability and thromboembolism associated with nephrotic syndrome develop secondary to several abnormalities in the clotting system. Mild thrombocytosis develops, and platelet adhesion and aggregation increase proportional to the magnitude of hypoalbuminemia. Antithrombin III is lost in the urine. Antithrombin III works with heparin to inhibit serine proteases (i.e., clotting factors II, IX, X, XI, and XII) and plays a vital role in modulating thrombin and fibrin production. Altered fibrinolysis and increases in the concentration of fibrinogen and clotting factors V, VII, VIII, and X may lead to a relative increase in clotting factors compared with regulatory proteins.

Systems Affected

• Renal/Urologic—proteinuria, initially. Often the underlying disease is progressive resulting in irreversible glomerular damage, loss of nephrons, azotemia, and chronic renal failure.

• Cardiovascular—hypoalbuminemia (i.e., edema and ascites), hypercholesterolemia/hyperlipidemia, hypertension, hypercoagulability, and thromboembolic disease

Genetics

• Familial glomerulonephritis has been reported in the breeds of Bernese mountain dog, samoyed, doberman pinscher, cocker spaniel, rottweiler, greyhound, and soft-coated wheaten terrier, and in cats.

• Familial amyloidosis has been reported in the breeds of Abyssinian, Oriental shorthair, and Siamese cats, and in Chinese shar-pei dogs.

Incidence/Prevalence N/A

Geographic Distribution N/A

SIGNALMENT

Species

More common in dogs than cats

Breed Predilection

• The golden retriever, miniature schnauzer, and long-haired dachshund, in addition to those breeds listed above, appear to be overrepresented in some glomerulonephritis studies.

• Beagle, collie, and Walker hound, in addition to those breeds listed previously, are reported to be at higher than average risk for amyloidosis.

Mean Age and Range

• Dogs with glomerulonephritis—mean age, 6.5-7.0 years (range, 0.8-17 years)

• Cats with glomerulonephritis—mean age at diagnosis, 4.0 years

• Most dogs and cats with amyloidosis are > 5 years old

Predominant Sex None

SIGNS

Historical Findings

• Signs associated with an underlying infectious, inflammatory, or neoplastic disease

• Acute dyspnea or severe panting resulting from a pulmonary thromboembolism in dogs (rare)

• Acute blindness because of retinal hemorrhage or detachment in dogs (rare)

Physical Examination Findings

• Edema and/or ascites (common)

• Retinal changes, including hemorrhage, detachment, and papilledema, indicating systemic hypertension in some animals

• Arrhythmia or murmur related to left ventricular hypertrophy secondary to hypertension

CAUSES

Glomerulonephritis and amyloidosis develop secondarily to chronic inflammatory conditions (e.g., infection, neoplasia, and immune-mediated disease). See chapters on glomerulonephritis and amyloidosis.

RISK FACTORS

See causes

 DIAGNOSIS

DIFFERENTIAL DIAGNOSIS

Proteinuria

• The most common cause of proteinuria is inflammatory urinary tract disease (e.g., bacterial cystitis/pyelonephritis, urolithiasis, and neoplasia). Inflammation of the urinary tract is usually associated with an active urine sediment (i.e., high numbers of RBC, WBC, epithelial cells, and bacteria observed in the urine sediment).

• Glomerulonephritis and amyloidosis often cause severe proteinuria with an inactive urine sediment (hyaline casts may be seen). Renal biopsy is the only accurate way to distinguish amyloidosis from glomerulonephritis.

Hypoalbuminemia

• Severe liver disease (e.g., hepatic cirrhosis)

• Protein-losing enteropathy (e.g., inflammatory bowel disease, lymphangiectasia, and neoplasia)

• Protein-losing nephropathy (e.g., amyloidosis and glomerulonephritis)

CBC/BIOCHEMISTRY/URINALYSIS

• Persistent, clinically important proteinuria with an inactive urine sediment (hyaline casts may be seen)

• Hypoalbuminemia

• Hypercholesterolemia

OTHER LABORATORY TESTS

Urine Protein/Creatinine Ratio

• Used to confirm and quantitate abnormal proteinuria

• The magnitude of proteinuria roughly correlates with the severity of glomerular lesions, making the urine protein/creatinine ratio useful in assessing response to treatment or progression of disease.

• If the glomerular disease progresses and causes loss of at least three quarters of the nephrons, the resulting low glomerular filtration usually reduces proteinuria.

Protein Electrophoresis

• Urine and serum protein electrophoresis may help identify the source of the proteinuria and establish a prognosis.

• Proteinuria associated with hemorrhage into the urinary tract may have an electrophoretic pattern similar to that of serum.

• Early glomerular damage usually results principally in albuminuria; however, with progression of the glomerular disease, an increasing amount of globulin may be lost as well.

• Markedly low serum albumin and a high serum concentration of the larger molecular weight proteins such as IgM suggest severe proteinuria and nephrotic syndrome.

IMAGING

• Protein-losing nephropathy does not cause specific changes on abdominal radiographs or ultrasonogram (thickened renal cortex and renal cortical hyperechogenicity may be observed in patients with severe amyloidosis); however, these tests are useful in ruling out other concurrent conditions.

• Dogs with pulmonary thromboembolism are usually dyspneic and hypoxic with minimal pulmonary parenchymal abnormalities on thoracic radiographs.

• Ultrasonography can be used to guide percutaneous renal biopsy.

OTHER DIAGNOSTIC PROCEDURES

• Renal biopsy—consider only after less invasive tests (e.g., CBC, serum biochemistry profile, urinalysis, and quantitation of proteinuria) have been completed and an assessment of blood clotting ability have been done. Histopathologic evaluation of renal tissue establishes a diagnosis (e.g., glomerulonephritis versus amyloidosis) and helps to formulate a prognosis.

• Blood pressure determination—in one study, 84% of dogs with glomerular disease (e.g., glomerulonephritis, glomerulosclerosis, and amyloidosis) were hypertensive.

TREATMENT

• Most can be treated as outpatients. Exceptions include severely azotemic or hypertensive patients and patients with thromboembolic disease.

• Activity should be restricted because of the possibility of thromboembolic disease.

• Sodium reduced, high-quality, low-quantity protein diet indicated.

• If the underlying cause can not be identified and corrected, glomerulonephritis and amyloidosis usually progress to chronic renal failure.

MEDICATIONS

DRUGS AND FLUIDS

Treatment of Hypertension

• If hypertension is not controlled by dietary sodium restriction, consider treatment with vasodilator.

• ACE inhibitor such as enalapril (0.5 mg/kg q24h) reduces glomerular capillary pressure, proteinuria, and incidence of glomerulosclerosis (some studies in rats). ACE inhibitor reduces glomerular capillary hydraulic pressure mainly by reducing postglomerular arteriolar resistance. Individual response to ACE inhibitors vary, and acute renal decompensation associated with hypotension is a potential adverse side effect.

Treatment of Edema and Ascites

• Cage rest and dietary sodium restriction

• Paracentesis and diuretics should be reserved for dogs and cats with respiratory distress and abdominal discomfort. Overzealous use of diuretics can cause dehydration and acute renal decompensation.

• Plasma transfusion provides only temporary benefit.

• It is important that dietary management include a reduced (not restricted) quantity of high-quality protein such as that in Hill's Pet Product's prescription diets canine and feline k/d. It is possible that normal or high dietary protein contributes to the progression of renal disease by causing glomerular hyperfiltration, increased proteinuria, and subsequently, glomerulosclerosis.

• The renin-angiotensin-aldosterone axis is modulated by dietary protein; angiotensin II may be responsible for the glomerular hyperfiltration mediated by dietary protein. Enalapril and low dietary protein have an additive antiproteinuric effect in rats. Enalapril attenuates hypercholesterolemia and glomerular injury in hyperlipidemic rats. Thus, besides reducing glomerular capillary hydraulic pressure, ACE inhibitors may have another mechanism by which they attenuate proteinuria.

Antithrombotic Treatment

• Prophylactic anticoagulant treatment may be beneficial in patients with clinically important proteinuria. Dogs with antithrombin III concentration < 70% of normal and fibrinogen concentration > 300 mg/dl have high risk for thrombus formation and are candidates.

• Coumadins are potent anticoagulants. Warfarin is highly protein bound, so its dosage must be individualized. An initial dosage of 0.22 mg/kg PO q24h is recommended for dogs. Prothrombin time (with the goal being to increase the baseline PT by 1.5 times) is the best laboratory test to monitor. If new drugs (especially highly protein-bound drugs like aspirin, which may displace coumadins from protein binding sites) are added to the treatment regimen, or if marked changes occur in serum albumin concentration, the patient's PT should be reevaluated.

• Low-dose aspirin (0.5 mg/kg PO q12h) is easily administered on an outpatient basis and does not require extensive monitoring as does warfarin treatment.

CONTRAINDICATIONS

Corticosteroids should not be used in azotemic patients.

PRECAUTIONS

• Dosages of highly protein-bound drugs (e.g., aspirin) may need to be adjusted as serum albumin concentrations change with treatment or progression of disease.

• Enalapril should be used with caution in azotemic patients.

POSSIBLE INTERACTIONS

See precautions

ALTERNATE DRUGS N/A

FOLLOW-UP

PATIENT MONITORING

• Urine protein/creatinine ratios, blood pressure, body weight, and serum urea nitrogen, creatinine, albumin, and electrolyte concentrations.

• Ideally, recheck examinations at 1, 3, 6, 9, and 12 months after initiation of treatment.

POSSIBLE COMPLICATIONS

Nephrotic syndrome
• Sodium retention and edema or ascites
• Hypercholesterolemia and hyperlipidemia
• Systemic hypertension
• Hypercoagulability and thromboembolic disease
Chronic renal insufficiency or failure

MISCELLANEOUS

ASSOCIATED CONDITIONS

Systemic hypertension
Hypercoagulability

AGE-RELATED FACTORS N/A

ZOONOTIC POTENTIAL N/A

PREGNANCY

High risk in patients with severe hypoalbuminemia or hypertension

SYNONYMS

• Glomerulopathy
• Protein-losing nephropathy

SEE ALSO

Glomerulonephritis, Amyloidosis, Proteinuria

ABBREVIATIONS

ACE = Angiotensin converting enzyme

References

Center SA, Smith CA, Wilkinson E, et al. Clinicopathologic, renal immunofluorescent, and light microscopic features of glomerulonephritis in the dog: 41 cases (1975-1985). J Am Vet Med Assoc 1987; 190:81-90.

Cook AK, Cowgill LD: Clinical and pathologic features of dogs with protein-losing glomerular disease (abstr). J Vet Int Med 1993;7:126.

DiBartola SP, Benson MD. Review: The pathogenesis of reactive systemic amyloidosis. J Vet Int Med 1989; 3:31-41.

Grauer GF. Glomerulonephritis. Sem Vet Med Surg (Small Anim) 1992;7:187-197.

Green RA, Russo EA, et al: Hypoalbuminemia-related platelet hypersensitivity in two dogs with nephrotic syndrome. J Am Vet Med Assoc 1985;186:485-488.

Author Gregory F. Grauer
Consulting Editors Larry G. Adams and Carl A. Osborne

NEPHROTOXICITY, DRUG INDUCED

BASICS

DEFINITION
Renal injury caused by a pharmacologic agent used to diagnose or treat a medical disorder

Pathophysiology
• Drugs can cause nephrotoxicosis by interfering with renal blood flow, glomerular function, or tubular function. • Many drugs are nephrotoxic because they are excreted from the body primarily by the kidneys. • Most nephrotoxic drugs cause proximal renal tubular necrosis. • If renal injury is severe, acute renal failure develops.

Systems Affected
• Renal/Urologic • If uremia develops, all body systems can be affected.

Genetics N/A

Incidence/Prevalence N/A

Geographic Distribution N/A

SIGNALMENT

Species
Seems more common in dogs than cats.

Breed Predilection N/A

Mean Age and Range
Any age, but old patients are more susceptible

Predominant Sex N/A

SIGNS

Historical Findings
• Polyuria and polydipsia • Inappetence • Depression • Vomiting • Diarrhea

Physical Examination Findings
• Dehydration • Oral ulcers • Foul smelling breath

CAUSES

Antimicrobial Drugs
• Aminoglycosides—all drugs in this class are potentially nephrotoxic, including neomycin, gentamicin, amikacin, kanamycin, and streptomycin. Nephrotoxicosis due to treatment with gentamicin occurs most often, probably because it is the most frequently used aminoglycoside. • Tetracyclines—outdated products can cause acquired Fanconi-like syndrome characterized by glucosuria, proteinuria, and renal tubular acidosis. Tetracyclines administered intravenously to dogs at high dosages (> 30 mg/kg) can cause acute renal failure.

Antifungal Drugs
Amphotericin-B is the only antifungal agent that causes clinically important nephrotoxicosis.

Antineoplastic Drugs
• Cisplatin is the only antineoplastic agent that causes clinically important nephrotoxicosis in dogs. • Doxorubicin may be associated with nephrotoxicosis in cats, but this is rarely of clinical importance.

Nonsteroidal Anti-Inflammatory Drugs (NSAIDS)
• Includes aspirin, ibuprofen, naproxen, piroxicam, and flunixin meglumine • Most likely to cause renal injury in patients with preexisting renal disease or those with concomitant dehydration or other causes of hypovolemia

Angiotensin Converting Enzyme (ACE) Inhibitors
• Includes captopril, benazapril, enalapril, and lisinopril • Most likely to cause acute renal failure in patients with hyponatremia, dehydration, or congestive heart failure.

Antiparasitic Drugs
Thiacetarsamide is the only antiparisitic drug that causes clinically important nephrotoxicosis.

Radiographic Contrast Agents
• Intravenous administration of radiographic contrast agents can cause acute renal failure, especially in patients with dehydration, hypovolemia, or hypotension associated with inhalation anesthesia.

RISK FACTORS
• Dehydration • Advanced age, probably because old patients have preexisting renal disease • Renal disease, whether inactive or active • Renal hypoperfusion; potential causes include any disorder associated with hypovolemia (e.g., vomiting, hemorrhage, and hypoadrenocorticism), low cardiac output (e.g., congestive heart failure, pericardial disease, cardiac arrhythmias, and inhalation anesthesia), or renal vasoconstriction (e.g., NSAID administration) • Electrolyte and acid/base abnormalities including hypokalemia, hyponatremia, hypocalcemia, and metabolic acidosis • Concurrent drug therapy—administration of furosemide increases the nephrotoxicosis of aminoglycosides. Treatment with cytotoxic drugs (e.g., cyclophosphamide) may increase nephrotoxic potential of other drugs. • Fever • Sepsis

DIAGNOSIS

DIFFERENTIAL DIAGNOSIS
• Must differentiate from other causes of acute renal failure including causes of acute tubular necrosis such as ethylene glycol toxicosis and renal ischemia and causes of nephritis such as leptospirosis • Most patients with drug-induced nephrotoxicosis have a history of recent treatment with a potentially nephrotoxic drug. Acute renal failure can occur several days after discontinuation of an aminoglycoside. • History should include determination of all drugs that have been administered to the patient, including over-the-counter preparations (e.g., aspirin, ibuprofen, and naproxen) and medications that have been prescribed for human use (e.g., piroxicam).

CBC/BIOCHEMISTRY/URINALYSIS
• Results of hemogram usually normal unless there are concomitant problems such as gastrointestinal hemorrhage associated with administration of NSAIDs. • Results of biochemical analysis are normal in the early stages of drug-induced nephrotoxicosis or reveal signs consistent with acute renal failure including azotemia, hyperphosphatemia, and metabolic acidosis. • Urinalysis may reveal low urine specific gravity, often < 1.025, proteinuria, glucosuria, or cylindruria.

OTHER LABORATORY TESTS
Serum aminoglycoside concentration useful for monitoring aminoglycoside administration to help prevent nephrotoxicity.

IMAGING N/A

OTHER DIAGNOSTIC PROCEDURES
Renal biopsy may be indicated to determine cause of acute renal failure and potential for reversibility, especially in patients that do not respond to treatment as expected.

TREATMENT

INPATIENT VERSUS OUTPATIENT
• Patients with acute renal failure are managed as inpatients.
• Patients that do not have azotemia and are able to eat and drink sufficiently to maintain hydration can be managed as outpatients.

ACTIVITY Reduce

DIET
• Outpatients can be fed their regular diet. • Dietary modification is indicated in patients with acute renal failure; oral feeding should be avoided until vomiting is controlled. When oral feeding is initiated, a moderately protein-restricted diet such as canine k/d (Hill's Pet Products, Topeka) may help control signs of uremia.

CLIENT EDUCATION
• Avoid unecessary stress (e.g., boarding and elective surgery) and provide unlimited access to clean, fresh water at all times. • If any signs of illness such as inappetence, vomiting, or diarrhea develop, the patient should be returned immediately for veterinary care to minimize worsening of renal function.

SURGICAL CONSIDERATIONS
Avoid elective surgery until renal disease is resolved.

MEDICATIONS

DRUGS AND FLUIDS
• 0.9% saline intravenously in patients with renal failure. Alternately, lactated Ringer's solution, but it contains a small amount of potassium, which may not be ideal in pa-

tients with acute renal failure and hyper-kalemia.
• Hydration deficits should be corrected rapidly (i.e., over 6-8 hours) to prevent further renal injury. Calculate volume of fluid to administer using the formula: volume (ml) = body weight (kg) x % dehydration x 1000 ml.
• In addition to correcting hydration deficits, administer maintenance requirements (66 ml/kglday) and replacement of ongoing losses caused by vomiting and diarrhea.

CONTRAINDICATIONS
Do not use furosemide to promote diuresis in patients with aminoglycoside nephrotoxicosis.

PRECAUTIONS
Avoid drugs that may worsen renal injury in patients with nephrotoxicosis including NSAIDs, vasodilators, and ACE inhibitors.

POSSIBLE INTERACTIONS N/A

ALTERNATE DRUGS N/A

 FOLLOW-UP

PATIENT MONITORING
• Weight of hospitalized patients several times daily to detect changes in fluid balance and adjust fluid therapy accordingly • Biochemical analysis and electrolytes every 1-2 days to evaluate severity of azotemia and detect electrolyte and acid/base abnormalities • Urinalysis in patients receiving aminoglycosides every 1-2 days to detect signs of worsening nephrotoxicosis such as glucosuria, increased proteinuria, and cylindruria • Urine output to determine if patient is polyuric or oliguric. Adjust fluid therapy on the basis of these findings and determine need for additional treatment to stimulate urine production.

PREVENTION/AVOIDANCE
• Avoid or correct risk factors that predispose to development of drug-induced nephrotoxicosis. • Monitor serum aminoglycoside concentration or perform frequent urinalysis while administering an aminoglycoside. • Do not administer furosemide with an aminoglycoside.

POSSIBLE COMPLICATIONS
Acute renal failure

EXPECTED COURSE AND PROGNOSIS
• Patients without azotemia may develop acute renal failure within several days, especially with aminoglycosides. • Renal injury caused by nephrotoxic drugs may lead to development of chronic renal failure months to years later.

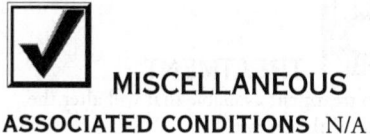 **MISCELLANEOUS**

ASSOCIATED CONDITIONS N/A

AGE RELATED FACTORS N/A

ZOONOTIC POTENTIAL N/A

PREGNANCY N/A

SYNONYMS N/A

SEE ALSO Renal failure, acute

ABBREVIATIONS
ACE = angiotensin converting enzyme
NSAIDs = nonsteroidal anti-inflammatory drugs

References
Brown SA, Barsanti JA, Crowell WA. Gentamicin-associated acute renal failure in the dog. J Am Vet Med Assoc 1985;186:686-690.
Brown SA, Barsanti JA. Gentamicin nephrotoxicosis in the dog. In: Kirk RW, ed. Current veterinary therapy IX. Philadelphia: WB Saunders, 1986:1146-1150.
Rubin SI. Nephrotoxicity of amphotericin B. In: Kirk RW, ed. Current veterinary therapy IX. Philadelphia: WB Saunders, 1986;1142-1146.
Rubin SI. Nonsteroidal antiinflammatory drugs, prostaglandins, and the kidney. J Am Vet Med Assoc 1986;188:1065-1068.

Author S. Dru Forrester
Consulting Editors Larry G. Adams and Carl A. Osborne

NEUROAXONAL DYSTROPHY

BASICS

OVERVIEW
• Inherited abiotrophies of neurons in diverse regions of the CNS, particularly the cerebellum and associated pathways • Several types have been described in dogs and cats. • Axonal spheroids are present throughout the CNS grey matter with the exception of the cerebral cortex. The most severe lesions are found in the Purkinje cells in the cerebellum.

SIGNALMENT
• Dogs—rottweiler, collie, chihuahua, and German shepherd dog • Domestic cats • Age at onset is breed-specific, ranging from 5 weeks (cats) to 1-2 years (rottweilers)

SIGNS
Deficits relate to the cerebellum—ataxia with progressive dysmetria and hypermetria of the limbs; increased patellar reflexes. • Loss of menace responses despite normal vision and facial nerve function • Mild intention tremor or head and neck dysmetria in some patients • Strength and proprioception normal

CAUSES AND RISK FACTORS
• Autosomal recessive inheritance in cats; similar mode of inheritance suspected in dogs • Breed predisposition

DIAGNOSIS

DIFFERENTIAL DIAGNOSIS
• Distemper encephalitis can be differentiated on the basis of the presence of systemic signs preceding or accompanying the neurologic deficits and on results of CSF analysis which are normal in animals with neuroaxonal dystrophy. • Cerebellar hypoplasia is apparent by 3-6 weeks of age and is not progressive. • Infectious encephalitides such as fungal, rickettsial, and protozoal diseases are differentiated on the basis of multisystemic signs, serologic testing, and CSF analysis. • Patients with cervical spinal cord disease have proprioceptive deficits and tetraparesis. • The diagnosis is by exclusion; it may not be possible to reach an antemortem diagnosis.

CBC/BIOCHEMISTRY/URINALYSIS
Results normal

OTHER LABORATORY TESTS N/A

IMAGING N/A

OTHER DIAGNOSTIC PROCEDURES
All antemortem diagnostic tests are normal.

TREATMENT
• No treatment available that will alter the course of the disease
• Most patients can be treated as an outpatient unless severe deficits preclude nursing care at home.
• Restrict activity to areas where a fall can be avoided (i.e., avoid stairs, swimming pool, etc).

MEDICATIONS

DRUGS AND FLUIDS N/A

CONTRAINDICATIONS/POSSIBLE INTERACTIONS N/A

FOLLOW-UP
• Although the disease progresses insidiously, by 6 years of age most rottweilers are severely affected. • The disease is not fatal but severely incapacitating.

MISCELLANEOUS

ABBREVIATION
CNS = central nervous system

Reference

De Lahunta A. Abiotrophy in domestic animals: A review. Can J Vet Res 1990;54:65-76.

Author Mary O. Smith
Consulting Editor Joane M. Parent

BASICS

OVERVIEW
• Nocardiosis is an uncommon infection of dogs or cats. The organism is a soil saprophyte that enters the body through contamination of wounds or by respiratory inhalation. A compromised immune system enhances the likelihood of infection.

SIGNALMENT Dogs or cats of any breed

SIGNS
• The predominant clinical sign depends on the site of infection. • The pleural form causes pyothorax, resulting in dyspnea, emaciation, and fever. • The cutaneous form results in chronic nonhealing wounds often accompanied by fistulous tracts. Extension of the infection may result in lymphadenopathy, draining lymph nodes, and osteomyelitis.
• The disseminated form usually begins in the respiratory tract and causes lethargy, fever, and weight loss. Cyclic fever may be a characteristic sign. Neurologic signs may develop as the CNS may be affected. Pleural and/or abdominal effusion may occur. This form is most common in young dogs.

CAUSES AND RISK FACTORS
• Nocardia asteroides (dogs and cats)
• Nocardia brasiliensis (cats only)
• Proactinomyces spp. (rare)

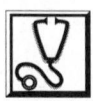

DIAGNOSIS

DIFFERENTIAL DIAGNOSIS
Cutaneous Form
• Actinomycosis • Atypical mycobacteriosis • Leprosy • Bite wound abscesses • Draining tracts resulting from foreign bodies
Pleural Form
• Bacterial pyothorax • Thoracic neoplasia • Chronic diaphragmatic hernia
Disseminated Form
• Systemic fungal infections • Feline infectious peritonitis

CBC/BIOCHEMISTRY/URINALYSIS
• Neutrophilic leukocytosis • Non-regenerative anemia of long-standing infections (anemia of chronic disease)
• Chemistries are normal usually, but hyper-gammaglobulinemia may be present in long-standing infections.

OTHER LABORATORY TESTS N/A

IMAGING
Radiographs may reveal pleural or peritoneal effusion, pleuropneumonia, or osteomyelitis.

OTHER DIAGNOSTIC PROCEDURES
• Cytologic examination of exudates stained with Romanowsky, Gram's, and modified acid-fast stains may give a rapid diagnosis.
• Cytology may reveal gram-positive branching filamentous rods and cocci. They cannot be distinguished cytologically from Actinomyces spp. • Culturing of the organism is diagnostic. It may be recovered by aerobic culturing on Sabouraud's medium.

GROSS AND HISTOPATHOLOGIC FINDINGS
• Nocardia asteroides produces a pyogranulomatous reaction that is more suppurative than infections by Actinomyces spp. Abscesses may be identified. • Nocardia brasiliensis causes a granulomatous reaction with extensive fibrosis. • Although the organism is usually present, it cannot be distinguished histopathologically from Actinomyces spp.

TREATMENT N/A

MEDICATIONS

DRUGS AND FLUIDS
• When the organism is cultured, antibiotic sensitivity testing should be performed and the antibiotic chosen accordingly.
• When culturing is not performed or is pending, sulfonamides and sulfonamide-trimethoprim combinations are good first choice drugs.

• Other antibiotics that are often effective include aminoglycosides (gentamicin and amikacin), tetracyclines (doxycycline and tetracycline hydrochloride, minocycline), erythromycin, and the combination of ampicillin or amoxicillin and erythromycin. Amoxicillin plus an aminoglycoside is a synergistic combination that may be considered in any serious infection when culturing is not possible or pending.
• The average treatment period is 6 weeks; however, medical treatment should extend several weeks past apparent remission of the disease.
• When feasible, surgical drainage should accompany medical therapy. Placement of a thoracostomy tube for pleural effusion is important. Surgical drainage and debridement of draining tracts and lymph nodes should be attempted. Care should be taken to identify the presence of foreign bodies during surgical exploration.

CONTRAINDICATIONS/POSSIBLE INTERACTIONS
Tetracyclines may cause fevers of up to 107° F in cats. This drug should be discontinued and replaced if fever increases during therapy.

FOLLOW-UP
Because of the potential for bone and CNS involvement, patients should be monitored carefully for fever, weight loss, seizures, dyspnea, and lameness the first year following apparently successful therapy.

MISCELLANEOUS

Reference
Greene CE. Bacterial diseases. In: Ettinger SJ, ed. Textbook of veterinary internal medicine. 4th ed. Philadelphia: WB Saunders, 1994:367-376.
Author Gary D. Norsworthy
Consulting Editor Fred W. Scott

OPHTHALMIA NEONATORUM

BASICS

OVERVIEW
Infection of the conjunctiva or cornea before or just after the separation of the eyelids in the neonate. Occurs in puppies and kittens. Associated with Staphylococcus spp. or Streptococcus spp. in both dogs and cats and with Herpesvirus in cats. Potentially vision-threatening. Source of infection is believed to be from a vaginal infection of the dam or from a nonhygienic environment at the time of birth

SIGNALMENT
• All breeds of cats and dogs before they open their eyelids (approximately 10-14 days postpartum) are susceptible.

SIGNS
• Upper and lower eyelids are still adherent (physiologic ankyloblepharon) and bulge outward due to the accumulation of debris and discharge within the conjunctival fornices and between the cornea and lids. • A mucoid to mucopurulent discharge may extrude through the medial canthus. • The cornea and conjunctiva may be ulcerated. • Adhesions (symblepharon) of the conjunctiva to the cornea or to other areas of conjunctiva (including that of the nictitans) may be present. • Perforation of the cornea with iris prolapse and collapse of the globe occurs occasionally.

CAUSES AND RISK FACTORS
• Vaginal infection in the dam near the time of birth • Unclean environment for the neonates

DIAGNOSIS

DIFFERENTIAL DIAGNOSIS
Neonates with entropion in whom the eyelids have already separated may have mucoid to mucopurulent discharge. The discharge or the entropic eyelids may obscure the view of the cornea and give the appearance of ankyloblepharon. These animals are older than 10-14 days and their eyelids can be everted to determine absence of ankyloblepharon.

CBC/BIOCHEMISTRY/URINALYSIS
Results are normal unless the animal is concurrently infected with a systemic disease.

OTHER LABORATORY TESTS
Immunofluorescent antibody tests for feline herpesvirus may be useful in kittens.

IMAGING N/A

OTHER DIAGNOSTIC PROCEDURES
• A full physical examination of the dam and neonate • Bacterial cultures of the neonate's ocular discharge and the dam's vaginal discharge • Fluorescein staining to look for evidence of corneal or conjunctival ulceration

TREATMENT
• Separation of the eyelids is the cornerstone of treatment. This can sometimes be accomplished by manual traction beginning at the medial canthus. Alternatively, a small blunt scissors blade or the blunt, butt-end of a scalpel blade can be introduced into the medial canthus and used to gently separate (not cut) the eyelids.
• The conjunctival sacs and cornea should be lavaged with warm saline to remove the discharge.
• Warm compresses may aid in separation of the eyelids and in keeping the eyelids from readhering.

MEDICATIONS

DRUGS AND FLUIDS
• Broad-spectrum, topically applied antibiotics such as neomycin, bacitracin, and polymixin B are applied q6h for at least 1 week. If results of bacterial culture are available, antibiotic choice is made on the basis of sensitivity testing.
• Systemic support should be administered to systemically ill neonates.

CONTRAINDICATIONS/POSSIBLE INTERACTIONS
• Do not use tetracycline in neonatal animals because of the risk of affecting bone or teeth. If Chlamydia is involved, topically applied chloramphenicol is the drug of choice.
• Topically applied corticosteroids are contraindicated.

FOLLOW-UP

PATIENT MONITORING
• Warm compresses may be necessary for a few days to keep the eyelids from readhering.
• Topically applied antibiotic should be continued for a minimum of 7 days. • Puppies or kittens not initially affected should be observed for occurrence of the condition and treated if appropriate.

PREVENTION/AVOIDANCE
• The external environment and the dam's nipples need to be kept clean. • Vaginal infection in the dam should be treated before delivery, if possible.

POSSIBLE COMPLICATIONS
• Severe keratitis with scarring and symblepharon. • Rupture of the cornea with secondary phthisis. Blindness may be irreversible.

MISCELLANEOUS

Reference
Williams MM. Neonatal ophthalmic disorders. In: Kirk RW, ed. Current veterinary therapy X. Philadelphia: WB Saunders, 1989:658–673.

Author Stephanie L. Smedes
Consulting Editor Paul E. Miller

BASICS

OVERVIEW
Inflammation of one or both optic nerves resulting in reduction of visual function. May be a primary disease or secondary to systemic CNS disease because optic nerve communicates with subarachnoid space.

SIGNALMENT
Primary optic neuritis is uncommon; usually effects dogs >3 years old.

SIGNS

Historical Findings
• Acute onset blindness • Partial visual deficits often overlooked

Physical Examination Findings
• Blindness • Pupils fixed and dilated (some animals may have intact but diminished pupillary light reflexes) • Optic disc swelling, focal hemorrhage, active or inactive chorioretinitis • Normal fundus with retrobulbar disease

CAUSES AND RISK FACTORS
• Idiopathic • Neoplasm (primary or metastatic) • Distemper in dogs • Infectious peritonitis in cats • Systemic mycoses • Toxoplasmosis • Neosporum caninum • Granulomatous meningoencephalomyelitis • Toxicity (e.g., lead)

DIAGNOSIS

DIFFERENTIAL DIAGNOSIS
• Animals with cortical blindness should have normal pupillary light reflex, normal results of fundic examination, and possibly neurologic deficits. • Dogs with sudden acquired retinal degeneration syndrome (SARDS)—minimal or absent pupillary light reflex, normal fundus, flat electroretinogram.

CBC/BIOCHEMISTRY/URINALYSIS
No specific abnormalities

OTHER LABORATORY TESTS
Specific viral, fungal, or protozoal serologic tests

IMAGING Neuroimaging (CT/MRI)

OTHER DIAGNOSTIC PROCEDURES
• CSF analysis • Visual evoked potentials

TREATMENT
• Treat underlying disease.
• Blindness may be permanent in animals with idiopathic optic neuritis.
• Clinical course is unpredictable.
• Flare-ups may occur if medication is inadequate.

MEDICATIONS

DRUGS AND FLUIDS
• Treat primary disease process when identifiable.
• Idiopathic cause—prednisone (2 mg/kg q12h for 14 days then 1mg/kg q12h for 14 days, then gradual reduction to maintenance dosage).

CONTRAINDICATIONS/POSSIBLE INTERACTIONS N/A

FOLLOW-UP
• Monitor clinical signs or visual evoked potentials if available. • Prognosis depends on underlying disease.

MISCELLANEOUS

ABBREVIATIONS
• CSF = cerebrospinal fluid
• CT = computed tomography
• MRI = magnetic resonance imaging

Reference
Braund KG. Clinical syndromes in veterinary neurology. 2nd ed. St. Louis: Mosby, 1994:213–214.
Author David Lipsitz
Consulting Editor Paul E. Miller

ORAL CAVITY TUMORS, UNDIFFERENTIATED MALIGNANT TUMORS

 BASICS

OVERVIEW

Oral cavity tumors, undifferentiated malignant tumors are highly aggressive, rapidly growing masses in the area of the hard palate, premaxilla, maxilla, or orbit. Most tumors are highly invasive to bone and are nonencapsulated with a smooth to slightly nodular surface (mistaken as benign). They may become ulcerated. Biopsy reveals an undifferentiated malignancy of undetermined histogenesis. Highly metastatic neoplasm with cervical lymphadenopathy is common.

SIGNALMENT

• All dogs < 2 years old range, 6-22 months • No sex predilection • Primarily a disease of large breeds

SIGNS

Historical Findings

• Halitosis • Excessive salivation • Dysphagia • Bloody oral discharge • Weight loss

Physical Examination Findings

• Facial deformity • Cervical lymphadenopathy in a few patients • Oral mass

CAUSES AND RISK FACTORS   N/A

 DIAGNOSIS

DIFFERENTIAL DIAGNOSIS

• Melanoma • Squamous cell carcinoma • Fibrosarcoma • Epulis • Abscess

CBC/BIOCHEMISTRY/URINALYSIS

• Results may be normal • Neutrophilic leukocytosis in some patients • Results of urinalysis normal

OTHER LABORATORY TESTS   N/A

IMAGING

• Skull radiography to detect bone invasion • Thoracic radiography to detect lung metastasis

OTHER DIAGNOSTIC PROCEDURES

• Carefully palpate regional lymph nodes (mandibular and retropharyngeal) • Cytologic examination rarely diagnostic • A large, deep tissue biopsy (down to bone) required to differentiate from other oral malignancies

 TREATMENT

• Surgical excision is usually ineffective because of extensive local disease or metastasis on examination.
• If surgery is attempted, radical excision is recommended (e.g., hemimaxillectomy) with margins of at least 2 cm into normal bone and soft tissues.
• Efficacy of inpatient radiotherapy is unreported; most undifferentiated tumors are poorly responsive.
• Efficacy of chemotherapy is unreported; most undifferentiated tumors are poorly responsive.
• Cause of death is related to local recurrence and secondary anorexia and cachexia.

ORAL CAVITY TUMORS, UNDIFFERENTIATED MALIGNANT TUMORS

MEDICATIONS

DRUGS AND FLUIDS N/A

CONTRAINDICATIONS/POSSIBLE INTERACTIONS N/A

FOLLOW-UP

• Thorough head and neck examination with survey thoracic radiography should be performed at 1, 2, 3, 6, 9, 12, 15, 18, and 24 months after treatment. • Most dogs have lymph node metastasis on examination.
• Most dogs are euthanatized within 30 days of diagnosis because tumor growth is progressive and uncontrolled.

MISCELLANEOUS

References

Patnaik AL, Lieberman PH, Erlandson RA, et al. A clinicopathologic and ultrastructural study of undifferentiated malignant tumors of the oral cavity in dogs. Vet Pathol 1986;23:170--175.
Author Kevin A. Hahn
Consulting Editor Wallace B. Morrison

ORGANOPHOSPHATE AND CARBAMATE TOXICITY

BASICS

DEFINITION
Toxicity caused by organophosphate or carbamate, common active ingredients in pet and premise flea and tick control products, and household and agricultural products. Examples of organophosphates used for flea and tick control include chlorpyrifos, diazinon, phosmet, fenthion, cythioate, and tetrachlorvinphos. Carbamates include carbaryl and propoxur for pets, carbofuran for agriculture, and methomyl for fly control.

Pathophysiology
Organophosphates and carbamates cause CNS effects by inhibiting cholinesterase, which hydrolyzes the neurotransmitter acetylcholine in nervous tissue, RBC, and muscle. Pseudocholinesterase is found in plasma, liver, pancreas, and nervous tissue, mainly in cats. Normally, cholinesterase hydrolyzes acetylcholine in the synaptic space, resulting in termination of neurotransmission. Cholinesterase inhibition allows acetylcholine accumulation at the postsynaptic receptor, which causes stimulation of effector organs. Spontaneous reactivation of cholinesterase after binding with organophosphates is very slow and, once aging occurs, virtually nonexistent. Carbamates reversibly bind cholinesterase.

Systems Affected
• Nervous—clinical signs result from overriding stimulation of parasympathetic pathways, but may also result from sympathetic stimulation. Acetylcholine stimulates nicotinic receptors of the somatic nervous system (muscle), parasympathetic preganglionic nicotinic and postganglionic muscarinic receptors, and sympathetic preganglionic nicotinic receptors. • Musculoskeletal—acetylcholine stimulates nicotinic receptors of the somatic nervous system (muscle).

Genetics
• Animals with inherently low cholinesterase activity are more susceptible to cholinesterase depression. • Cholinesterase activity in cats is more easily inhibited than that in dogs.

Incidence/Prevalence
Common small animal intoxicant

Geographic Distribution
More common in areas of high flea burden or agricultural regions

SIGNALMENT

Species
Cats are more susceptible than dogs.

Breed Predilections
Organophosphates are stored in fat and slowly released into the circulation. Breeds with lean body mass such as racing breeds and sight hounds, and longhair lean cats have more organophosphate compound available to inhibit cholinesterase.

Mean Age and Range N/A
Predominant Sex N/A
SIGNS

General Comments
Clinical signs result from excess parasympathetic stimulation.

Historical Findings
• Carbamates can cause rapid onset of seizures and respiratory failure, and should be treated aggressively without delay.
• Chronic anorexia, muscle weakness, and muscle twitching can occur in cats with or without episodes of acute toxicosis, and last for days to weeks.

Physical Examination Findings
• Hypersalivation • Vomiting • Diarrhea
• Miosis • Bradycardia • Depression
• Ataxia • Muscle tremors • Seizures
• Hyperthermia • Dyspnea • Respiratory failure • Death

CAUSES
Overdose of products containing organophosphate or carbamate

RISK FACTORS
• Concurrent exposure to organophosphate and carbamate compound • Treating cats with products intended for use in dogs only
• Topical application on pets of products meant for premise use • Allowing pets into rooms while the floors are still damp with organophosphate premise products
• Incorrect dilutions of insecticides

DIAGNOSIS

DIFFERENTIAL DIAGNOSIS
Clinical signs and amount of exposure should be consistent with toxicosis.

CBC/BIOCHEMISTRY/URINALYSIS
N/A

OTHER LABORATORY TESTS
Cholinesterase activity is reduced to < 25% of normal in whole blood, retina, and brain. Reactivation of carbamate inhibited cholinesterase can occur during transport and testing. Test for cholinesterase activity must be interpreted in context of amount of exposure, clinical signs, and time of onset of signs.

IMAGING N/A

OTHER DIAGNOSTIC PROCEDURES
• Tissue (e.g., brain, liver, kidney, and fat) or stomach content analysis for organophosphate or carbamate insecticide can indicate exposure, but negative results do not rule out toxicosis. • Fur or hair may contain sprays or dips.

GROSS AND HISTOPATHOLOGIC FINDINGS
• Insecticide granules or pieces of chewed containers may be in the gastrointestinal tract.

• Histopathologic lesions are rare. • Delayed neuropathy is not usually associated with commercially available organophosphates.

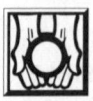

TREATMENT

INPATIENT VS OUTPATIENT
• Mild signs from exposure to flea and tick collars can be treated simply by removing the collar or brushing excess powder from the coat. • Animals with salivation, tremors, or dyspnea are treated as inpatients.

ACTIVITY N/A

DIET
Maintain nutritional and fluid requirements for chronically anorexic cats .

CLIENT EDUCATION
Caution owners that cats with chronic anorexia and weakness may need days to weeks of supportive care for full recovery.

SURGICAL CONSIDERATIONS
N/A

MEDICATIONS

DRUGS AND FLUIDS
• Diazepam (0.05-1.0 mg/kg IV) or phenobarbital (3.0-30 mg/kg IV to effect, low dosage in cats) and atropine sulfate (0.2 mg/kg, 1/4 IV, remaining SC, as needed) should be administered immediately. Atropine is repeated only as needed to control life-threatening clinical signs from muscarinic stimulation. • Oxygen may be indicated until respiration returns to normal. • Muscle fasciculations can be reduced by pralidoxime chloride (Protopam, Wyeth-Ayerst Laboratories, New York, NY; 10-15 mg/kg, IM or SC, q8h-q12h until recovery or discontinued after three doses due to a lack of response). Pralidoxime chloride is most beneficial when started within 24 hours of exposure. However, even several days after dermal organophosphate exposure, pralidoxime chloride may stimulate some anorexic cats (with or without tremors) to resume eating. Reconstituted bottles of pralidoxime chloride kept refrigerated and wrapped in tin foil have been successfully used for up to 2 weeks.
• For dermal exposure, bathe animal with a hand dishwashing detergent. • Emesis can be induced with 3% hydrogen peroxide (2.0 ml/kg, maximum 45 ml). When emesis is contraindicated, use gastric lavage with animal under sedation and endotracheal tube in place and a large bore stomach tube, followed by administration of activated charcoal (2.0 gm/kg PO or by stomach tube) mixed with sorbital as a cathartic (3 ml/kg of a 70% solution) in a water slurry. If animal has diarrhea, do not administer sorbital.

ORGANOPHOSPHATE AND CARBAMATE TOXICITY

CONTRAINDICATIONS
Phenothiazine tranquilizers may potentiate organophosphate toxicosis.

PRECAUTIONS
Avoid overuse of atropine, which can cause tachycardia, CNS stimulation, seizures, disorientation, drowsiness, and respiratory depression.

POSSIBLE INTERACTIONS N/A

ALTERNATE DRUGS N/A

FOLLOW-UP

PATIENT MONITORING
Monitor heart rate, respiration, and fluid and caloric intake.

PREVENTION/AVOIDANCE
• Follow directions on label. • Avoid use on sick or debilitated animals. • Avoid simultaneous use of organophosphate and carbamate products.

POSSIBLE COMPLICATIONS N/A

EXPECTED COURSE AND PROGNOSIS
• Good in animals with acute toxicity treated promptly • Chronic organophosphate toxicosis in cats may last for several weeks.

✓ MISCELLANEOUS

ASSOCIATED CONDITIONS N/A

AGE RELATED FACTORS N/A

ZOONOTIC POTENTIAL N/A

PREGNANCY N/A

SYNONYMS Organophosphate, carbamate

SEE ALSO Poisoning (Intoxication)

ABBREVIATION
CNS = central nervous system
RBC = red blood cells

References

Fikes JD. Feline chlorpyrifos toxicosis. In: Kirk RW, Bonagura JD eds. Current veterinary therapy XI. Philadelphia: WB Saunders, 1992;188-191.

Fikes JD. Organophophate and carbamate insecticides. Vet Clin North Am Small Anim Pract 1990; 20:353-367.

Authors Steven R. Hansen and Elizabeth A. Curry-Galvin

Consulting Editor Gary Osweiler

OSTEOCHONDRODYSPLASIA

BASICS

OVERVIEW

• Osteochondrodysplasia is a growth and developmental abnormality of cartilage and bone. It is a general term that encompasses many disorders involving bone growth. This condition results from delayed endochondral ossification. • The skeletal defects usually involve the appendicular skeleton and specifically the metaphyseal growth plates.
• Achondroplasia is a failure of cartilage growth and is characterized by a proportionate short-limbed dysplasia evident soon after birth. • Hypochondrodysplasia is a less severe form of achondrodysplasia. • Breeder selection of certain traits as desirable has resulted in the development of many achondroplastic and hypochondrodysplastic breeds.

SIGNALMENT

• Achondroplastic breeds: bulldog, Boston terrier, pug, Pekingese, Japanese spaniel, and shih tzu. • Hypochondroplastic breeds: dachshund, basset hound, beagle, Welsh corgi, Dandie Dinmont terrier, Scottish terrier, and Skye terrier. • Nonselected chondrodysplastic abnormalities have been reported in: Alaskan malamute, Samoyed, Laborador retriever, English pointer, Norwegian elkhound, Great Pyrenees, cocker spaniel, Scottish terrier and Scottish deerhound.
• Ocular-skeletal dysplasia has been diagnosed in Labrador retrievers and samoyeds.

SIGNS

Historical Findings
Owners present the animal because of obvious skeletal deformities or retarded growth.

Physical Examination Findings
• Deformities most often appear in the appendicular skeleton, but they may also occur in the axial skeleton. • Long bones appear shorter than normal and are often bowed.
• Major joints (elbow, stifle, carpus, tarsus) appear enlarged. • The radius and ulna are often more severely affected because of asynchronous growth. • Lateral bowing of the forelimbs, enlarged carpal joints, and valgus deformity of the paw. • Shortened maxilla (relative mandibular prognathism). • Spinal deviations because of hemivertebrae.
• Retinal dysplasia and partial to complete retinal detachment

CAUSES AND RISK FACTORS

• Autosomal dominant trait in achondrodysplastic and hypochondrodysplastic dogs.
• Simple autosomal recessive or polygenic trait in nonselected chondrodysplastic dogs.
• Littermates are often affected.

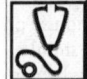

DIAGNOSIS

DIFFERENTIAL DIAGNOSIS

Premature closure of the ulnar or radial physes: history of trauma; only radius and ulna are affected; unilateral or bilateral abnormalities.

CBC/BIOCHEMISTRY/URINALYSIS
N/A

OTHER LABORATORY TESTS   N/A

IMAGING

• Radiographs of affected limbs: irregular flattening of the metaphysis, widening of the physeal line, retained endochondral cores and irregularities in ossification of the affected long bone; degenerative joint disease (DJD) and joint laxity due to abnormal stress and weight-bearing on the limbs. • Radiographs of the spine: hemivertebrae and wedge-shaped vertebrae.

OTHER DIAGNOSTIC PROCEDURES

Bone biopsy of growth plate: disorganization of the proliferative zone, abnormalities within the hypertrophic zone and abnormal formation of the primary and secondary spongiosa.

TREATMENT

• In certain breeds, achondrodysplasia may be considered a normal abnormality (chondrodystrophic breeds).
• Surgery is of little benefit in most dogs with nonselected chondrodysplasia.
• Corrective osteotomy to realign limb(s) or joint(s) may have limited benefit

MEDICATIONS

DRUGS AND FLUIDS

Palliative use of analgesics and anti-inflammatory drugs is warranted.

CONTRAINDICATIONS/POSSIBLE INTERACTIONS N/A

FOLLOW-UP

• Prognosis dependent on severity of involvement of appendicular skeleton. • Dam/sire breedings that result in offspring with deformities consistent with osteochondrodysplasia should not be repeated. • Breeding of affected animals is to be discouraged.

MISCELLANEOUS

SYNONYMS

Dwarfism

ABBREVIATIONS

DJD = degenerative joint disease

Reference

Sande RD, Bingel SA. Animal models of dwarfism. Vet Clin North Am (Small Anim Pract) 1982;13:71.

Author Peter D. Schwarz

Consulting Editor Peter D. Schwarz

OSTEOCHONDROSIS

BASICS

DEFINITION
Osteochondrosis (OC) is a pathologic process in growing cartilage. Its main feature is a disturbance of endochondral ossification that leads to excessive retention of cartilage.

Pathophysiology
• In animals with OC, the cells of the growth plates and of the immature articular joint cartilage do not differentiate normally. The process of endochondral ossification is retarded while cartilage continues to grow, resulting in abnormally thick regions that are less resistant to mechanical stress. • In immature joint cartilage where nutrition is maintained by diffusion of nutrients from the synovial fluid, excessive cartilage thickness results in impaired metabolism with degeneration and necrosis of the poorly supplied cartilage cells. A fissure can result within this thickened cartilage as a result of mechanical stress that eventually leads to the formation of a cartilage flap or osteochondritis dissecans (OCD). Clinical signs of lameness may occur at this point. • Lameness (pain) becomes evident once synovial fluid establishes contact with subchondral bone. Cartilage breakdown products released into the synovial fluid contribute to inflammation and pain. • In growth plates, retention of cartilage usually does not lead to necrosis, as seen in articular cartilage, probably due to better nutrition provided by vessels found within the cartilage. Instead of cartilage flaps, retention of cartilage in growth plates may lead to slippage and asymmetric growth. This is most marked in the distal ulnar physis. • The most commonly affected joints with OC are shoulder (caudocentral humeral head), elbow (medial humeral condyle), stifle (lateral > medial femoral condyle), and hock (medial > lateral ridge of the talus). Bilateral disease is common. • Other reported locations in which OC has been diagnosed include femoral head, dorsal rim of acetabulum, glenoid cavity of scapula, patella, distal radius, medial malleolus, cranial end-plate of sacrum, vertebral articular facets, and cervical vertebrae. • OC has been demonstrated clinically in horses, pigs, broiler chickens, turkeys, and humans.

Systems Affected Musculoskeletal

Genetics
Polygenetic transmission; expression is determined by an interaction of genetic and environmental factors. Heritability index varies with breed (0.25-0.45)

Incidence/Prevalence
Osteochondrosis is a common and serious problem in many breeds of dogs.

Geographic Distribution N/A

SIGNALMENT

Species Dogs

Breed Predilection
Large and giant breeds, especially great Dane, Labrador retriever, Newfoundland, rottweiler, Bernese mountain dog, English setter, and Old English sheepdog

Mean Age and Range
• Age of onset of clinical signs is typically 4-8 months • Age of diagnosis is generally between 4-18 months • Signs of degenerative joint disease (DJD) secondary to OC can occur at any age.

Predominate Sex
• Shoulder—male-female 2:1 • Elbow, stifle, and hock show no sex predilection

SIGNS

General Comments
Clinical signs are related to the joint(s) affected and the presence of concurrent DJD.

Historical Findings
• Lameness, sudden or insidious in onset, in one or more limbs that becomes worse after exercise is the most prominent finding. • A history of lameness for several week's to month's duration is common. • Lameness may be slight, moderate, or severe, with the dog supporting little weight on the affected limb.

Physical Examination Findings
• Pain usually can be elicited on palpation by flexing, extending, or rotating the involved joint. • Generally weight-bearing lameness • Joint effusion with capsular distension is common with OCD of the elbow, stifle, and hock. • Muscle atrophy of the affected limb is a consistent finding with chronic lameness. • Hock OCD—hyperextension of the tarsocrural joint

CAUSES
• Developmental • Nutritional

RISK FACTORS
• Feedings 3 times the recommended calcium intake • Rapid growth and weight gain

DIAGNOSIS

DIFFERENTIAL DIAGNOSIS
• Intraarticular (osteochondral) fractures • Elbow dysplasia (forelimb) • Panosteitis

CBC/BIOCHEMISTRY/URINALYSIS
N/A

OTHER LABORATORY TESTS N/A

IMAGING
• Standard craniocaudal and mediolateral radiographic views are necessary for all joints involved. • OC appears as a flattening of the subchonral bone or as a subchondral lucency. OC and OCD cannot be differentiated at this time. Sclerosis of the underlying bone is common in chronic OCD lesions and occasionally the flap is calcified, making it visible. • Calcified bodies (joint mice) within the joint indicate that the cartilage flap has been dislodged. • Radiograph contralateral joint for comparison to check for involvement. • Oblique views may improve visualization, especially for hock, elbow, and shoulder lesions. •"Skyline" views of the talar ridges are beneficial to identify medial or lateral lesions. • CT and MRI scans are useful to visualize extent of subchondral lesions; however; they are not reliable in detecting the presence of a loose cartilage flap.

Positive Contrast Arthrography
Useful for differentiating between OC and OCD of the shoulder

OTHER DIAGNOSTIC PROCEDURES
• Joint tap with analysis of synovial fluid is useful to confirm involvement of joint. Grossly, it should be straw colored with normal to low viscosity. Cytologic evaluation demonstrates < 10,000 nucleated cells/ml with more than 90% classified as mononuclear cells. • Arthroscopy can be used to differentiate OCD from OC and also for corrective treatment.

GROSS AND HISTOPATHOLOGIC FINDINGS
• Initially, the affected site in articular cartilage may appear yellowish. • There is retention of articular cartilage extending into subchondral bone surrounded by increased amount of trabecular bone • Clefts form between the underlying trabecular bone and the degenerated and necrotic deep layer of the overlying thickened (retained) cartilage.

TREATMENT

INPATIENT VERSUS OUTPATIENT
• OC is not a treatable condition.
• Surgery is required to usually treat OCD.

ACTIVITY
Restricted activity for both OC and OCD

DIET
• Weight control is important to reduce the load and therefore the stress on the affected joint(s).
• Restricted weight gain and growth in young dogs may reduce the incidence.

CLIENT EDUCATION
• Discuss the hereditability of the disease.
• Discuss the possibility of development of degenerative joint disease.
• Discuss the influence of excessive intake of nutrients that promote rapid growth.

SURGICAL CONSIDERATIONS
• OC is a nonsurgical condition. It may progress over time to OCD as the dog continues to grow.
• Shoulder—surgery is indicated for all OCD

lesions. Pain and lameness in a dog with radiographic evidence of OC is an indication for surgical exploration.
• Elbow—surgery is indicated for all OCD (OC) lesions and to assess for other conditions (see elbow dysplasia)
• Stifle—surgery is controversial because all dogs develop severe DJD even with surgery
• Hock—surgery to remove the osteochondral flap is controversial since all dogs develop severe DJD even with surgery. If warranted, surgery to reattach the flap to the underlying subchondral bone should be attempted.

MEDICATIONS

DRUGS AND FLUIDS
• Antiinflammatory (NSAIDs) and analgesic drugs can be used to symptomatically to treat associated DJD.
• These agents do not promote healing of the cartilage flap.

CONTRAINDICATIONS
Corticosteroids should be avoided because of the potential side effects and the articular cartilage damage associated with long-term use.

PRECAUTIONS
Gastrointestinal irritation may occur with the use of NSAIDs and may preclude their use in individual animals.

POSSIBLE INTERACTIONS N/A

ALTERNATE DRUGS
Chondroprotective drugs, such as polysulfated glycosaminoglycans, may be of benefit in limiting cartilage damage and degeneration. They also may help alleviate pain and inflammation.

FOLLOW-UP

PATIENT MONITORING
• If surgery is performed, activity should be limited for the first 4 weeks. • Early, active movement of the affected joint(s) is to be encouraged. • Yearly examinations are recommended to assess progression of DJD.

PREVENTION/AVOIDANCE
• Breeding of affected animals is to be discouraged. • Dam/sire breedings that result in offspring with OC (OCD) should not be repeated.

POSSIBLE COMPLICATIONS N/A

EXPECTED COURSE AND PROGNOSIS
• Shoulder—good to excellent prognosis for return to full function • Elbow, stifle, and hock—fair to guarded prognosis. Dependent on several factors—size of lesion (most important), presence of DJD, and age at time of diagnosis/treatment.

MISCELLANEOUS

ASSOCIATED CONDITIONS N/A

AGE RELATED FACTORS N/A

ZOONOTIC POTENTIAL N/A

PREGNANCY N/A

SYNONYMS N/A

SEE ALSO Elbow dysplasia

ABBREVIATIONS
OC = osteochondrosis
OCD = osteochondritis dissecans
DJD = degenerative joint disease
NSAID = nonsteroidal antiinflammatory drug

References

Olsson SE. Osteochondritis dissecans in dogs: a study of pathogenesis, clinical signs, pathologic changes, natural course and sequelae. J Am Vet Radiol Soc 1973;14:(1):4 (abst)..

Olsson SE. Lameness in the dog: a review of lesion causing osteoarthrosis of the shoulder, elbow, hip, stifle and hock joints. In: Proceedings Annu Meet Am Anim Hosp Assoc 1975;42:363-370.

Fox SM, Walker AM. The etiopathogenesis of osteochondrosis. Vet Med Feb 1993:116-122.

Author Peter D. Schwarz
Consulting Editor Peter D. Schwarz

OSTEOMYELITIS

BASICS

DEFINITION
Osteomyelitis is an acute or chronic inflammation of bone and the associated soft tissue elements of marrow, endosteum, periosteum and vascular channels that is caused usually by bacteria and rarely by fungi and other microorganisms.

Pathophysiology
• Hematogenously disseminated microorganisms may localize in metaphyseal bone of young animals and vertebrae of adults and cause osteomyelitis when local tissue defense mechanisms have been compromised.
• Direct inoculation of bone with pathogenic bacteria might not initiate osteomyelitis unless there is concurrent tissue injury, bone necrosis, sequestration, fracture instability, altered tissue defenses, foreign material, or surgical implants. Once bone infection is established, bacteria may persist by adhering to implants and sequestra. • Staphylococci and other bacteria produce slime that combined with host-derived proteins, cellular debris, and carbohydrate is called a biofilm. Biofilm enshrouds bacterial colonies, providing protection from antimicrobial drugs and host defenses. • Furthermore, biofilm induces some bacteria to transform to more virulent strains that are more resistant to antimicrobial drugs.
• Osteomyelitis is exacerbated by fracture instability. Resorption of bone resulting from infection and instability causes widening of the fracture gap and implant loosening, which consequently contributes to persistence of infection.

Systems Affected Musculoskeletal

Genetics N/A

Incidence/Prevalence
• The incidence of osteomyelitis following open reduction and internal fixation of closed fractures is usually less than 1%. • Osteomyelitis caused by trauma and open fracture is more common, but the true incidence is unknown. • Hematogenous osteomyelitis in young dogs is rare. • Discospondylitis in adult dogs and cats is uncommon. • Fungal osteomyelitis is uncommon.

Geographic Distribution
• Actinomyces bone infections in regions of sharp grass (California, Florida, and Australia) • Blastomycosis in central and eastern regions of United States, including the Great Lakes and the Mississippi and Ohio valleys • Coccidioidomycosis in southwestern United States, Mexico, and Central and South America • Histoplasmosis and the Ohio, Missouri, and Mississippi valleys and tributaries

SIGNALMENT

Species Dogs and cats

Breed Predilections
• German shepherds for Aspergillus osteomyelitis, possibly due to a breed-related immunodeficiency • Large-breed dogs for blastomycosis

Mean Age and Range
Hematogenous metaphyseal osteomyelitis in young growing dogs

Predominant Sex
Male dogs for posttraumatic osteomyelitis and blastomycosis

SIGNS

General Comments
• Acute postoperative wound infections after orthopoedic surgery may be indistinguishable from acute osteomyelitis, and may progress to chronic osteomyelitis. • Most patients with osteomyelitis are chronic at the time of presentation and diagnosis.

Historical Findings
• Episodes of lameness, draining tracts, persistent ulcers, previous trauma, fracture, or surgery in patients with posttraumatic osteomyelitis • Dogs with infections of the vertebrae or intervertebral discs may have hind limb weakness and difficulty in rising.
• Travel in regions endemic for mycotic infections may precede development of fungal osteomyelitis.

Physical Examination Findings
• Dogs with acute hematogenous osteomyelitis have sudden onset of systemic illness, pyrexia, lethargy, limb pain, and local signs of acute inflammation. • Chronic osteomyelitis is usually associated with chronic draining tracts, nonhealing ulcers, pain, and secondary muscle atrophy and joint stiffness. Unhealed fractures with concurrent infection may have instability, crepitus, and limb deformity.
• Fungal infections may produce limb swelling, lameness, and intermittently draining tracts. • Bone infections of the spine may cause pain and neurologic deficits, including paresis and paralysis.

CAUSES
• Open fractures and traumatic injuries • Open reduction and internal fixation of closed fractures • Elective orthopoedic surgery and prosthetic joint implants • Gunshot wounds and fractures • Penetrating foreign bodies • Bite and claw wounds • Extension to bone of soft tissue infections: periodontitis, rhinitis, otitis media, paronychia • Hematogenous infections • Staphylococci cause approximately 50% of bone infections, often as a monomicrobial infection. Polymicrobial infections are also common and may contain mixtures of aerobic gram-negative bacteria and sometimes anaerobic bacteria. Anaerobes are difficult to isolate, but are involved in up to 60% of bone infections. Anaerobes isolated include Actinomyces spp, Clostridium spp, Peptostreptococcus spp, Bacteroides spp, and Fusobacteria spp. • Fungal osteomyelitis may develop from infections with Coccidioides immitis, Blastomyces der-

matitidis, Histoplasma capsulatum, Cryptococcus neoformans, and Aspergillus spp.

RISK FACTORS
• Open fracture and bone contamination
• Soft tissue trauma • Bite and claw wounds
• Migrating foreign bodies • Orthopoedic surgery • Prosthetic orthopoedic implants
• Cortical bone allografts • Immunodeficiency

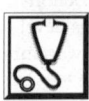

DIAGNOSIS

DIFFERENTIAL DIAGNOSIS
• Neoplasia • Bone cysts • Delayed fracture union as a result of instability • Hypertrophic osteodystrophy • Secondary hypertrophic osteopathy • Medullary bone infarction

CBC/BIOCHEMISTRY/URINALYSIS
Hemogram—inflammatory left shift usually only evident with acute osteomyelitis

OTHER LABORATORY TESTS
Serologic testing aids in confirmation of some fungal infections

IMAGING

Radiography
• With acute osteomyelitis, bone architecture is normal and only soft tissue swelling seen
• Signs of chronic osteomyelitis include sequestra (dead piece of cortical bone), reactive periosteal new bone, involucrum formation (shell of new bone surrounding sequestrum), and bone resorption. Resorption results in widening of fracture gaps, cortical thinning, generalized osteopenia, and implant loosening. • Contrast radiology may be useful in delineating sinuses and radiolucent foreign bodies. Water soluble contrast media is injected through a Foley catheter into sinuses.

Ultrasonography
Useful for localizing large accumulation of fluid and guiding fluid sampling by needle aspiration

Other Imaging Modalities
Scintigraphy with [99m]technetium-labeled methylene disphosphonate is highly sensitive for detecting skeletal lesions, but is generally not specific for osteomyelitis. However, scintigraphy with [111]Indium-labeled leukocytes is sensitive and specific for osteomyelitis. It is especially useful in detecting acute bone infections before radiologic signs appear and in differentiating infection from neoplasia.

OTHER DIAGNOSTIC PROCEDURES
• Aspirates of fluid or Jamshidi needle specimens of tissue, collected from the focus of infection by sterile techniques, are cultured aerobically and anaerobically. • Open surgical biopsy is indicated when needle aspirates are negative or when debridement is necessary for treatment. Samples of necrotic tissue, sequestra, implants, and foreign material are cultured aerobically and anaerobically.

Histopathologic examination of some of this tissue if fungal infection suspected, or to rule out neoplasia • Samples (fluid and tissue) for anaerobic culture must be placed immediately into appropriate media, such as reduced Cary-Blair anaerobic transport media
• Culturing pus from draining tracts is misleading, because of colonization of tracts by skin organisms and gram-negative bacteria
• Blood cultures may be positive with acute osteomyelitis

GROSS AND HISTOPATHOLOGIC FINDINGS

• Bone sequestration is virtually diagnostic for osteomyelitis • Inflammation and necrosis of bone and the adjacent tissues with pyogenic bacteria • Cytologic or histopathologic examination of smears or sections yields a diagnosis of fungal osteomyelitis in majority of cases. Special fungal stains (methenamine silver or PAS) aid in microorganism identification.

TREATMENT

INPATIENT VERSUS OUTPATIENT

• Hospitalization for surgical debridement of infection, drainage, culturing, irrigation, and wound management until infection begins to resolve
• Animals with infected fractures require hospitalization for surgical stabilization of the fracture.
• Long-term antimicrobial drug therapy is given orally on an outpatient basis.

ACTIVITY

Restricted if there is any danger of a pathologic fracture developing and in patients with unhealed fractures

DIET No restriction

CLIENT EDUCATION

Discuss the expense of treatment, the likelihood of recurrence, the problems with sequestration, the need for repeated surgical intervention, the long duration of therapy, and prognosis.

SURGICAL CONSIDERATIONS

• Surgical debridement, removal of sequestrum, and establishment of drainage indicated in chronic osteomyelitis
• With infected fractures, preexisting internal fixation implants are left in place while the fracture remains stable and healing is proceeding.
• Unstable implants are removed and the fracture stabilized with an external skeletal fixator
• Bone deficits filled with autologous cancellous bone graft after infection has abated and granulation tissue fills the wound

• Large segmental deficits in long bones can be bridged by Ilizarov technique of bone segment transport
• Because bacteria harbored by implant-associated biofilm leads to recurrence, all implants are removed once fractures are healed.
• Some cases of localized chronic osteomyelitis amenable to resolution by amputation (tail, digit, limb) or en bloc resection (sternum, thoracic wall, mandible, maxilla) and primary wound closure

MEDICATIONS

DRUGS AND FLUIDS

• Choice of antimicrobial drugs primarily depends on in vitro determination of susceptibility of microorganisms. Consider also possible toxicity, frequency and route of administration, and expense. Most antimicrobial drugs penetrate normal and infected bone well, but need to be given for 4-8 weeks.
• Most staphylococci isolated from osteomyelitis in dogs are S. intermedius that are resistant to penicillin because of b-lactamase production, but are highly susceptible to cloxacillin, amoxicillin-clavulanate, cefazolin, and clindamycin. Aminoglycosides and quinolones (ciprofloxacin and enrofloxacin) are effective against gram-negative aerobic bacteria. Quinolones can be given orally and are not nephrotoxic. To protect against resistance, quinolones should only be used for infections caused by gram-negative organisms or Pseudomonas spp that are resistant to other oral antimicrobial drugs.
• Continuous local delivery of antimicrobial drugs by antibiotic-impregnated methymethacrylate beads or implantable minipumps is indicated in management of chronic osteomyelitis
• Itraconazole (5-10 mg/kg, PO, q24h) given continuously may control disseminated aspergillosis for up to 2 years.

CONTRAINDICATIONS

Quinolones are not given to young animals because experimentally they induced articular cartilage lesions in immature dogs.

PRECAUTIONS

Aminoglycosides may cause nephrotoxicity, especially in animals that are dehydrated or have electrolyte losses or preexisting renal disease.

POSSIBLE INTERACTIONS N/A

ALTERNATE DRUGS

Alternative antimicrobial drugs are identified by repeating cultures and susceptibility determination if infections become unresponsive to initial regimen of antimicrobial drugs.

FOLLOW-UP

PATIENT MONITORING

Radiographic monitoring of bone healing every 4-6 weeks and reculturing of bone if persistent infection suspected

PREVENTION/AVOIDANCE N/A

POSSIBLE COMPLICATIONS

• Recurrence of infection • Chronic osteomyelitis may result in limb deformity, impaired function, fracture disease, or neurologic deficits. • Malignant neoplasia is a rare sequelae to chronic infection of fractures repaired by internal fixation.

EXPECTED COURSE AND PROGNOSIS

• Acute osteomyelitis and chronic bacterial discospondylitis may be cured by 4-8 weeks of antimicrobial drug therapy, provided there is limited bone necrosis and no fracture.
• Resolution of chronic osteomyelitis with antimicrobial drugs alone is unlikely when not accompanied by appropriate surgical treatment. • Recurrence of chronic osteomyelitis is evident with return of lameness or draining tracts. Recurrence can occur weeks, months, or years after the last treatment.
• Recurrence of infection may require repeated sequestrectomy, debridement, microbiologic culturing, drainage, fracture stabilization, bone grafting, or implant removal.

MISCELLANEOUS

ASSOCIATED CONDITIONS N/A

AGE RELATED FACTORS N/A

ZOONOTIC POTENTIAL N/A

PREGNANCY N/A

SYNONYM Bone infection

SEE ALSO

• Discospondylitis • Systemic mycoses

ABBREVIATIONS N/A

References

Johnson KA. Osteomyelitis. In: Birchard SJ, Sherding RG, eds. Saunders manual of small animal practice. Philadelphia: WB Saunders, 1994:1091-1095.

Wolfe AM, Troy GC. Deep mycotic diseases. In: Ettinger SJ, Feldman EC, eds. Textbook of veterinary internal medicine. 4th ed. Philadelphia: WB Saunders, 1995:439-463.

Author Kenneth A. Johnson
Consulting Editor Peter D. Schwarz

OSTEOSARCOMA

BASICS

DEFINITION
• A malignant neoplasm of the bone containing sarcomatous stroma and tumor osteoid
• The most common primary bone tumor seen in dogs • Poor prognosis because of the high rate of metastasis • Less commonly reported in cats, but cats are ranked third at risk after dogs and humans • Although distant metastasis can occur, the biologic behavior of osteosarcoma in cats is believed to be less aggressive than in dogs.

Pathophysiology
The tendency of osteosarcoma to occur in large and giant dogs and to occur in major weight-bearing bones and late-closing physes may point to repeated low-grade trauma as a cause. However, no pathophysiologic pathway has been identified. Osteosarcoma has also been reported in sites in which metallic implants have been used for fracture repair.

Systems Affected
• Musculoskeletal—appendicular more commonly affected than axial skeleton in dogs; axial skeleton more frequently affected than appendicular in cats, according to some reports; most common sites include the skull and other flat bones, followed by the humerus, femur, and tibia • Metastasis occurs primarily by the hematogenous route and is seen frequently in the lungs and in other bones. Lymphogenous spread is rare. • Extraskeletal sites, including skin, brain, and other tissues, occasionally affected

Genetics
• Although breed predilections do exist, there is no proven mode of inheritance. • Breed size and rate of maturity may be more important than breed or family line.

Incidence/Prevalence
• 80% of all primary bone tumors in dogs are osteosarcoma. • Osteosarcoma accounts for 2-7% of all malignancies in dogs and has been estimated to affect approximately 7.9/100,000 dogs annually. • Statistics for cats not available

Geographic Location N/A

SIGNALMENT

Species Dogs and cats

Breed Predilections
• Dogs—large and giant breeds
• Cats—domestic shorthair

Mean Age and Range
• Dogs—median age 7 years; reported in dogs as young as 6 months • Cats—generally older than dogs; no median age or range reported

Predominant Sex
• Dog—males more common except for Saint Bernard; a 1.2:1 male to female ratio reported in dogs with appendicular osteosarcoma • Cats—females appear to be more commonly affected

SIGNS

General Comments
• Swelling of a long bone at the metaphysis and associated pain and lameness • Clinical recognition of bone tumors affecting the axial skeleton more difficult. Localized swelling, a palpable mass, or other signs associated with the region (e.g., respiratory signs associated with large rib mass)

Historical Findings
• Dogs and cats often have lameness on examination believed by the owner to be caused by a known or unknown traumatic event.
• Lameness or swelling may also develop at a previously repaired fracture site. • Patients with bone metastasis beyond the primary site may have polyostotic lameness. • Neurologic signs may predominate in patients with a primary tumor or metastasis in the vertebrae.

Physical Examination Findings
• Affected limb visibly swollen in many patients • Pain often localized to the affected site. Lameness varies from mild to nonweight-bearing. • Lymphedema in animals with more advanced disease. Soft tissue involvement can be severe. • Pathologic fracture

CAUSES
• Unknown • Multiple, repeated minor trauma to major weight-bearing bones may be involved.

RISK FACTORS
• Large and giant breeds • Early onset of maturity • Previous fracture repair with metallic implant or history of ionizing radiation may predispose

DIAGNOSIS

DIFFERENTIAL DIAGNOSIS
• Other primary bone tumor • Metastatic lesion from another primary tumor source • Osteomyelitis, bacterial or fungal

CBC/BIOCHEMISTRY/URINALYSIS
Results usually normal

OTHER LABORATORY TESTS
Exogenous creatinine clearance may be of benefit in patients with possible renal dysfunction.

IMAGING

Radiographic Findings of Primary Tumor
• An anterior posterior and lateral view of the suspected lesion should be taken. Radiographically, bone density may be increased (proliferative, sclerotic, and osteoblastic lesions), decreased (lytic and osteoclastic lesions), or mixed (proliferative and lytic lesions). • In early stages, lysis or proliferation may be localized and minimal, later progressing to marked cortical destruction and extension of tumor into soft tissues. • A periosteal reaction with the often described "starburst"

pattern may be seen. This represents a response to injury and cannot be considered pathognomonic for tumor. • Codman's triangle represents an area of subperiosteal new bone formation that blends in with the reactive bone at the periphery of the tumor, giving the appearance of a "triangle" on radiographs. This is commonly seen, but is not diagnostic for osteosarcoma or other primary bone tumors. • Osteosarcoma does not typically cross a joint space. • Primary osteosarcoma is typically metaphyseal in location.

Thoracic Radiography
• Three views of the thorax, including right and left lateral and ventrodorsal, should be taken to evaluate for possible metastasis. • Approximately 5-10% of patients have evidence of metastasis at the time of diagnosis. • Metastatic osteosarcoma is not usually seen until the nodules are > 6-8 mm. Multiple discrete, round, dense nodules are seen. • In patients with rib osteosarcoma, findings include osteolysis and extrathoracic or intrathoracic mass often with secondary pleural effusion.

Nuclear Bone Scans
• Can detect bone and lung metastasis at earlier stages than plain radiography, but must be interpreted with caution, because sites of previous trauma or inflammation can be indistinguishable from cancer • Metastatic neoplasia found in 10-25% of patients

OTHER DIAGNOSTIC PROCEDURES

Bone Biopsy
• Can be performed under local or general anesthesia depending on the patient's demeanor and degree of pain • The most diagnostic site within the tumor is the center of the lesion. Peripheral biopsy often reveals only reactive bone. • Small biopsy samples may be misdiagnosed as other primary bone tumors.

GROSS AND HISTOPATHOLOGIC FINDINGS
• Grossly, mild to severe destruction of cortical bone • Histologically, abnormal formation of bone or osteoid tissue by tumor cells. The sarcoma cells are plump, polygonal to spindloid in shape, generally very cellular, often containing numerous mitotic figures.

TREATMENT

INPATIENT VERSUS OUTPATIENT
• The initial diagnostic workup, including the bone biopsy, can be done on an outpatient basis.
• Patients are hospitalized for surgery or limb-salvage procedures and the first chemotherapy treatment in dogs.
• Follow-up chemotherapy can be done on an outpatient basis.

ACTIVITY
Restricted only in perioperative period

DIET N/A

CLIENT EDUCATION

• Clients need to be carefully counseled on survival expectations.

• Discuss the need for early surgical and chemotherapeutic intervention for best outcome.

SURGICAL CONSIDERATIONS

Dogs—Appendicular Sites

• Amputation of the affected limb followed by chemotherapy considered the treatment of choice

• For forelimb tumors, a forequarter amputation is preferred. For rear limb tumors, disarticulation at the hip is preferred for femoral tumors; a midshaft femoral amputation can be considered for distal tibial tumors.

• Limb salvage—the primary tumor is surgically removed and replaced by a bone allograft. A bone plate then stabilizes the repair. Chemotherapy recommended after surgery or in patients undergoing amputation. Local chemotherapy implants appear to be improving median survivals in limb-spared patients.

Dogs—Axial Sites

• Skull sites—mandibulectomy or maxillectomy if feasible followed by chemotherapy

• Rib—chest wall resection (reconstruction often necessary) followed by chemotherapy

Cats—Appendicular Sites

Amputation treatment of choice. Chemotherapy not necessary due to low metastatic rate.

Cats—Axial Sites

Same as in dogs but often more difficult to obtain complete surgical resection

Inoperable Tumors

Radiotherapy often palliative

MEDICATIONS

DRUGS AND FLUIDS

• Cisplatin is currently the chemotherapy drug of choice in treating osteosarcoma in dogs. Chemotherapy helps prevent or delay the onset of distant metastasis, which is known to have occurred microscopically at the time of diagnosis in > 90% of patients.

• Cisplatin is given immediately after surgery

and then at 21-day intervals for a total of 4 treatments.

• Aggressive saline diuresis is given with treatment to help prevent renal toxicosis associated with cisplatin.

The following is one diuresis protocol commonly used:

• 18.3 ml/kg/hr 0.9% saline for 4 hours

• Cisplatin (70 mg/m^2) then diluted in saline in enough fluid to maintain same fluid rate to be delivered over 20 minutes

• After chemotherapy, diuresis continued at same rate for an additional 2 hours

• Vomiting or nausea during treatment can be controlled with butorphenol (4 mg/kg SQ)

CONTRAINDICATIONS

Patients with moderate to severe, preexisting renal disease may not be able to tolerate chemotherapy with platinum compounds.

PRECAUTIONS

• Chemotherapy requires special handling. OSHA regulations for handling cytotoxic drugs should be carefully followed.

• Aluminum or metal containing catheters should be avoided.

• Cisplatin is uniformly toxic to cats and should not be used.

POSSIBLE INTERACTIONS N/A

ALTERNATE DRUGS

• Similar survivals have been shown with carboplatin instead of cisplatin.

• Aggressive saline diuresis is not necessary with this drug. The recommended dosage is 300 mg/m^2 and is also given at 21-day intervals for total of 4 treatments.

• Carboplatin should be considered for patients with compromised renal function, although caution must still be used in these patients.

FOLLOW-UP

PATIENT MONITORING

• Local recurrence is possible with limb-salvage procedures; therefore, monitoring should include radiography of local site.

• Thoracic radiography should be done monthly for 3 months after surgery and then every third month thereafter.

PREVENTION/AVOIDANCE N/A

POSSIBLE COMPLICATIONS

• For limb salvage—local recurrence, infection, and implant failure • For amputation—arthritis in the hips or other joints may inhibit mobility in three-legged patients. Other complications are rare. • For all patients—primary complication is distant metastasis

• Hypertrophic osteopathy seen in some patients with lung metastasis

EXPECTED COURSE AND PROGNOSIS

Dogs

• Without treatment, metastasis to lungs or other bones, pathologic fracture, and diminished quality of life caused by local progression of disease develops within 4 months of diagnosis. • With amputation alone, median survival is 4 months. • With amputation or limb salvage plus cisplatin chemotherapy, median survival is 1 year. Survival rate of 2 years in approximately 30%.

Cats

The biologic behavior of osteosarcoma in cats is less aggressive than in dogs. With amputation alone, median survival of > 4 years has been reported.

MISCELLANEOUS

ASSOCIATED CONDITIONS N/A

AGE RELATED FACTORS N/A

ZOONOTIC POTENTIAL None

PREGNANCY

Breeding not recommended while patient undergoing chemotherapy

SYNONYMS

Osteogenic sarcoma

SEE ALSO

• Chondrosarcoma (Bone) • Fibrosarcoma (Bone) • Hemangiosarcoma (Bone)

ABBREVIATIONS None

Reference

LaRue SM, Withrow SJ. Tumors of the skeletal system. In: Withrow SJ, MacEwen EG, eds. Clinical veterinary oncology. Philadelphia: JB Lippincott, 1989:234.

Author Joyce E. Obradovich

Consulting Editor Wallace B. Morrison

OTITIS EXTERNA

BASICS

DEFINITION
Otitis externa is defined as inflammation of the external ear canal; otitis media, similarly, is defined as inflammation of the middle ear. Neither terms are diagnoses; they are descriptions of signs.

Pathophysiology
• Chronic inflammation within the external ear canal from any cause results in alterations in the normal environment of the canal. • The external ear canal is lined with epithelium containing modified apocrine (cerumen) glands. With chronic inflammation, these glands enlarge and produce excessive wax. • Epidermal and dermal thickening with fibrosis occurs; thickened canal folds effectively reduce canal width. • Calcification of auricular cartilage is an end-stage result of chronic inflammation. • Otitis media often results from the extension of otitis externa through a ruptured tympanum. Primary otitis media can occur from polyps or neoplasia within the middle ear.

Systems Affected
Nervous—with obstruction of the external canal, rupture of the tympanum and/or inflammation of the vestibulocochlear nerve. Vestibular—with inflammation of the vestibulocochlear nerve.

Genetics N/A

Incidence/Prevalence N/A

Geographic Distribution N/A

SIGNALMENT

Species Dogs and Cats

Breed Predilections
Pendulous-eared dogs, especially spaniels and retrievers; terriers, poodles, and other dogs with hirsute external canals are commonly reported.

Mean Age and Range N/A

Predominant Sex N/A

SIGNS

General Comments
• Otitis externa is often a secondary symptom of an underlying disease. • Infection results in the production of purulent and malodorous exudate. • Inflammation may result in exudation; however, pain and redness are most significant.

Historical Findings
• Pain, head shaking, scratching at the pinnae, and malodorous ears are common complaints. • Development of otitis media signs, such as a head tilt or incoordination, rarely occurs prior to signs of otitis externa.

Physical Examination Findings
• Pain and presenting examination are hallmarks of otitis externa. • Redness and swelling of the external canal are common. Canal obstruction by stenosis of the canal and fold swelling may occur. • Scaling and exudation may result in malodor and canal obstruction. • Holding the pinna down or voluntary tilting of the head is common in cats. • Vestibular signs, with head tilt, nystagmus, anorexia, ataxia, and infrequent vomiting indicates the development of otitis media/interna.

CAUSES

Predisposing Factors
• Abnormal or breed-related conformation of the external canal, including stenosis, hirsutism, and pendulous pinnae that restrict proper air flow into the canal. • Excessive moisture, due to swimming or to frequent cleanings with improper solutions, can lead to infections.

Primary Causes
• Parasites—Otodectes cynotis, Demodex spp., Sarcoptes and Notoedres, and Otobius megnini often induce otitis externa. • Hypersensitivities including atopy, food allergy, contact allergy and systemic or local drug reaction are the most common primary causes of otitis externa. • Foreign bodies, including plant awns, have a geographic prevalence. Other foreign bodies can also occur. • Obstructions due to neoplasia, polyps, cerumen gland hyperplasia, and accumulation of hair may be either a primary or a secondary event. • Keratinization disorders, including primary seborrhea, secondary seborrhea, and increased cerumen production result in functional obstruction of the ear canal. • Auto-immune diseases frequently affect the pinnae and less often, the external ear canal itself.

Perpetuating Factors
• Bacterial infection—the canine ear is most often infected by Proteus spp. and Pseudomonas spp. The feline ear more commonly contains coagulase-positive staphylococci. • Infections are often mixed with, or due entirely to Malassezia pachydermatis. Infections with other yeast or fungal species are possible, though rare. • Progressive changes, such as canal hypertrophy, cerumen gland hyperplasia and adenitis, fibrosis, and cartilage calcification cause recalcitrant otitis externa and prevent return to a normal ear canal even with proper treatment.

RISK FACTORS
Inappropriate treatment, excessively aggressive cleaning technique, and the presence of a predisposing or primary cause can increase the risk of developing otitis externa.

DIAGNOSIS

DIFFERENTIAL DIAGNOSIS N/A

CBC/BIOCHEMISTRY/URINALYSIS
Hemogram, serum chemistry profile, and urinalysis may indicate the presence of a primary underlying disease.

OTHER LABORATORY TESTS N/A

IMAGING
Bullae radiographs may assist in determining the presence or extent of otitis media.

OTHER DIAGNOSTIC PROCEDURES
• Skin scrapings from the pinna may reveal Demodex mites. • Skin biopsy from the pinna and canal may reveal the presence of an auto-immune disease, neoplasia, or cerumen gland hyperplasia. • Culture of aural exudate is rarely of assistance in devising a treatment plan, and should be reserved for cases of resistant infection. • Microscopic examination of aural exudate is the single most important diagnostic tool after complete examination of the ear canal. • The presence of a mite is a presumptive diagnosis. • The type of bacteria or yeast present assists in the choice of therapy. • The finding of white blood cells within the exudate indicates that active infection is present, and therefore systemic antibiotic therapy is warranted.

GROSS AND HISTOPATHOLOGIC FINDINGS N/A

TREATMENT

INPATIENT VERSUS OUTPATIENT
• Most patients can be treated as outpatients. • If vestibular signs are severe, hospitalization for fluid support may be necessary.

ACTIVITY No restrictions

DIET
No restrictions unless a food allergy is suspected.

CLIENT EDUCATION
Client education is crucial for the resolution of otitis externa and maintaining a healthy ear. Clients must always be instructed, by demonstration, in the proper method for cleaning ears. A handout with a diagram of the canine ear is helpful.

SURGICAL CONSIDERATIONS
• Surgery is indicated when the canal is severely stenotic or obstructed, or when neoplasia or a polyp is diagnosed.
• Severe, unresponsive otitis media may require a bullae osteotomy to permit drainage of infected exudate.
• Surgery is not indicated except in conjunction with the overall diagnosis and treatment of otitis externa. Lateral ear resection as well as ablation leave the pinnae intact. Therefore, if the primary disease process involves the pinnae (i.e. hypersensitivity, auto-immune disease), then disease and discomfort will persist.

MEDICATIONS

DRUGS AND FLUIDS

Systemic Medications

• Systemic medications should be directed at treating any underlying causes as well as relieving clinical disease associated with otitis externa.

• Systemic antibiotics are useful in severe cases of bacterial otitis externa and are mandatory in all cases in which the tympanum has ruptured, leading to otitis media.

• Appropriate antibiotics, to treat both otitis externa and media, include trimethoprim-potentiated sulfonamides (dosage varies by preparation), cephalexin (25 mg/kg q12h to q8h), enrofloxacin (2.5 mg/kg q12h), and clindamycin (10 mg/kg q12h).

• Systemic antifungals, such as ketoconazole (5 to 10 mg/kg q12h), can be used if overwhelming yeast or fungal infection is present.

• Systemic anti-inflammatory dosages of prednisone (0.25-0.5 mg/kg q12h) can reduce swelling and pain associated with otitis externa, as well as reduce the production of wax within the ear canal. Systemic corticosteroids should be used sparingly and for short durations only.

• Ivermectin is effective, both topically and systemically, for the treatment of various external ear parasites. Three subcutaneous injections of 300 µg/kg are administered at two week intervals.

Topical Medications

• Topical therapy of otitis externa is paramount for resolution and control of clinical disease. Three steps should be followed in the treatment of all cases of otitis externa:

1. The external ear canal should be completely cleaned of debris and foreign bodies. If correctly instructed, clients can effectively clean the ears of cooperative patients. Complete flushing of the external canal under general anesthesia should be reserved for uncooperative patients or for severely affected canals. However, treatment of otitis media often requires sedation and flushing in order to remove debris from the bullae.

2. Aggressive ear cleaning should be frequent during initial therapy (q12h to q24hr), and maintained once signs of otitis externa have resolved (q48h to once per week).

3. Appropriate topical medications should be applied frequently and in sufficient quanti-

tiy to permit complete treatment of the entire external canal.

• Commercial ear cleansers are highly effective combinations of ingredients for cleaning and disinfecting ear canals. Ingredients in these mixture perform the following functions: 1) Cerumenolytics, including dioctyl sodium sulfosuccinate (DSS) and carbamide peroxide, emulsify waxes to facilitate their removal. 2) Antiseptics, such as acetic acid and chlorhexidine gluconate, reduce or eliminate infectious organisms. 3) Astringents, such as isopropyl alcohol, boric acid, and salicylic acid, reduce the amount of moisture within the ear canal.

• Topical antibiotics, antifungals, and/or parasiticides should be used only when examination of aural exudates reveals the actual presence of infectious organism(s).

CONTRAINDICATIONS

• Ivermectin is not FDA-approved for treating the various ear mites in dogs and cats. Therefore, client disclosure and consent is paramount prior to administration of ivermectin. In addition, several breeds of dogs have shown increased sensitivity to this medication and should not be treated.

• Topical cleansers, other than sterile saline or dilute acetic acid, should not be used if the tympanum is ruptured. Topical medications should be used with caution in these cases because of their associated ototoxicity .

PRECAUTIONS

Extreme caution must be exercised when cleaning the external ear canals of all cats, and of dogs with severe and chronic otitis externa, because the tympanum can be easily ruptured. Post-flushing vestibular complications are common in cats and, although usually temporary, clients must be warned of possible complications and residual effects.

POSSIBLE INTERACTIONS

Several topical medications used for otitis externa infrequently induce contact irritation or allergic response. Therefore, re-evaluation is necessary in all worsening cases of otitis externa.

ALTERNATE DRUGS N/A

FOLLOW-UP

PATIENT MONITORING

• Frequent examinations are crucial to the resolution of ear disease. • Repeat exudate examinations can assist in monitoring infection course.

PREVENTION/AVOIDANCE

Routine ear cleaning by the client, in addition to control of underlying diseases, is required to maintain a healthy ear.

POSSIBLE COMPLICATIONS

Uncontrolled otitis externa can lead to otitis media, deafness, vestibular disease, cellulitis, facial nerve paralysis, progression to otitis interna, and rarely meningoencephalitis.

EXPECTED COURSE AND PROGNOSIS

• With proper therapy, most cases of otitis externa should resolve in 3-4 weeks. • Perpetuating factors, such as stenosis of the ear canal and calcification of the auricular cartilage will not resolve, and may result in recurrence of disease. • Otitis media may require six weeks or longer of systemic antibiotics, until all signs of vestibular disease have resolved and the tympanic membrane has healed.

MISCELLANEOUS

ASSOCIATED CONDITIONS N/A

AGE RELATED FACTORS N/A

ZOONOTIC POTENTIAL

Sarcoptes or Notoedres mite infestation and fungal infections are potential zoonoses, and must therefore be ruled out.

PREGNANCY

Systemic glucocorticoids should not be used during pregnancy, if possible.

SYNONYMS N/A

SEE ALSO N/A

ABBREVIATIONS N/A

Reference

Griffin CE. Otitis Externa and Otitis Media. In: Griffin CE, Griffin CE, Kwochka KW, et al., eds. Current veterinary dermatology: the science and art of therapy. St. Louis: Mosby Year Book, 1993.

Author Alexander H. Werner
Consulting Editor Lowell Ackerman

OTITIS MEDIA AND INTERNA

BASICS

DEFINITION
Otitis media/interna is an inflammation of the middle (otitis media) and inner (otitis interna) ears most commonly caused by bacterial infection.

Pathophysiology
Otitis media/interna most often arises from extension of infection of the external ear through the tympanic membrane but may extend from the oral and nasopharyngeal cavities via the eustachian tube. Otitis interna also can result from hematogenous spread of a systemic infection.

Systems Affected
• Nervous—the vestibulocochlear receptors in the inner ear and the facial nerve and sympathetic chain in the middle ear (peripheral) from extension of infection intracranially (central) • Ophthalmic (cornea and conjunctiva)—from exposure and/or lack of tear production after nerve damage • Gastrointestinal (taste)—from damage to the parasympathetic branch of the facial nerve (chordae tympani) supplying the ipsilateral rostral two thirds of the tongue

Genetics N/A

Incidence/Prevalence
Highest in association with otitis externa whether caused by bacteria or mites

Geographic Distribution N/A

SIGNALMENT

Species Dogs and cats

Breed Predilections
• Cocker spaniels and other long-eared breeds
• Poodles with chronic otitis or pharyngitis from dental disease

Mean Age and Range Any age

Predominant Sex N/A

SIGNS

General Comments
Clinical signs are related to the severity and extent of the infection and may range from none to those related to bulla discomfort and nervous system involvement.

Historical Findings
• The animal may have pain when opening the mouth, be reluctant to chew, or shake the head or paw at the affected ear. • The head tilts and the animal may lean, veer, or roll toward the side affected with peripheral vestibulitis. • With bilateral involvement, wide head excursions, truncal ataxia, and deafness may be observed. • Vomiting and nausea may be present during the acute phases. Vestibular deficits may be transient and episodic. • Saliva and food dropping from the corner of the mouth, an inability to blink, and an ocular discharge may be reported with facial nerve damage. • Anisocoria and/or protrusion of the third eyelid (Horner's syndrome) may be noted.

Physical Examination Findings
• Evidence of aural erythema, discharge, and thick and stenotic canals is supportive of otitis externa. • A gray, dull, opaque, and bulging tympanic membrane on otoscopic exam indicates a middle ear exudate. • Dental tartar, gingivitis, tonsillitis, or pharyngitis may be associated. • Ipsilateral mandibular lymphadenopathy can occur with severe infections. • Pain upon opening the mouth or bulla palpation may be detected. • A corneal ulcer may be caused by inability to blink or a dry eye.

Neurologic Examination Findings
• Depending on the severity, the middle ear (facial nerve and sympathetic chain) and/or the inner ear (vestibular apparatus and hearing receptors) are affected, damaging the associated neurologic structures. • If the vestibular portion of cranial verve (CN) VIII is affected, there is always an ipsilateral head tilt. There may be, but not necessarily, a nystagmus (resting or positional and rotatory or horizontal), vestibular strabismus (ipsilateral ventral deviation of eyeball with neck extension), and ipsilateral leaning, veering, falling, or rolling. Rarely, bilateral damage of CN VIII occurs. The animal is then reluctant to move and may stay in a crouched posture with wide head excursions. In these patients, the physiologic nystagmus is poor to absent. • With facial nerve damage, there is ipsilateral paresis/paralysis of the ear, eyelids, lips, and nares. There may be decreased tear production as indicated by the Schirmer tear test. With chronic facial nerve paralysis, there is contracture of the affected side of the face caused by of fibrosis of the denervated muscles. The deficits can be bilateral. • If the sympathetic chain is affected, Horner's syndrome develops. There should always be miosis of the affected pupil; however, there may or may not be protrusion of the third eyelid, ptosis, and enophthalmos.

CAUSES
• Bacteria are the primary etiologic agents. • Yeast infections (Malassezia spp., Candida spp.) and Aspergillus are other agents to be considered. • Mites predispose to secondary bacterial infections. • In unilateral cases, foreign bodies, trauma, polyps, and tumors (i.e., fibromas, squamous cell carcinoma, ceruminous gland carcinoma, and primary bone tumors) are possibilities.

RISK FACTORS
• Nasopharyngeal polyps and inner, middle, or outer ear neoplasia may predispose to bacterial infection. • Vigorous ear flush • Some ear cleaning solutions (e.g., chlorhexidine) are irritating to the middle and inner ear and should be avoided if the tympanum is ruptured. • Inhalant anesthesia and traveling by airplane may change middle ear pressures.

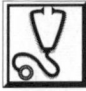

DIAGNOSIS

DIFFERENTIAL DIAGNOSIS
• Signs associated with congenital vestibular anomalies are present from birth. • Hypothyroidism may cause a polyneuropathy with a predilection for CN VII and VIII. There is inadequate elevation of thyroxine (T4) levels after a thyroid-stimulating hormone test. • Central vestibular diseases can usually but not always be differentiated based on the presence of depression/stupor and other brain stem signs. • Neoplasia and nasopharyngeal polyps are common causes of refractory and relapsing otitis media/interna and are diagnosed by imaging of the head. • Thiamine deficiency in cats typically results in bilateral central vestibular signs. A history of an all-fish diet or persistent anorexia helps in the diagnosis. • Metronidazole toxicity can produce bilateral central vestibular signs subsequent to high dosage or prolonged usage. Use of the drug combined with bilateral central vestibular signs is diagnostic. • Trauma is supported by the history and physical evidence of injury. • Idiopathic vestibular disease in older dogs and young to middle-aged cats, idiopathic facial paralysis, and idiopathic Horner's syndrome are diagnoses made by exclusion.

CBC/BIOCHEMISTRY/URINALYSIS
• There may be leukocytosis with a left shift. • The globulins may be high if the infection is chronic. • Urinalysis is usually normal unless the bacterial infection is hematogenous, whereby there may be pyuria and bacteruria.

OTHER LABORATORY TESTS
• Blood and/or urine cultures may be positive in cases with a hematogenous source of infection. • A low TSH response test supports a diagnosis of hypothyroidism.

IMAGING
• Bullae radiographs—the tympanic bullae may appear cloudy if exudate is present. Thickening of the bullae and petrous temporal bone may be observed in chronic cases. Lysis of the bone may be seen in severe cases of osteomyelitis. The radiographs may be normal. • CT and MRI show detailed evidence of fluid and soft tissue density within the middle ear and the extent of involvement of the adjacent structures. CT shows associated bony changes better than MRI.

OTHER DIAGNOSTIC PROCEDURES
• Myringotomy can be performed by inserting a spinal needle (2.5-3.5 in) through the otoscope and tympanic membrane to aspirate middle ear fluid for cytologic examination and culture and sensitivity. • Brain stem auditory evoked response (BAER) tests the functional integrity of the peripheral and central auditory pathways, detecting if there is associated hearing loss. • CSF analysis—neu-

trophilic pleocytosis and increased protein with intracranial extension of the infection. CSF culture and sensitivity should then be performed.

GROSS AND HISTOPATHOLOGIC FINDINGS

A purulent exudate within the middle ear cavity surrounded by a thickened bullae and microscopic evidence of degenerative neutrophils with intracellular bacteria is characteristic.

TREATMENT

• Patients with severe debilitating infections or neurologic signs should be admitted to the hospital.
• Stable patients can be discharged pending further diagnostics and surgery, if indicated.

ACTIVITY

If substantial vestibular signs, restrict activity to avoid injury.

DIET

• If vomiting from vestibulitis, withhold food and water for 12-24 hours.
• If severe disorientation, hand feed and water small amounts frequently with head elevated to avoid aspiration pneumonia.

CLIENT EDUCATION

• Most bacterial infections resolve with an early aggressive course of broad spectrum antibiotics and do not recur.
• Relapsing signs may occur and require surgical drainage when changes in the bony structures and/or middle ear effusion are evident on imaging studies.

SURGICAL CONSIDERATIONS

• Reserve surgery for relapsing or nonresponsive cases. The severity of the neurologic signs should not be used as an indication for surgical intervention because surgery is reserved for cases with evidence of middle ear exudate, osteomyelitis refractory to medical management, and nasopharyngeal polyps or neoplasia.
• Bullae osteotomy allows drainage of the middle ear cavity. Ear ablation through the horizontal ear canal is indicated when otitis media is associated with recurrent otitis externa or neoplasia.

• Cytologic examination and culture and sensitivity of middle ear effusion and histopathologic evaluation of samples of abnormal tissue should be performed at the time of surgery.

MEDICATIONS

DRUGS AND FLUID

• If concurrent otitis externa, the ear should be cultured and cleaned. Warm normal saline is preferred if the tympanum is ruptured. If a cleaning solution is used, a thorough flush should follow with normal saline. Drying of the ear canal is done with a cotton swab and low vacuum suction. Astringents such as Otic Domeboro® or boric acid can be effective.
• Topical water-based or ophthalmic antibiotic solutions such as chloramphenicol (Chlorosol) are preferred.
• Long-term (6-8 weeks) broad spectrum system antibiotic should be administered and selected based on culture and sensitivity, if available. Penicillinase-resistant penicillin and cephalosporins are good initial drugs.

CONTRAINDICATIONS

• Oil-based or irritating external ear preparations (e.g., chlorhexidine) should be avoided, as should aminoglycosides, when the tympanum is ruptured or there are associated neurologic deficits. They are toxic to inner ear structures.
• Topical and systemic corticosteroids are contraindicated with otitis media/interna as it may exacerbate the signs associated with an infection.

PRECAUTIONS

Avoid rigorous flush of external ear as this may result in or exacerbate signs of otitis media/interna.

POSSIBLE INTERACTIONS N/A

ALTERNATE DRUGS N/A

FOLLOW-UP

PATIENT MONITORING

Evaluation for resolution of signs should be performed in 10-14 days or sooner if the pet is deteriorating.

PREVENTION/AVOIDANCE

• Routine ear cleaning and dental prophylaxis may reduce the chances of infection. • When medical management is ineffective, a surgical evaluation for lateral ear resection should be explored.

POSSIBLE COMPLICATIONS

• Signs associated with vestibular and facial nerve damage or Horner's syndrome may remain. • Severe infections may spread to the brain stem. • Osteomyelitis of the petrous temporal bone and middle ear cavity effusion are common sequela to severe, chronic infections.

EXPECTED COURSE AND PROGNOSIS

Otitis media/interna usually is responsive to medical management. Improvement in vestibular signs takes 2-6 weeks, and is more rapid in smaller dogs and cats.

MISCELLANEOUS

ASSOCIATED CONDITIONS N/A

AGE RELATED FACTORS

Ear mites are more common in kittens and puppies.

ZOONOTIC POTENTIAL N/A

PREGNANCY N/A

SYNONYMS

Middle and inner ear infection

SEE ALSO

• Facial Nerve Paresis/Paralysis • Head Tilt • Horner's Syndrome • Otitis Externa

ABBREVIATIONS

BAER = brain stem auditory evoked response
CN = cranial nerve
CSF = cerebrospinal fluid

References

Bruyette DS, Lorenz MD. Otitis externa and media: diagnostic and medical aspects. Semin Vet Med Surg (Small Anim) 1993;8:3-9.
Schunk KL, Averill DR. Peripheral vestibular syndrome in the dog: a review of 83 cases. J Am Vet Med Ass 1983;182:1354-1358.

Author Richard J. Joseph
Consulting Editor Joane M. Parent

OVARIAN TUMORS

BASICS

OVERVIEW
• Epithelial (i.e., carcinoma), germ cell (i.e., dysgerminoma and teratoma), and sex-cord stromal (i.e., granulosa cell tumor, Sertoli-Leydig cell tumor, thecoma, and luteoma) tumors • Rare in dogs, but 40% are carcinomas, 10% are germ cell, and 50% are sex-cord tumors • Extremely rare in cats, but 15% are germ cell and 85% are sex cord tumors • Metastasis is common and hormone production is possible.

SIGNALMENT
• 0.5-1.2% of tumors in dogs and 0.7-3.6% of tumors in cats • Middle-aged to old animals • Teratoma develops in young animals.

SIGNS
• Tumors that produce steroid hormones can cause anestrus, persistent estrus, pyometra, gynecomastia, bilaterally symmetrical alopecia, pancytopenia, and masculinization.
• Ascites or pleural effusion in some patients
• Other signs associated with mass effects of the tumor

CAUSES AND RISK FACTORS
Intact sexual status

DIAGNOSIS

DIFFERENTIAL DIAGNOSIS
• Other causes of abdominal effusion • Other midabdominal mass

CBC/BIOCHEMISTRY/URINALYSIS
No consistent abnormalities

OTHER LABORATORY TESTS N/A

IMAGING
• Abdominal radiography may detect unilateral or bilateral midabdominal mass at the caudal pole of the kidney or effusion. • Abdominal ultrasound • Thoracic radiography

OTHER DIAGNOSTIC PROCEDURES
• Cytologic evaluation of pleural or abdominal fluid may be diagnostic for malignant effusion. • Histopathologic examination necessary for definitive diagnosis

TREATMENT
• Ovariohysterectomy the treatment of choice for solitary mass
• Peritoneal transplantation during surgical removal is possible.

MEDICATIONS

DRUGS AND FLUIDS

• Little information available on chemotherapy for ovarian tumors
• One patient treated successfully with cyclophosphamide, chlorambucil, lomustine, and bleomycin
• The author has used cisplatin chemotherapy successfully in three dogs with ovarian carcinoma.

CONTRAINDICATIONS/POSSIBLE INTERACTIONS

• Cisplatin should not be used in cats.
• Cisplatin should not be used in dogs with renal disease.

FOLLOW-UP

• Abdominal and thoracic radiography every 3 months to monitor for recurrence and metastasis. • Ovariohysterectomy for prevention • Prognosis guarded • Chemotherapy has the potential to lengthen survival.

MISCELLANEOUS

Pyometra, ovarian cysts, and cystic endometrial hyperplasia are associated with ovarian tumors.

Reference

Patnaik AK, Greenlee PG. Canine ovarian neoplasms: a clinicopathologic study of 71 cases including histology of 12 granulosa cell tumors. Vet Pathol 1987;24:509-514.

Author Terrance A. Hamilton
Consulting Editor Wallace B. Morrison

PANCREATITIS

BASICS

DEFINITION
Inflammatory disease of the pancreas temporally divided into acute and chronic types. Acute pancreatitis is inflammation of the pancreas that occurs abruptly with little to no permanent pathologic change. Chronic pancreatitis denotes continuing inflammatory disease that is often accompanied by irreversible morphologic change.

Pathophysiology
A variety of host defense mechanisms exist that normally prevent pancreatic autodigestion by the enzymes that it secretes. Under select circumstances, these natural defenses fail, and autodigestion occurs when these digestive enzymes are activated within acinar cells. Local and systemic tissue injuries are caused by the activity of released pancreatic enzymes and oxygen derived free radicals.

Systems Affected
• Gastrointestinal—altered gastrointestinal motility (ileus) because of regional chemical peritonitis; local or generalized peritonitis because of enhanced vascular permeability; hepatic lesions because of shock, pancreatic enzymes, inflammatory cellular infiltrates, and cholestasis • Renal/urologic—hypovolemia because of loss of gastrointestinal secretions, which may cause prerenal azotemia • Respiratory—pulmonary edema, pleural effusion, or pulmonary embolism in some animals • Cardiovascular—cardiac arrhythmias caused by release of myocardial depressant factor in some animals • Hemic/lymphatic/immune—disseminated intravascular coagulation (DIC) in some animals

Genetics N/A

Incidence/Prevalence
True incidence in dogs and cats is unknown. Up to 1% of normal dogs have histologic evidence of pancreatitis.

Geographic Distribution N/A

SIGNALMENT

Species Dogs and cats

Breed Predilections
• Miniature schnauzer, miniature poodle, cocker spaniel • Siamese cats

Mean Age and Range
• Acute pancreatitis is most common in middle-aged and older (> 7 years) dogs with a mean age on examination of 6.5 years. • Mean age for acute pancreatitis in cats is 7.3 years.

Predominant Sex Female (dogs)

SIGNS

General Comments
• Clinical signs in dogs are largely attributable to abnormalities involving the gastrointestinal tract. • Clinical signs in cats are more vague, nonspecific, and nonlocalizing.

Historical Findings
• Lethargy/depression common in both dogs and cats • Anorexia common to both species • Vomiting common in dogs due to acute inflammation; less common in cats • Dogs may exhibit abdominal pain by displaying abnormal postures. • Diarrhea more common in dogs than cats

Physical Examination Findings
• Severe lethargy often observed in both species • Dehydration common • Abdominal pain • Fluid distended bowel loops palpable in some animals • Mass lesions palpable in some dogs and cats • Fever common in dogs; both fever and hypothermia reported in cats • Icterus more common in cats than dogs • Less common systemic abnormalities include respiratory distress, bleeding disorders, and cardiac arrhythmias.

CAUSES
The inciting cause(s) of acute pancreatitis in both dogs and cats is usually unknown. The following etiologic factors should be considered: • Nutritional factors such as hyperlipoproteinemia • Pancreatic trauma and ischemia • Duodenal reflux • Drugs and toxins (see contraindications) • Pancreatic duct obstruction • Chronic renal disease • Hypercalcemia • Infectious agents (e.g., Toxoplasma and FIP virus)

RISK FACTORS
• Breed • Obesity in dogs • Presence of intercurrent disease in dogs such as diabetes mellitus, hyperadrenocorticism, chronic renal failure, and neoplasia • Recent drug administration • See causes.

DIAGNOSIS

DIFFERENTIAL DIAGNOSIS
• Differentiate acute pancreatitis from other causes of acute abdomen. • Perform a CBC, serum biochemical analysis, and urinalysis to rule out metabolic disease. • Perform abdominal radiography to rule out organ perforation; generalized loss of detail indicates abdominal effusion; screens patient for organomegaly, masses, radiopaque calculi, obstructive disorders, and radiopaque foreign bodies. • Perform abdominal ultrasound to eliminate mass and organomegaly. • Perform paracentesis and fluid analysis if the patient has effusion. • Specialized procedures as needed include gastrointestinal contrast radiography, excretory urography, and cytologic examination of fine needle aspirate.

CBC/BIOCHEMISTRY/URINALYSIS
• Hemoconcentration, leukocytosis with a left shift, and toxic neutrophils in many dogs • Cats more variable and may have neutrophilia (30%) and nonregenerative anemia (26%) • Prerenal azotemia, which usually reflects dehydration • Liver enzyme activities (e.g., ALT and ALP) often high as a conse-

quence of hepatic ischemia or exposure to pancreatic toxins • Hyperbilirubinemia more common in cats, caused by hepatocellular damage and intra- or extrahepatic biliary obstruction • Hyperglycemia in dogs and cats with necrotizing pancreatitis caused by hyperglucagonemia. Mild hypoglycemia in some dogs. Cats with suppurative pancreatitis may be hypoglycemic. • Hypercholesterolemia and hypertriglyceridemia common • Serum amylase and lipase activities high in some dogs but are nonspecific. Amylase and lipase activities are high in some animals with hepatic, renal, or neoplastic disease in the absence of pancreatitis. Dexamethasone administration may increase serum lipase concentrations in dogs. Lipase may be normal or high in cats. Amylase usually normal or low in cats. In general, lipase activity a more reliable marker for the diagnosis of pancreatitis. Normal plasma lipase activity does not rule out disease. • Results of urinalysis normal

OTHER LABORATORY TESTS

Trypsin-Like Immunoreactivity (TLI) Assay
• Serum TLI is pancreatic specific in origin and high serum concentrations are seen in some dogs and cats with pancreatitis. • Serum TLI tends to peak before and decrease more rapidly than amylase and lipase in dogs. • Reduction in glomerular filtration may cause serum TLI to rise. • Normal TLI assay does not rule out pancreatitis.

ELISA for Trypsinogen Activation Peptide (TAP)
• Acute pancreatitis stimulates the intrapancreatic activation of trypsinogens by the release of TAP into the serum. TAP is then eliminated from the body in the urine. • An ELISA assay has recently been developed for the detection of TAP in the urine but is not yet commercially available. • This assay appears to be a specific and rapid aid for the diagnosis of acute pancreatitis in dogs.

IMAGING

Abdominal Radiography
Finding may include:
• Increased soft tissue opacity in the right cranial abdominal compartment • Loss of visceral detail ("ground glass" appearance) because of abdominal effusion • Static gas pattern in the proximal duodenum • Widened angle between pyloric antrum and proximal duodenum • Delayed transit of contrast through the stomach and proximal small bowel

Thoracic Radiography
Note: Perform in patients with pulmonary complications.
Findings may include:
• Pulmonary edema • Pleural effusion • Changes suggesting pulmonary embolism

Ultrasonography
• Nonhomogeneous solid or cystic mass lesions indicate pancreatic abscess. • Loss of

normal pancreatic echogenicity in many animals • Peritoneal effusion and extrahepatic biliary obstruction in some animals

OTHER DIAGNOSTIC PROCEDURES

• Ultrasound guided needle-aspiration biopsy may confirm the diagnosis. • Laparotomy and pancreatic biopsy may be required to identify or confirm pancreatitis.

GROSS AND HISTOPATHOLOGIC FINDINGS

• Edematous pancreatitis—mild swelling • Necrotizing pancreatitis—grayish-yellow areas of pancreatic necrosis accompanied by various amounts of hemorrhage • Chronic pancreatitis—the pancreas is small in size, firm, gray, and irregular and may contain extensive adhesions to surrounding viscera • Microscopic changes include edema, parenchymal necrosis, and neutrophilic cellular infiltrate in animals with acute lesions. Chronic lesions show pancreatic fibrosis around ducts, ductal epithelial hyperplasia, and mononuclear cellular infiltrate.

TREATMENT

INPATIENT VERSUS OUTPATIENT

Patients should be hospitalized for initial medical management.

ACTIVITY Restricted

DIET

• Animals with acute pancreatitis should have all oral alimentation withheld (NPO) to reduce pancreatic secretions.
• Typical time period for NPO is 3-5 days. Failure to withhold oral intake for this minimum time may cause relapse. Once clinical signs resolve, small volumes of water should be offered. If tolerated, begin small, frequent feedings of a carbohydrate such as boiled rice. Gradually introduce to the diet a protein source of high biologic value such as cottage cheese or lean meat.
• Avoid high-protein and high-fat diets since they are major stimuli for pancreatic secretions. Low-fat prescription diets may be fed.
• Animals needing extended periods of NPO may require total parenteral nutrition.

CLIENT EDUCATION

• Discuss the need for extended hospitalization.
• Discuss the possibility of complications such as recurrence, diabetes mellitus, and pancreatic enzyme deficiency.

SURGICAL CONSIDERATIONS

• Surgery may be required to remove acute pancreatic abscess or devitalized tissue, which characterizes patients with necrotizing pancreatitis.
• Extrahepatic biliary obstruction caused by pancreatitis requires surgical correction.

MEDICATIONS

DRUGS AND FLUIDS

• Aggressive intravenous fluid therapy is a cornerstone of successful treatment. A balanced electrolyte solution such as lactated Ringer's solution is the first-choice rehydration fluid. The volume of rehydration fluid needed to correct initial fluids should be accurately calculated and given over a 4-6 hour period.
• Colloids (e.g., dextrans and hetastarch) may be needed to maintain pancreatic microcirculation.
• After replacement of deficits, additional fluids are given to match the patient's maintenance requirements and ongoing losses. Potassium chloride (KCl) supplementation is usually indicated because of potassium loss in the vomitus.

Drugs

• Corticosteroids indicated only in patients in shock
• Centrally-acting antiemetics indicated in patients with intractable vomiting—chlorpromazine (0.5 mg/kg q8h) and prochlorperazine (0.1 mg/kg q8h)
• Antibiotics used if patient has clinical or laboratory evidence of sepsis—penicillin G (20,000 units/kg q6h), ampicillin sodium (20 mg/kg q8h), and possibly aminoglycosides
• Analgesics may be required to relieve abdominal pain; butorphanol (0.4 mg/kg q8h SC) is effective in dogs and cats.

CONTRAINDICATIONS

• Avoid using anticholinergic drugs such as atropine. These drugs have variable effects on pancreatic secretion, and they cause generalized suppression of gastrointestinal motility, which can precipitate ileus.
• Avoid the use of azathioprine, chlorothiazide, estrogens, furosemide, tetracycline, and sulfamethazole.

PRECAUTIONS

• Use corticosteroids only in patients that are adequately hydrated because corticosteroids promote vasodilatation. Corticosteroids can exacerbate pancreatitis.
• Use phenothiazine antiemetics only in patients that are well-hydrated because these drugs have hypotensive properties.
• Use dextrans cautiously in patients with hemorrhagic pancreatitis because their use promotes bleeding.

POSSIBLE INTERACTIONS N/A

ALTERNATE DRUGS N/A

FOLLOW-UP

PATIENT MONITORING

• Evaluate patient's hydration status closely during first 24 hours of treatment. Assess results of physical examination, PCV, total plasma protein, BUN, body weight, and urine output twice daily. • Evaluate the effectiveness of fluid therapy after 24 hours and adjust flow rates and fluid composition accordingly. Repeat serum biochemical analysis to assess electrolyte and acid-base status.
• Repeat measurement of plasma enzyme concentrations (i.e., lipase or TLI) after 48 hours to evaluate the status of the pancreatic inflammatory process. • Closely monitor for systemic complications. Perform appropriate diagnostic tests as needed (see complications). • Continue NPO for at least 3-5 days. Gradually taper fluids down to maintenance requirements if possible. • Once clinical signs resolve, gradually introduce oral alimentation as described.

PREVENTION/AVOIDANCE

• Weight reduction if patient is obese • Avoid high-fat diets. • Avoid the use of drugs that may precipitate disease.

POSSIBLE COMPLICATIONS

Life-Threatening

• Pulmonary edema • Cardiac arrhythmias • Peritonitis • DIC • Hepatic lipidosis—cats • Failed response to supportive therapy

Non Life-Threatening

• Diabetes mellitus • Exocrine pancreatic insufficiency

EXPECTED COURSE AND PROGNOSIS

• A fair prognosis should be given to most patients with edematous pancreatitis. These patients usually respond to appropriate symptomatic treatment. Relapse or treatment failure is most commonly seen in animals given premature oral alimentation. • A more guarded to poor prognosis is warranted in patients with necrotizing pancreatitis and life-threatening complications.

MISCELLANEOUS

ASSOCIATED CONDITIONS N/A

AGE RELATED FACTORS N/A

ZOONOTIC POTENTIAL N/A

PREGNANCY N/A

SYNONYMS N/A

SEE ALSO

• Exocrine Pancreatic Insufficiency • Amylase/lipase • Diabetes Mellitus

ABBREVIATIONS

TAP = trypsinogen activation peptide
TLI = trypsin-like immunoreactivity

References

Strombeck DR, Guilford WG. Small animal gastroenterology. Davis, CA: Stonegate Publishing, 1990.

Author Albert E. Jergens
Consulting Editor Albert E. Jergens

PANNICULITIS

BASICS

OVERVIEW
Panniculitis is a term used to describe inflammation of the subcutaneous fat. It has multiple causes and is clinically seen as either a nodule or nodules or as draining tracts. It can be localized to one site (most common) or multifocal (rare).

SIGNALMENT
No age, breed, or sex predilections are seen in dogs or cats in general. For particular syndromes such as sterile nodular panniculitis, dachshunds are at increased risk, and miniature poodles and collies are also possibly predisposed.

SIGNS
• In localized and early multifocal panniculitis, intact nodules are freely movable under the skin. Since the location of the disease is under the skin it cannot be visualized clinically and can only be palpated under the surface of the skin. The subcutaneous nodules vary in texture from soft to firm. • The color of the nodules may be the same as normal skin or they may be yellow, brown or red. • In the multifocal form the overlying epidermis becomes necrotic and the lesions then ulcerate and are seen clinically as draining lesions. • In cases with chronic draining lesions, scar tissue forms in the areas of previous ulcerative lesions. Alopecia often occurs in the scarred areas.

CAUSES AND RISK FACTORS
• Trauma—foreign body, post–injection panniculitis (corticosteroid, other subcutaneous drugs) • Infectious—bacterial, fungal • Degenerative—idiopathic sterile nodular, sterile pedal • Immune–mediated—vaccine injection site, drug induced, systemic lupus erythematosus • Metabolic: pancreatitis • Nutritional—vitamin E deficiency in cats • Neoplastic—pancreatic carcinoma

DIAGNOSIS

DIFFERENTIAL DIAGNOSIS
• Lipom – needle aspirates show pure fatty tissue, no inflammatory cells; biopsy confirms the diagnosis. • Deep pyoderma – aspirates reveal pyogranulomatous reactions with both intra– and extracellular, coccoid shaped bacteria; biopsies and cultures confirm the diagnosis. • Cutaneous cysts – aspirates reveal amorphous debris and epidermal cells; biopsies confirm the diagnosis. • Cutaneous neoplasia – aspirates may be suggestive; biopsies confirm the diagnosis.

CBC/BIOCHEMISTRY/URINALYSIS
Mild to moderate leucocytosis and a mild non–regenerative anemia

OTHER LABORATORY TESTS
• Antinuclear antibody test (ANA) • Direct immunofluorescence • Serum protein electrophoresis

IMAGING N/A

OTHER DIAGNOSTIC PROCEDURES
• Needle aspirate biopsies – exudate containing inflammatory cells help rule out noninflammatory lesions like lipomas; organisms confirm infectious disease, while no organisms suggest a sterile condition and cultures are indicated to confirm. • Cultures – no growth would suggest sterile nodular panniculitis • Excision biopsy – deep excision biopsies that include the pannicular fat are the only way to confirm a diagnosis of panniculitis; skin punch biopsies are neither large enough nor deep enough to obtain a diagnostic sample.

GROSS AND HISTOPATHOLOGIC FINDINGS
• Any inflammation of the subcutaneous fat regardless of the cause looks the same histologically. The inflammatory reaction may be granulomatous, pyogranulomatous, necrotic, eosinophilic, or lymphoplasma–histiocytic.
• If the reaction is primarily lymphoplasma–histiocytic and other clinical signs suggest lupus dermatosis as a possible cause, (see SLE, autoimmune diseases) other diagnostic tests (ANA, and direct immunofluorescence) are needed to confirm.

TREATMENT
• Solitary lesions are cured by surgical excision.
• Multiple lesions require systemic medications.

MEDICATIONS

DRUGS AND FLUIDS

• For the idiopathic sterile nodular form – systemic glucocorticoids are used most often.

• For most cases of idiopathic sterile nodular panniculitis, treatment consists of prednisone at (1mg/lb/d) until lesions have regressed (3–8 weeks) then discontinue treatment. Most cases do not relapse and some go into long periods of remission. A few cases are recurrent and alternate day glucocorticoids or a combination of glucocorticoids and azathioprine (1mg/lb/d) may be helpful.

CONTRAINDICATIONS/POSSIBLE INTERACTION   N/A

FOLLOW-UP

Depends on the type of treatment – if long term glucocorticoid, immune modulating drugs, or both are used, appropriate monitoring of the CBC, chemistry screen and urinalysis are indicated (see treatment for autoimmune disease).

MISCELLANEOUS

References

Scott DW, Miller WH, Griffin CE. Muller and Kirk's small animal dermatology. 5th ed. WB Saunders, 1995;932.

Author David Duclos

Consulting Editor Lowell Ackerman

PANOSTEITIS

BASICS

DEFINITION
Panosteitis is a self-limiting, painful condition affecting one or more of the long bones in young, medium-to large-breed dogs characterized clinically by lameness and radiographically by high density of the marrow cavity.

Pathophysiology
• The etiology of panosteitis is unknown. • Attempts to isolate microorganisms have failed. Suggestions of metabolic, allergic, or endocrine aberrations are also without support. • Pain may be due to disturbance of endosteal and periosteal elements, vascular congestion, or high intramedullary pressure.

Systems Affected
Musculoskeletal—panosteitis causes lameness of variable intensity that may affect a single limb or become a "shifting leg lameness"

Genetics
There is no proven genetic transmission of panosteitis but the predominance of German shepherds in the affected population strongly suggests an inheritable basis for the disease.

Incidence/Prevalence
Although this is a common disease, there are no reliable estimates of incidence/prevalence.

Geographic Distribution N/A

SIGNALMENT

Species Dogs

Breed Predilections
German shepherds and German shepherd mix-breed dogs are most commonly affected. Cases involving other medium-to-large breeds are also commonly reported.

Mean Age and Range
Affected dogs are usually 5-18 months of age, but dogs as young as 2 months and as old as 5 years are affected.

Predominant Sex Male

SIGNS

Historical Findings
• There is no associated history of trauma. • Lameness of varying intensity usually involves the forelimbs initially, but may subsequently affect the hind limbs, producing a shifting leg lameness. • The dog may "carry" the affected leg. • Mild depression, inappetence, and weight loss may occur in severely affected patients.

Physical Examination Findings
• Painful response to deep palpation of the long bones (diaphysis) in an affected limb is a distinguishing characteristic. • Palpate firmly along the entire shaft of each bone while carefully avoiding any "pinching" or nearby muscle. • The ulna is the most frequently affected bone. • The radius, humerus, femur, and tib-

ia (listed in decreasing order of frequency) may also be affected either concurrently or subsequently. • There may be low-grade fever and muscle atrophy.

CAUSES Unknown

RISK FACTORS
Purebred German shepherds or mixed-breed dogs with German shepherd ancestry are at increased risk.

DIAGNOSIS

DIFFERENTIAL DIAGNOSIS
• Panosteitis may be found alone or can coexist with other juvenile orthopedic diseases. • Osteochondritis dissecans, fragmented medial coronoid process, ununited anconeal process, and hip dysplasia must be ruled out. • Fractures and ligamentous injuries from unobserved trauma must also be considered. • When there is shifting leg lameness, immune-mediated arthritides, Lyme disease, or bacterial endocarditis are possibilities.

CBC/BIOCHEMISTRY/URINALYSIS
• Early cases may show eosinophilia. • The results of other hematology tests, clinical chemistries, and urinalysis are usually normal.

OTHER LABORATORY TESTS N/A

IMAGING
• The presence of characteristic radiographic densities within the medulla of long bones confirms a diagnosis of panosteitis. Depending on the duration of the disease, radiographic lesions fall into three phases • Early phase—initially the trabecular pattern of the ends of the diaphysis becomes more prominent but may appear blurred. Granular opacities may be seen. • Middle phase—patchy sclerotic opacities appear first around the nutrient foramen and later throughout the diaphysis. The cortex becomes wider. The periosteum may also appear thickened and increased in opacity. • Late phase—during resolution, the overall opacity of the medullary canal diminishes again towards normal, although a coarse trabecular pattern and some granular opacity may remain. In some cases, there also may be a period in which the medullary canal becomes more lucent than normal.

OTHER DIAGNOSTIC PROCEDURES
N/A

GROSS AND HISTOPATHOLOGIC FINDINGS
• Biopsy or necropsy of affected dogs is rarely performed because of the excellent prognosis for recovery. There are no gross pathologic lesions. • Histologically, there is a degeneration of the marrow adipocytes surrounding the nutrient foramen followed by proliferation of vascular stromal cells within the marrow sinusoids. Osteoid formation and endosteal

new bone formation progress proximally and distally. Vascular congestion may accompany the proliferation of new bone, secondarily stimulating endosteal and periosteal reaction. Remodeling of the endosteum occurs during resolution, reestablishing the normal endosteal and marrow architecture.

TREATMENT

INPATIENT VERSUS OUTPATIENT
Dogs with panosteitis are treated as outpatients.

ACTIVITY
• Although limited activity has not been shown to hasten recovery, it does lessen the pain. • In moderate to severe cases, the pain associated with movement of an affected limb limits exercise and may cause muscle atrophy.

DIET N/A

CLIENT EDUCATION
• Ensure that the client is aware that a diagnosis of panosteitis does not eliminate the possibility of the dog developing other juvenile orthopedic diseases. • Signs of pain and lameness may last for several weeks. • Recurrence of clinical signs is common up to 2 years of age.

SURGICAL CONSIDERATIONS N/A

MEDICATIONS

DRUGS AND FLUIDS
• Nonsteroidal antiinflammatory drugs (NSAIDs) can be used to minimize pain and decrease inflammation. Symptomatic therapy has no bearing on the duration of disease. Aspirin, buffered or enteric coated (10-25 mg/kg, PO, q8h or q12h); phenylbutazone (3-7 mg/kg, PO, q8h, total dose < 800 mg/day); meclofenemic acid (0.5 mg/kg, PO, q12h); and piroxicam (0.3 mg/kg, PO, q24h for 3 days then every other day) are commonly used NSAIDs. • Antiinflammatory dosage of glucocorticoids, such as prednisone (0.1-0.5 mg/kg, PO), can be given. The potential side affects are well documented; therefore, low dose and alternate-day therapy is the goal if used chronically.

CONTRAINDICATIONS
Intolerance to NSAIDs is indicated by gastrointestinal upset and may preclude their use in individual patients.

PRECAUTIONS
• Most NSAIDs cause some degree of gastric ulceration. • Acetaminophen is unsuitable as an analgesic because of its potential for toxicity.

POSSIBLE INTERACTIONS

NSAIDs should not be used in conjunction with glucocorticoids because of the risk of gastrointestinal tract ulceration.

ALTERNATE DRUGS N/A

FOLLOW-UP

PATIENT MONITORING

Persistent lameness should be rechecked (at 2-4 week intervals) to detect more serious, concurrent, orthopedic problems.

PREVENTION/AVOIDANCE N/A

POSSIBLE COMPLICATIONS N/A

EXPECTED COURSE AND PROGNOSIS

Panosteitis is a self-limiting disease. Treatment is symptomatic and appears to have no influence on duration of clinical signs. Multiple limb involvement is common.

Although exceptional cases may persist for months, the duration of lameness in a typical case is a few days to several weeks.

MISCELLANEOUS

ASSOCIATED CONDITIONS N/A

AGE RELATED FACTORS

Panosteitis is typically a disease of immature and young dogs.

ZOONOTIC POTENTIAL N/A

PREGNANCY

Although females are reportedly more susceptible to panosteitis during estrus, there is no proven relationship between the disease and reproductive hormones or pregnancy.

SYNONYMS

• Enostosis • Fibrous osteodystrophy • Juvenile osteomyelitis • Eosinophilic panosteitis

SEE ALSO N/A

ABBREVIATIONS

NSAID = nonsteroidal antiinflammatory drug

References

Manly PA, Romich JA. Miscellaneous orthopedic diseases. In: Slatter DH, ed. Textbook of small animal surgery. 2nd ed. Philadelphia: WB Saunders, 1993:1984-1987.

Halliwell WH. Tumor-like lesions of bone. In: Bojrab MJ, ed. Disease mechanisms in small animal surgery. 2nd ed. Philadelphia: WB Saunders, 1993:932-933.

Brinker WO, Piermattei DL, Flo GL. Disease conditions in small animals. In: Handbook of small animal orthopedics and fracture treatment. 2nd ed. Philadelphia: WB Saunders, 1990:547-550.

Author Larry Carpenter
Consulting Editor Peter D. Schwarz

PAPILLEDEMA

BASICS

OVERVIEW
Swelling of optic disc secondary to high intracranial pressure. Swelling of the optic disc reflecting other pathologies (e.g., orbital disease) is referred to as optic disc edema.

SIGNALMENT N/A

SIGNS

Historical Findings
• Disc edema per se produces no visual deficits. • Cerebral signs.

Physical Examination Findings
• Neurologic signs • Elevation and hyperemia of optic nerve head • Blurring of optic disc margin • Filling in of physiologic cup

CAUSES AND RISK FACTORS
• Hydrocephalus • Hepatic encephalopathy • Neoplasm (primary or metastatic) • Distemper in dogs • Infectious peritonitis in cats • Systemic mycoses • Toxoplasmosis • Neosporum caninum • Granulomatous meningoencephalomyelitis • Trauma

DIAGNOSIS

DIFFERENTIAL DIAGNOSIS
Diseases that cause optic disc swelling (e.g., optic neuritis, congenital anomalies, and hyaline bodies)

CBC/BIOCHEMISTRY/URINALYSIS
No specific abnormalities

OTHER LABORATORY TESTS
Specific viral, fungal, or protozoal serologic tests

IMAGING
• Orbital ultrasound • Neuroimaging (CT/MRI)

OTHER DIAGNOSTIC PROCEDURES
CSF analysis (measure intracranial pressure)

TREATMENT
• Resolve cause of high intracranial pressure or orbital disease.
• Patients need critical monitoring.

MEDICATIONS

DRUGS AND FLUIDS
Treatment for CNS disease
• Mannitol—250mg/kg IV over 20 minutes, repeat as necessary
• Furosemide (Lasix)—1mg/kg q8h IV
• Hyperventilation—maintain arterial PCO_2 between 25-30 mmHg
• Corticosteroids—prednisone 0.5mg/kg q12h PO or dexamethasone SP 0.25 mg/kg q6h-q12h IV

CONTRAINDICATIONS/POSSIBLE INTERACTIONS
• Mannitol is contraindicated in animals with intracranial hemorrhage.
• Beware of brain herniation.
• Systemically administered corticosteroids should not be used unless infectious causes are ruled out.

FOLLOW-UP
Prognosis depends on underlying disease.

MISCELLANEOUS

Reference

Whiting AS, Johnson LN. Papilledema: Clinical clues and differential diagnosis. Am Fam Phys 1992;45:1125–1134.

Author David Lipsitz
Consulting Editor Paul E. Miller

BASICS

OVERVIEW
• Canine viral papillomas are benign tumors caused by canine oral papillomavirus (COPV). COPV is a member of the Papovaviridae family. The mucocutaneous tumors are benign and self-limiting. • Canine viral papillomatosis occurs in three forms: oral, ocular, and cutaneous. • Papillomas caused by COPV are typically multiple and occur in young dogs, whereas noninfectious papillomas are solitary and occur typically in older patients. • Tumors caused by COPV typically arise in patients 6 months to 4 years of age and spontaneously regress within 1-5 months. • Rarely, papillomas caused by COPV will undergo malignant transformation to squamous cell carcinoma. • Treatment is not usually required but may be needed if owners are particularly concerned or if tumors are causing obstruction or repeated trauma. Treatment modalities include surgical excision, cryosurgery, and electrosurgery. Crushing of several tumors may also stimulate regression.

SIGNALMENT
• Dogs only. Papillomaviruses are usually species specific.
• Affected animals are typically younger than 2 years of age with oral papillomas, 6 months to 4 years with ocular papillomas, and the age range for cutaneous papillomas caused by virus is uncertain.

SIGNS

Historical Findings
Owners may report difficulty eating or apparent discomfort.

Physical Examination Findings
• Vary with form of disease • Oral—halitosis, ptyalism, oral bleeding, and reluctance to eat may be noted. Lesions vary from smooth, white mucosal elevations to cauliflowerlike warts on the lip margins, oral mucosa, tongue, palate, pharynx, and epiglottis. Tumors (50-100) may be present at time of first diagnosis. • Ocular—wart lesions on conjunctiva, cornea, and eyelid margins • Cutaneous—papilloma site distribution is variable. Lesions have been noted on the lower extremities, foot pads, and subungually.

CAUSES AND RISK FACTORS
Risk factors not clearly identified. Recovered dogs appear to be immune.

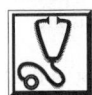

DIAGNOSIS

DIFFERENTIAL DIAGNOSIS
• Transmissible venereal tumor (TVT)
• Squamous cell carcinoma • Fibromatous epulis

CBC/BIOCHEMISTRY/URINALYSIS
Usually within normal limits unless dogs have become malnourished as a result of prolonged dysphagia

OTHER LABORATORY TESTS N/A

IMAGING N/A

OTHER DIAGNOSTIC PROCEDURES
• Rarely needed because gross appearance is pathognomonic. Biopsy will differentiate.
• Sedation and laryngeal exam may be needed to ensure patent airway in severely affected dogs.

GROSS AND HISTOPATHOLOGIC FINDINGS
• Gross appearance discussed above.
• Histopathology reveals layers of enlarged vacuolated wart cells surrounding an inner core of malpighian cells that may be normal in size and appearance. Few if any characteristics of malignancy are typically noted.

TREATMENT
• Treatment is rarely needed as disease is self-limiting.
• Surgical excision, cryosurgery, electrosurgery, or crushing of several tumors to stimulate immune response are all available options.
• Maintenance of environment and nutritional support are important factors in maintaining health of the patient while awaiting tumor remission.
• Patient should be kept apart from other susceptible animals because of the contagious nature of the lesions.

MEDICATIONS

DRUGS AND FLUIDS
• Systemic chemotherapy using vincristine, cyclophosphamide, doxorubicin, or bleomycin has been attempted with varying degrees of success. Chemotherapy usually is reserved for persistent papillomas that have failed to regress after more than 5 months.

CONTRAINDICATIONS/POSSIBLE INTERACTIONS
Autogenous wart vaccines have been recommended by some, but their efficacy is unknown.

FOLLOW-UP

PATIENT MONITORING
Respiration should be monitored and the patient admitted for further care if airway obstruction is suspected or confirmed.

PREVENTION/AVOIDANCE
Recovered animals are generally immune. Prevention involves limiting contact of susceptible animals with known carriers.

EXPECTED COURSE AND PROGNOSIS
Prognosis is good. Malignant transformation rate is low.

MISCELLANEOUS

ZOONOTIC POTENTIAL
None. Papillomaviruses are generally species specific.

ABBREVIATION
COPV = canine oral papillomavirus

Reference
Calvert CA. Canine viral papillomatosis. In: Greene CE, ed. Infectious diseases of the dog and cat. Philadelphia: WB Saunders, 1990:288-290.
Author Matthew S. Mellema
Consulting Editor Fred W. Scott

PARAGONIMIASIS

BASICS

OVERVIEW
• Paragonimus kellicotti, the lung fluke, is a trematode that may inhabit the lungs of a variety of mammals. • Paragonimus kellicotti is the only species of importance to dogs and cats in the United States.

SIGNALMENT
• Most common in cats, dogs, and other mammalian hosts 6 months of age and older. • No breed or gender has been recognized.

SIGNS
• Respiratory signs are typically mild and include a persistent cough. • Lung sounds are usually normal unless significant lung pathology exists. Clinical signs are likely to be more severe during the migratory and growth phases as the flukes establish themselves. • In animals with heavy infections, the slightest exertion will initiate a cough. Hemoptysis sometimes is seen at this stage. • Fatalities occur owing to pulmonary hemorrhage or secondary infection after simultaneous entry of a number of flukes into the lungs. • Pneumothorax may occur if subpleural cysts rupture.

CAUSES AND RISK FACTORS
• Like most flukes, the adult stage is not host-specific, with Paragonimus kellicotti found in a number of mammalian hosts. The mink is regarded as the preferred host, but reservoirs may include the muskrat, opossum, raccoon, skunk, bobcat, and fox. • Louisiana and the Great Lakes area have a high incidence of mammalian host infection, but Paragonimus kellicotti has been reported in most states in the eastern United States. • The life cycle—adult flukes in the lung release operculated eggs into the bronchial tree that are subsequently coughed up, swallowed, and shed in the feces. • After 2-3 weeks development within eggs in an aquatic environment, short-lived, ciliated miracidia emerge and must find a suitable snail intermediate within 24 hours or perish. Amphibious snails (Pomatiopsis spp.) serve as the first intermediate host. • Miracidia initiate a complex asexual reproductive phase in snail tissue and produce large numbers of free-swimming cercariae. Cercariae penetrate through the exoskeleton of the crayfish which is the second intermediate host, encyst as metacercaria, and await in-

gestion by the final host. • A number of species of crayfish (Cambarus spp.) may serve as second intermediate hosts. Metacercariae locate in crayfish heart muscle. Metacercariae become infective to the final host in a period of several weeks. An immature fluke is present within the cyst wall at this time. • After ingestion, metacercariae excyst in the small intestine, and young flukes penetrate the intestinal wall into the peritoneal cavity and migrate across the diaphragm to the pleural cavity. They migrate in lung tissue for 3-4 weeks before pairing up. Cysts are radiographically visible 4 weeks after infection. Mature flukes are found in fibrous pulmonary cysts 5-6 weeks after infection, at which time patency occurs. Cysts of Paragonimus usually are found close to the lung surface and appear as nodular, elevated masses of 1-2 cm beneath the pleura. Migration of young flukes through the pleura sometimes is marked by small hemorrhages that progress to small scars. During migration through the lung parenchyma, young flukes pair up and are generally found with two adults within individual cysts. Paragonimus are small, thick flukes, reddish-brown in the living state, and measure 1 by 0.5 cm.

DIAGNOSIS

DIFFERENTIAL DIAGNOSIS
• Based on clinical and radiographic findings • Differential diagnoses for the circumscribed, pulmonary, soft tissue densities include abscessation, primary or metastatic pulmonary neoplasia, and congenital pulmonary anomaly.

CBC/BIOCHEMISTRY/URINALYSIS
Eosinophilia; serum chemistry profile and urinalysis are unremarkable

OTHER LABORATORY TESTS N/A

IMAGING
Diagnosis can be made by thoracic radiography, particularly when eggs are not being passed. Fluke-containing cysts are seen as circumscribed, pulmonary, soft tissue densities. On rare occasions, cysts are radiolucent (appearance of an air bubble in the cyst). This "signet ring" appearance, when present, is pathognomonic for Paragonimus infection.

OTHER DIAGNOSTIC PROCEDURES
• Infections usually are diagnosed by finding the characteristic operculated egg using rou-

tine fecal flotation procedures (eggs of many fluke species sink in flotation solution) or fecal sedimentation procedures. • Paragonimus eggs are yellow-brown, and have an operculum set into a characteristic collarlike thickening. • Eggs also may be identified in aspirated fluid from transtracheal wash or tracheobronchial lavage via bronchoscopy.

TREATMENT
• Primary treatment is directed at killing the flukes contained within the pulmonary cysts. • Pulmonary lesions resolve within 2 months after successful therapy but will persist if the lesions are several years old.

MEDICATIONS

DRUGS AND FLUIDS
• Fenbendazole and albendazole are effective at the oral dose of 25 mg/kg q12h for 14-21 days. • Praziquantel is effective at a dosage of 25 mg/kg q8h IM, SC in the cat, for 2-3 days.

CONTRAINDICATIONS/POSSIBLE INTERACTIONS N/A

FOLLOW-UP
• Monitor by thoracic radiography and periodic fecal examinations. • Most cats and dogs show clinical improvement and reversal of the respiratory signs. • Nodular radiographic lesions resolve within 2 months after successful therapy.

MISCELLANEOUS

Reference

Bowman DD, Frongillo MK, Johnson RC, et al. Evaluation of praziquantel for treatment of experimentally induced paragonimiasis in dogs and cats. Am J Vet Res 1991;52:68-71.

Author Johnny D. Hoskins
Consulting Editors Lynelle Johnson and Bradley L. Moses

BASICS

OVERVIEW
• Phimosis—Inability to protrude the penis beyond the preputial orifice • Paraphimosis—penis protrudes from the preputial orifice and cannot be returned to its normal position

SIGNALMENT
Congenital preputial stenosis, possibly hereditary, has been observed in the German shepherd dog and golden retriever.

SIGNS
• Phimosis may be undetected until the dog is unsuccessful in attempts to copulate.
• Severe defects in the neonate interfere with urination or cause pooling of urine in the preputial cavity, which can cause balanoposthitis leading to septicemia. • Dogs with paraphimosis of short duration may not have any signs other than the dog's licking of an exteriorized penis. After some hours of exposure, ischemic necrosis and urethral obstruction can develop.

CAUSES AND RISK FACTORS
• Phimosis is caused by an abnormally small preputial orifice. Can be congenital or acquired (i.e., caused by injury or disease).
• May be associated with a persistent penile or preputial frenulum, a thin band of connective tissue joining the penis and prepuce along the ventral glans. • Paraphimosis is usually associated with erection or copulation. Hair surrounding the preputial orifice is trapped against surface of the penis, especially the bulbus glandis, and the penis cannot retract. • A moderately stenotic preputial orifice may contribute. • Can also be caused by injury, os penis fracture, and priapism (i.e., neurologic condition of persistent erection without sexual interest).

DIAGNOSIS

DIFFERENTIAL DIAGNOSIS
Paraphimosis—exposure of the glans penis caused by abnormality of the retractor penis muscles or preputial muscles, large preputial opening, and short prepuce.

TREATMENT
• Phimosis requires surgical enlargement of the preputial orifice. When the dog has a persistent penile frenulum, separate tissue holds the glans penis to the parietal lamina of the prepuce.
• Paraphimosis requires immediate treatment. After 24 hours, the tissue damage and urethral obstruction may require penile amputation. If urethral patency is in question, place an indwelling urinary catheter. Replacement of the penis in normal position is the goal.
• Remove foreign objects, lubricate the penis, apply compresses of hypertonic glucose solution, and surgically enlarge preputial orifice if necessary.
• An abdominal compression bandage and indwelling urinary catheter to maintain the penis within the prepuce may also reduce localized edema.

MEDICATIONS

DRUGS AND FLUIDS
Maintain treatment with antibiotic ointments to prevent adhesions between the penis and prepuce.

CONTRAINDICATIONS/POSSIBLE INTERACTIONS N/A

FOLLOW-UP N/A

MISCELLANEOUS

References

Phimosis

Burke TJ. Small animal reproduction and infertility. Philadelphia: Lea & Febiger, 1986.

Johnston SD. Disorders of the canine penis and prepuce. In: Morrow DA, ed. Current therapy in theriogenology 2. Philadelphia: WB Saunders, 1986;549-550.

Paraphimosis

Feldman EC, Nelson RW. Canine and feline endocrinology and reproduction. Philadelphia: WB Saunders, 1987.

Author Rolf E. Larsen

Consulting Editor Sara K. Lyle

PARVOVIRAL INFECTION—DOGS

BASICS

DEFINITION
• Canine parvovirus type 2 (CPV-2) infection is an acute systemic illness characterized by hemorrhagic enteritis. The disease is often fatal in pups, who may collapse in a "shock-like" state and die suddenly without enteric signs after only a brief period of malaise. The myocardial form, observed in pups during the early outbreaks when the dog population was fully susceptible, is now rare. Most pups are now protected against neonatal infection by maternal antibodies. • Monoclonal antibodies have revealed antigenic changes in CPV-2 since its emergence about 1978. The original virus is now virtually extinct in the domestic dog population. The viruses currently circulating in dogs, designated CPV-2a and CPV-2b, have remained genetically stable since 1984. However, the "new viruses" are more virulent than the original isolates and case mortality rates appear to be higher than in the earliest outbreaks. Most of the clinical literature is based on the response of dogs to CPV-2, and it should be reevaluated in light of the emergence and dominance of the newer types. As with rabies variants, the antigenic changes in CPV-2 have no effect on the ability of various vaccines to protect dogs.

Pathophysiology
• CPV-2 is closely related to feline panleukopenia virus (FPV) and several other parvoviruses that infect carnivores. Parvoviruses, including CPV-2, require actively dividing cells for growth. After ingestion of virus, the usual route, there is a 2 to 4-day period of viremia with concomitant growth in lymphatic tissues throughout the body and, by the third postinfection (PI) day, infection of the rapidly dividing crypt cells of the small intestine. • Viral shedding in the feces commences approximately 3-4 days after infection and reaches a peak about the time clinical signs first occur. Virus then ceases to be shed in detectable amounts by PI days 8-12. It is important, therefore, to collect feces for viral detection at the onset of clinical illness. • Absorption of bacterial endotoxins from the damaged intestinal mucosa are believed to play a role in CPV-2 disease.

Systems Affected
• Cardiovascular—seronegative pups infected shortly after birth • Lymphatic (lymphoid tissues)—thymus, lymph nodes, spleen, and Peyer's patches • Gastrointestinal—small intestinal crypt cells and adjacent mucosal epithelium

Genetics
Certain breeds appear to be especially susceptible; the genetic basis is unknown.

Incidence/Prevalence
The disease is most common in breeding kennels, animal shelters, pet emporiums, and wherever pups are reared. Incidence/prevalence rates vary.

Geographic Distribution   Worldwide

SIGNALMENT

Species
Both domestic and wild canids are susceptible.

Breed Predilections
Rottweilers, doberman pinschers, and English springer spaniels are reported to be at exceptional risk of severe disease.

Mean Age and Range
Most severe illness occurs in pups 6-16 weeks of age; however, illness may occur at any age.

Predominant Sex   N/A

SIGNS

General Comments
CPV-2 infection should be suspected whenever pups have an enteric illness, especially when there is sudden onset of apathy, vomiting, and loose stools with excessive mucus or blood.

Historical Findings
Sudden onset of bloody diarrhea, anorexia, and repeated episodes of vomiting. In breeding kennels, several littermate pups may become ill simultaneously or within a short period of time. Occasionally, one or two pups in a litter will have no or only mild signs followed by the death of littermates who, presumably, encounter greater amounts of virus.

Physical Examination Findings
• The incubation period and intensity of illness appear to be related to the viral dose and the antigenic type (CPV-2 versus CPV-2a, -2b). Pups infected with the prevalent viral types often die suddenly after a brief period of illness with or without bloody diarrhea. • Initial signs include depression, anorexia, and pyrexia. Repeated episodes of vomiting or retching are typical in severely affected dogs, commonly followed shortly by mucoid or hemorrhagic diarrhea. • Lymphopenia is characteristic of CPV-2 infection and may progress to absolute lymphopenia. In severely affected dogs, there may be neutropenia concurrent with the onset of intestinal damage. Leukocytosis and bone marrow hyperplasia are common during recovery. • Dehydration, weight loss, and abdominal discomfort are consistent features.

RISK FACTORS
• Dogs in animal shelters, pet shops, attendance at shows, or elsewhere dogs have congregated are at greatest risk. Pups less than 3 months of age are at high risk of severe infection. • Copathogens such as parasites, viruses, and certain bacterial species (e.g., Campylobacter spp., Clostridia difficile) have been hypothesized to exacerbate illness. • Severe, often fatal parvovirus infections have been demonstrated in pups exposed simultaneously to CPV-2 and canine coronavirus.

• Crowding and poor sanitation reduces the chances of successful immunization in kennels and animal shelters; however, there is no evidence of enhanced disease in individuals. • Certain distemper vaccines (e.g., the Rockborn strain) have been reported to increase risk of severe disease in pups exposed simultaneously to CPV-2 and distemper vaccines.

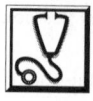

DIAGNOSIS

DIFFERENTIAL DIAGNOSIS
• Canine coronavirus infection • Salmonellosis, colibacillosis, and other enteric bacterial infections • Gastrointestinal foreign bodies • Gastrointestinal parasites (e.g., giardiasis) • Hemorrhagic gastroenteritis • Intussusception • Toxin ingestion

CBC/BIOCHEMISTRY/URINALYSIS
• Lymphopenia commonly occurs between PI days 4-6. It may be relative or, in severe cases, absolute. In some dogs, relative neutrophilia is observed. Leukopenia is a variable finding, although serial hemograms will detect leukopenia in most patients. Severe leukopenia is a poor prognostic sign. • Serum chemistry profiles help assess electrolyte disturbances (especially hypokalemia and hypoglycemia).

OTHER LABORATORY TESTS
Serologic tests are not diagnostic because dogs will have high titers from vaccination and/or maternal antibody.

IMAGING   N/A

OTHER DIAGNOSTIC PROCEDURES
• Samples for virus detection should be submitted during the acute phase of infection. Specimens should be shipped refrigerated, not frozen. • Virus may be detected in stool or intestinal content samples at the onset of disease and for 2-4 days afterwards by use of commercial solid-phase ELISA tests (e.g., CITE Test, IDDEX, Inc., Portland ME) or ImmunoComb (BIOGAL, Kibbutz Galed, Israel) in which sensitivity and specificity appear high. When blood is present in stools, results may be negative because of the presence of antibodies. Electron microscopy is another method of detecting virus during the early stages of infection. Virus also may be identified in tissue samples by immunofluorescence or immunoperoxidase staining.

GROSS AND HISTOPATHOLOGIC FINDINGS
• Gross changes include subserosal congestion and hemorrhage or frank hemorrhage into the intestinal lumen. In some dogs, the intestines are empty or contain yellow or blood-tinged fluid. Lymph nodes are often enlarged and edematous with hemorrhages in the cortex. Thymus atrophy is common in young dogs; only a remnant of the thymus may remain in some dogs that die.

Pulmonary edema and hydropericardium may be the only gross change in pups with myocarditis and acute heart failure. Pale streaks may be visible in the myocardium of pups with subacute heart failure. • Pups that die with the cardiac form typically have lesions of congestive heart failure. Focal areas of necrotic myocytes, edema and lymphocytic infiltration are common in the myocardium. Basophilic inclusions may be observed in pups that die acutely. In the more chronically affected, interstitial fibrosis and scarring are common.

TREATMENT

Treatment is symptomatic and supportive. Refer to section on treatment of acute gastroenteritis. Intensity of treatment depends on the gravity of signs on examination. Goals are to mollify the intestinal tract, restore and maintain fluid balance, and minimize fluid losses. Prompt and intensive care favors treatment success. Dietary restriction is important.

INPATIENT VERSUS OUTPATIENT
Inpatient treatment is usually recommended, especially with pups that have a severe depression and intractable vomiting and/or diarrhea. Pup isolation is essential; care must be exercised to prevent spread of CPV-2, a very stable virus.

ACTIVITY
Restricted activity until signs ameliorate

DIET
Food and water should be withheld for 12-24 hours. Maintain on IV or SC (if not vomiting) fluids and electrolytes. Highly digestible, low-fat nourishment is indicated in recovering pups.

CLIENT EDUCATION
Inform client of the need for thorough disinfection, especially if other dogs are on the premises. A 1:30 dilution of bleach (5% sodium hypochlorite) will destroy CPV-2 in a few minutes. Failure to maintain strict sanitation and, preferably, isolation until the pups

reach at least 3 months of age are hazards. Pups can be infected with virulent virus before any vaccine will engender immunity. CPV-2 is shed for less than 2 weeks after infection; a carrier state has not been demonstrated.

SURGICAL CONSIDERATIONS N/A

MEDICATIONS

Refer to section on treatment and management of acute gastrointestinal disease.

DRUGS AND FLUIDS
• Lactated Ringer's solution supplemented with potassium chloride and sodium bicarbonate (if acidosis) • Amino acids and 5% dextrose with bicarbonate if blood sugar level is below 60 • Other medications claimed beneficial include B-complex vitamins; if oral treatment is possible, Pepto-Bismol (1 ml/pound) may be given. Additional drugs that have been recommended by clinicians include parenteral administration of antibiotics (ampicillin and gentamicin), corticosteroids (dexamethasone or prednisolone), or antiemetics. Drugs that suppress intestinal motility are controversial and they should be used with discretion in dogs with CPV-2 infection.

CONTRAINDICATIONS N/A
PRECAUTIONS
Gentamicin can cause fatal renal toxicity in dehydrated or young pups. Examine for tubular casts in urine after 4-5 days of use.

POSSIBLE INTERACTIONS N/A
ALTERNATE DRUGS N/A

FOLLOW-UP

PATIENT MONITORING
Acutely ill pups should be monitored at frequent intervals until recovery seems likely.

PREVENTION/AVOIDANCE
• Inactivated and live vaccines are available for prophylaxis. • Inactivated vaccines engen-

der protection from disease but do not interrupt transmission. • Vaccination regimens should be determined by estimation of risk. • Immunization is uncertain if pups have maternal antibodies. • About 70-75% of pups vaccinated with efficacious products may be expected to develop immunity at 12 weeks of age. • Vaccination is not an effective control method in contaminated environments. • Vaccines differ in their capacity to immunize pups with maternal antibodies. • Control of CPV-2 requires efficacious vaccines, pup isolation, and stringent hygiene.

EXPECTED COURSE AND PROGNOSIS
The prognosis is good for pups surviving 3-4 days of illness.

ZOONOTIC POTENTIAL
Disease is restricted to dogs.

PREGNANCY
In utero infections have not been reported in field cases.

MISCELLANEOUS

SYNONYMS N/A

SEE ALSO
• Coronavirus Infection—Dogs • Acute Viral Gastroenteritis

ABBREVIATIONS
CPV-2 = canine parvovirus type 2
FPV = feline panleukopenia virus
PI = postinfection

References

Pollock RHV, Carmichael LE. Canine viral enteritis. In: Greene CE, ed. Infectious diseases of the dog and cat. Philadelphia: WB Saunders, 1990:268-279.

Pollock RHV, Parrish CR. Canine parvovirus. In: Olsen RG, Krakowa S, Blakeslee JR, eds. Boca Raton: CRC Press, 1985:145-177.

Author Leland Carmichael
Consulting Editor Fred W. Scott

PATELLAR LUXATION

BASICS

DEFINITION
Medial or lateral displacement of the patella from its normal anatomic position in the femoral trochlea

Pathophysiology
• The degree of skeletal disease varies between the mildest to the severest forms. • Common musculoskeletal changes include tibial rotation on its long axis, bowing of the distal and proximal tibia, shallow to absent femoral trochlea, dysplasia of the femoral and tibial epiphysis, and displacement of the quadriceps muscle group. • Because of the variable degree of clinical and pathologic changes, a system for classifying patellar luxations has been developed (grades I-IV).

Systems Affected   Musculoskeletal

Genetics
• Proposed are recessive, polygenic, and multifocal inheritance • Hereditary in Devon rex cats

Incidence/Prevalence
• Considered one of the most common stifle joint abnormalities in dogs. Greater than 75% of the diagnosed patellar luxations are medial. Bilateral involvement is seen 50% of the time. • Uncommon in cats; may be more common than suspected since most cats are not lame

Geographic Distribution   N/A

SIGNALMENT

Species
• Predominately dogs • Rarely cats

Breed Predilections
• Most common in toy and miniature dog breeds • Miniature and toy poodles, Yorkshire terriers, Pomeranians, Pekingese, Chihuahuas, and Boston terriers

Mean Age and Range
Clinical signs may develop soon after birth but generally after 4 months of age.

Predominant Sex
There appears to be a sex predilection; the risk of medial patellar luxation for females is one and a half times that for males.

SIGNS

General Comments
Clinical signs are dependent on the grade (severity) of luxation, amount of degenerative arthritis, chronicity of the disease, and the presence of other stifle joint abnormalities (i.e., cruciate ligament rupture).

Historical Findings
• Persistent abnormal hindlimb carriage and function in neonates and puppies • Occasional "skipping" or intermittent hindlimb lameness that worsens symptomatically in young to mature dogs • Sudden signs of lameness due to

minor trauma or worsening degenerative joint disease in older animals

Physical Examination Findings
• Grade I—the patella can be manually luxated; however, the patella reduces when pressure is released • Grade II—the patella can be manually luxated or it can spontaneously luxate with flexion of the stifle joint. The patella remains luxated until it is manually reduced or when the animal extends the joint and derotates the tibia in the opposite direction of luxation. • Grade III—the patella remains luxated most of the time but can be manually reduced with the stifle joint in extension. Flexion and extension of the stifle results in reluxation of the patella. • Grade IV—the patella is permanently luxated and cannot be manually repositioned. There may be up to 90° of rotation of the proximal tibial plateau. The femoral trochlear groove is shallow or absent, and there is displacement of the quadriceps muscle group in the direction of luxation. • The limb is intermittently carried with the stifle joint flexed (grades I and II). • Animals exhibit a crouching, bowlegged (genu varum), or knock-knee (genu valgum) stance for medial or lateral luxations, respectively (grades III and IV). Also, most of the body weight is transferred to the front limbs. • Pain can be elicited if chondromalacia of the patella or femoral trochlea is present.

CAUSES
• Congenital • Traumatic

RISK FACTORS
• Coxa vara (decrease in the femoral neck-femoral shaft axis) is associated with medial patellar luxations. • Coxa valga (increase in the femoral neck- femoral shaft axis) is associated with lateral patellar luxations. • Excessive anteversion (forward inclination of the femoral head and neck)

DIAGNOSIS

DIFFERENTIAL DIAGNOSIS
• Cranial cruciate ligament rupture can be differentiated on the basis of palpation by the presence of cranial drawer motion. Concurrent rupture of the cranial cruciate ligament is present in 15-20% of dogs with chronic patellar luxations. • Avulsion fracture of the tibial tubercle will cause laxity of the quadriceps mechanism, resulting in patella instability. • Rupture of the patellar tendon will result in proximal displacement of the patella and instability. • Malunion and malalignment of fractures of either the femur or tibia can result in displacement of the quadriceps muscle group.

CBC/BIOCHEMISTRY/URINALYSIS
N/A

OTHER LABORATORY TESTS   N/A

IMAGING
• Craniocaudal and mediolateral radiographs of the stifle joint are indicated for all animals with either grade III or IV patellar luxations. Radiographs that include the joint above (hip) and below (hock) are necessary to determine if excessive bowing and/or torsion of the femur and tibia is present. • Skyline radiographs of the femoral trochlea are useful to determine if it is shallow, flattened, or even convex.

OTHER DIAGNOSTIC PROCEDURES
Diagnosis of patellar luxation is based on historical findings, physical examination, and radiographs.

GROSS AND HISTOPATHOLOGIC FINDINGS

Gross Findings
Cartilage "wear" lesions of the patella and femoral trochlea; osteophytes at the joint capsule-bone interface; joint capsule redundancy on the side opposite of luxation; and fibrosis and contracture on the side of luxation

Microscopic
Cartilage fibrillation and loss of glycosaminoglycan content; synovitis

TREATMENT

INPATIENT VERSUS OUTPATIENT
• Grade I and some grade II patellar luxations can be treated conservatively on outpatient basis.
• Most grade II and almost all grades III and IV luxations should be surgically treated.

ACTIVITY
Normal to restricted activity depending on severity of luxation

DIET
Weight control is important to reduce the load and therefore the stress on the stifle joint.

CLIENT EDUCATION
• Discuss the heritability of the condition.
• Discuss the possibility of development of degenerative joint disease.
• Discuss the high risk of cranial cruciate ligament disease.
• Discuss the potential for the condition to worsen over time (i.e., grade I → grade II).

SURGICAL CONSIDERATIONS
• If bone deformity exists (i.e., shallow trochlea or tibial tubercle deviation), surgical bone reconstruction techniques are required.
• Trochleoplasty—arthroplastic procedure to deepen the trochlear sulcus. Recession sulcoplasty is the removal of hyaline cartilage and cancellous bone to deepen the sulcus. Fibrocartilage eventually resurfaces the trochlea. Recession sulcoplasty can also be the removal of a V-shaped wedge, preserving the hyaline cartilage. After deepening of the

trochlea, the osteochondral bone wedge is replaced, creating a new sulcus composed of hyaline cartilage. This method is preferred in most animals. Trochlear chondroplasty is useful only in young (< 6 months) animals. A cartilage flap is created, subchondral bone is removed beneath it, and the flap replaced to line the new sulcus. Hyaline cartilage is preserved to cover the bottom of the sulcus while fibrocartilage covers the sides.

• Transposition of the tibial tubercle is used to realign the longitudinal axis of the quadriceps mechanism so that it is centered over the femoral trochlea. The tibia tubercle is osteotomized and transposed opposite the direction of luxation. The tubercle is stabilized with pins and wire.

• Imbrication of the joint capsule and supporting soft tissues on the side opposite the luxation is done to help "pull" the patella over

• Desmotomy or releasing incision is made on the side toward which the patella is luxated

• Patellar and tibial antirotational suture ligaments are used to reinforce stretched supporting soft tissue structures

• Corrective osteotomies realign the longitudinal axis of the hindlimb

MEDICATIONS

DRUGS AND FLUIDS

Antiinflammatory and analgesic drugs can be used to symptomatically treat associated degenerative joint disease.

CONTRAINDICATIONS

Corticosteroids should be avoided because of the potential side effects and the articular cartilage damage associated with long-term use.

PRECAUTIONS

Gastrointestinal irritation may occur with the use of nonsteroidal antiinflammatory drugs (NSAIDs) and may preclude their use in individual animals.

POSSIBLE INTERACTIONS N/A

ALTERNATE DRUGS

Chondroprotective drugs, such as polysulfated glycosaminoglycans, may be of benefit in limiting cartilage damage and degeneration.

FOLLOW-UP

PATIENT MONITORING

• Early, active use of the limb is encouraged if a trochleoplasty technique has been performed. Exercise should be limited for 4 weeks, and jumping should be prevented.
• Yearly examinations are recommended to assess progression of disease.

PREVENTION/AVOIDANCE

• Breeding of affected animals is to be discouraged. • Dam/sire breedings that result in offspring with patellar luxations should not be repeated.

POSSIBLE COMPLICATIONS

• Recurrent patellar luxation after surgical stabilization has been reported as high as 48% • Recurrent luxations are generally of a lesser grade than the preoperative grade.

EXPECTED COURSE AND PROGNOSIS

• More than 90% of patients treated by surgery function well enough not to show lameness or clinical dysfunction. • Almost all stifle joints will have radiographic evidence of degenerative joint disease.

MISCELLANEOUS

ASSOCIATED CONDITIONS

Always look for cranial cruciate ligament disease.

AGE RELATED FACTORS N/A

ZOONOTIC POTENTIAL N/A

PREGNANCY N/A

SYNONYMS N/A

SEE ALSO Arthritis (Osteoarthritis)

ABBREVIATIONS

None

References

Willauer C, Vasseur P. Clinical results of surgical correction of medial luxation of the patella in dogs. Vet Surg 1987;16:31-36.

Arnoczky S, Tarvin G. Surgical repair of patella luxations and fractures. In: Bojrab MJ, ed. Current techniques in small animal surgery. 3rd ed. Philadelphia: Lea & Febiger, 1990;714-722.

Brinker WO, Piermattei DL, Flo GL. Patellar luxations In: Handbook of small animal orthopedics and fracture treatment. 2nd ed. Philadelphia: WB Saunders, 1990;377-397.

Author Peter D. Schwarz
Consulting Editor Peter D. Schwarz

PATENT DUCTUS ARTERIOSUS

BASICS

DEFINITION
Abnormal persistence of the normal fetal connection (ductus arteriosus) between the aorta and the pulmonary artery (PA)

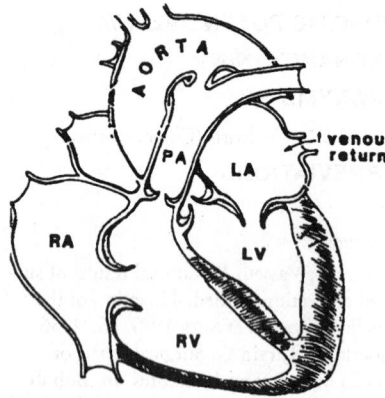

Pathophysiology
Animals with a small ductus have no important hemodynamic changes. As the size of the ductus increases, volume overload of the left ventricle develops, often resulting in left ventricular failure. In animals with large shunts through a patent ductus arteriosus (PDA), pulmonary hypertension frequently occurs. If the pulmonary vascular resistance exceeds the systemic vascular resistance, then the shunt will reverse and go from right to left. Right ventricular failure can result from the high afterload imposed upon it by pulmonary hypertension.

Systems Affected
• Cardiovascular due to volume overload caused by the shunt • Respiratory if pulmonary edema develops

Genetics
Hereditary in miniature poodles, transmitted as a polygenic trait

Incidence/Prevalence
• Congenital heart disease affects 8 per 1,000 live births; PDA is the most common congenital cardiac defect in dogs. • Actual incidence is probably higher because some defects cause neonatal death.

Geographic Distribution N/A

SIGNALMENT

Species Dogs and cats

Breed Predilections
Miniature poodle, German shepherd dog, collie, Pomeranian, Shetland sheep dog, toy breeds

Mean Age and Range
• Signs of left or right heart failure can occur at any age. Most animals develop severe clinical signs in the first 6–8 weeks of life.
• Dogs with a small defect often survive for several years. • Cats rarely survive to a few weeks of age.

Predominant Sex Female

SIGNS

General Comments
• Clinical signs related to the degree of shunting and may range from none to severe congestive heart failure (CHF) • Cats seldom display signs of cardiac failure until decompensation is advanced.

Historical Findings
• Coughing, labored breathing, exercise intolerance, and collapse, severity of which related to the degree of heart failure • Seizures and syncope often suggest right-to-left shunting PDA.

Physical Examination Findings
• Continuous type machinery murmur, a hallmark of left-to-right shunting PDA. This characteristic murmur is sometimes restricted to the cranial left heart base. • Water-hammer or bounding pulse revealed by palpation of the femoral artery. In animals with left-to-right shunting PDA, the pulse pressure is widened because of the drop in diastolic pressure through the ductus. • High systolic blood pressure from the volume overloaded left ventricle • Precordial thrill, which can be palpated over the cranial left heart base in most animals. The left apical impulse is prominent. The right apical impulse is more prominent in animals with a right-to-left shunting PDA. • Cyanosis. Common in animals with a right-to-left shunting PDA. Cyanosis is often limited to the caudal half of the body because of the location of the ductus, which is distal to the arteries supplying the head and forelimbs. • Animals with right-to-left shunting PDA usually do not have a murmur. A split second heart sound is often heard. Rarely, a diastolic murmur of pulmonic insufficiency is present because of pulmonary hypertension.

CAUSES
• Congenital defect • Hypoxia • Prostaglandins

RISK FACTORS
• Any condition causing hypoxia • Premature birth

DIAGNOSIS

DIFFERENTIAL DIAGNOSIS
• Aorticopulmonary window, a round or oval communication between the aorta and the main pulmonary artery close to their origin at the heart base • Concurrent aortic stenosis and insufficiency. The systolic murmur of aortic stenosis and the diastolic murmur of aortic insufficiency combine to mimic the machinery murmur of PDA. • Echocardiographic and angiocardiographic studies can be used to differentiate PDA from other congenital cardiac defects. • Continuous murmur developing in a mature animal not consistent with PDA

CBC/BIOCHEMISTRY/URINALYSIS
• Usually normal • Polycythemia; PCV > 60 in most animals with right-to-left shunting PDA

OTHER BLOOD TESTS N/A

IMAGING

Thoracic Radiographic Findings
• Dorsal ventral radiographs (following figure modified from Fox PR, ed. Canine and feline cardiology. New York: Churchill Livinstone, 1988) often reveal three bulges along the left cardiac silhouette: an aneurysmal bulge of the aortic arch (AO), a large pulmonary outflow tract (PA), and a large left auricle (L). • Mild to

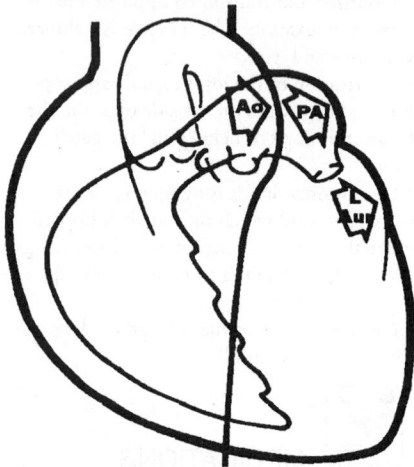

moderate left ventricular and left atrial enlargement in most animals • Overcirculation of the pulmonary vasculature in many animals • Severe cardiomegaly, pulmonary congestion, and pulmonary edema in animals with CHF • Right ventricular enlargement and prominent pulmonary arteries in animals with severe pulmonary hypertension

Echocardiographic Findings
• Reflects volume overload of the left side of the heart and includes left atrial dilation, left ventricular dilation, and normal to excessive wall motion • Ductus can be seen in some animals • Shunting of blood through the ductus detected by Doppler echocardiography in many animals • Contrast echocardiography (agitated saline injected into a peripheral vein during the ultrasound study) to confirm the presence of a right-to-left shunting PDA

Angiographic Findings
• Cardiac catheterization and angiocardiography rarely needed to confirm PDA • Selective angiocardiography by injection of contrast media into the ascending aorta may confirm left-to-right shunting PDA. The simultaneous filling of the main pulmonary artery and aorta is diagnostic for PDA. A main pulmonary artery contrast injection can be used to confirm the diagnosis of right-to-left shunting PDA. • Nonselective angiocardiography can be used to support the diagnosis of a right-to-left shunting PDA. This technique is of no value in the diagnosis of left-to-right shunts.

OTHER DIAGNOSTIC PROCEDURES

Electrocardiographic Findings
• Left ventricular and left atrial enlargement in most animals with PDA • Right ventricular hypertrophy in some animals with pulmonary hypertension • Atrial fibrillation and ventricular arrhythmias in some animals with CHF

Gross and Histopathologic Findings
• Left ventricular and atrial enlargement
• PDA with abnormal intima

TREATMENT

INPATIENT VERSUS OUTPATIENT
• Animals with CHF should be hospitalized for initial medical management.
• Stable animals can be discharged pending surgery.

ACTIVITY Restricted

DIET
Sodium restriction only if animal has CHF

CLIENT EDUCATION
• Serious complications expected in animals with uncorrected PDA
• Discuss hereditability of the defect.
• Discuss need for early surgical correction to improve long-term prognosis.
• Other cardiac defects may accompany PDA and not be detected until the PDA is ligated.

SURGICAL CONSIDERATIONS
• Every effort should be made to ligate left-to-right shunting PDA.
• Percutaneous catheter occlusion by use of Gianturco embolization coils is an alternative to duct ligation; available at a few referral centers
• In animals with mild to moderate left-sided heart failure, resolution of pulmonary edema must precede anesthesia and surgery.
• Stabilization of patients with severe heart failure should be attempted, but these animals are poor anesthetic risks.
• Correction of PDA contraindicated in animals with right-to-left shunting PDA. Acute right failure and death will occur, because the PDA functions as a relief valve for the right ventricle.

MEDICATIONS

DRUGS AND FLUIDS
• With unacceptable anesthetic or surgical candidates, medical management of heart failure indicated
• No drugs available that are effective in closing a patent ductus
• Animals with left ventricular failure treated with furosemide (1-2 mg/kg PO q6h-q12h), enalapril (0.5 mg/kg PO q12h-q24h), and often digoxin (0.22 mg/m²).

CONTRAINDICATIONS None

PRECAUTIONS
• Use of digoxin should be monitored by ECG; watch for clinical signs of toxicity.
• Use ACE inhibitors and digoxin cautiously if renal disease is present.

POSSIBLE INTERACTIONS N/A

ALTERNATE DRUGS N/A

FOLLOW-UP

PATIENT MONITORING
• Careful auscultation of the patient after surgery. If a murmur is present, evaluate for other cardiac defects. • Routine follow-up after shunt ligation, with careful auscultation at annual physical. If continuous murmur recurs, consider recannulization of the ductus.
• Animal with PDA that has not been closed should be followed more closely.

PREVENTION/AVOIDANCE
Do not breed affected animals.

POSSIBLE COMPLICATIONS
• Left heart failure • Pulmonary hypertension • Right heart hypertrophy and failure • Bacterial endocarditis • Cardiac arrhythmias (atrial fibrillation, ventricular arrhythmias) • Recannulization of ductus after ligation

EXPECTED COURSE AND PROGNOSIS
• Surgical results best if PDA is closed as soon as possible in the first few months of life (95% success rate) • Pups surviving beyond 6 to 8 weeks usually live to adulthood. • Animals

with severe heart failure are poor anesthetic risks. • A right-to-left shunting PDA cannot be surgically corrected. • Cats rarely survive more than few weeks of age. • Dogs with a small defect often survive for several years.

MISCELLANEOUS

ASSOCIATED CONDITIONS
Other cardiac defects

AGE RELATED FACTORS
Murmur present from birth

ZOONOTIC POTENTIAL N/A

PREGNANCY
• High risk in animals with a moderate to large ductus • High risk in animals with high pulmonary resistance and right-to-left shunting PDA

SYNONYMS
Aorticopulmonary shunt or communication

SEE ALSO
• Congestive Heart Failure, Left-sided
• Murmurs, Heart

ABBREVIATIONS
PDA = patent ductus arteriosus
CHF = congestive heart failure
ACE = angiotensin converting enzyme

References

Goodwin JK. Congenital heart disease. In: Miller MS, Tilley LP, eds. Manual of canine and feline cardiology. 2nd ed. Philadelphia:WB Saunders, 1995.

Edward J, Tilley LP. Congenital cardiac defects. In: Bojrab J, ed. Pathophysiology in small animal surgery. Philadelphia:Lea Febiger, 1981.

Liska W, Tilley LP. Patent ductus arteriosus.Vet Clin North Am (Small Anim Pract) 1979;9:195-206.

Tilley LP, Owens JM. Congenital heart defects. In: Manual of cardiology. New York:Churchill Livingstone, 1986.

Bonagura JD. Congenital heart disease. In: Ettinger, SJ, ed. Textbook of veterinary internal medicine. 3rd ed. Philadelphia:WB Saunders, 1989.

Authors Larry P. Tilley and Francis W. K. Smith, Jr.
Consulting Editors Larry P. Tilley and Francis W. K. Smith, Jr.

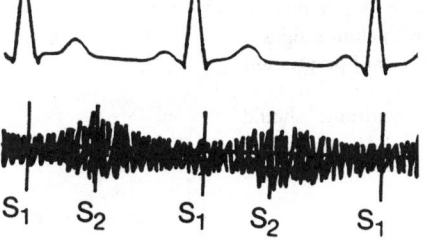

Figure. Continuous murmur in a poodle with a patent ductus arteriosus. (From Smith FWK Jr., Tilley LP. Rapid interpretation of heart sounds, murmurs, and arrhythmias. Baltimore: Williams & Wilkins, 1992, with permission.)

PECTUS EXCAVATUM

BASICS

OVERVIEW
• A deformity of the sternum and costal cartilages that results in a dorsal to ventral narrowing of the chest, primarily in the caudal aspect • May have secondary abnormalities of respiratory and cardiovascular function from restriction of ventilation and cardiac compression • Most cases are congenital • Acquired disease is seen in humans when large, negative, intrapleural pressures on compliant chest walls result in the collapse of the sternum and intercostal cartilages. • Concurrent cardiac defects are common. • Speculation exists in veterinary medicine that upper respiratory obstruction at a young age may cause abnormal respiratory gradients and subsequent pectus excavatum. • Some patients demonstrate the "swimmer syndrome," in which neonatal dogs lack the ability to posture properly and remain in sternal recumbency, which may lead to invagination of the sternum.

SIGNALMENT
• Dogs and cats • Brachycephalic breeds
• Most commonly presented between 4 weeks and 3 months of age

SIGNS
• Dyspnea, exercise intolerance, weight loss, hyperpnea, recurrent pulmonary infections, cough, vomiting, cyanosis, poor appetite, and episodes of mild upper respiratory disease
• A thoracic defect is easily palpated or seen on physical examination. • Respiratory problems are common (increased inspiratory effort, inspiratory stridor, moist rales if infection is present). • Cardiac murmurs associated with concurrent cardiac defects or compression of the heart are common.
• Heart sounds often are muffled, especially over the right hemithorax. • There is no correlation between severity of clinical signs and the severity of anatomic or physiologic abnormalities.
• "Swimmer's syndrome," in which the limbs are not adducted properly and ambulation is impaired, may be seen.

CAUSES AND RISK FACTORS
• A genetic predisposition may exist. • Puppies raised on surfaces with poor footing may be predisposed to "swimmer's syndrome."
• Dogs predisposed to respiratory obstructive processes

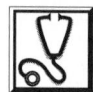

DIAGNOSIS

DIFFERENTIAL DIAGNOSIS
Numerous causes of dyspnea, cyanosis, hyperpnea, and/or cough must be entertained. Physical examination and radiographic evaluation enables the clinician to rule out the most common differentials:
• Tracheal malformations or collapse
• Cardiac disease • Electric cord bite
• Hemothorax • Pyothorax • Pneumonia
• Allergic bronchitis • Stenotic nares •
Elongated soft palate

CBC/BIOCHEMISTRY/URINALYSIS
N/A

OTHER LABORATORY TESTS N/A

IMAGING
• Radiographs confirm the diagnosis. Deformities that cause a decreased thoracic volume are readily noted. Cardiac malposition usually is seen, with the heart shifted to the left of midline and sometimes cranially. Cardiac enlargement may be detected. Lung fields may show evidence of concurrent disease. Shifting of the heart shadow to the left may expose the right hilus and encourage a diagnosis of pulmonary disease. • Echocardiography is indicated to fully evaluate cardiac status (eliminate primary cardiac disease and detect possible concurrent cardiac defects). Cardiac enlargement on radiographs may be attributed only to malpositioning.

OTHER DIAGNOSTIC PROCEDURES
N/A

TREATMENT
• Surgery is the only available treatment modality. The decision to repair deformities should be made on the basis of clinical signs of disease. Patients with mild disease (only a flat chest) may become normal without surgical intervention. Manual medial compression of the thorax by the owners or in the form of a splint is recommended. Animals with moderate or severe disease are surgical candidates. Frontosagittal and vertebral indexes provide objective criteria for determining severity.
• The technique for repair may be dictated by the age of the animal (young animals with a compliant sternum and ribs may do well with external coaptation; older animals with less compliant thoraces may need partial sternectomy).
• It appears that surgery does benefit patients with concurrent respiratory distress. The potential benefits of surgery for those lacking respiratory distress but with moderate or severe deformity is unknown. Asymptomatic animals have progressed to develop respiratory distress, and animals with clinical signs of disease have shown evidence of progression over time.
• Puppies with "swimmer's syndrome" should be placed on surfaces with excellent footing. Careful toggling of front and rear legs may improve adduction.
• Brachycephalic breeds with concurrent upper airway problems may benefit from therapy directed at these problems.

MEDICATIONS

DRUGS AND FLUIDS
Treat underlying or secondary medical conditions.

CONTRAINDICATIONS/POSSIBLE INTERACTIONS
Anesthesia will require constant monitoring, and respiratory support should be available.

FOLLOW-UP
• Examinations should be performed as dictated by the degree of clinical signs or when surgical intervention has been precluded.
• There are no specific actions that an owner can take to avoid this disease, though genetic factors may be involved in some animals.
• Progression of respiratory signs may occur in the asymptomatic or mildly symptomatic animal. • The prognosis in all patients is guarded and is dependent upon properly timed and expertly administered intervention.

MISCELLANEOUS

Reference

Boudrieau RJ, Fossum TW, Hartsfield SM, Hobson HP, Rudy RL. Pectus excavatum in dogs and cats. Compend Cont Ed Pract Vet 1990;12:341-355.
Author Justin H. Straus
Consulting Editors Lynelle Johnson and Bradley L. Moses

BASICS

OVERVIEW
• An inherited disorder characterized by leukocyte nuclear hyposegmentation in the presence of a mature coarse chromatin pattern. Limited breeding studies suggest autosomal dominant transmission of the anomaly.
• Heterozygous Pelger-Hüet (PH) anomaly usually encountered; neutrophils resemble bands and metamyelocytes • Heterozygous PH anomaly not associated with abnormalities of leukocyte function, immunodeficiency, or predisposition to infection • Homozygous form of PH anomaly is usually lethal in utero, but survivors may have leukocytes with round to oval nuclei on stained blood smear. Homozygous PH anomaly and chondrodysplasia reported in one stillborn kitten; not reported in dogs.

SIGNALMENT
Occurs in several breeds of dogs and domestic shorthair cats

SIGNS
Historical Findings
Parents or siblings also may have the anomaly.

Physical Examination Findings
None

CAUSES AND RISK FACTORS
Genetic defect with probable autosomal dominant transmission

DIAGNOSIS

DIFFERENTIAL DIAGNOSIS
• Severe inflammation or bacterial infection often associated with toxic change of neutrophils • FeLV or FIV infection in cats with altered cellular maturation • Drug-induced alterations in cellular morphology, especially encountered with use of sulfa drugs • Preleukemic maturation disturbances

CBC/BIOCHEMISTRY/URINALYSIS
• Serendipitous finding during WBC differential count • On stained blood smear, nuclear hyposegmentation of neutrophils (persistent left shift without toxic changes), eosinophils, basophils, and monocytes • On stained bone marrow smear, megakaryocytes may appear hypolobulated. • Hereditary nature of disease revealed by examination of blood smears from parents and siblings

OTHER LABORATORY TESTS
• Stained bone marrow smear reveals nuclear hyposegmentation of leukocytes and nuclear hypolobulation of megakaryocytes. • Blast cell count within reference intervals

IMAGING N/A

OTHER DIAGNOSTIC PROCEDURES
If relatives are unavailable for study, prospective test mating demonstrates hereditary nature of PH anomaly.

TREATMENT

No therapy is needed as anomaly is not associated with clinical disease

MEDICATIONS

DRUGS AND FLUIDS None
CONTRAINDICATIONS/POSSIBLE INTERACTIONS None

FOLLOW-UP

PATIENT MONITORING None

PREVENTION/AVOIDANCE
• Inform owner of PH anomaly to avoid unnecessary laboratory testing or inappropriate drug therapy in future. • Provide genetic counseling to eliminate trait from breeding animals. • Breed affected heterozygotes and select normal offspring for future matings to preserve desirable genetic lines.

POSSIBLE COMPLICATIONS
• When heterozygotes are bred, litter size may be reduced because homozygous PH anomaly usually is a lethal trait. • Association with chondrodysplasia in term homozygous offspring not yet confirmed

EXPECTED COURSE AND PROGNOSIS
Normal lifespan with heterozygous PH anomaly • Homozygous PH anomaly usually lethal (fetal resorption)

MISCELLANEOUS

ASSOCIATED CONDITIONS
Fetal resorption (homozygous embryos)

PREGNANCY
Fetal resorption (homozygous embryos)

ABBREVIATIONS
FeLV = feline leukemia virus
FIV = feline immunodeficiency virus
PH = Pelger-Hüet
WBC = white blood cells

Reference
Ettinger SJ, Feldman EC. Textbook of veterinary internal medicine. 4th ed. Philadelphia: WB Saunders, 1994.
Author Kenneth S. Latimer
Contributing Editor Alan H. Rebar

PEMPHIGOID

BASICS

OVERVIEW
Bullous pemphigoid is a rare, autoimmune vesiculobullous, severe ulcerative dermatosis of the skin and/or oral mucosa in dogs. Forms include: bullous (most commonly identified), and chronic pemphigoid (rare).

SIGNALMENT
• Breed predilection for collies, shetland sheepdogs and possibly doberman pinschers.
• No age or sex predisposition.

SIGNS

Bullous Pemphigoid
• Cutaneous lesions: transient blisters, crusts, epidermal collarettes, and ulcerations
• Widespread distribution: mucous membranes, head, neck, axillae, ventral abdomen/groin, and feet (nailbed involvement or footpad ulceration). The oral cavity and skin of the axillae and groin are most frequently involved. • Onset often acute with severe symptoms. • Systemic illness: anorexia, depression, febrile in severely affected dogs. • Pain and pruritus are variable.
• Symptoms similar to pemphigus vulgaris.

Chronic Pemphigoid
Chronic, clinically benign bullous pemphigoid consists of lesions confined to the axillae, groin or isolated mucocutaneous areas; exhibits a slow and chronic course.

CAUSES AND RISK FACTORS
Deposit of an autoantibody ("pemphigoid antibody") directed against the antigen at the basement membrane zone of skin and mucosa resulting in blister formation below the epidermis.

DIAGNOSIS

DIFFERENTIAL DIAGNOSIS
Pemphigus vulgaris, systemic lupus erythematosus, erythema multiforme, toxic epidermal necrolysis, drug eruption, mycosis fungoides, lymphoreticular neoplasia, hidradenitis suppurativa, and ulcerative stomatitis.

CBC/BIOCHEMISTRY/URINALYSIS
Routine hematology and serum biochemistry changes non-specific: leukocytosis, neutrophilia, mild nonregenerative anemia, hypoalbuminemia, and hyperglobulinemia.

OTHER LABORATORY TESTS
Antinuclear antibody (ANA), lupus erythematosus (LE) tests negative.

IMAGING   N/A

OTHER DIAGNOSTIC PROCEDURES
• Biopsies of lesions for histopathology: subepidermal vesicle formation with inflammatory infiltrates of granulocytes and mononuclear cells, but without acantholysis.
• Direct immunofluorescence of specimen from the basement membrane zone of the dermal-epidermal junction positive in 50-90% of cases; indirect immunofluorescence is usually negative. • Bacteriologic culture for identification and drug sensitivity of secondary bacteria.

TREATMENT
• Initially, may need to treat supportively as inpatient if serious systemic signs or secondary infections.
• Subsequent outpatient treatment with frequent hospital rechecks and monitoring.
• Lowfat diet to avoid pancreatitis secondary to corticosteroid and possible azathioprine therapy.
• Avoidance of sunlight as UV light may exacerbate lesions.

BULLOUS PEMPHIGOID
• Immunosuppressive agents.
• Antibiotics for common secondary bacterial infections.
• Gentle soaks/cleansing with antibacterial shampoos or povidone iodine and water.

CHRONIC PEMPHIGOID
• Immunosuppressive therapy.
• Topical or intralesional corticosteroids.

MEDICATIONS

DRUGS AND FLUIDS

Corticosteroids

Prednisone or prednisolone 1.1-3.3 mg/kg PO q12h (the higher doses probably necessary, but side effects are likely and need to be monitored).

Cytotoxic Agents

• A large number of patients require cytotoxic agents to achieve control of the disease owing to intolerable side effects of high dose corticosteroids or failure to achieve/maintain remission with glucocorticoids alone. In combination with corticosteroids, they can work synergistically with a reduction of side effects.
• Azathioprine (2.2 mg/kg PO q24h, then q48h.)
• Chlorambucil (0.1 mg/kg PO q24h, then q48h.)
• Cyclophosphamide (50 mg/m² BSA q48h.)
• 6-mercaptopurine (2.2 mg/kg PO q24h, then q48h.)
• Dapsone (1 mg/kg PO q8h, then as needed application limited).

Chrysotherapy with Prednisone

• Aurothioglucose 1 mg/kg IM (following a test dose of 1 or 5 mg the first week, and 2 or 10 mg the second week, for small dogs and dogs >25 kg, respectively; with a lag phase of 6-8 weeks) every 7 days, then every 14-30 days
• Aranofin 0.1-0.2 mg/kg PO q12h-q24h.

CONTRAINDICATIONS/POSSIBLE INTERACTIONS

• Corticosteroids may cause PU/PD/PP and temperament changes.
• Pancreatitis from corticosteroid and azathioprine therapy. • Leukopenia and thrombocytopenia from cytotoxic drugs.
• Nephrotoxicity from cytotoxic drugs and chrysotherapy.
• Hepatotoxicity from corticosteroids and cytotoxic drugs.
• Hemorrhagic cystitis from cyclophosphamide.
• Immunosuppression can predispose to demodex, cutaneous, and systemic fungal and bacterial infections.
• Dermatitis, stomatitis, and allergic reactions from chrysotherapy.

 FOLLOW-UP

PATIENT MONITORING

• Frequent outpatient recheck of signs of suppression/progression of disease, and for reports of medication side effects
• Frequent outpatient monitoring of routine hematology and serum biochemistry for medication side effects

EXPECTED COURSE AND PROGNOSIS

Bullous Pemphigoid

• Untreated bullous pemphigoid may be fatal. • Treatment must be aggressive and side effects may be significant. • Lifelong treatment and monitoring of side effects of medications is usually necessary for bullous pemphigoid. • Side effects of medications may impact quality of life. • Secondary infections cause morbidity and possible mortality.
• Some pets may not respond to therapy.
• Prognosis guarded

Chronic Pemphigoid

• Fair prognosis • This mild, chronic variant of the disease is treated with relatively low doses of systemic glucocorticoid, and some patients can be treated with topical glucocorticoids alone.

 MISCELLANEOUS

Reference

Ackerman LJ and Manning TO. Immune-mediated skin diseases. In: Morgan RV, ed. Handbook of small animal practice. 2nd ed. New York: Churchill Livingstone 1992;991-1004.
Author Margaret S. Swartout
Consulting Editor Lowell J. Ackerman

PEMPHIGUS

BASICS

DEFINITION
• Pemphigus is a group of uncommon autoimmune dermatoses characterized by varying degrees of ulceration, crusting, pustule and vescicle formation, which affect the skin and sometimes mucous membranes. • Pemphigus foliaceus is the most common type of pemphigus. • Pemphigus erythematosus is a relatively common form, and may be a more benign variant of pemphigus foliaceus, or represent a crossover syndrome of pemphigus and lupus erythematosus. • Pemphigus vulgaris is the second most common type of pemphigus and is the most severe. • Pemphigus vegetans is the rarest form, possibly a more benign variant of pemphigus vulgaris.

Pathophysiology
Tissue-bound autoantibody directed at interepidermal cell antigen is deposited within the intercellular spaces, causing epidermal cell separation and cell rounding (acantholysis). Severity of the ulceration and of the disease is related to depth of autoantibody deposition within the skin. Pemphigus foliaceus and pemphigus erythematosus are due to autoantibody at a superficial location in the epidermis. The lesions are less severe than for Pemphigus vulgaris, which is mediated by autoantibody deposition deeper in the skin, resulting in deeper ulcer formation.

Systems Affected
Skin/Exocrine - autoantibody is tissue-bound.

Genetics N/A

SIGNALMENT

Species
Dogs and cats are affected by all forms except pemphigus vegetans which is found only in dogs.

Breed Predilections
• Pemphigus foliaceus–Akita, bearded collie, chow chow, dachshund, doberman pinscher, Finnish spitz, Newfoundland, and schipperke • Pemphigus erythematosus–collie, German shepherd dog and shetland sheepdog.

Mean Age and Range
Usually occurs in middle-aged to older animals.

Predominant Sex N/A

SIGNS

Pemphigus Foliaceus
• Scales, crusts, pustules, epidermal colarettes, erosions, erythema, alopecia, and footpad hyperkeratosis with splitting; occasional vesicles are transient. • Common involvement of the head, ears and footpads; often becoming generalized. Mucosal and mucocutaneous lesions are uncommon.
• Frequent nipple and nail bed involvement in cats. • Sometimes lymphadenopathy, edema, depression, fever, and lameness if footpads involved. However, often in good health. • Variable pain and pruritus.
• Secondary bacterial infection possible.

Pemphigus Erythematosus
Symptoms as for pemphigus foliaceus, but lesions usually confined to head, face and footpads.

Pemphigus Vulgaris
• Ulcerative lesions, erosions, epidermal colarettes, blisters, and crusts; more severe than pemphigus foliaceus or pemphigus erythematosus. • Mucous membranes, mucocutaneous junctions, skin; may become generalized. Oral ulceration is frequent, and axillae and groin areas are often involved. • Positive Nikolsky sign (new or extended erosive lesion created when lateral pressure is applied to the skin near an existing lesion) • Variable pruritus and pain • Anorexia, depression and fever • Secondary bacterial infections common

Pemphigus Vegetans
Pustule groups become eruptive papillomatous lesions and vegetative masses which ooze; oral involvement has not been noted, and there is no systemic illness.

CAUSES N/A

RISK FACTORS N/A

DIAGNOSIS

DIFFERENTIAL DIAGNOSIS

Pemphigus Foliaceus
• Bacterial folliculitis • Dermatophytosis • Demodicosis • Candidiasis • Keratinization disorders • Lupus erythematosus • Pemphigus erythematosus • Subcorneal pustular dermatosis • Drug eruption • Zinc-responsive dermatitis • Dermatomyositis • Tyrosinemia • Mycosis fungoides • Lymphoreticular malignancies • Metabolic epidermal necrosis • Sterile eosinophilic pustulosis • Linear IgA dermatosis

Pemphigus Erythematosus
• Pemphigus foliaceus • Systemic lupus erythematosus • Discoid lupus erythematosus • Nasal pyoderma • Demodicosis • Dermatophytosis • Epidermolysis bullosa simplex • Uveodermatologic syndrome

Pemphigus Vulgaris
• Bullous pemphigoid • Systemic lupus erythematosus • Toxic epidermal necrolysis • Drug eruption • Mycosis fungoides • Lymphoreticular neoplasia • Ulcerative stomatitis causes • Erythema multiforme

Pemphigus Vegetans
• Pemphigus vulgaris • Bacterial folliculitis • Pemphigus foliaceus • Lichenoid dermatoses • Cutaneous neoplasia

CBC/BIOCHEMISTRY/URINALYSIS
Hematologic or serum biochemical abnormalities uncommon, though leukocytosis and hyperglobulinemia sometimes noted.

OTHER LABORATORY TESTS
ANA may be weakly positive in pemphigus erythematosus only.

IMAGING N/A

Other Diagnostic Procedures
Cytology of aspirates or impression smears of pustules or crusts may show acantholytic cells and neutrophils.

Gross and Histopathologic Findings
• Biopsies of lesional/perilesional skin submitted for histopathology show acantholysis and intraepidermal clefting, with microabscess or pustule formation, and surface acantholytic keratinocytes. • Location of epidermal lesions varies with disease:
• Pemphigus foliaceus and erythematosus—subcorneal or intragranular clefting and acantholysis. Pemphigus vulgaris and vegetans—suprabasilar clefting. • Immunopathology of biopsied skin via immunofluorescent antibody assays or peroxidase-antiperoxidase assays demonstrates positive staining in the intercellular spaces in 50-90 % of cases. • Results can be affected by concurrent or previous corticosteroid (or other immunosuppressive drug) administration. Indirect immunofluorescence is usually negative. Pemphigus erythematosus may demonstrate basement membrane stain as well as staining of the intercellular spaces.
• Bacteriologic culture for identification of secondary bacterial infections.

TREATMENT

INPATIENT VERSUS OUTPATIENT
• Initial inpatient supportive therapy, antibiotics and soaks may be needed for severely affected patients.
• Generally, outpatient treatment with initial frequent hospital rechecks; ultimately, less frequent hospital visits indicated when disease in remission and patient on maintenance medical regime.

ACTIVITY N/A

DIET
Low fat diet to avoid pancreatitis predisposed by corticosteroids and possible azathioprine therapy.

CLIENT EDUCATION
Avoidance of the sun is recommended, since ultraviolet light may exacerbate lesions.

SURGICAL CONSIDERATIONS N/A

MEDICATIONS

DRUGS AND FLUIDS

Pemphigus Vulgaris and Foliaceus
Corticosteroids
Prednisone/prednisolone administered 2.2-4.4 mg/kg/day PO divided q12h to initiate control, with a minimum maintenance of 0.5 mg/kg PO q48h. Dosage reductions should

be made at every 2-4 week intervals, by 5-10 mg/week.

Cytotoxic Agents

• More than half of dogs and cats treated need the addition of other immunomodulating drugs. These generally work synergistically with prednisone, thereby allowing reduction in dose and side effects of the corticosteroid.

• Azathioprine 2.2 mg/kg PO q24h (in dogs), then q48h (infrequently used in cats owing to potential for marked bone marrow suppression; feline dose 1 mg/kg q24h-q48h).

• Chlorambucil 0.1-0.2 mg/kg PO q24h, then q48h (often used in cats; used also in dogs).

• Cyclophosphamide 50 mg/m^2 PO BSA q48h (in dogs).

• Cyclosporine 15-27 mg/kg/day PO (limited application).

• Dapsone 1 mg/kg PO q8h, then as needed (dogs; limited application).

Chrysotherapy

• Often used in conjunction with prednisone

• Aurothioglucose 1 mg/kg IM (following a test dose of 1 or 5 mg the first week, and 2 or 10 mg the second week, for small dogs or dogs >25 kg, respectively; with a lag phase of 6-8 weeks) every 7 days, then every 14-30 days.

• Aranofin 0.1-0.2 mg/kg PO q12h-q24h.

Pemphigus Erythematosus and Vegetans

• Oral prednisone/prednisolone 1.1 mg/kg PO q24h, then q48 hrs, then to the lowest maintenance dose possible. May be stopped.

• Topical steroids may be sufficient in mild cases.

CONTRAINDICATIONS N/A

PRECAUTIONS

• Corticosteroids may cause PU/PD/PP, temperament changes, and diabetes mellitus

• Pancreatitis from corticosteroid and azathioprine therapy

• Leukopenia and thrombocytopenia from cytotoxic drugs and chrysotherapy

• Nephrotoxicity from cytotoxic drugs and chrysotherapy

• Hepatotoxicity from corticosteroids and cytotoxic drugs

• Hemorrhagic cystitis from cyclophosphamide

• Immunosuppression can predispose to demodex, cutaneous and systemic bacterial and fungal infections.

• Dermatitis, stomatitis, and allergic reactions from chrysotherapy.

POSSIBLE INTERACTIONS N/A

Alternate Medications

Alternative Corticosteroids

• Use if undesirable side effects of prednisone, or poor response to prednisone.

• Methylprednisolone (for those who tolerate prednisone poorly) 0.8 to 1.5 mg/kg PO q12h.

• Triamcinolone 0.2-0.3 mg/kg PO q12h, then 0.1-0.2 mg/kg q48h-q72h.

• Dexamethasone 0.1-0.2 mg/kg PO q12h, then 0.05-0.1 mg/kg q48h-q72h.

• Glucocorticoid pulse therapy (11 mg/kg methylprednisolone sodium succinate IV for three consecutive days to induce remission (limited application).

Topical Steroids

• Hydrocortisone cream

• More potent topical corticosteroids: 0.1% betamethasone valerate, fluocinolone acetonide, or 0.1% amcinonide q12h, then q24h-q48h

• Tetracycline and niacinamide both dosed at 500 mg PO q8h for dogs > 10 kg, and half doses for dogs < 10 kg (limited application).

FOLLOW-UP

PATIENT MONITORING

• Frequent outpatient recheck of symptoms to determine suppression/progression of disease, and for monitoring of medication side effects

• Frequent outpatient monitoring of routine hematology and serum biochemistry for medication side effects, especially in patients on high doses of corticosteroids, cytotoxic drugs, or chrysotherapy.

PREVENTION/AVOIDANCE N/A

POSSIBLE COMPLICATONS N/A

EXPECTED COURSE AND PROGNOSIS

Pemphigus Vulgaris And Foliaceus

• Aggressive therapy with corticosteroids and cytotoxic drugs needed. Patients may require medication for life. Patient monitoring will be necessary; side effects of medications may affect quality of life. • If untreated, these diseases (especially pemphigus vulgaris) may prove to be fatal. • Secondary infections cause morbidity and possible mortality, especially with pemphigus vulgaris. • Prognosis guarded

Pemphigus Erythematosus and Vegetans

• Relatively benign and self-limiting • Oral corticosteroids may eventually be tapered to low maintenance doses and even stopped in some patients. • If untreated, a chronic dermatosis will result, but systemic symptoms are rare. • Prognosis fair.

MISCELLANEOUS

References

Ackerman LJ, Manning TO. Immune-mediated skin diseases. In: Morgan RV, ed. Handbook of small animal practice. 2nd ed. New York: Churchill Livingstone, 1992;991-1004.

Angarano DW. Autoimmune dermatosis. In: Nesbitt GH, ed. Contemporary issues in small animal practice: dermatology. New York: Churchill Livingstone 1987;79-94.

Rosenkrantaz WS. Pemphigus foliaceus. In: Griffin CE, et al., eds. Current veterinary dermatology. St. Louis, MO: Mosby Year Book 1993;141-148.

Author Margaret S. Swartout

Consulting Editor Lowell Ackerman

PERIANAL FISTULA

 BASICS

OVERVIEW
Perianal fistula is characterized by multiple chronic fistulous tracts or ulcerating sinuses involving the perianal region. The cause is not known, but apocrine gland inflammation (hidradenitis suppurativa), impaction and infection of the anal sinuses and crypts, infection of the circumanal glands and hair follicles, and anal sacculitis have all been proposed. The gastrointestinal system becomes involved because of excessive scar tissue formation around the anus. Self-mutilation can also be a major problem associated with this disorder.

SIGNALMENT
• Dogs • German shepherd dog and Irish setter most commonly affected breeds • Mean age, 7 years (range, 7 months-12 years) • No gender predisposition reported, but sexually intact dogs have a higher prevalence • A genetic basis has been proposed, but not proven

SIGNS
• Vary with the severity and extent of involvement • Dyschezia, tenesmus, hematochezia, constipation, diarrhea, malodorous mucopurulent anal discharge, fecal incontinence, painful tail movements, licking and self-mutilation, anorexia, weight loss, reluctance to sit, posturing difficulties, and personality changes

CAUSES AND RISK FACTORS
• Proposed causes involve an inflammatory component • Low tail carriage and a broad tail base are risk factors predisposing the dog to inflammation and infection because of poor ventilation, accumulation of feces, moisture, and secretions • High density of apocrine sweat glands in the cutaneous zone of the anal canal of German shepherd dogs • Hidradenitis suppurativa may be associated with immune or endocrine dysfunction, genetic factors, and poor hygiene

 DIAGNOSIS

DIFFERENTIAL DIAGNOSIS
• Chronic anal sac abscess • Perianal adenocarcinoma that is ulcerated and draining • Rectal fistula

CBC/BIOCHEMISTRY/URINALYSIS
Results usually normal. Patients with inflammation may have an inflammatory leukogram.

OTHER LABORATORY TESTS   N/A

IMAGING   N/A

OTHER DIAGNOSTIC PROCEDURES
Presumptive diagnosis is based on clinical signs and results of physical examination. Definitive diagnosis is made by biopsy of the affected area.

 TREATMENT

Surgery is considered the most effective treatment. However, a tremendous amount of controversy exists as to which surgical method should be used, and none of those currently employed result in consistent resolution of the problem. Surgical options include electrosurgery, cryosurgery, surgical debridement with fulguration by chemical cautery, exteriorization and fulguration by electrocautery, surgical resection, radical excision of the rectal ring, tail setting, tail amputation, and laser surgery. Each technique has advantages and disadvantages that must be weighed when making a choice. The primary objective of surgery is the complete removal or destruction of diseased tissue while preserving normal tissue and function. Multiple procedures may be necessary for complete resolution.

MEDICATIONS

DRUGS AND FLUIDS

Medical treatment of perianal fistulas is usually unrewarding and can be detrimental by delaying more definitive treatment and allowing progression. Medical palliation involves clipping hair from the affected area, daily antiseptic lavage, systemic and topical antibiotics, hydrotherapy, elevation of the tail, and systemic corticosteroids.

CONTRAINDICATIONS/POSSIBLE INTERACTIONS

Corticosteroids are contraindicated when infection is possible.

FOLLOW-UP

• After surgery for appropriate healing, signs of recurrence, and associated complications
• Complications associated with the various surgical procedures include recurrence, failure to heal, dehiscence, tenesmus, fecal incontinence, anal stricture, and flatulence. The incidence of postoperative complications is directly related to severity of disease. • Prognosis is guarded for complete resolution except in mildly affected patients. Clients often become frustrated with the difficulty of attaining definitive resolution of this disorder.

MISCELLANEOUS

SYNONYMS

• Anal furunculosis • Perianal sinus

References

Matthiesen DT, Marretta SM. Diseases of the anus and rectum. In: Slatter D, ed. Textbook of small animal surgery. 2nd ed. Philadelphia: WB Saunders, 1993;627-644.

van Ee RT. Perianal fistulas. In: Bojrab MJ, ed. Disease mechanisms in small animal surgery. 2nd ed. Philadelphia: Lea & Febiger, 1993;285-286.

Author James L. Cook
Consulting Editor Brent D. Jones

PERICARDIAL EFFUSION

BASICS

DEFINITION
Abnormally high volume of fluid within the pericardial sac. Cardiac tamponade is a clinical result of hemodynamic compromise caused by pericardial effusion.

PATHOPHYSIOLOGY
As pericardial effusion accumulates, the elastic or stretching capabilities of the pericardial sac are exceeded. Further accumulations of pericardial effusion lead to high intrapericardial pressure. When intrapericardial pressure rises above cardiac diastolic filling pressure, cardiac tamponade occurs. The right atrium and right ventricle normally have the lowest cardiac filling pressure, and these chambers are predominantly affected in animals affected by cardiac tamponade. The resultant low reduction in cardiac filling (preload reduction) leads to diminished blood flow forward (low cardiac output). In animals with chronic disease, compensation for low cardiac output includes activation of compensatory mechanisms, which leads to fluid accumulation. Congestive signs are typically manifested as right-sided congestive heart failure.

SYSTEMS AFFECTED
• Cardiovascular—signs of low cardiac output and congestive heart failure • Hepatobiliary—chronic passive congestion with mildly to moderately high liver enzymes • Renal/urologic—prerenal azotemia

SIGNALMENT
• Dogs and cats • Middle-aged to old dogs are predisposed. • Golden retrievers and German shepherd dogs are predisposed to right atrial hemangiosarcoma and idiopathic effusion. • Male dogs are predisposed to idiopathic effusion.

SIGNS

General Comments
Chronic pericardial effusion often causes ascites without an important cardiac murmur.

Historical Findings
• Lethargy • Anorexia • Weakness • Exercise intolerance • Abdominal distension • Syncope or collapse

Physical Examination Findings
Acute Pericardial Effusion
• Pallor • Slow capillary refill time • Weak arterial pulses • Weakness, syncope, collapse • Tachypnea • Tachycardia
Chronic Pericardial Effusion:
• Jugular vein distension • Ascites • Muffled heart sounds • Weak arterial pulses • Pulsus paradoxus • Pallor • Slow capillary refill time • Weakness • Tachypnea • Tachycardia

CAUSES
• Neoplasia—hemangiosarcoma, heart-base tumor (chemodectoma), thyroid carcinoma, mesothelioma, metastatic neoplasia, and lymphoma (cats) • Idiopathic pericardial effusion (benign pericardial effusion or hemorrhagic pericardial effusion) • Coagulopathy—intoxication with vitamin K antagonist rodenticide, thrombocytopenia, or other coagulopathies • Infection—feline infectious peritonitis, coccidioidomycosis, and bacterial pericarditis • Congenital disorders —peritoneopericardial hernia • Left atrial tear or cardiac trauma • Congestive heart failure • Foreign body

RISK FACTORS N/A

DIAGNOSIS

DIFFERENTIAL DIAGNOSIS
• Includes congestive heart failure secondary to other causes (e.g., chronic valvular disease and cardiomyopathy), hepatic failure, abdominal neoplasm with hemorrhage, and protein-losing nephropathy or enteropathy. • A cardiac murmur or gallop is usually present in animals with heart failure caused by cardiomyopathy or valvular disease. • Other causes of ascites (e.g., hepatic failure, hypoproteinemia, intraabdominal neoplasia, and hemorrhage caused by coagulopathy) characteristically cause remarkable abnormalities on CBC and biochemistry profile and typically do not have jugular venous distension. Examination of the jugular vein can be extremely helpful in differentiating these conditions from heart failure.

CBC/BIOCHEMISTRY/URINALYSIS
• Complete blood count is usually normal. However, anemia may be present in animals with hemangiosarcoma, lymphoma, or coagulopathy. • Red cell morphology may be abnormal (e.g., nucleated red blood cells, schistocytes, and acanthocytes) and thrombocytopenia may be found in animals with hemangiosarcoma. • Biochemistry profile is often normal; however, mild to moderately high liver enzymes (in animals with chronic passive hepatic congestion), mild azotemia (typically pre-renal), and mild electrolyte abnormalities (e.g., hyponatremia, hypochloremia, and hyperkalemia) may be present. • Urinalysis is usually normal with normal renal concentrating ability, unless a diuretic has been administered.

OTHER LABORATORY TESTS
• Prolonged clotting times (eg, activated partial thromboplastin time and one-stage prothrombin time) are prolonged in animals with vitamin K antagonist rodenticide intoxication. • Feline infectious peritonitis titers may be high in cats. • Cats with lymphoma may be feline leukemia virus posititve.

IMAGING

Thoracic Radiographic Findings
• Mild to severe cardiac enlargement with the cardiac silhouette often globoid in appearance • Often, very sharp edges of the cardiac silhouette on the dorsoventral view because of lack of cardiac motion artifact • Mild to moderate pleural effusion in some animals • Ascites is many animals. • Large caudal vena cava in some animals

Echocardiography
• The superior diagnostic test to confirm pericardial effusion. • An echo-free space is clearly identified between the pericardium and the epicardial surface of the heart. • Often demonstrates the cause of pericardial effusion in animals with neoplasia (e.g., right atrial hemangiosarcoma and heart base tumor around aorta) or peritoneopericardial hernia

Pneumopericardiography
• This technique is inferior to echocardiography with respect to diagnostic accuracy. • Resulting images are often difficult to interpret without extensive experience with this technique.

OTHER DIAGNOSTIC PROCEDURES

Electrocardiographic Findings
• Sinus tachycardia in many animals, with ventricular or supraventricular arrhythmias occurring occasionally • Low voltage QRS complexes (< 1 mV in leads I, II, III, aVF, aVL, and aVR), ST segment elevation, and electrical alternans in some animals • Electrical alternans (Figure) is identified as a regular (1 to 1 or 2 to 1) variation in QRS-T wave height or morphology, which results from the heart swinging back and forth within the pericardial sac.

TREATMENT
When cardiac tamponade is present, immediate pericardiocentesis is indicated. For those uncomfortable with the technique of pericardiocentesis, referral to individuals with competence in this technique is strongly advised. Pericardiocentesis may need to be performed repeatedly, and surgery may be indicated in selected patients.

PERICARDIOCENTESIS
• Place the patient in sternal recumbency. Clip the haircoat on the right thorax between the 3rd and 8th intercostal space from above the costochondral junction ventrally to the sternum. The right side of the thorax is preferred over the left because of the diminished likelihood of coronary artery laceration. Simultaneous ECG monitoring is advised to detect arrhythmias resulting from contact between the needle or catheter and the myocardium. Echocardiography is useful to identify the best intercostal space for pericardiocentesis. In the absence of echocardiography, pericardiocentesis is performed at the 5th intercostal space just below the costochondral junction. A long (2 cm or longer), large (18 gauge or larger) catheter is advanced

into the pericardial sac after aseptic skin preparation and local anesthetic block with lidocaine. A small amount of clear pleural fluid may be obtained before advancement of the catheter into the pericardial sac. In dogs, pericardial effusion is usually hemorrhagic, although some animals have a serous or serosanguineous effusion. Remove as much effusion as possible. If arrhythmias develop, reposition the needle.

• Except in animals with active hemorrhage into the pericardial sac, the effusion obtained by pericardiocentesis should not clot and should have a PCV that is different than that of peripheral blood. The supernatant of the effusion is often xanthochromic.

SURGERY

• Pericardiectomy may be useful in the treatment of chemodectoma or heart-base tumor.
• Idiopathic pericardial effusion may respond to pericardiocentesis; however, pericardectomy is indicated in animals with recurrent idiopathic pericardial effusion.
• Surgery and chemotherapy are generally ineffective in the treatment of right atrial hemangiosarcoma.

MEDICATIONS

Drug therapy should not be used in place of pericardiocentesis.

DRUGS AND FLUIDS

• Unless the animal has marked dehydration, fluids are generally not required or recommended in animals with chronic pericardial effusion. Mild volume expansion may be useful in selected animals with acute pericardial effusion caused by intrapericardial hemorrhage—0.45 NaCI with 2.5% dextrose is preferred by some; infusion volume is usually one half of calculated maintenance fluid requirement.

• Administration of a diuretic may help reduce ascites; however, this can lead to progressive azotemia and renal dysfunction and worsen patient's weakness. Diuretics such as furosemide or spironolactone can be used if client refuses pericardiocentesis; however, low dosage should be used and with caution. In general, diuretics are not advised.
• Vitamin K is indicated for patients with rodenticide intoxication.
• Appropriate antibiotics are indicated to treat infection by susceptible organism causing infectious pericarditis.
• Chemotherapy may be useful to treat effusion caused by lymphosarcoma, but this treatment is usually ineffective in the treatment of atrial hemangiosarcoma and heart-base tumor.

CONTRAINDICATIONS

Digitalis, vasodilators, and angiotensin converting enzyme inhibitors have been reported to be relatively or absolutely contraindicated.

PRECAUTIONS

Diuretic administration often leads to weakness and prerenal azotemia.

POSSIBLE INTERACTIONS N/A

ALTERNATE DRUGS

• While generally ineffective, systemic or intrapericardial chemotherapy may be attempted to treat right atrial hemangiosarcoma.
• Corticosteroids, by systemic or intrapericardial administration, may be useful in selected animals with idiopathic pericardial effusion.

FOLLOW-UP

PATIENT MONITORING

• During the first 24 hours, ECG monitoring is advised because pericardiocentesis often leads to ventricular arrhythmias. • Pericardial

effusion may recur at any stage; however, follow-up examination and echocardiography at 10-14 days and every 2-4 months is recommended to detect idiopathic pericardial effusion.

POSSIBLE COMPLICATIONS

• Hypotension or shock • Pneumothorax, arrhythmias, and myocardial injury secondary to pericardiocentesis

MISCELLANEOUS

ASSOCIATED CONDITION

Hemangiosarcoma of the spleen

AGE-RELATED FACTORS

• Idiopathic pericardial effusion may be more common in middle-aged to elderly dogs
• Hemangiosarcoma and heart-base tumors are more common in elderly dogs

ZOONOTIC POTENTIAL

Coccidioidomycosis

PREGNANCY N/A

SYNONYMS

• Pericardial tamponade • Cardiac tamponade • Pericarditis

SEE ALSO See Causes

ABBREVIATIONS None

References

Miller MW, Sisson DD. Pericardial disorders. In: Ettinger SJ, Feldman EC, eds. Textbook of veterinary internal medicine. 4th ed. Philadelphia: WB Saunders, 1995;1032-1045.
Rush JE, Atkins CE. Pericardial diseases. In: Allen DG, ed. Small animal medicine. Philadelphia: JB Lippincott, 1991;309-321.
Author John E. Rush
Consulting Editors Larry P. Tilley and Francis W. K. Smith, Jr.

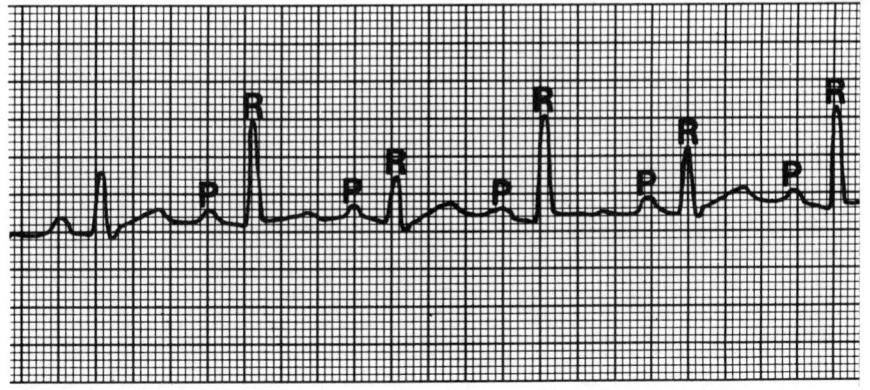

Sinus rhythm with electrical alternans. Heart rate is 150 beats/min. Electrical alternans is associated with pericardial effusion. (From Tilley LP. Essentials of canine and feline electrocardiography. 3rd ed. Williams & Wilkins, Baltimore: 1992, with permission).

PERICARDIODIAPHRAGMATIC HERNIA

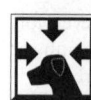

BASICS

OVERVIEW
• Embryologic malformation of the ventral midline allowing communication between the pericardial and peritoneal cavities. • May be associated with other congenital malformations including congenital malformations, sternal deformities (especially in cats), cranial abdominal hernia, and ventricular septal defects. • Signs may be caused by large amounts of abdominal viscera compressing the heart or lungs and incarceration of abdominal organs (e.g., liver and small bowel).

SIGNALMENT
• Dogs and cats • Age at which clinical signs first occur varies but does not commonly occur in the first year • Weimaraners may be predisposed. • No evidence that lesions are hereditary, but it has been reported in littermates.

SIGNS

General Comments
Dependent on the nature and amount of abdominal contents that are herniated.

Historical Findings
• Vomiting • Diarrhea • Weight loss • Abdominal pain • Coughing • Dyspnea

Physical Examination Findings
• Muffled heart sounds • Displaced or attenuated apical cardiac impulse • Palpable sternal deformity or cranial abdominal hernia • Cardiac tamponade and signs of right-sided congestive heart failure (rare)

CAUSES AND RISK FACTORS
• Embryologic malformation • Prenatal injury of the septum transversum and pleuroperitoneal folds

DIAGNOSIS

DIFFERENTIAL DIAGNOSIS
• Never an acquired traumatic defect because there is no natural direct communication between the peritoneal and pericardial cavities after birth. • Pericardial effusion

CBC/BIOCHEMISTRY/URINALYSIS
No associated hematologic or biochemical alterations

OTHER LABORATORY TESTS N/A

IMAGING
• Radiographic findings depend on size of defect and amount of herniated abdominal contents. Caudal heart border and diaphragm may overlap. An "empty" abdomen and possible multiple radiographic densities may be seen on thoracic radiographs. • Barium series may demonstrate bowel loops crossing the diaphragm and within the pericardial sac. • Nonselective angiography outlines the cardiac chambers within the large cardiac silhouette. • Echocardiography gives a definitive diagnosis.

OTHER DIAGNOSTIC PROCEDURES
ECG may show small complexes if abdominal contents have herniated or marked effusion is present.

TREATMENT
Surgical closure of the hernia after returning viable organs to their normal location is usually curative.

MEDICATIONS

DRUGS AND FLUIDS
• In most patients, myocardial contractility is unaffected and drugs for improving cardiac output are not indicated.
• Symptomatic treatment can be given based on nature and amount of abdominal contents that are herniated.

CONTRAINDICATIONS/POSSIBLE INTERACTIONS
• Drugs that reduce ventricular afterload (e.g., arteriolar vasodilators) or preload (e.g., venous dilators and diuretics) are not useful and can cause reduction of ventricular filling, hypotension, and low cardiac output.

FOLLOW-UP
• Prognosis after surgery is excellent in animals with no other significant congenital anomalies or complicating factors

MISCELLANEOUS

References
Miller MW. Pericardial disease. In: Miller MS, Tilley LP, ed. Manual of canine and feline cardiology. 2nd ed. Philadelphia: WB Saunders, 1995.
Author Larry P. Tilley
Consulting Editors Larry P. Tilley and Francis WK Smith, Jr.

BASICS

OVERVIEW
• Inflammatory condition of the parietal (pericardial sac) and/or visceral (epicardium) pericardium • Clinical syndromes caused by pericardial effusion, constrictive pericarditis, extension to surrounding tissues (pleural, myocardium), or an underlying disease process. • In dogs, pericarditis most commonly seen as idiopathic hemorrhagic pericarditis which is a mild inflammatory condition but can lead to pericardial effusion and tamponade.

SIGNALMENT
• Idiopathic hemorrhagic pericarditis more commonly seen in young to middle-aged, medium to large-breed dogs (e.g., great Pyrenees, great Dane, Saint Bernard, golden retriever). • Males predisposed • Other signalments depend on the underlying disease. • Cats rarely have signs of pericarditis on examination

SIGNS
• In dogs, the signs usually caused by low cardiac output and right heart failure secondary to cardiac tamponade—anorexia, weakness, collapse, ascites, dyspnea, diminished pulse strength, tachycardia, muffled heart sounds, jugular distension, and pulsation. • Similar signs are often present in animals with constrictive pericarditis and pericardial effusion; these conditions may coexist (constrictive-effusive pericarditis). A "pericardial knock" is occasionally heard in early diastole as ventricular end-diastolic pressure rises rapidly to a plateau.

CAUSES AND RISK FACTORS
• The cause of idiopathic hemorrhagic pericarditis is unknown. Causes of pericarditis in dogs include blunt or penetrating trauma and bacterial or fungal infection (e.g., tuberculosis, coccidioidomycosis, actinomycosis, nocardiosis, and infection with Pasteurella spp). • In cats, pericarditis is unusual but occurs as a consequence of trauma or infection. Associated infectious agents include feline infectious peritonitis virus, Staphylococcus aureus, Escherichia coli, Streptococcus , Actinomyces, Cryptococcus, and, possibly, Toxoplasma.

DIAGNOSIS

DIFFERENTIAL DIAGNOSIS
• Other causes of pericardial effusion (e.g., neoplasia, left atrial rupture, right-sided congestive heart failure, peritoneal-pericardial diaphragmatic hernia, and pericardial cysts) • Other causes of right-sided congestive heart failure (e.g., cardiomyopathy, myocarditis, tricuspid or pulmonary valve disease, and severe, left-sided congestive heart failure)

• Other causes of abdominal effusion (e.g., neoplastic effusion, hemorrhage, and hypoproteinemia caused by hepatic, renal, or gastrointestinal disease) • Other causes of weakened arterial pulses or collapse (e.g., cardiomyopathy, shock, hypoadrenocorticism, arrhythmias, saddle thrombus, and aortic stenosis) • Pericarditis may be masked by multisystemic signs relating to the underlying disease

CBC/BIOCHEMISTRY/URINALYSIS
Leukocytosis in some animals if a systemic inflammatory condition is present; this is not true in animals with idiopathic hemorrhagic pericarditis, however.

OTHER LABORATORY TESTS N/A

IMAGING
Thoracic Radiography
• Findings may suggest pericardial effusion (rounded cardiac silhouette), particularly in animals with chronic effusion allowing slow but marked expansion of the pericardium; the absence of this finding does not rule out pericardial effusion or pericarditis, however. Radiodense foreign objects may be seen. • Intrapericardial injection of gas after pericardiocentesis (pneumopericardiography) may also reveal space-occupying lesions; neoplastic lesions may be difficult to distinguish from granulomas or cysts.

Echocardiography
• Two-dimensional echocardiography preferred for evaluation of effusion, cardiac tamponade, and neoplasia

Cardiac Catheterization
• Constrictive pericardial physiology recognized by simultaneous pressure measurements in the right and left ventricles, which show pressure equalization of the two sides at a high end diastolic pressure. Atrial tracings show a rapid drop in pressure in early diastole followed by an early rise to plateau at a high - end diastolic pressure.

OTHER DIAGNOSTIC PROCEDURES
Electrocardiographic Findings
Small QRS complexes, electrical alternans, S-T segment elevation, and arrhythmias in some animals

Fluid Analysis
Cytologic examination of pericardial effusion not usually helpful because the most common types, neoplastic and idiopathic, cannot be differentiated this way. In the unusual circumstance of pericarditis, however, cytologic examination has the potential for revealing an etiologic agent and ruling out a suppurative process. Cytologic evaluation of effusion or pericardial biopsy provides the definitive diagnosis of pericarditis.

Other
• If an infectious agent is suspected, aerobic and anaerobic cultures of the effusion are indicated. • Histopathologic examination of the pericardium is imperative if thoracic exploratory surgery is performed.

TREATMENT
• Pericardiocentesis and partial pericardectomy to treat severe effusion. Medical treatment of congestive heart failure is ineffective unless primary heart disease is the cause of the effusion. Thoracic exploration with partial pericardectomy prevents effusions from limiting cardiac function and allows for surgical debridement, retrieval of specimens for histopathologic examination, removal of foreign objects, and evaluation for neoplastic or granulomatous disease.
• Constrictive pericarditis with extensive involvement of the epicardium may require epicardial stripping to relieve the constriction and relieve adhesions between the epicardium and pericardium. This is a difficult procedure with high mortality.

MEDICATIONS

DRUGS AND FLUIDS
• Treatment of infectious disease with chemotherapeutic agents determined through culture and sensitivity testing is paramount.
• Steroid administration in animals with idiopathic hemorrhagic pericarditis has been recommended, but efficacy is unknown.

CONTRAINDICATIONS/POSSIBLE INTERACTIONS
• Fluid therapy exacerbates heart failure if the latter is present.
• Diuretics and preload reducers are contraindicated in animals with cardiac tamponade. Removal of effusions and mechanical relief of constriction are required.
• Steroids may exacerbate an infection.

FOLLOW-UP
Pericardial effusion may recur if the pericardium is intact. Occasionally, clinically important pleural effusion may occur after pericardectomy. Therefore, follow-up with echocardiography or thoracic radiography is recommended.

MISCELLANEOUS

ABBREVIATIONS None

References
Miller MW, Sisson DD. Pericardial disorders. In: Ettinger SJ, Feldman EC, eds. Textbook of veterinary internal medicine. 4th ed. Philadelphia: WB Saunders, 1995.
Author Donald J. Brown
Consulting Editors Larry P. Tilley and Francis W. K. Smith, Jr.

PERINEAL HERNIA

 BASICS

OVERVIEW
• Results from a defect in the musculature of the pelvic diaphragm • Allows herniation of retroperitoneal fat or pelvic viscera through the pelvic diaphragm.

SIGNALMENT
• Much more common in dogs than cats.
• Almost exclusively (95%) in male dogs.
• Usually greater than 5 years of age. • Boston terriers, collies, boxers, Pekingese, and mongrels overrepresented.

SIGNS
• Fluctuant perineal swelling (uni- or bilateral) • Defect in pelvic diaphragm palpable per rectum. • Tenesmus • Stranguria/dysuria
• Painful defecation • Flatulence • Fecal or urinary incontinence (rare)

CAUSES AND RISK FACTORS
Ultimate cause is unknown. Suggested causes include:
• Congenital pelvic muscle weakness
• Gonadal hormone imbalance • Prostatic disease • Chronic constipation/tenesmus
• Concurrent rectal disease (deviation, sacculation, diverticulum)

 DIAGNOSIS

DIFFERENTIAL DIAGNOSIS
• Perianal or perineal neoplasia is usually a firm irregular swelling. • Anal sac disease (abscess, cellulitis) is usually painful and localized to the anal sacs.

CBC/BIOCHEMISTRY/URINALYSIS
• No consistent changes • Complete lab analysis is recommended to look for concurrent diseases in older patients. • May be azotemic if urinary obstruction due to bladder entrapment

OTHER LABORATORY TESTS N/A

IMAGING
• Plain radiographs document extent of rectal/colonic dilatation. • Contrast radiography differentiates rectal deviation from rectal sacculation or diverticulum.

OTHER DIAGNOSTIC PROCEDURES
N/A

 TREATMENT

• Not an emergency unless bladder herniation with urinary obstruction
• Surgery almost always indicated to reduce hernia and repair muscular defect
• Internal obturator flap herniorrhaphy technique has the lowest recurrence rate.
• Concurrent castration is generally recommended.
• High fiber diet to obtain a soft formed stool.
• Warn owners that underlying cause may not be corrected by surgery

MEDICATIONS

DRUGS AND FLUIDS

• Stool softeners should be used, as needed, to maintain a soft formed stool and thus reduce straining.
• Perioperative prophylactic antibiotics are justified. Choose for broad spectrum with activity against gram negative organisms.

CONTRAINDICATION/POSSIBLE INTERACTIONS N/A

FOLLOW-UP

• Early neutering of male dogs reduces risk.
• Immediate post-surgical complications include infection, fecal incontinence, sciatic nerve paralysis, and rectal prolapse.
• Overall recurrence rate 10–50% following repair

MISCELLANEOUS

ASSOCIATED CONDITIONS

• Megacolon • Prostatic disease

Reference

Dean PW, Bojrab MJ. Perineal hernia repair in the dog. In: Bojrab MJ, ed. Current Techniques in Small Animal Surgery. Philadelphia: Lea & Febiger, 1990:442–448.

Author Bradford C. Dixon
Consulting Editor Brent D. Jones

PERIPHERAL NEUROPATHIES (POLYNEUROPATHIES)

BASICS

DEFINITION
Diseases that affect many peripheral motor, sensory, autonomic, and/or cranial nerves in any combination.

Pathophysiology
Inherited or acquired; the primary pathologic process is destruction or degeneration of the ventral horn cells (neuronopathy), primary demyelination, or axonal degeneration (with secondary demyelination).

Systems Affected
• Nervous—primarily the peripheral nervous system, with possible involvement of the cranial nerves • Many other organ systems may be involved in the primary disease process that is causing the polyneuropathy.

Genetics
Most inherited polyneuropathies are inherited as autosomal recessive disorders. Spinal muscular atrophy in Brittany spaniels is an autosomal dominant disorder.

Incidence/Prevalence
• The inherited polyneuropathies are rare. • The actual incidence of peripheral nerve involvement in the metabolic and neoplastic diseases is unknown. • The inflammatory polyneuropathies are uncommon. The most frequently encountered is coonhound paralysis, which has a somewhat seasonal prevalence (highest in fall and early winter).

Geographic Distribution
• The distribution of coonhound paralysis is confined to North, Central, and parts of South America. • Distal denervating disease is the most common polyneuropathy in dogs in the United Kingdom, although it has not been reported elsewhere. • For all other polyneuropathies, there is no evidence of a geographical distribution.

SIGNALMENT

Species
Both inherited and acquired polyneuropathies are seen in dogs and cats.

Breed Predilections
Inherited Polyneuropathies
Spinal Muscular Atrophy
Brittany spaniels, Swedish Lapland dogs, English pointers, German shepherds, rottweilers • Cairn terriers (progressive neuronopathy)
Axonopathies
German shepherds (giant axonal neuropathy) • Boxers (progressive axonopathy) • Domestic shorthair cats (primary hyperoxaluria) • Dalmatians (laryngeal paralysis-polyneuropathy complex) • Birman cats (distal polyneuropathy) • Rottweilers (distal sensorimotor polyneuropathy)

Demyelination
Tibetan mastiffs (hypertrophic neuropathy)
Lysosomal Storage Diseases
• West highland white, cairn terriers, domestic kittens (globoid cell leukodystrophy) • Siamese and mixed-breed cats (GM1 gangliosidosis-type II) • Siamese cats (sphingomyelinosis) • English setters, Chihuahuas, Siamese cats (ceroid lipofuscinosis) • Longhair dachshunds, English pointers (sensory neuropathy)
Acquired Polyneuropathies
• Because of their use, coonhounds have a higher incidence of coonhound paralysis than other breeds. • Cats have a higher incidence of clinical diabetic polyneuropathy than dogs. • Insulinomas have a reported higher incidence in German shepherds, boxers, Irish setters, standard poodles, and collies.

Mean Age and Range
• Inherited polyneuropathies begin at less than 6 months of age. Exceptions include hyperchylomicronemia (usually > 8 months), hyperoxaluria (5-9 months), rottweiler distal polyneuropathy (> 1 year), giant axonal neuropathy (14-16 months), and the intermediate and chronic forms of spinal muscular atrophy in heterozygote Brittany spaniels (6-12 months) • Acquired polyneuropathies secondary to neoplasia and insulinoma-associated hypoglycemia tend to occur in middle-aged and older animals. Neospora polyradiculoneuritis is most commonly seen in dogs less than 6 months of age (highest incidence between 2-4 months).

Predominant Sex N/A

SIGNS

Historical Findings
• Most of the inherited motor and sensorimotor polyneuropathies have a slow progressive history of generalized weakness, muscle tremors, muscle atrophy, often with a plantigrade/palmigrade stance and gait. Sensory neuropathies may present with a history of self-mutilation or ataxia. Lysosomal storage diseases often have evidence of slowly progressive central nervous system involvement, including head tremors, ataxia, dysmetria, seizures, blindness, dementia, and depression. Hypertrophic neuropathy of German shepherds has a rapidly progressive history of generalized weakness (< 3 weeks). • Acquired polyneuropathies may have a rapidly progressive course of an initial stiff, stilted gait, leading to progressive generalized paresis or paralysis (coonhound paralysis, distal denervating disease) or a slowly progressive course of generalized weakness, muscle atrophy, and, in the distal polyneuropathies (diabetic cat), a plantigrade stance. Animals with dysautonomia primarily present with an acute onset (< 48 hours) of depression, anorexia, constipation, third eyelid protrusion, vomiting, and urinary incontinence. With metabolic polyneuropathies, the nonneurologic clinical signs associated with the initiating metabolic defect often are the primary reasons for presentation. With paraneoplastic polyneuropa-

thy, the primary tumor may be clinically absent at the time of presentation.

Physical Examination Findings
• The classic signs of motor and sensorimotor polyneuropathies are tetraparesis to tetraplegia, hypo- to areflexia, hypo- to atonia, and muscle atrophy. Muscle tremors are also common. • Sensory neuropathies demonstrate proprioceptive deficits, hypo- to anesthesia, without muscle atrophy or hyporeflexia (except in boxers). • Hypothyroidism has been associated with both a generalized polyneuropathy and laryngeal paralysis, megaesophagus, facial nerve paralysis, and peripheral vestibular disease. • Hepatosplenomegaly is a common finding in lysosomal storage diseases. • There may be evidence of neoplasia in paraneoplastic polyneuropathy. • Dysautonomic animals have a dry rhinarium, xerostomia, low tear production, bradycardia, and anal areflexia. • Primary hyperchylomicronemia often produces lipid granulomata, which can be palpated under the skin and in the abdomen. • Abdominal palpation may reveal enlarged, painful kidneys in cats with primary hyperoxaluria. • Cranial nerve abnormalities (including dysphonia or aphonia) are variable findings with polyneuropathies.

CAUSES

Acquired
• Immune—primary or secondary as may be seen with SLE or other immune diseases such as polymyositis, glomerulonephritis, polyarthritis, and pemphigus • Metabolic—diabetes mellitus in cats, hypothyroidism, and insulinoma. May be associated with (adeno) carcinomas, malignant melanoma, mast cell tumor, osteosarcoma, multiple myeloma, or lymphosarcoma. • Infectious—Neospora caninum and FeLV • Cancer drugs—vincristine, vinblastin, and colchicine • Toxic—thallium, organophosphates, carbon tetrachloride, and lindane • Idiopathic

RISK FACTORS
Development of the specific diseases (metabolic, immune, neoplastic) or exposure to specific drugs/toxins or etiologic factors (raccoon saliva) that have been associated with the development of polyneuropathies

DIAGNOSIS

DIFFERENTIAL DIAGNOSIS
• For acute poly(radiculo)neuropathies—botulism, tick paralysis, and acute disseminated or multifocal myelopathies • For chronic polyneuropathies—polymyopathy and chronic disseminated/multifocal myelopathies.

CBC/BIOCHEMISTRY/URINALYSIS
Standard laboratory tests do not reflect the presence of polyneuropathy but often indicate the possible underlying metabolic or neoplastic disease. High serum CK indicates an accompanying polymyopathy.

PERIPHERAL NEUROPATHIES (POLYNEUROPATHIES)

OTHER LABORATORY TESTS

None with respect to the actual polyneuropathy. Positive serology assists in the diagnosis of Neospora caninum and FeLV infection; low specific leukocyte lysosomal enzymes indicates specific storage diseases; plasma epinephrine and norepinephrine levels are low in dysautonomia; serum cholesterol, triglycerides, and very low density lipoprotein (VLDL) are increased in hyperchylomicronemia; hyperoxaluria and L-glyceric aciduria are seen in primary hyperoxaluria in cats; monoclonal gammopathy is present in multiple myeloma.

IMAGING

Thoracic and abdominal radiographs are important in the diagnosis of megaesophagus and in the demonstration of ileus, bladder atony, constipation, and delayed gastric emptying in dysautonomia. Radiography and ultrasound may help in the search for a neoplastic etiology.

OTHER DIAGNOSTIC PROCEDURES

Electrophysiology (including EMG, motor and sensory nerve conduction and action potential amplitudes, and late wave studies) is the cornerstone for diagnosing polyneuropathies. Lumbar CSF analysis is valuable in diagnosing nerve root involvement. Muscle biopsy confirms evidence of denervation (type I and II myofiber angular atrophy). Peripheral nerve biopsy further delineates the disease process.

GROSS AND HISTOPATHOLOGIC FINDINGS

Dependent on the specific polyneuropathy, varying degrees of axonal degeneration, demyelination, and/or neuronal cell body degeneration are seen. The anatomic distribution of the lesion along the peripheral nerves (proximal, distal, or widespread) is dependent on the polyneuropathy.

TREATMENT

INPATIENT VERSUS OUTPATIENT

• Most polyneuropathies can be treated as outpatients.
• Acute polyradiculoneuropathies should be observed closely in hospital for respiratory failure in the early progressive phase of disease.
• Animals with dysautonomia may require intensive IV fluid therapy and/or parenteral feeding.
• With paraneoplastic polyneuropathy, treatment of the primary tumor via surgery, chemotherapy, or radiation requires hospitalization.

ACTIVITY

No restrictions, if ambulatory. Physiotherapy is an excellent ancillary treatment in polyneuropathies.

DIET

• No special dietary management is necessary, except in patients with hyperchylomicronemia, unless megaesophagus or dysphagia is present.
• A low-fat diet alone can resolve the polyneuropathy of hyperchylomicronemia within 2-3 months.

CLIENT EDUCATION

Owners need to be aware that treatment of the primary etiology may not lead to reversal of the peripheral nerve sign, and, in some cases, deterioration will continue.

SURGICAL CONSIDERATIONS N/A

MEDICATIONS

DRUGS AND FLUIDS

• Most inherited polyneuropathies are untreatable.
• In most acquired polyneuropathies, the major aim is to treat the primary etiology, if identifiable, with the hope that the secondary polyneuropathy will improve or resolve after appropriate therapy. However, this does not always occur. Chronic progressive or relapsing polyneuropathies (most likely of immune origin) may be improved by the use of long-term immunosuppressive corticosteroid therapy (prednisone 1-2 mg/kg q12h), or by azathioprine (2.2 mg/kg once daily) or cyclophosphamide (50 mg/m² once daily q48h). However, the response of individual animals is variable. SLE-related polyneuropathy would be treated in the same manner.
• Immunosuppressive corticosteroid therapy may improve the polyneuropathy associated with neoplasia without specific action against the primary tumor.
• Neospora-associated polyradiculoneuritis is best treated with clindamycin (5.5 mg/kg PO q12h), although efficacy of treatment of this form of the disease is questionable.
• Dysautonomia also is treated symptomatically with IV fluid therapy (lactated Ringer's solution), artificial tears, metoclopramide (0.2-0.4 mg/kg PO q8h), bethanechol (0.5-2.5 mg SQ q12h or 2.5-10 mg PO q6h-q8h in cats; and 0.5-15 mg SQ bid or 2.5-30 mg PO q6h-q8h in dogs), and physostigmine eye drops.

CONTRAINDICATIONS

Corticosteroid therapy is contraindicated in neospora-associated polyradiculoneuritis and coonhound paralysis.

PRECAUTIONS N/A

POSSIBLE INTERACTIONS N/A

ALTERNATE DRUGS N/A

FOLLOW-UP

PATIENT MONITORING

Repeat neurologic examinations are the single most helpful tool in assessing the success or failure of therapy. Purely demyelinating polyneuropathies have a more rapid course of improvement than those involving axonal degeneration (the majority), which can take months for partial or complete recovery, if at all.

PREVENTION/AVOIDANCE

• For the inherited polyneuropathies or neospora polyradiculoneuritis (placental

transfer of the organism from the bitch), the owner should avoid future breeding.
• Contact with raccoons should be avoided in dogs with a previous history of coonhound paralysis.

POSSIBLE COMPLICATIONS

Continued neurologic deterioration is expected in many of the inherited polyneuropathies, and, therefore, eventual inability to successfully ambulate might be expected. Complications of any acute or chronic progressive polyneuropathy include severe muscle atrophy and resultant pressure sores, urinary tract infection, muscle fibrosis and contracture, and aspiration pneumonia.

EXPECTED COURSE AND PROGNOSIS

• Most of the inherited polyneuropathies have a poor to hopeless prognosis for any recovery of peripheral nerve function (except hyperchylomicronemia). • Acute polyradiculoneuritis (coonhound paralysis) has a good long-term prognosis, although it may take weeks to months before the animal is ambulatory. • Metabolic polyneuropathies also have a fair to good prognosis with successful treatment of the primary metabolic abnormality (insulinomas, however, have a high recurrence rate). • Most other acquired polyneuropathies will show continued deterioration, despite treatment attempts and, therefore, will have a guarded to poor prognosis. However, in some cases, progression can be slow and insidious over many months or years.

MISCELLANEOUS

ASSOCIATED CONDITIONS N/A

AGE RELATED FACTORS N/A

ZOONOTIC POTENTIAL N/A

PREGNANCY

Some of the metabolic causes for polyneuropathy have a significant impact on the pregnant animal. Treatment with high-dose corticosteroids and the other immunosuppressive agents is contraindicated in the pregnant animal.

SYNONYMS N/A

SEE ALSO

See causes.

ABBREVIATIONS

ANA = antinuclear antibody
CSF = cerebrospinal fluid
EMG = electromyography
SLE = systemic lupus erythematosus
TSH = thyroid stimulating hormone
VLDL = very low density lipoprotein

Reference

Duncan ID. Peripheral neuropathy in the dog and cat. Prog Vet Neurol 1991;2:111-128.

Author Paul A. Cuddon
Consulting Editor Joane M. Parent

PERIRENAL PSEUDOCYSTS

BASICS

OVERVIEW
Capsulogenic renal cyst, capsular cyst, pararenal pseudocyst, capsular hydronephrosis, perirenal cyst, and perirenal pseudocyst are terms used to describe renomegaly caused by accumulation of fluid between the kidney and its surrounding capsule. One or both kidneys are affected.

SIGNALMENT
• Primarily old male cats (> 8 years) • When detected in young cats, the disease is usually unilateral • Rare in dogs. The difference in prevalence between species may be related to the prominent network of subcapsular veins that are characteristic of feline kidneys.

SIGNS
• Maybe none • Nonpainful, large abdomen common • Signs of concomitant renal failure in some animals

CAUSES AND RISK FACTORS
• The cause of perirenal accumulation of fluid is not completely understood. It is a dynamic, not a static, process. • Evaluation of the pseudocyst fluid may be helpful in understanding the pathophysiologic mechanisms. • Accumulation of transudate type fluid may be caused by high capillary hydrostatic pressure or lymphatic obstruction. Some cats have histopathologic evidence of renal fibrosis; however, it has not been determined whether progressive renal parenchymal contraction occludes lymphatics and blood vessels, promoting transudation of fluid. • Perirenal accumulation of transudate can also result from ruptured renal cysts. • Accumulation of perirenal urine may indicate that the renal pelvis or proximal ureter has been disrupted. • Accumulation of blood in pseudocysts can result from external trauma, surgery, neoplastic erosion of blood vessels, rupture of aneurysms, coagulopathies, or paracentesis.

DIAGNOSIS

DIFFERENTIAL DIAGNOSIS
• Causes of renomegaly include renal neoplasia, hydronephrosis, polycystic kidney disease (common), feline infectious peritonitis, and mycotic or bacterial nephritis (less common). • Ascites and enlargement of other abdominal organs can cause nonpainful abdominal distension.

CBC/BIOCHEMISTRY/URINALYSIS
• Results unremarkable unless animal has renal insufficiency • Azotemia and inappropriately low urine specific gravity (<1.035) indicate concomitant renal failure.

OTHER LABORATORY TESTS None

IMAGING
• Renomegaly is commonly detected by survey radiography. • Excretory urography and ultrasonography delineate normal or small kidneys beneath an abnormally wide intracapsular space.

OTHER DIAGNOSTIC PROCEDURES
Examination of aspiration of intracapsular material may reveal a modified transudate (acellular, low-protein fluid), hemorrhage, or urine (fluid creatinine concentration several times higher than serum creatinine concentration).

TREATMENT
• Perirenal pseudocysts are not immediately life-threatening.
• In some animals, no treatment is needed; however, monitoring renal function is essential so that treatment can be considered if renal function declines.
• Capsulectomy or peritoneal fenestration is generally associated with a short-term favorable outcome. Long-term response has not been defined.
• Nephrectomy should be avoided to preserve maximal renal function.
• Decompression by paracentesis with a needle and syringe provides temporary relief.
• Pseudocysts usually refill in 1-2 weeks, at which time paracentesis can be repeated.
• Some patients require treatment for concomitant renal failure.

MEDICATIONS

DRUGS AND FLUIDS

Appropriate antimicrobic, (i.e., lipid soluble antibiotic chosen on the basis of antimicrobial susceptibility) should be considered if the pseudocyst becomes infected.

CONTRAINDICATIONS AND POSSIBLE INTERACTIONS N/A

FOLLOW-UP

• Patients should be monitored periodically (every 2-6 months) for development of renal failure. • The short-term prognosis appears to be favorable after capsulectomy in patients that have no evidence of renal dysfunction. • The long-term prognosis for patients with perirenal pseudocysts is not known because it has not yet been determined if perirenal pseudocysts are associated with underlying lesions in the renal parenchyma that may be progressive.

MISCELLANEOUS

Reference

Lulich JP, Osborne CA, Polzin DJ. Cystic diseases of the kidney. In: Osborne CA, Finco DR, eds. Canine and feline nephrology and urology. Philadelphia: Williams & Wilkins, [In press].

Authors Jody P. Lulich and Carl A. Osborne
Consulting Editors Larry G. Adams and Carl A. Osborne

PERITONITIS

BASICS

DEFINITION
Localized or generalized inflammation of the peritoneum, a serous membrane that lines the abdominal cavity and abdominal viscera. Generalized peritonitis is a serious and often fatal condition in small animals.

Pathophysiology
Insult to the peritoneum causes localized inflammation with cellular inflammation and fibrin production. In severe cases of generalized peritonitis, the peritoneum responds with increased vascular permeability, cellular infiltration with leukocytes and macrophages, and fibrin deposition. With increases in vascular permeability, interstitial fluid accumulates rapidly. Significant quantities of electrolytes, plasma proteins, and red blood cells can be lost as well. This may progress to hypovolemia, dehydration, severe hemoconcentration, septicemia, and metabolic alterations.

Systems Affected
• Gastrointestinal—peritoneum affected primarily • Cardiovascular • Renal—affected secondarily as a result of hemoconcentration, hypovolemia, and metabolic acidosis

SIGNALMENT
There is no sex, age, or breed predilection.

SIGNS
• Signs vary depending on the cause, duration, and severity of the peritonitis. General depression, vomiting, diarrhea, and fever are common but not specific for peritonitis. Shock, including dry mucous membranes, delayed capillary refill time, and cool extremities may be present. Occasionally an owner may describe an unusual posture (e.g., a "praying position"). • May manifest as profound shock.

CAUSES

Primary Peritonitis
• Primary peritonitis, often termed idiopathic, is uncommon. The causative agents, either bacteria or viruses, gain access to the peritoneal cavity by hematogenous spread. Examples include feline infectious peritonitis (FIP) and the occasional case of bacterial peritonitis associated with recognizable infection elsewhere, resulting from the same causative organism. • The organism may gain access to the peritoneum via the ovarian bursa and uterus. • Transmural migration of endogenous intestinal bacteria through the intestinal wall may occur as a result of localized ischemia or systemic shock. • Unlike secondary peritonitis, which often has an acute onset and serious systemic signs, primary peritonitis usually develops over a period of days to weeks. FIP signs may take months to become clinically evident. The gradual development of weakness, infected ascites, and ab-

dominal distension is common. Fever, abdominal pain, vomiting, and depression are less common in the early stages.

Secondary Peritonitis
• Secondary peritonitis is considerably more common than primary peritonitis and is defined as peritoneal inflammation secondary to disruption of the abdominal cavity or a hollow viscus. It may be associated with a surgical procedure or may occur after trauma or disease. It is the most common fatal complication of abdominal surgical treatment and diseases involving the abdominal organs. In dogs and cats, diffuse bacterial peritonitis commonly results in septic shock and, often, death. Causes of secondary peritonitis may be categorized as mechanical and foreign body, chemical, infectious, and miscellaneous.
• The most frequent lesion causing generalized peritonitis is surgical wound dehiscence, particularly of the gastrointestinal tract. Prevention of wound dehiscence of the gastrointestinal tract and other abdominal organs through gentle tissue handling and careful surgical technique is important. Early detection of postoperative complications by close monitoring is also important. • Trauma is the second most common cause of generalized peritonitis, with motor vehicle accidents and gunshot injuries frequently represented.
• Lesions of the abdominal organs are also an important cause of generalized peritonitis. In the gastrointestinal tract, neoplasia, intussusception, and gastric ulceration all may cause generalized peritonitis. Urinary bladder rupture, gallbladder rupture, gastric juice, pancreatic juice, and chyle may induce irritant damage.

RISK FACTORS
• Gastrointestinal surgery • Breeds at risk for gastric torsion/volvulous • Cats—risks associated with feline infectious peritonitis

DIAGNOSIS

DIFFERENTIAL DIAGNOSIS
• Must differentiate from other causes of abdominal pain or distension such as that caused by organ enlargement, neoplasia, cystic structures, pancreatitis, abdominal abscesses • Must differentiate from other causes of shock such as septic shock, hypovolemic shock, and bacteremia. • History of abdominal surgery, especially involving the intestinal tract, trauma, especially resulting from automobile accidents, or gunshot wounds should raise concerns about peritonitis.

CBC/BIOCHEMISTRY/URINALYSIS
• CBC—neutrophilia progressing to neutropenia. Severe hemoconcentration. • Biochemistry—hyperkalemia secondary to acidosis, shock, poor renal perfusion, and tissue necrosis is a fairly consistent finding. Hypoglycemia may occur early in septic pa-

tients caused by the presumed "insulinlike" effect of endotoxin. Electrolyte abnormalities vary depending on the etiology and duration of disease. Metabolic alterations, including metabolic acidosis, occur rapidly.

OTHER LABORATORY TESTS N/A

IMAGING
• Radiographic findings are inconsistent. Loss of normal detail or a "ground glass" appearance to the abdomen may indicate the presence of abdominal fluid. Free gas in the abdomen may be present; however, care must be taken to evaluate gas in light of recent abdominal surgery. A fluid line may be seen on a standing lateral radiographic view.
• The use of contrast radiography is generally not warranted and may complicate the clinical case if contrast material enters the peritoneal cavity because of intestinal leakage or spillage at surgery. • Ultrasonography has been shown to be useful in the diagnosis of pancreatitis, liver abscess, prostate abscess, ruptured gallbladder and presence of abdominal fluid.

OTHER DIAGNOSTIC PROCEDURES
• Paracentesis and diagnostic peritoneal lavage have been shown to be safe and reliable in evaluating the cause of peritonitis. The technique involves aseptic preparation of the paracentesis site. The urinary bladder is emptied and a 22-gauge hypodermic needle is inserted into the site through the skin and into the peritoneal cavity. Fluid is allowed to drip from the needle into a sterile collection tube. If no fluid is released, gentle suction can be applied to the needle using a 3-cc syringe. In the event of a negative tap, a four-quadrant tap should be performed. Punctures are made cranial and caudal to the umbilicus and lateral to the midline on each side.
• Diagnostic peritoneal lavage can be performed in patients suspected of having generalized peritonitis but who have a negative four-quadrant paracentesis. Twenty ml/kg body weight of warm saline is instilled into the peritoneum using an intravenous administration set, allowing the fluid to flow with gravity. The animal is carefully rolled from side to side to mix the fluid. A sample is then recovered for cytologic evaluation and for culture and sensitivity. The entire amount of fluid infused does not need to be recovered.
• Samples for cytology should be collected in a sterile ethylenediamine-tetraacetic acid (EDTA) tube. • Samples for culture and sensitivity should be collected in a clot tube.
• The diagnosis of bacterial peritonitis based on the presence of toxic degenerating neutrophils and intracellular bacteria is associated with 100% accuracy. • If chemical peritonitis is suspected, abdominal fluid creatinine and BUN (to detect urine leakage), amylase activity (for pancreatitis), alkaline phosphatase (for intestinal trauma), or bilirubin (for leakage of bile) should be evaluated.

TREATMENT

SURGICAL CONSIDERATIONS

• In generalized peritonitis, treatment will require surgery.

• The aim of surgery is to (1) identify and correct the underlying cause, (2) remove any foreign material from the peritoneal cavity, (3) provide adequate drainage and lavage of the peritoneal cavity, and (4) provide an avenue for nutritional support after surgery.

• The owner should be made aware that the fatality rate, even with surgery, may approach 70%.

• Exploratory laparotomy involves a ventral midline incision from xyphoid to pubis. A sample of abdominal fluid is obtained for culture and sensitivity testing. Wide and complete exploration is necessary to identify the source of contamination. Once found, the source of the problem is corrected or removed. Suture material is nonabsorbable monofilament or absorbable monofilament. Cat gut sutures are contraindicated. The abdominal cavity is thoroughly lavaged with 200-300 ml/kg warm, sterile saline or until the fluid returns with a clear appearance. Antiseptics in the fluid are not indicated and may impair normal metabolism.

• Intraoperative placement of a gastrotomy or enterostomy feeding tube is warranted to provide nutritional support postsurgically.

• Closure is either open or closed depending on the extent of the peritoneal contamination, the ability to remove the contamination, the severity of the patient's condition (more severe disease should be treated open), and whether or not continuation of septic processes is expected.

• If the abdomen is closed, it is done so routinely. If the decision is made to leave the abdomen open, partial closure is performed, followed by the application of a sterile laparotomy pad and bandage.

MEDICATIONS

DRUGS AND FLUIDS

• Hypovolemia/shock is treated with intravenous fluids to correct hypovolemia and metabolic changes (acidosis, electrolyte abnormalities). Volume replacement at a rate of up to 90 ml/kg is started based on extent of disease. Isotonic fluids such as lactated Ringer's or Normosol-R are expected recommended. If the patient is hypoglycemic, the use of 5% dextrose in a polyionic replacement fluid is indicated. Plasma and dextran solutions are the fluids of choice, because protein loss to the extravascular space is extensive.

• Infection-antibiotic therapy is warranted and should be started as soon as a diagnosis of peritonitis is made. The antibiotic should be broad spectrum and should be present at therapeutic levels in the peritoneal cavity. Aminoglycosides, ampicillin, and cephalosporins are good first choice antibiotics alone or in combination. Ultimately, antibiotic choice should be based on results of culture and sensitivity testing.

• Controversy exists regarding the use of corticosteroids in sepsis. Most authors agree that the properties of corticosteroids (stabilizing lysosomal membranes, decreasing vascular permeability, protection against endotoxin, restoration of intestinal wall permeabiltiy) make them a useful adjunct to therapy for peritonitis. Nonsteroidal antiinflammatory drugs have been documented to be beneficial in the treatment of peritonitis in dogs.

CONTRAINDICATIONS

The use of corticosterieods and nonsteroidal inflammatory medications (flunixin meglumine) is controversial.

PRECAUTIONS

Care should be taken to evaluate renal function and ensure adequate renal perfusion in patients treated with aminoglycosides.

POSSIBLE INTERACTIONS N/A

ALTERNATE DRUGS N/A

FOLLOW-UP

PATIENT MONITORING

• Feeding should begin via feeding tube after enterostomy or gastrotomy tube placement.

• Evaluation of serum albumin with replacement of protein losses if albumin falls below 2.0 gm/dl • Bandage changes should be continued at 24-hour intervals until successful management of open peritoneal drainage is attained (usually 4-5 days) followed by completion of abdominal closure.

POSSIBLE COMPLICATIONS

Death from septicemia, hypovolemia, and electrolyte disturbances occurs in a high percentage of patients.

MISCELLANEOUS

ASSOCIATED CONDITIONS N/A

AGE RELATED FACTORS N/A

ZOONOTIC POTENTIAL N/A

PREGNANCY N/A

SYNONYMS N/A

SEE ALSO N/A

ABBREVIATION

FIP = feline infectious peritonitis

References

Seim HB. Management of peritonitis. In: Bonagura JD, ed. Current veterinary therapy XII. Philadelphia: WB Saunders, 1995:764-770.

Crowe DT, Bjorling DE, Hosgood G, Salisbury K. Generalized peritonitis in dogs: 50 cases. JAVMA 1988;193:1448-1450.

Crowe DT, Bjorling DE. Peritoneum and peritoneal cavity. In: Slatter DH, ed. Textbook of small animal surgery. Philadelphia: WB Saunders, 1985:579-591.

Author David K. Rosen
Consulting Editor Fred W. Scott

PERSISTENT RIGHT AORTIC ARCH

BASICS

OVERVIEW
• Entrapment of the esophagus by a persistent right 4th aortic arch on the right, the base of the heart and pulmonary artery centrally, and ductus or ligamentum arteriosum on the left and dorsally • Causes megaesophagus cranial to the obstruction at the base of the heart

SIGNALMENT
Seen most commonly in the German shepherd, Irish setter, and Boston terrier

SIGNS
• Regurgitation of undigested solid food in animals < 6 months old • Malnourishment in many animals • Time between eating and regurgitation varies • Signs of aspiration pneumonia (e.g., cough and tachypnea or dyspnea) in some animals

CAUSES AND RISK FACTORS N/A

DIAGNOSIS

DIFFERENTIAL DIAGNOSIS
• Other vascular ring anomalies such as double aortic arch (rare) • Congenital megaesophagus • Stricture, diverticulum, or esophageal foreign body • Esophageal motility disorder in shar-pei

CBC/BIOCHEMISTRY/URINALYSIS
• Results usually normal • High WBC in some animals with aspiration pneumonia

OTHER LABORATORY TESTS N/A

IMAGING
• Thoracic radiographs show food-filled cranial esophagus or signs of aspiration pneumonia in some animals. • Contrast esophagram confirms megaesophagus extending to the heart base. • Fluoroscopy can be used to differentiate esophageal motility disorders.
• Angiography may be needed to differentiate between specific vascular ring anomalies.

OTHER DIAGNOSTIC PROCEDURES

Endoscopy
Esophagoscopy can be used to differentiate esophageal motility disorders.

TREATMENT
• Surgical correction of the vascular entrapment is indicated. Medical management of concurrent aspiration pneumonia may be necessary.
• Feeding procedures for megaesophagus may also be necessary.

MEDICATIONS

DRUGS AND FLUIDS

• Supportive care with oxygen may be needed in animal with aspiration pneumonia.
• Broad spectrum antibiotics such as enrofloxin (2.5 mg/kg q12h) and amoxicillin (10-15 mg/kg q12h) should be instituted in animals with aspiration pneumonia.

CONTRAINDICATIONS/POSSIBLE INTERACTIONS N/A

FOLLOW-UP

• Prognosis for resolution of the problem, even after surgery, is guarded to poor.
• Complications of malnourishment and aspiration pneumonia are common and severe.
• Esophageal function is often permanently compromised.

MISCELLANEOUS

SEE ALSO Double Aortic Arch

References

Jones BD. Diseases of the esophagus. In: Ettinger SJ, ed. Textbook of veterinary internal medicine. 3rd ed. Philadelphia: WB Saunders, 1989.
Olivier NB. Congenital heart disease in dogs. In: Fox PR, ed. Canine and feline cardiology. New York: Churchill Livingstone, 1988.
Author Carroll Loyer
Consulting Editors Larry P. Tilley and Francis W. K. Smith, Jr.

PHEOCHROMOCYTOMA

 BASICS

DEFINITION
A catecholamine-producing tumor of chromaffin cells of the adrenal medulla

Pathophysiology
• Pheochromocytomas can be benign or malignant. Clinical signs are caused by invasion by the tumor or overproduction of catecholamines. Local invasion may cause tumor thrombosis of the posterior vena cava, resulting in abdominal distension, ascites, or peripheral edema. Distant metastases to the lymphatics, lungs, liver, and kidneys may develop after invasion of the great vessels.
• Functional pheochromocytomas produce norepinephrine, both norepinephrine and epinephrine, or, less commonly, dopamine. Overproduction of catecholamines by a pheochromocytoma may be episodic or continuous depending on the secretory pattern of the tumor. Catecholamine excess may cause a myriad of physiologic changes, the most common of which is systemic hypertension. Although chronic episodic signs are most common, acute hypertensive crisis with cardiac arrhythmias can cause sudden collapse and death. Rupture of these highly vascular, intraabdominal tumors can cause acute hypovolemic shock.

Systems Affected
Cardiovascular—because of the hypertensive effects of catecholamines

Genetics
Pheochromocytoma may be inherited as an autosomal dominant trait in humans; heritability has not been determined in animals.

Incidence/Prevalance
Uncommon in dogs, rare in cats

Geographic Distribution N/A

SIGNALMENT

Species Dogs and (rarely) cats

Breed Predilections None

Mean Age and Range
10.5 years (3-15 years)

Predominant Sex None

SIGNS

General Comments
• Clinical signs are vague and may be associated with many other disease conditions.
• Clinical findings are variable and episodic because of intermittent catecholamine release from the tumor. • The tumor is uncommonly diagnosed antemortem. A high degree of clinical suspicion of disease is needed for diagnosis. Paroxysmal signs of systemic hypertension warrant further diagnostics.

Historical Findings
• Weakness, lethargy, anorexia, weight loss, and rapid respirations or panting may be re-
ported. • Owners may characterize clinical signs as episodic. • Observant owners may note flushing of the skin of the pinnae. • If hypertension is severe, epistaxis or neurologic signs may be seen.

Physical Examination
• Frequently nonspecific unless the patient is examined during a hypertensive episode • In only about 25% of patients is the tumor large enough to be palpable. If local invasion of the posterior vena cava has occurred, ascites, hindlimb edema, and distension of the caudal epigastric vessels may be observed. • Physical abnormalities associated with catecholamine excess vary. Affected dogs may be restless or irritable and exhibit flushing of the skin and mucous membranes. A bounding femoral pulse may be palpable. • Thoracic auscultation reveals tachypnea with increased bronchovesicular lung sounds, tachycardia or other arrhythmias, and cardiac murmurs in some patients. • Fundic examination may demonstrate retinal hemorrhage or detachment and associated blindness secondary to sustained hypertension. Mydriasis may also develop because of excessive sympathetic stimulation. • Abnormal neurologic signs such as seizures, nystagmus, and head tilt may develop secondary to cerebral hemorrhage.

CAUSES
Pheochromocytoma is a benign or malignant tumor of chromaffin cells of the adrenal medulla.

RISK FACTORS Unknown

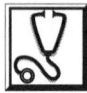 DIAGNOSIS

DIFFERENTIAL DIAGNOSIS
• Other causes of systemic hypertension (e.g., chronic renal disease, hyperthyroidism, acromegaly, and hyperadrenocorticism)
• Other metabolic or systemic disorders such as cardiovascular or pulmonary disease and neurologic disorders

CBC/BIOCHEMISTRY/URINALYSIS
• No consistent abnormalities • Hemoconcentration and mature neutrophilia may result from catecholamine excess. • Hypercholesterolemia has been reported in some patients and may be related to the effects of catecholamines on triglyceride lipase. • Proteinuria or hematuria may be observed in patients with hypertensive glomerulopathies.

OTHER LABORATORY TESTS

Catecholamine Concentrations
Assays for plasma or urinary catecholamines and their metabolites are technically difficult, expensive, and not readily available. Interpretation may be difficult because the release of catecholamines in patients with pheochromocytoma is episodic, and measured values may overlap with those of normal but otherwise stressed dogs. For this
reason, assessment of a 24-hour urine sample may be more diagnostic than testing a single serum sample.

Provocative Testing
Because of the difficulty obtaining and interpreting serum or urinary catecholamines, provocative tests have been developed that assess changes in blood pressure in response to catecholamine blockade or release. Phentolamine and clonidine have been used to block catecholamine effects, while histamine and glucagon have been used to stimulate catecholamine release. These drugs can cause profound hypotension and hypertension, respectively, and thus should be used with extreme caution.

IMAGING
• Abdominal radiography may reveal an adrenal mass, possibly calcified, displacing the adjacent kidney. If an abdominal mass is suspected, thoracic radiographs should be obtained to examine the lungs for metastatic disease. These are often nonspecific but may reveal cardiomegaly or pulmonary edema associated with heart failure. • Contrast radiography such as intravenous urography or venography may demonstrate displacement of a kidney or compression of the posterior vena cava by an adrenal mass. • Abdominal ultrasonography or computed tomography are more effective than plain radiography in demonstrating unilateral adrenomegaly and in detecting tumor invasion or distant metastasis.

OTHER DIAGNOSTIC PROCEDURES
• Arterial blood pressure measurement may document hypertension; however, because of the episodic release of catecholamines, multiple determinations may be necessary. • Electrocardiography may demonstrate cardiac arrhythmias, usually premature ventricular contractions.

GROSS AND HISTOPATHOLOGIC FINDINGS
• Pheochromocytoma is usually located in the retroperitoneal space associated within a single adrenal gland; however, it may be located along the aorta or its branches. These tumors tend to be vascular and invasive, making tumor dissection difficult. • Histopathologic assessment of malignancy of a pheochromocytoma is difficult. For optimal characterization, the use of Zenker's fixative is recommended.

 TREATMENT

INPATIENT VERSUS OUTPATIENT
Inpatient. Medical treatment is needed to stabilize the cardiovascular status of the patient before anesthesia and surgery.

ACTIVITY
Restrict activity to limit catecholamine release.

DIET

No special restrictions

CLIENT EDUCATION

• Pheochromocytomas should be treated aggressively because of the locally invasive nature of the tumor and the potential for metastases. Surgical resection can significantly prolong survival time, even in patients with advanced disease.

• Long-term prognosis depends on the presence of distant metastasis and concurrent disease.

SURGICAL CONSIDERATIONS

Anesthesia

Extreme care should be taken in the planning of anesthetic protocols for patients with pheochromocytoma to avoid inducing catecholamine release or potentiatiation. Atropine should be avoided since it potentiates the chronotropic effects of epinephrine. Glycopyrolate is preferred to reduce vagal tone. Xylazine may also enhance the sensitivity of the myocardium to catecholamine-induced arrhythmias. Ketamine raises the heart rate, blood pressure, and circulating catecholamine concentrations.

Recommended anesthetic protocols for patients with pheochromocytoma include premedication with low-dose acepromazine (0.025-0.05 mg/kg IM) since acepromazine can reduce catecholamine-induced arrhythymias.. Thiopental and thiamylal are usually satisfactory for induction of anesthesia. Although opiods such as oxymorphone can be used in patients with preexisting arrhythmias, morphine and meperidine can cause histamine release and are not recommended. Isoflurane is probably preferred to maintain anesthesia since it causes less sensitization of the myocardium to catecholamines than does halothane.

Intraarterial catheters for measuring blood pressure and a jugular catheter for monitoring central venous pressure (CVP) should be placed before induction. Throughout anesthesia, a balanced electrolyte solution should be administered to maintain CVP. During induction and maintenance of anesthesia, heart rate, ECG, arterial blood pressure, and body temperature should be constantly monitored. On induction, care should be taken to avoid excitement and hypoxia. Intubation can cause tachycardia and raise blood pressure. Potential intraoperative complications include hypovolemia secondary to hemorrhage, hypertension, and arrhythmias. Acute hypertension may develop when the tumor is manipulated, necessitating boluses of short

acting alpha-adrenergic blockers such as phentolamine (0.02-1.0 mg/kg IV). Small doses of the beta-adrenergic blocker propranalol (0.03-0.1 mg/kg IV) may be helpful in preventing ventricular arrhythmias. Lidocaine boluses (1.0-2.0 mg/kg IV) may be required to convert persistent ventricular arrhythmias.

Surgery

Adrenalectomy can be performed through a ventral midline laparotomy or a retroperitonal approach. The ventral approach allows more complete exposure of other abdominal glands and is preferred. Most tumors lie in the retroperitoneal space, in or around the adrenal gland or near the aorta. Although most pheochromocytomas are associated with only one gland, complete exploration of the abdomen is important. Tumor vascularity and potential for vena cava invasion necessitate caution in dissection.

A rapid fall in arterial pressure may occur on removal of the tumor, requiring aggressive fluid infusion. Marked blood loss associated with the resection may necessitate colloid administration or whole blood or plasma transfusion.

MEDICATIONS

DRUGS AND FLUIDS

• Presurgical medical management of catecholamine excess involves the use of alpha- and beta-adrenergic blocking agents.

• Phenoxybenzamine, a long-acting, alpha-adrenergic blocker should be administered (0.2-0.4 mg/kg PO q12h) for 10-14 days before surgery. A higher dosage (to 1.5 mg/kg) may be necessary to achieve the desired decrease in blood pressure.

• Beta-adrenergic blocking agents are used in conjunction with phenoxybenzamine to further control cardiac arrhythmias and hypertension; however, to avoid severe hypertension, use beta blockers only after adequate alpha-adrenergic blockade has been achieved with phenoxybenzamine. The beta blocker propranolol is most commonly used (0.15-0.5 mg/kg PO q8h).

• Long-term medical management may be necessary in patients with inoperable or metastatic tumors.

CONTRAINDICATIONS

See anesthetic considerations.

PRECAUTIONS

See anesthetic considerations.

POSSIBLE INTERACTIONS

See anesthetic considerations.

FOLLOW-UP

PATIENT MONITORING

• Arterial blood pressure closely for 24-48 hours after surgery

• Urinary catecholamines and their metabolites should return to normal within days of surgery if resection is adequate.

PREVENTION/AVOIDANCE N/A

POSSIBLE COMPLICATIONS

Potential postoperative complications include hemorrhage and associated hypotension or persistent hypertension. Persistent hypertension may indicate incomplete resection or metastatic disease.

EXPECTED COURSE AND PROGNOSIS

Complete resection of the tumor without evidence of metastases warrants a good prognosis.

MISCELLANEOUS

ASSOCIATED CONDITIONS

None

AGE RELATED FACTORS None

ZOONOTIC POTENTIAL N/A

PREGNANCY N/A

SYNONYMS N/A

SEE ALSO Hypertension, Systemic

ABBREVIATION

CVP = central venous pressure

References

Gilson SD, Withrow SJ, Orton EC, Twedt DC. Pheochromocytoma in the dog. A retrospective review of 50 cases. Vet Canc Soc Newsletter 1992;16:6-7.

Gilson SD, Withrow SJ, Orton EC. Surgical treatment of pheochromocytoma: technique, complications, and results in six dogs. Vet Surg 1994;23-195-200.

Trim CM. Anesthesia and the endocrine system. In: Slatter D, ed. Textbook of small animal surgery. 2nd ed. Philadelphia: WB Saunders, 1993:2290-2294.

Wheeler SL. Pheochromocytoma. In: Kirk RW, ed. Current veterinary therapy IX. Philadelphia: WB Saunders, 1986:977-981.

Author Leland Thompson

Consulting Editor Rhett Nichols

PHOSPHOFRUCTOKINASE DEFICIENCY

BASICS

OVERVIEW
• Phosphofructokinase (PFK) is the most important rate-controlling enzyme in glycolysis. RBC and intensely exercising skeletal muscle depend heavily on anaerobic glycolysis for energy.• PFK-deficient dogs have compensated hemolytic anemia and mild myopathy resulting from markedly reduced total PFK activity in both tissues. • Anemia develops because of insufficient ATP generation to maintain normal RBC shape, ionic composition, and deformability; another reason for the occurrence of anemia is that RBC from affected dogs are alkaline fragile and lyse when blood pH is slightly high.

SIGNALMENT
• In dogs, PFK deficiency is an inherited defect transmitted as an autosomal recessive trait.
• Occurs in English springer spaniels and American cocker spaniels • Homozygously affected animals generally not recognized as abnormal before 1 year of age

SIGNS
• Some animals exhibit mild clinical signs that go unrecognized for years; others regularly exhibit episodes of severe illness.
• Depression or weakness concomitant with episodes of red to brown pigmenturia. This hemoglobinuria is less likely to be recognized in female dogs, because of the sex difference in urination pattern. • Mild lethargy with slight fever during mild hemolytic episodes
• Marked lethargy, weakness, pale or icteric mucous membranes, mild hepatosplenomegaly, muscle wasting, and fever as high as 41°C may occur during severe hemolytic crises.
• Intravascular hemolysis can be caused by hyperventilation-induced alkalemia associated with exercise or excitement. • Signs of muscle dysfunction—usually limited to exercise intolerance and slightly decreased muscle mass, but muscle cramping and severe progressive myopathy can occur. • Heterozygous carrier animals appear clinically normal.

CAUSES AND RISK FACTORS
Deficiency of muscle-type subunit of PFK—markedly reduced total PFK activity in RBC as well as skeletal muscle

DIAGNOSIS

DIFFERENTIAL DIAGNOSIS
• Other causes of hemolytic anemia, such as immune-mediated hemolytic anemia, Heinz body anemia, pyruvate kinase deficiency
• PFK-deficient dogs should be Coombs' test negative, lack parasites or Heinz bodies in stained blood films, and lack evidence of disseminated coagulation or heartworm disease. PFK deficiency is differentiated from pyruvate kinase deficiency using specific enzyme assays or DNA tests.

CBC/BIOCHEMISTRY/URINALYSIS
• Affected dogs have persistent compensated hemolytic anemias. MCV—usually between 80 and 90 fl. Reticulocyte counts—generally between 10% and 30%. PCV values 30%-40%, except during hemolytic crises when PCV may decrease to 15% or less • Bilirubinuria that is often markedly high in male dogs. Hemoglobinuria occurs in association with episodes of intravascular hemolysis.
• Findings in serum of slightly high potassium, magnesium, calcium, urea, AST, total protein, and globulin. Serum CK, LDH, alkaline phosphatase, iron and bilirubin may be slightly to moderately high. Serum bilirubin may be markedly high in association with a hemolytic crisis; urea and creatinine may be markedly high if renal failure is present secondary to hemoglobin nephrosis or shock.

OTHER LABORATORY TESTS
• Measure RBC PFK activity to easily identify homozygous affected animals older than 3 months of age. • Heterozygous carrier dogs have approximately one half normal enzyme activity in RBC. • Perform DNA test using polymerase chain reaction technology to clearly differentiate normal and carrier animals of any age.

IMAGING N/A

OTHER DIAGNOSTIC PROCEDURES
N/A

TREATMENT
• Bone marrow transplantation is the only cure.
• Infrequently, affected dogs may die during hemolytic crisis as the result of anemia or renal failure.

MEDICATIONS

DRUGS AND FLUIDS
• To treat fever that often accompanies intravascular hemolysis and potentiates hemolytic crisis—aspirin (10 mg/kg PO q12h), or dipyrone (0.055 ml of 50% solution/kg SQ q8h)
• When intravascular hemolysis is severe—IV fluid therapy to minimize chances of acute renal failure
• Blood transfusions are usually not needed, but they should be given if the anemia becomes life-threatening.

CONTRAINDICATIONS/POSSIBLE INTERACTIONS N/A

FOLLOW-UP
Animals with this deficiency can have a normal lifespan, if they are properly managed.
• Owners should avoid placing affected dogs in stressful situations or subjecting them to strenuous exercise, excitement, or high environmental temperatures.

MISCELLANEOUS

ABBREVIATIONS
AST = aspartate aminotransferase
ATP = adenosine triphosphate
CK = creatine kinase
DNA = deoxyribonucleic acid
LDH = lactate dehydrogenase
MCV = mean corpuscular volume
PFK = phosphofructokinase
RBC = red blood cells

Reference

Giger U, Harvey JW. Hemolysis caused by phosphofructokinase deficiency in English springer spaniels: seven cases (1983-1986). J Am Vet Med Assoc 1987;191:453-459.
Author John W. Harvey
Consulting Editor Alan H. Rebar

BASICS

OVERVIEW
Stomach worm, Physaloptera spp, of dogs and cats. Acute gastritis caused by small number, even single, worm infections. No extraintestinal involvement. Infective larvae carried by coprophagous grubs, bugs, beetles.

SIGNALMENT
Dogs and cats. Any age and sex

SIGNS
• Small 2.5–5 cm worms with cuticular collars and spiralled tails seen in stomach, vomitus • Vomition

CAUSES AND RISK FACTORS
Physaloptera, spirurid worms, transmitted as infective larvae in coprophagous beetles, bugs or in transport hosts such as birds, rodents, frogs

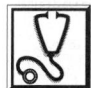

DIAGNOSIS

DIFFERENTIAL DIAGNOSIS
• Other spirurid infections, e.g., Spirocerca, the esophageal worm, produce similar eggs

and may cause a projectile vomition • Viral, bacterial infections • Foreign objects in the stomach • Noxious substances accidentally ingested

CBC/BIOCHEMISTRY/URINALYSIS
Usually normal

OTHER LABORATORY TESTS
Fecal examination for ovoid to ellipsoidal eggs 30–40 × 20 µm, thick-shelled, larvated

IMAGING
Abdominal radiography, including contrast studies to evaluate cause of vomiting

OTHER DIAGNOSTIC PROCEDURES
Endoscopy will allow visualization of worms

TREATMENT

With no migration beyond the stomach wall, use adulticide anthelmintics with release in stomach

MEDICATIONS

DRUGS AND FLUIDS
• Dichlorvos (Task, Task Tabs) 1 time or 2 weeks apart

• Fenbendazole (Panacur) q24h for 5 days
• Pyrantel pamoate (Nemex)
• Medication to reduce gastric irritation

CONTRAINDICATIONS/POSSIBLE INTERACTIONS
Organophosphate (dichlorvos) not to be given to heartworm positive dogs or cats

FOLLOW-UP

Fecal examination after 2 weeks to determine drug effect

MISCELLANEOUS

Reference

Corwin RM, Green SE. Gastrointestinal parasitism in the dog and cat. In: Jones BD, ed. Canine and feline gastroenterology. WB Saunders, 1986;487–509.

Author Robert M. Corwin
Consulting Editor Brent D. Jones

PLAGUE (YERSINIA PESTIS)

BASICS

OVERVIEW
• Yersinia pestis is a gram-negative, bipolar staining rod and member of the Enterobacteriaceae. • Plague occurs worldwide; cases found in the western United States—New Mexico, Arizona, California, Colorado, Idaho, Nevada, Oregon, Texas, Utah, Washington, Wyoming, and Hawaii • Y. pestis reservoir in wild rodents (sylvatic)—ground squirrels, prairie dogs, rabbits, bobcats, coyotes; cases common from May to October • Pathophysiology—fleas ingest blood meal from infected animal; blood clots and blocks gut of flea; flea bites next victim and regurgitates Y. pestis into skin; during a rapid course, the bacteria migrate from skin lymphatics to regional lymph node (LN), submandibular usually; bacteria survive phagocytosis (because of capsule protection) to multiply in LN; phagocytic cells rupture and bacteria are resistant to further phagocytosis; fever; painful lymphadenopathy occurs (bubo); intense local inflammation results in bubonic plague; intermittent bacteremia; LN may rupture; may become septicemic with or without LN involvement

SIGNALMENT
• Cats highly susceptible to infection and exhibit severe fatal disease with fever and lymphadenopathy • Dogs naturally resistant to infection; may exhibit mild febrile signs with depression only

SIGNS

Bubonic Plague
• Most common form in cats • Incubation period from 2-7 days after flea bite or after eating infected rodent • Duration of illness variable • Buboes occur on head and neck with marked lymphadenopathy; LN—submandibular, hemorrhagic, necrotic, edematous • If cat survives long enough, LN abscesses, ruptures, drains through fistulous tract to skin • Bacteremia occurs in acute stages; fever (103°-105° F) • Other systemic signs include depression, vomiting/diarrhea, dehydration, enlarged tonsils, anorexia, ocular discharge, weight loss, ataxia, coma, and oral ulcers.

Septicemic Plague
• Rare in cats • Septicemia without lymphadenopathy or abscess formation • Other signs same as for bubonic plague

CAUSES AND RISK FACTORS
• Hunter cats (outdoor) at greater risk of contacting wild rodent populations and rodent fleas • Travel with pet to endemic areas of country (western United States and Hawaii) • Homes with heavy flea infestation (lack of control in pets also) • Homes with large rodent populations nearby (e.g., garbage food source and wood piles in which they live)

DIAGNOSIS

DIFFERENTIAL DIAGNOSIS
Need to differentiate from fight wound abscess (P. multocida, S. aureus)

CBC/BIOCHEMISTRY/URINALYSIS
• CBC-leukocytosis; WBC show characteristics of an acute bacterial infection (vacuolation, toxic granules); in acute stages blood platelets, may be normal or low; with DIC (elevated fibrin degradation products [FDP]) • Chemistry profile—liver function tests elevated (serum aminotransferase, bilirubin)

OTHER LABORATORY TESTS
Serology (Communicable Disease Center [CDC] and/or state health departments)— cats and dogs develop high passive hemagglutinating (PHA) titers to fraction 1A (capsule antigen) 8-12 days postinfection; may see fourfold rise in titer between acute and convalescent serum samples; high titers persist greater than 1 year in surviving animals

IMAGING N/A

OTHER DIAGNOSTIC PROCEDURES
Culture isolation by reference laboratory of Y. pestis from antemortem clinical material (abscess, LN, peripheral blood) before treatment is given or from postmortem tissue (LN, abscess, liver, spleen) is definitive (large numbers of gram-negative coccobacilli with bipolar staining); FA test of these clinical materials or tissues is a quick presumptive method to identify infected animals

GROSS AND HISTOPATHOLOGIC FINDINGS
• Gross findings—few lesions in acutely ill cats; enlarged LNs (buboes) on head and neck; enlarged liver and spleen • LN shows destruction of normal architecture, hemorrhagic necrosis, extracellular bacteria.

TREATMENT
• Early treatment important; high mortality if not treated early • Treat on inpatient basis; good supportive nursing care important • High zoonotic potential—all personnel in contact with animal must use mask, gloves, gowns to avoid infection of staff, especially in patients with respiratory form; isolate patients • Treat animals for fleas.

MEDICATIONS

DRUGS AND FLUIDS
• Treat all suspect cases empirically until laboratory confirmation is obtained.

• Systemic antimicrobials—use in all patients except those with lung involvement (those should be euthanized because of high zoonotic potential); can use any of these drugs: tetracyclines (oxytetracyclines, tetracycline, chlortetracycline)—75 mg/kg/day PO q8h for 10 days; parenteral—15 mg/kg/day divided q12h doxycycline effectiveness not established for plague treatment; chloramphenicol—100-150 mg/kg/day PO divided q8h

CONTRAINDICATIONS/POSSIBLE INTERACTIONS N/A

ALTERNATE DRUGS
Gentamicin, trimethoprim-sulfamethoxazole, and kanamycin can be used if the above drugs cannot be used.

FOLLOW-UP

PATIENT MONITORING
DIC common later in infection if primarily not treated early

PREVENTION/AVOIDANCE
• Limit pet travel to plague endemic areas. • In endemic areas, keep the pet on a leash to limit/control exposure to wild rodents and their fleas. • Periodic flea control (spray or dust) of animal and house in plague endemic area • Neuter cats to limit their hunting behavior and wild rodent exposure. • Eliminate rodents and their habitats near houses and outbuildings (e.g., wood piles, garbage, trash piles). • Store food in rodent-proof containers.

EXPECTED COURSE AND PROGNOSIS
Prognosis poor if not treated early

MISCELLANEOUS

ZOONOTIC POTENTIAL
High; must not be mistaken for bite abscesses or tularemia

ABBREVIATIONS
LN = lymph node
FDP = fibrin degradation products

Reference
Rollag OJ, Skeels MR, Nims LJ, Thilsted JP, Mann JM. Feline plague in New Mexico: report of five cases. J Am Vet Med Assoc 1981;179:1381-1383.

Author Patrick L. McDonough
Consulting Editor Fred W. Scott

PLASMA CELL GINGIVITIS AND PHARYNGITIS—CATS

BASICS

OVERVIEW
• Infiltration of plasma cells and lymphocytes is the typical response to bacterial or other antigenic stimulation. The term feline adult-onset gingivostomatitis is probably more accurate for identifying the subset of cats with the lesions described below. • Several distinct clinical entities have commonly been grouped together in the past because of their similar histologic appearance. Every attempt should be made to differentiate these subgroups because their response to treatment and prognosis vary considerably.

SIGNALMENT
• Adult cats, young to middle-age • No sex predilection • Purebred cats are at increased risk for some forms of the feline gingivostomatitis complex but this does not appear to be case for the adult-onset form described here. • Incidence may be declining.

SIGNS
• Halitosis • Ptyalism • Pain on opening the mouth • Dysphagia (may pick up food and then drop it) • Anorexia • Weight loss • Bright red proliferative and friable lesions affecting the gingiva, oral mucosa and/or fauces • Plaque and calculus accumulation • Missing teeth • Dental resorptive lesions

CAUSES AND RISK FACTORS
• Etiology unknown • Bacteria associated with plaque-induced periodontal disease probably contribute to the antigenic response. The fact that the lesions in many cats which are unrespsonsive to other treatments heal following extraction of the teeth indicates that the bacteria associated with periodontal disease play an important role in the pathogenesis. • FeLV-infected cats with impaired immune systems are predisposed to increased incidence or severity of oral inflammation. • Chronic oral disease is a common manifestation of persistent FIV infection. The severity of the oral lesions tend to worsen as the immunosuppression progresses. • Feline calicivirus (FCV) is commonly found in the oral fluids of affected cats but its role in this disease is controversial. Persistent FCV viremia in FeLV and FIV infected cats with impaired immune systems may result in more severe lesions. • Oral lesions are common consequences of deficiencies in local or systemic immune systems.

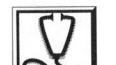

DIAGNOSIS

DIFFERENTIAL DIAGNOSIS
• Plaque induced gingivitis and periodontitis—lesions are typically not as severe or extensive, gingival recession and root exposure are common. • Pemphigus vulgaris—lesions at mucocutaneous junction and on the skin are common • Metabolic disease—renal and hepatic disease primarily

CBC/BIOCHEMISTRY/URINALYSIS
• CBC values vary widely • High globulin due to a polyclonal hypergammaglobulinemia is the most consistent abnormality.

OTHER LABORATORY TESTS
FeLV and FIV tests

IMAGING
Radiographic studies may show loss of teeth, periodontal bone loss, retained root fragments, or evidence of osteomyelitis.

OTHER DIAGNOSTIC PROCEDURES
Biopsies often show ulcerated, hyperplastic lesions with heavy infiltrations of plasma cells and lymphocytes.

TREATMENT

• No single treatment protocol is uniformly successful. Control of the oral flora by good oral hygiene and suppression of the inflammatory response are primary goals of treatment.
• The need for nutritional support should be anticipated in cats which are painful and anorexic.
• Owners should be cautioned that this is a frustrating problem to treat and may require drastic measures (i.e., complete dental extraction).
• Daily brushing or application of chlorhexidine solution or gel or an oral hygiene gel will help to control plaque and calculus accumulation.
• Thorough dental prophylaxis including supragingival and subgingival scaling, root planing and soft tissue debridement where indicated, followed by polishing and the application of topical fluoride.
• Teeth with dental resportive lesions should be restored or extracted. Extractions must be complete. All retained root tips should be removed.
• Refractory cases may benefit from extraction of the premolar and molar teeth. The canine teeth and incisors are also extracted if they are involved or if extraction of the premolars and molars does not resolve the inflammation. It is essential that the roots be removed entirely. Radiographic confirmation after extractions are completed is recommended.

MEDICATIONS

DRUGS AND FLUIDS

Antibiotics
• Typically cause temporary improvement with relapse when discontinued.

• Amoxicillin/clavulanate (12.5–25 mg/kg q12h PO) • Metronidazole (10 mg/kg q8 PO or 30mg/kg q24h PO)

Anti-inflammatory Drugs
• May be beneficial in immunocompetent patients who are responding to chronic bacterial and/or antigenic stimulation. Best response seen when combined with antibiotics.
• Glucocorticoids can be injected subgingivally (e.g., Triamcinolone—maximum 10 mg/cat) or given systemically (Prednisilone—1 mg/kg q12 PO for 2 weeks and then taper dose).

CONTRAINDICATIONS
Use of immunosuppressive agents in immunocompromised patients

PRECAUTIONS N/A

POSSIBLE INTERACTIONS N/A

ALTERNATE DRUGS
Aurothioglucose, azothiaprine, cyclophosphamide and cyclosporine have been used with variable success.

FOLLOW-UP

• The prognosis for complete resolution is guarded. Before undertaking extensive treatment the FeLV and FIV status should be established. • If good home care is probable, dental prophylaxis in conjunction with antibiotics and corticosteroids are a good initial approach. If improvement is seen but the inflamation persists another immunosuppressive agent such as aurothioglucose can be tried. • If home care is not possible or if the lesions severe, extraction should be considered early in the course of treatment.

MISCELLANEOUS

SYNONYMS
Feline lymphocytic-plasmacytic gingivitis, feline gingivostomatitis, feline adult-onset gingivostomatitis

ABBREVIATIONS
FeLV = feline leukemia virus
FIV = feline immunodeficiency virus
FCV = feline calicivirus

References
Pedersen NC. Inflammatory oral cavity diseases of the cat. Vet Clin N Amer Small Anim Pract 1992;22:13223–1345.
Author Eric R. Pope
Consulting Editor Brent D. Jones

PLASMACYTOMA, MUCOCUTANEOUS

 BASICS

OVERVIEW
• Tumor of plasma cell origin • Development is rapid. • May represent subtype of extramedullary plasmacytoma that is primary tumor of soft tissue origin or metastasis of primary osseous multiple myeloma

SIGNALMENT
• Most common in mixed-breed dogs and cocker spaniels • Both sexes affected equally • Mean and median age at diagnosis for dogs—9.7 and 10.5 years, respectively • Rare in cats

SIGNS
• Usually raised or ulcerated, solid nodule 0.25-6.0 cm in diameter • Plasmacytoma of the lips is typically small. • Usually solitary • Rarely polypoid • Common locations include mouth, feet, trunk, and ears • Occasionally occur with multiple myeloma or lymphosarcoma that develop together or at different times • Systemic signs rare

CAUSES AND RISK FACTORS
Unknown

 DIAGNOSIS

DIFFERENTIAL DIAGNOSIS
Biopsy distinguishes from other round cell tumors (e.g., lymphosarcoma, mast cell tumor, histiocytoma, and transmissible venereal tumor) and poorly differentiated, carcinoma, or amelanotic melanoma.

CBC/BIOCHEMISTRY/URINALYSIS
Results are usually normal unless patient has multiple myeloma or lymphosarcoma.

OTHER LABORATORY TESTS N/A

IMAGING N/A

OTHER DIAGNOSTIC PROCEDURES
• Cytologic examination of fine-needle aspirate reveals moderate to marked cellularity; individual tumor cells round to polyhedral with discrete margins and prominent anisocytosis and anisokaryosis; round to oval nuclei with fine to coarse chromatin and no visible nucleoli. Cytoplasm stains lightly basophilic. • Histologically, most tumors well-circumscribed and easily identifiable

 TREATMENT

• Tumors occasionally invasive, so aggressive surgical excision is recommended • Radiotherapy successful in some patients

 **MEDICATIONS**

DRUGS AND FLUIDS
Chemotherapy not recommended

CONTRAINDICATIONS/POSSIBLE INTERACTIONS N/A

 FOLLOW-UP

PATIENT MONITORING
Usually none unless accompanied by multiple myeloma or lymphosarcoma

EXPECTED COURSE AND PROGNOSIS
Excellent in most patients

 MISCELLANEOUS

ASSOCIATED CONDITIONS
• Multiple myeloma • Lymphosarcoma
• Some cats have systemic amyloidosis

Reference
Rakich PM, Latimer KS, Weiss R, Steffens WL. Mucocutaneous plasmacytomas in dogs. 75 cases (1980-1987). J Am Vet Med Assoc 1989;194:803-810.
Author Wallace B. Morrison
Consulting Editor Wallace B. Morrison

PLEURAL EFFUSION

BASICS

DEFINITION
Abnormal accumulation of fluid within the pleural cavity

PATHOPHYSIOLOGY
• More than normal production or less than normal resorption of fluid • Alterations in hydrostatic and oncotic pressures or vascular permeability and lymphatic function may contribute to fluid accumulation.

SYSTEMS AFFECTED
• Respiratory • Cardiovascular

SIGNALMENT N/A

SIGNS

General Comments
Clinical signs vary depending on the fluid volume, rapidity of fluid accumulation, and the underlying cause.

Historical Findings
• Dyspnea • Tachypnea • Orthopnea • Open-mouth breathing • Cyanosis • Exercise intolerance • Lethargy • Inappetence • Cough

Physical Exam Findings
• Dyspnea—respirations often shallow and rapid • Muffled or inaudible heart and lung sounds ventrally • Preservation of breath sounds dorsally • Dullness ventrally on thoracic percussion

CAUSES

High Hydrostatic Pressure
• Congestive heart failure (CHF) • Over-hydration • Neoplasia

Low Oncotic Pressure
Hypoalbuminemia—protein losing enteropathy, protein-losing nephropathy, and liver disease

Vascular or Lymphatic Abnormality
• Infectious (i.e., bacterial, viral, or fungal) • Neoplasia (e.g., mediastinal lymphosarcoma, thymoma, mesothelioma, primary lung, tumor, and metastatic disease) • Chylothorax (e.g., lymphangiectasia, CHF, cranial vena cava obstruction, neoplasia, fungal, heartworms, diaphragmatic hernia, lung lobe torsion, and trauma) • Diaphragmatic hernia • Hemothorax (e.g., trauma, neoplasia, and coagulopathy) • Lung lobe torsion • Pulmonary thromboembolism • Pancreatitis

RISK FACTORS N/A

DIAGNOSIS

DIFFERENTIAL DIAGNOSIS

Differentiating Similar Signs
Must differentiate from other causes of dyspnea including primary lung disease (e.g., pneumonia, neoplasia, and pulmonary fibrosis), pulmonary edema, and upper airway obstructions; thoracic auscultation and radiographs crucial in distinguishing these abnormalities

Differentiating Causes
• Historical or physical evidence of external trauma warrant consideration of hemothorax or diaphragmatic hernia. • Fever suggests an inflammatory, infectious, or neoplastic cause. • Murmurs, gallops, or arrhythmias combined with jugular venous distension or pulsation suggest an underlying cardiac cause. • Concurrent ascites suggests feline infectious peritonitis (FIP), CHF (mainly dogs), severe hypoalbuminemia, diaphragmatic hernia, disseminated neoplasia, or pancreatitis. • In cats, less than normal compressibility of the cranial thorax suggests a cranial mediastinal mass. • Concurrent ocular changes (e.g., chorioretinitis and uveitis) suggest FIP or fungal disease.

CBC/BIOCHEMISTRY/URINALYSIS
• Results of hemogram may be abnormal in animals with pyothorax, FIP, neoplasia, or lung lobe torsion. • Severe hypoalbuminemia (< approximately 1 g/dl to cause effusion) suggests protein-losing enteropathy, protein-losing nephropathy, or liver disease. • Hyperglobulinemia (polyclonal) suggests FIP.

OTHER LABORATORY TESTS
• Serologic tests for feline leukemia virus (if patient has mediastinal lymphosarcoma), feline immunodeficiency virus (if patient has pyothorax), and coronavirus (if patient has FIP) are available. • If cardiac disease is suspected, consider a heartworm test in dogs and cats and a thyroid and taurine evaluation in cats.

IMAGING

Radiographic Findings
• Used to confirm the presence of pleural effusion. • Should not be performed until after thoracocentesis in dyspneic patients with evidence of pleural effusion on physical examination. • Radiographic evidence of pleural effusion includes separation of lung borders away from the thoracic wall and sternum by fluid density in the pleural space, fluid-filled interlobar fissure lines, silhouette sign (i.e., loss or blurring of the cardiac and diaphragmatic borders), blunting of the lung margins at the costophrenic angles (ventrodorsal view), and widening of the mediastinum (ventrodorsal view). • Rounding of the caudal lung lobe borders (lateral view) most common in animals with fibrosing pleuritis caused by chylothorax, pyothorax, or FIP • Unilateral effusion most common in animals with chylothorax and pyothorax; hemothorax, pulmonary neoplasia, diaphragmatic hernias, and lung lobe torsion also causative • Evaluate post-thoracocentesis radiographs carefully for cardiomegaly, intrapulmonary lesions, mediastinal masses, diaphragmatic hernia, lung lobe torsion, and evidence of trauma (e.g., rib fractures). • Positive contrast peritoneography can be used to diagnose a diaphragmatic hernia.

• Thoracic duct can be evaluated by positive contrast lymphangiography.

Echocardiographic Findings
• Ultrasonographic evaluation of the thorax is recommended whenever cardiac disease, a diaphragmatic hernia, or cranial mediastinal mass is suspected. • Echocardiography is easiest to perform before thoracocentesis, provided the animal is stable.

Other Diagnostic Procedures
• Thoracocentesis allows characterization of the fluid type and determination of potential underlying cause. • Fluid analysis should include physical characteristics (i.e., color, clarity, odor, clots), total protein, total nucleated cell count, and cytologic examination. Table 1 provides characteristics of various pleural fluid types and their disease associations. • If infection suspected, perform a bacterial culture and sensitivity test and consider special stains (e.g., gram stain and acid-fast stain) of the fluid. • If FIP is suspected, consider protein electrophoresis of the fluid.
• If chyle is suspected, perform an ether clearance test or Sudan stain of the pleural fluid and triglyceride and cholesterol evaluations of the fluid and serum. • Exploratory thoracotomy may provide diagnostic biopsy specimens of lung, lymph nodes, or pleura.

TREATMENT
• Initial treatment is thoracocentesis to relieve respiratory distress.
• Preventing fluid reaccumulation requires treatment based on a definitive diagnosis.
• Most patients are hospitalized because they require intensive management such as indwelling chest tubes (e.g., patients with pyothorax) or thoracic surgery .
• Surgery is indicated for management of some neoplasias, diaphragmatic hernia repair, lymphangiectasia (i.e., thoracic duct ligation), foreign body removal, and lung lobectomy for lung lobe torsion.
• If the patient is stable after thoracocentesis, outpatient treatment may be possible for some diseases.

MEDICATIONS

DRUGS AND FLUIDS
• Treatment varies with specific disease
• Diuretics generally reserved for patients with diseases causing fluid retention and volume overload (e.g., CHF)

CONTRAINDICATIONS N/A

PRECAUTIONS
• Drugs that depress respirations or decrease blood pressure.

• Inappropriate use of diuretics predisposes the patient to dehydration and electrolyte disturbances without eliminating the effusion.

POSSIBLE INTERACTIONS N/A

ALTERNATE DRUGS N/A

FOLLOW-UP

PATIENT MONITORING

• Radiographic evaluation key to assessment of treatment in most patients.

POSSIBLE COMPLICATIONS

•Death due to respiratory compromise

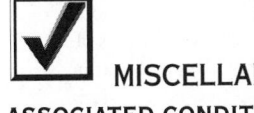

MISCELLANEOUS

ASSOCIATED CONDITIONS N/A

AGE RELATED FACTORS N/A

ZOONOTIC POTENTIAL N/A

PREGNANCY N/A

SYNONYMS

• Hydrothorax may be used for transudates and modified transudates. • Pyothorax = empyema = septic pleuritis

SEE ALSO

See causes

ABBREVIATIONS

CHF = congestive heart failure

FIP = feline infectious peritonitis

PMN = polymorphonuclear leukocytes or neutrophils

LSA = lymphosarcoma

References

Sherding RG. Disease of the pleural cavity. In: Sherding RG, ed. The cat: diseases and clinical management. 2nd ed. New York: Churchill & Livingstone, 1994:1053-1083.

Fossum TW. Pleural effusion. In: Birchard SJ, Sherding RG, eds. Saunders Manual of small animal practice. Philadelphia: WB Saunders, 1994;580-586.

Bauer T, Woodfield JA. Pleura and pleural space disorders. In: Ettinger SJ, Feldman EC, eds. Textbook of veterinary internal medicine. Vol 1, 4th ed. Philadelphia: WB Saunders, 1995;817-829.

Author Linda B. Lehmkuhl

Consulting Editor Larry P. Tilley and Francis W.K. Smith, Jr.

Table 1.

	Transudate	Modified Transudate	Nonseptic Exudate	Septic Exudate	Chyle	Hemorrhage
			Characterization of pleural fluid			
Color	Colorless to pale yellow	Yellow or pink	Yellow or pink	Yellow to red-brown	Milky white	Red
Turbidity	Clear	Clear to cloudy	Clear to cloudy; fibrin	Cloudy to opaque; fibrin	Opaque	Opaque
Protein (g/dl)	<1.5	2.5-5.0	3.0-8.0	3.0-7.0	2.5-6.0	>3.0
Nucleated cells/μl	<1,000	1,000-7,000 (LSA up to 100,000)	5,000-20,000 (LSA up to 100,000)	5,000-300,000	1,000-20,000	Similar to peripheral blood
Cytology	Mostly mesothelial cells	Mostly macrophages and mesothelial cells; few nondegenerate PMN; neoplastic cells in some cases	Mostly nondegenerate PMN and macrophages; neoplastic cells in some cases	Mostly degenerate PMN, also macrophages; bacteria	Small lymphocytes, PMN, and macrophages	Mostly RBC; macrophages with erythrophagocytosis
Disease associations	Hypoalbuminemia (protein-losing nephropathy, protein losing enteropathy, or liver disease); early CHF	CHF; neoplasia; diaphragmatic hernia pancreatitis	FIP; neoplasia; diaphragmatic hernia; lung lobe torsion	Pyothorax	Lymphangiectasia, CHF, cranial vena cava obstruction neoplasia, fungal, dirofilariasias, diaphragmatic hernia, lung lobe torsion, trauma	Trauma, coagulopathy, neoplasia, lung lobe torsion

Modified from Sherding RG. Diseases of the pleural cavity. In: Sherding RG, ed. The cat: diseases and clinical management. 2nd ed. New York: Churchill Livingstone, 1994;1061.

PNEUMOCYSTOSIS

 BASICS

OVERVIEW
• Pneumocystis carinii is a saprophytic inhabitant of the mammalian respiratory tract. The life cycle is completed in the alveolar spaces. It is classified by many as a protozoan but also exhibits properties of a fungus. • Clinical infections have been reported in dogs, but all reported infections in cats have been subclinical. Infections are usually confined to the respiratory tract, but a case of disseminated disease has been reported in the dog. • Transmission is from infected to susceptible animal within a species. Strain differences may account for the difficulty observed in interspecies transmission. • Any animal with documented pneumocystosis should have additional workup in an attempt to identify an underlying cause of immunosuppresssion.

SIGNALMENT
• Dogs. No clinical infections reported in cats. • Majority of reported cases have been in the dachshund breed at less than 6 months of age. These cases were suspected as having a congenital immunodeficiency. Clinical disease has also been reported in the shetland sheepdog. • Those with a predilection for impaired immunity would seem to carry an increased risk for overgrowth of the organism (e.g., the very young or very old patient).

SIGNS

Historical Findings
• Gradual weight loss (despite good appetite) and respiratory difficulty progressing over 1-4 weeks • Exercise intolerance often a primary complaint • Coughing may be seen • Vomiting and diarrhea also occasionally noted

Physical Examination Findings
• Dyspnea • Tachycardia • Marked dry respiratory sounds on thoracic auscultation • Poor condition • Cachexia • Cyanosis if infection is severe • Slight fever may be noted

CAUSES AND RISK FACTORS
• Immunodeficiency increases risk of infection. • Concurrent pulmonary disease increases risk of infection. • Stress, crowding, and immunossuppressive therapy have all been associated with outbreaks in humans and these factors may play a role in the activation of infection in cases in dogs as well.

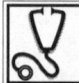 **DIAGNOSIS**

DIFFERENTIAL DIAGNOSIS
• Infectious tracheobronchitis • Bacterial and mycotic pneumonitis • Heart failure

CBC/BIOCHEMISTRY/URINALYSIS
• Changes are usually nonspecific. • Leukocytosis with neutrophilia and a left shift may be seen. • Eosinophilia and monocytosis may be seen. • Erythrocytosis may be seen secondary to chronic hypoxemia.

OTHER LABORATORY TESTS
• Arterial blood gases may reveal impaired gas exchange with hypoxemia, hypocapnia, and an increase in blood pH. • Antigens to P.carinii may be detected in sputum by ELISA or FA tests. • Serologic tests have been developed for human serum but are of uncertain value in canine patients.

IMAGING
• Thoracic radiograph findings may show a mixed alveolar and interstital lung pattern. Cor pulmonale may result in tracheal elevation, right-sided heart enlargement, and pulmonary arterial enlargement. • Other thoracic radiograph findings may include solitary lesions, unilateral changes, cavitary lesions, pneumothorax, or a lobar infiltrate.

OTHER DIAGNOSTIC PROCEDURES
• Pulse oximetry may reveal low arterial oxygen saturation.• Transtracheal aspiration, gastric contents, bronchoalveolar lavage, and oropharyngeal secretions may all reveal the organism. • Lung aspirate or lung biopsy are the most reliable diagnostic procedures, but also carry the greatest risk for complications. Impression smears may be made before tissue fixation.

GROSS AND HISTOPATHOLOGIC FINDINGS
• Lungs appear firm, consolidated, and pale brown or gray on gross inspection. Fluid is not expressed from cut lung surfaces and the lungs do not collapse when the chest cavity is opened. Small amounts of pleural fluid may be noted. Some degree of right heart enlargement may be found. • Histopathology reveals the alveolar spaces to be filled with amorphous, foamy, eosinophilic material. The material is described as having a honeycombed appearance. Macrophages but few neutrophils are typically seen. Alveolar septa may be thickened and fibrosed. Trophozoites and cyst stages may be identified.

 TREATMENT

• Supportive care, including supplemental oxygen in hypoxemic patients, is essential. • Because of frequency of underlying immunocompromise, isolation from other patients is advised. • Ventilatory support may be needed in severe cases. • Nebulization may provide some additional therapeutic benefits. • Activity restriction is advised.

MEDICATIONS

DRUGS AND FLUIDS
• Trimethoprim-sulfonamide 15mg/kg PO q6h × 2 weeks
• Pentamidine isethionate 4mg/kg IM q24h × 2 weeks
• Carbutamide 50mg/kg IM q12h × 3 weeks

CONTRAINDICATIONS/POSSIBLE INTERACTIONS
• Major side effects of pentamidine isethionate include impaired renal function, hepatic dysfunction, hypoglycemia, hypotension, hypocalcemia, urticaria, and hematologic disorders.
• Localized pain at the injection site has been noted.

FOLLOW-UP

PATIENT MONITORING
• Serial blood gases and thoracic radiographs are likely to provide valuable prognostic information and can be used to monitor response to therapy. • BUN and glucose should be checked daily if treatment with pentamidine isethionate is used. Treatment should be discontinued or dosage decreased if azotemia or other complications are noted. • Clinical course is variable. Monitor for resolution of the cough and dyspnea after treatment is initiated.

MISCELLANEOUS

ZOONOTIC POTENTIAL
There is little or no zoonotic potential.

Reference

Greene CE, Chandler FW. Pneumocystosis. In: Greene CE, ed. Infectious diseases of the dog and cat. Philadelphia: WB Saunders, 1990:854-861.

Author Matthew S. Mellema
Consulting Editor Fred W. Scott

PNEUMONIA, ALLERGIC—DOGS

BASICS

DEFINITION
The fully developed inflammatory response to antigens in lung parenchyma characterized by exudation of cells and fluid into lung interstitium, conducting airways, and alveolar spaces

Pathophysiology
• Although the evidence that hypersensitivity or allergic pneumonitis is an immunologic disorder is generally accepted, the immunologic mechanisms involved in the pathogenesis of the disease have not been clarified. • It is likely that characteristics of antigens, the host response, and the regulation of that response to the antigen determine the evolution of the disease. • Three disease patterns exist: eosinophilic pneumonitis, allergic bronchitis, and pulmonary eosinophilic granulomatosis.
• Antigens enter the lower respiratory tract primarily by the inhalation route and less commonly by the hematogenous route.
• Chronic exposure to antigens elicits a humoral and cellular immune response, and allergic or hypersensitivity pulmonary disorders are associated with an abnormal humoral antibody response, as well as a cell-mediated immunoregulatory defect. • IgE, IgG, and other immunoglobulin classes are involved. • Cell-mediated immunity is also altered with numbers of activated macrophages, T-lymphocytes, and depressed suppressor T-cell activity. • Inflammatory infiltration of lung interstitium and alveolar spaces occurs • In severe cases, marked granulomatous disease occurs. • In occult heartworm disease with pneumonitis, microfilaria become entrapped in the pulmonary circulation. • Another clinical variation is allergic bronchial disease in response to infection or colonization of the airways with a fungal organism, usually Aspergillus spp. • Mortality is associated with severe hypoxemia (low arterial oxygen concentration) and, rarely, severe hemoptysis.

Systems Affected
• Respiratory • Cardiovascular—cor pulmonale may develop

Genetics N/A

Incidence/Prevalence N/A

Geographic Distribution
Widespread

SIGNALMENT

Species Dog

Breed Predilection
None

Mean Age and Range
All ages can be affected.

Predominant Sex
No gender predilection

SIGNS
• Clinical signs are extremely variable, depending upon the severity of the disease.
• Cough (nonresponsive to antibacterial therapy) • Fever • Dyspnea • Abnormal breath sounds on auscultation • Increased intensity of bronchial breath sounds • Crackles
• Exercise intolerance • Anorexia • Lethargy
• Weight loss • Peripheral lymphadenopathy

CAUSES
• Aeroallergens (spores or hyphae from fungi and actinomycetes, pollen, insect antigens, etc.)
• Parasitic antigens (heartworm microfilaria)

RISK FACTORS
• Living in an endemic heartworm area without administering heartworm preventive medication • Living in a dusty or moldy environment

DIAGNOSIS

DIFFERENTIAL DIAGNOSIS
• Bacterial pneumonia • Viral pneumonia (canine distemper virus, canine adenovirus)
• Rickettsial pneumonia (ehrlichiosis, Rocky Mountain spotted fever) • Protozoal pneumonia (toxoplasmosis) • Parasitic pneumonia (capillariasis, paragonimiasis, dirofilariasis)
• Fungal pneumonia (histoplasmosis, blastomycosis, coccidioidomycosis, cryptococcosis)
• Infectious tracheobronchitis • Pulmonary abscess • Pleural infection (pyothorax)
• Bronchial foreign body • Chronic bronchitis • Congestive heart failure

CBC/BIOCHEMISTRY/URINALYSIS
• Complete blood count—inflammatory leukogram (neutrophilic leukocytosis with or without a left shift, eosinophilia, basophilia, or monocytosis) • Serum biochemical profile—hyperglobulinemia is suggestive of occult dirofilariasis

OTHER LABORATORY TESTS
• Arterial blood gas determination—arterial blood gas values correlate well with the degree of physiologic disruption and are a sensitive monitor of a patient's progress during treatment; $PaO_2 < 80$ torr on room air is mild to moderate hypoxemia; $PaO_2 < 60$ torr on room air is severe hypoxemia • Heartworm microfilaria and antigen tests—positive test suggests that clinical signs are a result of pulmonary hypertension associated with dirofilariasis or eosinophilic pneumonitis associated with microfilaria trapped in the lung is complicating the clinical condition. Thoracic radiographs will help document the severity of pulmonary hypertension and the presence or absence of interstitial pneumonitis. • Protein electrophoresis—a spike of beta globulin (hyperbetaglobulinemia) typically is found in patients with occult dirofilariasis

IMAGING
Radiography
• Variable findings depending on extent and severity of disease. • Eosinophilic pneumonitis—linear or miliary interstitial pattern that resembles changes seen with early pulmonary edema or fungal pneumonia. An alveolar pattern characterized by increased pulmonary densities with indistinct margins is only seen in severe cases. Dogs with dirofilariasis will show tortuous, enlarged pulmonary arteries and right-sided cardiomegaly. • Allergic or eosinophilic bronchitis—bronchial pattern with bronchi extending into the periphery of the lung (tram/railroad track and donut signs) • Eosinophilic granuloma—multiple nodular lesions of variable sizes in different lung lobes along with patchy, focal alveolar densities and tracheobronchial lymphadenopathy

OTHER DIAGNOSTIC PROCEDURES
• The definitive method of establishing a diagnosis is to obtain aspirates, washings, or brushings for cytologic examinations.
• Transtracheal washing • Bronchoscopy
• Bronchoalveolar lavage (with or without bronchoscope) • Fine-needle lung aspiration
• Intradermal skin testing may identify allergens in some patients • Fecal—negative routine flotation, direct smear, sediment examination, and Baermann's technique make respiratory parasitic infection less likely

GROSS AND HISTOPATHOLOGIC FINDINGS
Gross Findings
Diffuse, patchy, or nodular firm lesions, usually pale or mottled

Histopathologic Findings
• Eosinophilic, lymphocytic, and macrophage infiltration of alveolar walls and alveolar spaces
• As the disease progresses, the interstitial infiltrative process becomes fibrotic with obliteration of alveolar spaces; granulomas may be dispersed within the interstitial fibrosis.

TREATMENT

INPATIENT VERSUS OUTPATIENT
Treatment in the hospital is recommended if the patient is showing multisytemic signs such as anorexia, weight loss, or lethargy.

ACTIVITY
Restricted during treatment at home or in the hospital

DIET
Ensure normal intake.

CLIENT EDUCATION
Morbidity and mortality are associated with severe hypoxemia.

SURGICAL CONSIDERATIONS
Lung lobes with large granulomas can be removed.

MEDICATIONS

DRUGS AND FLUIDS
• Dehydration hinders mucociliary clearance and secretion mobilization.
• Maintenance of normal systemic hydration is an important therapeutic objective; use a balanced multielectrolyte solution.
• Heartworm adulticidal therapy should be initiated after the patient has been stabilized with corticosteroids and rest.
• Corticosteroids (prednisolone or prednisone 2-4 mg/kg/day until clinical signs begin to resolve and then dosage can be tapered)
• Intraconazole or ketaconazole can be used in patients with confirmed allergic bronchopulmonary fungal infection. This is a rare condition and antifungal drugs should only be used if the fungal infection is confirmed by cytologic examination or culture.

CONTRAINDICATIONS N/A

PRECAUTIONS N/A

POSSIBLE INTERACTIONS N/A

ALTERNATE DRUGS
Other immunosuppressive drugs such as cyclophosphamide, azothiaprine, mercaptopurine, etc. can be used in patients in which corticosteroids are contraindicated or have been ineffective.

FOLLOW-UP

PATIENT MONITORING
• Arterial blood gases are the most sensitive monitor of the patient's progress. • Auscultate patient thoroughly several times daily. • Thoracic radiographs will improve more slowly than the clinical appearance of the patient; they should not be used to routinely monitor progress unless the patient's condition deteriorates.

PREVENTION/AVOIDANCE
• Routine heartworm preventive medication
• Change dog's environment if an aeroallergen is suspected.

POSSIBLE COMPLICATIONS
Pulmonary thromboembolism in dogs treated with adulticides for dirofilariasis

EXPECTED COURSE AND PROGNOSIS
• Good prognosis if primary allergen is identified and eliminated. • If allergen is not identified, prognosis for control is good, though many dogs require long-term steroid therapy.
• Prognosis in heartworm infected dogs depends on severity of pulmonary hypertension, cor pulmonale, and thromboembolism.
• Prognosis in dogs with eosinophilic granulomatosis is guarded because many have progressive disease.

MISCELLANEOUS

ASSOCIATED CONDITIONS
Dirofilariasis, bronchopulmonary fungal infection

AGE RELATED FACTORS N/A

ZOONOTIC POTENTIAL N/A

PREGNANCY
The use of corticosteroids and other immunosuppressive drugs is contraindicated in pregnant animals.

SYNONYMS
• Allergic bronchitis • Chronic eosinophilic bronchitis • Bronchitic pulmonary eosinophilia • Allergic bronchopulmonary aspergillosis • Allergic alveolitis • Eosinophilic pneumonitis • Eosinophilic pneumonia • Hypersensitivity pneumonitis • Eosinophilic pulmonary granulomatosis • Extrinsic allergic alveolitis • Occult heartworm pneumonitis • Parasitic pulmonary eosinophilia • Pulmonary infiltrates with eosinophilia

SEE ALSO
• Cough • Dyspnea • Heartworm Disease • Respiratory Parasites • Lymphomatoid Granulomatosis

ABBREVIATIONS N/A
PaO$_2$ = arterial oxygen

References

Kuehn NF, Roudebush P. Allergic lung disease. In: Allen DG, ed. Small animal medicine. Philadelphia: JB Lippincott, 1991:423-432.

Bauer T. Pulmonary hypersensitivity disorders. In: Kirk RW, ed. Current veterinary therapy X. Philadelphia: WB Saunders, 1989:369-376.

Calvert CA. Eosinophilic pulmonary granulomatosis. In: Kirk RW, Bonagura JD, eds. Current veterinary therapy XI. Philadelphia: WB Saunders, 1992:813-816.

Calvert CA, Rawlings CA. Pulmonary manifestations of heartworm disease. Vet Clin N Am 1985;15:991-1009.

Hawkins EC. Tracheal wash and bronchoalveolar lavage in the management of respiratory disease. In: Kirk RW, Bonagura JD, eds. Current veterinary therapy XI. Philadelphia: WB Saunders, 1992:795-800.

Author Philip Roudebush
Consulting Editors Lynelle Johnson and Bradley L. Moses

PNEUMONIA, BACTERIAL

BASICS

DEFINITION
The fully developed inflammatory response to virulent bacteria in lung parenchyma characterized by exudation of cells and fluids into conducting airways and alveolar spaces

Pathophysiology
• Bacteria enter the lower respiratory tract primarily by the inhalation or aspiration routes and less commonly by the hematogenous route. • The normal tracheobronchial tree and lung are not continuously sterile. • Oropharyngeal bacteria frequently are aspirated and may be present for an unknown interval in the normal tracheobronchial tree and lung. • This microbial population has the potential to cause or complicate respiratory infection and clouds interpretation of airway and lung cultures. • Whether a respiratory infection will develop depends on the complex interplay of many factors, including size, inoculation site, virulence of the organism, and resistance of the host. • Respiratory virus infections alter bacterial colonization patterns, increase bacterial adherence to respiratory epithelium, and reduce mucociliary clearance and phagocytosis. This impairment of host defenses by the virus may allow resident bacteria to invade the lower respiratory tract. • Bacterial invasion of the lung incites an overt inflammatory reaction. • Exudative phase—inflammatory hyperemia and serous exudation of high protein fluid into interstitial and alveolar spaces • Leukocytic emigration phase—leukocytes infiltrate the airways and alveoli, resulting in consolidation, ischemia, tissue necrosis, and atelectasis as a consequence of bronchial occulusion, obstructive bronchiolitis, and impaired collateral ventilation • Mortality is associated with severe hypoxemia (low arterial oxygen concentration) and/or sepsis.

Systems Affected
Respiratory—primary or secondary infection

Incidence/Prevalence
Data not available

Geographic Distribution Widespread

SIGNALMENT

Species
More common in dogs than cats

Breed Predilection
Dogs—sporting dogs, hounds, working dogs, and mixed-breed dogs over 12 kg body weight

Mean Age and Range
Dogs—range 2 months to 15 years old; 45% less than 1 year old

Predominant Sex
Dogs—60% males

SIGNS
• Cough • Fever • Dyspnea • Abnormal breath sounds on auscultation—increased intensity or bronchial breath sounds; crackles; wheezes • Serous or mucopurulent nasal discharge • Anorexia • Lethargy • Weight loss • Exercise intolerance • Dehydration

CAUSES

Dogs
• Bordetella bronchiseptica and Streptococcus zooepidemicus are primary bacterial pathogens; most isolates in dogs with pneumonia are thought to be opportunisitic invaders. • A single bacterial pathogen is isolated in most patients but mixed infections are also common. • Gram-negative isolates predominate in both single and mixed infections. • Most common isolates from dogs with suspected bacterial pneumonia

Organism	% of Dogs
Bordetella bronchiseptica	7-22
Escherichia coli	17-29
Klebsiella	10-15
Pseudomonas	6-34
Staphylococcus	9-20
Streptococcus	15-27
Other	17-35

• Anaerobic bacteria are found in pulmonary abscesses and aspiration pneumonia. • Number of bacterial isolates per positive sample from dogs with suspected bacterial pneumonia

Number of bacteria	% of Dogs
1	58-60
2	22-23
3	11-16
> 4	2-7

Cats
Bacterial pathogens are poorly documented; Bordetella bronchiseptica and Pasteurella spp. are reported most frequently.

RISK FACTORS
• Preexisting viral, mycoplasmal, or fungal respiratory infection • Regurgitation, dysphagia, or vomiting • Reduced levels of consciousness (stupor, coma, anesthesia) • Thoracic trauma or surgery • Therapy with certain drugs (aspirin, digoxin) • Immunosuppressive therapy (anticancer chemotherapy, glucocorticoids) • Severe metabolic disorders (uremia, diabetes mellitus, hyperadrenocorticism) • Functional or anatomic disorders (tracheal hypoplasia, primary ciliary dyskinesia, cleft palate) • Intravenous catheter placement • Protein-calorie malnutrition

Immunodeficiency
• Phagocyte dysfunction (feline leukemia virus infection, diabetes mellitus) • Complement deficiency (rare) • Selective IgA deficiency • Combined T-cell and B-cell dysfunction (rare)

DIAGNOSIS

DIFFERENTIAL DIAGNOSIS
• Viral pneumonia (canine distemper virus, canine adenovirus, feline calicivirus) • Rickettsial pneumonia (ehrlichiosis, Rocky Mountain spotted fever) • Protozoal pneumonia (toxoplasmosis) • Parasitic pneumonia (capillariasis, paragonimiasis, aelurostrongylosis, dirofilariasis) • Fungal pneumonia (histoplasmosis, blastomycosis, coccidioidomycosis, cryptococcosis) • Bacterial or fungal rhinitis • Chronic sinusitis • Pharyngitis • Tonsillitis • Infectious tracheobronchitis • Pulmonary abscess • Pleural infection (pyothorax) • Bronchial foreign body

CBC/BIOCHEMISTRY/URINALYSIS
Complete blood count—inflammatory leukogram (neutrophilic leukocytosis with or without a left shift)

OTHER LABORATORY TESTS
• Arterial blood gas determination—arterial blood gas values correlate well with the degree of physiologic disruption and are a sensitive monitor of a patient's progress during treatment; $PaO_2 < 80$ torr on room air is mild to moderate hypoxemia; $PaO_2 < 60$ torr on room air is severe hypoxemia • Blood culture—may be helpful in identifying etiologic agent

IMAGING
• Thoracic radiographs—alveolar pattern characterized by increased pulmonary densities in which margins are indistinct and in which air bronchograms or lobar consolidation are seen. A patchy or lobar alveolar pattern may be present in a cranial ventral lung lobe distribution.

OTHER DIAGNOSTIC PROCEDURES
• The definitive method of establishing a diagnosis is to obtain aspirates, washings, or brushings for microbiologic and cytologic examinations. • Transtracheal washing • Bronchoscopy • Bronchoalveolar lavage (with or without bronchoscope) • Fine-needle lung aspiration • Fecal—negative routine flotation, direct smear, sediment examination, and Baermann's technique make respiratory parasitic infection less likely

GROSS AND HISTOPATHOLOGIC FINDINGS

Gross Findings
• Irregular consolidation in cranioventral regions • Consolidated lung varies from dark red to gray-pink to more gray, depending on the age and nature of the process. • Palpable firmness of the tissue is the single most important gross criterion.

Histopathologic Findings
• Nidus of inflammation is bronchiolar-alveolar junction • Early—bronchioles and adjacent alveoli are filled with neutrophils and an

admixture of cell debris, mucus, fibrin, and macrophages; necrotic to hyperplastic epithelium • Later—neutrophilic, fibrinous, hemorrhagic, or necrotizing inflammation, depending on virulence of bacteria and host response

TREATMENT

INPATIENT VERSUS OUTPATIENT
Treatment in the hospital is recommended if the patient is showing multisytemic signs such as anorexia, high fever, weight loss, or lethargy.

ACTIVITY
Restricted during treatment at home or in the hospital except as part of physiotherapy after aerosolization

DIET
Ensure normal intake with a diet high in protein and energy density; enteral or parenteral nutritional support is indicated in severely ill patients.

CLIENT EDUCATION
Morbidity and mortality are associated with severe hypoxemia and sepsis.

SURGICAL CONSIDERATIONS
Surgery (lung lobectomy) may be indicated in cases of pulmonary abscessation, bronchopulmonary foreign bodies with secondary pneumonia, or animals in which pneumonia unresponsive to conventional therapy is limited to one or two lung lobes.

MEDICATIONS

DRUGS AND FLUIDS
• Oral and parenteral antimicrobials are the principal therapy. • It is unrealistic to expect any single antibacterial to be routinely effective against the wide variety of organisms that cause bacterial pneumonia. • Initial choices of antibacterials can be based on the shape of bacteria noted on airway or lung cytologic preparations. • Substantially more patients recover if antibacterial therapy is administered according to culture results and in vitro susceptibility testing than if empirically administered. • Dehydration hinders mucociliary clearance and secretion mobilization.
• Maintenance of normal systemic hydration is an important therapeutic objective; use a balanced multielectrolyte solution.
• Nebulization with bland aerosols results in more rapid resolution of canine pneumonia if used in conjunction with physiotherapy and antibacterials. • Physiotherapy (mild forced exercise, chest wall coupage, tracheal manipulation to stimulate mild cough, postural drainage) should always be used immediately after aerosolization to enhance secretion clearance.

Antimicrobial Therapy
• Gram-positive cocci—ampicillin, amoxicillin, chloramphenicol, gentamicin, trimethoprim-sulfa, first-generation cephalosporin • Gram-negative rods—amikacin, chloramphenicol, gentamicin, trimethoprim-sulfa, fluroquinolones
• Bordetella—amikacin, chloramphenicol, tetracycline, gentamicin, kanamycin
• Anaerobes—ampicillin, amoxicillin, penicillin, clindamycin, second- or third-generation cephalosporins

CONTRAINDICATIONS
Anticholinergics and antihistamines may thicken secretions and, thus, inhibit mucokinesis and exudate removal from airways.

PRECAUTIONS
Antitussives should be used with caution and only for short intervals to control intractable cough. Use of potent, centrally-acting antitussives may inhibit mucokinesis and exudate removal from airways.

POSSIBLE INTERACTIONS   N/A

ALTERNATE DRUGS
Expectorants are recommended by some clinicians; however, there is no objective evidence that expectorants actually increase mucokinesis or mobilization of secretions.

FOLLOW-UP

PATIENT MONITORING
• Arterial blood gases are the most sensitive monitor of the patient's progress. • Auscultate the patient thoroughly several times daily.
• Thoracic radiographs will improve more slowly than the clinical appearance of the patient; they should not be used routinely to monitor progress unless the patient's condition deteriorates.

PREVENTION/AVOIDANCE
• Vaccination against upper respiratory viruses
• Vaccination against B. bronchiseptica if a dog is boarded or exposed to large numbers of other animals

POSSIBLE COMPLICATIONS
Young dogs infected with Bordetella bronchiseptica may develop chronic bronchitis.

EXPECTED COURSE AND PROGNOSIS
• Good prognosis if aggressive antibacterial and supportive therapy are initiated
• Prognosis is more guarded in young animals, those with immunodeficiency, and those that are debilitated or have severe underlying disease.

MISCELLANEOUS

ASSOCIATED CONDITIONS
• Bacterial pneumonia frequently occurs secondary to underlying metabolic diseases such as hyperadrenocorticism, diabetes mellitus, and uremia. • Bacterial pneumonia frequently occurs secondary to underlying functional or anatomic abnormalities such as cleft palate, tracheal hypoplasia, and primary ciliary dyskinesia.

AGE RELATED FACTORS
• Young animals may have a poorer prognosis and puppies often develop long-term complications such as chronic bronchitis. • Underlying functional and anatomic problems and immunodeficiencies should be suspected in young animals with pneumonia.

ZOONOTIC POTENTIAL   N/A
PREGNANCY
Bitches infected with Bordetella bronchiseptica may transmit the infection to puppies after they are born.

SYNONYMS N/A

SEE ALSO
See causes.

ABBREVIATIONS
PaO$_2$ = arterial oxygen

References
Roudebush P. Bacterial infections of the respiratory system. In: Greene CE, ed. Infectious diseases of the dog and cat. Philadelphia: WB Saunders, 1990:114-124.
Roudebush P. Infectious pneumonia. In: Kirk RW, Bonagura JD, eds. Current veterinary therapy XI. Philadelphia: WB Saunders, 1992:228-236.
Hawkins EC. Tracheal wash and bronchoalveolar lavage in the management of respiratory disease. In: Kirk RW, Bonagura JD, eds. Current veterinary therapy XI. Philadelphia: WB Saunders, 1992:795-800.
Author Philip Roudebush
Consulting Editors Lynelle Johnson and Bradley L. Moses

PNEUMONIA, FUNGAL

BASICS

DEFINITION
Inflammation of the pulmonary interstitial, lymphatic, and peribronchial tissues caused by deep mycotic infection

Pathophysiology
Mycelial fungal elements of dimorphic fungi are inhaled from contaminated soil. The organisms then colonize the lungs. At body temperature, the fungus grows in the yeast phase, and systemic dissemination often occurs. Clinical signs are determined by which organ systems are affected. Pulmonary interstitial involvement can cause in hypoxia while airway involvement may cause coughing. Cell-mediated immunity is important in response to infection. The normal response is characterized by pyogranulomatous inflammation.

Systems Affected
• Systemic mycoses affect multiple organ systems. The scope of this chapter is limited to respiratory involvement. • Blastomycosis—about 85% of dogs and cats have respiratory involvement. Diffuse interstitial or bronchial pneumonia is most common but solitary mass lesions may be seen. Tracheobronchial lymphadenopathy may contribute to cough. Nasal infection occasionally is seen. • Histoplasmosis—diffuse interstitial pneumonia is encountered, especially in cats. Perihilar or mediastinal lymphadenopathy often contributes to cough. • Coccidioidomycosis—diffuse interstitial or bronchial pneumonia is common. Perihilar or mediastinal lymphadenopathy is seen in most. • Cryptococcosis—nasal involvement is most common in cats. The lungs usually are subclinically affected by small, multifocal granulomas in dogs. • Aspergillosis—nasal disease is most common. Pneumonia is only seen in systemically affected animals.

Genetics
May be related to defects of cell-mediated immunity

Incidence/Prevalence
Dependent on geographic distribution

Geographic Distribution
• Blastomycosis—endemic in the southeastern and midwestern United States along the Mississippi, Ohio, Missouri, and Tennessee rivers and southern Great Lakes as well as the southern Midatlantic states • Histoplasmosis—similar to blastomycosis but more widely distributed. Pockets of disease in Texas, Oklahoma, and California. • Coccidioidomycosis—southwestern United States from Texas to California • Cryptococcosis and aspergillosis—seen sporadically throughout the United States

SIGNALMENT

Species
Dogs and cats (less common in cats except for cryptococcosis)

Breed Predilection
• Systemic mycoses—large-breed dogs kept outdoors or used for hunting or field trials. Doberman pinschers and rottweilers may be predisposed to more severe disseminated disease. • Cryptococcosis—cocker spaniels overrepresented • Systemic aspergillosis—German shepherds overrepresented

Mean Age and Range
Younger animals (< 4 years) are predisposed but any age may be affected.

Predominant Sex
Males are affected two to four times more often than females.

SIGNS

General Comments
Multisystemic illness is noted with the signs and symptoms, depending on the organ systems involved.

Historical Findings
• Chronic weight loss, inappetence, fever, and oculonasal discharge • Coughing may be a prominent sign but is inconsistently seen even in patients with marked pulmonary disease. • Dyspnea or exercise intolerance often is noted. Labored breathing is more common in cats. • Acute blindness or blepharospasm may be noted if the eyes are affected. • Cutaneous nodules usually are not noted until draining tracts appear. • Lameness is noted if the feet are affected or if osteomyelitis occurs.

Physical Examination Findings
• Depression and emaciation may be seen in chronic cases and fever is noted in about 50% of affected animals. • Dogs and cats with fungal pneumonia usually will have harsh, loud, breath sounds on auscultation. Crackles may be prominent, especially in cats. A cough may be induced on tracheal palpation. Severely affected dogs and cats will be dyspneic at rest. • Physical examination findings referable to other systems depend on the systems affected. Multiple subcutaneous nodules with draining tracts; uveitis and granulomatous retinal detachment are common in dogs and cats with blastomycosis. Severe pain caused by osteomyelitis is common in dogs with coccidioidomycosis. Emaciation and diarrhea (often bloody) is a prominent finding in dogs with histoplasmosis.

CAUSES
• Blastomyces dermatitidis—the lungs are the primary route of infection
• Histoplasma capsulatum—the lungs and, possibly, GI tract are the primary routes of infection • Coccidioides immitis—the lungs are the primary route of infection • Cryptococcus neoformans—the nasal cavity is the primary route of infection with direct extension into the eyes or CNS

RISK FACTORS
• Exposure to soils rich in organic matter, bird droppings, or other fecal matter may predispose the animal to blastomycosis, histo-

plasmosis, and cryptococcosis. • Coccidioidomycosis—environmental exposure to sandy, alkaline soil after periods of rainfall.
• Immunosuppression (especially poor cell-mediated immunity) may contribute to systemic spread of fungal infection. In cats, FeLV and FIV should be ruled out.
• Prednisone administration may significantly worsen the disease. • Antineoplastic chemotherapy; lymphoreticular neoplasia; or other infection such as ehrlichiosis

DIAGNOSIS

DIFFERENTIAL DIAGNOSIS
• Fungal pneumonias must be differentiated from other infectious, neoplastic, and immune-mediated multisystemic disease:
• Parasitic pneumonia or bacterial pneumonia
• Chronic bronchial disease/asthma in cats
• Metastatic neoplasia or lymphoreticular and histiocytic neoplasia • Eosinophilic lung disease • Lymphomatoid granulomatosis
• Idiopathic pyogranulomatous disease • FIP or other vasculitic disease • Pulmonary edema

CBC/BIOCHEMISTRY/URINALYSIS
• CBC—moderate leukocytosis with or without a left shift. Lymphopenia is common. Leukopenia may be seen with histoplasmosis. Thrombocytopenia and nonregenerative anemia are common. • Serum chemistry panel—hyperglobulinemia and hypoalbuminemia are common. Hypercalcemia may be seen in some affected dogs and cats. Liver enzymes are more likely to be high in patients with with histoplasmosis. • Urinalysis is usually normal. Proteinuria may be seen. Organisms may be seen (rarely) if the kidneys or lower urinary tract is affected.

OTHER LABORATORY TESTS
• Serologic testing—both false-positive and false-negative tests may be seen. A high incidence of seropositivity may represent previous or subclinical infection in endemic areas.
• A latex agglutination test for capsular antigen is a highly reliable test for cryptococcosis.
• Blood gases are useful for documenting the extent of respiratory dysfunction, and for following progression of disease or response to therapy.

IMAGING
• Radiography—diffuse, nodular, interstitial and peribronchial infiltrates. Nodular densities may coalesce to granulomatous masses with indistinct edges. Tracheobronchial lymphadenopathy is common. • Appendicular and/or axial skeleton—osteolysis with periosteal proliferation and soft tissue swelling
• Abdominal ultrasound may reveal granulomatous masses or enlarged lymph nodes.
• Ocular ultrasound may reveal a retrobulbar granulomatous mass.

OTHER DIAGNOSTIC PROCEDURES

• Impression smears or aspirates of skin nodules are most likely to yield organisms. • Fine needle aspirate of lung or bronchoalveolar lavage is more likely to be diagnostic than transtracheal aspirate. • Lymph node aspirate or biopsy • Vitreal aspirates • CSF tap in patients with cryptococcosis • Bone marrow, splenic or liver aspirate, or rectal cytology in cases of histoplasmosis • Biopsy may be needed.

GROSS AND HISTOPATHOLOGIC FINDINGS

Pyogranulomatous inflammation. Organisms usually are seen in patients with blastomycosis and cryptococcosis. They are sometimes difficult to find in animals with coccidioidomycosis and histoplasmosis.

TREATMENT

INPATIENT VERSUS OUTPATIENT

Dogs and cats that are still eating usually can be treated as outpatients. Inpatient evaluation and treatment is needed for the dehydrated, anorectic, or severely hypoxic animal.

ACTIVITY

Activity should be limited.

DIET

A high-protein, caloric-dense diet. For patients with histoplasmosis with marked gastrointestinal involvement, a highly digestible diet should be chosen.

CLIENT EDUCATION

• Only about 70% of dogs and a slightly smaller percentage of cats will likely respond to treatment. Prognosis depends upon the extent of disease and the immune status of the patient.
• Treatment is expensive and will likely be necessary for 2 months or longer.
• Areas in the environment of high organic matter or feces should be cleaned if possible.

SURGICAL CONSIDERATIONS N/A

MEDICATIONS

DRUGS AND FLUIDS

• Itraconazole (5-10 mg/kg PO daily with food) is the drug of choice.

• Amphotericin B (0.5 mg/kg [dog] or 0.25 mg/kg [cat] IV 3 times a week) to a total dose of 8 mg/kg if used alone or 4 mg/kg if used with an azole drug. It should be given in 200-500 ml of 5% dextrose preceded by saline diuresis. Amphotericin B is best used with itraconazole or ketoconazole in severely affected animals.
• Fluconazole (2.5-5 mg/kg PO daily) is the drug of choice for cryptococcosis and infections with CNS or urinary tract involvement.
• Supportive care should include fluids, potassium, oxygen, and antibiotics as needed.

CONTRAINDICATIONS

Corticosteroids

PRECAUTIONS

• The azole drugs should not be used in animals with severe liver disease.
• Amphotericin B should not be used in animals that are azotemic or dehydrated. It should be stopped if the BUN becomes greater than 50 mg/dl or the creatinine becomes greater than 3.0 mg/dl.
• Anorexia and higher liver enzymes are the most common adverse affects of itraconazole and the other azole drugs.

POSSIBLE INTERACTIONS

Antacids and anticonvulsants may reduce blood levels of itraconazole.

ALTERNATE DRUGS N/A

FOLLOW-UP

PATIENT MONITORING

• Liver enzymes should be evaluated monthly while patient is on itraconazole, fluconazole, or ketoconazole. • BUN and creatinine should be evaluated before each dose of amphotericin B. • Thoracic radiographs should be reevaluated before discontinuing therapy.

PREVENTION/AVOIDANCE

Monitor for signs of recurrence.

POSSIBLE COMPLICATIONS

• Blindness is usually permanent. • Renal failure from amphotericin B

EXPECTED COURSE AND PROGNOSIS

• A minimum of 2 months of therapy is required. Treatment should be continued until

1 month past disease remission, or in cryptococcosis, until the latex agglutination titer is < 1. • Approximately 70% will be cured with itraconazole treatment. Relapse may occur up to a year after treatment.

MISCELLANEOUS

ASSOCIATED CONDITIONS N/A

AGE RELATED FACTORS

Young animals are predisposed.

ZOONOTIC POTENTIAL

Infections in humans are primarily from a common environmental source. There is no direct transmission from animal to human except by penetrating wounds contaminated by the organism.

PREGNANCY

Fungal abortion is possible. Azole antifungals are teratogenic and should not be used in pregnant animals.

SYNONYMS N/A

SEE ALSO

• Blastomycosis • Histoplasmosis
• Coccidioidomycosis • Cryptococcosis
• Aspergillosis

ABBREVIATIONS N/A

References

Greene CE, ed. Infectious diseases of the dog and cat. Philadelphia: WB Saunders, 1990.
Wolf AM, Troy GC. Deep mycotic diseases. In: Ettinger SJ, Feldman EC, eds. Textbook of veterinary internal medicine. Philadelphia: WB Saunders, 1995:439-463.
Wolf AM. Antifungal agents. In: August JR, ed. Consultations in feline internal medicine 2. Philadelphia: WB Saunders, 1994.

Author Joseph Taboada
Consulting Editors Lynelle Johnson and Bradley L. Moses

PNEUMOTHORAX

BASICS

DEFINITION
• Pneumothorax is an accumulation of air or gas within the pleural space. • Classified as spontaneous (nontraumatic) or traumatic • Spontaneous pneumothorax may be primary (idiopathic) or secondary (resulting from underlying pulmonary disease). • Tension pneumothorax may have spontaneous or traumatic causes and results in a life-threatening increase in intrathoracic pressure.

Pathophysiology
• In the normal animal, the intrapleural space is a potential space, and intrapleural pressure is subatmospheric. A small amount of fluid within the normal pleural space forms a cohesive bond between the lungs and the thoracic wall. • When the intrapleural space becomes filled with air, as in pneumothorax, this cohesive bond is lost, and the normal elastic recoil of the lungs causes collapse from the thoracic wall as the thorax expands. • Respiratory compromise occurs secondary to 1) decreased tidal volume and hypoxia; 2) diffusion impairment; 3) ventilation to perfusion mismatch; and 4) intrapulmonary shunting of blood. • Initial physiologic responses—tachypnea (increased respiratory rate) followed by hyperventilation (increased rate and depth of respiration) will decrease arterial CO_2 and increase the arterial pH. As alveoli collapse, partial pressure of oxygen in the alveoli decreases, causing vasoconstriction, which reduces perfusion to poorly ventilated areas. • Generalized pulmonary hypoxic vasoconstriction and mechanical collapse of pulmonary vessels increases pulmonary arterial pressure and right heart work. As intrapleural pressure increases, compensatory mechanisms fail, arterial O_2 decreases, arterial CO_2 increases, the animal becomes severely acidotic, and death may ensue. • Tension pneumothorax—a flap of pulmonary parenchymal tissue acts as a one-way valve, allowing entry of air into the pleural space during inspiration, but preventing its escape during expiration. The thorax becomes fixed in maximal expansion, and the animal loses the ability to compensate. • Cardiovascular effects—decreased venous return secondary to loss of negative intrapleural pressure with compression and collapse of the venae cava

Systems Affected
• Respiratory • Cardiovascular

Genetics N/A

Incidence/Prevalence
• Traumatic pneumothorax is the most common type in dogs. • Traumatic pneumothorax occurs in 11-18 % of dogs and cats examined because of a history of vehicular trauma.

Geographic Distribution N/A

SIGNALMENT

Species Dogs and cats

Breed Predilections
Traumatic N/A

Spontaneous
• Rottweilers may be overrepresented. • Most affected dogs have a deep-chested conformation.

Mean Age and Range
Traumatic N/A

Spontaneous
Most common in middle-aged and old animals

Predominant Sex N/A

SIGNS

Historical Findings
Traumatic
Recent history of trauma and often acute dyspnea

Insidious or acute onset of clinical signs
• History may include clinical signs of dyspnea and high respiratory rate developing over days to months. • Low exercise tolerance
• May have had a history of previous lung or thoracic disease (secondary spontaneous pneumothorax)

Physical Examination Findings
General Comments
• Animals with pneumothorax will show various degrees of dyspnea, depending on the severity of lung collapse and the rate of progression of pneumothorax. • Tachypnea and anxiety are the most common examination findings. • Frothy blood may exude from the nose and mouth. • Cyanosis, pale mucous membranes, and open-mouth breathing in severe cases • Animals with tension pneumothorax may have a barrel-shaped thoracic cavity, minimal respiratory excursions, and tachycardia. • Abdominal breathing
• Auscultation—reduced vesicular lung sounds dorsally; heart sounds may be muffled
• Percussion—hyperresonant chest wall; tympanic with tension pneumothorax
Traumatic
• Open pneumothorax—external wounds of the thorax may be evident • Closed pneumothorax—signs of blunt trauma may be evident • Cervical subcutaneous emphysema may be seen in animals with laceration of the trachea or esophagus.

CAUSES

Traumatic
• External forces (gunshot, vehicular accidents, bite or stab wounds) • Iatrogenic—chest tube removal, thoracocentesis, thoracotomy complications, excessive positive pressure ventilation • Pneumomediastinum—esophageal perforation or tracheal laceration/avulsion may cause pneumothorax by rupture of mediastinal pleura

Spontaneous
• Primary—cause unknown; has not been well-documented in the dog or cat
• Secondary—destruction of pulmonary parenchyma, causing pulmonary cavitation and necrosis of visceral pleura (bullous emphysema, bacterial pneumonia, parasitic or mycotic granulomas, dirofilariasis, invasive thymoma, bronchogenic carcinoma, pulmonary abscess, foreign bodies, congenital pulmonary cysts)

RISK FACTORS

Traumatic
Free-roaming dogs or cats are more likely to sustain trauma.

Spontaneous
Previous pulmonary disease or pneumothorax

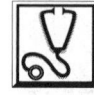

DIAGNOSIS

DIFFERENTIAL DIAGNOSIS
• Restrictive pulmonary diseases • Diaphragmatic hernia • Pleural effusion—hemothorax, chylothorax, pyothorax, and hydrothorax

CBC/BIOCHEMISTRY/URINALYSIS
• CBC—stress leukogram, and leukocytosis if secondary bacterial infection present
• Biochemistry—high liver enzymes secondary to trauma or hypoxia • Urinalysis—usually normal

OTHER LABORATORY TESTS
Arterial blood gas analysis may reveal hypoxemia, hypo- or hypercapnia, respiratory alkalosis, or respiratory or metabolic acidosis, depending on the magnitude of the pneumothorax and the ability of the animal to compensate.

IMAGING

Radiography
• Performed only after animal is stabilized
• Lateral and dorsoventral positioning may be less stressful. • Retraction of lung margins from thoracic wall with partial pulmonary collapse • On the lateral view, the heart appears elevated off the sternum. • Unilateral tension pneumothorax reveals mediastinal shift away from the side of high intrapleural pressure.
Traumatic
• Traumatic bullae or areas of consolidation (contusion) • Radiopaque, penetrating foreign objects (e.g., pellets, bullets) • Signs of trauma (pleural effusion, rib fractures)
Spontaneous
• Primary—infrequently, cavitary lesions, bullae, or subpleural blebs • Secondary—pulmonary parenchymal disease (pneumonia, neoplasia, dirofilariasis)

OTHER DIAGNOSTIC PROCEDURES
• Thoracocentesis is the diagnostic test of choice and should be performed as a therapeutic measure before other diagnostic tests in dyspneic animals. • Thoracoscopy—to

visualize the pleural space and pulmonary surface • Bronchoscopy—to locate lacerations of the trachea or main bronchi

GROSS AND HISTOPATHOLOGIC FINDINGS

• Dependent on the underlying cause
• Histopathologic examination of the lungs in a patient with bullous emphysema may reveal subpleural alveolar emphysema, pleural fibrosis, multifocal pulmonary atelectasis, smooth muscle hypertrophy of bronchioles, and bronchiolitis. • Gross inspection of the lungs may reveal pulmonary blebs.

TREATMENT

• In patients with traumatic pneumothorax, pleurocutaneous fistulae should be temporarily closed with sterile antibiotic ointment and gauze and closed surgically after patient stabilization.
• If dyspnea is not present and the patient is stable, evacuation of air is unnecessary (air will eventually be resorbed).
• If the animal is dyspneic, pleural air should be evacuated—needle thoracocentesis (butterfly catheter, three-way stop cock, and extension set) or tube thoracostomy for severe and active pneumothorax. Air should be evacuated at an aseptically prepared site of the dorsal two thirds of the thorax, between the seventh and ninth rib spaces. Tube thoracostomy is recommended if more than two thoracocenteses are necessary within 24 hours.
• Continuous negative-pressure pleural drainage by tube thoracostomy is recommended if pleural air rapidly reaccumulates.
• Heimlich valves have limitations because the flutter device often becomes occluded, and smaller patients may not generate enough intrathoracic pressure to evacuate the chest.
• Exploratory thoracotomy should be considered if pneumothorax and clinical signs persist for longer than 2-5 days, more than two episodes of pneumothorax recur after proper treatment, or if there is radiographic evidence for the source of the leakage that could be surgically resected (e.g., pulmonary blebs).
• Treatment of tension pneumothorax may require the use of a trocar into the pleural space to relieve increased intrapleural pressure before thoracostomy tube placement.

INPATIENT VERSUS OUTPATIENT

Inpatient care until stabilized

ACTIVITY

Cage rest is recommended to enhance healing of pulmonary tissue.

DIET N/A

CLIENT EDUCATION

Discuss clinical signs of pneumothorax recurrence and advise immediate return if seen.

SURGICAL CONSIDERATIONS

• The site of air leakage can be identified by flooding the pleural cavity with saline solution; confirmed by bubbles rising from the site of the fistula.
• Because the source of the bronchopleural fistula often is unknown and multiple lesions are common, median sternotomy often is necessary.
• Large lacerations may require sutures; neoplastic lesions usually require lobectomy; pulmonary blebs should be resected.
• Resection of apical blebs may prevent recurrence of spontaneous pneumothorax secondary to bullous emphysema.

MEDICATIONS

DRUGS AND FLUIDS

• Intravenous fluid therapy for patients in cardiovascular shock
• Oxygen administration for dyspneic and hypoxemic patients
• Drugs for primary causes of spontaneous pneumothorax (antibiotics for pneumonia, chemotherapy for neoplasia, adulticide therapy for dirofilariasis)
• If anesthetic agents are required, use drugs that allow rapid control of the airway by endotracheal intubation (e.g., ketamine and valium, thiobarbiturates).

CONTRAINDICATIONS

Heavy sedation should be avoided in critical patients.

PRECAUTIONS

Drugs that suppress respiration, such as narcotics, should be used with caution. Watch for signs of hypoventilation (increased $PaCO_2$, decreased PaO_2); positive pressure ventilation may be required.

POSSIBLE INTERACTIONS N/A

ALTERNATE DRUGS N/A

FOLLOW-UP

PATIENT MONITORING

• Respiratory rate and character, mucous membrane color, and heart rate should be monitored hourly for the first 24-48 hours. Pulse oximetry aids in continuous monitoring of hemoglobin oxygen saturation. • ECG monitoring is recommended in trauma cases.
• Serial radiographic evaluation and blood gas analyses reveal effectiveness of pleural air evacuation and reexpansion of lungs. Pulmonary bullae may become apparent.
• Thoracostomy tubes may be removed if 10 ml of air or less is removed in 12 hours.

PREVENTION/AVOIDANCE

• Prevent dogs from free-roaming. • Avoid excessively high airway pressures (> 25-30 cm of H_2O) during positive pressure ventilation to prevent barotrauma.

POSSIBLE COMPLICATIONS

Reexpansion pulmonary may occur; the incidence of this complication in veterinary patients is unknown.

EXPECTED COURSE AND PROGNOSIS

Traumatic

• Full recovery is expected with conservative management (thoracocentesis or thoracostomy tubes) in most patients. • Prognosis is good provided injury is not massive and recognition and treatment of pneumothorax is prompt.

Spontaneous

Recurrence rates of spontaneous pneumothorax are high (up to 100% treated by thoracocentesis alone; up to 81% treated with thoracostomy tubes); surgical treatment with pleurodesis is recommended to reduce the recurrence rate (25% treated with surgical resection of lesion) if pneumothorax does not resolve within 48 hours of conservative management.

MISCELLANEOUS

ASSOCIATED CONDITIONS N/A

AGE RELATED FACTORS N/A

ZOONOTIC POTENTIAL N/A

PREGNANCY N/A

SYNONYMS N/A

SEE ALSO

Thoracic Trauma

ABBREVIATIONS

PaO_2 = partial pressure of arterial oxygen
$PaCO_2$ = partial pressure of arterial carbon dioxide

References

Dramek BA, Caywood DD. Pneumothorax. Vet Clin N Am Sm Anim Pract 1987;17:285-300.
Bennett RA, Orton EC, Tucker A, Heiller CL. Cardiopulmonary changes in conscious dogs with induced progressive pneumothorax. Am J Vet Res 1989;50:280-284.
Holtsinger RH, Beale BS, Bellah JR, King RR. Spontaneous pneumothorax in the dog: a retrospective analysis of 21 cases. J Am Anim Hosp Assoc 1993;29:195-210.
Connolly JP. Hemodynamic measurements during a tension pneumothorax. Crit Care Med 1993;21:294-296.
Kramek BA, Caywood DD, O' Brien TD. Bullous emphysema and recurrent pneumothorax in the dog. J Am Vet Med Assoc 1985;186:971-974.

Author Cynthia Crager Ramsey
Consulting Editor Lynelle Johnson and Bradley L. Moses

POLIOENCEPHALOMYELITIS—CATS

BASICS

OVERVIEW
• Nonsuppurative meningoencephalomyelitis of unknown cause • Neurons in the thoracic spinal cord appear to be preferentially affected; lesions also located in cervical and lumbar spinal cord, brain stem, and cerebrum. • Axonal degeneration and demyelination in ventral and lateral funiculi of spinal cord occurs secondarily to neuronal necrosis.

SIGNALMENT
• Domestic shorthair cats and a few purebreds • 2 months-6.5 years • Females more commonly affected than males.

SIGNS
• Vary with location of CNS lesion • Chronic, progressive incoordination of hind or all four limbs • Seizures in a few patients

CAUSES AND RISK FACTORS
Viral cause suspected but not proven

DIAGNOSIS

DIFFERENTIAL DIAGNOSIS
Other Infectious Causes:
• FIP • Toxoplasmosis • Fungal infection • Bacterial infection

CBC/BIOCHEMISTRY/URINALYSIS
• Laboratory changes not well characterized. • Nonspecific changes (e.g., leukopenia and nonregenerative anemia) in rare patients

OTHER LABORATORY TESTS N/A

IMAGING N/A

OTHER DIAGNOSTIC PROCEDURES
• Mononuclear pleocytosis with mild to moderately high CSF protein (little data) • Serum or CSF antibody titers have not been thoroughly evaluated.

TREATMENT
• Treatment was not attempted in any of the reported cases. • Since the lesions are nonsuppurative, steroid administration may palliate clinical signs, at least temporarily.

MEDICATIONS

DRUGS AND FLUIDS N/A

CONTRAINDICATIONS/POSSIBLE INTERACTIONS N/A

FOLLOW-UP
N/A

MISCELLANEOUS

ABBREVIATIONS
CNS = Central nervous system
CSF = Cerebrospinal fluid

References
Vandevelde M, Braund KG. Polioencephalitis in cats. Vet Pathol 1979;16:420-427
Hoff EJ, Vandevelde M. Non-suppurative encephalomyelitis in cats suggestive of a viral origin. Vet Pathol 1981;18:170-180
Author Karen R. Dyer
Consulting Editor Joane M. Parent

BASICS

OVERVIEW
• Rare, polysystemic inflammatory disease associated with vasculitis of unknown cause, involving the small- and medium-sized arteries • The vascular lesions consist of intimal proliferation, vessel wall degeneration, necrosis and thrombosis. • Leads to loss of integrity of the vessel wall, petechial and ecchymotic hemorrhages, focal areas of tissue infarction and necrosis, aneurysm formation, and nodular swelling and thickening of the major arteries • Target organs in dogs are the kidneys, skin, mucous membranes, adrenal glands, meninges, gastrointestinal tract, connective tissue, myocardium, and the peripheral nervous system. • Classified as systemic necrotizing vasculitis

SIGNALMENT
Dogs and cats; rare in both

SIGNS

Historical Findings
Often nonspecific:
• Vomiting • Malaise • Weakness • Lethargy • Reluctance to walk • Vague pain • Weight loss

Physical Examination Findings
• Multisystem involvement • Skin ulceration, rashes • Ulceration of mucous membranes • Nasal discharge • Spinal pain • Cardiac failure • Renal failure, hematuria • Pyrexia • Joint pain • Seizures

CAUSES AND RISK FACTORS
• Deposition or formation of immune complexes in the walls of small- and medium-sized muscular arteries • The immune complexes elicit an inflammatory response. • In humans, classified among the immune-mediated collagen disorders • Possibly drug-induced

DIAGNOSIS

DIFFERENTIAL DIAGNOSIS
• Systemic lupus erythematosis • Staphylococcus hypersensitivity • Rheumatoid arthritis • Subacute endocarditis • Other necrotizing vasculitises are not characterized by granuloma formation.

CBC/BIOCHEMISTRY/URINALYSIS
• Leukocytosis with a left shift • Anemia • High BUN and creatinine • Hypergammaglobulinemia • Proteinuria

OTHER LABORATORY TESTS
Immune tests: antinuclear antibody, lupus erythematosis, rheumatoid factor

IMAGING N/A

OTHER DIAGNOSTIC PROCEDURES
• Histologic examination of biopsy specimens of the skin is necessary for diagnosis. The lesion is characterized by necrotizing inflammation in various stages involving small and medium muscular arteries. • Acute lesions involve the vessel wall and perivascular area and show infiltration of polymorphonuclear neutrophils. • Immunofluorescent antibody testing.

TREATMENT

Depends on extent and involvement of specific organs

MEDICATIONS

DRUGS AND FLUIDS
• Glucocorticoids
• Cyclophosphamide only if steroids fail.

CONTRAINDICATIONS/POSSIBLE INTERACTIONS N/A

FOLLOW-UP
• Monitor cardiac and renal functions • Monitor for infection • Monitor CBC if cyclophosphamide is used. • Educate owner regarding poor prognosis

MISCELLANEOUS

SEE ALSO Vasculitis

ABBREVIATIONS None

References

Ettingers SJ, ed. Textbook of veterinary internal medicine. 3rd ed. Philadelphia: WB Saunders, 1993.

Carpenter JL, Moore FM, Albert, DM. Polyarteritis nodosa and rheumatic heart disease in a dog. J Am Vet Med Assoc 1988;192:929.

Authors Larry P. Tilley and T. Arch Robertson

Consulting Editors Larry P. Tilley and Francis W.K. Smith, Jr.

POLYARTHRITIS, EROSIVE, IMMUNE-MEDIATED

BASICS

DEFINITION

Erosive polyarthritis is an immune-mediated inflammatory disease of joints that results in erosion of articular cartilage.

Pathophysiology

The pathogenesis of the erosive polyarthropathies involves a type III hypersensitivity reaction. Immune complexes form and become deposited within the synovial membrane. An inflammatory response and complement activation ensues. Destructive enzymes released from inflammatory cells, synoviocytes, and chondrocytes damage the articular cartilage, leading to erosive changes. Rheumatoid arthritis (RA) is associated with an abnormal antigenic response to host immunoglobulin. The offending antigen in erosive polyarthritis of Greyhounds (EPG) and feline chronic progressive polyarthritis (FCPP) are unknown.

Systems Affected

Musculoskeletal—diarthrodial joints

Genetics

Not known to be hereditary

Incidence/Prevalence

These diseases are rare.

Geographic Distribution   N/A

SIGNALMENT

Species

Dogs (RA, EPG), cats (FCPP)

Breed Predilections

• Small or toy breeds are more susceptible to RA. • Greyhounds are the only breed known to be susceptible to EPG.

Mean Age and Range

• Most dogs affected with RA are young or middle-aged (8 months to 8 years). • Young Greyhounds are more susceptible to EPG (3-30 months). • The onset of FCPP in most cats is at 1 1/2-4 1/2 years of age.

Predominant Sex

Male cats have been reported to be exclusively affected by FCPP.

SIGNS

General Comments

Clinical signs of nonerosive and erosive forms of immune-mediated polyarthritis can be similar initially. As erosive polyarthritis becomes chronic, it is easily distinguished.

Historical Findings

• Dogs and cats affected by immune-mediated arthritis typically show an acute onset of a single or multiple limb lameness. • The onset in cats may be more insidious. The lameness may shift from leg to leg. • Joint swelling may be evident, especially in the carpi and tarsi. • No history of trauma is usually present. • Other systemic clinical signs may also

be seen, including vomiting, diarrhea, anorexia, and pyrexia. These diseases are often cyclic and may appear to respond to antibiotic therapy when in actuality the disease may be spontaneously undergoing remission.

Physical Examination Findings

• Clinical signs include stiffness of gait, lameness, reduced range of motion, crepitus, and joint swelling and pain in one or more joints. • Depending on the duration of disease, joint instability and subluxation may be present. • Lameness can vary in severity from mild, weightbearing lameness to nonweightbearing lameness. • All diarthrodial joints can be affected; however, RA and FCPP have a predilection for the carpus, tarsus, and phalangeal joints. • The most common joints affected in dogs with EPG are the carpi, tarsi, elbow, stifle and hip.

CAUSES

• The cause of these diseases is unknown, but an immunologic mechanism is likely. • Mycoplasma spumans was cultured from one Greyhound with EPG; however, this organism has not been isolated in other dogs with the disease. • Feline leukemia (FeLV) and feline syncytium-forming (FeSFV) viruses have been linked to cats with FCPP.

RISK FACTORS   N/A

DIAGNOSIS

DIFFERENTIAL DIAGNOSIS

• Idiopathic polyarthritis • Infectious arthritis • Systemic lupus erythematosus • Reactive polyarthritis • Neoplasia

CBC/BIOCHEMISTRY/URINALYSIS

• Complete blood count, serum chemistries and urinalysis are usually normal. • The hemogram may show leukocytosis, neutrophilia, and hyperfibrinogenemia.

OTHER LABORATORY TESTS

• Rheumatoid factor is only positive in about 25% of cases of RA. • The Coomb's test and antinuclear antibody (ANA) titer are normal. • Serum titers for Borrelia, Ehrlichia, and Rickettsia should be normal. • Serological evidence of FeSFV can be found in all affected cats with FCPP; 50% or less of cats will also have exposure to FeLV.

IMAGING

Radiographic changes include joint capsular distension, osteophytosis, soft tissue thickening, narrowed joint spaces, and subchondral sclerosis in severe cases. Cyst-like lucencies can occasionally be seen in subchondral bone. Subluxation, luxation, and obvious joint deformity is evident in chronic cases.

OTHER DIAGNOSTIC PROCEDURES

• Arthrocentesis and synovial fluid analysis are essential for diagnosis. Synovial fluid typically appears cloudy with normal viscosity

and has a large number of nondegenerate neutrophils (20,000-200,000 cells/ ml). • Synovial fluid should be submitted for bacterial culture and sensitivity. • Biopsy of the synovial tissue is helpful in diagnosing these diseases and ruling out other arthritides or neoplasia.

GROSS AND HISTOPATHOLOGIC FINDINGS

• Erosion of articular cartilage is present, particularly near the periphery at synovial attachments. Eburnation and sclerosis of subchondral bone appears with full thickness cartilage loss in chronic cases. The synovial membrane is grossly thickened and may have villous projections. Granulation tissue (pannus) may invade the margins of articular cartilage. Enthesiophytes are found at joint capsular attachments and adjacent to the joint. • Histopathology of the synovial membrane typically shows villous synovial hyperplasia, hypertrophy, and a lymphoplasmacytic inflammatory infiltrate. • Synovial fluid appears cloudy and is increased in volume.

TREATMENT

INPATIENT VERSUS OUTPATIENT

Treatment of erosive polyarthropathies can often be frustrating and requires frequent follow-up evaluation. Cure is not expected; remission of disease is the goal.

ACTIVITY

Exercise should be limited to a level that minimizes aggravation of clinical signs.

DIET

Weight reduction will reduce the stress placed on affected joints.

CLIENT EDUCATION

A poor prognosis for cure and complete resolution should be given to owners.

SURGICAL CONSIDERATIONS

• Arthroplasty (total hip replacement, femoral head ostectomy) procedures can be performed. • Arthrodesis can be used in selective cases of joint pain and joint instability. Arthrodesis of the carpus generally yields the best result, while arthrodesis of the shoulder, elbow, stifle or hock gives less predictable results.

MEDICATIONS

DRUGS AND FLUIDS

• Use of nonsteroidal anti-inflammatory drugs (NSAIDs) to treat RA in dogs has been unrewarding. The recommended treatment is a combination of glucocorticoids (GCC) and cytotoxic drugs, such as cyclophosphamide, azathioprine, 6-mercaptopurine, and methotrexate. Glucocorticoids are used in combination with cytotoxic drugs due to their synergistic effect.

POLYARTHRITIS, EROSIVE, IMMUNE-MEDIATED

• Therapy is usually initiated with prednisone at 1.5-2.0 mg/kg, PO q12h for 10-14 days. If synovial fluid cell counts return below 4000 cells/ml and mononuclear cells predominate, the dose of prednisone can be slowly tapered over several weeks to 1.0 mg/kg, PO q48h. If clinical signs persist or synovial fluid analysis is abnormal, cytotoxic drugs should be started with prednisone.

• Cyclophosphamide is given at 2.5 mg/kg for dogs less than 10 kg, 2.0 mg/kg for dogs between 10 and 25 kg, and 1.75 mg/kg for dogs heavier than 50 kg. This dosage is given PO q24h for four consecutive days of each week.

• If azathioprine or 6- mercaptopurine are used, they are given at 2.0 mg/kg, orally for 14 - 21 days, PO q48h. Prednisone is given as with cyclophosphamide; however, it is given on alternating days with the thiopurine. Combination chemotherapy will usually induce remission within 2 to 16 weeks.

• Cytotoxic drugs are discontinued one to three months after remission is achieved; this is determined by resolution of clinical signs and confirmation of a normal synovial fluid analysis.

• Alternate day GCC therapy (prednisone, 1.0 mg/kg, orally) is generally successful in maintaining remission. If clinical signs or synovial effusion recurs, long-term cytotoxic drug therapy may be necessary.

• If clinical signs do not recur while on alternate day GCC for 2-3 months, the drug can be stopped.

• If clinical signs recur when GCC are stopped, treatment should continue; if remission does not ensue, long-term cytotoxic drug therapy may be necessary.

• Weekly injections of 1 mg/kg sodium aurothiomalate (chrysotherapy) has also been successful in alleviating symptoms of RA.

• Treatment of EPG has proved to be unrewarding. Antibiotics, NSAIDs, GCC, cytotoxic drugs and polysulfated glycosaminoglycan (Adequan) have failed to induce remission.

• Treatment of FCPP may help to slow progression. Prednisone (2 mg/kg, q12h) and cyclophosphamide (2.5 mg/kg q24h) are typically used as described above.

CONTRAINDICATIONS

• Cytotoxic drugs should not be used in animals with chronic infections or bone marrow suppression (cats with FCPP).

• Chrysotherapy is contraindicated in dogs with renal disease, due to nephrotoxicity.

PRECAUTIONS

• Long term administration of GCC can lead to Cushing's disease.

• Cytotoxic drugs frequently induce bone marrow suppression. Complete blood counts should be monitored for reductions in the leukocyte count to below 6000 cells/ml and platelet count to below 125,000 cells/ml; If this occurs, the dose of the cytotoxic drug should be reduced by one-fourth. If the leukocyte count falls below 4000 cells/ml and platelet count below 100,000 cells/ml, cytotoxic drugs should be discontinued for one week, then reinstituted at three fourths the normal dose when the leukocyte and platelet counts return to normal.

• The thiopurines (2-6 weeks) generally cause bone marrow suppression earlier than cyclophosphamide (several months).

• Use of cyclophosphamide should be limited to less than four months due to the possibility of developing a sterile hemorrhagic cystitis. If these signs occur, the drug should be discontinued at once.

POSSIBLE INTERACTIONS

None known

ALTERNATE DRUGS See above

 FOLLOW-UP

PATIENT MONITORING

Clinical deterioration indicates the need for a change in drug selection, or dosage or surgical intervention.

PREVENTION/AVOIDANCE N/A

POSSIBLE COMPLICATIONS N/A

EXPECTED COURSE AND PROGNOSIS

Progression of disease is likely and the long term prognosis is poor.

 MISCELLANEOUS

ASSOCIATED CONDITIONS N/A

AGE RELATED FACTORS N/A

ZOONOTIC POTENTIAL N/A

PREGNANCY N/A

SYNONYMS N/A

SEE ALSO N/A

ABBREVIATIONS

RA = rheumatoid arthritis
EPG = erosive polyarthritis of greyhounds
FCPP = feline chronic progressive polyarthritis
NSAID = nonsteroidal ani-inflammatory drug

References

Beale BS. Arthropathies. In: Bloomberg MS, Taylor RT, Dee J, eds. Canine sports medicine and surgery. Philadelphia: WB Saunders, in press

Goring RL, Beale BS. Immune mediated arthritides. In: Bojrab MJ, ed, Disease mechanisms in small animal surgery. Philadelphia: Lea and Febiger, 1993;742-750.

Pedersen NC. Joint diseases of dogs and cats. In: Ettinger SJ, ed. Textbook of veterinary internal medicine. 3rd ed. Philadelphia: WB Saunders, 1989;2329-2377.

Author Brian Beale
Consulting Editor Peter D. Schwarz

POLYARTHRITIS, NONEROSIVE, IMMUNE-MEDIATED

BASICS

DEFINITION

Nonerosive polyarthritis is an immune-mediated inflammatory disease of joints which does not cause erosive change. Nonerosive immune-mediated arthropathies include idiopathic polyarthritis, systemic lupus erythematosus (SLE), polyarthritis associated with chronic disease (chronic infectious, neoplastic or enteropathic disease), polyarthritis-polymyositis syndrome, polyarthritis-meningitis syndrome, polyarteritis nodosa, familial renal amyloidosis in Chinese shar pei dogs, lymphocytic-plasmacytic synovitis, villonodular synovitis, juvenile-onset polyarthritis of Akitas, and the proliferative form of feline chronic progressive polyarthritis (FCPP).

Pathophysiology

The pathogenesis involves a type III hypersensitivity reaction. Immune complexes form and become deposited within the synovial membrane. An inflammatory response and complement activation ensues leading to clinical signs of arthritis. In SLE patients, nuclear material from various cells becomes antigenic leading to formation of autoantibodies (antinuclear antibody).

Systems Affected

Musculoskeletal—diarthrodial joints

Genetics

Not known to be hereditary

Incidence/Prevalence

Idiopathic polyarthritis is the most common form of immune-mediated, nonerosive polyarthritis in dogs. The other forms are uncommon.

Geographic Distribution N/A

SIGNALMENT

Species Dogs and cats

Breed Predilections

• Idiopathic polyarthritis affects both large and small-dog breeds, but is more common in the former. It is uncommon in cats. Breeds that appear to be overrepresented include German shepherds, Doberman pinschers, retrievers, spaniels, pointers, toy poodles, Lhaso apsos, Yorkshire terriers, and Chihuahuas. • In contrast to rheumatoid arthritis, SLE has a tendency to affect larger-breed dogs. Breeds reported more often include collies, German shepherds, poodles, beagles, and Shetland sheepdogs. • Doberman pinschers appear to have a high sensitivity to developing polyarthritis secondary to administration of sulfa drugs. • Polyarthritis-meningitis syndrome has been reported in the Weimaraner, German shorthaired pointer, boxer, Bernese mountain dog, and Japanese Akita. • Amyloidosis and synovitis are prominent features of a syndrome affecting young shar pei dogs. • Juvenile-onset polyarthritis has been reported in akitas.

Mean Age and Range

Most dogs affected with nonerosive immune-mediated polyarthritis are young to middle-aged.

Predominant Sex

Male cats have been reported to be exclusively affected by FCPP.

SIGNS

General Comments

Clinical signs of nonerosive and erosive forms of immune-mediated polyarthritis can be similar initially. As erosive polyarthritis becomes chronic, it is easily distinguished.

Historical Findings

• Dogs and cats affected by immune-mediated arthritis typically show an acute onset of a single or multiple limb lameness. The lameness may shift from leg to leg. No history of trauma is usually present. • Other systemic clinical signs may also be present, including vomiting, diarrhea, anorexia, pyrexia, polyuria, polydipsia, or clinical signs associated with systemic infectious (e.g., pyometra, prostatitis, diskospondylitis) or neoplastic disease. • These diseases are often cyclic and may appear to respond to antibiotic therapy when in actuality the disease may be spontaneously undergoing remission. Some affected animals are being treated with antibiotics (sulfur-containing antibiotics) at the time arthritis ensues.

Physical Examination Findings

• Clinical signs include stiffness of gait, lameness, reduced range of motion, crepitus, and joint swelling and pain in one or more joints. • Lameness can vary in severity from mild, weightbearing lameness to nonweightbearing lameness. • All diarthrodial joints can be affected; however, most forms of nonerosive polyarthritis have a predilection for the stifle, elbow, carpus, and tarsus.

CAUSES

• The cause of most of these diseases is unknown, but an immunologic mechanism is likely. • Polyarthritis of chronic disease has been associated with antigenic stimulation in the presence of concurrent gastrointestinal disease, neoplasia, urinary tract infection, periodontitis, bacterial endocarditis, heartworm disease, pyometra, chronic otitis media or externa, fungal infections, and chronic Actinomyces infections. • Polyarthritis can occur secondary to a hypersensitivity reaction involving the deposition of drug-antibody complexes in blood vessels of the synovium. Antibiotics of the following classes have been suspected of initiating this syndrome: sulfas, cephalosporins, lincomycin, erythromycin, and penicillins. • Feline leukemia and feline syncytium-forming viruses have been linked to cats with FCPP.

RISK FACTORS N/A

DIAGNOSIS

DIFFERENTIAL DIAGNOSIS

• Early erosive polyarthritides • Infectious arthritis • Joint trauma • Polymyositis

CBC/BIOCHEMISTRY/URINALYSIS

• Complete blood count, serum chemistries, and urinalysis are usually normal. • The hemogram may show leukocytosis, neutrophilia, and hyperfibrinogenemia. • Hematologic abnormalities such as thrombocytopenia and hematolytic anemia are seen in only 10 to 20% of all patients with SLE.

OTHER LABORATORY TESTS

• Either a positive LE preparation or a positive ANA test should be seen in dogs with SLE. • Serum titers for Borrelia, Ehrlichia, and Rickettsia should be normal. • Serologic evidence of FeSFV can be found in all affected cats with FCPP; 50% or less of cats will also have exposure to FeLV.

IMAGING

The primary radiographic change associated with nonerosive polyarthritis is joint capsular distension and occasionally enthesiophytosis in prolonged or recurrent cases.

OTHER DIAGNOSTIC PROCEDURES

• Arthrocentesis and synovial fluid analysis are essential for diagnosis. Synovial fluid typically appears cloudy with normal viscosity and has a high number of nondegenerate neutrophils (20,000-200,000 cells/ ml). • Synovial fluid should be submitted for bacterial culture and sensitivity. • Synovial biopsy may be helpful for diagnosis.

GROSS AND HISTOPATHOLOGIC FINDINGS

The joint capsule may appear thickened and a synovial effusion is present. Synovial hypertrophy and hyperplasia are associated with mononuclear cell infiltrate. Neutrophils are also seen in the synovial tissues due to chemotaxis.

TREATMENT

INPATIENT VERSUS OUTPATIENT

Outpatient therapy is most common.

ACTIVITY

Exercise should be limited to a level that minimizes aggravation of clinical signs.

DIET

Weight reduction will reduce the stress placed on affected joints.

CLIENT EDUCATION

A poor prognosis for cure and complete resolution should be given to owners.

SURGICAL CONSIDERATIONS N/A

POLYARTHRITIS, NONEROSIVE, IMMUNE-MEDIATED

MEDICATIONS

DRUGS AND FLUIDS

• Glucocorticoids (GCC) are usually used for the initial treatment of immune-mediated nonerosive polyarthritis.

• If response is poor, combination chemotherapy using GCC and cytoxic drugs is started. Underlying causes of polyarthritis should be eliminated if possible (i.e. chronic disease, offending antibiotic). Complete remission is usually achieved; however, a recurrence rate of 30 to 50% can be expected once therapy is discontinued.

• Therapy is usually initiated with prednisone at 1.5 to 2.0 mg/kg, PO q12h for 10-14 days. If synovial fluid cell counts return below 4000 cells/ml and mononuclear cells predominate, the dose of prednisone can be slowly tapered over several weeks to 1.0 mg/kg, PO q48h. If clinical signs persist or synovial fluid analysis is abnormal, cytotoxic drugs should be started with prednisone. If clinical signs do not recur while on alternate day GCC therapy for two to three months, the drug can be discontinued. Cytotoxic drugs are used in combination with GCC due to their synergistic effect.

• The most commonly used cytotoxic drugs include cyclophosphamide and the thiopurines, azathioprine and 6-mercaptopurine. Cyclophosphamide is given at 2.5 mg/kg for dogs less than 10 kg, 2.0 mg/kg for dogs between 10 and 25 kg, and 1.75 mg/kg for dogs heavier than 50 kg. This dosage is given PO q24h for four consecutive days of each week. Prednisone is also given as described above; although some clinicians reduce the total daily dose by half.

• If azathioprine or 6- mercaptopurine is used, they are given at 2.0 mg/kg, PO q24h 14-21 days, then q48h. Prednisone is given as with cyclophosphamide; however, it is given on alternating days with the thiopurine. Remission usually occurs in 2 to 16 weeks.

• Cytotoxic drugs are discontinued one to three months after remission is achieved; this is determined by resolution of clinical signs and confirmation of normal synovial fluid analysis.

• Alternate-day GCC therapy (prednisone, 1.0 mg/kg, PO) is generally successful in maintaining remission.

• If clinical signs or synovial neutrophilia recur, long term cytotoxic drug therapy may be necessary. If clinical signs do not recur while on alternate-day GCC therapy for two to three months, the drug can be discontinued. If clinical signs recur when GCC are stopped, treatment should be extended; if remission does not ensue, long-term cytotoxic drug therapy may be needed.

• Treatment of FCPP may help to slow progression. Prednisone (2 mg/kg, q12h) and cyclophosphamide (2.5 mg/kg) are typically used as described above. Treatment of FCPP may help to slow progression. Prednisone (2 mg/kg, q12h) and cyclophosphamide (2.5 mg/kg) are typically used as described above.

CONTRAINDICATIONS

Cytotoxic drugs should not be used in animals with chronic infections or bone marrow suppression (cats with FCPP).

PRECAUTIONS

Long term administration of GCC can lead to iatrogenic Cushing's disease. Administration of cytotoxic drugs frequently induces bone marrow suppression. Complete blood counts should initially be monitored weekly (see polyarthritis, erosive).

POSSIBLE INTERACTIONS

None known

ALTERNATE DRUGS   See above

FOLLOW-UP

PATIENT MONITORING

Clinical deterioration indicates the need for a change in drug selection or dosage.

PREVENTION/AVOIDANCE   N/A

POSSIBLE COMPLICATIONS   N/A

EXPECTED COURSE AND PROGNOSIS

• Progression of disease is guarded with SLE and FCPP and good with most other nonerosive arthritides. • Recurrence is seen intermittantly.

MISCELLANEOUS

ASSOCIATED CONDITIONS   N/A

AGE RELATED FACTORS   N/A

ZOONOTIC POTENTIAL   N/A

PREGNANCY   N/A

SYNONYMS   N/A

ABBREVIATIONS

FCPP = feline chronic progressive polyarthritis
GCC = glucocorticoids
SLE = systemic lupus erythematosus

References

Beale BS. Arthropathies. In: Bloomberg MS, Taylor RT, Dee J, eds. Canine sports medicine and surgery. Philadelphia: WB Saunders, in press.

Goring RL, Beale BS. Immune-mediated arthritides. In: Bojrab MJ, ed. Disease mechanisms in small animal surgery. Philadelphia: Lea and Febiger, 1993;742-750.

Pedersen NC. Joint diseases of dogs and cats. In: Ettinger SJ, ed. Textbook of veterinary internal medicine. 3rd ed. Philadelphia: WB Saunders, 1989;2329-2377.

Author Brian Beale
Consulting Editor Peter D. Schwarz

POLYCYSTIC KIDNEY DISEASE

BASICS

OVERVIEW
Polycystic kidney disease is a disorder in which large portions of normally differentiated renal parenchyma are displaced by multiple cysts. Renal cysts develop in preexisting nephrons and collecting ducts. Both kidneys are invariably involved, probably because of the inherited nature of the disease.

SIGNALMENT
• Persian and other long-haired cats are affected more commonly than other breeds.
• Dog breeds affected include cairn terriers and beagles.

SIGNS
• Cysts often remain undetected until they have become of sufficient size and number to contribute to renal failure or abdominal enlargement. For these reasons, patients typically are clinically normal during initial stages of cyst formation and growth.
• Bosselated (lumpy) kidneys may be detected by abdominal palpation.
• Most renal cysts are not painful when palpated; however, acute secondary infection of cysts may be associated with rapid distension of the renal capsule and pain.

CAUSES AND RISK FACTORS
• The disease is believed to be an inherited process; however, lack of genealogic information often precludes a precise diagnosis of inherited disease in most adult dogs and cats with multiple renal cysts.
• The stimuli for renal cyst formation remains obscure; genetic, endogenous, and environmental factors appear to influence the process.
• Endogenous compounds hypothesized to stimulate cellular hyperplasia and contribute to cyst development include parathyroid hormone, vasopressin, cAMP, and endotoxins of enteric microbes.
• Cystogenic chemicals include diphenylthiazole, nordihydroguaiarectic acid, diphenylamine, trichlorophenoxyacetic acid, and long-acting corticosteroids.

DIAGNOSIS

DIFFERENTIAL DIAGNOSIS
• Other multicystic diseases of the kidneys
• Glomerulocystic disease of collie
• Renal cystadenocarcinoma associated with nodular fibrosis in German shepherd dogs
• Renal cysts associated with chronic renal failure or renal dysplasia
• Noncystic causes of renomegaly
• Renal neoplasia
• Hydronephrosis
• Perirenal pseudocysts
• Feline infectious peritonitis
• Mycotic or bacterial nephritis

CBC/BIOCHEMISTRY/URINALYSIS
• Results are usually unremarkable unless patient has renal insufficiency.
• Hematuria is rare.

OTHER LABORATORY TESTS
• Cyst fluid can be clear, cloudy, or hemorrhagic, and the fluid from different cysts in the same kidney can vary in character.
• Bacterial culture of cyst fluid is helpful to diagnosis concomitant infection.

IMAGING
Radiography
Survey radiography and intravenous urography are insensitive methods of confirming cystic disease.

Ultrasonography
• Reveals anechoic cavitating lesions characterized by sharply marginated smooth walls and distal enhancement which are diagnostic
• Reveals hypoechoic cystic cavities in some animals with cysts that have become infected with bacteria
• Used to detect cysts in other organs (e.g., liver), which is helpful in differentiating polycystic kidney disease from acquired multicystic disorders of the kidneys

OTHER DIAGNOSTIC PROCEDURES
Evaluation of fine needle aspirates of the kidney may allow differentiation of cystic disease from other diseases that cause renomegaly.

TREATMENT
• Polycystic kidney disease is usually not immediately life threatening; however, bacterial nephritis and cyst involvement warrants immediate measures to prevent sepsis and mortality.
• Spontaneous resolution of cysts has not been documented in dogs or cats. With time, most cysts increase in size and number, often compressing adjacent normal-functioning renal parenchyma.
• Elimination of renal cysts and associated renal parenchymal lesions is not yet feasible. Therefore, treatment is often limited to minimizing the pathophysiologic consequences of renal cyst formation (i.e., renal failure, renal infection, hematuria, and pain).
• Percutaneous aspiration of fluid from large renal cysts can be performed to minimize pain and compression of adjacent normal renal parenchyma. This procedure is impractical for kidneys with hundreds of cysts. Likewise, periodic aspiration of fluid (weekly to biweekly) is needed to maintain reduced cyst volume.
• Some patients may require treatment for concomitant renal failure.
• Nephrectomy should be avoided, but may be considered if infected cysts are associated with sepsis.

MEDICATIONS

DRUGS AND FLUIDS
• Bacterial infection of cysts has been observed in cats. Unless infection is accompanied by pyelonephritis, bacteria may not be observed in urine. Parenchymal infection should be considered when renal cysts are associated with renal pain, fever and even in absence of bacteriuria.
• Treatment of infected cysts requires special consideration. The acidic nature of cyst fluid and its containment by an epithelial barrier might inhibit the establishment of bactericidal concentrations of commonly used acidic antibiotics (e.g., cephalosporins and penicillins) within cysts lumens. Alkaline, lipid-soluble antibiotics (e.g., timethroprim-sulfonamide combinations, enrofloxacin, chloramphenicol, tetracycline, and clindamycin), which penetrate epithelial barriers and become ionized and trapped in cyst lumens, have been recommended for humans with infected cysts and should be considered for veterinary patients.

CONTRAINDICATIONS AND POSSIBLE INTERACTIONS NA

FOLLOW-UP
• Patients should be monitored every 2–6 months for associated disease (e.g., renal failure, renal infection, and pain).
• In the absence of sepsis, the short-term prognosis appears to be favorable without treatment.
• The long-term prognosis for patients with polycystic kidney disease often depends on the severity and progression of renal failure.

MISCELLANEOUS

Reference

Lulich JP, Osborne CA, Polzin DJ. Cystic diseases of the kidney. In: Osborne CA, Finco DR, eds. Canine and feline nephrology and urology. Philadelphia: Williams & Wilkins. In press.

Authors Jody P. Lulich and Carl A. Osborne
Consulting Editors Larry G. Adams and Carl A. Osborne

BASICS

OVERVIEW
Polycythemia vera is a myeloproliferative disorder.

SIGNALMENT
• Dogs and cats • Primarily old

SIGNS
• Signs are gradual in onset and run a chronic course • Depression • Anorexia • Weakness • High blood viscosity • Polydipsia and polyuria • Erythema of skin and mucous membranes • Dilated and tortuous retinal blood vessels • Splenomegaly and hepatomegaly uncommon

CAUSES AND RISK FACTORS
Unknown

DIAGNOSIS

DIFFERENTIAL DIAGNOSIS
• Severe dehydration • Renal neoplasia • Chronic pyelonephritis • Hyperadrenocorticism • Androgen stimulation • Pulmonary disease • Cardiac disease

CBC/BIOCHEMISTRY/URINALYSIS
• Absolute increase in RBC mass • Leukocytosis in 50% of dogs • Normal arterial PO_2

OTHER LABORATORY TESTS
Serum erythropoietin concentration is low to zero.

IMAGING
Thoracic radiography, electrocardiography, cardiac ultrasonography, abdominal radiography, renal ultrasonography, and intravenous pyelography are recommended to determine underlying cause

OTHER DIAGNOSTIC PROCEDURES
Cytologic examination of bone marrow and core biopsy may be diagnostic.

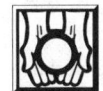

TREATMENT

• Phlebotomy and concurrent replacement with isotonic fluids intravenously for quick relief of signs during clinical crisis • Hydroxyurea to inhibit intracellular DNA synthesis and retard bone marrow proliferation

MEDICATIONS

DRUGS AND FLUIDS
• Hydroxyurea—40 to 50mg/kg divided twice daily and titrate to response and toxicity (dogs and cats) • Busulfan can be substituted for hydroxyurea; also requires careful monitoring for myelosuppression

CONTRAINDICATIONS/POSSIBLE INTERACTIONS
Hydroxyurea is potentially myelosuppressive. Frequent blood monitoring is advised.

FOLLOW-UP
Periodic recheck examinations including CBC and platelet count to monitor toxic effects on bone marrow

MISCELLANEOUS

ASSOCIATED CONDITIONS N/A

Reference

Morrison WB. Polycythemia. In: Ettinger SJ, Feldman EC, eds. Textbook of veterinary internal medicine. WB Saunders, 1994;197-199.

Author Wallace B. Morrison
Consulting Editor Wallace B. Morrison

PORTOSYSTEMIC SHUNT

 BASICS

DEFINITION

Vascular communications between the portal and systemic venous systems (usually between the portal vein and caudal vena cava) that allow access of portal blood to the systemic circulation without first passing through the liver. Portosystemic shunts in dogs and cats can be congenital or acquired. Congenital portosystemic shunts, the most common type, are anomalous embryonal vessels that occur as single shunts (either intrahepatic or extrahepatic). Acquired portosystemic shunts form in response to portal hypertension and typically are multiple extrahepatic shunts. Acquired portosystemic shunts usually occur secondary to chronic end-stage liver disease and will not be discussed further.

Pathophysiology

Clinical signs of hepatic encephalopathy develop as a result of inadequate hepatic clearance of enterically derived toxins. Impaired hepatic blood flow and lack of hepatotrophic factors result in a small liver. Urate urolithiasis, an important complication of portosystemic shunt, occurs because of high urinary excretion of ammonia and uric acid.

Systems Affected

• Nervous—hepatic encephalopathy • Gastrointestinal—vomiting and diarrhea • Renal/Urologic—ammonium urate urolithiasis

Genetics

The genetic basis is not understood, but affected lines have been recognized in miniature schnauzer, Irish wolfhound, old English sheepdogs, and Cairn terrier.

Incidence/Prevalence

Not known

Geographic Distribution N/A

SIGNALMENT

Species Dogs and cats

Breed Predilections

• Higher risk in purebreed than mixed-breed dogs, especially miniature schnauzers and Yorkshire terriers • Higher risk in mixed-breed than purebreed cats • Cats and small-breed dogs usually have an extrahepatic portosystemic shunt. • Large-breed dogs usually have an intrahepatic portosystemic shunt.

Mean Age and Range

• Clinical signs usually recognized in the first 6 months of life; most dogs are < 2 years old when diagnosed. • Some dogs with congenital portosystemic shunt are not diagnosed until later in life (5-10 years old). • Cats are older than dogs on initial examination.

Predominant Sex N/A

SIGNS

General Comments

• Clinical signs of portosystemic shunt are referable to the CNS, gastrointestinal system,

or urinary tract. • Signs of hepatic encephalopathy usually predominate and often wax and wane, temporarily improving with administration of broad-spectrum antibiotics and fluids. • Signs may be exacerbated by a protein-rich meal, gastrointestinal bleeding, or administration of methionine-containing drugs.

Historical Findings

Prolonged recovery after anesthesia, or excessive sedation after administration of tranquilizer or anticonvulsant .
CNS signs
• Anorexia • Lethargy • Episodic weakness • Ataxia • Head-pressing • Disorientation • Circling • Pacing • Behavioral changes • Blindness • Seizures • Coma • Hypersalivation (especially cats) • Bizarre aggressive behavior (more likely in cats than in dogs)
Gastrointestinal signs
• Vomiting (intermittent) • Diarrhea (intermittent) • Stunted growth or failure to gain weight
Urinary signs
• Polyuria and polydipsia • Pollakiuria • Dysuria • Hematuria (urolithiasis).

Physical Examination Findings

• May be unremarkable except for small body stature •The liver is not usually palpable because of its small size. • In animals with overt signs of hepatic encephalopathy, results of neurologic examination are consistent with diffuse cerebral disease. • Golden or copper-colored irises commonly seen in affected cats • Ascites and edema rare

CAUSES

• Congenital • Acquired secondary to portal hypertension

RISK FACTORS N/A

 DIAGNOSIS

DIFFERENTIAL DIAGNOSIS

• In animal with CNS signs, consider infectious diseases (e.g., feline infectious peritonitis, canine distemper, toxoplasmosis, and feline leukemia virus-related diseases), toxicity, hydrocephalus, idiopathic epilepsy, and metabolic disorders such as hypoglycemia. Neurologic and ophthalmic examinations, measurement of serum titers, electroencephalogram, and CSF tap may help to distinguish these disorders from portosystemic shunt. • In animal with gastrointestinal signs, consider gastrointestinal foreign body, parasites, dietary indiscretion or intolerance, chronic gastritis, and inflammatory bowel disease. • In animal with urinary signs, consider bacterial urinary tract infection or other causes of urolithiasis. • Primary liver disease can be differentiated by liver biopsy. • In young animals with clinical features consistent with portosystemic shunt but without a demonstrable shunt on portography or rectal portal scintigraphy, consider hepatic mi-

crovascular dysplasia or congenital urea cycle enzyme deficiency.

CBC/BIOCHEMISTRY/URINALYSIS

• Microcytosis, mild nonregenerative anemia, target cells, and poikilocytosis • Low BUN, hypoproteinemia (i.e., low albumin and globulin), hypoglycemia, hypocholesterolemia, normal to mildly high liver enzyme activity, and normal serum bilirubin concentration. Hypoproteinemia is less consistent in cats. • Dilute urine, ammonium biurate crystals; hematuria, pyuria, and proteinuria (urolithiasis)

OTHER LABORATORY TESTS

• Serum bile acids—fasting concentration often high but may be normal. Two-hour postprandial concentration consistently high, typically exceeding 100 umol/L. If postprandial concentration is consistently normal, a diagnosis of portosystemic shunt can be excluded. • Blood ammonia values are commonly high, although fasting values may be normal. The ammonia tolerance test is consistently abnormal.

IMAGING

Abdominal Radiographic Findings

• Most dogs with a congenital portosystemic shunt have microhepatica; this finding is less consistent in cats. • Mild renomegaly can be seen. • Ammonium urate calculi are not usually visible unless they contain magnesium and phosphate.

Abdominal Ultrasonographic Findings

• Portosystemic shunt can be visualized by an experienced operator. Intrahepatic portosystemic shunts are easier to identify than extrahepatic portosystemic shunts. • The kidney and bladder should be scanned for uroliths.

Portogram

A mesenteric portogram is the procedure of choice to characterize the type and anatomic location of a portosystemic shunt.

Rectal Portal Scintigraphy

Scintigraphy is a noninvasive alternative to portography that can demonstrate shunting, but does not provide reliable anatomic information. It is only available at referral centers.

OTHER DIAGNOSTIC PROCEDURES

Liver biopsy

GROSS AND HISTOPATHOLOGIC FINDINGS

• The liver is grossly small and smooth with microscopic features of hepatocyte atrophy, small or absent portal vessels, and lipogranulomas. • Microscopic abnormalities of the CNS are consistent with hepatic encephalopathy and include astrocytosis and polymicrocavitation.

 TREATMENT

INPATIENT VS OUTPATIENT

• Patients with signs of hepatic encephalopathy should be hospitalized for initial medical management.

• Stable patients may be released on medical management of hepatic encephalopathy pending surgery.

ACTIVITY Unrestricted

DIET Protein-restricted diet

CLIENT EDUCATION

• Discuss need for surgical ligation of portosystemic shunt.
• Discuss poor long-term prognosis without surgery (some dogs may be managed medically for months to years; cats are less likely to be controlled with medical treatment).
• Avoid feeding high-protein diets or snacks.

SURGICAL CONSIDERATIONS

• Total surgical ligation of a single portosystemic shunt is preferred; however, only partial ligation is often performed because of the risk of portal hypertension.
• Intrahepatic shunts are more difficult to correct than extrahepatic shunts.
• Control signs of hepatic encephalopathy medically before attempting surgical correction.
• Observe closely for 24-48 hours after surgery to detect signs of portal hypertension, which may require emergency surgery to remove the ligature. Other potential complications include intraoperative hypothermia and hypoglycemia, seizures, sepsis, portal vein thrombosis, acute pancreatitis, cardiac arrythmias, and hemorrhage.

MEDICATIONS

DRUGS AND FLUIDS

• Hepatic encephalopathy is treated with lactulose (0.25-0.5 mg/kg PO q6h-q8h) and an antibiotic such as neomycin (10-20 mg/kg PO q8h) or metronidazole (7.5 mg/kg PO q8h-q12h).

• For hepatic coma, discontinue oral medications and food, and give a retention enema q6h composed of neomycin (15 mg/kg) plus lactulose (diluted 1:2 with water; 50-200 ml total).
• For fluid therapy, give 0.9% saline or Lactated Ringer's solution supplemented with 2.5-5% dextrose and 20-30 mEq of KCl/L of maintenance fluid.

CONTRAINDICATIONS

• Avoid drugs that require liver metabolism.
• Avoid alkalinizing agents such as NaHCO3.

PRECAUTIONS

Sedative agents, especially benzodiazapines, may precipitate signs of hepatic encephalopathy.

POSSIBLE INTERACTIONS N/A

ALTERNATE DRUGS N/A

FOLLOW-UP

PATIENT MONITORING

Lactulose and neomycin (PO) and a protein-restricted diet are usually continued for at least 2 to 4 weeks after surgery, depending on individual response. On a long-term basis, many dogs do not require a special diet or medications, especially if a total ligation has been performed.

PREVENTION/AVOIDANCE N/A

POSSIBLE COMPLICATIONS

Only transient improvement in clinical signs may be seen if the portosystemic shunt recanulizes, or if acquired portosystemic shunts form secondary to surgically-induced portal hypertension.

EXPECTED COURSE AND PROGNOSIS

• Total shunt ligation is more likely to be associated with a good clinical outcome in both dogs and cats. • Hepatic function test values (e.g., serum bile acid concentration) often improve but do not return to normal, even in dogs that become clinically normal. • The prognosis in cats that undergo surgery is not as good as in dogs. Clinical signs may recur.

MISCELLANEOUS

ASSOCIATED CONDITIONS

Cryptorchidism

AGE-RELATED FACTORS

A good clinical outcome is more likely if surgery is performed when the patient is <1 year old.

ZOONOTIC POTENTIAL N/A

PREGNANCY N/A

SYNONYMS

• Portovascular anastomosis • Portocaval shunt

SEE ALSO

• Hypertension, Portal • Hepatic Encephalopathy

ABBREVIATIONS

BUN = blood urea nitrogen
CSF = cerebral spinal fluid
CNS = central nervous system

References

Johnson SE. Diseases of the liver. In: Ettinger, SJ, Feldman EC, eds. Textbook of veterinary internal medicine. 4th ed. Philadelphia: W.B. Saunders, 1994.

Author Susan E. Johnson
Consulting Editor Albert E. Jergens

POXVIRUS INFECTION—CATS

BASICS

OVERVIEW
• Member of the genus Orthopoxvirus, family Poxviridae • Enveloped DNA viruses; resistant to drying (viable for years) but readily inactivated by most disinfectants • Geographically limited to Eurasia • Relatively common

SIGNALMENT
• No age, sex, or breed predisposition • Domestic and exotic cats affected

SIGNS
• Multiple circular skin lesions are dominant feature • Usually develop on head, neck, or forelimbs • Primary lesions may be crusted papules, plaques, nodules, crateriform ulcers, or areas of cellulitis/abscessation • Secondary lesions, erythematous nodules that ulcerate and crust, are often widespread and develop after 1-3 weeks • Pruritus is variable. • Systemic signs (20%) may develop—anorexia, lethargy, pyrexia, vomiting, diarrhea, oculonasal discharge, conjunctivitis, and pneumonia

CAUSES AND RISK FACTORS
• Infection thought to be acquired during hunting; most common in young adults and active hunters, often from rural environment • Lesions often develop at the site of a bite wound (presumably inflicted by the prey animal carrying the virus) • Most cases occur in autumn when small wild mammals at maximum population and most active • Severe cutaneous and systemic signs with poor prognosis are frequently associated with immunosuppression (iatrogenic or resulting from coinfection with FeLV or FIV) • Cat-to-cat transmission is rare and causes only subclinical infection.

DIAGNOSIS

DIFFERENTIAL DIAGNOSIS
• Bacterial and fungal infections • Eosinophilic granuloma complex • Neoplasia (particularly mast cell tumor and lymphosarcoma) • Miliary dermatitis

CBC/BIOCHEMISTRY/URINALYSIS
N/A

OTHER LABORATORY TESTS N/A

IMAGING   N/A

OTHER DIAGNOSTIC PROCEDURES
• Virus isolation on scab material provides definitive diagnosis (90% positive) • Electron microscopy of extracts of scab, biopsy specimen, or exudate provides rapid presumptive diagnosis (70% positive) • Skin biopsy—characteristic histologic changes include epidermal hyperplasia and hypertrophy, multilocular vesicle and ulceration, large eosinophilic intracytoplasmic inclusion bodies • Serologic testing demonstrates rising titers (hemagglutination inhibition, virus neutralizing, complement fixation, or ELISA). Titers may remain elevated for months or years.

TREATMENT

• No specific treatment • Supportive treatment (antibiotics, fluids) when necessary • Elizabethan collar may be necessary to prevent self-induced damage.

MEDICATIONS

DRUGS AND FLUIDS
Antibiotics to prevent secondary infections

CONTRAINDICATIONS/POSSIBLE INTERACTIONS
Immunosuppressive agents (e.g., glucocorticoids or megesterol acetate) are absolutely contraindicated because these can induce fatal systemic disease.

FOLLOW-UP

• Most cats recover spontaneously in 1-2 months. • Healing may be delayed by secondary bacterial skin infection. • Prognosis is poor with severe respiratory or pulmonary involvement.

MISCELLANEOUS

• Rare human pox virus infections linked to contact with infected cats with skin lesions; therefore, use basic hygiene precautions (disposable gloves) when handling infected cats. • In humans—may cause painful skin lesion or severe systemic illness, particularly in very young, elderly, and those with preexisting skin condition or immune deficiency) • Natural reservoir hosts, possibly small rodents and cats, are infected incidentally. • No vaccine available, but use of vaccinia virus may be considered for valuable zoo collections; however its effects in nondomestic cats have not been investigated

Reference
Gaskell RM, Bennett M. Feline poxvirus infection. In: Chandler EA, Gaskell CJ, Gaskell RM, eds. Feline medicine and therapeutics. Oxford: Blackwell Scientific Publications, 1994:515-520.
Author J. Paul Woods
Consulting Editor Fred W. Scott

Prolapsed Gland of the Third Eyelid (Cherry Eye)

BASICS

OVERVIEW
A "cherry eye" is a prolapsed gland of the third eyelid. Normally, the gland of the third eyelid is anchored by a fibrous attachment to the periorbita beneath the third eyelid. In several breeds of dogs and cats, this attachment is weak, predisposing the animal to unilateral or bilateral prolapsed gland of the third eyelid.

SIGNALMENT
• Usually seen in young dogs (age 6 months to 2 years) of the following breeds: cocker spaniel, bulldog, beagle, bloodhound, lhasa apso, shih tzu, and other brachycephalic breeds • Rare in cats, but does occur in Burmese and Persian

SIGNS
• Appears as an oval, hyperemic mass protruding from behind the leading edge of the third eyelid • Can be unilateral or bilateral • Accompanying epiphora, hyperemic conjunctiva, or blepharospasm in some animals • Additional swelling and hyperemia caused by environmental irritation and desiccation of the exposed gland

CAUSES AND RISK FACTORS
Congenital weakness of the attachment of the gland of the third eyelid. The inheritance of this condition is not known.

DIAGNOSIS

DIFFERENTIAL DIAGNOSIS
• "Scrolled" or everted cartilage of the third eyelid—this is a condition seen in wiemaraners, great Danes, German short-haired pointers, and other breeds in which the T-shaped cartilage of the third eyelid is rolled away from the surface of the eye instead of conforming to the surface of the cornea. • Neoplasia of the third eyelid—neoplasms of the third eyelid are usually seen in older animals. Squamous cell carcinoma, lymphosarcoma, and fibrosarcoma may involve the third eyelid. An adenoma or adenocarcinoma may originate from the gland of the third eyelid. If a "cherry eye" is seen in an older animal (>7-9 years), a small incisional biopsy is indicated to differentiate neoplasm from prolapsed gland of the third eyelid. • Orbital fat prolapse—orbital fat can dissect anteriorly between the conjunctiva and globe. This occurs occasionally in the medial canthus and simulates a prolapsed gland of the third eyelid.

CBC/BIOCHEMISTRY/URINALYSIS
N/A

OTHER LABORATORY TESTS N/A

IMAGING N/A

OTHER DIAGNOSTIC PROCEDURES
N/A

TREATMENT
• Surgical replacement of the gland (see descriptions of the surgical techniques in the reference below). • Excision of the gland should be avoided because the gland of the third eyelid produces up to 50% of the aqueous tear film. • Animals that have had the gland of the third eyelid removed are at substantial risk for developing keratoconjunctivitis sicca (dry eye) at an older age. • An Elizabethan collar is recommended to prevent self trauma.

MEDICATIONS

DRUGS AND FLUIDS
Topically applied antiinflammatory medications can be used before and after surgery to lessen swelling of the gland.

CONTRAINDICATIONS/POSSIBLE INTERACTIONS N/A

FOLLOW-UP
• Depending on the surgical procedure used to replace the gland, a recurrence rate of 5-20% is common. Re-replacement of the gland is encouraged. • If only one gland is involved initially, the owners should be warned that the other gland may develop a prolapse and that no preventive procedure or medication exists.

MISCELLANEOUS

SYNONYMS Cherry eye

Reference

Stanley RG, Klaswan RL. Modification of the orbital rim anchorage method for surgical replacement of the gland of the third eyelid in dogs. J Am Vet Med Assoc 1984;205:1412–1414.

Author Brian C. Gilger

Consulting Editor Paul E. Miller

PROPTOSIS

BASICS

OVERVIEW
Forward displacement of the globe with the eyelids situated caudal to the eyeball. It is frequently associated with trauma to the head and usually occurs peracutely. It is potentially vision threatening and can cause bradycardia secondary to traction on the retrobulbar muscles and the associated oculocardiac reflex.

SIGNALMENT
• More common in brachiocephalic breeds; however, it can occur in any species or breed if the traumatic force is severe enough.

SIGNS
The globe is situated anterior to the eyelids, such that the eyelids are entrapped posterior to the eyeball.

Possible Accompanying Signs
• Abnormalities in pupil size (dilated or constricted) • Corneal ulceration and desiccation • Intraocular inflammation
• Fractures of the bony orbit or other parts of the skull • Subconjunctival or intraocular hemorrhage • Rupture of the globe • Brain trauma • Trauma to the contralateral eye
• Shock • Other signs associated with trauma

Associated Signs After Repositioning
• Dorso-lateral strabismus (caused by rupture of the inferior oblique and medial rectus muscles) • Blindness • Dilated pupil
• Decreased tear production • Corneal desiccation

CAUSES AND RISK FACTORS
• Trauma is the primary cause; in brachiocephalic breeds, the force necessary may be relatively minor, whereas in dolichocephalic and mesocephalic breeds, the degree of trauma required to cause proptosis is usually severe.
• Rarely, retrobulbar tumor or severe cellulitis or other infection can cause proptosis.

DIAGNOSIS

DIFFERENTIAL DIAGNOSIS
• Buphthalmia—enlargement of the globe. Rarely an acute phenomenon and the eyelids will be positioned correctly, albeit they may not be able to close completely over the enlarged globe. • Exophthalmia—also defined as forward displacement of the globe, but with the eyelids positioned correctly. This may be an acute situation, but it is rarely peracute. The eye cannot be retropulsed due to a mass-effect (i.e., neoplasia, retrobulbar polymyositis, infection, or cellulitis) in the retrobulbar tissues.

CBC/BIOCHEMISTRY/URINALYSIS
Normal unless proptosis is secondary to trauma

OTHER LABORATORY TESTS N/A

IMAGING
Skull radiographs might show fractures if proptosis is secondary to trauma.

OTHER DIAGNOSTIC PROCEDURES
N/A

TREATMENT
• Keep the cornea lubricated. • Assess the animal systemically before surgery on the globe. • As soon as possible, reposition the globe unless there is obvious infection, rupture, desiccation of the globe, or severing of the optic nerve. In these situations, the globe should be enucleated once the animal is stable. • Repositioning—accomplished by placing two or three temporary tarshorraphy mattress sutures through the eyelids, exiting at the lid margins, crossing across to the other lid, entering at the lid margin, and reversing the procedure. A lateral canthotomy may ease tension on the eyelids and allow easier suture placement. While protecting the globe (a lubricated scalpel blade handle can serve this function), the preplaced sutures are tied and the globe is repositioned. The lateral canthotomy is also sutured closed. • If proptosis is caused by a disease other than trauma, the primary condition should be treated.

MEDICATIONS

DRUGS AND FLUIDS

• Systemically and topically applied, broad-spectrum antibiotics are used until sutures are removed (usually sequentially rather than all at once and beginning in 10-14 days).
• Systemically administered corticosteroids are usually used at least initially. These may be continued on a chronic basis in animals with marked periorbital and retrobulbar swelling. • Topically applied corticosteroids may be used in animals with associated intraocular inflammation (uveitis) or hyphema, as long as no corneal or conjunctival ulcers exist. • Atropine is used in animals with intraocular inflammation or hyphema to relieve ciliary spasm and lower the risk of synechiae.
• Treat for shock if present.

CONTRAINDICATIONS/POSSIBLE INTERACTIONS

• Topically applied corticosteroids should not be used in ulcerated eyes. • Systemic corticosteroids should not be used in animals with retrobulbar infection.

 FOLLOW-UP

PATIENT MONITORING

Sutures are usually removed in 10-14 days, and the integrity of the globe, vision, and the cornea is reassessed at that time.

POSSIBLE COMPLICATIONS

• Most animals are left with a dorso-lateral strabismus, although this may improve with time. • Schirmer tear tests should be performed after surgery because some animals will have reduced tear production or neurotropic keratitis.

EXPECTED COURSE AND PROGNOSIS

• Most proptosed eyes can be salvaged; however, most animals with traumatic proptosis will be blind in that eye (more common in the dolichocephalic breeds than in the brachiocephalic breeds). • Normal appearing retinal vessels and optic nerve with normal intraocular pressure and a short time period from occurrence to repair indicate a comparatively favorable prognosis for maintaining vision. • The presence of a positive menace response or direct or consensual pupillary light reflex originating from the injured eye indicates a good prognosis for maintaining vision.
• Pupil size at the time of the injury is not necessarily an accurate prognostic indicator.

 MISCELLANEOUS

SEE ALSO

Orbital diseases (exophthalmus, enophthalmus, strabismus)

Reference

Slatter D. Fundamentals of veterinary ophthalmology. 2nd ed. Philadelphia: WB Saunders, 1990:537–540.
Author Stephanie L. Smedes
Consulting Editor Paul E. Miller

PROSTATIC CYSTS

 BASICS

OVERVIEW

Prostatic and periprostatic cysts are single or multiple, epithelial-lined, serosanguineous fluid-filled structures. The cysts are usually large and are found attached to or in the region of the prostate gland. Although the cause is rarely known, obstruction of prostatic ducts ("retention cyst"), expansion of microscopic cysts of benign prostatic hyperplasia and, rarely, resolution of a hematoma, have been considered.

SIGNALMENT

Adult male intact dogs; age range 2-12 years, mean age 7.5 years

SIGNS

- Dysuria
- Tenesmus
- Urethral discharge
- Abdominal distention

CAUSES AND RISK FACTORS

Androgenic hormones

 DIAGNOSIS

DIFFERENTIAL DIAGNOSIS

- Prostatic abscess
- Distended urinary bladder
- Prostatic neoplasia
- Results of cytologic examination of fluid and ultrasonographic examination usually rule out these diseases. Prostatic neoplasia is occasionally associated with cystic areas within the prostate. The cysts can become secondarily infected, so detection of bacteria should not be overinterpreted.

CBC/BIOCHEMISTRY/URINALYSIS

No abnormalities expected.

OTHER LABORATORY TESTS

- Cytologic examination of cyst fluid (often collected by ultrasound-guided, fine- needle aspiration) usually reveals serosanguineous fluid.
- The fluid should be cultured for bacteria, since it can become infected secondarily.

IMAGING

- Contrast urocystography and ultrasonography will differentiate intra-prostatic versus extra-prostatic locations.
- If calcified cysts are detected by survey radiography (rare), this finding is diagnostic for osteocollageous prostatic retention cyst.

OTHER DIAGNOSTIC PROCEDURES

N/A

 TREATMENT

- If cysts are large, infected, or causing clinical signs, complete surgical excision (if possible) is the treatment of choice. If surgical excision is not feasible, biopsy and marsupialization of the cyst wall is indicated. Concomitant castration is recommended to reduce the development of nonneoplastic prostatic disease.
- If the cysts are small, castration is the treatment of choice. Reevaluation after castration should be done to confirm resolution of the cyst(s).

MEDICATIONS

DRUGS AND FLUIDS N/A

CONTRAINDICATIONS/POSSIBLE INTERACTIONS N/A

FOLLOW-UP

• Ultrasonographic examination at 2-4 week intervals after castration to follow resolution of small cysts.

• Evaluation 2 weeks after surgery may be adequate if no complications arise. If a drainage procedure is used, periodic evaluations (biweekly after discharge from the hospital) are recommended.

• Postoperative urinary incontinence and ascending infection are common potential sequelae of marsupialization; therefore, a guarded prognosis is warranted if complete cyst resection is not possible.

MISCELLANEOUS

Reference

Weaver AD. Discrete prostatic (paraprostatic) cysts in the dog. Vet Rec 1978; 102:435-440.

Author Laine A. Cowan

Consulting Editors Larry G. Adams and Carl A. Osborne

PROSTATITIS AND PROSTATIC ABSCESS

BASICS

DEFINITION
Prostatitis is subdivided into acute bacterial prostatitis, chronic bacterial prostatitis, and prostatic abscess. Fungal and granulomatous prostatitis are extremely rare. Acute and chronic prostatitis refer to the inflammatory process and are differentiated by clinical signs. Prostatic abscess is intraprostatic parenchymal accumulation of purulent inflammatory reactants.

Pathophysiology
• Bacteria usually gain access to the prostate gland by ascending the urethra and overcoming the lower urinary tract host defense mechanisms. Most intact male dogs with bacterial urinary tract infection have the same bacteria present in the prostate gland. However, dogs with prostatic inflammation may have a prostatic infection without evidence of bacteria or inflammation in their urine.
• Incomplete resolution of acute bacterial prostatitis can lead to chronic bacterial prostatitis or abscess formation; however, most dogs with chronic bacterial prostatitis do not have a history of urinary tract or prostatic infection.
• Intraprostatic accumulation of prostatic secretions (e.g., in animals with cystic benign prostatic hyperplasia or squamous metaplasia) can become secondarily infected, resulting in chronic bacterial prostatitis or prostatic abscess.

Systems Affected
• Renal/Urologic—the remainder of the urinary tract can be infected by extension of the urinary tract infection.
• Reproductive—alterations in prostatic fluid in dogs with bacterial prostatitis can cause infertility.
• Gastrointestinal—dogs with acute bacterial prostatitis or abscess often have tenesmus when the prostate gland is large or tender.
• Hepatobiliary—some dogs with prostatic abscess have hyperbilirubinemia and high ALP. Liver alterations are probably caused by sepsis and the resulting cholestasis.
• Peritoneum—focal or generalized peritonitis can develop in animals with prostatic abscessation.

Genetics
No known genetic basis

Incidence/Prevalence
Since many dogs with chronic bacterial prostatitis are asymptomatic, the prevalence is difficult to determine. Among surveys of dogs with prostatic disease, infection was present in 40 %.

Geographic Distribution N/A

SIGNALMENT

Species
Dogs

Breed Predilections
Any breed can be affected. Higher prevalence is found in doberman pinschers than other breeds.

Mean Age and Range
• Dogs with bacterial prostatitis usually are middle-aged
• Mean age, 7-11 years, range, 1-16 years

Predominat Sex
Intact male dogs

SIGNS

Common Signs
• Lethargy
• Blood or pus dripping from the urethra independent of urination
• Tenesmus
• Pyrexia
• Pain

Less Common Signs
• Shock
• Stiff hind limb gait
• Preputial or hind limb edema
Clinical signs are useful in differentiating chronic bacterial prostatitis from acute bacterial prostatitis and prostatic abscess.
• Dogs with chronic bacterial prostatitis are often asymptomatic.
• Dogs with acute bacterial prostatitis are systemically ill, usually depressed and febrile, and the prostate gland is tender on palpation.
• Dogs with prostatic abscess usually have signs similar to those with acute bacterial prostatitis and prostatomegaly. Occasionally, these dogs may have extremes of signs, i.e., they can be asymptomatic or be in septic shock. Occasionally, prostatic abscess impinges on the urethra and causes stranguria.

CAUSES
• Bacterial urinary tract infection in an intact dog usually results in concomitant prostatic infection.
• Gonadal infection (e.g., Brucella canis) is less common than urinary tract infection.
• Systemic mycotic pathogens are rare.

RISK FACTORS
• Impaired host immunity (e.g., corticosteroid administration, diabetes mellitus, urinary retention, urolithiasis, and lower urinary tract anatomic abnormality)
• High urinary/urethral bacterial numbers (e.g., caused by catheterization)
• Intraprostatic accumulation of prostatic secretions, such as cystic benign prostatic hypertrophy or squamous metaplasia, may become infected secondarily.

DIAGNOSIS

DIFFERENTIAL DIAGNOSIS
• Noninfectious prostatic disease (e.g., benign prostatic hypertrophy, neoplasia, prostatic cysts, and periprostatic or perirectal masses or cysts)
• Disease that causes tenesmus (e.g., large intestinal disease)
• Rectal and abdominal palpation helps to localize the problem to the prostate gland. Benign prostatic hypertrophy, cysts, and neoplasia can be ruled out based on results of ultrasonography and cytologic examination or histopathologic evaluation of the prostate gland.

CBC/BIOCHEMISTRY/URINALYSIS
• Chronic bacterial prostatitis—hematuria, pyuria, and bacteriuria in some animals
• Acute bacterial prostatitis—pyuria and bacteriuria +/- hematuria in most animals; neutrophilic leukocytosis with or without a left shift and neutrophil toxicity
• Abscess—pyuria and bacteriuria, +/- hematuria in most animals; neutrophilic leukocytosis with a regenerative left shift, high ALP and bilirubin and hypoglycemia

OTHER LABORATORY TESTS
Prostatic fluid evaluation (i.e., cytologic examination and bacterial culture) confirms the diagnosis of bacterial prostatitis.

IMAGING
Ultrasonographic evaluation of the prostate gland helpful to noninvasively differentiate cavitary (i.e., abscess) from noncavitary (i.e., acute bacterial prostatitis and chronic bacterial prostatitis) bacterial prostatic diseases.

OTHER DIAGNOSTIC PROCEDURES
• In animals with acute bacterial prostatitis or prostatic abscessation, prostatic wash techniques must be used with caution because sepsis or abscess rupture can result.
• Examination of an ultrasound-guided, fine-needle aspiration of a cystic region in the prostate may be used to confirm an abscess if an ejaculate cannot be obtained; however, fine-needle aspiration can also rupture an abscess. If a prostatic abscess is suspected, percutaneous needle biopsy should be avoided.
• In dogs with prostatic abscess that is not systemically ill, a preoperative cystometrogram and urethral pressure profile may be helpful in obtaining baseline measurements if the dog develops urinary incontinence after surgery.

GROSS AND HISTOPATHOLOGIC FINDING
• Biopsies are rarely indicated in animals with acute bacterial prostatitis or chronic bacterial prostatitis.
• Acute bacterial prostatitis—purulent inflammation may be multifocal or centered on the acini or it may invade the stroma. If the prostatic ducts are occluded during resolution of the acute inflammation, multifocal, walled-off, chronic bacterial prostatitis may result. Alternatively, the acute inflammation may cause scarring.
• Chronic bacterial prostatitis—the disease process is usually focal or multifocal; therefore, the diagnostic histologic lesion may be missed if a small sample is obtained. The

typical eosinophilic staining of the columnar epithelium is lost. The acinar lumina and periacinar tissue contain debris and are infiltrated with various numbers of neutrophils and macrophages.
• Prostatic abscess—multifocal accumulations of purulent exudate are seen in the prostatic parenchyma.

TREATMENT

INPATIENT VERSUS OUTPATIENT
Dogs with chronic bacterial prostatitis are treated as outpatients. Hospitalization is required because dogs with acute bacterial prostatitis are systemically ill, and dogs with abscesses require surgery.

ACTIVITY
• No restrictions necessary
• Dogs may be infertile and should not be used for breeding until resolution of the infection.

DIET N/A

CLIENT EDUCATION
• Acute and chronic prostatitis can become recurrent problems (manifested as chronic bacterial prostatitis or abscess).
• Prostatic abscessation can be life-threatening (e.g., sepsis and shock).
• Postoperative urinary incontinence and recurrent infection are common, and repeat surgery may be necessary in dogs with prostatic abscess.

SURGICAL CONSIDERATIONS
• Penrose tube drainage, marsupialization, and partial or complete prostatectomy procedures have been recommended, the latter two requiring special surgical expertise. Preliminary reports on the use of an ultrasonic surgical aspirator (for subtotal prostatectomy in dogs with prostatic abscesses) are promising. Although surgical drainage is essential for treatment of prostatic abscess, problems are associated with each surgical option.
• Many of these dogs are poor anesthetic candidates because of sepsis.
• Dogs with prostatic infection should be castrated (after infection resolves in animals with acute bacterial prostatitis or chronic bacterial prostatitis) to lessen the likelihood of recurrence.

MEDICATIONS

DRUGS AND FLUIDS
• Patients with acute bacterial prostatitis or prostatic abscess usually require parenteral fluid support. If in shock, administer a shock dose (90 ml/kg for 1 hour) of isotonic fluids (0.9% NaCl or lactated Ringer's solution). If the patient is hypoglycemic, glucose should be added to the fluids. Treatment for septic shock (including flunixine and dexamethasone) may be necessary.
• In patients with chronic bacterial prostatitis, the chosen antibiotic must be able to en-

ter the prostatic lumen and must be chosen on the basis of in vitro susceptibility testing. Usually, trimethoprim/sulfonamides or fluoroquinolones are the drugs of choice (since *E. coli* is the most common organism). A minimum of 4 weeks of antimicrobial administration is necessary.
• In patients with acute bacterial prostatitis, a similar antimicrobial choice is appropriate while awaiting the results of the bacterial susceptibility. Penetration into the prostate gland is not as great a concern in these patients. Usually, a 3-week regimen is adequate.
• In patients with acute bacterial prostatitis and prostatic abscess, dogs are usually systemically ill and may be septic; parenteral antibiotics are indicated until the dog is stable. In dogs with prostatic abscess, a minimum of 8 weeks of antimicrobial administration is indicated.
• If the patient has tenesmus, a stool softeners such as psyllium can be used.

CONTRAINDICATIONS
Estrogens and androgens may cause prostatic squamous metaplasia or enlargement, respectively.

PRECAUTIONS
• In sensitive dogs, long-term sulfonamide administration may lead to keratoconjunctivitis sicca.
• An adverse reaction to sulfonamide drugs characterized by a cutaneous or lupus-like syndrome has occurred in a small number of doberman pinschers.

POSSIBLE INTERACTIONS None
ALTERNATIVE DRUGS
• If the bacteria are not sensitive to the drugs listed, other antimicrobials that enter the prostate gland include chloramphenicol, erythromycin, and clindamycin.
• Colloids ± hypertonic saline may be used for treatment of septic shock.

FOLLOW-UP

PATIENT MONITORING
• Because of the problem of recurrent infection, repeat prostatic fluid culture is indicated at 1, 4, and 8 weeks after completion of the antimicrobial regimen.
• Additionally, dogs treated for prostatic abscess should be reevaluated every 2 weeks until the problem resolves. Ultrasound imaging, urine analysis, prostatic fluid analysis, and a CBC usually indicated at each reevaluation.

PREVENTION/AVOIDANCE
Castration, by causing prostatic involution, is the best method of preventing recurrence.

POSSIBLE COMPLICATIONS
• Recurrent urinary tract infections
• Urinary incontinence (primarily associated with prostatic abscess)
• Infected stoma or edema (associated with some prostatic drainage procedures)

EXPECTED COURSE AND PROGNOSIS
• Other than the potential for recurrent prostatic infection, acute bacterial prostatitis and

chronic bacterial prostatitis usually respond well to treatment.
• Dogs with prostatic abscesses often need prolonged follow-up and reassessment.
• Some dogs that are incontinent immediately after surgery may regain partial or complete urinary control with drug therapy.

MISCELLANEOUS

ASSOCIATED CONDITIONS
Urinary tract infection, urocystolithiasis, and chronic glucocorticoid exposure (iatrogenic or hyperadrenocorticism) may be associated with chronic bacterial prostatitis.

AGE- RELATED FACTORS
Sexually mature dogs

ZOONOTIC POTENTIAL
Brucella canis has been isolated from dogs with prostatic infection (rare)

PREGNANCY N/A

SYNONYMS None

SEE ALSO
• Benign prostatic hyperplasia
• Dysuria and pollakiuria
• Hematuria
• Incontinence, urinary
• Lower urinary tract infection
• Prostatic cysts
• Prostatomegaly
• Pyelonephritis
• Pyuria
• Urine retention, functional
• Urinary tract obstruction

References

Krawiec DR, Heflin D: Study of prostatic disease in dogs: 177 cases (1981-1986) J Am Vet Med Assoc 1992; 200:1119-1122.

Mullen HS, Matthiesen DT, Scavelli TD: Results of surgery and postoperative complications in 92 dogs treated for prostatic abscessation by a multiplepenrose drain technique. J Am Anim Hosp Assoc 1990; 26:369-379.

Olson PN, Wrigley RH, Thrall MA, et al. Disorders of the canine prostate gland: pathogenesis, diagnosis, and medical therapy. Comp Cont Ed Pract Vet 1987; 9:613-624.

Feeney DA, Johnston GR, Klausner JS, et al. Canine prostatic disease—comparison of ultrasonographic appearance with morphologic and microbiologic findings: 30 cases (1981-1985). J Am Vet Med Assoc 1987; 190:1027-1034.

Rawlings CA, Crowell WA, Barsanti JA, et al. Intracapsular subtotal prostatectomyin normal dogs: use of an ultrasonic surgical aspirator. Vet Surg 1994; 23:182-189.

Author Laine A. Cowan

Consulting Editors Larry G. Adams and Carl A. Osborne

PROTEIN-LOSING ENTEROPATHIES

BASICS

DEFINITION
A group of diseases characterized by excessive loss of serum proteins into the intestinal tract. The diseases associated with protein-losing enteropathy (PLE) include primary gastrointestinal diseases as well as generalized disorders such as congestive heart failure, nephrotic syndrome, and metastatic neoplasia.

Pathophysiology
The intestines serve as a route for catabolism of serum proteins. The capillaries in the intestinal mucosa have large fenestrations which allow macromolecules to enter the interstitial space. Once serum proteins leak into the gastrointestinal tract through these fenestrations, the proteins are rapidly digested into constituent amino acids, and these amino acids can be reabsorbed and used for synthesis of new proteins. In the dog, two-thirds of normal protein loss occurs through the small intestine. If this normal protein loss is accelerated by mucosal disease processes or by obstruction of lymphatic outflow from the intestines, protein, including both albumin and globulins, is lost. In response to the increased protein loss through the intestines, the liver will increase production of albumin, but the liver is unable to increase albumin synthesis to more than twice normal production. When the protein loss exceeds protein synthesis, hypoproteinemia results. Hypoproteinemia causes decreased plasma oncotic pressure which alters body fluid hemodynamics, leading to peripheral edema or body cavity effusions.

Systems Affected
- Gastrointestinal - diarrhea, vomiting, ascites
- Skin/Exocrine - subcutaneous edema
- Respiratory - pleural effusion

Genetics
Breeds of dogs with a familial predisposition for intestinal lymphangiectasia include soft-coated Wheaten terriers, basenjis, and Lundehunds

Incidence/Prevalence
True incidence unknown

Geographic Distribution N/A

SIGNALMENT

Species
Dog and cat

Breed Predilection
Breeds of dogs with a familial predisposition for intestinal lymphangiectasia include soft-coated Wheaten terriers, basenjis, and Lundehunds, and an increased prevalence for intestinal lymphangiectasia has been reported in Yorkshire terriers

Mean Age And Range Any age

Predominant Sex None

SIGNS
Clinical signs are variable and often include:
- Diarrhea - chronic, intermittent of watery to semi-solid consistency • Lethargy • Weight loss • Ascites • Dependent edema • Respiratory difficulty from pleural effusion • Vomiting (uncommon) • Thickened bowel loops

CAUSES

Disorders of Lymphatics
- Intestinal lymphangiectasia • Neoplasia (lymphosarcoma) • Granuloma of the small bowel or mesentery • Congestive heart failure: constrictive pericarditis, Budd-Chiari syndrome

Diseases Associated With Increased Mucosal Permeability or Mucosal Ulceration
- Lymphoplasmacytic enteritis • Intestinal neoplasia: lymphosarcoma, carcinoma • Acute or chronic enteritis • Intussusception, especially chronic • Chronic foreign body • Ulcerative gastritis/enteritis • Histoplasmosis • Granulomatous enteritis • Intestinal parasitism: hookworms, whipworms, coccidia • Hemorrhagic gastroenteritis • Immune-mediated diseases: food allergies, eosinophilic gastroenteritis, gluten-induced enteropathies

RISK FACTORS
- Disorders of lymphatics • Heart disease • Gastrointestinal disease

DIAGNOSIS

DIFFERENTIAL DIAGNOSIS
- Must differentiate from other causes of hypoproteinemia and dependent edema. • Severe hepatic disease causing reduced hepatic synthesis of albumin. Globulins will often be normal or increased. • Glomerulonephritis or renal amyloidosis causing excessive loss of albumin. Proteinuria should be detected on urinalysis. • Acute or chronic blood loss. • Inadequate protein intake (i.e., starvation) is a rare cause of hypoproteinemia.

CBC/BIOCHEMISTRY/URINALYSIS
- Anemia may be present • Lymphopenia will be seen with lymphangiectasia. • Hypoalbuminemia and hypoglobulinemia (panhypoproteinemia) Hypocalcemia secondary to hypoalbuminemia • Hypocholesterolemia may be present • Urinalysis should be normal.

OTHER LABORATORY TESTS
- 3-5 fecal examinations should be performed to rule out parasitism, and they should be negative. Serum protein electrophoresis can be performed to quantitate and identify protein loss. Gastrointestinal protein loss will be characterized by loss of albumin and globulins. Liver disease will be characterized by low levels of albumin with normal or high globulins, and renal disease characteristically causes hypoalbuminemia with normal serum globulins. • Urine protein:creatinine ratio can be performed to rule-out proteinuria. • Serum bile acids (pre- and post-prandial) or an ammonia tolerance test can be performed to assess hepatic function. • Specific gastrointestinal function tests can be performed, including Sudan stains to detect steatorrhea, oral d-xylose test to detect poor absorption of carbohydrates, and plasma turbidity test to detect abnormal fat absorption. • Cytologic examination of feces and rectal mucosal smears may reveal histoplasmosis. • Definitive localization of protein loss through the gastrointestinal tract can be obtained through administration of ^{15}Cr-labelled albumin. • Fecal alpha$_1$-antiprotease, a plasma protein that resists proteolytic degradation in the gastrointestinal tract, concentration can be measured. The concentration should be high with PLE.

IMAGING
- Survey thoracic and abdominal radiographs are taken to rule out causes of PLE such as cardiac disease, fungal disease, and intestinal obstruction. • Cardiac ultrasound can be performed to rule out cardiac disease. • Upper gastrointestinal contrast study can be performed to look for infiltrative bowel diseases or masses.

OTHER DIAGNOSTIC PROCEDURES
- Endoscopy allows for mucosal visualization and biopsy. • Laparotomy allows for surgical biopsies of intestines and lymph nodes to be obtained.

TREATMENT

INPATIENT VERSUS OUTPATIENT
Usually outpatient

ACTIVITY
Normal

DIET
Diet is usually modified, depending on the underlying cause of PLE.

CLIENT EDUCATION
Owners should be prepared for long-term therapy as spontaneous cures are rare.

SURGICAL CONSIDERATIONS
Hypoalbuminemia increases post-operative morbidity due to slow wound healing. Some causes of PLE (e.g., intestinal neoplasia, intussusception, chronic foreign body) require surgical intervention.

MEDICATIONS

DRUGS AND FLUIDS
- Diuretics such as furosemide can be used to control edema and pleural effusion although they do not work well because of decreased plasma oncotic pressure.

• Plasma transfusions, dextrans or Hetastarch® can be given to increase plasma oncotic pressure when clinical signs from edema or effusion are severe. These agents are administered at a dose of 10-20 ml/kg intravenously.

• Anti-ulcer medications (e.g. cimetidine or ranitidine) can be used if gastric ulcers are present.

• Intestinal lymphangiectasia, the most common lesion in PLE, is treated by feeding a low-fat diet and by supplementing fat with medium-chain triglycerides (MCTs). Commercial sources of MCTs are MCT oil® (Mead Johnson, Evansville, IN) or Portagen® (Mead Johnson, Evansville, IN). Corticosteroids can be used if dietary therapy is unsuccessful or if no underlying cause for intestinal lymphangiectasia can be found.

• Intestinal lymphosarcoma treatment includes the use of chemotherapeutic agents.

• Lymphoplasmacytic enteritis treatment includes dietary modification and anti-inflammatory drugs. In addition, antibiotics such as metronidazole, sulfasalazine, or tylosin may be effective.

• Immune-mediated disease: Eosinophilic gastroenteritis is treated by feeding a hypoallergenic diet and by administering corticosteroids. Gluten-induced enteropathy is treated by feeding a high-protein diet with exclusion of glutens which are contained in wheat, rye, barley, oats, and buckwheat. Alternatively, corticosteroids or other immunosuppressive agents can be used.

CONTRAINDICATIONS N/A

PRECAUTIONS N/A

POSSIBLE INTERACTIONS N/A

ALTERNATE DRUGS N/A

 FOLLOW-UP

PATIENT MONITORING
Monitor body weight, serum protein concentration, and evidence of return of clinical signs (pleural effusion, ascites, edema) every 7-14 days.

PREVENTION/AVOIDANCE N/A

POSSIBLE COMPLICATIONS
• Respiratory difficulty from pleural effusion.
• Severe protein-calorie malnutrition.
• Intractable diarrhea. • Prognosis is guarded as primary disease often can not be cured.

EXPECTED COURSE AND PROGNOSIS
Varies considerably with underlying cause

 MISCELLANEOUS

ASSOCIATED CONDITIONS
Soft-coated Wheaten terriers may have protein-losing nephropathy in conjunction with PLE.

AGE RELATED FACTORS N/A

ZOONOTIC POTENTIAL
Histoplasmosis, hookworms, and coccidia are potentially zoonotic to humans.

PREGNANCY N/A

SYNONYMS N/A

SEE ALSO
See Causes

ABBREVIATIONS
PLE = protein losing enteropathy

References
Fossum TW, Sherding RG, Zack PM, et al. Intestinal lymphangiectasia associated with chylothorax in two dogs. J Am Vet Med Assoc 1987;190:61-64.
Fossum TW. Protein-losing enteropathy. Semin Vet Med Surg (Sm Anim) 1989;4:219-225.
Meschter CL, Rakich PM, Tyler DE. Intestinal lymphangiectasia with lipogranulomatous lymphangitis in a dog. J Am Vet Med Assoc 1987;190:427-430.
Tams TR, Twedt DC. Canine protein-losing gastroenteropathy syndrome. Compend Contin Educ Pract Vet 1981;3:105-114.
Author Mollyann Holland
Consulting Editor Brent D. Jones

PSEUDORABIES VIRUS INFECTION

BASICS

OVERVIEW
•Pseudorabies is an uncommon but highly fatal disease of dogs and cats, usually occurring in animals that have contact with swine. Pseudorabies is characterized by sudden death, often without characteristic signs, or with signs that include hypersalivation, intense pruritus, and neurologic signs.

SIGNALMENT
Domestic and exotic dogs and cats and other domestic animals, including swine, cattle, sheep, and goats. Farm dogs and cats primarily, with no breed or age predilection.

SIGNS
• Sudden death • Hypersalivation, rapid and labored breathing, fever, and vomiting • Neurologic signs, including depression and lethargy, ataxia, convulsions, reluctancy to move, recumbency, intense pruritus and self-mutilation, coma, and death

CAUSES AND RISK FACTORS
• An alphaherpesvirus, called pseudorabies virus (PRV) or herpesvirus suid. • Contact with swine • Eating contaminated, uncooked meat or offal from swine

DIAGNOSIS

DIFFERENTIAL DIAGNOSIS
• Rabies—in the "furious" form of rabies, dog or cat will attack anything that moves. No pruritus or sudden death. Immuno-fluorescent antibody test of brain is positive. • Canine distemper—no increased salivation, sudden death, or personality change. Respiratory and GI signs common. • Poisoning (organophosphate, lead, strychnine, inorganic arsenic)—no pruritus or personality change. • History of exposure to toxin, and signs consistent with toxicity

CBC/BIOCHEMISTRY/URINALYSIS
N/A

OTHER LABORATORY TESTS
Animal (rabbit) inoculation

IMAGING N/A

OTHER DIAGNOSTIC PROCEDURES
• Immunofluorescent antibody test of brain tissue • Histopathology of tissues reveal intranuclear inclusions in neurologic tissue • Viral isolation from affected tissues

TREATMENT
There is no treatment for this disease in dogs and cats, other than general supportive therapy.

MEDICATIONS

DRUGS AND FLUIDS
None specific. Treatment is not effective.

CONTRAINDICATIONS/POSSIBLE INTERACTIONS
None

FOLLOW-UP
Because of extremely high fatality rate, there generally is no follow-up.

MISCELLANEOUS
• Association with swine contact or ingestion of contaminated meat • Mild zoonotic potential from PRV

ABBREVIATIONS
PRV = pseudorabies virus

References

Gustafson DP. Pseudorabies (Aujeszky's disease, mad itch, infectious bulbar paralysis). In: Holzworth J, ed. Diseases of the cat. Philadelphia: WB Saunders, 1987:242-246.

Hawkins BA, Olson GR. Clinical signs of pseudorabies in the dog and cat: a review of 40 cases. Iowa State Univ Vet 1985;47(2):116-119.

Author Fred W. Scott

Consulting Editor Fred W. Scott

PUG ENCEPHALITIS (MENINGOENCEPHALITIS)

BASICS

OVERVIEW
• Sporadic disorder of pugs predominantly affecting the cerebral hemispheres and meninges • Causes seizure activity

SIGNALMENT
• Adolescent and mature dogs • Males and females

SIGNS
• Clinical signs refer to the cerebrum and meninges. • Seizure activity is by far the most common reason for examination. • Other common signs are abnormal mentation, circling, head pressing, and central blindness. • Cervical rigidity and resistance to passive head and neck movements also observed and reflect the meningeal • Two clinical courses—one that evolves acutely within 2 weeks and one that affects dogs for several months • The seizure history varies from infrequent, recurrent, single seizures to cluster seizures to status epilepticus. • Some dogs are normal between seizures.

CAUSES AND RISK FACTORS
• Activation of a latent canine herpesvirus type I infection after an initial neonatal infection has been speculated as a cause. • Genetic predisposition is likely.

DIAGNOSIS

DIFFERENTIAL DIAGNOSIS
• Infectious encephalitides can be differentiated by the frequent multisystemic involvement of these infections, hematologic testing, CSF analysis and culture, and serologic testing. • A brain tumor can be differentiated by CSF analysis and brain imaging. • Granulomatous meningoencephalitis can be differentiated by CSF analysis. • Metabolic encephalopathies can be differentiated on the basis of normal results of liver function tests and CSF analysis and normal blood glucose and blood urea concentrations. • Toxic encephalopathy can be differentiated by a history of access and CSF analysis.

CBC/BIOCHEMISTRY/URINALYSIS
Results normal

OTHER LABORATORY TESTS N/A

IMAGING N/A

OTHER DIAGNOSTIC PROCEDURES
• CSF analysis—pleocytosis with predominantly (70-98%) small lymphocytes and high protein concentration • Histopathologic findings—nonsuppurative necrotizing meningoencephalitis predominantly of the cerebral hemispheres and leptomeninges

TREATMENT
• Hospitalize for treatment
• Treat seizure activity rapidly and aggressively.
• Look for a treatable cause.

MEDICATIONS

DRUGS AND FLUIDS
• No effective treatment available according to the reported cases. However, the predominance of small lymphocytes on CSF analysis and clinical experience indicate that steroid administration may be beneficial, at least temporarily.
• Treatment with anticonvulsants may reduce severity and frequency of seizures.

CONTRAINDICATIONS/POSSIBLE INTERACTIONS N/A

FOLLOW-UP
• Acutely affected dogs with seizures and cerebral cortical abnormalities often progress to status epilepticus or coma within 7 days.
• Chronically affected dogs that have seizures but are normal interictally may live for 6 months or more if seizures are controlled by anticonvulsant therapy.

MISCELLANEOUS

Reference

Cordy DR, Holiday TA. A necrotizing meningoencephalitis of pug dogs. Vet Pathol 1989;26:191-194.

Author Susan M. Taylor
Consulting Editor Joane M. Parent

PULMONARY CONTUSIONS

BASICS

OVERVIEW
• Pulmonary contusions consist of hemorrhage in the lung parenchyma caused by tearing and crushing during direct trauma to the thorax. Relatively small volumes of blood in the lung may significantly compromise lung function by causing ventilation-perfusion mismatch. • In the shock patient with capillary damage, the hemorrhage may be accompanied by pulmonary edema after fluid resuscitation.

SIGNALMENT
Pulmonary contusions are seen in both dogs and cats, with no specific breed, age, or sex predilection.

SIGNS
• Historical findings consistent with blunt trauma • Tachypnea • Increased respiratory effort • Postural adaptations to respiratory distress • Cyanotic or pale mucous membranes • Auscultation of harsh bronchovesicular sounds or crackles • Expectoration of blood or blood-tinged fluid

CAUSES AND RISK FACTORS
• Blunt trauma • Motor vehicle accidents • Falls from a height • Abuse (beating) • Coagulopathy • Von Willebrand factor deficiency

DIAGNOSIS

DIFFERENTIAL DIAGNOSIS
• Hemothorax may cause dull lung sounds and pleural effusion on thoracic radiographs. • Pneumothorax may cause dull lung sounds and pleural air on thoracic radiographs. • Diaphragmatic hernia may be distinguished radiographically. • Coagulopathies may cause pulmonary hemorrhage. These can be distinguished by coagulation testing and platelet counts. • Acute onset of pulmonary hemorrhage can be a feature of some neoplasms such as hemangiosarcoma. • Acute onset of pulmonary hemorrhage occasionally occurs as a result of pulmonary infarction in patients with bacterial endocarditis or heartworm disease.

CBC/BIOCHEMISTRY/URINALYSIS
• Complete blood count may reveal anemia or mature neutrophilia. • Serum chemistry profile may demonstrate hypoproteinemia indicating blood loss or reveal damage to other organ systems. • Urinalysis usually is normal.

OTHER LABORATORY TESTS N/A

IMAGING
Thoracic radiographs should always be performed in trauma cases to rule out hemothorax, pneumothorax, or diaphragmatic hernia. If pulmonary contusions are present, there are usually patchy areas of alveolar pattern, which may be focal or asymmetrical.

OTHER DIAGNOSTIC PROCEDURES
• Transtracheal wash may demonstrate the presence of excessive numbers of erythrocytes and macrophages. • Pulse oximetry or arterial blood gas analysis may confirm the presence of hypoxemia.

TREATMENT
• Most patients with pulmonary contusions should be hospitalized for stabilization. They may have sustained injuries to other organ systems that also require diagnosis and treatment. Activity should be restricted, and such animals should be observed carefully for deterioration of respiratory function during the first 24 hours after the traumatic episode. Frequent ECG monitoring is also recommended because patients with thoracic trauma are at risk for traumatic myocarditis. • There is no medical treatment available that will cause resolution of pulmonary contusions. Management of such patients is therefore based on supportive care. The clinician should support respiratory function, stabilize cardiovascular function and resuscitate if necessary, and assess injuries to other organ systems.

MEDICATIONS

DRUGS AND FLUIDS

• Oxygen supplementation should be considered if hypoxia is present. The most severely affected animals may require intubation and positive pressure ventilation. • In the shock patient, fluid therapy may be required to support cardiovascular function. If possible, fluid therapy should be conservative because it may lead to deterioration of pulmonary function by exacerbating pulmonary edema. To minimize edema development, synthetic colloids should be considered if hypoproteinemia is present. • Blood or plasma transfusions should be considered if hemorrhage has resulted in anemia or if a coagulopathy is present. • Diuretics such as furosemide (0.5-2 mg/kg IV or IM) can be administered when hemorrhage is accompanied by edema and respiratory distress is severe.

CONTRAINDICATIONS/POSSIBLE INTERACTIONS

Diuretics are of no value in the early stages of pulmonary contusions and, in fact, can be harmful. By causing diuresis, diuretics decrease the intravascular volume, which is contraindicated in the shock patient. After fluid resuscitation, however, some pulmonary edema may accompany hemorrhage, and the edema may at that time be responsive to diuretics.

 FOLLOW-UP

PATIENT MONITORING

Should include observation of respiratory rate and effort, mucous membrane color, heart rate and pulse quality, auscultation, measurement of packed cell volume and total solids, and other parameters for 24 hours. Radiographs can be repeated in 48 hours to ensure that the contusions are resolving.

PREVENTION AND AVOIDANCE

Relies on appropriate restraint of the animal to prevent exposure to trauma

POSSIBLE COMPLICATIONS

• Development of bacterial pneumonia as a result of systemic immunosuppression, reduced pulmonary defenses, and aspiration of gastrointestinal tract contents • Development of a moist productive cough and failure to improve within 48 hours should provoke suspicion of pneumonia. • Less commonly, animals with severe shock may develop adult respiratory distress syndrome.

EXPECTED COURSE AND PROGNOSIS

• Most animals with pulmonary contusions show deterioration of respiratory function during the initial 12-24 hours after trauma, and then gradually improve. In general, clinical improvement in respiratory status occurs within 48 hours, with a more gradual resolution of radiographic lesions.
• If the animal has failed to improve after 48 hours, the clinician should evaluate the animal for complications or concurrent diseases.

 MISCELLANEOUS

ASSOCIATED CONDITIONS

• Fractured ribs • Flail chest • Ruptured trachea, bronchi, or esophagus • Cardiac arrhythmias (ventricular) • Other possible complications of trauma

Reference

Hackner SG. The emergency management of traumatic pulmonary contusions. Compend Cont Ed Pract Vet (in press).

Author Lesley G. King

Consulting Editors Lynelle Johnson and Bradley L. Moses

PULMONARY EDEMA

BASICS

DEFINITION
An accumulation of extravascular fluid in the pulmonary interstitial and alveolar spaces

PATHOPHYSIOLOGY
In normal lungs, fluid exudes from the pulmonary capillaries into the interstitial space and is returned to the circulation via the pulmonary lymphatic vessels. This dynamic process is dependent upon capillary and interstitial hydrostatic and oncotic pressures and upon capillary and alveolar epithelial permeability. When fluid formation exceeds fluid removal by the lymphatic vessels, pulmonary edema results. When edema becomes clinically important, pulmonary gas exchange is impaired and clinical signs develop.

SYSTEMS AFFECTED
• Pulmonary • Cardiovascular

SIGNALMENT
• Dogs and cats • Immature and mature animals with cardiac disease • Animals of any age affected by noncardiac causes.

SIGNS

General Comments
Clinical signs depend upon the cause and severity of edema and the rapidity of onset.

Historical Findings
• Tachypnea • Dyspnea • Dry cough (uncommon in cats) • Open mouth breathing (common in cats)

Physical Examination Findings
• No auscultable abnormalities • Crackles at end inspiration • Crackles and wheezes during inspiration and expiration • Pink tinged frothy secretions from nares and mouth (end stage) • Cardiac murmurs, gallops, and arrhythmias (animals with cardiogenic pulmonary edema)

CAUSES

High Capillary Hydrostatic Pressure
• Cardiogenic—cardiomyopathy (i.e., dilated, hypertrophic, intermediate, and restrictive), mitral valvular endocardiosis, ruptured chordae tendineae, thyrotoxicosis, endocarditis, aortic valve disease, patent ductus arteriosus, ventral septal defect, and arrhythmias • Non-cardiogenic—overzealous intravenous fluid administration

Low Capillary Oncotic Pressure
• Hypoproteinemia • Overzealous intravenous fluid administration

High Capillary or Alveolar Epithelial Permeability
• Pneumonia • Toxins (e.g., smoke, gastric contents, and snake venom) • Heatstroke, disseminated intravascular coagulation • Near drowning • Circulating endotoxins

High Negative Intrathoracic or Interstitial Pressure
Upper airway obstruction • Reexpansion of atelectatic lung

Unknown Mechanisms
Neurogenic (e.g., seizures, head trauma, and electrocution)

RISK FACTORS
Heart disease

DIAGNOSIS

DIFFERENTIAL DIAGNOSIS
• Must differentiate from other causes of coughing or dyspnea such as upper airway obstruction, tracheitis, bronchitis, pneumonia, heartworm disease, collapsing trachea, respiratory foreign body, and neoplasia. Thoracic radiographs and hematologic testing will help exclude these. • Many animals with cardiogenic pulmonary edema have other signs of heart disease (e.g., murmur, arrhythmias, and tachycardia). • The character of the cough (i.e., dry versus wet) and dyspnea (i.e., expiratory versus inspiratory) may better define the cause of the clinical signs.

CBC/BIOCHEMISTRY/URINALYSIS
• Helpful in evaluating noncardiogenic causes of pulmonary edema. • Generally normal in animals with cardiogenic edema. May see stress leukogram, prerenal azotemia, and high liver enzymes as a result of passive congestion.

OTHER LABORATORY TESTS
Arterial blood gas analysis documents hypoxemia, but this does not correlate well with the severity of pulmonary edema.

IMAGING

Thoracic Radiographic Findings
• Radiographic signs of pulmonary edema vary with the severity and cause of the edema. • An interstitial or alveolar lung pattern is characteristic of pulmonary edema. • Cardiogenic pulmonary edema often associated with cardiomegaly (most often left atrium or auricular appendage) and pulmonary venous enlargement. Early cardiogenic pulmonary edema in dogs is often situated in the hilar region. In animals with advanced heart failure, the edema becomes diffuse. The edema is usually symmetrical, but may start out in the right caudal lung lobe. In cats, pulmonary edema is usually patchy and diffuse. • Neurogenic pulmonary edema is often situated in the caudal lung field.

Echocardiography
May confirm cardiac disease, but it cannot identify pulmonary edema.

OTHER DIAGNOSTIC PROCEDURES
Pulmonary capillary wedge pressure, an indicator of left atrial pressure, can be measured

with a Swan Ganz catheter temporarily "wedged" in the pulmonary artery. High pressure (> 20-25 mmHg) is usually found in animals with cardiogenic pulmonary edema. Central venous pressure not always high in animals with left heart failure.

GROSS AND HISTOPATHOLOGIC FINDINGS N/A

TREATMENT
• If the animal has respiratory distress, minimal handling and supplemental oxygen (< 50%) are indicated. Diagnostics should be postponed until the animal's condition is more stable. Intubate and ventilate if necessary.
• If the animal is stable and the edema is not severe, treat as an outpatient.
• Cage rest or exercise restriction is recommended until the edema is resolved.
• The sodium content of the diet should be restricted (< 13 mg/kg/day; < 90 mg/100 grams of dry food) in patients with cardiogenic edema.

MEDICATIONS

DRUGS AND FLUIDS

To Reduce Edema
• Diuretics (e.g., furosemide and hydrochlorothiazide)
• Vasodilators (e.g., nitroglycerin, nitroprusside, and enalapril)

To Improve Oxygen Delivery to Alveoli (May Be Useful)
Bronchodilators (e.g., aminophylline, theophylline, terbutaline)

To Reduce Anxiety (Use Only If Necessary)
• Morphine (dogs only)
• Acepromazine
• Diazepam

To Increase Capillary Oncotic Pressure
• Plasma
• Intravenous colloids (e.g., dextran and hetastarch)

To Treat High Vascular Permeability
• Treat the underlying cause.
• Consider corticosteroids.

CONTRAINDICATIONS
• Unless specifically indicated, drugs with negative inotropic actions should not be used in animals with cardiogenic pulmonary edema.
• Morphine is contraindicated in animals with neurogenic pulmonary edema.

PRECAUTIONS
Reduced cardiac output, hypotension, and prerenal azotemia may occur with overzealous use of diuretic or vasodilator.

POSSIBLE INTERACTIONS N/A

ALTERNATE DRUGS

The addition of a thiazide diuretic to furosemide may be beneficial in animals with refractory cardiogenic pulmonary edema.

FOLLOW-UP

PATIENT MONITORING

Thoracic radiographs to assess treatment

POSSIBLE COMPLICATIONS

Cardiogenic Pulmonary Edema

• Often recurs since the inciting cause is rarely eliminated. • Response to treatment a good indicator of short-term prognosis. • Long-term prognosis guarded because of underlying disease.

MISCELLANEOUS

ASSOCIATED CONDITIONS N/A

AGE RELATED FACTORS N/A

ZOONOTIC POTENTIAL N/A

PREGNANCY N/A

SYNONYMS Pulmonary congestion

SEE ALSO

• Congestive Heart Failure, Left Sided
• Cough • Dyspnea • Pulmonary Edema, Noncardiogenic

ABBREVIATIONS

DIC= disseminated intravascular coagulation
PDA= patent ductus arteriosus
VSD= ventricular septal defect

References

Harpster N. Pulmonary edema. In: Kirk RW, ed. Current veterinary therapy X. Philadelphia: WB Saunders, 1989.

Kuehn NF, Roudebush P. Pulmonary edema. In: Allen DG, ed. Small animal medicine. Philadelphia: JB Lippincott, 1991.

Bonagura JD, Lehmkuhl LB. Fluid and diuretic therapy in heart failure. In: DiBartola SP, ed. Fluid therapy in small animal practice. Philadelphia: WB Saunders, 1992.

Ware W, Bonagura JB. Pulmonary edema. In: Fox PR, ed. Canine and feline cardiology. New York: Churchill Livingstone, 1988.

Author Patti S. Snyder
Consulting Editors Larry P. Tilley and Francis W. K. Smith, Jr.

PULMONARY EDEMA, NONCARDIOGENIC

BASICS

DEFINITION
Noncardiogenic pulmonary edema (NPE) is the accumulation of edema fluid in the pulmonary interstitium and alveoli in the absence of heart disease.

Pathophysiology
• The common etiology of all forms of NPE is increased pulmonary vascular permeability, which allows leakage of fluid into the interstitium and alveoli. If severe, this is followed by an inflammatory response and accumulation of neutrophils and macrophages in the interstitium and alveoli. In the most severely affected patients, the inflammatory changes are referred to as adult respiratory distress syndrome (ARDS).
• A variety of mechanisms may contribute to changes in pulmonary vascular permeability:
• Profound but transient increases in pulmonary arterial pressure caused by massive sympathetic discharge. Systemic release of catecholamines may lead to systemic vasoconstriction, which temporarily shunts blood into the pulmonary circulation and leads to transient pulmonary circulatory overload and endothelial damage. This mechanism probably occurs in neurogenic edema, electric cord bites, and upper airway obstruction.
• Increased intrathoracic negative pressure induced by inspiratory attempts against an airway obstruction • Pulmonary manifestation of a generalized inflammatory response (SIRS) that occurs in sepsis or pancreatitis
• All forms of NPE are similar, in that the inciting insult may trigger a cascade inflammatory response that often worsens over a 24-hour period. The severity of clinical manifestations is variable, ranging from mild to severe. The most seriously affected animals may progress from normality to death in as little as a couple of hours after the incident.

Systems Affected
• Respiratory • Hemic/lymphatic/immune—if severe and causing respiratory failure, this form of pulmonary edema may be associated with disseminated intravascular coagulation
• Cardiovascular—hypotension, tachycardia, and shock • Renal/urologic—acute renal failure

Genetics Unknown

Incidence/Prevalence Uncommon

Geographic Distribution N/A

SIGNALMENT

Species
Mainly dogs, occasionally cats

Breed Predilections
No specific breed predilection, although brachycephalic dogs are more prone to airway obstruction

Mean Age and Range
Higher incidence of NPE in puppies less than 1 year old associated with strangulation, head trauma, and electric cord bites; and in older animals associated with laryngeal obstruction and neoplasia

Predominant Sex None

SIGNS

General Comments
• Associated clinical findings vary depending on the underlying cause of noncardiogenic pulmonary edema. • Clinical findings also vary depending on the severity of pulmonary edema.

Historical Findings
• History of a predisposing cause (hit by car, electric cord bite) • Acute onset of dyspnea

Physical Examination Findings
• Dyspnea—increased respiratory rate and effort, open-mouthed breathing • Postural adaptations to respiratory distress, if severe
• Unwillingness to lie down • Pale or cyanotic mucous membranes • Auscultation may reveal harsh sounds (early/mild) or generalized crackles (late/severe) • Expectoration of pink froth or bubbles, and, if intubated, large volumes of bloody fluid may flow out through the endotracheal tube • Normal cardiac auscultation, although some have arrhythmias and most are tachycardic

CAUSES
• Upper airway obstruction (laryngeal paralysis, choke chain injury, mass, abscess, others)
• Electric cord bite • Acute neurologic disease (head trauma, prolonged seizures) • Smoke inhalation • Pancreatitis, sepsis, and endotoxemia; SIRS • Organ torsion • Anaphylaxis in cats

RISK FACTORS
• Hypoproteinemia • Crystalloid fluid resuscitation

DIAGNOSIS

DIFFERENTIAL DIAGNOSIS
• Cardiogenic pulmonary • Pulmonary infections such as bacterial, viral, or fungal pneumonia • Pulmonary neoplasia • Pulmonary hemorrhage • Pulmonary thromboembolism

CBC/BIOCHEMISTRY/URINALYSIS
• CBC usually demonstrates leukocytosis, but may reveal leukopenia and thrombocytopenia as a result of neutrophil sequestration in the lung and platelet consumption. • Serum chemistries usually are normal, although hypoalbuminemia may occur as a result of pulmonary protein loss, and mild hyperglycemia has been reported. • Urinalysis usually is normal.

OTHER LABORATORY TESTS
• Arterial blood gas analysis usually demonstrates mild to severe hypoxia and hypocapnia if severe hyperventiliation is present. The results are not specific to the disease process,

but instead give an indication of the severity of pulmonary dysfunction. • Coagulation testing may reveal mild to moderate prolongation of PT and PTT as a result of factor consumption and disseminated intravascular coagulation.

IMAGING
• Thoracic radiographs are vital. Early or mild disease may simply reveal an increased interstitial pattern. Animals with moderate or severe disease have alveolar infiltrates. The majority of animals with NPE have alveolar infiltrates in the dorsocaudal lung fields.
• Alveolar infiltrates may also involve all other lung fields and are often asymmetrical with predominant, right-sided involvement.
• Echocardiography may be used to rule out cardiogenic pulmonary edema.

OTHER DIAGNOSTIC PROCEDURES
• Pulmonary artery wedge pressure determination • Pulse oximetry

GROSS AND HISTOPATHOLOGIC FINDINGS
The lungs may be heavy, red or congested, fail to collapse, and exhibit a wet cut surface. Foam may be present in the major airways. Histopathologic is variable depending on the severity of the insult. Early or mildly affected patients may have eosinophilic amorphous material filling the alveoli or almost normal histopathology because the fluid is removed in processing. In severely affected patients that progress to ARDS, however, alveolar hyaline membranes, alveolitis, and interstitial inflammatory infiltrates with neutrophils and macrophages become evident, accompanied by atelectasis, vascular congestion and hemorrhage, and type II pneumocyte proliferation. Such inflammatory changes may be found a short time (hours) after a severe insult.

TREATMENT

INPATIENT VERSUS OUTPATIENT
This decision depends on the severity of clinical manifestation of respiratory dysfunction; mild cases may not require hospitalization. The decision also depends on the underlying cause of NPE (e.g., dogs with upper airway obstruction or severe seizures may require hospitalization to address those issues).

ACTIVITY
If the dog has moderate to severe hypoxia and respiratory distress, rest and minimal stress are vital to minimize oxygen requirements.

DIET N/A

CLIENT EDUCATION
The client must be informed of the possibility that the condition may worsen before improving. Severe cases of NPE that progress rapidly to fulminant pulmonary edema and respiratory failure are associated with a poor prognosis.

SURGICAL CONSIDERATIONS

Surgical considerations are only relevant to treatment of the underlying cause of NPE.

MEDICATIONS

• No specific treatment is available to correct the damaged endothelium in the pulmonary vasculature. Further, because a variety of different inflammatory mediators and cascades are involved in the generation of the inflammatory response, there is not a specific anti-inflammatory drug that can effectively block the inflammatory response and lead to resolution of the pulmonary edema.
• Every effort should be made to resolve and treat the underlying cause of NPE (e.g., by relief of an airway obstruction or treatment of sepsis).
• Generally, patients with mild to moderate involvement improve on their own within a short period of time (24-48 hours) and have complete resolution of pulmonary edema. Management of these patients primarily involves support of pulmonary and cardiovascular function while the lung repairs.
• Patients with severe edema are difficult to treat, and many die despite extensive supportive care.

DRUGS AND FLUIDS

• Oxygen therapy is vital in moderate to severe cases. Supplemental oxygen may be administered by means of masks or hoods, nasal catheters, or oxygen cages. The inspired oxygen concentration depends on the severity of disease in affected animals. Most do well on 40-50% oxygen, but those with severe edema may require 80-100% inspired oxygen to sustain life. Severely affected animals may require positive pressure ventilation and positive end-expiratory pressure.
• Fluid therapy with balanced electrolyte replacement solutions is required for dehydrated animals or those in shock. If hypoproteinemia is present, plasma or synthetic colloids should be administered to improve oncotic pressure and therefore minimize movement of fluid into the lungs.
Diuretics such as furosemide usually are administered to these patients but may be inef-

fective because edema is caused by changes in permeability rather than increased hydrostatic pressure. Furosemide bolus 0.5-2 mg/kg IV or IM, or as a continuous infusion at 0.1-1 mg/kg/hr
• Corticosteroids may be used in patients with upper airway obstruction to minimize swelling. They are generally ineffective for treatment of the pulmonary inflammatory response in these patients and may predispose to infectious complications such as bacterial pneumonia.
• Dexamethasone sodium phosphate 2-4 mg/kg IV single dose (shock/severe), 0.1-0.2 mg/kg IV (moderate/antiinflammatory)
• Prednisolone sodium succinate 5-11 mg/kg IV single dose (shock)

CONTRAINDICATIONS N/A

PRECAUTIONS

Excessive use of diuretics may lead to significant decreases in intravascular volume, with minimal resolution of NPE. Decreased intravascular volume may exacerbate cardiovascular collapse and shock.

POSSIBLE INTERACTIONS N/A

ALTERNATE DRUGS N/A

FOLLOW-UP

PATIENT MONITORING

• Observation of respiratory rate and pattern, and frequent auscultation (every 2-4 hours) for the first 24-48 hours, depending on severity of disease • Assessment of pulmonary function by pulse oximetry or arterial blood gas analysis initially every 2-4 hours if dyspnea is present • PCV and evaluation of mucous membranes, pulse quality, heart rate, and urine output every 2-4 hours to assess cardiovascular status and progression to shock

PREVENTION/AVOIDANCE

• Avoid contact with electric wires. • Correct airway obstruction. • Treat seizures or increased intracranial pressure.

POSSIBLE COMPLICATIONS

Usually none, if the animal recovers from the acute crisis

EXPECTED COURSE AND PROGNOSIS

Most patients recover within 24-72 hours, and require no specific therapy other than oxygen and fluid supplementation. The most severely affected patients may progress to ARDS, which is fatal. Overall survival rates for NPE vary from 80-100%. Long-term prognosis is excellent for patients that have recovered.

MISCELLANEOUS

ASSOCIATED CONDITIONS
ARDS

AGE RELATED FACTORS N/A

ZOONOTIC POTENTIAL N/A

PREGNANCY N/A

SYNONYMS
• Shock lung • Traumatic wet lung • Acute alveolar failure • Capillary leak syndrome • Progressive respiratory distress • Congestive atelectasis • Hemorrhagic lung syndrome

SEE ALSO N/A

ABBREVIATIONS
ARDS = adult respiratory distress syndrome
NPE = noncardiogenic pulmonary edema
PT = prothrombin time
PTT = partial thromboplastin time
SIRS = systemic inflammatory response syndrome

References
Kerr LY. Pulmonary edema secondary to upper airway obstruction in the dog: a review of nine cases. J Am Anim Hosp Assoc 1989;25:207-212.
Drobatz KJ, Concannon K. Noncardiogenic pulmonary edema. Comp Cont Ed Pract Vet 1994;16:333-346.
Drobatz KJ, Saunders HM, Pugh C, Hendricks JC. Noncardiogenic pulmonary edema 26 cases (1987-1993). In press.
Kolata RJ, Burrows CF. The clinical features of injury by chewing electrical cords in dogs and cats. J Am Anim Hosp Assoc 1981;17:219-222.
Author Lesley G. King
Consulting Editors Lynelle Johnson and Bradley L. Moses

PULMONARY FIBROSIS

BASICS

OVERVIEW
Fibrosis of the lung interstitium affects pulmonary mechanics, alters ventilation-perfusion ratios, and leads to chronic tachypnea. Fibrosis is the end result of previous lung injury and may be preceded by multifocal alveolitis. The initiating causes of alveolitis and lung fibrosis are not known; however, in human beings over 100 known agents can incite alveolar inflammation.

SIGNALMENT
• Older West Highland white terriers; other terriers • Any older dog and cat with severe, diffuse lung disease

SIGNS

Historical Findings
• Open-mouth breathing • Exercise intolerance • Cough

Physical Examination Findings
• Dyspnea • Increased respiratory rate and effort • Cyanosis • Auscultation—bilateral end-inspiratory and early-expiratory crackles

CAUSES AND RISK FACTORS
• Most cases are idiopathic. • Viral infections—canine distemper, adenovirus, and parainfluenza • Toxins or drugs—paraquat, kerosene, and nitrofurantoin • Oxygen toxicosis • Acute pancreatitis

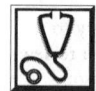

DIAGNOSIS

•DIFFERENTIAL DIAGNOSIS
• Generalized cardiogenic pulmonary edema is accompanied by cardiac disease and pulmonary venous distension. Response to diuretic therapy is expected. • Fungal pneumonia and metastatic neoplasia are also associated with an interstitial pattern and usually can be diagnosed by the results of transtracheal wash or bronchoalveolar lavage cytology and cultures. • Obesity, end-expiration, and poor film quality may all result in increased lung density.

CBC/BIOCHEMISTRY/URINALYSIS
N/A

OTHER LABORATORY TESTS N/A

IMAGING
Radiography—bilateral, diffuse increase in interstitial pattern; right-sided cardiomegaly may result from chronic lung disease

OTHER DIAGNOSTIC PROCEDURES
• Arterial blood gas measurements—hypoxemia, high alveolar-arterial oxygen difference • Bronchoalveolar lavage cytology—nontoxic neutrophil counts exceeding 20% of cells in dogs with alveolitis/fibrosis • Bacterial, mycoplasma, and fungal cultures—no growth • Open lung biopsy shows proliferative interstitial pneumonia. Proliferation of atypical and multinucleated alveolar epithelial cells, thickening of interalveolar septa, intraalveolar hemorrhage and edema, and intracapillary and intraalveolar fibrin deposits. Macrophages and alveolar epithelial cells in alveolar lumina. Masson trichrome staining reveals increase in interalveolar septal collagen.

TREATMENT
• Treat as inpatient if oxygen therapy needed. Because manifestations of pulmonary fibrosis do not occur until pulmonary gas exchange is severely compromised, the goals of treatment are to control signs and improve quality of life. • Obesity may impair diaphragmatic function, cause early small airway closure, and impede ventilation. Weight loss will lessen signs of respiratory impairment. • Exposure to dusts or fumes should be eliminated.

MEDICATIONS

DRUGS AND FLUIDS
• Immunosuppressive dosages of prednisone (1 mg/kg PO q12h for 2 weeks, then tapered over the next month) is recommended if underlying infection is not present. Most beneficial early in the course of disease. • Bronchodilators may lessen signs of disease. • Oxygen therapy during acute exacerbations

CONTRAINDICATIONS/POSSIBLE INTERACTIONS
• Steroids may predispose to overt infection and are not advised unless bacterial and fungal cultures are negative. • Beta blockers may cause bronchoconstriction. • Diuretics will reduce pulmonary clearance mechanisms as a result of airway dehydration and may predispose to infection.

FOLLOW-UP
• Monitor with serial arterial blood gas measurements and bronchoalveolar lavage cytologic examination of specimens. • Pulmonary fibrosis is a progressive condition with guarded prognosis. • Pulmonary hypertension and right heart failure may occur with any severe, chronic lung disease. • Bullous emphysema and spontaneous pneumothorax may occur as a result of severe alveolar damage.

MISCELLANEOUS

Reference
Bonagura JD, Hamlin RL, Gaber CE. Chronic respiratory disease in the dog. In: Kirk RW, ed. Current veterinary therapy X. Philadelphia: WB Saunders, 1989:361-368.

Author Rosemary A. Henik

Consulting Editors Lynelle Johnson and Bradley L. Moses

BASICS

OVERVIEW
• Pulmonary mineralizations include both calcification and ossification and may be generalized or localized. • Calcification may be dystrophic or metastatic. Dystrophic calcification occurs secondary to tissue degeneration or inflammation, whereas metastatic calcification occurs secondary to metabolic diseases. • Pulmonary ossification in the form of small, multiple nodules, which are called "osteomas," is common in normal dogs. • A small number of generalized pulmonary mineralizations of unknown cause have been reported in dogs and cats under descriptive terms, including pulmonary alveolar microlithiasis or "pumice-stone" lung, bronchiolar microlithiasis, and idiopathic pulmonary calcification or ossification.

SIGNALMENT Older dogs and cats

SIGNS

Historical Findings
• None if focal pulmonary mineralization is incidental finding • Exercise intolerance • Cough

Physical Examination Findings
• Dyspnea • Cyanosis • Abnormal breath sounds

CAUSES AND RISK FACTORS
• Mineralizations often are idiopathic.
• Metastatic calcification occurs secondary to metabolic diseases that induce high serum calcium concentration and/or bone resorption—hyperadrenocorticism, primary or secondary hyperparathyroidism, hypervitaminosis D, or renal failure • Hyperadrenocorticism may also cause dystrophic mineralization as a result of gluconeogenic and catabolic effects of high cortisol on proteins, resulting in calcium binding to the organic matrix of the abnormal proteins.

• Alveolar and bronchial microliths may be secondary to exudative or granulomatous lung diseases.

DIAGNOSIS

DIFFERENTIAL DIAGNOSIS
• Dystrophic calcification secondary to chronic pulmonary inflammatory disease • Atypical pulmonary neoplasia • Histoplasmosis or tuberculosis granulomas (usually with hilar lymph node calcification) • Alveolar microlithiasis • Barium sulfate aspiration • Interstitial pulmonary edema (will respond to diuretics and be differentiated by bone scintigraphy)

CBC/BIOCHEMISTRY/URINALYSIS
• Hypercalcemia if hyperparathyroidism, neoplasia, or hypervitaminosis D • Polycythemia as a result of chronic hypoxemia • Stress leukogram, decreased urine specific gravity, and elevated alkaline phosphatase may be seen in dogs with hyperadrenocorticism

OTHER LABORATORY TESTS
Arterial blood gas measurements—hypoxemia

IMAGING
Thoracic radiographs—generalized or localized, discrete or diffuse abnormalities, ranging from an unstructured interstitial pattern to mineralized nodules within pulmonary parenchyma

OTHER DIAGNOSTIC PROCEDURES
• Transtracheal wash or bronchoalveolar lavage cytology—inflammatory cells if underlying inflammation or infection; microliths appear as nonstaining crystalline concretions • Bacterial and fungal cultures— results depend on underlying cause of mineralization • Delayed bone phase scintigraphy using technetium Tc 99m methylene diphosphonate—generalized pulmonary uptake if sufficient osteoid is being produced • Lung biopsy—grossly, lungs are firm, noncompressible, and variably resistant to blunt dissection resulting from mineralizations

TREATMENT
• No treatment indicated if localized mineralization found in asymptomatic patient

MEDICATIONS

DRUGS AND FLUIDS
• Bronchodilators for relief of dyspnea and respiratory muscle fatigue • Furosemide, venodilators, and thoracocentesis to treat pleural effusion • Antimicrobials or antifungals if positive bacterial or fungal cultures, respectively
• Treatment for underlying metabolic disease (e.g., mitotane for hyperadrenocorticism, chemotherapy for neoplasia, etc.)

CONTRAINDICATIONS/POSSIBLE INTERACTIONS
Fluid loading may exacerbate dyspnea and right heart failure.

FOLLOW-UP
Pleural effusion, chronic obstructive bronchitis, or emphysematous bullae may occur as a result of severe, chronic pulmonary disease.

MISCELLANEOUS

Reference
Suter PF, Lord PF. Thoracic radiography: a text atlas of thoracic diseases of the dog and cat. Switzerland: PF Suter, 1984:582.
Author Rosemary A. Henik
Consulting Editors Lynelle Johnson and Bradley L. Moses

PULMONARY THROMBOEMBOLISM

BASICS

DEFINITION
Develops when a thrombus lodges in the pulmonary arterial tree and occludes blood flow to the lung served by that artery.

Pathophysiology
• Pulmonary thromboemboli associated with heartworm disease occur in situ in the pulmonary vessels. In most other instances, the origin of the thrombus is unclear. • Potential sites of origin include the right atrium, vena cava, jugular veins, and femoral or mesenteric veins. These venous thrombi are carried in the bloodstream to the lungs where they lodge in the pulmonary circulation. • Abnormal blood flow (stasis), vascular endothelial damage, and altered coagulability (hypercoagulable state) are believed to predispose to thrombus formation. • In most animals, pulmonary thromboembolism occurs as a complicating feature of another primary disease process.

Systems Affected
• Pulmonary—diminished pulmonary blood flow leads to arterial hypoxemia and dyspnea.
• Cardiovascular—pulmonary hypertension may result, leading to right ventricular enlargement and right ventricular failure.

Genetics N/A

Incidence/Prevalence
• Incidence and prevalence not known; however, the likelihood of pulmonary thromboembolism increases in animals with abnormal coagulation or with severe systemic disease. • Pulmonary thromboembolism is an uncommon diagnosis in dogs and a rare diagnosis in cats.

Geographic Distribution N/A

SIGNALMENT

Species Dogs and cats

Breed Predilections
No predisposition, although the disease may be more common in medium- and large-breed dogs.

Mean Age And Range
More frequently seen in mature and elderly dogs

Predominant Sex N/A

SIGNS

Historical Findings
• Often reflect the primary disease that has led to pulmonary thromboembolism. • Pulmonary thromboembolism is occasionally the reason for initial examination, and in such a patient, peracute dyspnea, collapse, cough or hemoptysis, weakness, and inability to sleep or get comfortable may be historical complaints.

Physical Examination Findings
• Tachypnea and dyspnea in most animals
• Tachycardia, weak arterial pulses, jugular vein distension, pale or cyanotic mucus membrane color, delayed capillary refill time, and split second heart sound in some animals

CAUSES
• Heartworm disease • Neoplasia • Hyperadrenocorticism (Cushing's disease) • Protein-losing nephropathy (renal loss of anti-thrombin III) • Cardiac disease • Immune-mediated hemolytic anemia • Pancreatitis
• Orthopedic trauma or surgery • Sepsis
• Severe systemic disease and disseminated intravascular coagulopathy • Liver disease

RISK FACTORS
• Coagulopathy, especially any hypercoagulable state • The diseases listed under "Causes" are associated. • Estrogen administration and airplane travel may be causative.

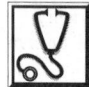

DIAGNOSIS

DIFFERENTIAL DIAGNOSIS
• Other diseases that cause clinically important dyspnea and hypoxemia without profound radiographic findings include upper airway obstruction, laryngeal paralysis, and diffuse airway disease processes (e.g., toxin inhalation and interstitial pneumonia).
• Upper airway obstruction often manifests as inspiratory dyspnea, and lung sounds are often loudest over the trachea or larynx.
• Pulmonary thromboembolism should be a leading diagnostic consideration in an animal with a disease known to be associated that has acute onset of dyspnea.

CBC/BIOCHEMISTRY/URINALYSIS
• Results often reflect the underlying disease
• Leukocytosis may develop

OTHER LABORATORY TESTS
• Coagulation profile may show high fibrin degradation products, high fibrinogen, or alterations in one-stage prothrombin time (PT) and activated partial thromboplastin time (PTT). • Arterial blood gases often demonstrate arterial hypoxemia (PaO_2 < 65 mmHg) and diminished $PaCO_2$ with respiratory alkalosis. • Metabolic and respiratory acidosis may develop in severely affected animals.

IMAGING

Thoracic Radiographic Findings
Normal or pulmonary artery enlargement or pruning, cardiomegaly, interstitial and alveolar lung patterns, small volume pleural effusion, or areas of regional hyperlucency

Echocardiographic Findings
Right ventricular enlargement, an enlarged pulmonary artery segment, or diminished size of the left ventricular cavity in some animals

Angiographic Findings and Radionuclide Studies
• A definitive diagnosis usually requires pulmonary angiography or a radionuclide study.
• Right-sided cardiac catheterization with pulmonary angiography may permit identification of an intravascular thrombus or regions of reduced pulmonary blood flow. In contrast, nonselective angiography has a low level of diagnostic success, especially in medium- and large-breed dogs • Combined ventilation and perfusion scans with radioisotopes permits identification of well ventilated lung regions that do not receive blood flow. When thoracic radiographs are nearly normal, a perfusion scan alone may be adequate..

OTHER DIAGNOSTIC PROCEDURES

Electrocardiography
• Animal with acute cor pulmonale—right axis deviation, P pulmonale, ST segment deviation, and large T waves • Arrhythmias

GROSS AND HISTOPATHOLOGIC FINDINGS
• Thrombi within the major branches of the pulmonary arteries in most animals. • In some animals, multiple smaller thrombi in small vessels of the pulmonary arteries eventually leading to marked respiratory dysfunction and death.

TREATMENT

INPATIENT VERSUS OUTPATIENT
• Individuals suspected of having pulmonary thromboembolism should always be treated as inpatients until hypoxemia is resolved.

ACTIVITY
• Restricted if pulmonary thromboembolism has been diagnosed to prevent worsening hypoxemia or syncope.

DIET N/A

CLIENT EDUCATION
• Pulmonary thromboembolism is often a fatal disease, and unless an underlying cause can be identified and corrected, further episodes of pulmonary thromboembolism are likely. Sudden death is not unusual in animals.
• Treatment with anticoagulant medications can lead to bleeding, and frequent reevaluation of clotting times (e.g., PT and PTT) is essential for successful management. Anticoagulant administration may be required for several months even after resolution of the disease that caused the pulmonary thromboembolism.

SURGICAL CONSIDERATIONS
• Surgery requires cardiopulmonary bypass and is not available at most institutions. Even if it were available, extrapolation from human literature suggests that there would be high surgical mortality

MEDICATIONS

The underlying disease should always be identified and treated. If this is unlikely to be successful, aggressive efforts to treat pulmonary thromboembolism will probably be in vain.

DRUGS AND FLUIDS

• Intravenous fluids should be administered cautiously, unless preexisting volume depletion is present, because they may contribute to the development of right-sided congestive heart failure.
• Heparin may be of some use in preventing further thrombi from developing. Low dosages are probably inadequate for management of confirmed pulmonary thromboembolism; a higher dosage (200 to 300 units/kg sc q8h) is indicated.
• Thrombolytic drug administration (e.g., streptokinase and tissue plasminogen activator) may also be useful. These drugs are expensive and carry a higher risk of causing bleeding complications.
• Coumadin is usually indicated for chronic treatment (0.1 mg/kg q24h) with dosage adjustments to maintain a PT of 1.5 to 2 times the baseline value.

CONTRAINDICATIONS N/A

PRECAUTIONS

• Aspirin use in critically ill animals may cause gastrointestinal ulceration and bleeding.
• Heparin, streptokinase, tissue plasminogen activator, and warfarin can all lead to hemorrhagic diathesis.
• Clinical experience suggests that the death rate from pulmonary thromboembolism is much higher than the complication rate from treatment with antithrombotic drugs.

POSSIBLE INTERACTIONS

• Coumadin interacts with a number of other drugs, and the degree of anticoagulation may change after initiation of these drugs. A review of the mechanism of action and pharmacology of the antithrombotic drugs is suggested before their clinical use.

ALTERNATE DRUGS N/A

FOLLOW-UP

PATIENT MONITORING

• Serial arterial blood gases may help determine improvement in respiratory function.
• PT should be monitored every 3 days initially to adjust the dosage of Coumadin to achieve a PT of 1.5 to 2 times the baseline value. International normalization ratios are recommended to minimize the effects of test kit variability on PT results. Once a effective dosage has been achieved (typically no sooner than 2 weeks) weekly PT can be monitored weekly.

PREVENTION/AVOIDANCE

• Activity may improve venous blood flow and prevent the development of venous thrombi in immobile animals with severe systemic disease. • Aspirin may have some role in preventing pulmonary thromboembolism, but it is inadequate as treatment • Heparin may be administered to animals predisposed to the development of pulmonary thromboembolism (200 units/kg IV initially and 75 units/kg SC q4h-q8h)

POSSIBLE COMPLICATIONS

• Clinically important bleeding complications may arise in animals treated with anticoagulant drugs. Bleeding may occur from any organ system. Active bleeding or anemia necessitating blood or plasma transfusion should be anticipated, and blood products should be readily available for use.

EXPECTED COURSE AND PROGNOSIS

Prognosis generally fair to poor and is dependent on resolution of the precipitating cause. For irreversible diseases (e.g., some neoplasias and advanced protein-losing nephropathy) the long term prognosis is poor. The prognosis is somewhat better for animals with trauma or sepsis.

MISCELLANEOUS

ASSOCIATED CONDITIONS

See Causes and Risk Factors

AGE RELATED FACTORS N/A

ZOONOTIC POTENTIAL N/A

PREGNANCY N/A

SYNONYMS

Pulmonary embolism

SEE ALSO

• Immune-Mediated Hemolytic Anemia
• Hyperadrenocorticism (Cushing's Disease)
• Nephrotic Syndrome • Heartworm Disease
• Sepsis • Disseminated Intravascular Coagulation

ABBREVIATIONS

PT = prothrombin time

References

LaRue MJ, Murtaugh RJ. Pulmonary thromboembolism in dogs: 47 cases (1986-1987) J Am Vet Med Assoc 1990;197:1368-1372.
Hawkins EC. Diseases of the lower respiratory system. In: Ettinger SJ, Feldman EC, eds. Textbook of veterinary internal medicine. 4th ed. Philadelphia: WB Saunders, 1995.

Author John E. Rush
Consulting Editors Larry P. Tilley and Francis W. K. Smith Jr.

PULMONIC STENOSIS

BASICS

DEFINITION
An abnormal narrowing of the pulmonary artery, usually at the valvular level

PATHOPHYSIOLOGY
No important hemodynamic changes in animals with mild pulmonic stenosis. In animals with moderate to severe stenosis, restriction of adequate blood flow to the lungs during exercise may occur. Tricuspid regurgitation and right heart failure may develop secondary to morphologic changes in the right ventricle.

SYSTEMS AFFECTED
• Cardiovascular—possible right heart failure, arrhythmias, or sudden death • Nervous—inadequate cerebral blood flow during exercise

GENETICS N/A

INCIDENCE/PREVALENCE
• Relatively common congenital defect in dogs • Very uncommon in cats

GEOGRAPHIC DISTRIBUTION N/A

SIGNALMENT

Species Dogs and cats

BREED PREDILECTION
Beagle, Chihuahua, cocker spaniel, English bulldog, Samoyed, schnauzer, terriers

Mean Age/Range
The diagnosis is usually made in young, asymptomatic animals on the basis of an auscultable murmur. Some animals may be diagnosed at a later age because of exercise intolerance or collapse.

Predominant Sex N/A

SIGNS

General Comments
Signs such as exercise intolerance and collapse and signs associated with right heart failure (e.g., ascites and pleural effusion) are related to the degree of stenosis

Historical Findings
• Exercise intolerance or syncope • Dyspnea or tachypnea • Abdominal distention

Physical Examination Findings
• A left basilar, systolic, harsh crescendo-decrescendo type murmur is characteristic. Differentiating between pulmonic stenosis and subaortic stenosis on the basis of murmur location is difficult. • A thrill is often palpable over the left heart base. • The precordial impulse may be prominent on the right side because of right ventricular hypertrophy.
• Femoral pulses are typically normal.
• Jugular distention or pulses may be present, especially in animals with tricuspid insufficiency. • A right thoracic systolic murmur may be ausculted if the animal has tricuspid valve insufficiency. • If right heart failure secondary to tricuspid insufficiency has devel-

oped, ascites may be observed. • Tachypnea and muffling of heart and lung sounds caused by pleural effusion may also be present.

CAUSES Congenital

RISK FACTORS N/A

DIAGNOSIS

DIFFERENTIAL DIAGNOSIS
• Subaortic stenosis • Atrial septal or ventral septal defect with relative pulmonic stenosis • Tetralogy of Fallot

CBC/BIOCHEMISTRY/URINALYSIS
Results usually normal

OTHER LABORATORY TESTS N/A

IMAGING

Thoracic Radiography
• Dorsoventral radiographs often show poststenotic bulge of the pulmonary artery visible at the 2 o'clock position. • The pulmonary vasculature is usually normal but may be underperfused in animals with severe disease.
• Right ventricular hypertrophy is usually not appreciated because it is concentric hypertrophy which cannot be seen on the radiographic cardiac silhouette. • If concurrent tricuspid regurgitation has occurred, animal may have severe right ventricular enlargement with or without pleural effusion .

Echocardiographic Findings
• Concentric hypertrophy of the right ventricle because of chronic pressure overload.
• Thickened right ventricular free wall and interventricular septum in proportion to the degree of stenosis • Abnormal pulmonic valve leaflets in most animals; thickened, poorly moving valve cusps; "doming" of the valve leaflets toward the pulmonary artery in some animals • Subvalvular and supravalvular lesions in some animals, either in tandem with the valvular lesion or, rarely, as isolated lesions • Large right atrium in some animals, especially if tricuspid regurgitation has developed. • Poststenotic dilation of the pulmonary artery in some animals • Spectral Doppler echocardiography documents and quantifies the degree of stenosis. A peak systolic gradient of 50 to 80 mm Hg is moderate pulmonic stenosis; measurements below or above these values are mild or severe stenosis, respectively. • Color and pulsed-wave Doppler echocardiography may document the degree of obstruction. • Doppler echocardiography documents concurrent tricuspid regurgitation or patent foramen ovale, if present.

Angiocardiographic Findings
• Selective angiography into the right ventricle confirms the obstruction and its degree and also documents tricuspid insufficiency.
• Nonselective angiography may show right ventricular hypertrophy.

Cardiac Catheterization Findings
• Rarely necessary to document pulmonic stenosis • A pressure pull-back from the pulmonary artery to the right ventricle documents and quantifies the degree of stenosis.

OTHER DIAGNOSTIC PROCEDURES

Electrocardiographic Findings
• Very helpful in distinguishing between pulmonic stenosis and subaortic stenosis • A right ventricular enlargement pattern in moderate to severe pulmonic stenosis

Gross and Histopathologic Findings
Right ventricular hypertrophy, with an abnormal and thickened pulmonic valve and poststenotic dilation of the main pulmonary artery

TREATMENT

INPATIENT VERSUS OUTPATIENT
Animals can be managed on an out-patient basis unless they are in severe right heart failure, in which case in-patient treatment is beneficial.

ACTIVITY
Restricted in symptomatic animals or those with severe disease; no restriction in asymptomatic animals or those with mild disease.

DIET
Sodium restricted only in animals with severe right heart failure.

CLIENT EDUCATION
• Animals with mild to moderate disase are typically asymptomatic with normal life-spans.
• Animals with severe disease warrant intervention to prevent right heart failure or sudden to death due to arrhythmias.
• Animals in right heart failure are very difficult to control and the prognosis is poor.

SURGICAL CONSIDERATIONS
• Currently, the procedure of choice to relieve the obstruction is balloon angioplasty—the obstruction is dilated by means of a balloon catheter. Morbidity and mortality is low, and results are generally favorable.
• If this procedure fails or is unavailable, surgery in animals with severe disease can be considered.
• Valvotomy, patch-graft, or inflow occlusion techniques may be attempted at referral centers. Morbidity and mortality with these procedures can be high, and will vary depending on surgeon and center.

MEDICATIONS

DRUGS AND FLUIDS
Right heart failure is very difficult to control; treatment with furosemide (2-4 mg/kg PO,

IV, IM q6h-q12h) and digoxin (0.22 mg/M^2 PO q12H) should be instituted.

CONTRAINDICATIONS
Arterial vasodilators (e.g., hydralazine, enalapril) are not indicated

PRECAUTIONS
Overzealous use of diuretics may cause weakness or increase frequency of syncope.

POSSIBLE INTERACTIONS N/A

ALTERNATE DRUGS N/A

FOLLOW-UP

PATIENT MONITORING
Repeat echocardiography is indicated to monitor the status of the right heart in animals with moderate to severe disease.

PREVENTION/AVOIDANCE
Do not breed affected animals.

POSSIBLE COMPLICATIONS
• Right heart failure • Syncope • Exercise intolerance • Arrhythmias • Sudden death

EXPECTED COURSE AND PROGNOSIS
• Animals with mild to moderate disease have a good prognosis for normal life with normal exercise. • Animals with severe disease have a guarded prognosis for exercise tolerance and may have a markedly reduced lifespan due to right heart failure or sudden death.

MISCELLANEOUS

ASSOCIATED CONDITIONS N/A

AGE RELATED FACTORS
The murmur is present from birth.

ZOONOTIC POTENTIAL N/A

PREGNANCY
Affected animals should not be bred.

SYNONYMS N/A

SEE ALSO
• Congestive Heart Failure, Right-Sided
• Murmurs

ABBREVIATIONS
None

References

Bonagura JD. Congenital heart disease. In: Ettinger SJ, ed. Textbook of veterinary internal medicine. 3rd ed. Philadelphia:WB Saunders, 1989.

Olivier NB. Congenital heart disease in dogs. In: Fox PR, ed. Canine and feline cardiology. New York: Churchill Livingstone, 1988.

Friedman WF. Congenital heart disease in infancy and childhood. In: Braunwald E, ed. Heart disease. 4th ed. Philadelphia: WB Saunders, 1992.

Author Carroll Loyer
Consulting Editors Larry P. Tilley and Francis W. K. Smith, Jr.

PUPPY STRANGLES

BASICS

OVERVIEW
- Juvenile cellulitis is an uncommon granulomatous and pustular disorder of puppies.
- The disorder is rarely seen in adult dogs.
- The face, pinnae, and submandibular lymph nodes are the most common sites
- The immunopathogenesis is unknown

SIGNALMENT
- Puppies are usually affected between the ages of 3 weeks to 4 months • Golden retrievers, daschunds, and gordon setters appear to be predisposed

SIGNS
- Acutely swollen face (eyelids, lips, and muzzle) • Submandibular lymphadenopathy
- Within 24-48 hours, a marked, pustular and exudative dermatitis develops that frequently fistulates • Purulent otitis externa
- Lesions often become crusted • Affected skin is usually painful • 50% of puppies may be lethargic • Anorexia, pyrexia, and a sterile suppurative arthritis develop in 25% of cases
- Rarely, a sterile pyogranulomatous panniculitis may develop over the trunk, preputial, or perianal area. These lesions may appear as fluctuant, subcutaneous nodules that fistulate.

CAUSES AND RISK FACTORS
- The cause and pathogenesis are unknown
- An immune dysfunction with a heritable cause is suspect.

DIAGNOSIS

DIFFERENTIAL DIAGNOSIS
- Staphylococcal dermatitis • Demodecosis
- Drug eruption • Deep fungal infection

CBC/BIOCHEMISTRY/URINALYSIS
N/A

OTHER LABORATORY TESTS   N/A

IMAGING   N/A

OTHER DIAGNOSTIC PROCEDURES

Cytology
Pyogranulomatous inflammation with no microorganisms. Neutrophils are nondegenerative

Culture
Cultures are usually negative; positive microbial culture is commonly seen with secondary bacterial contamination.

Biopsy
- Multiple, discrete or confluent granulomas and pyogranulomas consisting of clusters of large, epithelioid macrophages and neutrophils • Sebaceous glands and apocrine glands may be obliterated • Suppurative changes in the dermis predominate in later stages • Panniculitis

TREATMENT
- Early and aggressive therapy is indicated
- Scarring may be severe
- Topical therapy may be soothing and palliative as an adjunct therapy to corticosteroids

MEDICATIONS

DRUGS AND FLUIDS

• High doses of corticosteroids are required—1mg/lb divided q12h for at least 2 weeks. Treatment should not be tapered too rapidly.

• Rarely, resistant cases may occur which require chemotherapeutics.

• Dogs with panniculitis may require longer therapy

• Antibiotics should be used if there is evidence of secondary bacterial infection and as an adjunct therapy with immunosuppressive doses of steroids

CONTRAINDICATIONS/POSSIBLE INTERACTIONS N/A

 FOLLOW-UP

• Most cases do not recur • Scarring may be a problem, especially around the eyes

 MISCELLANEOUS

Reference

Scott, GH, Muller RW, Griffin CE. Muller and Kirk's small animal dermatology. 5th ed. Philadelphia: WB Saunders, 1995;938-941.

Author Karen Helton-Rhodes
Consulting Editor Lowell Ackerman

PYELONEPHRITIS

BASICS

DEFINITION
Pyelonephritis is a microbial colonization of the upper urinary tract including the renal pelvis, collecting diverticula, renal parenchyma, and ureters. Because pyelonephritis is not usually limited to the renal pelvis and parenchyma, a more descriptive term is upper urinary tract infection. This chapter is limited to bacterial pyelonephritis.

Pathophysiology
• Infection of any portion of the urinary tract usually requires some impairment of normal host defenses against urinary tract infection (see chapter on lower urinary tract infection). Normal host defenses include mucosal defense barriers, ureteral peristalsis, ureterovesical flap valves, and an extensive renal blood supply.
• Pyelonephritis usually occurs by ascension of the microbes causing lower urinary tract infection. In dogs and cats, hematogenous seeding of the kidneys does not usually cause pyelonephritis. Regardless of the route of infection, upper urinary tract infection is frequently accompanied by lower urinary tract infection.
• Pyelonephritis can develop secondarily to infection of metabolic nephroliths. Upper urinary tract infection by urease-producing bacteria can predispose to formation of struvite nephroliths.
• Obstruction of an infected kidney or ureter can cause septicemia (so-called urosepsis).

Systems Affected
• Renal/Urologic
• Pyelonephritis can cause urosepsis, thereby affecting any body system.

Genetics NA

Incidence/Prevalence
• Unknown
• Probably occurs much more commonly than is recognized clinically, because many animals with pyelonephritis are asymptomatic or have signs limited to lower urinary tract infection.

Geographic Distribution NA

SIGNALMENT

Species
Dogs affected more commonly than cats

Breed Predilections None

Mean Age and Range
• Mean age unknown
• Dogs of any age affected

Predominant Sex
• Sex distribution is unknown.
• In dogs, urinary tract infection affects females more than males.
• In cats, urinary tract infection is uncommon and occurs with similar frequency in males and females.

SIGNS
Many patients are asymptomatic or have signs of lower urinary tract infection only.

Historical Findings
• None
• Polyuria/Polydipsia (PU/PD)
• Abdominal or lumbar pain
• Signs associated with lower urinary tract infection (e.g., dysuria, pollakiuria, stranguria, hematuria, and malodorous or discolored urine)

Physical Examination Findings
• None
• Pain on palpation of the kidneys
• Fever

CAUSES
• Usually, ascending urinary tract infection caused by aerobic bacteria
• The most common isolates are *E. coli* and *Staphylococcus* spp. Other bacteria, including *Proteus, Streptococcus, Klebsiella, Enterobacter,* and *Pseudomonas,* that frequently infect the lower urinary tract may ascend into the upper urinary tract.
• Anaerobic bacteria, ureaplasma, and fungi rarely infect the upper urinary tract.

RISK FACTORS
• Ectopic ureters
• Vesicoureteral reflux
• Lower urinary tract infection
• Conditions that predispose to urinary tract infection (e.g., diabetes mellitus, hyperadrenocorticism, exogenous steroid administration, renal failure, urethral catheterization, urine retention, uroliths, urinary tract neoplasia, and perineal urethrostomy)
• In cats with experimentally induced lower urinary tract disease, indwelling urinary catheters combined with administration of exogenous steroids frequently resulted in pyelonephritis.

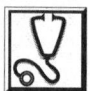

DIAGNOSIS

DIFFERENTIAL DIAGNOSIS
• The clinical diagnosis of pyelonephritis is usually presumptive based on results of CBC, biochemical analysis, urinalysis, urine culture, and diagnostic imaging. Definitive diagnosis is not usually required for planning treatment.
• Since many dogs and cats lack specific signs attributable to pyelonephritis, any patient with urinary tract infection could potentially have pyelonephritis. The best method for differentiating between upper and lower urinary tract infection is ultrasonography or excretory urography.
• One must consider the possibility of pyelonephritis since patients are frequently asymptomatic. Pyelonephritis should be considered as a differential diagnosis for dogs or cats with fever of unknown origin, PU/PD, chronic renal failure, or lumbar or abdominal pain.

CBC/BIOCHEMISTRY/URINALYSIS
• CBC results often normal in animals with chronic pyelonephritis. Leukocytosis and neutrophilia with a left shift are detected in some patients.
• Biochemistry results are usually normal unless chronic pyelonephritis leads to chronic renal failure (azotemia with an inappropriate urine specific gravity).
• Urinalysis reveals hematuria, pyuria, proteinuria, bacteriuria, and leukocyte casts in some animals. Leukocyte casts are diagnostic for renal inflammation and are usually the result of pyelonephritis. Dilute urine specific gravity observed in animals with nephrogenic diabetes insipidus. Absence of urinalysis abnormalities does not rule out pyelonephritis.

OTHER LABORATORY TESTS
Quantitative urine culture is done to confirm urinary tract infection. See chapter on lower urinary tract infection for interpretation. Dogs with chronic pyelonephritis may have a negative urine culture requiring multiple cultures to confirm urinary tract infection.

IMAGING
• Ultrasonography or excretory urography are the best methods for presumptively differentiating between upper and lower urinary tract infection. Experimentally, ultrasonography is more useful than excretory urography for identification of mild- to- moderate acute pyelonephritis.
• Ultrasonographic findings supportive of pyelonephritis include dilation of the renal pelvis and proximal ureter and a hyperechoic mucosal margin line within the renal pelvis or proximal ureter.
• Excretory urography reveals dilation and blunting of the renal pelvis with lack of filling of the collecting diverticula, dilation of the proximal ureter, reduced opacity of the nephrogram phase and of the contrast media in the collecting system in some animals.
• In animals with acute pyelonephritis, the kidneys may be large, whereas in animals with chronic pyelonephritis, the kidneys may be small with an irregular surface contour.
• Concomitant nephroliths detected in some animals by survey radiography, ultrasonography, or excretory urography

OTHER DIAGNOSTIC PROCEDURES
• Definitive diagnosis requires urine culture of specimen obtained from the renal pelvis or parenchyma or renal biopsy. Pyelocentesis can be performed percutaneously by ultrasound guidance or during exploratory surgery. Specimen for culture can be obtained from the renal pelvis (or from nephroliths) during nephrotomy.
• To confirm pyelonephritis, the biopsy specimen must include the renal cortex and medulla. Therefore, renal biopsy should be performed by open surgery and only if necessary. Pyelonephritis can have a patchy distribution and be missed by needle biopsy.

GROSS AND HISTOPATHOLOGIC FINDINGS

• Kidneys affected by chronic pyelonephritis have areas of infarction and scarring on the capsular surface in some animals. The renal pelvis and collecting diverticula may be dilated and distorted from chronic infection and inflammation. Purulent exudate is occasionally seen in the renal pelvis.
• Histologic findings include papillitis, pyelitis, interstitial nephritis, and leukocyte casts in tubular lumens.

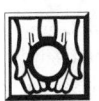

TREATMENT

INPATIENT VS OUTPATIENT

Outpatient unless animal has septicemia or renal failure

ACTIVITY Unlimited

DIET

Dietary modification is recommended in animals with concomitant chronic renal failure or nephrolithiasis.

CLIENT EDUCATION

• Unresolved chronic pyelonephritis may lead to chronic renal failure; diagnostic follow-up important to document resolution of pyelonephritis.
• In animals with nephroliths, resolution is unlikely unless the nephroliths are removed.

SURGICAL CONSIDERATIONS

• Obstruction of the upper urinary tract in a patient with pyelonephritis may result in urosepsis and should be corrected by surgery (or lithotripsy for nephroliths).
• Infected nephroliths can be surgically removed, medically dissolved (struvite), or fragmented by extracorporeal shock wave lithotripsy. Periprocedural antibiotics should be used to reduce the risk of urosepsis when manipulating infected nephroliths.

MEDICATIONS

DRUGS AND FLUIDS

• Antibiotic selection should be based on urine culture and sensitivity testing.
• Antibiotics should be bactericidal, achieve good serum and urine concentrations, and not be nephrotoxic.
• High serum and urine antibiotic concentrations do not necessarily ensure high tissue concentration in the renal medulla; therefore, chronic pyelonephritis may be difficult to eradicate.

• Orally administered antibiotics should be given at full therapeutic dosages for 4 - 6 weeks.
• Drugs that achieve good urine concentrations but poor serum concentrations (e.g., nitrofurantoin) should not be used.

CONTRAINDICATIONS

Aminoglycosides

PRECAUTIONS

Trimethoprim/sulfa combinations can cause side effects (e.g., keratoconjunctivitis sicca, blood dyscrasia, and polyarthritis) when administered for approximately 4 weeks.

POSSIBLE INTERACTIONS NA

ALTERNATE DRUGS NA

FOLLOW-UP

PATIENT MONITORING

Urine culture and urinalysis should be done during antibiotic administration (~ 5-7 days into treatment) and 1 and 4 weeks after antibiotics are finished.

PREVENTION / AVOIDANCE

Elimination of factors predisposing to urinary tract infection and correction of ectopic ureters

POSSIBLE COMPLICATIONS

Renal failure, recurrent pyelonephritis, struvite nephrolithiasis, septicemia, septic shock, and metastatic infection (eg, endocarditis and polyarthritis)

EXPECTED COURSE AND PROGNOSIS

• The prognosis for patients with pyelonephritis is fair to good with a return to normal health unless the animal also has nephrolithiasis, chronic renal failure, or some other underlying cause of urinary tract infection (e.g., obstruction or neoplasia).
• Established infection of the renal medulla may be difficult to resolve because of poor tissue penetration of antibiotics.
• The prognosis for patients with chronic renal failure caused by pyelonephritis is determined by the severity and rate of progression of the chronic renal failure.
• Recurrent pyelonephritis is likely if infected nephroliths are not removed.

MISCELLANEOUS

ASSOCIATED CONDITIONS

Hyperadrenocorticism, exogenous glucocorticoid administration, and diabetes mellitus are associated with lower urinary tract infection, which can ascend into the ureters and kidneys.

AGE-RELATED FACTORS NA

ZOONOTIC POTENTIAL NA

PREGNANCY

Use antibiotics that are safe for the pregnant bitch or queen.

SYNONYMS

Upper urinary tract infection, pyelitis

SEE ALSO

• Lower Urinary Tract Infection • Nephrolithiasis • Renal Failure, Chronic • Urinary Tract Obstruction • Urolithiasis, Struvite—Dogs • Urolithiasis, Struvite—Cats

ABBREVIATIONS

PU/PD = polyuria and polydipsia

References

Neuwirth L, Mahaffey M, Crowell W, et al. Comparison of excretory urography and ultrasonography for detection of experimentally induced pyelonephritis in dogs. Am J Vet Res 1993;54:660-669.

Lulich JP, Osborne CA. Bacterial infections of the urinary tract. In: Ettinger SJ, Feldman EC, eds. Textbook of veterinary internal medicine. 4th ed. Philadelphia: WB Saunders, 1995:1775-1788.

Lees GE, Forrester SD. Update: Bacterial urinary tract infections. In: Kirk RW, Bonagura JD, eds. Current veterinary therapy XI. Philadelphia: WB Saunders, 1992:909-914.

Lulich JP, Osborne CA. Fungal urinary tract infections. In: Kirk RW, Bonagura JD, eds. Current veterinary therapy XI. Philadelphia: WB Saunders, 1992:914-919.

Allen TA, Jaenke RS. Pyelonephritis in the dog. Compend Contin Ed Pract Vet 1985;7:421-428.

Author Larry G. Adams

Consulting Editors Larry G. Adams and Carl A. Osborne

PYLORIC STENOSIS

BASICS

DEFINITION
Pyloric stenosis or chronic hypertrophic pyloric gastropathy is an obstructive narrowing of the pyloric canal resulting from varying degrees of muscular hypertrophy or mucosal hyperplasia.

Pathophysiology
The disease can result from a congenital lesion composed primarily of hypertrophy of the smooth muscle or an acquired form characterized by three different types. The acquired form can be primarily circular muscle hypertrophy (Type 1), a combination of muscular hypertrophy and mucosal hyperplasia (Type 2), or primarily a result of mucosal hyperplasia (Type 3). The cause is unknown but proposed factors include increased gastrin levels which have a trophic effect on the muscle and mucosa or changes in the myenteric plexus that lead to chronic antral distention and its associated effects.

Systems Affected
• Gastrointestinal: chronic intermittent vomiting • Respiratory: if aspiration pneumonia develops • Musculoskeletal: weight loss

Genetics
Inheritance pattern is unknown.

Incidence and Prevalence Uncommon

Geographic Distribution N/A

SIGNALMENT

Species
More common in dogs. Rare in cats.

Breed Predilections
• Congenital: Brachycephalic breeds (boxer, Boston terrier, bulldog), Siamese cats
• Acquired: Lhasa apso, shih tzu, Pekingese, poodle

Mean Age
• Congenital: Shortly after weaning and up to one year of age • Acquired: 9.8 years of age

Predominant Sex
Twice as many males as females.

SIGNS

General Comments
• Clinical signs are related to the degree of pyloric narrowing. • Projectile vomiting is generally not a presenting complaint.

Historical Findings
• Chronic intermittent vomiting of undigested or partially digested food (rarely containing bile) within a few hours of eating.
• Congenital lesions begin to produce clinical signs shortly after weaning. • Frequency of vomiting increases with time. • Weight loss
• Lack of responsiveness to antiemetics or motility agents • Hematemesis • Anorexia

Physical Examination Findings
Most dogs are generally in good physical condition. However, some may present with weight loss or abdominal distention.

CAUSES
• Congenital or acquired • May be influenced by infiltrative mural diseases. • Chronic elevations in gastrin levels. • Neuroendocrine factors may play a role.

RISK FACTORS
Chronic stress, inflammatory disorders, chronic gastritis, gastric ulcers, and genetic predispositions are influential factors in the disease process in humans and may play a role in small animals.

DIAGNOSIS

DIFFERENTIAL DIAGNOSIS
• Gastric neoplasia (most common) • Foreign body • Granulomatous fungal disease
• Eosinophilic granuloma • Motility disorders
• Cranial abdominal mass

CBC/BIOCHEMISTRY/URINALYSIS
• Findings are variable depending on the degree and chronicity of obstruction. • Anemia if concurrent ulceration • Pre-renal azotemia if dehydration • Hypochloremia • Hypokalemia • Metabolic alkalosis or acidosis

OTHER LABORATORY TESTS N/A

IMAGING

Abdominal Radiographs
Normal to markedly enlarged stomach.

Upper GI Barium Contrast Study
• May display a "beak" sign created by pyloric narrowing allowing minimal barium to pass into the pyloric antrum. • Retention of the majority of barium in the stomach after four hours indicates delayed gastric emptying.
• Presence of intraluminal filling defects or pyloric wall thickening.

Fluoroscopy
Normal gastric contractility, however barium does not travel through the pylorus.

Other Diagnostic Procedures
Endoscopy allows evaluation of the mucosa for ulceration, hyperplasia, and mass lesions.

GROSS AND HISTOPATHOLOGIC FINDINGS
• Gross findings include focal to multifocal mucosal polyps, diffuse mucosal thickening, and pyloric wall thickening with variable degree of pyloric narrowing • Histologic examination reveals changes ranging from hypertrophy of the circular smooth muscle to hyperplasia of the mucosa and associated glandular structures. There is a wide spectrum of inflammatory cell infiltration.

TREATMENT

INPATIENT VERSUS OUTPATIENT
Patients should be evaluated and surgery scheduled at the earliest convenience.

ACTIVITY N/A

DIET
Highly digestible, low fat diet until surgical intervention.

CLIENT EDUCATION
Surgical treatment is highly successful, however, if clinical signs recur post-operatively, more aggressive surgical procedures may be indicated.

SURGICAL CONSIDERATIONS
• Surgical intervention is the treatment of choice. Goals involve establishing a diagnosis with histopathological samples, excision of abnormal tissue, and restoration of gastrointestinal function with the least radical procedure.
• Surgical procedures depend on the degree of obstruction:

1) Pyloromyotomy (Fredet-Ramstedt)
2) Pyloroplasty (Heineke-Mikulicz or antral advancement flap)
3) Gastroduodenostomy (Bilroth 1)
4) Gastrojejunostomy (Bilroth 2)

MEDICATIONS

DRUGS AND FLUIDS
• Isotonic saline administration with supplementation of chloride and potassium if indicated by physical examination and laboratory findings.
• Antiemetics and motility modifiers are generally ineffective.

CONTRAINDICATIONS
• If evidence of complete pyloric obstruction, metoclopromide should be avoided.
• Avoid anticholinergic agents due to their effects on gastrointestinal motility.

PRECAUTIONS N/A

POSSIBLE INTERACTIONS N/A

ALTERNATE DRUGS N/A

FOLLOW-UP

PATIENT MONITORING
The patient should be monitored post-operatively for recurrence of clinical signs due to an inadequate choice of surgical procedure.

PREVENTION AND AVOIDANCE N/A

Possible Complications
Post-operative surgical complications include recurrence of clinical signs, gastric ulceration, pancreatitis, bile duct obstruction, and incisional dehiscence with peritonitis.

Expected Course and Prognosis
• 85% of dogs show good to excellent results with resolution of clinical signs upon proper surgical intervention.
• Poor prognosis if gastric neoplasia (especially adenocarcinoma) is an underlying cause.

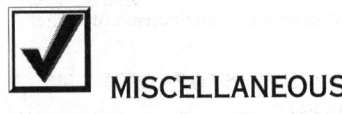 MISCELLANEOUS

ASSOCIATED CONDITIONS
Gastric ulceration

AGE RELATED FACTORS
• The occurrence of intermittent vomiting in young brachycephalic breeds upon weaning is indicative of congenital stenosis. • Chronic intermittent vomiting in adult (8-10 year old) small breed dogs supports a diagnosis of an acquired obstruction.

ZOONOTIC POTENTIAL None
PREGNANCY
High gastrin levels in pregnant females may predispose to the development of the syndrome.

SYNONYMS
• Chronic hypertrophic pyloric gastropathy
• Hypertrophic gastritis • Acquired antral pyloric hypertrophy • Chronic pyloric stenosis
• Gastric polyps

SEE ALSO
Adenocarcinoma, Stomach, Small and Large Intestines

References

DeNovo R. Antral pyloric hypertrophy syndrome. In: Kirk R, ed. Current veterinary therapy X. Philadelphia: WB Saunders, 1989.

Matthiesen D. Chronic gastric outflow obstruction. In: Slatter D, ed. Textbook of small animal surgery. 2nd ed. Philadelphia: WB Saunders, 1993.

Stanton M. Gastric outlet obstruction. In: Bojrab MJ, ed. Disease mechanisms in small animal surgery. 2nd ed. Philadelphia: Lea and Febiger, 1993.

Author James E. Williams, Jr.
Consulting Editor Brent D. Jones

PYODERMA

BASICS

DEFINITION
Bacterial infection of the skin.

Pathophysiology
Skin infections occur when the surface integrity of the skin has been broken, the skin has become macerated by chronic exposure to moisture, normal bacterial flora have been altered, circulation has been impaired, or immunocompentency has been compromised

Systems Affected Skin/Exocrine

Genetics N/A

Incidence/Prevalence
• Very common in dogs • Uncommon in cats

Geographic Distribution N/A

SIGNALMENT

Species Dogs and cats

Breed Predilections
• Breeds with short coats, skin folds or pressure callouses • The German shepherd dog develops a severe, deep pyoderma that may only partially respond to antibiotics and frequently relapses.

Mean Age and Range
Age of onset usually related to underlying cause

Predominant Sex N/A

SIGNS

General Comments
• Superficial pyodermas usually involve the trunk. The extent of the lesions may be obscured by the hair coat. • Deep pyodermas often affect the chin, bridge of the nose, pressure points and feet, or may be generalized.

Historical Findings
• Acute or gradual onset • Variable pruritus. The underlying cause may be pruritic or the staphlococcal infection itself may be pruritic. If the underlying cause is an allergy, the pruritus usually precedes the rash and the pruritus will not resolve with resolution of the pyoderma. Consider an underlying endocrine problem causing a relapsing pyoderma if the pruritus resolves with resolution of the pyoderma. • May be seasonal if the underlying cause is flea allergy or atopy. • If endocrine dysfunction is the underlying cause, symptoms such as polydipsia/polyuria, pendulous abdomen, lethargy, weight gain, or signs of feminization may be reported.

Physical Examination Findings
• Papules • Pustules • Hemorrhagic bullae • Crusts • Epidermal collarettes • Circular erythematous or hyperpigmented spots • Target lesions • Alopecia, moth-eaten hair coat • Scaling • Lichenification • Abscess • Furunculosis, cellulitis

CAUSES
• Most frequently caused by Staphylococcus

intermedius. In cats, Pasturella multocida is also an important pathogen. Deep pyodermas may be complicated by gram-negative organisms (E. coli, Proteus sp., Pseudomonas sp.) • Rarely caused by higher bacteria (Actinomyces, Nocardia, Mycobacteria, Actinobacillus).

RISK FACTORS
• Allergy (flea, atopy, food, contact) • Parasites (especially Demodex) • Fungal infection (dermatophyte) • Endocrine disease (hypothyroidism, hyperadrenocorticism, sex hormone imbalance) • Immune incompetency (glucocorticoids, young animals) • Seborrhea (acne, schnauzer comedo syndrome) • Conformation (short coat, skin folds) • Trauma (pressure points, grooming, scratching, rooting behavior, irritants) • Foreign body (foxtail, grass awn)

DIAGNOSIS

DIFFERENTIAL DIAGNOSIS
• The differential diagnosis for pustular disease is superficial staphylococcal pyoderma, dermatophytosis, demodicosis, pemphigus foliaceus and subcorneal pustular dermatosis. • The differential diagnosis for furunculosis is deep staphylococcal pyoderma, higher bacterial infection, demodicosis, dermatophytosis, opportunistic fungal infections, deep fungal infections, panniculitis, and zinc responsive dermatosis. • Superficial pyoderma in short-coated breeds is often misdiagnosed as urticaria because of acute onset of pruritic bumps.

CBC/BIOCHEMISTRY/URINALYSIS
• In superficial pyodermas the hemogram, serum chemistry profile and urinalysis can be normal or may reflect the underlying cause (anemia due to hypothyroidism, stress leukogram and high serum alkaline phosphatase due to Cushing's disease, eosinophilia due to parasitism). • Generalized deep pyodermas may show leukocytosis with a left shift and hyperglobulinemia in addition to changes related to the underlying cause.

OTHER LABORATORY TESTS N/A

IMAGING N/A

OTHER DIAGNOSTIC PROCEDURES
• Culture usually positive for Staphylococcus intermedius. Gram-negative organisms in addition to Staphylococci or higher bacteria may be cultured from deep pyodermas. Culturing the contents of an intact pustule gives the most reliable results. If no pustules are present, a punch biopsy obtained by sterile technique may be cultured. (More likely to get false negative results.) Culturing beneath a crust or culturing freshly expressed exudate from a draining tract may yield the pathogen or a contaminant. (Least reliable method.) If multiple organisms are cultured

with different antibiotic sensitivities, choose antibiotic on basis of staphylococcal susceptability. • Skin scraping, dermatophyte culture, intradermal allergy testing, hypoallergenic food trial, endocrine tests may identify the underlying cause. • Skin biopsy • Direct smear from intact pustule shows neutrophils engulfing bacteria. Cytology may differentiate pemphigus foliaceus (acantholytic keratinocytes) and deep fungal infections (blastomycosis, cryptococcosis) from pyodermas. • Cytology of tissue grains may identify filamentous organisms characteristic of higher bacteria.

GROSS AND HISTOPATHOLOGIC FINDINGS
• Subcorneal pustules, intraepidermal neutrophilic microabscesses, perifolliculitis, folliculitis, furunculosis, nodular to diffuse dermatitis, or panniculitis. The inflammatory reaction may be suppurative or pyogranulomatous. • Tissue grains within pyogranulomas are observed most often with Staphylococcus, Actinomyces, Actinobacillus and Nocardia. • Special stains may help identify gram-negative bacteria or acid fast organisms.

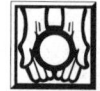

TREATMENT

INPATIENT VERSUS OUTPATIENT
Usually treated as outpatient except for patients with severe, generalized, deep pyodermas that may require intravenous fluids, parenteral antibiotics or daily whirlpool baths.

ACTIVITY No restriction

DIET
• Hypoallergenic diet if disease is secondary to food allergy; otherwise a high quality, well balanced dog food.
• High protein, poor quality "bargain" diets and excessive supplementation should be avoided.

CLIENT EDUCATION NA

SURGICAL CONSIDERATIONS
Fold pyodermas require surgical correction to prevent recurrence.

MEDICATIONS

DRUGS AND FLUIDS
• S. intermedius isolates are usually susceptible to cephalosporins, cloxacillin, oxacillin, methicillin, amoxicillin-clavulanate, erythromycin, and chloramphenicol. Somewhat less effective are lincomycin and trimethoprim-sulfonamide. Isolates are frequently resistant to amoxicillin, ampicillin, penicillin, tetracycline, and sulfonamides.
• Since most isolates of Staphylococcus and P. multocida are susceptible to amoxicillin - clavulanate, this antibiotic is generally effective for skin infections in cats.

• Superficial pyodermas initially may be treated empirically.

• Antibiotic therapy for recurrent, resistant or deep pyodermas should be based on culture and sensitivity testing.

CONTRAINDICATION

Steroids are contraindicated and will encourage resistance and recurrence even when used concurrently with antibiotics.

PRECAUTIONS

• Erythromycin, lincomycin and oxacillin may produce vomiting. Administer with small amount of food.

• Although isolates are frequently sensitive to gentamicin and kanamycin, renal toxicity of these drugs usually precludes their prolonged systemic use.

• Trimethoprim-sulfa has been associated with KCS, fever, hepatotoxicity, polyarthritis, and hematologic abnormalities.

• Chloramphenicol should be used with caution in cats and may cause mild, reversible anemia in dogs.

POSSIBLE INTERACTIONS

Trimethoprim-sulfa may result in low thyroid test results.

ALTERNATE DRUGS

• Ancillary therapy includes benzoyl peroxide or chlorhexidine shampoos to remove surface debris. Whirlpool baths are helpful in deep pyodermas to remove crusted exudate and encourage drainage.

• Staphage lysate, staphoid AB or autogenous bacterins may improve antibiotic efficacy and decrease recurrence in some cases.

 FOLLOW-UP

PATIENT MONITORING

Antibiotics should be continued for a minimum of 2 weeks beyond clinical cure. This time period is usually about 1 month for superficial pyodermas, and 2 to 3 months or longer for deep pyodermas.

PREVENTION/AVOIDANCE

• Routine bathing with benzoyl peroxide or chlorhexidine shampoos may help prevent recurrences. • Some cases that continue to relapse may be managed with long-term q24h antibiotic therapy. • Padded bedding may ease pressure point pyodermas.

POSSIBLE COMPLICATIONS

Bacteremia and septicemia

EXPECTED COURSE AND PROGNOSIS

Likely to be recurrent or nonresponsive if underlying cause is not identified and effectively managed.

 MISCELLANEOUS

ASSOCIATED CONDITIONS N/A

AGE RELATED FACTORS

• Impetigo affects young dogs prior to puberty in association with poor husbandry and often requires only topical therapy. • A superficial pustular dermatitis occurs in kittens in association with overzealous "mouthing" by the queen. • Pyoderma secondary to atopy usually begins at 1 to 3 years of age, while pyoderma secondary to endocrine disorders usually begin in middle adulthood.

ZOONOTIC POTENTIAL

• Cutaneus tuberculosis (rare) • The zoonotic potential of feline leprosy is unknown.

PREGNANCY N/A

SYNONYMS N/A

SEE ALSO

• Acne—Dogs • Acne—Cats • Dermatitis, Interdigital • Pododermatitis • Perianal Fistulae

References

Muller GH, Kirk RW, Scott DW. Small animal dermatology. 4th ed. Philadelphia: WB Saunders, 1989;244-287.

Author Ellen C. Codner

Consulting Editor Lowell Ackerman

PYOMETRA AND CYSTIC ENDOMETRIAL HYPERPLASIA

BASICS

DEFINITION
Cystic endometrial hyperplasia is a hormonally mediated, progressive pathologic change in the uterine lining. Pyometra develops secondary to cystic endometrial hyperplasia when bacterial invasion of the abnormal endometrium leads to intraluminal accumulation of purulent exudate.

Pathophysiology
Normal cycling bitches experience a 2-month diestrus, with ovarian secretion of progesterone after every estrus. Repeated exposure of the endometrium to high concentrations of estrogen followed by high concentrations of progesterone in the absence of pregnancy leads to cystic endometrial hyperplasia. Secretions formed are an excellent medium for growth of bacteria ascending from the vagina through the partially open cervix during proestrus and estrus. Bacteria involved are those of the normal vaginal flora; Escherichia coli is the most common isolate.

Systems Affected
• Reproductive • Renal/Urologic • Hemic/Lymphatic/Immune • Hepatobiliary

Genetics
No genetic predisposition known

Incidence/Prevalence
Most dogs and cats in the United States undergo elective ovariohysterectomy (OHE), precluding accurate assessment of incidence.

Geographic Distribution N/A

SIGNALMENT

Species
Dogs and cats > 6 years old

Breed Predilections N/A

Mean Age And Range
• Can also develop in younger animals, especially if they were treated with exogenous estrogen or progestogen. • In dogs usually diagnosed 1–12 weeks after estrus • In cats the onset relative to estrus is more variable. • No breed predisposition known. • Pyometra of the uterine stump in spayed animals can develop any time after OHE.

Predominant Sex N/A

SIGNS

Historical Findings
If the cervix is closed, animals are more likely to show signs of systemic illness, progressing to signs of septicemia and shock.

Physical Examination Findings
• Palpably large uterus—careful palpation of the abdomen may allow determination of uterine size. Overly aggressive palpation may induce uterine rupture. If the cervix is open, the uterus may not be palpably large. • Vaginal discharge—presence depends on cervical patency. The discharge is sanguinous to mucopurulent. • Depression and lethargy • Anorexia • Polyuria and polydipsia • Vomiting • Abdominal distension • Fever (variable)

CAUSES
• In dogs, this condition is caused by the unique, repeated exposure of the endometrium to estrogen, followed by exposure to progesterone. • In cats, it may be caused by estrogen at estrus, followed by a progestational phase caused by induction of ovulation by coitus or by other stimuli as yet undefined.

RISK FACTORS
• Older, nulliparous animals may be predisposed. • Pharmacologic use of estrogen ("mismate") shots during midestrus to early diestrus • No correlation exists between this condition and pseudopregnancy in dogs.

DIAGNOSIS

DIFFERENTIAL DIAGNOSIS
• Pregnancy • Other causes of polyuria and polydipsia such as diabetes mellitus, hyperadrenocorticism, and primary renal disease. • Severe vaginal disease

CBC/BIOCHEMISTRY/URINALYSIS
• Immature neutrophilia; more severe if the cervix is closed. • Mild, normocytic, normochromic anemia • Hyperglobulinemia and hyperproteinemia • Azotemia • ALT and ALP are high in patients with septicemia or severe dehydration. Electrolyte disturbances vary with the clinical course of the disease. • Urinalysis—urine collected by catheterization of the urinary bladder is least traumatic to collect and most diagnostically accurate.

OTHER LABORATORY TESTS
• Cytologic examination of vaginal discharge reveals regenerative polymorphonuclear cells and bacteria. This may be indistinguishable from the purulent discharge associated with vaginal disease (e.g., vaginitis, vaginal mass, foreign object, and vaginal anatomic anomaly). • Bacterial culture and sensitivity test of vaginal discharge. This is not helpful in confirming the diagnosis since bacteria cultured from the pyometra are usually normal vaginal flora. • Serologic testing for Brucella canis. The rapid slide agglutination test is used as a screen. The test is sensitive but not specific; if positive, recheck by an agar gel immunodiffusion test (Cornell University Diagnostic Laboratory, Ithaca, NY, 607 253–3900) or bacterial culture of whole blood, lymph node aspirate, or vaginal discharge.

IMAGING
• Radiography can be used to detect a large uterus and to rule out pregnancy after day 45 after ovulation or days 43 – 54 after breeding. In patients with pyometra, the uterus may appear as a distended, tubular structure in the caudal ventral abdomen. • Ultrasonography can be used to assess size of the uterus and the extent of cystic endometrial hyperplasia and to rule out pregnancy after day 20–24 after ovulation. The normal uterine wall is not visible as a distinct entity. Cystic endometrial hyperplasia and pyometra are associated with a thickened uterine wall and intraluminal fluid. Pregnancy and pyometra can occur together in dogs (rare).

OTHER DIAGNOSTIC PROCEDURES
Vaginoscopy. Only indicated in dogs with purulent vulvar discharge and no apparent uterine enlargement. Vaginoscopy allows determination of site of origin of the vaginal discharge. It is not possible in cats.

GROSS AND HISTOPATHOLOGIC FINDINGS
The endometrium in dogs and cats with cystic endometrial hyperplasia or pyometra is described as "cobblestone." The cystic endometrial surface is covered by malodorous, mucopurulent exudate. The endometrium is thickened because of increase in the size of endometrial glands and cystic gland distension.

TREATMENT

INPATIENT VERSUS OUTPATIENT
Pyometra is a life–threatening condition if the cervix is closed. Animals should be hospitalized, and supportive care with IV administration of fluids and antibiotics begun immediately. Choice of antibiotic is empirical pending results of bacterial culture and sensitivity test.

ACTIVITY N/A

DIET N/A

CLIENT EDUCATION
• The preferred treatment is OHE. Medical treatment is appropriate only for valuable breeding animals or those for whom the owner is willing to provide nonprogestational, estrus–suppressing drugs for life.
• Medical treatment of closed–cervix pyometra is associated with uterine rupture and peritonitis (see Medications – Precautions).
• Medical treatment probably does not cure underlying cystic endometrial hyperplasia in patients with either open– or closed–cervix pyometra but may enable some affected bitches to reproduce.

SURGICAL CONSIDERATIONS
OHE is the preferred treatment for patients with both open– and closed–cervix pyometra, since it is a chronic progressive disease. Be cautious during OHE of a bitch with closed–cervix pyometra, because the enlarged uterus may be very friable. If uterine rupture or leakage of purulent material from the uterine stump occurs, repeated lavage of the peritoneal cavity with sterile saline is indicated.

MEDICATIONS

DRUGS AND FLUIDS

• Prostaglandin F_{2a} (PGF_{2a}). Dosages given are recommended only for the native compound, because dosage for analogues is not well defined. Dogs—0.25 mg/kg SQ q24h for 2–7 days until the uterus nears normal size as determined by palpation, radiography, or ultrasound. If the animal is in a luteal phase (serum progesterone > 2 ng/ml), the dosage 0.25 mg/kg SQ q12h for 4 days can be used. Once-daily dosing causes smooth muscle contractions and subsequent uterine evacuation. Twice-daily dosing also causes luteolysis and a subsequent decrease in serum progesterone concentration. The animal should be reevaluated 2–4 weeks after PGF_{2a} has been discontinued. If the uterus has increased in size or the patient still has marked vaginal discharge, the protocol can be repeated. OHE should be performed in bitches refractory to prostaglandin. Cats—0.1–0.5 mg/kg SQ q24h for 2–5 days until the size of the uterus nears normal
• Antibiotics—all animals with pyometra should be treated with systemic antibiotics. Choice of antibiotic is empirical pending results of bacterial culture and sensitivity test. Common choices include ampicillin (20 mg/kg PO q8h) and enrofloxacin (Baytril) (2.5 mg/kg PO q12h).

CONTRAINDICATIONS

PGF_{2a} causes strong myometrial contractions which, in patients with closed–cervix pyometra, can cause uterine rupture or force purulent exudate through the uterine tubes causing secondary peritonitis.
Always rule out pregnancy before administering PGF_{2a} to a valuable breeding animal.

PRECAUTIONS

• PGF_{2a} is not approved for use in dogs and cats.
• Side effects of PGF_{-2a} are referable to contraction of smooth muscle and include hypersalivation, emesis, and defecation and, in cats, intense grooming of the flanks and vulva.

Side effects appear within minutes of injection of the drug and subside within 30-60 minutes. Severity of side effects diminshes throughout the treatment regimen. Side effects may be diminished by diluting the drug with an equal volume of sterile saline before injecting SQ and by walking dogs for 20-30 minutes after injection.

POSSIBLE INTERACTIONS N/A

ALTERNATE DRUGS

Drugs that enhance the immune response (e.g., estrogens) or induce myometrial contractility (e.g., oxytocin and ergot alkaloids) are unreliable. Antibiotics are not efficacious as sole treatment unless the uterus is normal in size and the serum progesterone is < 2 ng/ml.

FOLLOW-UP

PATIENT MONITORING

• Release the patient from the hospital when the uterus is near normal in size and clinical signs have lessened in severity or disappeared. Reevaluate in 2-4 weeks as described previously.
• Continue antibiotic administration for 3–4 weeks. • Vaginal discharge may persist for up to 4 weeks. • Serial CBCs—WBC count rises precipitously after OHE, because bone marrow continues to release polymorphonuclear neutrophils into the bloodstream, from which they can no longer enter the uterus, the "sink" of inflammation in this disease.

PREVENTION/AVOIDANCE

• At the next proestrus, obtain a specimen of the the anterior vagina for bacterial culture using a guarded culture swab. • Treat the bitch with an appropriate antibiotic for 3 weeks. • Breed in that season because 1) the gravid uterus may be less susceptible to re–infection, 2) the bitch has underlying cystic endometrial hyperplasia which will limit her breeding life, so it is best to get the desired number of pups from her as soon as possible, and 3) the bitch is not more likely to clear the disease spontaneously if allowed to cycle without being bred.

POSSIBLE COMPLICATIONS

The bitch may enter estrus after treatment earlier than anticipated if medical treatment has induced premature luteolysis.

EXPECTED COURSE AND PROGNOSIS

The bitch still has underlying cystic endometrial hyperplasia and so is predisposed to recurrence. She should be bred to the desired stud dogs in a timely manner, and undergo ovariohysterectomy as soon as her breeding life is over. The use of subfertile stud dogs is not recommended.

MISCELLANEOUS

ASSOCIATED CONDITIONS

Pyometra of the uterine stump in spayed animals can develop any time after OHE and may be associated with an ovarian remnant.

AGE RELATED FACTORS N/A

ZOONOTIC POTENTIAL N/A

PREGNANCY

Always rule out pregnancy before administering PGF_{2a} to a valuable breeding animal, because PGF_{2a} is an effective pregnancy terminating agent in dogs and cats.

SYNONYMS N/A

SEE ALSO N/A

ABBREVIATIONS

OHE = Ovariohysterectomy
PGF_{2a} = prostaglandin F2a
WBC = white blood cells

Reference

Hardy RM, Osborne CA. Canine pyometra: pathophysiology, diagnosis and treatment of uterine and extrauterine lesions. J Am Anim Hosp Assoc 1974;10:245–268.
Author Margaret V. Root
Consulting Editor Sara K. Lyle

PYOTHORAX

BASICS

DEFINITION
Accumulation of pus within the pleural cavity, usually associated with infection

Pathophysiology
Infectious pyothorax generally arises from transpulmonary, transesophageal, or transthoracic innoculation of bacteria into the pleural space with subsequent suppurative pleuritis. Commonly associated causes include inhalation of grass awns or other foreign objects or penetrating wounds to the thorax. Pyothorax secondary to systemic infection or pleuropneumonia is less common.

Systems Affected
• Respiratory • Hemic/lymphatic/immune
• Renal/urologic—protein-losing glomerulopathy

Genetics N/A

Incidence/Prevalence N/A

Geographic Distribution N/A

SIGNALMENT

Species Dogs and cats

Breed Predilections
• Hunting and sporting breeds • Domestic shorthaired cats

Mean Age and Range N/A

Predominant Sex N/A

SIGNS

General Comments
• Often insidious in nature, with few clinical signs until late in the course of disease
• Respiratory compromise often is not severe.

Historical Findings
• Reported signs include a decrease in performance, collapse after exercising, slow recovery, and weight loss and partial anorexia.
• Temporary improvement with antibiotic therapy • History of fights or puncture wounds should be confirmed.

Physical Examination Findings
• Tachypnea usually is apparent but may be mild and unassociated with dyspnea.
• Cachexia often is observed. • Cough may be present. • Pyrexia may or may not be present and is usually low-grade. • Thoracic auscultation may reveal muffled heart sounds, diminished lung sounds ventrally, and amplified lung sounds dorsally. • Cats may show few clinical signs before onset of apparently acute respiratory distress. • Injury to the thoracic wall may not be apparent or may be healed at the time of examination. Perform thorough palpation and inspection of the thorax for evidence of scarring or fibrosis.

CAUSES

Infectious
Actinomyces spp., Nocardia spp., Bacteroides spp., Corynebacterium, E. coli, fungal agents,

Streptococcus. The frequency of isolation of these organisms may vary geographically. Infections usually are polymicrobial.

Neoplastic
Intrathoracic tumors rarely cause pyothorax secondary to tumor necrosis.

RISK FACTORS
Hunting, field trials, and other strenuous outdoor sporting activities. Fighting in cats.

DIAGNOSIS

DIFFERENTIAL DIAGNOSIS
Other pleural effusions such as chylothorax, hemothorax, and transudative effusions. Examination of the fluid will help differentiate the etiology.

CBC/BIOCHEMISTRY/URINALYSIS

CBC
Severe neutrophilic leukocytosis with a left shift (usually regenerative) and monocytosis anemia of chronic disease. If substantial hemorrhage into the pleural cavity has occurred, a regenerative anemia may be seen.

Biochemistry
Often normal. May show hyperglobulinemia as a result of inflammation, hypoalbuminemia as a result of renal losses, and mild elevation in alkaline phosphatase. If other organs are secondarily infected (e.g., with pyelonephritis or hepatitis), organ-specific changes may be apparent.

Urinalysis
May show proteinuria if glomerulopathy has developed

OTHER LABORATORY TESTS
Fungal titers may be positive.

IMAGING

Radiography
• Reveals pleural effusion • Abscesses within the pulmonary parenchyma • Pleural fissure lines • The effusion may be bilateral or unilateral.

Ultrasound
Reveals pleural effusion. May show significant amount of fibrinous deposition in the pleural space.

OTHER DIAGNOSTIC PROCEDURES

Thoracocentesis
• Cytologic evaluation will confirm the diagnosis of pyothorax, as many effusions appear grossly hemorrhagic. Gram's stain may assist in early identification of pathogenic organisms. • The presence of "sulfa granules" (small accumulations of purulent debris) in the exudate is characteristic of infection with the filamentous organisms (Actinomyces, Nocardia).
• Organisms may be seen in the fluid samples, often within neutrophils.
• Degenerative neutrophils are abundant.

Microbiology
• All fluid samples should be cultured aerobically and anaerobically. Many of the filamentous, microaerophilic, and anaerobic organisms are slow-growing, so cultures should be maintained for 2-4 weeks. If "sulfa granules" are present in the sample, maceration of these granules may enhance the culturing of an organism, as bacteria are found in higher concentrations within these "granules."
• Culturing for fungal organisms depends on history and geographical location. • Urine samples should be cultured if pyelonephritis is suspected.

TREATMENT
• Treat like any abscess; drainage is critical. Without adequate drainage, resolution is highly unlikely.
• Continuous evacuation via tube thoracostomy with low-pressure suction through a large-bore (20-24 Fr), perforated tube. In compromised patients, general anesthesia may need to be replaced by other anesthetic or analgesic protocols.
• Drainage should be monitored by periodic thoracic radiograph to ensure that bilateral tube placement is not necessary, that tube placement is adequate, and that there is no pocketing or loculation of exudate or primary pulmonary pathology that may not have been apparent at the initial radiographic examination.
• Thoracic lavage (q6h-q8h) with warm, sterile saline may assist in breaking down consolidated debris. • Coupage (rapid thoracic percussion) may assist in removing consolidated debris. • Cultures should be repeated if the patient fails to improve.
• Thoracic drainage should be continued until net drainage is < 2-3 ml/kg/day and intracellular bacteria are no longer present on Gram's stain. Drainage may be slightly higher with red-rubber tubes because these are more irritant.
• CBC and albumin may be measured to monitor effectiveness of therapy. Renal protein loss usually resolves with treatment of the pyothorax and requires no specific therapy.

GROSS AND HISTOPATHOLOGIC FINDINGS
• Fibrinous and suppurative pleuritis, with or without pulmonary abscessation
• Glomerulonephritis

INPATIENT VERSUS OUTPATIENT
Patients often need to be hospitalized for several weeks.

ACTIVITY
• The patient should be encouraged to exercise lightly during the hospitalization period (10 minutes q6h-q8h) to promote ventilatory efforts and aid in breaking down pleural adhesions. • After discharge, gradual increase in exercise over 2-4 months is advised.

DIET
• High-calorie diet • Protein replacement usually is unnecessary.

CLIENT EDUCATION
The duration and expense of inpatient and outpatient treatment are considerable.

SURGICAL CONSIDERATIONS
• Surgery is associated with higher mortality and is contraindicated unless pulmonary abscessation, pleural fibrosis, lung lobe torsion, or extensive loculation of the pus is present, limiting effective thoracic drainage. • Surgery may be indicated if pus is restricted to mediastinum.

MEDICATIONS
DRUGS AND FLUIDS
Antimicrobials
• Determined by the in vitro sensitivity results of the culture • If the presence of a particular pathogen is suspected, therapy may be initiated based on common antibiotic sensitivities of particular organisms before obtaining culture results (e.g., Actinomyces spp. and Bacteroides [non-fragilis] spp. are often susceptible to amoxicillin; Nocardia spp. are often susceptible to potentiated sulfas).
• Trimethoprim-sulfa, aminoglycosides, and quinolones are largely ineffective in healing pyothorax. • Occasionally, multiple antibiotics may be needed. Metronidazole plus amoxicillin is a good combination in cats.
• Dosages are generally high (e.g., amoxicillin 40 mg/kg PO q8h) to allow adequate penetration into the pleural cavity. Treatment may need to be continued for several months or occasionally indefinitely.

Analgesics
Generally not required. Intrapleural anesthesia may be used with bupivicaine mixed with the lavage fluid if severe discomfort is present.

CONTRAINDICATIONS
Glucocorticoids and immunosuppressive agents should be avoided in infectious pyothorax.

PRECAUTIONS
Potentiated sulfas may be associated with keratoconjunctivitis sicca, polyarthropathies, hypothyroidism, thrombocytopenia, and anemia, especially with prolonged use.

POSSIBLE INTERACTIONS N/A

ALTERNATE DRUGS
If the primary organism is not known and culture and sensitivity results are pending, amoxicillin should be chosen because of its high efficacy against anerobic bacteria and low probability of complications or toxicity. Clindamycin may also be considered.

FOLLOW-UP
PATIENT MONITORING
• Net thoracic fluid production should be measured to detemine when thoracic drains may be removed. • Thoracic radiographs also should be evaluated to ensure adequate evacuation of fluid. • Once discharged, antibiotics should be continued for 1 month past the time when the patient is clinically normal, the hemogram is normal, and there is no radiographic evidence of fluid recurrence.
• Residual radiographic changes may be permanent, but fluid should be absent. • The patient should be assessed monthly via CBC and radiographs. • The average duration of antibiotic therapy is 3-4 months, but may continue for 6-12 months.

PREVENTION/AVOIDANCE
Avoid activity that predisposes to this disease (often not practical).

POSSIBLE COMPLICATIONS
• Complications of antibiotic therapy are described above. • Incorrect insertion of the drainage tube may prevent adequate drainage or produce pneumothorax. Too proximal a placement of the tube may place pressure on the brachial arteries and veins, resulting in unilateral limb edema or lameness. • Lung laceration during tube placement • Persistent, recurrent pyothorax as a result of compartmentalization of pus or premature discontinuation of treatment • Chronic fibrosing pleuritis and poor performance upon apparent recovery (pleural fibrosis sometimes can be successfully removed at surgery) • Persistent mediastinitis

EXPECTED COURSE AND PROGNOSIS
• Fair to excellent with aggressive management. Poor with repeated, intermittent antibiotic therapy only or with inadequate drainage. • Return to performance depends on chronicity of disease and level of management.

MISCELLANEOUS
ASSOCIATED CONDITIONS
• Occasionally, retroperitoneal abscessation and discospondylitis from migration of a foreign body through the diaphragm into the retroperitoneal space • Glomerulonephropathy

AGE RELATED FACTORS N/A

ZOONOTIC POTENTIAL
Fungal infections during in vitro isolation

PREGNANCY N/A

SYNONYMS
• Empyema • Suppurative pleuritis • Pleurisy

SEE ALSO
• Dyspnea and Tachypnea • Pleural Effusion
• Chylothorax

ABBREVIATIONS N/A

References

Roudebush P. Bacterial infections of the respiratory system. In: Greene C, ed. Infectious diseases of the dog and cat. Philadelphia: WB Saunders, 1990:114-121.

Hardie EM. Actinomycosis and nocardiosis. In: Greene C, ed. Infectious diseases of the dog and cat. Philadelphia: WB Saunders, 1990.

Marino DJ, Jaggy A. Nocardiosis. A literature review with selected case reports in two dogs. J Vet Int Med 1993;7:4-11.

McCurnin DM, Poffenbarger EM. Small animal physical diagnosis and clinical procedures. Philadelphia: WB Saunders, 1991:167-171.

Author Mark Rishniw
Consulting Editors Lynelle Johnson and Bradley L. Moses

PYRETHRIN AND PYRETHROID TOXICITY

BASICS

OVERVIEW

Natural pyrethrins are derived from Chrysanthemum cinerariaefolium and related plant species and synthetic pyrethroids such as allethrin, cypermethrin, permethrin, fenvalerate, and fluvalinate. Insecticidal compounds are commonly found in flea and tick control products.

These reversibly prolong sodium conductance in nerve axons, resulting in repetitive nerve discharges. This effect is enhanced in mammals with subnormal body temperatures and in cold blooded animals.

SIGNALMENT

• Adverse reactions occur more frequently in cats because of their inherently poor ability to metabolize many compounds. • Cats and small dogs have a relatively large body surface area compared with body mass, making it easier to overdose small pets with topical insecticides.

SIGNS

Clinical signs of toxicity range from mild hypersensitivity to acute anaphylactic, toxic, and idiosyncratic reactions.

Mild side effects:
• Hypersalivation • Paw flicking • Ear twitching • Mild depression • Vomiting or diarrhea in some animals

Moderate to serious signs from topical exposure or ingestion other than from grooming:
• Protracted vomiting and diarrhea
• Marked depression • Ataxia • Muscle tremors, which must be differentiated from paw flicking and ear twitching • Extreme dermal or oral overdose may cause seizures or death. • Cats are especially sensitive to concentrated permethrin-containing products labeled for use on dogs, and can develop muscle tremors, ataxia, seizures, and death within hours. • Allergic reactions can be manifested as urticaria, hyperemia, pruritis, anaphylaxis, shock, respiratory distress, and rarely, death.
• Cases involving death of a pet must be investigated including necropsy, histopathologic examination, and other diagnostic tests to rule out predisposing underlying conditions.

CAUSE AND RISK FACTORS

• Pets, especially cats that are sprayed in the face, may exhibit nonharmful salivation.
• Overall, cats are more sensitive because of less efficient metabolic pathways, extensive grooming habits, and long haircoats, which can retain large quantities of product when sprayed heavily. • Pets that have subnormal body temperatures after anesthesia or sedation are predisposed to adverse reactions, because the nervous system effects of pyrethrins and pyrethroids are enhanced at low temperatures. • Toxicosis can also result from the accidental or intentional use of dog-only products on cats, use of incorrectly diluted dips or sponge-ons, accidental ingestion of insecticides (i.e., other than grooming after correct product application), and the incorrect use of premise products on pets.
• Underlying disease conditions such as cardiomyopathy and hyperthyroidism can become clinical emergencies when pets are stressed by bathing, dipping, or spraying.

DIAGNOSIS

DIFFERENTIAL DIAGNOSIS

• All pesticides, medications, or other toxicants in the area as well as previous medical history or underlying conditions must be considered. • Before a tentative diagnosis of pyrethrin or pyrethroid insecticide toxicosis can be made, the exposure history including amount and frequency of product usage, type and severity of clinical signs, and onset and duration of clinical signs must be consistent.
• Specific rule-outs include organophosphate, carbamate, or d-limonene toxicosis, flea bite anemia, cardiomyopathy, or hyperthyroidism.

CBC/BIOCHEMISTRY/URINALYSIS

No specific abnormalities result from pyrethrin toxicity. However, in unusually severe cases, these tests are warranted to rule out underlying or predisposing conditions.

OTHER LABORATORY TESTS

• Analytical tests to detect pyrethrins in animal tissues or fluids are not generally available. Some synthetic pyrethroids can be detected in tissues to confirm exposure.
• Cholinesterase activity is not reduced by pyrethrins or pyrethroid insecticides. Whole blood cholinesterase determination is recommended, however, to rule-out exposure to organophosphate or carbamate insecticides.

IMAGING N/A

OTHER DIAGNOSTIC PROCEDURES
N/A

TREATMENT

• Adverse reactions to pyrethrins or pyrethroids are generally mild and self-limiting. Salivation, paw flicking, and ear twitching generally resolve without care. • Pets that have been saturated with spray products should be dried with a warmed towel from a clothes dryer and brushed out. If signs continue or progress to tremors and ataxia, the pet should be hospitalized and bathed with a hand dish washing detergent. • Maintenance of a normal body temperature is critical.

MEDICATIONS

DRUGS AND FLUIDS

• Tremors are managed with diazepam (0.05-1.0 mg/kg IV). • Seizures or unresponsive tremors are managed with phenobarbital (3.0-30 mg/kg IV to effect, low dosage in cats). • Fluid support with balanced electrolyte solution is recommended to treat seriously affected pets. • Topical decontamination procedures (e.g., detergent bath with a hand dish washing detergent) are used to treat pets exposed dermally. • For animals that have ingested large amounts or been overdosed by dermal application of a synthetic pyrethroid (eg, permethrin on cats), administer activated charcoal (2.0 gm/kg PO or by stomach tube) mixed with sorbital as a cathartic (3.0 ml/kg of a 70% solution) in a water slurry. Sorbital is available premixed with activated charcoal from some manufacturers. If the patient has diarrhea, isorbital should not be given. • Gastrointestinal decontamination is only warranted when large amounts of insecticide are taken orally; for example, when an undiluted bottle of dip is spilled and the contents are lapped up by a dog. If the pet is asymptomatic and ingestion took place within 1-2 hours, emesis can be induced with 3% hydrogen peroxide after feeding (2.0 ml/kg, maximum 45 ml). If the pet is symptomatic and ingestion took place within 1-2 hours, gastric lavage can be done with the animal under sedation and an endotracheal tube in place; use a large bore stomach tube and repeat flushings until clear water is seen draining from the stomach tube.

CONTRAINDICATIONS/POSSIBLE INTERACTIONS

• Atropine sulfate is not antidotal and its use should be avoided. • Excess use of atropine, such as may be indicated for organophosphate or carbamate toxicosis can cause tachycardia, CNS stimulation, disorientation, drowsiness, respiratory depression, and even seizures. • Avoid hypothermia.

FOLLOW-UP

Hypersalivation can recur when pets, especially cats, groom themselves for several days after the use of flea control products. Clinical signs from self-limiting hypersalivation to severe tremors or seizures requiring hospitalization generally resolve within 24-72 hours. Proper application of flea control products can greatly reduce the incidence of adverse reactions. Correct application amount of most sprays is 1-2 pumps of a typical trigger sprayer per pound of body weight. To reduce salivation by sensitive cats, spray products can be sprayed onto a grooming brush and evenly brushed through the haircoat. Dips must be diluted correctly and should be sponged onto the haircoat instead of applying by total body emersion. Premise products should not be applied topically unless labeled for such uses.

 MISCELLANEOUS

SEE ALSO

• Poisoning (Intoxication) • Organophosphate and Carbamate Toxicity

ABBREVIATION

CNS = central nervous system

Reference

Valentine WM. Pyrethrin and pyrethroid insecticides. In: Beasley VR, ed. Vet Clin North Am Small Anim Pract 1990; 20:375-382.

Authors Steven R. Hansen and Elizabeth A. Curry-Galvin

Consulting Editor Gary Osweiler

PYRUVATE KINASE DEFICIENCY

BASICS

OVERVIEW
• Red blood cells (RBC) require energy in the form of ATP for maintenance of shape and deformability, active membrane transport, partial synthesis of nucleotides, and synthesis of glutathione. Mature RBC lack mitochondria and depend on anaerobic glycolysis for ATP generation.
• Pyruvate kinase (PK) catalyzes an important rate-controlling, ATP-generating step in glycolysis; consequently, energy metabolism is markedly impaired in PK-deficient RBC, which results in shortened RBC lifespan and anemia. The bone marrow attempts to compensate by erythroid hyperplasia, with marked reticulocytosis in peripheral blood.

SIGNALMENT
• Autosomal recessive trait recognized in basenji, beagle, West Highland white terrier, cairn terrier, and American Eskimo dogs, and in Abyssinian cats. • Homozygously affected animals generally not recognized as abnormal until several months of age and may not be recognized until adulthood

SIGNS
• Exercise intolerance, pale mucous membranes, tachycardia, systolic heart murmurs, and often splenomegaly or hepatomegaly. Icterus is rarely seen. • Affected dogs may be slightly smaller than normal for their breed and age and may exhibit weakness and muscle wasting.
• Heterozygous carriers are asymptomatic.

CAUSES AND RISK FACTORS
• RBC from normal adult dogs exhibit only one PK isozyme, designated the R-type. PK deficiency in the basenji dog results from a single base deletion of the PK L-gene, which encodes for the L-type isozyme in hepatocytes and the R-type isozyme in RBC. • Specific molecular defects in other breeds of dogs and PK-deficient cats have not been reported.

DIAGNOSIS

DIFFERENTIAL DIAGNOSIS
• Other causes of hemolytic anemia, including autoimmune hemolytic anemia, hemo-
bartonellosis, babesiosis, Heinz body hemolytic anemia, microangiopathic hemolytic anemia, and phosphofructokinase (PFK) deficiency. • PK-deficient dogs should be Coombs' test negative, lack parasites or Heinz bodies in stained blood films, be seronegative for Babesia species, and lack evidence of disseminated intravascular coagulation or heartworm disease. • In contrast to PFK deficiency, PK-deficient dogs do not exhibit episodes of intravascular hemolysis and hemoglobinuria. These deficiencies are differentiated using specific enzyme assays or DNA tests.

CBC/BIOCHEMISTRY/URINALYSIS
• Macrocytic hypochromic anemia, with PCV values between 16% and 28% and uncorrected reticulocyte counts of 15%-50%
• Normal or slightly high leukocyte counts with a mature neutrophilia • Normal to slightly high platelet counts • Moderate to marked polychromasia, anisocytosis, and frequent nucleated RBC on stained blood films
• Poikilocytes in some animals, especially in splenectomized dogs • Possible abnormal clinical chemistry findings such as hyperferremia, mild hyperbilirubinemia, and slightly high ALT and alkaline phosphatase activities. Dogs with liver failure may have hypoalbuminemia. • Normal urinalysis, except for bilirubinuria in dogs

OTHER LABORATORY TESTS
• Measure low total RBC PK activity for diagnosis in cats and some dogs. Many affected dogs have normal or increased activities because of the expression of a M2 isozyme that does not normally occur in mature RBC. Heterozygous animals have approximately 50% of normal RBC PK activity. • Use additional assays (enzyme heat stability test, measurement of RBC glycolytic intermediates, electrophoresis of isozymes and enzyme immunoprecipitation) to reach a diagnosis in dogs whose total enzyme activity is not low.
• Use DNA diagnostic test for screening basenji dogs. If defect is identical in other dog breeds, this test could also be applied to those breeds.

IMAGING N/A

OTHER DIAGNOSTIC PROCEDURES
N/A

TREATMENT
Affected animals can only be cured by bone marrow transplantation.

MEDICATIONS

DRUGS AND FLUIDS
Although not adequately evaluated, long-term therapy with iron-chelating drugs such as deferoxamine mesylate might prolong the life expectancy of affected animals.

CONTRAINDICATIONS/POSSIBLE INTERACTIONS N/A

FOLLOW-UP
• Affected dogs develop hepatic iron overload, which can result in cirrhosis. Myelofibrosis and osteosclerosis also develop with age in dogs. As a result, most affected dogs die by 4 years of age as a result of bone marrow or liver failure. • Severe anemia with minimal reticulocytosis, abnormal liver function tests, and ascites secondary to hypoalbuminemia indicate the terminal stage of the disease in dogs.
• The long-term consequences of this deficiency in cats have yet to be determined.

MISCELLANEOUS

ABBREVIATIONS
ALT = alanine aminotransferase
ATP = adenosine triphosphate
DNA = deoxyribonucleic acid
PCV = packed cell volume
PFK = phosphofructokinase
PK = pyruvate kinase
RBC = red blood cells

Reference

Giger U, Noble NA. Determination of erythrocyte pyruvate kinase deficiency in basenjis with chronic hemolytic anemia. J Am Vet Med Assoc 1991;20:1755-1761.
Author John W. Harvey
Consulting Editor Alan H. Rebar

BASICS

OVERVIEW

• Caused by the zoonotic rickettsia Coxiella burnetii • Infection occurs most commonly by inhalation or ingestion of organisms while feeding on infected body fluids (urine, feces, milk, or parturient discharges), tissues (especially placenta), or carcasses of infected animal reservoir hosts (cattle, sheep, goats). Infection can occur after tick exposure (many species of ticks implicated). • Endemic worldwide • Lungs thought to be main portal of entry to systemic circulation. Replicates in vascular endothelium, causing widespread vasculitis, the severity of which depends on the pathogenicity of the strain of organism. Vasculitis results in necrosis and hemorrhage in lungs, liver, and CNS. After recovery, an extended latent period exists until chronic immune-complex phenomena develop. The organism is reactivated out of the latent state during parturition, resulting in large numbers entering the placenta, parturient fluids, urine, feces, and milk.

SIGNALMENT

Cats and dogs both infected.

SIGNS

Historical Findings

• Fever, lethargy, depression, and anorexia • Abortion (especially cats) • Ataxia and seizures (especially dogs)

Physical Examination Findings

• Most cases are asymptomatic. • Fever and depression • Multifocal neurologic signs (dogs)

DIAGNOSIS

DIFFERENTIAL DIAGNOSIS

• Other causes of abortion in the cat—infections (viral rhinotracheitis, panleukopenia, FeLV, toxoplasmosis, bacteria [including coliforms], Streptococci, Staphylococci, Salmonellae), fetal defects, maternal problems (nutrition, genital tract abnormalities), environmental stress, endocrine disorders (hypoluteidism) • Other causes of encephalitis in the dog

CBC/BIOCHEMISTRY/URINALYSIS

CBC, biochemical panel, and urinalysis findings are nonspecific.

OTHER LABORATORY TESTS

Serology (collect 2-3 ml serum, refrigerate) and organism isolation (collect tissue sample, (e.g., placenta, for animal inoculation, refrigerate). Tests available (New Mexico Department of Agriculture, Veterinary Diagnostic Services, 700 Camino de Salud NE, Albuquerque, NM 87106)

IMAGING N/A

OTHER DIAGNOSTIC PROCEDURES

N/A

TREATMENT

• Alert owner of possible zoonotic risk. Humans contract the disease by inhalation of infected aerosols (e.g., after parturition). Children commonly infected from ingestion of raw milk but are usually nonsymptomatic. Previous urban outbreaks have been related to exposure to infected cats. Incubation period from time of contact until the first signs of illness varies from 5-32 days. Person-to-person transmission is possible.
• Treat as an impatient to avoid zoonotic risk to owner. Gloves and masks should be worn when treating an infected animal or when attending an aborting cat.

MEDICATIONS

DRUGS AND FLUIDS

• Tetracycline (22 mg/kg PO q8h, for 2 weeks)

• Doxycycline (20 mg/kg PO q12h for 1 week) • Enrofloxacin (10 mg/kg PO q12h, for 1 week) should be effective but no clinical reports (effective in vitro)

CONTRAINDICATIONS/POSSIBLE INTERACTIONS N/A

FOLLOW-UP

Interpretation of success of therapy is difficult because many animals spontaneously improve anyway. However, even nonsymptomatic cases should be aggressively treated because of the zoonotic potential. The utility of predicting success of therapy based on serologic improvement is unknown.

MISCELLANEOUS

ZOONOTIC POTENTIAL

Q fever has major zoonotic potential. However, by the time a diagnosis is made in a cat or dog, human exposure and infection has occurred. Thus, owners or people in contact with the pet should be instructed to seek medical advice immediately.

Reference

Greene CE, Breitschwerdt EB. Rocky mountain spotted fever and Q fever. In: Greene CE, ed. Infectious diseases of the dog and cat. Philadelphia: WB Saunders, 1990;430-433.

Author Stephen C. Barr
Consulting Editor Fred W. Scott

RABIES

BASICS

DEFINITION
A severe, invariably fatal, viral polioencephalitis of warm-blooded animals and humans

Pathophysiology
Virus enters body through a wound (usually from a bite of rabid animal) or via mucous membranes, replicates in myocytes and spreads to the neuromuscular junction and neurotendinal spindles. The virus travels to the CNS via intraaxonal fluid within peripheral nerves, then spreads throughout the CNS, and finally spreads centrifugally within peripheral, sensory, and motor neurons.

Systems Affected
• Nervous—clinical encephalitis, either paralytic or furious • Salivary glands—contain large quantities of virus that is shed in saliva

Genetics None

Incidence/Prevalence
The overall prevalence of virus infection is low, but can be significant in enzootic areas. The incidence of disease within infected animals is high, approaching 100%. The prevalence is especially high in underdeveloped countries where vaccination of dogs and cats against rabies is not routinely carried out.

Geographic Distribution
Rabies is found worldwide, with the exception of a few areas, including the British Isles, Australia, New Zealand, Hawaii, Japan, and parts of Scandinavia. Species adapted strains of virus have specific geographic distributions within endemic countries.

SIGNALMENT

Species
Dogs, cats, humans, and all warm-blooded animals. In the United States four strains of virus are endemic within their respective populations: fox, raccoon, skunk, and bat. All four strains can be transmitted to dogs and cats.

Breed Predilections None

Mean Age and Range
None, but adult animals that come in contact with wildlife are most at risk

Predominant Sex None

SIGNS

General Comments
Three stages of disease occur in progression: 1) prodromal, 2) furious, and 3) paralytic. Signs are quite variable and atypical presentations are the rule rather than the exception.

Historical Findings
• Change in attitude—solitude; apprehension, nervousness, anxiety; unusual shyness or aggressiveness • Erratic behavior—biting or snapping, licking or chewing at sight of wound; biting at cage; wandering and roam-ing • Excitability, irritability, viciousness • Muscular incoordination, disorientation, seizures, paralysis • Change in tone of bark • Excess salivation or frothing

Physical Examination Findings
• All or some of the historical findings • Mandibular and laryngeal paralysis, with dropped jaw, inability to swallow, and hypersalivation • Fever

CAUSES
Rabies virus, a single-stranded RNA virus in the genus Lyssavirus, family Rhabdoviridae

RISK FACTORS
• Exposure to wildlife, especially skunks, raccoons, bats, and foxes • Lack of adequate vaccination against rabies • Bite or scratch wounds from unvaccinated dogs and cats or wildlife • Exposure to aerosols in bat caves • Use of modified live virus rabies vaccine in an immunocompromised animal

DIAGNOSIS

DIFFERENTIAL DIAGNOSIS
Any dog or cat showing unusual mood or behavior changes, or exhibiting any unaccountable neurological signs, must have rabies high up on the differential list. These cases must be handled with considerable care to prevent possible transmission of the virus to individuals caring for or treating the animal.

DIFFERENTIAL DIAGNOSIS
• Any neurological disease, such as brain tumor or viral encephalitis • Head wound—should identify lesions from wound • Laryngeal paralysis • Choking • Pseudorabies

CBC/BIOCHEMISTRY/URINALYSIS
Routine laboratory test results for rabies fail to provide any characteristic hematologic or biochemical changes.

OTHER LABORATORY TESTS N/A

IMAGING N/A

OTHER DIAGNOSTIC PROCEDURES
• Minimal increased protein and leukocyte counts may be detected in cerebrospinal fluid (CSF). • Direct immunofluorescent antibody (DFA) testing of nervous tissue—brain, head, or entire body of a small animal that has died or has been euthanized because of rabies should be chilled immediately and submitted to a state-approved laboratory for rabies diagnosis. Extreme care must be exercised in collecting, handling, and shipping these specimens. This test is rapid and sensitive. • Direct immunofluorescent antibody testing of dermal tissue—a skin biopsy of the sensory vibrissae of the maxillary area, including deeper subcutaneous hair follicles, can be submitted for DFA testing for rabies

GROSS AND HISTOPATHOLOGIC FINDINGS
• Gross pathological changes are generally absent, despite the dramatic neurological disease. • Histopathological findings are of an acute to chronic polioencephalitis. There is a gradual increase in the severity of the non-suppurative inflammatory process in the CNS as the disease progresses. Large neurons within the brain may contain the classic intracytoplasmic inclusions called Negri bodies.

TREATMENT
Strictly as inpatient

ACTIVITY
Confined to secured quarantine area with clearly posted signs indicating rabies case or suspect. Runs or cages should be locked with only designated person(s) having access to the animal. Feeding and watering should be done without opening cage or run door.

DIET
Soft, moist food, although most animals will not eat

CLIENT EDUCATION
Client must be thoroughly informed of the seriousness of rabies to the animal and the zoonotic potential. Clients should be queried as to their exposure (contact, bite, etc.) and strongly urged to see their physician immediately. Local public health official must be notified.

SURGICAL CONSIDERATIONS
Generally none. Skin biopsy may be helpful to establish antemortem diagnosis, but this must be confirmed by virus identification from CNS.

MEDICATIONS

DRUGS AND FLUIDS
There is no treatment for rabies. Once the diagnosis is certain, euthanasia is indicated.

CONTRAINDICATIONS
None

PRECAUTIONS
Rabies cases must be strictly quarantined and confined to prevent exposure to humans and other animals.

POSSIBLE INTERACTIONS N/A

ALTERNATE DRUGS N/A

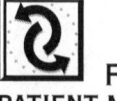

FOLLOW-UP

PATIENT MONITORING
• All rabies suspect cases should be securely isolated and monitored for any development of mood change, attitude change, or clinical signs that might suggest rabies. • An appar-

ently healthy dog or cat that bites or scratches an individual should be monitored for a period of 10 days. If no signs of illness occur in the animal within 10 days, there will have been no exposure of the person to rabies virus. Dogs and cats will not shed rabies virus more than 3 days before development of clinical disease. • An unvaccinated dog or cat that is bitten or exposed to a known rabid animal must be quarantined for up to 6 months or according to local or state regulations.

PREVENTION/AVOIDANCE

• All dogs and cats with any potential exposure to wildlife or other dogs should be vaccinated according to standard recommendations and state and local requirements. Cats and dogs should be vaccinated after 12 weeks of age, given a second vaccine 12 months later, and then every 3 years using a vaccine approved for 3 years. Cats should receive only inactivated vaccines. • Dogs and cats entering a rabies free country are quarantined for long periods, usually 6 months. • Any contaminated area, cage, food dish, or instrument must be thoroughly disinfected. A 1:32 dilution (4 ounces per gallon) of household bleach will quickly inactivate the virus.

POSSIBLE COMPLICATIONS

Complications caused by paralysis or attitude changes can occur.

EXPECTED COURSE AND PROGNOSIS

Prognosis is grave and almost invariably fatal. Nearly 100% of dogs and cats will succumb within 7-10 days.

MISCELLANEOUS

ASSOCIATED CONDITIONS None

AGE RELATED FACTORS

Any age can be affected.

ZOONOTIC POTENTIAL

Extreme potential for zoonosis. Humans must avoid being bitten by a rabid animal or an asymptomatic animal that is incubating the disease.

PREGNANCY

Infection during pregnancy will be fatal to dam.

SYNONYM Rage

SEE ALSO N/A

ABBREVIATIONS

RV = rabies virus
CNS = central nervous system
CSF = cerebrospinal fluid

References

Barr MC, Olsen CW, Scott FW. Feline viral diseases. In: Ettinger SJ, Feldman EC, eds. Veterinary internal medicine. Philadelphia: WB Saunders, 1995:409-439.

Clark KA, Eidson M, Jenkins SR, et al. Compendium of animal rabies control. J Am Vet Med Assoc 1994;204:173-176.

Eng TR, Fishbein DB, National Study Group on Rabies. Epidemiologic factors, clinical findings, and vaccination status of rabies in cats and dogs in the United States in 1988. J Am Vet Med Assoc 1990;197:201-209.

Greene CE, Dreesen DW. Rabies. In: Greene CE, ed. Infectious diseases of the dog and cat. Philadelphia: WB Saunders, 1990:365-383.

Krebs JW, Strine TW, Smith JS, Rupprecht CE, Childs JE. Rabies surveillance in the United States during 1993. J Am Vet Med Assoc 1994;205:1695-1709.

Author Fred W. Scott
Consulting Editor
Fred W. Scott

RECTAL AND ANAL PROLAPSE

BASICS

OVERVIEW
An anal prolapse (partial prolapse) is a protrusion of rectal mucosa through the external anal orifice. A double layer of the rectum which invaginates through the anal canal is a rectal prolapse (complete prolapse).

SIGNALMENT
• Any age, sex, or breed. • High prevalence for young, parasitized, dogs or cats with diarrhea

SIGNS
• Persistent tenesmus secondary to urogenital or distal gastrointestinal tract disease is common • Presence of tubular hyperemic mass protruding from the anus.

CAUSES AND RISK FACTORS
• Cystitis • Prostatitis • Dystocia • Perineal hernia • Prostatic hypertrophy • Colitis • Rectal foreign bodies • Proctitis • Rectal or anal tumors • Urolithiasis • Tenesmus following perineal or urogenital surgery

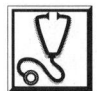

DIAGNOSIS

DIFFERENTIAL DIAGNOSIS
Rule out intussusception by passing a blunt probe between the mass and the anus. The probe should not penetrate more than 1-2 cm before contacting the fornix. If the probe passes easily 5-6 cm, then suspect prolapsed intussusception.

CBC/BIOCHEMISTRY/URINALYSIS
Nonspecific findings. Recommended to evaluate underlying disorders or abnormalities.

OTHER LABORATORY TESTS
Fecal examination warranted to rule out parasitism.

IMAGING N/A

OTHER DIAGNOSTIC PROCEDURES
• Colonoscopy may be helpful to evaluate recurrent prolapse for underlying cause.

• Viability of the prolapsed tissue must be assessed by surface appearance and tissue temperature. • Vital tissue: Swollen, hyperemic, exudes red blood from cut surface. • Responds to conservative massage and osmotic agents. • Devitalized tissue: Dark purple or black, exudes dark cyanotic blood, ulcerations present.

TREATMENT
• Identification and treatment of underlying cause is imperative.
• Conservative medical management consists of gentle replacement of prolapsed tissue through the anus with the use of lubricants. Adjunctive use of a purse string suture may aid in retention. Use of an epidural may facilitate treatment and relieve discomfort. Loperamide has been recommended to increase sphincter tone and decrease tenesmus. (Refer to references for techniques.)
• Colopexy is recommended for recurrent viable prolapses. (Refer to references for description of procedures.)
• When prolapse is devitalized, amputation and rectal anastomosis is recommended.

MEDICATIONS

DRUGS AND FLUIDS
• Loperamide - (0.1 mg/k) q8h
• Topical 50% Dextrose KY Jelly
• Appropriate anesthetic/analgesics as needed

CONTRAINDICATIONS/POSSIBLE INTERACTIONS N/A

FOLLOW-UP

PATIENT MONITORING
Purse string suture removal after 7-10 days

POSSIBLE COMPLICATIONS
• Recurrence (especially if uncontrolled underlying problem). • Anastomosis dehiscence within 5-7 days postoperatively • Postoperative rectal stricture

MISCELLANEOUS

References
Burrows CF, Ellison GE. Recto anal disease. In: Ettinger SJ, Feldman EC, eds. Textbook of veterinary internal medicine. 3rd ed. Philadelphia: WB Saunders 1989:1559-1568.

Matthiesen DT, Manfra-Marretta S. Diseases of the anus. In: Slatter DH, ed. Textbook of small animal surgery. 2nd ed. Philadelphia: WB Saunders 1993:627-645.

Author Michelle Joy Waschak
Consulting Editor Brent D. Jones

BASICS

OVERVIEW

Pathologic, fibrotic narrowing or constriction of the rectal canal. Excessive fibrous connective tissue formation occurs as the result of wound healing, chronic inflammation, or neoplastic invasion. Maturation of this scar tissue causes narrowing of the rectal luminal diameter. Gastrointestinal function is compromised because of outflow obstruction.

SIGNALMENT

• Dogs and cats • No age, breed, or gender predilection reported • No genetic basis reported

SIGNS

• Vary with the severity of the lesion • Dyschezia • Tenesmus • Constipation • Diarrhea • Secondary megacolon can develop

CAUSES AND RISK FACTORS

• Inflammatory—abscess, anal sacculitis, perianal fistulas, proctitis, foreign body, and prostatitis • Traumatic—lacerations • Neoplastic—rectal adenocarcinoma, leiomyoma, rectal polyps, prostatic adenocarcinoma, and others • Iatrogenic—rectal anastomosis, rectal mass excision, and rectal biopsy

DIAGNOSIS

DIFFERENTIAL DIAGNOSIS

Rectal stricture must be differentiated from rectal stenosis and functional constriction. Stenosis is partial obstruction of the rectal lumen, usually caused by intraluminal or extraluminal mass. Stenosis is the result of a space-occupying effect rather than a constrictive effect. Functional constriction occurs secondary to rectal spasms. Differentiate by rectal palpation and radiographic examination.

CBC/BIOCHEMISTRY/URINALYSIS

Results usually normal . Patients with inflammation may have an inflammatory leukogram.

OTHER LABORATORY TESTS N/A

IMAGING

Survey radiography and contrast studies (e.g., barium enema and barium gastrointestinal series) may reveal a consistent narrowing of the rectal luminal diameter. However, lesions in close proximity to the rectum may be difficult to delineate.

OTHER DIAGNOSTIC PROCEDURES

• Digital rectal palpation to characterize and determine the extent and location of the stricture • Proctoscopy may be useful for seeing stricture and procuring a biopsy specimen. • Biopsy of the lesion should be done to rule out neoplastic involvement.

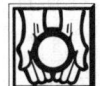

TREATMENT

• Histopathologic evaluation of the lesion should be performed before treatment. Resolution of the underlying cause of the stricture should precede treatment of the stricture when possible.
• Medical treatment is directed at palliation by the use of stool softeners and enemas.
• Surgical treatment ranges from bougienage for benign superficial strictures to partial or complete resection for more extensive lesions.
• Radiotherapy may be beneficial in the treatment of some neoplasms.

MEDICATIONS

DRUGS AND FLUIDS

• Appropriate prophylactic antimicrobial therapy has been advocated in conjunction with medical or surgical therapy.
• Corticosteroids (anti-inflammatory dosage) have been used to treat noninfectious inflammatory conditions and after bougienage.
• Antineoplastic chemotherapeutic agents may be indicated for various neoplasms.

CONTRAINDICATIONS/POSSIBLE INTERACTIONS

• Corticosteroids are contraindicated when infection is possible.
• Corticosteroids may have undesired affects on healing after surgical correction of the stricture.

FOLLOW-UP

• Patients are monitored for resolution or recurrence of clinical signs. Patients with neoplastic lesions are monitored for recurrence and metastatic disease. • Complications related to medical treatment include inefficacy, diarrhea, and side effects of any medications used. Surgical treatment can cause fecal incontinence, secondary stricture formation, and wound dehiscence. • The prognosis varies with the severity of the stricture. Patients with benign strictures that can readily be managed medically or with bougienage or resection may have a good long-term outcome. However, most patients with rectal stricture causing recognizable clinical signs have a guarded to poor prognosis for complete resolution.

MISCELLANEOUS

References

Matthiesen DT, Marretta SM. Diseases of the rectum and anus. In: Slatter D, ed. Textbook of small animal surgery. 2nd ed. Philadelphia: WB Saunders, 1993;627-644.

Niebauer GW. Rectoanal Disease. In: Bojrab MJ, ed. Disease mechanisms in small animal surgery. 2nd ed. Philadelphia: Lea & Febiger, 1993;271-284.

Author James L. Cook

Consulting Editor Brent D. Jones

RECTOANAL POLYPS

 BASICS

OVERVIEW
Benign growths of the anorectal mucosa classified as various histologic forms of adenoma

SIGNALMENT
• Middle-age to old animals • Males no more predisposed than females

SIGNS
• Blood-tinged or mucous-covered feces • Tenesmus • Soft, pedunculated and possibly friable mass may be seen or palpated rectally • Rectal or polyp prolapse

CAUSES/RISK FACTORS
Unknown

 DIAGNOSIS

DIFFERENTIAL DIAGNOSIS
• Adenocarcinoma, leiomyoma, and lymphosarcoma • Other causes of rectal prolapse

CBC/BIOCHEMISTRY/URINALYSIS
Results normal

OTHER LABORATORY TESTS N/A

IMAGING N/A

OTHER DIAGNOSTIC PROCEDURES
• Biopsy or cytologic examination of a rectal scrapping may help the initial diagnosis. • Histopathologic examination required for definitive diagnosis • Colonoscopy recommended to evaluate entire rectum and colon for additional polyps

 TREATMENT

Surgical excision is the treatment of choice. The mass may be exteriorized directly through the anus, or a dorsal rectal or ventral approach may be required. Since rectal polyps rarely invade the musularis mucosa, small or pedunculated tumors can be removed by local excision.

MEDICATIONS

DRUGS AND FLUIDS
• Appropriate perioperative antibiotics are recommended. • Stool softeners may help decrease tenesmus.

CONTRAINDICATIONS/POSSIBLE INTERACTIONS N/A

FOLLOW-UP

Reexamination of excision site 14 days after surgery and again at 3 and 6 months to ensure absence of recurrance or stricture

MISCELLANEOUS

SEE ALSO
• Rectal Prolapse • Adenocarcinoma, Anal Sac/Perianal/Rectal

Reference

Matthiesen DT, Manfra-Marretta S. Diseases of the anus. In: Slatter DH, ed. Textbook of small animal surgery. 2nd ed. Philadelphia: WB Saunders, 1993;627-645.
Author Michelle Joy Waschak
Consulting Editor Brent D. Jones

RENAL DISEASE, CONGENITAL AND DEVELOPMENTAL

BASICS

DEFINITION
• Functional or morphologic abnormality resulting from heritable (genetic) or acquired disease processes affecting differentiation and growth of the developing kidney before or shortly after birth • Renal agenesis is the complete absence of one or both kidneys.
• Renal dysplasia is disorganized development of renal parenchyma. • Renal ectopia is congenital malposition of one or both kidneys. Ectopic kidneys may be fused. • Tubulointerstitial nephropathy is a noninflammatory disorder of renal tubules and interstitium.
• Polycystic renal disease is characterized by formation of multiple, variable-sized cysts throughout the renal medulla and cortex.
• Renal telangiectasia is characterized by multifocal vascular malformations involving the kidneys and other organs. • Renal amyloidosis is the extracellular deposition of amyloid in glomerular capillaries, glomeruli, and medullary interstitium. • Nephroblastoma is a congenital renal neoplasm arising from the pluripotent metanephric blastema. • Multifocal renal cystadenocarcinoma is a hereditary renal neoplasm in dogs. • Fanconi's syndrome is a generalized renal tubular functional anomaly characterized by impaired reabsorption of glucose, phosphate, electrolytes, amino acids, and uric acid. • Primary renal glucosuria is an isolated functional defect in renal tubular reabsorption of glucose.
• Cystinuria is excessive urinary excretion of cystine, resulting from an isolated functional defect in renal tubular reabsorption of cystine and other dibasic amino acids. • Hyperuricuria is excessive urinary excretion of uric acid, sodium urate, or ammonium urate, resulting from impaired hepatic conversion of uric acid to allantoin and enhanced renal tubular secretion of uric acid. • Primary hyperoxaluria is a disorder characterized by intermittent hyperoxaluria, L-glyceric aciduria, oxalate nephropathy, and acute renal failure.
• Congenital nephrogenic diabetes insipidus is a disorder of renal concentrating ability, resulting from diminished renal responsiveness to antidiuretic hormone.

Pathophysiology
• Many congenital and developmental renal disorders are caused by genetic abnormalities, which disrupt the normal sequential and coordinated development and interaction of multiple embryonic tissues involved in formation of the mature kidney. • Congenital and developmental renal disorders may also be caused by nongenetic factors affecting the developing kidney before or shortly after birth.

Systems Affected   Renal/urologic

Incidence/Prevalence
Uncommon. However, disorders caused by genetic factors occur with higher frequency in related animals from more than one generation compared with the general population.

Geographic Distribution   N/A

SIGNALMENT

Species   Dogs and cats

Breed Predilections
Sporadic cases of congenital and developmental renal disease can occur without a familial predisposition in any breed of dog or cat .

Mean Age and Range:
Most patients are < 5 years old.

SIGNS

Historical Findings
• Findings indicating chronic renal failure
• Some glomerulopathies associated with abdominal distension, edema, or other signs of the nephrotic syndrome • Abdominal distenstion in some animals with polycystic kidneys or renal neoplasm • Hematuria in some animals with renal telangiectasia or renal neoplasm • Apparent abdominal pain in some animals with renal telangiectasia • Animals with unilateral renal agenesis, ectopic kidneys, and isolated renal tubular transport defects frequently asymptomatic

Physical Examination Findings
• Those associated with chronic renal failure
• Ascites or pitting edema in some patients with glomerulopathy or amyloidosis • Renomegally or abdominal mass lesions in some patients with polycystic kidneys, renal neoplasms, or fused ectopic kidneys • Renal pain in some patients with renal telangiectasia

CAUSES

Nonhereditary
• Infectious agents—feline panleukopenia virus and canine herpesvirus infection associated with renal dysplasia • Drugs—corticosteroids, diphenylamine, and biphenyls associated with polycystic kidneys; chlorambucil and sodium arsenate associated with renal agenesis. • Dietary factors—hypo- or hypervitaminosis A associated with renal ectopia

RISK FACTORS
See factors listed under Causes.

DIAGNOSIS

DIFFERENTIAL DIAGNOSIS
• Rule out noncongenital and nondevelopmental causes of primary renal disease. • Rule out nonrenal causes of hematuria, proteinuria, glucosuria, abdominal distension, and ascites.

CBC/BIOCHEMISTRY/URINALYSIS
• Nonregenerative anemia in animals with chronic renal failure • Azotemia and urine specific gravity < 1.030 in dogs and < 1.035 in cats, if renal failure develops

OTHER LABORATORY TESTS
Refer to chapters describing specific renal diseases, clinical problems, or laboratory test abnormalities.

IMAGING
Survey abdominal radiography, renal ultrasonography, and excretory urography—important means of identifying and characterizing congenital and developmental renal disorders.

OTHER DIAGNOSTIC PROCEDURES
Light microscopic evaluation of a kidney biopsy specimen should be considered in patients with morphologic or functional abnormalities of the kidney for which a definitive diagnosis has not been established by other, less invasive means.

GROSS AND HISTOPATHOLOGIC FINDINGS
• Congenital and developmental renal disorders may be associated with various combinations of primary, compensatory, and degenerative lesions. Conversely, some functional disorders may not be associated with alterations in renal morphology. • Renal dysplasia—end-stage kidneys. Primary lesions include immature ("fetal") glomeruli, persistent mesenchyme, persistent metanephric ducts, atypical tubular epithelium, and dysontogenic metaplasia. Primary lesions are usually associated with and may be obscured by secondary degenerative, inflammatory, and compensatory lesions. • Glomerulopathy—usually normal to small kidneys. Most hereditary glomerulopathies are characterized by primary membranoproliferative glomerulonephritis with variable degrees of tubulointerstitial disease. However, cystic atrophic membranous glomerulopathy is the characteristic lesion in affected rottweilers. • Tubulointerstitial nephropathy—end-stage kidneys. Renal lesions include periglomerular fibrosis, parietal epithelial cell hyperplasia and hypertrophy, interstitial fibrosis, and interstitial mononuclear cell infiltrate. • Polycystic renal disease and renal amyloidosis—see specific chapters.
• Renal telangiectasia—lesions include multiple, variable-sized, red-black, blood-filled nodules in the renal cortex and medulla, interstitial fibrosis, interstitial mononuclear cell infiltrate, and hydronephrosis. • Nephroblastoma—unilateral renal mass. Microscopically characterized by both embryonic mesenchymal and epithelial tissue components. • Multifocal renal cystadenocarcinoma—bilaterally large kidneys with irregular protruding cystic structures or multifocal neoplastic renal tubular epithelial cell proliferations. Often associated with cutaneous nodular dermatofibrosis and multiple uterine leiomyoma. • Renal ectopia—kidneys may be located in the retroperitoneal space of the pelvic canal, iliac fossa, or abdomen. Fused kidneys assume a variety of shapes. Horseshoe kidneys are symmetrically fused along the medial border of either pole. • Fanconi's syndrome—inconsistent microscopic findings of tubular atrophy, interstitial fibrosis, tubular cell karyomegally, and acute papillary necrosis. • Primary hyperoxaluria—large, irregularly-shaped kidneys. Microscopic lesions include renal tubular deposition of calcium

RENAL DISEASE, CONGENITAL AND DEVELOPMENTAL

oxalate crystals and variable interstitial and periglomerular fibrosis.

TREATMENT

• The nature of congenital and developmental renal disorders often precludes specific treatment. Supportive or symptomatic treatment may be of value in improving quality of life and minimizing progression in patients with renal dysfunction.
• Treatment options are based on clinical signs and appropriate laboratory evaluations.
• Refer to chapters describing specific renal diseases, clinical syndromes, clinical problems, and laboratory test abnormalities.

MEDICATIONS

DRUGS AND FLUIDS
Refer to chapters describing specific renal diseases, clinical syndromes, clinical problems, and laboratory abnormalities.

CONTRAINDICATIONS
Potentially nephrotoxic drugs (e.g., gentamicin) and anesthetic agents that impair renal function (e.g., methoxyflurane) should be avoided when possible.

PRECAUTIONS
Drugs requiring renal excretion should be avoided in patients with renal failure. If necessary, dosage regimens should be modified.

POSSIBLE INTERACTIONS N/A
ALTERNATE DRUGS N/A

FOLLOW-UP

PATIENT MONITORING
Refer to chapters describing specific renal diseases, clinical syndromes, clinical problems, or laboratory test abnormalitiesy.

PREVENTION/AVOIDANCE
Congenital and developmental renal disorders are irreversible. Therefore, control of lies in their prevention. Consideration should always be given to early identification and correction of predisposing factors (genetic and nongenetic) that may affect future offspring.

POSSIBLE COMPLICATIONS
• Acute or chronic renal failure • Nephrotic syndrome • Urolithiasis • Hydronephrosis • Urinary tract infection

EXPECTED COURSE AND PROGNOSIS
• Prognosis is highly variable and depends on the specific disorder, the extent of primary lesions, and the severity of renal dysfunction.
• Most congenital and developmental disorders are irreversible and may lead to advanced chronic renal failure. However, some patients with mild to moderate degrees of renal dysfunction may remain stable for long periods. • Animals with some disorders (e.g., unilateral renal agenesis, renal ectopia, cystinuria, hyperuricuria, and primary renal glucosuria) may remain asymptomatic unless complicated by urolithiasis, urinary tract infection, or other disease that promote a progressive renal dysfunction.

MISCELLANEOUS

ASSOCIATED CONDITIONS
• Polycystic renal disease associated with hepatic biliary cysts • Cystinuria and hyperuricuria associated with the formation of uroliths • Amyloidosis in shar-peis associated with intermittent pyrexia or swelling of the hocks • Renal neoplasm associated with hypertrophic osteoarthropathy, polycythemia, or other paraneoplastic syndrome

AGE RELATED FACTORS N/A
ZOONOTIC POTENTIAL N/A
PREGNANCY N/A

SYNONYMS
Familial renal disease, juvenile renal disease

SEE ALSO
• Amyloidosis • Anemia of Chronic Renal Disease • Fanconi's syndrome • Hematuria • Hyperparathyroidism, Renal Secondary • Nephrotic Syndrome • Oliguria/Anuria • Polycystic Kidneys • Polyuria/polydypsia • Renal Failure, Acute • Renal Failure, Chronic • Renal Tubular Acidosis • Renomegally • Urolithiasis, Cystine

ABBREVIATIONS N/A

References

Finco DR. Inherited and congenital renal disorders. In: Osborne CA, Finco DR, eds. Canine and feline nephrology and urology., 2nd ed. Philadelphia: Williams & Wilkins, 1996.

Kruger JM, Osborne CA, Lulich JP, et al. The urinary system. In: Hoskins JD, ed. Veterinary pediatrics, 2nd ed. Philadelphia: WB Saunders, 1996.

Authors John M. Kruger, Carl A. Osborne, and Scott D. Fitzgerald
Consulting Editors Larry G. Adams and Carl A. Osborne

RENAL FAILURE, ACUTE

 BASICS

DEFINITION
Acute renal failure (ARF) is a syndrome characterized by sudden onset of filtration failure by the kidneys, accumulation of uremic toxins, and dysregulation of fluid, electrolyte, and acid-base balance. it is potentially reversible if diagnosed quickly and treated aggressively. Although postrenal azotemia fulfills these criteria, the following discussion refers to intrinsic acute renal failure.

Pathophysiology
Acute renal failure is initiated by ischemia, nephrotoxins, or intrinsic renal disease. Renal excretory failure is perpetuated by multiple factors including (a) reduced glomerular surface area and permeability, (b) low renal blood flow, (c) intratubular obstruction by tubular debris, (d) cellular and interstitial edema, and (e) "backleak" of filtrate across damaged tubular epithelia. Resolution occurs by renal regeneration and repair.

Systems Affected
- Renal
- Gastrointestinal
- Nervous
- Respiratory
- Musculoskeletal
- Hemic/Lymph/Immune

Genetics N/A

Incidence/Prevalence
- Prevalence of ARF is substantially lower than that of chronic renal failure (CRF).
- Prevalence may increase in the fall and winter with greater exposure of animals to antifreeze containing ethylene glycol.

Geographic Distribution N/A

SIGNALMENT

Species Dogs and cats

Breed Predilections None

Mean Age and Range
Older animals at greater risk

Predominant Sex N/A

SIGNS

Historical Findings
Sudden onset of anorexia, listlessness, vomiting (± bloody), diarrhea (± bloody), halitosis, ataxia, seizures, known toxin exposure, recent medical or surgical conditions, and oliguria/anuria or polyuria.

Physical Examination Findings
Normal body condition and haircoat (no evidence of chronicity), depression, dehydration (sometimes overhydration), variable scleral injection, oral ulceration, glossitis, necrosis of the tongue, uremic breath, hypothermia, fever, tachypnea, bradycardia, nonpalpable urinary bladder, and large, painful, firm, kidneys.

CAUSES

Hemodynamic/Hypoperfusion
Shock, malignant hypertension, heart failure, thromboembolism (e.g., disseminated intravascular coagulation [DIC], vasculitis, and transfusion reaction), heatstroke, excessive vasoconstriction (e.g., administration NSAID), excessive vasodilation (e.g., administration ACE inhibitor or antihypertensive drug), and prolonged anesthesia

Nephrotoxic
Administration of antimicrobials (e.g., aminoglycoside, sulfonamide, and cephalosporin), Amphotericin B, chemotherapeutic agent (e.g., cisplatin and doxorubicin), thiacetarsamide, NSAID, radiographic contrast agent, ethylene glycol, heavy metal (e.g., lead, mercury, arsenic, and thallium), insect or snake venom, heme pigment, or calcium

Intrinsic and Systemic Disease
Leptospirosis, immune-mediated glomerulonephritis and arteritis, septicemia, DIC, hepatic failure, heat stroke, transfusion reaction, bacterial endocarditis, pyelonephritis, cortical necrosis, and lymphosarcoma

RISK FACTORS
- Endogenous—preexisting renal disease, dehydration, hypovolemia, hypotension, advanced age, concurrent disease, hyponatremia, hypokalemia, hypocalcemia, and acidosis
- Exogenous—drugs (e.g., furosemide, NSAID, prolonged anesthesia, and aminoglycoside), diet (e.g., low sodium, high or low protein), prolonged surgery, trauma, multiple organ disease, and high environmental temperature

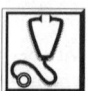 **DIAGNOSIS**

DIFFERENTIAL DIAGNOSIS
- Prerenal azotemia—oliguria, concentrated urine specific gravity (dogs, ≥ 1.030; cats, ≥ 1.035), correctable with fluid repletion
- Postrenal azotemia—anuria, dysuria, stranguria, large bladder, urethral obstruction, and uroperitoneum
- CRF—polyuria, polydipsia, chronic history of illness, loss of body condition, and anemia
- Prerenal-on-CRF- Clinical and laboratory features of CRF but partially correctable with fluid repletion
- Prerenal-on-ARF—cute onset uremia, partially correctable with fluid repletion
- Hypoadrenocorticism—hyponatremia, hyperkalemia, and "flat" ACTH stimulation test
- Pancreatitis—markedly high serum lipase, cranial abdominal pain, large nonhomogeneous pancreas (ultrasound), high trypsin-like immunoreactivity, hyperbilirubinemia, and high liver enzyme activity
- Heptatorenal syndrome—clinical and laboratory evidence of hepatic failure

CBC/BIOCHEMISTRY/URINALYSIS
- Normal or high PCV, variable leukocytosis, and lymphopenia
- Progressive (moderate to severe) increases in BUN, creatinine, and phosphate, variably high potassium and glucose, and variably low bicarbonate and calcium
- Inability to concentrate urine (≥ 1.020), mild- to- moderate proteinuria, glucosuria, variably high number of casts, WBC, RBC, and tubular epithelial cells, variable bacteriuria, and crystalluria (calcium oxalate)

OTHER LABORATORY TESTS
- Enzymuria—high urinary gamma-glutamyl transpeptidase, N-acetyl-beta-D-glucosaminidase predicts early nephrotoxic tubular damage in some animals
- Metabolic acidosis is common; mixed disorders may occur.
- Leptospirosis titer—≥ 1:3,200 or rising if animal infected
- Ethylene glycol concentration—positive if animal poisoned

IMAGING
- Routine and contrast radiography—in animals with acute respiratory failure (ARF), kidneys are normal to large with smooth contours
- Ultrasonography—hyperechoic kidneys suggest ethylene glycol toxicity

OTHER DIAGNOSTIC PROCEDURES
- Catheterize to monitor urine output—helps establish the diagnosis and formulates treatment and prognosis: anuria, ≤ 0.1 ml/kg/hr; oliguria, ≤ 0.25 ml/kg/hr; nonoliguria, ≥ 2 ml/kg/hr
- Percutaneous renal biopsy—helps establish the cause, severity, and potential reversibility of injury. Later in the course of disease (4-6 weeks), it may help predict ongoing renal repair and permanence of renal damage.

GROSS AND HISTOPATHOLOGIC FINDINGS
ARF is characterized by nephrosis or nephritis, interstitial edema, and lack of interstitial fibrosis. The subacute stage is characterized by attenuated epithelium, interstitial fibrosis and mineralization, cellular infiltration, and variable tubular regeneration.

 TREATMENT

GENERAL TREATMENT PRINCIPLES
Eliminate inciting insults. Discontinue nephrotoxic drugs. Established and maintain hemodynamic stability. Ameliorate life-threatening fluid imbalances, biochemical abnormalities, and uremic toxicities. Induction of emesis, gastric lavage, and administration of activated charcoal, cathartics, and specific antidotes should be instituted in animals with acute poisoning. Early hemodialysis can be used to eliminate dialyzable toxins.

INPATIENT VERSUS OUTPATIENT
Inpatient

ACTIVITY N/A

DIET
- Restrict oral intake until vomiting subsides. For most patients, endogenous fat stores supply requisite calories during early phases of

dietary restriction; thereafter moderately protein restricted diets or enteral feeding solutions are used to control azotemia and supply caloric requirements
• Parenteral nutrition (vomiting animals)—caloric requirements provided by 30-50% dextrose and 20% emulsified lipid solution; protein requirements (dogs, 3-4 gm/100 kcal; cats, 5-6 gm/100 kcal) provided by 8.5% amino acid mixture via central venous catheter
• Enteral feeding (anorectic, nonvomiting animals)—caloric and protein requirements supplied by blended commercial prescription diet (e.g., Hill's Pet Products, Prescription Diet Feline and Canine k/d; Waltham, Canine Medium Protein Diet or Feline and Canine Low Protein Diet) or commercial formulated liquid diet (e.g., Renal Care). Enteral feedings can be force-fed or given by nasoesophageal, pharyngostomy, gastrostomy, or enterostomy tube.

CLIENT EDUCATION
Inform clients of the poor prognosis for complete recovery, potential for morbid complications of treament (e.g., fluid overload, sepsis, and multiple organ failure), requirement and expense of prolonged hospitalization, alternatives to conventional medical management (i.e., peritoneal dialysis, hemodialysis, and renal transplantation), and zoonotic potential of leptospirosis.

SURGICAL CONSIDERATIONS
For animals (particularly cats) with fulminating ARF, renal transplantation may provide long-term survival.

MEDICATIONS
DRUGS AND FLUIDS
Alterations in Extracellular Fluid Volume
• Hypovolemia—correct estimated fluid deficits with normal (0.9%) saline or balanced polyionic solution within 4-6 hours. Blood losses should be replaced by whole blood transfusion. Once the patient is hydrated, ongoing fluid requirements are provided by 5% dextrose for insensible requirements (approximately 20-25 ml/kg/day) and balanced electrolyte solution equal to urinary and other losses (i.e., vomiting and diarrhea).
• Hypervolemia—stop fluid administration and eliminate excess fluid by diuretic administration or dialysis

Inadequate Urine Production
• Ensure patient is fluid volume replete. Provide additional isonatric fluid to achieve mild (3-5%) volume expansion. Failure to induce diuresis by fluid replacement indicates severe parenchymal damage or underestimation of fluid deficit. If fluid replete, administer diuretics and/or dopamine.
• Hypertonic mannitol (10-20%)—0.5-1.0 gm/kg IV over 15-30 minutes; if effective, continue as intermittent IV bolus q 4h-q6h or 1.0-2.0 mg/kg/min IV CRI; if ineffective, discontinue.

• Furosemide (alternative or subsequent to mannitol)—2-6 mg/kg IV; if effective, continue q8h; if ineffective, discontinue or combine with dopamine.
• Dopamine—1-5 mcg/kg/min IV in 5% dextrose as CRI; synergistic with furosemide; if effective, continue as CRI; if ineffective, combine with furosemide or discontinue.
• If these treaments fail to induce diuresis within 4-6 hours, consider dialysis.

Acid-Base Disorders
Administer bicarbonate if serum bicarbonate is ≤ 15 mEq/L. Bicarbonate replacement (mEq) = [(bicarbonate deficit) X body weight (kg) X 0.3]; give half IV over 30 minutes and the remainder over 4-6 hours; then reassess.

Hyperkalemia
See potassium, hyperkalemia

Vomiting
• NPO until vomiting subsides
• Reduce gastric acid production—cimetidine (2.5-5.0 mg/kg IV q8h-q12h) or ranitidine (2 mg/kg IV q8h-q12h) or omeprazole (0.7-2.0 mg/kg PO q24h [dogs])
• Mucosal protectant—sucralfate (0.5-1.0 gm PO q 6-8 hours)
• Antiemetics—metoclopramide (0.2-0.5 mg/kg IV or IM q6h-q8h)

CONTRAINDICATIONS
Avoid nephrotoxic agents

PRECAUTIONS
Modify dosages of all drugs requiring renal metabolism or elimination.

POSSIBLE INTERACTIONS
Metoclopramide may impair the effects of dopamine.

ALTERNATE DRUGS
• Control of vomiting—chloropromazine (0.5 mg/kg IM q6h-q12h), prochlorperazine (0.1-0.2 mg/kg IM q6h-q8h), or trimethobenzamide (3.0 mg/kg IM q 6h-q8h) can be used to treat protracted vomiting but is associated with CNS depression, vasodilatation, and hypotension.

Peritoneal or Hemodialysis
• Dialysis can stabilize the patient until renal function is restored. Without dialysis, most oliguric animals die before renal repair can occur.
• Specific indications include severe oliguria or anuria, life-threatening fluid overload, life-threatening electrolyte or acid base disturbance, BUN ≥ 100 mg/dl, serum creatinine ≥ 10 mg/dl, clinical course refractory to conservative treament for more than 24 hours, and poisoning with a dialyzable toxin.

FOLLOW-UP
PATIENT MONITORING
Assess fluid, electrolyte, and acid-base balances, body weight, urine output, and clinical status daily.

PREVENTION/AVOIDANCE
Anticipate the potential for ARF in patients that are hemodynamically unstable, receiving nephrotoxic drugs, have multiple organ failure, or are undergoing prolonged anesthesia and surgery. Maintenance of hydration, mild saline volume expansion, and administration of mannitol may be preventative.

POSSIBLE COMPLICATIONS
Seizures, coma, cardiac arrhythmias, congestive heart failure, pulmonary edema, uremic pneumonitis, gastrointestinal bleeding, hypovolemic shock, sepsis, cardiopulmonary arrest, and death

EXPECTED COURSE AND PROGNOSIS
• Nonoliguric ARF is a milder form of disease than oliguric. Recovery may occur over 3-6 weeks, but the prognosis remains guarded to unfavorable.
• Oliguric ARF predicts extensive renal injury, is difficult to manage, and has a poor prognosis for recovery. Recovery is signaled by a sudden (and often excessive) increase in urine production and a sluggish and incomplete return of renal function over 4-12 weeks. Dialysis extends the potential for renal regeneration and repair.
• Anuric ARF is generally fatal. Dialysis is required for renal repair. Recovery of renal function is usually incomplete.
• Oligo-anuric ARF with multiple organ failure is uniformly fatal.

MISCELLANEOUS
AGE-RELATED FACTORS N/A
ZOONOTIC POTENTIAL
Leptospirosis has infectious and zoonotic potential. Avoid contact with infective urine.
PREGNANCY
ARF is a rare complication of pregnancy in animals. Acute metritis, pyometra, and postpartum sepsis or hemorrhage promotes ARF.
SYNONYMS
Acute tubular necrosis, acute uremia, lower nephron nephrosis, and vasomotor nephropathy
SEE ALSO
• Oliguria and Anuria • Creatinine and BUN—Azotemia and Uremia • Renal Failure, Chronic

ABBREVIATIONS
ARF = acute renal failure; CRF = chronic renal failure
CRI = continuous-rate-infusion
DIC = disseminated intravascular coagulation
NSAID = nonsteroidal anti-inflammatory drugs
ACE = angiotensin-converting enzyme

References
Grauer GF, Lane IF. Acute renal failure. In: Ettinger SJ, Feldman EC, eds. Textbook of veterinary internal medicine. 4th ed. Philadelphia: WB Saunders 1995:1720-1733.
Author Larry D. Cowgill
Consulting Editors Larry G. Adams and Carl A. Osborne

RENAL FAILURE, CHRONIC

BASICS

DEFINITION
Renal failure (azotemia and urine specific gravity < 1.030 in dogs and < 1.035 in cats) results from primary renal disease that has persisted for months to years. Chronic renal failure is characterized by irreversible renal dysfunction that tends to deteriorate progressively over months to years.

Pathophysiology
Greater than approximately 75% reduction in functional renal mass results in impaired urine concentrating ability (leading to polyuria and polydipsia [PU/PD]) and retention of nitrogenous waste products of protein catabolism (leading to azotemia). Severe chronic renal failure results in uremia. Low erythropoietin and calcitriol production by the kidneys results in hypoproliferative anemia and renal secondary hyperparathyroidism, respectively.

Systems Affected
• Renal/Urologic—impaired renal function leading to PU/PD and signs of uremia
• Nervous, gastrointestinal, musculoskeletal, and other body systems secondarily affected by uremia

Genetics
Inherited in the following breeds (mode of inheritance known or suspected indicated in parentheses):
• Abyssinian cats (autosomal dominant with incomplete penetrance)
• Persian cats (autosomal dominant)
• Bull terrier (autosomal dominant)
• Cairn terrier (autosomal recessive)
• German shepherd dog (autosomal dominant*)
• Samoyed (X-linked dominant)

Incidence/Prevalence
Reportedly 9 cases per 1000 dogs examined and 16 cases per 1000 cats examined. Prevalence increases with age—in animals >15 years of age, reportedly 57 per 1000 dogs examined and 153 per 1000 cats examined.

Geographic Distribution N/A

SIGNALMENT

Species
Dogs and cats

Breed Predilections
All breeds of dogs and cats are affected. Familial renal disease resulting in chronic renal failure has been reported in the following breeds: basenji, beagle, bull terrier, cairn terrier, chow, cocker spaniel, doberman pincher, German shepherd, lhasa apso, miniature schnauzer, Norwegian elkhound, rottweiler, samoyed, Chinese shar pei, shih tzu, soft-coated wheaten terrier, standard poodle and Abyssinian cat.

Mean Age and Range
• Mean age at diagnosis is approximately 7 years in dogs and 9 years in cats.
• Animals of any age can be affected, but prevalence increases with increasing age.

Predominant Sex
None

SIGNS

General Comments
Clinical signs are related to the severity of renal dysfunction and presence or absence of complications such as hypertension. Cats with mild chronic renal failure may be asymptomatic. An animal with stable chronic renal failure may decompensate resulting in a uremic crisis.

Historical Findings
• Polyuria/Polydipsia (less frequent in cats than dogs)
• Anorexia
• Lethargy
• Vomiting
• Weight loss
• Nocturia
• Constipation
• Diarrhea
• Acute blindness (because of hypertension)
• Seizures or coma (late)
• Cats may also have ptyalism and muscle weakness with cervical ventroflexion (because of hypokalemic myopathy)

Physical Examination Findings
• Small, irregular kidneys (or large kidneys secondary to polycystic kidney disease or lymphoma)
• Dehydration
• Cachexia
• Mucuos membrane pallor
• Oral ulceration
• Uremic breath odor
• Constipation
• Hypertensive retinopathy
• Renal osteodystrophy

CAUSES
Most cases are idiopathic, and the disease is termed chronic generalized nephropathy. Known causes include familial and congenital renal disease, nephrotoxins, hypercalcemia, hypokalemic nephropathy, glomerulonephritis, amyloidosis, pyelonephritis, polycystic kidney disease, nephroliths, chronic urinary obstruction, drugs, lymphoma, FIP (cats) and, possibly, diabetes mellitus.

RISK FACTORS
Aging, hypercalcemia, hypokalemia (cats), hypertension, urinary tract infection (urinary tract infection), and diabetes mellitus.

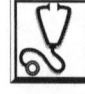
DIAGNOSIS

DIFFERENTIAL DIAGNOSIS
• See chapter on Polyuria/Polydypsia for differential diagnosis

• Differential diagnosis for azotemia include causes of prerenal and postrenal azotemia, acute renal failure, and hypoadrenocorticism.
• Prerenal azotemia—characterized by azotemia with urine specific gravity > 1.030 in dogs and > 1.035 in cats.
• Postrenal azotemia—characterized by azotemia with obstruction or rupture of the excretory system.
• Acute renal failure—differentiated from chronic renal failure by normal renal size, cylinduria, lack of indications of chronicity (e.g., nonregenerative anemia and renal secondary hyperparathyroidism), and recent nephrotoxin exposure or hypotensive episode.
• Hypoadrenocorticism—characterized by hyponatremia/hyperkalemia with decreased cortisol response to ACTH-stimulation test.

CBC/BIOCHEMISTRY/URINALYSIS
• Nonregenerative anemia
• Azotemia (high BUN and creatinine), hyperphosphatemia, acidosis (low total CO_2), hyperamylasemia, hyperlipasemia, hypercalcemia or hypocalcemia, and hypokalemia or hyperkalemia
• Urine specific gravity < 1.030 in dogs and < 1.035 in cats; mild proteinuria

OTHER LABORATORY TESTS
• High serum parathyroid hormone to document renal secondary hyperparathyroidism
• Bone marrow examination to rule out other causes of nonregenerative anemia

IMAGING
• Abdominal radiographs demonstrate small kidneys (or large kidneys secondary to polycystic kidney disease or lymphoma)
• Ultrasound demonstrates small kidneys and hyperechoic renal parenchyma with less apparent distinction between the cortex and medulla in some animals. Animals with lymphomahave renomegaly with hypoechoic renal parenchyma. See also congenital/developmental renal disorders, pyelonephritis, nephrolithiasis, hydronephrosis, and polycystic kidneys.

OTHER DIAGNOSTIC PROCEDURES
• Direct or indirect blood pressure determinations indicated to detect hypertension
• Urine protein/creatinine ratio to determine magnitude of proteinuria
• Renal biopsy helpful in selected patients to document underlying cause of chronic renal failure, especially in animals with glomerular disease, familial renal disease, lymphoma, or FIP. However, in most dogs and cats with chronic renal failure, renal biopsy is not indicated.

GROSS AND HISTOPATHOLOGIC FINDINGS
• Gross findings—small kidneys have a lumpy or granular surface. The renal capsule is frequently adhered to the renal parenchyma.
• Histopathologic findings—frequently nonspecific; chronic generalized nephropathy or end-stage kidneys. Findings are specific for

diseases causing chronic renal failure in some patients.

TREATMENT

INPATIENT VERSUS OUTPATIENT
Animals with compensated chronic renal failure may be managed as outpatients; however, animals with a uremic crisis should be managed as inpatients.

ACTIVITY Unrestricted

DIET
• Reduced dietary protein, phosphorus, and sodium with adequate buffering capacity (alkalinizing diet)
• Free access to fresh water at all times

CLIENT EDUCATION
• Disease tends to progress to terminal chronic renal failure over months to years
• Discuss heretability of familial renal disease

SURGICAL CONSIDERATIONS
• Avoid hypotension during anesthesia to prevent additional renal injury.
• Renal transplantation has been successfully performed in cats with chronic renal failure.

MEDICATIONS

DRUGS AND FLUIDS

Uremic Crisis
• Correct fluid and electrolyte deficits with intravenous fluid therapy (e.g., lactated Ringer's solution)
• Cimitidine (dogs, 10 mg/kg IV initial dose followed by 5 mg/kg IV q8h-q12h; cats, 2.5-5 mg/kg IV q8 h-q12h) to minimize nausea and vomiting
• Potassium chloride IV or oral potassium gluconate PO (2-6 mEq/cat/day) as needed to correct hypokalemia

Compensated Chronic Renal Failure
• Cimitidine (dogs, 5 mg/kg PO q8h-q12h; cats, 2.5-5 mg/kg q8h-q12h) to minimize nausea
• Potassium gluconate (2-6 mEq PO/cat/day) as needed to correct hypokalemia
• Intestinal phosphate binders (e.g., aluminum carbonate, 30-100 mg/kg/day PO with meals) as needed to correct hyperphosphatemia (see renal secondary hyperparathyroidism)
• Calcitriol (see renal secondary hyperparathyroidism)
• Erythropoietin (see anemia of chronic renal disease)
• ACE inhibitors (e.g., enalapril 0.5 mg/kg PO q24h) as needed for hypertension
• Subcutaneous fluid therapy (daily or every other day) may be beneficial in animals with moderate to severe chronic renal failure.
• Oxazepam (2.5 mg/cat PO) as needed to increase appetite

CONTRAINDICATIONS
Avoid nephrotoxic drugs (aminoglycosides, cisplatin, amphotericin B) and corticosteroids in patients with chronic renal failure.

PRECAUTIONS
• Reduce dosage or prolong dosaging interval of drugs eliminated by the kidneys, including cimitidine, enalapril, ranitidine, and metaclopramide.
• Use ACE inhibitors with caution in patients with chronic renal failure. Monitor patient for worsening of azotemia or proteinuria.
• Use caution with NSAIDs in patients with chronic renal failure.

POSSIBLE INTERACTIONS
Cimitidine and trimethoprim can cause artifactual increases in the serum creatinine concentration by reducing tubular secretion in dogs with chronic renal failure.

ALTERNATE DRUGS
• Ranitidine (0.5-2 mg/kg PO or IV q12h) can be used instead of cimitidine to treat uremic gastritis.
• Metaclopramide (0.2-0.4 mg PO or SQ q6h-8qh) can be used in addition to H_2-receptor antagonists to treat uremic vomiting.
• Hemodialysis is available at selected referral hospitals.

FOLLOW-UP

PATIENT MONITORING
Dogs and cats with chronic renal failure should be monitored at regular intervals, depending on treatment and severity of chronic renal failure. Monitoring should initially be weekly for animals receiving calcitriol or erythropoietin. Animals with mild- to- moderate chronic renal failure should be reevaluated every 1 to 3 months.

PREVENTION / AVOIDANCE
Do not breed animals with familial renal disease.

POSSIBLE COMPLICATIONS
• Systemic hypertension
• Uremic stomatitis
• Gastroenteritis
• Anemia
• Secondary urinary tract infection

EXPECTED COURSE AND PROGNOSIS
• Short-term prognosis depends on severity of chronic renal failure.
• Long-term prognosis is guarded to poor because chronic renal failure tends to be progressive over months to years.

MISCELLANEOUS

ASSOCIATED CONDITIONS
• Hyperthyroidism in cats
• Urinary tract infection
• Systemic hypertension

AGE- RELATED FACTORS
Increased incidence of chronic renal failure in older animals. Normal renal function decreases with aging.

ZOONOTIC POTENTIAL None

PREGNANCY
Animals with mild chronic renal failure may maintain pregnancy. Animals with moderate- to- severe chronic renal failure may be infertile or have spontaneous abortion. Breeding not recommended in females with chronic renal failure.

SYNONYMS
Kidney failure, chronic renal disease

SEE ALSO
• Acute Renal Failure • Anemia of Chronic Renal Disease • Creatinine and Blood Urea Nitrogen (BUN)-Azotemia and Uremia
• Congenital/Developmental Renal Disorders
• Hypertension, Systemic • Hydronephrosis
• Nephrolithiasis • Polycystic Kidneys
• Polyuria/Polydypsia • Pyelonephritis
• Hyperparathyroidism, Renal Secondary
• Urinary Tract Obstruction

ABBREVIATIONS
ACE = angiotensin-converting enzyme
FIP = feline infectious peritonitis
NSAIDs = non-steroidal anti-inflammatory drugs
PU/PD = polyuria/polydipsia
RSHPTH = renal secondary hyperparathyroidism,

References

Polzin DJ, Osborne CA, Bartges JW, James KM, Churchill JA. Chronic renal failure. In: Ettinger SJ, Feldman EC, editors. Textbook of veterinary internal medicine. 4th ed. Philadelphia: WB Saunders, 1995.1734-1760.

Polzin DJ, Osborne CA, Adams LG, Lulich JP. Medical management of feline chronic renal failure. In: Kirk RW, Bonagura JD, eds. Current veterinary therapy XI. Philadelphia: WB Saunders, 1992:848-853.

Brown SA, Barsanti JA, Finco DR. Medical management of canine chronic renal failure. In: Kirk RW, Bonagura JD, eds. Current veterinary therapy XI. Philadelphia: WB Saunders, 1992:842-847.

DiBartola SP. Familial renal disease in dogs and cats. In: Ettinger SJ, Feldman EC, eds. Textbook of veterinary internal medicine. 4th ed. Philadelphia: WB Saunders, 1995:1796-1801.

Gregory CR. Renal transplantation in cats. Compend Contin Ed Pract Vet 1993;15:1325-1339.

Author Larry G. Adams
Consulting Editors Larry G. Adams and Carl A. Osborne

RENAL TUBULAR ACIDOSIS

BASICS

OVERVIEW
Renal tubular acidosis is a rare syndrome that refers to the development of metabolic acidosis caused by either reduced bicarbonate reabsorption from the proximal renal tubule (proximal or type 2 renal tubular acidosis) or reduced hydrogen ion secretion in the distal tubule (distal or type 1 renal tubular acidosis). Proximal renal tubular acidosis has not been documented as an isolated entity in dogs but has been observed as part of Fanconi's syndrome. The following discussion is limited to distal renal tubular acidosis.

SIGNALMENT
• Reported in 5 dogs and 3 cats
• No apparent breed or sex predilection
• Age range at time of diagnosis, 1 to 8 years

SIGNS
• Anorexia and lethargy most common
• Other signs depend on the presence or absence of associated diseases (eg, pyelonephritis):
  • Panting
  • Weakness (related to hypokalemia)
  • Polyuria
  • Polydipsia
  • Vomiting
  • Weight loss
  • Hematuria
  • Dysuria (related to urolithiasis)
  • Fever

CAUSES AND RISK FACTORS
• Associated with distal renal tubular acidosis in human beings: primary (i.e., inherited), secondary to other inherited diseases (e.g., Ehlers-Danlos syndrome), toxins and drugs (e.g., amphotericin B), altered calcium metabolism causing nephrocalcinosis (e.g., hypervitaminosis D), autoimmune and hypergammaglobulinemic disorders (e.g., multiple myeloma and systemic lupus erythematosus), and tubulointerstitial nephropathy.
• In cats, distal renal tubular acidosis has been associated with pyelonephritis (two cases) and hepatic lipidosis (one case)

• In dogs, distal renal tubular acidosis has been associated with struvite urolithiasis (one case) and experimentally induced renal ischemia (one case).

DIAGNOSIS

DIFFERENTIAL DIAGNOSIS
Consider other diseases that can cause normal anion gap metabolic acidosis (e.g., diarrhea).

CBC/BIOCHEMISTRY/URINALYSIS
• Vary depending on associated diseases
• Hypokalemia (because of increased renal excretion) in some animals; may be severe enough to cause muscle weakness
• Alkaline urine pH (> 6.0 assuming urinary tract infection is absent)

OTHER LABORATORY TESTS
Blood gas analysis and evaluation of serum electrolytes reveals normal anion gap metabolic acidosis.

IMAGING N/A

OTHER DIAGNOSTIC PROCEDURES
The key diagnostic feature is normal anion gap metabolic acidosis accompanied by an inappropriately alkaline urine pH (> 6.0). In some animals in which a nonrenal cause of normal anion gap metabolic acidosis cannot be found and the urine pH is < 6.0, an acid load may be required to document distal renal tubular acidosis. This is done by administering ammonium chloride (200 mg/kg PO, dogs). The bladder is drained at hourly intervals. The urine pH (as measured by a pH meter) should decrease to < 6.0 within 3 hours. Caution should be exercised in administering this test to animals with severe acidosis.

TREATMENT
• Treatment is individualized depending on the nature and severity of associated conditions.
• The amount of bicarbonate needed to resolve the metabolic acidosis associated with distal renal tubular acidosis is less than that needed to resolve the acidosis associated with proximal renal tubular acidosis.

• Hypokalemia may resolve with bicarbonate administration alone or potassium supplementation may be required.

MEDICATIONS

DRUGS AND FLUIDS
• Sodium bicarbonate—1 to 2 mEq/kg/day PO
• Potassium supplementation if hypokalemia is not corrected by sodium bicarbonate

CONTRAINDICATIONS/POSSIBLE INTERACTIONS NA

FOLLOW-UP
• Serial blood gas analysis is done every 3 to 5 days until blood gases and acid-base status have normalized.
• Administer serum electrolytes, particularly potassium, as needed.
• The long-term prognosis depends on the nature and severity of associated conditions. The prognosis may be reasonably good in animals that do not have other diseases and respond well to bicarbonate. However, there is little information on the long-term course of this disease.

MISCELLANEOUS

SEE ALSO
• Acidosis, Metabolic
• Potassium, Hypokalemia

Reference

Mueller DL, Jergens AE. Renal tubular acidosis. Compendium on Continuing Education 1991;13:435-444.

Author Darcy H. Shaw

Contributing Editors Larry G. Adams and Carl A. Osborne

BASICS

OVERVIEW

• Genus in the family Reovirus • Non-enveloped, double-stranded RNA virus
• Name is an acronym (respiratory enteric orphan + virus) and denotes that the virus is isolated from respiratory and enteric tracts and not associated with any known disease (hence orphan) • Ubiquitous in geographic distribution and host range, including humans and virtually every species of mammal

SIGNALMENT N/A

SIGNS

Dogs

Conjunctivitis, rhinitis, tracheobronchitis (minor role), pneumonia, diarrhea, and encephalitis (rare)

Cats

• Respiratory illness, conjunctivitis, gingivitis, and ataxia • Generally mild disease • Similarly to rotavirus and coronavirus, reovirus infects mature epithelial cells on luminal tips of the intestinal villi causing destruction of these cells and resulting in villous atrophy. The loss of absorptive capability and loss of brush border enzymes (e.g., disaccharidases) leads to osmotic diarrhea.

CAUSES AND RISK FACTORS

• Predominately excreted from respiratory and digestive tract; therefore, acquired by inhalation and oral ingestion • Reovirus infection is common, but a specific disease has not been reproduced • Infections by other viral pathogens have been observed repeatedly and it has been speculated that reovirus may have an immunosuppressive effect that may promote infection by other viral pathogens.

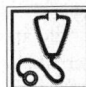

DIAGNOSIS

DIFFERENTIAL DIAGNOSIS

• Canine viral enteritis—canine parvovirus, canine coronavirus, canine astrovirus, canine calicivirus, canine herpesvirus, canine distemper virus, and canine rotavirus • Canine infectious tracheobronchitis—canine parainfluenza, Bordetella bronchiseptica, mycoplasmas, and canine adenovirus-1, canine adenovirus-2, canine herpesvirus, canine distemper virus • Feline upper respiratory disease—feline rhinotracheitis virus, feline calicivirus, chlamydia, mycoplasma, and bacterial infection

CBC/BIOCHEMISTRY/URINALYSIS

Noncontributory

OTHER LABORATORY TESTS N/A

IMAGING N/A

OTHER DIAGNOSTIC PROCEDURES

• Virus isolation—cytopathic effect is slow to develop • Histopathology—large intracytoplasmic inclusion bodies

TREATMENT

Doubtful whether reovirus is an important pathogen; therefore vaccines have not been developed and other control measures have been ignored

MEDICATIONS

DRUGS AND FLUIDS N/A

CONTRAINDICATIONS/POSSIBLE INTERACTIONS N/A

FOLLOW-UP N/A

MISCELLANEOUS

ZOONOTIC POTENTIAL

• Infection can spread among individuals of the same or different species. • The role, if any, that animals serve as a reservoir for the virus or as a possible source of human infection is unknown. • In people, by early childhood the vast majority demonstrate serologic evidence of past reovirus infection yet difficult to link reoviruses to disease • Majority of human reovirus infections must be asymptomatic or blend imperceptibly with minor respiratory and gastrointestinal illness of infancy and early childhood.

References

Thein P, Scheid R. Mammalian reoviral infections. In: Steele JH, ed. Viral zoonoses, vol II. CRC handbook series in zoonoses, section B. Boca Raton: CRC Press, 1981:191-216.

Pedersen NC. Feline infectious diseases. Goleta, CA: American Veterinary Publications, 1988:69-70.

Author J. Paul Woods
Consulting Editor Fred W. Scott

RESPIRATORY DISTRESS SYNDROME, ACUTE

BASICS

DEFINITION
• Adult respiratory distress syndrome (ARDS) refers to life-threatening, acute, respiratory failure caused by heterogenous acute lung injury and noncardiogenic pulmonary edema.
• ARDS is characterized by the following criteria: 1) normal pulmonary capillary wedge pressure, 2) impaired pulmonary compliance, 3) refractory hypoxemia, 4) radiographic findings consistent with diffuse bilateral pulmonary infiltration, and, in severely affected animals, 5) acute pulmonary arterial hypertension.

Pathophysiology
• No single mechanism is responsible for ARDS, but rather a complex series of interacting events and factors. • Initially, noncardiogenic pulmonary edema is caused by pulmonary capillary endothelial injury. Fluid and proteins leak into gas exchange areas of the lung, causing stiff lungs with low functional and residual capacity, impaired respiratory compliance, and severe hypoxemia.
• There are numerous causes of noncardiogenic pulmonary edema. • Inflammatory mediators injure the alveolar-capillary membrane, causing exudation of proteins that can inactivate surfactant and damage type II pneumocytes. Surfactant deficiency decreases lung compliance and leads to atelectasis, causing maldistribution of ventilation and right-to-left shunting with areas of low ventilation and perfusion. • Vasoconstriction and widespread occlusion of pulmonary microvasculature causes pulmonary hypertension, which may lead to right ventricular dysfunction.
• Patients may die of refractory hypoxemia or, more frequently, of secondary sepsis or multiple system organ failure.

Systems Affected
• Respiratory—acute respiratory distress
• Other systems may be affected, dependent on the inciting cause of ARDS and development of multiple system organ failure.

Genetics Unknown

Incidence/Prevalence Unknown

Geographic Distribution N/A

SIGNALMENT
Species Dogs and cats

Breed Predilections N/A

Mean Age and Range Not reported

Predominant Sex N/A

SIGNS

General Comments
• Symptoms of ARDS appear 1-96 hours after the predisposing event, usually within 12-48 hours (depending on the inciting cause of ARDS). • First stage—gradual onset of tachypnea and shallow breathing related to impaired functional residual capacity and pulmonary compliance • Second stage—apparent stabilizing of the condition, mild atelectasis, and early signs of diffuse interstitial pulmonary infiltrates may be seen on thoracic radiographs • Third stage—signs of respiratory insufficiency characterized by hyperventilation, tachycardia, pulmonary crackles • Terminal stage—persistent, severe hypoxemia (despite administration of 100% oxygen), tachypnea, and cyanosis

Historical Findings
Variable depending on the inciting cause

Physical Examination Findings
Severe respiratory distress—tachypnea, dyspnea, cyanosis

CAUSES
• Bacterial (especially gram-negative) septicemia, viral infections (parvoviral enteritis), and other severe infections • Aspiration pneumonia • Massive trauma, lung contusion • Hypotension • Thromboembolic disease • Burns • Pancreatitis • Massive transfusion • Uremia • Eclampsia • Central nervous system disease • Radiation • Smoke/noxious gas inhalation • High inspired oxygen fractions (oxygen toxicity) • Near drowning • Pulmonary infection (viral, bacterial, mycoplasma, fungal) • Drug ingestion (acetylsalicylic acid, heroin, methadone, barbiturates, or propoxyphene) • Paraquat ingestion • Peritonitis

RISK FACTORS
• Sepsis syndrome • Circulating endotoxin and increased tumor necrosis factor (TNF) • Sustained shock • Thrombocytopenia • Aspiration of gastric contents • Lung contusion • Multiple transfusions • Multiple fractures

DIAGNOSIS

Patients with serious underlying disease, particularly trauma or sepsis, that develop respiratory distress, refractory hypoxemia, and radiographic alveolar and interstitial infiltrates in the absence of heart disease are presumed to have ARDS.

DIFFERENTIAL DIAGNOSIS
• Cardiogenic pulmonary edema • Pneumonitis • Pulmonary contusion/hemorrhage

CBC/BIOCHEMISTRY/URINALYSIS
Variable abnormalities will be revealed by CBC, biochemical profile, and urinalysis depending on the inciting cause of the ARDS. In early stages of ARDS, neutropenia and thrombocytopenia are observed, caused by sequestration into the lungs.

OTHER LABORATORY TESTS
• Arterial blood gas analysis reveals persistent, severe hypoxemia despite oxygen administration. Hypercapnia occurs late in the course of ARDS and is an ominous prognostic sign.
• The alveolar-arterial oxygen gradient is significantly widened (> 30 mm Hg, inspiring room air) as a result of intrapulmonary shunting and ventilation-perfusion mismatch (normal < 10 mm Hg, inspiring room air).

IMAGING

Radiography
• Signs of ARDS usually precede radiographic changes by as much as 12-24 hours, and radiographic findings may correlate poorly with physiological status. • Early radiographic findings include fine interstitial infiltrates, which may progress to diffuse alveolar and interstitial infiltrates. • Cardiac silhouette usually is normal.

Echocardiography
• Should be performed to rule out cardiogenic pulmonary edema • May reveal moderately decreased fractional shortening in patients with septicemia-induced ARDS

OTHER DIAGNOSTIC PROCEDURES
• Cardiac catheterization—pulmonary artery pressure determination (high), pulmonary capillary wedge pressure determination (normal or low) • Lung compliance will be impaired, evidenced by increased airway pressures during positive pressure ventilation.

GROSS AND HISTOPATHOLOGIC FINDINGS
• Dependent on the primary cause of ARDS
• Lungs are usually deep red, firm, heavy, and appear wet. • Severe interstitial and alveolar edema with a membrane of proteinaceous material in alveoli

TREATMENT
Resolution of ARDS and survival are contingent on the ability to maintain adequate tissue oxygenation, providing time for reversal of the primary disease process and repair of pulmonary endothelial and epithelial defects.

INPATIENT VERSUS OUTPATIENT
Inpatient care

ACTIVITY
Cage confinement to reduce oxygen requirements

DIET
• Nutritional support is extremely important to restore positive nitrogen balance, increase respiratory muscle strength, and reduce susceptibility to pulmonary infection.
• Enteral feeding is preferred over parenteral feeding if the former is possible.
• Diets high in carbohydrates may increase carbon dioxide production, which can overwhelm the compromised respiratory system and cause progressive hypercapnia and respiratory acidosis.

CLIENT EDUCATION
Advanced medical care required, cost of therapy, poor prognosis

SURGICAL CONSIDERATIONS
May be indicated for inciting cause (repair trauma, remove foci of infection)

MEDICATIONS

DRUGS AND FLUIDS
• Mechanical ventilation is recommended to overcome hypoxemia and to reduce the excessive work of breathing. Positive end-expiratory pressure (PEEP) of 5-15 cm H_2O offers the greatest potential to reverse alveolar flooding and ventilation-perfusion mismatching.
• If positive pressure ventilation cannot be provided, supplemental oxygen should be provided by oxygen cage or nasal catheter.
• To optimize oxygen transport, hemoglobin should be maintained at normal values by packed red blood cell or whole blood transfusion.
• The use of antiinflammatory drugs (corticosteroids) is controversial; benefits have not been documented.
• Fluids (crystalloid and colloid) should be administered to maintain proper fluid balance and oxygen delivery.
• Intravenous furosemide and vasodilators (e.g., nitroprusside) may be administered if the pulmonary capillary wedge pressures increase.
• Broad-spectrum antimicrobial therapy if bacterial infection is present.

CONTRAINDICATIONS N/A

PRECAUTIONS
• Excessive diuretic use may decrease blood volume and left ventricular preload, causing reduced cardiac output.
• The usefulness of intravenously infused vasodilators is limited because their effects are not limited to the pulmonary vasculature. Systemic hypotension is an unwanted side effect. Furthermore, intravenously infused vasodilators can significantly increase intrapulmonary shunting by vasodilating vessels to areas of poor ventilation, leading to a severely reduced PaO_2.

POSSIBLE INTERACTIONS N/A

ALTERNATE DRUGS N/A

FOLLOW-UP

PATIENT MONITORING
• Frequent arterial blood gas analyses, particularly once positive pressure ventilation is established, are required to assess adequacy of oxygenation and fluid therapy and the progression of pulmonary disease. Repeated alveolar-arterial oxygen gradients and hypoxemia scores (PaO_2/F_1O_2) can be used to monitor progression or improvement in oxygenation.
• Pulmonary artery, central venous, and pulmonary capillary wedge pressures should be monitored with a pulmonary artery catheter if available. • Placement of an indwelling Foley urinary catheter to monitor urine output and calculation of "ins and outs" can prevent overhydration. • Pulse oximetry may be used to continuously monitor hemoglobin oxygen saturation. • Monitor for multiple system organ failure. Clinical signs include jaundice, gastrointestinal hemorrhage, or signs of disseminated intravascular coagulation.
• Repeated biochemical profiles and coagulation profiles may detect early organ failure.

PREVENTION/AVOIDANCE
• Early and aggressive therapy for sepsis syndrome • Use of inline micropore filters will reduce the incidence of microembolization when large volumes of stored blood are administered. • Proper immobilization of long bone fractures may decrease the incidence of fat embolization. • Carefully monitor all trauma patients for clinical signs of progressive hypoxia for at least 24-48 hours.

POSSIBLE COMPLICATIONS
Sepsis is frequently a secondary complication of ARDS.

EXPECTED COURSE AND PROGNOSIS
• Most patients are expected to die despite aggressive therapy. • In human beings, mortality rates of 16 to 90 % are reported. • In human beings with ARDS, unfavorable prognostic factors include sepsis, thrombocytopenia, multiple organ involvement (multiple system organ failure), and renal failure; patients who remain acidemic on mechanical ventilation; patients requiring > 50 % inspired oxygen concentration to maintain adequate oxygenation; pulmonary hypertension; decreased diastolic blood pressure

MISCELLANEOUS

ASSOCIATED CONDITIONS
• Disseminated intravascular coagulation and shock have been shown to correlate with ARDS. • Multiple system organ failure may develop in patients with ARDS, secondary to impaired oxygenation of multiple organs, or from activation of inflammatory cells and their mediators in the liver, kidneys, gastrointestinal tract, brain, and heart. Respiratory dysfunction may be just one aspect of a more generalized inflammatory process that causes injury to capillary endothelial beds.

AGE RELATED FACTORS
Unknown in veterinary medicine

ZOONOTIC POTENTIAL N/A

PREGNANCY N/A

SYNONYMS
• Shock lung • Traumatic wet lung • Posttraumatic pulmonary insufficiency • Stiff lung • Adult pulmonary distress syndrome • Acute lung injury • Noncardiogenic pulmonary edema • Posttraumatic atelectasis • Posttraumatic massive pulmonary collapse • Congestive atelectasis • Adult hyaline membrane disease • Capillary leak syndrome • Posttransfusion lung • Microembolism syndrome

SEE ALSO
• Pulmonary Edema, Noncardiogenic
• Dyspnea and Tachypnea

ABBREVIATIONS
ARDS = adult respiratory distress syndrome
IL-1 = interleukin-1
$PaCO_2$ = partial pressure of arterial carbon dioxide
PaO_2 = partial pressure of arterial oxygen
PAF = platelet activating factor
PEEP = positive end-expiratory pressure
TNF = tumor necrosis factor

References

Turk J, Miller M, Brown T, et al. Coliform septicemia and pulmonary disease associated with canine parvoviral enteritis: 88 cases (1987-1988). J Am Vet Med Assoc 1990;196:771-773.

Zachariades N, Agouridakis P, Parker J. The adult respiratory distress syndrome: a review. J Oral Maxillofac Surg 1993;51:402-407.

Parent C, King LG, et al. Clinical and clinicopathologic findings in dogs with actue respiratory syndrome: 19 cases (1985-1993). J Am Vet Med Assoc 1996;208:1419.

Author Cynthia Crager Ramsey
Consulting Editors Lynelle Johnson and Bradley L. Moses

RESPIRATORY PARASITES

BASICS

DEFINITION
Helminths and arthropods that reside in the respiratory tract or pulmonary vessels of dogs and cats

Pathophysiology
Infestation with parasites causes irritant allergic rhinitis, bronchitis, pneumonitis, or arteritis, depending on the location of the organism within the respiratory system.

Systems Affected
• Respiratory • Cardiovascular • Hepatic—with hepatopulmonary migration of some parasites

Genetics N/A

Incidence/Prevalence
Variable—depends on parasite

Geographic Distribution
• Pneumonyssus caninum—worldwide • Filaroides osleri—worldwide • Filaroides hirthi—North America • Filaroides milksi—North America, Europe • Aelurostrongylus abstrusus—worldwide • Capillaria aerophila—North America • Crenosoma vulpis—worldwide • Angiostrongylus vasorum—Europe, Africa, Asia • Dirofilaria immitis— worldwide • Paragonimus kellicotti—North America

SIGNALMENT

Species Dogs and cats

Breed Predilections
Outdoor animals

Mean Age and Range N/A

Predominant Sex N/A

SIGNS
Three basic categories: upper respiratory, lower respiratory, vascular (depends on location and lifestyle of parasite)

General Comments
• Often insidious and chronic, with few clinical signs • Respiratory compromise often is not severe.

Historical Findings
• Upper respiratory parasites (URP)—reported signs include sneezing, nasal discharge (serous, sanguinous), reverse sneezing, nasal irritation/rubbing • Lower respiratory parasites (LRP)—chronic coughing, nonresponsive to symptomatic therapy • Respiratory vascular parasites (RVP)—chronic coughing, fatigue, weight loss, tachypnea; living in or traveling through endemic heartworm area

Physical Examination Findings
• URP—findings similar to historical findings; variable clinical signs • LRP—elicitable cough; occasionally, harsh lung sounds; often cause coughing in cats • RVP—elicitable cough; may have heart murmur; occasional split second heart sound (with pulmonary hypertension); see Heartworm Disease

CAUSES
• URP—Pneumonyssus caninum (Pneumonyssoides caninum, nasal mites) Capillaria aerophila, Crenosoma vulpis • LRP, dogs—Filaroides osleri (Oslerus osleri), Filaroides hirthi, Filaroides milksi, Capillaria aerophila, Crenosoma vulpis, Paragonimus kellicotti (lung fluke); cats—Aelurostrongylus abstrusus, Capillaria aerophila (rare), Paragonimus kellicotti • RVP, dogs—Dirofilaria immitis (heartworm), Angiostrongylus vasorum; cats—Dirofilaria immitis (heartworm)

RISK FACTORS
• Depends on parasites—some have intermediate/paratenic hosts that are ingested by the definitive host, which may increase risk in scavenging animals • Crenosoma vulpis—snails • Paragonimus kellicotti—snails, crab, crayfish • Aelurostrongylus abstrusus—snails and slugs; transport hosts—rodents, frogs, lizards, birds • Dirofilaria immitis—mosquitoes • Multianimal households with unhygenic living conditions—allows fecooral or direct contact transmission

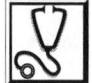

DIAGNOSIS

DIFFERENTIAL DIAGNOSIS
• URP—other causes of epistaxis, rhinitis, or sinusitis (infectious, neoplastic, allergic) • LRP—allergic bronchitis (nonparasitic), chronic bronchitis, infectious tracheobronchitis, allergic pneumonitis, bronchopneumonia, granulomatous pneumonia, pulmonary granulomatosis, hepatopulmonary migration of enteric helminths • RVP—pneumonitis, pulmonary arterial hypertension, pneumonia, severe left heart failure, right heart failure

CBC/BIOCHEMISTRY/URINALYSIS
• Hemogram—variable responses; may show eosinophilia, basophilia (especially with heartworm), neutrophilia, or monocytosis • Biochemistry—often normal; may show elevations in liver enzymes with some parasites during early stages as a result of hepatic migration if burden is substantial • Urinalysis—normal; may see proteinuria in patients with heartworm disease

OTHER LABORATORY TESTS
• Hematologic examination for microfilaria—Difil test, Knott test • Serologic testing—antigen detection via ELISA for dirofilaria (CITE-test, Dirocheck, VetRed)

IMAGING
Radiography
• Often unrewarding • Generalized interstitial pattern • Tortuous pulmonary arteries and right heart enlargement with RVP • Granulomatous masses or cystic bullae (especially right caudal lobe) with Paragonimus

Echocardiography
Echocardiography may be helpful with RVP;

worms may be visualized within main pulmonary artery and right ventricle.

OTHER DIAGNOSTIC PROCEDURES
• Examination of sputum may reveal eggs or larvae (L1). • Fecal examination—lung flukes may shed eggs into the feces. Lungworm eggs usually hatch within the respiratory system, so larval extraction from feces via Baermann method is necessary. Angiostrongylus eggs and larvae can be found in feces.

Rhinoscopy/Bronchoscopy
• URP—examination via retrograde pharyngo/rhinoscopy with antegrade flushing of anesthetic gas often allows visualization of nasal mites. Retrograde nasal lavage and cytological examination of fluid also may be helpful. • LRP—tracheal and bronchial parasites and parasitic nodules may be visualized and occasionally surgically removed for definitive identification. BAL may allow extraction of larvae or worms from alveoli. • RVP—serologic, fecal, and radiographic examination are diagnostic • Anthelmintic response—therapeutic trial may be attempted

GROSS AND HISTOPATHOLOGIC FINDINGS
• URP—nasal mites or worms may be found in sinuses and nasal cavity • LRP—pulmonary nodules may be seen throughout parenchyma or within bronchi • RVP—heartworms may be seen within pulmonary vessels and cardiac chambers. Arteritis of end arteries and arterioles with myointimal proliferation may be present. Thromboemboli also may be seen.

TREATMENT

INPATIENT VERSUS OUTPATIENT
• Treatments for URP and LRP can be done on an outpatient basis, although repeated examinations may be necessary to monitor response to therapy.
• Heartworm adulticide therapy usually requires hospitalization.

ACTIVITY
• No restrictions unless severe pulmonary dysfunction is present in patients with URP and LRP
• Restricted after heartworm therapy

DIET
No special restrictions

CLIENT EDUCATION
• Treatment response and duration vary between URP, LRP, and heartworm disease.
• There is risk of recurrence in dogs that maintain lifestyles conducive to transmission of the parasites (e.g., hunting and sporting dogs, multidog households).

SURGICAL CONSIDERATIONS N/A

MEDICATIONS

DRUGS AND FLUIDS

Anthelminthics
• Few studies confirm efficacy—most data is anecdotal
• Pneumonyssus caninum—ivermectin 200-400 μg/kg SQ or PO; 2 treatments 2 weeks apart. (Note: Ivermectin is not registered for use in dogs at this dosage. This dosage is contraindicated in collies, collie breeds, and Australian shepherds because of high incidence of toxicity in these breeds.) If ivermectin is contraindicated, pyrethrin/pyrethroid inhalation (Shelltox ministrips) may be tried.
• Aelurostrongylus abstrusus—fenbendazole 50 mg/kg PO q24h for 4 days; repeat after 10 days. Ivermectin 200 μg/kg SQ q24h for 3 days or PO for 5 days. (Note: Ivermectin is not registered for use in cats.)
• Other URP and LRP—fenbendazole 50-100 mg/kg PO q24h for 7-14 days or longer if there is evidence of persistent infestation. Ivermectin has also been used with variable success at 200 μg/kg weekly for 2-4 treatments.
• Crenosoma vulpis has been reported to be susceptible to diethylcarbamazine (dosage unknown).
• Paragonimus kellicotti—praziquantel 25 mg/kg PO or SQ for 2 days; fenbendazole 50-100 mg/kg PO q24h for 10-14 days
• Angiostrongylus vasorum—mebendazole for 5 days (dosage unknown)
• Dirofilaria immitus—see Heartworm Disease for details

Antiinflammatory Agents
Generally not required and may reduce efficacy of anthelminthic

CONTRAINDICATIONS
Ivermectin is not registered for use in dogs or cats other than for heartworm prophylaxis in dogs. It is contraindicated at dosages greater than 50 μg/kg in breeds with known increased sensitivity (e.g., collies, collie breeds, and Australian shepherds).

PRECAUTIONS
Caution is recommended when considering ivermectin therapy. After administering ivermectin at the dosages listed above (200 μg/kg), observation of the patient for adverse side effects is advised for 4-6 hours.

POSSIBLE INTERACTIONS N/A

ALTERNATE DRUGS N/A

FOLLOW-UP

PATIENT MONITORING
• Serial fecal Baermann larval extractions or examination for eggs. Note that some anthelminthics may suppress egg or larval production in some species. • Repeated radiographic examination may aid in assessing efficacy of therapy for LRP. • Resolution of clinical signs is suggestive of response to therapy, but does not indicate complete clearance of parasites. • If peripheral eosinophilia was present initially, this may subside with therapy. • See Heartworm Disease for recommendations concerning dirofilariasis.

PREVENTION AND AVOIDANCE
• Avoid activity that predisposes to infestations (often not practical). • Avoid contact with wildlife reservoirs (especially wild canids). • Consider prophylactic therapy for heartworm.

POSSIBLE COMPLICATIONS
• Imidazole anthelminthics are relatively non-toxic in dogs and cats. • Chronic pulmonary damage is possible with persistent and heavy LRP burdens. • Infestations are rarely fatal. • Pulmonary hypertension and right heart failure may occur with heartworm disease (see Heartworm Disease for further details). • Angiostrongylus infestations may result in coagulopathies.

EXPECTED COURSE AND PROGNOSIS
• Fair to excellent with aggressive management, but is quite variable • Return to performance depends on chronicity of disease and level of chronic pulmonary damage by LRP. • Recurrence is possible.

MISCELLANEOUS

ASSOCIATED CONDITIONS N/A

AGE RELATED FACTORS N/A

ZOONOTIC POTENTIAL N/A

PREGNANCY N/A

SYNONYMS
• Lungworm infestation (Aelurostrongylus, Angiostrongylus, Capillaria, Crenosoma, Filaroides, Paragonimus) • Nasal mite infestation (Pneumonyssus caninum) • Heartworm disease, dirofilariasis (Dirofilaria immitus)

SEE ALSO
• Heartworm Disease • Pneumonia, Allergic • Paragonimiasis

ABBREVIATIONS
URP = upper respiratory parasite
LRP = lower respiratory parasite
RVP = respiratory vascular parasite

References
Urquhart GM, Armour J, Duncan JL, et al. Veterinary parasitology. Longman Scientific & Technical, Longman Group UK Ltd, 1987.
Foreyt WJ. Veterinary parasitology reference manual. Board of Regents, Pullman, Wash: Washington State University, 1989.
Soulsby EJL. Helminths, arthropods and protozoa of domesticated animals. 7th ed. Philadelphia: Lea & Febiger, 1982.
American Heartworm Society. Recommendations for the diagnosis and management of heartworm (Dirofilaria immitis) Infection. 1992.
Marks SL, Moore MP, Rishniw M. Pneumonyssus caninum: the canine nasal mite. Comp Cont Educ 1994;16:577-582.
Author Mark Rishniw
Consulting Editors Lynelle Johnson and Bradley L. Moses

RETAINED PLACENTA

 BASICS

OVERVIEW
• Placenta retained beyond the immediate postpartum period in the bitch. Placentae are usually passed within 15 minutes of birth of a puppy. • Queens may retain placentae for days without signs of illness. • Extremely uncommon in the bitch and queen • Bitches can develop acute metritis secondary to retained placenta.

SIGNALMENT
• Bitch within a few days postpartum • Most common in toy dog breeds • Rare in the queen

SIGNS

Historical Findings
• Recent parturition • Continued vulvar discharge of lochia • Owner may be aware of number of placentae passed; this is not always reliable.

Physical Examination Findings
Green lochia vulvar discharge • Palpation of firm mass in uterus, but this is not always possible

CAUSES AND RISK FACTORS
• Toy breed • Large litter size • Dystocia

 DIAGNOSIS

DIFFERENTIAL DIAGNOSIS
• Postpartum metritis. Physical examination and vaginal cytologic examination show no signs of infection in patients with uncomplicated retained placenta. Metritis can develop in conjunction. • Retained fetus. Radiography or ultrasonography will differentiate.

CBC/BIOCHEMISTRY/URINALYSIS
Results usually normal in patients with uncomplicated retained placenta

OTHER LABORATORY TESTS
Vaginal cytologic examination reveals parabasal epithelial cells, +/– erythrocytes, and biliverdin clumps.

IMAGING
Ultrasonography reveals echogenic but non-fetal mass within the uterus.

OTHER DIAGNOSTIC PROCEDURES
Celiotomy/hysterotomy required for diagnosis in some patients

 TREATMENT

• Treatment of healthy bitches and queens is minimal and on an outpatient basis
• Owner should be instructed to monitor temperature and observe for signs of systemic illness.
• Ovariohysterectomy is curative and should be considered if breeding is not a consideration.
• Surgical removal of retained placenta indicated if medical treatment is unsuccessful and the bitch develops metritis.

MEDICATIONS

• With known or suspected retained placenta in a healthy bitch or queen— oxytocin (dogs, 0.5 U/kg up to 20 U IM; cats, 0.5-3.0 U IM) • If metritis occurs, treat accordingly (see Metritis)

CONTRAINDICATIONS/POSSIBLE INTERACTIONS

Progestational drugs should not be given.

FOLLOW-UP

• Monitor temperature and physical condition • Acute metritis can develop in the bitch if the placenta is not passed. • If metritis does not develop, the prognosis for future reproduction is good. • If metritis develops, the prognosis for future reproduction is fair to poor, but the prognosis for recovery is fair to good with treatment.

MISCELLANEOUS

Reference

Feldman EC, Nelson RW. Canine and feline endocrinology and reproduction. Philadelphia: WB Saunders, 1987:444, 537.

Author Joni L. Freshman

Consulting Editor Sara K. Lyle

RETINAL DEGENERATION

BASICS

DEFINITION
Degeneration of the retina from any cause, inherited or acquired. Inherited retinal degenerations (generalized progressive retinal atrophy [PRA]) are a group of progressive retinal diseases that can be subdivided into photoreceptor degenerations, which begin after the retina matures, and photoreceptor dysplasias, which begin before the retina fully develops (< 12 weeks).

Pathophysiology
• A variety of inherited defects, including reduced rod outer segment production and abnormal cyclic nucleotide metabolism, have been found in animals with PRA. Metabolic defects have also been described in animals with retinal degeneration secondary to retinal pigment epithelial or choroidal disease (i.e., central PRA, ornithine deficiency, and the mucopolysacharidoses). • Degeneration can be idiopathic or secondary to diffuse or focal inflammation and scarring (i.e., chorioretinitis), nutritional deficiency, or previous retinal detachment.

Systems Affected Ophthalmic—eye

Genetics
Dogs
• PRA—autosomal recessive in most breeds, especially the collie, Irish setter, miniature poodle, cocker spaniel, Labrador retriever, and many others • Central progressive retinal atrophy (central PRA)—autosomal dominant with incomplete penetrance in the Labrador retriever. Inheritance of other breeds not determined • Neuronal ceroid lipofuscinosis—autosomal recessive (proven or presumed) in most breeds studied
• Hemeralopia—autosomal recessive cone dysplasia in the Alaskan malamute, undetermined inheritance in the miniature poodle
Cats
• Rod-cone dysplasia—autosomal dominant in the Abyssinian (clinical signs at 4 months)
• Rod-cone degeneration—autosomal recessive in the Abyssinian (clinical signs at 2 years). Isolated reports of both dominant and recessive inheritance in young Persian and domestic shorthair cats • Gyrate atrophy—autosomal recessive (ornithine aminotransferase deficiency)

Incidence/Prevalence
The prevalence of hereditary retinal degenerations is greater in dogs than in cats. Taurine deficiency is uncommon in cats because cat foods are now appropriately supplemented.

Geographic Distribution
Central PRA is more common in dogs from Europe than from the United States.

SIGNALMENT

Species Dogs and cats

Breed Predilections
Dogs, Hereditary
• Early onset PRA—Irish setter, collie, Norwegian elkhound, miniature schnauzer, Belgian shepherd • Late onset PRA—miniature/toy poodle, American and English cocker spaniel, Labrador retriever, Tibetan terrier, miniature longhaired dachshund, akita, samoyed • Central PRA—Labrador, golden retriever, border collie, collie, shetland sheepdog, briard, and others • Neuronal ceroid lipofuscinosis—English setter, dalmatian, Tibetan terrier, and collie • Sudden acquired retinal degeneration (SARD)—Brittany spaniels, miniature schnauzer, and dachshunds predisposed
Cats, Hereditary
Abyssinian, Siamese, Persian, domestic shorthair

Mean Age and Range
• Early PRA and dystrophies—3-4 months to 2 years • Late PRA—clinical signs occur > 4-6 years • SARD—middle to old-aged animals

Predominant Sex
• PRA—none, except possibly X-linked recessive in Siberian husky • SARD—70% of affected animals are female

SIGNS

Historical Findings
• PRA—a gradually progressing nyctalopia (night blindness) that ultimately affects vision in bright light. The owners may notice dilated pupils or brighter tapetal reflex at night. A dog with PRA may appear to become acutely blind when it finally becomes totally blind or if it is moved to unfamiliar surroundings. In animals with hemeralopia (rare), the cones degenerate and day-vision is lost. • Central PRA (rare in the U.S.)—central vision is lost, although the dog may never become completely blind. Affected dogs (especially hunting dogs) may have difficulty locating stationary objects in bright light. • SARD—lose vision in 1-4 weeks and are often polyuric, polydipsic, and polyphagic.

Physical Examination Findings
• Severe degeneration impairs or nearly abolishes the direct and contralateral consensual pupillary light reflexes. Degeneration of the retina manifests as tapetal hyperreflectivity and nontapetal depigmentation or hyperpigmentation and, eventually, retinal blood vessel attenuation and optic nerve atrophy.
• Many affected dogs with PRA develop cataracts. • Dogs with SARD may be obese, may have hepatomegaly, and the pupillary light reflexes may be slow or absent.
• Taurine deficient retinopathy in cats—hyper-reflectivity begins as a spot in superiotemporal fundus (area centralis) in both eyes; subsequently, a superionasal spot appears; with progression of disease, a horizontal band forms superior to the optic nerve; finally, diffuse degeneration and hyper-reflec-

tivity develop. • Post-inflammatory retinal scars—typically, focal or multifocal lesions manifest as areas of tapetal hyper-reflectivity or hyperdepigmentation.

CAUSES

Degenerative
PRA is genetic and affects both eyes symmetrically. Retinal and optic nerve atrophy occur in animals with chronic or uncontrolled glaucoma. Retinal degeneration can occur secondary to scarring from previous multifocal or diffuse retinal detachment or inflammation.

Anomalous
Rod-cone photoreceptor dysplasias are genetically inherited and affect both eyes. Some dysplasias may be multifocal and nonblinding, i.e., in English springer spaniel and Labrador retriever.

Metabolic
Mucopolysaccharidosis in mixed-breed dog and Siamese and domestic shorthair cats. Deficiency of ornithine aminotransferase, a mitochondrial enzyme, causes progressive and total "gyrate" atrophy of choroid and retina.

Neoplastic
Scars from previous retinal detachment or neoplastic cell infiltrate

Nutritional
Severe deficiency of vitamin E or A may cause partial or complete retinal degeneration in dogs and cats (seen experimentally). Taurine deficiency causes retinal degeneration and dilated cardiomyopathy in cats.

Infectious/Immune
See retinal detachment

Idiopathic
SARD in dogs; one possible case has been reported in a cat

Toxic
Idiosyncratic reaction to griseofulvin in cats induces diffuse retinal inflammation and subsequent atrophy. Concurrent administration of ketamine hydrochloride and methylnitrosourea in cats induces diffuse degeneration.

RISK FACTORS
• Ocular disease, (e.g., cataracts, posterior segment inflammation, and glaucoma)
• Taurine deficient diet (dog food fed to cats) • Inherited retinal degenerations in related animals

DIAGNOSIS

DIFFERENTIAL DIAGNOSIS (SEE BLIND QUIET EYE)

Acute Vision Loss
In animals with SARD, optic neuritis, retinal detachment or unrecognized PRA, or glaucoma, the pupillary light reflex is slow or absent, whereas in animals with rapidly developing diabetic cataracts or visual cortex disease, the pupillary light reflex is normal.

Slowly Progressive Visual Loss
Ophthalmic examination permits differentiation of PRA, cataracts, severe corneal disease (e.g., pigmentation, scarring, or edema), chronic retinitis, chorioretinitis, or vitreal inflammation (i.e., posterior uveitis).

CBC/BIOCHEMISTRY/URINALYSIS

• Results are usually normal unless the degeneration is secondary to a systemic disease. • Dogs with SARD may have laboratory results consistent with hyperadrenocorticism and possibly may have this disease.

OTHER LABORATORY TESTS

• SARD—ACTH stimulation and dexamethasone suppression tests confirm and help localize central versus adrenal hyperadrenocorticism. • Cats with diffuse degeneration—Taurine concentration, especially if cat has dilated cardiomyopathy; serum and urinary (may collect on dry filter paper) ornithine concentration are high in cats with ornithine aminotransferase deficiency.

IMAGING

• Thoracic radiographs and cardiac ultrasound may be indicated in cats with suspected taurine deficient retinal degeneration. • Abdominal radiographs and ultrasound may be indicated in dogs with SARD. • Computed tomography or MRI may be useful for localizing and identifying causes of central blindness, i.e., optic nerve damage, cortical blindness, and SARD in animal with pituitary adenoma.

OTHER DIAGNOSTIC PROCEDURES

• Complete ophthalmoscopic examination. • Electroretinography confirms blindness caused by retinal degeneration when it is not apparent on ophthalmoscopy. Severe degeneration yields minimal or no response (e.g., animals with SARD and late PRA), whereas in animals with optic neuritis and CNS blindness, the electroretinogram is normal.

GROSS AND HISTOPATHOLOGIC FINDINGS

Thin retina. Edges of focal retinal scars are sharply delineated and the course of blood vessels is not altered. Hyperpigmented areas associated with post-inflammatory scars or central PRA. Histologic characteristics of end-stage retinal degenerations are marked photoreceptor atrophy and generalized reduction in retinal cell density. In animals with central PRA, lipopigment accumulates in the neuroepithelium.

TREATMENT

INPATIENT VERSUS OUTPATIENT
Outpatient

ACTIVITY See client education

DIET
Cat diets should contain 500-750 ppm taurine.

CLIENT EDUCATION

• If patient is visually impaired, inform the client that the condition is irreversible but nonpainful. • Blind dogs should be watched or kept on a leash outside if they are not in fenced yards or if they are in an area with a pool. Balls with bells inside can be used as toys. Dogs memorize their environment, and, unless the family moves or rearranges the furniture, most blind animals function well. The occasional older blind pet with problems such as hearing loss or senility may not adapt well to blindness. Also, behavioral changes such as increased aggression or reduced activity may occur when animals become blind. Animals with only one blind eye can function normally. • Blind cats may adapt better than dogs but should probably be kept indoors.

SURGICAL CONSIDERATIONS
Surgery is not indicated in animals with blind, nonpainful eyes.

MEDICATIONS

DRUGS AND FLUIDS

• No effective medical treatment currently exists for retinal degeneration. • In cats with ornithine aminotransferase deficiency, pyridoxine supplementation may increase activity of the enzyme, but it has not clinically arrested or reversed retinal degeneration.
• Adequate dietary taurine may halt the progression of the taurine deficient retinopathy.

CONTRAINDICATIONS N/A

PRECAUTIONS
Cataract surgery should not be performed in animals that have retinal degeneration; thus, electroretinography is useful to avoid unnecessary surgery.

POSSIBLE INTERACTIONS N/A

ALTERNATE DRUGS N/A

FOLLOW-UP

PATIENT MONITORING

• Serial fundic examinations (i.e., at 3-6 month intervals) confirm progressive degeneration if the diagnosis is in doubt. Retinas of dogs with SARD develop obvious signs of degeneration over several weeks. • If cataracts develop and progress in animals with PRA, watch for painful complications such as glaucoma and uveitis.

PREVENTION/AVOIDANCE
Do not breed animals suspected of having inherited PRA. Known carriers (e.g., an offspring of an affected animal) also should not be bred.

POSSIBLE COMPLICATIONS
• Cataracts • Glaucoma • Uveitis • Ocular trauma associated with visual impairment • Obesity secondary to reduced activity

EXPECTED COURSE AND PROGNOSIS

• Inherited PRA progresses to cause complete blindness. Progression is often slow, so animal can adapt to visual loss. The condition is nonpainful. • Degeneration from previous inflammation or trauma usually does not progress unless a systemic disease causes persistent (e.g., uveodermatologic syndrome) or recurrent (e.g., blastomycosis and toxoplasmosis) ocular inflammation.
• SARD causes irreversible blindness. • In cats, if taurine deficiency was transient, the degeneration may halt at any stage (e.g., a horizontal hyper-reflective band over the optic nerve).

MISCELLANEOUS

ASSOCIATED CONDITIONS
SARD may be associated with adrenal or pituitary hyperadrenocorticism.

AGE RELATED FACTORS N/A

ZOONOTIC POTENTIAL N/A

PREGNANCY N/A

SYNONYMS

• PRA, progressive retinal atrophy, progressive rod-cone degeneration, retinal atrophy, retinal degeneration, retinal dystrophy, and dysplasia. • Taurine deficient retinopathy was previously called feline central retinal degeneration.

SEE ALSO

• Retinal Detachment • Blind Quiet Eye

ABBREVIATIONS

• PRA = progressive retinal atrophy
• SARD = sudden acquired retinal degeneration

References

Gelatt KN, ed. Veterinary ophthalmology. 2nd ed. Philadelphia: Lea & Febiger, 1991.
Millichamp NJ, Dziezyc J, eds. Small animal ophthalmology: Vet Clin North Am Small Anim Pract 1990:20.

Author Patricia J. Smith
Consulting Editor Paul E. Miller

RETINAL DETACHMENT/INFLAMMATION

BASICS

DEFINITION
Any separation of the neural retina from the neuroepithelium (RPE) of the retina at the outer segment-neuroepithelium interface

Pathophysiology
The potential space between the RPE and neural retina in which fluid or exudates accumulate is referred to as the subretinal space. It is useful to characterize a retinal detachment by its etiopathogenesis, which is one or a combination of rhegmatogenous (retinal tear), subretinal exudation, or traction.

Rhegmatogenous
A tear that may be related to age, cataracts, or retinal degeneration allows vitreous to move into the subretinal space and results in detachment. This is probably the predominant type that occurs after cataract surgery. Some vitreous abnormality (e.g., liquefaction) is usually required to cause a retinal detachment from a tear.

Exudative
Fluid accumulates in the subretinal space because of breakdown of the blood-retinal barrier. Fluid may be serous, hemorrhagic, or exudative (e.g., granulomatous in animals with blastomycosis chorioretinitis). Hematogenous pathogenetic factors are common. Vasculitis, hypertension, and hyperviscosity may cause serous retinal detachment with or without hemorrhage.

Traction
Traction on the retina, usually by fibrous or fibrovascular tissue, raises the retina from the underlying RPE. Occurs after trauma or inflammation.

Systems Affected
• Opthalmic—retina • Nervous—vision can be severely compromised or permanently lost

Genetics
Relates to cause. For example, dogs with hereditary cataracts or lens luxations may develop retinal detachment.

Incidence/Prevalence
In dogs and cats, exudative retinal detachments are most common. Rhegmatogenous detachments are more common in dogs because of the greater prevalence of cataracts and cataract surgery.

Geographic Distribution N/A

SIGNALMENT

Species Dogs and cats

Breed Predilections
• Relates to cause. Terrier breeds are predisposed to primary lens luxation, which may contribute to retinal tear and detachment with or without surgery.

Mean Age and Range
• Relates to cause. More common in older animals because cataracts and systemic diseases such as neoplasia are often age-related

Predominant Sex N/A

SIGNS
• Blindness or reduced vision. • Dilated pupil with slow or no pupillary light reflex. • Blood vessels or a membrane is usually observed easily through the pupil just behind the lens. • Vitreous abnormalities such as liquefaction, hemorrhage, or syneresis (liquefaction) are often present. • Interruption or alteration of course of blood vessels due to retinal elevation. If subretinal fluid is clear, vessels may cast shadows upon the tapetum or RPE. • Active chorioretinitis has indistinct margins, exhibits tapetal hyporeflectivity or white-gray color in the nontapetum, and will alter the course of blood vessels. • In cats with ophthalmomyiasis, internal curvilinear tracts from migrating larvae are evident. • Underlying systemic disease may cause other signs.

CAUSES
Bilateral retinal detachment or retinal inflammation suggests a systemic problem.

Degenerative
End-stage progressive retinal atrophy (retinal degeneration).

Anomalous
Optic nerve colobomas (e.g., collie eye anomaly), multiple ocular anomalies in akita or any breed, severe retinal dysplasia (e.g., oculoskeletal dysplasia in Labrador retriever, English springer spaniel, and Bedlington terrier), and RPE dysplasia in Australian shepherd. Any young animal with congenital ocular defect may have congenital or juvenile retinal detachment.

Metabolic
• Systemic hypertension, hyperviscosity, polycythemia, and hypoxia with hemorrhagic complications. • Dogs—renal failure, pheochromocytoma, hypothyroidism, hypercholesterolemia, and hyperproteinemia as in animals with multiple myeloma. • Cats—renal failure with secondary hypertension is probably one of the most common causes in cats. Hyperthyroidism may cause secondary hypertension.

Neoplastic
Any primary or metastatic neoplasm. Commonly associated with multiple myeloma, lymphosarcoma, granulomatous meningoencephalitis, and large ocular masses (e.g., ciliary body adenocarcinoma or melanoma).

Infectious
• Infectious retinitis or chorioretinitis may cause focal or diffuse retinal detachment. • Infection may extend from or to the CNS.

Causes of Chorioretinitis in Dogs
• Viral—canine distemper • Bacterial—any septicemia or bacteremia, leptospirosis, brucellosis • Rickettsial—ehrlichiosis, Rocky Mountain spotted fever, borrelia • Fungal—aspergillosis, blastomycosis, coccidioidomycosis, histoplasmosis, cryptococcosis • Algal—geotrichosis, prototheosis • Parasitic—ocular larval migrans (Strongyles, Ascarids, Baylisascaris), toxoplasmosis, leishmaniasis, neospora

Causes of Chorioretinitis in Cats
• Viral—feline leukemia, feline immunodeficiency, and feline infectious peritonitis • Bacterial—any septicemia or bacteremia • Fungal—cryptococcosis, histoplasmosis • Parasitic—toxoplasmosis, ophthalmomyiasis interna, ocular larval migrans

Immune Mediated/Inflammatory
• Immune complex disease can cause vasculitis or inflammation that may result in exudative retinal detachment or chorioretinitis. • Immune-mediated thrombocytopenia can cause hemorrhage. • Dogs—systemic lupus erythematosus and uveodermatologic syndrome. • Cats—periarteritis nodosa and systemic lupus erythematosus.

Idiopathic
• If all other causes are ruled out, including retinal tears • Reported in giant-breed dogs

Trauma
• Bilateral retinal detachment related to trauma probably never occurs. • Penetrating injury or foreign body that causes retinal tears or intraocular hemorrhage may cause partial or complete retinal detachment. • Severe blunt trauma with inflammatory or hemorrhage. • Surgical trauma may contribute to retinal tearing.

Toxic
• Idiosyncratic reactions to drugs, e.g., trimethoprim-sulfa in dogs, griseofulvin in cats. • Ethylene glycol toxicity has induced retinal detachment and chorioretinitis in dogs and cats.

RISK FACTORS
• Old age • Hypermature cataracts • Luxated lenses • Extracapsular or intracapsular lens extraction

DIAGNOSIS

DIFFERENTIAL DIAGNOSIS
• Ophthalmic examination usually sufficient for a diagnosis of retinal detachment or inflammation • Blindness or impaired vision—optic neuritis, glaucoma, cataracts, progressive retinal atrophy, sudden acquired retinal detachment, CNS disease • Dilated pupil with slow or absent pupillary light reflexes—glaucoma, oculomotor nerve lesion, optic neuritis, progressive retinal atrophy, sudden acquired retinal detachment • Membrane or vessels associated with or behind lens—persistent tunica vasculosa lentis, persistent pupillary membranes, fibrovascular membrane secondary to intraocular neoplasia, inflammation

CBC/BIOCHEMISTRY/URINALYSIS
• Results typically normal if the problem is confined to the eye • Abnormalities consistent with an associated systemic disease process

OTHER LABORATORY TESTS
Additional tests depend on suspected systemic problem:
• Protein electrophoresis • Documentation of Bence-Jones protein in urine • Coagulation profile • Bacterial culture of ocular or body fluids • Thyroid hormone measurement (cats) • Serologic testing for the infectious diseases listed in causes

IMAGING
• Thoracic radiograph to search for lymphadenopathy, metastatic disease, or infiltrates consistent with infectious agents. • Radiographs of the spine may reveal bony changes consistent with discospondylitis or multiple myeloma. • Ocular ultrasound identifies retinal detachments and also intraocular masses and sometimes lens luxations. It is especially helpful if the ocular media is not clear.
• Cardiac ultrasound may be indicated in cats with hypertensive retinopathy.

OTHER DIAGNOSTIC PROCEDURES
• Single or repeated blood pressure measurement may reveal hypertension. Mean arterial pressure in dogs and cats is usually < 160 mm Hg. • Binocular indirect ophthalmoscopy.
• CSF tap is indicated if signs of CNS disease or optic neuritis are present. • Vitreocentesis may be performed if other diagnostic tests have failed to yield an etiologic agent and an infectious agent or neoplasia is suspected. Vitreocentesis can aggravate the inflammation or induce hemorrhage that may lessen the chance of the retina reattaching and restoring vision.

GROSS AND HISTOPATHOLOGIC FINDINGS
The retina is separated from the retinal pigmented epithelium and the underlying choroid. Masses or subretinal exudate may be seen. Histologic appearance depends on the cause. A chronic detachment results in retinal atrophy and a tombstone appearance to the RPE.

 TREATMENT

INPATIENT VERSUS OUTPATIENT
Depends on physical condition of the animal. In most cases, outpatient.

ACTIVITY
Restrict activity until reattachment has occurred or if the animal is irreversibly blind.

DIET N/A

CLIENT EDUCATION
• Chorioretinitis may be a sign of systemic disease, so diagnostic testing is important. Retinal detachment associated with lens luxation or cataract surgery has a bilateral potential, so both eyes should be observed closely.
• Retinal detachments may be reversible with return of vision, if the underlying cause is treated and detachment has not been present for a long time. Prognosis for vision is thus guarded. • Blind pets, especially cats, can adapt remarkably well and live a good quality life (see retinal degeneration).

SURGICAL CONSIDERATIONS
• Rhegmatogenous detachments can be surgically repaired, but this is performed only at a few institutions and is costly. • Laser retinopexy may reverse retinal detachments associated with optic disk colobomas in dogs with collie eye anomaly.

 MEDICATIONS

DRUGS AND FLUIDS
• Underlying systemic causes should be identified and treated appropriately
• Diuretics may or may not help promote subretinal fluid absorption.
• If systemic mycosis is ruled out and the detachment is believed to be immune-mediated in nature, systemically administered prednisone (2 mg/kg divided q12h for 3-5 days, then tapering) may facilitate retinal reattachment.
• Anti-inflammatory doses of prednisone (0.5 mg/kg then tapering) may be useful in patients with multifocal chorioretinitis.

CONTRAINDICATIONS
Systemically administered corticosteroids should not be used unless systemic mycosis is ruled out.

PRECAUTIONS N/A

POSSIBLE INTERACTIONS N/A

ALTERNATE DRUGS
• Chemotherapeutic agents are suggested for treatment of neoplastic conditions, e.g., lymphosarcoma or multiple myeloma.
• Uveodermatologic syndrome sometimes requires azathioprine in addition to steroids to control inflammation.

 FOLLOW-UP

PATIENT MONITORING
As appropriate for underlying cause and type of medical treatment.

PREVENTION/AVOIDANCE N/A

POSSIBLE COMPLICATIONS
Permanent blindness, cataracts, glaucoma, chronic ocular pain, and death if secondary to a systemic disease process.

EXPECTED COURSE AND PROGNOSIS
• Prognosis for vision in animals with complete retinal detachment is guarded. Retinal degeneration that may cause blindness even if reattachment occurs develops in days to weeks (earlier with exudative versus serous detachments). If the underlying cause is removed and reattachment occurs, vision may return. • Focal or multifocal chorioretinitis does not markedly impair vision but will leave scars. • Systemic disease or neoplasia with ocular manifestations may influence the prognosis for life.

 MISCELLANEOUS

ASSOCIATED CONDITIONS
Systemic disease

AGE RELATED FACTORS N/A

ZOONOTIC POTENTIAL
Toxoplasmosis may be transmitted to humans if animals are shedding oocysts in feces.

PREGNANCY N/A

SYNONYMS
Chorioretinitis or retinochoroiditis

SEE ALSO Retinal degeneration

ABBREVIATIONS N/A

References
Gelatt KN ed. Veterinary ophthalmology. 2nd Ed. Philadelphia: Lea & Febiger, 1991.
Millichamp NJ, Dziezyc J, eds. Small animal ophthalmology. Vet Clin North Am Small Anim Pract 1990;20:564–877.
Author Patricia J. Smith
Consulting Editor Paul E. Miller

RHABDOMYOMA

BASICS

OVERVIEW
Rhabdomyoma is an extremely rare, benign, striated muscle tumor that occurs only half as frequently as its malignant counterpart. Most are found in the heart and are probably congenital. Examples of extracardiac rhabdomyomas are very rare, but they have been reported in the tongue in dogs and pinna in cats.

SIGNALMENT
• No sex or breed predilections identified
• Extracardiac rhabdomyoma affects mostly middle-aged animals.

SIGNS
Physical Examination Findings
• None in animals with cardiac rhabdomyoma • Animals with an extracardiac tumor have localized swelling.

CAUSES AND RISK FACTORS
Unknown

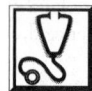

DIAGNOSIS

DIFFERENTIAL DIAGNOSIS
Cardiac Rhabdomyoma
• Rhabdomyosarcoma • Lymphosarcoma
• Hemangioma or hemangiosarcoma
• Fibroma or fibrosarcoma • Chondroma
• Myxoma • Myxofibroma • Mesothelioma
• Neurofibroma • Teratoma • Lipofibroma
• Lymphangioendothelioma • Radiographs

generally reveal soft tissue density and are of no major benefit in extracardiac rhabdomyoma. • Mixed spindle cell sarcoma

Extracardiac Rhabdomyoma
• Rhabdomyosarcoma • Lipoma or liposarcoma • Mast cell tumor • Fibrosarcoma • Nonneoplastic, inflammatory disease

CBC/BIOCHEMISTRY/URINALYSIS
Results normal

OTHER LABORATORY TESTS N/A

IMAGING
Echocardiography in a patient with cardiac rhabdomyoma may reveal a pedunculated mass or an infiltrative mass most often affecting the cardiac ventricles. The interventricular septum appears to be the most common site.

OTHER DIAGNOSTIC PROCEDURES
• ECG reveals arrhythmias in some patients.
• Radiography generally reveals soft tissue density and are not helpful in patients with extracardiac rhabdomyoma. • Cytologic examination of aspirate suggests a mesenchymal neoplasm in some patients but usually does not afford a definitive diagnosis. • Histologic examination and possibly electron microscopy required for definitive diagnosis; tumor may be difficult to differentiate from other "eosinophilic granular cell" neoplasms.

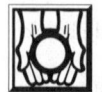

TREATMENT
• None available for cardiac rhabdomyoma
• Surgical excision for extracardiac rhabdomyoma

MEDICATIONS

DRUGS AND FLUIDS N/A

CONTRAINDICATIONS/ POSSIBLE INTERACTIONS N/A

FOLLOW-UP
• Follow-up evaluations monthly for the first 3 months, then at 3-6 month intervals for 1 additional year • Cardiac decompensation progressing to congestive heart failure develops in some patients with cardiac rhabdomyoma.

MISCELLANEOUS
Congenital rhabdomyoma of the heart exhibits no potential for malignant transformation.

Reference
Moulton JE: Tumors in domestic animals. 3rd ed. Berkeley, CA: University of California Press, 1990.
Author James P. Thompson
Consulting Editor Wallace B. Morrison

BASICS

OVERVIEW
• A malignant tumor derived from striated muscle • Typically shows diffuse, infiltrative, and poorly circumscribed growth characteristics • Exhibits aggressive and widespread metastasis to regional lymph nodes and visceral sites, including lungs, liver, and spleen

SIGNALMENT
• No sex or breed predilection • Tumors originate from skeletal muscles • Typically develop in old animals

SIGNS

Physical Examination Findings
• Large, diffuse, soft tissue mass of skeletal muscle • May exhibit metastasis within the primary muscle, permitting the identification of multiple nodules

CAUSES AND RISK FACTORS
Unknown

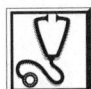

DIAGNOSIS

DIFFERENTIAL DIAGNOSIS
• Fibrosarcoma • Mast cell neoplasia • Rhabdomyoma • Lipoma, infiltrative lipoma, or liposarcoma

CBC/BIOCHEMISTRY/URINALYSIS
Results normal

OTHER LABORATORY TESTS N/A

IMAGING
Radiography reveals dense, soft tissue mass

OTHER DIAGNOSTIC PROCEDURES
• Cytologic examination of aspirate reveals a malignant mesenchymal neoplasm in some patients but usually does not afford a definitive diagnosis. • Incisional biopsy usually required for diagnosis

GROSS AND HISTOPATHOLOGIC FINDINGS
• Large, pleomorphic, elongated tumor cells which may show cross-striation and eosinophilic cytoplasm • Immunohistology or electron microscopy may be required for definitive diagnosis.

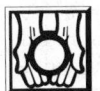

TREATMENT

• The characteristic invasiveness makes complete surgical excision extremely difficult.
• Amputation of an affected limb should be considered.
• Treatment methods other than surgical excision have not been described, and no studies of outcome of surgical excision have been published.
• Radiotherapy may be applicable in patients with incompletely excised tumors, but therapeutic results have not been described.

MEDICATIONS

DRUGS AND FLUIDS
• Chemotherapy may provide palliation for animals with widespread neoplasia. No specific regimens have been evaluated; however, the following 21-day protocol may be attempted: doxorubicin 20 mg/m^2 IV (cats) or 30 mg/m^2 IV (dogs) day 0 of treatment; cyclophosphamide 50 mg/m^2 PO days 3, 4, 5, and 6 of treatment; vincristine 0.5 mg/m^2 IV days 7 and 14 of treatment.

• The tumor is considered chemotherapy resistant if it fails to reduce in size after two cycles of this protocol.

CONTRAINDICATION/POSSIBLE INTERACTIONS
Chemotherapy with the above protocol may be myelosuppressive and cause gastrointestinal toxicity. Careful monitoring is very important. Do not use this protocol without chemotherapy experience.

FOLLOW-UP
Physical examination and possibly thoracic radiography and abdominal ultrasound monthly for 3 months after surgical excision and every 3-6 months thereafter

MISCELLANEOUS
• May be associated with hypoglycemia • See also urinary bladder rhabdomyosarcoma

Reference
Theilen GH, Madewell BR. Veterinary cancer medicine. 2nd ed. Philadelphia: Lea & Febiger, 1987.
Author James P. Thompson
Consulting Editor Wallace B. Morrison

RHABDOMYOSARCOMA, URINARY BLADDER

 BASICS

OVERVIEW
• A malignant tumor derived from pluripotent or striated myoblastic cells of mesenchymal origin that surround the developing Müllerian or Wolffian ducts • Commonly referred to as "botryoid" (i.e., grapelike appearance) rhabdomyosarcoma or embryonal rhabdomyosarcoma • Constitutes < 1% of all bladder tumors

SIGNALMENT
• Most occur in female, large-breed dogs < 18 months of age • Saint Bernard may be overrepresented

SIGNS

Physical Examination Findings
Signs consistent with lower urinary tract disease predominate—hematuria, stranguria, pollakiuria, and, possibly, urine retention

CAUSES AND RISK FACTORS
Unknown

 DIAGNOSIS

DIFFERENTIAL DIAGNOSIS
• Bacterial cystitis • Urocystolithiasis
• Transitional cell carcinoma • Squamous cell carcinoma • Fibroma or fibrosarcoma
• Bladder polyps • Granulomatous urethritis

CBC/BIOCHEMISTRY/URINALYSIS
• CBC and biochemistry results usually normal • Urinalysis shows hematuria in most patients. • Cytologic examination of urine sediment exhibits cellular pleomorphism and cross-striations consistent with rhabdomyosarcoma in some patients.

OTHER LABORATORY TESTS N/A

IMAGING
• Bladder ultrasonography or double contrast cystourethrography • Intravenous pyleography to evaluate any trigonal mass and to assess the ureters and renal pelves

OTHER DIAGNOSTIC PROCEDURES
N/A

 TREATMENT

• Invasiveness makes surgical excision extremeiy difficult.
• Surgical resection may be enhanced by bladder submucosal saline injection to aid in establishing a dissection plane.

MEDICATIONS

DRUGS AND FLUIDS
• Adjuvant chemotherapy recommended to assist in control or elimination of residual neoplastic disease after surgical resection. The following 21-day cycle has been used successfully: doxorubicin 30 mg/m^2 IV day 0 of treatment; cyclophosphamide 50 mg/m^2 PO days 3, 4, 5, and 6 of treatment.
• A total of four cycles of chemotherapy should be administered; tumor cell growth indicates clear evidence of chemotherapy resistance.

CONTRAINDICATIONS/POSSIBLE INTERACTIONS
Chemotherapy can be toxic. Seek advice before initiating treatment if you are unfamiliar with cytotoxic drugs.

FOLLOW-UP
• Evaluation every 21 days during chemotherapy and every 3-6 months thereafter • Evaluations should include a physical examination, CBC, serum biochemistry profile, and urinalysis. • Schedule thoracic radiography and abdominal ultrasonography every 3-6 months during the first year after surgery.

MISCELLANEOUS
• Hypertrophic osteopathy associated with this tumor in some patients • Metastasis common • Many patients have concurrent bacterial cystitis; antibiotics should be chosen on the basis of bacterial culture and sensitivity testing.

Reference
Senior DF, et al. Successful treatment of botryoid rhabdomyosarcoma in the bladder of a dog. J Am Anim Hosp Assoc 1993;29:386-390.

Author James P. Thompson
Consulting Editor Wallace B. Morrison

RHINITIS AND SINUSITIS

BASICS

DEFINITION
Rhinitis is inflammation of the mucous membrane of the nose. Sinusitis is inflammation of the associated paranasal sinuses. The term rhinosinusitis has been coined, as one rarely occurs without the other.

Pathophysiology
Rhinosinusitis may be acute or chronic, non-infectious or infectious. Animals with chronic disease usually present for veterinary care. All causes often are complicated by opportunistic, secondary microbial invasion. The associated mucosal vascular congestion and friability, excessive mucus gland secretion, neutrophil chemotaxis, and nasolacrimal duct obstruction lead to the clinical signs of congestion, obstructed airflow, sneezing, epistaxis, nasal discharge (mucopurulent), and epiphora. Turbinate and facial bone destruction may occur with neoplastic or fungal disease.

Systems Affected
• Respiratory—nasolacrimal drainage
• Nervous

Genetics Unknown

Incidence/Prevalence
Viral upper respiratory tract (URT) infection is common in cats, nasal tumors and foreign bodies occur occasionally, and primary bacterial rhinosinusitis is rare.

Geographic Distribution N/A

SIGNALMENT

Species Dogs and cats

Breed Predilections
Brachycephalic cats are more prone than others to chronic viral rhinitis.

Mean Age and Range
• Infectious, foreign body, and congenital disease in young dogs and cats • Allergic rhinitis in middle-aged animals • Tumor and dental disease in old animals

Predominant Sex N/A

SIGNS

Historical Findings
Sneezing, nasal discharge, and pawing at the nose are most commonly reported by the owner. Anosmia and inappetance is common in cats with sinusitis.

Physical Examination Findings
• Nasal discharge—unilateral suggests foreign body, tooth root abscess, or neoplasm
• Epistaxis—suggests fungal or neoplastic disease, although tooth root abscesses may bleed
• Diminished nasal airflow—unilateral or bilateral • Ocular discharge—serous from nasolacrimal obstruction; mucoid from viral or chlamydial rhinitis • Mandibular lymphadenopathy • Frontal and facial bone deformity from fungal or neoplastic disease

CAUSES

Infectious Causes
• Viral—herpes (FVH-1) and calicivirus (FCV) in cats; herpes, adenovirus (types I and II), and parainfluenza viruses in dogs
• Chlamydia psittaci in cats • Fungal—Cryptococcus neoformans most common in cats, Aspergillus fumigatus in dogs. Blastomycosis, rhinosporidiosis, and penicilliosis occur rarely. • Bacterial—primary bacterial rhinosinusitis is rare. Often secondary to a breach of the mucosal barrier from trauma, foreign body, or viral infection. Pasteurella multocida is common in both species; Bordetella bronchiseptica occurs in dogs. Staphylococcus, Pseudomonas, and E. coli have been cultured. • Parasitic—Cuterebriasis in cats; Pneumonyssus caninum in dogs (often reverse sneezing)

Noninfectious Causes
• Less common than infectious • Foreign bodies—mostly inhaled vegetable matter (grass, seeds), penetrating objects (bullets, teeth from fights), or objects refluxed from the nasopharynx (sticks) • Allergic or irritant rhinitis from inhaled pollen, molds, dusty litters, or cigarette smoke • Dental disease—periapical abscesses of the canine incisors (carnassial abscesses generally fistulate laterally through cheek) • Oronasal fistulas—congenital palatal defects or fistulas from extraction of canine incisors • Neoplasia—nasal lymphoma is the most common in cats, with or without FIV. Adenocarcinoma is the most common nasal tumor of dogs. Squamous cell carcinoma, osteosarcoma, chondrosarcoma, and fibrosarcoma also may occur.

RISK FACTORS
• Dolichocephalic dogs prone to fungal and neoplastic disease • Brachycephalic cats more prone to chronic viral rhinosinusitis • Toy breed dogs prone to severe periodontal disease

DIAGNOSIS

DIFFERENTIAL DIAGNOSIS
• Epistaxis • Coagulopathy • Hypertenson

CBC/BIOCHEMISTRY/URINALYSIS
• Hemogram may reflect chronic inflammation, blood loss anemia • Serum chemistry panel and urinalysis usually normal

OTHER LABORATORY TESTS
• FeLV and FIV serologic tests-associated immunosuppression possible • Serum Aspergillus titers

IMAGING

Radiography
Skull series must be taken with general anesthesia. Intraoral dental films are excellent for cats and toy breed dogs. Nonscreen films for table-top techniques. All animals with nasal discharge (hemorrhagic, mucous, serous) will have fluid density obscuring the nasal detail. Bony lysis or proliferation of the turbinate and facial bones is the most important radiographic finding, and is consistent with fungal and neoplastic invasion. Assessment of the apical roots of the canine incisors is also important. Rarely can soft tissue masses be visualized with standard radiographs.

OTHER DIAGNOSTIC PROCEDURES

Cytology
Simple nasal swabs or flushes rarely yield diagnostic samples. Generally requires a traumatic flush technique such as passing a bevel-pointed, stiff, polypropylene urinary catheter nasally, rapidly inserting the point into the area of interest, and flushing out the debris. New methylene blue used to identify the capsule of C. neoformans.

Blind Biopsy
Core biopsy specimens may be harvested with a modified urinary catheter as described above or with a Tru-Cut biopsy needle passed nasally. Small alligator or endoscopic clamshell biopsy forceps may also be used to grasp tissue. Coagulation studies (activated clotting and mucosal bleeding time) should be done before sampling.

Endoscopy
Rostral rhinoscopy with an otoscope speculum only provides a view of the most rostral rhinarium, rarely a site of lesions. A small bore, rigid, fiberoptic arthroscope or cystoscope, especially with continuous saline flushing through the sheath, provides excellent visualization to the level of the ethmoid turbinates. Allows for visual guidance of biopsy or foreign body retrieval instruments. Caudal rhinoscopy involves using a dental mirror and rostral retraction of the soft palate with a spay hook. Retroflexing a flexible bronchoscope can provide visual inspection of the nasopharynx to the level of the caudal choanae and allows for directed biopsy of any lesions. Neoplasms generally are visualized as space-occupying masses protruding out between turbinals. Destructive rhinitis, characterized by loss of the scroll-like turbinate structure, is typically found in patients with chronic rhinitis secondary to foreign body or tooth root abscess, and with aspergillus. Fungal plaques may be seen.

Exploratory Rhinotomy
The most invasive, but also most informative, diagnostic procedure. Ventral rhinotomy provides excellent exposure and cosmesis in dogs. Dorsal rhinotomy and frontal sinusotomy used in cats and brachycephalic dogs. May harvest culture and biopsy samples.

TREATMENT

INPATIENT VERSUS OUTPATIENT
The form of treatment depends on the cause.

ACTIVITY No change

DIET
No change

CLIENT EDUCATION
• In patients with chronic sinusitis (viral), cure is unlikely. Control of more severe clinical signs with medication, or possibly surgery, is the goal. Therapy is likely lifelong.
• Discuss the contagious potential of some of the infectious causes.

SURGICAL CONSIDERATIONS
• Rhinotomy and turbinectomy in refractory patients to remove infected tissues or foreign bodies
• Nasopharyngeal polyp removal in cats
• Extraction when tooth root abscess identified
• Radiation therapy generally offers good palliation for nasal tumors in dogs and cats. Orthovoltage radiation therapy must be preceded by tumor debulking. Cobalt and megavoltage irradiation are effective alone.
• Mesenchymal neoplasms (osteosarcoma, etc.) carry a poor prognosis, with or without surgical excision.

MEDICATIONS

DRUGS AND FLUIDS
• In most patients, irrespective of the underlying etiology, response to antibiotics is seen. Secondary bacterial infection may cause many clinical signs. Relapse is inevitable with cessation of therapy. Systemic antibiotic therapy (4-6 weeks) may be indicated to help prevent deep colonization by the resident flora. In some patients, low-dose, once-daily treatment may be continued indefinitely to maintain remission. This should never be advised as a substitute for a thorough diagnostic evaluation. Antibiotics may be based upon nasal culture or empirically chosen (first-generation cephalosporins, trimethoprim sulfadioxine, or chloramphenicol). Tetracycline is used if chlamydia is suspected.
• Corticosteroids and antihistamines in patients with allergic rhinitis

• Nasal lymphoma is treated chemotherapeutically as any multicentric lymphoma. Systemically administer itraconazole to treat cryptococcus in cats and aspergillus in dogs. Local flushing of enilconazole or clotrimazole administered via surgically placed tubing in the frontal sinus in aspergillus and penicillium infections in dogs.

CONTRAINDICATIONS N/A

PRECAUTIONS N/A

POSSIBLE INTERACTIONS
• Potential hepatopathies with systemic antifungals • Tetracyclines can damage the tooth buds in young animals.

ALTERNATE DRUGS N/A

FOLLOW-UP

PATIENT MONITORING
Mostly clinical assessment and monitoring for relapse of clinical signs

PREVENTION/AVOIDANCE
Isolation and separation of chronic viral carriers

POSSIBLE COMPLICATIONS
Relapse and lack of response

EXPECTED COURSE AND PROGNOSIS
• Prognosis depends on etiology and chronicity. • Trauma and foreign body, good to excellent • Viral infections, fair to good, although many cats become chronically infected • Fungal infection, guarded to fair, depending on invasiveness (i.e., grave with CNS signs) and the immunocompetence of the host • Neoplasms, grave to poor, although cats with lymphoma may survive 8-10 months with chemotherapy

MISCELLANEOUS

ASSOCIATED CONDITIONS N/A

AGE RELATED FACTORS
• Most of the infectious causes occur in young animals. • Neoplasms more common in old animals.

ZOONOTIC POTENTIAL
None documented for any of the fungal rhinitides

PREGNANCY
Antifungal drugs teratogenic

SYNONYMS N/A

SEE ALSO
• Epistaxis • Nasal Discharge (Sneezing, Reverse Sneezing, Gagging) • Nasopharyngeal polyps • Nasopharyngeal Stenosis • Trachealbronchitis, Infectious • Fungal Infections

ABBREVIATION
URT = upper respiratory tract

References

August JR. Chronic sneezing. In: August JR, ed. Consultations in feline medicine. 2nd ed. Philadelphia: JB Lippincott, 1994:273-277.

Bedford PGC. Diseases of the nose and throat. In: Ettinger SJ, ed. Textbook of veterinary internal medicine. 3rd ed. Philadelphia: WB Saunders, 1989:768-794.

Kuehn NF, Roudebush P. Nasal discharge. In: Allen DG, ed. Small animal medicine. 1991:383-395.

Roudebush P. Bacterial infections of the respiratory system. In: Greene CE, ed. Infectious diseases of the dog and cat. Philadelphia: WB Saunders, 1990:114-117.

Author Robert Mason

Consulting Editors Lynelle Johnson and Robert L. Moses

RHINOSPORIDIOSIS

 BASICS

OVERVIEW

Rhinosporidiosis is a rare and chronic infection of the mucous membranes of dogs. It generally forms a cauliflowerlike mass that protrudes from the nostril.

SIGNALMENT

• It has been reported in 13 dogs, 7 of which were males. There does not appear to be a breed predilection. • It has not been reported in cats. • There is worldwide distribution of the organism, but endemic areas are reported to be in Argentina, Sri Lanka, and India.
• Most infections in dogs in the United States are reported in the southern states. • It is suspected that stagnant fresh water and arid environmental conditions increase the likelihood of occurrence.

SIGNS

• The most common site of infection is the anterior nasal cavity. • The predominant clinical signs include sneezing, epistaxis, and stertorous breathing. • Generally, a mass protrudes from the nostril. It is usually single and polypoid and may be lobulated or sessile.
• White or yellowish superficial flecks may be seen on the surface of the mass. These are fungal sporangia. • It has also been reported to infect the vagina, penis, conjunctival sac, and the ears in humans.

CAUSES AND RISK FACTORS

Rhinosporidium seeberi

 DIAGNOSIS

DIFFERENTIAL DIAGNOSIS

• Nasal neoplasia • Nasal inflammatory polyp

CBC/BIOCHEMISTRY/URINALYSIS

Usually normal

OTHER LABORATORY TESTS

MAGING

Radiographs of the nasal cavity are generally normal because the mass is located in the anterior nasal cavity and does not invade the turbinates.

OTHER DIAGNOSTIC PROCEDURES

Impression smears from the nasal mass that are stained with new methylene blue stain may reveal the organism.

GROSS AND HISTOPATHOLOGIC FINDINGS

• Histopathologic examination of the mass reveals papillomatous hyperplasia and ulceration of the epithelium accompanied by fibrovascular stroma. • Identification of the organism in histopathologic specimens is diagnostic. • If organisms are released into the surrounding tissues, an intense inflammatory reaction will be apparent.

 TREATMENT N/A

MEDICATIONS

• Surgical excision of the mass is the treatment of choice. This may be accomplished via an approach through the external nares or rhinotomy.

• Failure to remove the entire mass will likely result in regrowth.

DRUGS AND FLUIDS

Dapsone has been used to treat humans, but its use has only been reported in one dog. Favorable response was reported, but the drug was not curative.

CONTRAINDICATIONS/POSSIBLE INTERACTIONS

• Side effects from the use of dapsone in dogs are reported to be hepatotoxicity, anemia, neutropenia, thrombocytopenia, gastrointestinal signs, and skin reactions.

• There is no known risk of transmission to humans by handling of infected dogs. However, this organism is infectious to humans.

FOLLOW-UP

Because of the difficulty of removing the entire mass via an approach through the external nasal orifice, a patient treated in this manner should be monitored closely for regrowth.

MISCELLANEOUS N/A

Reference

Wolf AM. Deep mycotic diseases. In: Ettinger SJ, ed. Textbook of veterinary internal medicine. 4th ed. Philadelphia: WB Saunders, 1994:439-463.

Author Gary D. Norsworthy
Consulting Editor Fred W. Scott

RHINOTRACHEITIS—CATS

BASICS

DEFINITION
A common, acute, herpesvirus disease of domestic and exotic cats characterized by sneezing, rhinitis, conjunctivitis, ulcerative keratitis, and fever

Pathophysiology
Feline rhinotracheitis (FVR) results from an acute, cytolytic infection of respiratory or ocular epithelial cells after oral, intranasal, or conjunctival exposure to feline herpesvirus type 1 (FHV-1).

Systems Affected
• Respiratory—rhinitis with sneezing and serous to purulent nasal discharge usually occur • Tracheitis with coughing can occur, as can chronic sinusitis as a sequela to FVR. • Ophthalmic—conjunctivitis with swollen conjunctiva and serous to purulent ocular discharge. Ulcerative keratitis with or without panophthalmitis can be a sequela in some cats. • Reproductive—infection of unvaccinated, pregnant cats can result in fetal infection in utero, with severe neonatal herpetic infection

Genetics N/A

Incidence/Prevalence
The incidence and prevalence of FHV-1 infection are high, especially in multicat facilities and adoption shelters. Cats that have recovered from infection will be latent carriers of the virus in nerve ganglia, especially in the trigeminal ganglion.

Geographic Distribution Worldwide

SIGNALMENT

Species Cats

Breed Predilections
All breeds are susceptible to FHV-1 infection.

Mean Age and Range
Young kittens are most often affected. Cats of all ages can develop clinical disease.

Predominant Sex No sex predilection

SIGNS

Historical Findings
• Acute onset with paroxysmal sneezing • Watery eyes with blepharospasm, usually bilateral • Partial to complete anorexia • Recurring mild upper respiratory infection in older cats • Abortion

Physical Examination Findings
• Fever, often pronounced • Acute rhinitis with serous to mucopurulent to purulent nasal discharge, sometimes blood-tinged • Acute conjunctivitis with serous to mucopurulent to purulent ocular discharge and blepharospasm • Chronic and/or reoccurring rhinitis and sinusitis with purulent nasal discharge • Ucerative herpetic keratitis, sometimes with descemetocele or panophthalmitis

CAUSES
• Feline herpesvirus type 1 (FHV-1), an alphaherpesvirus • Only one serotype of FHV-1 is known.

RISK FACTORS
• Lack of vaccination against FHV-1 • Crowding of cats in multicat facilities • Poor ventilation • Stress, both physical (cold) or psychological (introduction of new cats into household) • Queening and raising kittens often will result in a carrier queen infecting her kittens about 5 weeks of age. • Other infectious diseases, especially feline calicivirus infection, feline immunodeficiency virus infection, or feline leukemia virus infection

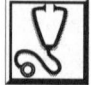

DIAGNOSIS

DIFFERENTIAL DIAGNOSIS
• Feline calicivirus infection—less sneezing and ocular involvement, ulcerative stomatitis common, pneumonia common, does not produce ulcerative keratitis • Feline chlamydiosis—tends to produce chronic conjunctivitis, often unilateral; longer incubation period (7-10 days), may have pneumonitis and intracytoplasmic inclusions in conjunctival scrapings; responds to some antibiotics such as tetracycline • Bacterial upper respiratory infections such as bordetellosis, haemophilus infection, or pasteurellosis—less nasal or ocular involvement; tend to respond to antibiotic therapy • Toxoplasmosis—pneumonia often present. No upper respiratory signs usually.

CBC/BIOCHEMISTRY/URINALYSIS
Laboratory tests usually are not helpful in diagnosing FVR. Transient mild leukopenia often occurs followed by leukocytosis caused by secondary bacterial infections.

OTHER LABORATORY TESTS
Serology on paired serum samples to detect rising antibody titers (limited value)

IMAGING N/A

OTHER DIAGNOSTIC PROCEDURES
• Immunofluorescent assay of nasal and/or conjunctival scrapings for detection of FHV-1 antigen • Viral isolation from pharyngeal swab sample • Conjunctival smears stained to detect intranuclear inclusion bodies

GROSS AND HISTOPATHOLOGIC FINDINGS
• Gross findings include evidence of ocular and nasal discharge (often purulent), mucosal edema of upper respiratory epithelium, sinusitis, and ulcerative keratitis with possible panophthalmitis in some cats. Tracheitis may be present in some cats as well. • Microscopic findings include submucosal edema with inflammatory cell infiltrates of upper respiratory and conjunctival tissues, focal necrosis of mucosa, chronic sinusitis, and intranuclear inclusion bodies in epithelial cells.

TREATMENT

INPATIENT VERSUS OUTPATIENT
Outpatient treatment unless severely affected

ACTIVITY
Patient should be restricted from contacting other cats during the acute infection to prevent spread of the virus to healthy cats.

DIET
Diet should not be altered unless in an attempt to entice the cat to eat special diets such as baby food.

CLIENT EDUCATION
Stress the importance of adequate vaccination and early (4-5 weeks of age) vaccination in breeding catteries. Early weaning may prevent transmission of virus from carrier queens to kittens in future litters.

SURGICAL CONSIDERATIONS
• Intratracheal tube may be needed in severely affected cats. • Insertion of an intranasal or a pharyngostomy feeding tube also may be indicated.

MEDICATIONS

DRUGS AND FLUIDS
• Broad spectrum antimicrobial therapy (amoxicillin, 22 mg/kg PO q12h) to treat secondary bacterial infections • Eye ointments that contain antibiotics may be indicated. • Fluid therapy as indicated, including tap water given by intranasal tube • Pediatric nasal decongestant drops, 0.25% oxymetazoline Hcl (Afrin Pediatric Nasal Drops), to decrease nasal discharge; give 1 drop/day into one nostril • Antiviral ophthalmic ointments or drops (Herplex, Vira-A) may be indicated to treat or prevent ulcerative keratitis • Systemic antiviral compounds to treat herpesvirus infections may be helpful, although not routinely used or needed. • Conjunctival vaccination with an intranasal-approved FHV-1 vaccine may be helpful in cats with chronic keratitis to enhance the local immune response.

CONTRAINDICATIONS
Corticosteroids given systemically can cause a recrudescence of FHV infection in carrier cats. Eye ointments with corticosteroids, but without antiviral compounds, may predispose to the development of ulcerative keratitis.

PRECAUTIONS None

POSSIBLE INTERACTIONS None

ALTERNATE DRUGS
Various antiviral drugs (e.g., phosphonoformate and acyclovir) have been studied for possible parenteral therapy of FVR with less

than ideal results. Feline interferon may eventually be shown to have some efficacy against FHV-1.

FOLLOW-UP

PATIENT MONITORING
• Appetite • Clear nasal exudate regularly.

PREVENTION/AVOIDANCE
• Routine vaccination with a MLV or inactivated vaccine will prevent development of severe clinical disease, although vaccination will not prevent infection and local viral replication with shed of virus. • Vaccination protocols will vary depending on the population of cats. Routine vaccination starts at 8-10 weeks of age with a second vaccine given 3-4 weeks later, and annual booster vaccinations are recommended. In breeding catteries where respiratory disease is a problem, kittens should be vaccinated earlier using one of two alternate protocols. • First, FHV/FCV/FPV vaccination is started at 4-5 weeks of age with the vaccine repeated at 3-4 week intervals until 12 weeks of age. Second, many breeders are vaccinating litters of kittens at 10-14 days of age with a single dose/litter of FHV/FCV vaccine approved for intranasal use, then vaccinating the cats parenterally at 6, 10, and 14 weeks of age with a triple or polyvalent vaccine.

POSSIBLE COMPLICATIONS
• Chronic sinusitis with sneezing and nasal discharge • Herpetic ulcerative keratitis
• Scarring and closure of the lacrimal duct with chronic ocular discharge

EXPECTED COURSE AND PROGNOSIS
• FVR generally runs a course of 7-10 days. Some cats may have only a mild ocular/nasal discharge with sneezing for 1-2 days, while other cats may become chronic and have clinical disease for weeks. • The prognosis for FVR cats is generally good, although some chronic sequela may occur. Mortality is generally very low or negligible except in very young kittens.

MISCELLANEOUS

ASSOCIATED CONDITIONS
FVR often occurs with feline calicivirus infection or various bacterial infections.

AGE RELATED FACTORS
FVR usually occurs in kittens 6-12 weeks of age, although infection can occur at any age.

ZOONOTIC POTENTIAL None

PREGNANCY
Unvaccinated pregnant cats that become infected with FHV-1 often will transmit the virus to the kittens in utero, resulting in abortion or neonatal FVR.

SYNONYMS
• Feline herpesvirus infection • "Rhino"
• "Coryza"

SEE ALSO
Calicivirus—Cats

ABBREVIATIONS
FVR = feline viral rhinotracheitis
FHV-1 = feline herpesvirus type 1
FCV = feline calicivirus
FPV = feline parvovirus

References

Barr MC, Olsen CW, Scott FW. Feline viral diseases. In: Ettinger SJ, Feldman EC, eds. Veterinary internal medicine. Philadelphia: WB Saunders, 1995:409-439.

Ford RB. Role of infectious agents in respiratory disease. Vet Clin North Am (Small Anim Pract) 1993;23:17-35.

Ford RB, Levy JK. Infectious diseases of the respiratory tract. In: Sherding RG, ed. The cat: diseases and clinical management. New York: Churchill Livingstone, 1994:489-500.

Pedersen NC. Feline herpesvirus type-1 infection. In: Pratt PW, ed. Feline infectious diseases. Goleta, CA: American Veterinary Publications, 1988:21-28.

Author Fred W. Scott
Consulting Editor Fred W. Scott

ROCKY MOUNTAIN SPOTTED FEVER

BASICS

DEFINITION
Rocky mountain spotted fever (RMSF) is a tick-borne rickettsial disease caused by Rickettsia rickettsii. It affects dogs and is considered the most important rickettsial disease in humans.

Pathophysiology
• Transmission occurs via the saliva of a vector (the American dog tick, Dermacentor variabilis, found east of the Great Plains, or the wood tick, Dermacentor andersoni, found from the Cascades to the Rocky Mountains) or blood transfusion. Ticks need to be attatched for 5-20 hours to infect a host (humans, dogs, and cats) or reservoir hosts (rodents and dogs). Incubation period varies from 2 days to 2 weeks. • Once in a host, the organism invades and multiplies in vascular endothelium. The resulting widespread vasculitis in organs with endarterial circulation causes most clinical signs and results from microvascular hemorrhage, platelet aggregation (thrombocytopenia), vasoconstriction and increased vascular permeability, increased plasma loss into the interstitial space (organ swelling), hypotension, and eventually DIC and shock.

Systems Affected
• Multisystemic involvement • Hemic/lymphatic/immune—bleeding tendencies from thrombocytopenia, vasculitis, lymphadenopathy, splenomingaly • Musculoskeletal—joint pain • Ophthalmic—conjunctivitis, scleral injection • Nervous—stupor, seizures, vestibular deficits, coma, cervical pain • Respiratory—dyspnea, cough • Skin/exocrine—edema of extremities, face • Cardiovascular

Genetics N/A

Incidence/Prevalence
• Occurs during tick season between late March until the end of September • The overall prevalence of infections in ticks is less than 2%. • Prevalence varies between geographic localities.

Geographic Distribution
Americas. No accurate prevalence figures for dogs but similar distribution as for humans in which most cases occur on the eastern seaboard states (especially the Carolinas), states in or near the Mississippi river valley, and south central states (Texas, Oklahoma, Kansas).

SIGNALMENT
Purebred dogs seem more prone to developing clinical illness than mixed breeds. German shepherds have a higher prevalence than other breeds. No age or sex predilection.

SIGNS

Historical Findings
• Fever (occurs within 2-3 days of tick attachment) • Lethargy, depression, anorexia • Swelling (edema) of lips, scrotum, prepuce, ears, extremities • Stiff gait (especially in dogs with scrotal or prepucial swelling) • Spontaneous bleeding (sneezing, epistaxis) • Respiratory distress • Neurologic signs (ataxia, head tilt) • Ocular pain

Physical Examination Findings
• Both clinical and subclinical illness occurs. • Clinical forms are variable in severity, lasting for 2-4 weeks if untreated. • Ticks may still be present in acute cases. • Pyrexia • Cutaneous lesions, including edema of face, limbs, prepuce, scrotum • Conjunctivitis, scleral injection • Respiratory signs (dyspnea, exercise intolerance resulting from pneumonitis) with increased bronchovesicular sounds • Generalized lymphadenopathy • Neurologic signs (vestibular dysfunction, altered mental status, seizures) • Myalgia/arthralgia • Petechia, ecchymoses (occular, oral, genital regions) in 20% of patients • Hemorrhagic diathesis (epistaxis, melena, hematuria) in severely affected animals • Cardiac arrhythmias (sudden death) • DIC and death (from shock) in severe acute cases

CAUSES N/A

RISK FACTORS
Exposure to ticks

DIAGNOSIS

DIFFERENTIAL DIAGNOSIS
• Canine ehrlichiosis (Erhlichia canis). Not seasonal. Clinically can be indistinguishable from RMSF (especially acute cases). Differentiate serologic testing. Both RMSF and ehrlichiosis respond to same treatment. • Immune-mediated thrombocytopenia. Not usually associated with fever or lymphadenopathy. Serologic testing used to best distinguish from ehrlichiosis. Often treat for both until have titers back. • Systemic lupus erythematosus. Antinuclear antibody test usually negative in ehrlichiosis. Serologic testing can be diagnostic. • Multiple myeloma. Differentiated from chronic ehrlichiosis by serologic testing to distinguish cause of hyperglobulinemia. • Chronic lymphocytic leukemia (CLL). Differentiated from chronic ehrlichiosis by lymphocytosis, cytology of bone marrow, serologic testing. • Brucellosis as a cause of scrotal edema. Serologic testing can be diagnostic.

CBC/BIOCHEMISTRY/URINALYSIS
CBC—thrombocytopenia with megathrombocytosis, mild anemia (normochromic, normocytic), mild leukopenia (early in infection), leukocytosis (and monocytosis) as disease becomes more chronic • Biochemistry—usually nonspecific changes, including mild increases in ALT, ALP, BUN, creatinine, total bilirubin (rare); hypercholesterolemia consistently found (cause unknown); hypoalbuminemia (resulting from vascular endothelial damage); azotemia; hyponatremia, hypochloremia, metabolic acidosis • Urinalysis—proteinuria (with or without azotemia) as a result of glomerular/tubular damage; hematuria (coagulation defects)

OTHER LABORATORY TESTS
Serum titers take 2-3 weeks to rise so may be negative in very acute cases. Perform paired titers 3 weeks apart, which show a fourfold increase between acute and convalescent titers. Paired titers avoid misdiagnosis because of considerable cross-reactivity with other rickettsial organisms. High titers can be detected for up to a year after treatment of the disease.

IMAGING N/A

OTHER DIAGNOSTIC PROCEDURES
• Direct immunofluorescence test of skin biopsies (obtained by local anesthesia and punch biopsies) from affected lesions can detect rickettsial antigens as early as 3-4 days postinfection. • CSF is often normal but might show an increase in protein and nucleated cells.

GROSS AND HISTOPATHOLOGIC FINDINGS
• Grossly, widespread petechia, splenomegally, generalized hemorrhagic lymphadenopathy. • Histologogically, necrotizing vasculitits with perivascular cell infiltration (mononuclear and neutrophilic). Vascular lesions are most promenant in the skin, kidneys, myocardium, meninges, retina, pancreas, gastrointestinal tract, urinary bladder. Hepatic and focal myocardial necrosis, nodular gliosis in the brain, and interstitial pneumonia are common. Special stains are needed to identify organisms.

TREATMENT

INPATIENT VERSUS OUTPATIENT
Because progression to shock and severe CNS disease can be rapid, patients should be hospitalized until stable and show a response to treatment.

ACTIVITY
Restricted

DIET N/A

CLIENT EDUCATION
Good prognosis in acute cases with appropriate and prompt therapy. Response occurs within hours of treatment. If treatment is not instituted until CNS signs occur or later in the disease process, mortality will be high. Dogs with CNS signs can die within hours.

SURGICAL CONSIDERATIONS
If surgery is needed for other reasons, blood transfusion may be needed to correct anemia and/or thrombocytopenia.

MEDICATIONS

DRUGS AND FLUIDS

• Doxycycline, a synthetic derivative of tetracycline, is the drug of choice (10 mg/kg, q12h, PO, for 10 days) and can be given intravenously for 5 days if the dog is vomiting. Oxytetracycline and tetracycline (22 mg/kg, q8h, PO, for 14 days) are also effective and less expensive.

• In puppies under 6 months of age, chloramphenicol (20 mg/kg, q8h, PO, for 14 days) is recommended to avoid yellow discoloration of erupting teeth caused by tetracyclines. However, owners should be warned (chloramphenicol's public health risks) because it directly interferes with heme and bone marrow synthesis. Similarly its use should be avoided in dogs with thrombocytopenia, pancytopenia, or anemia.

• Enrofloxacin (3 mg/kg, q8h, PO, for 7 days) is also effective. Avoid use in young dogs because articular cartilage damage can occur (preceded by lameness). Gastrointestinal upsets (vomiting, anorexia) can also occur.

• Balanced electrolyte solution is indicated in dehydrated animals but must be used cautiously because of increased vascular permeability and expanded extracellular fluid volume (exacerbating cerebral and pulmonary edema).

• Blood transfusion is indicated in anemic animals. Platelet-rich plasma or a blood transfusion is indicated in animals with hemorrhage resulting from thrombocytopenia.

CONTRAINDICATIONS

• Do not use tetracyclines (or derivatives) in dogs under 6 months of age because permanent yellowing of the teeth will occur.

• Do not use tetracyclines in dogs with renal insufficiency.

• Doxycycline may be used because it can be excreted via the gastrointestinal tract.

PRECAUTIONS

If serologic confirmation of infection is desired by running a posttreatment titer (i.e., treatment is initiated before a titer has developed), avoid chloramphenicol, which reduces serologic titers to a greater extent than tetracyclines.

POSSIBLE INTERACTIONS N/A

ALTERNATE DRUGS N/A

FOLLOW-UP

• Early antibiotic treatment will reduce the fever, albumin extravasation, and improve attitude in dogs within 24-48 hours. Repeat platelet count every 3 days after initiating antirickettsial agent until it increases into normal range. Platelet counts should return to normal within 2-4 days after initiating treatment. • Although serologic titers are reduced in treated dogs as opposed to untreated dogs, titers will remain positive during convalescence. Naturally infected dogs never seem to become reinfected.

PREVENTION/AVOIDANCE

Control tick infestation on dogs using dips or sprays containing dichlorvos, chlorfenvinphos, dioxathion, propoxur, or carbaryl. Flea and tick collars may reduce reinfestation but their reliability is unproven. Avoid tick-infested areas. Tick eradication in the environment is impossible because the organism is maintained in rodents and other reservoir hosts. If ticks are removed from the dogs by hand, use gloves (see zoonosis), and ensure tick mouth parts are removed, because a foreign body reaction is likely to result if they are left in place.

POSSIBLE COMPLICATIONS N/A

EXPECTED COURSE AND PROGNOSIS

Acute cases have an excellent prognosis with appropriate treatment. Dogs with CNS disease have a poor prognosis.

MISCELLANEOUS

ASSOCIATED CONDITIONS N/A

AGE RELATED FACTORS N/A

ZOONOTIC POTENTIAL

The incidence in people seems to be dropping with approximately 300 cases of RMSF reported per year from mid-1992 to mid-1993 in the United States (previous years had shown up to 1000 cases/year). Young adults and children are mainly infected. People can become infected from ticks that are transfered from dogs, but not from dogs directly. People can become infected when removing infected ticks from dogs. Major clinical signs in humans mimic those in dogs but mainly include fever and headaches. Neurologic signs occur later in illness. A skin rash is appreciated only in 50% of patients. Treatment with tetracyclines results in a rapid recovery.

PREGNANCY N/A

SYNONYMS N/A

SEE ALSO N/A

ABBREVIATIONS

DIC = disseminated intravascular coagulation
CLL = chronic lymphocytic leukemia
CSF = cerebrospinal fluid
RMSF = Rocky Mountain spotted fever

Reference

Greene CE, Breitschwerdt EB. Rocky Mountain spotted fever and Q fever. In: Greene CE, ed. Infectious diseases of the dog and cat. Philadelphia: WB Saunders, 1990;419-430.

Greene CE, Burgdorfer W, Cavagnolo R, et al. Rocky Mountain spotted fever in dogs and its differentiation from canine ehrlichiosis. J Am Vet Med Assoc 1985;186:465-472.

Hibler SC, Hoskins JD, Greene CE. Rickettsial infections in dogs part I. Rocky Mountain potted fever and Coxiella infections. Comp Con Ed Pract Vet 1985;7:856-865.

Breitschwerdt EB, Davidson MG, Aucoin DP, et al. Efficacy of chloramphenicol, enrofloxacin, and tetracycline for treatment of experimental Rocky Mountain spotted fever in dogs. Antimicrob Agents Chemother 1991;35:2375-2381.

Breitschwerdt EB, Walker DH, Levy MG, et al. Clinical, hematologic, and humoral immune response in female dogs inoculated with Rickettsia rickettsii and Rickettsia montana. Am J Vet Res 1988;49:70-76.

Author Stephen C. Barr
Consulting Editor Fred W. Scott

RODENTICIDE ANTICOAGULANT POISONING

BASICS

DEFINITION
Coagulopathy caused by reduced vitamin K_1 dependent clotting factors in the circulation after exposure to anticoagulant rodenticides.

Pathophysiology
Anticoagulant rodenticides inhibit vitamin K_1 epoxide reductase, DT diaphorase, and possibly other enzymes involved in the reduction of vitamin K_1 epoxide to vitamin K_1. Vitamin K_1 is necessary for carboxylation of clotting factors II, VI, IX and X. The uncarboxylated clotting factors cannot bind calcium, and therefore are unable to participate in clot formation.

Systems Affected
Hemic/lymphatic/immune—depletion of activated clotting factors, causing hemorrhage

Genetics N/A

Incidence/Prevalence
Common in small animal medicine because many baits are sold over the counter and widely used in homes.

Geographic Distribution
None because of widespread marketing of anticoagulant rodenticide products

SIGNALMENT

Species Dogs and cats

Breed Predilection N/A

Mean Age and Range N/A

Predominant Sex N/A

SIGNS

General Comments
Anticoagulant rodenticide exposure may be slightly more prevalent in the spring and fall when rodenticide products are put out.

Historical Findings
• Usage of anticoagulant rodenticides
• Dyspnea • Bleeding

Physical Examination Findings
Hematomas, often ventral • Hematoma at venipuncture site • Muffled heart or lung sounds • Pale mucous membranes
• Lethargy • Depression

CAUSES
• The disease is caused by exposure to anticoagulant rodenticide products. • The first generation coumarin anticoagulants (eg, warfarin) have been largely replaced by more potent, second generation active ingredients (eg, brodifacoum, bromadiolone, diphacinone, and chlorphacinone.)

RISK FACTORS
• Small doses over several days are more dangerous than a single large dose. Either type of exposure can cause toxicosis. • Secondary toxicosis by consumption of poisoned rodents by pets is not likely.

DIAGNOSIS

DIFFERENTIAL DIAGNOSES
• Disseminated intravascular coagulopathy
• Congenital clotting factor deficiencies

CBC/BIOCHEMISTRY/URINALYSIS
Anemia if animal has marked hemorrhage

OTHER LABORATORY TESTS
• ACT > 150 seconds supports coagulopathy
• Prolonged PT and PTT support exposure to rodenticide • Analysis of blood or liver for anticoagulant rodenticides to confirm exposure to a specific product

IMAGING
Radiography of the thorax can be used to detect hemothorax or hemopericardium.

OTHER DIAGNOSTIC PROCEDURES
Thoracentesis of dyspneic animals may confirm hemothorax.

GROSS AND HISTOPATHOLOGIC FINDINGS
• Free blood in the thoracic cavity, lungs, and abdominal cavity is common. • Less frequently seen is hemorrhage into the cranial vault, gastrointestinal tract, and urinary tract. This occurs both subcutaneously, and intramuscularly.

TREATMENT

INPATIENT VS OUTPATIENT
• In an acute crisis, animals should be treated as inpatients. • Once the coagulopathy is stabilized, animals are frequently treated as outpatients.

ACTIVITY
The animal should be kept confined during the early stages, because activity enhances blood loss.

DIET
Not recognized to have an important effect on this disease.

CLIENT EDUCATION
Explain to the owner that re-exposure will be a serious problem.

SURGICAL CONSIDERATIONS
• Thoracentesis may be important to remove free thoracic blood, which causes dyspnea and respiratory failure. • The coagulopathy must be corrected before surgery.

MEDICATIONS

DRUGS AND FLUIDS
• The drug of choice is vitamin K_1 (2.5 to 5.0 mg/kg PO q24h 5 days to 6 weeks, depending on the specific product involved.)
• Bioavailability of vitamin K_1 is enhanced by the concurrent feeding of a small amount of fat, such as canned dog food. • Fresh whole blood or plasma transfusion may be required in patients that are hemorrhaging.

CONTRAINDICATIONS
Anaphylactic reactions have been reported if vitamin K_1 is given intravenously, so this practice is discouraged.

PRECAUTIONS
Avoid unnecessary surgical procedures and parenteral injections.

POSSIBLE INTERACTIONS
Sulfonamides and phenylbutazone may displace anticoagulant rodenticides from plasma binding sites, leading to more free toxicant and toxicosis.

ALTERNATE DRUGS
Vitamin K_3 is not efficacious in the treatment of anticoagulant rodenticide toxicosis, and thus its use is contraindicated.

FOLLOW-UP

PATIENT MONITORING
ACT and PT

PREVENTION/AVOIDANCE
Do not allow animals access to anticoagulant rodenticides.

POSSIBLE COMPLICATIONS
Secondary bacterial pneumonia after intrapulmonary hemorrhage in some animals

EXPECTED COURSE AND PROGNOSIS
• If the animal survives the first 48 hours of acute coagulopathy, the prognosis improves.
• Continue vitamin K_1 administration for up to 3-4 weeks if second generation anticoagulants are the likely source of toxicosis. • PT or ACT should be monitored for 3-5 days after treatment is discontinued.

RODENTICIDE ANTICOAGULANT POISONING

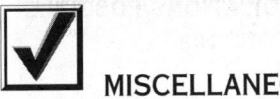

MISCELLANEOUS

ASSOCIATED CONDITIONS
N/A

AGE RELATED FACTORS N/A

ZOONOTIC POTENTIAL N/A

PREGNANCY
Chlorophacinone can pass into amniotic fluid, and then be passed on to the pups of an exposed pregnant bitch; similar concerns for passage of affected milk to pups

SYNONYMS N/A

SEE ALSO
Poisoning (Intoxication)

ABBREVIATIONS
ACT = activated clotting time
PT = prothrombin time
PPT = partial thromboplastin time

References
Murphy M and Gerken D. The anticoagulant rodenticides. In: Kirk RW and Bonagura J. eds. Current veterinary therapy X. Philadelpia: WB Saunders, 1989; 143-146.

Author Michael J. Murphy
Consulting Editor Gary Osweiler

ROTAVIRUS INFECTIONS

BASICS

OVERVIEW
• Genus within the family Reoviridae
• Nonenveloped, double-stranded RNA virus, relatively resistant to environmental destruction (acid and lipid solvents) • Unique double capsid protects virus from inactivation in the upper GI tract • Named rota (Latin), meaning wheel, after the shape of the capsid • Wide host range, identified in almost every species investigated • The most significant cause of severe gastroenteritis in young children (< 2 years) and animals throughout the world

SIGNALMENT
• Dogs—diarrhea reported in pups < 12 weeks old; most in pups < 2 weeks old
• Cats—kittens and young cats (< 6 months of age) more susceptible to infection

SIGNS
• Dogs—most infections subclinical or limited to relatively mild, nonspecific watery to mucoid diarrhea, anorexia, and lethargy, although rare fatalities reported • Cats—primarily subclinical or mild diarrhea; however, with coinfections or in stressed conditions, more severe clinical disease may occur

CAUSES AND RISK FACTORS
• Transmitted by fecal-oral contamination
• Infect mature epithelial cells on luminal tips of the intestinal villi, causing swelling, degeneration, and desquamation. The denuded villi contract, resulting in villous atrophy with loss of absorptive capability and loss of brush border enzymes (e.g., disaccharidases), leading to osmotic diarrhea.

DIAGNOSIS

DIFFERENTIAL DIAGNOSIS
• Canine viral enteritis—canine parvovirus, canine coronavirus, canine astrovirus, canine calicivirus, canine herpes virus, canine dis-

temper virus, canine reovirus • Feline viral enteritis—feline parvovirus (feline panleukopenia virus), feline leukemia virus, feline coronavirus, feline astrovirus, feline calicivirus • Other causes of enteritis—bacteria (e.g., Salmonella, Campylobacter, Clostridium), fungi, protozoa, parasitic, foreign bodies, intussusception, allergies, and toxicants

CBC/BIOCHEMISTRY/URINALYSIS
Noncontributory

OTHER LABORATORY TESTS   N/A

IMAGING   N/A

OTHER DIAGNOSTIC PROCEDURES
• Direct electron microscopy—to detect the virus in the feces (rapid, lack of sensitivity)
• Immunoelectron microscopy—more sensitive and specific than direct electron microscopy (not commonly available) • ELISA—to detect common group rotaviral antigen in feces (Rotazyme, Abbott Laboratories, North Chicago, IL) • Histology—swollen, small intestinal villi with mild infiltration by macrophages and neutrophils (virus detected by fluorescent antibody test) • Virus isolation
• Polymerase chain reaction—in future
• Serology—not recommended because most animals (e.g., 85% of dogs) carry antibodies as a result of previous exposure or from passive antibody immunization transfer from the bitch or queen (must demonstrate fourfold difference in acute and convalescent serum samples)

TREATMENT
• Symptomatic for diarrhea (fluids, electrolytes, and dietary restriction)
• Principal protection probably antibodies present in milk of immune bitch or queen

MEDICATIONS

DRUGS AND FLUIDS
Antibiotic therapy not indicated

CONTRAINDICATIONS/POSSIBLE INTERACTIONS N/A

FOLLOW-UP N/A

MISCELLANEOUS

ZOONOTIC POTENTIAL
• Rotaviruses are not host-specific, thus a puppy or kitten with rotaviral enteritis may pose a potential human health hazard, particularly for infants. • Care should be exercised when handling fecal material from a diarrheic pet. • In people, rotavirus diarrheal disease in infants has high morbidity and low mortality attributed to fluid therapy in developed countries, whereas in developing countries, rotaviruses are usually the leading cause of life-threatening diarrhea in infants and young children.

References
Pollock RVH, Carmichael LE. Canine rotavirus infection. In: Greene CE, ed. Infectious diseases of the dog and cat. Philadelphia: WB Saunders, 1990:283-284.
Pedersen NC. Feline rotavirus. In: Appel M, ed. Virus infections of carnivores. New York: Elsevier Science Publishers, 1987:259-260.
Author J. Paul Woods
Consulting Editor Fred W. Scott

ROUNDWORMS (ASCARIASIS)

BASICS

OVERVIEW
Ascariasis of dogs, especially pups, is caused by Toxocara canis and of cats by Toxocara cati with both host species infected by Toxascaris leonina. These are relatively large robust worms of up to 10–12 cm length so that distension of the small intestine often leads to colic, interference with gut motility, and inability to utilize food. Because of transplacental transmission to fetuses, pups may be born with a developing worm burden. Over first month of life, infected neonatal pups may rapidly debilitate with abdominal pain, prior to appearance of eggs in stools. Kittens may be similarly affected by transcolostral transmission. Older pups and kittens may become infected by ingestion of infective eggs disseminated on premises by dams with postgestational infections. Toxascaris may be transmitted by eggs or by predation of transport hosts (rodents) infected with dormant infective larvae.

SIGNALMENT
Dogs and cats. especially clinically important in pups and kittens

SIGNS

Historical Findings
• Abdominal distension • Colicky pain • Cachexia • Not nursing or eating • Scanty feces • Coughing due to larval migration that induces eosinophilic response • Whole litter may be affected

Physical Examination Findings
• Weakness, loss of condition, cachexia • Abdominal distension with intestines palpable

CAUSES AND RISK FACTORS
• Toxocara infection • Infected bitch or queen • Food or environment contaminated with feces • Concurrent enteric infections

DIAGNOSIS

DIFFERENTIAL DIAGNOSIS
• Hookworm infection • Strongyloides infection

CBC/BIOCHEMISTRY/URINALYSIS
May have eosinophilia

OTHER LABORATORY TESTS
• Fecal egg exam of pups, kittens > 3 weeks of age • Toxocara egg spherical with pitted outer shell membrane, single dark cell (zygote filling interior), 80–85 μm (T. canis), ~75 μm(T. cati) • Toxascaris egg ovoid with smooth exterior shell membrane, 1- or 2-cell not filling interior, light cytoplasm, 80 x 70 μm

IMAGING N/A

OTHER DIAGNOSTIC PROCEDURES
Necropsy findings of siblings that have died of similar signs

TREATMENT
• Treat acute cases as in-house patients to deworm and to supplement with intravenous feeding
• Alert client about possibility of sudden death or long debilitation
• Treat bitch, queen with adulticide/larvicide anthelmintic (fenbendazole) to decrease likelihood of subsequent litter and mature maternal infections

MEDICATIONS

DRUGS AND FLUIDS
• Adulticide/larvicide anthelmintic for pup or kitten and for dam • Supplemental intravenous feedings

Dog
• Adulticide/larvicide anthelmintics include: fenbendazole (Panacur) in food q24h for 5 days, milbemycin oxime (Interceptor) tabs by body weight monthly • Adulticide anthelmintics include: dichlorvos (Task for mature or Task Tabs for pups) twice monthly, febantel + praziquantel (Vercom) twice monthly, ivermectin + pyrantel pamoate (Heartgard-30 Plus) monthly • pyrantel pamoate (Nemex) twice monthly

CONTRAINDICATIONS/POSSIBLE INTERACTIONS
Organophosphates (dichlorvos) are contraindicated in heartworm-positive dogs and cats

FOLLOW-UP
Monitor fecal egg counts post-treatment

MISCELLANEOUS

ZOONOTIC POTENTIAL
Yes - Visceral larval migrans occurs following ingestion of infective ova.

AGE RELATED FACTORS
Greater clinical concern in neonates

SYNONYMS
Ascariasis

Reference
Bowman, DD ed. Georgi's parasitology for veterinarians. 6th ed. Philadelphia: WB Saunders, 1994;203–206

Author Robert M. Corwin
Consulting Editor Brent D.Jones

SALIVARY MUCOCELE

BASICS

OVERVIEW

Salivary mucocele is a collection of mucoid saliva caused by salivary gland leakage, the result of damage to the salivary tissue which incites an inflammatory reaction. The saliva follows the path of least resistance until it exits the body or becomes contained by normal or inflammatory tissue. The gastrointestinal system is affected because of dysphagia or anorexia due to pain, inflammation, or obstruction. The respiratory system can be affected because of upper airway obstruction. This is the most common clinical condition of the salivary gland.

SIGNALMENT

• Dogs and cats • Breeds that may have a relatively higher prevalence are the German shepherd dog and toy and miniature poodle • No age or gender predisposition reported • No genetic basis reported

SIGNS

• Vary with the severity and location of the lesion • Sublingual gland most frequently affected • Painful or nonpainful swelling • Dysphagia • Anorexia • Hemorrhage • Stridor • Dyspnea

CAUSES AND RISK FACTORS

• Traumatic—blunt trauma, penetrating foreign body, and bite wound • Inflammatory —sialoadenitis and foreign body • Secondary to adjacent disease (e.g., carnassial abscess and neoplasia)

DIAGNOSIS

DIFFERENTIAL DIAGNOSIS

Salivary mucocele must be differentiated from sialoadenitis, sialolith, compartment syndrome, salivary neoplasia, congenital branchial cleft cyst, and lymphadenopathy. Diagnosis made by examination of fine needle aspirate, biopsy, or sialography.

CBC/BIOCHEMISTRY/URINALYSIS

Results usually normal. Patients with an inflammatory cause may have an inflammatory leukogram.

OTHER LABORATORY TESTS N/A

IMAGING

Contrast sialography confirms the diagnosis but can be difficult and time-consuming and is often unnecessary.

OTHER DIAGNOSTIC PROCEDURES

• Palpate to characterize and determine the extent and location of the mucocele • Examination of a fine needle aspirate reveals grey-gold or blood-tinged viscid mucus. Mucus-specific stains (e.g., periodic acid-Schiff) help to confirm the diagnosis. • Biopsy of appropriate tissues is beneficial in ruling out neoplasia and branchial cleft cysts.

TREATMENT

• Immediate drainage by aspiration or lancing may be necessary in a patient with mucoceles causing respiratory compromise.
• Periodic drainage may be appropriate in patients that are poor anesthetic candidates. Drainage is rarely curative, because the mucocele usually returns to its former size within weeks.
• Definitive treatment includes drainage or resection of the mucocele in conjunction with removal of the damaged salivary gland. The submandibular and sublingual glands are always resected together because of their proximity.
• A surgical alternative to resection is marsupialization or redirection of salivary flow.

Recurrence is more likely with marsupialization than with resection.

MEDICATIONS

DRUGS AND FLUIDS N/A

CONTRAINDICATIONS/POSSIBLE INTERACTIONS N/A

FOLLOW-UP

• Monitor for swallowing abnormalities in the immediate postoperative period. Episodes of dysphagia are uncommon and usually transient. • Recurrence occurs in less than 5% of patients and is caused by incomplete resection, resection of the wrong gland, or iatrogenic damage to the contralateral gland. • Prognosis in dogs without concurrent disease in which complete resection is accomplished is good.

MISCELLANEOUS

References

Harvey CE. The tongue, lips, cheeks, pharynx, and salivary glands. In: Slatter D, ed. Textbook of small animal surgery. 2nd ed. Philadelphia: WB Saunders, 1993.

Harvey CE. Salivary gland disorders. In: Bojrab MJ, ed. Disease mechanisms in small animal surgery. 2nd ed. Philadelphia: Lea & Febiger, 1993.

Author James L. Cook

Consulting Editor Brent D. Jones

BASICS

OVERVIEW
• Infection with a rickettsia of the genus Neorickettsia • Small intestinal epithelium and associated lymphoid tissue; eventually systemic

Incidence/Prevalence
Northern pacific rim of the United States

SIGNALMENT

Species
Cats not susceptible

Breed Predilections
None

Mean Age and Range
All ages

Predominant Sex
Both sexes

SIGNS
Acute enteritis, diarrhea, vomiting, enlarged lymph nodes, severe nasal discharge (occasionally), and high body temperature

CAUSES AND RISK FACTORS
• Ingestion of raw fish containing the trematode vector or this rickettsia • Eating raw fish

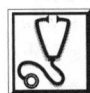

DIAGNOSIS

DIFFERENTIAL DIAGNOSIS
•Poisoning, parvovirus, and distemper

CBC/BIOCHEMISTRY/URINALYSIS
No specific findings

OTHER LABORATORY TESTS N/A

IMAGING N/A

OTHER DIAGNOSTIC PROCEDURES
• Giemsa-stained aspirate of enlarged lymph node to reveal intracytoplasmic rickettsial bodies • Fecal examination to reveal eggs of the trematode, Nanophyetus salmincola

GROSS AND HISTOPATHOLOGICAL FINDINGS
• Changes in lymphoid tissues—enlarged, yellowish, prominent white foci • Intestinal contents frequently contain free blood.

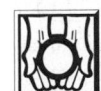

TREATMENT
• Hospitalize acutely ill animals.
• Inform owner of necessity to act quickly and consider other pets that may have eaten the same fish. There is no risk to humans reported.

MEDICATIONS

DRUGS AND FLUIDS
• Oxytetracycline (7 mg/kg IV q8h for 3 days), tetracyline (22 mg/kg PO q8h for 3 days), chloramphenicol, sulfonamide
• Supportive therapy, including fluids with electrolytes and basic measures to control diarrhea, are essential.
• Animal should be treated with praziquanel (10-30 mg/kg, SQ, once) to remove flukes.
• Whole blood transfusions if large blood loss through diarrhea

FOLLOW-UP
Monitor hydration, electrolytes, acid base, and temperature.

EXPECTED COURSE AND PROGNOSIS
Animals likely to succumb within 5-10 days of infection unless treated. With aggressive diagnosis and treatment, prognosis reasonable.

MISCELLANEOUS

ASSOCIATED CONDITIONS
• The Elokomin fluke fever agent is a similar rickettsia causing a more mild form of the disease. • Infection with N. salmonicola does not itself cause severe clinical disease.
Authors Dwight Bowman and Edward Pearce
Consulting Editor Fred W. Scott

SALMONELLOSIS

BASICS

DEFINITION
Salmonellosis is a bacterial disease that causes enteritis, septicemia, and abortions and is caused by many different serotypes of Salmonella. Disease spans subclinical infections (carrier states; salmonella shed in stool) to mild, moderate, and severe clinical cases in neonatal and stressed adult dogs and cats. Subclinical infections are more common than clinical disease, which itself is rare. Clinical salmonellosis is more common in young cats and dogs and in those adults subject to stress conditions (overcrowding, hospitalization, dietary changes, transportation, immunosuppressive/cytotoxic/antimicrobial drugs).

Pathophysiology
Salmonella, a gram-negative bacterium, colonizes the small intestine (ileum), adheres to and invades the enterocytes, and eventually enters and multiplies in the lamina propia and local mesenteric lymph nodes. Cytotoxin (cell death) and enterotoxin (increases cAMP) are produced, inflammation occurs, and prostaglandins synthesis ensues with a resulting secretory diarrhea and mucosal sloughing. In uncomplicated gastroenteritis, the salmonellae are stopped at the mesenteric LN stage and the animal has only diarrhea, vomiting, and dehydration. More serious disease occurs if bacteremia and septicemia follow the gastroenteritis; focal extraintestinal infections (abortion, joint disease) or endotoxemia may result, leading to organ infarction, generalized thrombosis, DIC, and death. Some animals recover from the septicemic form but suffer prolonged recovery as a result of their debilitated state.

Systems Affected
• Gastrointestinal—enterocolitis, inflammation, mucosal sloughing, secretory diarrhea
• Systemic disease (e.g., bacteremia, focal infections, septicemia)—multiorgan infarction, thrombosis, abscesses, meningitis, osteomyelitis, abortion

Genetics
Little is known of the genetic susceptibility of salmonellosis in dogs and cats.

Incidence/Prevalence
True incidence is unknown. Most infections are subclinical.
Dogs
• Clinical disease most often is seen in young and pregnant dogs. • Fecal/rectal swab survey of clinically "normal" domestic pet dogs—1-30% positive • Fecal/rectal swab survey of boarder kennels—16.7% • Fecal/rectal swab survey of vet hospitals—21.5% • Abattoir survey of mesenteric LN—4.5-26%
Cats
• High natural resistance to salmonellosis; "stressed" hospitalized cats at high risk of infection • Fecal survey of "normal" cats—1-18% • Fecal survey of random source research colony cats—10.6% • Abattoir survey of mesenteric LN—2.5%

Geographic Distribution Worldwide

SIGNALMENT

Species
Dogs and cats

Mean Age and Range
Dogs
Clinical disease is manifest in neonatal/immature puppies and in pregnant bitches; most adult carrier dogs are clinically normal.
Cats
Adult cats are highly naturally resistant to salmonella infections unless "stressed" by overcrowding, dietary changes, transport, and hospitalization.

Predominant Sex N/A

SIGNS

General Comments
• Host animal condition increase susceptibility—immune status (immature or suppressed), age (neonatal/aged), upset GI tract microbial flora (antimicrobial treatment)
• Environmental stress factors increase susceptibility—crowding, unsanitary conditions, hospitalization (surgery, anesthesia, feed/water changes, travel, antibiotics) • Alteration of indigenous/normal microbial flora of the GI tract.

Historical Findings
• Diarrhea, vomiting, fever, malaise, anorexia, vaginal discharge/abortion (dog) • Chronic febrile illness—persistent fever, anorexia, malaise without diarrhea

Physical Examination Findings
Spectrum of Clinical Manifestations in Dogs and Cats
• Asymptomatic carrier states—no clinical signs • Gastroenteritis—anorexia, malaise/lethargy, depression, fever (102-104° F), diarrhea with mucus and/or blood, progressive dehydration, abdominal pain, tenesmus, pale mucous membranes, mesenteric lymphadenopathy, and weight loss • Gastroenteritis with bacteremia with or without septicemia and focal extraintestinal infections—if septicemia/septic shock/endotoxemia, will see pale mucous membranes, weakness, cardiovascular collapse, tachycardia, and tachypnea • Focal extraintestinal infections—conjunctivitis, uterus/abortion, cellulitis, and pyothorax
• Note: cats may exhibit syndrome of a chronic febrile illness (without GI signs)—persistent fever, prolonged illness with vague, nonspecific clinical signs, and left shift on leukogram • Recovering cases may exhibit chronic intermittent diarrhea for up to 3-4 weeks and shed salmonella in stool for 6 weeks or longer (ileum and ileocecal LNs are colonized with salmonella).

CAUSES
• Any one of more than 2000 serotypes of salmonellae • Two or more simultaneous salmonella serotypes in a host animal is not uncommon.

RISK FACTORS

Disease Agent
Salmonella serotype, its virulence factors, infectious dose, and route of exposure

Host Factors That Increase Susceptibility to Disease
• Age (neonatal/young dogs and cats; immature immune system) • Overall health status (debilitated young animals or adults, other concurrent disease, parasitism; young animals with an immature GI tract with poorly developed normal microbial flora)

Environmental Factors
• Coprophagia spreads infection. • Dehydrated (dry) dog and cat feed known to harbor salmonellae; "pressed" foods such as kibble and dog biscuits are usually not as risky • Grooming habits of dogs and cats result in salmonella contaminated hair coat, which contaminates cage or run environment and feed and water dishes. • Research colony cats/dogs, boarded animals, shelter/pound animals; overcrowded housing; unsanitary conditions; exposure to other infected (or carrier) animals; buildup of Salmonella in the environment; more efficient fecal-oral cycling; high opportunity for fecal exposure; "stress" factors
Hunting/Stray Dogs and Cats
• Scavenging for food; exposure to garbage, contaminated food/water, dead animals
• Exposure to other infected (or carrier) animals
Hospitalized Dogs and Cats
Nosocomial exposure (plus stress) or activation (by stress) of preexisitng asymptomatic (carrier) salmonella infection

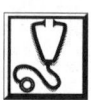

DIAGNOSIS

DIFFERENTIAL DIAGNOSIS
• Acute gastroenteritis (dog and cat)—vomiting, diarrhea • Infectious enteritis (need serology and/or culture to differentiate etiologies)—viral gastroenteritis, feline panleukopenia, FeLV, FIV, feline enteric coronavirus, canine enteric coronairus, canine parvovirus, rotavirus, canine distemper • Bacterial gastroenteritis—E. coli, Campylobacter jejuni, Yersinia enterocolitica • Bacterial overgrowth syndrome—Clostridium difficile, Cl. perfringens • Parasites—helminths (hookworms, ascarids, whipworms, Strongyloides), Protozoa (Giardia, Coccidia, Cryptosporidia), Rickettsiae, salmon poisoning • Acute gastritis—erosions or ulcers • Dietary-induced distress—overeating, abrupt changes, starvation, thirst, allergy or food intolerance, indiscretions (foreign material, garbage) • Drug- or toxin-induced distress • Extraintestinal disorders/metabolic disease

CBC/BIOCHEMISTRY/URINALYSIS

Hematology Profile
CBC-variable, depending on stage of illness—neutropenia initially, left shift with toxic neutrophils, nonregenerative anemia, lymphopenia, thrombocytopenia

Chemistry Profile
Hypoalbuminemia, electrolyte imbalances

OTHER LABORATORY TESTS N/A

IMAGING N/A

OTHER DIAGNOSTIC PROCEDURES
Note: Use of antimicrobials in a patient before sampling may produce a false-negative culture result.
• Fecal/rectal culture—salmonella positive (special media needed) • Fecal leukocytes—positive • Bacteremia/septicemia/DIC—blood culture are salmonella positive. Joint fluid may be culture positive for salmonella. • Subclinical carrier states—chronic, intermittent fecal culture positive for salmonella (> 6 weeks)

GROSS AND HISTOPATHOLOGIC FINDINGS
• Gross lesions seen only in severely affected cases • Cultures of ileum, mesenteric LN, liver/spleen, and bone marrow are salmonella positive.

TREATMENT

INPATIENT VERSUS OUTPATIENT
• Outpatient for uncomplicated gastroenteritis (without bacteremia) and carrier states
• Inpatient for bacteremia/septicemia states and for gastroenteritis in neonatal/immature animals that are rapidly debilitated by diarrhea

ACTIVITY
• All patients in the acute stages of disease may be shedding large numbers of Salmonellae in their stool; animals should be isolated when in the hospital area.
• Acutely ill animals, bacteremic/septicemic, and chronically ill animals should have restricted activity with cage rest, monitoring, and warmth.

DIET
Restrict food 24-48 hours, then gradually introduce a highly digestible, low-fat diet .

CLIENT EDUCATION
In the acute stages of disease, pets may be shedding large numbers of salmonellae in their stool; need for frequent hand washing; restrict access to the animal

SURGICAL CONSIDERATIONS N/A

MEDICATIONS

DRUGS AND FLUIDS
Appropriate therapy varies according to severity of illness (assess percentages of dehydration, body weight, ongoing fluid loss, shock,

PCV/total protein, electrolytes, acid-base status.

Asymptomatic "Carrier" State
Antimicrobials are contraindicated; in human medicine, clearing of carrier states demonstrated with quinolone drugs; more controlled trials in animals are needed

Uncomplicated Gastroenteritis (Vomiting and Diarrhea without Systemic Signs)
• Antimicrobials are not indicated.
• Treat signs; supportive care; fluid and electrolyte replacement
• Parenteral, balanced, polyionic isotonic solution (lactated Ringer's)
• Oral fluids—hypertonic glucose solutions (for secretory diarrhea)
• Plasma transfusions if serum albumin < 2 g/dl
• Locally acting intestinal adsorbents and protectants

Neonates, Aged, and Debilitated Animals (Severe Bloody Diarrhea and Systemic Signs of Septicemia and Shock [Endotoxic] with or without Diarrhea)
• Plasma transfusions; glucocorticoids shown to reduce mortality in endotoxic shock
• Antimicrobial therapy indicated (must do culture and susceptibility testing/MICs to assess drug resistance problems)
• Trimethoprim-sulfa—15 mg/kg PO or SQ q12h
• Enrofloxacin—5 mg/kg PO or IM q12h
• Norfloxocin—22 mg/kg PO q12h
• Chloramphenicol—dogs, 50 mg/kg PO, IV, IM, or SQ q8h; cats, 50 mg/kg total PO, IV, IM, or SQ q12h

CONTRAINDICATIONS None

PRECAUTIONS
• Be cautious when using chloramphenicol and trimethoprim/sulfa in neonatal and pregnant dogs and cats.
• Avoid use of fluoroquinolones in pregnant, neonatal, or growing animals (medium-sized dogs less than 8 months of age and large or giant breeds less than 12-18 months of age) because of cartilage lesions.

POSSIBLE INTERACTIONS N/A

ALTERNATE DRUGS N/A

FOLLOW-UP

PATIENT MONITORING
• Repeat fecal culture monthly for few months to assess development of carrier state
• Monitor patient's contacts at risk of secondary spread of infection; contact veterinarian if animal shows signs of recurring disease

PREVENTION/AVOIDANCE
• Keep animals healthy—proper nutrition, no raw meat, and vaccinate for other infectious diseases • Frequent cleaning and disinfection; good sanitation of cages, runs, feed/water dishes • Proper storage of feed and feed utensils • Reduce overcrowding of animals in pounds, shelters, kennels, catteries,

and research colonies. • Isolate and screen/monitor for sickness in new additions to household, kennels, etc., before mixing with other animals

POSSIBLE COMPLICATIONS
• Spread of infection not uncommon within household to other animals or humans
• Development of chronic infection with diarrhea • Recurrence of disease with stress

EXPECTED COURSE AND PROGNOSIS
• Uncomplicated gastroenteritis—prognosis is excellent; frequently the case is self-limited; animals recover with good nursing care; recovered animals may shed salmonella intermittently for months or longer as a "recovered carrier" • Neonatal/aged/stressed animals can develop septicemia and systemic disease that can be severe and debilitating and lead to death if untreated.

MISCELLANEOUS

ASSOCIATED CONDITIONS N/A

AGE RELATED FACTORS
Clinical disease frequently seen in neonatal and aged animals.

ZOONOTIC POTENTIAL
• High zoonotic potential, especially in children, elderly, immunosuppressed, and antimicrobial users. • Acutely ill animals shed large numbers of salmonellae in stool.
• Grooming habits allow rapid contamination of animal's fur and environment.
• Isolation is needed.

PREGNANCY
• Pregnancy may complicate salmonellosis.
• Abortion may be a sequellae to infection.
• Antimicrobial therapy must take into account the effect on the fetus.

SYNONYM
Songbird fever

SEE ALSO N/A

ABBREVIATION
LN = lymph node

References
Morse EV, Duncan MA. Canine salmonellosis: prevalence, epizootiology, signs, and public health significance. J Am Vet Med Assoc 1975;167:817-820.
Dow SW, Jones RL, Henik RA, Husted PW. Clinical features of salmonellosis in cats: six cases (1981-1986). J Am Vet Med Assoc 1989;194:1464-1466.
Author Patrick L. McDonough
Consulting Editor Fred W. Scott

SARCOPTIC MANGE

BASICS

OVERVIEW

• A nonseasonal, intensely pruritic, highly contagious parasitic skin disease of dogs caused by infestation with the mite, Sarcoptes scabiei var. canis. • The mites burrow through the stratum corneum and cause intense pruritus by mechanical irritation, production of irritating byproducts, and secretion of allergenic substances that produce a hypersensitivity reaction in sensitized dogs.

SIGNALMENT

• Seen in dogs of all ages and breeds • In multiple dog households, more than one dog usually show symptoms.

SIGNS

• Nonseasonal, extremely intense pruritus.
• Alopecia and erythematous rash on elbows, hocks, ventral abdomen, and chest.
• Lesions on ear margins range from barely perceptible scaling to alopecia or crusts. The ear canals are not affected. • With chronicity; periocular and trunkal alopecia; secondary crusts, excoriations, and pyoderma may develop. Possible peripheral lymphadenopathy. • Frequently bathed dogs may present with chronic pruritus but have no skin lesions. • Minimal or no response to antiinflammatory doses of steroids.

CAUSES AND RISK FACTORS

Previous exposure to a carrier dog 2-6 weeks before the development of symptoms
• Living outside (roaming dogs) • Boarded at kennel • Visits to veterinarian's office
• Visits to groomer • Residence at animal shelter

DIAGNOSIS

DIFFERENTIAL DIAGNOSIS

• Flea allergic dermatitis • Food allergy
• Contact allergy • Atopy • Demodicosis
• Pyoderma • Pelodera dermatitis

CBC/BIOCHEMISTRY/URINALYSIS
N/A

OTHER LABORATORY TESTS   N/A

IMAGING   N/A

OTHER DIAGNOSTIC PROCEDURES

• Positive pinnal-pedal reflex; rubbing the ear margin between your thumb and forefinger should induce the dog to scratch with his ipsilateral hind leg (unless he's very nervous). • Superficial skin scrapings (mites and ova are extremely difficult to find; false negative results are common). • Fecal flotation occasionally reveals mites or ova. • Favorable response to scabicidal treatment. So that you don't miss a potentially curable disease, any dog with clinical signs suggestive of sarcoptic mange should be treated for scabies, even if skin scrape results are negative.

TREATMENT

• Any dog with nonseasonal pruritus that responds poorly to steroids should be treated with a scabicide (even if skin scrape results are negative) to definitively rule out sarcoptic mange.
• When scabicidal dips are used the entire dog must be treated (treatment failures are often linked to the owner's reluctance to apply dip to the dog's face and ears) and the dog can not be allowed to get wet between treatments.
• All in-contact dogs should be treated, even those with no clinical signs because they may be asymptomatic carriers and it can take 1 month for their clinical signs to develop.

MEDICATIONS

DRUGS AND FLUIDS

Treatment choices include:
• Antiseborrheic shampoo bath followed by total body treatment with 2% lime sulfur solution (LymDip), mercaptomethyl phtalimide (Paramite), or malathion dip once weekly for 2 weeks beyond remission or for a minimum of 5 weeks.
• Antiseborrheic shampoo bath followed by total body treatment with amitraz (Mitaban) 5.3 cc/gal water three times at 1-2 week intervals. (This is not an FDA approved treatment for sarcoptic mange.)
• Ivermectin (Ivomec), 0.2-0.3 mg/kg PO or SQ twice, two weeks apart. (This is extralabel use and is not approved by the FDA for treatment of sarcoptic mange)
• Some dogs benefit from prednisone therapy,

0.5 mg/kg q 12 hr for the first week of treatment.
• Antibiotics for secondary pyoderma may be needed for 2-3 weeks.

CONTRAINDICATIONS/POSSIBLE INTERACTIONS

Ivermectin should be used with extreme caution in collies, shetland sheepdogs, old English sheepdogs, Australian shepherds, and their crossbreeds because ivermectin toxicity is more likely to occur in herding-type breeds.

FOLLOW-UP

Response to treatment should be seen within 2 weeks. If none is seen, make sure the treatment protocol is being followed.

MISCELLANEOUS

ASSOCIATED CONDITIONS

• Sarcoptic mange can resemble pruritic impetigo in young puppies. • Always consider sarcoptic mange as a possible cause of pruritus in an allergic dog that is no longer responding to corticosteroid therapy.

ZOONOTIC POTENTIAL

Sarcoptic mange is zoonotic. People that come in close contact with an affected dog may develop a pruritic, papular rash on their arms, chest, or abdomen. Human lesions are usually transient and should resolve spontaneously after the affected dog(s) have been treated. If the lesions on people persist, advice from a human dermatologist should be sought.

References

Muller GH, Kirk RW, Scott DW. Small animal dermatology. 4th ed. Philadelphia: WB Saunders, 1989;396-404.
Griffin CE. Scabies. In: Griffin CE, Kwochka KW, Macdonald JM, eds. Current veterinary dermatology: the science and art of therapy. St. Louis: Mosby Year Book, 1993:85-89.
Author Linda Medleau
Consulting Editor Lowell Ackerman

BASICS

OVERVIEW
Thoracic limb extensor hypertonia associated with hind limb paralysis after acute spinal cord lesion caudal to the cervical intumescence in dogs

SIGNALMENT
Any dog suffering from a severe thoracolumbar spinal cord injury

SIGNS
• The forelimbs, although rigidly extended, have normal gait and postural reactions since no lesions are located at the cervical intumescence or above. • Hind limb signs vary depending on the severity and location of the thoracolumbar cord lesion; usually upper motor neuron in type, but can be lower motor neuron

CAUSES AND RISK FACTORS
• The posture is caused by the interruption of the activity of the "border cells," interneurons in the lumbar spine that have an ascending inhibitory action on the forelimb extensor motor neurons. • Road accident and intervertebral disc disease are the two most common causes.

DIAGNOSIS

DIFFERENTIAL DIAGNOSIS
• In animals with decerebrate rigidity, all four limbs are rigid and upper motor neuron dysfunction is present in all limbs. Consciousness is affected (ie, stupor to coma). • In animals with decerebellate rigidity, the forelimbs are rigid but the hind limbs are flexed. • Postural reactions are normal to abnormal; consciousness is normal to abnormal; other signs of cerebellar disease are characteristic (eg, intention tremor and loss of menace). • Animals with cervical spinal cord injury may have extensor tone in the forelimbs but also have deficits in voluntary movements; postural reactions and reflexes are present in all four limbs.

CBC/BIOCHEMISTRY/URINALYSIS
N/A

OTHER LABORATORY TESTS N/A

IMAGING
Radiology including myelography to demonstrate the thoracolumbar lesion

OTHER DIAGNOSTIC PROCEDURES
CSF analysis to demonstrate the thoracolumbar lesion

TREATMENT
• Treatment directed toward the underlying thoracolumbar lesion
• No specific treatment is available, but the condition resolves if adequate spinal cord function is restored.

MEDICATIONS

DRUGS AND FLUIDS
As indicated for underlying spinal cord disease

CONTRAINDICATIONS/POSSIBLE
INTERACTIONS N/A

FOLLOW-UP
The posture may persist for days to weeks. It is not an indication for a hopeless prognosis. If treatment is applied rapidly and aggressively, the patient may recover, especially if the dogs has pain perception caudal to the lesions.

MISCELLANEOUS

Reference
de Lahunta A. Veterinary neuroanatomy and clinical neurology. 2nd ed. Philadelphia: WB Saunders, 1983:185-186.
Author Mary O. Smith
Consulting Editor Joane M. Parent

SCHWANNOMA

BASICS

OVERVIEW
Schwannoma is a nerve sheath tumor occurring most commonly in the brachial plexus.

SIGNALMENT
• Middle-aged to old dogs • Males may have a slightly higher risk than females. • Cats rarely affected

SIGNS
• Chronic, progressive forelimb lameness the most common owner complaint • Muscle atrophy and axial pain also reported. • Some affected animals chew at the affected limb, presumably because of abnormal sensation secondary to the tumor. • Ipsilateral Horner's syndrome can develop secondarily to involvement of the sympathetic nerve fibers arising from the most cranial thoracic nerves.
• Occasionally, a palpable axillary mass

CAUSES AND RISK FACTORS
None identified

DIAGNOSIS

DIFFERENTIAL DIAGNOSIS
• Other neoplasms (e.g., lymphosarcoma, neurofibroma, and neurofibrosarcoma)
• Traumatic injury to the brachial plexus
• Intervertebral disc disease

CBC/BIOCHEMISTRY/URINALYSIS
Results usually normal

OTHER LABORATORY TESTS N/A

IMAGING
• Survey radiography of the spine may reveal widened intervertebral foramina at the site of the tumor. • Myelography should be performed to assess extent of spinal cord involvement as well as to locate nerve roots • CT scan and MRI provide much greater detail for identifying nerve root tumors

OTHER DIAGNOSTIC PROCEDURES
Electromyography may reveal denervation to the affected area.

TREATMENT

• Surgical excision the treatment of choice. Affected nerves are discolored, firm, and large.
• Excision of the affected area may achieve a viable limb and excellent quality of life if involvement is minimal. Patients with extensive lesions may need to be treated aggressively by amputation. Involvement of the spinal cord necessitates a laminectomy to relieve compression. Recurrence is common.
• Radiotherapy is another treatment option. However, little data exists on effectiveness.

MEDICATIONS

DRUGS AND FLUIDS
• Corticosteroids may help to temporarily reduce peritumoral edema and relieve clinical signs.
• Successful chemotherapy has not been described.

CONTRAINDICATIONS/POSSIBLE INTERACTIONS N/A

FOLLOW-UP

EXPECTED COURSE AND PROGNOSIS
• Recurrence after surgical excision common
• This tumor tends to be slow growing and slow to metastasize. • Prognosis poor

MISCELLANEOUS

ASSOCIATED CONDITIONS N/A

AGE RELATED FACTORS N/A

ZOONOTIC POTENTIAL N/A

PREGNANCY N/A

Reference
Steinberg, HS Brachial plexus injuries and dysfunctions. Vet Clin North Am 1988;18:565-580.
Author Ruthanne Chun
Consulting Editor Wallace B. Morrison

BASICS

OVERVIEW
• An inflammatory disease process directed against the cutaneous adnexal structures.
• The disease may be genetically inherited or immune-mediated. Initial defect may be a keratinization disorder or an abnormality in lipid metabolism.

SIGNALMENT
• Young adult to middle-aged dogs • Two forms of disease: one occurring in long-coated breeds and one in short-coated breeds
• Predisposed breeds: standard poodle, akita, Samoyed and vizsla

SIGNS
Long-Coated Breeds
• Symmetrical, partial alopecia • Dull brittle hair • Tightly adherent silver-white scale
• Follicular casts around hair shaft • Small tufts of matted hair • Lesions often first observed along dorsal midline • Secondary bacterial folliculitis, pruritus, and malodor develop in severely affected animals • Akitas often more severely affected

Short-Coated Breeds
• Moth-eaten, circular, or diffuse alopecia
• Mild scaling • Affects the trunk, head, and ears • Secondary bacterial folliculitis is rare

CAUSES AND RISK FACTORS
Mode of inheritance is being studied

 DIAGNOSIS

DIFFERENTIAL DIAGNOSIS
• Primary seborrhea • Bacterial folliculitis
• Demodicosis • Dermatophytosis • Endocrine skin disease

CBC/BIOCHEMISTRY/URINALYSIS
N/A

OTHER LABORATORY TESTS N/A

IMAGING N/A

OTHER DIAGNOSTIC PROCEDURES
Differentiate by age, breed, response to systemic antibiotics, skin scraping, dermatophyte culture, endocrine function tests and skin biopsies with special stains for bacteria and fungi

GROSS AND HISTOPATHOLIGIC FINDINGS
• Nodular granulomatous to pyogranulomatous inflammatory reaction at the level of the sebaceous glands. • Orthokeratotic hyperkeratosis and follicular cast formation. More prominent in long-coated breeds. • Complete loss of sebaceous glands with periadnexal fibrosis in advanced cases. • Destruction of entire hair follicle and adnexal unit rarely seen.

 TREATMENT

• Clinical signs may wax and wane irrespective of treatment.
• Controlled studies have not been done to document efficacy of any therapy.
• Treatment results have been extremely variable.
• Akitas are the breed most refractory to treatment.
• Response to therapy may vary depending on severity of disease at the time of diagnosis.

 **MEDICATIONS**

DRUGS AND FLUIDS
• 50-75% mixture of propylene glycol and

water applied as spray q24h to affected areas.
• Soak affected areas in baby oil for 1 hour, followed with multiple shampoos to remove oil and scales.
• 1 extra strength Derm Cap® and 500 mg evening primrose oil q12h PO. Possible side effects include vomiting, diarrhea, flatulence.
• Isotretinoin (Accutane) 1 mg/kg q12h PO. Reduce to 1 mg/kg q24h after one month and to 1 mg/kg q48h after two months. Continue as needed for maintenance.
• Cyclosporine (Sandimmune) 5 mg/kg q12h PO. Side effects include vomiting, diarrhea, gingival hyperplasia, hirsutism, papillomatous skin lesions, increased incidence of infections, nephrotoxicity, and hepatotoxicity.
• Bactericidal antibiotics and Sulf-Oxydex shampoo indicated for secondary bacterial folliculitis.

 FOLLOW-UP

Owners of affected dogs are urged to register their dog so that mode of inheritance can be determined.

 MISCELLANEOUS

Reference

Rosser EJ. Sebaceous adenitis. In: Griffin CE, Kwochka KW, MacDonald JM Current Veterinary Dermatology. St Louis, MO: Mosby Year Book, 1993;211-214.
Author Ellen C. Codner
Consulting Editor Lowell Ackerman

SEMINOMA

BASICS

OVERVIEW
Seminoma is usually a benign unilateral, solitary tumor of the testis. It is often difficult to palpate—one in nine dogs > 4 years old have a seminoma and 71% are not detected by physical examination.

SIGNALMENT
• Usually affects old male dogs • Mean age of 10 years • No breed predisposition

SIGNS
• Usually none • Rarely associated with feminization from estrogen excess (see Sertoli Cell Tumor)

CAUSES AND RISK FACTORS
Cryptorchidism

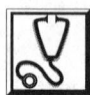

DIAGNOSIS

DIFFERENTIAL DIAGNOSIS
• Sertoli cell tumor • Interstitial cell tumor

CBC/BIOCHEMISTRY/URINALYSIS
Results usually normal unless the patient has evidence of male feminization syndrome.

OTHER LABORATORY TESTS N/A

IMAGING
• Tumors < 3 cm diameter usually hypoechoic on ultrasound • Tumors > 5 cm diameter usually have mixed echo pattern on ultrasound

OTHER DIAGNOSTIC PROCEDURES
N/A

TREATMENT
• Castration and histopathologic examination
• Radiotherapy reported effective in patients with seminoma and regional metastasis

MEDICATIONS

DRUGS AND FLUIDS N/A

CONTRAINDICATIONS/POSSIBLE INTERACTIONS N/A

FOLLOW-UP

PATIENT MONITORING
Recovery usually complete after castration

PREVENTION/AVOIDANCE N/A

POSSIBLE COMPLICATIONS
None likely

EXPECTED COURSE AND PROGNOSIS
• Usually excellent after castration • Tumor usually has benign behavior but some metastasize to regional lymph nodes, visceral organs, lungs, and other sites.

MISCELLANEOUS

ASSOCIATED CONDITIONS
• Most tumors are < 2 cm diameter. • Prostate disease, perianal adenoma, and perineal hernia may accompany seminoma. • One third of seminomas found in a cryptorchid testis • Extrascrotal seminomas more common in the right testis

AGE RELATED FACTORS
Usually affects middle-aged and older dogs

ZOONOTIC POTENTIAL N/A

PREGNANCY N/A

Reference
McDonald RK, Walker M, Legendre AM, et al. Radiotherapy of metastatic seminoma in the dog. J Vet Int Med 1988;2:103-107.
Author Wallace B. Morrison
Consulting Editor Wallace B. Morrison

BASICS

OVERVIEW
Common testicular tumor in dogs

SIGNALMENT
Old male dogs

SIGNS
• Unilaterally large testicle with atrophy of the unaffected testicle • Feminization syndrome with gynecomastia, galactorrhea, atrophy of penis, pendulous prepuce, attraction to other male dogs, and standing in the female position to urinate • Squamous metaplasia of the prostate and prostatomegaly develops in some animals. • Dermatologic changes, including nonpruritic alopecia, thinning of the haircoat, and hyperpigmentation • Abdominal mass if animal is cryptorchid • Location can be inguinal

CAUSES AND RISK FACTORS
Cryptorchidism

DIAGNOSIS

DIFFERENTIAL DIAGNOSIS
• Interstitial cell tumor • Seminoma • Hyperadrenocorticism • Hypothyroidism

CBC/BIOCHEMISTRY/URINALYSIS
Severe bone marrow suppression associated with hyperestrogenism

OTHER LABORATORY TESTS   N/A

IMAGING
Variable echotexture on ultrasound

OTHER DIAGNOSTIC PROCEDURES
• Serum estradiol concentration high in most patients • Serum progesterone concentration high in most patients

TREATMENT
Castration and histopathologic examination

MEDICATIONS   N/A

DRUGS AND FLUIDS   N/A

CONTRAINDICATIONS   N/A

POSSIBLE INTERACTIONS   N/A

FOLLOW-UP   N/A

PATIENT MONITORING   N/A

PREVENTION/AVOIDANCE   N/A

POSSIBLE COMPLICATIONS
None unless associated with surgery or estrogen excess

EXPECTED COURSE AND PROGNOSIS
• Good in most patients • Guarded if severe cytopenias develop because of hyperestrogenism

MISCELLANEOUS

ASSOCIATED CONDITIONS
• Cryptorchid testicles are 13-13.6 times more likely to develop neoplasia than are scrotally located testicles. • Sertoli cell tumor is more likely to have an abdominal location than other testicular tumors. High testicular temperature in the abdominal location may destroy spermatogenic cells and leave sertoli cells unregulated. 25-29% of dogs with sertoli cell tumor develop male feminization syndrome. • About 70% of intraabdominal testicular tumors in dogs are associated with male feminization syndrome. • Approximately 10-14% of sertoli cell tumors behave in a malignant fashion and metastasize to regional lymph nodes and other abdominal and thoracic organs. • Hyperestrogenism can cause hematopoietic failure.

AGE RELATED FACTORS
Common in old male dogs

ZOONOTIC POTENTIAL   N/A

PREGNANCY   N/A

Reference

Metzger FL, Hattel AL, White DG. Hematuria, hyperestrogenemia, and hyperprogesteronemia due to a sertoli-cell tumor in a bilaterally cryptorchid dog. Canine Pract 1993;18:32-35.

Author Wallace B. Morrison
Consulting Editor Wallace B. Morrison

SEXUAL DEVELOPMENT DISORDERS

 BASICS

DEFINITION

Errors in the establishment of chromosomal, gonadal, or phenotypic sex cause abnormal sexual differentiation. Individuals are examined with a variety of patterns from ambiguous genitalia to apparently normal genitalia with sterility.

Pathophysiology

Normal sexual differentiation can be described in three sequential steps—establishment of chromosomal sex, development of gonadal sex, and development of phenotypic sex. Chromosomal sex is established at fertilization (either XX or XY).

Abnormalities of Chromosomal Sex

• XXY syndrome (Klinefelter's syndrome)—79, XXY; hypoplastic testes; phenotypic male (normal to hypoplastic genitalia); dogs and cats (some tortoiseshell males) • XO syndrome (Turner's syndrome)—77, XO; dysgenetic ovaries; phenotypic female; infantile genitalia; dogs and cats • XXX syndrome—79, XXX; ovaries without follicles; female phenotype; high follicle stimulating hormone and luteinizing hormone; dogs • True hermaphrodite chimera—XX/XY or XX/XXY; ovarian and testicular tissue; phenotypic sex depends on amount of testicular tissue; dogs and cats • XX/XY chimera with testes and XY/XY chimera—vary from phenotypic female with abnormal genitalia to male with possible fertility; dogs and cats (some tortoiseshell males) • Gonadal differentiation is determined by the sex chromosome constitution. The gene Sry normally located on the Y chromosome encodes a protein that initiates testis differentiation. In individuals lacking Sry , ovarian differentiation occurs.

Disorders Characterized by Disagreement of Chromosomal Sex and Gonadal Sex

• XX sex reversal: XX true hermaphrodite—ovaries and testes; phenotypic female or partially masculinized female phenotype; varies from normal to abnormal vulva and normal-sized to large clitoris, uterus, oviducts, epididymis, and vas deferens; rarely fertile • XX males—testes, usually cryptorchid; epididymis, vas deferens, prostate, and uterus; hypoplastic penis and prepuce; dogs only • Determination of phenotypic sex (differentiation of the tubular reproductive tract and external genitalia) depends on gonadal sex. The basic embryonic plan is female; only if testes are present and capable of secreting müllerian inhibiting substance and testosterone is the development of the male phenotype possible. Abnormalities of phenotypic sex (chromosomal and gonadal sex agree, but internal or external genitalia are ambiguous) include female pseudohermaphrodite—XX; ovaries; masculinized genitalia ranging from

mild clitoral enlargement to nearly normal male genitalia; caused by sex steroid administration during pregnancy; dogs only • Male pseudohermaphrodite—XY; testes; internal or external genitalia female to some degree • Persistent müllerian duct syndrome (PMDS)—all wolffian and müllerian duct derivatives present; usually normal penis, prepuce, and scrotum; dogs and cats • Hypospadias—abnormal location of urinary orifice (varies from glans penis to perineum); external genitalia unambiguous; dogs • Testicular feminization—XY; testes (often abdominal); no wolffian or müllerian duct derivatives; vulva externally; cats

Systems Affected

• Reproductive—anomalies of the gonads, tubular tract, and external genitalia • Renal/urologic—occasionally affected (e.g., incontinence, hematuria, and cystitis)

Genetics

• Abnormalities of chromosomal sex usually are caused by random events during gamete formation or early embryonic development. • Abnormalities of gonadal sex—XX sex-reversal in the American cocker spaniel is inherited as an autosomal recessive trait. Similar familial disorders reported in the German shorthaired pointer, English cocker spaniel, beagle, Chinese pug, Kerry blue terrier, and weimaraner, but breeding trials are necessary to confirm the mode of inheritance. • Abnormalities of phenotypic sex—PMDS in the miniature schnauzer is inherited as an autosomal recessive trait with expression limited to XY individuals. Hypospadias is considered inherited in the Boston terrier. Testicular feminization, reported only in cats, is probably X-linked.

Incidence/Prevalence

In the general dog and cat populations, these abnormalities are rare. However, in affected breeds, the inherited abnormality can be common within families or even within the breed as a whole.

Geographic Distribution N/A

SIGNALMENT

Species Dogs and cats

Breed Predilections

American cocker spaniel, English cocker spaniel, beagle, German shorthaired pointer, weimaraner, Chinese pug, Kerry blue terrier, basset hound, miniature schnauzer, and Boston terrier

Mean Age and Range

Because all of these disorders are congenital, defects are present at birth; however, individuals with normal external genitalia may not be identified until reaching breeding age or at routine gonadectomy.

Predominant Sex

Disorders are seen in both phenotypic females and males.

SIGNS

General Comments

Historical and physical examination findings vary greatly depending on the type of disorder of sexual differentiation. The following lists include possible clinical findings in animals with any of the disorders; not all are seen with one specific disorder.

Historical Findings

• Failure to cycle • Infertility and sterility (male or female) • Vulva or prepuce and penis of abnormal size, shape, or location • Abnormal location of urine stream • Males attracted to other males • Urinary incontinence • Vulvar discharge

Physical Examination Findings

• Vulva normal or hypoplastic • Clitoris large, os clitoris • Perivulvar dermatitis and vulvar discharge • Testes scrotal, unilateral, or bilateral cryptorchid • Penis and prepuce normal or hypoplastic • Urethral meatus normal or abnormal location • Dermatologic signs of hyperestrogenism in males • Abdominal mass

CAUSES

• Congenital (heritable or nonheritable) • Exogenous steroid hormone administration during gestation

RISK FACTORS

Androgen or progestogen administration during pregnancy (female pseudohermaphrodite)

 DIAGNOSIS

DIFFERENTIAL DIAGNOSIS

Individuals with Unambiguous Genitalia

• Infertility (female)—rule out male infertility, mistimed breeding, subclinical cystic endometrial hyperplasia, and hypothyroidism • Failure to cycle (female)—rule out silent heat, hypothyroidism, hypercortisolism, and previous gonadectomy • Infertility (male)—rule out female infertility, mistimed breeding, exogenous drug use affecting fertility, orchitis or epididymitis, testicular degeneration or hypoplasia, and prostatitis

CBC/BIOCHEMISTRY/URINALYSIS

• Results usually normal • Results of urinalysis reveal evidence of cystitis in some animals with anatomic abnormalities that affect the location of the urethral meatus.

OTHER LABORATORY TESTS

• In general, concentrations of sex steroid hormones (e.g., progesterone, testosterone, and estradiol) are below the normal range; however, with some of the mild disorders (individuals not sterile), concentrations are normal. • Karyotyping is required to define chromosomal sex.

IMAGING

• Routine radiography and ultrasonography may be of diagnostic value in phenotypic females or males in which an abdominal mass (e.g., testicular neoplasia) is suspected, or in phenotypic males with signs referable to pyometra (uterus present with female pseudohermaphrodite or PMDS) • Contrast studies of the lower urogenital tract can be useful in diagnosing female pseudohermaphrodites.

OTHER DIAGNOSTIC PROCEDURES
N/A

GROSS AND HISTOPATHOLOGIC FINDINGS

In all patients, a precise description of the external genitalia is needed with particular attention given to the size and location of the vulva or prepuce, presence of the clitoris or penis, and position of the urinary orifice. In most patients (in which abnormalities of chromosomal sex are not identified), exploratory laparotomy is required to determine the location and morphology of the gonads and internal genitalia. Histopathologic examination of all tissues removed is paramount to defining the type of disorder. Gonads vary from a nearly normal architecture to dysgenetic or a combination of ovotestis. It is also essential to describe the components of the müllerian and/or wolffian duct system, if present.

TREATMENT

INPATIENT VERSUS OUTPATIENT
Except for individuals requiring exploratory laparotomy, outpatient status is sufficient.

ACTIVITY N/A

DIET N/A

CLIENT EDUCATION
Owners should be advised to remove affected or carrier individuals from the breeding program if disorders with a known or suspected heritable basis are documented.

SURGICAL CONSIDERATIONS
Gonadectomy and hysterectomy (if a uterus is present) recommended

MEDICATIONS

DRUGS AND FLUIDS N/A

CONTRAINDICATIONS
Avoid androgen or progestogen use during pregnancy.

PRECAUTIONS N/A

POSSIBLE INTERACTIONS N/A

ALTERNATE DRUGS N/A

FOLLOW-UP

PATIENT MONITORING N/A

PREVENTION/AVOIDANCE
Sterilization and removal of carrier animals with heritable disorders from the breeding program

POSSIBLE COMPLICATIONS
Infertility, sterility, urinary tract problems (e.g., incontinence and cystitis), testicular neoplasia, and pyometra

EXPECTED COURSE AND PROGNOSIS N/A

MISCELLANEOUS

ASSOCIATED CONDITIONS N/A

AGE RELATED FACTORS
In individuals not diagnosed at an early age, pyometra (e.g., animal with PMDS and female pseudohermaphrodite) or testicular neoplasia (e.g., animals with PMDS, Tfm, and XX sex-reversal)

ZOONOTIC POTENTIAL N/A

PREGNANCY N/A

SYNONYMS
• Hermaphrodites • Pseudohermaphrodites • Intersexes • Klinefelter's syndrome • Turner's syndrome

SEE ALSO
Cryptorchidism

ABBREVIATION
PMDS = persistent müllerian duct syndrome

References

Meyers-Wallen VN. Genetics of sexual differentiation and anomalies in dogs and cats. J Reprod Fert Suppl 1993;47:441-452.

Meyers-Wallen VN, Patterson DF. Disorders of sexual development in dogs and cats. In: Current veterinary therapy X. Philadelphia: WB Saunders, 1989:1261-1269.

Meyers-Wallen VN, Patterson DF. Disorders of sexual development in the dog. In: Current therapy in theriogenology. 2nd ed. Philadelphia: WB Saunders, 1986:567-574.

Authors Sara K. Lyle and Vickie N. Meyers-Wallen

Consulting Editor Sara K. Lyle

SHAKER DOG (WHITE SHAKER SYNDROME)

BASICS

OVERVIEW
Whole body tremor

SIGNALMENT
• Most often seen in young to middle-aged dogs with white hair coats (eg, Maltese and West Highland white terrier), but can be seen in dogs with a variety of coat colors • Both sexes affected

SIGNS
• Diffuse body tremoring • Initially, clinical signs can be confused with signs of apprehension or hypothermia.

CAUSES AND RISK FACTORS
Most often associated with mild inflammatory CNS disease

DIAGNOSIS

DIFFERENTIAL DIAGNOSIS
Rule out other causes of weakness, apprehension, hypothermia, and seizure.

CBC/BIOCHEMISTRY/URINALYSIS
Results usually normal

OTHER LABORATORY TESTS N/A

IMAGING N/A

OTHER DIAGNOSTIC PROCEDURES
CSF analysis—mild (< 20 WBC x 10 /L) monocytic or lymphocytic pleocytosis with normal protein content in most patients; can be normal

TREATMENT
As inpatient or outpatient

MEDICATIONS

DRUGS AND FLUIDS
• Corticosteroids given to reduce the inflammatory response; most patients have clinical improvement in 3-7 days
• Give prednisolone or prednisone (1-2 mg/kg divided q12h) for the first 1-2 weeks.
• Depending on clinical response, the steroid dosage can be tapered slowly. Assess patient periodically for clinical deterioration. If corticosteroid dosage is reduced too rapidly, clinical signs may recur, necessitating reinduction of the initial dosage. Most often, a taper over 4-6 months is appropriate. Many do not require further treatment.
• In some dogs, recurrence necessitates reinstitution of corticosteroids.

• A small percentage of dogs require every other day, low-dose corticosteroids indefinitely to maintain remission.

CONTRAINDICATIONS/POSSIBLE INTERACTIONS
Corticosteroids may be contraindicated if the patient has infectious encephalitis.

FOLLOW-UP
Weekly evaluations for approximately 1 month, then monthly until corticosteroids are discontinued

MISCELLANEOUS

SYNONYMS
• Shaker syndrome • Idiopathic cerebellitis

Reference
Bagley RS, Kornegay JN, Wheeler SJ, Plummer SB, Cauzinille L. Generalized tremors in Maltese: Clinical findings in seven cases. J Am Anim Hosp Assoc 1993,29:141-145.
Author Rodney S. Bagley
Consulting Editor Joane M. Parent

BASICS

OVERVIEW
• A systemic autoimmune disease characterized by keratoconjunctivitis sicca, xerostomia, and lymphoplasmacytic adenitis • Underlying mechanism unknown; however, autoantibodies directed against glandular tissues have been identified • Often occurs with other autoimmune or immune-mediated diseases such as rheumatoid arthritis and pemphigus

SIGNALMENT
• Higher incidence in several canine breeds—English bulldog, West Highland white terrier, and miniature schnauzer • Chronic disease of adult dogs • None in cats

SIGNS

Historical Findings
• Adult onset • Conjunctivitis and keratitis
• Keratitis sicca most prominent clinical feature

Physical Examination Findings
• Blepharospasm • Conjunctival hyperemia
• Corneal lesions (opacity to ulceration)
• Gingivitis • Stomatitis

CAUSES AND RISK FACTORS
• Possible genetic predisposition in breeds with increased incidence • Occurs concurrent with other immune-mediated and autoimmune diseases

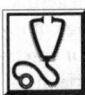

DIAGNOSIS

DIFFERENTIAL DIAGNOSIS
• Other causes of keratoconjunctivitis sicca, such as canine distemper, trauma, and drug toxicities • Keratoconjunctivitis sicca associated with other immune-mediated diseases, such as atopy, lymphocytic thyroiditis, polymyositis, systemic lupus erythematosus, rheumatoid arthritis, and pemphigoid diseases

CBC/BIOCHEMISTRY/URINALYSIS
Normal findings

OTHER LABORATORY TESTS
• Hypergammaglobulinemia noted on serum protein electrophoresis • Positive antinuclear antibody test • Positive lupus erythematosus cell test • Positive rheumatoid factor test
• Positive indirect fluorescent antibody test for autoantibodies

IMAGING N/A

OTHER DIAGNOSTIC PROCEDURES
Schirmer tear test (0-5 mm/min)

GROSS AND HISTOPATHOLOGIC FINDINGS
Histopathologic changes of salivary gland include lymphoplasmacytic adenitis; conjunctival biopsies reveal conjunctivitis.

TREATMENT
• Treatment approach directed at controlling keratoconjunctivitis sicca
• Any concurrent diseases must be medically managed; medical therapy may include anti-inflammatory or immunosuppressive drugs.
• Surgical management of keratoconjunctivitis sicca indicated in animals that fail to respond to medical treatment

MEDICATIONS

DRUGS AND FLUIDS
Topical tear preparations
• Appropriate topical antibiotic therapy for secondary bacterial infections

• Immunosuppressive or anti-inflammatory therapy
• For more aggressive medical therapy and surgical intervention, see Keratoconjunctivitis sicca (KCS).

CONTRAINDICATIONS/POSSIBLE INTERACTIONS
Use of topical steroids in acute keratoconjunctivitis sicca may result in corneal ulceration and is therefore not recommended.

FOLLOW-UP
• Reexamine patient weekly until keratoconjunctivitis sicca is controlled. Additional follow-up may be indicated to manage underlying or concurrent disease. • Monitor patients who are on immunosuppressive therapy every other week for possible side effects. • Prognosis is variable and dependent on the presence or absence of concurrent disease.

MISCELLANEOUS

SEE ALSO
Keratoconjunctivitis Sicca (KCS)

Reference
Quimby FW, Schwartz RS, Poskitt T, et al. A disorder of dogs resembling Sjögren's syndrome. Clin Immunol Immunopathol 1979;12:471-476.
Author Paul W. Snyder
Consulting Editor Alan H. Rebar

SMALL INTESTINAL BACTERIAL OVERGROWTH

BASICS

DEFINITION
A condition of the canine duodenum or jejunum in which there are drastically increased numbers of bacteria present in the fasting state. Any bacterial species may be present, and there are usually multiple species found. At least in some dogs, it seems that the species present may change with time. Intestinal bacterial overgrowth (IBO) is currently defined by finding (10^4 anaerobic and/or (10^5 total bacterial CFUs/ml of lasting intestinal fluid. There may be a difference between IBO (having too many bacteria) and the disease syndrome of IBO (having too many bacteria plus having clinical signs of small intestinal disease). IBO is different than colonization of the alimentary tract by a known pathogenic bacteria with virulence factors (e.g., Salmonella sp, Campylobacter jejuni) or overgrowth of toxigenic Clostridium perfringens in the colon.

Pathophysiology
Bacteria are constantly ingested with food and/or saliva and most are destroyed by the stomach's low pH and/or by anti-bacterial factors in the small intestine (e.g., pancreatic enzymes). Those bacteria which are not destroyed are eliminated from the small intestine by normal intestinal motility. When natural defenses are inadequate and excessive numbers of bacteria persist in the upper small intestine, they may cause pathologic changes even though they are not obligate pathogens. Deconjugation of bile acids, dehydroxylation of fatty acids, formation of alcohols, and destruction of brush border enzymes are a few of the proported pathologic mechanisms. Anaerobic bacteria (e.g., Bacteroides sp and Clostridium sp) are generally thought to be more likely to cause problems than some of the aerobic bacteria. In some cases, IBO may cause protein-losing enteropathy.

Systems Affected
• Gastrointestinal • Hepatobiliary—Portal vein carries substances (e.g., bacterial toxins) from the small intestines into the liver.

Genetics
A genetic basis has not been established. However, some breeds (e.g., German shepherds) appear to be at increased risk.

Incidence/Prevalence Unknown

Geographic Distribution N/A

SIGNALMENT
Species
• Dog • We do not know if IBO exists in cats and, if it does exist, how it compares to the syndrome in dogs is not known. Some clinically normal cats have been found to have (10^5 bacteria/ml in their small intestines.

Breed Predilections
Subjectively, German shepherds and shar peis appear to have a higher than expected incidence of IBO.

Mean Age and Range
IBO has been identified in dogs < 1 year of age and > 8 years of age.

Predominant Sex None

SIGNS
General Comments
When IBO causes disease, it causes signs of small intestinal dysfunction which may wax and wane

Historical Findings
• The principal sign of disease is weight loss, which may occur in spite of a reasonable appetite. • Small intestinal diarrhea (e.g., no mucus or blood in the feces, no tenesmus) is common but not invariable. • Vomiting and borborygmus may occur.

Physical Examination Findings
• Poor physical condition is the principal sign • Diarrhea • Intestinal thickening is not expected, unless there are other, concurrent intestinal diseases. • Other typical signs of infection (e.g., fever, depression) are not expected.

CAUSES
Most cases are idiopathic. The following are known causes, but are not responsible for the majority of cases diagnosed in dogs.
• Altered small intestinal anatomy (i.e., blind or stagnant loops, partial obstruction)
• Exocrine pancreatic insufficiency (EPI)
• Hypochlorhydria or achlorhydria (spontaneous or iatrogenic)

RISK FACTORS
Suspected risk factors include serum IgA deficiency and intestinal disease (e.g., IBD, dietary intolerance, parasites) which affects local defense mechanisms

DIAGNOSIS

DIFFERENTIAL DIAGNOSIS
• Maldigestion (EPI) • Malabsorption due to any cause (IBD, alimentary lymphosarcoma, dietary intolerance/allergy), whether protein-loosing or not, IBD especially may mimic and/or be associated with IBO. • Intestinal parasites (especially Giardia).

CBC/BIOCHEMISTRY/URINALYSIS
Usually normal although some animals will be hypoalbuminemic. Hypoalbuminemia suggests that the intestinal disease is severe and warrants an aggressive diagnostic and therapeutic approach.

OTHER LABORATORY TESTS
• Serum folate may be high and cobalamin concentrations may be low in dogs with IBO. However, while the specificity of these abnormalities for IBO appears to be high, the sensitivity of these tests for IBO is dubious. It is clear that some dogs with symptomatic IBO have normal serum folate and cobalamin concentrations. • Breath hydrogen analysis is seldom done outside of institutions. It appears to have some false negative and false positive results.

IMAGING
Finding an intestinal mass or particular obstruction may explain why IBO is present. These are not present in most dogs with IBO.

OTHER DIAGNOSTIC PROCEDURES
• Quantitated culture of aerobic and anaerobic bacteria from fasted, upper intestinal fluid is the ``gold standard'' for diagnosis of IBO. However, this test is difficult to perform outside of an institution and false negatives are believed to occur (i.e., one may culture fluid from an unaffected portion of an affected dog's small intestine). • Therapeutic trial for IBO. This is advantageous in that it is simple and inexpensive. The main drawback is difficulty in interpreting the results. A dog may have more than one disease present at the time of presentation (e.g., IBD plus IBO, dietary intolerance plus IBO) and failure of the patient to clinically respond to antibiotics may lead the clinician to wrongly believe that IBO is absent. It might also be possible to be using the wrong antibiotics in a particular patient.

GROSS AND HISTOPATHOLOGIC FINDINGS
• There are rarely any visible signs suggestive of IBO. • Histopathology and cytology of intestinal mucosa are very insensitive for detecting IBO (i.e., one does not see bacteria, neutrophils, or inflammatory infiltrates).

TREATMENT

INPATIENT VERSUS OUTPATIENT
Usually outpatient.

ACTIVITY N/A

DIET
A highly digestible diet which is restricted in fat is desired. Antigen-restricted diets are recommended if concurrent dietary intolerance/allergy is suspected.

CLIENT EDUCATION
Although the patient may respond in days (i.e., the diarrhea may stop), one must be prepared to treat IBO for at least 3-4 weeks before saying that the therapy is ineffective.
• There may be concurrent diseases present (e.g., IBD, EPI, dietary intolerance/allergy, alimentary tract neoplasia, cardial obstruction) which must also be treated.

SURGICAL CONSIDERATIONS
Surgery is only indicated if there is a partial obstruction, a diverticuli, or an intestinal mass. This is rarely the case in dogs with IBO.

SMALL INTESTINAL BACTERIAL OVERGROWTH

MEDICATIONS

DRUGS AND FLUIDS

• Broad-spectrum, orally administered antibiotics that kill aerobic and anaerobic bacteria are preferred. Since the species of bacteria present in the intestine can apparently change with time in at least some affected animals, a culture and sensitivity are not necessarily useful unless the patient has failed to respond to previous, appropriate therapy.

• Tetracycline (22 mg/kg PO q12h) or tylosin (10-40 mg/kg/day divided q12h) are good initial choices. If tetracycline is used, do not administer it with food lest calcium in the diet chelate the tetracycline and render it ineffective. The preparation of tylosin used is usually a powder designed to be used in poultry or pigs. This powder is usually administered in the food. Because tylosin is so safe, even for long-term use, one may approximate the dose by giving 1/4 tsp q12h to dogs (> 15 kg, 1/8th tsp to dogs from 7–15 kg, and 1/16th tsp to dogs < 7 kg. • Drugs which do not kill anaerobic bacteria (e.g., neomycin) are much less effective in most cases.

• Metronidazole has been used to treat IBO because of its activity against anaerobic bacteria. However, metronidazole is also effective in some dogs with IBD because of it's effect on the immune system. Therefore, successful therapy with this drug may reflect underlying IBD or IBO or both. Furthermore, metronidazole has not seemed as effective as tetracycline in some cases.

• In dogs with EPI plus IBO, appropriate supplementation of pancreatic enzymes with a low fat diet is usually sufficient. However, if enzyme replacement and a low fat diet does not resolve the diarrhea and/or weight loss, then concurrent antibiotic therapy for IBO may be needed.

CONTRAINDICATIONS None

PRECAUTIONS

Tetracycline must be used carefully in dogs with significant hepatic disease as it may make the hepatic disease worse in rare individuals.

POSSIBLE INTERACTIONS N/A

ALTERNATE DRUGS

A variety of other antibiotics may be tried. Amoxicilin (22 mg/kg PO q12h) or chloramphenicol (25 mg/kg PO q8h) are often acceptable. However, the public health concerns of chloramphenicol (i.e., fatal, aplastic anemia in people) must be explained to the clients.

FOLLOW-UP

PATIENT MONITORING

Body weight and, in hypoproteinemic patients, the serum albumin concentration are the most important parameters to monitor. If they are improving, then the clinician is doing the right thing for the patient. Optimally, the diarrhea should also resolve. However, if the diarrhea persists despite an improved body weight and/or increased serum albumin concentration (that is not due to dehydration), then one should look for other, concurrent intestinal diseases.

PREVENTION/AVOIDANCE N/A

POSSIBLE COMPLICATIONS

While unproven, IBO may predispose to or cause IBD in some dogs.

EXPECTED COURSE AND PROGNOSIS

The best results occur if the animal is untreated before severe secondary intestinal disease (see below) occurs.

MISCELLANEOUS

ASSOCIATED CONDITIONS

• It is uncertain whether IBO can cause IBD or if IBD can predispose the animal to IBO. However, there is at least one case reported in which therapy for IBO seemed to alleviate the IBD. The implication is that IBO might be responsible for causing IBD in some patients.

• Consider the possibility of concurrent EPI, especially in German shepherd dogs.

AGE RELATED FACTORS N/A

ZOONOTIC POTENTIAL N/A

PREGNANCY

Avoid use of tetracyclines during pregnancy

SYNONYMS None

SEE ALSO

• Inflammatory Bowel Disease • Exocrine Pancreatic Insufficiency • Lymphosarcoma • Giardia

ABBREVIATIONS

CFU = colony forming units
EPI = exocrine pancreatic insufficiency
IBD = inflammatory bowel disease
IBO = intestinal (small) bacterial overgrowth

References

Leib MS. Stagnant loop syndrome in the dog and cat. Sem Vet Med Surg 1987;2(4): 257–265.

Rutgers HC, Batt RM, Kelly DF. Lymphocytic-plasmacytic enteritis associated with bacterial overgrowth in a dog. J Am Vet Med Assoc 1988;192(12):1739–1742.

Willard MD, Simpson RB, Fossum TW, et al. Characterization of naturally developing small intestinal bacterial overgrowth in 16 German shepherd dogs. J Am Vet Med Assoc 1994;204(8):1201–1206.

Williams DA, Batt RM, McLean L. Bacterial overgrowth in the duodenum of dogs with exocrine pancreatic insufficiency. J Am Vet Med Assoc 1987;191(2):201–206.

Author Michael D. Willard
Consulting Editor Brent D. Jones

SMOKE INHALATION

 BASICS

OVERVIEW

• Smoke inhalation injury occurs by three major processes: 1) direct heat damage to the upper airway and nasal mucosa, 2) inhaled carbon monoxide, which decreases tissue oxygen delivery by preferentially binding to hemoglobin, and other inhaled toxins (oxidants, aldehydes), which directly irritate the airway, and 3) inhaled particulate matter that adheres to the airways and alveoli. • In individual patients, the extent of damage varies depending on the exposure and the material that was burning. Severe lung injury can occur in dogs and cats with little cutaneous or oral evidence of burning. Initial reactions in the lung include bronchoconstriction, airway edema, and mucous production, followed by an inflammatory response and fluid accumulation as a result of high capillary permeability. Superimposed bacterial infections are a common cause of morbidity late in the disease. Thus, most animals show progression of lung dysfunction in the initial 2-3 days after exposure to smoke.

SIGNALMENT N/A

SIGNS

• Historical findings are consistent with exposure to smoke. • The animal may have a smoky odor. • Tachypnea and increased depth of respiration • Inspiratory effort suggestive of upper airway obstruction by edema • Postural adaptations to respiratory distress • Mucous membranes may be cherry red from carbon monoxyhemoglobin or they may be pale or cyanotic. • Auscultation of wheezes, harsh bronchovesicular sounds, or crackles • Cough

CAUSES AND RISK FACTORS

Exposure to smoke, usually trapped in burning buildings

 DIAGNOSIS

DIFFERENTIAL DIAGNOSIS N/A

CBC/BIOCHEMISTRY/URINALYSIS

• Complete blood count may reveal neutrophilia. The presence of neutropenia is a poor prognostic sign, indicating neutrophil sequestration in the lung. • Serum chemistry profile may reveal hypoxic damage to other organ systems such as the kidney or liver. • Urinalysis usually is normal.

OTHER LABORATORY TESTS N/A

IMAGING

Thoracic radiographs should always be performed to establish a baseline of expectation that pulmonary function will deteriorate. Findings vary from normality to a bronchointerstitial or alveolar pattern. Cranioventral alveolar infiltrates suggest aspiration pneumonia.

OTHER DIAGNOSTIC PROCEDURES

• Transtracheal wash should be performed for cytologic examination and culture if there is a suspicion of superimposed bacterial tracheobronchitis or pneumonia. Cytologic examination usually reveals excessive mucous, neutrophils, and alveolar macrophages with an acute suppurative reaction. Bacteria may be seen, but the absence of obvious bacteria does not rule out the presence of bacterial infection. • Pulse oximetry or arterial blood gas analysis may confirm the presence of hypoxemia, but will be of less value in the presence of carbon monoxyhemoglobin.

 TREATMENT

Initial management involves stabilization of respiratory function and establishment of a patent airway. Animals with severe upper airway edema or obstruction may require intubation or tracheostomy. Supportive care should be provided through the acute phase, with careful monitoring to detect complications.

MEDICATIONS

DRUGS AND FLUIDS

• Oxygen should be administered immediately after rescue from the fire in order to displace carbon monoxide from hemoglobin. Oxygen should be administered at the highest available concentration, for at least an hour, by mask, hood, cage, or nasal line.
• In the shock patient, fluid therapy may be required to support cardiovascular function. To minimize pulmonary edema, fluid therapy should be conservative if possible, and synthetic colloids should be used if hypoproteinemia is present. Patients with extensive dermal burns usually have considerable losses of fluid and protein from the skin surface and therefore may have high fluid requirements.
• Blood or plasma transfusions should be considered if necessary.
• Broad-spectrum antibiotics should be considered after appropriate bacterial cultures have been performed, if bacterial infection is suspected.
• Diuretics such as furosemide (0.5-2 mg/kg IV or IM) can be administered if edema is severe, although they are usually of little benefit.
• A single early dose of corticosteroids may help to decrease airway edema in patients with severe edema.

CONTRAINDICATIONS/POSSIBLE INTERACTIONS

• Diuretics may cause diuresis and decrease the intravascular volume without a major beneficial effect on airway or pulmonary edema.
• Corticosteroids should only be used if absolutely necessary, because they may predispose the patient to bacterial infection.

FOLLOW-UP

PATIENT MONITORING

Should include observation of respiratory rate and effort, mucous membrane color, heart rate and pulse quality, auscultation, measurement of packed cell volume and total solids, and other parameters for 24-72 hours. Radiographs should be repeated in 48 hours to ensure that the condition is resolving and to monitor for bacterial pneumonia.

PREVENTION AND AVOIDANCE N/A

POSSIBLE COMPLICATIONS

Development of bacterial tracheobronchitis or pneumonia as a result of systemic immunosuppression and reduced pulmonary defenses, including poor mucociliary clearance. Development of a moist productive cough, fever, and failure to improve within 48 hours should provoke suspicion of pneumonia. Animals with severe systemic inflammatory response syndrome may develop adult respiratory distress syndrome (ARDS).

EXPECTED COURSES AND PROGNOSIS

Most animals with smoke inhalation deteriorate during the initial 24-48 hours after trauma and then gradually improve, unless they develop bacterial pneumonia or ARDS. The presence of severe burns or organ injury is associated with a poor prognosis.

MISCELLANEOUS

ABBREVIATIONS

ARDS = adult respiratory distress syndrome

Reference

Saxon WD, Kirby R. Treatment of acute burn injury and smoke inhalation. In: Kirk RW, Bonagura JD, eds. Current veterinary therapy XI, small animal practice. Philadelphia: WB Saunders, 1992:146-154.

Author Lesley G. King
Consulting Editors Lynelle Johnson and Bradley L. Moses

...KE VENOM TOXICITY

CORAL SNAKES

BASICS

OVERVIEW
Two clinically important coral snakes of North America:
Micrurus fulvius fulvius—Eastern coral snake; range: North Carolina to the north, southern Flordia to south and the Mississippi River to the west
Miicrurus fulvius tenere—Texas coral snake; range: west of Mississippi in Arkansas, Louisiana, and Texas
Coral snakes belong to the family Elapidae, having fixed front fangs.
The color pattern consists of bands fully encircling the body of red, yellow, and black. Coral snakes can be distinguished from the harmless tricolored kingsnakes by the arrangement of these colored bands. If yellow (caution) and red (danger) color bands touch, then stay clear.
Coral Snakes have a relatively small head with a black snout and round pupils.
Bites are relatively uncommon due to the snakes reclusive behavior and nocturnal habits.
Bites often occur on the lip.
Onset of clinical signs maybe delayed several hours (up to 18 hours) after envenomation. Victims develop bulbar paralysis, with respiratory collapse as the primary cause of death.

SIGNALMENT Dogs and cats

SIGNS
• Bulbar paralysis affecting cranial motor nerves, respiratory tract, and skeletal muscles causing an acute flaccid quadraplegia.
• Salivation caused by dysphagia • Dyspnea
• Dysphonia • Hyporeflexive spinal reflexes

CAUSES AND RISK FACTORS
Size of the snake

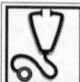

DIAGNOSIS

DIFFERENTIAL DIAGNOSIS
• Myesthenia Gravis • Botulism • Polyradiculoneuritis • Tick bite paralysis

CBC/BIOCHEMISTRY/URINALYSIS
• Hemolysis • RBC burring • High CPK in some animals • Hemoglobinuria

OTHER LABORATORY TESTS N/A

IMAGING N/A

OTHER DIAGNOSTIC PROCEDURES N/A

TREATMENT
• Hospitalize for a minimum of 48 hours.
• Specific antivenin is available (Antivenin [Micrurus fulvius], equine origin, Wyeth) with cross reactivity for both Eastern and Texas Coral snakes. • First aid measures should be avoided generally. The most effective first aid is rapid transport to a veterinary facility for antivenin administration. DO NOT WAIT FOR ONSET OF CLINICAL SIGNS! • If antivenin is not available, provide ventilatory support for several days in a critical care facility .

MEDICATIONS

DRUGS AND FLUIDS
• Antivenin administration is indicated if the history includes recent coral snake interaction and the animal has puncture wounds, or if the clinical signs are consistent with coral snake envenomation. • Administer 1-2 vials of specific antivenin (Micrurus fulvius, Wyeth). Additional vials may be necessary.

(Administration technique same as for pit viper antivenin). • The same precautions as for pit viper antivenin administration should be observed (see pit viper antivenin reactions).
• Broad-spectrum antibiotic for 7-10 days

CONTRAINDICATIONS/POSSIBLE INTERACTIONS
Corticosteriods not indicated

FOLLOW-UP
Clinical signs can last up to 1-1 1/2 weeks.

MISCELLANEOUS

ABBREVIATIONS
CPK = creatine phosphokinase
RBC = red blood cells

References
Peterson M, Meerdink G. Venomous bites and stings. Kirk, ed. Current veterinary therapy X. Philadelphia: WB Saunders, 1989.
Author Michael E. Peterson
Consulting Editor Gary Osweiler

SNAKE VENOM TOXICITY

PIT VIPERS
• Crotalus sp.—rattlesnakes • Sistrurus sp.—pigmy rattlesnakes and massassauga • Agkistrodon sp.—copperheads and cotton mouth water moccasins

BASICS

OVERVIEW
Pit vipers have retractable fangs, a heat seeking "pit" between the nostril and eye, and a triangular-shaped head. They are found throughout the continental United States. They have been considered hematoxic, but several species have subpopulations with lethal neurotoxic components (e.g., the Mojave rattlesnake). Eighty-five per cent of animals bitten by a pit viper have altered laboratory values and clinically important swelling. The venom consists of enzymes and nonenzymatic polypeptides. The enzymes include hyaluronidase and phospholipase A, which cause local tissue injury. Other enzymes interfere with the coagulation cascade, causing major coagulation defects. The nonenzymatic polypeptides affect the cardiovascular and respiratory systems. Severe hypotension results from pooling of blood within the splanchnic (dogs) or pulmonary (cats) vessels and fluid loss from the vascular compartment secondary to severe pereipheral edema.

Generally severity of venom toxicity is ranked 1. rattlesnake. 2. moccasin, and 3. copperhead.

SIGNALMENT Dogs and cats

SIGNS

Historical Findings
• Outdoors, rural setting • Owner saw bite or heard snake.

Physical Examination Findings
• Clinical signs may be delayed for 8 hours after envenomation. • Puncture wounds • Local tissue swelling • Pain surrounding bite site • Ecchymosis/petechiation of tissues and mucus membranes • Shock, hypotension, tachycardia, and shallow respiration • Bruising, with possible necrosis and sloughing of bite site tissue • Depression and lethargy • Nausea and excessive salivation • Location of bites—head and forelimbs in most animals

CAUSES AND RISK FACTORS

Snake Associated Risks
• Toxic peptide fraction in relation to the enzyme fraction—comparatively high in spring and low in fall • Venom production since last bite • Age—very young snakes have high peptide fractions • Aggressiveness and motivation of the snake

Victim Associated Risks
• Site of the bite • Size of the victim • Elapsed time between bite and initiation of treatment • Activity level of victim after the bite (activity increases absorption of venom.)

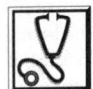

DIAGNOSIS

DIFFERENTIAL DIAGNOSIS
• Angioedema secondary to insect envenomation • Blunt trauma • Penetrating wound, animal bite, or penetration of foreign body • Draining abscess

CBC/BIOCHEMISTRY/URINALYSIS
• Hemoconcentration • Burring of RBC within first 24 hours • Thrombocytopenia • WBC normal • Hypokalemia • High CPK • Hematuria or myoglobinuria

OTHER LABORATORY TESTS
• ACT, PT, and PTT prolonged in some animals • FDP high in some animals

IMAGING N/A

OTHER DIAGNOSTIC PROCEDURES
ECG may detect ventricular arrhythmia, especially in severely depressed patients.

TREATMENT
• Tissue reaction around the bite site is not a reliable indicator of systemic toxicity. • Bite location may affect uptake of venom; bites to tongue and torso are of major concern.
• First aid measures should be limited to calming the patient and transporting quickly to a veterinary facility.

MEDICATIONS

DRUGS AND FLUIDS
• Crystalloid fluids IV • Antivenin (Antivenin [Crotalidae] Polyvalent, equine origin, Ft. Dodge or Wyeth) • Antivenin (1 vial) mixed with 200 ml crystalloid. Administer slowly IV with careful monitoring of the inner pinna for onset of hyperemia (indicator of possible allergic reaction). If allergic reaction occurs, antivenin should be stopped and diphenhydramine given. After 5 minutes, antivenin infusion is restarted at a slower rate.

CONTRAINDICATIONS/POSSIBLE INTERACTIONS
• Corticosteriods are of no value. • Dimethyl sulfoxide (DMSO) enhances the uptake and spread of the venom. • Heparin should not be used.

FOLLOW-UP
• Repeat laboratory analysis 6 hours after admission to the hospital. • Clinical signs can last up to 1 to 1 1/2 weeks.

MISCELLANEOUS

ABBREVIATIONS
ACT = activated clotting time
CPK = creatine phosphokinase
ECG = electrocardiogram
FDP = fibrin degradation products
PT = prothombin time
PTT = partial thromboplastin time
RBC = red blood cells
WBC = white blood cells

References
Peterson M, Meerdink G. Venomous bites and stings. Kirk, ed. Current veterinary therapy X. 1989.

Author Michael E. Peterson
Consulting Editor Gary Osweiler

SPERMATOCELE/SPERM GRANULOMA

 BASICS

OVERVIEW

• Spermatocele—a cystic distension of the efferent ductules or epididymis containing spermatozoa, usually associated with loss of patency of the duct. • Sperm granuloma—the granulomatous inflammatory reaction that develops when spermatozoa escape from the efferent ductules or epididymal duct into the surrounding tissue. Clinically important when bilateral obstruction of the duct system leads to azoospermia.

SIGNALMENT N/A

SIGNS

• Suspected whenever an azoospermic dog has normal-sized testicles • Rarely associated with pain or visible or palpable lesions

CAUSES AND RISK FACTORS

Trauma causing a break in the epididymal duct releases sperm antigens into the surrounding tissue. • Adenomyosis, the invasion of the epithelial lining cells of the epididymis into the muscular layers, may be a factor and is associated with excess estrogenic stimulation. • Epithelial hyperplasia of the epididymis may be a precursor of adenomyosis. Hyperplasia is not often seen in dogs < 2.5 years old, but some degree is seen in 75% of dogs > 7.75 years old. Risk increases with age.

 DIAGNOSIS

DIFFERENTIAL DIAGNOSIS

• In dogs with azoospermia—testicular degeneration, hypoplasia, and retrograde ejaculation • In dogs with scrotal signs (e.g., pain and palpable lesions)—epididymitis, orchitis, and scrotal dermatitis

CBC/BIOCHEMISTRY/URINALYSIS

Urinalysis (cystocentesis) after ejaculation to rule out retrograde ejaculation

OTHER LABORATORY TESTS

Assay for canine follicle stimulating hormone (FSH). High concentration is associated with degeneration and hypoplasia. Normal concentration in azoospermic dogs with normal-sized testicles is associated with bilateral blockage of the epididymis or retrograde ejaculation.

IMAGING N/A

OTHER DIAGNOSTIC PROCEDURES

• If testicular biopsy by surgical means is attempted, the epididymis can be seen. Spermatoceles appear as yellow cysts within the epididymis. • Histologic examination of testicular specimen demonstrating complete spermatogenesis in an azoospermic dog indicates blockage.

 TREATMENT

• Azoospermic dogs rarely recover spontaneously.
• Bilateral blockage of the epididymis is probably not treatable except by microsurgical anastomosis of the ductus deferens to the cystic structure or patent segment of the epididymis. Few attempts have been made to perform this procedure in dogs.

MEDICATIONS

No medication is recognized as effective in unblocking the duct system.

DRUGS AND FLUIDS N/A

CONTRAINDICATIONS/POSSIBLE INTERACTIONS N/A

 FOLLOW-UP N/A

 MISCELLANEOUS

Reference

Althouse GC, Evans LE, Hopkins SM. Episodic scrotal mutilation with concurrent bilateral sperm granuloma in a dog. J Am Vet Med Assoc 1993;202:776-778.

Author Rolf E. Larsen

Consulting Editor Sara K. Lyle

SPIDER VENOM TOXICITY

BLACK WIDOW SPIDER (LATRODECTISM SP.)

BASICS

OVERVIEW:
• Females are toxic. They are 2-2.5 cm in length, shiny black, with a red or orange hour-glass mark on the ventral abdomen. Immature females are brown with red to orange stripes that change into the hour-glass shape as the female darkens to black and ages. Some bites may be "dry " with no venom injected. Latrodectus species are found in every state in the United States except Alaska; often found around buildings and human habitation. • Venom contains alpha-latrotoxin, a potent neurotoxin. The toxin opens cation selective channels at the presynaptic nerve terminal, causing massive release of acetylcholine and norepinephrine, which causes sustained muscular spasms.

SIGNALMENT Dogs and cats

SIGNS

Historical Findings
• Sudden onset of clinical signs • Onset of signs may be delayed several days in animals with mild envenomation.

Physical Examination Findings
Dogs:
• Progressive muscle fasciculations • Severe pain, cramping of large muscle masses, and abdominal rigidity without tenderness
• Marked restlessness, writhing, and contorted spasms • Hypertension and tachycardia should be anticipated. • Bronchorrhea, hypersalivation, hyperesthesia, lymph node tenderness, regional numbness, and facial swelling ("Latrodectus facies") in some dogs
• Rhabdomyolysis is possible.
Cats:
• Early, marked paralytic signs • Severe

pain manifested by howling and loud vocalizations • Excessive salivation and restlessness • Vomiting (vomiting up the spider is not unusual) • Diarrhea • Muscle tremors, cramping, ataxia, and inability to stand, which becomes adynamic and atonic
• Respiratory collapse • Death without antivenin

CAUSES AND RISK FACTORS
• Very young or old age increases risk.
• Hypertensive heart disease increases risk.

DIAGNOSIS

DIFFERENTIAL DIAGNOSIS
• Back pain from disc disease • Acute abdomen

CBC/BIOCHEMISTRY/URINALYSIS
• Leukocytosis • Albuminuria • High CPK if patient has severe muscle spasms

OTHER LABORATORY TESTS
Result of stool hemoccult test normal

IMAGING
Abdominal radiographs normal

OTHER DIAGNOSTIC PROCEDURES
N/A

TREATMENT
• Admit to hospital for supportive care.
• Monitor respiratory status.

MEDICATIONS

DRUGS AND FLUIDS
• Antivenin (Lyovac [Latrodectus] antivenin, equine origin, Merck, Sharpe and Dohm); given slowly IV diluted in crystalloid solution 1 vial to 100 ml fluids. Monitor the inner ear

pinna for evidence of hyperemia as an indicator of allergic response to antivenin. Usually one vial is sufficient for response within 30 minutes. • If allergic reaction occurs, stop antivenin infusion, give diphenhydramine and restart infusion of antivenin at slower rate after a 5 to 10-minute wait. With proper use of the antivenin, reactions are rare.
• Envenomation in cats is usually fatal without antivenin. • Muscle spasms and severe pain may be controlled with careful IV administration of narcotics or benzodiazepines. Use lowest effective dosage to avoid respiratory depression. • Treat intractable hypertension with sodium nitroprusside. • Methocarbomol (Robaxin) relieves muscle spasms, but has no effect on hypertension or respiratory depression.

CONTRAINDICATIONS/POSSIBLE INTERACTIONS
Fluids administered IV when patient has hypertension

FOLLOW-UP
• Weekly monitoring of the wound site should be performed until healed.
• Prognosis uncertain for days • Weakness, fatigue, and insomnia may persist for months.

MISCELLANEOUS

ABBREVIATION
CPK = creatine phosphokinase

Reference
Peterson ME, Meerdink G. Venomous bites and stings. In: Kirk RW, ed. Current veterinary therapy X. Philadelphia: WB Saunders, 1989:177-186.
Author Michael E. Peterson
Consulting Editor Gary Osweiler

BROWN RECLUSE FAMILY
(LOXOSCELES SPECIES)

BASICS

OVERVIEW
Brown spiders are 8 to 15 mm in body size, with legs 2-3 cm long; violin-shaped pattern on cephalothorax with the neck of the fiddle extending caudally; found throughout the southern states of the United States and up the Mississippi river valley to southern Wisconsin. They are active at night, and bites are usually caused by the spider becoming trapped in bedding.

Induces necrotic arachnidism, an indolent dermatonecrotic lesion mediated by the venom enzyme sphingomyelinase D, direct hemolysis of erythrocytes, platelet aggregation, renal failure, coagulopathy, and death.

SIGNALMENT Dogs and cats

SIGNS
• Local pain and stinging which may last 6-8 hours, followed by pruritus and soreness
• The classic "target lesion" is an ischemic area with a dark central eschar on an uneven erythematous background. • At 2-5 weeks after the bite, the central eschar may slough, leaving a deep, non- healing ulcer that usually spares muscle tissue. • Less common are hemolytic anemia with hemoglobinuria in the first 24 hours. • Other possible systemic manifestations within the first 2 or 3 days after envenomation are fever, chills, rash, weakness, leukocytosis, nausea, and arthalgias.

CAUSES AND RISK FACTORS N/A

DIAGNOSIS

DIFFERENTIAL DIAGNOSIS
• Bacterial or mycobacterial infection, decubitus ulcer, and third-degree burn
• Hemolytic anemia, jaundice, thrombocytopenia, ehrlichiosis, and RBC parasitism

CBC/BIOCHEMISTRY/URINALYSIS
• Anemia, leukocytosis, and thrombocytopenia • Hemoglobinuria

OTHER LABORATORY TESTS
Coagulation profile may reveal prolonged clotting times.

IMAGING N/A

OTHER DIAGNOSTIC PROCEDURES
N/A

TREATMENT
• Mild, local envenomation usually responds to cool compresses. • Necrotic lesions may need debridement after erythema has subsided. • Severe envenomation may require skin grafting after the lesion has reached full maturity.

MEDICATIONS

DRUGS AND FLUIDS
• Dermatonecrotic lesions can be treated with Dapsone (1 mg/kg q8h for 10 days), a leukocyte inhibitor, to minimize the inflammatory component of the envenomation. Repeat if needed. (Note: dosage is for dogs; author has no experience with cats).
• Administer antibiotics to patients not being treated with dapsone. • Supportive care should include fluid therapy, presumptive treatment of bacterial superinfection, and rarely, blood transfusion.

CONTRAINDICATIONS
• Dapsone can cause hypersensitivity and methemoglobinemia in animals with G-6-PD deficiency. • Heat should not be used because it exacerbates the condition.

FOLLOW-UP
Weekly monitoring of the wound site until healed

MISCELLANEOUS

ABBREVIATION
RBC = red blood cells

Reference

Peterson ME, Meerdink G. Bites and stings of venomous animals. In: Kirk RW, ed. Current veterinary therapy X. Philadelphia: WB Saunders Co, 1989;177-186.
Author Michael E. Peterson
Consulting Editor Gary Osweiler

SPONDYLOSIS DEFORMANS

BASICS

OVERVIEW
• Degenerative, noninflammatory condition of the vertebral column characterized by the production of osteophytes along the ventral, lateral, and dorsolateral aspects of the vertebral endplates • Most common location in dogs is the thoracolumbar spine in the area of the anticlinal vertebra and the upper lumbar vertebrae. In cats, the thoracic vertebrae are more commonly affected.

SIGNALMENT
• Commonly seen in large-breed dogs, especially German shepherd; also boxer, Airedale terrier, and cocker spaniel • Reported in 68% of asymptomatic domestic cats • Occurrence increases with age—50% of dogs by 6 years and 75% by 9 years • Females > males

SIGNS
• Patients are typically asymptomatic; therefore, lesions of minor clinical importance
• Pain may follow fracture of bony spurs or bridges.

Historical Findings
• Stiffness • Restricted motion • Pain

Physical Examination Findings
Neurologic deficits referable to the spinal cord or nerve root compression are unusual.

CAUSES AND RISK FACTORS
• Repeated microtrauma • Major trauma

DIAGNOSIS

DIFFERENTIAL DIAGNOSIS
• Discospondylitis is differentiated from spondylosis by radiographic evidence of endplate lysis. • Spinal osteoarthritis is a degeneration of the articular facet joints.

CBC/BIOCHEMISTRY/URINALYSIS
Results normal

OTHER LABORATORY TESTS N/A

IMAGING
Spinal radiography initially shows osteophytes as triangular projections several millimeters from the edge of the vertebral body. With progression, they appear to bridge the intervertebral space. True ankylosis is rare.

OTHER DIAGNOSTIC PROCEDURES
In unusual cases, myelography and computed tomography or magnetic resonance imaging required to demonstrate an atypical dorsal osteophyte compressing the spinal cord or nerve roots or encroaching on critical soft tissue structures

TREATMENT
• Inform owner that spondylosis deformans is usually an asymptomatic, incidental finding and is probably not responsible for the clinical signs.
• If the patient has back pain or neurologic deficits, neurodiagnostic evaluation of the spine should be done in consideration of surgical intervention.
• If spondylosis is the cause of pain, can treat as outpatient with strict rest and analgesic administration or possibly acupuncture
• If the patient is obese, a weight reduction program is advised.

MEDICATIONS

DRUGS AND FLUIDS
• Nonsteroidal antiinflammatory drugs (NSAIDs) are preferred to steroids in dogs unless the patient has neurologic deficits because of fewer side effects.
• Administer NSAIDs after feeding and in combination with an antacid (cimetidine 6-10 mg/kg q8h or ranitidine 1-2 mg/kg q12h) or a gastrointestinal protector (Mesoprostel 3-5 ug/kg) to reduce the possibility of gastrointestinal ulceration.
• Use judiciously (i.e., only when the animal is exhibiting signs).

ALTERNATE DRUGS
• Phenylbutazone—11-22 mg/kg (maximum daily dose of 80 mg)
• Naproxen—2 mg/kg q24h (maximum daily dose of 75 mg)
• Ibuprofen—6-10 mg/kg q24h
• Other NSAIDs should be used cautiously since they cause gastrointestinal ulceration.
• Acetaminophen (Tylenol)—5 mg/kg q12h

Dogs
Buffered, enteric-coated aspirin such as Ascriptin or Ecotrin (10-20 mg/kg q8h-q12h)

Cats
• Aspirin—a baby aspirin or 1/4 of a 325-mg aspirin tablet q 3 days can be administered safely in adult cats for analgesia
• Prednisone—0.5-1.0 mg/kg divided q12h and taper to alternate days or less if possible

CONTRAINDICATIONS/POSSIBLE INTERACTIONS
• Do not use acetaminophen (Tylenol) in cats.
• Avoid prolonged administration or combinations of NSAIDs and steroids because of risk of gastrointestinal ulceration.

FOLLOW-UP
• Gradually return the animal to normal activity after signs have subsided for several weeks. • Relapse can occur with strenuous activity.

MISCELLANEOUS

ABBREVIATIONS
CT = computed tomography
MRI = magnetic resonance imaging
NSAID = nonsteroidal antiinflammatory drug

Reference
Romatowski J. Spondylosis deformans in the dog. Compend Cont Educ Pract Vet 1986;8:531-536.
Author Richard J. Joseph
Consulting Editor Joane M. Parent

BASICS

OVERVIEW

A zoonotic fungal disease that may affect the integument, lymphatics, or be generalized. It is caused by the virtually ubiquitous dimorphic fungus Sporothrix schenckii, which typically infects via direct inoculation. Apparently, direct inoculation is not a requirement in all cases.

SIGNALMENT

Seen in cats, dogs, and humans.

SIGNS

Historical Findings

• Previous trauma or puncture wound in the affected area is a variable finding. • Poor response to previous antibacterial therapy.

Physical Examination Findings

• The cutaneous form in the dog is associated with numerous nodules which may drain or crust typically affecting the head or trunk. In the cat, the lesions often initially appear as wounds or abscesses mimicking wounds associated with fighting and can be found on the head, lumbar region, or distal limbs. • The cutaneolymphatic form is usually an extension of the cutaneous form, which spreads via the lymphatics resulting in the formation of new nodules and draining tracts or crusts. Lymphadenopathy is common. • The disseminated form is associated with the systemic signs of malaise and fever. The potential of an underlying immunosuppressive disease should be considered as a contributing factor.

CAUSES AND RISK FACTORS

• Animals exposed to soil rich in decaying organic debris appear to be predisposed. • In dogs, puncture wounds associated with foreign bodies provide an increased opportunity for infection. In roaming cats, cat scratches provide a similar opportunity.

DIAGNOSIS

DIFFERENTIAL DIAGNOSIS

• Various bacterial and fungal diseases should be considered when patient presents with the symptoms of a nodular granulomatous disease and draining tracts. • Neoplastic conditions • Parasitic infections (Demodex or pelodera)

CBC/BIOCHEMISTRY/URINALYSIS

N/A

OTHER LABORATORY TESTS N/A

IMAGING N/A

OTHER DIAGNOSTIC PROCEDURES

• It is important to note that this is a zoonotic disease and proper precautions should be taken to prevent infection. An absence of a break in the skin does not protect against the disease. • Cytology of the exudate and staining is often the only test necessary to confirm an infection in the cat. The cigar- to round-shaped yeast may be found intracellularly or free in the exudate. In dogs, special fungal stains (PAS or GMS) may aid in the diagnosis, but a negative finding does not rule out the disease. • Cultures of the deeply affected tissue often require surgery to obtain an adequate sample and a special note to the laboratory listing sporotrichosis as a differential diagnosis. Secondary bacterial infections are common.

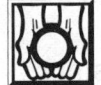

TREATMENT

The zoonotic nature of sporotrichosis should be considered when treating an animal with this disease. In some situations, outpatient treatment may be considered.

MEDICATIONS

DRUGS AND FLUIDS

• Supersaturated solution of potassium iodide (SSKI) is the treatment of choice. Dogs: 40 mg/kg q8h PO with food. Cats: 20 mg/kg PO q12h with food. This drug should be continued for 30 days after resolution of the clinical lesions. In the dog, if signs of iodism are noted (dry hair coat, excessive scales, nasal or ocular discharge, vomiting, depression or collapse), the drugs should be discontinued for one week. If the symptoms were mild, it may be reinitiated at the same dose. If the symptoms are severe or recurrent, other drugs should be considered. In the cat, the symptoms of iodism (depression, vomiting, anorexia, twitching, hypothermia, and cardiovascular collapse) are more common and this drug should be discontinued. Drugs other than SSKI should then be initiated.
• Ketoconazole and itraconazole have shown encouraging results in the treatment of this as well as other fungal diseases in cats and dogs. The ketoconazole dose in dogs is 15mg/kg q12h PO (preferably with an acidic meal such as tomato juice) until one month after clinical resolution. Resolution should occur within approximately 3 months. Side effects

are relatively mild with anorexia being the most common. Acute hepatopathy, pruritus, alopecia, and lightening of the hair color have also been reported. In cats, the ketoconazole dose is 5-10 mg/kg q12-24h PO (also preferably with an acidic meal) for one month beyond clinical cure. Gastrointestinal disturbances are more commonly seen in cats as are other side effects such as depression, fever, jaundice, and neurological signs. It is sometime necessary to alternate drugs when treating cats with this disease.

CONTRAINDICATIONS/POSSIBLE INTERACTIONS N/A

FOLLOW-UP

PATIENT MONITORING

Reevaluations are recommended every 2-4 weeks to monitor clinical signs and side effects associated with treatment.

PREVENTION/AVOIDANCE

Although difficult, it is helpful to determine the source of the original infection to prevent repeat infections.

EXPECTED COURSE AND PROGNOSIS

Failure of response to therapy should not be unexpected. If this occurs, alternative treatment or combined treatment regimens (SSKI and ketoconazole) should be considered. Itraconazole remains relatively untested but promising in the treatment of this disease.

MISCELLANEOUS

AGE RELATED FACTORS

In dogs, the disease occurs more commonly in hunting dogs because of the increased likelihood of puncture wounds associated with thorns or splinters. In cats, intact male cats that roam outdoors and fight are predisposed to puncture wounds and acquiring the disease from their opponents.

ZOONOTIC POTENTIAL

This disease is zoonotic and proper precautions and client education is of paramount importance.

Reference

Scott DW, Miller WH, Griffin CE. Muller & Kirk's small animal dermatology. 5th ed. Philadelphia: WB Saunders, 1995:364-368.
Author Dunbar Gram
Consulting Editor Lowell Ackerman

SQUAMOUS CELL CARCINOMA, DIGIT

BASICS

OVERVIEW
Squamous cell carcinoma of the digit is a malignant tumor arising from the subungual epithelium. It is the most common digital tumor in dogs.

SIGNALMENT
• Large breeds and black dogs are predisposed, particularly the standard poodle and Labrador retriever. • Median age is 10 years but this tumor can occur in dogs as young as 4 years old. • Rare in cats

SIGNS
• Swelling of the digit is the reason for examination. • Ulceration in some animals • Multiple digits rarely affected • Lymph node and lung metastasis are reported but are uncommon at the time of examination.

CAUSES AND RISK FACTORS
• Cause unknown • Hereditary factors and black skin pigmentation are risk factors.

DIAGNOSIS

DIFFERENTIAL DIAGNOSIS
• Nail bed infection • Other tumors (e.g., melanoma, soft tissue sarcomas, and mast cell tumor)

CBC/BIOCHEMISTRY/URINALYSIS
Results normal

OTHER LABORATORY TESTS N/A

IMAGING
• Thoracic radiographs important to rule out metastatic disease; results typically normal at the time of diagnosis • Radiographs of the affected foot reveal lysis of the third phalanx of the affected digit in 75% of patients.
• Wedge biopsy of abnormal tissue required to confirm the diagnosis

OTHER DIAGNOSTIC PROCEDURES
Lymph node biopsy

TREATMENT
Amputation of the affected digit at the level of the metacarpal (or metatarsal) phalangeal joint the treatment of choice

MEDICATIONS

DRUGS AND FLUIDS N/A

CONTRAINDICATIONS/POSSIBLE INTERACTIONS
N/A

FOLLOW-UP
• If surgical excision is complete, and no evidence of metastatic disease is seen at the time of surgery, the 1- and 2-year survival rates after amputation of the digit are 76% and 43%, respectively. • Recurrence not anticipated • Metastasis uncommon • Chemotherapy not recommended after surgery

MISCELLANEOUS

Reference
O'Brien MG, Berg J, Engler SJ. Treatment by digital amputation of subungual squamous cell carcinoma in dogs: 21 cases (1987-1988). J Am Vet Med Assoc 1992;201:759-761.

Author Robyn E. Elmslie
Consulting Editor Wallace B. Morrison

SQUAMOUS CELL CARCINOMA, EAR

BASICS

OVERVIEW
Squamous cell carcinoma is a malignant tumor arising from the squamous epithelium of the skin of the pinnae. Occasionally the ear canal is involved. It is most common in animals that have had high exposure to sunlight.

SIGNALMENT
• Common tumor in cats with white or light-colored fur and skin • Mean age at time of diagnosis, 12 years(range, 7-24 years) • Rare in dogs

SIGNS
• Lesions develop slowly over months to years. • Precancerous stage characterized by crusty eczematous lesions of the edge of the pinnae that flare up and regress repeatedly • Proliferation and ulceration of the ear signal the true cancerous phase. The ear becomes extensively disfigured if left untreated. • Metastatic disease uncommon

CAUSES AND RISK FACTORS
• Prolonged sunlight exposure is an important cause. • White fur and light skin pigmentation are risk factors.

DIAGNOSIS

DIFFERENTIAL DIAGNOSIS
• Classic clinical findings facilitate differentiation of this disease from other neoplastic conditions. • Lesions on the pinnae are caused by vasculitis or cryoglobulinemia resemble squamous cell carcinoma in some patients.

CBC/BIOCHEMISTRY/URINALYSIS
Results normal

OTHER LABORATORY TESTS N/A

IMAGING
Thoracic radiographs and cytologic examination of lymph nodes required to rule out metastatic disease.

OTHER DIAGNOSTIC PROCEDURES
• Histologic examination of the lesions of the pinnae are required for confirmation of the diagnosis. • Most squamous cell carcinomas of the skin are very invasive but very slow to metastasize. • Squamous cell carcinoma is distinguished microscopically by groups of epithelial cells and keratinizing cells forming keratin "pearls."

TREATMENT
• Aggressive surgical excision is required. The pinnae must be amputated below the demarcation of unhealthy tissue.
• Histologic evaluation of surgical margins is essential to assess completeness of surgical excision.
• Photodynamic therapy is an alternative to amputation of the pinnae. Results are less predictable with this form of treatment, and more than one treatment is often required.
• Cryosurgery is successful for the treatment of small lesions.
• Hyperthermia is reported to be beneficial.

MEDICATIONS

DRUGS AND FLUIDS
• Etretinate has been used successfully to prevent progression of precancerous lesions.
• Bleomycin has been used systemically to treat advanced squamous cell carcinoma. The benefit of chemotherapy has yet to be established.

CONTRAINDICATIONS/POSSIBLE INTERACTIONS N/A

FOLLOW-UP
• Limiting sun exposure may prevent development of new lesions. • Sunscreen and tattooing are also useful to prevent development of new lesions. • Early treatment of crusting lesions on the ears by cryosurgery or surgical excision is recommended. • Prognosis is good if complete surgical excision is achieved.

MISCELLANEOUS

ABBREVIATIONS N/A

Reference
Dorn CR, Taylor D. Sunlight exposure and the risk of developing cutaneous and oral squamous cell carcinoma in white cats. J Natl Cancer Inst 1971;46:1073-1078.
Author Robyn E. Elmslie
Consulting Editor Wallace B. Morrison

SQUAMOUS CELL CARCINOMA, GINGIVA

BASICS

OVERVIEW

Squamous cell carcinoma of the gingiva causes progressive, rapid (weeks) local invasion of neoplastic epithelial cells within in the oral cavity in dogs and cats. It is the most common oral malignancy in cats and second most common in dogs. The squamous cell carcinoma is highly invasive to bone with a nonencapsulated, raised, irregular, ulcerated, or necrotic surface. Metastasis is rare, with spread to lymph nodes more common than the lungs. Cause of death is secondary to local recurrence and cachexia.

SIGNALMENT

• Mean age of dogs, 10.5 years (range, 3 to 15 years) • No sex or breed predilection
• More common in medium- and large-breeds dogs than small • The most common site is the rostral mandible.

SIGNS

Historical Findings

• Excessive salivation • Dysphagia • Halitosis
• Weight loss

Physical Examination Findings

• Loose teeth • Bloody oral discharge • Facial deformity • Cervical lymphadenopathy in a few patients • Reactive hyperplasia (> 50%); metastatic tumor (< 50%)

CAUSES AND RISK FACTORS N/A

DIAGNOSIS

DIFFERENTIAL DIAGNOSIS

• Amelanotic melanoma • Fibrosarcoma

• Epulis • Abscess • Benign polyp • Plasmacytoma • Eosinophilic granuloma • Undifferentiated oral malignancy

CBC/BIOCHEMISTRY/URINALYSIS

Results usually normal

OTHER LABORATORY TESTS N/A

IMAGING

• Skull radiography • Thoracic radiography to detect pulmonary metastasis (uncommon)

OTHER DIAGNOSTIC PROCEDURES

A large, deep tissue biopsy (down to bone) required for diagnosis

TREATMENT

• Radical surgical excision required (ie, partial mandibulectomy or maxillectomy) and usually well-tolerated by patients
• 1-year survival after excision in dogs—25% to 45%
• 2 year-survival after excision in dogs—20% to 35%
• Median survival after excision in dogs—from 7-11 months. Survival improves when excisional margins are free of neoplastic cells.
• Mean and medial survival in dogs after excision and radiotherapy—7 and 8 months, respectively; range, 0-27 months
• Mean and median survival in cats after excision—2.5 and 14 months, respectively; range, 0-36 months
• Median survival after excision and radiotherapy in cats—14 months (range, 1-36 months)
• Outpatient chemotherapy with cisplatin or doxorubicin is palliative in dogs
• Cause of death related to local recurrence and secondary anorexia and cachexia.

MEDICATIONS

DRUGS AND FLUIDS N/A

CONTRAINDICATIONS/POSSIBLE INTERACTIONS

• Chemotherapy can be toxic. Seek advice if unfamiliar with cytotoxic drugs.
• Never use cisplatin in cats.

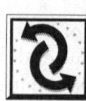

FOLLOW-UP

• Repeat head and neck examination by survey thoracic radiography at 1, 2, 3, 6, 9, 12, 15, 18, and 24 months after treatment • The overall prognosis is poor in cats because most are locally invasive and diagnosed late in the course of disease.

MISCELLANEOUS

References

Oakes MG, Lewis DD, Hedlund CS, et al. Canine oral neoplasia. Comp Cont Ed Pract Vet 1993;15:15-31.

Author Kevin A. Hahn
Consulting Editor Wallace B. Morrison

BASICS

OVERVIEW
• Very rare as primary lung tumor • Bronchial epithelial origin that has undergone squamous metaplasia

SIGNALMENT
• No breed predilection • Dogs—mean age, 11 years • Cats—mean age, 12 years

SIGNS

Historical Findings
• None in some animals • Harsh, nonproductive cough • Dyspnea • Lethargy or exercise intolerance • Cachexia and weight loss

Physical Examination Findings
• Tachypnea • Wheeze • Hemoptysis • Hypertrophic osteopathy • Neuromyopathy and paraplegia • Digital lesions (metastasis) in cats

CAUSES AND RISK FACTORS
74% of dogs with a primary lung tumor come from an urban environment.

DIAGNOSIS

DIFFERENTIAL DIAGNOSIS
• Bronchogenic cysts • Bullae and blebs • Abscesses • Paragonimus • Eosinophilic lung disease • Other primary lung neoplasm • Metastatic pulmonary neoplasm • Aspiration pneumonia

CBC/BIOCHEMISTRY/URINALYSIS
• Neutrophilic leukocytosis • Hypercalcemia (rare)

OTHER LABORATORY TESTS N/A

IMAGING
• Most common appearance on survey thoracic radiography is a solitary mass arising from a single focus. • Margins well-circumscribed and sharp demarcation from other surrounding normal parenchyma

OTHER DIAGNOSTIC PROCEDURES
• Cytologic examination may provide tentative diagnosis • Tissue biopsy for definitive diagnosis

TREATMENT
• Wide and complete resection of the affected lung lobe offers the best opportunity for long-term control.
• Examine tracheobronchial lymph nodes.
• Manually palpate all remaining lung lobes.
• High metastatic potential, especially if regional lymph nodes are positive

MEDICATIONS

DRUGS AND FLUIDS
Outpatient treatment with cisplatin chemotherapy (60 mg/m^2 IV q3wk-q4wk) reported with unclear results of efficacy

CONTRAINDICATIONS/POSSIBLE INTERACTIONS
• Chemotherapy can be toxic. Seek advice before treatment if you are unfamiliar with cytotoxic drugs.
• Renal damage and bone marrow suppression are possible.
• Cisplatin should never be used in cats.

FOLLOW-UP
• Head and neck examination by survey thoracic radiography at 1, 2, 3, 6, 9, 12, 15, 18, and 24 months after treatment
• If left untreated or patient has evidence of metastatic disease, survival usually < than 3 months; normal-sized lymph nodes at surgery indicate better prognosis
• More than 90% of primary lung squamous cell carcinomas metastasize through lymphatic vessels, airways, hematogenously, or transpleurally.
• Usually advanced in cats when diagnosis is made

MISCELLANEOUS

Reference
Ogilvie GK, Weigel RM, Hasckek WM, et al. Prognostic factors for tumor remission and survival in dogs after surgery for primary lung tumor: 76 cases (1975-1985). J Am Vet Med Assoc 1989;195:106-108.

Author Kevin A. Hahn
Consulting Editor Wallace B. Morrison

SQUAMOUS CELL CARCINOMA, NASAL AND PARANASAL SINUSES

BASICS

OVERVIEW
• Arise from the surface epithelium • Slowly progressive (months) • Some patients have cranial extension and seizures

SIGNALMENT
• More common in dogs than cats • Median age of affected dogs, 9.5 years (3-16 years) • Prevalence in dogs and cats, 0.3%-8% of all tumors • Accounts for 28.5% of all nasal neoplasms in dogs

SIGNS

Historical Findings
• Intermittent and progressive unilateral to bilateral epistaxis • Sneezing • Seizures secondary to cranial invasion

Physical Examination Findings
• Purlient or bloody nasal discharge • Facial deformity or exophthalmia

CAUSES AND RISK FACTORS N/A

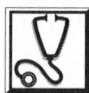

DIAGNOSIS

DIFFERENTIAL DIAGNOSIS
• Viral infection rhinitis (cats) • Aspergillosis (dogs) • Cryptococcosis (cats) • Foreign body • Trauma • Tooth root abscess • Oronasal fistula • Coagulopathy

CBC/BIOCHEMISTRY/URINALYSIS
Results usually normal

OTHER LABORATORY TESTS N/A

IMAGING
• Skull radiographs reveal a typical pattern of asymmetrical destruction of caudal turbinates with superimposition of a soft tissue mass. Fluid density may be observed in the frontal sinuses secondary to outflow obstruction.
• Thoracic radiographs to detect pulmonary metastasis • Computed tomography or magnetic resonance imaging are the best methods to observe integrity of cribiform plate or orbital invasion.

OTHER DIAGNOSTIC PROCEDURES
• Deep tissue biopsy is definitive. • Bacterial culture and sensitivity rarely helpful • Visualization by rhinoscopy often obscured by exucade

TREATMENT
• Surgery alone is not curative.
• Turbinectomy can be performed before external (teletherapy) or internal (brachytherapy) irradiation.
• Rhinitis developing after turbinectomy and radiotherapy usually subsides in 1-2 months.
• Radiotherapy, with or without surgery, provides the best clinical control in dogs.
• Chemotherapy can be palliative.

MEDICATIONS

DRUGS AND FLUIDS N/A.

CONTRAINDICATIONS/POSSIBLE INTERACTIONS N/A.

FOLLOW-UP
• Repeat examination with survey thoracic radiography at 1, 2, 3, 6, 9, 12, 15, 18, and 24 months after treatment • Skull radiography, computed tomography, magnetic resonance imaging when signs recur • Median survival if left untreated, 3-5 months • One-year survival with radiotherapy, 38-57% in dogs and cats; 2-year survival, 30-48%
• Median survival in dogs, 8-25 months
• Median survival in cats, 1-36 months
• Median survival in dogs after cisplatin treatment, 22 weeks • Local recurrence common with extension to the brain • Secondary fungal rhinitis occurs in some patients after turbinectomy.

MISCELLANEOUS
Keratinizing and nonkeratinizing forms are reported. • Transitional (intermediate) cell carcinoma in a nonkeratinizing form classified as undifferentiated

Reference
Theon AP, Peaston AE, Madewell BR, et al. Irradiation of nonlymphoproliferative neoplasms of the nasal cavity and paranasal sinuses in 16 cats. J Amer Vet Med Assoc 1994;204:78-83
Author Kevin A. Hahn
Consulting Editor Wallace B. Morrison

SQUAMOUS CELL CARCINOMA, NASAL PLANUM

BASICS

OVERVIEW
• Malignant tumor of epithelial cells of the nasal planum • Locally invasive and rarely metastasizes

SIGNALMENT
• Common in cats; rare in dogs • Mean age cats, 8.5 - 12.1 years • Mean age dogs, 9-10 years • No reported sex or breed predilection in cats or dogs • Lightly pigmented nose

SIGNS
• May begin as superficial crusting and scabbing, progress to carcinoma in situ, and develop into superficial and then invasive, erosive carcinoma • Slow progression

CAUSES AND RISK FACTORS
Exposure to ultraviolet light and absence of protective pigment

DIAGNOSIS

DIFFERENTIAL DIAGNOSIS
Biopsy differentiates from immune-mediated disease, the eosinophilic granuloma complex, and other neoplasms.

CBC/BIOCHEMISTRY/URINALYSIS
Results usually normal

OTHER LABORATORY TESTS N/A

IMAGING N/A

OTHER DIAGNOSTIC PROCEDURES
Fluorescent nuclear antibody and cytology of large lymph nodes to detect metastasis

TREATMENT
• Superficial tumors can be treated by surgery, cryosurgery, irradiation, or photodynamic therapy.
• Etretinate is useful in some patients with early, precancerous lesions.
• Invasive tumors require radical surgical excision and adjunctive radiotherpy.

MEDICATIONS

DRUGS AND FLUIDS
Chemotherapy not yet evaluated

CONTRAINDICATIONS/POSSIBLE INTERACTIONS N/A

FOLLOW-UP

PATIENT MONITORING
• Physical examination and thoracic radiography at 1, 3, 6, and 12 months after treatment • Biopsy any suspicious lesion

PREVENTION/AVOIDANCE
• Limit sun exposure, especially between the hours of 10:00 am and 2:00 pm. • Yearly tattoos on nonpigmented areas may be helpful. • Sunscreens ineffective

POSSIBLE COMPLICATIONS N/A

EXPECTED COURSE AND PROGNOSIS
• Mean survival time in cats treated by radiotherapy alone, 17.7 months (1-year survival, 61.5%, with 81.8% recurrence) • Mean survival time in cats treated by surgery alone, 18 months with 37.5-50%. recurrence • Eight dogs treated by radiotherapy alone had 100% recurrence with a mean time to recurrence, 2.9 months. • Surgery alone in dogs can be curative unless disease is advanced. • Prognosis good for small, noninvasive tumors and guarded for invasive tumors

MISCELLANEOUS

ASSOCIATED CONDITIONS
Secondary bacterial infection

AGE RELATED FACTORS None

ZOONOTIC POTENTIAL None

PREGNANCY N/A

Reference
Withrow SJ. Tumors of the respiratory system. In: Withrow SJ, MacEwen EG, eds. Clinical veterinary oncology. Philadelphia: JB Lippincott, 1989;215-218.
Author Joanne C. Graham
Consulting Editor Wallace B. Morrison

SQUAMOUS CELL CARCINOMA, SKIN

BASICS

DEFINITION
• Squamous cell carcinoma of the skin is a malignant tumor of squamous epithelium.
• Bowen's disease, which is multicentric squamous cell carcinoma in situ, was recently identified as a new disease in cats.

Pathophysiology
• Unknown • Can metastasize anywhere

Systems Affected
Skin/exocrine—skin and metastatic sites

Genetics
Unknown

Incidence/Prevalence
Represents 9-25% of all skin tumors in cats and 4-18% of all skin tumors in dogs

Geographic Distribution
More prevalent in sunny climates and high altitudes (high ultraviolet light exposure)

SIGNALMENT

Species Dogs and cats

Breed Predilection
• No breed predilection reported in cats, but affected cats often have light or unpigmented skin. • Scottish terrier, Pekingese, boxer, poodle, Norwegian elkhound, Dalmatian, beagle, whippet, and white English bull terrier may be predisposed. • Large-breed dogs with black skin and haircoats may be predisposed to multiple squamous cell carcinoma involving the digits.

Mean Age and Range
• Dogs, 9 years • Cats, 9-12.4 years

Predominant Sex None

SIGNS

Historical Findings
• Crusts, ulcer, or mass that may have been present for months and unresponsive to conservative treatment. • Cats with Bowen's disease have a different history. The skin becomes pigmented then an ulcer forms in the center. This is followed by a painful scabby lesion that may expand peripherally.
• Squamous cell carcinoma of the lips, nose, and pinna may start out as a shallow crusting lesion that progresses to a deep ulcer.
• Tumors involving the facial skin in cats may become invasive. • Tumors involving the nail beds in dogs generally invade underlying bone.

Physical Examination Findings
• Proliferative or erosive skin lesions • Most commonly seen on nasal planum, eyelids, lips, and pinna in cats; and toes, scrotum, nose, legs, and anus in dogs. • Dalmatian, beagle, whippet, and white English bull terrier may be predisposed to squamous cell carcinoma of the flank and abdomen. • Cats with Bowen's disease may have 2 to > 30 lesions

on the head, digits, neck, thorax, shoulders, and ventral abdomen. Hair in the lesion epilates easily and crusts cling to the epilated hair shaft.

CAUSES
• Unknown • Exposure to ultraviolet irradiation in sunlight

RISK FACTORS
• Prolonged exposure to ultraviolet light and light or nonpigmented skin • Previous thermal injury (burn scar)

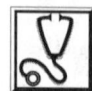

DIAGNOSIS

DIFFERENTIAL DIAGNOSIS
• The disease is misdiagnosed as draining abscesses or infected wounds on the basis of gross appearance. • Squamous cell carcinoma of digit is sometimes confused with nail bed infection and osteomyelitis. • Biopsy distinguishes from eosinophilic granuloma complex, immune-mediated disease, mast cell tumor, and cutaneous lymphosarcoma.

CBC/BIOCHEMISTRY/URINALYSIS
Results usually normal

OTHER LABORATORY TESTS None

IMAGING
• Thoracic radiography to detect lung metastasis • Abdominal radiography to evaluate and monitor sublumbar lymph nodes if clinically relevant • Radiography of extremities in patients with digital squamous cell carcinoma to determine extent of underlying bone involvement

OTHER DIAGNOSTIC PROCEDURES
• Cytologic examination of fine-needle aspirate to evaluate large lymph nodes for metastasis • Biopsy needed to confirm diagnosis

GROSS AND HISTOPATHOLOGIC FINDINGS

Gross Findings
• The tumors are ulcerative (most common) or proliferative. Ulcers may appear shallow and crusted and progress to deep craters. Proliferative tumors may have a cauliflower-like appearance and may ulcerate and bleed easily.
• The lesions of Bowen's disease are painful ulcers that scab over and expand peripherally to reach more than 4 cm in diameter.

Histopathologic Findings
• Cords or irregular masses of epidermal cells infiltrating into the dermis and subcutis
• Large numbers of "horn (keratin) pearls" In well-differentiated tumors • Other common features include desmosomes and mitotic figures. • In patients with Bowen's disease, dysplastic, highly ordered keratinocytes proliferate replacing normal epidermis but do not penetrate the basement membrane into the surrounding dermis.

TREATMENT
• Treat superficial tumors by surgery, cryosurgery, photodynamic therapy, or irradiation.
• The topical use of synthetic retinoids may be useful in the treatment of early superficial lesions.
• Invasive tumors require aggressive surgical excision or radiotherapy.
• Digits with tumors should be amputated.
• Tumors involving the pinna may require partial or total pinna resection.
• Nasal planum removal is recommended for invasive tumors of the nares.
• Radiotherapy is recommended for inoperable tumors or as adjunct to surgery.

INPATIENT VERSUS OUTPATIENT
Patients with invasive tumors should be treated as inpatients while undergoing treatment.

ACTIVITY
• Restriction dictated by the location of the tumor and the type of treatment.
• In general, limit activity until sutures are removed if surgery has been done.

DIET Normal

CLIENT EDUCATION
• Clients should be informed of the benefit of early diagnosis and treatment.
• Risk factors associated with the development of the tumor (ultraviolet light exposure) should be discussed.

SURGICAL CONSIDERATIONS
• Wide surgical excision the treatment of choice
• Skin flaps and body wall reconstruction required in some animals

MEDICATIONS

DRUGS AND FLUID
• Adjunctive chemotherapy is recommended if surgical excision is incomplete, the mass is nonresectable, or if patient has metastasis.
• Cisplatin and mitoxantrone have been reported to induce partial and complete remissions, generally of short duration, in a small number of animals.

CONTRAINDICATIONS
• Cisplatin causes severe hydrothorax, pulmonary edema, and death in cats and should not be used in this species.
• Cisplatin is potentially nephrotoxic and contraindicated in dogs with concurrent renal disease.

PRECAUTIONS
Veterinarians administering chemotherapeutics should follow guidelines and protocols published on the safe use of these drugs and should be familiar with potential side effects.

POSSIBLE INTERACTIONS None
ALTERNATIVE DRUGS None

FOLLOW-UP

PATIENT MONITORING
• Physical examination and radiography at 1, 3, 6, and 12 months after treatment or if the owner thinks the tumor is recurring
• Thoracic and abdominal radiography at each recheck examination (if the lesion is on the caudal portion of the animal)

PREVENTION/AVOIDANCE
• Limit sun exposure, especially between the hours of 10:00 am and 2:00 pm. • Yearly tattoos on nonpigmented areas may be helpful.
• Sunscreens are usually licked off by the animal but may be helpful in some areas (e.g., pinna).

POSSIBLE COMPLICATIONS N/A

EXPECTED COURSE AND PROGNOSIS
• The prognosis is good for animals with superficial lesions that receive appropriate treatment. • Invasive lesions and those involving the nail bed or digit warrant a guarded prognosis.

MISCELLANEOUS

ASSOCIATED CONDITIONS None

AGE RELATED FACTORS None

ZOONOTIC POTENTIAL None

PREGNANCY None

SYNONYMS None

SEE ALSO
Squamous Cell Carcinoma, Nasal Planum

ABBREVIATIONS None

References

Susaneck SJ, Withrow SJ. Tumors of the skin and subcutaneous tissues. In: Withrow SJ, MacEwen EG, editors. Clinical veterinary oncology. Philadelphia: J.B. Lippincott Company, 1989:139-155.

Himsel CA, Richardson RC, Craig JA. Cisplatin chemotherapy for metastatic squamous cell carcinoma in two dogs. J Am Vet Med Assoc 1986;189:1575-1578.

O'Brien MG, Berg J, Engler SJ. Treatment by digital amputation of subungual squamous cell carcinoma in dogs: 21 cases (1987-1988). J Am Vet Med Assoc 1992;201:759-761.

Marks S. Clinical evaluation of etretinate (Tegison®) for the treatment of preneoplastic and early neoplastic cutaneous squamous cell carcinoma in dogs. Veterinary Cancer Society Newsletter 1990;14:4-5.

Peaston AE, Leach MW, Higgins RJ. Photodynamic therapy for nasal and aural squamous cell carcinoma in cats. J Am Vet Med Assoc 1993;202:1261-1265.

Author Joanne C. Graham
Consulting Editor Wallace B. Morrison

SQUAMOUS CELL CARCINOMA, TONGUE

BASICS

OVERVIEW
• Rare tumor that occurs more commonly in cats than dogs • In cats, most commonly located on the ventrolateral surface of the body of the tongue at the level of the reflection of the frenulum • In dogs, most commonly located on the dorsum of the tongue • Most tumors grow rapidly. • Highly metastatic by way of lymphatic vessels to regional lymph nodes and lung (37-43% at examination)

SIGNALMENT
• Most dogs and cats middle-aged or old (> 7 years) • No breed predilection in dogs

SIGNS

Historical Findings
• Dysphagia • Excessive salivation • Excessive oral bleeding • Dyspnea • Anorexia • Weight loss • Dehydration

Physical Examination Findings
Oropharyngeal mass

CAUSES AND RISK FACTORS
Unknown

DIAGNOSIS

DIFFERENTIAL DIAGNOSIS
• Abscess • Foreign body • Other lingual tumor

CBC/BIOCHEMISTRY/URINALYSIS
Variable (results may be normal)

OTHER LABORATORY TESTS N/A

IMAGING
• Survey thoracic radiography to detect pulmonary metastasis • Survey radiography of the oral cavity and pharynx rarely demonstrates evidence of bone invasion.

OTHER DIAGNOSTIC PROCEDURES
• Extensive physical examination of the cervical region • Cytologic examination may suggest diagnosis. • Deep tissue biopsy necessary for definitive diagnosis

TREATMENT
• Most tumors are inoperable; however, aggressive surgical excision is palliative in some patients.
• Postsurgical aftercare by owner often required
• A partial glossectomy can be performed on the rostral half (mobile tongue) or longitudinal half of the tongue (up to 40-60% removed); however, more than 50% of patients have incomplete surgical margins.
• Response to radiotherapy poor (< 7 weeks)
• Chemotherapy infrequently reported. One dog survived 27 months after incomplete resection and treatment with mitoxantrone.

MEDICATIONS

DRUGS AND FLUIDS   N/A

CONTRAINDICATIONS/POSSIBLE INTERACTIONS N/A

FOLLOW-UP
• Head and neck examination by survey thoracic radiography at 1, 2, 3, 6, 9, 12, 15, 18, and 24 months after treatment • Few survive more than 6 months after diagnosis. • 1-year survival after surgical excision is < 25%.
• Complete resection with clean surgical margins provides the best potential for long-term control. • Local recurrence common with regional extension to tongue, pharynx, and lymph nodes

MISCELLANEOUS

Reference

Carpenter LG, Withrow SJ, Powers BE, et al. Squamous cell carcinoma of the tongue in 10 dogs. J Amer Anim Hosp Assoc 1993;29:17-24.
Author Kevin A. Hahn
Consulting Editor Wallace B. Morrison

BASICS

OVERVIEW
• Rapid and progressive local invasion of cords of neoplastic squamous epithelium arising from the tonsillar fossa into tonsillar lymphoid tissue • Local extension common • Quick to metastasize to lymph nodes (> 98%) and lung (> 63%) • Composes nearly 20-25% of all oral tumors and 50% of all intraoral tumors of dogs and cats • Commonly unilateral, affecting the right more than the left tonsil

SIGNALMENT
• Most affected dogs and cats middle-aged or old (range, 2.5-17 years) • No known breed prevalence

SIGNS

Historical Findings
• Dysphagia • Excessive salivation • Excessive oral bleeding • Anorexia • Weight loss

Physical Examination Findings
• Oropharyngeal mass • Cervical lymphadenomegaly • Dyspnea

CAUSES AND RISK FACTORS
• Exact cause unknown • Ten times more common in animals living in an urban versus a rural environment

DIAGNOSIS

DIFFERENTIAL DIAGNOSIS
• Lymphoma • Abscess • Salivary gland tumor • Metastatic neoplasm • Other neoplasia • Tonsillitis

CBC/BIOCHEMISTRY/URINALYSIS
Results usually normal

OTHER LABORATORY TESTS N/A

IMAGING
• Thoracic radiography to detect metastasis • Cervical radiography to evaluate retropharyngeal lymph nodes

OTHER DIAGNOSTIC PROCEDURES
Tissue biopsy

TREATMENT

• Not curable with surgery because of early metastasis
• Tonsillectomy, when done, should be bilateral. May be helpful in animals with airway obstruction.
• Cervical lymphadenectomy rarely is curative and should only be performed for diagnosis or before adjuvant therapy.
• Response to regional radiotherapy poor (< 7 weeks)
• No general recommendations regarding effective chemotherapy can be made.
• Anecdotal reports of cisplatin or bleomycin used with limited success
• Grave prognosis warranted due to extensive local disease and high rate of metastasis
• Cisplatin chemotherapy

MEDICATIONS

DRUGS AND FLUIDS N/A

CONTRAINDICATIONS/POSSIBLE INTERACTIONS N/A.

FOLLOW-UP

• Head and neck examination by survey thoracic radiography at 1, 2, 3, 6, 9, 12, 15, 18, and 24 months after treatment • Local recurrence common with regional extension to tongue, pharynx, and lymph nodes • Median survival in dogs after localized radiotherapy, 110 days • Median survival in dogs after systemic chemotherapy, 60-130 days • Median survival in dogs after localized radiotherapy combined with systemic chemotherapy (e.g., doxorubicin and cisplatin), 270 days
• Metastasis the leading cause of death regardless of treatment in < 1 year • 1-year survival after surgical excision, < 10%

MISCELLANEOUS

Reference
Brooks MB, Matus RE, Leifer CE, et al. Chemotherapy versus chemotherapy plus radiotherapy in the treatment of tonsillar squamous cell carcinoma in the dog. J Vet Int Med 1988;2:206-211.
Author Kevin A. Hahn
Consulting Editor Wallace B. Morrison

STEROID HEPATOPATHY

BASICS

DEFINITION
A reversible vacuolar hepatopathy caused by high glucocorticoid activity (either endogenous or exogenous) with resulting increases in serum hepatic enzyme concentrations.

Pathophysiology
Glucocorticoids cause reversible glycogen accumulation in the hepatocytes within 2-3 days after administration. Cellular swelling follows, resulting in hepatomegaly and, possibly, impaired hepatic function. Dogs have marked variation in sensitivity to glucocorticoids depending on individual sensitivity, pharmacologic type, pharmacologic preparation (e.g., repositol versus short–acting), route of administration, and duration of glucocorticoid administration. Short-term administration of a low dose may cause steroid hepatopathy in some patients, while high doses and long-term administration are necessary to cause similar changes in other dogs. Steroids given by injection usually cause earlier and more severe lesions than those given orally. Topical, ocular, and aural glucocorticoid administration can also cause steroid hepatopathy. Cats are less commonly affected than dogs.

Systems Affected
• Hepatobiliary—variable impairment of hepatic function • Other effects relate to the multisystemic effects of glucocorticoids.

Genetics N/A

Incidence/Prevalence
• One of the most commonly seen hepatopathies, occurring in 33% of dogs undergoing hepatic biopsy. Many additional cases are diagnosed by laboratory evaluation and never undergo hepatic biopsy. • Uncommon in cats

Geogrpahic Distribution N/A

SIGNALMENT

Species
Common in dogs, but uncommon in cats

Breed Predilections
Breeds predisposed to hyperadrenocorticism (i.e., dachshund, poodle, beagle, boxer, Boston terriers, and German shepherd dog) are likely to develop steroid hepatopathy.

Mean Age and Range
• Dogs with steroid hepatopathy caused by spontaneous hyperadrenocorticism are usually middle–aged to older dogs (more than 75% > 9 years old). • Dogs with steroid hepatopathy caused by iatrogenic glucocorticoid administration can be any age.

SIGNS

Predominant Sex N/A

General Comments
• Usually related to the multisystemic effects of glucocorticoids • Animals rarely show signs of hepatic disease or failure.

Historical Findings
Signs of glucocorticoid excess include
• Polyuria/polydipsia • Polyphagia • Endocrine alopecia • Abdominal distension • Muscle weakness • Panting • Lethargy

Physical Examination Findings
• Hepatomegaly • Other findings relate to glucocorticoid excess rather than to hepatic disease, and include endocrine alopecia, hyperpigmentation, and a pendulous abdomen. These signs vary depending on the severity and duration of excess glucocorticoid activity.

CAUSES
• Iatrogenic glucocorticoid administration • Spontaneous hyperadrenocorticism (either pituitary dependent or functional adrenal mass).

RISK FACTORS
• Pharmacologic doses of glucocorticoids • Breed at risk for hyperadrenocorticism • Spontaneous (either pituitary dependent or functional adrenal mass) hyperadenocorticism

DIAGNOSIS

DIFFERENTIAL DIAGNOSIS
• Most other hepatopathies can be confused with steroid hepatopathy, especially those that cause hepatomegaly and high serum hepatic enzyme activities. These other hepatic diseases include passive congestion, neoplasia (either primary or metastatic to the liver), hepatic or biliary cysts, inflammatory disease, hepatopathy secondary to anticonvulsant administration, and vacuolar hepatopathy secondary to diabetes mellitus. • The features that distinguish steroid hepatopathy from other hepatopathies include the presence of normal serum total bilirubin concentration, normal to mild abnormalities in hepatic function tests (such as serum bile acid concentration), a homogeneous appearing liver on ultrasonography, characteristic morphologic findings on hepatic biopsy , and abnormal specialty tests that evaluate pituitary-adrenocortical function. • If laboratory and clinical signs are compatible with steroid hepatopathy or the animal is asymptomatic, hyperadrenocorticism should be ruled out before hepatic biopsy.

CBC/BIOCHEMISTRY/URINALYSIS
• Stress leukogram in some animals (variable) • Markedly high serum ALP and GGT activities • Mild to moderately high serum ALT and AST activities • The activity of serum GGT usually parallels that of serum ALP, and serum GGT activity cannot be used to distinguish steroid hepatopathy from other hepatobiliary diseases. • Serum albumin and bilirubin concentrations are normal. • High serum total bilirubin concentration effectively eliminates steroid hepatopathy from the differential diagnosis of primary hepatobiliary disease.

OTHER LABORATORY TESTS
• Serum bile acids can be normal or slightly to moderately high (up to approximately 75 uM/L). Marked increases in serum bile acid concentration are unlikely to result from steroid hepatopathy. • Blood ammonia concentration and the ammonia tolerance test are usually normal in animals with steroid hepatopathy. • The isoenzyme of serum ALP differs from the isoenzyme of serum ALP induced by biliary stasis. This isoenzyme is referred to as the steroid–induced isoenzyme of serum ALP. However, this isoenzyme is variably high in animals with many primary hepatobiliary diseases and, therefore, measurement of its activity is not useful for diagnosing steroid hepatopathy. • In animals with spontaneous hyperadrenocorticism, the ACTH stimulation test, low-dose dexamethasone suppression test, and urine cortisol:creatinine ratio are often confirmatory. In animals with iatrogenic glucocorticoid administration, the ACTH stimulation test is blunted, characterized by a low post–ACTH serum cortisol concentration.

IMAGING
• Abdominal radiographs usually reveal hepatomegaly. • Hepatic ultrasonography usually reveals a diffusely large, homogeneous liver that is hyperechogenitic.

OTHER DIAGNOSTIC PROCEDURES
• If a diagnosis of steroid hepatopathy is uncertain, hepatic biopsy is warranted and serves to distinguish steroid hepatopathy from other hepatic diseases. • Hepatic biopsy methods include percutaneous and ultrasound–guided techniques, laparoscopy, and laparotomy. • A diagnosis of steroid hepatopathy by hepatic biopsy may suggest unsuspected hyperadrenocorticism, and further laboratory testing to diagnose this condition may be warranted.

GROSS AND HISTOPATHOLOGIC FINDINGS
• Gross findings vary and can include a normal- appearing liver, mild to moderate hepatomegaly, mild surface irregularity, and loss of the normal lobular pattern. • Histopathologic abnormalities usually are pathognomonic and include marked vacuolization and ballooning of hepatocytes in a centrilobular or diffuse distribution. Mild hepatic necrosis may also be observed..

TREATMENT

INPATIENT VS OUTPATIENT
Outpatients

ACTIVITY Normal activity

DIET Normal diet

CLIENT EDUCATION

• Clients should understand that clinical signs are related to the multisystemic effects of glucocorticoids and that impaired hepatic function is uncommon.

• Glucocorticoid administration should be discontinued if at all possible. If this is not possible, impaired hepatic function is a minor concern.

SURGICAL CONSIDERATIONS

Surgery is usually not required except in cushingoid animals with resectable, functional, adrenocortical mass.

MEDICATIONS

DRUGS AND FLUIDS

Hyperadrenocorticism should be treated medically once a diagnosis is confirmed. Drugs used to treat hyperadrenocorticism include mitotane (Lysodren®) and ketoconazole.

CONTRAINDICATIONS N/A

PRECAUTIONS

• Glucocorticoids should be administered cautiously to all patients, and especially those at risk for steroid hepatopathy.

• Alternate-day glucocorticoid administration reduces the severity of steroid hepatopathy as well as other side effects caused by these drugs.

• All hepatotoxic drugs (including anticonvulsants such as phenobarbital) should be used with caution in patients with steroid hepatopathy.

POSSIBLE INTERACTIONS N/A

ALTERNATE DRUGS

• If clinical signs (eg, lethargy, polyuria/polydipsia, and abdominal distension) persist in a patient receiving glucocorticoid for immune-mediated disorders, alternative immune-modulating drugs may be substituted. These include azathioprine (Imuran®), cyclophosphamide (Cytoxan®), and chlorambucil (Leukeran®).

• Other drugs used to treat hyperadrenocorti-

cism include cyproheptadine, bromocriptine, metyrapone, and L–Deprenyl.

FOLLOW-UP

PATIENT MONITORING

• The degree of hepatomegaly should be monitored by abdominal palpation and abdominal radiography.

• Serum biochemical profile should demonstrate serum activities of ALP, GGT, ALT, and AST returning to normal.

• In animals with hyperadrenocorticism, an ACTH stimulation test should be used to monitor efficacy of treatment.

PREVENTION/AVOIDANCE

Administration of glucocorticoids should be avoided if at all possible. When steroids need to be used for prolonged periods, taper to the lowest effective alternate-day dose.

POSSIBLE COMPLICATIONS

Numerous and relate to the multisystemic effects of glucocorticoids.

EXPECTED COURSE AND PROGNOSIS

• Some animals show minimal changes in serum hepatic enzyme activities and hepatic morphology after chronic glucocorticoid administration. Other animals show high serum hepatic enzyme activities and hepatic morphologic changes that persist for weeks after a single dose of glucocorticoid. • The laboratory and hepatic morphologic changes seen with steroid hepatopathy are completely reversible when the source of excess glucocorticoids is removed.

MISCELLANEOUS

ASSOCIATED CONDITIONS

• Spontaneous hyperadrenocorticism (pituitary or adrenal dependent) • Diabetes mellitus • Pulmonary thromboembolism • Urinary tract infection • Myopathy • Neuropathy

AGE RELATED FACTORS

Dogs with steroid hepatopathy caused by spontaneous hyperadrenocorticism are usually middle–aged to older (> 75% > 9 years old).

ZOONOTIC POTENTIAL N/A

PREGNANCY

Animals with glucocorticoid excess often have reproductive failure characterized by testicular atrophy or abnormal estrus cycle activity.

SYNONYMS

• Glucocorticoid hepatopathy • Corticosteroid hepatopathy

SEE ALSO Hyperadrenocorticism

ABBREVIATIONS

ALP = alkaline phosphatase
ALT = alanine aminotransferase
AST = aspartate transaminase
GGT = gamma glutamyl transferase

References

Strombeck DR, Guilford WG. Small animal gastroenterology. 2nd ed. Davis, CA: Stonegate Publishing Company, 1990:629–647.

Feldman EC. Hyperadrenocorticism. In: Ettinger SJ, Feldman EC, eds. Textbook of veterinary internal medicine. 4th ed. Philadelphia: WB Saunders, 1995: 1538–1578.

Johnson SE. Pathophysiology, laboratory diagnosis, and diseases of the liver. B. Diseases of the liver. In: Ettinger SJ, Feldman EC, eds. Textbook of veterinary internal medicine. 4th ed. Philadelphia: WB Saunders, 1995:1313–1357.

Author Keith P. Richter
Consulting Editor Albert E. Jergens

STORAGE DISEASES, GLYCOGEN

BASICS

OVERVIEW
Glycogen storage disease is an inherited disorder of carbohydrate metabolism characterized by abnormal accumulation of glycogen in tissues. The clinical result of this disorder is hypoglycemia and secondary compensatory changes in amino acid, lipid, and purine metabolism, which account for most of the clinical and biochemical abnormalities. The primary tissues affected are the liver, heart, brain, skeletal muscle, and kidneys. In humans, 11 distinct types of glycogen storage disease are described; however, to date, only 3 have been reported in dogs and cats, type II and VII (dogs) and type IV (cats).

SIGNALMENT
• Dogs and cats are both affected, but the disease is rare. • Because this is a heritable disease of metabolism, it is usually only observed in puppies and kittens; however, if the defect is detected early or is not severe, the animal will survive to adulthood. • No known sex predilection • Affected breeds include German shepherd dog and Norwegian forest cat. • In humans, a genetic basis has been proven for several of these defects, but in dogs and cats the molecular basis for these metabolic defects is not known.

SIGNS

General Comments
Signs are often vague and nonspecific, and depend on which defect in carbohydrate metabolism the patient has.

Historical findings
• Growth failure • Poor development of muscles • Syncope • Seizures

Physical Examiniation Findings
• Hepatomegaly • Large abdomen • Tachypnea • Tachycardia • Weakness • Bleeding diathesis

CAUSES/RISK FACTORS
• Reduced or absent enzyme protein, destabilization of enzyme protein (results in degradation), and deficiency of enzyme translocase, resulting in inability to transport enzyme protein through the cell organelle processing • Enzymes known to be absent or abnormal in patients with human glycogen storage disease include glucose-6-phosphatase, amylo-1, 6-glucosidase, phosphorylase, phosphorylase b, phosphofructokinase, and cAMP dependent kinase.

DIAGNOSIS

DIFFERENTIAL DIAGNOSIS
In general, a degree of clinical suspicion is required to make the diagnosis.
• Metabolic storage diseases of other types (e.g., lysosomal storage disease and mucopolysaccharidosis) • Congenital or developmental anomaly • Neonatal hypoglycemia syndrome • Fading kitten/puppy syndrome

CBC/BIOCHEMISTRY/URINALYSIS
• Nonregenerative anemia and low hemoglobin concentration • Hypoglycemia, especially with short (< 4h) fast, the most consistent abnormality • High BUN, creatinine, ALT, AST, and ALP, and low albumin.
• Proteinuria, hematuria, and isosthenuria in some patients

OTHER LABORATORY TESTS
• Platelet function testing (i.e., buccal mucosal bleeding time) may reveal platelet function abnormality. • A specific enzymatic activity assay of the enzyme in question in leukocytes, liver cells, and muscle cells

IMAGING
• Imaging studies can be used to provide additional evidence of liver disease, but will not provide a definitive diagnosis of glycogen storage disease. • Radiology—hepatomegaly, splenomegaly, and reduced abdominal detail. Cardiomegaly may be observed in older patients. • Ultrasonography—hepatomegaly, splenomegaly, and reduced echogenicity of the hepatic parenchyma may be seen associated with the hepatocellular glycogen deposits. Cardiomyopathy may be detected in older patients.

OTHER DIAGNOSTIC PROCEDURES
Liver or muscle biopsy are required to reach a definitive diagnosis in most patients.

GROSS AND HISTOPATHOLOGIC FINDINGS
The hepatocytes are distended with cytosolic glycogen, and the surrounding sinusoids are compressed from the massive glycogen accumulation.

TREATMENT
The main objective of treatment is to control hypoglycemia, thus minimizing clinical manifestations and secondary biochemical abnormalities. This can be accomplished by feeding a high carbohydrate/low fat diet frequently (every 1-3 hours). The congenital nature of the disease makes diagnosis and treatment difficult, and it is often diagnosed at necropsy. General supportive care, in addition to nutritional management, is necessary. In humans, gene therapy is being explored and may soon become the definitive therapy.

MEDICATIONS

DRUGS AND FLUIDS
Fluid administration may be required in puppies and kittens too weak to eat. Dextrose containing solutions are best (e.g., lactated Ringer's solution with 5% dextrose), and may be given intraosseously if necessary.

CONTRAINDICATIONS/ POSSIBLE INTERACTIONS N/A

FOLLOW-UP
Routine monitoring of hydration status, growth of animal, and blood glucose concentration

MISCELLANEOUS

SEE ALSO
• Storage Disease, Lysosomal • Mucopolysaccharidosis

ABBREVIATIONS
ALP =alkaline phosphatase
ALT = alanine aminotransferase
AST = aspartate aminotransferase
BUN = blood urea nitrogen

References
Glycogen storage diseases. In: Ettinger SW, ed. Small animal internal medicine. Philadelphia: WB Saunders, 1989.
Author Debra L. Zoran
Consulting Editor Albert E. Jergens

BASICS

OVERVIEW
• Rare inherited disorders caused by partial or complete deficiency of a lysosomal enzyme or an enzyme-activator protein which leads to intracytoplasmic accumulation (storage) of the substrate of that enzyme • Storage products can be proteins, carbohydrates, or lipids. • Many different types reported in both dogs and cats

SIGNALMENT
Several breeds are susceptible:
• Dogs—German shorthaired pointer, English setter, beagle, cairn terrier, bluetick hound, West Highland terrier, and Sidney silky terrier • Cats—Siamese, Korat, and domestic shorthair • Most affected in animals <1 year old • Inheritance usually autosomal recessive or X-linked

SIGNS
• Many organ systems are affected, but neurologic signs tend to predominate. • Animals usually are normal at birth, but fail to thrive and manifest a variety of neurologic signs within the first few months of life, suggesting multifocal neurologic disease. • Signs of cerebellar dysfunction are common, but patients can have many other signs including ataxia, exercise intolerance, seizures, behavioral changes, and visual deficits. • Severity of enzyme deficiency varies, so patients have various degrees of severity of clinical signs. • Carrier animals can be affected with a milder form of the disease. • Some patients have other signs such as organomegaly or skeletal malformations.

CAUSES AND RISK FACTORS
• A genetic deletion or mutation that causes an absolute or partial deficiency of a lysosomal enzyme or activator protein, or deficient production of enzymes that do not have normal biological activity • Susceptible breeds

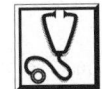

DIAGNOSIS

DIFFERENTIAL DIAGNOSIS
• Patients with metabolic encephalopathy usually have episodic clinical signs, and results of hemogram, biochemistry analysis, and urinalysis are often diagnostic. • Toxicities can be ruled in by the acute onset of the clinical signs and a history of exposure. • Patients with cerebellar hypoplasia have onset of signs at 3-6 weeks of age and the disease is nonprogressive. • Patients with cerebellar abiotrophy have deficits limited to the cerebellum. In early stages of both diseases, it may be difficult to differentiate one from the other without specific tests. • Infectious meningoencephalomyelitis such as FIP is differentiated by CSF analysis and possibly other signs such as chorioretinitis.

CBC/BIOCHEMISTRY/URINALYSIS
• Cytoplasmic vacuolation of lymphocytes in some patients • Abnormal accumulation of substances (eg, oligosaccharide in alpha mannosidosis) in urine in some patients

OTHER LABORATORY TESTS N/A

IMAGING N/A

OTHER DIAGNOSTIC PROCEDURES
Specific diagnosis is made by demonstrating low enzyme activity in preparations of serum, brain, viscera, leukocytes, or skin fibroblasts.

TREATMENT
• Generally as outpatient unless severe deficits preclude nursing care at home

• The animal's activity needs to be restricted to safe areas. Avoid stairs.
• Insure proper intake of food—animals often debilitated
• Bone marrow transplantation has been used experimentally with some success in human medicine.
• Only primary treatment is preventative through control of breeding and genetic counseling.
• Animals may be at high risk of developing secondary infection and should be closely monitored; initiate appropriate treatment if infection develops.

MEDICATIONS

DRUGS AND FLUIDS
Intravenous administration of fluids if the patient is dehydrated

CONTRAINDICATIONS/POSSIBLE INTERACTIONS N/A

FOLLOW-UP
These diseases are progressive and ultimately fatal.

MISCELLANEOUS
Pedigree analysis of affected animals may be useful in diagnosis and is important for identification of potential carrier animals.

Reference
Jolly RD. Lysosomal storage diseases. Neuropathol Appl Neurobiol 1978;4:419-427.
Author Mary O. Smith
Consulting Editor Joane M. Parent

STRONGYLOIDIASIS

BASICS

OVERVIEW
Neonatal infection of paramucosa of small intestine by Strongyloides canis and S. felis (stercoralis) associated with an acute to chronic diarrhea. Transcolostral transmission to neonates, skin penetration by infective larvae, or ingestion of infective larvae. Infection may persist by autoinfection. Relatively host-specific; possibly transmissible to humans. Also Strongyloides tumefaciens in cats causing adenomatous mass in colon.

SIGNALMENT
• Dogs and cats. • Neonatal diarrhea of pups and kittens with transcolostral transmission

SIGNS

Historical Findings
• Neonatal diarrhea or constipation
• Dermatitis

Physical Examination Findings
• Debilitated pups, kittens • Dermatitis

CAUSES AND RISK FACTORS
• Transcolostral transmission • Possibility of autoinfection • Skin penetration by infective larvae

DIAGNOSIS

DIFFERENTIAL DIAGNOSIS
• Toxocara infections • Viral infections
• No colostrum

CBC/BIOCHEMISTRY/URINALYSIS
Normal for age

OTHER LABORATORY TESTS
Fecal examination for small (~50 μm length) larvated eggs

IMAGING N/A

OTHER DIAGNOSTIC PROCEDURES
N/A

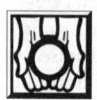

TREATMENT
• An adulticide/larvicide recommended for neonatal infection of small intestine with possible respiratory migration by infective larvae.

MEDICATIONS

DRUGS AND FLUIDS
• Fenbendazole (Panacur) 50mg/kg q24h PO for 5 days as a paste or a suspension given by stomach tube
• Ivermectin 50 μg/kg PO 1 time (extra-label use) • Fluid therapy might be warranted

CONTRAINDICATIONS/POSSIBLE INTERACTIONS
• Difficulty with administration of efficacious anthelmintic

FOLLOW-UP
Fecal examination for Strongyloides larvae or eggs posttreatment

MISCELLANEOUS

ZOONOTIC PORTENIAL Yes

Reference
Bowman DD. Georgi's parasitology for veterinarians. 6th ed. Philadelphia: WB Saunders, 1994;154–58.
Author Robert M. Corwin
Consulting Editor Brent D. Jones

BASICS

OVERVIEW

Strychnine is a potent, seizurogenic alkaloid toxin derived from the seeds of Strychnos nux-vomica and S. ignatii. It is used to control rats, moles, gophers, and predators. Absorption is rapid and onset of clinical signs occurs in 10-120 minutes. The toxin reversibly blocks the binding of the inhibitory neurotransmitter glycine, resulting in an unchecked reflex stimulation. It is eliminated as hepatic metabolites and the parent compound in the urine. The cause of death is apnea and hypoxia due to rigidity of the muscles of respiration. Baits containing > 0.5% strychnine are limited to use by certified applicators. Baits containing less than 0.5% strychnine are available to the general public.

SIGNALMENT

Poisoning is seen in birds, mammals, and other vertebrates.

SIGNS

• Violent tetanic seizures, which can be initiated by physical, visible, or auditory stimuli • Extensor rigidity • Muscle stiffness • Opisthotonus • Tachycardia and hypertension • Hyperthermia • Acidosis (metabolic and respiratory) • Apnea and hypoxia • Vomiting (rare)

CAUSES AND RISK FACTORS

• Malicious poisonings are still fairly common. • Poisoning by direct exposure to baits is more common in dogs than other species. • Relay toxicoses by the ingestion of poisoned rodents and birds has occurred. • Lethal dose in dogs, > 0.2 mg/kg • LD50 in cats, 0.5 mg/kg

DIAGNOSIS

DIFFERENTIAL DIAGNOSES

• Lead, nicotine, amphetamine, metaldehyde, chocolate, zinc phosphide, tremorgenic mycotoxin, antidepressant, 4-aminopyridine, cocaine, pyrethrin/pyrethroid, 1080 (fluroacetate), caffeine, LSD, organochlorine insecticide • Uremia, hepatic failure, neoplasia, hypoglycemia, encephalitides, heat stroke, trauma, ischemia, and tetanus

CBC/BIOCHEMISTRY/URINALYSIS

• Acidosis • High CPK and lactic dehydrogenase • Myoglobinuria

OTHER LABORATORY TESTS

Analysis of stomach content, liver, kidneys, and urine for strychnine. The kidneys and urine can be negative if the animal dies too rapidly.

IMAGING N/A

OTHER DIAGNOSTIC PROCEDURES

Inducing a seizure with a stimulus IS NOT DIAGNOSTIC of strychnine toxicosis and could be lethal.

GROSS AND HISTOPATHOLOGIC FINDINGS

• Gross and histopathologic findings associated with trauma from the seizure activity • Baits can frequently be found in the stomach content. They may be color coded red or green.

TREATMENT

GENERAL LIFE SUPPORT

• Primary goal is to prevent asphyxia and control seizures. • Complete anesthesia and artificial respiration may be required. • Up to 48 hours of in-hospital treatment may be required. • The patient should be kept in a quiet, dimly lighted room.

DECONTAMINATION

• Decontamination lessens the duration and severity of signs. • Gastric or enterogastric lavage lessens absorption. • Fluid diuresis enhances elimination. • Emesis should not be induced unless it is within minutes of ingestion and the animal is asymptomatic.

MEDICATIONS

DRUGS AND FLUIDS

Decontamination

• Activated charcoal (2 gm/kg PO) • Cathartic-sorbitol (2.1 gm/kg PO) or magnesium sulfate (0.5 gm/kg PO)

Seizure control

• Diazepam (may not be effective) • Pentobarbital to effect • Glycerol guiacolate (110 mg/kg PO repeat as needed) • Methocarbamol (150 mg/kg PO repeat at 90 mg/kg as needed) • Inhalation anesthesia

Diuresis

• Normal saline with 5% mannitol (7 mg/kg/hr) • Urinary acidification with ammonium chloride (150 mg/kg) will increase elimination.

CONTRAINDICATIONS/POSSIBLE INTERACTIONS

• DO NOT acidify with ammonium chloride if the patient is acidotic • DO NOT use ketamine. • DO NOT use morphine.

FOLLOW-UP

• Monitor for secondary renal damage from myoglobinuria and possible tubular cast development. • Guarded prognosis until seizures are controlled, but good prognosis once seizures are controlled.

MISCELLANEOUS

SEE ALSO

Poisoning (Intoxication)

ABBREVIATION

CPK = creatine phosphokinase

Reference

Osweiler GD. Strychnine poisoning. In: Kirk RW, ed. Current veterinary therapy VIII. Philadelphia: WB Saunders, 1983:98-100.
Author Jeffrey O. Hall
Consulting Editor Gary Osweiler

SUBINVOLUTION OF PLACENTAL SITES

BASICS

OVERVIEWS
• Failure or delay of normal postpartum uterine involution • Eosinophilic masses of collagen at placental sites fail to slough at 3 to 4 weeks postpartum. • Fetal trophoblastic cells fail to regress normally; instead, they invade the maternal myometrium. • Cause of events unknown; hormonal or uterine causes are not suspected

SIGNALMENT
• Documented only in dogs • Bitches < 3 years • Seen with first litter • No breed predilection

SIGNS

Historical Findings
• Animal examined 6-12 weeks postpartum
• Serosanguineous vulvar discharge beyond 6 weeks postpartum • No systemic signs

Physical Examination Findings
• Serosanguineous vulvar discharge • Firm, spherical structure within uterus on abdominal palpation

CAUSES AND RISK FACTORS
• Cause of events unknown • Hormonal causes unlikely since only some of placental sites may be involved • Uterine disease unlikely since first litter prevalence is high.

DIAGNOSIS

DIFFERENTIAL DIAGNOSIS
• Metritis—vaginal cytologic and physical examinations differentiate • Vaginitis—vaginal cytologic examination differentiates • Vaginal neoplasia—vaginal cytologic examination and vaginal endoscopy differentiate • Uterine neoplasia—ultrasonography or exploratory laparotomy differentiate • Cystitis—vaginal cytologic examination and urinalysis differentiate
• Coagulopathy—clotting times differentiate
• Trauma • Endogenous estrogen stimulation

such as might be seen in a bitch with an extremely shortened interestrous interval • Exogenous estrogen stimulation

CBC/BIOCHEMISTRY/URINALYSIS
• Results usually normal • Serology for B. Canis negative

OTHER LABORATORY TESTS N/A

IMAGING
Uterine ultrasonograpy reveals focal uterine wall thickening along with a lumen containing echogenic fluid.

OTHER DIAGNOSTIC PROCEDURES
• Vaginal cytologic examination—key for diagnosis. Results reveal erythrocytes, parabasal epithelial cells, and the pathognomonic trophoblastic cells (not always found.) • Grossly the sites are characterized by a thickened, hemorrhagic area that may be nodular. • Definitive diagnosis relies on histopathologic examination revealing eosinophilic collagen masses with trophoblasts extending into the myometrium.
• Guarded vaginal culture if vaginal cytologic examination or hemogram supports a diagnosis of secondary metritis

TREATMENT
• Outpatient treatment is typical.
• Spontaneous remission occurs before or at next cycle.
• Owner should be aware of rare possibility of excessive hemorrhage and taught to monitor mucous membrane color.
• Ovariohysterectomy is curative and treatment of choice if future breeding not desired.
• Surgical curetagge of subinvoluted sites may also be performed.
• Treatment is reserved for the rare patient that develops anemia, metritis, or peritonitis.

MEDICATIONS

DRUGS AND FLUIDS
• Drug therapy is generally not successful.

• Severely affected patients may require blood transfusion (rare).

CONTRAINDICATIONS/POSSIBLE INTERACTIONS
• Ecbolics can cause uterine rupture.
• Progestational drugs increase the risk of metritis, which may mimic pyometra.

FOLLOW-UP

PATIENT MONITORING
• Mucous membrane color and amount of discharge • PCV if anemia is a concern
• Changes in discharge color or odor plus vaginal cytologic examination and culture to diagnose secondary infection

POSSIBLE COMPLICATIONS
• Infection, blood loss anemia, uterine rupture (all rare) • Spontaneous resolution is the norm. • Recurrence is not expected.

EXPECTED COURSE AND PROGNOSIS
Prognosis for future reproduction is excellent in animals with spontaneous resolution.

MISCELLANEOUS

References

Wheeler SL. Subinvolution of placental sites in the bitch. In: Morrow DA, ed. Current therapy in theriogenology 2. Philadelphia: WB Saunders, 1986;513-515.

Johnston SD. Subinvolution of placental sites. In: Kirk RW, ed. Current veterinary therapy IX. Philadelphia: WB Saunders, 1986;1231-1233.

Author Joni L. Freshman
Consulting Editor Sara K. Lyle

BASICS

OVERVIEW

• Malignant neoplasm believed to arise from primitive mesenchymal precursor cells outside the synovial membrane and bursa and not the synovial membrane • Histologically characterized as having two cellular elements, epitheloid and fibroblastic • Highly invasive locally • Most commonly occurs in the stifle, elbow, carpal, tibiotarsal, and phalangeal joints • Clinical stage and histologic grade important influence on survival • Metastasis detected in up to 22% of patients on examination; 41% of dogs ultimately develop metastasis.

SIGNALMENT

• Large-breed dogs, most commonly mixed breed with golden retriever overrepresented in some studies • Median age 9 years; range, 3-13 years • Rarely reported in cats

SIGNS

Historical Findings

• Lameness • Visible or palpable mass • Weight loss • Anorexia • Many patients typically have clinical signs for several months to years before diagnosis.

Physical Examination Findings

• Palpable mass associated with a joint, with swelling typically involving both sides of the joint • Primarily found in extremities • Regional lymph nodes large or normal • Pain on palpation of affected joint common

CAUSES AND RISK FACTORS

Unknown

DIAGNOSIS

DIFFERENTIAL DIAGNOSIS

• Osteoarthritis • Sarcoma or carcinoma arising from soft tissue region of the joint • Osteomyelitis (fungal or bacterial) • Primary bone tumor • Villonodular synovitis

CBC/BIOCHEMISTRY/URINALYSIS

Results usually normal

OTHER LABORATORY TESTS N/A

IMAGING

• Radiographs of primary lesion may only show soft tissue mass. • Bone or subchondral lysis usually involves both bones of the joint, unlike that seen in patients with primary bone tumor. • A periosteal reaction is seen on radiographs in some patients. • Thoracic radiography to detect metastasis

OTHER DIAGNOSTIC PROCEDURES

• Biopsy of suspected tumor. Include wedge biopsy of soft tissue mass as well as Jamshidi biopsy of affected bone. It is not necessary to enter the joint. • Cytologic evaluation of regional lymph nodes when possible

TREATMENT

• Amputation currently the treatment of choice—forequarter amputation for tumors of forelimb; coxofemoral disarticulation for tumors of stifle; proximal femoral amputation for tumors of or below tibial tarsal joint • Median survival with amputation alone— 36 months for patients with invasive tumors without regional lymph node involvement or distant metastasis • Anecdotal reports of long-term survival in patients with inoperable tumors treated by chemotherapy (doxorubicin HCL and cyclophosphamide) without surgery • Local resection followed by radiotherapy to the tumor bed beneficial in humans—not yet explored in animals • Metastasis primarily to lungs and regional nodes • Stump recurrence occasionally seen

MEDICATIONS

DRUGS AND FLUIDS

Although doxorubicin HCL and cyclophosphamide are used to treat patients with inoperable cancer, no evidence supports the use of chemotherapy after amputation.

FOLLOW-UP

• Thoracic radiography and careful physical examination (especially regional lymph nodes) monthly for 3 months followed by every third month thereafter for 2 years • Prognosis excellent for patients with localized disease treated by amputation • Prognosis poor for patients with tumors and regional lymph node involvement or distant metastasis and tumors of high histologic grade

MISCELLANEOUS

ABBREVIATIONS None

Reference

Vail DM, Powers BE, Getzy DM, et al. Evaluation of prognostic factors for dogs with synovial sarcoma: 36 cases (1986-1991). J Am Vet Med Assoc 1994;205:1300-1307.

Author Joyce E. Obradovich

Consulting Editor Wallace B. Morrison

TAPEWORMS

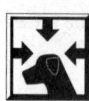

BASICS

OVERVIEW
Tapeworm infections of small intestine with Taenia spp, esp. T. pisiformis of dogs and T. taeniaeformis of cats, and Dipylidium caninum of dogs and cats. Taeniids are transmitted by predation of rabbits or rodents; Dipylidium is flea-vectored with flea maggots picking up tapeworm eggs in dog or cat feces and transmitted by adult fleas when ingested by dogs or cats. No apparent harm done to host; may have perianal pruritus.

SIGNALMENT
Dogs and cats

SIGNS
• Chains of segments or single segments on feces; rectangular (Taenia) or beadlike (Dipylidium) • Dragging or rubbing anus on the ground due to perianal pruritus with Dipylidium • Segments pasted to perianal skin

CAUSES AND RISK FACTORS
• Eating viscera of rabbits, rodents for taeniid infections • Fleas in environment for Dipylidium infections

DIAGNOSIS

DIFFERENTIAL DIAGNOSIS
Anal gland impaction

CBC/BIOCHEMISTRY/URINALYSIS
Normal

OTHER LABORATORY TESTS N/A

IMAGING N/A

OTHER DIAGNOSTIC PROCEDURES
• Scotch tape pressed to perianal skin for Dipylidium egg packets; single egg ~50 μm diameter, pale yellow, hexacanth embryo
• Taenia eggs spherical, brown, ~30–35 μm, hexacanth embryo (6 apparent hooks on embryo)

OTHER TESTS
Check perianal glands

TREATMENT
• Treat as outpatient
• Discuss need for flea control to prevent recurrence of Dipylidium

MEDICATIONS

DRUGS AND FLUIDS
• Fenbendazole (Panacur) effective at 50mg/kg q24h PO for 5 days for taeniid infections
• Febantel (Vercom) 10 mg/kg q24h PO for 3 days effective for taeniid infections
• Praziquantel (Droncit) 5 mg/kg PO once for Taenia, Dipylidium
• Epsiprantel (Cestex) 5.5mg/kg PO for dogs, 2.8mg/kg PO cats for Taenia, Dipylidium

• Flea control is necessary for control of Dipylidium

CONTRAINDICATIONS/POSSIBLE INTERACTIONS
Do not use praziquantel or epsiprantel for puppies or kittens less than 4 weeks old

FOLLOW-UP
Fecal examination for tapeworm segments

MISCELLANEOUS

ZOONOTIC POTENTIAL
Humans can become infected with Dipylidium caninum following ingestion of infected fleas.

Reference
Bowman DD. Georgi's parasitology for veterinarians. 6th ed. Philadelphia: WB Saunders, 1994;137–150.

Author Robert M. Corwin
Consulting Editor Brent D. Jones

BASICS

OVERVIEW
• Taurine is an amino acid that has many biological roles in many different tissues. Its highest concentrations are in the heart, retina, central nervous system, leukocytes and skeletal muscles. One of taurine's best defined functions is conjugation of bile in mammals.
• Taurine deficiency has been associated with reversible myocardial failure and central retinal degeneration in the cat. Taurine is a dietary essential amino acid in the cat because cats lack the ability to synthesize taurine from other amino acids. • Taurine deficiency has been associated with a reversible myocardial failure in dogs and foxes.

SIGNALMENT
• Cats—uncommon because commercially available cat food is no longer deficient in taurine • Dogs—American cocker spaniels, possibly golden retrievers

SIGNS
See Cardiomyopathy, Dilated (cats and dogs).

CAUSES AND RISK FACTORS
• Cats fed a vegetarian diet or home-cooked diet that may be taurine deficient. • The cause or risk factors associated with myocardial taurine deficiency in dogs are not known.

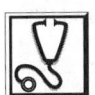

DIAGNOSIS

DIFFERENTIAL DIAGNOSIS
Idiopathic dilated cardiomyopathy
See Cardiomyopathy, Dilated (cats and dogs).

CBC/BIOCHEMISTRY/URINALYSIS
No characteristic abnormalities

OTHER LABORATORY TESTS
• Plasma or whole blood taurine concentrations less than 25 nmoles/ml is considered too low in dogs and cats. This assay is performed at a limited number of institutions.
• Prolonged fasting in cats has been associated with a low plasma taurine level.

IMAGING
See Cardiomyopathy, Dilated (cats and dogs)

OTHER DIAGNOSTIC TESTS
Endomyocardial biopsy with quantitative taurine analysis may help confirm taurine deficiency, although the risk and cost of the procedure typically outweighs the benefit.

TREATMENT
Conventional heart failure therapy is used in addition to the taurine supplementation.

MEDICATIONS

DRUGS AND FLUIDS

Taurine Supplementation
• Cats—250 mg PO bid
• Dogs—250-500 mg PO bid
• In the American cocker spaniel, carnitine supplementation is also recommended.

CONTRAINDICATIONS/POSSIBLE INTERACTIONS
No recognized adverse effects or interactions are known.

FOLLOW-UP
• Repeat echocardiogram in 3-6 months after initiating taurine supplementation to determine efficacy of therapy. • If after this period of time no significant improvement is seen in contractility, you may wish to discontinue the supplementation.

MISCELLANEOUS
• Taurine supplements are available over-the-counter in most health food stores. • Taurine supplementation is relatively inexpensive compared to carnitine supplementation.

References
Kramer GA, Kittleson MD, Fox PR, Lewis J, Pion PD. Plasma taurine concentrations in normal and in dogs with heart disease. J Vet Intern Med 1995;9(4):253-258.
Pion PD, Kittleson MD, Rogers QR, et al. Myocardial failure in cats associated with low plasma taurine: a reversible cardiomyopathy. Science 1987;237:764-768.

Author Terri C. DeFrancesco
Consulting Editors Larry P. Tilley and Francis W. K. Smith, Jr.

TESTICULAR DEGENERATION AND HYPOPLASIA

BASICS

OVERVIEW
• Hypoplasia is used to describe a variety of histologic lesions thought to be congenital (though not often obvious until after puberty) or heritable. • Degeneration implies histologic changes in the testes after puberty and can be differentiated from testicular hypoplasia by the increased thickness of the basement membrane in the degenerated testis.

SIGNALMENT
• Any age or breed • Young, azoospermic, never-fertile dogs with small testes may be hypoplastic. • Old azoospermic or oligospermic, previously-fertile dogs with small testes are probably suffering from testicular degeneration.

SIGNS
• Rarely any specific signs in dogs with hypoplasia other than small testes • In dogs with degeneration, any previous scrotal or testicular lesion can be related.

CAUSES AND RISK FACTORS
• Degeneration—heat, irradiation, metals (e.g., lead salts, cadmium, and organic mercurial compounds), nitrogen-containing and halogenated compounds, a variety of other toxins, orchitis, steroid hormones (e.g., the estrogen secreted by a sertoli cell tumor) and other hormonal abnormalities such as hypothyroidism, hypocortisolism, and hyperadrenocorticism. Increasing age (6.3% of beagles maintained to 7.75 years had incomplete spermatogenesis) and arterial sclerosis. Some chemotherapeutic agents (e.g., cimetadine, ketoconazole, and nitrofurans). • Hypoplasia—Klinefelter's syndrome (i.e., extra X chromosome) and hypogonadotropic hypogonadism (can be acquired from traumatic or neoplastic lesion of the pituitary gland)

DIAGNOSIS

DIFFERENTIAL DIAGNOSIS
Spermatocele, sperm granuloma, orchitis, neoplasia, and ejaculatory failure (e.g., retrograde).

CBC/BIOCHEMISTRY/URINALYSIS
N/A

OTHER LABORATORY TESTS
To differentiate from blockage (spermatocele), use canine follicle stimulating hormone (FSH) assay. High FSH concentration indicates incomplete spermatogenesis associated with hypoplasia or degeneration.

IMAGING N/A

OTHER DIAGNOSTIC PROCEDURES
• Testicular biopsy in patients with azoospermia—fine needle to identify presence of long spermatids and spermatozoa, trucut for tissue plug, and open incisional for the most complete histopathologic diagnosis; tissue for sectioning should be fixed in Bouin's or Zenker's fixative. • Normal spermatogenesis indicates blockage in azoospermic dogs. • Basement membrane thickness differentiates hypoplasia from degeneration. • Karyotype identifies dogs with extra X chromosome or other numerical or structural chromosome anomaly.

TREATMENT

• When degeneration is linked to pituitary, adrenal gland, thyroid gland, or other metabolic disruption, correction of underlying cause is the goal.
• In the absence of a specific diagnosis, gonadotropic hormones are sometimes tried with rare anecdotal success.
• Semen analysis should be performed at least 60 days after correcting the underlying cause before reversibility can be assessed.

MEDICATIONS

DRUGS AND FLUIDS
• Human chorionic gonadotropin 500 IU SQ 2 times/week
• Equine chorionic gonadotropin (PMSG) 20 IU/kg SQ 3 times/week.

CONTRAINDICATIONS/POSSIBLE INTERACTIONS N/A

FOLLOW-UP N/A

MISCELLANEOUS

References

McEntee K. Reproductive pathology of domestic animals. San Diego: Academic Press. 1990.

Feldman EC, Nelson RW. Canine and feline endocrinology and reproduction. Philadelphia: WB Saunders, 1987.

Author Rolf E. Larsen
Consulting Editor Sara K. Lyle

BASICS

OVERVIEW
• Clostridium tetani is an obligate, anaerobic, spore-forming, gram-positive rod found in soil and as part of the normal bacterial flora of the intestinal tract of mammals; predilection for contaminated, necrotic, anaerobic wounds (puncture, surgery, lacerations, burns, frostbite, open fractures, abrasions)

Pathophysiology
• Germinating spores in wounds produce potent exotoxin tetanospasmin (tetanus toxin) • Tetanus is found worldwide, especially in the tropics. • Tetanus spores are resistant to disinfectants and to the effects of environmental exposure.

SIGNALMENT
• Tetanus occurs occasionally in the dog. • Rarely in cats

SIGNS
• Appear a few days to few months after spores enter wound (fracture, surgery, puncture) • Necrotic wound often apparent on exam. Note: wound may have healed over!

Physical Examination Findings
Localized Tetanus
• Mild rigidity of muscles or leg nearest the site of spore inoculation (wound) • Stiffness of (hind) limbs; stilted gate • Mild weakness and incoordination • Can resolve spontaneously (reflecting partial immunity to tetanospasmin) or can be prodromal to generalized tetanus (occurring when enough toxin gains access to CNS)
Progressive/Generalized Tetanus
• Tail stretches out • Progressive tetany of muscles to point of "sawhorse" appearance • Convulsions (clonic) of limbs; whole body convulsions (opisthotonus) • Pain during contractions • Difficulty breathing (dyspnea) • Eyelids retract (visus sardonicus) • Wrinkled forehead • Erect ears • Grinning appearance (commissure of lips retracted) • Third eyelid falls (prolapse) when head is touched • Recession of eyeballs within orbit (enophthalmos) • Difficulty opening jaws (lockjaw, trismus), salivation, difficulty eating (dysphagia) • Fever • Painful urination (dysuria) and constipation • Stimulation (sudden movement, sound, touch) causes tetanic muscle spasms. • Death occurs during spasm of laryngeal and respiratory muscles resulting in fatal acute asphyxia or when respiratory muscles are sufficiently paralyzed.

CAUSES AND RISK FACTORS
• Unattended wounds (punctures, surgical, compound bone fractures) create portal of entry for spores. • Outdoor pets greater opportunity for acquiring wounds

DIAGNOSIS

DIFFERENTIAL DIAGNOSIS
Differentiate from intoxications mimicking tetanus (i.e., lead and strychnine poisoning).

CBC/BIOCHEMISTRY/URINALYSIS
• CBC—initial leukopenia switches to moderate leukocytosis; then a gradual return to "normal" range • Chemistry profile—some increase in AST, CPK, and LDH as a result of muscle damage during later stages of disease • Urinalysis—essentially normal except high myoglobin from muscles damaged by constant excitation

OTHER LABORATORY TESTS
• Serology—antitetanus antibody often undetectable in serum of patients • Culture—attempt to culture wounds for C. tetani or detect toxin in serum or wounds (by mouse neutralization) are usually unrewarding; CSF and blood cultures for bacterial pathogens of meningitis

IMAGING N/A

OTHER DIAGNOSTIC PROCEDURES N/A

TREATMENT
• Good supportive, constant nursing care is important on inpatient basis for prolonged period (3-4 weeks); care is expensive. Prognosis dependent on number of factors—the more toxin bound to nerves, the poorer the prognosis; better prognosis if remove source of additional toxin by debriding wound, etc.
• Assess airway and ventilation; may be necessary to perform endotracheal intubation; tracheostomy may be necessary later
• Keep patient in darkened, quiet area; do not disturb; keep on soft bedding; prevent decubital ulcers
• Debride wound to remove necrotic tissue, irrigate with physiologic salt solution, provide drainage; expose to air
• Place soft, small bore nasal feeding tube and feed gruel mixed with water

MEDICATIONS

DRUGS AND FLUIDS
• Administer adequate fluid (lactated Ringer's) to remove products of muscle spasms (myoglobin).
• Tranquilize (acetylpromizine) or sedate (diazepam) to control tetany and decrease rigidity.
• Test for hypersensitivity reaction; then administer human tetanus immunoglobulin (TIG = 500-3000 U IM at multiple sites, especially proximal to wound) or equine tetanus antitoxin (10,000 U IV).
• Administer adsorbed tetanus toxoid IM
• Administer penicillin systemically and locally into the wound (20,000 IU/kg q12h for 5 days; use crystalline penicillin on the first day and procaine penicillin thereafter). Note: Antibiotics have no effect against toxin that is already bound to nerves!

CONTRAINDICATIONS/POSSIBLE INTERACTIONS
• Glucocorticoids • Atropine • Narcotics

FOLLOW-UP

PATIENT MONITORING
•Prevent skin breakdown (ulcers) and peripheral nerve palsies by cautious moving of stabilized patient; monitor blood pressure and electrocardiogram.

PREVENTION/AVOIDANCE
• Vaccinate with tetanus toxoid. • Prevent skin wound trauma (clean runs and yards of wire, glass, etc.). • Early and thorough wound irrigation with hydrogen peroxide, debridement, draining, especially in known tetanus-prone wounds • Administer penicillin for a minimum of 3 days for all deep contaminated wounds.

POSSIBLE COMPLICATIONS N/A

EXPECTED COURSE AND PROGNOSIS
Course of recovery is slow; requires rehabilitation to regain full use of limbs; unattended disease usually has fatal outcome

MISCELLANEOUS

ZOONOTIC POTENTIAL
No zoonotic potential; however, tetanus spores are ubiquitous in environment

Reference
Matthews BR, Forbes DC. Tetanus in a dog. Can Vet J 1985;26:159-161.
Author Patrick L. McDonough
Consulting Editor Fredric W. Scott

TETRALOGY OF FALLOT

BASICS

OVERVIEW
• Consists of a ventricular septal defect (VSD), pulmonic stenosis, and an overriding aorta and right ventricular hypertrophy. The aorta straddles the malalignment VSD (Figure). The VSD is usually large, having an area that equals or exceeds that of the open aortic valve. • The hemodynamics of this malformation are determined primarily by the size of the VSD and the severity of right ventricular outflow tract obstruction. A large VSD allows equilibration of left and right ventricular pressures; shunt direction is then determined by the relationship between peripheral vascular resistance and the resistance to right ventricular ejection. Severe right ventricular outflow tract obstruction results in a right-to-left shunt. In this case, cyanosis and compensatory erythrocytosis are prominent clinical features. • An uncommon congenital defect, but the most common congenital cardiac malformation causing cyanosis in dogs and cats.

SIGNALMENT
• Dogs and cats. Uncommon in both species • English bull dogs and keeshond predisposed

SIGNS

Historical Findings
• Weakness • Syncope • Shortness of breath

Physical Examination Findings
• A systolic ejection murmur caused by right ventricular outflow tract obstruction in most animals. Some animals with hyperviscosity and severe pulmonary stenosis do not have murmurs. • Cyanosis in most animals. The degree of cyanosis depends on the direction and volume of shunt. If the degree of right ventricular outflow tract obstruction is mild, the direction of the shunt may be left to

right. In this case, cyanosis is absent and the pathophysiology is that of an isolated VSD. • Arterial pulses usually normal • Congestive heart failure occurs rarely, possibly because the right ventricle can unload into the left.

CAUSES AND RISK FACTORS
Congenital. Polygenic inheritance of a continuum of conotruncal defects that includes tetralogy of Fallot has been shown in keeshonds. Genetic and environmental factors probably contribute to development of naturally occurring tetralogy of Fallot.

DIAGNOSIS

DIFFERENTIAL DIAGNOSIS
• Pulmonic stenosis, aortic stenosis, ventricular septal defect, and atrial septal defect all can cause left basilar ejection quality murmurs. • Animals with severe pulmonic stenosis and a right-to-left atrial level shunt may have similar findings on physical examination. • Other anatomic right-to-left shunts (patent ductus arteriosus or VSD with pulmonary hypertension) do not cause murmurs. Differential cyanosis is observed if a PDA shunts right to left.

CBC/BIOCHEMISTRY/URINALYSIS
• Compensatory erythrocytosis if the shunt is right to left. • Other clinicopathologic findings usually normal

OTHER LABORATORY TESTS N/A

IMAGING

Thoracic Radiographic Findings
• Variable degree of right ventricular enlargement • The ascending aorta may be prominent. • The pulmonary vessels are small.

Echocardiographic Findings
• Right ventricular hypertrophy • Large VSD visualized directly • Straddling of the VSD by

the aorta • Contrast echocardiography delineates a right-to-left shunt.

Angiocardiography
• Reveals the malalignment VSD, right ventricular hypertrophy, pulmonic stenosis, and direction of shunt. • Nonselective angiography may confirm the diagnosis in small animals.

Oximetry
Used to confirm the presence of peripheral desaturation of hemoglobin

OTHER DIAGNOSTIC PROCEDURES

Electrocardiographic Findings
• Right ventricular hypertrophy pattern in most dogs and cats • Various intraventricular conduction disturbances have been observed in cats.

TREATMENT
• Most animals can be treated as outpatients. Exercise restriction recommended. Definitive surgical correction requires cardiopulmonary bypass. Palliative surgical procedures that enhance pulmonary blood flow have been attempted . • Erythrocytosis is treated by periodic phlebotomy to maintain a PCV of 62-68%.

MEDICATIONS

DRUGS AND FLUIDS
Nonselective beta adrenergic antagonists such as propranolol may be palliative. These drugs act as negative inotropes and prevent the physiologic drop in peripheral vascular resistance that occurs during exercise. These hemodynamic effects serve to limit right-to-left shunting. Propranolol may also have a favorable effect on the oxyhemoglobin dissociation curve.

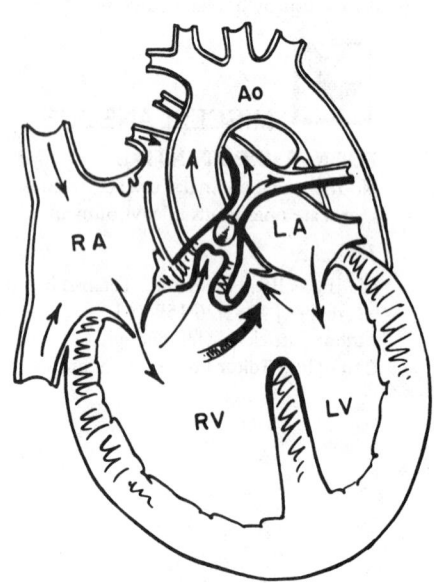

Classic tetralogy of Fallot. RA = right atrium, LA = left atrium, RV = right ventricle, LV = left ventricle, AO = aorta. (From Roberts W. Adult congenital heart disease. Philadelphia: F.A. Davis Co., 1987, with permission.)

CONTRAINDICATIONS/POSSIBLE INTERACTIONS

Vasodilators contraindicated

FOLLOW-UP

• PCV should be monitored every 1-3 months • Breeding of affected animals not advised • Bacterial endocarditis, neurologic complications associated with erythrocytosis, arrhythmias, and sudden death are potential sequelae. • The prognosis is poor. Most animals with clinical signs live less than 1 year, although survivals > 3 years have been documented.

MISCELLANEOUS

ABBREVIATIONS

VSD = ventricular septal defect
PCV = packed cell volume

Reference

Bonagura JD. Congenital heart disease. In: Ettinger SJ, ed. Textbook of veterinary internal medicine. 3rd ed. Philadelphia: WB Saunders, 1989.
Author Jonathan A. Abbott
Consulting Editors Larry P. Tilley, Francis W. K. Smith, Jr.

THROMBOCYTOPATHIES

 BASICS

OVERVIEW
Acquired or hereditary defects that can affect any of the main functions of the platelets, including activation, adhesion, and aggregation

SIGNALMENT
• Acquired defects can occur in any breed of dog or cat • Von Willebrand's disease (VWD) has been reported in many breeds of dogs and rarely cats (see chapter on Von Willebrand's disease).• Canine thrombasthenic thrombopathia occurs in otter hounds. • Basset hound hereditary thrombopathia is widespread in the basset hound breed. • Spitz thrombopathia is characteristic • Platelet function defect in grey collies with cyclic hematopoiesis • Chediak-Higashi syndrome occurs in cats.

SIGNS
• Spontaneous bleeding in some animals, often associated with mucosal surfaces • Frequent epistaxis • Auricular hematomas in basset hound hereditary thrombopathia • Prolonged bleeding in some animals during diagnostic or surgical procedures

CAUSES AND RISK FACTORS
Acquired
• Use of drugs, including anesthetics, antibiotics, antihistamines, anti-inflammatories, and heparin. • Nonsteroidal anti-inflammatory drugs (eg, aspirin) inhibit platelet function by preventing the formation of thromboxane A2, a potent platelet agonist. • Secondary to systemic disease such as renal azotemia, pancreatitis, liver disease, and neoplastic disorders (both hematopoietic and nonhematopoietic neoplasms)

Hereditary
• VWD occurs because of a deficiency of von Willebrand's factor (VWF), which is critical for platelet adhesion. • Canine thrombasthenic thrombopathia in otter hounds is due to a deficiency of the platelet glycoproteins necessary for fibrinogen-induced aggregation. • Basset hound hereditary thrombopathia and Spitz thrombopathy are platelet aggregation defects. • Aggregation defect due to lack of normal constituents in platelet-dense granules results in cyclic hematopoiesis in grey collies and Chediak-Higashi syndrome.

 DIAGNOSIS

DIFFERENTIAL DIAGNOSIS
Other acquired or hereditary bleeding disorders characterized by bleeding that is more severe than the bleeding seen in most cases of acquired or hereditary platelet function defects

CBC/BIOCHEMISTRY/URINALYSIS
• Anemia, if bleeding is severe—may be regenerative or nonregenerative depending on the duration of bleeding • Low platelet counts in some otter hounds with thrombasthenic thrombopathy • Giant platelets in some dogs with thrombasthenic thrombopathy • Large pink cytoplasmic granules in granulocytes with or without monocytes in cats with Chediak-Higashi syndrome • Lack of specific changes in the biochemical profile

OTHER LABORATORY TESTS
• Von Willebrand's factor (VWF) assays in animals with suspected VWD • Thyroid function evaluation in dogs with suspected VWD—concurrent hypothyroidism in some animals • Platelet function testing in select laboratories to characterize hereditary platelet function defects • Coagulation tests including PT and PTT to eliminate disseminated intravascular coagulation, or presence of a vitamin K antagonist. APTT test may be prolonged in some animals with VWD.

IMAGING N/A

Other Diagnostic Procedures
Mucosal bleeding time—to document platelet function defects

 TREATMENT

• In many animals, spontaneous bleeding that is not life-threatening occurs. If a factor such as VWF is low, give whole blood or plasma (cryoprecipitate of fresh frozen plasma is preferred) to replace the deficient factor. • Restrict activity during a bleeding episode. • If a hereditary defect is identified, do not use the animal for breeding. • Before surgery, identify animals with platelet function defects using mucosal bleeding time or cuticle bleeding time—enables preparation for excessive bleeding during the procedure. • In animals with acquired platelet disorders, treat the underlying disease process, or remove the offending drug to resolve platelet dysfunction.

MEDICATIONS

DRUGS AND FLUIDS

• Give 1-deamino-(8-D-arginine)-vasopressin (DDAVP) (0.3-3 µg/kg) to dogs with VWD during a bleeding episode. Administration of this drug to normal dogs increases the VWF.
• Give DDAVP to normal dogs 30 minutes before collection of blood for transfusion to dogs with VWD.
• Provide thyroid supplementation in dogs with hypothyroidism and concurrent VWD (efficacy of this treatment has been questioned).
• Other inherited disorders are not easily treated.

CONTRAINDICATIONS/POSSIBLE INTERACTIONS

Do not use nonsteroidal anti-inflammatory drugs because they inhibit platelet function.

FOLLOW-UP

Take special precautions when performing surgical procedures on these animals. • Make owner aware that fatal bleeds are possible, but in most platelet function defects, they occur infrequently.

MISCELLANEOUS

SEE ALSO

Von Willebrand's disease

ABBREVIATIONS

DDAVP = 1-deamino-8-D-arginine vasopressin
PT = prothrombin time
PTT = partial thromboplastin time
VWD = Von Willebrand's disease
VWF = Von Willebrand factor

Reference

Reagan WJ, Rebar AH. Platelet disorders. In: Ettinger SL, Feldman EC, eds. Textbook of veterinary internal medicine. Philadelphia: WB Saunders Company, 1994.

Author William J. Reagan
Editor Alan H. Rebar

THROMBOCYTOPENIA, PRIMARY IMMUNE MEDIATED

BASICS

DEFINITION
Immune-mediated destruction of platelets

Pathophysiology
Autoimmune process in which antibodies develop against platelet antigens. Antibodies bind to the antigen on the platelet surface, and then the antibody-coated platelets are prematurely removed from the circulation by the macrophage phagocytic system.

Systems Affected
If the platelet count is low enough (< 40,000/μl) hemorrhage can occur into any organ system. Systems commonly recognized as affected clinically include integumentary, gastrointestinal, respiratory, and urinary.

Genetics N/A

Incidence and Prevalence
In a recent study at North Carolina State Veterinary Teaching Hospital, 5.2% of dogs admitted to the hospital had thrombocytopenia. In patients with thrombocytopenia, 2.8% were thought to have primary immune-mediated thrombocytopenia. In similar studies in cats, 1.2% had thrombocytopenia, and 2% of these were thought to have immune-mediated thrombocytopenia.

Geographic Distribution N/A

SIGNALMENT

Species
• Dogs • Rare in cats

Breed Predilection
• Cocker spaniel, poodle, Old English sheepdog, and, possibly, German shepherd • No known breed predilection in cats

Mean Age and Range
• Mean age in dogs, 6-7 years • Age range in dogs, 7 months to 14 years

Predominant Sex
More common in female dogs

SIGNS

Historical Findings
• Hemorrhages in the skin and mucous membranes • Excessive hemorrhage associated with a mild traumatic event • Spontaneous epistaxis • Vomiting blood • Blood in the stool • Lethargy, weakness, and collapse • Bleeding less commonly seen in cats

Physical Examination Findings
• Petechial and ecchymotic hemorrhages in the skin and mucous membranes • Epistaxis • Melena, hematochezia, or hematemesis • Hematuria • Pale mucous membranes • Lethargy, weakness, and collapse • Scleral and retinal hemorrhages and hyphema • Dyspnea • Heart murmur • Neurologic signs

CAUSES Idiopathic

RISK FACTORS Unknown

DIAGNOSIS

DIFFERENTIAL DIAGNOSIS
• Disseminated intravascular coagulation. To rule out, perform coagulation profile • Blood loss as a result of trauma or secondary to vitamin K antagonist (thrombocytopenia is mild) • Low platelet production (thrombocytopenia is usually moderate to severe) • Evaluate animal for other cytopenias such as nonregenerative anemia and leukopenia, and perform examination of bone marrow aspirate and core biopsy to identify the type of primary bone marrow disease. • Myeloproliferative disorders and FeLV infection commonly cause thrombocytopenia in cats. FIV sometimes causes thrombocytopenia. Perform FeLV and FIV tests to rule out these diseases. • Hepatomegaly and splenomegaly (mild thrombocytopenia) • Secondary immune-mediated thrombocytopenia. Clinical and laboratory findings are identical to those of primary immune-mediated thrombocytopenia. Causes of the former include drugs, neoplasms, infectious diseases (e.g., ehrlichiosis, FeLV infection, and, probably, Rocky Mountain spotted fever), and immune-mediated diseases such as systemic lupus erythematosis and immune-mediated hemolytic anemia. Perform serum titers to rule out ehrlichiosis and Rocky Mountain spotted fever. Perform ANA test for systemic lupus erythematosis. Evaluate blood film for spherocytes and agglutination to help determine if patient has immune-mediated hemolytic anemia. • Thrombocytopenia develops secondarily to many infectious diseases.

CBC/BIOCHEMISTRY/URINALYSIS
• In most patients, severe thrombocytopenia (platelet count < 20,000/μl); not uncommon to see platelet counts in the 1000-5000/μl range • Mild to moderate anemia often with hypoproteinemia. If there has been enough time for the bone marrow to respond, the anemia is regenerative. • Neutrophilia in some patients • Hematuria

OTHER LABORATORY TESTS
• Antiplatelet antibody test—if positive and other causes of thrombocytopenia are ruled out, it strongly supports the diagnosis. False-negatives do occur. • Antimegakaryocyte antibody test—if positive and other causes of thrombocytopenia are ruled out, it strongly supports the diagnosis. False-negatives do occur. This test may be less sensitive than the antiplatelet antibody test. • Mean platelet volume. Microthrombocytosis (mean platelet volume, < 5.4 fl) has been documented in some patients and usually is seen early in the disease process. As the disease progresses, the platelets increase in size resulting in macrothrombocytosis.

IMAGING
Used to rule out other causes of thrombocytopenia

OTHER DIAGNOSTIC PROCEDURES
Bone marrow aspiration with or without core biopsy. Cytological evaluation of the bone marrow is helpful to make sure that thrombocytopenia is not caused by low production. If megakaryocytes are readily observed, then low production of platelets is unlikely. Selective immune-mediated destruction of megakaryocytes is rare. Erythroid and megakaryocytic hyperplasia is seen in some patients.

GROSS AND HISTOPATHOLOGIC FINDINGS
• Petechial and ecchymotic hemorrhages in the mucous membranes, skin, and serosal surfaces • Hemorrhage into any organ, especially the gastrointestinal, respiratory, and urinary systems • Possibly, erythroid and megakaryocytic hyperplasia in the bone marrow

TREATMENT

INPATIENT VERSUS OUTPATIENT
If the patient has severe hemorrhage, stabilize and then treat as an outpatient.

ACTIVITY Restricted

DIET N/A

CLIENT EDUCATION
• Animals with severe hemorrhage should be brought to the hospital for monitoring and treatment. • Fatal hemorrhage is more likely if exercise is not restricted.

SURGICAL CONSIDERATIONS
Splenectomy may be done in cases that are refractory to medical treatment.

MEDICATIONS

DRUGS AND FLUIDS
• Prednisone or prednisolone (1-2mg/kg PO q12h for at least 2 weeks or until marked improvement in the platelet count is seen). Once the platelet count is within the normal reference range, the dosage should be gradually tapered over weeks to months.
• Dexamethasone can be used initially (0.1-0.2 mg/kg IV q12h).
• If the patient is unresponsive to corticosteroid, vincristine can be added (0.02-0.03 mg/kg or 0.5-0.75 mg/m² IV once a week).
• In addition to the vincristine or alternatively to the vincristine, cyclophosphamide can be added (2.2 mg/kg or 50 mg/m² PO q24h 3-4 days per week).
• Blood transfusions if the anemia is severe and causing clinical signs
• Platelet-rich plasma may be given if available.

THROMBOCYTOPENIA, PRIMARY IMMUNE MEDIATED

CONTRAINDICATIONS None

PRECAUTIONS
• If glucocorticoid-associated, gastric ulceration develops, drugs such as sucralfate can be used
• Long-term treatment with corticosteroids can cause iatrogenic hyperadrenocorticism.
• Cyclophosphamide can cause bone marrow suppression and sterile hemorrhagic cystitis.
• Vincristine is irritating if injected perivascularly. It can also cause constipation, peripheral neuropathy, and bone marrow suppression.

POSSIBLE INTERACTIONS N/A

ALTERNATE DRUGS
• Dogs—danazole (5 mg/kg PO q12h) can be used concurrently with glucocorticoids. Do not use danazole in cats. • Dogs—azathioprine (2 mg/kg or 50 mg/m² PO q24h-q48h) can be used to maintain remission.

FOLLOW-UP

PATIENT MONITORING
Platelet count daily until the count is >50,000/μl and then weekly until the count returns to the normal range (in some patients the count will not return to the normal range). If the owner notices severe bleeding, the patient should be brought in for evaluation.

PREVENTION/AVOIDANCE
Minimize stress that may initiate recurrence.

POSSIBLE COMPLICATIONS
Severe hemorrhage and death

EXPECTED COURSE AND PROGNOSIS
If the thrombocytopenia is severe and cannot be quickly improved by immunosuppressive therapy, animals may succumb as a result of fatal hemorrhage. Approximately 25% of patients referred to a veterinary teaching hospital died or were euthanatized. Of the patients that survived, approximately 50% had acute disease requiring only one course of immunosuppressive drugs, and 50% had chronic disease that recurred months to years later. In patients with acute disease that respond to corticosteroids, the platelet count increases in several days.

MISCELLANEOUS

ASSOCIATED CONDITIONS
Immune-mediated hemolytic anemia

AGE RELATED FACTORS None

ZOONOTIC POTENTIAL None

PREGNANCY
Use of immunosuppressive drugs may cause damage to the fetus.

SYNONYMS
• Idiopathic thrombocytopenia purpura • Idiopathic immune-mediated thrombocytopenia

SEE ALSO
Thrombocytopenia

ABBREVIATIONS
FeLV = feline leukemia virus
FIV = feline immunodeficiency virus

References

Reagan WJ, Rebar AH. Platelet disorders. In: Ettinger SL, Feldman EC, eds. Textbook of veterinary internal medicine. Philadelphia: WB Saunders, 1994.

Thompson JP. Immunologic diseases. In: Ettinger SL, Feldman EC, eds. Textbook of veterinary internal medicine. Philadelphia: WB Saunders, 1994.

Rosenthal RC. Chemotherapy. In: Ettinger SL, Feldman EC, eds. Textbook of veterinary internal medicine. Philadelphia: WB Saunders, 1994.

Williams DA, Maggio-Price L. Canine idiopathic thrombocytopenia: clinical observations and long-term follow-up in 54 cases. J Am Vet Med Assoc 1984;185:660-663.

Couto CG. Hematology and immunology. In: Nelson RW, Couto CG, eds. Essentials of small animal internal medicine. St Louis: Mosby, 1992.

Author William J. Reagan
Consulting Editor Alan H. Rebar

THYMOMA

BASICS

OVERVIEW
Originates from thymic epithelium and is infiltrated with mature lymphocytes

SIGNALMENT
• Rare in dogs and cats • Occurs most commonly in medium- and large-breed dogs
• Dogs—mean age, 9 years • Cats—mean age, 10 years

SIGNS
• Coughing • Tachypnea • Dyspnea • Swelling of the head, neck, or front limbs (ie, anterior caval syndrome) • Muscle weakness and megaesophagus caused by myasthenia gravis

DIAGNOSIS

DIFFERENTIAL DIAGNOSIS
• Lymphoma • Branchial cyst • Ectopic thyroid carcinoma • Chemodectoma

CBC/BIOCHEMISTRY/URINALYSIS
Lymphocytosis in a few patients

OTHER LABORATORY TESTS N/A

IMAGING N/A

OTHER DIAGNOSTIC PROCEDURES
• Thoracic radiographs reveal a cranial mediastinal mass, pleural effusion, and megaesophagus in some patients. • Cytologic examination shows mature lymphocytes and epithelial cells. • Evaluate for myasthenia gravis if the patient has signs of muscle weakness, dysphagia, or regurgitation.

TREATMENT
• Treat as inpatient
• Surgical excision the treatment of choice. Thymoma tends to be highly invasive and difficult to resect in dogs, but less invasive and easier to remove in cats.
• Use an intercostal approach for small masses and a sternotomy for large masses.
• Radiotherapy of potential benefit by reducing the lymphoid component of the mass

MEDICATIONS

DRUGS AND FLUIDS
• Little information available on chemotherapy
• Prednisone (20 mg/m² q48h) and cyclophosphamide (50-100 mg/m² q48h) have been used in a very limited number of patients. Two patients had a partial remission.
• Myasthenia gravis treated with prednisone and anticholinesterase drugs until the tumor can be removed

CONTRAINDICATIONS/POSSIBLE INTERACTIONS
Immunosuppressive drugs should not be used to treat myasthenia gravis if the patient has aspiration pneumonia.

FOLLOW-UP
• Thoracic radiography every 3 months to monitor for recurrence • Cure possible if tumor is surgically resectable • Prognosis is poor for patient with nonresectable thymoma

MISCELLANEOUS
About 20-40% of animals with thymoma are also diagnosed with nonthymic tumors, polymyositis, and other autoimmune diseases.

Reference

Atwater SW, Powers BE, Park RD, et al. Thymoma in dogs: 23 cases (1980-1991). J Am Vet Med Assoc 1994;205:1007-1013.

Author Terrance A. Hamilton
Consulting Editor Wallace B. Morrison

TICK BITE PARALYSIS

BASICS

DEFINITION
Flaccid, lower motor neuron paralysis caused by salivary neurotoxins from certain species of female ticks

Pathophysiology
The tick injects salivary neurotoxins that probably interfere with the depolarization acetylcholone release mechanism in the presynaptic nerve terminal, leading to reduction in the release of acetylcholone. This effect is strongly temperature dependent with Ixodes holocyles tick infestation. One adult tick is sufficient to cause neurologic signs, but a large larval or nymphal Ixodes tick infestation can also induce signs. Signs do not occur until 6-9 days after initial tick attachment. Not all infested animals develop tick paralysis and not all adult female ticks produce the toxins.

Systems Affected
• Nervous—the peripheral nervous system and the neuromuscular junction are most affected by the neurotoxin. Cranial nerves can become involved, including the vagal, facial, and trigeminal nerves. The sympathetic nervous system is also affected in animals with Ixodes tick paralysis. • Respiratory—may be involved due to paralysis of the intercostal muscles and diaphragm. The caudal brainstem respiratory center may be affected in animals with Ixodes tick paralysis.

Genetics No genetic basis

Incidence/Prevalence
Tick paralysis is somewhat seasonal in both North America and Australia (ie, more prevalent in the summer months). In the warmer climates of the southern areas of the United States and northern Australia, tick paralysis becomes a year-round problem. The overall incidence of this disease is low in the United States. Austrailia has a higher incidence.

Geographic Distribution
• In the United States, Dermacentor variabilis has a wide distribution over the eastern two-thirds of the country, as well as in California and Oregon. D. andersonii is found from the Cascades to the Rocky Mountains. Amblyomma americanum is found from Texas and Missouri to the Atlantic Coast. Amblyomma maculatum prefers the high temperature and humidity associated with the Atlantic and Gulf of Mexico seaboards. • In Australia, cases of Ixodes tick paralysis are limited to the coastal areas of eastern Australia and are especially associated with areas of bush and scrub.

SIGNALMENT

Species
• Australia—dogs and cats • United States—dogs; cats appear to be resistant

Breed Predilections N/A

Mean Age and Range N/A
Predominant Sex N/A

SIGNS

Historical Findings
A history of the animal walking in a wooded area approximately 1 week before the onset of signs. The onset of neurologic signs is gradual, starting with unsteadiness and weakness in the pelvic limbs.

Neurologic Examination Findings
• Once neurologic signs appear, there is rapid ascending lower motor neuron paresis to paralysis. Animals become recumbent in approximately 1-3 days, with hypo- to areflexia and hypo- to atonia. Pain sensation is preserved. Cranial nerve dysfunction is not a prominent feature, but some animals have facial weakness and reduced jaw tone. Some animals have dysphonia and dysphagia early in the course of disease. Although uncommon in the United States, respiratory paralysis can occur in severely affected animals. Urination and defecation are usually normal. • In animals with Ixodes tick paralysis, the neurologic signs are much more severe and rapidly progressive. The ascending motor weakness can progress to paralysis within a few hours. Sialosis, megaesophagus, and vomiting or regurgitation are characteristic. The sympathetic nervous system effects of the Ixodes neurotoxin include mydriatic and poorly responsive pupils, hypertension, tachyarrhythmias, high pulmonary capillary hydrostatic pressure, and pulmonary edema. Involvement of the caudal medullary respiratory center is additive to the peripheral pulmonary changes, causing progressive fall in respiratory rate without a change in tidal volume, resulting in hypoxia, hypercapnia, and respiratory acidosis. Respiratory muscle paralysis is much more prevalent in animals with Ixodes tick paralysis, and dogs and cats progress to dyspnea, cyanosis, and respiratory paralysis within 1-2 days if not treated.

CAUSES

United States
• Dermacentor variabilis (common wood tick) • Dermacentor andersonii (Rocky Mountain wood tick) • Amblyomma americanum (Lone Star tick) • Amblyomma maculatum (Gulf Coast tick)

Australia
Ixodes holocyclus—secretes a far more potent neurotoxin compared with that of the North American species

RISK FACTORS
None, other than being in environments that harbor the aforementioned ticks

DIAGNOSIS

DIFFERENTIAL DIAGNOSIS
• Botulism • Acute polyneuropathy • Coonhound paralysis • Acute polyradiculoneuritis • Distal denervating disease

• Generalized (diffuse) or multifocal myelopathy

CBC/BIOCHEMISTRY/URINALYSIS
N/A

OTHER LABORATORY TESTS
In severely affected animals, arterial blood gas analysis may reveal low PaO_2, high $PaCO_2$, and a low pH.

IMAGING
In animals with Ixodes tick paralysis, thoracic radiography may reveal megaesophagus.

OTHER DIAGNOSTIC PROCEDURES
• Thorough search for a tick—areas that should be searched are the head, neck, body and limbs, ear canals, mouth, rectum, vagina, prepuce, and in-between the digits and foot pads. If a tick is found, it should be immediately removed. • Electrodiagnostics—electromyelogram reveals normal insertion activity and an absence of spontaneous myofiber activity (no fibrillations and positive sharp waves). There is also a lack of motor unit action potentials. Motor nerve stimulation is followed by either a dramatic decrease in amplitude or a complete absence of compound muscle action potentials.

GROSS AND HISTOPATHOLOGIC
FINDINGS N/A

TREATMENT

INPATIENT VERSUS OUTPATIENT
• Dogs with neurologic dysfunction suggestive of tick paralysis should be hospitalized until either a tick is found and removed or appropriate treatment to kill a hidden tick is performed. • In-hospital supportive care is essential until the dog begins to show signs of recovery. Animals with hypoventilation and hypoxia should be placed in an oxygen cage. • Artificial ventilation is necessary for animals in respiratory failure.

ACTIVITY
• The animal should be kept in a quiet environment. • Animals with Ixodes tick paralysis should be kept in a cool, air-conditioned area because the toxin is temperature sensitive. Avoid activity to prevent increase in body temperature.

DIET
Food and water should be withheld if animals have dysphagia or vomiting/regurgitation.

CLIENT EDUCATION
• Good nursing care is essential, although the dog's recovery is rapid after removal of ticks (United States). • Clients should be warned that in animals with Ixodes tick paralysis, signs often continue to worsen despite tick removal, and thus more aggressive treatment to neutralize the toxin needs to be undertaken.

SURGICAL CONSIDERATIONS N/A

MEDICATIONS

DRUGS AND FLUIDS

• If the offending tick cannot be found, tick elimination can be achieved by dipping the dog in an insecticidal bath. This is often all that is needed to treat dogs with tick paralysis in the United States. Intravenous fluid therapy is generally not required unless recovery is prolonged. In Australia, circulating toxin needs to be neutralized by IV administration of hyperimmune serum (0.5-1 mg/kg), depending on the severity of the clinical signs.

• If signs are severe, phenoxybenzamine, an alpha-adrenergic antagonist (1 mg/kg diluted in saline and given slowly IV over 20 minutes) appears to be beneficial in relieving the sympathetic effects of the toxin. Acepromazine can be used as an alternate drug (0.5-1 mg/kg IV) because it also has alpha-adrenergic effects.

CONTRAINDICATIONS

Drugs that interfere with neuromuscular transmission are contraindicated (ie, tetracyclines, aminoglycosides, and procaine penicillin). In patients with Ixodes tick paralysis, atropine is contraindicated if the animal is in the advanced stages of disease or has marked bradycardia.

PRECAUTIONS

If fluids are administered intravenously to animals with Ixodes tick paralysis, they should be given at a very slow rate to avoid further complications of pulmonary congestion.

POSSIBLE INTERACTIONS N/A

ALTERNATE DRUGS N/A

FOLLOW-UP

PATIENT MONITORING

• Reassessment of neurologic status after tick removal at least daily should show rapid improvement in muscle strength in animals with the North American form of the disease.

• Animals with Ixodes tick paralysis need continuous, intensive monitoring of neurologic status as well as respiratory and cardiovascular function, even after tick removal, because of the residual effect of the Ixodes neurotoxin.

PREVENTION/AVOIDANCE

• Vigilantly check for ticks after exposure (at least every 2-3 days) because the signs do not occur for 4-6 days after tick attachment.

• Weekly insecticidal baths or the use of insecticide impregnated collars helps. • Short-term acquired immunity develops after exposure to Ixodes neurotoxin.

POSSIBLE COMPLICATIONS

No long-term complications if the animal survives the acute effects of the toxin

EXPECTED COURSE AND PROGNOSIS

• North American tick paralysis—if the tick(s) is removed, prognosis good to excellent, with recovery occurring in 1-3 days

• Isodes tick paralysis—prognosis often guarded, with recovery more prolonged. Untreated animals die within 1-2 days.

MISCELLANEOUS

ASSOCIATED CONDITIONS N/A

AGE RELATED FACTORS N/A

ZOONOTIC POTENTIAL

Humans can also succumb to tick paralysis (especially in Australia) by being bitten by the same ticks. However, animals with tick paralysis cannot transmit the disease to humans.

PREGNANCY Unknown

SYNONYM Tick bite paralysis

SEE ALSO

• Periperal Neuropathies (Polyneuropathies)
• Coonhound Paralysis

ABBREVIATIONS

N/A

References

Malik R, Farrow BRH. Tick paralysis in North America and Australia. Vet Clin North Am (Small Anim Pract) 1991;21: 157-171.

Braund KG. Clinical syndromes in veterinary neurology. 2nd ed. St. Louis: Mosby, 1994:273-274.

Ilkiw JE. Tick paralysis in Australia. In: Kirk RW, ed. Current veterinary therapy VIII. Philadelphia: WB Saunders, 1983:691-693.

Author Paul A. Cuddon
Consulting Editor Joane M. Parent

TICKS AND TICK CONTROL

BASICS

DEFINITION
Dogs and cats may be parasitized by hard ticks of the family Ixodidae. These ectoparasites which feed only on the blood of their hosts are arthropods, closely related to scorpions, spiders and mites. Ticks have a great potential to act as vectors of protozoa, fungi, bacteria, viruses, rickettsiae, filarial nematodes and spirochetes.

PATHOPHYSIOLOGY
• Hard ticks have four life stages: egg, larva, nymph, and adult. Larvae and nymphs must feed to repletion prior to detaching and molting. As adult female ticks engorge, they may increase their weight by more than 100 fold and after detachment may lay thousands of eggs. • Blood loss anemia may result from heavy infestations. • Damage to the integument occurs as tick mouth parts cut through the host's skin. Tick bites are generally painless but local irritation and infection may occur. • Salivary secretion of neurotoxins may lead to systemic signs (tick paralysis) and local action of salivary contents may cause impaired hemostasis and immune suppression. • Pathogens may be acquired when ticks feed on infected reservoir hosts (often rodents and small feral mammals). In some cases transovarial transmission of pathogens occurs and infected eggs will hatch and produce infected larvae. The greatest potential for systemic disease occurs when infections acquired in early life stages are transmitted to new hosts when the next stage feeds. Transmission of pathogens and toxins often requires periods of attachment from hours to days and the essentially painless bite of ticks allows feeding times of adequate duration. • Tick-borne pathogens may affect virtually any organ system.

Systems Affected
• Skin/Exocrine • Hemic/Lymphatic/ Immune • Nervous

Incidence/Prevalence N/A

Geographic Distribution
Strong geographic specificities exist for some tick species and hence geographic prevalence of associated diseases exist. Lyme borreliosis is associated with populations of Ixodes scapularis in the midwest, northeast and parts of the southeast and Ixodes pacificus in western costal states. Canine ehrlichiosis is most common in the southeast although its tick vector, Rhipicephalus sanguineus, has been found throughout the continental United States.

SIGNALMENT
Tick parasitism is often considered to be most common in large, hunting breeds of dogs which are likely to come in contact with environments harboring questing ticks. However, the encroachment of tick populations into suburban environments as well as

the expansion of the suburban environment into surrounding forests, prairies and coast line areas has placed domestic animals in close contact with ticks. While cats are thought to be fastidious groomers and quite efficient at removing ticks, tick attachment and subsequent tick-vectored diseases are routinely diagnosed in felines.

Species Dogs and Cats

Breed Predilections N/A

Mean Age and Range N/A

Predominant Sex N/A

SIGNS

Physical Examination Findings
Presence of attached ticks or tick feeding cavities from which ticks have detached may be seen on the skin. Signs of associated tickborne diseases (borreliosis, ehrlichiosis, babesiosis, rocky mountain spotted fever, and others) vary with the organ system(s) affected. In some cases, irritation caused by ticks and subsequent self trauma may lead to pyotraumatic dermatitis (hot spots) in dogs.

CAUSES
Direct contact with questing ticks may result in tick parasitism. While ticks do not jump or fly, they are attracted to hosts by motion, variation in light patterns, warmth, and presence of carbon dioxide.

DIAGNOSIS

Diagnosis of tick parasitism is made by examining the skin for presence of attached ticks or for tick feeding cavities left by replete ticks as they detach. Diagnosis of tick-borne diseases is made by evaluating epidemiologic considerations for each disease, history of tick parasitism, and complete clinical evaluation of ill individuals.

DIFFERENTIAL DIAGNOSIS N/A

CBC/BIOCHEMISTRY/URINALYSIS

OTHER LABORATORY TESTS N/A

IMAGING N/A

OTHER DIAGNOSTIC PROCEDURES N/A

TREATMENT

Ticks should be removed as soon as possible to limit time available for neurotoxin or pathogen transmission. Most efficient removal is accomplished with fine pointed tweezers. Ticks are grasped close to the skin and gently pulled free. Species with short, strong mouth parts (e.g., Dermacentor) usually pull free with host skin attached; species with long, fragile mouth parts (e.g., Ixodes) often leave fragments embedded in the feeding cavity. In either case, washing

with soap and water is generally sufficient to prevent local inflammation of secondary infection

INPATIENT VERSUS OUTPATIENT
Outpatient

ACTIVITY N/A

DIET N/A

CLIENT EDUCATION
Application of hot matches, Vaseline or other materials to ticks not only fails to cause tick detachment but allows for longer periods of attachment and feeding.

SURGICAL CONSIDERATIONS N/A

MEDICATIONS

DRUGS AND FLUIDS N/A

CONTRAINDICATIONS N/A

PRECAUTIONS N/A

ALTERNATE DRUGS N/A

FOLLOW-UP

PATIENT MONITORING N/A

PREVENTION/AVOIDANCE
• Tick avoidance requires avoiding environments that harbor ticks. Because ticks may survive on many intermediate hosts, and because suburban living has brought pets into environments frequented by these intermediate hosts, avoidance may be difficult for all but pets kept strictly indoors or for city dwellers. • A unique tick collar (Preventic Collar) for dogs contains amitraz which acts to prevent attachment of new ticks and to induce ticks already attached to detach. • Permethrin spray may be used in dogs as a tick repellent as well as a tick killer. • Ticks may be killed by bathing, spraying, or powdering affected dogs and cats with appropriate organophosphate or pyrethrin containing products. • Canine Lyme disease may be prevented by immunization with bacterin. Dogs should be vaccinated during puppy immunizations to maximize antibody production prior to parasitism by ticks infected with Borrelia burgdorferi.

POSSIBLE COMPLICATIONS N/A

EXPECTED COURSE AND PROGNOSIS N/A

MISCELLANEOUS

ASSOCIATED CONDITIONS N/A

AGE RELATED FACTORS N/A

ZOONOTIC POTENTIAL
• Ticks may parasitize many different species

of mammals, birds and reptiles at different stages in their developmental cycles. Infections acquired in early life stages may be transmitted when ticks feed again in the next stage. • If humans are parasitized they may be exposed to borreliosis, ehrlichiosis, babesiosis, spotted fever, or tick paralysis.

PREGNANCY N/A

SYNONYMS Acariasis

SEE ALSO
• Lyme Disease (Borreliosis) • Ehrlichiosis

• Babesiosis • Rocky Mountain Spotted Fever • Tick Bite Paralysis

ABBREVIATIONS N/A

References

Levy SA, Lissman BA, Ficke CM. Performance of a Borrelia burgdorferi bacterin in borreliosis—endemic areas. J Am Vet Med Assoc 1993;202:1834-1838

Sonenshine DE. Biology of ticks. New York: Oxford University Press, 1991.

Sonenshine DE. Biology of ticks. New York: Oxford University Press, 1993;2.

Author Steven A. Levy
Consulting Editor Lowell Ackerman

TOAD VENOM TOXICITY

 BASICS

OVERVIEW
The two species of primary concern are the Colorado River toad (Bufo alvarius) and the marine toad (Bufo marinus). Marine toad is the most toxic, but either can be fatal. Toads are most active during periods of high humidity; the "monsoon" season of late summer in the desert southwest (Colorado River toads). Most encounters occur during the evening, night, or early morning hours. Toads produce toxin from the parotid glands, a defensive toxin that is rapidly absorbed across the victim's mucus membranes. The toxin contains several major components including these catecholamines: indole alkyl amines, cardiac glycosides, and non-cardiac sterols. The indole alkyl amines are similar to the street drug "LSD."

SIGNALMENT
Primarily dogs; rarely, ferrets and cats

SIGNS

Historical Findings
• Moist, warm, outside environment
• Animal outside • Rapid onset of clinical signs

Physical Examination Findings
• Profuse hypersalivation • Hyperexcitation with vocalization • Often, brick red buccal mucus membranes • Hyperthermia
• Collapse • Marked cardiac ventricular arrhythmia (less frequent in animals with Colorado River Toad intoxication) • Crying and pawing at the mouth • Ataxia or stiff gaited • Seizures • Cyanosis • Dyspnea

CAUSES AND RISK FACTORS
• Living in proximity to toads • Animal going outside

 DIAGNOSIS

DIFFERENTIAL DIAGNOSIS
Caustics or other oral irritants

CBC/BIOCHEMISTRY/URINALYSIS
Serum potassium high in some animals

OTHER LABORATORY TESTS N/A

IMAGING N/A

OTHER DIAGNOSTIC PROCEDURES
ECG may reveal ventricular arrhythmias.

 TREATMENT

• Decontamination—flush mouth with copious quantities of water for 5 to 10 minutes.
• If victim is hyperthermic (> 105 F), proceed with cool bath. Remove from cool bath once temperature reaches 103 F. • Marine toad intoxication is a medical emergency; many bitten animals die. Rapid evaluation of cardiac activity is necessary. • Animals with Colorado River toad intoxication are usually normal within 30 minutes of onset of treatment and, with treatment, fatalities are relatively uncommon. • The risk of secondary heatstroke cannot be underestimated in these patients.

MEDICATIONS

DRUGS AND FLUIDS

• Atropine (0.04 mg/kg IM SC) reduces the amount of salivation and helps prevent aspiration. Should be used if patient exhibits bradycardia, heart block, or other sinoatrial node alterations because of digitalis-like effect of the toad toxin. • Propranolol (Inderal; 2 mg/kg IV); see contraindications; rapid administration may be required to combat cardiac arrhythmias; can be repeated in 20 minutes. In patient with persistent arrhythmias, continuous IV infusion of propranolol may be required (0.02 -0.2 mg/kg). • Anesthesia with pentobarbital increases canine tolerance to Bufo toad intoxication.

CONTRAINDICATIONS/POSSIBLE INTERACTIONS

• Patients with cardiac disease or bronchial asthma may not tolerate the high dose of propranolol that is generally recommended to treat toad toxicity-induced arrhythmias. In these patients, administer propranolol at 0.5 mg/kg as a slow IV bolus while monitoring the cardiac rhythm. Stop the injection when the cardiac rhythm normalizes. • Anesthetics such as pentobarbital may depress function of an already compromised myocardium, and should be used with caution.

FOLLOW-UP

Continuous ECG monitoring is recommended until the patient is fully recovered.

MISCELLANEOUS

ABBREVIATIONS

ECG = electrocardiogram

Reference

Palumbo NE, Perri SF. Toad poisoning. In: Kirk RW, ed. Current veterinary therapy VIII. Philadelphia: WB Saunders, 1983:160-162.

Author Michael E. Peterson
Consulting Editor Gary Osweiler

TOXOPLASMOSIS

BASICS

DEFINITION
Toxoplasma gondii is an obligate intracellular coccidian protozoan parasite that infects nearly all mammals. Felidae, including domestic cats, are the definitive hosts; all other warm-blooded animals are intermediate hosts.

Pathophysiology
The severity and manifestations of clinical illness depend on the location and degree of tissue injury caused by tissue cysts. Infection acquired by ingestion of tissue cysts or oocysts results in spread of organisms to extraintestinal organs via blood or lymph, resulting in focal necrosis to many organs (heart, eye, central nervous system). This acute disseminated infection is rarely fatal. Chronically, tissue cysts form to produce low grade disease that usually is not clinically apparent unless immunosuppression or concomitant illness allows T. gondii to proliferate and cause an acute inflammatory response. Clinical toxoplasmosis is often associated with other infections causing severe immunosuppression such as canine distemper, feline infectious peritonitis, and feline leukemia virus infections.

Systems Affected
• Multisystemic—clinical toxoplasmosis is more commonly recognized in cats than dogs, but the systems affected are usually the same • Approximately 80% of cats with toxoplasmosis will have evidence of intraocular inflammation, most commonly uveitis.

Genetics N/A

Incidence/Prevalence
Approximately 30% of cats and up to 50% of people are serologically positive for T. gondii. However, as most animals with toxoplasmosis are asymptomatic, clinical disease is uncommon.

Geographic Distribution
Worldwide

SIGNALMENT
• Cats are symptomatic more commonly than dogs. No breed predilections. • In one study, mean age of infection in cats was 4 years, with a range from 2 weeks to 16 years. More male cats have been reported with the disease than females.

SIGNS

General Comments
• Signs are determined mainly by site and extent of organ damage. • Signs can be acute (occurring at the time of initial infection) or from reactivation of encysted infection (chronic) caused by immunosuppression.

Historical Findings
• Nonspecific signs of lethargy, depression, anorexia • Weight loss • Fever • Other signs determined by site and extent of organ injury

• Ocular discharge, photophobia, miotic pupils (cats) • Respiratory distress
• Neurologic signs (ataxia, seizures, tremors, paresis/paralysis, cranial nerve deficits)
Digestive tract signs (vomiting, diarrhea, abdominal pain, jaundice) • Stillborn kittens

Physical Examination Findings
Cats
• Most severe in transplacentally infected kittens, which may be stillborn or die before weaning. Signs (anorexia, lethargy, high fevers unresponsive to antibiotics) in surviving kittens reflect necrosis/inflammation of lungs (dyspnea, increased respiratory noises), liver (icterus, abdominal enlargement from ascites), and CNS (encephalopathic).
• Postnatal acquired infections result most commonly in respiratory and gastrointestinal signs (anorexia, lethargy, high fevers unresponsive to antibiotics, dyspnea, weight loss, icterus, vomiting, diarrhea, abdominal effusion); less than 10% of cats show neurologic signs (blindness, stupor, incoordination, circling, torticollis, anisocoria, seizures). Ocular signs are common and relate to uveitis (aqueous flare, hyphema, mydriasis), iritis, detached retina, iridocyclitis, and keratic precipitates. • Can have a rapid course in acutely affected cats with CNS and/or respiratory involvement, or slow course in cats with reactivation of chronic infection.
Dogs
• Young dogs usually are afflicted by generalized infection, resulting in fever, weight loss, anorexia, tonsillitis, dyspnea, diarrhea, and vomiting. • Older dogs tend to develop localized infections mainly associated with neural and muscular systems. Neurologic signs are quite variable usually reflecting diffuse neurologic inflammation: seizures, tremors, ataxia, paresis, paralysis, muscle weakness, and tetraparesis. • Ocular involvement is rare in the dog. Signs are similar to those found in the cat. • Cardiac involvement occurs but usually is not clinically apparent.

CAUSES N/A

RISK FACTORS
Conditions causing immunosuppression such as feline leukemia virus, feline immunodeficiency virus, feline infectious peritonitis, hemobartonellosis, canine distemper, glucocorticoid or antitumor chemotherapy may predispose to infection with T. gondii or reactivation of a chronic T. gondii infection.

DIAGNOSIS

DIFFERENTIAL DIAGNOSIS
Cats
• Intraocular disease (anterior uveitis)––FIP, FeLV, FIV, immune-mediated, trauma, lens-induced, and corneal ulceration with reflex uveitis. • Dyspnea (respiratory signs)—asth-

ma, cardiogenic, pneumonia (bacterial, fungal, parasitic), neoplasia, heartworm disease, pleural disease (effusions), diaphragmatic hernia, chest wall injury. Neurologic signs—causes of meningoencephalitis, including viral (FIP, rabies, pseudorabies), fungal (cryptococcosis, blastomycosis, histoplasmosis), parasitic (cuterebriasis, coenurosis, aberrant heartworm migration), bacterial, and idiopathic disease (feline polioencephalomyelitis).

Dogs
Often associated with other immunosuppressive diseases such as distemper; thus, signs of distemper are apparent. Neurologic signs usually in very young dogs. Must be differentiated from Neospora caninum infection (both produce CNS and neuromuscular disease). Consider other conditions causing multifocal neurologic signs, including infectious/inflamatory toxicity and metabolic diseases.

CBC/BIOCHEMISTRY/URINALYSIS
CBC
• Most cats show mild normocytic normochromic anemia. • Approximately 50% of infected cats with severe disease have leukopenia; mainly as a result of lymphopenia, some have neutropenia alone or in addition to lymphopenia and a degenerative left shift. Leukocytosis may occur during recovery.

Biochemistry
Significant increases in ALT and AST in most patients. Approximately 25% of cats have icterus. Most have hypoalbuminemia. Cats that develop pancreatitis as a result of toxoplasmosis often have mildly low serum calcium concentrations; amylase levels are unreliable

Urinalysis
Mild proteinuria in a small proportion of cats. Bilirubinuria, especially in icteric cats.

OTHER LABORATORY TESTS
Serology
• IgM, IgG, and antigen serum titers give the most definitive information from one sample; a follow-up sample 3 weeks after the first will provide more complete information as to the type of infection (active, recent, chronic). Titers are available from Veterinary Diagnostic Laboratory, College of Veterinary Medicine, Colorado State University, Fort Collins, CO 80523. • IgM—single serologic titer of choice for diagnosis of active infection. Elevated 2 weeks postinfection (usually coincides with onset of clinical signs), persists for a maximum of 3 months, then falls. A prolonged titer may indicate reactivation or delay in antibody class shift from IgM to IgG (a result of immunosuppression from FeLV or FIV infection or steroid therapy). • IgG—titers rise 2-4 weeks postinfection and persist beyond a year. Thus, a single high IgG titer is not diagnostic for active infection. A fourfold increase in IgG titer over a 3-week period suggests active infection. • Antigen—positive 1-4 weeks postinfection. However, as it re-

mains positive during active or chronically persistent infection, measurement does not give much more information than antibody titers.

IMAGING
• A mixed pattern of patchy alveolar and interstitial pulmonary infiltrates may be seen on thoracic radiographs. • Pleural and abdominal effusions and hepatomegaly also may be seen.

OTHER DIAGNOSTIC PROCEDURES

CSF Analysis
High leukocyte count (both mononuclear cells and neutrophils) and protein in encephalopathic animals

Cytology
• Tachyzoites rarely may be detected in body fluids during acute infection (CSF, transtracheal washings, pleural or peritoneal effusions). • Fecal examination (Sheather's sugar solution) may be diagnostic • Fecal oocyst shedding rarely occurs during clinical disease. • Oocysts may be detected on routine fecal examinations in asymptomatic cats but are morphologically indistinguishable from Hammondia spp. and Besnoitia. Mouse inoculation is needed to distinguish between these organisms.

GROSS AND HISTOPATHOLOGIC FINDINGS
Gross—necrotic foci (up to 1 cm) most often seen in the liver, pancreas, mesenteric lymph nodes, and lungs. Necrosis of the brain (1 cm areas of discoloration) can be seen. Ulcers and granulomas may be present in the stomach and small intestine.

TREATMENT

INPATIENT VERSUS OUTPATIENT
Most can be treated as outpatients. Pneumonic and debilitated animals should be supported until stabilized.

ACTIVITY
Restricted

DIET N/A

CLIENT EDUCATION
Prognosis is guarded in cats needing therapy because response to therapy is inconsistent. Worse prognosis in neonates and the severely immunocompromised.

SURGICAL CONSIDERATIONS N/A

MEDICATIONS

DRUGS AND FLUIDS
• Clindamycin (25-50 mg/kg per day, divided into 2 doses, PO or IM) for at least 2 weeks after clinical signs clear • Uveitis may be concurrently treated with 1% prednisone drops, topically q8h for 2 weeks.

CONTRAINDICATIONS None

PRECAUTIONS
Side effects of clindamycin can include anorexia, vomiting, and diarrhea (dose-dependent).

POSSIBLE INTERACTIONS N/A

ALTERNATE DRUGS
Sulfadiazine (30 mg/kg, PO, q12h) in combination with pyrimethamine (0.5 mg/kg, PO, q12h) for 2 weeks. Can cause depression, anemia, leukopenia, and thrombocytopenia, especially in cats. Bone marrow suppression can be corrected by supplementing the animal's diet with folinic acid (5 mg/day) or brewer's yeast (100 mg/kg/day).

FOLLOW-UP

PATIENT MONITORING
Examine 2 days after initiation of clindamycin as clinical signs (fever, hyperesthesia, anorexia, uveitis) should have begun to resolve. Uveitis should resolve completely within 1 week of initiating treatment. • Examine 2 weeks after initiation of clindamycin to assess neuromuscular deficits, which should partially resolve (some deficits will always remain as a result of permanent CNS or peripheral neuromuscular damage). • Reexamine 2 weeks after owner feels signs have completely resolved (other than neuromuscular deficits) to assess discontinuing clindamycin.

PREVENTION/AVOIDANCE
• Prevent cats from eating raw meat, bones, viscera, or unpasteurized milk (especially goat milk), or from eating mechanical vectors (flies, cockroaches). Meat may be eaten if well-cooked. • Prevent cats from free roaming to hunt prey (birds, rodents) or to enter buildings where food-producing animals are housed.

POSSIBLE COMPLICATIONS N/A

EXPECTED COURSE AND PROGNOSIS
Because of the varied response to drug treatment, prognosis has to be guarded. In acute cases, prompt and aggressive therapy often is successful. Residual deficits (especially neurologic) cannot be predicted until after a course of therapy. • Ocular disease usually responds to appropriate therapy. • Severe muscular or neurologic disease usually results in chronic debility.

MISCELLANEOUS

ASSOCIATED CONDITIONS
• Distemper in young dogs • FeLV, FIP, FIV in cats

AGE RELATED FACTORS N/A

ZOONOTIC POTENTIAL
• T. gondii is of considerable zoonotic potential.
• A healthy cat with a positive T. gondii antibody titer poses little danger to its owner. A cat with no antibody titer is at more risk of becoming infected, shedding oocysts in the feces, and constituting a risk to its owner. To avoid contact with oocysts or tissue cysts:
• Do not feed raw meat. • Wash hands and surfaces (cutting boards) after preparing raw meat. • Boil drinking water if the source is unreliable. • Keep sandboxes covered to prevent cats defecating in them. • Wear gloves when gardening. • Wash hands and vegetables before eating to avoid contact with oocyst soil contamination. • Empty cat litter boxes daily (oocysts need 24 hours at least to become infective). • Disinfect litter boxes with boiling water. • Control stray cat population to avoid oocyst contamination of environment.
• Pregnant women should avoid all contact with a cat excreting oocysts in its feces, avoid contact with soil and cat litter, and not handle or eat raw meat (meat cooked to 150° F will kill T. gondii).

PREGNANCY
• Parasitemia during pregnancy can cause spread of tachyzoites to the fetus. However, as in people, parasitemia and therefore transmission to the fetus probably does not occur unless first-time infection of the dam occurs during pregnancy. • Placental transmission is rare.

SYNONYMS N/A

SEE ALSO N/A

ABBREVIATIONS
ALT = alanine aminotransferase
AST = aspartate aminotransferase
CNS = central nervous system
CLL = chronic lymphocytic leukemia
FeLV = feline leukemia virus
FIP = feline infectious peritonitis
FIV = feline immunodeficiency virus
IgG = immunoglobulin G
IgM = immunoglobulin M

References

Dubey JP, Greene CE, Lappin MR. Toxoplasmosis. In: Greene CE, ed. Infectious diseases of the dog and cat. Philadelphia: WB Saunders, 1990.

Dubey JP, Carpenter JL. Histologically confirmed clinical toxoplasmosis in cats: 100 cases (1952-1990). J Am Vet Med Assoc 1993;203:1556-1566.

Dubey JP. Toxoplasmosis. J Am Vet Med Assoc 1994;205:1593-1598.

Author Stephen C. Barr
Consulting Editor Fred W. Scott

TRACHEAL COLLAPSE—DOGS

BASICS

DEFINITION
•Tracheal collapse is a condition characterized by a dynamic reduction in the luminal diameter of the large, conducting airway as a result of weakening of cartilaginous support of the trachea. Redundancy of the dorsal tracheal membrane may further compromise the width of the lumen and compound the clinical signs. Compression of the trachea or bronchi as a result of hilar lymphadenopathy, left atrial enlargement, or external masses is not considered part of the condition described here.

Pathophysiology
• Tracheal cartilages from dogs with tracheal collapse have been shown to be hypocellular. • Lack of chondroitin sulfate and/or decreased glycoproteins within the cartilage matrix results in a reduction in bound water and loss of turgidity in the cartilage. • Abnormalities in the cartilage structure may represent degenerative changes secondary to long-standing small airway disease, or they may result from defects of chondrogenesis associated with primary genetic or nutritional abnormalities. • Abnormal pressure gradients develop along the trachea during respiration, which lead to dynamic collapse of the airway. • The weakened cartilage allows flattening of the tracheal ring structure, and the trachea collapses, typically in a dorsoventral direction. • Increased tension on the trachealis dorsalis muscle or neurogenic atrophy of the muscle causes stretching of the dorsal tracheal membrane with protrusion into the airway lumen. • Chronic pressure fluctuations within the airway lead to perpetuation of small airway disease and more widespread pulmonary dysfunction. • Mechanical trauma to the tracheal mucosa from collapse of the dorsal tracheal membrane during coughing exacerbates airway edema and inflammation and may lead to pseudomembrane formation.

Systems Affected
• Respiratory—signs from upper airway disorders, such as everted saccules, laryngeal paralysis, and elongated soft palate, may be worsened by severe or protracted dyspnea; lower respiratory tract infection or inflammation are more likely a result of poor tracheal clearance of secretions and bacteria • Cardiovascular—if the combination of pulmonary diseases is severe enough to lead to pulmonary hypertension • Nervous—when syncope develops from hypoxia or a vasovagal reflex associated with cough

Genetics Unknown

Incidence/Prevalence
Unknown, although the disorder is commonly diagnosed clinically

Geographic Distribution Worldwide

SIGNALMENT

Species Primarily dogs, rarely cats

Breed Predilections
Miniature poodle, Yorkshire terrier, chihuahua, Pomeranian, other small and toy breeds

Mean Age and Range
Middle-aged to elderly with onset of signs from 4-14 years of age. A congenital form also may be observed.

Predominant Sex N/A

SIGNS

General Comments
Clinical signs usually are worsened by excitement, heat, humidity, exercise, or obesity.

Historical Findings
• A dry "honking" cough is classically described for tracheal collapse. • A chronic history of intermittent coughing or difficulty breathing may be reported. • Retching is often noted, resulting from an attempt to clear the larynx of pulmonary secretions.
• Tachypnea, exercise intolerance, and/or respiratory distress commonly are reported.
• Cyanosis or syncope may be found in severely affected individuals.

Physical Examination Findings
• Tracheal sounds may be wheezing or musical. • Enhanced tracheal sensitivity generally is present. • An end-expiratory snap may be heard when large segments of the airway collapse on forceful expiration. • Cervical tracheal collapse is present with inspiratory dyspnea, while intrathoracic collapse may be associated with expiratory dyspnea. • Wheezes or crackles indicate the presence of small airway disease. • Mitral insufficiency murmurs often are found as a result of the commonality of both cardiac and respiratory disease in small-breed dogs. • The heart rate generally is normal or decreased for the breed of dog. • A pronounced second heart sound is suggestive of elevated pulmonary arterial pressures.
• Hepatomegaly has been reported (etiology unknown).

CAUSES
• Congenital/nutritional/familial defects or failures of chondrogenesis • Chronic small airway disease

RISK FACTORS
• Obesity • Pulmonary infection • Upper airway obstruction

DIAGNOSIS

DIFFERENTIAL DIAGNOSIS
• Chronic bronchitis • Congestive heart failure • Laryngeal paralysis • Laryngeal mass • Pneumonia—viral, bacterial, fungal, allergic, or parasitic • Intratracheal mass or foreign body • Cervical or mediastinal mass • Infectious tracheobronchitis • Bronchiectasis

CBC/BIOCHEMISTRY/URINALYSIS
• Minimum data base to assess general health • CBC—inflammatory leukogram (secondary to chronic stress of low-grade pneumonia); polycythemia may be found when chronic obstructive pulmonary disease is present

OTHER LABORATORY TESTS
• Arterial blood gases can be used to assess the degree of respiratory dysfunction. • Calculating the alveolar-arterial oxygen difference ($DA\text{-}a\ O_2$) from blood gas data will differentiate the pulmonary contribution to hypoxemia from that associated with upper airway obstruction. • $DA\text{-}a\ O_2 = PAO_2 - PaO_2$ where $PAO_2 = 0.21\ x\ (PB - PH_2O) - PaCO_2/0.8$ (normal < 15; PB = barometric pressure; PH_2O = water vapor pressure [47 at 37° C] and $PaCO_2$ from blood gas data)

IMAGING

Radiography
• Tracheal collapse can be identified by radiography in the majority (60%) of patients. • Inspiratory films will show cervical tracheal collapse. • Expiratory films are useful for outlining intrathoracic tracheal collapse. Collapse of the mainstem bronchus and ballooning of the cervical trachea also may be seen. • Bronchitis, pneumonia, and bronchiectasis may be identified. • Right-sided heart enlargement may be found secondary to chronic pulmonary disease. Breed conformation may confound interpretation of the cardiac silhouette.

Fluoroscopy
Dynamic collapse of the trachea and/or dorsal tracheal membrane may be more easily identified after induction of cough.

OTHER DIAGNOSTIC PROCEDURES

Bronchoscopy
• The severity of tracheal collapse can be graded (1-4) and small airway disease identified. • Grade 1—almost normal, slightly pendulous trachealis muscle • Grade 2—reduction of the tracheal lumen by 50% • Grade 3—reduction of the tracheal lumen by 75% with the trachealis muscle almost brushing the tracheal cartilage • Grade 4—tracheal cartilages are flattened, < 10% of the lumen may be visible, a double lumen may be seen when the trachealis muscle contacts the ventral surface of the trachea • Samples should be submitted for bacterial culture/sensitivity and cytology to guide therapy.

GROSS AND HISTOPATHOLOGIC FINDINGS
• The trachealis muscle is greatly elongated and the cartilages are flattened. • Tracheal inflammation or pseudomembrane formation may be evident. • Hypocellularity of the cartilage with decreased glycoproteins and chondroitin sulfate is noted microscopically.

• Variable changes associated with chronic obstructive pulmonary disease may be noted.

TREATMENT

INPATIENT VERSUS OUTPATIENT
• Stable patients can be discharged on appropriate therapy. • Severely dyspneic patients may require oxygen therapy or heavy sedation.

ACTIVITY
Severely limited pending stabilization

DIET
The majority of affected dogs will improve by achieving weight loss.

CLIENT EDUCATION
• Obesity, overexcitement, and humid conditions can cause a crisis. • Harnesses should be used in place of collars.

SURGICAL CONSIDERATIONS
Early intervention in selected cases (primarily cervical tracheal collapse) by a skilled surgeon may improve quality of life when adequate stablization of the airway can be achieved and when chronic pulmonary changes do not limit resolution of disease.

MEDICATIONS

DRUGS AND FLUIDS
• Sedation and cough suppression may be achieved with butorphanol (0.05 mg/kg IV, SC q6h).
• The addition of acepromazine (0.025 mg/kg SC) may enhance sedative effects.
• Narcotic cough suppressants such as butorphanol (0.5-1.0 mg/kg PO q6h-q12h) or hydrocodone (0.22 mg/kg PO q6h-q12h) are effective for chronic therapy.
• Some dogs may respond to Choledyl elixir (1 cc/4.5 kg q8h) despite inadequate theophylline levels.
• Theo-dur sustained release tablets (20 mg/kg q12h) or Slo-bid (25 mg/kg) are recommended to dilate the smaller airways and decrease pressure gradients along the trachea.
• Prednisone (0.5-1.0 mg/kg q12h tapered to q48h) may aid in reducing tracheal or bronchial inflammation.

CONTRAINDICATIONS
None

PRECAUTIONS
• Theo-dur tablets should be used, not sprinkles or capsules.
• Generic slow-release theophylline products should not be substituted because of erratic pharmacokinetics.
• Long-term steroid use should be avoided because of the propensity for weight gain or diseases associated with steroid excess.

POSSIBLE INTERACTIONS
• Primarily with theophylline
• Theophylline metabolism is increased by concurrent treatment with ketoconazole and phenobarbital. Inadequate plasma levels result.
• Metabolism is decreased by flouroquinolones (Baytril), erythromycin, cimetidine, beta blockers, steroids, mexiletine, and thiabendazole. Toxic plasma levels results, causing gastrointestinal upset, nervousness, or tachycardia.
• Changes in drug pharmacokinetics associated with congestive heart failure, cor pulmonale, and liver disease necessitate a reduction in dosage.

ALTERNATE DRUGS
Robitussin DM has offered palliation in some patients.

FOLLOW-UP

PATIENT MONITORING
• Weight • Exercise tolerance • Arterial blood gases

PREVENTION/AVOIDANCE
• Avoid obesity in breeds commonly afflicted.
• Avoid heat and humidity.

POSSIBLE COMPLICATIONS
Intractable dyspnea leading to respiratory failure.

EXPECTED COURSE AND PROGNOSIS
• Prognosis may be based on bronchoscopic evidence of airway obstruction. • Various combinations of medical therapy, in conjunction with weight control, should be tried to provide palliation. • Surgery may benefit some patients, primarily those with cervical tracheal collapse.

MISCELLANEOUS

ASSOCIATED CONDITIONS
• Chronic bronchitis • Laryngeal paralysis
• Everted laryngeal saccules • Pulmonary hypertension • Affected breeds commonly are afflicted with mitral insufficiency, which can complicate the diagnosis.

AGE RELATED FACTORS N/A

ZOONOTIC POTENTIAL N/A

PREGNANCY N/A

SYNONYMS N/A

SEE ALSO
Bronchitis, Chronic

ABBREVIATIONS
DA–aO$_2$ = alveolar-arterial oxygen difference
PAO$_2$ = alveolar oxygen
PaO$_2$ = arterial oxygen
PB = barometric pressure
PH$_2$O = water vapor pressure
PaCO$_2$ = arterial carbon dioxide

References
Hedlund CS. Tracheal collapse. Prob Vet Med 1991;3:229.
Done SH, Drew RA. Observations on the pathology of tracheal collapse in dogs. J Small Anim Pract 1976;17:783.
White RAS, Williams JM. Tracheal collapse—is there really a role for surgery? A survey of 100 cases. J Small Animal Pract 1994;35:191-196.
Tangner CH, Hobson HP. A retrospective study of 20 surgically managed cases of collapsed trachea. Vet Surg 1982;11:146-149.
McKiernan BC. Current uses and hazards of bronchodilator therapy. In: Kirk RW, Bonagura JD, eds. Current veterinary therapy XI, small animal practice. Philadelphia: WB Saunders, 1992:660-668.

Author Lynelle Johnson
Consulting Editors Lynelle Johnson and Bradley L. Moses

TRACHEOBRONCHITIS, INFECTIOUS—DOGS

 BASICS

DEFINITION
•Any contagious respiratory disease of dogs that is manifested by coughing and seemingly not caused by canine distemper (CD) is referred to as infectious tracheobronchitis.

Pathophysiology
In most dogs, the pathogenesis of infectious tracheobronchitis involves an initiating injury of the respiratory epithelium and/or viral infection followed by invasion of the damaged tissue by bacterial, fungal, mycoplasmal, parasitic, or other virulent organisms, resulting in further damage and clinical signs.

Systems Affected
Respiratory—primarily affected unless associated with sepsis or congenital anomalies

Genetics N/A

Incidence/Prevalence
Infectious tracheobronchitis occurs most commonly where dogs of varying ages and susceptibility congregate, often under less than ideal hygienic conditions in some pet shops, humane society shelters, research facilities, and boarding and training kennels.

Geographic Distribution Worldwide

SIGNALMENT

Species Dogs

Breed Predilections
Any dog breed may be affected.

Mean Age and Range
• Most severe in puppies that are 6 weeks to 6 months old and among puppies under less than ideal hygienic conditions in some pet shops, humane society shelters, research facilities, and boarding and training kennels.
• May occur in dogs of all ages and often occurs with preexisting, subclinical airway disease (e.g., congenital anomalies, chronic bronchitis, bronchiectasis).

Predominant Sex
Equal occurrence between the sexes

SIGNS

General Comments
Clinical signs are related to the degree of respiratory tract damage and age of the affected dog (may range from an uncomplicated cough to severe, life-threatening pneumonia).

Historical Findings
After exposure, clinical signs may be mild or nonexistent in the affected dog or severe as seen in dogs with pneumonia. It usually is apparent that most viral, bacterial, and mycoplasmal agents spread rapidly from seemingly healthy dogs to others in the same environment.

Physical Examination Findings
• The most characteristic sign of uncomplicated infectious tracheobronchitis is a cough in an otherwise healthy animal. The cough

usually begins approximately 4 days after exposure to the infecting agent(s). • The cough is usually dry and hacking, soft and dry, moist and hacking, or paroxysmal, followed by gagging or expectoration of mucus. Excitement, exercise, changes in temperature or humidity of the inspired air, or gentle pressure on the trachea will induce a paroxysm of coughing. • Severe infectious tracheobronchitis is an entirely different disease. A constant, low-grade or fluctuating fever (103-104° F) may be present and the affect on appetite tends to be severe. When present, the cough is moist and productive. Other clinical signs may include nasal discharge, lethargy, anorexia, dyspnea, and exercise intolerance. Lung sounds often are normal, but an increased intensity of normal lung sounds, crackle, or, less frequently, wheezes may be detected.

CAUSES
• Incriminated viral causes include CD, canine adenovirus type 2 (CAV-2), canine parainfluenza (CPI), canine adenovirus type 1 (CAV-1), canine reovirus-1, canine reovirus-2, canine reovirus-3, and canine herpesvirus. CAV-2 and CPI virus may damage the respiratory epithelium to such an extent that invasion by various bacteria and/or mycoplasmas results in severe airway disease. • Many different bacteria may contribute to clinical signs of infectious tracheobronchitis. Bordetella bronchiseptica, in the absence of other respiratory pathogens, produces clinical signs that are indistinguishable from other bacterial causes of infectious tracheobronchitis. It is likely that Pseudomonas, Escherichia coli, Klebsiella, Pasteurella, Streptococcus, and Mycoplasma and other bacterial species are equally capable of causing signs of infectious tracheobronchitis.

RISK FACTORS
• Less than ideal hygienic conditions of some pet shops, humane society shelters, research facilities, and boarding and training kennels
• Coexisting subclinical airway disease (e.g., congenital anomalies, chronic bronchitis, bronchiectasis)

 DIAGNOSIS

DIFFERENTIAL DIAGNOSIS
• The diagnosis usually is established provisionally by eliminating the noninfectious causes of coughing. The differential diagnosis for infectious tracheobronchitis for determining a specific infectious agent is difficult. A case history that reveals a source of exposure is important. The dog's vaccination status is also important. • See Cough.

CBC/BIOCHEMISTRY/URINALYSIS
• Early mild leukopenia (5000-6000 cells/dl) may be present, suggesting a viral etiology. Neutrophilic leukocytosis with a left shift is frequently found in dogs with severe pneu-

monia. • Serum chemistry profile and urinalysis usually are normal.

OTHER LABORATORY TESTS
Arterial blood gas analysis may be useful in dogs with pneumonia.

IMAGING

Radiography
• In most dogs with uncomplicated infectious tracheobronchitis, thoracic radiographs are unremarkable and are of value primarily for ruling out noninfectious causes of a cough.
• Thoracic radiographs may demonstrate an interstitial and alveolar lung pattern with a cranioventral distribution, typical of bacterial pneumonia; a diffuse interstitial lung pattern, typical of viral pneumonia; or a mixed lung pattern (i.e., combination of alveolar, interstitial, and peribronchial lung patterns).

OTHER DIAGNOSTIC PROCEDURES
If severe infectious tracheobronchitis is suspected, transtracheal washing or tracheobronchial lavage via bronchoscopy should be done. The identification of the antimicrobial sensitivity pattern of cultured bacteria aids significantly in providing an effective treatment plan.

GROSS AND HISTOPATHOLOGIC FINDINGS
• Though CPI causes few to no clinical signs, the lungs of infected dogs 6-10 days after exposure may contain petechial hemorrhages that are evenly distributed over the surfaces. CPI is detected by immunofluorescence in columnar epithelial cells of the bronchi and bronchioles 6-10 days after aerosol exposure.
• Lesions associated with CAV-2 infections are confined to the respiratory system. Large intranuclear inclusion bodies are found in bronchial epithelial cells and alveolar septal cells. Although the clinical signs associated with CAV-2 tend to be mild and short-lasting, the lesions persist for at least a month after infection. • In bordetellosis and severe bacterial infections, there is evidence of purulent bronchitis, tracheitis, and rhinitis with hyperemia and enlargement of the bronchial, mediastinal, and retropharyngeal lymph nodes. Large numbers of gram-positive or gram-negative organisms may be seen microscopically in the mucus of the tracheal and bronchial epithelium.

 TREATMENT

INPATIENT VERSUS OUTPATIENT
• Outpatient therapy is strongly recommended for dogs with uncomplicated infectious tracheobronchitis. All treatment can be given at home by the owner after the initial examination is completed.
• Inpatient therapy is strongly recommended for dogs with complicated infectious tracheobronchitis and/or pneumonia.

ACTIVITY
- Enforce rest for at least 14-21 days for uncomplicated infectious tracheobronchitis.
- Enforce rest for at least the duration of radiographic evidence of pneumonia.

DIET
Good quality canned or dry dog food

CLIENT EDUCATION
- Isolation of dog affected with infectious tracheobronchitis from other animals is to be encouraged. Infected dogs may transmit the agent(s) before onset of clinical signs and afterward until immunity is developed.
- Affected dogs with uncomplicated infectious tracheobronchitis should respond to treatment in 10-14 days. (See patient monitoring.)
- Once infections spread in a kennel, they can be controlled by evacuation for 1 or 2 weeks and disinfection with commonly used chemicals such as sodium hypochlorite (1:30 dilution), chlorhexidine, or benzalkonium.

SURGICAL CONSIDERATIONS N/A

MEDICATIONS

DRUGS AND FLUIDS
- Initial treatment of uncomplicated infectious tracheobronchitis is amoxicillin/clavulanate or trimethoprim/sulfonamide combinations.
- In severe cases, gentamicin or amikacin and a first-generation cephalosporin or enrofloxacin usually is effective.
- Antimicrobial therapy may be continued for at least 10 days beyond radiographic resolution.
- Because some antimicrobials may not reach adequate therapeutic concentrations in the lumen of the lower respiratory tract, oral or parenteral administration may have limited effectiveness against Bordetella bronchiseptica and some resistant bacterial species. Nebulization with kanamycin (250 mg), gentamicin (50 mg), or polymyxin B (333,000 IU) may eliminate Bordetella bronchiseptica when administered daily for 3-5 days.
- Suppression of dry, nonproductive cough can be achieved with cough medications such as butorphanol (0.05-0.1 mg/kg PO 2-3 times a day) or hydrocodone bitartrate (0.22 mg/kg PO 2-4 times a day).
- Maintenance of adequate hydration is important for the healing process. Steam or cold mist vaporizers may provide symptomatic relief. Airway hydration can be maximized by nebulization three times a day with normal saline solution, followed by coupage therapy.
- Bronchodilators may be used to control bronchospasm that is usually clinically apparent by wheezing.

CONTRAINDICATIONS
Cough suppressants should not be used in animals with pneumonia.

PRECAUTIONS None

POSSIBLE INTERACTIONS N/A

ALTERNATE DRUGS N/A

FOLLOW-UP

PATIENT MONITORING
- Affected dogs with uncomplicated infectious tracheobronchitis should respond to treatment in 10-14 days. A diagnosis of uncomplicated infectious tracheobronchitis should be questioned when the dog continues to cough 14 days or more after establishment of an adequate treatment plan. • In severe cases, thoracic radiography should be repeated until at least 14 days beyond resolution of all clinical signs.

PREVENTION/AVOIDANCE
- Shedding of the causative agent(s) of infectious tracheobronchitis in respiratory secretions of dogs that are asymptomatic undoubtedly accounts for the persistence of this problem in kennels, animal shelters, boarding facilities, and veterinary hospitals. • Viral and bacterial vaccines are now available to control the principal agents involved in infectious tracheobronchitis. • Puppies can be vaccinated intranasally (Intra-Trac-II, Schering-Plough Animal Health; Naramune-2, Bio-Ceutic Laboratories; Bronchi-Shield, Fort Dodge Laboratories) as early as 2-4 weeks of age without interference from maternal antibody, followed by annual revaccination. Mature dogs can receive a one-dose intranasal vaccination at the same time as their puppies or at the time they receive their annual vaccinations. • Other infectious tracheobronchitis vaccines available include inactivated Bordetella bronchiseptica parenteral vaccine (CoughGuard B or CoughGuard BP, SmithKline Beecham Animal Health; Bronchicine, Fermenta Animal Health). Parenteral vaccines are administered as two doses, 2-4 weeks apart. Puppies younger than 4 months of age should be revaccinated after reaching the age of 4 months. Initial vaccination of puppies with parenteral vaccines is recommended at or about 6-8 weeks of age.

POSSIBLE COMPLICATIONS N/A

EXPECTED COURSE AND PROGNOSIS
- The natural course of uncomplicated infectious tracheobronchitis, if untreated, tends to be 10-14 days. Simple restriction of exercise and prevention of excitement will shorten the course of the disease.
- The typical course of severe infectious tracheobronchitis ranges from 2-6 weeks. The dogs that die often have developed severe pneumonia that affects multiple lung lobes.

MISCELLANEOUS

ASSOCIATED CONDITIONS
May accompany other respiratory tract anomalies

AGE RELATED FACTORS
Most severe in puppies that are 6 weeks to 6 months old and among puppies from commercial pet shops and humane society shelters

ZOONOTIC POTENTIAL None

PREGNANCY
High risk in dogs on extensive medical therapy; especially risky for the developing puppies

SYNONYMS
Uncomplicated infectious tracheobronchitis is often referred to as "kennel cough."

SEE ALSO
See causes.

ABBREVIATIONS
CD = canine distemper
CPI = canine parainfluenza
CAV-1 = canine adenovirus type 1
CAV-2 = canine adenovirus type 2

References

Bemis DA. Bordetella and mycoplasma respiratory infection in dogs. Vet Clin N Am Small Anim Pract 1992;22:1173-1186.

Ford RB, Vaden SL. Canine infectious tracheobronchitis. In: Greene CE, ed. Infectious diseases of the dog and cat. Philadelphia: WB Saunders, 1990:259-265.

Hoskins JD, Taboada J. Specific treatment of infectious causes of respiratory disease in dogs and cats. Vet Med 1994:443-452.

Padrid P. Chronic lower airway disease in the dog and cat. Prob Vet Med 1992;4:320-344.

Author Johnny D. Hoskins
Consulting Editors Lynelle Johnson and Bradley L. Moses

TRANSITIONAL CELL CARCINOMA, RENAL, BLADDER, URETHRA

BASICS

DEFINITION
Malignancy arising from the transitional epithelium of the kidney, ureters, urinary bladder, and urethra

Pathophysiology
The entire urinary bladder wall may become thickened and indurated, resulting in reduced capacity. Patients with urethral involvement may have incontinence or obstruction. Ureteral obstruction or invasion by the tumor often causes hydroureter, hydronephrosis, and renal failure.

Systems Affected
Renal/Urologic
• Urinary bladder—the trigone is the most commonly affected site in dogs. A site predilection has not been identified in cats.
• Urethra—second most common site in dogs. Some patients have local invasion leading to urinary obstruction. • Vagina—transitional cell carcinoma occurring primarily in the vagina of dogs has been reported
• Kidneys—primary renal transitional cell carcinoma has been reported
Metastatic Sites
• Metastatic disease to regional lymph nodes and lungs is common. Metastases may also occur in bone. • Paraneoplastic—transitional cell carcinoma has been associated with hypertrophic osteopathy.

Genetics N/A

Incidence/Prevalence
• < 1% of all reported malignancies in dogs
• Rare in cats

Geographic Distribution N/A

SIGNALMENT
Middle-aged to old, spayed female, small-breed dogs are most commonly affected.

Species Dogs and cats

Breed Predilections
Scottish terrier, West Highland white terrier, Shetland sheepdog, Eskimo dog, dachshund

Mean Age and Range
Approximately 8 years; range, 1-15+ years (dogs)

Predominant Sex Female

SIGNS

General Comments
• Signs similar to those of urinary tract infection • Malignant epithelial cells may be identified in urine after resolution of the urinary tract infection. • Epithelial cells displaying criteria of malignancy may be identified on routine urinalysis in an animal with no overt clinical signs.

Historical Findings
• Hematuria, pollakiuria, stranguria, and dysuria or urinary incontinence most common

complaints • Signs may resolve temporarily with antibiotic administration

Physical Examination Findings
• Usually normal • Sublumbar lymphadenomegaly identified on rectal palpation in some patients

CAUSES
• Dogs—obesity, exposure to environmental carcinogens, chronic exposure to flea control products, and cyclophosphamide administration are all reported risk factors • Role of chronic urinary tract infection and inflammation unknown • Cats—unknown

RISK FACTORS
Dogs—obesity, exposure to flea control products, and long-term cyclophosphamide administration

DIAGNOSIS

DIFFERENTIAL DIAGNOSIS
• Urinary tract infection • Urolithiasis • Other neoplasms (e.g., squamous cell carcinoma, leiomyoma, leiomyosarcoma, rhabdomyosarcoma, lymphosarcoma, and transmissible venereal tumor) • Vaginitis and prostatitis

CBC/BIOCHEMISTRY/URINALYSIS
• Hemogram may or may not show signs of inflammation. • Test for high BUN and creatinine. • Urinalysis often reveals epithelial cells with multiple criteria of malignancy such as anisocytosis, anisokaryosis, high nuclear to cytoplasmic ratio, and deeply staining cytoplasm. Caution should be used against over interpreting cytologic findings if inflammation is also present.

OTHER LABORATORY TESTS
Urine culture and sensitivity testing indicated because concurrent urinary tract infection is common

IMAGING

THORACIC RADIOGRAPHY
Metastatic patterns include multiple, well-defined interstitial nodules, interstitial pattern more pronounced than normal, and alveolar infiltrates. Up to 37% of dogs have metastatic disease at the time of examination.

ABDOMINAL RADIOGRAPHY
Medial iliac lymphadenomegaly in some patients

OTHER DIAGNOSTIC PROCEDURES

Double Contrast Cystography
• Space-occupying lesion, usually at trigone of bladder • Depending on the primary site, an intravenous pyelogram, voiding urethrogram, or vaginogram may be indicated.

Ultrasonography
Helpful in identifying and monitoring disease within the bladder, urethra, kidney, and prostate

GROSS AND HISTOPATHOLOGIC FINDINGS
• Irregular to diffuse thickening of urinary bladder mucosa, most often within the trigonal region • Metastasis to regional lymph nodes, lungs, and bones (especially rib lesions) possible

TREATMENT
Radiotherapy (intraoperative) has been reported to achieve longer survival times and better local control than most chemotherapies. However, it was associated with urinary bladder stricture and fibrosis and urinary incontinence in treated dogs and is not recommended.

INPATIENT VERSUS OUTPATIENT
• Initial workup and diagnosis takes 1-2 days.
• Stable patients need not be hospitalized.

ACTIVITY Normal

DIET Normal

CLIENT EDUCATION
• Long-term prognosis poor
• Palliation often attainable
• Disease not usually surgically resectable
• Chemotherapy the treatment of choice
• Recurrence

SURGICAL CONSIDERATIONS
• Transitional cell carcinoma is a highly exfoliative malignancy. If surgical resection is attempted, all surgical instruments and gloves should be replaced after touching the tumor.
• Up to 50% of the urinary bladder can be resected with minimal loss of function.
• Wide surgical margins should be taken.

MEDICATIONS

DRUGS AND FLUIDS
• Cisplatin frequently used
• Piroxicam (0.3 mg/kg PO q24h with food) also reported to have activity against this tumor

CONTRAINDICATIONS
• Cisplatin should be avoided in patients with preexisting renal insufficiency or the development of renal insufficiency.
• Cisplatin should not be used in cats—may cause fatal pulmonary edema
• Piroxicam should be avoided in animals with known gastrointestinal erosions or ulcerations or renal insufficiency.
• The benefits and side effects of piroxicam in cats have not been evaluated.

PRECAUTIONS
• Dogs being treated with cisplatin should be monitored for renal insufficiency.
• Animals with transitional cell carcinoma may be predisposed to renal damage either because of hydroureter and hydronephrosis,

pyelonephritis secondary to chronic urinary tract infection associated with the tumor, or primary renal transitional cell carcinoma. Cisplatin should be avoided in these patients. • Piroxicam should not be used with other NSAIDs. Owners should watch for signs of gastrointestinal upset such as inappetance, vomiting, diarrhea, and melena.

POSSIBLE INTERACTIONS

Cisplatin should not be used concurrently with other nephrotoxic drugs (e.g., aminoglycoside antibiotics).

ALTERNATE DRUGS

• Carboplatin suggested to have activity by small studies; however, larger case series have not supported earlier findings
• Intravesicular treatment with thiotepa has been reported; however, because of the large tumor burden by the time of diagnosis, this treatment is not a good option in animals with transitional cell carcinoma.

FOLLOW-UP

PATIENT MONITORING

Double contrast cystography or ultrasonographic examination every 4-6 weeks

PREVENTION/AVOIDANCE N/A

POSSIBLE COMPLICATIONS

• Urethral or ureteral obstruction and renal failure • Metastatic disease to regional lymph nodes, lungs, or bone • Urinary incontinence • Recurrent urinary tract infection • Myelosuppression or gastrointestinal toxicity associated with chemotherapy

EXPECTED COURSE AND PROGNOSIS

• Progressive disease likely • Long-term prognosis grave—most dogs survive 4-6 months with treatment • Median survival in patients treated with cisplatin—approximately 180 days (range, 36-589) • Median survival in patients treated by piroxicam alone—approximately 181 days (range, 28-720+)

MISCELLANEOUS

ASSOCIATED CONDITIONS

Recurrent urinary tract infection common

AGE RELATED FACTORS N/A

ZOONOTIC POTENTIAL N/A

PREGNANCY N/A

SYNONYMS N/A

SEE ALSO N/A

ABBREVIATIONS

NSAIDs = nonsteroidal antiinflammatory drugs

References

Norris AM, Laing EJ, Valli VEO, et al. Canine bladder and urethral tumors: a retrospective study of 115 cases (1980-1985). J Vet Int Med 1992;6:145-153.

Knapp DW, Richardson RC, Chan TCK, et al. Piroxicam therapy in 34 dogs with transitional cell carcinoma of the urinary bladder. J Vet Int Med 1994;8:273-278.

Moore AS, Cardona A, Shapiro W, et al. Cisplatin (cisdiamminedichloroplatinum) for treatment of transitional cell carcinoma of the urinary bladder or urethra. A retrospective study of 15 dogs. J Vet Int Med 1990;4:148-152.

Shapiro W, Kitchell BE, Fossum TW, et al. Cisplatin for treatment of transitional cell and squamous cell carcinomas in dogs. J Am Vet Med Assoc 1988;193:1530-1533.

Chun R, Knapp DW, Widmer WR, et al. Pilot study of carboplatin. In: Proceedings, 13th Annu Conf Vet Cancer Soc 1993:53-54.

Author Ruthanne Chun
Consulting Editor Wallace B. Morrison

TRANSMISSABLE VENEREAL TUMOR

BASICS

OVERVIEW
• Sexually transmitted, naturally occurring tumor • Appears to be more common in temperate areas and large cities

SIGNALMENT
Young, intact dogs of either sex

SIGNS
• Red, friable, lobulated mass on the mucosa of the vagina or penis. The oral mucosa may also be affected. • Owners may report blood dripping from the prepuce or vagina. • Excessive licking of the genital area may be reported. • Tumor protrusion may be noticed by the owner.

CAUSES AND RISK FACTORS
• Direct transplantation of tumor cells onto abraded mucosa, either by coitus or oral transmission • Intact, free-roaming dogs are at greater than average risk.

DIAGNOSIS

DIFFERENTIAL DIAGNOSIS
• Other neoplasms • Vaginal hyperplasia

CBC/BIOCHEMISTRY/URINALYSIS
• Results of CBC and biochemical analysis normal • Examination of free catch urine reveals hematuria and abnormal cells in some patients

OTHER LABORATORY TESTS N/A

IMAGING N/A

OTHER DIAGNOSTIC PROCEDURES
• Examination of impression smears or aspirate of the tumor reveals homogenous sheets of round to oval cells with prominent nucleoli, scant cytoplasm, and multiple clear cytoplasmic vacuoles. • Biopsy

TREATMENT
• May spontaneously regress but treatment recommended
• Surgical excision of small tumors often followed by recurrence
• Radiotherapy reported to be curative after 1 treatment
• Medical treatment reported to be curative

MEDICATIONS

DRUGS AND FLUIDS
Vincristine administration reported to be curative (0.5-0.7 mg/m^2 IV once weekly for 2 weeks beyond complete resolution of gross disease)

CONTRAINDICATIONS/POSSIBLE INTERACTIONS
• Myelosuppression secondary to vincristine administration
• Tissue sloughing if extravasated
• Chemotherapy can be cytotoxic. Seek advice before initiating treatment if unfamiliar with cytotoxic drugs.

FOLLOW-UP

PATIENT MONITORING
CBC and platelet count before each treatment

PREVENTION/AVOIDANCE
• Spay or neuter • Prevent animals from roaming free.

POSSIBLE COMPLICATIONS
Tumor recurrence possible secondary to incomplete remission or reexposure

EXPECTED COURSE AND PROGNOSIS
• Excellent response to medical treatment
• Excellent prognosis

MISCELLANEOUS

ASSOCIATED CONDITIONS N/A

AGE RELATED FACTORS N/A

ZOONOTIC POTENTIAL N/A

PREGNANCY N/A

Reference

Brown NO, Calvert C, MacEwen EG. Chemotherapeutic management of transmissible venereal tumors in 30 dogs. J Am Vet Med Assoc 1980;176:983-986.
Author Ruthanne Chun
Consulting Editor Wallace B. Morrison

BASICS

OVERVIEW
• Traumatic myocarditis is the term applied to the syndrome of arrhythmias that sometimes complicates blunt trauma. The term, however, is a misnomer, because myocardial lesions (if present) are more likely to take the form of necrosis than inflammation. • Direct cardiac injury is not essential to the development of posttraumatic arrhythmia; extracardiac conditions are likely to be of equal or greater etiologic importance. • Ventricular arrhythmias occur in most animals. Ventricular rhythms that complicate blunt trauma are often relatively slow and become apparent only during pauses in the sinus rhythm. These are most appropriately referred to as accelerated idioventricular rhythm (AIVR). The QRS complexes are wide and bizarre; the rate is generally > 100 bpm but < 160 bpm. Usually, these rhythms are electrically and hemodynamically benign. • Dangerous ventricular tachycardias can also complicate blunt trauma and can also evolve from seemingly benign AIVR, compromising perfusion and placing the animal at risk for sudden death.

SIGNALMENT Dogs, rarely cats.

SIGNS
Historical Findings
• Trauma, most often as the result of road accidents. • Arrhythmias often noticed 24-48 hours after trauma sustained.

Physical Examination Findings
• Arrhythmias may be inapparent if the rate of an AIVR closely matches the sinus rate.
• Rapid, irregular rhythms in some animals
• Signs of poor peripheral perfusion (e.g., weakness, pale mucous membranes, and weak femoral pulses) in animals with ventricular rhythms that are rapid and poorly tolerated

CAUSES AND RISK FACTORS
• Blunt trauma • Hypoxia • Autonomic imbalance • Electrolyte derangements • Acid-base disturbances

DIAGNOSIS

DIFFERENTIAL DIAGNOSIS
AIVR should be differentiated from ventricular tachycardia. AIVR are usually initiated by late diastolic ventricular (escape) complexes or fusion complexes, and the heart rate is generally between 100 and 160 bpm. In contrast, ventricular tachycardia is usually initiated by a ventricular premature complex and affected animals have heart rates exceeding 160 bpm.

CBC/BIOCHEMISTRY/URINALYSIS
• Creatine kinase, liver enzymes, and lactic dehydrogenase often high because of organ trauma • Electrolyte derangements (particularly hypokalemia and hypomagnesemia) predispose to ventricular arrhythmia

OTHER LABORATORY TESTS N/A

IMAGING
Thoracic Radiographic Findings
Evidence of trauma, including pneumothorax, rib fractures, and pulmonary contusion in some animals

OTHER DIAGNOSTIC TESTS
Electrocardiographic Findings
• Ventricular arrhythmias, as previously discussed • Atrial fibrillation (rare)

TREATMENT
• Extracardiac conditions including pain, electrolyte derangements, and hypoxia, which can predispose to ventricular arrhythmia, should be treated if possible.
• Thoracic radiographs should be evaluated in all animals with blunt trauma. Disorders such as pneumothorax should be identified and remedied.
• The need for antiarrhythmic therapy is predicated by clinical signs and the electrocardiographic character of the arrhythmia. Pharmacologic suppression of AIVR usually unnecessary.

MEDICATIONS

DRUGS AND FLUIDS
• Fluid therapy for shock
• Rapid ventricular rhythms associated with hemodynamic compromise treated first with lidocaine (2 mg/kg boluses IV). A total of 8 mg/kg can be administered over 10-12 minutes. Start a lidocaine infusion (25-75 (μg/kg/min) once the rhythm is stabilized with lidocaine boluses.
• If the administration of lidocaine fails to result in conversion to sinus rhythm, try procainamide, beta blockers such as esmolol or propranolol, or even class III agents such as bretyllium.
• DC conversion while animal is under anesthesia or heavy sedation can be considered to treat rapid, hemodynamically unstable, ventricular rhythms that do not respond to drug therapy.
• Antiarrhythmic agents not necessarily benign; they can worsen existing arrhythmias and provide a substrate for the development of new arrhythmias (proarrhythmia). The relative risk or benefit to the animal must be carefully weighed at every step.

CONTRAINDICATIONS/POSSIBLE INTERACTIONS N/A

FOLLOW-UP
• ECG monitoring of animals with arrhythmias is recommended. Generally, the arrhythmias that complicate blunt trauma are self limiting and resolve within 48-72 hours.
• If antiarrhythmic therapy is deemed necessary, it can often be discontinued after 2-5 days. • Although dangerous arrhythmias occasionally complicate blunt trauma, the prognosis is usually associated with the severity of extra-cardiac injury.

MISCELLANEOUS

SEE ALSO
• Shock • Idioventricular Rhythm
• Ventricular Tachycardia

ABBREVIATIONS
AIVR = accelerated idioventricular rhythm
DC = direct current

Reference
Abbott JA. Traumatic myocarditis. In: Bonagura JD, ed. Current veterinary therapy XII. Philadelphia: WB Saunders, 1995.
Author Jonathan A. Abbott
Consulting Editors Larry P. Tilley and Francis W. K. Smith, Jr.

TRIGEMINAL NEURITIS

BASICS

OVERVIEW
• Acute onset of inability to close the jaw
• Bilateral involvement of trigeminal nerves
• Bilateral nonsuppurative neuritis, demyelination, and, in a few patients, fiber degeneration of all branches of trigeminal nerve and ganglion

SIGNALMENT
• Primarily adult dogs • Rare in cats

SIGNS
• Acute onset of a dropped jaw • Inability to close the mouth • Drooling • Difficulty in prehending food • Messy eating • No apparent deficits in sensory perception • Swallowing intact

CAUSES AND RISK FACTORS
• Unknown • Possibly immune-mediated

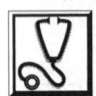

DIAGNOSIS

DIFFERENTIAL DIAGNOSIS
• Must be differentiated from musculoskeletal disorders of the temporomandibular joints and jaw. History of trauma and pain and the physical examination findings help rule in/out these disorders. • Rabies should always be considered initially until the clinician has accumulated sufficient evidence to rule it out. • Neoplastic involvement of both mandibular nerves secondary to myelomonocytic leukemia, lymphosarcoma, and neurofibrosarcoma has been reported but usually does not have an acute onset. • One should not confuse masticatory muscle myositis with trigeminal neuritis; the former causes trismus and a jaw that is difficult to open.

CBC/BIOCHEMISTRY/URINALYSIS
Results usually normal

OTHER LABORATORY TESTS N/A

IMAGING N/A

OTHER DIAGNOSTIC PROCEDURES
• No specific test is diagnostic for this disorder. • Tests to rule out the differentials listed (eg, skull radiography, examination of bone marrow aspirate, and muscle biopsy)

TREATMENT
• Treat as an outpatient if the owner is able to assist the animal when eating and drinking.
• Because of the animal's inability to prehend and move food and water to the throat, the animal must be helped eating and drinking. Animals can lap and swallow pureed food offered by a large syringe placed in the corner of mouth with the head slightly elevated.

MEDICATIONS

DRUGS AND FLUIDS
• Subcutaneously administered fluids may be necessary in some patients to maintain hydration.
• Pharyngostomy or gastrotomy tubes are rarely necessary to maintain adequate food intake.
• Antiinflammatory dosage of corticosteroids may speed recovery.

CONTRAINDICATIONS/POSSIBLE INTERACTIONS
Use steroids with caution because dehydration may develop from steroid-induced polyuria and polydipsia in a patient that relies on his owner for water intake.

FOLLOW-UP
• Self-limiting disorder • Full recovery in 2-4 weeks • Occasional masticatory muscle atrophy but without trismus

MISCELLANEOUS

Reference
de Lahunta A. Veterinary neuroanatomy and clinical neurology. 2nd ed. Philadelphia: WB Saunders, 1983:110.
Author T. Mark Neer
Consulting Editor Joane M. Parent

BASICS

OVERVIEW
• Francisella tularensis is a small gram-negative coccobacillus (type A—more virulent, found in rabbits and ticks; Type B—waterborne, found in rodents and ticks) • Also called rabbit fever, deerfly fever, market men's disease; disease in North America, principally of wild lagamorphs (cottontail, jack, snowshoe) and rodents (moles, squirrels, muskrats, beavers) • Tularemia widely distributed; mostly a disease of northern hemisphere; absent from United Kingdom, Africa, South America, Australia; most United States cases found in Missouri, Alaska, Oklahoma, South Dakota, Tennessee, Kansas, Colorado, Illinois, Utah, and Maine • Peak occurrence late spring, June through August, and in December

Pathophysiology
• Dog or cat comes into contact with or ingests tissue or body fluids of an infected mammal or water; or is bitten by bloodsucking arthropod (tick) or flies, mites, midges, fleas, or mosquitos; low numbers needed to infect cat through skin, airways, or conjunctivally; GI tract requires larger number of organisms to infect. Over 3-5 days after skin contact, F. tularensis multiplies locally (papule), ulceration 2-4 days later; spreads via lymphatics to regional lymph node (LN), bacteremia, septicemia (lung, liver, spleen, LN, bone marrow); focal necrosis in liver/spleen with neutrophil response, lymphocytes, macrophages; granuloma develops; casentes and/or abscesses. • Francisella is facultative intracellular parasite and survives and grows in liver. Ingestion route may involve lymphadenopathy of cervical and mesenteric LN followed by septicemic spread.

SIGNALMENT
• Disease in cats occurs only occasionally
• Dogs relatively resistant to infection

SIGNS
• Cats usually have ticks; are hunter cats
• Distribution of lesions: face, oral, tonsilar ulceration, diffuse intestinal lesions, lymphadenopathy, oropharyngeal and GI tract indicate ingestion as route of infection
• Acute disease occurs 2-7 days after contact with Francisella. • Sudden onset of anorexia, lethargy • Fever (40-41° C) • Enlarged palpable submandibular and cervical LN; depending on stage of disease also tender abdomen, palpable mesenteric LN, hepatomegaly
• Multifocal white patches/ulcers along glossopalatine arches and tongue • Mucous membranes icteric • No diarrhea or vomiting
• Francisella biogroups may all infect cats but may differ in virulence; possible for a mild infection to occur in some cats

CAUSES AND RISK FACTORS
• Hunter/outdoor cats in tularemic endemic areas at greater risk of contacting infected wildlife, dust, soil, and water • Heavy tick infections in cats • Presence of infected wildlife in the area of hunting activity

DIAGNOSIS

DIFFERENTIAL DIAGNOSIS
• In any acute disease state manifested by acute lymphadenopathy, malaise, oral ulceration, and fatal outcome, tularemia should be considered. • Bubonic plague (Y. pestis)—seen in western United States • Pseudotuberculosis (Y. pseudotuberculosis)—usually see vomiting and diarrhea

CBC/BIOCHEMISTRY/URINALYSIS
CBC—initially severe panleukopenia; later leukocytosis with left shift, toxic neutrophils, thrombocytopenia • Serum chemistry profile—hyperbilirubinemia, hyponatremia, hypoglycemia, and elevated alanine transaminase • Urinalysis—bilbirubinuria, hematuria

OTHER LABORATORY TESTS
Serology with tube agglutination or ELISA possible but difficult to do except in reference laboratory

IMAGING N/A

OTHER DIAGNOSTIC PROCEDURES
• Francisella difficult to see on Gram's stained direct smear of lesion or biopsy
• Cultural isolation by reference laboratory of blood, pleural fluid, LN aspirate onto cysteine/cystine containing media necessary for recovery of Francisella; not recoverable on routine laboratory media. Extreme caution is needed when working with infection specimens or isolates. • Direct FA of clinical materials/tissues is a rapid assay of infection status of patient

GROSS HISTOPATHOLOGIC FINDINGS
Gross pathologic findings—multifocal white patches/ulcers along glossopalatine arches and tongue; oral, tonsilar ulceration; lymphadenopathy of cervical/retropharyngeal/submandibular LN with abscessation; diffuse intestinal lesions; mesenteric lymphadenopathy, splenomegaly and hepatomegaly; mucus membranes icteric

TREATMENT
• Early treatment important; high mortality if not treated early
• Prognosis poor if mesenteric LN are palpable
• Treat on inpatient basis with good nursing care
• High zoonotic potential—all personnel in contact with patient or body fluids must use face mask, gloves, and gowns to avoid infection; patients must be isolated
• Treat animal for ectoparasites

MEDICATIONS

DRUGS AND FLUIDS
• Treat all cases empirically until laboratory confirmation obtained
• Drug of choice in humans for tularemia is streptomycin (15-20 mg/kg/day) or gentamicin (5 mg/kg/day) with dosage adjustments for renal insufficiency; third generation cephalosporins are also useful; chloramphenicol and tetracycline are both bacteriostatic for Francisella and treatment with these drugs may result in high rate of relapse after treatment. Little information is available on the efficacy of antimicrobials in treating tularemia in cats because of high mortality if cases not treated early. Amoxicillin (PO dosage—20 mg/kg q8h for 5-7 days; IM/SC dosage—20 mg/kg q12h for 5 days) has been used successfully in combination with gentamicin (IM/SQ dosage—4.4 mg/kg q12h once and then q24h thereafter until a clinical response or until 7 days) in treating tularemia in cats if treated early.

CONTRAINDICATIONS/POSSIBLE INTERACTIONS

FOLLOW-UP

PATIENT MONITORING
Severe, rapidly fatal infection in cats; treatment, in order to be effective, must be rapid; DIC reactions can occur late in the infectious process

PREVENTION/AVOIDANCE
• Limit pet travel into tularemia endemic areas. • In endemic areas, confine pets to control exposure to and ingestion of wildlife and their ectoparasites (ticks). • Periodic ectoparasite control (spray or dust) of animal, pastures in endemic areas • Neuter cats to limit their hunting behavior and wildlife exposure.
• Take precautions to limit contamination of food and water with carcasses of infected wildlife.

EXPECTED COURSE AND PROGNOSIS
Prognosis poor if not treated early

MISCELLANEOUS
Zoonotic potential is high; must not be mistaken for bite abscess in cats or plague

ABBREVIATION
LN = lymph node

Reference
Rohrbach BW. Tularemia. JAVMA 1988;193:428-432.
Author Patrick L. McDonough
Consulting Editor Fred W. Scott

TUMORAL CALCINOSIS

 BASICS

OVERVIEW
Ectopic deposition of calcium salts in soft tissue and in periarticular areas

SIGNALMENT
• Usually young, large-breed dogs • More than half of the reported patients are German shepherd dogs < 2 years old.

SIGNS
• One or more hard, well-circumscribed, nonpainful swellings in the cervical region, foot pads, or mouth • No clinical signs unless location interferes with function

CAUSES AND RISK FACTORS
• Cause and pathogenesis obscure • Several theories advanced but none satisfactorily explains development in all anatomic areas

 DIAGNOSIS

DIFFERENTIAL DIAGNOSIS
• Mineralized neoplasm • Mineralized abscess

CBC/BIOCHEMISTRY/URINALYSIS
Results normal

OTHER LABORATORY TESTS N/A

IMAGING
Radiography reveals calcified mass

OTHER DIAGNOSTIC PROCEDURES
N/A

 TREATMENT
•Surgical excision recommended

MEDICATIONS

DRUGS AND FLUIDS N/A

CONTRAINDICATIONS/POSSIBLE INTERACTIONS N/A

 FOLLOW-UP

PATIENT MONITORING
Usually not required

PREVENTION/AVOIDANCE N/A

POSSIBLE COMPLICATIONS
Usually none

EXPECTED COURSE N/A

PROGNOSIS
Usually good after surgical excision

 MISCELLANEOUS

ASSOCIATED CONDITIONS
Identical lesions are seen in patients with chronic renal failure, uremia, and primary hyperparathyroidism.

AGE RELATED FACTORS
Unknown

ZOONOTIC POTENTIAL N/A

PREGNANCY N/A

SYNONYMS
Synonyms include lipocalcinosis, calcinosis circumscripta, apocrine cystic calcinosis, tumoral lipocalcinosis, and hip stone.

Reference

Marks SL, Bellah JR, Wells M. Resolution of quadriparesis caused by cervicaltumoral calcinosis in a dog. J Am Anim Hosp Assoc 1992;27:72-76.

Author Wallace B. Morrison

Consulting Editor Wallace B. Morrison

UROLITHIASIS, CALCIUM OXALATE

BASICS

DEFINITION

Formation of calcium oxalate calculi within the urinary tract and the associated clinical condition

Pathophysiology

Presence of hypercalciuria, hyperoxaluria, hypocitraturia, and defective crystal growth inhibitors

Hypercalciuria

In dogs, normocalcemic hypercalciuria is thought to result from either intestinal hyperabsorption of calcium (so-called *absorptive hypercalciuria*) or reduced renal tubular reabsorption of calcium (so-called *renal-leak hypercalciuria*). Hypercalcemic hypercalciuria results from excessive glomerular filtration of mobilized calcium, which overwhelms normal renal tubular reabsorptive mechanisms (so-called *resorptive hypercalciuria* since excessive bone resorption is associated with high serum calcium concentrations).

Hyperoxaluria

In humans, hyperoxaluria is associated with inherited abnormalities of excessive oxalate synthesis (i.e., primary hyperoxaluria), excess consumption of foods containing high quantities of oxalate or oxalate precursors, pyridoxine deficiency, and disorders associated with fat malabsorption.

Hypocitraturia

Urine citrate is an inhibitor of calcium oxalate urolith formation. By complexing with calcium ions to form the relatively soluble salt of calcium citrate, citrate reduces the quantity of calcium available to bind with oxalate. In normal dogs, acidosis is associated with low urinary citrate excretion, whereas alkalosis promotes urinary citrate excretion.

Defective Crystal Growth Inhibitors

In addition to urinary concentration of calculogenic minerals, large molecular weight proteins in urine, such as nephrocalcin, have a profound ability to enhance solubility of calcium oxalate. Preliminary studies of urine obtained from dogs with calcium oxalate uroliths have revealed that nephrocalcin lacked appropriate numbers of carboxyglutamic acid residues compared with nephrocalcin isolated from normal dog urine.

Systems Affected

Renal/Urologic

Genetics   NA

Incidence/Prevalence

In dogs, calcium oxalate accounts for approximately 30–35% of the uroliths removed from the lower urinary tract and 40% of the uroliths removed from the upper urinary tract. In cats, calcium oxalate accounts for approximately 45–50% of the uroliths removed from the lower urinary tract and 50% of the uroliths retrieved from the upper urinary tract.

Geographic Distribution

Ubiquitous

SIGNALMENT

Species   Dogs and cats

Breed Predilections

• Dogs—in a large study, 44% of calcium oxalate uroliths were from three breeds, i.e., miniature schnauzer, lhasa apso, and Yorkshire terrier • Cats—the two pure breeds of cat with the greatest number were Himalayan (9%) and Persian (9%)

Mean Age And Range

• All ages of dogs and cats are affected. • Dogs—55% from 5-12 years • Cats—53% from 4-9 years

Predominant Sex

Mostly male dogs (73%) and male cats (55%)

SIGNS

General Comments

• None in some animals • Depend on location, size, and number of uroliths • Animals with nephroliths are typically asymptomatic but may have ureteral obstruction and hydronephrosis.

Historical Findings

Typical signs of urocystoliths or urethroliths include pollakiuria, dysuria, and hematuria.

Physical Examination Findings:

• Detection of urocystoliths or urethroliths by abdominal or rectal palpation; failure to palpate uroliths does not exclude them from consideration • A thickened and contracted bladder wall palpable in some animals, especially in cats • Large urinary bladder if animal has complete urethral obstruction

CAUSES

See Pathophysiology section

RISK FACTORS

• Excessive dietary calcium, protein, sodium, and vitamin D promote hypercalciuria. • Additional dietary oxalate (e.g., chocolate and peanuts) and ascorbic acid promote oxalate excretion. • Exogenous or endogenous exposure to high concentration of glucocorticoids promotes calcium excretion. • Furosemide promotes hypercalciuria.

DIAGNOSIS

DIFFERENTIAL DIAGNOSIS

• Other common causes of hematuria, dysuria, and pollakiuria with or without urethral obstruction including urinary tract infection and lower urinary tract neoplasia • Other common radiodense uroliths including those composed of magnesium ammonium phosphate and calcium phosphate silica (dogs)

CBC/BIOCHEMISTRY/URINALYSIS

• Results usually unremarkable • Urine sediment evaluation may reveal calcium oxalate crystals. • Hypercalcemia or azotemia (rare)

OTHER LABORATORY TESTS

Quantitative mineral analysis of urolithsis retrieved during voiding, by voiding urohydropropulsion, by aspiration into a urinary catheter, by cystoscopy, or cystotomy.

IMAGING

• Calcium oxalate uroliths are radiodense and may be detected by survey radiography. • Intravenous urography or ultrasonography may be required to verify ureteral obstruction.

OTHER DIAGNOSTIC PROCEDURES

NA

GROSS AND HISTOPATHOLOGIC FINDINGS   NA

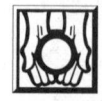

TREATMENT

INPATIENT VERSUS OUTPATIENT

• Retrograde urohydropropulsion is done to flush urethral stones back into the urinary bladder or voiding urohydropropulsion to eliminate bladder and urethral stones can be performed on an outpatient basis. • Shock wave lithotripsy and surgery require short periods of hospitalization.

ACTIVITY

During the period of tissue repair after surgery, activity level should be reduced.

DIET

• Dissolution of calcium oxalate uroliths with specials diets has not been reported. • Hypercalcemia in cats without evidence of hyperparathyroidism or malignancy is sometimes minimized by use of Prescription Diet Feline w/d (Hill's).

CLIENT EDUCATION

• Urolith removal does not alter the factors responsible for their formation. Therefore, eliminating risk factors is necessary to minimize recurrence. • Approximately 60% of dogs with a normal serum calcium concentration reform uroliths within 3 years. • Patients with hypercalcemia typically will reform uroliths at a faster rate.

SURGICAL CONSIDERATIONS

• Medical dissolution of calcium oxalate uroliths remains a goal for the future. • Consider surgical removal of uroliths from patients with obstruction or dysuria that cannot be removed by nonsurgical methods (e.g., voiding urohydropropulsion and catheter retrieval) or if clinical signs can not be alleviated by flushing the urolith back into the urinary bladder. • Shock wave lithotripsy is an alternative to surgery for removal of nephroliths and ureteroliths. • Parathyroidectomy should be considered in patients with primary hyperparathyroidism and hypercalcemia.

MEDICATIONS

DRUGS AND FLUIDS
No effective drugs available for dissolving calcium oxalate uroliths

CONTRAINDICATIONS
None

PRECAUTIONS
Steroids and furosemide promote calciuria

POSSIBLE INTERACTIONS N/A

ALTERNATE DRUGS N/A

FOLLOW-UP

PATIENT MONITORING
• Postsurgical radiographs are essential to verify complete urolith removal. • Abdominal radiography should be done every 3-6 months to reveal urolith recurrence early and prevent repeat surgery. Small uroliths can be removed easily by voiding urohydropropulsion or catheter retrieval.

PREVENTION/AVOIDANCE
• If patient is hypercalcemic, correct underlying cause. • If patient is normocalcemic, consider diet with reduced calcium, oxalate, sodium, and protein that do not promote formation of acidic urine (Prescription Diet Canine u/d, Prescription Diet Feline k/d, or Prescription Diet Feline w/d, Hill's Pet Products). Ideally, the diet should contain additional water (canned diets) and citrate and have adequate phosphorus and magnesium. Avoid supplementation with vitamins C and D. • Reevaluate patient 2-4 weeks after initiation of diet therapy to verify ameliora-

tion of crystalluria. If calcium oxalate crystalluria persists, consider additional potassium citrate (75 mg/kg PO q 12 h). Vitamin B$_6$ (2-4mg/kg PO q 24h-q48h) may be helpful to minimize oxalate excretion.

POSSIBLE COMPLICATIONS
• Urocystoliths can pass into and obstruct the urethra in male dogs, especially if the patient is dysuric; this can be managed by retrograde urohydropropulsion. • Dogs that do not consume their daily requirement of the urolith prevention diet can develop various degrees of protein calorie malnutrition. • Diet associated hyperlipidemia develops in some patients. Miniature schnauzers with hereditary hyperlipidemia and predisposition to pancreatitis can develop pancreatitis when consuming the prevention diet, in which case Prescription Diet Canine w/d (Hill's) can be used as an alternative diet. This diet should be supplemented with potassium citrate as needed to maintain a urine pH of approximately 7.0.

EXPECTED COURSE AND PROGNOSIS
Approximately 60% of dogs with normal serum calcium concentration reform uroliths in 3 years. Treatment to minimize recurrence is helpful. Comparable data is not available for cats. Patients with hypercalcemia typically reform uroliths at a faster rate.

MISCELLANEOUS

ASSOCIATED CONDITIONS
Any condition predisposing to hypercalciuria (e.g., hyperadrenocorticism, acidemia, hypervitaminosis D, and hyperparathyroidism) or hyperoxaluria (e.g., vitamin B$_6$ deficiency,

hereditary hyperoxaluria, and ingestion of chocolate and peanuts)

AGE RELATED FACTORS
Rare in young animals

ZOONOTIC POTENTIAL
None

PREGNANCY
Diets used to prevent calcium oxalate uroliths are not appropriate for pregnant animals.

SYNONYMS
Oxalate urolithiasis

SEE ALSO
Crystalluria

ABBREVIATIONS
None

References

Lulich JP, Osborne CA, Smith CL. Canine calcium oxalate urolithiasis: risk factor management. In: Kirk RW, Bonagura JD, eds. Current veterinary therapy XI. Philadelphia: WB Saunders, 1992;892-899.

Lulich JP, Osborne CA, Felice L. Calcium oxalate urolithiasis: cause, detection and control. In: August JR, ed. Consultations in feline internal medicine. Philadelphia: WB Saunders, 1994;343-349.

Thumchai R, Lulich JP, Osborne CA, et al. Epizootiology evaluation of 3498 feline uroliths: 1982-1992 (submitted for publication).

Lulich JP, Osborne CA. Voiding urohydropropulsion: a nonsurgical technique for removal of urocystoliths. In: Bonagura JD, Kirk RW, eds. Current veterinary therapy XII. Philadelphia: WB Saunders, 1995;1003-1006.

Authors Jody P. Lulich and Carl A. Osborne
Consulting Editors Larry G. Adams and Carl A. Osborne

UROLITHIASIS, CALCIUM PHOSPHATE

BASICS

OVERVIEW
• The formation of calcium phosphate calculi within the urinary tract and the associated clinical condition • Calcium phosphate uroliths represent 1-2 % of uroliths from dogs and cats submitted to laboratories for analysis. • Calcium phosphate uroliths are commonly called apatite uroliths. Hydroxyapatite and carbonate apatite are the most common forms. Brushite and whitlockite are less common forms. • A greater percentage of calcium phosphate uroliths are found in the kidneys compared with the urinary bladder.

SIGNALMENT
• Dogs and cats • Rarely detected in animals < 1 year old • No other distinguishing trends for breed, age, and gender in dogs or cats

SIGNS
• Depend on location, size, and number of uroliths • None in some animals • Typically, pollakiuria, dysuria, and hematuria. • Animals with nephroliths typically asymptomatic but may have hydronephrosis

CAUSES AND RISK FACTORS
• Calcium phosphate commonly found as a minor component of struvite and calcium oxalate uroliths • Pure calcium phosphate uroliths usually associated with metabolic disorders such as primary hyperparathyroidism, renal tubular acidosis, and excessive dietary calcium and phosphorus

DIAGNOSIS

DIFFERENTIAL DIAGNOSIS
• Other common causes of hematuria, dysuria, and pollakiuria with or without urethral obstruction include urinary tract infection and lower urinary tract neoplasia.

• Magnesium ammonium phosphate, calcium oxalate, and silica are other common radiodense uroliths.

CBC/BIOCHEMISTRY/URINALYSIS
• Results usually unremarkable • Hypercalcemia or azotemia rarely detected • Postrenal azotemia in some animals with complete obstruction • Amorphous crystals revealed by urine sediment evaluation in some animals. Brushite (calcium hydrogen phosphate dihydrate) forms elongated, lath-shaped crystals.

OTHER LABORATORY TESTS
Quantitative analysis of retrieved uroliths necessary to confirm their mineral composition

IMAGING
Radiodense uroliths often detected by survey radiography

OTHER DIAGNOSTIC PROCEDURES
N/A

TREATMENT
• Medical dissolution of calcium phosphate uroliths remains a goal for the future.
• Surgery can be considered for removal of clinically active uroliths.
• Nonsurgical methods of removing uroliths from the lower urinary tract include voiding urohydropropulsion, aspiration into a urinary catheter, and lithotripsy.
• Correction of hyperparathyroidism or other causes of hypercalcemia should minimize further urolith formation.

MEDICATIONS

DRUGS AND FLUIDS
No effective medications for dissolving calcium phosphate uroliths available

CONTRAINDICATIONS/POSSIBLE INTERACTIONS N/A

FOLLOW-UP

PATIENT MONITORING
• Radiography after surgery to verify complete urolith removal is essential. • Abdominal radiography every 3-4 months to enhance early detection of urolith recurrence and prevent the need for repeat surgery • Small uroliths easily removed by voiding urohydropropulsion or catheter retrieval

PREVENTION/AVOIDANCE
• A diet formulated to prevent formation of calcium oxalate uroliths may help prevent recurrence. Prescription Diet Canine U/D (Hill's) is formulated to reduce calcium excretion and is also phosphorus restricted.
• Because of the high moisture content of canned foods and their tendency to promote a dilute urine, canned diets may be more effective than dry diets in preventing recurrence.

MISCELLANEOUS

SYNONYMS
Apatite uroliths

Reference
Lulich JP, Osborne CA, Bartges JW, et al. Canine lower urinary tract disorders. In: Ettinger SJ, Feldman EC, eds. Textbook of veterinary internal medicine. Philadelphia: WB Saunders, 1995;1833-1861.
Authors Jody P. Lulich and Carl A. Osborne
Consulting Editors Larry G. Adams and Carl A. Osborne

BASICS

OVERVIEW
• The formation of polycrystalline concretions (ie, uroliths, calculi, or stones) composed of cystine in the excretory system .
• Occurs in dogs and cats with cystinuria, which is an inborn error of metabolism characterized by abnormal transport of cystine, a nonessential sulfur-containing amino acid composed of two molecules of cysteine, and other amino acids by the renal tubules.
• Cystine is normally present in low concentrations in plasma. It is freely filtered at the glomerulus and most is actively reabsorbed in the proximal tubules. Unlike normal dogs, cystinuric dogs reabsorb a much smaller proportion of the amino acid from glomerular filtrate. Some dogs may even have net cystine secretion. • Cystine is relatively insoluble in acid urine but becomes more soluble in alkaline urine. • Unless protein intake is severely restricted, cystinuric dogs have no detectable abnormalities associated with amino acid loss, with the exception of formation of cystine uroliths. The exact mechanism of cystine urolith formation is unknown. Because not all cystinuric dogs form uroliths, cystinuria is a predisposing rather than a primary cause of cystine urolith formation. • The precise mode of inheritance of cystinuria in dogs is unknown; however, both sex-linked and autosomal recessive patterns have been suggested.

SIGNALMENT
• Dogs and cats • Dogs—adult males primarily affected (mean age at diagnosis, 3- 5 years), but females also affected. • Many breeds affected, especially dachshund, English bulldog, and Newfoundland. • Cats—primarily adult males and females (mean age at diagnosis, 4 years). Most commonly recognized in domestic shorthair and Siamese breeds.

SIGNS
• None in some animals • Depend on location, size, and number of uroliths • Typical signs urocystoliths include pollakiuria, dysuria, and hematuria. • Typical signs of urethroliths include pollakiuria, dysuria, and sometimes voiding of small smooth uroliths. Complete outflow obstruction may cause postrenal uremia. • Animals with nephroliths typically show no signs, but may have hydronephrosis and renal insufficiency.

CAUSES AND RISK FACTORS
• Cystinuria is a risk factor for cystine urolithiasis. • Breed predisposition (ie, dachshund, English bulldog, and Newfoundland) • In animals with previous history of cystine urolithiasis, uroliths recur within 6 – 12 months after surgery without prophylaxis. • Urolith formation enhanced by acid urine

pH, highly concentrated urine, and incomplete and infrequent micturition.

DIAGNOSIS

DIFFERENTIAL DIAGNOSIS
• Uroliths mimic other causes of pollakiuria, dysuria, hematuria, and outflow obstruction.
• Differentiate from other types of uroliths, especially ammonium urate in English bulldogs, by urinalysis, radiography, and quantitative analysis of voided or retrieved uroliths.

CBC/BIOCHEMISTRY/URINALYSIS
• Cystine crystals are six-sided and are insoluble in acetic acid. • Positive urine cyanide-nitroprusside test

OTHER LABORATORY TESTS
• Urine amino acid profile—reveals abnormal quantities of cystine and, in some dogs and cats, lysine, arginine, and ornithine
• Quantitative mineral analysis of uroliths retrieved during voiding, by voiding urohydropropulsion, or by aspiration into a urinary catheter

IMAGING
• Radiography—cystine uroliths are radiolucent to slightly radiopaque with a smooth to slightly irregular surface. • Ultrasonography can be used to detect uroliths.

OTHER DIAGNOSTIC PROCEDURES
None

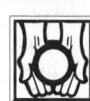

TREATMENT
• Medical dissolution of canine uroliths by a combination of N- (2-mercaptopropionyl) - glycine (2-MPG) and dietary management. Prescription Diet Canine u/d (Hill's Pet Products) reduces urinary excretion of cystine, promotes formation of alkaline urine, and reduces urine concentration. This diet is used in conjunction with 2-MPG for urolith dissolution. It is often effective alone in preventing recurrence of cystine uroliths.
• Removal of small urocystoliths by voiding urohydropropulsion or surgery

MEDICATIONS

DRUGS AND FLUIDS

Urine Alkalinizers
• Consider in patients that have acid urine despite dietary management and control of urease-positive urinary tract infection.
• Data derived from studies in cystinuric humans suggest that dietary sodium may enhance cystinuria. Therefore, potassium citrate may be preferable to sodium bicarbonate as a urine alkalinizer. A sufficient quantity of potassium citrate (40 – 75 mg/kg q12h) should be given to sustain a urine pH of 7.5.

Thiol-Containing Drugs
• 2-MPG reduces the urine concentration of cystine by combining with cysteine to form cysteine-2-MPG (which is more soluble than cystine).
• 2-MPG (Thiola-Mission Pharmacal; 15 – 20 mg/kg PO q12h) can be given to dissolve canine cystine uroliths in dogs in conjunction with dietary management. In our hospital, mean dissolution time was 10 weeks (range 2 – 30 weeks).
• 2-MPG can be given at a lower dosage (5 – 10 mg/kg PO q12h) to prevent recurrent canine cystine uroliths in dogs if dietary management is not optimal.
• Drug-induced adverse events associated with 2-MGP are uncommon in dogs; they include Coomb's positive spherocytic anemia, thrombocytopenia, and high hepatic enzyme activity.
• 2-MPG has not been evaluated in cystinuric cats.

FOLLOW-UP
• Prevention of recurrence with dietary management or 2-MPG • Monitor urolith dissolution at 30-day intervals by urinalysis and survey or contrast radiography. Although cystine uroliths tend to recur, recurrence does not occur in all cystinuric dogs and cats.

MISCELLANEOUS

Reference
Osborne CA, Lulich JP, Bargtes JW, et al. Canine and feline urolithiasis: relationship of etiopathogenesis to treatment and prevention. In: Osborne CA, Finco DR, eds. Canine and feline nephrology and urology. Philadelphia: Williams & Wilkins, [In press].

Authors Carl A. Osborne and Jody P. Lulich
Consulting Editors Larry G. Adams and Carl A. Osborne

UROLITHIASIS, STRUVITE—CATS

 **BASICS**

DEFINITION

Struvite uroliths and struvite urethral plugs have physical and probably etiopathogenic differences and, therefore, these terms should not be used as synonyms. Struvite uroliths are polycrystalline concretions composed primarily of magnesium ammonium phosphate and smaller quantities of matrix. Struvite urethral plugs are commonly composed of large quantities of matrix mixed with magnesium ammonium phosphate. Some urethral plugs are composed primarily of organic matrix, sloughed tissue, blood, and inflammatory reactants.

Pathophysiology
• See Urolithiasis, Struvite—Dogs
• The most commonly encountered form of naturally occurring urethral plugs in cats contain relatively large quantities of matrix in addition to minerals, especially struvite. The specific causes and composition of urethral plug matrix have not been identified. One hypothesis is that plug matrix occurs as a sequela to urinary tract infection, especially that cause by viruses.

Systems Affected
Renal/urologic—upper and lower urinary tract

Genetics N/A

Incidence/Prevalence
• The prevalence has been declining in the past decade because of the formulation of special diets designed to dissolve and prevent this type of stone.
• Currently, struvite composes less than half of uroliths in the lower urinary tract. of cats. Of these, 95% are sterile.
• Struvite has been detected in only about 5% of nephroliths in cats.
• Struvite remains the most common mineral in matrix-crystalline urethral plugs.

Geographic Distribution N/A

SIGNALMENT

Species
Cats (see Urolithiasis, Struvite—Dogs)

Breed Predilections
None

Mean Age and Tange
• Any age affected but the disease is most common in young adults.
• Immature cats are affected by infection-induced struvite uroliths but not by sterile struvite uroliths.

Predominant Sex
• Struvite uroliths are more common in females.
• Struvite urethral plugs affect males almost exclusively.

SIGNS

General Comments
• None in some cats
• Depends on location, size, and number of uroliths

Historical Findings
• Typical signs of urocystoliths include pollakiuria, dysuria, and hematuria.
• Typical signs of urethroliths include pollakiuria, dysuria, and sometimes voiding of small smooth uroliths.
• Signs of postrenal uremia (e.g., anorexia and vomiting) are found in some cats with outflow tract obstruction.
• Manifestations of renal insufficiency (e.g., polyuria and polydypsia) are found in some cats with nephroliths.
• Signs typical of outflow obstruction (e.g., dysuria, large urinary bladder, and signs of postrenal azotemia) are found in cats with struvite urethral plugs.

Physical Examination Findings
• A thickened, firm, contracted bladder is found in some cats with urocystoliths.
• Detection of urocystoliths by palpation is unreliable.
• Urethral plugs or uroliths may be detected by examination of the distal penis and penile urethral. Outflow obstruction results in a large urinary bladder and signs of postrenal uremia.

CAUSES
See pathophysiology

RISK FACTORS
• Probable risk factors for formation of sterile struvite uroliths include mineral composition, energy content, and moisture content of the diet, urine alkalinizing metabolites in the diet, quantity of diet consumed, ad libitum versus meal feeding schedule, formation of concentrated urine, and retention or urine. Elimination or control of these risk factors may result in dissolution of sterile struvite uroliths and prevention of their recurrence.
• Probable risk factors for infection-induced struvite urolithiasis include urinary tract infection by urease-producing microbial pathogen, abnormality in local host defenses (including perineal urethrostomy) that allows bacterial urinary tract infection to develop, and the quantity of urea (the substrate of urease) excreted in the urine.
• The normal small diameter of the distal urethra in male cats predisposes them to obstruction with plugs and uroliths.

 DIAGNOSIS

DIFFERENTIAL DIAGNOSIS
• Uroliths mimic other causes of pollakiuria, dysuria, hematuria, and outflow obstruction.
• Differentiate struvite uroliths and urethral plugs from other types of uroliths by signalment, urinalysis, urine culture, radiography, and quantitative analysis of voided or retrieved uroliths or plugs.

CBC/BIOCHEMISTRY/URINALYSIS
• Complete outflow obstruction may cause postrenal azotemia (azotemia with urine specific gravity >1.035).
• Magnesium ammonium phosphate crystals typically appear as colorless, orthohombic (having three unequal axes intersecting at right angles), coffin-like prisms. They often have three to six or more sides.
• Quantitative bacterial urine culture (preferably with specimen obtained by cystocentesis) should be done.

OTHER LABORATORY TESTS
• Quantitative mineral analysis is done of uroliths and urethral plugs retrieved during voiding, by voiding urohydropropulsion, by aspiration into a urinary catheter, or by cystoscopy.
• Bacterial culture is done of inner portions of infection-induced struvite uroliths.

IMAGING

Radiography
• Struvite uroliths are radiodense and may be detected by survey radiography. Some struvite urethral plugs are detected by survey radiography.
• Contrast urethrocystography is helpful in identifying the site of urethral obstruction and presence of urethral strictures.

Ultrasonography
• Detect presence of uroliths within the urinary tract.
• Determines precise location, size, and number of uroliths. The size and number are not a reliable index of probable efficacy of dissolution therapy.

OTHER DIAGNOSTIC PROCEDURES
None

GROSS AND HISTOPATHOLOGIC FINDINGS
Urethral plugs may contain RBC, WBC, transitional epithelial cells, and bacteria or viruses in addition to matrix and minerals.

 TREATMENT

INPATIENT VERSUS OUTPATIENT
• Retrograde urohydropropulsion to eliminate urethral stones, lavage to remove urethral plugs, voiding urohydropropulsion to eliminate bladder and urethral stones, and surgery require short periods of hospitalization.
• Medical dissolution of struvite uroliths is an outpatient strategy.

ACTIVITY
If dietary management is used, monitor outdoor activity.

DIET
• Dissolution of sterile and infection-induced struvite urocystoliths and nephroliths can be accomplished by feeding a calculolytic diet (Prescription Diet Feline s/d; Hills' Pet Products).

• Continue the diet for 1 month after survey radiographic evidence of urolith dissolution.

• Struvite crystalluria can be minimized by feeding a magnesium-restricted, urine acidifying diet.

CLIENT EDUCATION

• If dietary management is used, limit access to other foods and treats.

• Short-term (weeks to months) treatment with a calculolytic diet (Feline s/d) ± antibiotics as needed is effective in dissolving struvite uroliths. Avoid feeding calculolytic diets to immature cats.

• Owners of cats with infection-induced struvite urocystoliths must comply with dosage schedule for antibiotics.

SURGICAL CONSIDERATIONS

• Ureteroliths cannot be dissolved. Consider surgery for persistent ureteroliths associated with morbidity.

• Urethroliths can not be medically dissolved. Consider voiding urohydropropulsion or antegrade urohydropropulsion to induce urethroliths or urethral plugs to pass. Alternatively, move urethroliths into the bladder by retrograde urohydropropulsion.

• Immovable urethroliths, recurrent urethral plugs, or strictures of the distal urethra may require perineal urethrostomy.

• Nephroliths causing outflow obstruction or associated with nonfunctioning kidneys can not be dissolved medically.

• Consider surgical correction if uroliths are obstructing urine outflow or if correctable abnormality predisposing to recurrent urinary tract infection is identified by radiography or other means.

• Uroliths and urethral plugs should be localized before considering surgical correction.

MEDICATIONS

DRUGS AND FLUIDS

•Dietary dissolution of infection-induced urocystoliths or nephroliths requires oral administration of appropriate antibiotics, chosen on the basis of bacterial culture and antimicrobic susceptibility tests. Antibiotics must be given at therapeutic dosages until there is eradication of urinary tract infection and no radiographic evidence of uroliths.

CONTRAINDICATIONS

Urine acidifiers should not be given to azotemic patients or immature cats.

PRECAUTIONS

Azotemic patients are at higher risk than other animals for adverse drug events.

POSSIBLE INTERACTIONS None

ALTERNATIVE DRUGS None

FOLLOW-UP

PATIENT MONITORING

Monitor rate of urolith dissolution at monthly intervals by urinalysis, urine bacterial culture, and survey or contrast radiography.

PREVENTION/AVOIDANCE

• Recurrent sterile struvite uroliths can be prevented by use of magnesium-restricted, acidifying diet or urine acidifier. Do not administer urine acidifier with acidifying diet.

• Monitor patients whose urine has been acidified and change management protocol if persistent calcium oxalate crystalluria develops. In patients at risk for both struvite and calcium oxalate crystalluria, focus on prevention of calcium oxalate uroliths (see urolithiasis, calcium oxalate). Although struvite uroliths can be medically dissolved, recurrent calcium oxalate uroliths can not be dissolved.

• Infection-induced struvite urolithiasis can be prevented by eradicating and controlling urinary tract infection. Use of magnesium-restricted, acidifying diets is an ancillary method of prevention.

POSSIBLE COMPLICATIONS

• Urocystoliths can pass into and obstruct the urethra in male cats, especially if the patient is persistently dysuric. Urethral obstruction can be managed by retrograde urohydropropulsion. Dysuria can be minimized by treatment of bacterial urinary tract infection and by administration of an anticholinergic drug (eg, propantheline bromide 7.5 mg PO q3days).

• An indwelling urethral catheter can cause bacterial urinary tract infection and urethral stricture.

EXPECTED COURSE AND PROGNOSIS

In our hospital, the mean time for dissolution of sterile urocystoliths is 1 month (range, 2 weeks-5 months), and for infection-induced struvite urocystoliths it is 10 weeks (range, 9-12 weeks).

MISCELLANEOUS

ASSOCIATED CONDITIONS

Any disease that predisposes to bacterial urinary tract infection

AGE- RELATED FACTORS

Infection-induced struvite is the most common urolith in immature cats. Sterile struvite is rare in immature cats.

ZOONOTIC POTENTIAL

None

PREGNANCY N/A

SYNONYMS

FUS, feline urologic disease, feline lower urinary tract disease

SEE ALSO

• Urolithiasis, Struvite—Dogs
• Lower Urinary Tract Infection
• Nephrolithiasis

ABBREVIATIONS

MAP = magnesium ammonium phosphate

References

Osborne, CA, Kruger, JM, Lulich JP, et al. Disorders of the feline lower urinary tract. In: Osborne CA, Finco DR, eds. Canine and feline nephrology and urology. Philadelphia: Williams & Wilkins, In press.

Osborne, CA, Kruger, JM, Lulich JP, et al. Feline lower urinary tract diseases. In: Ettinger SJ, Feldman EC, eds. Textbook of veterinary internal medicine. 4th ed. Philadelphia: WB Saunders, 1995:1805-1832.

Osborne CA, Kruger JM, Lulich JP, et al. Feline matrix-crystalline urethral plugs: A unifying hypothesis of causes. J Small Anim Pract 1992;33:172-177.

Authors Carl A. Osborne, John M. Kruger, and Jody P. Lulich

Consulting Editors Larry G. Adams and Carl A. Osborne

UROLITHIASIS, STRUVITE—DOGS

BASICS

DEFINITION
The most common type of mineral encountered in uroliths of the lower urinary tract in dogs is magnesium ammonium phosphate hexahydrate (MAP), or struvite. Struvite composes approximately 40% of nephroliths in dogs.

Pathophysiology
Infection-Induced Struvite
• Urine must be supersaturated with MAP for struvite uroliths to form, which is associated with urinary tract infection by urease-producing microbes, alkaline urine, genetic predisposition, and diet.
• In animals affected by urinary tract infection caused by urease-producing microbes (especially *Staphylococcus, Proteus,* and *Ureaplasma*) and their urine contains a sufficient quantity of urea, the result is a unique combination of concomitant high concentrations of ammonium and carbonate (CO_3^{2-}) in an alkaline environment. These conditions favor formation of uroliths containing struvite ($MgNH_4 PO_4 6H_2O$), calcium apatite $[Ca_{10}(PO_4)_6(OH_2)_2]$, and carbonate apatite $[Ca_{10}(PO_4)_6 CO_3]$.
• Consumption of dietary protein in excess of the daily requirement for anabolism results in excess formation of urea from catabolism of amino acids. Hyperammonuria, hypercarbonaturia, and alkaluria mediated by microbial urease depends on the quantity of urea (the substrate of urease) in the urine.
• Abnormal urinary excretion of minerals is not required for initiation and growth of infection-induced struvite uroliths. However, metabolic and anatomic abnormalities may indirectly induce formation of struvite uroliths by predisposing the animal to urinary tract infection.
Sterile Struvite
Dietary or metabolic factors may be involved in the genesis of sterile struvite uroliths, but the mechanism of sterile struvite urolith formation in dogs is not clear.

Systems Affected
Renal/urologic

Genetics
• The high prevalence of struvite uroliths in some breeds of dogs such as the miniature schnauzer suggests a familial tendency. We hypothesize that susceptible miniature schnauzers inherit an abnormality of local host defenses of the urinary tract that increases their susceptibility to urinary tract infection.
• Sterile struvite uroliths have been encountered in a family of English cocker spaniels.

Incidence/Prevalence
Struvite uroliths account for approximately 55% of stones affecting the canine lower urinary tract and 40% of stones affecting the upper urinary tract in dogs.

Geogrphic Distribution
Ubiquitous

SIGNALMENT

Species
Dogs (see Urolithiasis, Struvite—Cats)

Breed Predilections
• Miniature schnauzer, dachshund, poodle, Scottish terrier, beagle, Pekingese, Welsh corgi
• Any breed can be affected.

Mean Age and Range
• Mean age, 6 years; range, <1 to > 16 years
• Most uroliths in immature dogs are infection-induced struvite.

Predominant Sex
More common in females (70%) than males (30%)

SIGNS

General Comments
• None in some animals
• Signs depend on location, size, and number of uroliths.

Historical Findings
• Typical signs of urocystoliths include pollakiuria, dysuria, and hematuria.
• Typical signs of urethroliths include pollakiuria, dysuria, and sometimes voiding of small smooth uroliths.
• Nephroliths are associated with manifestations of renal insufficiency in some animals.
• Obstruction to urine outflow in animals with bacterial urinary tract infection can cause generalized pyelonephritis and septicemia.

Physical Examination Findings
• Uroliths may be palpated in the urinary bladder and urethra.
• Obstruction of the urethra may cause enlargement of the urinary bladder.
• Obstruction of a ureter may cause enlargement of the associated kidney.
• Complete urine outflow obstruction combined with bacterial infection may cause ascending urinary tract infection, signs of renal failure, and signs of septicemia.

CAUSES
• Urinary tract disorder that predisposes to infection by urease producing bacteria, fungal pathogen, or ureaplasma in patients whose urine contains a large quantity of urea.
• Specific causes of sterile struvite uroliths are unknown.

RISK FACTORS
• Exogenous or endogenous exposure to high concentrations of glucocorticoids—predisposes animal to bacterial urinary tract infection
• Abnormal retention of urine
• Alkaline urine reduces the solubility of struvite

DIAGNOSIS

DIFFERENTIAL DIAGNOSIS
• Uroliths mimic other causes of pollakiuria, dysuria, hematuria, and outflow obstruction.
• Differentiate from other types of uroliths are done by signalment, urinalysis, urine culture, radiography, and quantitative analysis of voided or retrieved uroliths.

CBC/BIOCHEMISTRY/URINALYSIS
• Quantitative bacterial urine culture (preferably obtained by cystocentesis)
• Magnesium ammonium phosphate crystals typically appear as colorless, orthorhombic (having three unequal axes intersecting at right angles), coffin-like prisms. They often have three to six or more sides and oblique ends.
• Complete outflow obstruction can cause postrenal uremia.

OTHER LABORATORY TESTS
• Bacterial culture of inner portions of infection-induced struvite uroliths
• Quantitative mineral analysis of uroliths retrieved during voiding, by voiding urohydropropulsion, by aspiration into a urinary catheter, or by cystoscopy

IMAGING
• Struvite uroliths are radiodense and may be detected by survey radiography.
• Ultrasonography can be used to detect uroliths.
• Determine precise location, size, and number of uroliths. The size and number of uroliths are not a reliable index of probable efficacy of dissolution treatment.

OTHER DIAGNOSTIC PROCEDURES
N/A

GROSS AND HISTOPATHOLOGIC FINDINGS N/A

TREATMENT

INPATIENT VERSUS OUTPATIENT
• Retrograde urohydropropulsion to eliminate urethral stones, voiding urohydropropulsion to eliminate bladder and urethral stones, shock-wave lithotripsy, and surgery require short periods of hospitalization.
• Medical dissolution of struvite uroliths is an outpatient strategy.

ACTIVITY
If dietary management is used, monitor outdoor activity.

DIET
• Dissolution of infection-induced and sterile struvite urocystoliths and nephroliths can be accomplished by feeding the animal a calculolytic diet (Prescription Diet Canine s/d; Hill's Pet Products).
• Continue the diet for 1 month beyond survey radiographic evidence of urolith dissolution.
• Avoid protein-restricted diets in patients with protein-calorie malnutrition. The calculolytic diet is designed for short-term (weeks to months) dissolution rather than long-term (months to years) prophylaxis. If used, moni-

tor the patient for protein malnutrition. Avoid prolonged feeding of a calculolytic diet to immature dogs.

CLIENT EDUCATION
• If dietary management is used, limit access to other foods and treats.
• Short-term treatment with a calculolytic diet and administration of antibiotics has been effective in dissolving struvite uroliths.
• Comply with dosage schedule for antibiotics.

SURGICAL CONSIDERATIONS
• Ureteroliths cannot be dissolved. Consider surgery or shock-wave lithotripsy to treat persistent ureteroliths associated with morbidity.
• Urethroliths can not be medically dissolved. Consider voiding (antegrade) urohydropropulsion to induce urethroliths to pass. Alternatively, move urethroliths into the bladder by retrograde urohydropropulsion.
• Immovable urethroliths may require urethrotomy or urethrostomy.
• Nephroliths causing outflow obstruction and those associated with nonfunctioning kidneys cannot be dissolved medically.
• Consider surgical correction if uroliths are obstructing urine outflow or if correctable abnormalities predisposing to recurrent urinary tract infection are identified by radiography or other means.

MEDICATIONS

DRUGS AND FLUIDS
• Dietary dissolution of infection-induced urocystoliths or nephroliths requires oral administration of appropriate antibiotics chosen on the basis of bacterial culture and antimicrobic susceptibility tests. Antibiotics must be given at therapeutic dosages until there is eradication of urinary tract infection and no radiographic evidence of uroliths.
• Patients with infection-induced struvite urocystoliths associated with persistent urinary tract infection by urease- producing bacteria that are refractory to dietary and antibiotic dissolution can be given acetohydroxamic acid (Lithostat, Mission Pharmacal, 12.5 mg/kg PO q12h). Acetohydroxamic acid is a urease inhibitor that blocks hydrolysis of urea to ammonia.

CONTRAINDICATIONS
Acetohydroxamic acid is teratogenic and should not be given to pregnant dogs.

PRECAUTIONS
Prolonged administration of acetohydroxamic acid at a high dosage induces abnormalities in bilirubin metabolism in some dogs and may induce reversible hemolytic anemia.

POSSIBLE INTERACTIONS None
ALTERNATIVE DRUGS N/A

FOLLOW-UP

PATIENT MONITORING
Monitor rate of urolith dissolution monthly by urinalysis, urine culture, and survey or contrast radiography.

PREVENTION/AVOIDANCE
• Infection-induced struvite urolithiasis can be prevented by eradicating and controlling urinary tract infection. Use of a magnesium-restricted, acidifying diet is an ancillary method of prevention.
• Recurrent sterile struvite uroliths can be prevented by use of an acidifying, magnesium-restricted diet (Prescription Diet Canine c/d, Hills) or urine acidifier.
• Monitor for calcium oxalate crystalluria in patients whose urine has been acidified. Change management protocol if persistent calcium oxalate crystalluria develops.
• In patients at risk for both struvite and calcium oxalate crystalluria, focus on prevention of calcium oxalate uroliths. Whereas struvite uroliths can be medically dissolved, recurrent calcium oxalate uroliths cannot be dissolved.

POSSIBLE COMPLICATIONS
• Urocystoliths can pass into and obstruct the urethra of male dogs, especially if the patient is persistently dysuric. Urethral obstruction can be managed by retrograde urohydropropulsion. Dysuria can be minimized by treatment of bacterial urinary tract infection and administration of anticholinergic drugs (e.g., propantheline).
• Dogs that do not consume their daily requirement of the calculolytic diet may develop various degrees of protein calorie malnutrition. This can be prevented by proper calculation of the daily requirement and adjusting the quantity of diet fed on the basis of physical examination findings.
• Diet-associated polyuria is associated with various degrees of urinary incontinence in neutered female dogs with a predisposition to estrogen responsive incontinence.

EXPECTED COURSE AND PROGNOSIS
• In our hospital, the mean time for dissolution of infection-induced urocystoliths is 3 months (range, 2 weeks to 7 months), for infection-induced struvite nephroliths it is 6 months (range, 2 to 10 months), and for sterile struvite urocystoliths it is 6 weeks (range, 4 to 12 weeks).
• Owner compliance with diet management is suggested by reduced serum urea concentration ($\leq$ 10 mg/dl) and a low urine specific gravity (1.004 to 1.014).
• If uroliths become larger during dietary management or do not become smaller after

approximately 4 to 8 weeks, alternative methods should be considered. Difficulty in inducing complete dissolution of uroliths should prompt consideration that (1) the wrong mineral component was identified, (2) the nucleus is of different mineral composition than other portions of the urolith, and (3) the owner is not complying with medical recommendations.

MISCELLANEOUS

ASSOCIATED CONDITIONS
Any disease that predisposes an animal to bacterial urinary tract infection

AGE- RELATED FACTORS
Infection-induced struvite is the most common urolith in immature dogs.

ZOONOTIC POTENTIAL
None

PREGNANCY
• Acetohydroxamic is teratogenic.
• The calculolytic diet is not designed to sustain pregnancy.

SYNONYMS
Phosphate calculi, infection stones, urease stones, and triple-phosphate stones

SEE ALSO
• Lower Urinary Tract Infection
• Nephrolithiasis
• Pyelonephritis

ABBREVIATIONS
MAP = magnesium ammonium phosphate
AHA = acetohydroxamic acid

References

Osborne, CA, Lulich JP, Bartges JW, et al. Canine and feline urolithiasis: Relationship of etiopathogenesis to treatment and prevention. In: Osborne CA, Finco DR, eds. Canine and feline nephrology and urology. Philadelphia: Williams & Wilkins. In press.

Lulich JP, Osborne CA. Voiding urohydropropulsion: a nonsurgical technique for removal of urocystoliths. In: Bonagura JD, Kirk RW, eds. Current veterinary therapy. XII., Philadelphia: WB Saunders. In press.

Authors Carl A. Osborne, Jody P. Lulich, and David J. Polzin

Consulting Editors Larry G. Adams and Carl A. Osborne

UROLITHIASIS, URATE

BASICS

DEFINITION
Uroliths composed of uric acid, sodium urate, or ammonium urate.

Pathophysiology
• Impaired conversion of uric acid to allantoin causes high concentration of uric acid in serum and urine.

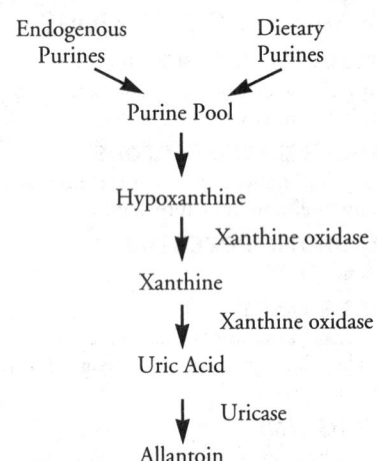

Endogenous Purines — Dietary Purines

Purine Pool

Hypoxanthine

Xanthine oxidase

Xanthine

Xanthine oxidase

Uric Acid

Uricase

Allantoin

• Animals with portosystemic shunt may develop ammonium urate uroliths because of impaired metabolism of uric acid and ammonia.

Systems Affected
Renal/urologic

Genetics N/A

Incidence/Prevalence
Approximately 7% of uroliths retrieved from dogs and cats.

Geographic Distribution N/A

SIGNALMENT

Species Dogs and cats

Breed Predilections
Dalmatian, English bulldog, and breeds at risk for portosystemic shunt (i.e., miniature schnauzer and Yorkshire terrier)

Mean Age and Range
• Mean age in animals without portosystemic shunt is 3.5 years (range, 0.5 to > 10 yrs)
• Mean age in animals with portosystemic shunt is < 1 year (range: 0.1 to >10 yrs).

Predominant Sex
• More common in male dogs without portosystemic shunt
• No sex predilection in dogs with portosystemic shunt or cats

SIGNS

Historical Findings
• Hematuria
• Dysuria
• Possible hepatoencephalopathy in animals with portosystemic shunt

Physical Examination Findings
• Urethral obstruction
• No signs in some animals

CAUSES
Rule out portosystemic shunt

RISK FACTORS
• High purine intake (glandular meat)
• Persistent aciduria in a predisposed animal.

DIAGNOSIS

DIFFERENTIAL DIAGNOSIS
Other causes of lower or upper urinary tract disease

CBC/BIOCHEMISTRY/URINALYSIS
• Aciduria
• Urate crystalluria
• Azotemia in animals with urinary outflow obstruction
• Low BUN in animals with portosystemic shunt

OTHER LABORATORY TESTS
High bile acids if animals with portosystemic shunt

IMAGING
• Urate uroliths may be radiolucent and, therefore, intravenous pyelogram (IVP) to detect nephroliths or double contrast cystography to detect urocystoliths may be necessary.
• Microhepatica in animals with portosystemic shunt
• Ultrasonography may reveal small uroliths and portosystemic shunts

OTHER DIAGNOSTIC PROCEDURES
N/A

GROSS AND HISTOPATHOLOGIC FINDINGS N/A

TREATMENT

INPATIENT VERSUS OUTPATIENT
Urethral or ureteral obstruction may require inpatient treatment. Dissolution of urate uroliths can be done on outpatient basis.

ACTIVITY
Usually not restricted, except after surgery

DIET
For dissolution and prevention, a low-purine, urine alkalinizing diet

CLIENT EDUCATION
Recurrence of uroliths is possible.

SURGICAL CONSIDERATIONS
• Cystotomy, urethrotomy, or nephrotomy to remove uroliths
• Portosystemic shunt ligation

MEDICATIONS

DRUGS AND FLUIDS
• Crystalloids for rehydration

• Allopurinol (15 mg/kg PO q12h), a xanthine oxidase inhibitor, for dissolution (see algorithm 1)

CONTRAINDICATIONS N/A

PRECAUTIONS
Allopurinol is contraindicated in animals with renal failure.

POSSIBLE INTERACTIONS
Skin eruption with use of allopurinol and ampicillin

ALTERNATE DRUGS N/A

FOLLOW-UP

PATIENT MONITORING
See algorithm 2

PREVENTION/AVOIDANCE
Low-purine, urine alkalinizing diet

POSSIBLE COMPLICATIONS
• Urethral obstruction
• Uroliths may recur.

EXPECTED COURSE AND PROGNOSIS
Medical dissolution takes an average of 8 weeks.

MISCELLANEOUS

ASSOCIATED CONDITIONS
Portosystemic shunt

AGE-RELATED FACTORS N/A

ZOONOTIC POTENTIAL N/A

PREGNANCY
Low-protein diet is not recommended for pregnant or lactating animal.

SYNONYMS N/A

SEE ALSO
• Urolithiasis, Xanthine
• Portosystemic Shunt

ABBREVIATIONS
BUN = blood urea nitrogen

References
Bartges JW, Osborne CA, Felice LJ. Canine Xanthine Uroliths: Risk Factor Management. In: Kirk RW, Bonagura, JD, eds. Current veterinary therapy XI. Philadelphia: WB Saunders, 1992: 900-905.
Osborne CA, Lulich JP, Bartges JW, Polzin DJ. Metabolic uroliths in cats. In: Kirk RW, Bonagura JD, eds. Current veterinary therapy XI. Philadelphia: WB Saunders, 1992: 906-910.

AUTHOR Joseph W. Bartges
CONSULTING EDITORS Larry G. Adams and Carl A. Osborne

Figure 1. Algorithm for Treatment of Urate Urocystolithiasis

Dysuria, pollakiuria, hematuria

No urethral obstruction
• Double contrast cystography
• Urethrography

Urethral obstruction
• Retrograde urohydropropulsion

Urocystolith size and number

Less than distended
urethral diameter
• Voiding urohydropropulsion

Urocystoliths greater than
distended urethral diameter

All uroliths retrieved
• Refer to prevention algorithm

All uroliths not retrieved

Dissolution treatment:
• Diet: restricted purine and
  urine alkalinizing
• Allopurinol 15 mg/kg PO q12h

Cystotomy and postoperative
double contrast cystography

All uroliths retrieved
• Refer to prevention
  algorithm

4 weeks:
• Urinalysis
• Double contrast cystography

All uroliths not retrieved

Urocystoliths not present
• Refer to prevention algorithm

Urocystoliths present

Decrease in size
and/or number
• Continue therapy

No change or increase
in size and/or number

Urocystoliths not retrieved
• Cystotomy
• Double contrast cystography

Urocystoliths retrieved and analyzed

Urate
• Increased allopurinol
  dose by 10-25%

Xanthine

Uroliths

No uroliths
• Refer to prevention
  algorithm

Stop allopurinol, continue diet, wait 1-2 months,
repeat double contrast cystogram, retrieve uroliths
and analyze.
If urate, begin allopurinal at 25% dosage reduction

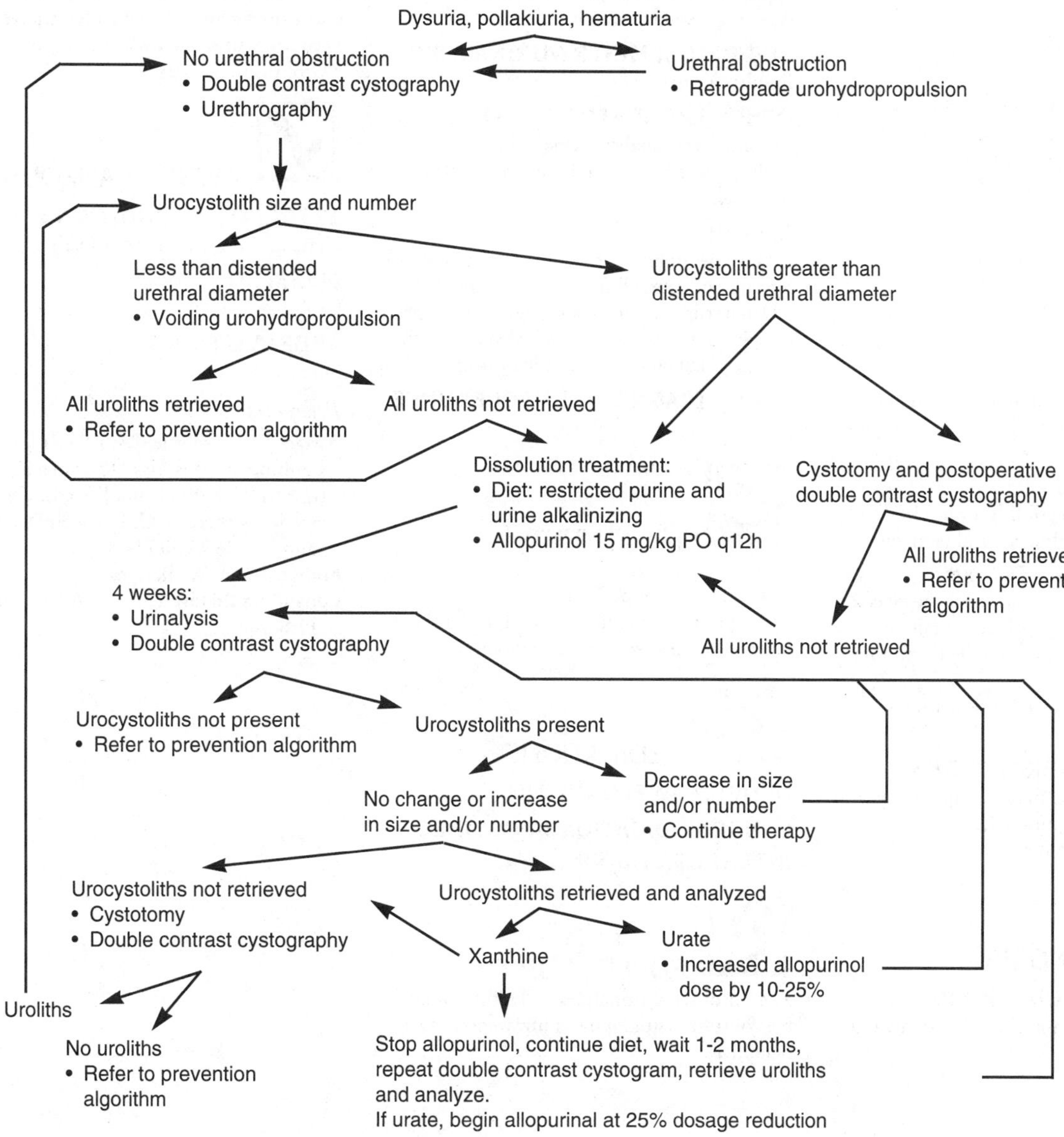

Figure 2. Algorithm for Prevention of Urate Urocystolithiasis

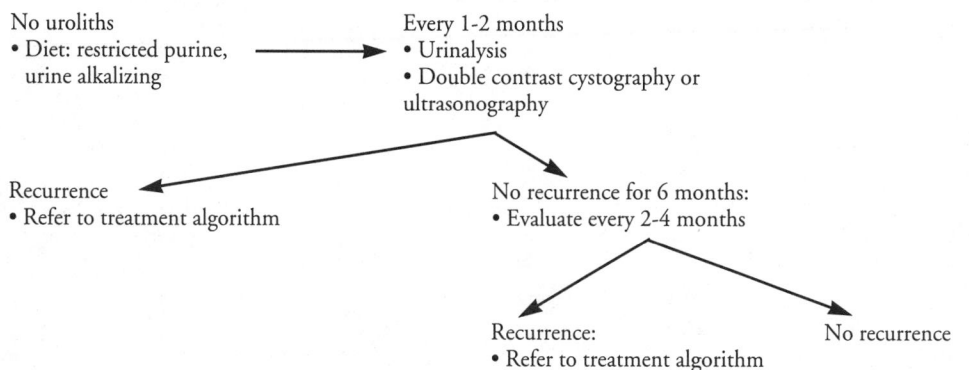

No uroliths
• Diet: restricted purine,
  urine alkalizing

Every 1-2 months
• Urinalysis
• Double contrast cystography or
  ultrasonography

Recurrence
• Refer to treatment algorithm

No recurrence for 6 months:
• Evaluate every 2-4 months

Recurrence:
• Refer to treatment algorithm

No recurrence

UROLITHIASIS, XANTHINE

BASICS

OVERVIEW
Xanthine is converted to uric acid by xanthine oxidase. Impaired conversion by allopurinol may cause hyperxanthinemia, xanthinuria, and xanthine uroliths.

SIGNALMENT
• Dogs and cats receiving allopurinol.
• Naturally occurring xanthine uroliths have been observed in young cats.

SIGNS

General Comments
Signs are related to anatomic location(s) of urolith(s). Affected animals may be asymptomatic.

Historical Findings
Typical signs of urocystoliths or urethroliths include pollakiuria, dysuria, and hematuria.

Physical Examination Findings
• Urocystoliths or urethroliths may be detected on abdominal or rectal palpation; failure to palpate uroliths does not exclude them from consideration.
• Large bladder if urethral obstruction is complete.

CAUSES AND RISK FACTORS
• Allopurinol administration, especially accompanied by high purine diet
• Hereditary xanthinuria

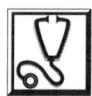

DIAGNOSIS

DIFFERENTIAL DIAGNOSIS
• Other causes of lower or upper urinary tract disease

• Differentiate from other types of uroliths—xanthine uroliths are radiolucent; xanthine crystals are yellow-brown, spherical

CBC/BIOCHEMISTRY/URINALYSIS
Results normal

OTHER LABORATORY TESTS
Quantitatively analyze urine sediment or uroliths. Xanthine crystals are yellow-brown, spherical.

IMAGING
• Xanthine uroliths are radiolucent and therefore are not detected on survey radiographs.
• Double contrast cystography, intravenous pyelography, or ultrasonography will identify uroliths and their location within the urinary tract.

OTHER DIAGNOSTIC PROCEDURES
N/A

TREATMENT
• Surgical removal
• Discontinue allopurinol.
• Low purine diet reduces amount of xanthine in urine and plasma. See urate urolithiasis.

MEDICATIONS

DRUGS AND FLUIDS N/A
CONTRAINDICATIONS/POSSIBLE INTERACTIONS N/A

FOLLOW-UP
• Monitor serial urinalyses and results of double contrast cystography or intravenous pyelography.

• If attempting to dissolve urate uroliths, discontinue allopurinol for 1-2 months and decrease dosage by 25% when reinstituted. Feed low-purine diet when using allopurinol.
• Uroliths may recur.

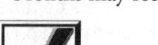

MISCELLANEOUS

ASSOCIATED CONDITIONS
Urate urolithiasis, nephrolithiasis

SEE ALSO
Urolithiasis, Urate

ABBREVIATIONS
None

References
Bartges JW, Osborne CA, Felice LJ. Canine xanthine uroliths: risk factor management. In: Kirk RW, Bonagura JD, eds. Current veterinary therapy XI. Philadelphia: WB Saunders, 1992:900-905.
Author Joseph W. Bartges
Consulting Editors Larry G. Adams and Carl A. Osborne

BASICS

OVERVIEW
• Failure of the uterine muscles to expel fetuses • Primary uterine inertia—the uterine muscles do not contract normally at parturition due to failure of the muscles to respond to hormonal stimuli, lack of the development of receptors, or an actual lack or failure of release or imbalance of hormones. • Also seen in very nervous animals, especially small breeds. • Obesity and lack of exercise one of the main causes of primary inertia • Uterine contractions may not be induced in a large breed dog with an abnormally small litter • Secondary uterine inertia (when a pup is not delivered within 2 hours) may develop during a prolonged parturition or after dystocia with subsequent uterine muscle failure (see Dystocia).

SIGNALMENT
Seen in some small breeds and nervous, obese, older, underexercised females and, possibly, small litters in all breeds

SIGNS
• Primary uterine inertia—lack of onset of parturition at the end of gestation and the animal is bright and alert • Vaginoscopy may detect that cervical dilation has occurred, and a small green–tinged vaginal discharge may be seen. • Secondary uterine inertia—animal usually has prolonged dystocia or, in some animals, 1 or 2 normal deliveries after which labor ceases even though more fetuses are in the uterus

CAUSES AND RISK FACTORS
• Primary uterine inertia—see overview • Secondary uterine inertia—obstruction in the reproductive tract so that the fetus cannot be expelled or absolute or relative fetal oversize. Other causes include fetal deficiency of adrenocorticoid hormone and faulty fetal presentation, position, and posture. • Progesterone administration will mimic condition.

DIAGNOSIS

DIFFERENTIAL DIAGNOSIS
• Pseudopregnancy (primary inertia) • Obstructive dystocia (secondary inertia)

CBC/BIOCHEMISTRY/URINALYSIS
• Results normal for a pregnant animal with primary inertia and may be useful if cesarean section is indicated • Serum calcium and blood glucose may be low in patients with secondary inertia.

OTHER LABORATORY TESTS
If more than 24 hrs have elapsed since the prepartum drop in rectal temperature or serum progesterone is < 2 ng/ml for 36 hours and labor has not started, a presumptive diagnosis of uterine inertia can be made.

IMAGING
• Radiography to determine the number and disposition of the fetus(es) • Ultrasonography to assess fetal stress and viability

OTHER DIAGNOSTIC PROCEDURES
N/A

TREATMENT
• True primary uterine inertia may not respond to medical treatment and therefore a cesarean section is indicated.
• Medical treatment is contraindicated in patients with obstructive dystocia and, on rare occasions, uterine rupture.
• Small doses of oxytocin induce more effective uterine contractions.

MEDICATIONS

DRUGS AND FLUIDS
• Oxytocin—total dose of 1–2 IU (small breeds), 3–4 IU (medium–sized breeds), or 5–6 IU (large breeds), SC or IM, and can be repeated in 45 minutes. If no progress is made after 2–3 injections, surgery is indicated.
• Calcium—given slowly as a 2–10 ml bolus of 10% calcium gluconate IV; must be stopped immediately if cardiac arrhythmias are detected.
• Glucose—10–20% dextrose in a slow IV infusion
• Another method that may work is to add 5–10 IU of oxytocin to a liter of 5% dextrose and administer this combination intravenously at a maintenance dosage rate. If effective contractions do not occur within 10–15 minutes, surgery is indicated. If contractions are induced, wait 1–1 1/2 hrs before surgery is performed.

CONTRAINDICATIONS/POSSIBLE INTERACTIONS
• Obstructive dystocia or uterine rupture (rare) • Overtreatment with oxytocin induces nonproductive tetanic contractions.

FOLLOW-UP

PATIENT MONITORING
• If medical treatment does work, make sure that all placentae are passed and dam should be evaluated for endocrine and reproductive tract disease, which may have predisposed the bitch to inertia. • Prognosis for puppy survival is good if treatment is instituted on the date of expected parturition. • Primary uterine inertia may recur at subsequent parturition dates

POSSIBLE COMPLICATIONS
Death of pups if too much time elapses from time that labor should have started until treatment is initiated.

MISCELLANEOUS

AGE RELATED FACTORS
Relatively older bitches are more prone to developing uterine inertia.

SEE ALSO
Dystocia

References

Johnston SD. Parturition and dystocia in the bitch. In: Morrow DA, ed. Current therapy in theriogenology 2. Philadelphia: WB Saunders, 1986;500–501.

Feldman EC, Nelson RW. Canine female reproduction. Canine and feline endocrinology and reproduction. Philadelphia: WB Saunders, 1987;399–480.

Author Klaas Post
Consulting Editor Sara K. Lyle

UVEAL MELANOMA—CATS

BASICS

OVERVIEW
The terms iris melanoma, uveal melanoma, and diffuse iris melanoma of cats are used interchangeably in the literature. These are the most common intraocular tumors in cats, and they usually arise from the anterior iridal surface with extension to the ciliary body and choroid. Unlike intraocular melanomas in dogs, those in cats tend to be flat and diffuse in appearance rather than nodular. The tumor has a benign clinical and histologic appearance initially, but a unique feature is that metastatic disease can develop up to several years later. Uveal melanomas in cats metastasize to regional lymph nodes, numerous visceral organs (especially those in the abdominal cavity), lungs, and less commonly, the skeleton.

SIGNALMENT
No sex or breed predisposition. Any age adult cat can be affected.

SIGNS
Historical Findings
Affected cat is often examined because of iris color change or when secondary glaucoma results in mydriasis or buphthalmia.

Physical Examination Findings
• The iris surface is hyperpigmented.
• Lesions are focal to diffuse, usually flat, slowly progressive, and may involve one or both eyes. • In cats with advanced disease, pigmented tumor cells can often be seen in the aqueous, and the iris is homogeneously thickened. • Drainage angle infiltration may occur and result in secondary glaucoma.

CAUSES AND RISK FACTORS N/A

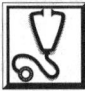

DIAGNOSIS

DIFFERENTIAL DIAGNOSIS
• Uveal melanoma most closely resembles iridal color change that results from chronic anterior uveitis. • Limbal melanomas have benign behavior and tend to be focal, superiorly located, flat to slightly raised limbal masses that do not invade the uveal tract unless they are very large. • "Freckles" on the surface of the iris that do not appear to change over time may be benign pigmented lesions but are more likely variants of iris melanoma.
• Heterochromia irides is a congenital, nonprogressive alteration in iridal pigmentation.

CBC/BIOCHEMISTRY/URINALYSIS
Normal

OTHER LABORATORY TESTS N/A

IMAGING
Thoracic radiographs and abdominal ultrasonography are helpful in determining the extent of metastatic disease. These imaging tests are recommended presurgically and every 6 months after the diagnosis of uveal melanoma.

OTHER DIAGNOSTIC PROCEDURES
• Complete ophthalmic examination, including tonometry and gonioscopy, is indicated.
• Fine needle aspiration of the iridal surface ("vacuuming") has been advocated for cytologic confirmation. Iridal biopsy may also be performed, but neither of these tests has been shown to be beneficial in staging the disease. Melanoma cells may appear in the iridocorneal angle and ciliary venous plexus, even when small, superficial, freckle-like masses are identified, and the eye is enucleated early. This finding suggests that metastasis can occur before development of invasive melanoma and secondary glaucoma.

TREATMENT
Although it is controversial, the author recommends enucleation to lessen the likelihood of metastasis. This is often difficult for the owner to accept because the eye is visual and asymptomatic. Gentle enucleation technique has been advised because enucleation has been associated with metastasis in human studies. Although no controlled or long term follow-up studies have been done, LASER (diode) photoablation has been used to treat freckle-like lesions with apparent success.

MEDICATIONS

DRUGS AND FLUIDS N/A

CONTRAINDICATIONS/POSSIBLE INTERACTIONS N/A

FOLLOW-UP
• If surgical options are declined, quarterly monitoring of intraocular pressure is advised to check for glaucoma. Mild elevation of intraocular pressure can be treated with carbonic anhydrase inhibitors (e.g., methazolamide approximately 6 mg q12h-q24h PO). Secondary glaucoma is best controlled by enucleation.
• Prognosis is guarded, even with enucleation, because metastasis may not become apparent for several years. Regional lymph nodes, lungs, and abdominal viscera are common sites for metastasis and should be monitored periodically.

MISCELLANEOUS

Reference
Dubielzig RR. Ocular neoplasia in small animals. Vet Clin North Am Small Anim Pract 1990;20:837–848.
Author Denise M. Lindley
Consulting Editor Paul E. Miller

BASICS

OVERVIEW
Melanomas of the anterior uvea (i.e., iris and ciliary body) and posterior uvea (i.e., choroid) are the most common primary intraocular neoplasm in dogs. Tumors are usually benign, unilateral, and most often affect the anterior uvea. Anterior uveal melanomas have a 4% rate of vascular metastasis to lungs and viscera. Choroidal melanomas do not metastasize. However, benign uveal melanomas often are destructive to the eye.

SIGNALMENT
• Average age of dogs with anterior uveal melanoma is 8-10 years, and of dogs with choroidal melanoma, 6.5 years. An age range of 2 months to 17 years is reported. • No breed or sex predilection exists.

SIGNS

Anterior Uveal Melanoma
• Pigmented scleral or corneal mass • Pigmented mass visible in the anterior chamber or posterior to the pupillary margin • Irregular pupil • Uveitis • Glaucoma • Hyphema • No vision loss (unless the mass obstructs the pupil or glaucoma has developed)

Choroidal Melanoma
• Diagnosis is often missed because of tumor location. • Funduscopy reveals a posterior segment mass.

CAUSES AND RISK FACTORS
• Idiopathic • Potential transformation of flat, pigmented iris "freckles" into melanomas

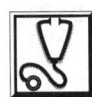

DIAGNOSIS

DIFFERENTIAL DIAGNOSIS
• Nonneoplastic uveal proliferations: iris freckles are not raised, diffuse iris hyperpigmentation secondary to chronic uveitis • Uveal cysts—these transilluminate and may move freely within the eye; melanomas do not. • Granulomatous masses • Ocular perforation with uveal prolapse • Other ocular neoplastic conditions • Outward scrolling of pupillary margin due to uveitis (ectropion uvea)

CBC/BIOCHEMISTRY/URINALYSIS
Usually normal

OTHER LABORATORY TESTS N/A

IMAGING Ultrasonography

OTHER DIAGNOSTIC PROCEDURES
• Slit lamp biomicroscopy to determine size and location of mass • Transillumination of mass • Tonometry • Indirect ophthalmoscopy • Gonioscopy to evaluate drainage angle for tumor extension • Examination of fine needle aspirate (infrequent)

GROSS AND HISTOPATHOLOGIC FINDINGS
• Biopsy of melanoma is not practical; pathologic findings are restricted to the enucleated globe. • Two cell types are usually seen: 1) plump cells filled with melanin, and 2) spindle cells. These usually have a benign appearance and low mitotic index (< 2 mitotic figures per high power field). The most reliable criterion for malignancy is the mitotic index, with clinically malignant tumors having a mitotic index of at least 4. • When submitting eyes for histologic evaluation, request bleached tissue sections and mitotic index.

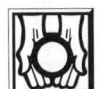

TREATMENT
• Because of the benign nature of most uveal melanomas, many clinicians opt for monitoring eyes (every 3-6 months) and do not enucleate unless the following occur: the size of the mass increases rapidly, the eye cannot be salvaged, the mass spreads diffusely within the eye, visual function is significantly impaired, extraocular invasion is present, secondary complications occur (e.g., glaucoma, signs of pain, and hemorrhage).
• If enucleation is needed, use gentle surgical technique to prevent showering of tumor cells into the vascular circulation. If extrascleral extension is present, the entire orbital contents should be exenterated.
• Other surgical treatments (rarely used): sector iridectomy and iridocyclectomy if discrete, small masses. Laser treatment of small iris tumors is a recently developed procedure.

MEDICATIONS

DRUGS AND FLUIDS N/A

CONTRAINDICATIONS/POSSIBLE INTERACTIONS N/A

FOLLOW-UP
• If the mitotic index is high or the patient has extrascleral, vascular, or optic nerve extension, then thoracic and abdominal radiography or ultrasonography is recommended postoperatively and at 6-month intervals during the next 12 months. • The enucleation site should be evaluated for tumor recurrence.

MISCELLANEOUS

Reference
Wilcock BP, Peiffer RL. Morphology and behavior of primary ocular melanomas in 91 dogs. Vet Pathol 1986;23:418.
Author Terri L. McCalla
Consulting Editor Paul E. Miller

UVEODERMATOLOGIC SYNDROME

BASICS

OVERVIEW
• This is a rare syndrome similar to Vogt-Koyanagi-Harada syndrome in man. • It is considered to be an autoimmune disorder resulting in concurrent granulomatous uveitis and depigmenting dermatitis.

SIGNALMENT
This disease has been reported in dogs (especially akitas, samoyeds and Siberian huskies) but does not appear to have any age or sex predilections.

SIGNS
• Sudden onset uveitis with concurrent or subsequent leukoderma of the nose, lips, eyelids.
• The footpads, scrotum, anus, and hard palate may also be affected by the depigmentation. Occasionally, ulcerations may also develop.

CAUSES AND RISK FACTORS
• The syndrome is felt to have an autoimmune etiology. Antiretinal antibodies have been found in affected dogs. • Exposure to sunlight can exacerbate the symptoms.

DIAGNOSIS

DIFFERENTIAL DIAGNOSIS
• The various immune-mediated skin diseases such as the pemphigus complex of diseases, systemic lupus erythematosis and discoid lupus erythematosis should be included as differential diagnoses. • Neoplasia and numerous other inflammatory and infectious skin diseases that can cause depigmentation should also be considered. • Skin biopsies, negative ANA titers and a normal retinal examination help to differentiate these diseases from uveodermatologic syndrome.

CBC/BIOCHEMISTRY/URINALYSIS
CBC, serum chemistries and urinalysis are usually normal

OTHER LABORATORY TESTS N/A

IMAGING N/A

OTHER DIAGNOSTIC PROCEDURES
• Biopsy and dermatopathology are best interpreted by by a veterinarian with experience in detecting the sometimes subtle differences in pathologic patterns. Early lesions reveal a lichenoid interface pattern with large histiocytes and pronounced pigmentary incontinence. • Hydropic degeneration of the epidermal basal cell is rare.

TREATMENT

• Aggressive and rapid initiation of immunosuppressive therapy is recommended to prevent formation of posterior synechiae and secondary glaucoma, cataracts or blindness.
• Retinal exams are the most important means of monitoring progress because improvement in dermatologic lesions may not reflect the retinal pathology.

MEDICATIONS

DRUGS AND FLUIDS
• Initially high doses of prednisone (1.1-2.2mg/kg q12h-q24h P0) and azathioprine (1.5-2.5 mg/kg q24h PO) are recommended. The dosages and frequencies should be tapered to an every other day basis for chronic use.
• Topical or subconjunctival steroids and cycloplegics may be indicated if anterior uveitis is present.

CONTRAINDICATIONS/POSSIBLE INTERACTIONS
The potential side effects of prednisone and azathioprine (anemia, leukopenia, thrombocytopenia, elevated serum alkaline phosphatase levels, vomiting and pancreatitis) warrant biweekly serum chemistries and CBCs including platelet counts initially. This can be decreased after the condition has stabilized and the dose and frequency have been tapered.

FOLLOW-UP

• Weekly or biweekly examinations including retinal evaluations is recommended initially along with the previously discussed tests used to monitor for side effects associated with therapeutics. The retinal exams are an important means of monitoring the disease because improvement in dermatologic lesions may not indicate improvement in the retinal lesions. • The azathiprine may be discontinued after a few months of therapy, but the prednisone may be necessary indefinitely.
• Some cases may improve with the initial use of prednisone alone, but the potential sequelae of delayed aggressive therapy warrants the additional use of azathioprine.

MISCELLANEOUS

Reference
Scott DW, Miller WH, Griffen CE. Small animal dermatology. 5th ed. Philadelphia: WB Saunders, 1995.
Author Dunbar Gram
Consulting Editor Lowell Ackerman

BASICS

OVERVIEW
• Vaccination can induce sarcoma in cats (primarily fibrosarcoma) at injection sites.
• Also associated with FeLV vaccination.
• The time between vaccination and tumor development can be as short as several months.

SIGNALMENT
Recognized only in cats

SIGNS

Physical Examination Findings
Firm, painless, subcutaneous swelling located at a previous vaccination site

CAUSES AND RISK FACTORS
• Unknown; but aluminum hydroxide, an adjuvant in many vaccines, has been suggested as a possible cause • The prevalence of fibrosarcoma in cats is low; estimated at 20/100,000 cats. • The risk for cats developing fibrosarcoma from a single FeLV or rabies vaccination in the cervical or interscapular region is about 50% higher than that for cats not receiving a vaccine at that site. • The risk for cats given 2 vaccinations is approximately 125% higher, and the risk for cats given 3 or 4 vaccinations is approximately 175% higher.

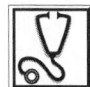

DIAGNOSIS

DIFFERENTIAL DIAGNOSIS
• Vaccine-associated Arthus reaction • Subcutaneous abscess • Mast cell neoplasia • Epidermal inclusion cyst • Sebaceous gland adenoma or adenocarcinoma • Apocrine gland adenoma or adenocarcinoma • Pilomatrixoma

CBC/BIOCHEMISTRY/URINALYSIS
Results normal

OTHER LABORATORY TESTS N/A

IMAGING
Regional and thoracic radiography to determine extent of disease and lung metastasis

OTHER DIAGNOSTIC PROCEDURES
• Cytologic examination of aspirate suggests mesenchymal neoplasia in some patients.
• Biopsy necessary for definitive diagnosis

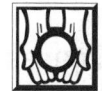

TREATMENT
• Wide surgical resection necessary because of invasiveness of this tumor
• Radiotherapy indicated if surgical removal is incomplete
• Chemotherapy may provide palliation in patients with nonresectable tumors. No specific regimens have been evaluated; however, the following 21-day protocol may be useful: doxorubicin (20 mg/m^2 IV) day 0 of treatment; cyclophosphamide (50 mg/m^2 PO) days 3, 4, 5, and 6 of treatment. Repeat cycle every 21 days for 5 cycles. If there is no response after 2 cycles, the tumor is considered chemotherapy resistant.

MEDICATIONS

DRUGS AND FLUIDS N/A

CONTRAINDICATIONS/POSSIBLE INTERACTIONS N/A

FOLLOW-UP
• Evaluations monthly for the first 3 months after surgical resection, then every 3 months for the remainder of the first year • Response to chemotherapy by CBC and platelet count before each treatment

MISCELLANEOUS
• Veterinarians should administer different vaccines at different sites. • Owners should be informed of benefits and risks of administering vaccines. • Vaccines should be administered in sites amenable to surgical resection (rear limb) in case a neoplasm develops.
• Other sarcomas associated with vaccination include malignant fibrous histiocytoma, osteosarcoma, rhabdomyosarcoma, and chondrosarcoma.

ABBREVIATION
FeLV = feline leukemia virus

Reference
Kass PH, et al. Epidemiologic evidence for a causal relation between vaccination and fibrosarcoma tumorigenesis in cats. J Am Vet Med Assoc 1993;203:396-405.
Author James P. Thompson
Consulting Editor Wallace B. Morrison

VAGINAL HYPERPLASIA AND PROLAPSE

 BASICS

OVERVIEW
• Protrusion of spherical or donut-shaped mass from vulva during proestrus or estrus
• Type I—slight eversion of the vaginal floor but no protrusion through the vulva. • Type II—vaginal tissue prolapses through the vulvar opening • Type III—donut-shaped eversion of the entire vaginal wall, including the urethral orifice. The urethral orifice can be seen ventrally on the prolapsed tissue. • Exaggerated response of vaginal mucosa to estrogen. Despite the name, the change seen histopathologically is consistent with edema rather than hyperplasia or hypertrophy. • Severe prolapse can affect the urethra and prevent normal urination.

SIGNALMENT
• Young (< 3 years), large-breed bitches
• Breeds predisposed—Labrador and Chesapeake Bay retriever, boxer, bulldog, mastiff, German shepherd dog, St. Bernard, Airedale terrier, and weimeraner • Hereditary component probable

SIGNS

Historical Findings
• Onset of proestrus or estrus; rarely seen at parturition • Licking vulvar area, failure to allow copulation, dysuria • Previous occurrence

Physical Examination Findings
• Protrusion of round, tongue-shaped or donut-shaped tissue mass from the vulva
• Vaginal examination locates the lumen and urethral orifice. In bitches with types I and II, the vaginal lumen is dorsal to the prolapse, whereas in those with type III, it is central to the prolapse. The urethral orifice is ventral to the prolapse with all three types. • Tissue may be dry or necrotic.

CAUSES AND RISK FACTORS
• Estrogen stimulation • Genetic predisposition

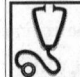 **DIAGNOSIS**

DIFFERENTIAL DIAGNOSIS
• Vaginal polyp. Vaginal examination differentiates. • Vaginal neoplasia (e.g., transmissible veneral tumor and leimyoma.) Signalment, stage of cycle, and vaginal examination differentiate.

CBC/BIOCHEMISTRY/URINALYSIS
N/A

OTHER LABORATORY TESTS N/A

IMAGING N/A

OTHER DIAGNOSTIC PROCEDURES
In old bitch, biopsy differentiates from neoplasia

 TREATMENT

• Outpatient unless patient has urethral obstruction
• Breeding possible by artificial insemination
• Prolapsed tissue must be kept clean and lubricated with sterile water-soluble lubricant
• Elizabethan collar and clean indoor environment to minimize tissue trauma
• Owner must monitor patient's ability to urinate
• Regression usually begins in late estrus and should be resolved during early diestrus.
• 66% recurrence at next cycle
• Ovariohysterectomy prevents recurrence and may hasten resolution.
• Severely affected patients require surgical reduction or resection; if possible, surgery should be scheduled when the mass is beginning to regress; 25% recurrence at next cycle.

MEDICATIONS

DRUGS AND FLUIDS

Gonadotrophic-releasing hormone 2.2 (µg/kg IM) or human chorionic gonadotrophin (1000 IU IM) if breeding not planned that cycle may hasten ovulation and resolution. These treatments will not be effective if given after ovulation.

CONTRAINDICATIONS/POSSIBLE INTERACTIONS

Avoid progestational drugs because they can induce pyometra.

 FOLLOW-UP

• Monitor health of prolapsed tissue. • Ovariohysterectomy is recommended because of the genetic component and likelihood of recurrence. • Prognosis good for recovery with medical treatment unless the urethra is involved • Prognosis good with surgical intervention if prolapse is severe

 MISCELLANEOUS

References

Wykes PM. Disease of the vagina and vulva in the bitch. In: Morrow DA, ed. Current therapy in theriogenology 2. Philadelphia: WB Saunders, 1986;476-481.

Johnston SD. Vaginal prolapse. In: Kirk RW, ed. Current veterinary therapy X. Philadelphia: WB Saunders, 1989;1302-1305.

Author Joni L. Freshman
Consulting Editor Sara K. Lyle

VAGINITIS

BASICS

DEFINITION
Inflammation of the vagina or vestibule

Pathophysiology
Primary bacterial or viral vaginitis is not common and most patients have a predisposing factor such as an anomaly, chemical irritation, neoplasia, vaginal trauma, or foreign body associated with the discharge. The uterus, clitoris, perivulvar skin, and urinary tract are also sources of discharge that may be confused with vaginitis.

Systems Affected Urogenital

Genetics N/A

Incidence/Prevalence
Not common, but reported as 7 out of 1000 patients in a 5-year period.

Geographic Distribution N/A

SIGNALMENT

Species Primarily dogs

Breed Predilections None

Mean Age and Range
Anomalies and prepubertal vaginitis are suspect in prepubertal bitches, but vaginitis can occur in bitch of any age, breed, or ovarian status.

Predominant Sex N/A

SIGNS

Historical Findings
• Discharge from the vulva • Pollakiuria • Vaginal licking • "Spotting" • "Scooting" • Attracting males

Physical Examination Findings
• Discharge from the vagina • Possibly, inflamed vulva and vagina

CAUSES
• Prepubertal vagina • Foreign body • Urinary tract infection • Vaginal trauma • Urine or feces contamination in patient with congenital anomaly • Acquired problem can incite vaginitis. • Urine contamination in patient with ectopic ureters • Incontinence due to "hypoestrogenism" • Vaginal neoplasia—transmissible venereal tumor, leiomyoma. • Bacterial—Pasteurella, Strepococcus, E. coli, Pseudomonas, Mycoplasma, Chlamydia, and Brucella canis • Viral—Herpes • Vaginal hematoma • Vaginal abscess • Exogenous androgens • Vestibulovaginal stricture • Zinc toxicity has been reported

RISK FACTORS
• Clitoral hypertrophy caused by exogenous androgens • Alteration of normal vaginal flora by administration of prophylactic antibiotics allowing overgrowth of pathogens • Anomalies in prepubertal bitches

DIAGNOSIS

DIFFERENTIAL DIAGNOSIS
• History and signalment establish risk of anomaly and the possibility of prepubertal vaginitis • Normal serosanguinous discharge during proestrus and sometimes into estrus • Slight purulent exudate may be normal in early diestrus; neutrophils are usually seen on cytologic examination • Normal postpartum discharge for up to 6-8 weeks. An odorless, dark brown or bloody discharge in substantial amounts is normal for about 4 weeks postpartum. • Subinvolution of placental sites (SIPS) if discharge lasts longer than 6-8 weeks postpartum • Urinary tract infection • Foreign body • Pyometra • Metritis • Retained placentas • Clitoral hypertrophy • Embryonic or fetal death • Urine or feces contamination caused by congenital anomaly or acquired condition • Perivulvar dermatitis can appear as vaginal discharge. • Urine contamination in patient with ectopic ureters or incontinence due to 'hypoestrogenism.' • Normal mucus discharge during pregnancy • Vaginal neoplasia—transmissible venereal tumor, leiomyoma. • Vaginal trauma. • Vaginal hematoma. • Vaginal abscess. • Ovarian neoplasia • Zinc toxicity

CBC/BIOCHEMISTRY/URINALYSIS
• Results usually normal • Voided urine samples may contain inflammatory cells.

OTHER LABORATORY TESTS
• Serum progesterone concentration determines whether the bitch is in diestrus. A slight diestrual discharge can be normal, but high progesterone increases the possibility of pyometra or pregnancy. • Rapid slide agglutination test helps rule out Brucella canis.

IMAGING
Contrast radiography of the vagina helps rule out vaginal neoplasia, foreign body, and vestibulovaginal, urethrovaginal, and rectovaginal stricture.

OTHER DIAGNOSTIC PROCEDURES
• Vaginal culture by use of a guarded culturette—perform before any other vaginal procedure is done. Only 5% of clinically normal bitches cultured repeatedly had negative cultures. The most common vaginal isolates from normal and infertile bitches are Pasteurella and Streptococci, with Escherichia coli and Staphylococci less common. The most common mixed culture in normal and infertile bitches is Pasteurella, Streptococci, and E. coli The most common pure culture in normal and infertile bitches is Pasteurella. More organisms are usually grown during estrus than at other stages of estrus, but the types do not change. • Vaginal cytologic examination to determine if the discharge is pus, blood, or feces. Septic inflammation is seen in older bitches with vaginitis. The ex-

tent of the cornification determines the estrogen influence and helps establish whether the bitch is in proestrus or estrus and if the discharge might be normal. • Vaginoscopy to detect anomaly, bands, mass, foreign body, hematoma, abcess, and an inflamed vagina or vestibule. An endoscope may be needed to see the anterior vagina. The cervix can not usually be seen by endoscopy, except possibly in large dogs. Fluid emanating from the uterus can be differentiated from vaginal and vestibular sources by observing the most cranial origin of the discharge. • A digital examination of the vagina to help identify vaginal anomalies such as bands, stricture, and, persistent hymen. Tumors can also be palpated. • Biopsy of vaginal masses to rule out neoplasia

GROSS AND HISTOPATHOLOGIC FINDINGS N/A

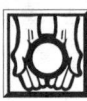

TREATMENT

INPATIENT VERSUS OUTPATIENT
Outpatient

ACTIVITY Need not be altered

DIET Need not be altered

CLIENT EDUCATION
• Prepubertal vaginitis normally resolves after the first estrus and antibiotic therapy is not needed.
• Vaginitis in adults is oftentimes associated with a correctable predisposing factor.
• Ovariohysterectomy and isolation of animals infected by Brucella canis
• Remove exogenous androgens and estrogens.

SURGICAL CONSIDERATIONS
• Remove or treat inciting causes (e.g., foreign body, neoplasia, anomaly, and urinary tract infection).
• Vaginectomy has been used in refractory patients.

MEDICATIONS

DRUGS AND FLUIDS
Primary vaginitis—administration of appropriate systemic antibiotic normally eradicates susceptible bacteria in 24 hours. Vaginal douches of 0.05% chlorhexidine, 0.5% povidone-iodine, or 0.2% nitrofurazone twice daily until the discharge resolves reported to be beneficial

CONTRAINDICATIONS
Many antibiotics are contraindicated in pregnancy.

PRECAUTIONS
Estrogens given during diestrus increase the risk of pyometra.

POSSIBLE INTERACTIONS
- Exogenous estrogen administered during diestrus
- Exogenous androgen

ALTERNATE DRUGS
Prepubertal vaginitis—estrus induction with Diethylstilbestrol may be helpful in refractory patients, although long-term effects have not been documented.

FOLLOW-UP

PATIENT MONITORING
- Reexamine prepubertal bitch after the first estrus or physical maturity. • Reexamine older bitch with no predisposing factors after a 14-day course of antibiotics. • If condition persists, reevaluate for an underlying cause, another cause, or perform another vaginal bacterial culture and sensitivity test.

PREVENTION/AVOIDANCE N/A

POSSIBLE COMPLICATIONS N/A

EXPECTED COURSE AND PROGNOSIS
- Prepubertal vaginitis normally resolves after the first estrus. • Vaginitis in adults usually resolves if the causative factor is removed; however, antibiotic therapy and vaginal douches may hasten recovery to within 2 weeks if the condition is uncomplicated chronic vaginitis.

MISCELLANEOUS

ASSOCIATED CONDITIONS N/A

AGE RELATED FACTORS
Puppies—prepubertal vaginitis, anomalies, and ectopic ureters

ZOONOTIC POTENTIAL
Brucella canis is rare in patients with vaginitis but should be considered.

PREGNANCY
Many antibiotics are contraindicated during pregnancy (see Drug Formulary)

SYNONYMS N/A

SEE ALSO See Causes

ABBREVIATIONS
SIPS = subinvolution of the placental sites

References

Bjurstrom L, Linde-Forsberg C. Long-term study of aerobic bacteria of the genital tract in breeding bitches. Am J Vet Res 1992;53:665-669.

Holt PE, Sayle B. Congenital vestibulo-vaginal stenosis in the bitch. J Small Anim Pract 1988;22:67-75.

Johnson CA. Diagnosis and treatment of chronic vaginitis in the bitch. Vet Clin North Am Small Anim Pract 1991;21:523-531.

Strom B, Linde-Forsberg C. Effects of ampicillin and trimethoprim-sulfamethoxazole on the vaginal bacterial-flora of the bitches. Am J Vet Res 1993;54:891-896.

van Duijkeren E. Significance of the vaginal bacterial flora in the bitch: a review. Vet Rec 1992;131:367-369.

Wykes PM, Soderberg SF. Disorders of the canine vagina. In: Morgan RV, ed. Handbook of small animal practice. 2nd ed. New York: Churchill Livingstone, 1992:661-666.

Author Bruce E. Eilts
Consulting Editor Sara K. Lyle

VASCULITIS

BASICS

OVERVIEW
• Inflammation of the blood vessels caused by endothelial injury or extension of adjacent inflammation or infection • Endothelial damage by infectious agent, parasite infestation, endotoxin, or immune complex deposition initiates local inflammation, neutrophil accumulation, and complement activation. Neutrophils release lysosomal enzymes leading to necrosis of vessel wall, thrombosis, and hemorrhage. In humans and dogs with polyarteritis nodosa, intimal proliferation and vessel wall degeneration and necrosis predominate, which lead to hemorrhage, thrombosis, and necrosis of involved vessels and adjacent tissues in most patients • Nondermal vasculitis (e.g., renal, hepatic, and serosal surfaces of body cavities) may be the mechanism leading to the development of clinically-apparent signs of systemic disease (e.g., polyarthritis and proteinuria) without causing obvious external lesions

SIGNALMENT   Dogs and cats

SIGNS

Historical Findings:
• Administration of provocative drug (e.g., penicillin, sulfonamides, streptomycin, and hydralazine) in sensitized animal • Exposure to ticks • Poor dirofilariasis prophylaxis in endemic area

Physical Examination Findings:
• Swelling • Ulceration • Necrosis of affected skin, especially mucous membranes, mucocutaneous junctions, pinnae edges, and footpads • Systemic signs reflecting organ involvement (e.g., hepatic, renal, and CNS) • Systemic signs of illness (e.g., lethargy, lymphadenopathy, pyrexia, vague signs of pain, and weight loss) • Cutaneous lesions of polyarteritis nodosa (subcutaneous nodules—less common in dogs than in people) • Signs associated with underlying infectious or immune-related disease (e.g., thrombocytopenia and polyarthropathy)

CAUSES AND RISK FACTORS

Infectious
• Parasitic (i.e., heart and pulmonary arteries)—Dirofilaria immitis, Angiostrongylus vasorum • Viral—e.g., feline infectious peritonitis and canine corona virus infection • Ricketsial—e.g., Rocky Mountain spotted fever and ehrlichiosis • Bacterial—sepsis

Immune-Related
• Systemic lupus erythematosus • Rheumatoid arthritis-like arthropathy • Lupus-like drug re-

action (e.g., to hydralazine, procainamide, and phenytoin in humans) • Type III hypersensitivities (e.g., to food, sulfonamides, and penicillin) • Polyarteritis nodosa • Neoplasia • Uremia

DIAGNOSIS

DIFFERENTIAL DIAGNOSIS
• Cutaneous signs developing after administration of medication implicates drug reaction (usually not immediate, may develop after days or weeks). • Vasculitis associated with polyarthropathy and pyrexia implicates immune or infectious cause. • Cold hemagglutinin disease suggested by distribution of cyanotic or necrotic lesions (nose, ears, toes, tail tip, prepuce) and history of exposure to cold.

CBC/BIOCHEMISTRY/URINALYSIS
• Results consistent with underlying infectious disease

OTHER LABORATORY TESTS
• Serologic tests may aid diagnosis of tick-related (i.e., ricketsial) disease • Antinuclear antibody test positive in patient with systemic lupus erythematosus, may be positive in patients with other systemic illnesses • Occult heartworm test positive in animal with dirofilariasis • Angiostrongylus infestation diagnosed by fecal examination and cytologic examinaiton of tracheal wash

IMAGING
• Radiographs helpful in diagnosis of dirofilariasis and Angiostrongylus infection

OTHER DIAGNOSTIC PROCEDURES
• Skin biopsy with specimen taken at edge of developing lesion may be diagnostic for presence of vasculitis but may not reveal cause. • Immunofluorescence test of skin biopsy specimen may rule out pemphigus and pemphigoid diseases. • If allergic response is suspected, resolution of signs upon discontinuation of suspect medication or food supports diagnosis.

TREATMENT
• Treatment of vasculitis most often involves resolution of underlying condition and supportive care.
• In animals with untreatable or unknown underlying condition, glucocorticoid, treatment with immunosuppressive (e.g., cyclophosphamide, azathioprine) and other drugs (e.g., dapsone and sulfasalazine) are occasionally effective, but clinical trials of efficacy have not been reported in animals.

MEDICATIONS

DRUGS AND FLUIDS
• Infectious or immune-related—treat underlying disease (see specific condition); supportive care
• Lupus-like drug reactions—discontinue drug; supportive care
• Type III hypersensitivity—discontinue drug; supportive care
• Polyarteritis nodosa—glucocorticoids and cyclophosphamide (unknown value)
• "Idiopathic" vasculitis—if most other causes have been ruled out, administer dapsone (1 mg/kg PO q8h for 14 days, then 1 mg/kg PO q12h for 14 days, then 1 mg/kg PO q24h; may eventually be decreased to q48h to maintain remission); alternative—sulfasalazine (45 mg/kg PO q8h). Neither drug's effectiveness is well-documented.

CONTRAINDICATIONS / POSSIBLE INTERACTIONS
• Do not administer sulfasalazine to animals who are sensitive to sulfonamides.

FOLLOW-UP
• Animals undergoing treatment with dapsone—monitor CBC and liver enzymes for side effects (e.g., hemolytic anemia, methemoglobinemia, and hepatopathy) • Animals undergoing treatment with sulfasalazine—monitor for keratoconjunctivitis sicca, blood dyscrasias, and hepatopathy

MISCELLANEOUS

SYNONYMS
• Angitis

SEE ALSO
• Leukocytoclastic Vasculitis • Lupus Erythematosus, Systemic • Pemphigus • Polyarteritis Nodosa • Vasculitis, Cutaneous

ABBREVIATIONS
ANA = antinuclear antibody
CNS = central nervous system
SLE = systemic lupus erythematosus

Reference
Suter PF, Fox PR. Peripheral vascular disease. In: Ettinger SJ, Feldman EC, eds. Textbook of veterinary internal medicine. 4th ed. Philadelphia: WB Saunders, 1995.

Author Rebecca L. Stepien

Consulting Editors Larry P. Tilley and Francis W. K. Smith, Jr.

BASICS

OVERVIEW
• Vasculitis is defined as an inflammation of blood vessels with a neutrophilic (leukocytoclastic/non-leukocytoclastic), lymphocytic, rarely eosinophilic or granulomatous or mixed cell type. • Pathomechanisms include type III (immune complex) reaction and type I (immediate) reactions.

SIGNALMENT
• Any age, breed or sex may be affected, but dachsunds and rottweilers may be predisposed. • The signalment also varies dependent on etiology.

SIGNS
• Palpable purpura, hemorrhagic bullae, necrosis and "punched-out" ulcers may be present. These usually involve the extremities (paws, pinnae, lips, tail and oral mucosa) and may or may not be painful. • Anorexia, depression, pyrexia, pitting edema of the extremities, polyarthropathy and myopathy may also be present dependent on the underlying cause.

CAUSES AND RISK FACTORS
Systemic lupus erythematosus, cold agglutinin disease, frostbite, disseminated intravascular coagulopathy, lymphoreticular neoplasia, drug reactions, post-vaccine, spider bites, immune-mediated disease, erythema nodosum-like panniculitis, rheumatoid arthritis, Rocky Mountain spotted fever and staphylococcal hypersensitivity

DIAGNOSIS

DIFFERENTIAL DIAGNOSIS
• See causes and risk factors. • Other differential diagnoses may include ear margin seborrhea, chemical and thermal burns, toxic epidermal necrolysis, erythema multiforme and sepsis. These are primarily differentiated on the basis of biopsy of representative lesions and histopathology.

CBC/BIOCHEMISTRY/URINALYSIS
Complete blood count, chemistry screen and urinalysis are usually normal.

OTHER LABORATORY TESTS
• In cases of sepsis, disseminated intravascular coagulation, systemic lupus erythematosus, Rocky Mountain spotted fever and rheumatoid arthritis, abnormalities may be present. • Serologic testing for parasitic and infectious disease should be considered in high-risk areas. • Immunodiagnostics such as antinuclear antibody titer, Coomb's test and cold agglutinin tests should also be considered.

IMAGING N/A

OTHER DIAGNOSTIC PROCEDURES
• Skin scrapings should be taken for possible demodicosis (with secondary sepsis). • A biopsy should be taken and submitted for histopathology to determine if vasculitis is indeed present. This should be taken from an early lesion. Histopathologic finding are variable dependent on the underlying etiology but usually include neutrophilic (leukocytoclastic/non-leukocytoclastic), lymphocytic, eosinophilic or granulomatous or mixed cells in and around the vessels. Vascular necrosis and fibrin thrombi may be prominent. Perivascular hemorrhage and edema may occur. • If vasculitis is present and there is evidence of systemic disease on the complete blood count, chemistry screen or urinalysis, then representative cultures (blood, urine, skin, etc.) should be performed.

TREATMENT
• Treatment of the underlying disease is the first priority in clinical management. If no systemic abnormalities are present, these cases may be treated as outpatients with no alterations in food/water intake. If systemic disease is present, inpatient care must be recommended.
• The owner must be aware that the prognosis is guarded until an etiology is found. Then the prognosis is based on the etiology.

MEDICATIONS
• While awaiting histopathology results and if no drug reaction is suspected, antibiotics are the first line of therapy.
• Once vasculitis is determined to be present and an underlying cause is found, the specific underlying disease should be appropriately treated.

DRUGS AND FLUIDS
• If immune-mediated disease is present with concurrent vasculitis, then prednisone should be administered (2-4 mg/kg q24h.)

• If no underlying etiology is found or prednisolone alone is not working, then dapsone (1 mg/kg q8h) or sulfasalazine (20-40 mg q8h) may be tried.

CONTRAINDICATIONS/POSSIBLE INTERACTIONS
• Dapsone and sulfasalazine would not be recommended if there is pre-existing renal or hepatic disease or pre-existing blood dyscrasias.
• Sulfasalazine would not be recommended with pre-existing or borderline keratoconjunctivitis sicca and should be used with caution in cats. Sulfasalazine may displace highly protein bound drugs such as methotrexate, warfarin, phenylbutazone, thiazide diuretics, salicylates, probenicid, and phenytoin. Antacids decrease the bioavailability of sulfonamides. Sulfasalazine may decrease the bioavailability of folic acid or digoxin. Ferrous sulfate or other iron salts may decrease blood levels of sulfasalazine if administered concurrently.

FOLLOW-UP
• Patients receiving prednisolone or dapsone should be monitored every 2 weeks initially with a complete blood count, chemistry screen and urinalysis. If a specific underlying disease is found, then it should be monitored appropriately. • If no underlying disease is found, vasculitis may be difficult to treat and the prognosis is guarded.

MISCELLANEOUS
• Corticosteroids and dapsone should not be used in pregnant animals. • Sulfasalazine should only be used during pregnancy when absolutely necessary.

Reference
Mueller GH, Kirk RW, Scott DW, eds. Small animal dermatology. 4th ed. Philadelphia: WB Saunders, 1989.
Author Karen A. Kuhl
Consulting Editor Lowell Ackerman

VENTRICULAR SEPTAL DEFECT

BASICS

DEFINITION
An anomalous communication between the two ventricles (figure). The defect may be in the inlet, outlet, muscular, or membranous septum. Most ventricular septal defects (VSD) in small animals are perimembranous and subcristal.

Pathophysiology
• The presence of a VSD results in a pulmonary systemic shunt. The direction and volume of the shunt is determined by the size of the defect, the relationship of the pulmonary and systemic vascular resistances, and the presence of other anomalies. • Most VSD in veterinary patients are small and therefore restrictive—i.e., the difference between left and right ventricular pressures is maintained. VSD of moderate size have an area that exceeds 40% of the area of the open aortic valve. They are only partially restrictive and result in various degrees of right ventricular hypertension. Large VSD have an area that is as great or greater than the aorta. They are nonrestrictive, and right ventricular pressure is necessarily systemic. Only moderate and large defects impose a pressure load upon the right ventricle. • In a patient with normal resistance to right ventricular ejection, the direction of the shunt is left-to-right. This increases pulmonary venous return and imposes a volume load on the left atrium and ventricle. With large shunts, left ventricular congestive failure can develop. • Generally, the left ventricle unloads into the pulmonary arterial system during systole. Unless the defect is of moderate or large size, the right ventricle is spared.

Systems Affected
• Pulmonary, if congestive heart failure (CHF) develops • Cardiovascular—theoretically, a large shunt could result in pulmonary vascular disease, pulmonary hypertension, and shunt reversal (i.e., Eisenmenger's syndrome). This is uncommon in small animals. If shunt reversal occurs, it usually does so early in life.

Genetics
Breed predispositions are recognized. Genetic transmission has not been established.

Incidence/Prevalence
VSD is one of the most common congenital cardiac malformations in cats; less common in dogs.

Geographic Distribution N/A

SIGNALMENT
Species Dogs and cats

Breed Predilections
English bulldog and, possibly, Brittany spaniel, chow chow, Newfoundland, and samoyed

Mean Age and Range
Most defects are detected by routine examination of puppies and kittens.

Predominant Sex N/A

SIGNS

Historical Findings
• Most patients are asymptomatic. • Clinical signs of left ventricular failure include dyspnea, exercise intolerance, syncope, and cough.

Physical Examination Findings
• Systolic murmur with a restrictive VSD. Typically, the murmur is loud, band shaped, and heard best over the right hemithorax. A softer, mid-systolic murmur of functional pulmonic stenosis may be heard over the left heart base. A diastolic decrescendo murmur results if the presence of the VSD leads to poor support of the noncoronary aortic valve leaflet and aortic regurgitation. Patients with right-to-left shunts generally do not have murmurs. • A split second heart sound in some animals • Femoral pulses are usually normal. • Mucous membranes are pink unless the presence of pulmonary hypertension causes a right-to-left shunt and arterial hypoxemia. • Tachycardia, dyspnea, and crackles may be evident if left ventricular failure occurs.

CAUSES
Ventricular septal defects are congenital and may have a genetic basis.

RISK FACTORS N/A

DIAGNOSIS

DIFFERENTIAL DIAGNOSIS
• Other congenital cardiac malformations that cause systolic murmurs include atrioventricular valve dysplasia, aortic or pulmonary stenosis, and complex malformations such as Tetralogy of Fallot. • The "to-and-fro" murmur that results when aortic valve regurgitation complicates a VSD must be distinguished from the continuous murmur of patent ductus arteriosus. • Generally, diagnosis of congenital cardiac malformations requires echocardiographic evaluation.

CBC/BIOCHEMISTRY/URINALYSIS
• Results usually normal • The uncommon event of right-to-left shunting results in compensatory erythrocytosis. • Patients with severe CHF may have prerenal azotemia.

OTHER LABORATORY TESTS N/A

IMAGING

Thoracic Radiography
• Radiographic appearance is determined by the size and direction of the shunt. Thoracic radiographs may be normal if the VSD is small. Larger defects cause various degrees of left or even generalized cardiac enlargement. Pulmonary hyperperfusion with prominence of the main pulmonary artery segment may be apparent. Congestive heart failure is manifest as pulmonary edema. • Right-sided cardiomegaly in patients with right-to-left shunts. The pulmonary arteries are abnormally large proximally but attenuated distally. The pulmonary veins are small because of reduced pulmonary perfusion.

Echocardiography
• Two-dimensional echocardiographic study may demonstrate left atrial enlargement with left ventricular dilation and hypertrophy. Systolic myocardial function is usually preserved. Right ventricular hypertrophy is apparent only if the defect is large or the VSD is one aspect of a complex malformation. The defect can sometimes be seen directly. Echocardiographic images must be evaluated critically; the artifact of "septal drop-out" is very common. • Generally, the diagnosis is confirmed by Doppler interrogation of the interventricular septum. If the defect is restrictive, a discrete, high velocity systolic jet is revealed by spectral Doppler. The shunt may be directly seen by color-flow Doppler. • Contrast echocardiography may be helpful in the diagnosis of a right-to-left VSD.

Cardiac Catheterization
Selective cardiac catheterization allows one to visualize the defect by contrast radiography as well as calculate the shunt fraction (QP/QS) and pulmonary vascular resistance.

OTHER DIAGNOSTIC PROCEDURES

Electrocardiographic Findings
• Evidence of left atrial enlargement, left ventricular hypertrophy, or even right ventricular hypertrophy in some animals • A right ventricular enlargement pattern in most animals if the shunt is right-to-left due to the presence of pulmonary hypertension or pulmonic stenosis.

GROSS AND HISTOPATHOLOGIC FINDINGS
The degree of chamber enlargement and hypertrophy is determined by the size of the defect. Pulmonary edema is seen in animals with congestive failure.

TREATMENT

INPATIENT VERSUS OUTPATIENT
Clinical signs are related to CHF. Most patients can be treated as outpatients.

ACTIVITY
Exercise should be restricted if animal has CHF; exercise of asymptomatic patients with small defects need not be restricted.

DIET
Moderate sodium restriction is recommended for patients with CHF.

CLIENT EDUCATION
Definitive surgical correction is not widely available. If CHF develops, it is terminal even with palliative care.

SURGICAL CONSIDERATIONS

Definitive surgical correction of the defect during cardiopulmonary bypass is recommended for moderate and large defects in which the QP/QS exceeds 2. Cardiopulmonary bypass is presently performed at a small number of veterinary centers. Pulmonary artery banding can be considered as a palliative procedure for patients with moderate or large shunts and CHF.

MEDICATIONS

DRUGS AND FLUIDS

• Furosemide, enalapril, and digoxin are recommended for animals with CHF (see CHF, left-sided).
• The use of ACE inhibitors should be considered for patients with echocardiographic evidence of left atrial and ventricular volume overload, even in the absence of clinical signs.

CONTRAINDICATIONS

Caution must be exercised if vasodilators are used in patients with complex malformations that include stenotic lesions.

PRECAUTIONS

ACE inhibitors and digoxin must be used cautiously if patient has renal dysfunction.

POSSIBLE INTERACTIONS N/A

ALTERNATE DRUGS N/A

FOLLOW-UP

PATIENT MONITORING

Periodic echocardiographic or radiographic evaluation is suggested for patients with no clinical signs.

PREVENTION/AVOIDANCE

Breeding of affected animals is not recommended .

POSSIBLE COMPLICATIONS

• Left ventricular congestive failure • Bacterial endocarditis • Pulmonary hypertension • Arrhythmias

EXPECTED COURSE AND PROGNOSIS

Patients with small shunts may live a normal lifespan. Isolated, restrictive VSD usually do not cause clinical signs. The presence of concurrent anomalies such as pulmonic stenosis or aortic insufficiency worsens the prognosis. Patients with overt CHF may live 6-18 months with medical treatment. The development of pulmonary hypertension and shunt reversal is uncommon.

MISCELLANEOUS

ASSOCIATED CONDITIONS

• The VSD may be one component of complex malformations such as tetralogy of Fallot. • Aortic valve insufficiency resulting from a poorly supported aortic valve leaflet complicates the condition in some patients. • Inlet VSD in cats may be associated with an atrial septal defect and tricuspid valve dysplasia as part of an endocardial cushion defect.

AGE RELATED FACTORS

The murmur of VSD becomes apparent shortly after birth when pulmonary vascular resistance drops.

ZOONOTIC POTENTIAL N/A

PREGNANCY

High risk in patients with large defects. Breeding of affected animals is not recommended .

SYNONYMS

Interventricular septal defect.

SEE ALSO

• Congestive Heart Failure, Left Sided
• Tetralogy of Fallot

ABBREVIATIONS

ACE = angiotensin converting enzyme
CHF = congestive heart failure
VSD = ventricular septal defect

References

Bonagura JD. Congenital heart disease. In: Ettinger SJ, ed. Textbook of veterinary internal medicine. 3rd ed. Philadelphia: WB Saunders, 1989;976-1030.

Fox PR. Congenital feline heart disease. In: Fox PR, ed. Canine and feline cardiology. New York: Churchill Livingstone, 1988;391-408.

Olivier NB. Congenital heart disease in dogs. In: Fox PR, ed. Canine and feline cardiology. New York: Churchill Livingstone, 1988;357-390.

Author Jonathan A. Abbott
Consulting Editors Larry P. Tilley, Francis W. K. Smith, Jr.

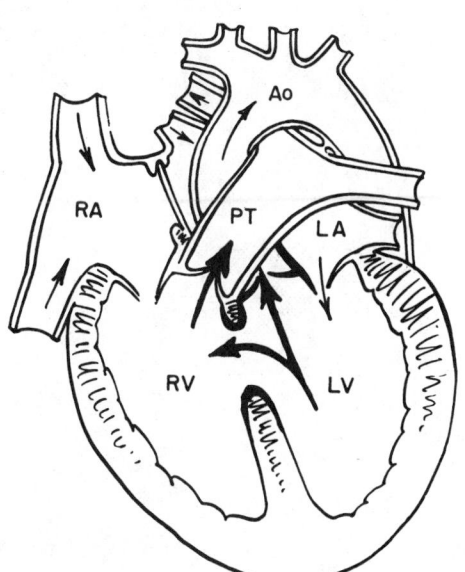

Figure. Ventricular Septal Defect. The defect is an unobstructed communication. Right ventricular hypertrophy and pulmonary hypertension are associated. Left-to-right shunting is shown. RA = right atrium, LA = left atrium, RV = right ventricle, LV = left ventricle, AO = aorta, PT = pulmonary trunk. (From Roberts W. Adult Congenital Heart Disease. Philadelphia: FA Davis, 1987, with permission.)

VESICOURACHAL DIVERTICULA

 BASICS

OVERVIEW

Vesicourachal diverticula is a common congenital anomaly of the urinary bladder that occurs when the portion of the urachus (i.e., a fetal conduit that allows passage of urine from the bladder to the placenta) located at the bladder vertex fails to close. The result is a blind diverticulum of variable size that protrudes from the bladder vertex. Other characteristics include the following:
• Congenital microscopic diverticula are microscopic lumens that may persist at the bladder vertex.
• Acquired macroscopic diverticula develop in patients with microscopic diverticula after the onset of concurrent but unrelated acquired lower urinary tract disease. Presumably, urethral obstruction or detrusor hyperactivity induced by inflammation causes high intraluminal pressure and subsequent enlargement of microscopic diverticula.
• Congenital macroscopic diverticula, most likely caused by impaired urine outflow, develop before or soon after birth and persist indefinitely.

SIGNALMENT

• Dogs and cats
• Frequently encountered in cats with acquired lower urinary tract disease
• Twice as common in male cats compared with female cats
• No breed or age predisposition

SIGNS

• Usually none
• Hematuria, dysuria, pollakiuria, or signs of urethral obstruction observed in some patients with concurrent acquired lower urinary tract disease

CAUSES AND RISK FACTORS

• The cause(s) of congenital microscopic and macroscopic diverticula are unknown.
• Congenital microscopic diverticula are risk factors for development of acquired macroscopic diverticula.
• Diseases associated with high bladder intraluminal pressure (e.g., bacterial urinary tract infection, uroliths, urethral plugs, and idiopathic disease) are risk factors for acquired macroscopic diverticula.

 DIAGNOSIS

DIFFERENTIAL DIAGNOSIS

• Persistent (or patent) urachus is characterized by inappropriate loss of urine through the umbilicus.
• Persistent urachal ligaments are nonpatent fibrous remnants of the urachus connecting the bladder vertex to the umbilicus.
• Urachal cysts are focal accumulations of fluid in isolated segments of a persistent urachus.

CBC/BIOCHEMISTRY/URINALYSIS

• Abnormal findings relate to the underlying disorder that causes vesicourachal diverticula, unless complicated by concurrent acquired lower urinary tract disease.
• Abnormal findings related to secondary urinary tract infection.

OTHER LABORATORY TESTS N/A

IMAGING

• Congenital and acquired macroscopic diverticula are best identified by positive contrast urethrocystography.
• Radiographs obtained with the bladder completely and then partially distended by contrast medium may facilitate detection of small diverticula.

OTHER DIAGNOSTIC PROCEDURES
N/A

GROSS AND MICROSCOPIC FINDINGS

• Extramural macroscopic diverticula appear as convex or conical projections from the bladder vertex.
• Intramural microscopic diverticula appear as transitional, epithelium-lined lumens persisting at the bladder vertex from the level of the submucosa to subserosa.

 TREATMENT

• Many macroscopic diverticula in cats (and probably dogs) are acquired and self–limiting if the underlying disease is eliminated.
• Treatment should be directed toward eliminating underlying cause(s) of lower urinary tract disease.
• Diverticulectomy should be considered if a macroscopic diverticulum persists in a patient with persistent or recurrent bacterial urinary tract infection despite appropriate antimicrobial therapy.

MEDICATIONS

DRUGS AND FLUIDS NA

CONTRAINDICATIONS/POSSIBLE INTERACTIONS NA

FOLLOW-UP

PATIENT MONITORING

If bacterial urinary tract infection persists or recurs despite proper antimicrobial therapy, the status of the diverticulum should be reevaluated by contrast radiography.

PREVENTION/AVOIDANCE

Avoid diagnostic procedures or treatment that alters normal host urinary tract defenses and predispose to urinary tract infection.

EXPECTED COURSE AND PROGNOSIS

• Congenital diverticula are usually clinically silent unless complicated by concurrent lower urinary tract disease.

• Acquired macroscopic diverticula typically heal within 2 to 3 weeks after amelioration of clinical signs of lower urinary tract disease.

• Diverticulectomy and appropriate antimicrobial therapy usually resolves recurrent urinary tract disease in patients with persistent congenital macroscopic diverticula.

MISCELLANEOUS

ASSOCIATED CONDITIONS

• Persistent congenital macroscopic diverticula are potential risk factors for recurrent urinary tract infection.

• Acquired macroscopic diverticula are typically encountered in patients with concurrent lower urinary tract disease.

Reference

Osborne CA, Johnston GR, Kruger JM, et al. Etiopathogenesis and biological behavior of feline vesicourachal diverticula. Vet Clin North Am Small Anim Pract 1987;17:697.

Authors John M. Kruger and Carl A. Osborne

Consulting Editors Larry G. Adams and Carl A. Osborne

VESTIBULAR DISEASE, GERIATRIC—DOGS

BASICS

DEFINITION
Acute nonprogressive disturbance of the peripheral vestibular system in old dogs

Pathophysiology
• Unknown. Abnormal flow of the endolymphatic fluid in the semicircular canals of the inner ear secondary to disturbance in production, circulation, or absorption of the fluid is suspected. Intoxication of the vestibular receptors and inflammation of the vestibular portion of the vestibulocochlear nerve (CN VIII) are other possibilities. • Often incorrectly referred to as a "stroke" (canine geriatric vestibular disease is neither central in location nor suspected to be vascular or ischemic in origin)

Systems Affected
Nervous—peripheral vestibular system

Genetics N/A

Incidence/Prevalence
• Common, sporadic, acquired disease of old dogs • No incidence/prevalence reported

Geographic Distribution N/A

SIGNALMENT

Species Dogs

Breed Predilections
• None reported • Seems to occur more frequently in medium to large breeds

Mean Age and Range
Geriatric; no specific age range reported but patients are usually > 8 years old

Predominant Sex N/A

SIGNS

General Comments
Clinical signs are strictly those of peripheral vestibular dysfunction. In severely affected animals, the clinician must be careful not to incorrectly attribute the signs (especially the gait) to a CNS location.

Historical Findings
Sudden onset of imbalance, disorientation, reluctance to stand, and, in most patients, head tilt and irregular eye movements. These signs may be preceded or accompanied by nausea and vomiting.

Neurologic Examination Findings
• Mild to marked head tilt that is directed toward the side of the lesion. In a few dogs, the disease is bilateral with erratic side-to-side movements of the head with or without mild head tilt in the direction of the more severely affected side. • Abnormal nystagmus (resting or positional) in the early stages in most dogs, which is either horizontal or rotatory with the fast phase always in a direction opposite to the head tilt. If involvement is bilateral, the abnormal nystagmus may be mild and the physiologic eye movements (e.g., normal vestibular nystagmus and conjugate eye movements) depressed or absent. • Mild to marked disorientation and vestibular ataxia with a tendency to lean or fall in the direction of the head tilt. In severely affected dogs, the patient is reluctant to stand, making assessment of the gait difficult. If the patient can stand, strength and proprioception are normal. A base wide stance is especially noticeable in dogs with bilateral involvement.

CAUSES Unknown

RISK FACTORS N/A

DIAGNOSIS

DIFFERENTIAL DIAGNOSIS
• The primary factor distinguishing geriatric vestibular disease from other causes of peripheral vestibular disease in dogs is the acute onset and rapid improvement without specific treatment. • Otitis media and interna are the most challenging differentials but can be distinguished if the patient has concurrent ipsilateral facial (CN VII) paresis or paralysis, deafness, or Horner's syndrome. Otitis externa with ruptured tympanic membrane supports otitis media and interna. • Ototoxic drugs eliminated by history • Trauma can cause similar acute changes but is usually ruled out by history, results of physical examination, and other neurologic deficits. • Hypothyroid neuropathy is not as acute in onset and is associated with clinical signs of hypothyroidism and possible CN VII deficit.

CBC/BIOCHEMISTRY/URINALYSIS
• Results generally normal • Hemoconcentration secondary to dehydration • Unrelated concurrent disorders (e.g., renal and hepatic disease) associated with old age may cause other laboratory abnormalities.

OTHER LABORATORY TESTS N/A

IMAGING
• Usually none • Radiographs of bullae may be required to rule out otitis media and interna.

OTHER DIAGNOSTIC PROCEDURES
Brain auditory evoked response— may be helpful to rule out otitis media and interna, since only the vestibular portion of the CN VIII is affected in dogs with geriatric vestibular disease

GROSS AND HISTOPATHOLOGIC FINDINGS None reported

TREATMENT

INPATIENT VERSUS OUTPATIENT
• Most dogs treated as outpatients • Severely affected dogs who cannot ambulate or require intravenous fluid support should be hospitalized during the initial stages of the disease.

ACTIVITY
Restrict activity as required by the degree of disorientation and vestibular ataxia.

DIET
No diet modification is required unless the patient has nausea, vomiting, and severe disorientation; if so, oral intake is withheld initially.

CLIENT EDUCATION
The initial signs can be alarming and incapacitating, but the prognosis for rapid improvement and recovery is excellent.

SURGICAL CONSIDERATIONS N/A

MEDICATIONS

DRUGS AND FLUIDS
• Treatment is supportive, including rehydration and maintenance fluids if required. • Sedation (e.g., diazepam) occasionally is required in dogs with severe disorientation and ataxia. • Antiemetic drugs or drugs against motion sickness (e.g., diphenhydramine) beneficial in some patients • Glucocorticoids do not alter the course of the disease and are not recommended, especially in old patients whose fluid intake may be low. • When otitis media and interna cannot be ruled out, antibiotic administration is advisable.

CONTRAINDICATIONS N/A

PRECAUTIONS N/A

POSSIBLE INTERACTIONS N/A

ALTERNATE DRUGS N/A

FOLLOW-UP

PATIENT MONITORING
• Neurologic examination of outpatient 2-3 days later to confirm stabilization and initial improvement • Discharge inpatient pending ability to ambulate and resumption of eating and drinking.

PREVENTION/AVOIDANCE N/A

POSSIBLE COMPLICATIONS
Fluid and electrolyte imbalances and decompensation of renal insufficiency (if present) may follow vomiting and insufficient fluid and food intake.

EXPECTED COURSE AND PROGNOSIS
• Improvement of clinical signs starts within approximately 72 hours with resolution of vomiting and improvement of nystagmus and vestibular ataxia • Gradual improvement of the head tilt and ataxia occurs over the next 7-10 days. If this does not occur, the animal should be evaluated for other causes of peripheral vestibular disease. • Most dogs return

to normal within 2-3 weeks. A mild head tilt may persist. • Rarely, patients experience mild, brief recurrence of signs with stress such as anaesthesia. • Repeat episodes can occur on the same or opposite side but are uncommon.

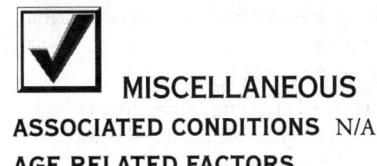

MISCELLANEOUS

ASSOCIATED CONDITIONS N/A

AGE RELATED FACTORS
Only geriatric dogs affected

ZOONOTIC POTENTIAL N/A

PREGNANCY N/A

SYNONYMS
• Canine idiopathic vestibular disease • Old dog vestibular syndrome

SEE ALSO
• Head Tilt (Vestibular Disease) • Otitis Media and Interna

ABBREVIATIONS
BAER = brain auditory evoked response
CGVD = canine geriatric vestibular disease

References
de Lahunta A. Veterinary neuroanatomy and clinical neurology. 2nd ed. Philadelphia: WB Saunders, 1983:238.
Oliver JE, Lorenz MD. Handbook of veterinary neurology. 2nd ed. Philadelphia: WB Saunders, 1993:212-216.
Parent JM, Cochrane SM. Head tilt. In: Allen DG, ed. Small animal medicine. Philadelphia: JB Lippincott, 1991:753-759.
Author Susan M. Cochrane
Consulting Editor Joane M. Parent

VESTIBULAR DISEASE, IDIOPATHIC—CATS

BASICS

DEFINITION
Acute nonprogressive disturbance of the peripheral vestibular system

Pathophysiology
Unknown. An abnormal flow of the endolymphatic fluid in the semicircular canals of the inner ear, secondary to a disturbance in the production, circulation, or absorption of the fluid, is suspected. Intoxication of the vestibular receptors or inflammation of the vestibular portion of the vestibulocochlear nerve (CN VIII) are other possibilities.

Systems Affected
Nervous—peripheral vestibular system

Genetics N/A

Incidence/Prevalence
• Common, sporadic acquired disease in cats
• No specific incidence/prevalence reported

Geographic Distribution N/A

SIGNALMENT

Species Cats

Breed Predilections N/A

Mean Age and Range
Any age, but rarely observed in cats < 1 year old

Predominant Sex N/A

SIGNS

General Comments
Clinical signs limited to those associated with peripheral vestibular disturbance

Historical Findings
Sudden onset of severe disorientation, falling and rolling, leaning, vocalizing, and crouched posture with tendency to panic when picked up

Neurologic Examination Findings
• Head tilt that is always towards the side of the lesion. Occasionally, the disease is bilateral with wide, side-to-side excursion of the head, with or without a mild tilt toward the most severely affected side. • Resting nystagmus, usually horizontal but can be rotatory in the fast phase, always in a direction opposite to the head tilt. If the disease is bilateral, the abnormal nystagmus is mild or absent, and the cat has diminished to absent physiologic vestibular nystagmus. • Vestibular ataxia with tendency to roll and fall toward the side of the head tilt. Preservation of strength and normal proprioception. If the disease is bilateral, the cat is reluctant to ambulate and prefers to stay in a crouched posture or with wide abduction of the limbs.

CAUSES
• Cause unknown • Previous upper respiratory tract infection is suspected in some patients, but the relationship to the vestibular disease is not confirmed. Limited necropsy data shows no evidence of inflammation.

RISK FACTORS
Some investigators report a higher number of cases in the summer and early fall than other seasons, possibly after outbreaks of upper respiratory disease, but this has not been proven. The disease is not restricted to this time of the year.

DIAGNOSIS

DIFFERENTIAL DIAGNOSIS
• Diagnosis made on the basis of peripheral vestibular signs that improve rapidly without specific treatment • Otitis media and interna (e.g., bacterial and parasitic) are the most challenging differentials; these can be distinguished by concurrent ipsilateral facial nerve (CN VII) paresis or paralysis, Horner's syndrome, deafness, ruptured tympanic membrane, otitis externa, and radiographic changes in tympanic bulla. • Nasopharyngeal polyp(s) also cause unilateral and bilateral peripheral vestibular signs; but, as in cats with otitis media or interna, other signs of tympanic bulla involvement are characteristic. Also, signs are not as acute and severe at onset of disease. • Blue-tailed lizard ingestion in southeastern United States is thought to produce an acute, unilateral, peripheral vestibular syndrome similar to idiopathic vestibular disease. Vomiting, salivation, irritability, and trembling are signs. Most cats recover without specific treatment. • Aminoglycoside toxicity, especially streptomycin in cats, can cause acute unilateral or bilateral peripheral vestibular syndrome or hearing loss. The history reveals use of the drug.

CBC/BIOCHEMISTRY/URINALYSIS
Results normal

OTHER LABORATORY TESTS
None required

IMAGING
• None usually necessary • Radiographs of tympanic bullae may occasionally be required to rule out otitis media and interna.

OTHER DIAGNOSTIC PROCEDURES
• Brain auditory evoked response—may help rule out other causes such as otitis media and interna and nasopharyngeal polyps • This disease is limited to the vestibular apparatus, so the hearing is intact.

GROSS AND HISTOPATHOLOGIC FINDINGS
None reported

TREATMENT

INPATIENT VERSUS OUTPATIENT
• Most cats treated as outpatients
• Severely affected cats may require a short period of hospitalization for supportive care.

ACTIVITY
Restricted according to the degree of disorientation and ataxia

DIET
No specific diet changes or restrictions required. Patients initially are reluctant to eat and drink, possibly because of the disorientation or nausea.

CLIENT EDUCATION
Despite initial alarming and incapacitating signs, the prognosis for rapid and complete recovery is excellent.

SURGICAL CONSIDERATIONS N/A

MEDICATIONS

DRUGS AND FLUIDS
• Treatment is supportive. Intravenous or subcutaneous fluid initially required in a few cats.
• Sedation (e.g., diazepam and acepromazine) required if the disorientation and rolling are severe
• Antiemetic drugs and drugs against motion sickness usually ineffective
• Glucocorticoids do not alter the course of the disease and are not recommended.
• Some authors advocate the use of antibiotics in the acute phase if otitis media and interna cannot be ruled out.

CONTRAINDICATIONS N/A
PRECAUTIONS N/A
POSSIBLE INTERACTIONS N/A
ALTERNATE DRUGS N/A

FOLLOW-UP

PATIENT MONITORING
• Repeat neurologic examination of outpatient in approximately 72 hours to confirm stabilization and initial improvement.
• Discharge inpatient pending ability to ambulate and resumption of eating and drinking.

PREVENTION/AVOIDANCE N/A

POSSIBLE COMPLICATIONS
• Uncommon • Dehydration and electrolyte imbalance (rare)

EXPECTED COURSE AND PROGNOSIS
• Marked improvement especially in the resting nystagmus within 72 hours, with progressive improvement of the gait and head tilt. Patients usually normal within 2-3 weeks.
• The head tilt is the final sign to resolve. A mild residual head tilt may remain. • If the signs do not improve rapidly, other causes of vestibular disease should be pursued. • Mild head tilt and ataxia may temporarily return with stress such as general anesthesia. • Rarely recurs

☑ MISCELLANEOUS

ASSOCIATED CONDITIONS N/A

AGE RELATED FACTORS N/A

ZOONOTIC POTENTIAL N/A

PREGNANCY N/A

SYNONYMS
• Feline vestibular syndrome • Idiopathic vestibular neuropathy

SEE ALSO
• Head Tilt (Vestibular Disease)
• Otitis Media and Interna

ABBREVIATIONS None

References

de Lahunta A. Veterinary neuroanatomy and clinical neurology. Philadelphia: WB Saunders, 1983:238-255.

Oliver JE, Lorenz MD. Handbook of veterinary neurologic diagnosis. Philadelphia: WB Saunders, 1993:212-216.

Parent JM, Cochrane SM. Head tilt. In: Allen DG, ed. Small animal medicine. Philadelphia: JB Lippincott, 1991:753-759.

Author Susan M. Cochrane

Consulting Editor Joane M. Parent

VITAMIN A TOXICITY

 BASICS

OVERVIEW
Hypervitaminosis A is a skeletal disease that occurs from excessive intake of vitamin A. High concentration inhibits both intramembranous and endochondral ossification, which results in dystrophic calcification of the skeleton.

SIGNALMENT
• Cats from 2 to 9 years old • No breed or gender predilection has been recognized.

SIGNS

Historical Findings
• Clinical and radiographic changes and dietary history (eg, administering liver or cod liver oil) • Daily diet high in liver or vitamin A supplement for > 14 weeks

Examination Findings
• Lethargy • Anorexia • Resentment of handling • Marsupial-like sitting position with the forelimbs raised • Weight-bearing lameness, most notable in the forelimbs as the osseous proliferation impinges on spinal nerves • Cutaneous hyper- or hyposensitivity over the cervical and forelimb regions • Cervical, joint, and spinal stiffness • Unkempt haircoat from inability to groom • Constipation • Weight loss

CAUSES AND RISK FACTORS
• Feeding large amounts of raw liver, usually beef or sheep liver • Excessive intake of vitamin A supplement (eg, cod liver oil can contain >1,000 IU/ml of vitamin A)

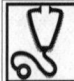 **DIAGNOSIS**

DIFFERENTIAL DIAGNOSIS
Differentials are osteomyelitis, multiple cartilaginous exostoses, and neoplasia.

CBC/BIOCHEMISTRY/URINALYSIS
• Neutrophilic leukocytosis with stress leukogram • Stress-induced hyperglycemia

OTHER LABORATORY TESTS N/A

IMAGING
• Radiographic findings • New bone formation involving the cervical vertebrae (often extending from C_1-T_2,) the sternum, and the costal cartilages • New periosteal bone formation on bone metaphyses or surrounding joints • Bony arthrodesis of joints

OTHER DIAGNOSTIC PROCEDURES
N/A

 TREATMENT

• Remove excess vitamin A from the diet.
• Young animals show permanent retardation of long bone length; appositional bone formation returns to normal.

MEDICATIONS

DRUGS AND FLUIDS
• Stop feeding raw liver or vitamin A supplement and use balanced commercial cat diet.
• Analgesics intended for cats should be used as required.

CONTRAINDICATIONS/POSSIBLE INTERACTIONS
Avoid NSAIDs in cats.

FOLLOW-UP

• Mature cats show reversal of most signs except those related to bony arthrodesis.
• Skeletal improvement is detected by radiographic and clinical changes. • Plasma concentrations of vitamin A decrease to normal within a few weeks of dietary change, but vitamin A content of liver may remain high for years.

MISCELLANEOUS

ABBREVIATIONS
NSAIDs = nonsteroidal antiinflammatory drugs

SEE ALSO
Poisoning (Intoxication)

References

Fry PD. Hypervitaminosis A in the cat. Vet Intl 1989;1:16-31.

Goldman AL. Hypervitaminosis A in a cat. J Am Vet Med Assoc 1992;200:1970-1972.

Seawright AA, English PB. Hypervitaminosis A and deforming cervical spondylosis of the cat. J Comp Pathol 1967;77:29-39.

Author Johnny D. Hoskins
Consulting Editor Gary Osweiler

VITAMIN D TOXICITY

BASICS

DEFINITION
Hypervitaminosis D is the abnormal accumulation of vitamin D in the body, most commonly the result of ingestion of vitamin D-containing rodenticides or over-supplementation of vitamins or vitamin D-containing preparations.

Pathophysiology
Ingested cholecalciferol, a fat soluble vitamin, is absorbed through chylomicrons and transported to the liver where it is metabolized to 25-hydroxycholecalciferol, the major circulating metabolite of vitamin D. Further metabolism of 25-hydroxycholecalciferol occurs in the kidneys where calcitriol is produced. Cholecalciferol and 25-hydroxycholecalciferol have limited biological activity; calcitriol is the most potent cholecalciferol metabolite in terms of enhancing calcium resorption from bone and intestinal calcium uptake. After excessive ingestion, cholecalciferol and other vitamin D metabolites abnormally increase intestinal absorption of calcium, stimulate bone resorption, and increase the renal tubular reabsorption of calcium, resulting in hypercalcemia (serum calcium > 12 mg/dl) and associated dystrophic calcification.

Systems Affected
• Renal/Urologic—dystrophic calcification of the kidneys • Gastrointestinal—dystrophic calcification • Cardiovascular—dystrophic calcification • Nervous—abnormal neurologic function because of altered calcium homeostasis and hypercalcemia

Genetics N/A

Incidence/Prevalence
Cholecalciferol-based rodenticide toxicosis is a common cause of poisoning in dogs and cats. Actual incidence is unknown.

Geographic Distribution N/A

SIGNALMENT

Species Dogs and cats

Breed predilections
• No breed predilection has been observed, although small dogs (adult body weight < 12 kg) make up most of reported canine cases.
• Toxicosis resulting from inappropriate, chronic, over-supplementation of vitamin D by owners has been reported in giant-breed dogs.

Mean age and range All ages

Predominant sex N/A

SIGNS

General Comments
• The diagnosis depends on history of exposure to a potentially toxic amount of vitamin D, development of associated clinical signs, and high vitamin D blood concentration and/or hypercalcemia. • Clinical signs generally develop within 12-36 hours after ingestion of cholecalciferol.

Historical Findings
• Vomiting • Depression • Anorexia • Polydipsia • Polyuria • Diarrhea.

Physical Examination Findings
• Gastrointestinal and pulmonary hemorrhage apparently because of dystrophic calcification in some animals. • Renal pain on palpation • Bradycardia or other cardiac arrhythmia

CAUSES
• The most common cause is the ingestion of excessive vitamin D, usually in the form of cholecalciferol-based rodenticides or vitamin supplements. The NRC daily recommended requirement of vitamin D for growing dogs is 22 IU/kg. • Daily administration of vitamin D (2,000-4,000 IU/kg for 1-2 weeks) can cause toxicosis. • Cholecalciferol-containing (0.075%) rodenticides have been marketed under the brand names Quintox®, Rampage®, Ortho Rat-B-Gone®, and Ortho Mouse-B-Gone®. Toxicoses in dogs after the ingestion of 2-3 mg cholecalciferol/kg has been reported.

RISK FACTORS
Animals with preexisting renal disease may be predisposed.

DIAGNOSIS

DIFFERENTIAL DIAGNOSIS
• Cholecalciferol-based rodenticide poisoning must be considered in the list of differential diagnoses for hypercalcemia. Other potential causes of hypercalcemia include normal juvenile hypercalcemia, cancer-associated (paraneoplastic) hypercalcemia, hypoadrenocorticism, primary renal failure, primary hyperparathyroidism, hemoconcentration (hyperproteinemia), and disuse osteoporosis.
• Gastrointestinal and pulmonary hemorrhage sometimes occur as an apparent result of dystrophic calcification; this should not be misdiagnosed as anticoagulant rodenticide toxicosis when the identity of a rodenticide ingested is in question.

CBC/BIOCHEMISTRY/URINALYSIS
• Hypercalcemia (serum calcium > 12 mg/dl), hyperphosphatemia, hyperproteinemia, and azotemia. Hyperphosphatemia and hypercalcemia develop within 12 and 24 hours, respectively, after ingestion. • Baseline serum calcium determination is recommended for all potentially affected animals. Baseline measurement serves as the basis for comparison with subsequent measurements. Calcium measurements are likely to be within normal limits for up to several hours after ingestion, even when potentially lethal doses are consumed.
• Hyposthenuria (Uspg 1.001-1.007), proteinuria, and glucosuria in some animals; urine sediment—leukocytes, erythrocytes, and casts in variable numbers in some animals.
• Metabolic acidosis in some animals

OTHER LABORATORY TESTS
• Total kidney calcium concentration high in some animals • High serum concentration of cholecalciferol and its primary metabolites, 25- hydroxycholecalciferol, 24,25-dihydroxy-cholecalciferol, and 1,25-dihydroxy-cholecalciferol, support a diagnosis of hypervitominosis D.

IMAGING
Mineralization of the kidneys, gastrointestinal tract, lungs, and other organs seen on radiographs in some animals.

OTHER DIAGNOSTIC PROCEDURES
Electrocardiographic abnormalities (e.g., bradycardia) in some animals

GROSS AND HISTOPATHOLOGIC FINDINGS
• Diffuse hemorrhage in the gastric mucosa, duodenum, and jejunum in some animals
• Necrosis and mineralization of the myocardium and of the arterial intima. Mineralization of glomerular capillary walls, renal cortical tubular basement membranes, Bowman's capsules, and stomach mucosa has been described.

TREATMENT

INPATIENT VERSUS OUTPATIENT
• Treatment of accidental vitamin D supplement ingestions < 25,000 IU/kg is not required.
• Initial treatment can be administration of an emetic by the owner. Specific emetics recommended for home use by the owner include syrup of ipecac (dogs,1-2 ml/kg; cats, 3.3 ml/kg) and 3% hydrogen peroxide (5-25 ml/ 5 kg). Vomiting usually starts within 5-15 minutes. If the animal has not vomited by 15 minutes, a single repeat dose is recommended. Owners should be forewarned that prolonged vomiting and depression may occur. Emetic administration by owners is indicated for minimal exposure and for animals for which there would be a substantial delay in transporting to a veterinarian.
• Asymptomatic animals that have ingested a potentially toxic dose of vitamin D should be examined; baseline serum biochemical analysis should be done and decontamination of gastrointestinal tract initiated. • Animals displaying clinical signs consistent with hypervitaminosis D should be hospitalized until serum calcium has normalized.

ACTIVITY N/A

DIET
A low calcium diet; milk, other dairy products, and calcium supplements are contraindicated.

CLIENT EDUCATION
• Owners should be encouraged to prevent any additional exposure to animals or children in their home environment.

• Discuss need for aggressive treatment aimed at decontamination of the gastrointestinal tract and control of hypercalcemia.

SURGICAL CONSIDERATIONS N/A

MEDICATIONS

DRUGS AND FLUIDS
• For decontamination of the gastrointestinal tract to reduce cholecalciferol absorption—administer an emetic and activated charcoal with a saline or osmotic cathartic. Apomorphine for dogs (0.03 mg/kg, IV; 0.04 mg/kg, IM); xylazine is somewhat effective in cats (1.1 mg/kg, IM or SQ). Activated charcoal powder (1-4 g/kg) combined with a saline cathartic (magnesium or sodium sulfate, 250 mg/kg PO) as a suspension in water (10 × volume) administered orally or by gastric tube.
• Correct fluid and electrolyte imbalances. Calciuresis may be enhanced by administering 0.9% sodium chloride IV. Early diuresis is strongly recommended for immature animals, animals with preexisting renal disease, and all animals that have ingested amounts likely to cause renal damage.

To reduce the hypercalcemic state:
• Furosemide (2-5 mg/kg PO q8h-q12h)
• Prednisone (2 mg/kg PO q12h)
• Salmon calcitonin (4-6 IU/kg SC q2h-q3h until serum calcium concentration normalizes). Higher calcitonin dosage (up to 10 to 20 IU/kg) may be required in refractory animals.
• Maintenance after calcium concentration has stabilized—furosemide (2- 4.5 mg/kg PO q8h-q12h) and prednisone (2 mg/kg PO q12h)
• In severely uremic or hypercalcemic animals, peritoneal dialysis with a calcium-free dialysate solution can be used to lower serum calcium concentration even if other methods have failed.
• Seizure control, treatment of arrhythmias, and other symptomatic treatment required in rare cases

CONTRAINDICATIONS
• Do not use calcium-containing fluids.

PRECAUTIONS
• Emetic administration is contraindicated if the animal is convulsing. Xylazine may aggravate respiratory depression and result in vagal mediated slowing of the heart rate. The α2 - antagonist, yohimbine (cat/dog: 0.1 mg/kg, IV), has been used effectively to reverse xylazine induced depression, bradycardia, and hypotension.
• Constipation is occasionally associated with the administration of activated charcoal. Owners should be warned of the possibility of dark black stools and diarrhea.
• Adrenocortical suppression is not expected to occur with this dosage of prednisone. However, to lessen the likelihood of acute adrenocortical insufficiency, a gradual tapering dosage of the prednisone should be administered toward the end of the 2- to 4-week treatment period.

POSSIBLE INTERACTIONS N/A
ALTERNATIVE DRUGS N/A

FOLLOW-UP

PATIENT MONITORING
• Serum calcium and BUN should be determined at 1, 2, and 3 days after clinically important exposure. If the animal has hypercalcemia (serum calcium > 12 mg/dl) or remains symptomatic, further diuresis and other additional treatment is indicated. • Vitamin D-induced hypercalcemia often persists for several weeks necessitating long-term management.

PREVENTION/AVOIDANCE
Restrict access to cholecalciferol-based rodenticides.

POSSIBLE COMPLICATIONS
• Animal may be prone to chronic renal failure. • Subclinical renal, cardiovascular, and gastrointestinal damage caused by dystrophic calcification in some animals

EXPECTED COURSE AND PROGNOSIS
Depends on severity and duration of the hypercalcemia. Animals that do not have hypercalcemia have an excellent prognosis. Unresponsive hypercalcemia after aggressive treatment is associated with a poor prognosis.

MISCELLANEOUS

ASSOCIATED CONDITIONS N/A

AGE RELATED FACTORS
Must distinguish from normal juvenile hypercalcemia

ZOONOTIC POTENTIAL
None. Human poisoning also possible.

PREGNANCY
Teratogenic effects (e.g., aortic and cardiac lesions) have been reported in humans and rodents.

SYNONYMS
Cholecalciferol toxicosis

SEE ALSO
• Hypercalcemia • Poisoning (Intoxication)

ABBREVIATIONS
BUN = blood urea nitrogen
NRC = National Research Council

References

Dorman DC. Anticoagulant, cholecalciferol and bromethalin-based rodenticides. Vet Clin North Am Small Anim Pract 1990;20:339-352.

Livezy KL, Dorman DC, Hooser SB, and Buck WB. Hypercalcemia induced by vitamin D_3 toxicosis in two dogs. Comp Anim Pract 1991;16:26-32.

Gunther R, Felice LJ, Nelson RK, and Franson AM. Toxicity of a vitamin D_3 rodenticide to dogs. J Am Vet Med Assoc 1988;193:211-214.

Moore FM, Kudisch M, Richter K, Faggella A. Hypercalcemia associated with rodenticide poisoning in three cats. J Am Vet Med Assoc 1988;193:1099-1100.

Author David Dorman
Consulting Editor Gary D. Osweiler

VON WILLEBRAND'S DISEASE

BASICS

DEFINITION
Von Willebrand disease (vWD) is a complex inherited defect of hemostasis related to defects in synthesis or function of von Willebrand factor. It is the most common inherited bleeding disorder in dogs.

Pathophysiology
Von Willebrand factor (vWF) is a large, multimeric glycoprotein that consists of identical subunits that are synthesized mostly by endothelial cells. vWF circulates in the plasma as a macromolecular complex with factor VIII and is required for platelet adhesion to subendothelium and for stabilizing and preventing rapid clearance of factor VIII from the circulation. Various defects in the vWF gene may cause deficient synthesis of vWF or production of dysfunctional or unstable forms of vWF. These defects may cause platelet function defects and delayed coagulation of blood.

Systems Affected
Hemic/lymph/immune—bleeding diathesis with hemorrhages seen in a variety of organs but especially at surgical sites and mucosal surfaces

Genetics
vWD is an autosomal trait in dogs. In most dogs, the defect follows a pattern of incomplete dominance, although the disease has been described as autosomal recessive in the Scottish terrier and Chesapeake Bay retriever.

Incidence/Prevalence
The prevalence of a low concentration of vWF is extremely variable in different breeds, with estimates of 68-73% in the Doberman pinscher, 18-28% in the Shetland sheepdog, and 16-30% in the Scottish terrier.

Geographic Distribution N/A

SIGNALMENT

Species
• Dogs • Rare in cats

Breed Predilections
Von Willebrand disease has been described in at least 54 breeds of dogs. Breeds with a known high prevalence of the defect include the Airedale terrier, bassett hound, dachshund, Doberman pinscher, German shepherd, golden retriever, keeshond, Manchester terrier, miniature schnauzer, Pembroke Welsh corgi, rottweiler, Shetland sheepdog, Scottish terrier, and standard poodle.

Mean Age and Range
Present from birth

Predominant Sex
Both males and females are affected.

SIGNS

General Comments
vWD can be subclinical or manifested as a bleeding diathesis most commonly as a consequence of surgery, toenail clipping, or some form of injury.

Historical Findings
• Previous abnormal bleeding associated with teething or disproportionate hemorrhage associated with minor injury • Many dogs survive ear cropping or tail docking without serious bleeding.

Physical Examination Findings
• Gastrointestinal bleeding • Hematuria
• Bleeding around gums at teething • Epistaxis
• Vaginal or penile bleeding • Petechiae are uncommon despite the presence of a platelet function defect.

CAUSES
vWD often is divided into three classifications:
• Type I—low vWF concentration but with all sizes of multimers detected. This is the most common pattern. Clinical severity varies. It is typical of the Doberman pinscher, Airedale, and the one third of shelties with detectable vWF. • Type II—selective depletion of high molecular weight multimers. This is an uncommon form described in a family of German shorthaired pointers.
• Type III—severe deficiency of vWF with virtual undetectable multimers of vWF. This is typical of the defect in the Scottish terrier, Chesapeake Bay retriever, and about two thirds of affected Shetland sheepdogs.

RISK FACTORS
Hypothyroidism may exacerbate the bleeding tendency in animals with vWD.

DIAGNOSIS

DIFFERENTIAL DIAGNOSIS
• Classic hemophilia—defective synthesis of factor VIII is usually associated with much lower factor VIII activity and with a more severe bleeding tendency with spontaneous hemorrhages in body cavities, deep muscle masses, and joints • Other inherited or acquired hemostatic defects

CBC/BIOCHEMISTRY/URINALYSIS
• Anemia, which is proportional to the degree of blood loss • Neutrophilia and mild left shift secondary to hemorrhage • Mild reticulocytosis • Platelet count is normal.

OTHER LABORATORY TESTS
• PT is normal; APTT in all but those with severe deficiency of vWF is normal. • vWF assay—the test of choice for diagnosis of vWD. The normal range of vWF is reported as 60-172% of normal reference pools of dogs. The reference method is the Laurell rocket electroimmunoassay, but a reliable ELISA method has recently been developed and is commercially available (Zymtec, Iatric Corporation, 2330 South Industrial Park Avenue, Tempe, AZ). Values of < 7% vWF indicate either a homozygous defect or severe (penetrant) heterozygous animal. Dogs with vWF concentration between 7-50% are usually heterozygous and vary from asymptomatic carriers to bleeders.

IMAGING N/A

OTHER DIAGNOSTIC PROCEDURES
The buccal mucosa bleeding time may be useful in predicting bleeding problems in dogs suspected of having vWD. The use of a gauze strip tied around the maxilla to cause venous engorgement in the folded back upper lip increases the sensitivity of the buccomucosal method. Nevertheless, the bleeding time does not identify all animals at risk for abnormal bleeding after surgery.

GROSS AND HISTOPATHOLOGIC FINDINGS
Hemorrhage is the only abnormality associated with vWD. It can occur at any site but most commonly occurs at sites of injury and mucosal surfaces.

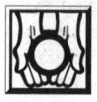

TREATMENT

INPATIENT VERSUS OUTPATIENT
After surgery in dogs with vWD, the animal should be monitored for abnormal bleeding for at least 48 hours before release from the hospital.

ACTIVITY
Usually it is not necessary to limit the activity of dogs with vWD because of the low frequency of spontaneous hemorrhages.

DIET N/A

CLIENT EDUCATION
• The pattern of inheritance should be explained to owners with discussion of the options for screening related animals for the defect. Carriers generally have an intermediate concentration of vWF.
• In regard to animals that have had bleeding episodes, the owner should be informed of early signs that indicate bleeding and instructed on preparations for early treatment with fresh frozen plasma.

SURGICAL CONSIDERATIONS
Steps should be taken to minimize the risk of bleeding problems in patients undergoing elective surgery.

MEDICATIONS

DRUGS AND FLUID
Fresh plasma in patients without anemia and fresh whole blood in patients with anemia are the practical treatments of choice. Transfusion with blood or plasma at 22 ml/kg generally is successful in controlling bleeding in affected dogs; favorable responses are seen at a lower dosage in some dogs. In contrast to classic hemophilia, control of the bleeding usually is achieved with a single transfusion.

CONTRAINDICATIONS

Drugs such as aspirin, phenothiazine tranquilizers, and antiinflammatory agents, which are known to inhibit platelet function, should be avoided.

PRECAUTIONS N/A

POSSIBLE INTERACTIONS N/A

ALTERNATE DRUGS

• There is some evidence that thyroid supplementation decreases the bleeding tendency and may increase the vWF concentration in hypothyroid dogs.

• Desmopressin acetate (1µg/kg SQ) has been shown to increase the vWF concentration and shorten the bleeding time in some dogs with von Willebrand's disease and may be helpful in reducing the risk of bleeding associated with surgery. This should not be viewed as an equal alternative to plasma transfusion, which is the most effective method of treating bleeding episodes.

FOLLOW-UP

PATIENT MONITORING

Observe closely for hemorhage associated with trauma or surgical procedures.

PREVENTION/AVOIDANCE

Inherited disorder. Avoid breeding affected animals. Pretreatment with desmopressin acetate (DDAVP) may prevent excessive bleeding during surgery.

ALTERNATE DRUGS N/A

POSSIBLE COMPLICATIONS

Hemorrhage

EXPECTED COURSE AND PROGNOSIS

vWD may be subclinical or manifested as a bleeding diathesis most commonly as a consequence of surgery, toenail clipping, or some form of injury. Course and prognosis vary with concentration of vWF.

MISCELLANEOUS

ASSOCIATED CONDITIONS N/A

AGE RELATED FACTORS

Bleeding tendency declines with age.

ZOONOTIC POTENTIAL N/A

PREGNANCY

Risk of bleeding at parturition

SYNONYMS None

ABBREVIATIONS

APTT = activated partial thromboplastin time
PT = prothrombin time
vWD = von Willebrand's disease
vWF = von Willebrand factor

References

Brooks M, Dodds WJ, Raymond SL. Epidemiologic features of von Willebrand's disease in Doberman pinchers, Scottish terriers, and Shetland sheepdogs: 260 cases (1984-1988). J Am Vet Med Assoc 1992;200:1123-1127.

Dodds WJ. Hemostasis. In: Kaneko JJ, ed. Clinical biochemistry of domestic animals. New York: Academic Press, 1989:274-315.

Johnson GS. Canine von Willebrand's disease. In: Feldman BF, ed. Hemostasis. Vet Clin North Am Small Anm 1988;18:195-229.

Kraus KH, Johnson GS. Von Willebrand's disease in dogs. In: Kirk RW, Bonagura JD, eds. Current veterinary therapy X. Philadelphia: WB Saunders, 1989:446-451.

Raymond SL, Jones DW, Brooks MB, Dodds WJ. Clinical and laboratory features of a severe form of von Willebrand disease in shetland sheepdogs. J Am Vet Med Assoc 1990;197:1342-1346.

Author Gary J. Kociba
Consulting Editor Alan H. Rebar

WHIPWORMS

 BASICS

Trichuris vulpis, the whipworm, in the cecum of dogs (T. campanula, cats) may cause bloody diarrhea, enteritis (cecitis). Usually not patent with eggs in feces until 3 months; may be clinical earlier than patency (90 days). Infective eggs ingested to establish cecal infection. No extraintestinal migration. Eggs persist in environment for months to years.

SIGNALMENT
Dogs of any age

SIGNS
• Bloody diarrhea • Acute to chronic debilitation

CAUSES AND RISK FACTORS
• Ingestion of infective trichurid eggs from contaminated environment • Eggs persist in environment as in soil for months to years

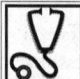 **DIAGNOSIS**

DIFFERENTIAL DIAGNOSIS
• Bacterial (spirochaetal) infections of cecum • Hookworm infection • Capillarid infections with eggs similar in appearance but smaller

CBC/BIOCHEMISTRY/URINALYSIS
Normal

OTHER LABORATORY TESTS
Fecal flotation: Trichurid eggs ovoid with prominent bipolar plugs, brown color, single cell (zygote) within egg shell membranes; 90 x 45 µm

IMAGING N/A

OTHER DIAGNOSTIC PROCEDURES
N/A

 TREATMENT

• Benzimidazoles, organophosphates, pyrantel pamoate effective in whipworm removal; may need to re-treat in 1–2 months
• Generally treat as outpatients

MEDICATIONS

DRUGS & FLUIDS

• Fenbendazole (Panacur) 50mg/kg q24h for 5 days; may need second course of treatment
• Dichlorvos (Task) twice 3–4 weeks apart
• Pyrantel pamoate (Nemex) at 15 mg/kg for dogs; may need second course of treatment

CONTRAINDICATIONS/POSSIBLE INTERACTIONS

• Organophosphates (dichlorvos) not to be used for dogs not determined free of heartworm infection
• Do not give dichlorvos concurrently with other organophosphates such as insecticides

 FOLLOW-UP

Fecal examination for trichurid eggs 3–4 weeks following treatment

 MISCELLANEOUS

SYNONYMS

Trichuriasis

ABBREVIATIONS

Reference

Bowman DD, Georgi's parasitology for veterinarians. 6th ed. Philadelphia: WB Saunders, 1994;226–229.

Author Robert M. Corwin
Consulting Editor Brent D. Jones

WOBBLER SYNDROME (CERVICAL VERTEBRAL INSTABILITY)

BASICS

DEFINITION
• Wobbler syndrome is a term loosely used to encompass compressive spinal cord lesions affecting the cervical spine (primarily caudal) in large- and giant-breed dogs. • Basically two types of compressive disease are described: 1) disk related disease in mature dogs arising from type II disk herniation with accompanying vertebral ligamentous hypertrophy, presumably caused by joint instability—C5-6 and C6-7 are primarily involved but C3-4 and C4-5 can be, and 2) vertebral related disease in young dogs arising from developmental abnormalities causing malformation and malarticulation of the spinal column—all cervical joints can be affected.

Pathophysiology
Compression of the cervical spinal cord

Systems Affected Nervous

Genetics
No inheritance specifically identified but many factors may be under genetic control

Incidence/Prevalence
• Reported in numerous breeds of large dogs • Old Doberman pinschers (disk related disease) and young Great Danes (vertebral related disease) are predisposed.

Geographic Distribution N/A

SIGNALMENT

Species Dogs

Breed Predilections
• Disk related disease—Doberman pinschers • Vertebral related disease—Great Danes

Mean Age and Range
• Disk related disease—mature, (≥ 2 years old; most patients > 5 years • Vertebral related disease—young, generally < 2 years old

Predominant Sex N/A

SIGNS

General Comments
Clinical signs highly variable depending on the degree of compression and duration of lesion

Historical Findings
Acute or chronic onset and progressive or nonprogressive nature

Physical Examination Findings
• Variable neck pain • Difficulty rising to a standing posture • Variable muscle atrophy, especially in forelimbs • Worn toenails • Ataxia involving all four limbs but to a lesser degree in the forelimbs; normal, decreased, or absent postural reactions in all four limbs; lower motor neuron or upper motor neuron in forelimbs and upper motor neuron signs in hind limbs; pain perception intact in most patients

CAUSES
• Disk related disease—disk degeneration or

vertebral instability • Vertebral related disease—nutritionally related malformation or malarticulation

RISK FACTORS
• Disk related disease—none specifically identified • Vertebral related disease—large, fast-growing dogs

DIAGNOSIS

DIFFERENTIAL DIAGNOSIS
• Disk related disease—trauma, diskospondylitis, primary disk disease, neoplasia, and inflammatory spinal cord diseases are differentiated by breed incidence, results of CSF analysis, and radiographic studies • Vertebral related disease—same as above plus juvenile orthopaedic disease

CBC/BIOCHEMISTRY/URINALYSIS
Results usually normal

OTHER LABORATORY TESTS N/A

IMAGING

Survey Cervical Radiography
• Disk related disease—may be normal or show narrowing of the disk space suggesting disk herniation • Vertebral related disease—may show abnormal articular facet shape or density, subluxation, malformed vertebral bodies, stenosis of the vertebral canal, and misshapen dorsal spinal processes

Myelography
• Disk related disease—soft tissue compression of the spinal cord by the dorsal annulus of the disk, dorsal longitudinal ligament, and dorsal ligamentum flavum • Vertebral related disease—compression of the spinal cord due to proliferation of the articular facets, remodeling of vertebral bodies, and other bony causes of stenosis of the spinal canal

OTHER DIAGNOSTIC PROCEDURES
CSF analysis—may be normal or show high protein due to compressive degeneration of the spinal cord

GROSS AND HISTOPATHOLOGIC FINDINGS
• White and gray matter necrosis at the level of compression • Wallerian-type degeneration of white matter above and below compression

TREATMENT

INPATIENT VERSUS OUTPATIENT
These patients are surgical candidates necessitating hospitalization.

ACTIVITY
Should be limited to avoid exacerbation of the condition

DIET
• Disk related disease—N/A
• Vertebral related disease—discontinue ex-

cessive use of dietary supplements and control food intake

CLIENT EDUCATION
• Depending on the chronicity of the disease, neurologic deficits may remain. In these patients, aim treatment at stopping progression. • Physiotherapy usually required to maximize return of function

SURGICAL CONSIDERATIONS

Decompression
• Ventral spondylectomy best suited for solitary lesions compressing from the floor of the spinal canal, such as occurs in dogs with disk related disease
• Dorsal laminectomy best in dogs with multiple sites of involvement or in which compression is mainly from the roof of the spinal canal; applies in disk related and developmental types of diseases

Fenestration
Indicated in disk-type of disease to prevent additional sites of involvement

Stabilization/Fusion
Controversy about use in disk related caudal cervical compression. Advocates argue that primary lesion is instability, which should be stabilized. Opponents argue that stabilization without decompression does nothing for the compressive lesion and actually may precipitate additional damage at the disk spaces on either side of the fused space.

MEDICATIONS

DRUGS AND FLUIDS
• Glucocorticosteroids in combination with surgery the most advantageous therapeutic approach
• Glucocorticosteroid administration alone only useful in mildly affected patients

CONTRAINDICATIONS N/A

PRECAUTIONS
Observe for signs of gastroenteritis and cystitis

POSSIBLE INTERACTIONS N/A

ALTERNATE DRUGS N/A

FOLLOW-UP

PATIENT MONITORING
Neurologic examinations as necessary to evaluate response to treatment

PREVENTION/AVOIDANCE
Limit running and jumping.

POSSIBLE COMPLICATIONS
In animals with disk related type of disease, adjacent sites may become involved.

EXPECTED COURSE AND PROGNOSIS
• Acute history—immediate aggressive treat-

WOBBLER SYNDROME (CERVICAL VERTEBRAL INSTABILITY)

ment necessary for best outcome • Chronic progressive history—the earlier in the course of disease surgery is performed, the better the outcome. Paralyzed dogs often cannot be helped.

MISCELLANEOUS

ASSOCIATED CONDITIONS N/A

AGE RELATED FACTORS
• Disk related disease—old dogs
• Developmental related disease—young dogs

ZOONOTIC POTENTIAL N/A

PREGNANCY N/A

SYNONYMS
• Disk related disease—cervical vertebral instability, spondylolisthesis, vertebral subluxation, caudal cervical spondylopathy, cervical spondylopathy • Vertebral related disease—vertebral stenosis, cervical vertebral stenotic myelopathy, cervical spondylopathy

SEE ALSO
• Intervertebral Disk Disease • Osteochondrosis

ABBREVIATION
CSF = cerebrospinal fluid

References

Braund KG. Degenerative and developmental diseases. In: Oliver JE, Hoerlein BF, Mayhew IG, eds. Veterinary neurology. Philadelphia: WB Saunders, 1987:185-215.

Oliver JE, Lorenz MD. Handbook of veterinary neurologic diagnosis. 2nd ed. Philadelphia: WB Saunders, 1991:180-185.

de Lahunta A. Veterinary neuroanatomy and clinical neurology. 2nd ed. Philadelphia: WB Saunders, 1983:195-204.

Author Patricia J. Luttgen
Consulting Editor Joane M. Parent

ZINC TOXICITY

BASICS

OVERVIEW
Toxicity from the ingestion of zinc ointment or zinc containing objects, which causes severe intravascular hemolysis and gastrointestinal irritation. Multiple organ failure (e.g., renal, hepatic, and cardiac), disseminated intravascular coagulation (DIC), and cardiopulmonary arrest may occur.

SIGNALMENT
Most frequently reported in dogs

SIGNS
• Pale mucous membranes • Hemoglobinuria • Hematuria • Anorexia
• Vomiting • Diarrhea • Icterus

CAUSES AND RISK FACTORS
Ingestion of zinc-containing objects:
• Nuts from transport cages • Zinc plumbing nuts • Zinc oxide ointment • Zinc game pieces from board games • Pennies minted after 1982

DIAGNOSIS

DIFFERENTIAL DIAGNOSIS
• Autoimmune hemolytic anemia • Babesia
• Onion toxicity • Caval syndrome • The presence of a radiographically apparent, metallic object in the gastrointestinal tract is strongly supportive of zinc toxicity and may help differentiate from other diseases.

CBC/BIOCHEMISTRY/URINALYSIS
• Severe intravascular hemolytic anemia
• High nucleated RBC counts • Basophilic stippling • Target cells • Polychromasia

• Azotemia and high ALP and ALT may indicate multiple organ failure.

OTHER LABORATORY TESTS
• High serum zinc concentration (normal in dogs, 0.7 – 2.0 ug/ml) • Coagulation panel may indicate DIC.

IMAGING
Metallic object in the gastrointestinal tract may be seen on abdominal radiographs.

OTHER DIAGNOSTIC PROCEDURES
ECG may reveal arrhythmias and ST segment abnormalities.

TREATMENT
Rapid removal of the zinc object by endoscopy or laparotomy is imperative.

MEDICATIONS

DRUGS AND FLUIDS
• Maintain hydration since acute renal failure is a serious sequelae of zinc toxicity.
• Severe intravascular hemolysis may necessitate blood transfusion.
• If patient has DIC, administer heparin (150 units/kg SC q6h).
• H2 receptor blockers (e.g., cimetidine, ranitidine) may be useful to reduce stomach acidity and the rate of release of zinc.
• CaEDTA (100 mg/kg diluted in 5% dextrose and divided into 4 doses a day, SC) may be given for zinc chelation.

CONTRAINDICATIONS/POSSIBLE INTERACTIONS
Avoid aminoglycoside antibiotics and other potential nephrotoxins because of risk of acute renal failure.

FOLLOW-UP
• Multiple organ failure and cardiopulmonary arrest are potential outcomes; however, rapid removal of the source of zinc may provide progressive improvement over 48-72 hours, and complete recovery can occur.
• Monitor patient by ECG for evidence of arrhythmias and ST segment alteration.
• Monitor coagulation profile, BUN, creatinine, ALP, and ALT for the first 72 hours after removal of zinc. • Provide client education about the hazards of ingestion of zinc-containing objects (especially pennies printed after 1982) and avoiding use of zinc oxide ointments.

MISCELLANEOUS

SEE ALSO
Poisoning (Intoxication)

ABBREVIATIONS
ALP = alkaline phosphatase
ALT = alanine transaminase
BUN = blood urea nitrogen
DIC = disseminated intravascular coagulation
ECG = electrocardiogram
RBC = red blood cells

Reference
Ogden L. Zinc Toxicosis. In: Kirk RW, Bonagura JD, eds. Current veterinary therapy XI. Philadelphia:WB Saunders, 1992:197-200.
Author Kathryn M. Meurs
Consulting Editor Gary D. Osweiler

APPENDIX I

NORMAL REFERENCE RANGES FOR LABORATORY TESTS

Table I-A.

Normal Hematologic Values			
Test	Units	Dogs	Cats
WBC	10 × 3/mm³	8.0–17.0	4.2–17.5
RBC	10 × 6/mm³	5.00–8.10	5.24–10.89
Hemoglobin	g/dl	12.0–18.0	9.0–16.7
Hematocrit	%	37.0–55.0	29.2–51.7
MCV	fl	60.0–77.0	41.0–56.2
MCH	pg	20.0–25.0	13.0–18.0
MCHC	%	32.0–36.0	29.5–34.8
Platelet count (automated)	10 × 3/mm³	200–500	170–600
Platelet count (manual)	10 × 3/mm³	200–500	300–700
Neutrophils	%	60–70	35–75
	Absolute	3600–13100	1925–14825
Bands	%	0–4	0–3
	Absolute	0–680	0–585
Lymphocytes	%	12–30	20–55
	Absolute	720–5100	1100–7000
Monocytes	%	3–10	1–4
	Absolute	180–1350	55–780
Eosinophils	%	2–10	2–12
	Absolute	120–750	110–750
Basophils	%	0–1	0–1
	Absolute	0–170	0–190
Retic ulocyte count	%	0.0–1.0	0.0–1.0
Corrected	%	0.0–1.0	0.0–1.0
Absolute	/mm³	0–80000	0–50000

From Abbott 3500 Hematology Analyzer; IDEXX Veterinary Services/Vetlab, Inc., Ft. Worth, TX.
It is important to realize that normal values vary among individual laboratories.

Table I-B.

Normal Biochemical Values

Test	Units	Dogs	Cats
Urea nitrogen (BUN)	mg/dl	10-26	15-34
Creatinine	mg/dl	0.5-1.3	1.0-2.2
BUN-creatinine ratio		5-35	7-36
Cholesterol	mg/dl	112-358	82-218
Glucose	mg/dl	60-115	60-130
Alkaline phosphatase (ALP)	IU/L	8-76	0-62
Alanine aminotransferase (ALT)	IU/L	6-70	28-76
Aspartate aminotransferase (AST)	IU/L	10-43	12-40
Total protein	g/dl	5.0-7.2	5.8-8.5
Albumin	g/dl	3.1-4.5	2.4-4.1
Globulin	g/dl	1.9-4.3	2.3-5.0
A-G ratio		0.6-1.1	0.5-1.1
Sodium	mEq/L	142-150	147-162
Potassium	mEq/L	4.0-5.4	3.7-5.2
Sodium-potassium ratio		> 27.0	> 27.0
Chloride	mEq/L	105-117	114-126
Total CO_2	mEq/L	15-23	13-25
Anion gap	mEq/L	15-25	15-25
Calcium	mg/dl	9.2-11.2	7.2-11.4
Phosphorus	mg/dl	2.3-5.5	3.0-7.0
Total bilirubin	mg/dl	0.0-0.6	0.0-0.4
Direct bilirubin	mg/dl	0.0-0.1	0.0-0.1
Indirect bilirubin	mg/dl	0.0-0.5	0.0-0.3
Lactate dehydrogenase (LDH)	IU/L	17-193	46-350
Creatine kinase (CK or CPK)	IU/L	8-216	54-440
Gamma glutamyl transferase (GGT)	IU/L	0-8	0-1
Uric acid	mg/dl	0.0-0.5	0.0-0.2
Amylase	IU/L	350-1650	550-1450
Lipase	U/L	0-375	0-115
Magnesium	mEq/L	1.5-2.0	1.6-2.1
Triglycerides	mg/dl	21-87	34-98
Bile acids:			
Fasting	µmol/L	0.0-5.0	0.0-5.0
Postprandial	µmol/L	3.9-12.7	5.0-10.0
Random	µmol/L	0.0-12.7	0.0-10.0
Total iron	µg/dl	54-196	68-215
Unsaturated iron binding capacity	µg/dl	127-340	105-205
Total iron binding capacity	µg/dl	277-428	170-400

From Hitachi Chemistry Analyzer; IDEXX Veterinary Services/Vetlab, Inc., Ft. Worth, TX.
It is important to realize that normal values vary among individual laboratories.

Table I-C.

Conversion Table for Hematologic Units

| | Example values | | Conversion factors | |
Analyte	Traditional	SI*	Traditional to SI	SI to Traditional
Hemoglobin	15.0 g/dl	150 g/L	10	0.1
HCT or PCV	45%	0.45 L/L	0.01	100
Erythrocytes	$6.0 \times 10^6/mm^3$	$6.0 \times 10^{12}/L$	10^6	10^{-6}
MCV	$75 \mu^3$	75 fl	No change	No change
MCH	25 μμg	25 pg	No change	No change
MCHC	33 g/dl	330 g/L	10	0.1
WBC	$15.0 \times 10^3/mm^3$	$15.0 \times 10^9/L$	10^6	10^{-6}
Platelets	$250 \times 10^3/mm^3$	$250 \times 10^9/L$	10^6	10^{-6}

* Système International d'Unités
Modified from Appendices. In: Bonagura JD, ed. Current veterinary therapy XII. Philadelphia: WB Saunders, 1995:1397 (with permission).

Table 1-D.

Conversion Table for Clinical Biochemical Units

Analyte	Traditional unit (with examples)	Conversion factor	SI unit (with examples)
Alanine aminotransferase	0-40 U/L	1.00	0-40 U/L
Albumin	2.8-4.0 g/dl	10.0	28-40 g/L
Alkaline phosphatase	30-150 U/L	1.00	30-150 U/L
Ammonia	10-80 μg/dl	0.5871	5.9-47.0 μmol/L
Amylase	200-800 U/L	1.00	200-800 U/L
Aspartate aminotransferase	0-40 U/L	1.00	0-40 U/L
Bile acids (total)	0.3-2.3 μg/ml	2.45	0.74-5.64 μmol/L
Bilirubin	0.1-0.2 mg/dl	17.10	2-4 μmol/L
Calcium	8.8-10.3 mg/dl	0.2495	2.20-2.58 mmol/L
Carbon dioxide	22-28 mEq/L	1.00	22-28 mmol/L
Chloride	95-100 mEq/L	1.00	95-100 mmol/L
Cholesterol	100-265 mg/dl	0.0258	2.58-5.85 mmol/L
Copper	70-140 μg/dl	0.1574	11.0-22.0 μmol/L
Cortisol	2-10 μg/dl	27.59	55-280 nmol/L
Creatine kinase	0-130 U/L	1.00	0-130 U/L
Creatinine	0.6-1.2 mg/dl	88.40	50-110 μmol/L
Fibrinogen	200-400 mg/dl	0.01	2.0-4.0 g/L
Folic acid	3.5-11.0 μg/L	2.265	7.93-24.92 nmol/L
Glucose	70-110 mg/dl	0.05551	3.9-6.1 mmol/L
Iron	80-180 μg/dl	0.1791	14-32 μmol/L
Lactate	5-20 mg/dl	0.1110	0.5-2.0 mmol/L
Lead	150 μg/dl	0.04826	7.2 μmol/L
Lipase Sigma Tietz (37° C)	≤ 1 ST U/dl	280	≤ 280 U/L
Lipase Cherry Crandall (30° C)	0-160 U/L	1.00	0-160 U/L
Lipids (total)	400-850 mg/dl	0.01	4.0-8.5 g/L
Magnesium	1.8-3.0 mg/dl	0.4114	0.80-1.20 mmol/L
Mercury	≤ 1.0 μg/dl	49.85	≤ 50 nmol/L
Osmolality	280-300 mOsm/kg	1.00	280-300 mmol/kg
Phosphorus	2.5-5.0 mg/dl	0.3229	0.80-1.6 mmol/L
Potassium	3.5-5.0 mEq/L	1.0	3.5-5.0 mmol/L
Protein (total)	5-8 g/dl	10.0	50-80 g/L
Sodium	135-147 mEq/L	1.00	135-147 mmol/L
Testosterone	4.0-8.0 mg/ml	3.467	14.0-28.0 nmol/L
Thyroxine	1-4 μg/dl	12.87	13-51 nmol/L
Triglyceride	10-500 mg/dl	0.0113	0.11-5.65 mmol/L
Urea nitrogen	10-20 mg/dl	0.3570	3.6-7.1 nmol/L
Uric acid	3.6-7.7 mg/dl	59.44	214-458 μmol/L
Urobilinogen	0-4.0 mg/dl	16.9	0.0-6.8 μmol/L
Vitamin A	90 μg/dl	0.03491	3.1 μmol/L
Vitamin B$_{12}$	300-700 ng/L	0.738	221-516 pmol/L
Vitamin E	5.0-20.0 mg/L	2.32	11.6-46.4 μmol/L
D-xylose	30-40 mg/dl	0.06666	2.0-2.71 mmol/L
Zinc	75-120 μg/dl	0.1530	11.5-18.5 μmol/L

From Appendices. In: Bonagura JD, ed. Current veterinary therapy XII. Philadelphia: WB Saunders, 1995:1401 (with permission).

APPENDIX II

ENDOCRINE TESTING

Table II-A.

Endocrine Function Testing Protocols

ADRENAL GLAND DISORDERS

ACTH STIMULATION TEST

Dogs

Administer 20 IU ACTH gel IM or 0.25 mg synthetic ACTH IV or IM (Cortrosyn, Organon Pharmaceuticals, West Orange, NJ).
ACTH Gel
Serum samples should be obtained before and 2 hours after injection of ACTH for cortisol assay.
Synthetic ACTH
Serum samples should be obtained before and 1 hour after injection of ACTH for cortisol assay.

Cats

Administer 0.125 mg synthetic ACTH IV. Serum samples should be obtained before and 1 hour after injection of ACTH for cortisol assay.

Interpretation

Screening for Cushing's Disease
An exaggerated response to ACTH is consistent with Cushing's disease. High normal cut-off values differ slightly between laboratories.
Screening for Hypoadrenocorticism
Pre- and post-cortisol determinations < 1 µg/dl (30 nmol/L) is consistent with hypoadrenocorticism.
Monitoring Mitotane or Ketoconazole Therapy for Cushing's Disease
Pre- and post-cortisol determinations should be within the normal basal cortisol range.

LOW-DOSE DEXAMETHASONE SUPPRESSION TEST (LDDST)

Dogs

Administer 0.015 mg/kg dexamethasone (Azium) IV or IM. Obtain serum samples before and 4 and 8 hours after injection of dexamethasone for cortisol assay.

Cats

Administer 0.1 mg/kg dexamethasone (Azium) IV or IM. Obtain serum sample before and 4 and 8 hours after injection of dexamethasone for cortisol assay.

Interpretation

Three Basic Patterns
Lack of Suppression
All cortisol values remain above 1 µg/dl (30 nmol/L). This pattern is consistent with Cushing's disease.
Suppression
Cortisol values fall below 1 µg/dl (30 nmol/L) at 4 and 8 hours. This pattern suggests that the animal does not have Cushing's disease.
Escape from Suppression
Cortisol value falls below 1 µg/dl (30 nmol/L) at 4 hours and rises above 1 µg/dl at 8 hours. This pattern is consistent with pituitary-dependent Cushing's disease.

HIGH-DOSE DEXAMETHASONE SUPPRESSION TEST (HDDST)

Administer 1 mg/kg dexamethasone (Azium) IV or IM. Obtain serum samples before and 4 and 8 hours after injection of dexamethasone for cortisol assay.

Interpretation

Any cortisol determination that falls below 1.5 µg/dl (45 nmol/L) at any point during the 8-hour testing period is considered suppression. Suppression after a high dose of dexamethasone is consistent with pituitary-dependent Cushing's disease. Lack of suppression (all cortisol values remain above 1.5 µg/dl) is diagnostic of a pituitary or adrenal tumor.

THYROID GLAND DISORDERS

TSH STIMULATION TEST

Administer 0.5 U/kg TSH (maximum dose 5 U) IV. Obtain serum samples before and 6 hours after injection of TSH for T_4 determination.

Interpretation

Post-TSH T_4 levels < 3 µg/dl (35 nmol/L) is consistent with hypothyroidism.

TRH STIMULATION TEST

Administer 0.1 mg/kg TRH IV. Obtain serum samples before and 4 hours after TRH injection for T_4 determination.

Interpretation

An increase in T_4 concentration < 50% after TRH administration is consistent with hypothyroidism.

T_3 SUPPRESSION TEST

Obtain a blood sample for determination of T_4 and T_3. The serum is removed and kept refrigerated or frozen. Administer T_3 (Cytomel, Smith, Kline, and French Laboratories) PO at a dosage of 25 µg/cat q8h for 2 days. On the morning of the third day, administer 25 µg of T_3, and 2-4 hours later obtain a second blood sample for T_3 and T_4 determinations. The basal (day 1) and postoral T_3 serum samples should be submitted to the laboratory together to avoid interassay variation.

Interpretation

Serum T_4 concentration after administration of T_3 > than 1.5 µg/dl (20 nmol/L) is consistent with hyperthyroidism.

GASTRINOMA

SECRETIN STIMULATION TEST

Administer 2 units of secretin/kg IV. Take blood samples before administration of secretin and then 2, 5, 10, 15, and 30 minutes later. Assay the samples for gastrin.

Interpretation

Dogs with gastrinomas have a rise in gastrin levels after the injection of secretin. In three reported cases, two dogs had a rise in gastrin levels 2 times baseline 5 minutes after secretin injection, and one dog had a rise in gastrin levels 1.4 times baseline 5 minutes after secretin injection. Normal dogs have a decline in gastrin levels after administration of secretin.

CALCIUM CHALLENGE TEST

Administer 2 mg/kg of calcium gluconate IV over a 1-minute period or administer 5 mg/kg of calcium gluconate as an IV infusion over several hours.

Obtain a blood sample before calcium administration and then 15, 30, 60, 90, and 120 minutes after the calcium administration. Assay the samples for gastrin.

Interpretation

Two reported patients with gastrinoma had a doubling of the gastrin level 60 minutes after the calcium infusion.

SEX HORMONE DISORDERS

GN-RH STIMULATION TEST

Administer 0.5-1.0 µg of Gn-RH/kg IM. Obtain blood samples before Gn-RH administration and 1 hour later. Assay blood samples for testosterone.

Interpretation

Normal dogs have baseline testosterone levels between 0.5-5 ng/ml, and after administration of Gn-RH the testosterone levels rise above 5 ng/ml. Animals with hypoandrogenism have lower values.

HCG STIMULATION TEST

Administer 44 IU of hCG/kg IM. Obtain blood samples before hCG administration and 4 hours later. Assay blood samples for testosterone.

Interpretation

Normal dogs have baseline testosterone levels between 0.5-5 ng/ml, and after administration of hCG the testosterone levels rise above 5 ng/ml. Animals with hypoandrogenism have lower values.

DIABETES INSIPIDUS

MODIFIED WATER DEPRIVATION TEST

Rule out other causes of polyuria and polydipsia (especially hyperadrenocorticism). Begin water restriction 3 days before abrupt water deprivation.

Day 1	130-165 ml/kg/day
Day 2	100-125 ml/kg/day
Day 3	65-70 ml/kg/day (normal maintenance requirement)

The morning of the fourth day, discontinue food and water. Start the test. Weigh the patient and empty the bladder. Weigh at 1-2 hour intervals. Monitor carefully for dehydration and depression. When 5% of body weight is lost or azotemia develops, empty the bladder and check urine specific gravity. Consider plasma vasopressin determination at this point.

Interpretation

If the urine specific gravity is > 1.025 (dogs) or > 1.030 (cats), stop the test. The patient does not have diabetes insipidus. If the urine specific gravity is not > 1.025 (dogs) or > 1.030 (cats), administer 0.55 U/kg aqueous vasopressin IM (maximum dose 5 U). Empty the bladder and check urine specific gravity at 30, 60, and 120 minutes postadministration. If urine specific gravity increases < 10%, nephrogenic diabetes insipidus is indicated; if it increases 10-50%, partial central diabetes insipidus is indicated; if it increases 50-800%, complete central diabetes insipidus is indicated.

Table II-B.

Tests of the Endocrine System*			
Hormone	Unit	Dogs	Cats
Adrenocorticotrophic hormone, basal (ACTH, plasma)	pmol/L	2-15	1-20
Aldosterone† (plasma)			
Basal	pmol/L	14-957	194-388
Post-ACTH	pmol/L	197-2103	277-721
Cortisol (serum or plasma, urine)			
Basal	nmol/L	25-125	15-150
Post-ACTH	nmol/L	200-550	130-450
Post–low-dose dexamethasone (0.01 or 0.015 mg/kg)	nmol/L	≤ 40	≤ 40
Post–high-dose dexamethasone (0.1 or 1.0 mg/kg)‡	nmol/L	≤ 40	≤ 40
Urinary cortisol-creatinine ratio	$\times 10^{-6}$	8-24†, 10§	—
Insulin, basal (serum)	pmol/L	35-200	35-200
Intact parathormone† (serum)	pmol/L	2-13	0-4
Progesterone (serum or plasma, female)	mmol/L	≤ 3.0 in anestrus, proestrus 50-220 in diestrus, pregnancy	≤ 3.0 in anestrus, proestrus 50-220 in diestrus, pregnancy
Testosterone (serum or plasma, male)	nmol/L	1-20	1-20
Thyroxine (T_4, serum)			
Basal	nmol/L	12-50	10-50
Post–thyroxine-stimulating hormone (TSH)	nmol/L	> 45	> 45
Triiodothyronine (T_3) suppression‖	nmol/L	–	≤ 20
Triiodothyronine, basal (T_3, serum)	nmol/L	0.7-2.3	0.5-2.0

*Prepared with the assistance of ME Peterson, The Animal Medical Center, New York, NY. Unless indicated otherwise, values in this table are adapted from Kemppainen RJ, Zerbe CA. Common endocrine diagnostic tests: normal values and interpretations. In: Kirk RW, ed. Current veterinary therapy X. Philadelphia: WB Saunders, 1989:961-968. Hormone determinations are variable between laboratories. The laboratory performing the analysis should provide reference values. Before submitting samples for hormone determinations, consult the laboratory for sample specifications, use of anticoagulants, and sample preservation. General sampling conditions are discussed in Reimers TJ. Guidelines for collection, storage, and transport of samples for hormone assay. In: Kirk RW, ed. Current veterinary therapy X. Philadelphia: WB Saunders, 1989:968-973. Factors that affect serum thyroid and adrenocortical hormone concentrations in dogs are discussed in Reimers TJ, Lawler DF, Sutaria PM, Correa MT, Erb HN. Effects of age, sex, and body size on serum concentrations of thyroid and adrenocortical hormones in dogs. Am J Vet Res 1990;51:454.

†Provided by RF Nachreiner, Animal Health Diagnostic Laboratory, Endocrine Diagnostic Section, Michigan State University.

‡This test is used after adrenocortical hyperfunction has been confirmed. It is used to differentiate adrenal tumor (where no suppression is seen) from pituitary-dependent cases (where suppression occurs but is variable).

§From Stolp R, Rijnberk A, Meiher JC, Croughs RJM. Urinary corticoids in the diagnosis of canine hyperadrenocorticism. Res Vet Sci 1983;34:141. Rijnberk A, van Wees A, Mol JA. Assessment of two tests for the diagnosis of canine hyperadrenocorticism. Vet Rec 1988;122:178-180.

‖From Peterson ME, Ferguson DC. Thyroid diseases. In: Ettinger SJ, ed. Textbook of veterinary internal medicine. Diseases of the dog and cat. 3rd ed. Philadelphia: WB Saunders, 1989:1632-1675.

From appendices In Bonagura J, ed. Kirk's current veterinary therapy XII. Philadelphia: WB Saunders, 1995;1410 (with permission).

Table II-C.

Conversion Table for Hormone Assay Units

Hormone	Unit		Conversion factors	
	Traditional	SI	Traditional to SI	SI to Traditional
Aldosterone	ng/dl	pmol/L	27.7	0.036
Corticotrophin (ACTH)	pg/ml	pmol/L	0.22	4.51
Cortisol	µg/dl	mmol/L	27.59	0.36
β-endorphin	pg/ml	pmol/L	0.289	3.43
Epinephrine	pg/ml	pmol/L	5.46	0.183
Estrogen (estradiol)	pg/ml	pmol/L	3.67	0.273
Gastrin	pg/ml	ng/L	1.00	1.00
Glucagon	pg/ml	ng/L	1.00	1.00
Growth hormone (GH)	ng/ml	µg/L	1.00	1.00
Insulin	µU/ml	pmol/L	7.18	0.139
α-melanocyte–stimulating hormone (α-MSH)	pg/ml	pmol/L	0.601	1.66
Norepinephrine	pg/ml	nmol/L	0.006	169
Pancreatic polypeptide (PP)	mg/dl	mmol/L	0.239	4.18
Progesterone	ng/ml	mmol/L	3.18	0.315
Prolactin	ng/ml	µg/L	1.00	1.00
Renin	ng/ml//hr	ng/L/s	0.278	3.60
Somatostatin	pg/ml	pmol/L	0.611	1.64
Testosterone	ng/ml	nmol/L	3.47	0.288
Thyroxine (T_4)	µg/dl	nmol/L	12.87	0.078
Triiodothyronine (T_3)	ng/dl	nmol/L	0.0154	64.9
Vasoactive intestinal polypeptide (VIP)	pg/ml	pmol/L	0.301	3.33

Contributed by ME Peterson, The Animal Medical Center, New York, NY.
From Appendices. In: Bonagura JD, ed. Current veterinary therapy XII. Philadelphia: WB Saunders, 1995:1411 (with permission).

APPENDIX III

APPROXIMATE NORMAL RANGES FOR COMMON MEASUREMENTS IN DOGS AND CATS

	Dog	Cat
Heart rate (bpm)	60-180	140-220
Capillary refill time	< 2 sec	< 2 sec
Body temperature	99.5-102.5° F	100.5-102.5° F
	37.5-39.2° C	38.1-39.2° C
Mean arterial pressure (mm Hg)	90-120	100-150
Blood volume (ml/kg)	75-90	47-66
Cardiac output		
(ml/kg/min)	100-200	167±39
(L/M²/min)	4.72 ± 1.09	
Systemic resistance		
(mm Hg/ml/kg/min)	0.64 ± 0.16	
(dynes/sec/cm)	2162 ± 458	
Mean pulmonary arterial pressure (mm Hg)	14 ± 3	
Central venous pressure (cm H_2O)	3 ± 4	
Pulmonary artery occlusion pressure (mm Hg)	5 ± 2	
Urine output	1-2 ml/kg/hr	1-2 ml/kg/hr
Breathing rate (breaths/min)	10-30	24-42
Minute ventilation (ml/kg/min)	170-350	200-350
Oxygen delivery		
(ml/kg/min)	29 ± 8	
(ml/M²/min)	815 ± 234	
Oxygen consumption		
(ml/kg/min)	4-11	3-8
(ml/M²/min)	198 ± 53	
Arterial Po_2 (mm Hg)	85-105	100-115
Arterial So_2	> 95	> 95
Arterial Pco_2 (mm Hg)	30-44	28-35
Arterial pH	7.36-7.46	7.34-7.43
Bicarbonate (mEq/L)	20-25	17-21
Base deficit (mEq/L)	0 to −4	−1 to −8
Total plasma proteins (g/dl)	6.0-8.0	6.8-8.3
Albumin (g/dl)	2.5-3.5	1.9-3.9
Packed cell volume (%)	37-55	29-48
Hemoglobin (g/dl)	12-18	9-15.1
Sodium (mEq/L)	145-154	151-158
Potassium (mEq/L)	4.1-5.3	3.6-4.9
Chloride (mEq/L)	105-116	113-121
Total CO_2 (mEq/L)	16-26	15-21

Modified from Aldrich J, Haskins SC. Monitoring the critically ill patient. In: Current veterinary therapy XII. Philadelphia: WB Saunders, 1995;98-105 (with permission).

APPENDIX IV

CLINICAL TOXICOSIS—SYSTEMS AFFECTED AND CLINICAL EFFECTS

Neurological Toxicants

Excitation or simulation of nervous system
  Amphetamine
  Aminopyridine
  Caffeine
  Cyanide
  Ergot (Claviceps spp.)
  Fluoroacetate
  Lead
  Metaldehyde
  Moonseed (Menispermum canadense)
  Mycotoxins
  Nicotine
  Organochlorine insecticides
  Organophosphate insecticides
  Phenols and chlorophenols
  Strychnine
  Theobromine
  Theophylline
  Water hemlock (Cicuta spp.)
Depression, coma
  Alcohols
  Antihistamines
  Barbiturates
  Carbon monoxide
  Hydrocarbons, aliphatic
  Hydrocarbons, aromatic
  Hydrocarbons, halogenated
  Lead
  Mercury
  Morphine derivatives
  Salicylates
  Snake venoms
Loss of motor control
  Botulinum
  Buckeye (Aesculus spp.)
  Carbon disulfide
  Curare
  Ergot
  Ethylene glycol
  Hexachlorophene
  Lead
  Nicotine
  Organophosphates
  Triaryl phosphates
Autonomic stimulation
  Atropine
  Carbamate insecticides
  Fly mushroom (Amanita muscaria)
  Organophosphate insecticides
Behavioral changes
  Belladonna alkaloids
  Ergot
  Lead
  Lysergic acid diethylamide (LSD)
  Marijuana
  Morning glory
  Nutmeg
  Opium derivatives
  Organochlorine insecticides
  Periwinkle
  Peyote

Gastrointestinal Toxicants

Stomatitis, pharyngitis
  Acids and alkalies
  Aldehydes
  Chromium salts
  Fertilizer
  Mercuric salts
  Detergents
  Petroleum distillates
  Phenol
Salivation
  Amanita muscaria
  Ammonia
  Cresol
  Metaldehyde
  Nicotine
  Organophosphates
  Thallium
Dry mouth
  Amphetamine
  Antihistamine
  Atropine
  Belladonna
  Opiates
Gastroenteritis
  Amanita spp.
  Antimony
  Arsenic
  Barium
  Bismuth
  Cantharidin
  Copper salts
  Croton oil
  Detergents, soaps, sanitizers
  Digitalis toxins
  Iron
  Lead
  Mercury
  Mushrooms
  Phenoxy herbicides
  Phosphorus
  Plants (see Appendix VI)
  Staphylococcus toxin
  Thallium
  Zinc phosphide

Hepatotoxins

Acetaminophen
Aflatoxin
Amanita phalloides
Blue-green algae
Coal tar derivatives
Copper
Halogenated hydrocarbons
Iron
Petroleum distillates
Phosphorus

Nephrotoxins

Inadvertent nephrotoxins
  Aldehydes
  Amanita mushrooms

Arsenic
Bismuth
Cadmium
Cresols
Dichromate
Ethylene glycol
Halogenated hydrocarbons
Mercury
Ochratoxin
Oxalates
Petroleum distillates
Phenols
Thallium
Turpentine
Volatile oils (e.g., penny-royal oil or oil of juniper)
Nephrotoxic drugs
  Acetaminophen
  Amphotericin B
  Bacitracin
  Gentamicin
  Kanamycin
  Neomycin
  Polymyxin B
  Sulfonamides
  Vancomycin

Blood Toxicants

Methemoglobin
  Acetaminophen
  Aniline derivatives
  Chlorate
  Copper
  Methylene blue
  Nitrite
  Nitrobenzene
Hemolysis
  Acetaminophen*
  Aniline
  Arsine
  Chlorates
  Copper
  Methylene blue*
  Nitrobenzene
  Onions
  Snake venoms
  Turpentine
  Red maple leaves
Aplastic anemia, leukopenia, thrombocytopenia
  Arsenicals
  Aspirin
  Benzene
  Chloramphenicol
  Cytostatic agents
  Estrogens
  Phenylbutazone
  Toluene
  Trichlorethylene
Coagulopathy
  Aflatoxin
  Aspirin
  Coumarin rodenticides

*Especially in cats

Phosphorus
Sulfonamides

Cardiovascular Toxicants

Tachycardia and arrhythmias
  Adrenalin
  Aminophylline
  Amphetamine
  Aminoglycoside antibiotics
  Atropine
  Caffeine
  Cyanide
  Dinitrophenol
  Fluorocarbons
  Nicotine
  Thallium
Bradycardia
  Barium
  Cardiac glycosides
  Digitalis
  Morphine
  Opiates
  Oleander
  Red squill
Myocardial damage
  Amanita phalloides
  Barium
  Carbon monoxide
  Oleander
  Phosphorus
  Thallium
Vascular necrosis
  Ergot
  Lead
  Mercury
  Selenium

Respiratory Toxicants

Air pollutants (nitrogen dioxide, sulfur dioxide)
Allergens
Ammonia
ANTU rodenticide
Chlorine
Gasoline, kerosene
Organophosphate insecticides
Ozone
Paraquat herbicide
Thallium

Ocular Toxicants

Mydriasis
  Amanita mushrooms
  Atropine
  Belladonna
  Methanol
Miosis
  Heroin
  Morphine
  Nicotine
  Organophosphates
Optic neuropathy
  Arsenicals
  Lead
  Mercury
  Methanol
  Thallium
  Vitamin A

General Signs

Fever
  Atropine
  Carbon monoxide
  Dinitrophenol
  Lead
  Metaldehyde
  Organochlorine insecticides
Hypothermia
  Alcohol
  Arsenic
  Barbiturates
  Heroin
  Morphine
  Oxalates
  Phenols
Cyanosis
  Carbon dioxide
  Hydrogen sulfide
  Nitrite
  Paraquat
Pink skin color
  Arsenic
  Carbon monoxide
  Cyanide
  Mercury
  Thallium

From Osweiler G. A brief guide to clinical toxicosis in small animals. In: Kirk RW, ed. Current veterinary therapy IX. Philadelphia: WB Saunders, 1986:132-135 (with permission).

APPENDIX V

TOXIC AGENTS AND THEIR SYSTEMIC ANTIDOTES—DOSAGE AND METHOD OF TREATMENT

Toxic agent	Systemic antidote	Dosage and method of treatment
Acetaminophen	N-acetylcysteine (Mucomyst, Mead Johnson)	150 mg/kg loading dose PO or IV, then 50 mg/kg q4h for 17-20 additional doses
Amphetamines	Chlorpromazine	1 mg/kg IM or IV; administer only half dosage if barbiturates have been given; blocks excitation
Arsenic, mercury, and other heavy metals except cadmium, lead, silver, selenium, and thallium	Dimercaprol (BAL, Hynson, Wescott & Dunning)	10% solution in oil; give small animals 2.5-5.0 mg/kg IM q6h for 2 days then q12h for the next 10 days or until recovery. (Note: With severe acute poisoning, 5 mg/kg should be given only on the first day.)
	D-penicillamine (Cuprimine, Merck)	Developed for chronic mercury poisoning, now seems most promising drug; no reports on dosage in animals; give 3-4 mg/kg q6h
Atropine, belladonna alkaloids	Physostigmine salicylate	0.1-0.6 mg/kg (do not use neostigmine)
Barbiturates	Doxapram	2% solution; give small animals 3-5 mg/kg IV only (0.14-0.25 ml/kg); repeat as necessary. (Note: The above is reliable only when depression is mild; in animals with deeper levels of depression, ventilatory support [and oxygen] is preferable.)
Bromides	Chlorides (sodium or ammonium salts)	0.5-1.0 g PO daily for several days; hasten excretion
Carbon monoxide	Oxygen	Pure oxygen at normal or high pressure; artificial respiration; blood transfusion
Cholecalciferol	Calcitonin (Calcimar, Rorer Pharm)	4 IU/kg SC or IM q8h-q12h
Cholinergic agents	Atropine sulfate	0.02-0.04 mg/kg, as needed
Cholinesterase inhibitors	Atropine sulfate	0.2 mg/kg, repeated as needed for atropinization; treat cyanosis (if present) first; blocks only muscarinic effects; atropine in oil may be injected for prolonged effect. Avoid atropine intoxication!
Cholinergic agents and cholinesterase inhibitors (organophosphates, some carbamates; but not carbaryl, dimethan, or carbam piloxime)	Pralidoxime chloride (2-PAM)	5% solution; 20-50 mg/kg IM or by slow IV (0.2-1.0 mg/kg) injection (maximum dose is 500 mg per minute), repeat as needed; 2-PAM alleviates nicotinic effect and regenerates cholinesterase; morphine, succinylcholine, and phenothiazine tranquilizers are contraindicated
Copper	D-penicillamine (Cuprimine)	See arsenic
Coumarin-derivative anticoagulants	Vitamin K$_1$ (AquaMEPHYTON, 5-mg capsules or 1% emulsion, Merck; Vita K1, 25-mg capsules, Eschar)	Give 3-5 mg/kg SC or PO per day with canned food; treat 7 days for warfarin-type, treat 21-30 days for second-generation anticoagulant rodenticides; oral therapy more effacious than parenteral
	Fresh whole blood, fresh plasma, or fresh frozen plasma	Blood transfusion, 10-25 ml/kg, as required
Curare	Neostigmine methylsulfate	Solution: 1:5000 or 1:2000 (1 ml = 0.2 or 0.5 mg/ml); dosage is 0.005 mg/5 kg SC; follow with IV injection of atropine (0.04 mg/kg)
	Edrophonium chloride (Tensilon, Roche)	1% solution; give 0.05-1.0 mg/kg IV
	Ventilatory support	
Cyanide	Methemoglobin (sodium nitrite is used to form methemoglobin)	1% solution of sodium nitrite; dosage is 16 mg/kg IV (1.6 ml/kg)
	Sodium thiosulfate	Follow with 20% solution of sodium thiosulfate at dosage of 30-40 mg/kg (0.15-0.2 ml/kg) IV; if treatment is repeated, use only sodium thiosulfate. (Note: both of the above may be given simultaneously as follows: 0.5 ml/kg of combination consisting of 10 g sodium nitrite, 15 g sodium thiosulfate distilled water q.s. to 250 ml; dosage may be repeated once; if further treatment is required, give only 20% solution thiosulfate at 0.2 ml/kg.)
Digitalis glycosides, oleander, and Bufo toads	Potassium chloride	Dogs: 0.5-2.0 g PO in divided doses or, in serious cases, as diluted solution given IV by slow drip (ECG monitoring is essential)
	Diphenylhydantoin	25 mg per minute IV, until ventricular arrhythmias are controlled
	Propranolol (β-blocker)	0.5-1.0 mg/kg IV or IM as needed to control cardiac arrhythmias (ECG monitoring is essential)
	Atropine sulfate	0.02-0.04 mg/kg as needed for cholinergic and arrhythmia control
Fluoride	Calcium borogluconate	3-10 ml of 5-10% solution
Fluoroacetate (Compound 1080)	Glyceryl monoacetin (Sigma)	0.1-0.5 mg/kg IM hourly for several hours (total 2-4 mg/kg), or diluted (0.5-1.0% solution IV; danger of hemolysis); monoacetin is available only from chemical supply houses
	Acetamide	Animal may be protected if acetamide is given before or simultaneously with Compound 1080 (experimental)
	Pentobarbital	May protect against lethal dose (experimental). (Note: all treatments are generally unrewarding.)
Hallucinogens (LSD, phencyclidine hydrochloride [PCP])	Diazepam (Valium, Roche)	As needed—avoid respiratory depression (2-5 mg/kg)
Heparin	Protamine sulfate	1% solution; give 1.0-1.5 mg by slow IV injection to antagonize each 1 mg of heparin; reduce dose as time increases between heparin injection and start of treatment (after 30 minutes give only 0.5 mg)
Iron salts	Deferoxamine mesylate (Desferal, Ciba)	Dosage for animals not yet established; dosage for humans is 5 g of 5% solution PO, then 20 mg/kg IM q4h-q6h; in case of shock, dosage is 40 mg/kg by IV drip over 4-hour period; may be repeated in 6 hours, then 15 mg/kg by drip q8h

Toxic Agents and Their Systemic Antidotes—Dosage and Method of Treatment (cont'd)

Lead	Calcium disodium edetate (CaEDTA)	Maximum safe dosage is 75 mg/kg per 24 hours (only for severe case); EDTA is available in 20% solution; for IV drip, dilute in 5% glucose to 0.5%; for IM, add procaine to 20% solution to give 0.5% concentration of procaine
	EDTA and BAL	BAL is given as 10% solution in oil (a) In severe cases (CNS involvement with > 100 μg lead per 100 g whole blood), give 4 mg/kg BAL only as initial dose; follow after 4 hours, and q4h for 3-4 days, with BAL and EDTA (12.5 mg/kg) at separate IM sites; skip 2 or 3 days and then treat again for 3-4 days; (b) In subacute cases with < 100 μg lead per 100 g whole blood, give only 50 mg EDTA/kg per 24 hours for 3-5 days;
	Penicillamine (Cuprimine, Merck)	(c) May use after either treatment (a) or (b) with 100 mg/kg per day PO for 1-4 weeks
	Thiamine hydrochloride	Experimental to treat CNS signs; 5 mg/kg IV q12h for 1-2 weeks; give slowly and watch for untoward reactions
Metaldehyde	Diazepam (Valium, Roche)	2-5 mg/kg IV to control tremors
	Triflupromaize	0.2-2.0 mg/kg IV
	Pentobarbital	To effect
Methanol	Ethanol	Give 1.1 g/kg (4.4 ml/kg) of 25% solution IV; then give 0.5 g/kg (2.0 ml/kg) q4h for 4 days; to prevent or correct acidosis, use sodium bicarbonate 0.4 g/kg IV; activated charcoal, 5 g/kg PO if within 4 hours of ingestion
Methemoglobinemia-producing agents (nitrites, chlorates)	Methylene blue (not recommended for cats)	1% solution (maximum concentration); give by slow IV injection, 8.8 mg/kg (0.9 ml/kg), and repeat if necessary; to prevent fall in blood pressure in cases of nitrite poisoning, use a sympathomimetic drug (ephedrine or epinephrine)
Morphine and related drugs	Naloxone hydrochloride (Narcan, Endo)	0.1 mg/kg IV; do not repeat if respiration is not satisfactory
	Levallorphan tartrate (Lorfan, Roche)	Give IV 0.1-0.5 ml of solution containing 1 mg/ml. (Note: use either of the antidotes only in acute poisoning. Ventilatory support may be indicated. Activated charcoal is also indicated.)
Oxalates	Calcium	10% solution of calcium gluconate IV; give 3-20 ml (to control hypocalcemia)
Phenothiazine	Methamphetamine hydrochloride (Desoxyn, Abbot)	0.1-0.2 mg/kg; treatment for hypovolemic shock may be required.
	Diphenhydramine hydrochloride	For CNS depression, 2-5 mg/kg IV to treat extrapyramidal signs
Phytotoxins and botulin	Antitoxins not available commercially (attempt to obtain through Centers for Disease Control)	As indicated for specific antitoxins; examples of phytotoxins: ricin, abrin, robin, crotin
Plants		Treat signs as necessary (see appendix VI)
Red squill	Atropine sulfate, propranolol, potassium chloride	As for digitalis and oleander
Snake bite		
Rattlesnake Copperhead Water moccasin	Antivenin (Wyeth), Trivalent Crotalidae (Fort Dodge)	Caution: equine origin; administer 1-2 vials IV, slowly, diluted in 250-500 ml of saline or lactated Ringer's solution; also administer antihistamines; corticosteroids are contraindicated
Coral snake	(Wyeth)	Caution: equine origin; may be used as with pit viper antivenin
Spider bite		
Black widow	Antivenin (Merck)	Caution: equine origin; administer IV undiluted
	Dantrolene sodium (Dantrium, Norwich-Eaton)	For neurologic signs, 1 mg/kg IV, followed by 1 mg/kg PO q4h
Brown recluse	Dapsone	1 mg/kg q12h for 10 days
Strontium	Calcium salts	Usual dose of calcium borogluconate
	Ammonium chloride	0.2-0.5 g PO 3-4 times daily
Strychnine and brucine	Pentobarbital	Give IV, to effect; higher dose is usually required than that required for anesthesia; place animal in warm, quiet room
	Amobarbital	Give slowly IV, to effect; duration of sedation is usually 4-6 hours
	Methocarbamol (Robaxin, Robins)	10% solution; average first dosage is 149 mg/kg IV (range, 40-300 mg); repeat half dosage as needed
	Glyceryl guaiacolate (Geocolate, Summit Hill Labs)	110 mg/kg IV, 5% solution; repeat as necessary
	Diazepam (Valium, Roche)	2-5 mg/kg; controls convulsions
Thallium	Diphenylthiocarbazone	Dogs: 70 mg/kg PO q8h for 6 days; hastens elimination but is partially toxic
	Prussian blue	0.2 mg/kg PO in 3 divided doses daily
	Potassium chloride	Give simultaneously with thiocarbazone or Prussian blue, 2-6 g PO daily in divided doses

IM = intramuscularly; IV = intravenously; PO = orally; SC = subcutaneously; q = every; h = hour; q.s. = sufficient quantity; ECG = electrocardiogram; CNS = central nervous system.

From Bailey EM Jr, Garland T. Toxicologic emergencies. In: Murtaugh RJ, Kaplan PM, eds. Veterinary emergency and critical care medicine. St. Louis: Mosby, 1992:443-446.

APPENDIX VI

TOXIC PLANTS AND THEIR CLINICAL SIGNS—ANTIDOTES AND TREATMENT

Plant and characteristics	Clinical signs	Antidotes and treatment
Angel's trumpet (Datura spp.) Garden annual with white trumpet-shaped flowers Whole plant toxic; highest in seeds	Thirst, GI atony, disturbed vision, delirium, hallucinations	Parasympathomimetic drugs
Autumn crocus (Colchicum autumnale) Houseplant Whole plant toxic; highest in bulbs	Burning sensation in throat and mouth, thirst, nausea, diarrhea	Fluids; analgesics and atropine to alleviate colic and diarrhea
Azalea (Rhododendron spp.) Garden, landscape plant Leaves and flowers are toxic Honey made from flower nectar is toxic	Burning sensation in mouth, salivation, emesis, diarrhea, muscular weakness, dimness of vision, bradycardia, arrhythmia, hypotension EMERGENCY CONDITION	Do not use emetics. Use activated charcoal. Fluid replacement and respiratory support are required. Treat heart block with isoproterenol.
Belladonna lily (Amaryllis spp.) Garden, potted plant Bulbs are most toxic	Nausea, diarrhea, hypotension, depression, liver damage	Gastric lavage, charcoal, fluids, and supportive treatment
Bittersweet (Celastrus spp.) Weed, vine with red berries Immature fruits are toxic	Gastric irritation, fever, diarrhea	Fluids
Bleeding heart (Dicentra spp.) Garden, woods, potted plant Toxicity of roots > leaves	Vomiting, diarrhea, convulsions or paralysis	Fluids and seizure control
Castor bean (Ricinus communis) Garden annual, grows to 2 m Seeds are 1 cm, dark and light mottled, and highly toxic	Latent period; colic, emesis, diarrhea, thirst	Emesis, charcoal, fluids, and electrolytes
Chinaberry tree (Melia azedarach) Ornamental tree in temperate to subtropical areas Fruit and bark are most toxic	Faintness, ataxia, mental confusion, intense gastritis, emesis, diarrhea	Fluid and electrolyte replacement
Christmas rose (Helleborus niger) Houseplant Entire plant is toxic	Pain in mouth and abdomen, nausea, emesis, colic, diarrhea, arrhythmia, hypotension	Gastric lavage or emesis; activated charcoal or saline cathartics to decontaminate the GI tract
Daphne (Daphne mezereum) Landscape shrub Entire plant is toxic	Vesication and edema of the lips and oral cavity, salivation, thirst, abdominal pain, emesis, hemorrhagic diarrhea	Fluid and electrolyte replacement
Delphinium or larkspur (Delphinium spp.) Outdoor garden, mountains; tall with blue flowers Toxicity of seeds > leaves	Trembling, ataxia, weakness, salivation	GI detoxication; physostigmine to treat muscarinic signs
English holly (Ilex spp.) Landscape plant Fruit is toxic	Nausea, vomiting, diarrhea	Fluid and electrolyte replacement
English ivy (Hedera helix) Houseplant Fruit and leaves	Salivation, thirst, emesis, gastroenteritis, diarrhea, dermatitis	Corticosteroids to treat dermal response; treat other signs symptomatically
Foxglove (Digitalis purpurea) Outdoor gardens Entire plant (especially leaves)	Nausea, emesis, abdominal pain, diarrhea, bradycardia, arrhythmia with prolonged P-R interval and hyperkalemia	GI decontamination with activated charcoal or saline cathartics. Treat hyperkalemia and give lidocaine for ventricular arrhythmia.
Golden chain (Laburnum anagyroides) Landscape tree with long chains of yellow flowers Entire plant is toxic	Emesis, depression, weakness, incoordination, mydriasis, tachycardia	GI decontamination with lavage or emesis followed by activated charcoal
Horse chestnut or buckeye (Aesculus spp.) Landscape or forest tree; palmate leaves Nuts and twigs most toxic	Gastroenteritis, diarrhea, dehydration, electrolyte imbalance	Fluid and electrolyte replacement, demulcents, and therapy for gastroenteritis
Iris or flag (Iris spp.) Perennial garden flower Rootstock most toxic	Colic, nausea, vomiting, diarrhea	Fluid and electrolyte replacement

Toxic Plants and Their Clinical Signs—Antidotes and Treatment (continued)

Plant and characteristics	Clinical signs	Antidotes and treatment
Irish potato (Solanum tuberosum) Vegetable garden Vines, green skin, and sprouts are toxic	Colic, diarrhea, salivation, ataxia, weakness, bradycardia, hypotension. Signs may vary from atropine-like to cholinsterase inhibition. Use antitdotes accordingly and with caution.	GI decontamination. If atropine-like signs predominate, use physostigmine. If salivation and diarrhea are present, use atropine cautiously.
Jack-in-the-pulpit (Arisaema triphyllum) Woods and gardens of temperate zones Entire plant is toxic	Glossitis, pharyngitis, oral inflammation, edema, salivation	Irrigate mouth with water. Cool liquids or demulcents held in mouth may relieve signs.
Lantana (Lantana camara) Garden and wild in mild temperate to tropical areas; bright orange and yellow flowers Foliage and immature berries are toxic	Weakness, lethargy, vomiting, diarrhea, mydriasis, bradypnea. Advanced signs are cholestasis, bilirubinemia, and photosensitization.	GI decontamination, fluids, and respiratory support. Protect from sunlight and treat for hepatic insufficiency.
Lily, including Easter lily, tiger lily (Lilium spp.); daylily (Hemerocallis spp.)	Depression, oliguria, renal failure in cats as a result of toxic tubular necrosis	Prompt GI decontamination and supportive therapy for renal failure. Toxin presently is unknown.
Lily of the valley (Convallaria majalis) Garden ornamental Toxicity of seeds and flowers > leaves	Colic, vomiting, diarrhea, bradycardia, arrhythmia	Decontaminate GI tract with lavage and charcoal. Avoid emetics. Lidocaine to treat ventricular arrhythmias; treat as for other digitalis glycoside overdose, including correction of hyperkalemia.
Lupine (Lupinus spp.) Garden ornamental Toxicity of seeds > leaves	Salivation, ataxia, seizures, dyspnea	GI decontamination, control seizures
Mistletoe (Phoradendron spp.) Parasitic shrub on other trees Access to pets in homes at holiday time Leaves, stems, and berries are moderately toxic	Emesis, colic, diarrhea, mydriasis, hypovolemia	Fluid and electrolyte replacement; demulcents for gastroenteritis
Monkshood (Aconitum spp.) Perennial garden ornamental Entire plant is toxic	Glossitis, pharyngitis, salivation, nausea, emesis, impaired vision, bradycardia	GI decontamination, fluid and electrolyte replacement. Manage similar to digitalis glycoside overdose, with caution about potassium administration.
Moonseed (Menispermum canadense) Woody vine of forests Fruit is most toxic	Convulsions	Maintain airway and support respiration as needed. Control seizures with least medication possible (e.g., diazepam).
Morning glory (Ipomoea purpurea and I. tricolor) Garden annual, potted plant Seeds most toxic Occasionally used as hallucinogen	Nausea, mydriasis, hallucinations, decreased reflexes, diarrhea, hypotension	Activated charcoal, dark quiet surroundings, tranquilize with diazepam
Mountain laurel (Kalmia spp.) Native of eastern and southeastern woods, mountains Leaves and flowers are toxic Honey from nectar also toxic	Oral irritation, salivation, emesis, diarrhea, weakness, impaired vision, bradycardia, hypotension, AV block	Emetics are contraindicated. Use activated charcoal, fluid replacement, and respiratory support as needed. Isoproterenol to treat AV block as needed.
Narcissus, daffodil, jonquil (Narcissus spp.) Garden ornamental bulb Bulb is most toxic	Nausea, emesis, hypotension, diarrhea	Gastric lavage, charcoal, fluid replacement, supportive treatment for gastroenteritis
Nettle (Urtica diocia) Garden weed Hairs on leaves contain toxin that enters skin on contact	Oral irritation and pain, salivation, swelling and edema of nose and peri-ocular areas or other areas of skin contact	Antihistamines and atropine may control appropriate signs. Local or systemic antiinflammatory supportive therapy to treat affected contact areas.
Oleander (Nerium oleander) Landscape shrub 1-3 m tall Whole plant is extremely toxic	Nausea, early signs of vomiting, colic, diarrhea; bradycardia and arrythmia with hyperkalemia develop soon after EMERGENCY CONDITION	Gastric lavage or induced emesis; activated charcoal or saline cathartics. Treat as for digitalis glycoside overdose, including correction of hyperkalemia. Lidocaine or other appropriate drugs for arrhythmia.
Philodendron (Monstera and Philodendron spp.) Houseplant Leaves are slightly to moderately toxic	Painful irritation, edema of lips, mouth, tongue, and throat; reported nephrotoxic to cats	Cool liquids or demulcents held in mouth may aid relief.
Poinsettia (Euphorbia pulcherrima) Garden or potted plant especially at Christmas holidays Sap of stem and leaves is midly to moderately irritant or toxic	Irritation of mouth; may cause vomiting, diarrhea, and dermatitis	Demulcents and fluids to prevent dehydration
Rhubarb (Rheum rhaponicum) Garden plant Raw or canned Leaves are high in oxalates	Vomiting, diarrhea, and, occasionally, icterus. Renal failure develops from oxalate nephrosis.	Early GI decontamination is important. Demulcents and fluid replacement. Treat possible oxalate nephrosis.

Toxic Plants and Their Clinical Signs—Antidotes and Treatment (continued)

Plant and characteristics	Clinical signs	Antidotes and treatment
Rosary pea or precatory bean (Abrus precatorius) Native of Caribbean islands Seeds (when broken or chewed) are highly toxic Illegal to import into United States	Nausea, vomiting, diarrhea, weakness, tachycardia, possible renal failure, coma, death	Emesis or lavage followed with charcoal, demulcents, fluids, and electrolytes. Vitamin C may improve survival.
Thorn apple or jimsonweed (Datura stramonium) Annual weed, some species are ornamental (D. metel) Entire plant is toxic, but seeds are most toxic and available Relatively common drug abuse plant used as hallucinogen	Thirst, disturbances of vision, delirium, mydriasis, gastrointestinal atony. Signs similar to atropine overdose.	Parasympathomimetic drug (e.g., physotigmine)
Tobacco (Nicotiana tabacum) Garden plant, weed, cigarettes Whole plant is toxic	Rapid onset of salivation, nausea, emesis, tremors, incoordination, and ataxia, followed by collapse and respiratory failure EMERGENCY CONDITION	Assist ventilation and vascular support first to save the animal. After respiration support, decontaminate the GI tract with lavage and activated charcoal.
Wisteria (Wisteria spp.) Woody vine or shrub with blue to white legume flowers Entire plant is toxic	Nausea, abdominal pain, prolonged vomiting	Antiemetics and fluid replacement therapy
Yellow jessamine (Gelsemium sempervirens) Mild temperate to subtropical climates Yellow trumpet-shaped flowers grow on evergreen vines	Abdominal pain, bradypnea, paresis, seizures, hypothermia	Symptomatic and supportive therapy of respiration and cardiovascular function. GI decontamination and fluid replacement therapy.
Yew (Taxus cuspidata and T. baccata) Evergreen landscape shrub with two-ranked flat needle Whole plant (except ripe fruit) is toxic	Acute onset or sudden death. Affected animals show trembling, muscle weakness, dyspnea, collapse, arrhythmia, and heart block.	Symptomatic and supportive therapy of respiration and cardiovascular function. GI decontamination and fluid replacement therapy.

Contributed by Gary Osweiler, College of Veterinary Medicine, Iowa State University, Ames, IA.

DRUG FORMULARY
Mark G. Papich

(Only systemic drugs are listed; topicals, dermatologics, ointments, ophthalmic and otic treatments, vaccines, and nutritional supplements are not included.)

Drug doses are, in most cases, specified for use in either dogs or cats. When no designation is given, the dose is that commonly used for both dogs and cats.

Unless otherwise noted, the dose listed is a recommendation for both dogs and cats.

Many of the drugs and doses listed are unapproved for veterinary use. Dosing information and indications for unapproved drugs are listed as a guide only. The authors do not advocate use of unapproved drugs when equivalent approved veterinary drugs exist.

For many of the drugs listed in this Formulary, adequate safety and efficacy studies have not been performed in cats and dogs. Doses and indications listed in this Formulary were derived from the most current available information at the time of publication. Adverse effects and precautions listed include only some of those that are possible, or that may have been reported in people. The authors are not responsible for adverse effects or toxicity occurring in patients when drugs are used according to the guidelines used in this formulary.

For drugs listed in this Formulary, brand names may be listed as examples only. Other brand names may exist and by listing a particular brand name the authors are not advocating one

Drug name	Pharmacology and category of use	Precautions	Dosing information and comments	Other names	Formulations available	Dosage
Acepromazine	Phenothiazine tranquilizer. Inhibits action of dopamine as neurotransmitter. Used for sedation and preanesthetic purposes.	Causes sedation. May lower seizure threshold and causes alpha-adrenergic blockade. Produces extrapyramidal side effects in some individuals.	Usually used as preanesthetic in combination with other drugs. When used as preanesthetic, dose is ordinarily 0.02-0.2 mg/kg IM, SC, IV.	PromAce, many generics	5, 10, 25 mg tablets; 1, 10 mg/ml injections	Dogs: 0.56-1.13 mg/kg IM, SC, IV; 0.56-2.25 mg/kg PO q6-8h. Cats: 1.13-2.25 mg/kg IM, SC, IV.
Acetaminophen	Analgesic agent. Exact mechanism of action is not known. *Not* a prostaglandin synthesis inhibitor.	Well tolerated in dogs at doses listed. High doses have caused liver toxicity. Do *not* administer to cats.	Many OTC formulations available. Acetaminophen with codeine may have greater analgesic efficacy in some animals.	Tylenol, many generics	120, 160, 325, 500 mg tablets	Dogs: 15 mg/kg PO q8h. Cats: not recommended.
Acetaminophen with codeine	Same as above, except the opiate codeine is added to enhance analgesia	See codeine and acetaminophen.	See codeine and acetaminophen.	Tylenol with codeine, others	Oral solution, tablets	Follow dosing recommendations for codeine.
Acetazolamide	Carbonic anhydrase inhibitor and diuretic. Used primarily to lower intraocular pressure. See dichlorphenamide.	Use cautiously in any animal sensitive to sulfonamides. Can produce hypokalemia in some patients. Do not use in patients with acidemia.	Usually used to treat glaucoma in combination with other agents	Diamox	125, 250 mg tablets	5-10 mg/kg PO q8-12h. Glaucoma: 4-8 mg/kg PO q8-12h.
Acetylcysteine	Decreases viscosity of secretions. Used as mucolytic agent in eyes and in bronchial nebulizing solutons. However, as a donator of sulfhydral group, used as antidote for intoxications (e.g., acetaminophen toxicosis in cats).	May cause sensitization with prolonged topical administration. May react with certain materials in nebulizing equipment.	Available as agent for decreasing viscosity of respiratory secretions, but most common use is as a treatment for intoxications	Mucomyst	20% solution	Antidote: 140 mg/kg (loading dose) PO, IV, then 70 mg/kg q4h for 5 doses. Eyes: 2% solution topically q2h.
Acetylsalicylic acid	See aspirin.					
ACTH	See corticotropin.					
Actinomycin D	See dactinomycin.					
Activated charcoal	See charcoal, activated.					
Adequan	See polysulfated glycosaminoglycan (PSGAG).					
Albendazole	Benzimidazole antiparasitic drug. Inhibits glucose uptake in parasites.	Wide margin of safety	Used primarily as antihelmintic, but also has demonstrated efficacy for giardiasis	Valbazen	113.6 mg/ml suspension	25-50 mg/kg PO q12h. Giardia: 25 mg/kg q12h for 2 days.
Albuterol	Beta-2 (β_2) adrenergic agonist. Bronchodilator. Stimulates β_2 receptors to relax bronchial smooth muscle. May also inhibit resease of inflammatory mediators, especially from mast cells.	Causes excessive β-adrenergic stimulation at high doses (tachycardia, tremors). Arrhythmias occur at toxic doses. Avoid use in pregnant animals.	Doses are primarily derived from extrapolation of human dose. Well-controlled efficacy studies in veterinary medicine are not available. Onset of action is 15-30 minutes; duration of action may be as long as 8 hours.	Proventil, Ventolin	Tablets, oral solution, syrup, injection, inhalation solution, aerosol	20-50 mcg/kg up to 4 times a day
Allopurinol	Decreases production of uric acid by inhibiting enzymes responsible for uric acid	May cause skin reactions (hypersensitivity)	Used in humans primarily for treating gout. In animals, used to decrease formation of uric acid uroliths.	Lopurin, Zyloprim	100, 300 mg tablets	10 mg/kg q8h, then reduce to 10 mg/kg q24h

Drug name	Pharmacology and category of use	Precautions	Dosing information and comments	Other names	Formulations available	Dosage
Alumunium carbonate gel	Antacid (neutralizes stomach acid) and phosphate binder in intestine	Generally safe. May interact with other drugs administered PO.	Antacid doses are designed to neutralize stomach acid, but duration of acid suppression is short.	Basalgel	Capsules (equivalent to 500 mg aluminum hydroxide)	10-30 mg/kg PO q8h (with meals)
Aluminium hydroxide gel	Antacid (neutralizes stomach acid) and phosphate binder in intestine	Generally safe. May interact with other drugs administered PO.	Antacid doses are designed to neutralize stomach acid, but duration of acid suppression is short.	Amphogel	64 mg/ml oral suspension; 600 mg tablet	10-30 mg/kg PO q8h (with meals)
Amikacin	Aminoglycoside antibacterial drug. Inhibits protein synthesis. See gentamicin.	May cause nephrotoxicosis with high doses or prolonged therapy. May also cause ototoxicity and vestibulotoxicity. See gentamicin.	Once-daily doses are designed to maximize peak-MIC ratio. Consider therapeutic drug monitoring for chronic therapy. See gentamicin.	Amiglyde-V, Amikin	50, 250 mg/ml injections	6.5 mg/kg IV, IM, SC q8h or 20 mg/kg IV, IM, SC q24h
Aminopentamide	Antidiarrheal drug. Anticholinergic (blocks acetylcholine at parasympathetic synapse).	Use cautiously in animals with GI stasis or when anticholinergic drugs are contraindicated (e.g., glaucoma).	Dosing guidelines based on manufacturer's recommendation	Centrine	0.2 mg tablet; 0.5 mg/ml injection	Dogs: 0.01-0.03 mg/kg IM, SC, PO q8-12h. Cats: 0.1 mg/cat IM, SC, PO q8-12h.
Aminophylline	Bronchodilator	Causes excitement and possible cardiac effect with high concentrations	See theophylline. Therapeutic drug monitoring is recommended for chronic therapy.	Many	100, 200 mg tablets; 25 mg/ml injection	Dogs: 10 mg/kg PO, IM, IV q8h. Cats: 6.6 mg/kg PO q12h.
6-aminosalicylic acid	See mesalamine and olsalazine.					
Amitraz	Antiparasitic drug for ectoparasites. Used for treatment of mites, including Demodex. Inhibits monoamine oxidase in mites.	Causes sedation in dogs (alpha-2 agonist), which may be reversed by yohimbine or atipamezole. When high doses are used, other side effects reported include pruritus, polydipsia/polyuria, bradycardia, hypothermia, hyperglycemia and (rarely) seizures.	Manufacturer's dose should be used initially. But, for refractory cases, this dose has been exceeded to produce increased efficacy. Doses that have been used include 0.025, 0.05, and 0.1% concentration applied 2 times a week and 0.125% solution applied to half the body every day for 4 weeks to 5 months.	Mitaban	10.6 ml concentrated dip (19.9%)	10.6 ml per 7.5 L water (0.025% solution). Apply 3-6 topical treatments every 14 days.
Amitriptyline	Tricyclic antidepressant drug. Used in humans to treat anxiety and depression. Used in animals to treat variety of behavioral disorders. Action is via inhibition of uptake of serotonin at presynaptic nerve terminals.	Multiple side effects are associated with tricyclic antidepressants such as antimuscarinic effects (dry mouth, rapid heart rate) and antihistamine effects (sedation). High doses can produce life-threatening cardiotoxicity.	Doses are primarily based on empiricism. There are no controlled efficacy trials available for animals.	Elavil	10, 25, 50, 75, 100, 150 mg tablets; 10 mg/ml injection	Dogs: 1-2 mg/kg PO q12-24h. Cats: 5-10 mg/day PO.
Ammonium chloride	Urine acidifier	Do not use in patients with systemic acidemia. May be unpalatable when added to some animals' food.	Doses are designed to maximize urine acidifying effect.	Generic	Crystals	Dogs: 100 mg/kg PO q12h. Cats: 800 mg/cat (approx. 1/4 to 1/3 tsp) mixed with food daily.
Amoxicillin trihydrate	Beta-lactam antibiotic. Inhibits bacterial cell wall synthesis. Generally broad spectrum activity, but resistance is common.	Use cautiously in animals allergic to penicillin-like drugs.	Dose requirements vary depending on susceptibility of bacteria.	Amoxi-Tabs, Amoxi-drops, Amoxil, others	50, 100, 200, 400 mg tablets; 50 mg/ml oral suspension	6-20 mg/kg PO q8-12h
Amoxicillin/clavulanic acid	Beta-lactam antibiotic and betalactamase inhibitor (clavulanic acid)	Same as amoxicillin	Same as amoxicillin	Clavamox	62.5, 125, 250, 375 mg tablets; 62.5 mg/ml suspension	Dogs: 12.5-25 mg/kg PO q12h. Cats: 62.5 mg/cat PO q12h.

1182

Drug name	Pharmacology and category of use	Precautions	Dosing information and comments	Other names	Formulations available	Dosage
Amphotericin B	Antifungal drug. Fungicidal for systemic fungi (damages fungal membranes).	Produces a dose-related nephrotoxicosis. Also produces fever, phlebitis, and tremors.	Administer IV via slow infusion and monitor renal function closely. When preparing IV solution, do not mix with electrolyte solutions; use D5W, for example. Administer NaCl fluid loading before therapy. One study administered this drug SC (Aust Vet J 1996;73:124).	Fungizone	50 mg injectable vial	0.5 mg/kg IV (slow infusion) q48h, to a cumulative dose of 4-8 mg/kg
Ampicillin	Beta-lactam antibiotic. Inhibits bacterial cell wall synthesis.	Use cautiously in animals allergic to penicillin-like drugs.	Dose requirements vary depending on susceptibility of bacteria. Absorbed approximately 50% less compared to amoxicillin when administered PO.	Omnipen, Principen, others	250, 500 mg capsules; 125, 250, 500 mg vials (ampicillin sodium)	20-40 mg/kg PO q8h; 10-20 mg/kg IV, IM, SC q6-8h (ampicillin sodium)
Ampicillin & Sulbactam	Same mechanism as ampicillin-clavulanate	Same as ampicillin-clavulanate		Uhasyn	2:1 combination injection	10-20 mg/kg IV or IM q8h
Ampicillin trihydrate	Beta-lactam antibiotic. Inhibits bacterial cell wall synthesis.	Use cautiously in animals allergic to penicillin-like drugs.	Absorption is slow and may not be sufficient for acute serious infection.	Polyflex	10, 25 mg vials for injection	6.5-10 mg/kg IM, SC q12h
Amprolium	Antiprotozoal drug. Antagonizes thiamine in parasites. Used for treatment of coccidiosis, especially in puppies.	Toxicity observed only at high doses (CNS signs resulting from thiamine deficiency)	Usually administered as feed-additive to livestock. For dogs, 30 ml of 9.6% amprolium has been added to 3.8 L of drinking water for control of coccidiosis.	Amprol, Corid	9.6% (9.6 g/100 ml) oral solution; soluble powder	1.25 g of 20% amprolium powder to daily feed or 30 ml of 9.6% amprolium solution to 3.8 L of drinking water for 7 days
Antacid drugs	See aluminum hydroxide, magnesium hydroxide, and calcium carbonate.					
Apomorphine hydrochloride	Emetic drug. Causes emesis via dopamine release or direct effects on CRTZ.	Produces emesis before serious adverse effects occur. Use cautiously in cats that may be sensitive to opiates.	May be difficult to obtain from manufacturer. Consult local poison center or pharmacist for availability.	Generic	6 mg tablet	0.02-0.04 mg/kg IV, IM; 0.1 mg/kg SC; or instil 0.25 mg in conjunctiva of eye (dissolve 6 mg tablet in 1-2 ml of saline)
Ascorbic acid	Vitamin. Used as acidifier.	Toxicity only at very high doses	Primarily used as nutritional supplement, but high doses have been used for treatment of certain diseases.	Vitamin C	Various forms	100-500 mg/animal/day (diet supplement); 100 mg/animal q8h (urine acidification)
L-asparaginase	Anticancer agent. Used in lymphoma protocols. Depletes cancer cells of asparagine and interferes with protein synthesis.	Hypersensitivity, alleric reactions	Usually used in combination with other drugs in cancer chemotherapy protocols	Elspar	10,000 U per vial for injection	400 U/kg IV, IP, IM weekly
Aspirin	Nonsteroidal antiinflammatory drug. Antiinflammatory action is generally considered to be caused by inhibition of prostaglandins. Used as analgesic, antiinflammatory, and antiplatelet drug.	Narrow therapeutic index. High doses frequently cause vomiting. Other gastrointestinal effects can include ulceration and bleeding. Cats are susceptible to salicylate intoxication because of slow clearance. Use cautiously in patients with coagulopathies because of platelet inhibi*	Analgesic and antiinflammatory doses have primarily been derived from empiricism. Antiplatelet doses are lower because of prolonged effect of aspirin on platelets. Buffered forms of aspirin or administration with food may decrease stomach irritation. Enteric-coated formulations are not recommended for dogs and cats.	Many generic and brand names (Bufferin, Ascriptin)	81, 325 mg tablets	Mild analgesia (dogs): 10 mg/kg q12h. Antiinflammatory: 20-25 mg/kg q12h (dogs); 10-20 mg/kg q48h (cats). Antiplatelet: 5-10 mg/kg q24-48h (dogs); 80 mg q48h (cats).

Drug name	Pharmacology and category of use	Precautions	Dosing information and comments	Other names	Formulations available	Dosage
Astemizole	Antihistamine (H_1 blocking) drug. Primarily used for allergic disease; in humans, used as adjunct for asthma. This is one of the second-generation antihistamines, which usually do not have the side effect of sedation as compared to other antihistamines.	Adverse effects have not been reported in small animals, but cardiotoxicity is a potential problem with high doses.	Available as tablets and oral suspension. Doses are primarily derived from extrapolation from human dose. Efficacy trials and dose titrations have not been performed.	Hismanal	10 mg tablet	Dogs: 0.2 mg/kg PO q24h (up to 1.0 mg/kg q12h)
Atenolol	Beta-adrenergic blocker. Relatively selective for β_1 receptor. Used primarily as an antiarrhythmic or in other cardiovascular conditions to slow sinus rate.	Bradycardia and heart block are possible. May produce bronchospasm in sensitive patients.	Dosing precautions are similar to other β-blocking drugs. Atenolol is reported to be less affected by changes in hepatic metabolism than other β-blockers.	Tenormin	25, 50, 100 mg tablets; 25 mg/ml oral suspension; 0.5 mg/ml ampules for injection	Dogs: 6.25-12.5 mg/dog q12h (or 0.25-1.0 mg/kg q12-24h). Cats: 6.25-12.5 mg/cat q24h.
Atracurium	Neuromuscular blocking agent (nondepolarizing). Competes with acetylcholine at neuromuscular end plate. Used primarily during anesthesia or other conditons in which it is necessary to inhibit muscle contractions.	Produces respiratory depression and paralysis. Neuromuscular blocking drugs have no effect on analgesia.	Administer only in situations in which careful control of respiration is possible. Doses may need to be individualized for optimum effect. Do not mix with alkalinizing solutions or lactated Ringer's solution.	Tracurium	10 mg/ml injection	0.2 mg/kg IV initally, then 0.15 mg/kg every 30 minutes or IV infusion at 3-8 µg/kg/minute
Atipamezole HCL	α_2-antagonist. Used to reverse α_2 agonists such as medetomidine.			Antisedan	5 mg/ml injection	Inject volume equal to that of medetomidine
Atropine	Anticholinergic agent (blocks acetylcholine effect at muscarinic receptor), parasympatholytic. Used primarily as adjunct to anesthesia or other procedures to increase heart rate and decrease respiratory and gastrointestinal secretion. Also used as antidote for organophosphate intoxication.	Potent anticholinergic agent. Do not use in patients with glaucoma, intestinal ileus, gastroparesis, or tachycardia. Side effects of therapy include xerostomia, ileus, constipation, tachycardia, and urine retention.	Used ordinarily as adjunct with anesthesia or other procedures. Do not mix with alkaline solutions.	Generic	400, 500, 540 µg/ml injections; 15 mg/ml injection	0.02-0.04 mg/kg IV, IM, SC q6-8h; 0.2-0.5 mg/kg (as needed) for organophosphate and carbamate toxicosis
Auranofin (triethylphosphine gold)	Used for gold therapy (crysotherapy). Mechanism of action is unknown, but may relate to immunosuppressive effect on lymphocytes. Used primarily for immune-mediated diseases.	Adverse effects include dermatitis, nephrotoxicity, and blood dyscrasias.	Use of this drug has not been evaluated in veterinary medicine. No controlled clinical trials are available to determine efficacy in animals. It has been suggested that this product (oral) is not as effective as injectable products such as aurothioglucose.	Ridaura	Capsules 3 mg	0.1-0.2 mg/kg PO q12h
Aurothioglucose	Used for gold therapy (crysotherapy). Mechanism of action is unknown, but may relate to immunosuppressive effect on lymphocytes. Used primarily for immune-mediated diseases such as dermatologic disease.	Adverse effects include dermatitis, nephrotoxicity, and blood dyscrasias.	Use of this drug has not been evaluated in veterinary medicine. No controlled clinical trials are available to determine efficacy in animals. This drug is often used in combination with other immunosuppressive drugs such as corticosteroids.	Solganol	50 mg/ml injection	Dogs < 10 kg: 1 mg IM first week, 2 mg IM second week, 1 mg/kg/week maintenance. Dogs > 10 kg: 5 mg IM first week, 10 mg IM second week, 1 mg/kg/week maintenance. Cats: 0.5-1 mg/cat IM every 7 days.

Drug name	Pharmacology and category of use	Precautions	Dosing information and comments	Other names	Formulations available	Dosage
Azathioprine	Thiopurine immunosuppressive drug. Inhibits T-cell lymphocyte function. This drug is metabolized to 6-mercaptopurine, which may account for immunosuppressive effects. Used to treat various immune-mediated disease.	Bone marrow suppression is the most serious concern. Cats particularly are susceptible. There has been some association with development of pancreatitis when administered with corticosteroids.	Usually used in combination with other immunosuppressive drugs, such as corticosteroids, to treat immune-mediated disease. Some evidence suggests that it is contraindicated in cats because of bone-marrow effects. Doses of 2.2 mg/kg have produced toxicity in cats.	Imuran	50 mg tablet; 10 mg/ml for injection	Dogs: 2 mg/kg PO q24h initially, then 0.5-1 mg/kg q48h. Cats: 1.5-3.125 mg/cat q48h.
Azithromycin	Azalide antibiotic. Similar mechanism of action as macrolides (erythromycin), which is to inhibit bacteria protein synthesis via inhibition of ribosome. Spectrum is primarily gram-positive.	Has not been in common use in veterinary medicine to establish adverse effects. Vomiting is likely with high doses. Diarrhea may occur in some patients.	Azithromycin may be better tolerated than erythromycin. Primary difference from other antibiotics is the high intracellular concentrations achieved.	Zithromax	250 mg capsules	Dogs: 10 mg/kg PO once every 5 days or 3.3 mg/kg once daily for 3 days. Cats: 5 mg/kg PO every other day.
AZT	See zidovudine.					
Bactrim	Sulfamethoxazole and trimethoprim. See trimethoprim-sulfonamide combinations.					
BAL	See dimercaprol.					
Benazapril	ACE inhibitor. See captopril for details. Used for vasodilation and treatment of heart failure.	See captopril. May cause azotemia in some patients; carefully monitor patients receiving high doses of diuretics. Use cautiously with other hypotensive drugs and diuretics. NSAIDs may decrease vasodilating effects	Approved dose is based on use in dogs in Europe and Canada. Other drugs used for treatment of heart failure may be used concurrently. With all ACE inhibitors, monitor electrolytes and renal function 3-7 days after initiating therapy and periodically thereafter	Lotensin	5, 10, 20, 40 mg tablets	0.25-0.5 mg/kg q24h PO
Betamethasone	Potent, long-acting corticosteroid. Antiinflammatory and immunosuppressive effects are approximately 30 times more than cortisol. Antiinflammatory effects are complex, but primarily via inhibition of inflammatory cells and suppression of expression of inflammatory mediators. Used in treatment of inflammatory and immune-mediated disease.	Side effects from corticosteroids are many and include polyphagia, polydipsia/ polyuria, and HPA-axis suppression. Adverse effects include gastrointestinal ulceration, hepatopathy, diabetes, hyperlipidemia, decreased thyroid hormone, decreased protein synthesis and wound healing, and immunosuppression.	Dosing schedules are based on desired effect. Antiinflammatory effects are seen at doses of 0.1-0.2 mg/kg; immunosuppressive effects at 0.2-0.5 mg/kg.	Celestone	Acetate/sodium phosphate injection	0.1-0.2 mg/kg PO q12-24h
Bethanechol	Muscarinic, cholinergic agonist. Parasympathomimetic. Stimulates gastric and intestinal motility, but primarily used to increase contraction of urinary bladder.	High doses of cholinergic agonists will increase motility of gastrointestinal tract and cause abdominal discomfort and diarrhea. Can cause circulatory depression in sensitive animals.	Administer injection SC only, not IV. Doses are derived from extrapolation of human doses or via empiricism. There are no well-controlled efficacy studies available for veterinary species.	Urecholine	5, 10, 25, 50 mg tablets; 5 mg/ml injection	Dogs: 5-15 mg/dog PO q8h. Cats: 1.25-5 mg/cat PO q8h.
Bisacodyl	Laxative/cathartic. Acts via local stimulation of gastrointestinal motility, most likely by irritation of bowel. Used primarily as laxative or for procedures in which bowel evacuation is necessary.	Avoid use in patients with renal disease. Avoid overuse.	Available as OTC tablet. Doses are derived from extrapolation of human doses or via empiricism. There are no well-controlled efficacy studies available for veterinary species. Onset of action is approximately 1 hour.	Dulcolax	5 mg tablet	5 mg/animal PO q8-24h

Drug name	Pharmacology and category of use	Precautions	Dosing information and comments	Other names	Formulations available	Dosage
Bismuth subsalicylate	Antidiarrhea agent and gastrointestinal protectant. Precise mechanism of action is unknown, but antiprostaglandin action of salicylate component may be beneficial for enteritis. Bismuth component is efficacious for treating infections caused by spirochaete bacteria (Helicobacter gastritis).	Adverse effects are uncommon; however, salicylate component is absorbed systemically and overuse should be avoided in animals that cannot tolerate salicylates (such as cats and animals allergic to aspirin). Owners should be warned that bismuth will discolor stools.	Available as OTC product. Doses are derived from extrapolation of human doses or via empiricism. There are no well-controlled efficacy studies available for veterinary species.	Pepto-Bismol	Oral suspension (262 mg/15 ml or 525 mg/ml in extra strength formulation); 262 mg tablet	1-3 ml/kg/day (in divided doses) PO
Bismuth subcarbonate	Same as for bismuth subsalicylate					0.3-3.0 g PO q4h
Bleomycin	Anticancer antibiotic agent. Used for treatment of various sarcomas and carcinomas. Exact mechanism of action is unknown, but may bind to DNA and prevent synthesis.	Causes local reaction at site of injection. Causes pulmonary toxicity as well as fever and chills in humans, but side effects are not well documented in veterinary species.	Injectable solution usually used in combination with other anticancer agents. Consult anticancer protocols for details regarding use.	Blenoxane	15 U vials for injection	10 U/m² IV or SC for 3 days, then 10 U/m² weekly (maximum cumulative dose 200 U/m²)
Bromide	See potassium bromide.					
Bunamidine hydrochloride	Used as anticestodal agent. Primarily to treat tapeworm infections in dogs and cats. Mechanism of action is to damage integrity of protective integument on parasite.	Vomiting and diarrhea have occurred after use. Avoid use in young animals.	Do not break tablets. Administer tablets on empty stomach. Do not feed for 3 hours after adminstration.	Scolaban	400 mg tablet	20-50 mg/kg PO
Bupivacaine	Local anesthetic. Inhibits nerve conduction via sodium channel blockade. Longer acting and more potent than lidocaine or other local anesthetics.	Adverse effects rare with local infiltration. High doses absorbed systemically can cause nervous system signs (tremors and convulsions). After epidural administration respiratory paralysis is possible with high doses.	Used for local infiltration or infusion into epidural space	Marcaine	0.25, 0.5% solution injections	0.22-0.3 ml epidural
Buprenorphine	Opioid analgesic. Partial µ-receptor agonist, κ-receptor antagonist. More potent than morphine (25-50 times).	Adverse effects are similar to other opiate agonists. Respiratory depression can occur with high doses. Dependency can develop with chronic use.	Used for analgesia, often in combination with other analgesics or in conjunction with general anesthesia. Longer acting than morphine. Not reversed by naloxone.	Temgesic	0.3 mg/ml	Dogs: 0.005-0.02 mg/kg IV, IM q4-8h. Cats: 0.005-0.01 mg/kg IV, IM q4-8h.
Buspirone	Antianxiety agent. Acts to block release of serotonin by binding to presynaptic receptors. In veterinary medicine has been primarily used for treatment of urine spraying in cats.	Some cats show increased aggression; some cats show increased affection toward owners.	Some efficacy trials suggest effectiveness for treating urine spraying in cats. There may be a lower relapse rate compared to other drugs.	BuSpar	5, 10 mg tablets	2.5-5 mg/cat PO q24h (may be increased to twice daily for some cats)
Busulfan	Anticancer agent. Bifunctional alkylating agent and acts to disrupt DNA of tumor cells. Used primarily for lymphoreticular neoplasia.	Leukopenia is the most severe side effect.	Usually used in combination with other anticancer agents. Consult specific protocol for details.	Myleran	2 mg tablet	3-4 mg/m² PO q24h

Drug name	Pharmacology and category of use	Precautions	Dosing information and comments	Other names	Formulations available	Dosage
Butorphanol	Opioid analgesic. κ-receptor agonist and weak μ-receptor antagonist. Butorphanol is used for perioperative analgesia, for chronic pain, and as an antitussive agent.	Adverse effects are similar to other opioid analgesic drugs. Sedation is common at analgesic doses. Respiratory depression can occur with high doses.	Often used in combination with anesthetic agents or in conjunction with other analgesic drugs	Torbutrol, Torbugesic	1, 5, 10 mg tablets; 0.5, 10 mg/ml injections	Antitussive (dogs): 0.055 mg/kg SC q6-12h or 0.55 mg/kg PO. Preanesthetic (dogs): 0.2-0.4 mg/kg IV, IM, SC (with acepromazine); Analgesia (cats): 0.4 mg/kg SC q6h; 0.2 mg/kg IV q6h; Dogs: 0.2-0.8 mg/kg IV, SC q2-6h.
Calcitriol	Used to treat calcium deficiency and diseases such as renal osteodystrophy and hypocalcemia associated with hypoparathyroidism. Not indicated as vitamin D supplement. Action is to increase calcium absorption in intestine.	Overdose can result in hypercalcemia.	Doses should be adjusted in each patient according to response and monitoring calcium plasma concentration.	Rocaltrol, Calcijex	0.25, 0.5 mg capsules (Rocaltrol); 1, 2 mcg/ml injections (Calcijex)	2.5-3 ng/kg (0.0025-0.003 mcg/kg) PO q24h
Calcium carbonate	Used as oral calcium supplement for hypocalcemia. Used as antacid to treat gastric hyperacidity and gastrointestinal ulcers. Neutralizes stomach acid. Also used as intestinal phosphate binder for hyperphosphatemia.	Few side effects. Increased calcium concentrations are possible. Avoid use with oral fluoroquinolones (e.g., ciprofloxacin, enrofloxacin) as it may decrease their absorption.	Doses are primarily derived from extrapolation of human doses. When used as calcium supplement, doses should be adjusted according to serum calcium concentrations.	Many, Titralac, Tums, generic	Tablet, oral suspension (e.g., 650 mg tablet contains 260 mg calcium ion)	5-10 ml of oral solution PO q4-6h. Phosphate binder: 60-100 mg/kg/day PO in divided doses.
Calcium chloride	Calcium supplement. Used in acute situations to supplement as electrolyte replacement or as a cardiotonic.	Overdose with calcium is possible. Do not administer IV solution SC or IM because it may cause tissue necrosis.	Injection is 27.2 mg (1.36 mEq of calcium ion) per ml. Usually used in emergency situations. Intracardiac administration has been performed, but avoid injections into the myocardium.	Generic 10% solution	10% solution	0.1-0.3 ml/kg IV (slowly)
Calcium citrate	Calcium supplement. Used in treatment of hypocalcemia, such as with hypoparathyroidism.	Hypercalcemia possible with oversupplementation	Doses should be adjusted according to serum calcium concentration.	Citracal (OTC)	950 mg tablet (contains 200 mg calcium ion)	Cats: 10-30 mg/kg PO q8h (with meals)
Calcium disodium EDTA	See edetate calcium disodium.					
Calcium gluconate	Calcium supplement. Used in treatment of hypocalcemia, such as with hypoparathyroidism. Used in electrolyte deficiency.	Hypercalcemia possible with oversupplementation.	Injection is 97 mg (9.5 mg [0.47 mEq] of calcium ion) per ml. 500 mg tablet contains 45 mg of calcium ion. Avoid administration of IV solution IM or SC because it will cause tissue necrosis.	Kalcinate, generic (10% solution)	10% injection	0.5-1.5 ml/kg IV (slowly)
Calcium lactate	Generally same comments as for other calcium supplements.		Calcium lactate contains 130 mg of calcium ion per g.	Generic	OTC tablets	Dogs: 0.5-2.0 g/dog/day PO (in divided doses). Cats: 0.2-0.5 g/cat/day PO (in divided doses).

Drug name	Pharmacology and category of use	Precautions	Dosing information and comments	Other names	Formulations available	Dosage
Captopril	Angiotensin-converting enzyme (ACE) inhibitor. Inhibits conversion of angiotensin I to angiotensin II. May have other vasodilating properties. Generally used to treat hypertension and congestive heart failure.	Hypotension possible with excessive doses. May cause azotemia in some patients, especially when administered with potent diuretics (furosemide). Use cautiously with diuretics and potassium supplements. NSAIDs may diminish antihypertensive effect.	Monitor patients carefully to avoid hypotension. With all ACE inhibitors, monitor electrolytes and renal function 3-7 days after initiating therapy and periodically thereafter. Use of captopril has been replaced by enalapril in many patients.	Capoten	25 mg tablet	Dogs: 0.5-2 mg/kg PO q8-12h. Cats: 3.12-6.25 mg/cat PO q8h.
Carbenicillin	Beta-lactam antibiotic. Inhibits bacterial cell wall synthesis. Active against Pseudomonas and other gram-negative bacteria.	Use cautiously in patients sensitive to penicillins (e.g., allergy).	Carbenicillin injection often is administered with an aminoglycoside. Do not mix with aminoglycosides prior to administration or inactivation will result.	Geopen, Pyopen	1, 2, 5, 10, and 30-gram vials for injection	40-50 mg/kg (up to 100 mg/kg IV, IM, SC q6-8h)
Carbenicillin indanyl sodium	Same as for carbenicillin. Primary use is for treating infections of lower urinary tract.	Same as carbenicillin	Oral formulation of carbenicillin, but attains concentrations that are only sufficient for treating urinary tract infections. Do not use for systemic infections.	Geocillin	500 mg tablets	10 mg/kg PO q8h
Carbimazole	Antithyroid drug similar to methimazole, but with perhaps fewer side effects	See methimazole.	Used in Europe. Clinical experience in United States is limited.	Neomercazole	Available in Europe	Cats: 5 mg/cat PO q8h (induction), followed by 5 mg/cat PO q12h
Carboplatin	Anticancer agent. Used for treating various carcinomas. Action is similar to cisplatin. See cisplatin for further details.	May cause anemia, leukopenia, or thrombocytopenia. Carboplatin may induce renal toxicity. Do not administer to cats.	Available for reconstitution for injection. Do not use with administration sets containing aluminum, because of incompatibility. Usually administered in specific anticancer protocols. Fluid-loading patients before infusion may decrease risk of nephrotoxicity.	Paraplatin	50, 150 mg vials for injection	Dogs: 300 mg/m^2 IV every 3-4 weeks
Carprofen	Analgesic agent. Used primarily for treatment of musculoskeletal pain. Although considered an NSAID, mechanism of action apparently does not involve prostaglandin synthesis.	Appears to cause less incidence of gastrointestinal ulceration and vomiting than other NSAIDs	Doses are based on early clinical investigations in dogs with arthritis.	Zinecarp (in Europe)	Tablets (not yet available in United States)	Dogs: 2.2 mg/kg PO q12h. Cats: doses not available.
Cascara sagrada	Stimulant cathartic. Action is believed to be by local stimulation of bowel motility. Used as laxative to treat constipation or evacuate bowel for procedures.	Overuse can cause electrolyte losses.	Available in various OTC products	Many brands (e.g., Nature's Remedy)	Many OTC formulations	Dogs: 1-4 ml/dog/day PO. Cats: 0.5-1.5 ml/cat/day.
Castor oil	Stimulant cathartic. Action is believed to be by local stimulation of bowel motility. Used as laxative to treat constipation or evacuate bowel for procedures.	Overuse can cause electrolyte losses. Castor oil has been known to stimulate premature labor in pregnancy.	Available as OTC product	Generic	Oral liquid	Dogs: 8-30 ml/day PO. Cats: 4-10 ml/day PO.

Drug name	Pharmacology and category of use	Precautions	Dosing information and comments	Other names	Formulations available	Dosage
Cefaclor	Cephalosporin antibiotic. Action is similar to other β-lactam antibiotics, which is to inhibit synthesis of bacterial cell wall leading to cell death. Cephalosporins are divided into first, second, or third generation depending on spectrum of activity. Consult package insert or specific reference for spectrum of activity of individual cephalosporin. Cefaclor is a second-generation cephalosporin.	All cephalosporins are generally safe; however, sensitivity can occur in individuals (allergy). Rare bleeding disorders have been known to occur with some cephalosporins.	Used primarily when resistance has been demonstrated to first-generation cephalosporins	Ceclor	250, 500 capsule; 25 mg/ml oral suspension	4-20 mg/kg PO q8h
Cefadroxil	See cefaclor. Cefadroxil is a first-generation cephalosporin.	See cefaclor. Cefadroxil has been known to cause vomiting after PO administration in dogs.	Spectrum of cefadroxil is similar to other first-generation cephalosporins. For susceptibility test, use cephalothin as test drug.	Cefa-Tabs, Cefa-Drops	50 mg/ml oral suspension; 50, 100, 200, 1,000 mg tablets	Dogs: 22 mg/kg PO q12h. Cats: 22 mg/kg PO q24h.
Cefazolin sodium	See cefadroxil. Cefazolin is a first-generation cephalosporin.	See cefaclor. For cefazolin, use cephalothin to test susceptibility.	First-generation cephalosporin commonly used as injectable drug for prophylaxis for surgery and as acute therapy for serious infections.	Ancef, Kefzol, generic	50, 100 mg per 50 ml for injection	20-35 mg/kg IV, IM q8h. Perisurgical use: 22 mg/kg q2h (during surgery).
Cefixime	See cefaclor. Cefixime is a third-generation cephalosporin.	See cefaclor.	Although not approved for veterinary use, pharmacokinetic studies in dogs have provided recommended doses.	Suprax	20 mg/ml oral suspension; 200, 400 mg tablets	10 mg/kg PO q12h. Cystitis: 5 mg/kg PO q12-24h.
Cefotaxime	See cefaclor. Cefotaxime is a third-generation cephalosporin.	See cefaclor.	Third-generation cephalosporin used when resistance encountered to first- and second-generation cephalosporins	Claforan	500 mg, 1, 2, 10 g vials for injection	Dogs: 50 mg/kg IV, IM, SC q12h. Cats: 20-80 mg/kg IV, IM q6h.
Cefotetan	See cefaclor. Cefotetan is a second-generation cephalosporin.	See cefaclor.	Second-generation cephalosporin similar to cefoxitin, but may have longer half-life in dogs	Cefotan	1, 2, 10 g vials for injection	30 mg/kg IV, SC q8h
Cefoxitin sodium	See cefaclor. Cefoxitin is a second-generation cephalosporin. May have increased activity against anaerobic bacteria.	See cefaclor.	Second-generation cephalosporin often used when activity against anaerobic bacteria is desired	Mefoxin	1, 2, 10 g vials for injection	30 mg/kg IV q6-8h
Ceftiofur	See cefaclor. Ceftiofur is a unique cephalosporin that does not fit into a distinct generation, but some properties are similar to 3rd generation class.	See cefaclor. Ceftiofur is primarily used only for urinary tract infections.	Available as powder for reconstitution before injection. After reconstitution, stable for 7 days when refrigerated, 12 hours at room temperature, or 8 weeks frozen.	Naxcel (Excenel in Canada)	50 mg/ml injection	2.2-4.4 mg/kg SC q24h (for urinary tract infections)
Cephalexin	See cefaclor. Cephalexin is a first-generation cephalosporin.	See cefaclor. For cephalexin, use cephalothin to test susceptibility.	Although not approved for veterinary use, trials show efficacy for treating pyoderma in dogs.	Keflex, generic forms	250, 500 mg capsules; 250, 500 mg tablets; 100 mg/ml, 125, 250 mg per 5 ml oral suspension	10-30 mg/kg PO q6-12h. Pyoderma: 22-35 mg/kg PO q12h.

Drug name	Pharmacology and category of use	Precautions	Dosing information and comments	Other names	Formulations available	Dosage
Cephalothin sodium	See cefaclor.	See cefaclor.	First-generation cephalosporin. Used as test drug for susceptibility tests of other first-generation cephalosporins.	Keflin	1, 2 g vials for injection	10-30 mg/kg IV, IM q4-8h
Cephapirin	See cefaclor. Cephapirin is a first-generation cephalosporin.	See cefaclor.	See cephalothin.	Cefadyl	500 mg, 1, 2, 4 g vials for injection	10-30 mg/kg IV, IM q4-8h
Cephradine	See cefaclor. Cephapirin is a first-generation cephalosporin.	See cefaclor.	See cephalothin.	Velosef	250, 500 mg capsules; 250, 500 mg, 1, 2 g vials for injection	10-25 mg/kg PO q6-8h
Charcoal, activated	Adsorbent. Used primarily to adsorb drugs and toxins in intestine to prevent their absorption.	Not absorbed systemically. Safe for administration.	Available in variety of forms; usually used as treatment of poisoning. Many commercial preparations contain sorbitol, which acts as flavoring agent and promotes intestinal catharsis.	ActaChar, Charcodote, Toxiban, generic	Oral suspension	1-4 gm/kg PO (granules); 6-12 ml/kg (suspension)
Chlorambucil	Cytotoxic agent. Acts in similar manner as cyclophosphamide as alkylating agent. Used for treatment of various tumors and immunosuppressive therapy.	Myelosuppression is possible. Cystitis does not occur with chlorambucil as with cyclophosphamide.	Consult anticancer drug protocol for specific regimens.	Leukeran	2 mg tablet	2-6 mg/m^2 or 0.1-0.2 mg/kg PO q24h initially, then q48h
Chloramphenicol and chloramphenicol palmitate	Antibacterial drug. Mechanism of action is inhibition of protein synthesis via binding to ribosome. Broad spectrum of activity.	Bone marrow suppression is possible with high doses or prolonged treatment (especially in cats). Avoid use in pregnant or neonatal animals. Interactions with other drugs (e.g., barbiturates) possible because chloramphenicol will inhibit hepatic microsomal enzymes.	Chloramphenicol use based on susceptibility data. Chloramphenicol palmitate requires active enzymes and should not be administered to fasted (or anorectic) animals.	Chloromycetin, generic forms	30 mg/ml oral suspension (palmitate); 250 mg capsule; 100, 250, 500 mg tablets	Dogs: 40-50 mg/kg PO q8h. Cats: 12.5-20 mg/kg PO q12h.
Chloramphenicol sodium succinate	Injection form of choramphenicol. Converted by liver to parent drug.	Same as chloramphenicol	Injectable solution converted to chloramphenicol by hepatic metabolism	Chloromycetin, generic	Injection	Dogs: 40-50 mg/kg IV, IM q6-8h. Cats: 12.5-20 mg/cat IV, IM q12h.
Chlorothiazide	Thiazide diuretic. Inhibits sodium reabsorption in distal renal tubules. Used as diuretic and antihypertensive. Since it decreases renal excretion of calcium, it also has been used to treat calcium-containing uroliths.	Do not use in patient with elevated calcium. May cause electrolyte imbalance such as hypokalemia.	Not as effective as high-ceiling diuretics (such as furosemide)	Diuril	250, 500 mg tablets; 50 mg/ml oral suspension; injection	20-40 mg/kg PO q12h
Chlorpheniramine maleate	Antihistamine (H1 blocker). Blocks action of histamine on receptors. Also may have direct antiinflammatory action. Use most often to prevent allergic reactions. Used for pruritus therapy in dogs and cats.	Sedation is most common side effect. Antimuscarinic effects (atropine-like effects) also are common.	Chlorpheniramine is included as ingredient in many OTC cough/cold and allergy medications.	Chlortrimeton, Phenetron, others	4, 8 mg tablets	Dogs: 4-8 mg/dog PO q12h (up to a maximum of 0.5 mg/kg q12h). Cats: 2 mg/cat PO q12h.

Drug name	Pharmacology and category of use	Precautions	Dosing information and comments	Other names	Formulations available	Dosage
Chlorpromazine	Phenothiazine tranquilizer/antiemetic. Inhibits action of dopamine as neurotransmitter. Most often used as central antiemetic. Also used for sedation and preanesthetic purposes.	Causes sedation. May lower seizure threshold and causes alpha-adrenergic blockade. Produces extrapyramidal side effects in some individuals.	Used for vomiting caused by toxins, drugs, or gastrointestinal disease.	Thorazine	25 mg/ml injection solution	0.5 mg/kg IM, SC q6-8h (before cancer chemotherapy administer 2 mg/kg SC q3h)
Chlortetracycline	Tetracycline antibacterial drug. Inhibits bacterial protein synthesis by interfering with peptide elongation by ribosome. Bacteriostatic agent with broad spectrum of activity.	Avoid use in young animals; may bind to bone and developing teeth. High doses have caused renal injury.	Broad spectrum antibiotic. Used for routine infections and intracellular pathogens.	Generic	Powder	25 mg/kg PO q6-8h
Chorionic gonadotropin	See gonadotropin.					
Cimetidine	Histamine-2 antagonist (H$_2$ blocker). Blocks histamine stimulation of gastric parietal cell to decrease gastric acid secretion. Used to treat ulcers and gastritis.	Adverse effects usually seen only with decreased renal clearance. In humans, CNS signs may occur with high doses. May increase concentrations of other drugs used concurrently (e.g., theophylline) because of inhibition of hepatic enzymes.	Precise doses needed to treat ulcers have not been established. Doses are derived from gastric secretory studies.	Tagamet (OTC and prescription)	100, 150, 200, 300 mg tablets; 60 mg/ml injection	10 mg/kg IV, IM, PO q6-8h (in renal failure, administer 2.5-5 mg/kg IV, PO q12h)
Ciprofloxacin	Fluoroquinolone antibacterial. Acts to inhibit DNA gyrase and inhibit cell DNA and RNA synthesis. Bactericidal. Broad antimicrobial activity.	Avoid use in dogs 4 weeks to 7 months of age. High concentrations may cause CNS toxicity, especially in animals with renal failure. Use cautiously in epileptic patients. Causes occasional vomiting.	Doses are based on plasma concentrations needed to achieve sufficient plasma concentration above MIC. Efficacy studies have not been performed in dogs or cats. IV solution should be given slowly.	Cipro	250, 500, and 750 mg tablet. 2 mg/mL injection.	5-15 mg/kg PO, IV q12h
Cisapride	Prokinetic agent. Stimulates gastric and intestinal motility by either acetylcholine action, activity on serotonin receptors, or direct effect on smooth muscle. Used for gastric reflux, gastroparesis, ileus, and constipation.	Contraindicated in patients with gastrointestinal obstruction	Doses are based on extrapolation from human doses, experimental studies, and anecdotal evidence. Efficacy studies have not been performed in dogs or cats.	Propulsid (Prepulsid in Canada)	10 mg tablet	Dogs: 0.1-0.5 mg/kg PO q8-12h. Cats: 2.5-5 mg/cat PO q8-12h. (As much as 1 mg/kg q8h has been administered to cats.)
Cisplatin	Anticancer agent. Used for treating various solid tumors, including osteosarcoma. Action is believed to be similar to bifunctional alkylating agents and interrupts replication of DNA in tumor cells.	Nephrotoxicity is the most limiting factor to cisplatin therapy. Cats are sensitive to cisplatin. Vomiting may occur in dogs with administration. Transient thrombocytopenia may occur in dogs.	To avoid toxicity, fluid loading before administration using sodium chloride should be performed. Antiemetic agents are often administered before therapy to decrease vomiting.	Platinol	1 mg/ml injection	60-70 mg/m^2 IV every 3-4 weeks (administer aggressive fluid diuresis with therapy).
Clavamox	See amoxicillin/clavulanic acid.					
Clavulanic acid	See amoxicillin/clavulanic acid.					

Drug name	Pharmacology and category of use	Precautions	Dosing information and comments	Other names	Formulations available	Dosage
Clemastine	Antihistamine (H1 blocker). Blocks action of histamine on tissues. Used primarily for treatment of allergy. Some evidence suggests that clemastine is more effective than other antihistamines for pruritus in dogs.	Sedation is the most common side effect.	Used for short-term treatment of pruritus in dogs. May be more efficacious when combined with other antiinflammatory drugs. Tavist syrup contains 5.5% alcohol.	Tavist, Contac 12 hr. allergy and generic.	1.34 mg tablets (OTC) 2.64 mg tablets (Rx) (1 mg tablets in Canada); 0.134 mg/ml syrup	Dogs: 0.05 mg/kg PO q12h
Clindamycin	Antibacterial drug of the lincosamide class (similar in action to macrolides). Inhibits bacterial protein synthesis via inhibition of bacterial ribosome. Bacteriostatic with spectrum of activity primarily against gram-positive bacteria and anaerobes.	Generally well tolerated in dogs and cats. Oral liquid product may be unpalatable to cats. Lincomycin and clindamycin may alter bacterial population in intestine and cause diarrhea; for this reason, do not administer to rodents or rabbits.	Most doses are based on manufacturer's drug approval data and efficacy trials. See dosing column for specific guidelines for different infections.	Antirobe, Cleocin	25 mg/ml oral liquid; 25, 75, 150 mg capsule; 150 mg/ml injection (Cleocin)	Dogs: 11 mg/kg PO q12h or 22 mg/kg PO q24h. Cats: 5.5 mg/kg q12h or 11 mg/kg q24h (Staphylococcal infections); 11 mg/kg q12h or 22 mg/kg PO q24h (anaerobic infections). Toxoplasmosis: 12.5 mg/kg PO q12h (in divided treatments) for 4 weeks.
Clofazimine	Antimicrobial agent used to treat feline leprosy. Slow bactericidal effect on Mycobacterium leprae.	Adverse effects have not been reported in cats. In humans, the most serious adverse effects are gastrointestinal.	Doses are based on empiricism or extrapolation of human studies.	Lamprene	50, 100 mg capsules	Cats: 1 mg/kg PO (up to a maximum of 4 mg/kg/day)
Clomipramine	Tricyclic antidepressant (TCA). Used in humans to treat anxiety and depression. Used in animals to treat variety of behavioral disorders, including obsessive-compulsive disorders. Action is via inhibition of uptake of serotonin at presynaptic nerve terminals.	Multiple side effects are associated with tricyclic antidepressants such as antimuscarinic effects (dry mouth, rapid heart rate) and antihistamine effects (sedation). High doses can produce life-threatening cardiotoxicity.	Doses are primarily based on empiricism. There are no controlled efficacy trials available for animals. There may be a 2-4 week delay after initiation of therapy before beneficial effects are seen.	Anafranil	10, 25, 50 mg tablets	1 mg/kg/day PO (up to a maximum dose of 3 mg/kg/day PO)
Clonazepam	Benzodiazepine. Action is to enhance inhibitory effects of GABA in central nervous system. Used for antiseizure action, sedation, and treatment of some behavioral disorders.	Side effects include sedation and polyphagia. Some animals may experience paradoxical excitement.	Doses are based primarily on reports from human medicine, empiricism, or experimental studies. No clinical efficacy studies have been performed in dogs or cats.	Klonopin	0.5, 1, 2 mg tablets	0.5 mg/kg PO q8-12h
Clorazepate	Benzodiazepine. Action is to enhance inhibitory effects of GABA in central nervous system. Used for antiseizure action, sedation, and treatment of some behavioral disorders.	Side effects include sedation and polyphagia. Some animals may experience paradoxical excitement.	Doses are based primarily on reports from human medicine, empiricism, or experimental studies. No clinical efficacy studies have been performed in dogs or cats. Clorazepate tablets degrade quickly in presence of light, heat, or moisture. Keep in original packaging or in tightly sealed container.	Tranxene	3.75, 7.5, 11.25, 15, 22.5 mg tablets	2 mg/kg PO q12h
Cloxacillin	Beta-lactam antibiotic. Inhibits bacterial cell wall synthesis. Spectrum is limited to gram-positive bacteria, especially staphylococci.	Use cautiously in animals allergic to penicillin-like drugs.	Doses based on empiricism or extrapolation from human studies. No clinical efficacy studies available for dogs or cats. Administer on empty stomach if possible.	Cloxapen, Orbenin, Tegopen	250, 500 mg capsules; 25 mg/ml oral solution	20-40 mg/kg PO q8h

Drug name	Pharmacology and category of use	Precautions	Dosing information and comments	Other names	Formulations available	Dosage
Codeine	Opiate agonist. Mechanism is similar to morphine, except with approximately one tenth the potency of morphine. See morphine for further details.	See morphine.	Doses listed for analgesia are considered initial doses; individual patients may need higher doses depending on degree of tolerance or pain threshold.	Generic	15, 30, 60 mg tablets; 5 mg/ml syrup	Analgesia: 0.5-1 mg/kg PO q 6-8h. Antitussive: 0.1-0.3 mg/kg PO q6-8h.
Colchicine	Antiinflammatory agent. Used primarily to treat gout. In animals, used to decrease fibrosis and development of hepatic failure (possibly by inhibiting formation of collagen).	Do not administer to pregnant animals. Adverse effects are not well documented in animals. Colchicine may cause dermititis in humans.	Doses based on empiricism. There are no well-controlled efficacy studies in veterinary species.	Generic	0.5, 0.6 mg tablets; injection	0.01-0.03 mg/kg PO q24h
Colony-stimulating factor	Stimulates granulocyte development in bone marrow. Used primarily to regenerate blood cells to recover from cancer chemotherapy or other therapy.		Doses are based on limited experimental information performed in dogs (JAVMA 1992;200: 1957).	Amgen		2.5 mcg/kg SC q12h
Corticotropin (ACTH)	Used for diagnostic purposes to evaluate adrenal gland function. Stimulates normal synthesis of cortisol from adrenal gland.	Adverse effects unlikely when used as single injection for diagnostic purposes.	Doses established by measuring normal adrenal response in animals.	Acthar	40 U/ml gel	Response test: Collect pre-ACTH sample and inject 2.2 IU/kg IM. Collect post-ACTH sample in 2 hours in dogs and at 1 and 2 hours in cats.
Cosequin	Cosequin is brand name for combination of glucosamine HCL and chondroitin sulfate. According to manufacturer these compounds stimulate synthesis of synovial fluid and inhibit degradation and improve healing of articular cartilage. Used primarily for degenerative joint disease.	Adverse effects have not been reported, although hypersensitivity is possible.	Doses are based primarily on empiricism and manufacturer's recommendations. No published trials of efficacy are available.	Cosequin	Regular strength (RS) and double strength (DS) capsules	Dogs: 1-2 RS capsules per day; 2-4 capsules of DS for large dogs. Cats: 1 RS capsule daily.
Cosyntropin	Cosyntropin is a synthetic form of corticotropin (ACTH) used for diagnostic purposes only. In humans it is preferred over corticotropin because it is less allergenic.	Same as for corticotropin	Same as for corticotropin. Use for diagnostic purposes only; not intended for treatment of hypoadrenocorticism.	Cortrosyn	250 µg per vial	Response test: Collect pre-ACTH sample and inject 0.25 mg IV in dogs and 0.125 mg IV in cats. Collect post-ACTH sample at 1 hour.
Cyanocobalamin (vitamin B$_{12}$)	Vitamin B analogue	Adverse effects are rare except in high overdoses.	Same as for other vitamin B preparations	Many	100 µg/ml injection	Dogs: 100-200 µg/day PO. Cats: 50-100 µg/day PO.
Cyclophosphamide	Cytotoxic agent. Bifunctional alkylating agent. Disrupts base-pairing and inhibits DNA and RNA synthesis. Cytotoxic for tumor cells and other rapidly dividing cells. Used primarily as adjunct for cancer chemotherapy and as immunosuppressive therapy.	Bone marrow suppression is most common adverse effect. Can produce severe neutropenia (that usually is reversible). Vomiting and diarrhea may occur in some patients. Dogs are susceptible to bladder toxicity (sterile hemorrhagic cystitis). May cause hair loss when used in some chemotherapeutic protocols.	Cyclophosphamide is usually administered with other drugs (other cancer drugs in cancer protocols or corticosteroids when used for immunosuppressive therapy). Consult specific anticancer protocols for specific regimens.	Cytoxan, Neosar	25 mg/ml injection; 25, 50 mg tablets	Anticancer: 50 mg/m^2 PO once daily 4 days per week or 150-300 mg/m^2 IV and repeat in 21 days. Immunosuppressive therapy: 50 mg/m^2 (approx. 2.2 mg/kg) PO q48h or 2.2 mg/kg once daily 4 days per week. Cats: 6.25-12.5 mg/cat once daily 4 days per week.

Drug name	Pharmacology and category of use	Precautions	Dosing information and comments	Other names	Formulations available	Dosage
Cyclosporine	Immunosuppressive drug. Depresses T lymphocytes.	Can cause vomiting, diarrhea, and anorexia. Nephrotoxicity may occur. In comparison to other immunosuppressive drugs, does not cause myelosuppression. Cimetidine, erythromycin, or ketoconazole may increase cyclosporine concentrations when used concurrently.	Adjust dose via monitoring if possible. Although topical drugs are not listed in this table, cyclosporine has been used successfully as topic treatment for keratoconjunctivitis sicca.	Sandimmune, Optimmune (ophthalmic)	100 mg/ml oral solution; 25, 100 mg capsules; 0.2% ointment; 50 mg/ml injection	Dogs: 10 and up to 17 mg/kg PO q24h. Cats: 10 mg/kg PO q12h.
Cyproheptadine	Phenothiazine with antihistamine and antiserotonin properties. Used as appetite stimulant (probably by altering serotonin activity in appetite center).	May cause increased appetite and weight gain	Clinical studies have not been performed in veterinary medicine. Use is based primarily on empiricism and extrapolation from human results. Syrup contains 5% alcohol.	Periactin	4 mg tablet; 2 mg/5 ml syrup	Antihistamine: 1.1 mg/kg PO q8-12h. Appetite stimulant: 2 mg/cat PO.
Cytarabine (cytosine arabinoside)	Anticancer agent. Exact mechanism is not known. Probably inhibits DNA synthesis. Used for lymphoma and leukemia protocols.	Bone marrow suppression. Causes vomiting and nausea.	Consult anticancer protocols for precise dosing regimens.	Cytosar	100 mg vial	Dogs (lymphoma): 100 mg/m^2 IV, SC once daily or 50 mg/m^2 twice daily for 4 days. Cats: 100 mg/m^2 once daily for 2 days.
Dacarbazine	Anticancer agent. Monofunctional alkylating agent. Used for melanoma.	Leukopenia, nausea, vomiting, and diarrhea. Do not use in cats.	Consult anticancer protocol for specific regimens.	DTIC	200 mg vial for injection	200 mg/m^2 IV for 5 days every 3 weeks or 800-1,000 mg/m^2 IV every 3 weeks
Danazol	Gonadotropin inhibitor. Suppresses LH and FSH and estrogen synthesis. In humans, used for endometriosis. May reduce destruction of platelets or RBC in immune-mediated disease.	May cause signs similar to other adrogenic drugs. Adverse effects have not been reported in animals. Gonadotropin inhibitor.	When used to treat autoimmune disease, usually used in conjunction with other drugs (e.g., corticosteroids)	Danocrine	50, 100, 200 mg capsules	5-10 mg/kg PO q12h
Dantrolene	Muscle relaxant. Inhibits calcium leakage from sarcoplasmic reticulum. In addition to muscle relaxation, it has been used for malignant hyperthermia. Also has been used to relax urethral muscle in cats.	Muscle relaxant can cause weakness in some animals.	Doses have been primarily extrapolated from experimental studies or human studies. No clinical trials available in veterinary medicine. Studies in which dantrolene relaxed urethra in cats used 1 mg/kg IV.	Dantrium	100 mg capsule	Dogs: 1-5 mg/kg PO q8h. Cats: 0.5-2 mg/kg PO q12h.
Dapsone	Antimicrobial drug used primarily for treatment of mycobacterium. May have some immunosuppressive properties or inhibit function of inflammatory cells. Used primarily for dermatologic diseases in dogs and cats.	Hepatitis and blood dyscrasias may occur. Toxic dermatological reactions have been seen in humans. Do not administer with trimethoprim (may increase blood concentrations).	Doses are derived from extrapolation of human doses or empiricism. No well-controlled clinical studies have been performed in veterinary medicine.	Generic	25, 100 mg tablets	1.1 mg/kg PO q8-12h

Drug name	Pharmacology and category of use	Precautions	Dosing information and comments	Other names	Formulations available	Dosage
Darbazine (prochlor-perazine and isopropamide)	Combination product. Prochlorperazine is a central-acting dopamine antagonist (antiemetic); iso-propamide is an anti-cholinergic drug (at-ropine-like effects). Used primarily to control vomiting in animals.	Side effects are at-tributed to each com-ponent. Prochlor-perazine produces phenothiazine-like ef-fects. See acepro-mazine. Isopro-pamide produces antimuscarinic ef-fects. See atropine. Use of antimuscarinic drugs is contraindi-cated in animals with gastroparesis and should be used cau-tiously in animals with diarrhea.	Doses are based on manufacturer's recommendations.	Darbazine	Capsules No. 1, 2, and 3	Dogs and cats: 0.14-0.2 ml/kg SC q12h. Dogs 2-7 kg: 1-#1 capsule PO q12h. Dogs 7-14 kg: 1-#2 capsule PO q12h. Dogs > 14 kg: 1-#3 capsule PO q12h.
Deferoxamine	Chelating agent with strong affinity for di- and trivalent cations. Used to treat acute iron toxicosis. Indicated in cases of severe poisoning. Deferoxamine also has been used to chelate aluminum and facilitate removal.	Adverse effects have not been reported in animals. Allergic re-actions and hearing problems have oc-curred in humans.	100 mg of deferox-amine binds 8.5 mg of ferric iron. Monitor serum iron concentra-tions to determine severity of intoxica-tion and success of therapy. Contact local poison control center for guidance. Successful therapy is indicated by monitor-ing urine color (orange-rose color change to urine indi-cates chelated iron is being eliminated).	Desferal	500 mg vial for injec-tion	10 mg/kg IV, IM q2h for two doses, then 10 mg/kg q8h for 24 hours
Deprenyl (L-deprenyl)	See selegiline.					
Desmopressin acetate	Synthetic peptide similar to antidiuretic hormone (ADH). Used as replacement therapy for patients with diabetes in-sipidus. Desmopressin also has been used for treatment of patients with mild to moderate von Willebrand dis-ease before surgery or other procedures that may cause bleeding.	No side effects re-ported. In humans, it rarely causes throm-botic events.	Desmopressin is used only for central diabetes insipidus. It is ineffective for treat-ment of nephrogenic diabetes insipidus or polyuria from other causes. Intranasal product has been ad-ministered as eye drops in dogs (JAV-MA 1994;205:170).	DDAVP	100 µg/ml injection; desmopressin ac-etate nasal solution (0.01% metered spray)	Diabetes insipidus: 2-4 drops (2 mg) q12-24h intranasally or in eye. Von Willebrand dis-ease: 1 µg/kg (0.01 ml/kg) SC, IV diluted in 20 ml of saline ad-ministered over 10 minutes.
Desoxycortico-sterone pivalate	Mineralocorticoid. Used for adrenocorti-co insufficiency (hy-poadrenocorticism). No glucocorticoid activity.	Excessive mineralo-corticoid effects with high doses	Initial dose based on studies performed in clinical patients. Individual doses may be based on monitor-ing electrolytes in patients.	DOCP, DOCA pivalate	Injection	1.5-2.2 mg/kg IM every 25 days
Detomidine	Alpha-2 (α_2) adrener-gic agonist. More po-tent and more specif-ic than xylazine. Used primarily for anesthe-sia and analgesia.	Potent alpha-2 ago-nist. Produces seda-tion and ataxia. Cardiac depression, heart block, and hy-potension possible with high doses.	Doses have not been established for small animals; used primar-ily for horses.	Dormosedan	10 mg/ml injection	Doses have not been established for small animals.
Dexamethasone	Corticosteroid. Dexamethasone has approximately 30 times the potency of cortisol. Multiple anti-inflammatory effects. See betamethasone.	Multiple side effects. See betamethasone.	Doses are based on severity of underlying disease. See betamethasone.	Azium, generic	2 mg/ml sodium phosphate (5 mg/ml) solution; 0.25, 0.5 mg tablets	Antiinflammatory: 0.1-0.2 mg/kg IV, IM, PO q12-24h. Shock, spinal injury: 2.2-4.4 mg/kg IV.

Drug name	Pharmacology and category of use	Precautions	Dosing information and comments	Other names	Formulations available	Dosage
Dextran	Synthetic colloid used for volume expansion. High molecular weight fluid replacement. Primarily used for acute hypovolemia and shock.	Only limited use in veterinary medicine and adverse effects have not been reported. In humans, coagulopathies are possible because of decreased platelet function. Anaphylactic shock also has occurred.	Used primarily in critical care situations. Delivered slowly via constant rate infusion. Monitor patient's cardiopulmonary status carefully during administration.	Dextran 70, Gentran 70	250, 500, 1,000 ml injectable solution	10-20 ml/kg IV to effect
Dextromethorphan	Centrally-acting antitussive drug. Shares similar chemical structure as opiates, but does not affect opiate receptors. Appears to directly affect cough receptor.	Adverse effects not reported in veterinary medicine. High overdose may cause sedation.	Many OTC preparations that may contain other ingredients (e.g., antihistamines, decongestants, and acetaminophen)	Benylin, others	Syrup; capsules; tablets; many OTC products	0.5-2 mg/kg PO q6-8h
Dextrose solution 5%	Sugar added to fluid solutions. Isotonic.	High doses produce pulmonary edema.	Commonly used fluid solution administered via constant rate infusion. *Not* a maintenance solution.	D5W	Fluid solution for IV administration	40-50 ml/kg IV q24h
Diazepam	Benzodiazepine. Central-acting CNS depressant. Mechanism of action appears to be via potentiation of GABA-receptor mediated effects in CNS. Used for sedation, anesthetic adjunct, anticonvulsant, and behavioral disorders. Diazepam metabolized to desmethyldiazepam (nordiazepam) and oxazepam.	Sedation is the most common side effect. May cause paradoxical excitement in dogs. Causes polyphagia. In cats, fatal hepatic necrosis has been reported.	Clearance in dogs is many times faster than in humans (half-life in dogs less than 1 hour). Requires frequent administration. For treatment of status epilepticus, may be administered IV or rectally. Avoid IM administration.	Valium, generic	2, 5 mg tablets; 5 mg/ml solution for injection	Preanesthetic: 0.5 mg/kg IV. Status epilepticus: 0.5 mg/kg IV, 1 mg/kg rectal, repeat if necessary. Appetite stimulant (cat): 0.2 mg/kg IV.
Dichlorophene	Vermiplex. See toluene.					
Dichlorphenamide	Carbonic anhydrase inhibitor. Diuretic. Acts to inhibit enzyme that forms hydrogen and bicarbonate ions. Reduces plasma bicarbonate concentration, producing systemic metabolic acidosis and alkaline diuresis. Primarily used to treat glaucoma.	Sulfonamide derivative. Use cautiously in animals sensitive to sulfonamides. Hypokalemia may occur in some patients. Severe metabolic acidosis is rare.	Dichlorphenamide is not used as diuretic but is most commonly employed to treat glaucoma. May be combined with other antiglaucoma agents.	Daranide	50 mg tablet	3-5 mg/kg PO q8-12h
Dichlorvos	Antiparasitic drug used primarily to treat hookworms, roundworms, and whipworms. Kills parasites by anticholinesterase action.	Do not use in heartworm-positive patients. Overdoses can cause organophosphate intoxication. (Treat with 2-PAM, atropine.)	Doses are based on manufacturer's recommendations.	Task	10, 25 mg tablets	Dogs: 26.4-33 mg/kg PO. Cats: 11 mg/kg PO.
Dicloxacillin	Beta-lactam antibiotic. Inhibits bacterial cell wall synthesis. Spectrum is limited to gram-positive bacteria, especially staphylococci.	Use cautiously in animals allergic to penicillin-like drugs.	Doses based on empiricism or extrapolation from human studies. No clinical efficacy studies available for dogs or cats. Administer on empty stomach if possible.	Dynapen	125, 250, 500 mg capsules; 12.5 mg/ml oral solution	11-55 mg/kg PO q8h

Drug name	Pharmacology and category of use	Precautions	Dosing information and comments	Other names	Formulations available	Dosage
Diethylcarbamazine (DEC)	Heartworm preventative. For action, see piperazine.	Safe in all species. Reactions can occur in animals with positive microfilaria.	Doses based on manufacturer's recommendations. Specific protocols for heartworm administration may be based on region of country.	Caricide, Filaribits	50, 60, 180, 200, 400 mg chewable tablets	Heartworm prophylaxis: 6.6 mg/kg PO q24h
Diethylstilbestrol (DES)	Synthetic estrogen compound. Used for estrogen replacement in animals. DES is most commonly used to treat estrogen-responsive incontinence in dogs. Also has been used to induce abortion in dogs.	Side effects may occur that are caused by excess estrogen. Estrogen therapy may increase risk of pyometra and estrogen-sensitive tumors.	Doses listed are for treating urinary incontinence and vary depending on response. Titrate dose to individual patients. Although used to induce abortion, it was *not* efficacious in one study that administered 75 µg/kg.	DES, generic	1, 5 mg tablets; 50 mg/ml injection	Dogs: 0.1-1.0 mg/dog PO q24h. Cats: 0.05-0.1 mg/cat PO q24h.
Digitoxin	Cardiac ionotropic agent. Increases cardiac contractility and decreases heart rate. Mechanism is via inactivation of cardiac muscle sodium-potassium ATPase. Beneficial effects for heart failure may occur via neuroendocrine effects (alters sensitivity of baroreceptors).	Digitalis glycosides have narrow therapeutic index. May cause variety of arrhythmias in patients (e.g., heart block and ventricular tachycardia). Causes vomiting, anorexia, and diarrhea. Adverse effects potentiated by hypokalemia and reduced by hyperkalemia. Some breeds of dogs (Dobermans) and cats more sensitive to adverse effects.	Used in heart failure for ionotropic effect and to decrease heart rate. Used in supraventricular arrhythmias to decrease ventricular response to atrial stimulation. May be used with other cardiac drugs. Monitor concentrations in patients to determine optimum therapy.	Crystodigin	0.05, 0.1 mg tablets	0.02-0.03 mg/kg PO q8h
Digoxin	Cardiac glycoside. See digitoxin.	See digitoxin.	Monitor patients carefully. Optimum plasma concentration is 1-2 ng/ml. Adverse effects common at concentration above 3.5 ng/ml. When dosing, calculate dose on lean body weight. Doses should be 10% less for elixir because of increased absorption.	Lanoxin, Cardoxin	0.0625, 0.125, 0.25 mg tablets; 0.05, 0.15 mg/ml elixir	Dogs: 0.22 mg/m² PO q12h (subtract 10% for elixir). Dogs (rapid digitalization): 0.0055-0.011 mg/kg IV q1h to effect. Cats 2-3 kg: 0.0312 mg PO q48h. Cats 4-5 kg: 0.0312 mg PO q24h. Cats > 6kg: 0.0312 mg PO q12h.
Dihydrotachysterol (vitamin D)	Vitamin D analogue. Used as treatment of hypocalcemia, especially that associated with hypothyroidism. Vitamin D promotes absorption and utilization of calcium.	Overdose may cause hypercalcemia. Avoid use in pregnant animals because it may cause fetal abnormalities. Use cautiously with high doses of calcium-containing preparations.	Available as oral solution, tablets, and capsules. Doses for individual patients should be adjusted by monitoring serum calcium concentrations.	Hytakerol, DHT	0.125 mg tablet; 0.5 mg/ml oral liquid	0.01 mg/kg/day PO. Acute treatment: administer 0.02 mg/kg initially, then 0.01-0.02 mg/kg PO q24-48h thereafter.
Diltiazem	Calcium-channel blocking drug. Blocks calcium entry into cells via blockade of slow channel. Produces vasodilation and negative chronotropic effects.	Hypotension, cardiac depression, bradycardia, and AV block. May cause anorexia in some patients.	Diltiazem preferred over verapamil in patients with heart failure because of less cardiac suppression. Note that in cats, when using sustained release form (XR or CD), doses are higher but administered once daily.	Cardizem, Dilacor	30, 60, 90, 120 mg tablets; 50 mg/ml injection	Dogs: 0.5-1.5 mg/kg PO q8h. Cats: 1.75-2.4 mg/kg PO q8h. Dilacor XR or Cardizem CD dose is 10 mg/kg PO q24h.
Dimenhydrinate	Antihistamine drug. See chlorpheniramine.	See chlorpheniramine.	See chlorpheniramine. There have been no clinical studies on the use of dimenhydrinate. It is primarily used empirically for treatment of vomiting.	Dramamine (Gravol in Canada)	Tablets; injection	4-8 mg/kg PO, IM, IV q8h. Cats: 12.5 mg PO, IM, IV q8h.

Drug name	Pharmacology and category of use	Precautions	Dosing information and comments	Other names	Formulations available	Dosage
Dimercaprol (BAL)	Chelating agent. Used to treat lead, gold, and arsenic toxicity.	Adverse effects not reported in veterinary medicine. In humans, sterile abscesses occur at injection site. High doses have caused seizures, drowsiness, and vomiting.	Use as soon as possible after intoxicant exposure. Alkalinization of urine will increase toxin removal. For lead intoxication, may be used with edetate calcium.	BAL in oil	Injection	4 mg/kg IM q4h
Dinoprost tromethamine	See prostaglandin $F_{2\alpha}$ 5 mg/ml injection.					
Dioctyl calcium sulfosuccinate	See docusate calcium.					
Dioctyl sodium sulfosuccinate	See docusate sodium.					
Diphenhydramine	Antihistamine. See chlorpheniramine.	See chlorpheniramine.	Antihistamine used primarily for allergic disease in animals	Benadryl	Available OTC; 2.5 mg/ml elixir; 25, 50 mg capsules; 50 mg/ml injection	2-4 mg/kg mg/kg IV, IM, PO q6-8h. Dogs: 25-50 mg/dog IV, IM, PO q8h.
Diphenoxylate	Opiate agonist. Stimulates smooth muscle segmentation in intestine as well as electrolyte absorption. Used for acute treatment of nonspecific diarrhea.	Adverse effects have not been reported in veterinary medicine. Diphenoxylate is poorly absorbed systemically and produces few systemic side effects. Excessive use can cause constipation.	Doses are based primarily on empiricism or extrapolation of human dose. Clinical studies have not been performed in animals. Contains atropine but dose is not high enough for significant systemic effects.	Lomotil	2.5 mg	Dogs: 0.1-0.2 mg/kg PO q8-12h. Cats: 0.05-0.1 mg/kg PO q12h.
Diphenylhydantoin	See phenytoin.					
Diphosphonate disodium edidronate	See etidronate disodium.					
Dipyridamole	Platelet inhibitor. Mechanism of action is attributed to increased levels of cAMP in platelet, which decreases platelet activation. Indicated primarily to prevent thromboembolism.	Adverse effects have not been reported in animals.	Used primarily in humans to prevent thromboembolism. Use in animals has not been reported. When used in humans, it is combined with other antithrombotic agents (e.g., warfarin).	Persantine	25, 50, 75 mg tablets; 5 mg/ml injection	4-10 mg/kg PO q24h
Dipyrone	No longer available commercially. (Previous use in animals was 28 mg/kg IV, IM, SC q8h.)					
Disopyramide	Class I antiarrhythmic agent. Depresses myocardial electrophysiological conduction rate.	Adverse effects have not been reported in animals. High doses may cause cardiac arrhythmias.	Not commonly used in veterinary medicine. Other antiarrhythmic drugs are preferred.	Norpace (Rhythmodan, Canada)	100, 150 mg capsules. (10 mg/mL injection, Canada only.)	6-15 mg/kg PO q8h
Disophenol Withdrawn from market by manufacturer.						
Dithiazine iodide	Microfilaricidal drug for dogs. Also effective for hookworms, roundworms, and whipworms.	Adverse effects are rare. Causes vomiting in some dogs. Causes discoloration of feces.	Before ivermectin and similar drugs, this was the only microfilaricidal agent for dogs. Not commonly used.	Dizan	10, 50, 100, 200 mg tablets.	Heartworms: 6.6-11 mg/kg PO q24h for 7-10 days. For other parasites: 22 mg/kg PO
Divalproex sodium	Depakote, Epival. Equivalent to valproic acid. See valproic acid.					

Drug name	Pharmacology and category of use	Precautions	Dosing information and comments	Other names	Formulations available	Dosage
Dobutamine	Adrenergic agonist. Action is primarily to stimulate myocardium via action on cardiac beta-1 (β_1) receptors. Increases heart contraction without increase in heart rate. Some action may occur via alpha receptors. Primarily used for acute treatment of heart failure.	May cause tachycardia and ventricular arrhythmias at high doses or in sensitive individuals	Dobutamine has a very rapid elimination half-life (minutes) and therefore must be administered via carefully monitored constant rate infusion. When mixing, avoid alkalinizing solutions. Administer in 5% dextrose solution (250 mg in 1 L 5% dextrose).	Dobutrex	250 mg per 20 ml vial for injection	Dogs: 2.5-20 mcg/kg/min IV infusion. Cats: 1-5 mcg/kg/min IV infusion.
Docusate calcium	Stool softener (surfactant). Acts to decrease surface tension to allow more water to accumulate in the stool.	No adverse effects reported in animals. In humans, high doses have caused abdominal discomfort.	Doses are based on extrapolations from humans or empiricism. No clinical studies reported for animals. Docusate calcium products may contain stimulant cathartic phenolphthalein, which should be used cautiously in cats.	Surfak, Doxidan	60 mg tablet; many others	Dogs: 50-100 mg PO q12-24h. Cats: 50 mg PO q12-24h.
Docusate sodium	See docusate calcium.	See docusate calcium.	See docusate calcium.	Colace, Doxan, Doss, many OTC brands	50, 100 mg capsules; 10 mg/ml liquid	Dogs: 50-200 mg PO q8-12h. Cats: 50 mg PO q12-24h.
Domperidone	Motility modifier (similar to metoclopramide)	See metoclopramide.	Not available in United States, only in Canada	Motilium	Not available in United States	2-5 mg/animal PO
Dopamine	Adrenergic agonist. Action is primarily to stimulate myocardium via action on cardiac beta-1 (β_1) receptors. There is some suggestion that dopamine increases renal perfusion via action on renal dopaminergic receptors; however, clinical evidence for beneficial effect is lacking.	May cause tachycardia and ventricular arrhythmias at high doses or in sensitive individuals.	Dopamine has a very rapid elimination half-life (minutes) and therefore must be administered via carefully monitored constant rate infusion. When mixing, avoid alkalinizing solutions. Administer in 5% dextrose solution or LRS (40 mg in 500 ml of fluid).	Intropin	40, 80, 160 mg/ml	2-10 mcg/kg/min IV infusion
Doxapram	Respiratory stimulant via action on carotid chemoreceptors and subsequent stimulation of respiratory center. Used to treat respiratory depression or to stimulate respiration postanesthesia. May also increase cardiac output.	Adverse effects not reported in animals. Cardiovascular effects and convulsions have occurred with high doses in humans. Contraindicated in newborn infants because it contains benzyl alcohol as vehicle.	Used for short-term treatment only	Dopram	20 mg/ml injection	5-10 mg/kg IV. Neonate: 1-5 mg SC, sublingual, or via umbilical vein.
Doxorubicin	Anticancer agent. Acts to intercalate between bases on DNA, disrupting DNA, and RNA synthesis in tumor cell. Doxorubicin also may affect tumor cell membranes. Used for treatment of various neoplasia, including lymphoma.	Most common acute effect is anorexia, vomiting, and diarrhea. Dose-related toxicity also includes bone marrow suppression, hair loss (in certain breeds), and cardiotoxicity. Cardiotoxicity limits the total dose administered (usually do not exceed 200 mg/m²).	Regimen listed may differ for various tumors. Consult specific anticancer protocol for guidelines. Dose must be infused IV (over 20-30 minutes). Animals may require antiemetic and antihistamine before therapy. Monitor ECG during therapy.	Adriamycin	2 mg/ml injection	30 mg/m² IV every 21 days

Drug name	Pharmacology and category of use	Precautions	Dosing information and comments	Other names	Formulations available	Dosage
Doxycycline	Tetracycline antibiotic. Mechanism of action of tetracyclines is to bind to 30S ribosomal subunit and inhibit protein synthesis. Usually bactericidal. Broad spectrum of activity, including bacteria, some protozoa, Rickettsia, and Ehrlichia.	Severe adverse reactions not reported with doxycycline. Tetracyclines in general may cause renal tubular necrosis at high doses. Tetracyclines can affect bone and teeth formation in young animals. Tetracyclines bind to calcium-containing compounds, which decreases oral absorption.	Many pharmacokinetic and experimental studies have been conducted in small animals, but no clinical studies. Ordinarily considered the drug of choice for Rickettsia and Ehrlichia infections in dogs. Doxycycline IV infusion is stable for only 12 hours at room temperature and 72 hours if refrigerated.	Vibramycin, generic forms	10 mg/ml oral suspension; 100 mg tablet; 100 mg injection vial	3-5 mg/kg PO, IV q12h or 10 mg/kg PO q24h Rickettsia in dogs: 5 mg/kg q12h
Edetate calcium disodium (CaNa$_2$EDTA)	Chelating agent. Indicated for treatment of acute and chronic lead poisoning. Sometimes used in combination with dimercaprol (BAL).	No adverse effects reported in animals. In humans, allergic reactions (release of histamine) occurs after IV administration.	May be used with dimercaprol. Equally effective when administered IV or IM, but IM injection may be painful. Ensure adequate urine flow before the first dose.	Calcium disodium versenate	20 mg/ml injection	25 mg/kg SC, IM, IV q6h for 2-5 days
Edrophonium	Cholinesterase inhibitor. Causes cholinergic effects by inhibiting metabolism of acetylcholine. Very short acting and ordinarily is only used for diagnostic purposes (e.g., for myasthenia gravis). Also has been used to reverse neuromuscular blockade of nondepolarizing agents (pancuronium).	Short acting and side effects are minimal. Excessive muscarinic/cholinergic effects may occur with high doses (counteract with atropine).	Usually used only for determination of diagnosis of myasthenia gravis. Too short acting to be used for therapy.	Tensilon, others	10 mg/ml injection	Dogs: 0.11-0.22 mg/kg IV. Cats: 2.5 mg/cat IV.
Enalapril	ACE inhibitor. See captopril for details. Used for vasodilation and treatment of heart failure.	See captopril. May cause azotemia in some patients; carefully monitor patients receiving high doses of diuretics. Use cautiously with other hypotensive drugs and diuretics. NSAIDs may decrease vasodilating effects.	Doses are based on clinical trials conducted in dogs by manufacturer. For dogs, start with once daily administration and increase to q12h if needed. Other drugs used for treatment of heart failure may be used concurrently. With all ACE inhibitors, monitor electrolytes and renal function 3-7 days after initiating therapy and periodically thereafter.	Enacard, Vasotec	2.5, 5, 10, 20 mg tablets	Dogs: 0.5 mg/kg PO q12-24h. Cats: 0.25-0.5 PO mg/kg q12-24h.
Enflurane	Inhalant anesthetic	Adverse effects (not related to anesthesia) not reported in animals.	Titrate dose for each individual with anesthetic monitoring.	Ethrane	Inhalation	Induction: 2-3% Maintenance: 1.5-3%
Enilconazole	Azole antifungal agent (for topical use only). Like other azoles, inhibits membrane synthesis (ergosterol) in fungus. Highly effective for dermatophytes.	Administered topically. Adverse effects have not been reported.	Imaverol is available only in Canada as 10% emulsion. In the United States, Clinafarm EC is available for use in poultry units as 13.8% solution. Dilute solution to at least 50:1 and apply topically every 3-4 days for 2-3 weeks. Enilconazole also has been instilled as 1:1 dilution into nasal sinus for nasal aspergillosis.	Imaverol, ClinaFarm-EC	10%, 13.8% emulsion	Nasal aspergillosis: 10 mg/kg q12h instilled into nasal sinus for 14 days (10% solution diluted 50/50 with water). Dermatophytes: Dilute 10% solution to 0.2% and wash lesion with solution 4 times at 3-4 day intervals.

Drug name	Pharmacology and category of use	Precautions	Dosing information and comments	Other names	Formulations available	Dosage
Enrofloxacin	Fluoroquinolone antibacterial drug. Acts via inhibition of DNA gyrase in bacteria to inhibit DNA and RNA synthesis. Bactericidal. Broad spectrum of activity.	Adverse effects include seizures in epileptic animals, arthropathy in dogs 4-28 weeks of age, and vomiting in dogs and cats at high doses. May increase concentrations of theophylline if used concurrently. Coadministration with divalent and trivalent cations (e.g., sucralfate) may decrease absorption.	Doses recommended by manufacturer (2.5 mg/kg q12h) effective for most sensitive bacteria or urinary tract infections. For bacteria with higher MIC (e.g., above 0.1 mg/ml), higher doses may be needed (5 µg/kg q24h); for MIC of 0.5 µg/ml, doses of 10-20 mg/kg q24h may be necessary. Solution for IM injection has been IV administered safely.	Baytril	68, 22.7, 5.7 mg tablets; 22.7 mg/ml injection	2.5 mg/kg PO, IM q12h (up to 10 mg/kg q24h) and 20 mg/kg for MIC of 5 µg/ml
Ephedrine	Adrenergic agonist. Agonist on alpha and beta-1 adrenergic receptors, but not beta-2 receptors. Used as vasopressor (e.g., administered during anesthesia). Central nervous system stimulant. Also has been used to treat urinary incontinence because of action on bladder sphincter muscle.	Adverse effects related to excessive adrenergic activity (e.g., peripheral vasoconstriction and tachycardia)	Used primarily in acute situations to increase blood pressure and urinary incontinence in dogs	Many, generic	25, 50 mg/ml injections	Urinary incontinence: 4 mg/kg or 12.5-50 mg/dog PO q8-12h; 2-4 mg/kg for cats. Vasopressor: 0.75 mg/kg IM, SC (repeat as needed).
Epinephrine	Adrenergic agonist. Nonselectively stimulates alpha (α) and beta (β) adrenergic receptors. Used primarily for emergency situations to treat cardiopulmonary arrest and anaphylactic shock.	Overdose will cause excessive vasoconstriction and hypertension. High doses can cause ventricular arrhythmias. When high doses are used for cardiopulmonary arrest, an electrical defibrillator should be available.	Doses are based on experimental studies, primarily in dogs. Clinical studies are not available. IV doses are ordinarily used, but endotracheal administration is acceptable when intravenous access is not available. Intraosseous route also has been used and doses are equivalent to IV. When endotracheal route is used, the dose is higher and duration of effect may be longer than IV administration. There appears to be no advantage to intracardiac injection compared to IV administration.	Adrenaline, generic forms	1 mg/ml (1:1,000) injection solution	Cardiac arrest: 10-20 µg/kg IV or 200 µg/kg intratracheal (may be diluted in saline before administration). Anaphylactic shock: 2.5-5 µg/kg IV or 50 µg/kg intratracheal (may be diluted in saline).
Epsiprantel	Anticestodal agent (similar to praziquantel)	See praziquantel.	See praziquantel.	Cestex	Coated tablet	Dogs: 5.5 mg/kg PO. Cats: 2.75 mg/kg PO.
Ergocalciferol (vitamin D₂)	Vitamin D analogue. Used for vitamin D deficiency and as treatment of hypocalcemia, especially that associated with hypothyroidism. Vitamin D promotes absorption and utilization of calcium.	Overdose may cause hypercalcemia. Avoid use in pregnant animals because it may cause fetal abnormalities. Use cautiously with high doses of calcium-containing preparations.	Should not be used for renal hypoparathyroidism because of inability to convert to active compound. Available as oral solution, tablets, capsules, and injection. Doses for individual patients should be adjusted by monitoring serum calcium concentrations.	Calciferol, Drisdol	400 U tablet (OTC); 50,000 U tablet (1.25 mg); 500,000 U/ml (12.5 mg/ml) injection	500-2000 U/kg/day PO

Drug name	Pharmacology and category of use	Precautions	Dosing information and comments	Other names	Formulations available	Dosage
Erythromycin	Macrolide antibiotic. Inhibits bacteria by binding to 50S ribosome and inhibiting protein synthesis. Spectrum of activity limited primarily to gram-positive aerobic bacteria. Used for skin and respiratory infections.	Most common side effect is vomiting (probably caused by cholinergic-like effect). May cause diarrhea in some animals. Do not administer PO to rodents or rabbits.	There are several forms of erythromycin, including the ethylsuccinate and estolate esters and stearate salt for PO administration. There is no convincing data to suggest that one form is absorbed better than another and one dose is included for all. Only erythromycin gluceptate and lactate are to be administered IV.	Many brands, generic	250 mg capsule or tablet	10-20 mg/kg PO q8-12h
Erythropoietin	Hematopoietic growth factor that stimulates erythropoiesis. Human recombinant erythropoietin. Used to treat nonregenerative anemia (Compend Cont Education 1992;14:25-34).	Since this product is a human-recombinant product, it may induce local and systemic allergic reactions in animals. Delayed anemia may occur because of cross-reacting antibiodies against animal erythropoietin (reversible when drug is withdrawn).	Use has been based on clinical reports in dogs and cats. The only form currently available is a human recombinant product.	Epogen, epoetin alfa	2,000 U/ml injection	35 U/kg IV, SC 3 times per week (adjust dose to hematocrit of 0.30-0.34)
Esmolol	Beta-blocker. Selective for beta-1 receptor. The difference between esmolol and other beta-blockers is the short duration of action. Indicated for short-term control of heart rate and arrhythmias.	Same as other precautions for beta-blockers. See propranolol.	Indicated for short-term IV therapy only. Doses are based primarily on empiricism or extrapolation of human dose. No clinical studies have been reported in animals.	Brevibloc	10 mg/ml injection	500 µg/kg IV, which may be given as 0.05-0.1 mg/kg slowly every 5 minutes or 50-200 µg/kg/min infusion
Estradiol cypionate (ECP)	Semisynthetic estrogen compound. Used primarily to induce abortion in animals.	High risk of endometrial hyperplasia and pyometra. High doses can produce leukopenia, thrombocytopenia, and fatal aplastic anemia.	Ordinarily, 22 µg/kg is administered once IM during days 3-5 of estrus or within 3 days of mating. However in one study, a dose of 44 µg/kg was more efficacious than 22 µg/kg when given during estrus or diestrus.	ECP, Depo-Estradiol, generic	2 mg/ml injection	Dogs: 22-44 µg/kg IM (total dose not to exceed 1.0 mg). Cats: 250 µg/cat IM between 40 hours and 5 days of mating.
Etidronate disodium	Bisphosphonate drug. Used to treat osteoporosis and hypercalcemia. Decreases bone turnover, inhibits osteoclast activity, retards bone resorption, and decreases rate of osteoporosis.	Adverse effects not reported for animals. In humans, gastrointestinal problems are common.	At high doses may inhibit mineralization of bone. In humans, alendronate has replaced etidronate because of side effects.	Didronel	200, 400 mg tablets; 50 mg/ml injection	Dogs: 5 mg/kg/day PO. Cats: 10 mg/kg/day PO.
Etretinate	Used for treatment of idiopathic seborrhea (JAVMA 1992;201: 419). Normalizes epidermal differentiation.	Do *not* use in pregnant animals. Causes major fetal abnormalities. In male dogs, causes spermatogenic arrest with chronic administration. Side effects resemble hypervitaminosis A (signs related to mucocutaneous, musculoskeletal, and central nervous system).	Limited use in dogs. Doses are based primarily on empiricism and extrapolation from human doses.	Tegison	10, 25 mg capsules	Dogs: 1 mg/kg/day PO (with food). Dogs < 15 kg: 10 mg/dog PO q24h. Dogs > 15 kg: 10 mg/dog PO q12h. Cats: 2 mg/kg/day.

Drug name	Pharmacology and category of use	Precautions	Dosing information and comments	Other names	Formulations available	Dosage
Famotidine	H$_2$ receptor antagonist. See cimetidine for details.	See cimetidine.	See cimetidine. Clinical studies for famotidine have not been performed, therefore optimal dose for ulcer prevention and healing are not known.	Pepsid	10 mg tablet; 10 mg/ml injection	0.5 mg/kg IM, SC, PO q12-24h
Fenbendazole	Benzimidazole antiparasite drugs. See albendazole.	Safe in all species. No known contraindications.	Dose recommendations are based on clinical studies by manufacturer.	Panacur, SafeGuard	22.2% (222 mg/g) Panacur granules; 100 mg/ml liquid	50 mg/kg/day PO for 3 days
Fentanyl	Synthetic opiate analgesic. Approximately 80-100 times more potent than morphine. See morphine for more details.	Adverse effects similar to morphine	Doses are based on empiricism and experimental studies. No clinical studies have been reported. In addition to fentanyl injection, transdermal fentanyl is available. See below.	Sublimaze, generic	250 mg per 5 ml injection	0.02-0.04 mg/kg IV, IM, SC or 0.01 mg/kg IV, IM, SC (with acetylpromazine or diazepam). Analgesia: 0.01 mg/kg.
Fentanyl, transdermal	Same as for fentanyl. Transdermal fentanyl incorporates fentanyl into adhesive patches applied to skin of dogs and cats. Studies have determined that patches release sustained levels of fentanyl for 72-108 hours in dogs and cats. One 100 µg/hr patch is equivalent to 10 mg/kg of morphine IM every 4 hours.	Adverse effects have not been reported. However, if adverse effects are observed (e.g., respiratory depression, excess sedation, excitement in cats), remove patch and, if necessary, administer naloxone.	Patches available in sizes of 25, 50, 75, and 100 µg/hr. Patch size is related to release rate of fentanyl. Studies have determined that 25 µg/hr patches are appropriate for cats; 50 µg/hr patches are appropriate for dogs 10-20 kg. Follow manufacturer's recommendations carefully when applying patches.	Duragesic	25, 50, 75, 100 µg/hr patch	Dogs 10-20 kg: 50 µg/hr patch every 72 hours. Cats: 25 µg patch every 96 hours.
Ferrous sulfate	Iron supplement	High doses cause stomach ulceration.	Recommendations are based on dose needed to increase hematocrit.	Many OTC brands	Many	Dogs: 100-300 mg/dog PO q24h. Cats: 50-100 mg/cat PO q24h.
Fluconazole	Azole antifungal drug. Similar mechanism as other azole antifungal agents. Inhibits ergosterol synthesis in fungal cell membrane. Fungistatic. Efficacious against dermatophytes and variety of systemic fungi.	Adverse effects have not been reported from fluconazole administration. Compared to ketoconazole, has less effect on endocrine function. However, increased liver enzyme plasma concentrations and hepatopathy are possible.	Doses for fluconazole are primarily based on studies performed in cats for treatment of cryptococcosis. Efficacy for other infections has not been reported. The primary difference between fluconazole and other azoles is that fluconazole attains higher concentrations in the central nervous system.	Diflucan	50, 100, 200 mg tablets; 10, 40 mg/ml oral suspension; 2 mg/ml IV injection	Cats: 50 mg/cat PO q12h
Flucytosine	Antifungal drug. Used in combination with other antifungal drugs for treatment of cryptococcosis. Action is to penetrate fungal cells and is converted to fluorouracil, which acts as antimetabolite.	Adverse effects have not been reported in animals.	Flucytosine is used primarily to treat cryptococcosis in animals. Efficacy is based on flucytosine's ability to attain high concentrations in CSF. Flucytosine may be synergistic with amphotericin B.	Ancobon	250 mg capsule; 75 mg/ml oral suspension	25-50 mg/kg PO q6-8h (up to a maximum dose of 100 mg/kg PO q12h)

Drug name	Pharmacology and category of use	Precautions	Dosing information and comments	Other names	Formulations available	Dosage
Fludrocortisone	Mineralocorticoid. Used as replacement therapy in animals with adrenal atrophy/adrenocortical insufficiency. Has high potency of mineralocorticoid activity compared to glucocorticoid activity.	Adverse effects are primarily related to glucocorticoid effects with high doses.	Dose should be adjusted by monitoring patient response (i.e., monitoring electrolyte concentrations). In some patients, it is administered with a glucocorticoid and sodium supplementation.	Florinef	100 µg (0.1 mg) tablets	Dogs: 0.2-0.8 mg/dog, or 0.02 mg/kg, PO q24h. Cats: 0.1-0.2 mg PO q24h.
Flumethasone	Potent glucocorticoid antiinflammatory drug. Potency is approximately 15 times that of cortisol. See dexamethasone for additional details.	See dexamethasone.	See dexamethasone. Doses are based on severity of underlying disease. See dose table.	Flucort	Tablets	Dogs: 0.0625-0.25 mg/day IV, IM, SC, PO. Cats: 0.03-0.125 mg/day IV, IM, SC, PO. Antiinflammatory: 0.15-0.3 mg/kg IV, IM, SC, PO q12-24h.
Flumazenil	Benzodiazepine receptor antagonist. Used as reversal agent after benzodiazepine administration in humans (not commonly used in veterinary medicine).	No adverse effects reported in animals. .	Used primarily to block effects of benzodiazepine drugs. May be used to treat toxicity caused by high doses of benzodiazepines (e.g., diazepam). Although used experimentally for hepatic encephalopathy, it is not recommended for this use.	Romazicon	100 µg/ml (0.1 mg/ml) injection	0.2 mg IV (total dose) as needed
Flunixin meglumine	NSAID. Acts to inhibit cyclooxygenase enzyme (COX) that synthesizes prostaglandins. Other antiinflammtory effects may occur (such as effects on leukocytes) but have not been well characterized. Used primarily for short-term treatment of moderate pain and inflammation.	Most severe adverse effects related to gastrointestinal system. Causes gastritis and gastrointestinal ulceration with high doses or prolonged use. Renal ischemia has also been documented. Therapy in dogs should be limited to 4 consecutive days. Avoid use in pregnant animals near term. Ulcerogenic effects are potentiated when administered with corticosteroids.	Not approved for small animals, but has been shown in experimental studies to be an effective prostaglandin synthesis inhibitor. Approved for use in small animals in Europe.	Banamine	250 mg packet granules; 10, 50 mg/ml injection	1.1 mg/kg IV, IM, SC once or 1.1 mg/kg/day PO 3 days per week. Ophthalmic: 0.5 mg/kg IV once.
5-fluorouracil	Anticancer agent. Antimetabolite. Action is via inhibition with nucleic acid synthesis.	Causes mild leukopenia and thrombocytopenia. Central nervous system toxicity. Do not use in cats.	Used in anticancer protocols. Consult anticancer treatment protocol for precise dosage and regimen.	Fluorouracil	50 mg/ml vial	Dogs: 150 mg/m² once per week IV. Cats: Do not use.
Fluoxetine	Antidepressant drug. Used to treat behavioral disorders such as obsessive-compulsive disorders. Mechanism of action appears to be via selective inhibition of serotonin reuptake and down regulation of 5-HT1 receptors.	Fewer adverse effects (especially antihistamine and antimuscarinic effects) compared to other antidepressant drugs. Adverse effects have not been reported in animals.	Use of fluoxetine in animals is largely experimental. Doses have been derived empirically and use is based primarily on anecdotal experience. Because of long half-life, accumulation in plasma may take several days to weeks.	Prozac	10, 20 mg capsules; 4 mg/ml oral solution	Dose not established (approx. 1 mg/kg PO q24h)
Follicle-stimulating hormone (FSH)	See urofollitropin.					
Furazolidone	Oral antiprotozoal drug with activity against Giardia. May have some activity against bacteria in intestine. Not used for systemic therapy.	Adverse effects not reported in animals. In humans, mild anemia, hypersensitivity, and disturbance of intestinal flora have been reported.	Clinical studies have not been reported for animals. Doses and recommendations are based on extrapolation from humans.	Furoxone	100 mg tablet	4 mg/kg PO q12h for 7-10 days

Drug name	Pharmacology and category of use	Precautions	Dosing information and comments	Other names	Formulations available	Dosage
Furosemide	Loop diuretic. Inhibits sodium and water transport in ascending loop of Henle, which produces diuresis. Also may have vasodilating properties, increasing renal perfusion and decreasing preload.	Adverse effects primarily are related to diuretic effect (loss of fluid and electrolytes).	Recommendations are based on extensive clinical use of furosemide in animals.	Lasix, generic	12.5, 20, 50 mg tablets; 10 mg/ml oral solution; 50 mg/ml injection	Dogs: 2-6 mg/kg IV, IM, SC, PO q8-12h (or as needed). Cats: 1-4 mg/kg IV, IM, SC, PO q8-24h.
Gemfibrozil	Cholesterol lowering agent	Adverse effects have not been reported in animals.	Used primarily in humans to treat hyperlipidemia. Clinical studies have not been performed in animals.	Lopid	300 mg capsule; 600 mg tablet	7.5 mg/kg PO q12h
Gentamicin	Aminoglycoside antibiotic. Action is to inhibit bacteria protein synthesis via binding to 30S ribosome. Bactericidal. Broad spectrum of activity (except streptococci and anaerobic bacteria).	Nephrotoxicity is the most dose-limiting toxicity. Ensure that patients have adequate fluid and electrolyte balance during therapy. Ototoxicity and vestibulotoxicity also are possible. When used with anesthetic agents, neuromuscular blockade is possible. Do not mix in vial or syringe with other antibiotics.	Dosing regimens are based on sensitivity of organisms. Some studies have suggested that once daily therapy (combining multiple doses into a single daily dose) is as efficacious as multiple treatments. Nephrotoxicity is increased with persistently high trough concentrations.	Gentocin	50, 100 mg/ml solution for injection	Dogs: 2-4 mg/kg q6-8h, or 6-10 mg/kg IV, IM, SC q24h.. Cats: 3 mg/kg IV, IM, SC q8h or 9 mg/kg q24h.
Glibenclamide	British name for glyburide					
Glipizide	Sulfonylurea oral hypoglycemic agent. Used as oral treatment in the management of diabetes mellitus. Increases secretion of insulin from pancreas, probably by interacting with sulfonylurea receptors on beta-cells.	Adverse effects have not been reported in animals. In humans, increased cardiac mortality is possible. Causes hypoglycemia. Many drug interactions have been reported in humans. It is not known if these occur in animals. Use cautiously with beta-blockers, antifungal drugs, anticoagulants, fluoroquinolones, sulfonamides, and others (consult package insert).	Oral hypoglycemic agents are successful in humans only for non–insulin-dependent diabetes. There has been only limited use in animals. Similar drugs include acetohexamide, chlorpropamide, glyburide, gliclazide, and tolazamide.	Glucotrol	5, 10 mg tablets	0.25-0.5 mg/kg PO q12h
Glyburide	Sulfonylurea hypoglycemic agent. See glipizide.	See glipizide.	See glipizide	Diabeta, Micronase, Glynase	1.25, 2.5, 5 mg tablets	0.2 mg/kg PO daily
Glycopyrrolate	Anticholinergic drug. For mechanism, see atropine. Glycopyrrolate may have less effect on central nervous system compared to atropine because of lower CSF levels. May have longer duration of action than atropine.	Adverse effects attributed to antimuscarinic (anticholinergic) effects. See atropine.	Glycopyrrolate is often used in combination with other agents, particularly anesthetic drugs.	Robinul-V	0.2 mg/ml injection	0.005-0.01 mg/kg IV, IM, SC
Glucosamine	Combined with chrondroitin sulfate in cosequin. See cosequin.					

Drug name	Pharmacology and category of use	Precautions	Dosing information and comments	Other names	Formulations available	Dosage
Gold sodium thiomalate	Gold therapy. For mechanism, see aurothioglucose.	See aurothioglucose.	Clinical studies have not been performed in animals. Efficacy and safety of this product are not available for animals. Aurothioglucose generally is used more often than Myochrysine.	Myochrysine	Injection	1-5 mg IM first week, then 2-10 mg IM second week, then 1 mg/kg IM once per week maintenance
Gold therapy	See aurothioglucose, gold sodium thiomalate, or auranofin.					
Golytely	Oral solution for producing catharsis	See polyethylene glycol electrolyte solution.				
Gonadorelin (Gn-RH, LH-RH)	Stimulates synthesis and release of luteinizing hormone (LH) and to a lesser degree, follicle-stimulating hormone (FSH). Used to induce luteinization.	Adverse effects have not been reported in animals.	Gonadotropin has been used to manage various reproductive disorders. Consult specific reference on reproductive problems in animals to guide therapy.	Factrel	50 µg/ml injection	Dogs: 50-100 µg/dog/day IM q24-48h. Cats: 25 µg/cat IM once.
Gonadotropin, chorionic (hCG)	Action of hCG is identical to that of luteinizing hormone (LH). Used to induce luteinization in animals.	Adverse effects have not been reported in animals.	Consult specific reference on reproductive problems in animals to guide therapy.	Profasi, Pregnyl, generic, APL	5, 10, 20 thousand U injections	Dogs: 22 U/kg IM q24-48h or 44 U IM once. Cats: 250 U/cat IM once.
Gonadotropin-releasing hormone	See gonadorelin.					
Griseofulvin (microsize)	Antifungal drug. Incorporates into skin layers and inhibits mitosis of fungi. Antifungal activity is limited to dermatophytes.	Adverse effects in animals include teratogenicity in cats, anemia and leukopenia in cats, anorexia, depression, vomiting, and diarrhea. Do not administer to pregnant cats.	A wide range of doses have been reported. Doses listed here represent the current consensus. Griseofulvin should be administered with food to enhance absorption.	Fulvicin U/F	125, 250, 500 mg tablets; 25 mg/ml oral suspension; 125 mg/ml oral syrup	50 mg/kg PO q24h (up to a maximum dose of 110-132 mg/kg/day in divided treatments)
Griseofulvin (ultramicrosize)	Same as above	Same as above	Same as above. Ultramicrosize is absorbed to a greater extent and doses should be less than microsize.	Fulvicin P/G, Gris-PEG	100, 125, 165, 250, 330 mg tablets	30 mg/kg/day PO in divided treatments
Growth hormone (hGH)	Growth hormone. Used to treat growth hormone deficiencies.	Growth hormone is diabetogenic in all animals. Excess growth hormone causes acromegaly.	Limited clinical experience in animals			0.1 U/kg 3 times per week for 4-6 weeks
Halothane	Inhalant anesthetic. Exact mechanism of action unknown.	Adverse effects related to anesthetic effects (e.g., cardiovascular and respiratory depression). Hepatotoxicosis has been reported in humans.	Use of inhalant anesthetics requires careful monitoring. Dose is determined by depth of anesthesia.	Fluothane	250 ml bottle	Induction: 3%. Maintenance: 0.5-1.5%.
Heparin sodium	Anticoagulant. Potentiates anticoagulant effects of antithrombin III. Used primarily for prevention of thrombosis.	Adverse effects caused by excessive inhibition of coagulation (bleeding).	Dose adjustments should be performed by monitoring clotting times. For example, dose is adjusted to maintain APTT to 1.5-2 times normal.	Liquaemin (United States), Hepalean (Canada)	1,000, 10,000 U/ml injections	100-200 U/kg IV loading dose, then 100-300 U/kg SC q6-8h. Low dose prophylaxis (dogs and cats): 70 U/kg SC q8-12h.
Hetastarch	See hydroxyethyl starch (HES).					
Hycodan	See hydrocodone bitartrate.					

Drug name	Pharmacology and category of use	Precautions	Dosing information and comments	Other names	Formulations available	Dosage
Hydralazine	Vasodilator. Antihypertensive. Used to dilate arterioles and decrease afterload. Primarily used for treatment of congestive heart failure and other cardiovascular disorders characterized by high peripheral vascular resistance.	Adverse effects attributed to excess vasodilation. Monitor patients for hypotension. May dangerously decrease cardiac output. Allergic reactions (lupus-like syndrome) have been reported in humans and are related to acetylator status, but have not been reported in animals.	Use in heart failure may accompany other drugs such as digoxin and diuretics. It is advised to monitor patient for hypotension to adjust dosage.	Apresoline	10 mg tablet; 20 mg/ml injection	Dogs: 0.5 mg/kg (initial dose); titrate to 0.5-2 mg/kg PO q12h. Cats: 2.5 mg/cat PO q12-24h.
Hydrocodone bitartrate	Opiate agonist. Used primarily for antitussive action. See codeine. Hycodan contains homatropine, but other combinations may contain guaifenesin or acetaminophen.	See codeine.	Hydrocodone is combined with atropine in the product Hycodan. Atropine can decrease respiratory secretions, but probably does not have significant clinical effects at doses in this preparation (1.5 mg homatropine per 5 mg tablet).	Hycodan	5 mg tablet 1mg/ml syrup	Dogs: 0.22 mg/kg PO q4-8 h. Cats: No dose available.
Hydrochlorothiazide	Thiazide diuretic. Inhibits sodium reabsorption in distal renal tubules. Used as diuretic and antihypertensive. Since they decrease renal excretion of calcium, they also have been used to treat calcium-containing uroliths.	Do not use in patient with elevated calcium. May cause electrolyte imbalance such as hypokalemia.	Not as potent as loop diuretics (such as furosemide). Clinical efficacy has not been established in veterinary patients.	HydroDIURIL, generic	10, 100 mg/ml oral solution; 25, 50, 100 mg tablets	2-4 mg/kg PO q12h
Hydrocortisone	Glucocorticoid antiinflammatory drug. Hydrocortisone has weaker antiinflammatory effects and greater mineralocorticoid effects compared with prednisolone or dexamethasone. See dexamethasone for further details. Also used for replacement therapy.	Adverse effects are attributed to excessive glucocorticoid effects. See betamethasone.	Dose requirements are related to severity of disease.	Cortef	10 mg tablet	Replacement therapy: 1-2 mg/kg PO q12h. Antiinflammatory: 2.5-5 mg/kg PO q12h.
Hydrocortisone sodium succinate	Same as hydrocortisone, except that this is a rapid-acting injectable product	Same as hydrocortisone	Same as hydrocortisone	Solu-Cortef	Injection	Shock: 50-150 mg/kg IV. Antiinflammatory: 5 mg/kg IV q12h.
Hydroxyethyl starch (HES)	Synthetic colloid volume expander (used in same manner as dextran). Used primarily to treat acute hypovolemia and shock.	Only limited use in veterinary medicine, therefore adverse effects have not been reported. May cause allergic reactions. Coagulopathies rare at usual doses.	Used in critical care situations. Infused via constant rate infusion. HES appears to be more effective and produces fewer side effects than dextran. Infuse slowly.	HES, Hetastarch	Injection	10-20 ml/kg IV to effect
Hydroxyurea	Antineoplastic agent. Used in combination with other anticancer modalities for treatment of certain tumors. Has been used to treat polycythemia vera.	Only limited use in veterinary medicine. No adverse effects have been reported. In humans, hydroxyurea causes leukopenia, anemia, and thrombocytopenia.	Limited use in veterinary medicine	Hydrea	500 mg capsule	Dogs: 50 mg/kg PO once daily, 3 days per week. Cats: 25 mg/kg PO once daily, 3 days per week.

Drug name	Pharmacology and category of use	Precautions	Dosing information and comments	Other names	Formulations available	Dosage
Hydroxyzine	Antihistamine of the piperazine class. Used primarily to treat pruritus in animals.	Side effects of therapy are related primarily to antihistamine effects. Sedation occurs in some animals.	Clinical studies have shown hydroxyzine to be somewhat effective for treatment of pruritus in dogs.	Atarax	10, 25, 50 mg tablets; 2 mg/ml oral solution	Dogs: 1-2 mg/kg IM, PO q6-8h. Cats: Safe dose not established.
Ibuprofen	Nonsteroidal antiinflammatory drug. See flunixin meglumine.	Safe doses have not been established for dogs and cats. Vomiting, severe gastrointestinal ulceration, and hemorrhage have been reported in dogs.	Avoid use, especially in dogs.	Motrin, Advil, Nuprin	200, 400, 600, 800 mg tablets	Safe dose not established
Imipenem	Beta-lactam antibiotic with broad spectrum activity. Action is similar to other beta-lactams. See amoxicillin. Imipenem is the most active of all beta-lactams. Used primarily for serious, multiply-resistant infections.	Adverse have not been reported in animals. Allergic reactions may occur with beta-lactam antibiotics. With rapid infusion or in patients with renal insufficiency, neurotoxicity may occur (seizures).	Doses and efficacy studies have not been determined in animals. Recommendations are based on studies performed in humans and extrapolation from humans. Reserve the use of this drug for only resistant, refractory infections. Observe manufacturer's instructions carefully for proper administration.	Primaxin	250 mg injection	3-10 mg/kg IV, IM q6-8h
Imipramine	Tricyclic antidepressant (TCA). Used in humans to treat anxiety and depression. Used in animals to treat variety of behavioral disorders, including obsessive-compulsive disorders. Action is via inhibition of uptake of serotonin at presynaptic nerve terminals.	Multiple side effects are associated with tricyclic antidepressants such as antimuscarinic effects (dry mouth and rapid heart rate) and antihistamine effects (sedation). High doses can produce life-threatening cardiotoxicity.	Doses are primarily based on empiricism. There are no controlled efficacy trials available for animals. There may be a 2-4 week delay after initiation of therapy before beneficial effects are seen.	Tofranil	12.5 mg/ml injection; 10, 25, 50 mg tablets	2-4 mg/kg q12-24h
Indomethacin	NSAID. See flunixin meglumine.	Causes severe gastrointestinal ulceration and hemorrhage in dogs. Do not use.	Do not use in dogs.	Indocin		Safe dose not established
Insulin, regular crystalline	Insulin has multiple effects associated with utilization of glucose. Used to treat insulin-dependent diabetes mellitus in dogs and cats.	Adverse effects primarily related to overdoses (hypoglycemia)	Doses should be carefully adjusted in each patient, depending on response. Monitor plasma/serum glucose concentrations.		100 U/ml injection	Ketoacidosis: Animals < 3 kg, 1 U/animal IM initially, then 1 U/animal q1h; Animals 3-10 kg, 2 U/animal initially, then 1 U/animal q1h; animals > 10 kg, 0.25 U/kg initially, then 0.1 U/kg q1h.
Insulin, lente	Same as above	Same as above	Same as above-preferred to NPH in cats		100 U/ml injection	Same as for NPH insulin
Insulin, NPH isophane	Same as above	Same as above	Same as above		100 U/ml injection	Dogs < 15 kg: 1 U/kg SC q12-24h (to effect). Dogs > 25 kg: 0.5 U/kg SC q12-24h (to effect). Cats: 0.25-0.5 U/kg q12h.
Insulin, ultrlente	Same as above	Same as above	Same as above-preferred to NPH in cats		100 U/ml injection	Same as NPH insulin except administer q24h in most animals.
Interferon (interferon α, HuIFN-α)	Human interferon. Used to stimulate the immune system in patients.	Adverse effects have not been reported in animals.	Doses and indications for animals have primarily been based on extrapolation of human recommendations or limited experimental studies (JAVMA 1991;199:1477). To prepare, add 3 million U to 1 L sterile saline and divide into aliquots and freeze. Thaw as needed for 30 U/ml solution.	Roferon	3 million U per vial	Cats: 10,000 U/kg SC q12h or 30 U PO once daily for 7 days and repeated every other week

Drug name	Pharmacology and category of use	Precautions	Dosing information and comments	Other names	Formulations available	Dosage
Iodide	See potassium iodide.					
Ipecac syrup	Emetic drug. For emergency treatment of poisoning. Active ingredient is thought to be emetine.	No adverse effects with acute therapy for poisoning. Chronic administration can lead to myocardial toxicity.	Available as nonprescription drug. Onset of vomiting may require 20-30 minutes.	Ipecac	Oral solution (30 ml bottle)	Dogs: 3-6 ml PO. Cats: 2-6 ml PO.
Iron	See ferrous sulfate.					
Isoflurane	Inhalant anesthetic. See halothane.	See halothane.	See halothane.	Aerrane	100 ml bottle	Induction: 5%. Maintenance: 1.5-2.5%.
Isoproterenol	Adrenergic agonist. Stimulates both beta-1 (β_1) and beta-2 (β_2) adrenergic receptors. Used to stimulate heart (inotropic and chronotropic). Also used to relax bronchial smooth muscle for acute treatment of bronchoconstriction.	Adverse effects related to excessive adrenergic stimulation and are seen primarily as tachycardia and tachyarrhythmias.	Short half-life. Must be infused via constant rate infusion or repeated if administered IM or SC. Recommended for short-term use only.	Isuprel	0.2 mg/ml ampules for injection	10 µg/kg IM, SC q6h or dilute 1 mg in 500 ml of 5% dextrose or Ringer's solution and infuse IV 0.5-1 ml/min (1-2 µg/min) or to effect
Isosorbide dinitrate	Nitrate vasodilator. Causes vasodilation via generation of nitric oxide. Relaxes vascular smooth muscle, especially venous. Reduces preload in patients with congestive heart failure. In humans, it is primarily used to treat angina.	Adverse effects are primarily related to overdoses that produce excess vasodilation and hypotension. Tolerance may develop with repeated doses.	Generally, doses are titrated to individual patients, depending on response.	Isordil, Isorbid, Sorbitrate	2.5, 5, 10, 20, 30, 40 mg tablets	2.5-5 mg/animal PO q12h or 0.22-1.1 mg/kg PO q12h
Isotretinoin	Keratinization stabilizing drug. Isotretinoin reduces sebaceous gland size, inhibits sebaceous gland activity, and decreases sebum secretion. In humans, it is primarily used to treat acne. In animals, has been used to treat sebaceous adenitis.	Absolutely contraindicated in pregnant animals. Adverse effects not reported for animals, although experimental studies have demonstrated that it can cause focal calcification (such as in myocardium and vessels).	Use in veterinary medicine is confined to limited clinical experience and extrapolation from human reports.	Accutane	10, 20, 40 mg capsules	1-3 mg/kg/day PO (up to a maximum recommended dose of 3-4 mg/kg/day)
Itraconazole	Azole (triazole) antifungal drug. See ketoconazole for mechanism of action. Active against dermatophytes and systemic fungi, including Blastomyces and Coccidioides.	Adverse effects have not been reported in animals. Itraconazole is better tolerated than ketoconazole. However, vomiting and hepatotoxicosis are possible.	Doses are based on limited studies in animals in which itraconazole has been used to treat blastomycosis in dogs. Other uses or doses are based on empiricism or extrapolation from human literature.	Sporanox	100 mg capsule	Dogs: 2.5 mg/kg PO q12h to 5 mg/kg q24h. Cats: 5 mg/kg PO q12h.

Drug name	Pharmacology and category of use	Precautions	Dosing information and comments	Other names	Formulations available	Dosage
Ivermectin	Antiparasitic drug. Neurotoxic to parasites by potentiating effects of inhibitory neurotransmitter GABA.	Toxicity may occur at high doses and in species in which ivermectin crosses blood-brain barrier (collie breeds). Toxicity is neurotoxic and signs include depression, ataxia, difficulty with vision, coma, and death. Ivermectin appears to be safe for pregnant animals. Do not administer to animals less than 6 weeks of age.	Doses vary depending on use. Heartworm prevention is lowest dose; other parasites require higher doses. Heartguard is only form approved for small animals; for other indications, large animal injectable products are often administered PO, IM, or SC to small animals. For demodex therapy it is advised to start with 100 µg/kg/day and increase dose by 100 µg/kg/day to 600 µg/kg/day.	Heartguard, Ivomec, Eqvalan liquid	1% injectable solution; 10 mg/ml oral solution, paste; 68, 136, 272 µg tablets	Heartworm preventative (dogs): 6 µg/kg PO every 30 days. Microfilaricide (dogs): 50 µg/kg PO 2 weeks after adulticide therapy. Ectoparasite therapy: 200-300 µg/kg IM, SC, PO. Endoparasites: 200-400 µg/kg SC, PO weekly. Demodex therapy: 600 µg/kg/day PO for 60-120 days.
Kanamycin	Aminoglycoside antibiotic. See gentamicin and amikacin for details.	Shares same properties with other aminoglycosides. See amikacin and gentamicin.	See gentamicin.	Kantrim	200, 500 mg/ml injections	10 mg/kg IV, IM, SC q6-8h
Kaopectate (kaolin and pectin)	Antidiarrheal compound. Kaolin may act as adsorbent for endotoxins and pectin may protect intestinal mucosa.	Side effects are uncommon.	Efficacy has not been established for treatment of diarrhea in animals.	Kaopectate	12 oz oral suspension	1-2 ml/kg PO q2-6h
Ketamine	Anesthetic agent. Exact mechanism of action is not known, but appears to act as dissociative agent. Ketamine has little analgesic activity. Rapidly metabolized and eliminated in most animals.	Causes pain with IM injection. Tremors, spasticity, and convulsive seizures have been reported. Increases cardiac output compared to other anesthetic agents. Do not use in animals with head injury because it may elevate CSF pressure.	Often used in combination with other anesthetics and anesthetic adjuncts such as xylazine, acepromazine, or diazepam. IV doses generally less than IM doses.	Ketalar, Ketavet, Vetalar	100 mg/ml injection solution	Dogs:5.5-22 mg/kg IV, IM (recommend adjunctive sedative or tranquilizer treatment). Cats: 2-25 mg/kg IV, IM (recom-mend adjunctive sedative or tranquilizer treatment).
Ketoconazole	Azole (imidazole) antifungal drug. Similar mechanism of action as other azole antifungal agents. Inhibits ergosterol synthesis in fungal cell membrane. Fungistatic. Efficacious against dermatophytes and variety of systemic fungi, including Blastomyces and Coccidioides.	Adverse effects in animals include dose-related vomiting, diarrhea, and hepatic injury. Do not administer to pregnant animals. Ketoconazole causes endocrine abnormalities, most specifically inhibition of cortisol synthesis. Ketoconazole will inhibit metabolism of other drugs (anticonvulsants, cyclosporine, and cisapride).	Oral absorption depends on acidity in stomach. Do not administer with antisecretory drugs or antacids. Because of endocrine effects, ketoconazole has been used for short-term treatment of hyperadrenocorticism.	Nizoral	200 mg tablets; 100 mg/ml oral suspension (only in Canada)	Dogs: 10-15 mg/kg PO q8-12h. Malassezia canis infection: 10 mg/kg PO q24h or 5 mg/kg q12h. Cats: 5-10 mg/kg PO q8-12h. Hyperadrenocorticism (dogs): 15 mg/kg PO q12h.
Ketoprofen	Nonsteroidal antiinflammatory drug. See flunixin meglumine.	All NSAIDs share similar adverse effect of gastrointestinal toxicity. See flunixin. Ketoprofen has been administered for 5 consecutive days in dogs without serious adverse effects. Most common side effect is vomiting.	Although not approved in the United States, ketoprofen is approved for small animals in other countries. Doses listed are based on approved use in those countries.	Orudis-KT (OTC tablet), Ketofen (injection)	12.5 mg tablet (OTC); 100 mg/ml injection	1 mg/kg PO q24h (up to 5 days)

Drug name	Pharmacology and category of use	Precautions	Dosing information and comments	Other names	Formulations available	Dosage
Ketorolac tromethamine	Nonsteroidal antiinflammatory drug (NSAID). Used for short-term relief of pain and inflammation. Acts by inhibiting cyclooxygenase enzyme (COX).	Use has not been evaluated clinically in dogs or cats. Use cautiously. NSAIDs may cause gastrointestinal ulceration.	Available as 10 mg tablet and 1.5% injection. Safe and effective clinical doses have not been established for dogs and cats. Doses have been extrapolated from use in humans.	Toradol	10 mg tablet; 10 mg/ml injection	Dogs: 0.5 mg/kg PO, IM, IV
L-dopa	See levodopa.					
Lactated Ringer's solution	Fluid solution for replacement. IV administration.	Administer IV fluids only in carefully monitored patients.	Fluid requirements vary depending on animal's needs (replacement versus maintenance). Consult fluid therapy reference for optimum rate. Rate listed here is for maintenance and shock.	Many	250, 500, 1,000 ml bags	Maintenance: 40-50 ml/kg/day IV. Shock therapy: Dogs: 90 ml/kg IV. Cats: 60-70 ml/kg IV.
Lactulose	Laxative. Produces laxative effect by osmotic effect in colon. Lactulose also has been used for treatment of hyperammonemia (hepatic encephalopathy) because it decreases blood ammonia concentrations via lowering pH of colon; thus ammonia in colon is not as readily absorbed.	Excessive use may cause fluid and electrolyte loss.	In veterinary medicine, clinical studies to establish efficacy are not available.	Chronulac, generic	10 g per 15 ml	Constipation: 1 ml per 4.5 kg PO q8h to effect. Hepatic encephalopathy: 0.5 ml/kg q8h PO (dogs); 2.5-5 ml/cat PO q8h (cats).
Leucovorin (folinic acid)	Reduced to folic acid, which is available for purine and thymidine synthesis. Used as antidote for folic acid antagonists.		Used primarily as rescue for overdoses of folic acid antagonists (methotrexate). Clinical studies have not been reported in veterinary medicine.	Wellcovorin, generic	5, 10, 15, 25 mg tablets; 3, 5 mg/ml injections	With Methotrexate administration: 3 mg/m^2 IV, IM, PO. Antidote for pyrimethamine toxicosis: 1 mg/kg PO q24h.
Levamisole	Antiparasitic drug of the imidazothiazole class. Mechanism of action a result of neuromuscular toxicity to parasites. Levamisole has been used for endoparasites in dogs and as microfilaricide. In humans, levamisole is used as immunostimulant to aid in treatment of colorectal carcinoma and malignant melanoma.	May produce cholinergic toxicity. May cause vomiting in some dogs.	In heartworm-positive dogs, it may sterilize female adult heartworms. Levamisole has also been used as an immunostimulant; however, clinical reports of its efficacy are not available.	Levasole, Tramisol, Ergamisol	0.184 g bolus; 11.7 g per 13 g packet; 50 mg tablet (Ergamisol)	Hookworms (dogs): 5-8 mg/kg PO once (up to 10 mg/kg PO for 2 days). Microfilaricide: 10 mg/kg PO q24h for 6-10 days. Immunostimulant: 0.5-2 mg/kg PO 3 times per week. Cats: 4.4 mg/kg PO once. Lungworms: 20-40 mg/kg PO q48h for 5 treatments.
Levodopa (L-dopa)	Converted to dopamine after crossing blood-brain barrier. Stimulates CNS dopamine receptors. In humans, used for treating Parkinson's disease. In animals, has been used for treating hepatic encephalopathy.	Adverse effects in animals have not been reported. In humans, dizziness, mental changes, difficult urination, and hypotension are among the reported adverse effects.	Clinical studies have not been reported in veterinary medicine. Titrate dose for each patient.	Larodopa, L-dopa	100, 250, 500 mg tablets or capsules	Hepatic encephalopathy: 6.8 mg/kg initially, then 1.4 mg/kg q6h

Drug name	Pharmacology and category of use	Precautions	Dosing information and comments	Other names	Formulations available	Dosage
Levothyroxine sodium	Replacement therapy for treating patients with hypothyroidism. Levothyroxine is T_4, which is converted in most patients to the active T_3.	High doses may produce thyrotoxicosis, which is uncommon (as compared to humans). Patients receiving corticosteroids may have decreased ability to convert T_4 to T_3.	Thyroid supplementation should be guided by testing to confirm diagnosis and postmedication monitoring to adjust dose.	Soloxine, Thyro-Tabs, Synthroid	0.1-0.8 mg tablets (in 0.1 mg increments)	Dogs: 22 µg/kg PO q12h (adjust dose via monitoring). Cats: 10-20 µg/kg/day PO (adjust dose via monitoring).
Lidocaine	Local anesthetic. See bupivicaine for mechanism of action. Lidocaine is also used commonly for acute treatment of cardiac arrhythmias. Class I antiarrhythmic. Decreases phase 0 depolarization without affecting conduction. Not useful for supraventricular arrhythmias.	High doses cause central nervous system effects (tremors, twitches, and seizures). Lidocaine can produce cardiac arrhythmias, but has greater effect on abnormal cardiac tissue than normal tissue. Cats are more susceptible to adverse effects.	When used for local infiltration, many formulations contain epinephrine to prolong activity at injection site. Avoid epinephrine in patients with cardiac arrhythmias.	Xylocaine	5, 10, 15, 20 mg/ml injections	Anti-arrhythmic (dogs): 2-4 mg/kg IV (to a maximum dose of 8 mg/kg over 10-minute period); 25-75 µg/kg/min IV infusion; 6 mg/kg IM q1.5h. Cats: 0.25-0.75 mg/kg IV slowly.
Lincomycin	Lincosamide antibiotic. Similar in mechanism to clindamycin and erythromycin. Spectrum includes primarily gram-positive bacteria. Used for pyoderma and other soft-tissue infections.	Adverse effects uncommon. Lincomycin has caused vomiting and diarrhea in animals. Do not administer orally to rodents and rabbits.	Action of lincomycin and clindamycin are similar enough that clindamycin can be substituted for lincomycin.	Lincocin	100, 200, 500 mg tablets	15-25 mg/kg PO q12h. Pyoderma: Doses as low as 10 mg/kg q12h have been used.
Liothyronine	Thyroid supplement. Liothyronine is equivalent to T_3.	Adverse effects have not been reported. See levothyroxine.	See levothyroxine. Doses of liothyronine should be adjusted on the basis of monitoring T_3 concentrations in patients.	Cytobin, Cytomel	60 µg tablet	4.4 µg/kg PO q8h T_3 suppression test: In cats, collect presample for T_4 and T_3, administer 25 µg q8h for 7 doses, then collect postsamples for T_3 and T_4 after last dose.
Lisinopril	ACE inhibitor. See captopril for details. Used for treatment of congestive heart failure and hypertension.	See captopril for details. Lisinopril has not been used extensively in animals to document adverse effects. Lisinopril appears to be better tolerated than captopril.	Clinical studies using lisinopril in animals have not been reported. See comments for captopril and enalapril. With all ACE inhibitors, monitor electrolytes and renal function 3-7 days after initiating therapy and periodically thereafter.	Prinivil, Zestril	2.5, 5, 10, 20, 40 mg tablets	Dogs: 0.5 mg/kg PO q24h. Cats: No dose established.
Lithium carbonate	Stimulates granulopoiesis and elevates neutrophil pool in animals. In humans, it is used for treatment of depression. Central nervous system effect is related to decreased concentrations of neurotransmitters.	Adverse effects have not been reported in animals. In humans, cardiovascular problems, drowsiness, and diarrhea are among the adverse effects.	Use in animals is not common. It has been used experimentally to increase neutrophils after cancer therapy.	Lithotabs	150, 300, 600 mg capsules; 300 mg tablets; 300 mg per 5 ml syrup	Dogs: 10 mg/kg PO q12h. Cats: Not recommended.
Lomotil	See diphenoxylate.					

Drug name	Pharmacology and category of use	Precautions	Dosing information and comments	Other names	Formulations available	Dosage
Loperamide	Opiate agonist. Stimulates smooth muscle segmentation in intestine as well as electrolyte absorption. Used for acute treatment of nonspecific diarrhea.	Adverse effects have not been reported in veterinary medicine. Diphenoxylate is poorly absorbed systemically and produces few systemic side effects. Excessive use can cause constipation.	Doses are based primarily on empiricism or extrapolation of human dose. Clinical studies have not been performed in animals.	Imodium	2 mg tablet; 0.2 mg/ml oral liquid	Dogs: 0.1-0.2 mg/kg PO q8-12h. Cats: 0.08-0.16 mg/kg PO q12h.
Lufenuron	Antiparasitic. Used for controlling fleas in animals. Inhibits development in hatching fleas.	Adverse effects have not been reported. Appears to be safe during pregnancy and in young animals.	Lufenuron may control flea development with administration once every 30 days in animals.	Program	45, 90, 135, 204.9, 409.8 mg tablets; 270 mg suspension	Dogs: 10 mg/kg PO, q30days. Cats: 30 mg/kg PO, q30 days.
Luteinizing hormone	See gonadorelin.					
Magnesium citrate	Saline cathartic. Acts to draw water into small intestine via osmotic effect. Fluid accumulation produces distension, which promotes bowel evacuation. Used for constipation and bowel evacuation before certain procedures.	Adverse effects have not been reported in animals; however, fluid and electrolyte loss can occur with overuse. Magnesium accumulation may occur in patients with renal impairment. Magnesium-containing cathartics decrease oral absorption of ciprofloxacin and other fluoroquinolones.	Commonly used to evacuate bowel before surgery or diagnostic procedures. Onset of action is rapid.	Citroma, CitroNesia (Citro-Mag in Canada)	Oral solution	2-4 ml/kg PO
Magnesium hydroxide	Same as magnesium citrate. Magnesium hydroxide also is used as oral antacid to neutralize stomach acid.	Same as magnesium citrate	See magnesium citrate.	Milk of Magnesia	Oral liquid	Antacid: 5-10 ml/kg PO q4-6h. Cathartic: 15-50 ml/kg PO (dogs); 2-6 ml/cat PO q24h (cats).
Magnesium sulfate	Same as magnesium citrate	See magnesium citrate.	See magnesium citrate.	Epsom salts	Crystals, many generic preparations	Dogs: 8-25 g/dog PO q24h. Cats: 2-5 g/cat PO q24h.
Mannitol	Hyperosmiotic diuretic. Increases plasma osmolality, which draws fluid from tissues to plasma. Antiglaucoma agent. Used for treatment of edema and reducing intraocular pressure. Mannitol also has been used to promote urinary excretion of certain toxins.	Causes fluid and electrolyte imbalance. Do not use in dehydrated patients. Use cautiously when intracranial bleeding is suspected because it may increase bleeding.	Use only in patients in which fluid and electrolyte balance can be monitored. Discard unused portions of prepared solution.	Osmitrol	5-25% solution for injection	Diuretic: 1 g/kg IV 5-25% solution to maintain urine flow. Glaucoma or CNS edema: 0.25-2 g/kg IV 15-25% solution over 30-60 minutes (repeat in 6 hours if necessary).
MCT oil	Medium chain triglycerides. Used to treat hepatic encephalopathy.	Adverse effects not reported in veterinary medicine. May cause diarrhea in some patients.	Results of clinical trials using MCT oil have not been reported. Many enteral feeding formulas contain MCT oil (many polymeric formulations).	MCT oil (many sources)	Oral liquid	1-2 ml/kg daily (in food)
Mebendazole	Benzimidazole antiparasitic drug. See albendazole.	Adverse effects are rare. Occasional vomiting and diarrhea in dogs. Some reports suggest idiosyncratic hepatic reactions in dogs.	Dose recommendations are based upon clinical studies performed by the manufacturer.	Telmintic	Each gram of powder contains 40 mg.	22 mg/kg (with food) q24h for 3 days

Drug name	Pharmacology and category of use	Precautions	Dosing information and comments	Other names	Formulations available	Dosage
Meclizine	Antiemetic and antihistamine. Used for treatment of motion sickness. Action may be caused by central anticholinergic actions. Also may suppress chemoreceptor trigger zone (CRTZ).	Adverse effects have not been reported in animals. Anticholinergic (atropine-like) effects may cause side effects.	Results of clinical studies in animals have not been reported. Use in animals is based on experience in humans or anecdotal experiences in animals.	Antivert, generic	12.5, 25, 50 mg tablets	Dogs: 25 mg PO q24h. Motion sickness: Administer 1 hour before traveling. Cats: 12.5 mg PO q24h.
Meclofenamic acid (meclofenamate sodium)	Nonsteroidal antiinflammatory drug. Used for treatment of arthritis and other inflammatory disorders. See flunixin.	Adverse effects have not been reported in animals, but adverse effects common in other NSAIDs are possible. See flunixin.	Results of clinical studies in animals have not been reported. Use in animals is based on experience in humans or anecdotal experiences in animals. Administer with food.	Arquel, Meclofen	50, 100 mg capsules	Dogs: 1 mg/kg/day PO for up to 5 days
Medetomidine	Alpha-2 adrenergic agonist. See xylazine. Used primarily as sedative, anesthetic adjunct, and analgesia.	Alpha-2 agonists decrease sympathetic output. Cardiovascular depression may occur. Causes initial vasoconstriction and bradycardia.	May be used for sedation, analgesia, and minor surgical procedures. Should be reversed with equal volume of atipamezole (Antisedan).	Domitor	Injection 1.0 mg/ml	0.01-0.08 mg/kg IV, IM 750 mcg/m^2 IV or 1,000 mcg/m^2 IM
Medium chain triglycerides	See MCT oil.					
Medroxyprogesterone acetate	Progestin hormone. Derivative of acetoxyprogesterone. In animals, used as progesterone hormone treatment to control estrus cycle. Also used for management of some behavioral and dermatologic disorders (such as urine spraying in cats and alopecia).	Adverse effects include polyphagia, polydipsia, adrenal suppression (cats), increased risk of diabetes, pyometra, diarrhea, and increased risk of neoplasia.	Clinical studies in animals primarily have focused on reproductive and behavioral use. Medroxyprogesterone acetate may have fewer side effects than megestrol acetate.	Injection (Depo-Provera); tablets (Provera)	150, 400 mg/ml suspension injections; 2.5, 5, 10 mg tablets	1.1-2.2 mg/kg IM every 7 days. Behavioral disorders: 10-20 mg/kg SC.
Megestrol acetate	See medroxyprogesterone acetate.	See medroxyprogesterone acetate.	See medroxyprogesterone acetate.	Ovaban	5 mg tablets	Proestrus: 2 mg/kg PO q24h for 8 days. Anestrus: 0.5 mg/kg PO q24h for 30 days. Behavioral disorders: 2-4 mg/kg q24h for 8 days (reduce dose for maintenance). Dermatologic therapy or urine spraying (cats): 2.5-5 mg/cat PO q24h for 1 week, then reduce to 5 mg once or twice per week. Suppress estrus (cats): 5 mg/cat/day for 3 days, then 2.5-5 mg once per week for 10 weeks.
Melarsomine	Organic arsenical compound used for heartworm therapy. Heartworm adulticide. Arsenicals alter glucose uptake and metabolism in heartworms.	Adverse effects include pulmonary thromboembolism (7-20 days after therapy), anorexia (13% incidence), injection site reaction or myositis (32% incidence), and lethargy or depression (15% incidence). Causes elevations of hepatic enzymes. High doses (3 times) can cause pulmonary inflammation and death. If high doses are administered, dimereaprol (3 mg/kg IM) may be used as antidote.	Dose regimens are based on severity of heartworm disease. Consult current reference to determine class of disease (class 1-4). Class 1 and 2 are least severe. Class 4 is most severe and should not be treated with adulticide before surgery. Avoid human exposure. (Wash hands after handling or wear gloves.) Do not freeze reconstituted solutions.	Immiticide	25 mg/ml injection (after reconstitution, retains potency for 24 hours)	Administer via deep intramuscular injection. Class 1-2 (dogs): 2.5 mg/kg/day for 2 consecutive days. Class 3 (dogs): 2.5 mg/kg once, then, in 1 month, 2 additional doses 24 hours apart.

Drug name	Pharmacology and category of use	Precautions	Dosing information and comments	Other names	Formulations available	Dosage
Melphalan	Anticancer agent. Alkylating agent, similar in action to cyclophosphamide.	Adverse effects related to its action as an anticancer agent. Causes myelosuppression.	Used to treat multiple myeloma and certain carcinomas	Alkeran	2 mg tablets	1.5 mg/m² or 0.1-0.2 mg/kg PO q24h for 7-10 days (repeat every 3 weeks)
Meperidine	Synthetic opioid agonist with activity primarily at the μ-opiate receptor. Similar in action to morphine, except with approximately one seventh the potency (75 mg IM or 300 mg PO has similar potency as 10 mg morphine).	Side effects similar to other opiates. See morphine.	Although comparative clinical studies have not been conducted in animals, meperidine is considered an effective analgesic in dogs and cats, but with short duration.	Demerol	50, 100 mg tablets; 10 mg/ml syrup; 25, 50, 75, 100 mg/ml injections	Dogs: 5-10 mg/kg IV, IM (as needed; as often as every 2-3 hours). Cats: 3-5 mg/kg IV, IM (as needed or every 2-4 hours).
Mepivacaine	Local anesthetic. See bupivacaine. Medium potency and duration of action compared to bupivacaine.	See bupivacaine.	See bupivacaine.	Carbocaine	10 mg/ml injection	Variable dose for local infiltration or epidural injection
6-mercaptopurine	Anticancer agent. Antimetabolite agent that inhibits synthesis of purines in cancer cells.	Many side effects are possible that are common to anticancer therapy (many of which are unavoidable), including bone marrow suppression and anemia.	Used for various forms of cancer, including leukemia and lymphoma. Consult specific anticancer protocol for specific regimen.	Purinethol	50 mg tablet	50 mg/m² PO q24h
Mesalamine	5-aminosalicylic acid. Used as treatment of colitis. Action is not precisely known, but suppresses inflammation in colon. Component of sulfasalazine.	See sulfasalazine. Mesalamine alone has not been associated with side effects in animals.	Mesalamine use has not been reported in animals from clinical trials; however, it has been used as a substitute for sulfasalazine in animals that cannot tolerate sulfonamides.	Asacol, Mesasal, Pentasa	400 mg tablet; 250 mg capsule	Veterinary dose has not been established. The usual human dose is 400-500 mg q6-8h. See sulfasalazine and osalazine.
Metamucil	Bulk-forming laxative containing psyllium. See psyllium for details.					
Metaproterenol	Beta-adrenergic agonist. Beta-2 (β_2) specific. Used primarily for bronchodilation. See albuterol for further details.	Adverse effects related to excessive beta-adrenergic stimulation. See albuterol.	Results of clinical studies in animals have not been reported. Use in animals (and doses) is based on experience in humans or anecdotal experience in animals. Beta-2 agonists also have been used in humans to delay labor (inhibit uterine contractions).	Alupent, Metaprel	10, 20 mg tablets; 5 mg/ml syrup; inhalers	0.325-0.65 mg/kg PO q4-6h
Methazolamide	Carbonic anhydrase inhibitor. Produces less diuresis than others. See dichlorphenamide and acetazolamide.	Use cautiously in patients sensitive to sulfonamides. See acetazolamide and dichlorphenamide.	Used to treat glaucoma in patients. May be used with other glaucoma agents. See acetazolamide and dichlorphenamide.	Neptazane	25, 50 mg tablets	2-4 mg/kg (to a maximum dose of 4-6 mg/kg) PO q8-12h

Drug name	Pharmacology and category of use	Precautions	Dosing information and comments	Other names	Formulations available	Dosage
Methenamine hippurate	Urinary antiseptic. Converted to formaldehyde in acidic urine to produce an antibacterial/antifungal effect. Active against a wide range of bacteria. Resistance does not develop. Less effective against Proteus, which produces an alkaline urine pH. Not effective for systemic infections.	Although formaldehyde formation in bladder may be irritating, in humans, high doses were required (> 8 g/day). In animals, no adverse effects have been reported.	Results of clinical studies in animals have not been reported. Use in animals is based on experience in humans or anecdotal experience in animals. Urine must be acidic for methenamine to convert to formaldehyde (monitor pH periodically). pH below 5.5 is optimal. Supplement with ascorbic acid or ammonium chloride to lower pH.	Hiprex	1 g tablets	Dogs: 500 mg/dog PO q12h. Cats: 250 mg/cat PO q12h.
Methenamine mandelate	Urinary antiseptic. See methenamine hippurate.	See methenamine hippurate	See methenamine hippurate.	Mandelamine	1 g tablet; granules for oral solution; 50, 100 mg/ml oral suspension	10-20 mg/kg PO q8-12h
Methimazole	Antithyroid drug. Used for treating hyperthyroidism, primarily in cats. Action is to serve as substrate for thyroid peroxidase and decrease incorporation of iodide into throsine molecules.	In humans, it has caused agranulocytosis and leukopenia. Well tolerated in dogs.	Use in cats is based on experimental studies in hyperthyroid cats. For the most part, methimazole has replaced propylthiouracil for use in cats.	Tapazole	5, 10 mg tablets	Cats: 5 mg/cat PO q8-12h for induction, then 2.5-5 mg/cat PO q8-12h
dl-methionine	See racemethionine.					
Methocarbamol	Skeletal muscle relaxant. Depresses polysynaptic reflexes. Used for treatment of skeletal muscle spasms.	Causes some depression and sedation of the central nervous system	Results of clinical studies in animals have not been reported. Use in animals (and doses) is based on experience in humans or anecdotal experience in animals.	Robaxin-V	500, 750 mg tablets; 100 mg/ml injection	44 mg/kg PO q8h on the first day, then 22-44 mg/kg PO q8h
Methohexital	Barbiturate anesthetic. See thiopental for details. Methohexital is about 2-3 times more potent than pentothal, but with shorter duration.	See thiopental.	See thiopental	Brevital	0.5, 2.5, 5 g vials for injection	3-6 mg/kg IV (give slowly to effect)
Methotrexate	Anticancer agent. Used for various carcinomas, leukemia, and lymphomas. Action is via antimetabolite action. Analogue of folic acid that binds dihydrofolate reductase. Inhibits DNA, RNA, and protein synthesis. In humans, methotrexate is also commonly used for autoimmune diseases such as rheumatoid arthritis.	Anticancer drugs cause predictable (and sometimes unavoidable) side effects that include bone marrow suppression, leukopenia, and immunosuppression. Hepatotoxicity has been reported in humans from methotrexate therapy. Concurrent use with NSAIDs may cause severe methotrexate toxicity. Do not administer with pyrimethamine, trimethoprim, or sulfonamides.	Use in animals has been based on experimental studies. There is only limited clinical information available. Consult specific anticancer protocols for precise dosage and regimen.	MTX, Mexate, Folex, Rheumatrex, generic	2.5 mg tablets; 2.5, 25 mg/ml injections	2.5-5 mg/m² PO q48h (dose depends on specific protocol). Dogs: 0.3-0.5 mg/kg IV once per week. Cats: 0.8 mg/kg IV every 2-3 weeks.
Methoxamine	Adrenergic agonist. Sympathomimetic. Alpha-1 (α_1) adrenergic agonist. Specific for alpha-1 receptors.	Adverse effects related to excessive stimulation of alpha-1 receptor (prolonged peripheral vasoconstriction). Reflex bradycardia may occur.	Used primarily in critical care patients or during anesthesia to increase peripheral resistance and increase blood pressure. Short onset and duration of action.	Vasoxyl	20 mg/ml injection	200-250 µg/kg IM or 40-80 µg/kg IV

Drug name	Pharmacology and category of use	Precautions	Dosing information and comments	Other names	Formulations available	Dosage
Methoxyflurane	Inhalant anesthetic. See halothane.	See halothane. Methoxyflurane has been reported to cause hepatic injury in animals. Labeling recommendations in some countries state that flunixin should not be administered to animals receiving methoxyflurane anesthesia.	See halothane.	Metofane	4 oz bottle	Induction: 3%. Maintenance: 0.5-1.5%.
Methylene blue 0.1%	Antidote for intoxication. Used to treat methemoglobinemia. Acts as reducing agent to reduce methemoglobin to hemoglobin.	Methylene blue can cause Heinz body anemia in cats, but is safe when used at therapeutic doses listed here.	Comparison of effects for intoxication has only been performed in experimental effects. One study demonstrated that acetylcysteine produced the best response; methylene blue also was helpful in some cats (AJVR 1995;56:1529).	Generic, new methylene blue	1% solution (10 mg/ml)	1.5 mg/kg IV slowly
Methylprednisolone	Glucocorticoid antiinflammatory drug. See betamethasone.	Same as other glucocorticoids. See betamethasone. Manufacturer suggests that methylprednisolone causes less PU/PD than prednisolone.	Use of methylprednisolone is similar to other corticosteroids. Dose adjustment should be made to account for difference in potency. See dose section.	Medrol	2, 4, 8, 18, 32 mg tablets	See doses for prednisolone. (Methylprednisolone has potency that is 1.25 times prednisolone.)
Methylprednisolone acetate	Depot form of methylprednisolone. Slowly absorbed from IM injection site, producing glucocorticoid effects for 3-4 weeks in some animals. Used for intralesional therapy, intraarticular therapy, and inflammatory conditons.	Many adverse effects possible from use of corticosteroids. See betamethasone.	Use of methylprednisolone acetate should be evaluated carefully because one injection will cause glucocorticoid effects that persist for several days to weeks.	Depo-Medrol	20, 40 mg/ml suspension for injection	Dogs: 1 mg/kg IM every 1-3 weeks. Cats: 10-20 mg/cat IM every 1-3 weeks.
Methylprednisolone sodium succinate	Same as methylprednisolone, except that this is a water-soluble formulation intended for acute therapy when high IV doses are needed for rapid effect. Used for treatment of shock and CNS trauma.	Adverse effects are not expected from single administration; however, with repeated use, other side effects are possible. See betamethasone.	Results of clinical studies in animals have not been reported. Use in animals (and doses) is based on experience in humans or anecdotal experience in animals.	Solu-Medrol	125, 500 mg vials for injection	Emergency use: 30 mg/kg IV and repeat at 15 mg/kg in 2-6 hours. Replacement or antiinflammatory therapy: See prednisolone.
4-methylpyrazole	Antidote for ethylene glycol (antifreeze) intoxication. Inhibits dehydrogenase enzyme that converts ethylene glycol to toxic metabolite.	Adverse effects have not been reported.	Used for emergency management of intoxication. Experimental studies have demonstrated effectivess in dogs, but in cats ethanol is more effective.	5% solution	5% solution	20 mg/kg IV initially, then 15 mg/kg at 12- and 24-hour intervals and 5 mg at 36 hours.
Methyltestosterone	Anabolic androgenic agent. Used for anabolic actions or testosterone hormone replacement therapy (androgenic deficiency). Testosterone has been used to stimulate erythropoiesis.	Adverse effects caused by excessive androgenic action of testosterone. Prostatic hyperplasia is possible in male dogs. Masculinization can occur in female dogs. Hepatopathy is more common with oral methylated testerone formulations.	See also testosterone cypionate and testosterone propionate. Use of testosterone androgens has not been evaluated in clinical studies in veterinary medicine. Use is based primarily on experimental evidence or experiences in humans.	Android, generic	10, 25 mg tablets	Dogs: 5-25 mg/dog PO q24-48h. Cats: 2.5-5 mg/cat PO q24-48h.

Drug name	Pharmacology and category of use	Precautions	Dosing information and comments	Other names	Formulations available	Dosage
Metoclopramide	Prokinetic drug. Antiemetic. Stimulates motility of upper gastrointestinal tract and centrally-acting antiemetic. Action is to inhibit dopamine receptors and enhance action of acetylcholine in gastrointestinal tract. Used primarily for gastroparesis and treatment of vomiting.	Adverse effects are primarily related to blockade of central dopaminergic receptors. Adverse effects similar to what is reported for phenothiazines (e.g., acepromazine) have been reported in addition to behavioral changes. Do not use in epileptic patients or with diseases caused by gastrointestinal obstruction.	Results of clinical studies in animals have not been reported. Use in animals (and doses) is based on experience in humans or anecdotal experience in animals.	Reglan, Maxolon (Maxeran in Canada)	10, 5 mg tablets; 1 mg/ml oral solution; 5 mg/ml injection	0.2-0.5 mg/kg IV, IM, PO q6-8h (or 1-2 mg/kg/day via continuous IV infusion)
Metoprolol tartrate	Adrenergic blocking agent. Beta-1 (β_1) adrenergic blocker. Similar properties to propranolol, except that metoprolol is specific for β_1 receptor. Used to control tachyarrhymias and slow heart rate.	Adverse effects are primarily caused by excessive cardiovascular depression (decreased inotropic effects). May cause heart block. Use cautiously in animals prone to bronchoconstriction.	Results of clinical studies in animals have not been reported. Use in animals (and doses) is based on experience in humans or anecdotal experience in animals.	Lopressor	50, 100 mg tablets; 1 mg/ml injection	Dogs: 5-50 mg/dog PO (0.5-1.0 mg/kg) q8h. Cats: 2-15 mg/cat PO q8h.
Metronidazole	Antibacterial and antiprotozoal drug. Disrupts DNA in organism via reaction with intracellular metabolite. Action is specific for anaerobic bacteria. Resistance is rare. Active against some protozoa, including Giardia.	Most severe adverse effect is caused by toxicity to CNS. High doses have caused lethargy, CNS depression, ataxia, vomiting, and weakness. Metronidazole may be mutagenic. Fetal abnormalities have not been demonstrated in animals with recommended doses, but use cautiously during pregnancy. Cats find broken tablets unpalatable.	Metronidazole is one of the most commonly used drugs for anaerobic infections. Although it is effective for giardiasis, other drugs used for Giardia include albendazole, fenbendazole, and quinacrine. CNS toxicity is dose related. Maximum dose that should be administered in any species is 50-65 mg/kg per day.	Flagyl, generic	250, 500 mg tablets; 50 mg/ml suspension; 5 mg/ml injection	Anaerobes: 10 mg/kg q8h or 15 mg/kg q12h (dogs); 10-25 mg/kg PO q24h (cats). Giardia: 12-15 mg/kg PO q12h for 8 days (dogs); 17 mg/kg (1/3 of a 250 mg tablet per cat) q24h for 8 days (cats).
Mexiletine	Antiarrhythmic drug. Used for ventricular arrhythmias. Mechanism of action is to block fast sodium channel. Class IB antiarrhythmic agent.	May produce arrhythmias. Use cautiously in animals with liver disease.	Results of clinical studies in animals have not been reported. Use in animals (and doses) is based on experience in humans or anecdotal experience in animals.	Mexitil	150, 200, 250 mg capsules	Dogs: 5-8 mg/kg PO q8-12h (use cautiously)
Mibolerone	Androgenic steroid. Used to suppress estrus.	Do not use in Bedlington terriers. Do not use with perianal adenoma or carcinoma. Many bitches show clitoral enlargement or discharge from treatment. Do not use in cats.	Treatment ordinarily is initiated 30 days before onset of estrus. Its use is not recommended for more than 2 years.	Cheque-drops	55 µg/ml oral solution	Dogs: 2.6-5 µg/kg/day PO. Dogs 0.45-11.3 kg: 30 µg. Dogs 11.8-22.7 kg: 60 µg. Dogs 23-45.3 kg: 120 µg. Dogs > 45.8 kg: 180 µg. Cats: Safe dose not established.
Midazolam	Benzodiazepine. Action is similar to other benzodiazepines. See diazepam. Used as anesthetic adjunct.	Precautions similar to other benzodiazepines. See diazepam.	Routine clinical use is not common. Clinical trials have not been reported. Contrary to other benzodiazepines, midazolam can be administered IM.	Versed	5 mg/ml injection	0.1-0.25 mg/kg IV, IM or 0.1-0.3 mg/kg/hour IV infusion

Drug name	Pharmacology and category of use	Precautions	Dosing information and comments	Other names	Formulations available	Dosage
Milbemycin oxime	Antiparasitic drug. Action is similar to ivermectin. Acts as GABA agonist in nervous system of parasite. Used as heartworm preventative, miticide, and microfilaricide.	In susceptible dogs (collie breeds), milbemycin may cross the blood-brain barrier and produce central nervous system toxicity (depression, lethargy, and coma). At doses used for heartworm prevention, this effect is less likely.	Doses vary depending on parasite treated. Consult dose column. Treatment of Demodex requires high dose administered daily (JAVMA 1995;207:1581).	23, 11.5, 5.75, 2.3 mg tablets	Interceptor	Microfilaricide: 0.5 mg/kg. Demodex: 2 mg/kg PO q24h for 60-120 days. Heartworm prevention: 0.5 mg/kg PO every 30 days.
Milk of Magnesia	See magnesium hydroxide.					
Mineral oil	Lubricant laxative. Increases water content of stool. Used to increase passage of feces for treatment of impaction and constipation.	Adverse effects have not been reported. Chronic use may decrease absorption of fat-soluble vitamins.	Use is empirical. No clinical results reported.	Generic	Oral liquid	Dogs: 10-50 ml/dog PO q12h. Cats: 10-25 ml/cat PO q12h.
Minocycline	Tetracycline antibiotic. Similar to doxycycline in pharmacokinetics. See doxycycline.	See doxycycline. Adverse effects have not been reoported for minocycline. Oral absorption is not affected by calcium products as with other tetracyclines.	Minocycline has received little attention for clinical use in North America. Clinical use has not been reported, but properties are similar to doxycycline.	Minocin	50, 100 mg tablets; 10 mg/ml oral suspension	5-12.5 mg/kg PO q12h
Misoprostol	Prostaglandin E_2 analogue. Prostaglandins provide a cytoprotective role in the gastrointestinal mucosa. Misoprostol is used to prevent gastritis and ulcers associated with NSAID (aspirin drug) therapy.	Adverse effects are caused by effects of prostaglandins. Most common side effects are gastrointestinal discomfort, vomiting, and diarrhea. Do not administer to pregnant animals; may cause abortion.	Doses and recommendations are based on clinical trials in which misoprostol was administered to prevent gastrointestinal mucosal injury caused by aspirin.	Cytotec	0.1 mg (100 µg), 0.2 µg (200 mg) tablets	Dogs: 2-5 µg/kg PO q6-8h. Cats: Dose not established.
Mithramycin	See plicamycin (Mithracin).					
Mitotane (o, p'-DDD)	Adrenocortical cytotoxic agent. Causes suppression of adrenal cortex. Used to treat adrenal tumors and pituitary-dependent hyperadrenocorticism (PDH).	Adverse effects, especially during induction period, include lethargy, anorexia, ataxia, depression, and vomiting. Corticosteroid supplementation (e.g., hydrocortisone or prednisolone) may be administered to minimize side effects.	Dose and frequency often are based on patient response. Adverse effects are common during initial therapy. Administration with food increases oral absorption. Maintenance dose should be adjusted on the basis of periodic cortisol measurements and ACTH stimulation tests. See also Vet Record 1988;122:486.	Lysodren, o, p'-DDD	500 mg tablet	PDH: 50 mg/kg/day PO (in divided doses) for 5-10 days, then 50-70 mg/kg/week PO. Adrenal tumor: 50-75 mg/kg/day PO for 10 days, then 75-100 mg/kg/week.
Mitoxantrone	Anticancer antibiotic. Similar to doxorubicin in action. See doxorubicin. Used for leukemia, lymphoma, and carcinomas.	As with all anticancer agents, certain adverse effects are predictable and unavoidable and related to drug's action. Mitoxantrone produces myelosuppression, vomiting, anorexia, and gastrointestinal upset, but may be less cardiotoxic than doxorubicin.	Proper use of mitoxantrone usually follows a specific anticancer protocol. Consult specific protocol for dosing regimen.	Novantrone	2 mg/ml injection	Dogs: 6 mg/m^2 IV every 21 days. Cats: 6.5 mg/m^2 IV every 21 days.

Drug name	Pharmacology and category of use	Precautions	Dosing information and comments	Other names	Formulations available	Dosage
Morphine	Opioid agonist and analgesic. Prototype for other opioid agonists. Action of morphine is to bind to μ- and κ-opiate receptors on nerves and inhibit release of neurotransmitters involved with transmission of pain stimuli (such as substance P). Morphine also may inhibit release of some inflammatory mediatiors. Central sedative and euphoric effects related to mu-receptor effects in brain.	Like all opiates, side effects from morphine are predictable and unavoidable. Side effects from morphine administration include sedation, constipation, and bradycardia. Respiratory depression occurs with high doses. Tolerance and dependence occurs with chronic administration. Cats are more sensitive to excitement than other species.	Effects from morphine administration are dose-dependent. Low doses (0.1-0.25 mg/kg) produce mild analgesia. Higher doses (up to 1 mg/kg) produce greater analgesic effects and sedation. Usually morphine is administered IM, IV, or SC; however, delayed-release tablets have been used in dogs experimentally at higher doses (1-3 mg/kg q12h). Epidural administration has been used for surgical procedures.	Generic	1, 15 mg/ml injections; 30, 60 mg delayed-release tablets	Dogs: 0.1-1 mg/kg IV, IM, SC (as needed every 4-6 hours). Epidural: 0.1 mg/kg. Cats: 0.1 mg/kg IM, SC (as needed).
Moxidectin	Antiparasitic drug. Neurotoxic to parasites by potentiating effects of inhibitory neurotransmitter GABA.	Toxicity may occur at high doses and in species in which ivermectin crosses blood-brain barrier (Collie breeds). Toxicity is neurotoxic and signs include depression, ataxia, difficulty with vision, coma, and death.	Similar use as ivermectin	Cydectin	Injection	Heartworm prevention: 3 μg/kg. Endoparasites (dogs): 25-300 μg/kg.
Myochrysine	See gold sodium thiomalate.					
Nalorphine	Opiate antagonist. Used to reverse effects from opiate agonists (such as morphine). See naloxone.	See naloxone.	See naloxone. Administer as indicated in dose section, but no more than 5 mg per dose. Duration is 2-3 hours, then it may have to be readministered.	Nalline	5 mg/ml injection	0.44 mg/kg IV, IM, SC (1 mg for every 10 mg of morphine)
Naloxone	Opiate antagonist. Used to reverse effects from opiate agonists (such as morphine). Naloxone may be used to reverse sedation, anesthesia, and adverse effects caused by opiates.	Adverse effects are not reported. Tachycardia and hypertension have been reported in humans.	Administration may have to be individualized based on patient response. Naloxone's duration of action is short in animals (60 minutes) and may have to be repeated.	Narcan	20, 400 μg/ml injections	0.01-0.04 mg/kg IV, IM, SC, as needed to reverse opiate
Naltrexone	Opiate antagonist. Similar to naloxone except that it is longer acting and administered PO. Used in humans for treatment of opiate dependence. In animals it has been used for treatment of some obsessive-compulsive behavioral disorders.	Adverse effects have not been reported in animals.	Treatment for obsessive-compulsive disorders in animals has been reported with naltrexone. Relapse rates may be high.	Trexan	50 mg tablet	Behavioral disorders: 2.2 mg/kg PO q12h

Drug name	Pharmacology and category of use	Precautions	Dosing information and comments	Other names	Formulations available	Dosage
Nandrolone deconate	Anabolic steroid. Derivative of testosterone. Anabolic agents are designed to maximize anabolic effects while minimizing androgenic action. See methyltestosterone. Anabolic agents have been used to reverse catabolic conditions, increase weight gain, increase muscle in animals, and stimulate erythropoiesis.	Adverse effects from anabolic steroids can be attributed to the pharmacologic action of these steroids. Increased masculine effects are common. Increased incidence of some tumors have been reported in humans. 17α-methylated oral anabolic steroids (oxymetholone, stanozolol, and oxandrolone) are associated with hepatic toxicity.	Results of clinical studies in animals have not been reported. Use in animals (and doses) is based on experience in humans or anecdotal experience in animals.	Deca-Durabolin	50, 100, 200 mg/ml injecton	Dogs: 1-1.5 mg/kg/week IM. Cats: 1 mg/cat/week IM.
Naproxen	Nonsteroidal antiinflammatory drug (NSAID). Action is similar to other NSAIDS (see Flunixin).	Naproxen is a potent NSAID. Adverse effects attributied to GI toxicity are common to all NSAIDs. See flunixin. Naproxen has produced serious ulceration in dogs because elimination in dogs is many times slower than in humans or horses.	Results of clinical studies in animals have not been reported. Use in animals (and doses) is based on pharmacokinetic studies in experimental animals. Caution when using the OTC formulation designed for humans because the tablet size is much larger than safe dose for dogs.	Naprosyn, Naxen, Aleve (OTC)	220 mg tablet (OTC), 25 mg/ml liquid suspension, 250, 375, 500 mg tablets, and 275, 550 mg tablets.	5 mg initially, then 2 mg/kg q48h
Neomycin	Aminoglycoside antibiotic. For mechanism and other effects see gentamicin and amikacin. Neomycin differs from other aminoglycosides because it is only administered topically or orally. Systemic absorption is minimal from oral absorption.	Although oral absorption is so minimal that systemic adverse effects are unlikely, some oral absorption has been demonstrated in young animals (calves). Alterations in intestinal bacterial flora from therapy may cause diarrhea.	Neomycin is primarily used for oral treatment of diarrhea. Efficacy for this indication (especially for nonspecific diarrhea) is questionable. Used for treatment of hepatic encephalopathy.	Biosol	500 mg bolus; 200 mg/ml oral liquid	10-20 mg/kg PO q6-12h
Neostigmine bromide and neostigmine methylsulfate	Anticholinesterase drug. Cholinesterase inhibitor. Inhibits breakdown of acetylcholine at synapse. Antimyasthenic drug. Used primarily for treatment of myasthenia gravis or as an antidote for neuromuscular blockade caused by nondepolarizing neuromuscular blocking drugs.	Adverse effects are related to drug's pharmacological effects: excessive cholinergic stimulation (muscarinic effects), including diarrhea, salivation, respiratory problems, vomiting, CNS effects, muscle twitching, or weakness. Atropine is used to treat overdose.	Compared to other drugs in this class (e.g., pyridostigmine), produces more severe muscarinic effects. Neostigmine has been used for diagnostic purposes also. See edrophonium. When injected for treatment of myasthenia, or diagnosis, it is recommended to use atropine to counteract side effects.	Prostigmin, Stiglyn	15 mg tablet (neostigmine bromide); 0.25, 0.5 mg/ml injection (neostigmine methylsulfate)	Antimyasthenic: 2 mg/kg/day PO (in divided doses, to effect). 10 μg/kg IM, SC, as needed. Antidote for curiform block: 40 μg/kg IM, SC. Diagnostic aid for myasthenia gravis: 40 μg/kg IM or 20 μg/kg IV.
Nifedipine	Calcium-channel blocking drug. See diltiazem. Action is similar to other calcium-channel blocking drugs, except nifedipine is more specific for vascular smooth muscle than cardiac tissue. Used for smooth muscle relaxation and vasodilation.	Adverse effects have not been reported in veterinary medicine. Most common side effect is hypotension.	Use of nifedipine is limited in veterinary medicine. Other calcium-channel blockers (such as diltiazem) are used more frequently. In humans, the dose is 10 mg three times a day and increased in 10 mg increments to effect.	Adalat, Procardia	10, 20 mg capsules	Dose not established.

Drug name	Pharmacology and category of use	Precautions	Dosing information and comments	Other names	Formulations available	Dosage
Nitrates	See nitroglycerin and isosorbide dinitrate.					
Nitrofurantoin	Antibacterial drug. Urinary antiseptic. Action is via reactive metabolites that damage DNA. Therapeutic concentrations are reached only in the urine.	Adverse effects include nausea, vomiting, and diarrhea. Turns urine brown. Do not administer during pregnancy.	Two dosing forms exist. Microcrystalline is rapidly and completely absorbed. Macrocrystalline (Macrodantin) is more slowly absorbed and causes less gastrointestinal irritation. Urine should be at acidic pH for maximum effect.	Furadantin, Macrodantin	25, 50, 100 mg capsules; 50, 100 mg tablets; 5 mg/ml oral suspension	4 mg/kg PO q8h
Nitroglycerin	Nitrate. Nitrovasodilator. Relaxes vascular smooth muscle (especially venous) via generation of nitric oxide and cyclic-GTP synthesis. Used primarily in heart failure to reduce preload or decrease pulmonary hypertension. In humans, used to treat angina pectoris.	Adverse effects from nitrates are related to their pharmacologic action. Most significant adverse effect is hypotension. Methemoglobinemia can occur with accumulation of nitrites.	Tolerance can develop with repeated, chronic use. Use should be intermittent for optimum effect. Nitroglycerin has high presystemic metabolism and oral availability is poor. When using ointment, 1 inch of ointment ≈ 15 mg.	Nitrol, Nitrobid, Nitrostat	0.5, 0.8, 1, 5, 10 mg/ml injections; 2% ointment; 0.2 mg/hour patch (transdermal systems)	Dogs: 4-12 mg (up to 15 mg) topically q12h. Cats: 2-4 mg (1/4 inch of ointment per cat) topically q12h.
Nitroprusside	Nitrate vasodilator. See nitroglycerin.	See nitroglycerin.	See nitroglycerin. Nitroprusside is administered via IV infusion. IV solution should be delivered in 5% dextrose solution. Protect from light. Discard solution if color change is observed. Titrate dose carefully in each patient.	Nitropress	50 mg vial for injection	1-10 µg/kg/min IV infusion
Nizatidine	Histamine H_2 blocking drug. See cimetidine. Same as cimetidine, except up to 10 times more potent.	See cimetidine and ranitidine. Side effects from nizatidine have not been reported for animals.	Results of clinical studies in animals have not been reported. Use in animals (and doses) is based on experience in humans or anecdotal experience in animals.	Axid	150, 300 mg capsules	5 mg/kg PO q24h
Norfloxacin	Fluoroquinolone antibacterial drug. Same action as ciprofloxacin, except spectrum of activity is not as broad as with ciprofloxacin and enrofloxacin.	Adverse effects have not been reported in animals. Some effects are expected to be similar to ciprofloxacin and enrofloxacin administration.	Use in animals (and doses) is based on pharmacokinetic studies in experimental animals, experience in humans, or anecdotal experience in animals.	Noroxin	400 mg tablets	22 mg/kg PO q12h
o, p'-DDD	See mitotane (Lysodren).					
Omeprazole	Proton pump inhibitor. Omeprazole inhibits gastric acid secretion by inhibiting the K^+/H^+ pump. Omeprazole is more potent and longer acting than most available antisecretory drugs. Used for treatment and prevention of gastrointestinal ulcers.	Side effects have not been reported in animals; however, in humans, there is concern about hypergastrinemia with chronic use. Do not administer with drugs that depend on acid stomach for absorption (e.g., ketoconazole).	Because of omeprazole's potency and accumulation in gastric cells, infrequent administration is possible. Lansoprazole is a newer drug of this class but has not been used in animals.	Prilosec (formerly Losec)	20 mg capsule	Dogs: 20 mg/dog PO once daily or 0.7 mg/kg q24h. Cats: Not recommended.

Drug name	Pharmacology and category of use	Precautions	Dosing information and comments	Other names	Formulations available	Dosage
Ondansetron	Antiemetic drug. Ondansetron's action is to inhibit action of serotonin (blocks 5-HT$_3$ receptors). Used primarily to inhibit vomiting associated with chemotherapy.	Ondansetron's adverse effects have not been reported in animals. Some effects may be indistinguishable from concurrent cancer drugs.	Ondansetron has been used infrequently in veterinary medicine because of its expense. Granisetron is a similar drug not yet evaluated in veterinary medicine.	Zofran	4, 8 mg tablets; 2 mg/ml injection	0.5-1.0 mg/kg 30 minutes before administration of cancer drugs
Ormetoprim	Trimethoprim-like drug used in combination with sulfadimethoxine. See Primor.					
Olsalazine	Antiinflammatory drug for treating colitis. Two molecules of aminosalicylic acid joined by an azobond. See mesalamine.	See mesalamine.	See mesalamine. Olsalazine is used in patients that cannot tolerate sulfasalazine.	Dipentum	500 mg tablet	Dose not established. (The usual human dose is 500 mg twice daily.)
Oxacillin	Beta-lactam antibiotic. Inhibits bacterial cell wall synthesis. Spectrum is limited to gram-positive bacteria, especially staphylococci.	Use cautiously in animals allergic to penicillin-like drugs.	Doses based on empiricism or extrapolation from human studies. No clinical efficacy studies available for dogs or cats. Administer on empty stomach if possible.	Prostaphlin, generic	250, 500 mg capsules; 50 mg/ml oral solution	22-40 mg/kg PO q8h
Oxazepam	Benzodiazepine. Central-acting CNS depressant. Mechanism of action appears to be via potentiation of GABA-receptor mediated effects in CNS. Used for sedation and to stimulate appetite.	Sedation is most common side effect. Causes polyphagia. In cats, fatal hepatic necrosis has been reported from diazepam.	Doses based on empiricism. There have been no clinical trials in veterinary medicine.	Serax	15 mg tablet	Appetite stimulant: 2.5 mg/cat PO
Oxtriphylline	Choline theophyllinate. Methylxanthine bronchodilator. Mechanism similar to theophylline.	See theophylline.	Adverse effects similar to theophylline. See theophylline. Some formulations (Theocon) contain oxtriphylline and guaifenesin. When administering slow-release tablet, do not crush tablet.	Choledyl-SA	400, 600 mg tablet; oral solutions and syrup available in Canada, but not United States	Dogs: 47 mg/kg (equivalent to 30 mg/kg theophylline) PO q12h
Oxybutynin chloride	Anticholinergic agent. Inhibits smooth muscle spasms via blocking action of acetylcholine. Used primarily to increase bladder capacity and to decrease spasms of urinary tract.	Adverse effects are related to anticholinergic effects (see atropine), but are less frequent compared to other anticholinergic drugs. Administer physostigmine for overdose.	Results of clinical studies in animals have not been reported. Use in animals (and doses) is based on experience in humans or anecdotal experience in animals.	Ditropan	5 mg tablet	Dogs: 5 mg/dog PO q6-8h

Drug name	Pharmacology and category of use	Precautions	Dosing information and comments	Other names	Formulations available	Dosage
Oxymetholone	Anabolic steroid. See nandrolone. There are no differences in efficacy among the anabolic steroids.	See nandrolone.	See nandrolone.	Anadrol	50 mg tablet	1-5 mg/kg/day PO
Oxymorphone	Opioid agonist. Action is similar to morphine, except that oxymorphone is 10-15 times more potent than morphine.	See morphine.	See morphine. There is some evidence that oxymorphone may have fewer cardiovascular effects compared to morphine.	Numorphan	1.5, 1 mg/ml injections	0.1-0.2 mg/kg IV, SC, IM (as needed); redose with 0.05-0.1 mg/kg q1-2h. Preanesthetic: 0.025-0.05 mg/kg IM, SC.
Oxytetracycline	Tetracycline antibiotic. See tetracycline.			Terramycin	250 mg capsules; 100, 200 mg/ml injections	7.5-10 mg/kg IV q12h; 20 mg/kg PO q12h
Oxytocin	Stimulates uterine muscle contraction via action on specific oxytocin receptors. Used to induce or maintain normal labor and delivery in pregnant animals. Does not increase milk production, but will stimulate contraction leading to milk ejection.	Adverse effects are uncommon if used carefully. Fetal stress and progression of normal labor should be monitored closely.	Used to induce labor. In humans, oxytocin is administered via injection, constant IV infusion, and intranasal solution.	Pitocin, Syntocinon (nasal solution), generic	10, 20 U/ml injection; 40 U/ml nasal solution	Dogs: 1-5 U IM, IV (repeat every 30 minutes for primary inertia). Cats: 0.5 IM, IV (maximum dose is 3 U/cat).
2-PAM	See pralidoxime chloride.					
Pancreatic enzyme	See pancrelipase (Viokase).					
Pancrelipase	Pancreatic enzyme. Used to treat pancreatic exocrine insufficiency. Provides lipase, amylase, and protease.	Adverse effects have not been reported.		Viokase	16,800 U lipase, 70,000 U protease, 70,000 U amylase per 0.7 g; capsules; tablets, powder	Mix 2 tsp powder with food per 20 kg body weight or 1-3 tsp per 0.45 kg of food.
Pancuronium bromide	Nondepolarizing neuromuscular blocker. See atricurium.	See atricurium.	See atricurium.	Pavulon	1, 2 mg/ml injections	0.1 mg/kg IV or start with 0.01 mg/kg and additional 0.01 mg/kg doses every 30 minutes
Paregoric	Paregoric (opium tincture) is an outdated product used to treat diarrhea. Paregoric contains 2 mg of morphine in every 5 ml of paregoric.	See opiates (such as morphine).	Use of paregoric has been replaced by more specific products such as loperamide or diphenoxylate.	Corrective mixture	2 mg morphine per 5 ml of paregoric	0.05-0.06 mg/kg PO q12h
D-penicillamine	Chelating agent for lead copper, iron, and mercury. Used primarily in animals for treatment of copper toxicity and hepatitis associated with accumulation of copper. It also has been used to treat cystine calculi. Penicillamine has been used in humans to treat rheumatoid arthritis.	Do not use in pregnant animals. In humans, allergic reactions have been reported as well as agranulocytosis and anemia.	Administer on an empty stomach (2 hours before meals).	Cuprimine, Depen	125, 250 mg capsules; 250 mg tablets	10-15 mg/kg PO q12h
Penicillin G benzathine	All benzathine penicillin G is combined with procaine penicillin G in commercial formulation.	See other forms of penicillin G.	Benzathine is not recommended for therapy because concentrations are too low to be therapeutic.	Benza-Pen and other names	150,000 U/ml combined with 150,000 µml of procaine penicillin.	24,000 U/kg IM q48h

Drug name	Pharmacology and category of use	Precautions	Dosing information and comments	Other names	Formulations available	Dosage
Penicillin G potassium and penicillin G sodium	Beta-lactam antibiotic. Action is similar to other penicillins (see amoxicillin). Spectrum of penicillin G is limited to gram-positive bacteria and anaerobes.	Same as other penicillins. See amoxicillin.	See other penicillins (amoxicillin).	Many	5-20 million U vials	20,000-40,000 U/kg IV, IM q6-8h
Penicillin G procaine	Same as other forms of penicillin G, except procaine penicillin is absorbed slowly, producing concentrations for 12-24 hours after injections.	Same as other penicillins. See amoxicillin.	Same as other penicillins (amoxicillin). Avoid SC injection with procaine penicillin G.	Generic	300,000 U/ml suspension	20,000-40,000 U/kg IM q12-24h
Penicillin V	Oral penicillin. Otherwise same as other penicillins.	Same as other penicillins (see amoxicillin)	Same as other penicillins (amoxicillin). Penicillin V should be administered on an empty stomach for maximum absorption. (250 mg = 400,000 U.)	Pen-Vee	250, 500 mg tablets	10 mg/kg PO q8h
Pentazocine	Synthetic opiate analgesic. Partial agonist (similar to buprenorphine or butorphanol).	Adverse effects similar to other opiates. See butorphanol or morphine.	See other opiates.	Talwin-V	30 mg/ml injection	Dogs: 1.65-3.3 mg/kg IM q4h. Cats: 2.2-3.3 mg/kg IV, IM, SC.
Pentobarbital	Short-acting barbiturate anesthetic. Action is via nonselective depression of central nervous system. Pentobarbital usually is used as IV anesthetic. Duration of action may be 3-4 hours.	Adverse effects are related to anesthetic action. See thiopental. Cardiac and respiratory depression are common.	Pentobarbital has narrow therapeutic index. When administering IV, inject first half of dose initially, then remainder of calculated dose gradually until anesthetic effect is achieved.	Nembutal, generic	50 mg/ml	25-30 mg/kg IV
Pentoxifylline	Methylxanthine. Pentoxifylline is used primarily as a rheological agent in humans (increases blood flow through narrow vessels). It may have antiinflammatory action via inhibition of cytokine synthesis. Used in dogs for some dermatoses.	May cause similar signs as other methylxanthines. See theophylline. Nausea and vomiting have been reported in humans.	Results of clinical studies in animals have not been reported. Use in animals (and doses) is based on experience in humans or anecdotal experience in animals.	Trental	400 mg tablet	Dose not established. Human dose is 400 mg PO 2-3 times per day.
Pepto-Bismol	See bismuth subsalicylate.					
Phenobarbital	Long-acting barbiturate. See other barbiturates (thiopental). Phenobarbital's major use is as an anticonvulsant in which it potentiates inhibitory actions of GABA.	Adverse effects are dose related. Phenobarbital causes polyphagia, sedation, ataxia, and lethargy. Some tolerance develops to side effects after initial therapy. Hepatotoxicity has been reported in some dogs receiving high doses.	Phenobarbital doses should be carefully adjusted via monitoring serum/plasma concentrations. Optimum range for therapeutic effect is 15-40 μg/ml.	Luminal, generic	15, 30, 60, 100 mg tablets; 130 mg/ml injection; 10 mg/ml oral solution	Dogs: 2-8 mg/kg PO q12h. Cats: 1-2 mg/kg PO q12h. Status epilepticus: 15-200 mg/animal IV (to effect).
Phenoxybenzamine	Alpha-1 (α_1) adrenergic antagonist. Binds alpha-1 receptor on smooth muscle, causing relaxation. Potent vasodilator. Used primarily to treat peripheral vasoconstriction. In some animals it has been used to relax urethral smooth muscle.	Causes prolonged hypotension in animals. Use carefully in animals with cardiovascular compromise.	Results of clinical studies in animals have not been reported. Use in animals (and doses) is based on experience in humans or limited experimental experience in animals.	Dibenzyline	10 mg capsule	Dogs: 0.25 mg/kg PO q8-12h or 0.5 mg/kg q24h. Cats: 2.5 mg/cat PO q8-12h or 0.5 mg/cat q12h. (In cats, doses as high as 0.5 mg/kg IV have been used to relax urethral smooth muscle.)

Drug name	Pharmacology and category of use	Precautions	Dosing information and comments	Other names	Formulations available	Dosage
Phentolamine	Nonselective alpha (α) adrenergic blocker. Vasodilator. Blocks stimulation of alpha receptors on vascular smooth muscle. Primarily used to treat hypertension.	May cause excess hypotension with high doses or in animals that are dehydrated. May cause tachycardia.	Results of clinical studies in animals have not been reported. Use in animals (and doses) is based on experience in humans or anecdotal experience in animals. Titrate dose for each patient to produce desired vasodilation.	Regitine (Rogitine in Canada)	5 mg vials for injection	0.02-0.1 mg/kg IV
Phenylbutazone	Nonsteroidal antiinflammatory drug (NSAID). See flunixin. Phenylbutazone is used primarily for arthritis and various forms of musculoskeletal pain and inflammation.	Phenylbutazone is generally well tolerated in dogs, but there is no data for cats. Possible adverse effects include gastrointestinal toxicity. See flunixin. Do not administer injectable formulation IM. Phenylbutazone causes bone marrow depression in humans, which also is possible in dogs.	Doses are based primarily on manufacturer's recommendations and clinical experience. There have been no comparative trials demonstrating efficacy of one NSAID over another.	Butazolidin, generic	100, 200, 400 mg, 1 g tablets; 200 mg/ml injection	Dogs: 15-22 mg/kg PO, IV q8-12h (44 mg/kg/day; 800 mg maximum). Cats: Not recommended.
Phenylephrine	Specific adrenergic agonist. Specific for alpha-1 receptor. Same as methoxamine.	Same as methoxamine	Same as methoxamine. Phenylephrine also is used commonly as topical vasoconstrictor (as in nasal decongestants).	Neo-Synephrine	10 mg/ml injection; 1% nasal solution	0.01 mg/kg IV every 15 minutes; 0.1 mg/kg IM, SC every 15 minutes
Phenylpropanolamine	Adrenergic agonist. Used as decongestant, bronchodilator, and to increase tone of urinary sphincter. See ephedrine and pseudoephedrine.	Adverse effects are attributed to excess stimulation of adrenergic (alpha and beta) receptors. See ephedrine. Side effects include tachycardia, cardiac effects, CNS excitement, restlessness, and appetite suppression.	Phenylpropanolamine is available in variety of dose forms, usually used for treatment of cough/colds in humans. Many preparations contain other ingredients.	Dexatrim, Propagest, others	15, 25, 30, 50 mg tablets	1.5-2 mg/kg PO q12h
Phenytoin	Anticonvulsant. Depresses nerve conduction via blockade of sodium channels. Also classified as class I antiarrhythmic. Commonly used as anticonvulsant in humans, but not effective in dogs and not used in cats.	Adverse effects include sedation, gingival hyperplasia, skin reactions, and CNS toxicity. Do not administer to pregnant animals.	Because of short half-life and poor efficacy in dogs and questionable safety in cats, other anticonvulsants are used as first choice before phenytoin.	Dilantin	30, 125 mg/ml oral suspension; 30, 100 mg capsules; 50 mg/ml injection	Antiepileptic (dogs): 20-35 mg/kg q8h. Antiarrhythmic: 30 mg/kg PO q8h or 10 mg/kg IV over 5 minutes.
Physostigmine	Cholinesterase inhibitor. Antidote for anticholinergic intoxication, especially intoxication that exhibits CNS signs. Major difference between physostigmine and neostigmine or pyridostigmine is that physostigmine crosses blood-brain barrier and the others do not.	Adverse effects have been attributed to excessive cholinergic effects; treat overdoses with atropine.	Physostigmine is indicated primarily only for treatment of intoxication. For routine systemic use of anticholinesterase drug, neostigmine and pyridostigmine have fewer side effects. When used, frequency of dose may be increased based on observation of effects.	Antilirium	1 mg/ml injection	0.02 mg/kg IV q12h
Phytonadione	See vitamin K$_1$.					

Drug name	Pharmacology and category of use	Precautions	Dosing information and comments	Other names	Formulations available	Dosage
Phytomenadione	See vitamin K$_1$.					
Piperazine	Antiparasitic compound. Produces neuromuscular blockade in parasite through inhibition of neurotransmitter, which causes paralysis of worms. Used primarily for treatment of helminth (ascarids) infections.	Remarkably safe in all species	Used to treat all species for roundworms	Many	860 mg powder; 140 mg capsule; 170, 340, 800 mg/ml oral solution	44-66 mg/kg PO once
Piroxicam	Nonsteroidal antiinflammatory drug (NSAID) of the oxicam class. Clinical effects are similar to other NSAIDs. See aspirin and flunixin.	Elimination of piroxicam is slow. Use cautiously in dogs. Adverse effects are primarily gastrointestinal toxicity (ulcers). See flunixin.	Piroxicam is primarily used to treat arthritis and other musculoskeletal conditions, but there are reports of its activity for treating certain tumors (e.g., transitional cell carcinoma of bladder).	Feldene, generic	10 mg capsule	Dogs: 0.3 mg/kg PO q48h. Cats: Dose not established.
Pitressin (ADH)	See vasopressin and desmopressin.					
Plicamycin (mithramycin)	Anticancer agent. Action is to combine with DNA in presence of divalent cations and inhibit DNA and RNA synthesis. Lowers serum calcium. Used to treat carcinomas and hypercalcemia.	Adverse effects have not been reported in animals. In humans, hypocalcemia and gastrointestinal toxicity have been reported. Do not use with drugs that may increase the risk of bleeding (e.g., NSAIDs, heparin, or anticoagulants).	Results of clinical studies in animals have not been reported. Use in animals (and doses) is based on experience in humans or anecdotal experience in animals.	Mithracin	2.5 mg injection	Antineoplastic: 25-30 µg/kg/day IV (slow infusion) for 8-10 days. Antihypercalcemic: 25 µg/kg/day IV (slow infusion) over 4 hours.
Polyethylene glycol electrolyte solution	Saline cathartic. See magnesium citrate. Nonabsorbable compounds that increase water secretion into bowel via osmotic effect. Used for bowel evacuation before surgical or diagnostic procedure.	Water and electrolyte loss with high doses or prolonged use. See magnesium citrate.	Used primarily to evacuate bowel as preparation for procedures	Golytely	Oral solution	25 ml/kg PO; repeat in 2-4 hours
Polysulfated glycosaminoglycan (PSGAG)	Large molecular weight compounds similar to normal constituents of healthy joints. Chondroprotective. Inhibits enzymes that may degrade articular cartilage. Used primarily to treat or prevent degenerative joint disease.	Adverse effects are rare. Allergic reactions are possible. PSGAG has heparin-like effects and may potentiate bleeding problems in some animals.	Doses are derived from empirical evidence and some experimental studies in dogs. See Compen Cont Educat 1994;16:501 or JAVMA 1994;204:1245. Although effective for acute arthritis, may not be as effective for chronic arthropathy.	Adequan	100, 250 mg/ml injections	2-4 mg/kg SC, IM once or twice weekly
Potassium bromide	Anticonvulsant. Anticonvulant action is to stabilize neuronal cell membranes. Bromide ordinarily is used in patients refractory to phenobarbital.	Adverse effects are related to high levels of bromide. Signs of toxicosis are CNS depression, weakness, and ataxia. Consider using sodium bromide in patients with hypoadrenocorticism.	Bromide usually is administered in combination with phenobarbital. Monitor serum bromide concentrations to adjust dose. Concentrations should be 1-2 mg/ml. (100-200 mg/dL). Diets high in chloride will cause shorter half-life and need for higher dose.	No commercial formulation	Usually prepared as oral solution	Dogs: 30-40 mg/kg PO q24h. Loading doses of 300 mg/kg divided over 3 days have been administered.

Drug name	Pharmacology and category of use	Precautions	Dosing information and comments	Other names	Formulations available	Dosage
Potassium chloride	Potassium supplement. Used for treatment of hypokalemia. Usually added to fluid solutions.	Toxicity from high potassium concentrations can be dangerous. Hyperkalemia can lead to cardiovascular toxicity (bradycardia and arrest) and muscular weakness. Oral potassium supplements can cause nausea and stomach irritation.	1 g potassium chloride provides 13.41 mEq potassium. When potassium is supplemented in fluids, do not administer at a rate faster than 0.5 mEq/kg/hr.	Generic	Various concentrations for injection (usually 2 mEq/ml); oral suspension; oral solution	0.5 mEq potassium/ kg/day or supplement 10-40 mEq/500 ml of fluids, depending on serum potassium concentration.
Potassium citrate	Same as potassium chloride	Same as potassium chloride	1 g potassium citrate provides 9.26 mEq potassium.	Generic, Urocit-K	5 mEq tablet (some forms are in combination with potassium chloride)	2.2 mEq per 100 kiloCalories of energy per day PO or 50-75 mg/kg PO q12h
Potassium gluconate	Same as potassium chloride	Same as potassium chloride	1 g potassium gluconate provides 4.27 mEq potassium.	Kaon, Tumil-K, generic	2 mEq tablet; 500 mg tablets; Kaon elixir is 20 mg/15 ml elixir	Dogs: 0.5 mEq/kg PO q12-24h. Cats: 2-6 mEq/day.
Pralidoxime chloride (2-PAM)	Used for treatment of organophosphate toxicosis	Adverse effects have not been reported.	When treating intoxication, consult poison control center for precise guidelines.	2-PAM, Protopam chloride	50 mg/ml injection	20 mg/kg q8-12h (initial dose IV slow or IM)
Praziquantel	Antiparasitic drug. Action on parasites related to neuromuscular toxicity and paralysis via altered permeability to calcium. Used primarily to treat infections caused by tapeworms.	Vomiting occurs at high doses. Anorexia and transient diarrhea have been reported. Safe in pregnant animals.	Dose recommendations are based on label dose supplied by the manufacturer.	Droncit	23, 34 mg tablets; 56.8 mg/ml injection	Dogs < 6.8 kg: 7.5 mg/kg PO once. Dogs > 6.8 kg: 5 mg/kg PO once. Dogs ≤ 2.3 kg: 7.5 mg/kg IM, SC once. Dogs 2.7-4.5 kg: 6.3 mg/kg IM, SC once. Dogs ≥ 5 kg: 5 mg/kg IM, SC once. Cats: 5 mg/kg IM, SC. Cats < 1.8 kg: 6.3 mg/kg PO once. Cats > 1.8 kg: 5 mg/kg PO once. Paragonimus: 25 mg/kg q8h for 2 days.
Prazocin	Alpha-1 (α_1) adrenergic blocker. Relaxes smooth muscle, especially of vasculature. Used as vasodilator and to relax smooth muscle (occasionally urethral muscle).	High doses cause vasodilation and hypotension.	Titrate dose to needs of individual patient. Results of clinical studies in animals have not been reported. Use in animals (and doses) is based on experience in humans or anecdotal experience in animals.	Minipress	1, 2, 5 mg capsules	0.5-2 mg/animal (1 mg per 15 kg) PO q8-12h
Prednisolone	Glucocorticoid antiinflammatory drug. Potency is approximately 4 times that of cortisol. See betamethasone for details on other glucocorticoids.	All glucocorticoids produce expected (and sometimes unavoidable) side effects. See betamethasone for partial list of side effects.	Doses for prednisolone are based on severity of underlying condition.	Delta-cortef, many others	5 mg tablet	Antiinflammatory: 0.5-1 mg/kg IV, IM, PO q12-24h initially, then taper to q48h. Immunosuppressive: 2.2-6.6 mg/kg/day IV, IM, PO initially, then taper to 2-4 mg/kg q48h. Shock, spinal trauma: See prednisolone sodium succinate.
Prednisolone sodium succinate	Same as prednisolone, except that this is a water-soluble formulation intended for acute therapy when high IV doses are needed for rapid effect. Used for treatment of shock and CNS trauma. See also methylprednisolone sodium succinate.	Adverse effects are not expected from single administration; however, with repeated use, other side effects are possible. See betamethasone.	See prednisolone.	Solu-Delta-Cortef	100, 200 mg vials for injection	Shock: 15-30 mg/kg IV; repeat in 4-6 hours. CNS trauma: 15-30 mg/kg IV; taper to 1-2 mg/kg q12h.

Drug name	Pharmacology and category of use	Precautions	Dosing information and comments	Other names	Formulations available	Dosage
Prednisone	Same as prednisolone, except that after administration, prednisone is converted to prednisolone	Same as prednisolone	Same as prednisolone	See prednisolone.	1, 5, 10, 20, 40, 50 mg tablets; 1, 5 mg/ml oral solution; 10, 40 mg/ml injections	Same as prednisolone
Primidone	Anticonvulsant. Primidone is converted to phenylethylmalonamide and phenobarbital both of which have anticonvulsant activity, but most of activity (85%) is probably a result of phenobarbital. See phenobarbital for more details.	Adverse effects are same as phenobarbital. Primidone has been associated with idiosyncratic hepatotoxicity in dogs. Although some labels caution its use in cats, one study in experimental cats determined that it is safe if used at recommended doses.	See phenobarbital. When monitoring therapy with primidone, phenobarbital plasma concentrations should be measured to estimate anticonvulsant effect.	Mylepsin, Neurosyn (Mysoline in Canada)	50, 250 mg tablets	8-10 mg/kg PO q8-12h as initial dose, then adjust via monitoring to 10-15 mg/kg q8h
Primor (ormetoprim and sulfadimethoxine)	Antibacterial drug. Ormetoprim inhibits bacterial dihydrofolate reductase; sulfonamide competes with PABA for synthesis of nucleic acids. Bactericidal/bacteriostatic. Broad antibacterial spectrum and active against some coccidia.	Several adverse effects have been reported from sulfonamides. See trimethoprim and sulfonamides. No adverse effects reported from ormetoprim.	Doses listed are based on manufacturer's recommendations. Controlled trials have demonstrated efficacy for treatment of pyoderma on once per day schedule.	Primor	Combination tablet (ormetoprim and sulfadimethoxine)	27 mg/kg PO on first day, followed by 13.5 mg/kg q24h
Procainamide	Antiarrhythmic drug. Class I antiarrhythmic used primarily for treatment of ventricular arrhythmias. Action is to inhibit sodium influx into cardiac cell via sodium channel blockade.	Adverse effects include cardiac arrhythmias, cardiac depression, tachycardia, and hypotension. In humans, procainamide produces hypersensitivity effects (lupus-like reactions), but these have not been reported in animals. Cimetidine may increase plasma concentrations.	Since animals do not produce active metabolite (N-acetyl procainamide) dose may be higher to control some arrhythmias compared to humans. Monitor plasma concentrations during chronic therapy (effective plasma concentrations in experimental dogs are 20 µg/ml). In animals, there is no evidence that slow-release oral formulations produce longer duration of sustained blood concentrations.	Pronestyl, Procan-SR generic	250, 375, 500 mg tablets, capsules; 100, 500 mg/ml injections 500, 750, 1000 mg sustained release tablets	Dogs: 10-30 mg/kg PO q6h (SR q8h PO 5-15 mg/kg q6h IM; 2 mg/kg IV over 3-5 min. up to total dose of 20 mg/kg q6h. 25-50 µg/kg/min IV infusion. Cats: 3-8 mg/kg IM, PO q6-8h.
Prochlorperazine	Phenothiazine. Central-acting dopamine (D2) antagonist. Used for sedation, tranquilization, and as antiemetic. Antiemetic action also may be related to alpha-2 and muscarinic blocking effects.	Causes sedation and other side effects attributed to other phenothiazines. See acepromazine.	Used primarily as antiemetic in animals. Clinical trials are not available; doses are based primarily on extrapolation and anecdotal experience.	Compazine	5, 10, 25 mg tablets (prochlorperazine maleate); 5 mg/ml injection (prochlorperazine edisylate)	0.1-0.5 mg/kg q6-8h IM SC
Progesterone, repositol	See medroxyprogesterone acetate (Depo-Provera).					
Promethazine	Phenothiazine with strong antihistamine effects. Used for treatment of allergy and as antiemetic (motion sickness).	Adverse effects include sedation and antimuscarinic (atropine-like) effects. Both phenothiazine effects (see acepromazine) and anticholinergic (see atropine) effects are possible in some patients.	Results of clinical studies in animals have not been reported. Use in animals (and doses) is based on experience in humans or anecdotal experience in animals.	Phenergan	6.25, 25 mg per 5 ml syrup; 12.5, 25, 50 mg tablets; 25, 50 mg/ml injections	0.2-0.4 mg/kg IV, IM, PO q6-8h (up to a maximum dose of 1 mg/kg)

Drug name	Pharmacology and category of use	Precautions	Dosing information and comments	Other names	Formulations available	Dosage
Propantheline bromide	Anticholinergic (antimuscarinic) drug. Blocks acetylcholine receptor to produce parasympatholytic (atropine-like) effects. See atropine. Used to decrease smooth muscle contraction and secretion of gastrointestinal tract. Also used to treat vagal-mediated cardiovascular effects.	Side effects are attributed to excess anticholinergic (antimuscarinic) effects. See atropine. Treat overdoses with physostigmine.	Propantheline has not been evaluated in clinical trials in animals, but is often the drug of choice for oral therapy in cases where an anticholinergic effect is desired.	Pro-Banthine	7.5, 15 mg tablets	0.25-0.5 mg/kg PO q8-12h
Propiopromazine	Phenothiazine sedative. Also has antiemetic and antihistaminic actions.	See other phenothiazines (acepromazine).	Results of clinical studies in animals have not been reported. Use in animals (and doses) is based on experience in humans or anecdotal experience in animals.	Tranvet, Largon	20 mg/ml injection	1.1-4.4 mg/kg q12-24h
Propofol	Anesthetic. Used for induction or producing short-term general anesthesia. Mechanism of action is not well defined but may be barbiturate-like.	Adverse effects attributed to general anesthetic properties. Propofol causes respiratory depression.	Propofol is primarily used for general anesthesia or adjunct for general anesthesia. Propofol's advantage over other agents is smooth, rapid recovery. Use strict aseptic technique for administration.	Diprivan	10 mg/ml injection	6.5 mg/kg IV (slowly)
Propranolol	Beta (β) adrenergic blocker. Nonselective for beta-1 and beta-2 adrenergic receptors. Class II antiarrhythmic. Used primarily to decrease heart rate, cardiac conduction, tachyarrhythmias, and blood pressure.	Adverse effects related to beta-1 blocking effects on heart. Causes cardiac depression and decreases cardiac output. Beta-2 blocking effects can cause bronchoconstriction. Decreases insulin secretion.	Usually dose is titrated according to patient's response. Start with low dose and increase gradually to desired effect. Clearance relies on hepatic blood flow; use cautiously in animals with impaired hepatic perfusion.	Inderal	10, 20, 40 mg tablet; 1 mg/ml injection	Dogs: 20-60 µg/kg IV over 5-10 minutes; 0.2-1 mg/kg PO q8h (titrate dose to effect). Cats: 0.4-1.2 mg/kg (2.5-5 mg/cat) PO q8h.
Propylthiouracil (PTU)	Antithyroid drug. See methimazole. Compared to methimazole PTU inhibits conversion of T_4 to T_3.	Adverse effects in cats include hemolytic anemia, thrombocytopenia, and other signs of immune-mediated disease (JAVMA 1984;184:806).	Use of PTU in most cats has been replaced with methimazole.	Generic, Propyl-Thyracil	50, 100 mg tablets	11 mg/kg PO q12h
Prostaglandin $F_{2\alpha}$	Prostaglndin induces leutolysis. Has been used to treat open pyometra in animals. Use for inducing abortion has been questioned.	Side effects include vomiting, diarrhea, and abdominal discomfort.	Use in treating pyometra should be monitored carefully.	Lutalyse	Injection	Pyometra: 0.1-0.2 mg/kg SC once daily for 5 days (dogs); 0.1-0.25 mg/kg SC once daily for 5 days (cats). Abortion: 25-50 mg/kg IM q12h (dogs); 0.5-1 mg/kg IM for 2 injections (cats).
Pseudoephedrine	Adrenergic agonist. Similar to ephedrine and phenylpropanolamine in action. Used to increase peripheral resistance, as a decongestant, and in animals to treat urinary incontinence.	Side effects attributed to adrenergic effects include excitement, rapid heart rate, and arrhythmias. See ephedrine and phenylpropanolamine.	Although clinical trials have not been conducted for comparison, it is believed that pseudoephedrine's action and efficacy are similar to ephedrine and phenylpropanolamine.	Sudafed, many others (some formulations have other ingredients)	30, 60 mg tablets; 120 mg capsule; 6 mg/ml syrup	0.2-0.4 mg/kg (or 15-60 mg/dog) PO q8-12h

Drug name	Pharmacology and category of use	Precautions	Dosing information and comments	Other names	Formulations available	Dosage
Psyllium	Bulk-forming laxative. Used for treatment of constipation and bowel evacuation. Action is to absorb water and expand to provide increased bulk and moisture content to the stool, which encourages normal peristalsis and bowel motility.	Adverse effects have not been reported in animals. Intestinal impaction can occur with overuse or in patients with inadequate fluid intake.	Results of clinical studies in animals have not been reported. Use in animals (and doses) is based on experience in humans or anecdotal experience in animals.	Metamucil, others	Powder	1 tsp per 5-10 kg (added to each meal)
Pyrantel pamoate	Antiparasitic drug. Acts to block ganglionic neurotransmission via cholinergic action.	No adverse effects have been reported.	Dose recommendations are based on the manufacturer's recommendations.	Nemex, Strongid	Paste; 50 mg/ml suspension	Dogs: 5 mg/kg PO once; repeat in 7-10 days. Cats: 20 mg/kg PO once.
Pyridostigmine bromide	Anticholinesterase. Same as neostigmine, except that pyridostigmine has longer duration of action.	Same as neostigmine, except that adverse effects may persist longer. Since this product contains bromide, use cautiously in patients already receiving bromide (such as potassium bromide for epilepsy).	Same as neostigmine	Mestinon, Regonol	12 mg/ml oral syrup; 60 mg tablet; 5 mg/ml injection	Antimyasthenic: 0.02-0.04 mg/kg IV q2h or 0.5-3 mg/kg PO q8-12h. Antidote (curariform): 0.15-0.3 mg/kg IM, IV.
Pyrimethamine	Antibacterial, antiprotozoal drug. Acts to antagonize dihydrofolate reductase enzyme to inhibit synthesize reduced folate and nucleic acids. Activity of pyrimethamine is greater against protozoa than bacteria.	Adverse effects in animals have not been reported.	Used either alone or in combination with sulfonamides	Daraprim	25 mg tablet	Dogs: 1 mg/kg PO q24h for 14-21 days (5 days for Neosporum caninum). Cats: 0.5-1 mg/kg PO q24h for 14-28 days.
Quibron	See theophylline.					
Quinacrine	Outdated antimalarial drug. Used occasionally for treatment of protozoa (Giardia). Inhibits nucleic acid synthesis in parasite.	Side effects are common. Vomiting occurs after oral administration.	Doses listed are for treatment of Giardia.	Atabrine		Dogs: 6.6 mg/kg PO q12h for 5 days. Cats: 11 mg/kg PO q24h for 5 days.
Quinidine gluconate	Antiarrhythmic drug. Class I antiarrhythmic. Action is to inhibit sodium influx via blockade of sodium channels. Used to treat ventricular arrhythmias and, occasionally, atrial fibrillation.	Side effects with quinidine are more common than procainamide and include nausea and vomiting. Adverse effects include hypotension and tachycardia (as a result of antivagal effect). Coadministration with digoxin may increase digoxin concentrations.	Quinidine is not used as commonly as other class I antiarrhythmic drugs. *Doses calculated according to amount of quinidine base in each product.*	Quiniglute, Duraquin	324 mg tablet; 80 mg/ml injection	Dogs: 6-20 mg/kg IM q6h; 6-20 mg/kg PO q6-8h (of base) 324 mg quinidine gluconate = 202 mg quinidine base.
Quinidine sulfate	Same as quinidine gluconate	Same as quinidine gluconate	*Doses calculated according to amount of quinidine base in each product.*	Cin-Quin, Quinora	100, 200, 300 mg tablets; 200, 300 mg capsules; 200 mg/ml injection	Dogs: 6-20 mg/kg PO q6-8h (of base); 5-10 mg/kg IV 300 mg quinidine sulfate = 250 mg quinidine base.
Quinidine polygalacturonate	Same as quinidine gluconate	Same as quinidine gluconate	*Doses calculated according to amount of quinidine base in each product.*	Cardioquin	275 mg tablet	Dogs: 6-20 mg/kg PO q6h (of base); 275 mg quinidine polygalacturonate = 167 mg quinidine base

Drug name	Pharmacology and category of use	Precautions	Dosing information and comments	Other names	Formulations available	Dosage
Racemethionine (dl-methionine)	Urinary acidifer. Lowers urinary pH. Also has been used to protect against acetaminophen overdose in humans by restoring hepatic concentrations of glutathione. In humans, it also is used to treat dermatitis caused by urinary incontinence (reduces urine ammonia).	Adverse effects have not been reported. Do not use in patients with metabolic acidosis or hepatic function impairment. Do not use in young cats.	Uroeze, Methio-Form	Generic tablets	500 mg tablet; powders added to animal's food	Dogs: 150-300 mg/kg/day PO. Cats: 1-1.5 g/cat PO (added to food each day).
Ranitidine	H$_2$ antagonist. See cimetidine for details. Same as cimetidine except 4-10 times more potent and longer acting.	See cimetidine. Ranitidine may have fewer effects on endocrine function and drug interactions compared to cimetidine.	See cimetidine. Pharmacokinetic information in dogs suggests that ranitidine may be administered less often than cimetidine to achieve continuous suppression of stomach acid secretion.	Zantac	75, 150, 300 mg tablets; 150, 300 mg capsules; 25 mg/ml injection	Dogs: 2 mg/kg IV, PO q8h. Cats: 2.5 mg/kg IV q12h ; 3.5 mg/kg PO q12h.
Retinoids	See isotretinoin (Accutane), retinol (Aquasol-A), or etretinate (Tegison).					
Retinol	See vitamin A (Aquasol-A).					
Riboflavin (vitamin B$_2$)	See vitamin B$_2$.					
Rifampin	Antibacterial. Action is to inhibit bacterial RNA synthesis. Spectrum of action includes staphylococci, mycobacteria, and streptococci. Used in humans primarily for treatment of tuberculosis.	Adverse effects not reported in animals; however, in humans, hypersensitivity and flu-like symptoms are reported. Multiple drug interactions are possible (e.g., with barbiturates, chloramphenicol, and corticosteroids). Consult package insert.	Results of clinical studies in animals have not been reported. Use in animals (and doses) is based on experience in humans or anecdotal experience in animals. Rifampin is highly lipid-soluble and has been used to treat intracellular infections. Administer on an empty stomach.	Rifadin	150, 300 mg capsules	10-20 mg/kg PO q24h
Ringer's solution	IV solution for replacement	Monitor pulmonary pressure when infusing high doses.	When administering IV fluid solution, carefully monitor rate and electrolyte concentrations.	Generic	250, 500, 1000 ml bags for infusion	40-50 ml/kg/ day IV, SC, IP
Salicylate	See acetylsalicylic acid (aspirin).					
Selegiline (Deprenyl)	Action is to inhibit specific monoamine oxidase (MAO type B). Specifically, it appears to inhibit degredation of dopamine in central nervous system. In people it is primarily used to treat Parkinson's disease and other neurodegenerative diseases (in combination with levodopa). In dogs, it has been used to treat problems such as cognitive dysfunction in geriatric dogs (with and without housetraining problems) and pituitary-dependent Cushing's disease (not effective for other fiorms of Cushing's disease).	Adverse effects have not been reported in dogs; however, amphetamine-like signs can be produced in experimental animals.	Results of clinical studies in animals have not been reported. However, experimental studies in animals, including dogs, indicates that cognitive dysfunction in aged dogs and PDH Cushing's Syndrome may be responsive to drugs such as selegiline that increase dopamine levels.	Deprenyl, l-deprenyl, Eldepryl (in Canada Anipryl)	5 mg tablet . (In Canada, available as 2, 5, and 15 mg. tablets).	Dogs: Begin with 1 mg/kg q24h PO. If there is no response within 2 months increase dose to maximum of 2mg/kg q24 PO. Cats: Dose not established.

Drug name	Pharmacology and category of use	Precautions	Dosing information and comments	Other names	Formulations available	Dosage
Senna	Laxative. Acts via local stimulation or via contact with intestinal mucosa.	Adverse effects not reported for animals.	Doses and indications are not well established for veterinary medicine. Use is strictly through anecdotal experience.	Senokot	Granules in concentrate; syrup	Cats: 5 ml/cat q24h (syrup); 1/2 tsp per cat q24h with food (granules)
Septra (sulfmethoxazole and trimethoprim)	See trimethoprim and sulfonamides (Tribrissen).					
Sodium bicarbonate	Alkalizing agent. Antacid. Used to treat systemic acidosis or to alkalize urine. Increases plasma and urinary concentrations of bicarbonate.	Adverse effects attributed to alkalizing activity. When administered PO, interaction may occur to decrease absorption of other drugs (partial list includes anticholinergic drugs, ketoconazole, fluoroquinolones, and tetracyclines).	When used for systemic acidosis, doses should be adjusted on basis of blood gas measurements or assessment of acidosis. Doses vary depending on underlying condition. See dose section. 8.5 % solution = 1 mEq/ml of sodium bicarbonate.	Generic, baking soda, soda mint	325, 520, 650 mg tablets; injections of various strengths (4.2-8.4%); 1 mEq/ml	Acidosis: 0.5-1 mEq/kg IV. Renal failure: 10 mg/kg PO q8-12h. Alkalization of urine: 50 mg/kg PO q8-12h. (1 tsp ≈ 2 g.)
Sodium chloride (0.9%)	Sodium chloride is used for IV infusion as replacement fluid.	Not a balanced electrolyte solution. Long-term infusion may cause electrolyte imbalace.	Rate of infusion varies depending on patient needs.	Generic	500, 1000 ml infusions	40-50 ml/kg/day IV, SC, IP
Sodium chloride (7.5%)	Concentrated sodium chloride used for acute treatment of hypovolemia.	Not a balanced electrolyte solution. Long-term infusion may cause electrolyte imbalace.	Hypertonic saline is used for short-term infusion for rapid replacement of vascular volume.	Generic	Infusion	2-8 ml/kg IV
Sodum iodide (20%)	Used to treat iodine deficiency	Overuse causes iodism (burning of mouth, gastric irritation, and skin lesions).		Iodopen, generic	100 µg elemental iodide (118 µg sodium iodide) per ml injection	20-40 mg/kg PO q8-12h
Sodium thiomalate	See gold sodium thiomalate.					
Sotalol	Nonspecific beta (β_1, β_2) adrenergic blocker. Action is similar to propranolol. In addition to being a class II antiarrhythmic drug, sotalol has some class III activity.	Adverse effects have not been reported for animals, but are expected to be similar to propranolol.	Sotalol is not used as commonly as propranolol and little clinical information has accumulated regarding its use.	Betapace	80, 160, 240 mg	Dogs: 1-2 mg/kg PO q12h
Spironolactone	Potassium-sparing diuretic. Action is to interfere with sodium reabsorption in distal renal tubule. Spironolactone competitively inhibits the action of aldosterone. Used for treating high blood pressure and congestion caused by heart failure.	Can produce hyperkalemia in some patients. Do not use in dehydrated patients. NSAIDs may interfere with action. Avoid supplements that are high in potassium.	Spironolactone usually is used with diuretic agent when used for congestive heart failure.	Aldactone	25, 50, 100 mg tablets	2-4 mg/kg/day PO or 1-2 mg/kg q12h
Stanozolol	Anabolic steroid. See nandrolone. (There are no established differences in efficacy among the anabolic steroids.)	See nandrolone.	See nandrolone.	Winstrol-V	50 mg/ml injection; 2 mg tablet	Dogs: 1-4 mg/dog PO q12h; 25-50 mg/dog/week IM. Cats: 1 mg/cat PO q12h; 25 mg/cat/week IM.

Drug name	Pharmacology and category of use	Precautions	Dosing information and comments	Other names	Formulations available	Dosage
Sucralfate	Gastric mucosa protectant. Antiulcer agent. Action of sucralfate is to bind to ulcerated tissue in gastrointestinal tract to aid healing of ulcers. There is some evidence that sucralfate may act as a cytoprotectant (via prostaglandin synthesis). Used to treat or prevent ulcers.	Adverse effects have not been reported. Not absorbed systemically. Sucralfate may decrease absorption of other PO administered drugs (fluoroquinolones and tetracyclines).		Carafate (Sulcrate in Canada)	1 g tablets; 200 mg/ml oral suspension	Dogs: 0.5-1 g PO q8-12h. Cats: 0.25 g PO q8-12h.
Sufentanil citrate	Opiod agonist. Action of fentanyl derivatives is via mu-receptor. See fentanyl and morphine. Sufentanil is 5-7 times more potent than fentanyl (13-20 µg of sufentanil produce analgesia equal to 10 mg of morphine).	Adverse effects are similar to other opiates. See morphine.	When used for anesthesia, often animals are premedicated with acepromazine or benzodiazepine.	Sufenta	50 µg/ml injection	2 µg/kg IV, (up to a maximum dose of 5 µg/kg)
Sulfadiazine	Sulfonamides compete with PABA for enzyme that synthesizes dihydrofolic acid in bacteria. Synergistic with trimethoprim. Broad spectrum of activity, including some protozoa. Bacteriostatic.	Adverse effects associated with sulfonamides include allergic reactions, type-II and III hypersensitivity, hypothyroidism (with prolonged therapy), keratoconjunctivitis sicca, and skin reactions.	Usually, sulfonamides are combined with trimethoprim or ormetoprim in 5:1 ratio. There is no clinical evidence that one sulfonamide is more or less toxic or efficacious than another sulfonamide.	Generic	500 mg tablet	100 mg/kg IV, PO (loading dose), followed by 50 mg/kg IV, PO q12h. See trimethoprim.
Sulfadimethoxine	See sulfadiazine.	See sulfadiazine.	See sulfadiazine.	Albon, Bactrovet, generic	125, 250, 500 mg tablets; 400 mg/ml injection; 50 mg/ml suspension	55 mg/kg PO (loading dose), followed by 27.5 mg/kg PO q12h. See Primor.
Sulfamethazine	See sulfadiazine.	See sulfadiazine.	See sulfadiazine.	Many brands (e.g., Sulmet)	30 g bolus	100 mg/kg PO (loading dose), followed by 50 mg/kg PO q12h
Sulfamethoxazole	See sulfadiazine.	See sulfadiazine.	See sulfadiazine.	Gantanol	500 mg tablet	100 mg/kg PO (loading dose), followed by 50 mg/kg PO q12h. See Bactrim and Septra.
Sulfasalazine (sulfapyridine and mesalamine)	Sulfonamide and anti-inflammatory drug. Used for treatment of colitis. Sulfonamide has little effect; salicylic acid (mesalamine) has antiinflammatory effects. See mesalamine.	Adverse effects are all attributed to sulfonamde component. See sulfadiazine. Keratoconjunctivitis sicca has been reported.	Usually used for treatment of idiopathic colitis. Often combined with dietary therapy.	Azulfidine (Salazopyrin in Canada)	500 mg tablet	10-30 mg/kg PO q8-12h. See mesalamine and olsalazine.
Sulfisoxazole	See sulfadiazine. Sulfisoxizole is primarily used only for treating urinary tract infections.	See sulfadiazine.	See sulfadiazine.	Gantrisin	500 mg tablet; 500 mg per 5 ml syrup	Urinary tract infections: 50 mg/kg PO q8h
Tamoxifen	Nonsteroid estrogen receptor blocker. Also has weak estrogenic effects. Tamoxifen also may also increase release of Gn-RH. Used as adjunctive treatment for certain tumors.	Adverse effects have not been thoroughly documented in animals. However, in humans, tamoxifen causes increased tumor pain. Do not use in pregnant animals. Reacts with antiulcer drugs.	Consult specific anti-cancer protocols for doses and regimens.	Nolvadex	10 mg tablet (tamoxifen citrate)	10 mg PO q12h (human dose)

Drug name	Pharmacology and category of use	Precautions	Dosing information and comments	Other names	Formulations available	Dosage
Taurine	Nutritional supplement for cats. Used in prevention and treatment of ocular and cardiac disease (cardiomyopathy) caused by taurine deficiency.	Adverse effects have not been reported.	Routine supplementation with taurine may not be necessary in cats that are receiving a balanced diet.	Generic	Powder	Dogs: 500 mg PO q12h. Cats: 250 mg/cat PO q12h.
Telezol	See tiletamine.					
Terbutaline	Beta-adrenergic agonist. Beta-2 (β_2) specific. Used primarily for bronchodilation. See albuterol for further details.	Adverse effects related to excessive beta-adrenergic stimulation. See albuterol.	Used primarily for bronchodilation. May be administered PO, IM, or SC. Terbutaline (and other beta-2 agonists) have also been used in humans to delay labor (dose in humans is 2.5 mg PO q6h).	Brethine, Bricanyl	2.5, 5 mg tablets; 1 mg/ml injection (equivalent to 0.82 mg/ml)	Dogs: 2.5 mg/dog (or 0.2 mg/kg) SC, PO q8h. Cats: 0.1 mg/cat SC q12h or 0.625 mg/cat PO.
Terfenadine	Antihistamine (H_1 blocking drug). Second-generation antihistamine. Similar to other antihistamines (such as chlorpheniramine), except sedation is not as common.	Adverse effects were reported in a dog that ingested 45 mg/kg. Sedation and other side effects are not as common as first-generation antihistamines. In humans, cardiotoxicity have been reported with high doses. Administration with cimetidine may increase concentrations.	Results of clinical studies in animals have not been reported. Use in animals (and doses) is based on experience in humans or anecdotal experience in animals. Most common use in animals is for treatment of allergic skin disease.	Seldene	60 mg tablet	4.5-10 mg/kg PO q12h
Testosterone cypionate	Testosterone ester. See methyltestosterone. Testosterone esters are administered PO to avoid first-pass effects.	See testosterone and methyltestosterone.	See methyltestosterone.	Andro-Cyp, Andronate, Depo-Testosterone, other forms	100, 200 mg/ml injections	1-2 mg/kg IM every 2-4 weeks. See methyltestosterone.
Testosterone propionate	Testosterone injection. See methyltestosterone.	See testosterone and methyltestosterone.	See methyltestosterone.	Testex (Malogen in Canada)	100 mg/ml injection	0.5-1 mg/kg IM 2-3 times per week
Tetracycline	Tetracycline antibiotic. Mechanism of action of tetracyclines is to bind to 30S ribosomal subunit and inhibit protein synthesis. Usually bactericidal. Broad spectrum of activity, including bacteria, some protozoa, Rickettsia, and Ehrlichia.	Severe adverse reactions not reported with doxycycline. Tetracyclines in general may cause renal tubular necrosis at high doses. Tetracyclines can affect bone and teeth formation in young animals. Tetracyclines bind to calcium-containing compounds, which decreases oral absorption.	Pharmacokinetic and experimental studies have been conducted in small animals, but no clinical studies.	Panmycin	250, 500 mg capsules; 100 mg/ml suspension	15-20 mg/kg PO q8h; 4.4-11 mg/kg IV, IM q8h
Thenium closylate	Antiparasitic drug. Used to treat hookworms (Ancylostoma and Uncinaria).	Tablet is bitter if coating is broken. May cause occasional vomiting after PO administration.	Doses listed are based on recommendations from manufacturer.	Canopar	500 mg tablets	Dogs > 4.5 kg: 500 mg PO once; repeat in 2-3 weeks. Dogs 2.5-4.5 kg: 250 mg q12h for one day; repeat in 2-3 weeks.

Drug name	Pharmacology and category of use	Precautions	Dosing information and comments	Other names	Formulations available	Dosage
Theophylline	Methylxanthine bronchodilator. Mechanism of action is unknown but may be related to increased cyclic AMP or antagonism of adenosine. There appears to be antiinflammatory action as well as bronchodilating action.	Adverse effects include nausea, vomiting, and diarrhea. With high doses, tachycardia, excitement, tremors, and seizures are possible. Cardiovascular and CNS adverse effects appear to be less frequent in dogs than humans.	Plasma concentrations of theophylline should be monitored in patients receiving chronic therapy to maintain plasma concentrations between 10 and 20 μg/ml. Doses for slow-release tablets are unique for each product. See theophylline, sustained-release and aminophylline.	Many brands, generic	100, 125, 200, 250, 300 mg tablets; 27 mg per 5 ml oral solution, elixir; 5% dextrose injection	Dogs: 9 mg/kg PO q6-8h. Cats: 4 mg/kg PO q8-12h.
Theophylline, sustained-release	Same as theophylline	Same as theophylline	Same as theophylline	Theo-Dur, Slo-Bid Gyrocaps	100, 200, 300, 450 mg tablets (Theo-Dur); 50-200 mg capsules (Slo-Bid)	Dogs: 20 mg/kg q12h (Theo-Dur); 30 mg/kg q12h (Slo-Bid); Cats: 25 mg/kg PO q24h at night (Theo-Dur and Slo-Bid).
Thiabendazole	Benzimidazole anthelmintic. See fenbendazole and albendazole.	Adverse effects are uncommon.	Ordinarily administered to horses and cattle. Experience in small animals is limited.	Omnizole, Equizole	2 or 4 g per oz (30 ml) suspension, liquid	Dogs: 50 mg/kg q24h for 3 days; repeat in 1 month. Respiratory parasites: 30-70 mg/kg PO q12h. Cats (Strongyloides): 125 mg/kg q24h for 3 days.
Thiacetarsamide sodium	Organic arsenical used for treatment of heartworm infections. Adulticide.	Adverse effects are common, especially anorexia, vomiting, and hepatic injury. Pulmonary thromboembolism may occur as consequence of heartworm kill.	Thiacetarsamide is administered via 4 injections over 2 days; however, if severe adverse effects are observed, discontinue regimen. See melarsomine.	Caparsolate	10 mg/ml	Dogs: 2.2 mg/kg IV twice daily for 2 days Cats: Not recommended
Thiamine (vitamin B_1)	Vitamin B_1 is used for treatment of vitamin deficiency.	Adverse effects are rare because water-soluble vitamins are easily excreted. Riboflavin may discolor the urine.	Vitamin B supplements often are administered in combination.	Bewon and others.	250 μg per 5 ml elixir; tablets of various sizes (5-500 mg); 100, 500 mg/ml injections	Dogs: 10-100 mg/dog/day PO. Cats: 5-30 mg/cat/day PO (up to a maximum dose of 50 mg/cat/day).
Thiamylal sodium	Ultra-short–acting barbiturate. See thiopental. Thiamylal is the thiobarbiturate analog of secobarbital.	See thiopental.	See thiopental.	Surital, Bio-Tal	Mix to various concentrations from 5-40 mg/ml for injection.	Dogs: 8-10 mg/kg IV in incremental doses up to 20 mg/kg (4% solution). Cats: Same as dogs (2% solution).
Thioguanine (6-TG)	Anticancer agent. Antimetabolite of purine analog type. Inhibits DNA synthesis in cancer cells.	Adverse effects, as with any anticancer drugs, are expected. See mercaptopurine. Immunosuppression and leukopenia are common.	Thioguanine is often combined with other agents for treatment of cancer. Consult specific reference on cancer therapy for guidance.	Generic	40 mg tablet	40 mg/m^2 PO q24h
Thiomalate sodium	See gold sodium thiomalate.					
Thiopental sodium	Ultra-short–acting barbiturate. Used primarily for induction of anesthesia or for short duration of anesthesia (10-15 minutes). Anesthesia is produced by central nervous system depression, without analgesia. Anesthesia is terminated by redistribution in the body.	Adverse effects are related to the anesthetic effects of the drug. Severe adverse effects are caused by respiratory and cardiovascular depression. Overdoses are caused by rapid or repeated injections. Avoid extravasation outside of vein.	Therapeutic index is low. Use only in patients in which it is possible to monitor cardiovascular and respiratory functions. Often administered with other anesthetic adjuncts.	Pentothal	Various size vials from 250 mg to 10 g (mix to desired concentration)	Dogs: 10-25 mg/kg IV (to effect). Cats: 5-10 mg/kg IV (to effect).

Drug name	Pharmacology and category of use	Precautions	Dosing information and comments	Other names	Formulations available	Dosage
Thiotepa	Anticancer agent. Alkylating agent of the nitrogen mustard type (similar to cyclophosphamide). Used for various tumors, especially malignant effusions.	Adverse effects are similar to other anticancer agents and alkylating drugs (many of which are unavoidable). Bone marrow suppression is the most common effect.	One should consult specific cancer chemotherapy protocol for guidance on administration. Thiotepa usually is administered directly in body cavities.	Generic	15 mg injection (usually in solution of 10 mg/ml)	0.2-0.5 mg/m² weekly or daily for 5-10 days IM, intracavitary, or intratumor
Thyroid hormone	See levothyroxine and liothyronine.					
Thyrotropin, thyroid-stimulating hormone (TSH)	Thyroid stimulating hormone is used for diagnostic testing. Stimulates normal secretion of thyroid hormone.	Adverse reactions rare. In humans, allergic reactions have occurred.	To prepare solution, add 2 ml NaCl to 10 U vial. Reconstituted solutions retain potency for 2 weeks at 2-8° C. Consult testing laboratory for specific guidelines for thyroid testing.	Thytropar	10 U vial	Dogs: Collect baseline sample, followed by 0.1 U/kg IV (maximum dose is 5 U); collect post-TSH sample at 6 hours. Cats: Collect baseline sample, followed by 2.5 U/cat IM; collect post-TSH sample at 8-12 hours.
Ticarcillin	Beta-lactam antibiotic. Action similar to ampicillin/amoxicillin. Spectrum similar to carbenicillin. Ticarcillin is primarily used for gram-negative infections, especially those caused by Pseudomonas.	Adverse effects are uncommon; however, allergic reactions are possible. High doses can produce seizures and decreased platelet function. Do not combine in same syringe or vial with aminoglycosides.	Ticarcillin is synergistic with, and often combined with, aminoglycosides (e.g., amikacin and gentamicin). Lidocaine (1%) may be used for reconstitution to decrease pain from IM injection.	Ticar, Ticillin	6 g per 50 ml vial; 1, 3, 6, 20, 30 g vials	33-50 mg/kg IV, IM q4-6h
Ticarcillin and clavulanate	Same as ticarcillin, except clavulanic acid has been added to inhibit bacterial beta-lactamase and increase spectrum.	Same as ticarcillin	Same as ticarcillin	Timentin	3 g per vial for injection	Same as ticarcillin (Dose according to ticarcillin component.)
Tiletamine and zolazepam	Anesthetic. Combination of tiletamine (dissociative anesthetic agent similar in action to ketamine) and zolazepam (benzodiazepine similar in action to diazepam). Produces short duration (30 minutes) of anesthesia.	Wide margin of safety. Side effects include excessive salivation (may be antagonized with atropine), erratic recovery, and muscle twitching.	Administer by deep IM injection. Consult manufacturer's package insert for dosing information for dogs and cats.	Telezol, Zoletil	50 mg of each component per ml	5-7 mg/kg IM
Tobramycin	Aminoglycoside antibacterial drug. Similar mechanism of action and spectrum as amikacin and gentamicin.	Adverse effects are similar to those of amikacin and gentamicin.	Dosing requirements vary depending on bacterial susceptibility. See dose schedules for gentamicin and amikacin.	Nebcin	40 mg/ml injection	2-4 mg/kg IV, IM, SC q8h
Tocanide	Antiarrhythmic drug. Considered an oral analog of lidocaine. Class I-B antiarrhythmic.	In dogs, anorexia and gastrointestinal toxicity have been reported. Arrhythmias, nausea, vomiting, trembling and ataxia are also possible.	Results of clinical studies in animals have not been reported. Use in animals (and doses) is based on experience in humans or anecdotal experience in animals. Therapeutic plasma concentrations are 6-10 μg/ml.	Tonocard	400, 600 mg tablets	Dogs: 15-20 mg/kg PO q8h. Cats: No dose established.
Triamcinolone	Glucocorticoid antiinflammatory drug. See betamethasone for details. Triamcinolone's potency approximates methylprednisolone (about 5 times cortisol and 1.25 times prednisolone).	Adverse effects are similar to other corticosteroids. See betamethasone.	See prednisolone.	Aristocort, generic	1, 2, 4, 8, 16 mg tablets; 10 mg/ml injection	Antiinflammatory: 0.5-1 mg/kg PO q12-24h; taper dose to 0.5-1 mg/kg PO q48h

Drug name	Pharmacology and category of use	Precautions	Dosing information and comments	Other names	Formulations available	Dosage
Triamcinolone acetonide	Same as triamcinolone, except that injectable suspension is slowly absorbed from IM or intralesional injection site. Used for intralesional therapy of tumors and similar purposes as methylprednisolone acetate.	See methylprednisolone acetate. When used for ocular injections, there is some concern that granulomas may occur at injection site.	See prednisolone.	Vetalog	2, 6 mg/ml suspension injections; 0.5, 1.5 mg tablets	0.1-0.2 mg/kg IM, SC; repeat in 7-10 days. Intralesional: 1.2-1.8 mg (or 1 mg for every cm diameter of tumor) every 2 weeks.
Triamterene	Potassium-sparing diuretic. Similar action as spironolactone, except that spironolactone has competitive inhibiting effect of aldosterone, triamterene does not.	See spironolactone.	Little clinical experience available for triamterene. There is no convincing evidence that triamterene is more effective than spironolactone.	Dyrenium	50, 100 mg capsules.	1-2 mg/kg q12h PO
Tribrissen	See trimethoprim sulfonamides.					
Trientine hydrochloride	Chelating agent. Used to chelate copper when penicillamine cannot be tolerated in a patient.	Adverse effects have not been reported in animals.	Used only in patients that cannot tolerate penicillamine. Generally induces less cupriuresis than penicillamine.	Syprine	250 mg capsule	10-15 mg/kg PO q12h
Trifluoperazine	Phenothiazine. Used for treatment of anxiety, to produce sedation, and as an antiemetic. Action is believed to be via antagonism of dopamine (similar to acepromazine); antiemetic action may be via antimuscarinic action.	Adverse effects not reported in animals, but are expected to be similar to other phenothiazines. See acepromazine, prochlorperazine.	Results of clinical studies in animals have not been reported. Use in animals (and doses) is based on experience in humans or anecdotal experience in animals.	Stelezine	10 mg/ml oral solution; 1, 2, 5, 10 mg tablets; 2 mg/ml injection	0.03 mg/kg IM q12h
Triflupromazine	Phenothiazine. Similar action as other phenothiazines (see trifluperazine and acepromazine), except triflupromazine may have stronger antimuscarinic activity than other phenothiazines. Used for antiemetic action.	Adverse effects have not been reported in animals. Possible adverse effects include anticholinergic effects.	Seme as trifluperazine	Vesprin	10, 20 mg/ml injections	0.1-0.3 mg/kg IM, PO q8-12h
Triiodothyronine	See liothyronine.					
Trimeprazine tartrate	Phenothiazine with antihistamine activity (similar to promethazine). Used for treating allergies and motion sickness.	Adverse effects are similar to promethazine.	There is evidence that trimeprazine is more effective when combined with prednisone for treatment of pruritus. Combination product is Temaril-P.	Temaril (Panectyl in Canada)	2.5 mg per 5 ml syrup; 2.5 mg tablet	0.5 mg/kg PO q12h
Trimethobenzamide	Antiemetic. Mechanism action is not understood.	Adverse effects have not been reported in animals.	Efficacy as antiemetic has not been reported in animals.	Tigan, others	100 mg/ml injection; 100, 250 mg capsules	Dogs: 3 mg/kg IM, PO q8h. Cats: Not recommended.
Trimethoprim sulfonamides (sulfadiazine or sulfamethoxazole)	Combination antibacterial drug. For action of sulfonamide, see sulfadiazine. For action of trimethoprim, see ormetoprim. Together, the combination is synergistic with a broad spectrum of activity.	Adverse effects primarily caused by sulfonamide component. See sulfadiazine.	Dosage recommendations vary. There is evidence that 30 mg/kg/day is efficacious for pyoderma; for other infections, 30 mg/kg twice daily has been recommended.	Tribrissen, others	30, 120, 240, 480, 960 mg tablets	15 mg/kg PO q12h or 30 mg/kg PO q12-24h. Toxoplasma: 30 mg/kg PO q12h.

Drug name	Pharmacology and category of use	Precautions	Dosing information and comments	Other names	Formulations available	Dosage
Tripelennamine	Antihistamine (H1) blocker. Similar in action as other antihistamines. See chlorpheniramine. Used to treat allergic disease.	Adverse effects similar to other antihistamines. See chlorpheniramine. Members of this class (ethanolamines) have greater antimuscarinic effects than other antihistamines.	There are no clinical reports of use in veterinary medicine. No evidence that it is more efficacious than other drugs in this class.	Pelamine, PBZ	25, 50 mg tablets; 20 mg/ml injection	1 mg/kg PO q12h
TSH (thyroid-stimulating hormone)	See thyrotropin.					
Tylosin	Macrolide antibiotic. See erythromycin for mechanism of action and spectrum.	May cause diarrhea in some animals. Do not administer PO to rodents or rabbits.	Tylosin is rarely used in small animals. Powdered formulation (tylosin tartrate) has been administered on food for control of signs of colitis in dogs. Tablets used for colitis in Canada.	Tylocine, Tylan	Soluble powder (tablets for dogs in Canada)	7-15 mg/kg PO q8h. Colitis: 40-80 mg/kg/day (with food).
Urofollitropin (FSH)	Stimulates ovulation. Contains FSH. In humans, it is used in combination with hCG to stimulate ovulation and induce pregnancy.	Side effects have not been reported in animals. In humans, thromboembolism or severe ovarian hyperstimulation syndrome has been reported.	Results of clinical studies in animals have not been reported. Use in animals is based on experience in humans.	Metrodin	75 U per vial for injection	Doses have not been established.
Ursodiol (ursodeoxycholate)	Anticholelithic. Used for treatment of liver diseases. Increases bile flow. In humans, used to prevent or treat gallstones.	Adverse effects not reported in animals. May cause diarrhea.	Results of clinical studies in animals have not been reported. Use in animals (and doses) is based on experience in humans or anecdotal experience in animals. Administer with meals.	Actigall	300 mg capsule	10-15 mg/kg PO q24h
Valproic acid	Anticonvulsant. Used, usually in combination with phenobarbital, to treat refractory epilepsy in animals. Action is not known, but may increase GABA concentrations in the CNS.	Adverse effects have not been reported in animals, but hepatic failure has been reported in humans. Sedation may be seen in some animals. Do not use in pregnant animals. May cause bleeding if used with drugs that inhibit platelets.	Valproic acid is listed here with divalproex. Divalproex is composed of both valproic acid and sodium valproate. Equivalent oral doses of divalproex sodium and valproic acid deliver equivalent quantities of valproate ion.	Depakene (valproic acid), Depakote (divalproex; Epival in Canada)	125, 250, 500 mg tablets (Depakote); 250 mg capsule; 50 mg/ml syrup (Depakene)	Dogs: 60-200 mg/kg PO q8h or 25-105 mg/kg/day PO when administered with phenobarbital
Vancomycin	Antibacterial drug. Mechanism of action is to inhibit cell wall and cause bacterial cell lysis (via different mechanism as betalactams). Spectrum includes staphylococci, streptococci, and enterococci (but not gram-negative bacteria). Used primarily for treatment of resistant staphylococcus and enterococci.	Adverse effects have not been reported in animals. Administer IV; causes severe pain and tissue injury if administered IM or SC. Do not administer rapidly; use slow infusion if possible (e.g., over 60 minutes). Adverse effects in humans include renal injury (more common with older products that contained impurities) and histamine release.	Vancomycin use is not common in animals; however, it is valuable for treatment of enterococci or staphylococci that are resistant to other antibiotics. Doses are derived from pharmacokinetic studies in dogs.	Vancocin	0.5-10 g vials for injection	Dogs: 15 mg/kg IV infusion q6h
Vasopressin (ADH)	Antidiuretic hormone. Vasopressin is used for treatment of polyuria caused by central diabetes insipidus. Not effective for polyuria caused by renal disease.	Adverse effects have not been reported. Allergic reactions have been reported in humans. Increase in blood pressure has been reported in humans.	Doses are adjusted on the basis of monitoring of water intake and urine output. See desmopressin.	Pitressin	20 U per ml (aqueous)	Aqueous: 10 U IV, IM.

Drug name	Pharmacology and category of use	Precautions	Dosing information and comments	Other names	Formulations available	Dosage
Verapamil	Calcium-channel blocking drug. Blocks calcium entry into cells via blockade of slow channel. Produces vasodilation and negative chronotropic effects.	Hypotension, cardiac depression, bradycardia, and AV block. May cause anorexia in some patients.	Diltiazem preferred over verapamil in patients with heart failure because of less cardiac suppression. Oral formulation not absorbed sufficiently (of the active stereoisomer) for adequate effects.	Calan, Isoptin	40, 80, 120 mg tablets; 2.5 mg/ml injection	Dogs: 0.05 mg/kg IV every 10-30 minutes (maximum cumulative dose is 0.15 mg/kg); oral dose is not established. Cats: 1.1-2.9 mg/kg PO q8h.
Vinblastine	Similar to vincristine. Sometimes used as an alternative to vincristine. Do not use to increase platelet numbers (may actually cause thrombocytopenia).	Does not produce neuropathy as vincristine, but there may be a higher incidence of myelosuppression. Causes tissue necrosis if injected outside vein.	Vinblastine is used in cancer chemotherapy protocols for various tumors. Consult specific chemotherapy protocol for regimens.	Velban	1 mg/ml injection	2 mg/m² IV (slow infusion) once per week
Vincristine	Anticancer agent. Vincristine causes arrest of cancer cell division by binding to microtubules and inhibiting mitosis. Used in combination chemotherapy protocols. Vincristine also increases numbers of functional circulating platelets and is used for thrombocytopenia.	Generally well tolerated. Less myelosuppressive than other anticancer drugs. Neuropathy has been reported, but is rare. Constipation can occur. Very irritating to tissues. Avoid extravasation outside vein during administration.	Vincristine is used in cancer chemotherapy protocols for various tumors. Consult specific chemotherapy protocol for regimens.	Oncovin, Vincasar, generic	1 mg/ml injection	Antitumor: 0.5-0.7 mg/m² IV or 0.025-0.05 mg/kg once per week. Thrombocytopenia: 0.02 mg/kg IV once per week.
Viokase	See pancrelipase.					
Vitamin A (retinoids)	Used to treat vitamin A deficiency. See also isotretinoin (Accutane) or etretinate (Tegison) for analogues used for other conditions.	Excessive doses can cause bone or joint pain and dermatitis.	Dosing of vitamin is expressed as U or retinol equivalents (RE) or mg of retinol. One RE equals 1 mg of retinol. One RE of vitamin A is equal to 3.33 U of retinol.	Aquasol-A	5,000 U (1,500 RE) per 0.1 ml oral solution; 10,000, 25,000, 50,000 U tablets	625-800 U/kg PO q24h (see dosing information section)
Vitamin B₁	See thiamine.					
Vitamin B₂ (riboflavin)	Used to treat Vitamin B₂ deficiency	Adverse effects are rare because water-soluble vitamins are easily excreted. Riboflavin may discolor the urine.	Not necessary to supplement in animals with well-balanced diets	Riboflavin	10-250 mg tablets	Dogs: 10-20 mg/day PO. Cats: 5-10 mg/day PO.
Vitamin B₁₂ (cyanocobalamin)	Vitamin B₁₂ is used to treat deficiencies. Conditions caused by deficiency may include anemia.	Adverse effects are rare because water-soluble vitamins are easily excreted.	Not necessary to supplement in animals with well-balanced diets	Cyanocobalamin	25-1000 μg tablets; injections	Dogs: 100-200 μg/day PO. Cats: 50-100 μg/day PO.
Vitamin C (ascorbic acid)	Used to treat vitamin C deficiency and occasionally used as urine acidifier. Insufficient data to show that ascorbic acid is effective for preventing cancer or cardiovascular disease.	Adverse effects have not been reported in animals. High doses may increase risk of oxalate stones in bladder.	Not necessary to supplement in animals with well-balanced diets	See ascorbic acid.	Tablets of various sizes; injection	100-500 mg/day
Vitamin D	See dihydrotachysterol or ergocalciferol.					
Vitamin E (alpha-tocopherol)	Vitamin considered as antioxidant. Used as supplement and treatment of some immune-mediated dermatoses.	Side effects have not been reported.	Vitamin E has been proposed as treatment for a wide range of human illnesses, but evidence for efficacy in animals is lacking.	Aquasol E, generic	Wide variety of capsules, tablets, oral solutions (e.g., 1000 U per capsule)	100-400 U PO q12h. Immune-mediated skin disease: 400-600 U PO q12h.

Drug name	Pharmacology and category of use	Precautions	Dosing information and comments	Other names	Formulations available	Dosage
Vitamin K₁ (phytonadione, phytomenadione)	Vitamin K₁ used to treat coagulopathies caused by anticoagulant toxicosis (warfarin or other rodenticides). Anticoagulants deplete vitamin K in the body, which is essential for synthesis of clotting factors.		Consult poison control center for specific protocol if specific rodenticide is identified. Use vitamin K₁ for acute therapy because it is more highly bioavailable. Administer with food to enhance absorption. Phytonadione and phytomenadione are synthetic lipid-soluble forms of vitamin K₁. Menadiol is vitamin K₄, which is converted in the body to vitamin K₃ (menadione).	AquaMEPHYTON (injection), Mephyton (tablets), Veta-K1 (tablets)	2, 10 mg/ml injections; 5, 25 mg tablets	Short-acting rodenticides: 1 mg/kg/day, IM, SC, PO for 10-14 days. Long-acting rodenticides: 2.5-5 mg/kg/day, IM, SC, PO for 3-4 weeks.
Warfarin	Anticoagulant. Depletes vitamin K, which is responsible for generation of clotting factors. Used to treat hypercoagulable disease and prevent thromboembolism.	Adverse effects are attributable to decreased clotting. Other drugs (including aspirin, chloramphenicol, phenylbutazone, ketoconazole, and cimetidine) may potentiate warfarin's action.	Warfarin response is individualistic. For optimum therapy, adjust dose by monitoring clotting time. For example, in some patients dose is adjusted to maintain PT to 1.5-2 times normal (or INR of 2-3). Consult specific reference for guidance (Current Veterinary Therapy XII, page 868).	Coumadin, generic	1, 2, 2.5, 4, 5, 7.5, 10 mg tablets	Dogs: 0.1-0.2 mg/kg PO q24h. Cats (thromboembolism): Start with 0.5 mg per day and adjust dose based on clotting time assessment.
Xylaxine	Alpha-2 (α₂) adrenergic agonist. Used primarily for anesthesia and analgesia.	Produces sedation and ataxia. Cardiac depression, heart block, and hypotension possible with high doses. Produces emesis after IV injection, especially in cats.	Often used in combination with other drugs (e.g., ketamine).	Rompun	20, 100 mg/ml injections	Dogs: 1.1 mg/kg IV; 2.2 mg/kg IM. Cats: 1.1 mg/kg IM (emetic dose is 0.4-0.5 mg/kg IV).
Yohimbine	Alpha-2 (α₂) adrenergic antagonist. Used primarily to reverse actions of xylazine or detomidine.	High doses can cause tremors and seizures.	Reverses signs of sedation and anesthesia caused by alpha-2 agonists	Yobine	2 mg/ml injection	0.11 mg/kg IV or 0.25-0.5 mg/kg SC, IM
Zidovudine (AZT)	Antiviral drug. In humans, used to treat AIDS. In animals, has been experimentally used for treatment of FeLV and FIV viral infection in cats.	Anemia and leukopenia	At this time, experience with using AZT for treating viral disease in animals is largely experimental or anecdotal. Consult a more detailed reference for guidance (Feline Pract 1995;23:16).	Retrovir	10 mg/ml syrup; 10 mg/ml injection	Cats: 5-10 mg/kg PO, SC q12h (doses as high as 30 mg/kg/day also have been used)
Zolazepam	See tiletamine and zolazepam.					

Key to abbreviations:

IM	Intramuscular	OTC	Over the counter (without prescription)
IP	Intraperitoneal	PO	per os (oral)
IV	Intravenous	SC	Subcutaneous
		U	Units

APPENDIX VIII

CONVERSION TABLE OF WEIGHT TO BODY SURFACE AREA (IN SQUARE METERS) FOR DOGS

kg	m²		kg	m²
0.5	0.06		26.0	0.88
1.0	0.10		27.0	0.90
2.0	0.15		28.0	0.92
3.0	0.20		29.0	0.94
4.0	0.25		30.0	0.96
5.0	0.29		31.0	0.99
6.0	0.33		32.0	1.01
7.0	0.36		33.0	1.03
8.0	0.40		34.0	1.05
9.0	0.43		35.0	1.07
10.0	0.46		36.0	1.09
11.0	0.49		37.0	1.11
12.0	0.52		38.0	1.13
13.0	0.55		39.0	1.15
14.0	0.58		40.0	1.17
15.0	0.60		41.0	1.19
16.0	0.63		42.0	1.21
17.0	0.66		43.0	1.23
18.0	0.69		44.0	1.25
19.0	0.71		45.0	1.26
20.0	0.74		46.0	1.28
21.0	0.76		47.0	1.30
22.0	0.78		48.0	1.32
23.0	0.81		49.0	1.34
24.0	0.83		50.0	1.36
25.0	0.85			

Although the above chart was compiled for dogs, it can also be used for cats. More precise values are represented in the formula BSA in $m^2 = (K \times W^{2/3}) \times 10^{-4}$; where m^2 = square meters, BSA = body surface area, W = weight in g, and K = constant of 10.1 in dogs and 10.0 in cats.

From Ettinger SJ. Textbook of veterinary internal medicine. Diseases of the dog and cat. 2nd ed. Philadelphia: WB Saunders, 1975:146.

APPENDIX IX

HOTLINES EVERY VETERINARIAN SHOULD KNOW

Veterinary product failure and adverse reaction reporting
  Veterinary Practitioners' Reporting Program—800-487-7776
  US Pharmacopeia: To report or request reporting forms for product quality problems, medication mishaps, and adverse reactions regarding drugs, biologics, chemicals, pesticides, medical devices, and other products used for companion, food, zoo, and exotic animals (reports may be submitted anonymously)

FDA/CMV: drugs, devices, animal feeds—301-594-1751 (weekdays, 7 am to 4 pm, ET) and 301-594-0797 (after hours)
  Line for health professionals to report adverse events, particularly with drugs (collect; after hours, record a message)

USDA: Veterinary Biologics and Diagnostics Hotline—800-752-6255 (weekdays, 7:30 am to 4 pm, CT; message service available other hours)
  A 24-hour hotline to report adverse reactions involving veterinary diagnostic and biologic products

FDA Medical Advertising Line—800-AD-US-FDA (800-238-7332)
  Assists health professionals seeking interpretive information on FDA policy

National Animal Poison Control Center hotlines
  800-548-2423—Fee $30 per case unless product is covered by a sponsoring company; credit cards only; with the 800 access only, follow-up calls are included; 900-680-0000—Fee $20 for first 5 minutes, $2.95 for each additional minute ($20 minimum); if product is covered by a sponsoring company, call will be switched to the 800 line and no fee charged

USDA voice response service—800-545-8732
  Up-to-date interstate shipping regulations, emergency notices, and animal care regulations for shipping pets on airlines; available 24 hours a day, including weekends and holidays, with a touch-tone phone

DEA toll-free number for Office of Diversion Control, Registration Section—800-882-9539
  A registration assistant is available from 8:30 am to 5 pm, ET, or leave a voice-mail message to request registration and order forms

Impaired veterinarians information line—800-248-2862, ext. 252 or 800-321-1473
  Information on and referrals for assistance with chemical impairment; sponsored by the AVMA

Pet loss support hotlines (grief counseling)
  916-752-4200—Staffed by University of California-Davis veterinary students; weekdays, 6:30 pm to 9:30 pm, PT
  904-392-4700, then dial 1 and 4080—Staffed by University of Florida veterinary students; weekdays, 7 pm to 9 pm, ET
  517-432-2696—Staffed by Michigan State University veterinary students; Tuesday to Thursday, 6:30 pm to 9:30 pm, ET
  708-603-3994—Staffed by Chicago VMA veterinarians and staff. Leave voice-mail message; calls will be returned 7 pm to 9 pm, CT (long-distance calls will be returned collect)
  540-231-8038—Staffed by Virginia-Maryland Regional College of Veterinary Medicine; Tuesday, Thursday, 6 pm to 9 pm, ET
  614-292-1823—Staffed by Ohio State University veterinary students; Monday, Wednesday, Friday, 6:30 pm to 9:30 pm, ET; voice-mail messages will be returned, collect, during operating hours
  508-839-7966—Staffed by Tufts University veterinary students; Tuesday, Thursday, 6 pm to 9 pm, ET; voice-mail messages will be returned daily, collect outside Massachusetts

HEMOPET—714-252-8455
  A national, full-service, nonprofit blood bank and educational network for animals, in Irvine, Calif; accessible 24 hours

Animal Blood Bank Hotline—800-243-5759
  A 24-hour hotline that focuses on transfusion medicine (particularly blood component therapy), recommending dosages and infusion rates, at no cost to caller

Eastern Veterinary Blood Bank—800-949-EVBB (800-949-3822)
  A 24-hour, commercial blood bank that focuses on transfusion medicine; gives recommendations and referrals to distribution centers when it cannot ship the requested product; for complicated cases, offers a paid consultation service; available to callers nationwide except in California and Oregon

Compiled by the Publications Division, American Veterinary Medical Association. Phone numbers current as of May 14, 1996. From JAVMA 1996;209:32 (with permission).

Index

Note: Page numbers followed by a "t" denote tables.

Hone Your Animal Instincts

Lumb and Jones' Veterinary Anesthesia, 3rd edition

John C. Thurmon, DVM, MS PhD, William Tranquilli, DVM, MS, and G. John Benson, DVM, MS

All anesthesia techniques currently used in veterinary medicine are covered, including topics such as laboratory and exotic animals, local anesthesia and regional anesthesia. Each of the 26 chapters is organized so that species-specific and organ-specific information can be easily accessed and understood. The contributors list is a virtual "who's who" of veterinary anesthesia.

1996/928 pages/568 illustrations/08238-8

Diseases of Cage and Aviary Birds

Walter J. Rosskopf, DVM and Richard W. Woerpel, DVM

This clinically specific resource emphasizes practical approaches to avian medicine and surgery. Unique chapters on wild birds, explicit coverage of clinical laboratory procedures and interpretation, and general avian care make this volume particularly helpful for the entire health care team.

1996/1100 pages/829 illustrations/07382-6

Practical Veterinary Ultrasound

Robert E. Cartee, DVM, MS, Barbara A. Selcer, DVM, MS, Judith A. Hudson, DVM, MS, PhD, Susan T. Finn-Bodner, DVM, MS, Mary B. Mahaffey, DVM, MS, Pamela L. Johnson, DVM, and Ken W. Marich

Here's the first practical, clinical guide to the use of ultrasound in a wide range of animals including exotics. The distinguished contributors, including anatomists, radiologists, and surgeons, present thorough information on physics and instrumentation.

This book is both a complete textbook on veterinary ultrasonography and a thorough diagnostic guide.

1995/352 pages/435 illustrations/01483-8

Biology and Medicine of Rabbits and Rodents, 4th ed.

J. E. Harkness, DVM and J. E. Wagner, DVM

This heavily revised edition contains updated clinical and scientific information on a full range of topics and coverage for each animal: rabbits, guinea pigs, hamsters, gerbils, mice and rats. Drs. Harkness and Wagner include vital information on: clinical pathology, blood collection, analgesia and analgesics, radiography, biology, and diseases.

1995/382 pages/29 illustrations/03919-9

Canine and Feline Nephrology and Urology

Carl A. Osborne, DVM, PhD and Delmar R. Finco, DVM, PhD

These acclaimed authors have created a clinically-specific and absolutely definitive management guide for urologic and nephrologic conditions in dogs and cats. You'll find extensive coverage of: physical and clinical laboratory assessment, endoscopic procedures, pharmacologic and dietary management, surgical indications, prognosis, and complications of treatment.

1996/960 pages/528 illustrations/0-683-06666-8

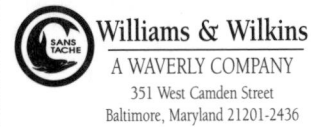

Williams & Wilkins
A WAVERLY COMPANY
351 West Camden Street
Baltimore, Maryland 21201-2436

Yes, I want to add these great veterinary resources to my library. Please send me:

___ Cartee: Practical Veterinary Ultrasound 01483-8..........................$65.00
___ Harkness: Biol & Med of Rabbits & Rodents, 4th ed. 03919-9.....$34.95
___ Osborne: Canine and Feline Neph and Urol 06666-8.................$105.00
___ Rosskopf: Diseases of Cage and Aviary Birds 07382-6...................$99.00
___ Thurmon: Lumb and Jones' Vet Anesth, 3rd ed. 08238-8...........$85.00

Phone orders accepted 24 hours a day, 7 days a week (US and Canada).
If not completely satisfied, return within 30 days (U.S. and Canada only).

To order Call:
Toll Free 800-638-0672
FAX: 1-800-447-8438

Outside the US and Canada, FAX 410-528-8550 for purchasing information.

INTERNET
E-mail: custserv@wwilkins.com
Home page: http://www.wwilkins.com

Payment options:

☐ Check enclosed (Plus $5.00 handling)

☐ Bill me (plus postage and handling)

☐ Charge my credit card (plus postage and handling)

☐ MasterCard ☐ VISA ☐ Am Express ☐ Discover

card # _____exp. date _____

signature/p.o.# _____

name _____

address _____

city/state/zip _____

your telephone # _____fax # _____

your specialty/profession _____e-mail address_____

CA, IL, MA, MD, NY, and PA residents please add state sales tax.
Prices subject to change without notice.
Prices are in U.S. dollars.

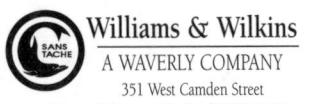

Williams & Wilkins
A WAVERLY COMPANY
351 West Camden Street
Baltimore, Maryland 21201-2436

Printed in US   96
TILLEYINS   >   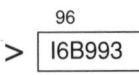   A